# PHARMACOTHERAPEUTICS

**a primary care clinical guide**

# PHARMACOTHERAPEUTICS

## a primary care clinical guide

**Ellis Quinn Youngkin, PhD, RNC, ARNP**
Professor and Graduate Program Coordinator
College of Nursing
Women's Health Care Nurse Practitioner
University Student Health Services
Florida Atlantic University
Boca Raton, Florida

**Kathleen J. Sawin, DNS, RN, CS, FAAN**
Certified Family and Pediatric Nurse Practitioner
Associate Professor
School of Nursing
Medical College of Virginia Campus
  of Virginia Commonwealth University
Richmond, Virginia
Postdoctoral Fellow
School of Nursing, Indiana University
Indianapolis, Indiana

**Jeanette F. Kissinger, EdD, RN, CS**
Professor Emeritus, School of Nursing
Medical College of Virginia Campus
  of Virginia Commonwealth University
Certified Adult Nurse Practitioner
Wellness Associates
Richmond, Virginia

**Debra S. Israel, PharmD, BCPS**
Clinical Coordinator
Seton Hospital System
Austin, Texas

APPLETON & LANGE
Stamford, CT

Copyright © 1999 by Appleton & Lange
A Simon & Schuster Company

www.appletonlange.com

99  00  01  02  03  /  10  9  8  7  6  5  4  3  2  1

Prentice Hall International (UK) Limited, *London*
Prentice Hall of Australia Pty. Limited, *Sydney*
Prentice Hall Canada, Inc., *Toronto*
Prentice Hall Hispanoamericana, S.A., *Mexico*
Prentice Hall of India Private Limited, *New Delhi*
Prentice Hall of Japan, Inc., *Tokyo*
Simon & Schuster Asia Pte. Ltd., *Singapore*
Editora Prentice Hall do Brasil Ltda., *Rio de Janeiro*
Prentice Hall, *Upper Saddle River, New Jersey*

**Library of Congress Cataloging-in-Publication Data**

Pharmacotherapeutics : a primary care clinical guide / [edited by]
  Ellis Q. Youngkin . . . [et al.].
      p.    cm.
    ISBN 0-8385-7681-8 (pbk. : alk. paper)
    1. Chemotherapy.  2. Pharmacology.  I. Youngkin, Ellis Quinn.
    [DNLM:  1. Drug Therapy—methods.  2. Pharmaceutical Preparations—
administration & dosage.  3. Primary Health Care—methods.  WB
330P5352  1999]
RM262.P466  1999
615.5′8—dc21
DNLM/DLC
for Library of Congress                                                                98-26172
                                                                                            CIP

*Cover Art:* Photomicrograph of a crystalline lattice of acetylsalicylic acid (aspirin).
Copyright © Dennis Kunkel, PhD, University of Hawaii.

Editor-in-Chief: Sally J. Barhydt
Production Service: Andover Publishing Services
Cover Design: Mary Skudlarek
Interior Design: Angela Foote

ISBN 0-8385-7681-8

90000

9 780838 576816

PRINTED IN THE UNITED STATES OF AMERICA

# DEDICATIONS

This book is dedicated to the following very important people who supported and loved us during the past months of preparation:

To my dear husband of 38 years, Carroll Youngkin, who has willingly helped me with a multitude of activities related to the book—typing, copying, stapling, stamping, mailing, and more—as well as patiently supporting the long hours of reading and writing. I love you. And to his mother, Marian Youngkin, who is like a mother to me. And to my dear children, Dottie Kouba and Glenn Youngkin, their spouses, Chris Kouba and Suzanne Youngkin; and our wonderful grandchildren: Valarie Quinn Kouba, Julianne Elizabeth Kouba, Emily Rose Kouba, and Grant McDaniel Youngkin. **EQY.**

To my mother, Annabelle Roth Sawin, my children Marc and Melissa Hedahl and our families from California to Massachusetts and North Dakota to South Carolina who have always been there for me to multiply my joys and divide my challenges. **KJS.**

Many thanks go to my loving family, colleagues, students, and friends who were part of the potter's wheel that shaped my life, but I dedicate my efforts in this book to my grandchildren, John and Elizabeth Fairey, whose unconditional love for "Nana K" is truly a gift from God. **JFK.**

To my husband, Lonny, for his support and understanding; to my children, Matthew, Rachel, and Sarah, whose presence brings me immeasurable joy; and to my mother, Ondree Lerman Israel, who continues to inspire me. **DSI.**

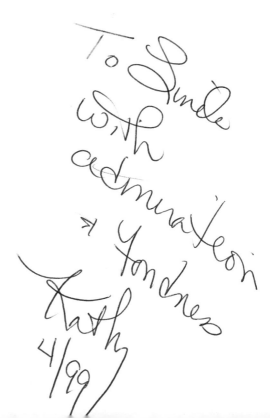

# CONTENTS

**UNIT I    PRINCIPLES OF PHARMACOTHERAPY**..........................**1**

1. **Introduction to Pharmacotherapy**......**3**
   *Ellis Quinn Youngkin, Kathleen J. Sawin, Jeanette F. Kissinger, and Debra S. Israel*

2. **Pharmacokinetics and Pharmacodynamics**............................**7**
   *Ginette A. Pepper*

3. **Pharmacotherapeutic Impact of Renal or Hepatic Dysfunction**..........**45**
   *Thomas J. Comstock*

**UNIT II    GENERAL ISSUES**...............**57**

4. **Safety in Pharmacotherapy**...............**59**
   *Lea Ann Hansen*

5. **Psychological, Sociological, and Cultural Factors**...................................**65**
   *Jeanette F. Kissinger and Kathleen J. Sawin*

6. **Regulatory Control of Drugs**............**79**
   *Gene White*

7. **Pharmacotherapy Resources for the Provider**..................................**85**
   *Geneva Briggs*

8. **Adverse Drug Events and Drug Interactions**......................................**97**
   *Geneva Briggs*

9. **Evaluating Patient Self-Care and Over-the-Counter Drugs**.................**111**
   *Karen D. Rich*

10. **Herbal Therapies for Common Health Problems**..............................**127**
    *Ellis Quinn Youngkin and Debra S. Israel*

11. **Immunizations**.................................**151**
    *Debra K. Hearington*

**UNIT III    SPECIAL ISSUES AND PATIENT POPULATIONS**....................**179**

12. **Pediatric Issues**...............................**181**
    *Katharine A. Gracely-Kilgore*

13. **Geriatric Issues**...............................**199**
    *Geneva Briggs*

14. **Individuals with Disabilities**............**205**
    *Stephanie G. Metzger*

15. **Migrant and Homeless Populations**.....................................**219**
    *Sandra L. Graves*

16. **Individuals with Chronic Pain**........**227**
    *Cynthia J. Simonson and Lori W. Lush*

17. **Pregnancy and Lactation**.................**239**
    *Laurie A. Buchwald*

18. **Contraceptives**..............................**255**
    *Catherine Berardelli and Vivien E. James*

19. **Menopause and Hormonal Replacement Therapy**.....................**289**
    *Susan Rawlins and Robert L. Martin*

**UNIT IV    PHARMACOTHERAPY FOR COMMON PRIMARY CARE DISORDERS**.........................................**307**

20. **Cardiovascular Disorders**...............**309**
    *Judith Bunnell Sellers and Mary L. Brubaker*

21. **Upper Respiratory Disorders**.........**369**
    *Constance R. Uphold and Thomas E. Johns*

22. **Lower Respiratory Disorders** .........393
    *Kathleen M. Tauer and Lauwana E. Hollis*

23. **Eye Disorders** .................................473
    *Joanne K. Singleton
    and Robert V. DiGregorio*

24. **Ear Disorders** .................................485
    *Jeanette F. Kissinger, Kathleen J. Sawin,
    and Debra S. Israel*

25. **Gastrointestinal Disorders** ..............495
    *Patricia J. Kelly and Candice Smith-Scott*

26. **Musculoskeletal Disorders**..............527
    *Sharon L. Sheahan, Aimee Gelhot, and
    Angela B. Hoth*

27. **Dermatologic Disorders**...................569
    *Candace M. Burns and Douglas F. Covey*

28. **Hematologic Disorders** ...................605
    *Margaret A. Fitzgerald*

29. **Neurologic Disorders** .......................621
    *Jessie Drew-Cates and Robert A. Gross*

30. **Endocrine Disorders: Thyroid
    and Adrenal Conditions** ..................683
    *Jeanne Archer and Michael S. Monaghan*

31. **Endocrine Disorders:
    Diabetes Mellitus**............................709
    *Martha J. Price and Daniel Kent*

32. **Obesity** .............................................731
    *Ellis Quinn Youngkin
    and Jeanette F. Kissinger*

33. **Mental Health Disorders** ................747
    *B. J. Landis and Stephen G. Bryant*

34. **Urinary Tract Disorders
    and Male Sexual Dysfunction** .........801
    *Linda D. Scott and David H. Nelson*

35. **Gynecologic Disorders and
    Female Sexual Dysfunction**.............835
    *Linda O. Morphis and M. Sharm Steadman*

36. **Sexually Transmitted Diseases,
    Vaginitis, and Pelvic
    Inflammatory Disease** .....................863
    *Susan Rawlins, Robert L. Martin,
    and Mai Duong*

37. **Immune System Disorders:
    HIV/AIDS, Mononucleosis,
    and Allergic Responses** ...................897
    *C. Fay Parpart, Mary S. Peery,
    and Kathleen J. Sawin*

**UNIT V   TABLES OF
PHARMACOTHERAPEUTIC
AGENTS**.................................................923

Table 100   **Anti-infective Agents** ........931
Table 200   **Cardiovascular Agents** ....1034
Table 300   **Central Nervous System
            (CNS) Agents**...................1088
Table 400   **Eye and Ear
            Preparations**....................1257
Table 500   **Gastrointestinal
            Agents**.............................1286
Table 600   **Hormones and
            Synthetic Substances** ......1327
Table 700   **Respiratory Agents** .........1389
Table 800   **Topical Preparations** ......1427
Table 900   **Urinary Tract
            Products** .........................1476
Table 1000  **Miscellaneous Agents** .....1479
Table 1100  **Vitamins, Minerals,
            and Trace Elements** .......1488

*Index*.................................................................1497

# CONTRIBUTORS

**Jeanne Archer, PhD, RN, APN**
University of Arkansas
School of Nursing
Little Rock, Arkansas

**Catherine Berardelli, PhD, RN, CS, FNP**
University of New England
Westbrook College Campus
Portland, Maine

**Geneva Briggs, PharmD, BCPS**
Clinical Associate
MedOutcomes, Inc
Richmond, Virginia

**Mary L. Brubaker, PharmD, FASHP, BCPS, BCNSP, CHES**
Clinical Assistant Professor
Northern Arizona University
Department of Nursing
Flagstaff, Arizona

**Stephen G. Bryant, PharmD**
Professor of Psychiatry and Pharmacology
The University of Texas Medical Branch
Galveston, Texas

**Laurie A. Buchwald, MS, RNC, WHNP, CFNP**
Women's Health Nurse Practitioner
Family Nurse Practitioner
Obstetrics and Gynecology of Radford
Radford, Virginia

**Candace M. Burns, PhD, ARNP**
Associate Professor
Director, Interdisciplinary Dual Degree
    Program in Adult Health/Occupational
    Health Nursing
University of South Florida College of Nursing
Tampa, Florida

**Thomas J. Comstock, PharmD**
Associate Professor
Department of Pharmacy and Pharmaceutics
Medical College of Virginia Campus of Virginia
    Commonwealth University
Richmond, Virginia

**Douglas F. Covev, PharmD, MHA**
Clinical Specialist/Ambulatory Care
Tampa Veterans' Hospital and Clinic
Tampa, Florida

**Robert V. DiGregorio, PharmD**
Associate Professor of Pharmacy Practice
Arnold & Marie Schwartz College of
    Pharmacy
Long Island University
Brooklyn, New York

**Jessie Drew-Cates, PhD, CFNP, CRRN**
St. Mary's Hospital Brain Injury Rehabilitation
Adjunct Assistant Professor, School of Nursing
Instructor, School of Medicine
University of Rochester
Rochester, New York

**Mai Duong, PharmD**
Clinical Specialist
Parkland Health & Hospital System
Dallas, Texas

**Margaret A. Fitzgerald, MS, CS-FNP**
President
Fitzgerald Health Education Associates
Andover, Massachusetts

**Aimee Gelhot, PharmD**
Ambulatory Care Specialist
Assistant Professor
College of Pharmacy
University of Kentucky
Lexington, Kentucky

**Katharine A. Gracely-Kilgore, RN, MSN, CPNP, PNP, CS**
Pediatrics
MCV Physicians in the Park at Stony Park
Richmond, Virginia

**Sandra L. Graves, MS, RN, CFNP**
Comprehensive Health Investment Project of
    Richmond
Richmond, Virginia

**Robert A. Gross, MD, PhD**
Associate Professor of Neurology, and of
    Pharmacy, and Physiology
Strong Epilepsy Center and University of
    Rochester School of Medicine
Rochester, New York

**Lea Ann Hansen, PharmD**
Associate Professor of Pharmacy
Medical College of Virginia Hospitals of
    Virginia Commonwealth University
Richmond, Virginia

**Debra K. Hearington, MS, RN, C-PNP**
School of Nursing
Medical College of Virginia Campus of Virginia
    Commonwealth University
Richmond, Virginia

**Lauwana E. Hollis, PharmD**
Assistant Clinical Professor
School of Pharmacy
Clinical Instructor
School of Nursing
Medical College of Virginia Campus of Virginia
    Commonwealth University
Richmond, Virginia

**Angela B. Hoth, PharmD**
Clinical Pharmacist
Iowa City Veterans Administration Medical
    Center
Adjunct Assistant Professor
College of Pharmacy
University of Iowa
Iowa City, Iowa

**Vivien E. James, PharmD**
Assistant Professor, Pharmacy and
    Pharmaceutics
School of Pharmacy
Medical College of Virginia Campus of Virginia
    Commonwealth University
Richmond, Virginia

**Thomas E. Johns, PharmD, BCPS**
Clinical Specialist, Infectious Diseases
Clinical Assistant Professor
College of Pharmacy
University of Florida
Gainesville, Florida

**Patricia J. Kelly, PhD, RN, FNP**
Family Nurse Practitioner
Department of Pediatrics
Division of Community Pediatrics
University of Texas Health Science Center at
    San Antonio
San Antonio, Texas

**Daniel Kent, BSPharm, CDE**
Clinical Diabetes Specialist II
Group Health Cooperative of Puget Sound
Seattle, Washington

**B. J. Landis, PhD, APN**
Director of Nursing Education
Family Nurse Practitioner
Area Health Education Center-Fort Smith
Fort Smith, Arkansas

**Lori W. Lush, PharmD**
Senior Editor
Medical Education Systems, Inc.
Acworth, Georgia

**Robert L. Martin, PharmD, BCPS**
Assistant Director—Pharmacy Services
Parkland Health & Hospital System
Dallas, Texas

**Stephanie G. Metzger, MS, RN, CS, PNP**
Rehabilitation Coordinator/Pediatric Nurse
    Practitioner
Children's Hospital
Clinical Faculty, School of Nursing
Medical College of Virginia Campus of Virginia
    Commonwealth University
Richmond, Virginia

**Michael S. Monaghan, PharmD, BCPS**
Associate Professor
Department of Pharmacy Practice
School of Pharmacy and Allied Health
    Professions
Creighton University
Omaha, Nebraska

**Linda O. Morphis, MN, RNCS**
Women's Health Nurse Practitioner
Clinical Assistant Professor
University of South Carolina College of
    Nursing
Columbia, South Carolina

**David H. Nelson, R.PH**
Washoe Medical Center
Assistant Professor
Orvis School of Nursing
University of Nevada
Reno, Nevada

**C. Fay Parpart, RN, MS, ANP, OCN**
HIV Nurse Practitioner
Stamford Health Systems
Stamford, Connecticut

**Ginette A. Pepper, PhD, RN, APN, FAAN**
University of Colorado Health Sciences Center
School of Nursing
Denver, Colorado

**Mary S. Peery, PharmD**
Medical College of Virginia Hospital of Virginia
    Commonwealth University
Richmond, Virginia

**Martha J. Price, DNSc, ARNP, CDE**
Diabetes Nurse Consultant
Center for Health Studies
Seattle, Washington

**Susan Rawlins, MS, RNC**
Director
Women's Health Care Nurse Advanced
    Practitioner Program
University of Texas Southwestern Medical
    Center at Dallas
Dallas, Texas

**Karen D. Rich, PharmD**
Assistant Professor
Department of Pharmacy and Pharmaceutics
Medical College of Virginia Campus of Virginia
    Commonwealth University
Richmond, Virginia

**Linda D. Scott, DNS, RN, CFNP**
Assistant Professor
University of Alabama
Capstone College of Nursing
Tuscaloosa, Alabama

**Judith Bunnell Sellers, DNSc, FNP, RNC**
Northern Arizona University
Department of Nursing
Flagstaff, Arizona

**Sharon L. Sheahan, PhD, CFNP**
Associate Professor of Nursing
University of Kentucky
Lexington, Kentucky

**Cynthia J. Simonson, RN, MS, CS, AOCN**
Adult Nurse Practitioner
Oncology Clinical Nurse Specialist
Massey Cancer Center
Medical College of Virginia Hospitals of
    Virginia Commonwealth University
Richmond, Virginia

**Joanne K. Singleton, PhD, RN, CS, FNP**
Assistant Professor
Pace University
Lienhard School of Nursing
New York, New York

**Candice Smith-Scott, PharmD**
Associate Clinical Professor
St. John's University
Jamaica, New York

**M. Sharm Steadman, PharmD, FASHP**
Associate Professor
Family and Preventive Medicine
University of South Carolina School of Medicine
Columbia, South Carolina

**Kathleen M. Tauer, MS, RN, CPNP**
University Student Health Services
Virginia Commonwealth University
Richmond, Virginia

**Constance R. Uphold, PhD, ARNP, RNC**
Associate Professor, College of Nursing
University of Florida
Nurse Fellow, Gainesville Veterans Affairs
    Medical Center
Gainesville, Florida

**Gene White, RPH, JD**
Associate Professor Emeritus
School of Pharmacy
Medical College of Virginia Campus of Virginia
    Commonwealth University
Richmond, Virginia
Adjunct Faculty of Pharmacy
Shenandoah University
Winchester, Virginia

# REVIEWERS

**Alan P. Agins, PhD**
Executive Director, PRN Associates
Continuing Nursing Education Specialist
Crozet, Virginia

**Jean Krajicek Bartek, PhD, ARNP**
Associate Professor
University of Nebraska Medical Center
College of Nursing and College of Medicine
  (Pharmacology)
Omaha, Nebraska

**Marjorie A. Maddox, ARNP, ANP-C**
*Formerly:* Associate Professor of Nursing
Coordinator of the ANP Graduate Courses
University of Louisville
Louisville, Kentucky

**Susan E. Malecha, BS Pharmacy, PharmD**
Drug Information Specialist
Chicago, Illinois

**Bonita McCormack, MSN, RNCS, ANP**
Chief of Nursing
Harvard University Health Services
Cambridge, Massachusetts

**Nancy Okamoto, RNCS, MS, NP**
Student Health Service
City College, San Francisco
San Francisco, California

**Mary Ann Scoloveno, EdD, PNP, RN**
Associate Professor
Rutgers, The State University of New Jersey
College of Nursing
Newark, New Jersey

# PREFACE

*Pharmacotherapeutics: A Primary Care Clinical Guide* is the result of our vision to create a pharmacotherapeutics text in primary care that provides the information needed by the clinician to choose the correct drug for therapy and monitor the results for effectiveness and safety. We conceived the idea for the book after hearing from practitioners across the country that such a book was needed. We thought that this type of book, properly developed with an interdisciplinary team, might also be useful to other primary care providers.

Fulfilling this vision involved the extraordinary efforts of 52 very knowledgeable and established professionals in nursing, pharmacology, pharmacy, and medicine. Most of the chapters, especially those in Unit IV on specific conditions and disorders, were written by a team consisting of a nurse practitioner and a doctor of pharmacy, pharmacist, or other professional prepared in pharmacology or pharmacy. This collaboration provides contemporary and accurate management regimen options and logical monitoring information with factors such as patient-related variables (age, organ function, concomitant disease states, etc.) and drug-related variables (toxicity, monitoring parameters, interactions, costs, etc.) as considerations. It is our belief that the members of an interdisciplinary team all share the responsibility for the therapeutic outcomes of our patients.

The book is aimed at the practicing primary care clinician or the graduate student who will be a practitioner in primary care. It is designed to be a clinical reference from which information may be easily retrieved, with enough depth for efficacy and safety. A major concern with a pharmacotherapy book is that new drugs are constantly made available. We hope the reader will use the book for guidance for therapy even as it "ages," and will be stimulated to keep abreast of the newest therapies, using additional research to discern if they are truly the safest, the best, and the most economical for the patient.

We attempt to maintain a focus on more common conditions that must be managed in primary care practice, and so the book delves into selected areas of tertiary care only where hospitalization is indicated as a condition worsens or complexity increases. Supporting data, found in the first three units of the book, aid the provider in implementing care from a more holistic viewpoint. We recognize that some approaches may vary from those with which the reader is familiar, but this diversity should serve to stimulate the clinician to compare regimens and anticipate outcomes while deciding on the therapy best suited for the particular patient in a specific situation.

The book is divided into five units:

**Unit I. Principles of Pharmacotherapy.** Principles of pharmacokinetics and pharmacodynamics as well as the impact of drugs on renal and hepatic dysfunction are presented in this section, in which we put particular focus on the importance of underlying concepts in basic pharmacology.

**Unit II. General Issues.** Issues presented in this section include patient safety, psychological, sociological, and cultural factors, legal considerations, pharmacotherapy resources for providers, adverse drug events and drug interactions, evaluation of over-the-counter therapies, herbal therapies, and immunizations.

**Unit III. Special Issues and Patient Populations.** This section provides insights for pharmacotherapy of children, the elderly, people with disabilities, migrant and homeless populations, individuals with chronic pain, and pregnant and lactating women. Contraception, menopause, and hormonal replacement therapy are also covered. More than ever, special populations require special care measures, and we want the practicing provider to have increased understanding in these areas.

**Unit IV. Pharmacotherapy for Common Primary Care Disorders.** Chapters in this unit address commonly encountered conditions and disorders across the age span in primary care. Diagnoses and conditions are categorized by systems. Although for each condition we assume the provider has reached an established, accurate diagnosis and is at the point of making an appropriate pharmacotherapeutic selection, definitions, epidemiologic and etiologic data, as well as history, physical examination, and diagnostic assessment findings are provided. A template is used for each condition for this section of the book to aid the reader in finding information consistently. By using this format, we intend to emphasize the necessity in primary care of looking at short-term management of conditions while still considering long-term goals in treating the patient. We focus on considerations such as when first line therapies would not be appropriate or when non-pharmacologic therapies should be tried first; in other words, we look holistically at the patient's care on a long timeline.

**Unit V. Tables of Pharmacotherapeutic Agents.** These comprehensive drug tables, from antibiotics to miscellaneous agents, are referenced throughout Unit IV. The tables provide information to guide the reader in the specific details about drugs that may be considered for therapy: drug and dosage forms, spectrum of activity and usual dosage range, administration issues and drug-drug drug-food interactions, common adverse drug reactions and pharmacokinetics, contraindications, pregnancy category, and lactation issues. Also included are tables of fat- and water-soluble vitamins and major and trace minerals.

The reader is reminded that the scope of prescribing varies for advanced practice nurses and physician assistants from state to state, and that the individual provider is responsible for knowing the legal limits of the scope of practice for the state in which he or she is practicing. With the advent of telemedicine and distance learning, this reminder may apply to more than one state as clinicians cross state lines to practice. Additionally, providers must constantly stay abreast of new standards based on evolving knowledge for practice. Readers are urged to recognize that this book is as current as possible, considering that new drugs are being continuously approved and removed from the market. Thus it is up to each practitioner to keep apprised of the newest drug additions and deletions for safe practice.

As you read and use this book, we hope you find that it enhances your practice, and we urge you to send us ideas to improve future editions.

We want this book to be a valuable resource to you in the ever-changing health care world in which we all live.

## ACKNOWLEDGMENTS

We wish to extend heartfelt thanks to our excellent contributing authors for their fine chapters. With their individual and collective expertise and hard work, the book has evolved as an expression of true collaborative efforts. We extend sincere thanks to Niels Buessem and his staff for their fine development and production support; to the fine staff at Appleton & Lange for their consistently helpful and excellent work in the publication of this book; and to Sally Barhydt, our wonderful editor-in-chief, whose support and confidence in us helped us complete this project. A special thank you goes to the PharmDs who developed the extensive tables of drugs: Steven Eggleston, Cathy Mather, and Karen Tisdel; and to our own co-author, Deb Israel, for her superior work in reviewing and polishing them into useful references. A special thanks also is sent to Elizabeth Chisholm and Susan Faison, who as baccalaureate nursing students at Virginia Commonwealth University School of Nursing helped ensure that we had current literature resources. We want to direct a large measure of appreciation to the students and preceptor colleagues we work with who make our professions possible and who give so generously to the development of our next generation of clinicians. Last, but certainly not least, deep appreciation goes to our families and friends who have encouraged us and withstood the pressures of deadlines in the years of preparation. During the process of writing this book, we and our families had two retirements, five births, two young adults launched, and five position changes, and we survived. We celebrate the unveiling of this book—healthy, settled, safe, and certainly relieved. We wish you all health and love.

**Ellis Quinn Youngkin**
**Kathleen J. Sawin**
**Jeannette F. Kissinger**
**Debra S. Israel**

*Cover art:* Photomicrograph of a crystalline lattice of acetylsalicylic acid (aspirin).

Aspirin was first used by Hippocrates in the 5th century to treat aches and pains. From the first commercial processing of the drug in 1893 to 1897 when Bayer and Company named the product aspirin, this bitter powder from the bark of the willow tree has come a long way. Aspirin continues to be commonly used for headaches, muscular pain, toothaches, arthritis, and menstrual pain; it also relieves fever and reduces inflammation. By the end of the 20th century, aspirin had new roles in preventive medicine by reducing the risk of strokes and heart attacks as well as preventing certain types of cataracts. There is also preliminary evidence that aspirin may help prevent colorectal cancer and Alzheimer's disease. As with most drugs, these benefits come with risks of side effects, including nausea, heartburn, stomach pain, and ulcer formation. High doses of aspirin may also cause ringing in the ears, and renal and hepatic damage may occur with prolonged use. Given its past and current uses and future uses that are yet to be defined, aspirin truly represents a "prototype" drug.

# I

# PRINCIPLES OF PHARMACOTHERAPY

# 1

# INTRODUCTION TO PHARMACOTHERAPY

*Ellis Quinn Youngkin, Kathleen J. Sawin, Jeanette F. Kissinger, and Debra S. Israel*

How often does the practitioner wish there were a resource that would assist with questions such as:

- Which pharmacotherapy would be best for this condition?
- If the patient has these particular personal characteristics, would this medication be preferred over that one?
- What outcome should be expected if this medication is used, and how soon?
- What if the outcome is not as expected, and a change in pharmacotherapy is indicated? What should be used next?
- What are the concerns that should be kept in mind when using a particular pharmacotherapy?
- What should the patient and family be told about using this drug?

These are but a few of the questions that arise in making pharmacotherapy decisions. Situations like the following raise such questions:

- Ms. E. brings Bryan, a 10-year-old Caucasian boy, to your office with complaints of a runny nose, itchy eyes, and constant postnasal drip. What is the safest, most effective treatment for Bryan?
- Mr. T., a 65-year-old African-American man, has hypertension that is not responding to the calcium channel blocker you prescribed. What is the best course of medication change or addition?
- Ms. J., a 48-year-old Hispanic woman, has hot flashes that are keeping her awake at night. She

is still having some periods, but they are somewhat irregular. She was diagnosed with essential hypertension 2 years ago. She was doing well on her medications but ran out 3 weeks ago. Her blood pressure is elevated significantly today. What pharmacotherapies are indicated?

- Ms. N., a 19-year-old Asian woman, presents with burning with urination, frequency, and hematuria. The urine test indicates significant infection. She is allergic to sulfa and nitrofurantoin. This is her third urinary tract infection (UTI) in 18 months. What further information do you need to prescribe an effective medication? Does Ms. N. need any further diagnostic tests? A referral to a urologist?
- Mr. P., a 68-year-old Indian man with asthma, calls complaining of more difficulty breathing. He is using several inhalers—a steroid, a long-acting bronchodilator, and a short-acting bronchodilator—but states these are not working as well as they used to. Is Mr. P.'s use of the inhalers correct and timely? Is he taking any cultural treatments for his asthma?
- Ms. G., a 20-year-old Caucasian woman, is 8 weeks pregnant. She has been diagnosed with trichomonas vaginitis and complains of severe pruritis. What are the treatment options at this stage of pregnancy?

Literally thousands of drugs are available today to the clinician and the patient for wellness and illness care, either over-the-counter or by prescription. If this thought is not daunting enough to the clinician, reflect on the myriad concerns and considerations surrounding safe and correct drug therapy. Attaining desired therapy outcomes depends on the interactions and influences of hundreds of variables. Everything possible must be taken into consideration from the route of administration and expected action of the drug to political, legal, economic, and ethical concerns, to interactions between the therapy and other drugs, foods, herbs, and legal and nonlegal substances, as well as environmental toxins. In addition, the patient's hereditary disease background and personal characteristics, such as age, sex, race, culture, beliefs, physical factors such as weight, illness status, family influences, and education and learning style must be factored in. Even the biologic rhythm of the person in relation to the specific drug is becoming an important variable.

With such an array of influences challenging the clinician with each drug therapy decision, the primary goal of a clinical guidebook is for it to be logically and efficiently useful in practice. Thus, this book is intended first to be a practical, easy-to-use resource for the clinician, and second to be a learning tool for advanced practice professional students. The major thrust of the book is to present information on pharmacotherapeutic management of commonly encountered conditions in primary care practice with an emphasis on monitoring therapy outcomes. Table 1–1 gives definitions for common terms frequently encountered in this text.

## PLANNING FOR PHARMACOTHERAPY AND THE PHARMACEUTICAL PROCESS

A plan for rational drug therapy requires the following preparatory steps, all of which are necessary in deciding on pharmacotherapy (Melmon & Morrelli, 1978):

1. Diagnosing the condition accurately. If a diagnosis cannot be made, in fact, the other steps become more important. This book will not deal with the process of diagnosis; it assumes an accurate diagnosis has been made.
2. Knowing the disease pathophysiology. Understanding the abnormalities of anatomy and physiology of a disease is necessary to understanding drug actions and in determining drug selection.
3. Knowing basic pharmacology and pharmacokinetics of drugs in both normal and ill individuals. According to experts, it is essential to understand four processes for knowledgeable pharmacotherapy (DiPiro et al., 1992) These are:

Pharmaceutical process: Knowing if and how the drug is being administered to the patient requires knowledge of drug bioavailability and whether the patient is actually taking the drug. The provider needs to know the chemical and physical properties of the drug and drug forms and dosages, and may need to incorporate methods to enhance compliance.

Pharmacokinetic process: Knowing if the drug is reaching the site intended for action includes absorption, distribution, metabolism, and elimination data about the drug for a specific patient and that patient's own variables, such as weight, sex, and medical history.

Pharmacodynamic process: Knowing if the drug is causing the pharmacologic effects on the cellular or organ structures, for example, the effect of an antihypertensive agent on blood pressure.

Pharmacotherapeutic process: Knowing if the effect is therapeutic, that is, whether the pathophysiologic process has been altered in a beneficial way or not. This book primarily addresses pharmaceutical and pharmacokinetic processes in Units I and II and pharmacodynamic and pharmacotherapeutic processes in

### TABLE 1–1.  DEFINITIONS OF TERMS

*Pharmaceutic* or *pharmaceutical:* relating to pharmacy or to pharmaceutics.
*Pharmaceutics:* the science of pharmaceutical systems, that is, preparations, dosage forms, and so on. A synonym is *pharmacy.*
*Pharmacodynamics:* the study of drug actions on the living organism.
*Pharmacognosy:* a branch of pharmacology concerned with the physical characteristics and botanical sources of crude drugs.
*Pharmacokinetic:* relating to the disposition of drugs in the body.
*Pharmacokinetics:* movements of drugs within biologic systems as affected by uptake, distribution, elimination, and biotransformation.
*Pharmacologic or pharmacological:* relating to pharmacology or to the composition, properties, and actions of drugs.
*Pharmacology:* the science concerned with drugs and their sources, appearance, chemistry, actions, and uses.
*Pharmacotherapy:* the treatment of disease by means of drugs.

*Source: Adapted from McDonough Jr., J. T. (Ed.) (1994). Stedman's Concise Medical Dictionary (2nd ed.). Baltimore: Williams & Wilkins.*

Units III through V, although some overlap occurs in Units II through V based on chapter objectives.

4. Applying knowledge of diagnosis, pathophysiology, and basic pharmacology and pharmacokinetics of drugs to the care of the patient. This means taking into account all relevant patient variables that may affect the pharmacotherapeutic choice. Everything from inherited factors such as race to acquired factors such as culture and nutritional habits must be considered.

5. Expecting specific therapeutic outcomes based upon relationships between variables for the individual patient. This requires determining which effects will be monitored to see if therapy has been effective or not. For example, certain symptoms would be expected to disappear by a specified time, or certain lab data would be expected to change. The outcomes that are desired are presented; the choice of therapy is based upon these in relation to the other patient variables.

6. Determining a therapeutic plan when deciding on pharmacotherapy. The drug is chosen because it is indicated for the diagnosis, is appropriate in its action for the problem and for expected outcomes, is based on scientific knowledge of pharmaceutical and pharmacokinetic processes, can be monitored based on anticipated outcomes, and can be evaluated based on measurable results.

## SELECTING THE BEST PHARMACOTHERAPEUTIC REGIMEN FOR THE CONDITION

Again, the assumption is that the correct diagnosis has been made before the most appropriate drug can be selected. An inadequate or incorrect diagnosis can result in incorrect or no therapy. Risks and benefits of each drug considered for therapy must be weighed (DiPiro et al, 1997). Contraindications, interactions with drugs, other substances, or food, potential for toxicity, potential for complications caused by patient factors, possibility of hypersensitivity, and predictability of adverse effects must be considered.

Specific information about each drug in a class is presented in the drug tables in Unit V of this book. Cross-references to these tables appear throughout the text. Drug tables are arranged alphabetically by classifications and alphabetically by generic drug names within the tables. The index of the book indicates where the classification table is found and where the

drug is listed in Unit V. For convenience the index lists both generic and trade names.

When the final drug choice is made, the specific regimen is determined. This includes dose per each 24 hours, interval between doses, length of total therapy, route and method of administration, and form of drug to enhance adherence by the patient (DiPiro et al, 1997). Since this book focuses on outpatient, ambulatory care, it will be the patient's or caretaker's responsibility (once the provider has selected the drug regimen and the pharmacist has filled the prescription) to be sure the drug therapy is delivered on time and in a correct dose and manner. If an essential part of monitoring and evaluation requires knowledge by the patient and/or caretaker, the clinician must be sure this knowledge is correctly understood. Other measures for monitoring and evaluation will require gathering subjective information by history and performing diagnostic tests and/or physical examination measures for objective data. Definitive alternative plans must be made in case of adverse effects or unmet therapeutic goals. Quality care can be maintained only through monitoring of patient outcomes.

In conclusion, pharmacotherapy requires careful prerequisite planning in order to select and implement the appropriate therapy for a given condition with a specific individual who has numerous influencing variables. Improving or maintaining the quality of life for the patient is a guiding objective. In addition, effective pharmacotherapy requires meticulous monitoring and evaluation based on measurable, expected outcomes in order to provide continuing therapy, alter the therapy, or take other appropriate action for effective therapeutic management of the patient and the condition. This book provides insights into pharmacotherapy management for selected populations and conditions in primary care.

## REFERENCES

DiPiro, J. T., Talbert, R. L., Hayes, P. E., Yee, G. C., Matzke, G. R., & Posey, L. M. (Eds.) (1992). *Pharmacotherapy: A pathophysiologic approach* (2nd ed.). New York: Elsevier.

DiPiro, J. T., Talbert, R. L., Yee, G. C., Matzke, G. R., Wells, B. G., & Posey, L. M. (Eds.). (1997). *Pharmacotherapy: A pathophysiologic approach* (3rd ed.). Stamford, CT: Appleton & Lange.

Melmon, K. L., & Morrelli, H. F. (Eds.). (1978). Clinical pharmacology basic principles in therapeutics (p. 3). New York: Macmillan.

# 2

# PHARMACOKINETICS AND PHARMACODYNAMICS

*Ginette A. Pepper*

The study of the interaction of drugs and other chemicals with living systems is *pharmacology*, which is a broad field of knowledge with several subdivisions. *Pharmacokinetics* focuses on changes in the concentrations of drugs over time resulting from absorption, distribution, metabolism, and excretion. *Pharmacodynamics* is the science of the molecular interactions of drugs with receptors and the subsequent reactions that result in the clinically observed drug response. Some other subdivisions of pharmacology are *toxicology* (the effects and detection of and antidotes for poisons and overdoses of drugs), *pharmacogenetics* (the relationship of genetics to variations in drug response), *pharmaceutics* (the compounding and preparation of dosing units), and *chronopharmacology* (the relationship of biologic rhythms to variations in drug response). Pharmacology, a scientific field, is distinguished from *pharmacy*, which is a practice discipline, just as sociology is a scientific field and social work is a practice discipline. The safe and effective use of drugs in the prevention, diagnosis, and treatment of disease and modification of physiologic functions such as reproduction, is the applied field of *pharmacotherapeutics*. Practice disciplines involved in pharmacotherapeutics include medicine, nursing, pharmacy, dentistry, veterinary medicine, podiatry, and all others involved in prescribing, dispensing, administering, and monitoring drug therapy and informing patients about their medications.

## VARIABILITY IN DRUG RESPONSE

If all patients with a particular diagnosis were identical, pharmacotherapeutics would require little more than application of a universal protocol. Because factors such as age, gender, race, body build, organ function, diet, genetic inheritance, concurrent medications, and comorbidity can alter the pharmacokinetics and pharmacodynamics of drugs, the clinician optimally individualizes drug therapy based upon his or her understanding of how these variables affect drug response. The understanding of pharmacokinetic and pharmacodynamic variability can guide the prescriber in the selection of drug, dosage, form, route, frequency, and titration, as well as in patient education and monitoring of drug therapy. For example, recognizing that a patient with renal impairment taking digoxin would be at risk for accumulation of this renally excreted drug, the prescriber should reduce the dosage or extend the dosing interval and educate the patient to detect and report symptoms of toxicity. Figure 2–1 illustrates that the relationship between administration of a drug and the response to the drug is determined by three phases of drug action: pharmaceutics, pharmacokinetics, and pharmacodynamics. Anything that modifies one of the phases of drug action can affect drug response, as manifested by the intended therapeutic effects and unintended adverse effects. The purposes of this chapter are to

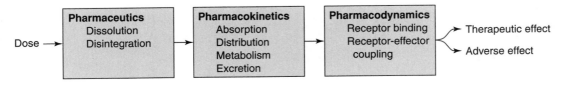

**Figure 2–1.** Phases of drug action.

**Source:** Modified from Pepper, G. A. and Wiener, M. B. (1985). Biophysical and psychosocial principles of drug action. In M. B. Wiener and G. A. Pepper (Eds), *Clinical pharmacology and therapeutics in nursing (2nd ed.)*. New York: McGraw-Hill, p. 56.

define the processes of each phase of drug action, to describe what factors modify the processes, to identify how the processes are measured, and to discuss the clinical implications of alterations in the phases of drug action.

## PLASMA PROFILE

Figure 2–2 illustrates the typical graphic representation of the plasma concentration of drugs over time after oral drug administration. This plasma profile reflects important clinical markers of the pharmaceutic and pharmacokinetic phases. During the absorptive phase of the curve, the *onset* of drug action occurs when the concentration of drug in the plasma $(C_p)$ first exceeds the minimum effective concentration, and the peak of drug action occurs when the highest plasma concentration (sometimes referred to as the $C_{max}$ or maximum concentration) is attained. The elimination phase of the curve is characterized by *termination* of the drug's effect when the plasma concentration falls below the minimum effective concentration. The *duration* of drug action is the time during which the plasma concentration exceeds the minimum effective concentration. *Toxicity* occurs when the plasma concentration exceeds the toxic level. The *therapeutic range* reflects the target serum concentrations for optimal drug response. This range is large in drugs with a wide margin of safety and small in drugs with a narrow margin of safety. An important parameter of the plasma profile commonly used in pharmaceutic and pharmacokinetic research studies is the *area under the*

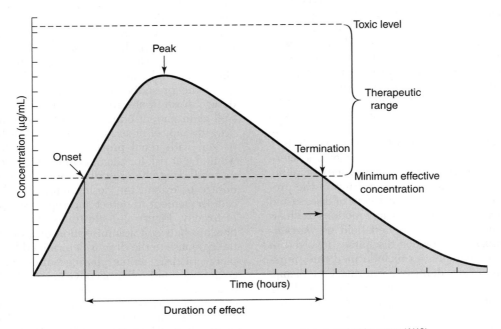

**Figure 2–2.** Plasma profile for a single dose. Shaded area represents area under the curve (AUC).

*curve* (AUC). Usually derived from computer calculations, the area under the curve is a measure of total exposure to the drug. Conceptualizing how unique variables alter the plasma profile can provide the clinician with guidance for individualizing pharmacotherapeutic decisions. For example, if taking a drug with food increases the rate of absorption, it can be anticipated that the peak concentration would be higher and the drug effect would be more intense for a shorter period of time.

## PHARMACEUTIC PHASE

The pharmaceutic phase involves the liberation of the drug from the dosing unit. Because a drug must be in solution to be absorbed and safely distributed in the body, the pharmaceutic phase is called the *rate-limiting step* of drug action; that is, the onset of the drug's effect can occur no faster than the rate at which the drug is released into solution from the product. Liquid dosing forms, such as injectables and elixirs, are already in solution and are immediately available for absorption and transport. The pharmaceutic phase for solid oral preparations, such as tablets and capsules, requires a two-step process: (1) disintegration into smaller particles and (2) dissolution of the particles so molecules of the diluent and drug intermingle in the solution. This phase is comparable to dissolving sugar cubes in tea. The cube must first disintegrate into sugar granules, and then the granules dissolve in the tea. The amount of fluid and intensity of stirring will influence how readily the sugar dissolves. Similarly, the fluid ingested with a drug and the motility of the gut will promote drug dissolution. Diseases or drugs that reduce gut motility will slow the liberation of drugs from solid preparations. Although they appear to be liquid, suspensions are actually particles of the drug suspended in liquid, so drugs in suspension must dissolve before they are available for absorption.

## IMMEDIATE-RELEASE PREPARATIONS

How a medication is compounded by the manufacturer determines the release characteristics of the drug product and onset of drug action, as illustrated in Figure 2–3. The preparation may be produced to speed the dissolution of the drug, frequently by formulation of the drug as a salt. For example, naproxen is available in tablet form as naproxen (Naprosyn) and as the salt, naproxen sodium (Aleve, Anaprox), which is more rapidly released from the tablet and has a faster onset. The dosage of naproxen sodium is 10% greater due to the weight of the sodium (200 mg of naproxen is equivalent to 220 mg of naproxen sodium). The Naproxen oral suspension and naproxen suppositories share the slower-release characteristics and dose of the naproxen tablets. Figure 2–3a compares the plasma profiles of a hypothetical drug with its more rapidly released salt, revealing that the peak concentration is higher and the onset and time to peak effect are twice as rapid for the salt form. Solutions for injection or topical use may also be formulated as salts or compounds to ensure solubility, which is especially important for intravenous or ophthalmic administration in which crystals or particles in the solution can have serious consequences.

Liberation of a drug from a dosing unit may also be modified to minimize adverse effects. Nitrofurantoin capsules (Macrodantin) contain macrocrystals of the drug which slow dissolution and absorption, causing less gastrointestinal irritation than the microcrystals in nitrofurantoin tablets and suspensions (Furadantin, others). Drugs such as bisacodyl (Dulcolax, others) are enteric-coated to prevent dissolution of the tablet in the acid environment of the stomach, reducing gastric irritation, nausea, and vomiting, but delaying drug onset (Fig. 2–3b). However, decreased production of hydrochloric acid, which occurs with aging, some diseases, and drugs for peptic ulcer disease (histamine blockers, antacids, and proton pump inhibitors), can increase the pH of the stomach enough to promote premature dissolution of enteric-coated drugs in the stomach.

Dosing systems that target delivery of the drug directly to the receptors in high concentrations provide minimal absorption and very low systemic drug concentrations. Topical decongestant sprays such as oxymetazoline (Afrin, others) are delivered directly to the site of action in the nasal mucosa and have few of the cardiac and central nervous system adverse effects of the oral decongestants such as phenylpropanolamine and pseudoephedrine (Sudafed, others). Similarly, metered dose inhalers for corticosteroids provide the advantages of steroid treatment of asthma without the serious metabolic effects of oral therapy.

(a) Comparison of drug with its salt

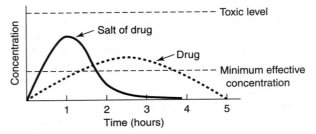

(b) Enteric coated tablet

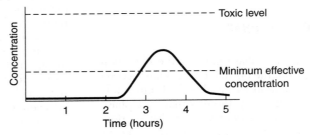

(c) Short-acting preparation dosed 4 times daily

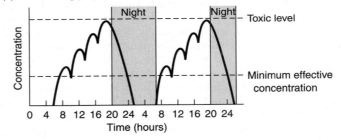

(d) Sustained release preparation

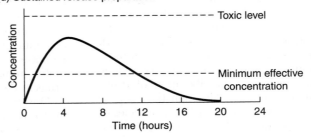

(e) Controlled release transdermal system

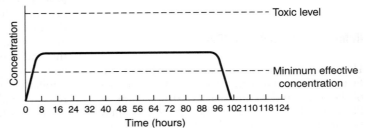

**Figure 2–3.** Plasma profiles for various pharmaceutic preparations.

## PROLONGED-RELEASE PREPARATIONS

When immediate-release preparations are used, there are fluctuations in drug concentration over the span of a dosing interval, resulting in peaks in drug concentration that can approach toxic concentrations and trough plasma concentrations below the minimum effective concentration, especially during the night, when the drug is not administered (Fig. 2–3c). Prolonged-release formulations decrease the required frequency of dosing, improving both convenience and compliance. Further, the decreased fluctuation in plasma concentrations can enhance therapeutic benefit. For example, research studies have suggested that immediate-release calcium channel blockers such as nifedipine (Adalat, Procardia) may be associated with increased incidence of coronary heart events compared to prolonged-release formulations (Adalat CC, Procardia XL), because the rapid absorption and sudden onset of hypotension can trigger reflex sympathetic stimulation. Additionally, plasma concentrations of the shorter-acting immediate-release calcium channel blockers are low in the early morning hours, providing no protection during the period of highest incidence of coronary events, and patients are more likely to omit doses of drugs requiring multiple daily doses (*Ad Hoc* Committee, 1997; Furberg & Psaty, 1996; Pepper, 1997*a*).

The first prolonged-release formulations consisted of capsules containing coated pellets of medication that dissolved at various rates depending on the amount of coating. The delayed dissolution of pellets prolongs the liberation of the drug and extends the duration of action (Fig. 2–3*d*). In prolonged-release intramuscular injectables, the drug is combined with an oil- or water-insoluble substance, called *depot* injections. Examples of these products, which are injected at intervals of a week to months and gradually release the drug, are penicillin G benzathine (Bicillin L-A), medroxyprogesterone acetate suspension (Depo-Provera), and haloperidol decanoate (Haldol LA). Recently, the development of prolonged-release dosage forms has focused on drug-polymer systems using either a *matrix* or *reservoir* configuration. These polymers are synthetically produced chains of molecules. In matrix systems molecules of the drug are bound to the polymers and released as the polymer dissolves or is hydrated; examples are delayed-release verapamil tablets (Calan SR, Isoptin SR) and morphine (MS Contin). Reser-

voir systems contain a pool of the drug surrounded by a rate-limiting polymeric membrane that controls the release of the drug. Products using a reservoir system (Fig. 2–3e) include oral extended-release tablets of nifedipine (Procardia XL), as well as transdermal fentanyl (Duragesic), nitroglycerin (Nitro-Dur, others), and clonidine (Catapres-TTS).

Many abbreviations, suffixes, and terms are used by manufacturers for prolonged-release dosage forms, such as sustained-release (SR), delayed-release, extended-release, controlled-release (CR, CD, CC), transdermal systems (TDS, TTS), and long-acting (LA, XL), so the nomenclature for these forms can be quite confusing. Because prolonged-release tablets and capsules contain 2–4 times as much medication as an immediate-release form of the drug, it is essential that both patients and clinicians distinguish these products.

## BIOEQUIVALENCE

Although pharmaceutically equivalent drugs contain identical amounts of the active drug, the excipients or inactive ingredients such as buffers, fillers, coloring, and flavoring in a tablet may differ widely from one manufacturer to another. These ingredients and the manufacturing process can cause clinical variability in the rate and extent of liberation of a drug from the dosing unit and its subsequent absorption. During the 1970s, studies showed that the digoxin tablets made by different manufacturers and even different lot numbers from the same manufacturer had as much as twofold differences in the area under the curve. This much variability could have harmful effects, especially for a drug like digoxin that has a narrow therapeutic range. Federal legislation passed in the 1980s mandated that manufacturers demonstrate that generic drugs are bioequivalent to the innovator drug, which is generally the first brand of a drug to be marketed. Although most generic drugs on the market have proven bioequivalence to the innovator, some drug groups such as hormones, oral and transdermal extended-release products, and a few older drugs do not have bioequivalence among manufacturers. Most agents are legally required to demonstrate bioequivalence within the range of −20%–+25% of the innovator, since experts have judged that this difference in the plasma concentration of a drug will not cause clinically detectable differences. Some researchers and clinicians have argued that this much difference may be clinically significant for some populations and diseases, such as the very young, the very old, and patients who are very difficult to regulate on cardiac, psychiatric, or other drugs. Clinicians should also note that bioequivalence has not yet been established for most drugs among the same strengths of different dosage forms; that is, a 40-mg capsule may not yield the same plasma profile as a 40-mg tablet, although a requirement for standardization among dosage forms is being considered. Food and Drug Administration (FDA) information on bioequivalence is published annually in the USPDI Volume III (1998) titled *Approved Drug Products and Legal Requirements*.

## CLINICAL IMPLICATIONS OF PHARMACEUTICS

When taking oral medications including liquids and suspensions, patients should ingest a full glass of water, which promotes the dissolution of drugs and their passage into the stomach. Generally, medications prescribed to be taken at bedtime should be taken at least 30 min before retiring, since an upright position aids the transport of medication into the stomach. Erosive esophagitis has resulted when drugs such as alendronate (Fosamax) or tetracycline were used without these precautions. Suspensions must be shaken before measurement to disperse the drug particles equally throughout the liquid, whereas solutions do not require agitation. Clinicians need to be mindful that patients with conditions that slow peristalsis, such as diabetic gastroparesis, or those taking anticholinergic drugs may have delayed or decreased drug absorption, especially for poorly soluble drugs such as digoxin (Lanoxin, others) or phenytoin (Dilantin, others). Similarly, it should be noted that enteric-coated medications might not afford protection against gastrointestinal irritation if the patient is taking antiulcer medications. Prescribers familiar with the range of dosage forms available and the plasma profile for each can provide alternatives that enhance the efficacy of drug therapy.

Patients must be well educated when a prolonged-release drug is substituted for immediate-release forms, as there have been numerous incidents of drug toxicity in patients taking prolonged-release preparations on a schedule appropriate for immediate-release form. The prohibition against crushing or chewing pro-

longed-release forms should also be emphasized. Some matrix forms are scored and may be divided without danger, but reservoir preparations must remain intact. Prescribers and patients should consult the pharmacist for proper use of dosage forms. Used transdermal patches must be disposed of in a location where pets or children cannot access the used product. Some reservoir systems such as the gastrointestinal system (GITS) used for nifedipine extended-release tablets (Procardia XL) may appear intact in the stool. Patients should be reassured that this is normal and that the drug has actually been released and absorbed.

Generally, it is recommended that immediate-release forms of a drug should be used to titrate the dosage of a drug, with the switch to an extended-release preparation being made after the optimal daily dosage has been identified, although some calcium channel blockers may be an exception (Pepper, 1997a). If a patient's response to a medication suddenly changes, the clinician should inquire whether there has been a prescription refill, since the pharmacist may have substituted a generic equivalent. For some patients the legal variability in bioequivalence can manifest as changes in disease control. In these cases and when the products are not bioequivalent, the prescriber can specify that the prescription be filled using a consistent manufacturer. This may be done by indicating the brand or manufacturer on the prescription and writing "DAW" (dispense as written) or "PBO" (prescribed brand only) or by communicating with the pharmacist orally or in writing of the need for consistent products. It is not essential that the drug be the innovator brand, which is often more expensive. Rather, it is important that the product used to titrate to optimal dosage is also used for maintenance therapy. Working together, the pharmacist and prescriber can ensure both quality and cost control.

## BIOTRANSPORT

Drug molecules must cross biologic membranes to reach the sites of action and sites where they will undergo the pharmacokinetic processes. The transport of chemicals across biologic membranes is called *biotransport*. How readily a drug crosses membranes is determined by the characteristics of biologic membranes and the characteristics of the particular drug molecule. *Biologic membranes* are composed of layers of individual cells, and drugs must usually pass through the cells to cross the membranes. Surrounding each cell is the *cell membrane*, consisting of a double layer of phospholipids oriented so that the lipid portions of the molecule are surrounded by the phosphate-containing portion of the molecule. Figure 2–4 shows several types of proteins embedded in the lipid bilayer. Some proteins form channels through which ions can traverse the membrane rapidly. Other proteins are carriers, capable of binding to a chemical and transporting it across the membrane. Drug receptors are also located on proteins embedded in membranes. Unless it can pass through a channel or is one of the few chemicals transported by a carrier, a drug must dissolve in the lipid layer as it crosses the cell membrane.

Features of drugs that affect their ability to cross membranes are size, lipid solubility, polarity, and ionization. Small molecules cross membranes more readily than large molecules. In fact, molecules with molecular weights in excess of 1000 are usually too large to be used as drugs because they cannot cross biologic membranes to access sites of action. Drugs which are lipid-soluble (*lipophilic*) dissolve easily in the lipid layer of the cell membrane and cross biologic membranes readily. Drugs which are water-soluble (*hydrophilic*) do not dissolve easily in the lipid layer and cross membranes poorly, if at all. *Polarity* and *ionization* are characteristics that make drugs hydrophilic (see Figure 2–5). Polar molecules have an uneven distribution of charge, with the positive and negative charges congregating at different parts of the molecule. However, polar molecules do not have a net charge. Ions are molecules that have a net charge, either positive or negative, which is represented by the

plus or minus sign in the chemical formula, such as the bicarbonate ion ($HCO_3^-$) or calcium ion ($Ca^{2+}$). In general, polar molecules and ions do not cross biologic membranes.

Many drugs are weak acids or weak bases. Acids and bases exist in ionized or nonionized states, depending upon the pH of the solution. Acids are molecules which can release a proton ($H^+$), becoming ionized with a net negative charge. Bases are molecules that can accept a proton, resulting in a positively charged ion. The ionized and nonionized forms of the acid (or base) are at equilibrium in a solution of a given pH, with some portion of total number of molecules in the ionized state and some portion in the nonionized state. Only drug molecules that are nonionized cross biologic membranes, but when the nonionized molecules cross the membrane, some of the remaining ionized drug molecules become nonionized to maintain the equilibrium. Acids in acid environments are predominantly in the nonionized form and cross biologic membranes rapidly. For example, acetylsalicylic acid (aspirin) is primarily nonionized in the acid environment of the stomach and is readily absorbed. Acids in alkaline environments are predominantly ionized, so the majority of the aspirin molecules in the small intestine cannot cross biologic membranes. However, even enteric-coated aspirin, which does not dissolve until it reaches the small intestine, is almost completely absorbed, because the small portion of aspirin that is nonionized is rapidly absorbed. Eventually, because of the shift of ionized aspirin to nonionized aspirin to maintain equilibrium, virtually all of the aspirin is absorbed. Conversely, bases in alkaline environments are pre-

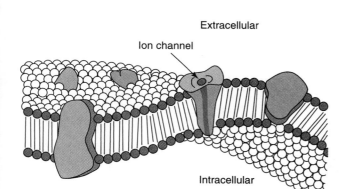

Extracellular

Ion channel

Intracellular

**Figure 2–4.** Structure of the cell membrane. The cell membrane is a double layer of phospholipid molecules with the highly polar phosphate heads of the molecules oriented outward and the nonpolar chains of fatty acids inside the membrane. Embedded in the membrane are proteins which include transport carriers, ion channels, and receptors.

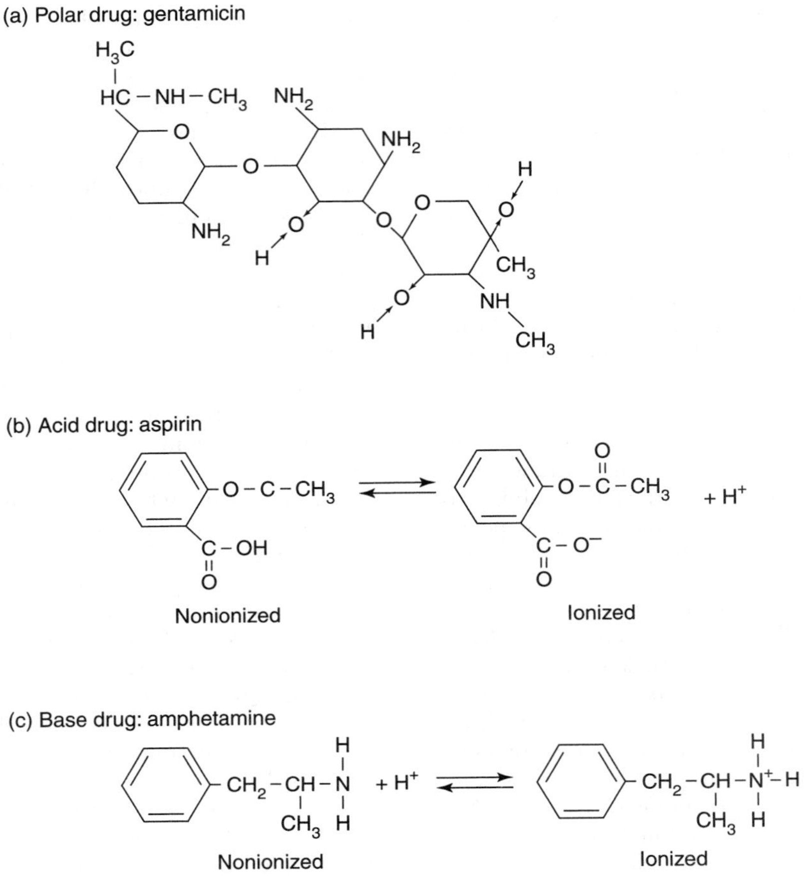

(a) Polar drug: gentamicin

(b) Acid drug: aspirin

Nonionized                                              Ionized

(c) Base drug: amphetamine

Nonionized                                              Ionized

**Figure 2–5.** Hydrophilic drug molecules. (a) Polar molecule. Oxygen atoms in the -OH groups of the structure of gentimicin attract electons (schematically represented by arrows), displacing the center of negative charge from the center of positive charge, resulting in a polar molecule. (b) Acid molecule. Aspirin is an acid that becomes ionized when it releases the protein ($H^+$), resulting in a net negative charge. (c) Base molecule. Amphetamine is a base that becomes polarized when it accepts a proton ($H^+$), resulting in a net positive charge.

dominantly nonionized; bases in acid environments are predominantly ionized. A base such as amphetamine in the stomach will be mainly in the ionized state and will have negligible absorption, but in the small intestine, it is absorbed rapidly.

## Mechanisms of Biotransport

Figure 2–6 shows four major mechanisms by which chemicals cross biologic membranes: filtration, pinocytosis, carrier-mediated transport,

and passive diffusion. Two types of drug interactions, competition for protein carriers, and ion trapping, are related to these mechanisms.

*Filtration.* In filtration, the drug passes through channels or pores in the cell membrane, or passes through the gaps between cells. Only very small molecules can cross by filtration through cell membranes, but if small enough, even polar molecules or ions such as potassium or lithium can cross by this mechanism. Filtration is also the mechanism by which drugs exit the vascula-

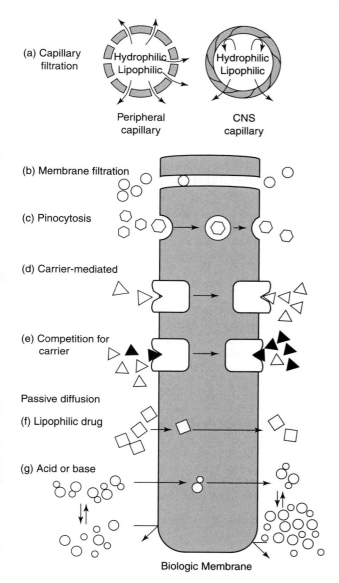

(a) Capillary filtration

Peripheral capillary

CNS capillary

(b) Membrane filtration

(c) Pinocytosis

(d) Carrier-mediated

(e) Competition for carrier

Passive diffusion

(f) Lipophilic drug

(g) Acid or base

Biologic Membrane

**Figure 2–6.** Mechanisms of biotransport. (a) Both lipophilic and hydrophilic drugs can filter out of peripheral capillaries, but drugs exiting central nervous system (CNS) capillaries must be lipophilic to pass through cells. (b) Small molecules can filter through channels in cell membranes. Larger and polar molecules can cross by (c) pinocytosis and (d) carrier-mediated transport, but (e) competition for the protein carrier can impair transport. (f) Lipophilic drugs diffuse through membranes readily, but (g) only ionized forms of acids and bases can cross membranes.

ture, since the epithelial cells that form the walls of the capillaries have gaps between them and all but the largest molecules readily exit. However, in some parts of the body, such as the brain, the cells of the capillaries have very tight junctures with no gaps between cells, and drugs cannot exit these capillaries by filtration.

**Pinocytosis.** In pinocytosis the cell wall engulfs the molecule, and it is transferred across the membrane in a vacuole. It is thought that antibodies cross the placenta by pinocytosis, transferring im-

munity from mother to infant. Currently pinocytosis is not significant in biotransport of drugs, but ongoing research suggests that in the future it may be possible to chemically induce pinocytosis by cell membranes. This would allow large molecules like heparin to be taken orally or facilitate the entry of macromolecules such as the missing enzyme in phenylketonuria into cells.

**Carrier-mediated Transport.** Drugs can be transported across biologic membranes by protein carrier molecules embedded in the cell membrane. Carrier-mediated transport has been proposed as the mechanism for transport of some drugs during absorption from the gastrointestinal tract, into the brain, and into cells. The elimination of drugs by active transport into the kidney tubule using protein carriers is called tubular secretion. When drugs are transported across membranes by protein carriers, it is possible that two drugs, or a drug and an endogenous chemical (ie, one that naturally occurs in the body) will use the same carrier protein. The concurrent presence of both molecules may overwhelm the carrier mechanism and result in decreased transfer of one or both substances. For example, levodopa competes with amino acids for carrier transport during absorption in the gastrointestinal tract, so taking levodopa with protein foods can cause erratic absorption. Instructing the patient to take levodopa with low-protein meals may help to stabilize the response to therapy.

***Passive Diffusion.*** In passive diffusion chemicals cross through the lipid bilayer of the cell membrane. Because passive diffusion is the major mechanism of drug biotransport, most drugs are relatively small molecules that are nonpolar and lipid-soluble, or are acids or bases that are nonionized at some physiologic pH. Polar or ionized drugs can be effective if administered parenterally. For example, the antibiotic gentamicin is a polar molecule (molecular weight 1500) that is administered intravenously for systemic infections because it is not absorbed orally unless there are lesions in the gastrointestinal tract.

Passive diffusion, as well as filtration, is driven by the concentration gradient, with drug molecules moving from areas of highest concentration to areas of lower concentration. If a biologic membrane intervenes between areas of different concentration of the drug, the drug moves "down" the gradient through the membrane until the concentration is equal on the two sides of the biologic membrane. When blood containing a drug passes through tissues with lower concentration than that in the plasma, drug molecules exit the blood vessels into the tissues. Thus, a drug does not usually accumulate in greater concentration on one side of a biologic membrane unless it is actively transported by a carrier-mediated mechanism. However, drugs that are acids or bases can accumulate unequally on either side of a membrane if there is a different pH on each side of the membrane. This phenomenon is called *ion trapping* or *pH partitioning*. For example, am-

phetamine molecules, which are nonionized in the alkaline pH of the plasma, become more ionized when they are filtered or diffused into the mammary gland, since human milk is slightly more acidic than plasma. The ionized drug becomes trapped in the milk because it cannot diffuse back across membranes. Thus, drugs that are bases can occur in higher concentration in the milk than in the maternal plasma.

## PHARMACOKINETIC PHASE

The pharmacokinetic phase has been described as what the body does to the drug during its sojourn in the organism. The processes of pharmacokinetics are absorption, distribution, metabolism, and excretion. The concentration of a drug available at the site of action over time depends upon these four processes, so the duration of action and magnitude of the drug's effect are governed by pharmacokinetics. Any alteration in the fundamental chemical or physiologic mechanisms underlying a pharmacokinetic process due to age, gender, disease, drug interaction, or other source of variation can modify the time-concentration relationship of the plasma profile. When this occurs, patient response to the drug, either therapeutic or adverse, can be altered. Although the pharmacokinetic processes of absorption, distribution, metabolism, and excretion actually occur simultaneously, with changes in one process affecting other processes, they are best learned as discrete sequential events.

### ABSORPTION

Absorption is defined as the passage of the drug from the site of administration into the systemic circulation. Drugs administered intravenously are delivered directly into the systemic circulation, bypass the absorptive process, and are totally and immediately absorbed. The rate and extent of absorption of drugs delivered by other routes of administration are influenced by four physical or physiologic mechanisms: (1) surface area, (2) contact time, (3) concentration gradient, and (4) presystemic metabolism.

#### Surface Area

The rate and completeness of absorption are proportional to the area of the absorptive surface. The reason that enteric-coated aspirin is well-absorbed in the small intestine, where most of this acid drug is ionized, is that the small intestine has a large absorptive surface that rapidly absorbs the nonionized aspirin. Because the absorptive surface of the lungs is even larger, drugs delivered through the lungs, such a nicotine in cigarette smoke, achieve high peak levels very rapidly. Transdermal nicotine skin patches release the nicotine at a steady rate, which does not produce a plasma profile at all similar to that for the actual smoking of cigarettes. Other delivery systems for nicotine, such as nasal sprays, which more closely mimic the rapid peak in the plasma profile of smoking, are being tested for effectiveness in promoting smoking cessation.

## Contact Time

Contact time is the duration that the drug is contiguous to an absorptive surface. Conditions that alter peristalsis affect contact time for oral drugs. For example, diarrhea can curtail drug and nutrient absorption. The administration technique, such as how long a transdermal patch is worn, whether an ointment is wiped off after application, or how long the breath is held after a metered dose inhaler, affects the contact time of topical drugs.

## Concentration Gradient

The concentration gradient drives the movement of a drug by passive diffusion through biologic membranes. For example, a drug moves out of the reservoir in a transdermal skin patch into the dermal tissues and then into the circulation as it moves down the concentration gradient. A good blood supply to the site of drug administration sweeps the drug molecules away once they enter the circulation, thereby maintaining the concentration gradient that sustains absorption until virtually all of the drug has crossed into the circulation.

## Presystemic Metabolism

Before a drug enters the systemic circulation, there are a number of sites illustrated in Figure 2–7 where it may be metabolized to an inactive metabolite. Some drugs are destroyed by the acid in the stomach. Penicillin G is an example of an acid-labile drug; only 30–40% of an orally administered dose will be absorbed because the rest is destroyed by stomach acid. If penicillin G is taken with food, which stimulates the release

of additional stomach acid, the absorption may be decreased to 20%. Drugs can also be metabolized by bacteria in the small intestine. Digoxin undergoes presystemic metabolism by intestinal bacteria, and toxicity can be triggered by antibiotic therapy that kills intestinal bacteria, because more of the digoxin is available for absorption. The venous circulation for most of the intestinal tract, excluding the mouth and lower one third of the rectum, passes first through the portal circulation into the liver, where toxins and impurities ingested with food are eliminated, before the portal blood merges with the systemic circulation in the inferior vena cava. Drugs can be metabolized on this initial pass through the liver, a phenomenon known as *first-pass metabolism*. Drugs susceptible to the first-pass effect (listed in Table 2–1) will have marked differences between oral and parenteral dosages. For example, 60 mg of morphine administered orally is required to achieve the pain relief given by 10 mg parenterally, since the majority of morphine is lost through first-pass metabolism. In addition, drugs that undergo first-pass metabolism often have variable dosage requirements among individuals because the genetic variability in drug-metabolizing enzymes causes variation in drug absorption from person to person.

## Factors That Alter Absorption

Any condition that alters surface area, contact time, concentration gradient, or presystemic metabolism can affect absorption. The route of administration is a major variable in absorption. Intramuscular injection yields a faster onset and shorter duration than subcutaneous injection because muscular anatomy is characterized by flat planes of muscle tissue that promote the spread of the injected drug across a larger absorptive surface area. Further, the greater blood flow to muscles than to subcutaneous tissue promotes the concentration gradient. Exercise can increase the absorption of a drug injected into a muscle or subcutaneous tissue of an extremity by increasing blood flow, just as hypoperfusive states resulting from shock or vascular and cardiac diseases can decrease absorption of injected drugs. Sublingual, lingual (metered dose spray), and buccal administration are advantageous for drugs that undergo first-pass metabolism. Nitroglycerin is used to treat acute anginal attacks by these routes, which not only bypass its extensive first-pass metabolism, but also promote the rapid absorption essential for immediate onset.

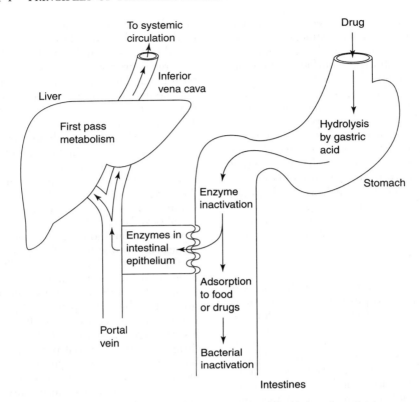

**Figure 2–7.** Presystemic metabolism. Drugs can be metabolized before absorption is complete by gastric acid, bacterial action in the intestine, and enzymes in the intestine or cell wall. The first pass effect involves metabolism as drugs absorbed into the portal circulation pass through the liver before entering the systemic circulation.

Rectal administration also may bypass first-pass metabolism, but rectal absorption is erratic due to the small absorptive surface area and tendency for the drug to ascend into segments subject to first-pass metabolism.

Acute or chronic malabsorptive diseases alter oral drug absorption by affecting the amount or integrity of the absorptive surface and by altering contact time through changes in peristalsis. Liver disease can decrease first-pass metabolism so that a greater portion of the administered dosage reaches the systemic circulation. Topical or transdermal absorption is increased in the presence of a rash, sunburn, or irritation, since the blood flow to the absorptive surface is increased. The effects of pregnancy and age on drug absorption are complex and of limited clinical significance, except decreased first-pass metabolism in the elderly, which probably contributes to high plasma concentrations of some drugs in these populations (see Chap. 13).

## Absorption Drug Interactions

Mechanisms of drug interaction that alter absorptive processes include chelation, adsorption, alteration of peristalsis, alteration of hydrochloric acid production, alteration of intestinal flora, and competition for protein carriers. Coadministration of tetracycline or ciprofloxacin (Cipro) with food or medication that contains a divalent cation ($Ca^{2+}$, $Mg^{2+}$, $Fe^{2+}$) or trivalent cation ($Fe^{3+}$, $Al^{3+}$) results in the formation of an insoluble chelate that prevents the absorption of the antibiotic. The therapeutic benefit of cholestyramine (Questran), attapulgite (Kaopectate) or kaolin and pectin (Kaopectolin) is due to the ability of these agents to adsorb (attract and combine with) toxins and chemicals like cholesterol, preventing their absorption. These adsorbent agents also decrease the absorption of drugs such as digoxin and diuretics. Either increased or decreased gastrointestinal peristalsis affects drug absorption. The prokinetic agents

## TABLE 2–1. DRUGS WITH EXTENSIVE FIRST-PASS METABOLISM

| Drug | Oral Bioavailability, F |
| --- | --- |
| Diltiazem (Cardizem) | 0.44 |
| Imipramine (Tofranil) | 0.40 |
| Isosorbide dinitrate (Isordil) | 0.22 |
| Labetalol (Normodyme, Trandate) | 0.18 |
| Lidocaine (Xylocaine) | 0.35 |
| Meperidine (Demerol) | 0.52 |
| Metoprolol (Lopressor) | 0.38 |
| Morphine | 0.24 |
| Nifedipine (Procardia) | 0.50 |
| Nortriptyline (Aventyl, Pamelor) | 0.51 |
| Propranolol (Inderal) | 0.26 |
| Verapamil (Isoptin, Calan) | 0.22 |

comparing the area under the curve of the plasma profile for oral administration (or another route) to the area under the curve for intravenous administration, which represents complete absorption. The abbreviation for bioavailability is F for fraction of the drug absorbed, but bioavailability is often reported as the percentage absorbed. Drugs with significant first-pass metabolism (listed in Table 2-1) have low bioavailability, because the drug is metabolized before it reaches the systemic circulation. Other drugs with low bioavailability are those with poor solubility, which retards dissolution, and drugs susceptible to other types of presystemic metabolism.

## DISTRIBUTION

Distribution is defined as the transport of drugs to sites of action and elimination, as well as storage of the drug in the organism. Figure 2–8 represents how potential distribution space for a drug is conceptualized as containing a central compartment consisting of the plasma and a peripheral compartment consisting of the rest of the extracellular fluid and tissues. Drugs that distribute primarily to the central compartment circulate through the kidneys and liver frequently and thus are subject to elimination, whereas drugs stored in the peripheral compartment may persist for weeks. Physiologic mechanisms that determine the distribution characteristics of a drug are (1) blood flow, (2) special membrane barriers, (3) plasma protein binding, and (4) amount and characteristics of storage tissues.

### Blood Flow

Once drug molecules enter the systemic circulation, they are initially distributed to organs in proportion to blood flow to the organ. Since the brain receives 20% of cardiac output even though it is less than 5% of body mass, its potential exposure to drugs is considerable. When short-acting barbiturates are administered intravenously for the induction of anesthesia, the patient falls asleep rapidly because of the initial exposure from the intravenous bolus, but will awaken in a few minutes unless other anesthetics are administered. The half-life of these agents averages over 20 h, so it is not the elimination of the drug that causes the termination of effect. Rather it is the *redistribution phenomenon* that occurs when the concentration of drug

metoclopramide (Reglan) and cisapride (Propulsid) speed intestinal transit and decrease the absorption of many drugs. Drugs with anticholinergic properties (eg, tricyclic antidepressants, phenothiazines, antihistamines, antiparkinsonian agents, antispasmodics) slow peristalsis, which delays gastric emptying and prolongs intestinal transit time. Because little absorption occurs in the stomach, delayed gastric emptying delays drug onset. Once the drug passes into the intestine, contact time is increased by the slowed peristalsis, which enhances overall absorption. Changes in stomach pH alter the absorption of drugs such as the antifungal ketoconazole (Nizoral), which requires a low pH for absorption and may be poorly absorbed when antiulcer drugs that decrease stomach acidity are given concurrently. Since bacteria in the intestines metabolize digoxin and other drugs presystemically, broad-spectrum antibiotic therapy can increase drug absorption and lead to toxicity. Competition for the protein carrier for transport across absorptive surfaces is a rare drug interaction; the erratic absorption of levodopa in competition with amino acids is the most significant example. Chelation, adsorption, competition for protein carriers, and alteration of gastric acidity with antacids require the interacting drugs to be present in the stomach at the same time. Therefore, timing of drug administrations as far apart as possible will minimize these interactions, but this strategy is ineffective for other types of drug interactions.

### Bioavailability

The measure of liberation and absorption of drugs is bioavailability, which is computed by

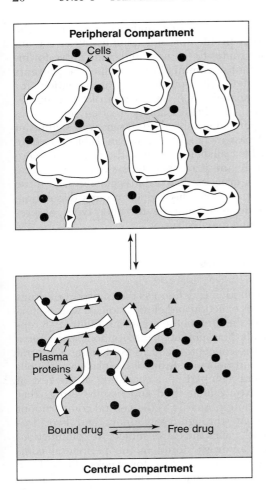

**Figure 2–8.** Conceptual distribution compartments. The distribution spaces for drugs are conceptualized as a central compartment (also called plasma compartment) and the peripheral compartment (also called tissue compartment). In the plasma compartment are a drug (●) which is 80% plasma protein bound and a drug (▲) that is 30% bound. In the peripheral compartment the lipophilic drug (●) is sequestered in the lipid membranes, while the hydrophilic drug (▲) distributes to extracellular fluid.

molecules distributed to the brain from the initial bolus is higher than that in the plasma, so the molecules move out of the brain and are redistributed to organs with lower blood flow. Blood flow is also critical during antibiotic therapy. If the site of the infection is well perfused, the antibiotic is more effective than if blood flow is restricted by peripheral vascular disease or some other condition.

## Special Membrane Barriers

A number of membrane barriers have been identified that restrict the passage of chemicals, including the placental barrier, the blood-testicular barrier, and the blood-milk barrier. The blood-brain barrier is a function of the anatomy of capillaries in the brain which have tight junctures between the cells, rather than the gaps that characterize other capillaries. Glia, the connective tissues of the brain, also play a role in limiting access of chemicals to the brain. Drug molecules must pass through the cells to gain access to the central nervous system, and only lipophilic substances achieve significant concentrations in the brain. This can be a problem when there is an infection of brain tissue, because most antibiotics are hydrophilic. However, meningitis causes vasodilation of the capillaries and increases penetration of hydrophilic drugs. To circumvent the blood brain barrier, drugs can be administered directly into the cerebrospinal fluid or administered as precursors that can cross the blood-brain barrier. For example, precursor therapy is used in Parkinson's disease, which is associated with reduced concentrations of dopamine in certain areas of the brain. Dopamine is a polar molecule that cannot cross the blood-brain barrier and causes marked cardiovascular effects in the peripheral tissues. The precursor levodopa, crosses the blood-brain barrier and is converted to dopamine by the enzyme dopa decarboxylase. Unfortunately, levodopa is also converted to dopamine by dopa decarboxylase in peripheral tissues, resulting in adverse cardiovascular effects. Combining levodopa and an inhibitor of dopa decarboxylase that does not cross the blood-brain barrier in the combined product, carbidopa-levodopa (Sinemet) results in a beneficial effect in the brain with decreased dosage requirements, because levodopa is converted to dopamine in the brain, but not in the peripheral tissues where dopa decarboxylase is inhibited.

## Plasma Protein Binding

Figure 2–8 illustrates that many drugs are transported in plasma bound to proteins, which increases their water solubility and renders them pharmacologically inactive. That is, as long as the drug is bound to plasma protein, it is pharmacodynamically inert because it cannot exit the vascular space to get to receptors and it is pharmacokinetically inert because it cannot be metabolized or excreted. The drug in the plasma exits in an equilibrium of bound and free drug. Highly bound drugs have greater than 90% of the drug in the plasma bound to plasma protein and less than 10% as the pharmacologically active free drug. Warfarin (Coumadin) is an example of a highly bound drug with 98% of the drug bound to plasma albumin. The 2% free warfarin molecules interact with receptors in the liver to alter production of clotting factors, but are also eliminated by metabolism. Then 2% of the remaining drug in the body is freed from the albumin to react with receptors and be metabolized. Thus, plasma protein binding can act as the body's physiologic sustained-release mechanism. If warfarin were not protein-bound, it would be too toxic to use clinically unless given by intravenous infusion. Plasma proteins which bind drugs include albumin, globulins, and lipoproteins (Table 2–2). Albumin binds acidic drugs at several different binding sites, whereas $\alpha_1$-acid glycoprotein (AAG) binds bases. Most drugs that are highly bound concentrate in the plasma compartment, because the plasma protein binding sequesters the drug in the blood vessels.

## Tissue Storage

Drug molecules not bound to plasma proteins can distribute to the peripheral compartment.

Hydrophilic drugs distribute to the lean mass which includes the extracellular water, intracellular water, and the muscles. Lipophilic drugs distribute to lipids in cell membranes and adipose tissue, which can store the drug and gradually release it over time. Drugs can also be stored by being bound to other peripheral tissues. For example, digoxin binds to protein in muscles. The amount of tissue influences how much drug can be stored. Obese patients have greater capacity to store lipophilic drugs, and patients with muscle wasting have decreased digoxin storage potential. This depot storage of drugs prolongs their duration of action, because the molecules are in the peripheral compartment and not subject to metabolism and excretion.

## Factors That Alter Distribution

Age, gender, disease, and nutrition are variables that alter drug distribution by affecting blood flow, special barriers, plasma protein binding, and tissue storage. The distribution of cardiac output, competence of the blood-brain barrier, amount and capacity of plasma proteins to bind drugs, and body composition vary with developmental stage and pregnancy, resulting in age-related differences in drug distribution. Gender

## TABLE 2–2. EXTENT AND PRIMARY SITE OF BINDING TO PLASMA PROTEINS

| Albumin | Percentage Bound | $\alpha_1$-acid Glycoprotein | Percentage Bound | Lipoproteins | Percentage Bound |
|---|---|---|---|---|---|
| Amoxicillin | 18 | Bupavicaine | 98 | Amitriptyline | |
| Aspirin | 49 | Disopyramide | | (Elavil) | 95 |
| Chlorpropamide (Diabinese) | 96 | (Norpace) | * | Nortriptyline | |
| Diazepam (Valium) | 99 | Imipramine (Tofranil) | 90 | (Pamelor) | 92 |
| Fluoxetine (Prozac) | 98 | Lidocaine | 70 | | |
| Glipizide (Glucotrol) | 98[†] | Prazosin (Minipress) | 95 | | |
| Ibuprofen (Motrin) | 99 | Propranolol (Inderal) | 87 | | |
| Meperidine (Demerol) | 58 | Quinidine | 87 | | |
| Phenobarbital | 51 | Verapamil (Calan) | 90 | | |
| Phenytoin (Dilantin) | 89 | | | | |
| Simvastatin (Zocor) | 95 | | | | |
| Sulfamethoxazole (in Bactrim, Septra) | 62 | | | | |
| Tetracycline | 65 | | | | |
| Tolbutamide (Orinase) | 96 | | | | |
| Valproic acid (Depakene, Depakote) | 93 | | | | |
| Warfarin (Coumadin) | 98 | | | | |

*Binding varies by concentration.
[†]Nonionic binding; does not displace other albumin-bound drugs.

differences in drug distribution due to body composition commence at puberty and account for substantial variability in drug response. Women have less lean mass and greater fat mass than men. A woman taking an identical "dose" of ethanol as a man of the same weight would have a higher blood level of the drug because ethanol is distributed to lean mass, which constitutes a smaller percentage of the total weight of women. Diseases that cause fluid retention change the distribution of drugs by increasing total body water. Nephrotic syndrome depletes plasma albumin, and uremia impairs the binding of drugs because the waste products accumulated in plasma bind to albumin, decreasing binding sites available for drugs. Although it is known that $\alpha_1$-acid glycoprotein is increased in inflammatory diseases and cancer, the effect of these changes on drug binding and clinical response has not been established. Undernutrition and overnutrition also affect body composition and the amount of plasma albumin available to bind drugs.

## Distribution Drug Interactions

The number of binding sites on plasma protein is limited, so two drugs that bind to the same site on plasma protein compete for binding if they are present in the plasma simultaneously. Competition for plasma protein binding can also occur between a drug and an endogenous substance such as bilirubin, which is highly bound to albumin. Newborns receiving sulfonamides have developed kernicterus when bilirubin displaced from binding sites by the sulfonamides was deposited in the brain. The immediate effect of adding a highly protein bound drug to the regimen of a patient already taking another drug bound to the same site is a magnified effect of one or both drugs, because there is a greater free drug concentration available to interact with receptors. Figure 2–9 shows that over time the free drug is subject to increased elimination and the initial concentration of free drug will be restored, reducing the total drug (bound drug + free drug) concentration. Therefore, the clinical effects of competition for plasma protein binding are usually self-limiting and of short duration. However, if the interaction involves a highly plasma protein bound drug with a narrow therapeutic range or if the elimination of the free drug is impaired by organ disease or drug interaction, drug toxicity can develop. Further, this drug interaction must be considered in the interpretation of laboratory assays for plasma concentrations of drugs ("blood levels"). Since these assays measure the total drug level in the plasma, the plasma concentration may appear subtherapeutic due to the accelerated excretion of free drug, even though the remaining free drug is sufficient to control the disease clinically. If the clinician fails to recognize the drug interaction and does not ascertain that the clinical

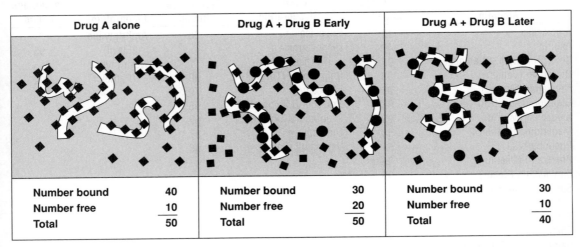

| Drug A alone | | Drug A + Drug B Early | | Drug A + Drug B Later | |
|---|---|---|---|---|---|
| Number bound | 40 | Number bound | 30 | Number bound | 30 |
| Number free | 10 | Number free | 20 | Number free | 10 |
| Total | 50 | Total | 50 | Total | 40 |

**Figure 2–9.** Competition for protein binding. When present alone, Drug A (■) is 80% bound to plasma protein. Addition of Drug B (●) which is avidly bound to the same sites on plasma protein causes competition and release of Drug A, doubling the concentration of its free fraction and increasing its clinical effect. Over time the increased free Drug A is eliminated and the free drug concentration returns to baseline. Although the total drug is less, only the pharmacologically inert bound drug is decreased.

response to the drug is appropriate, raising the dosage to achieve the "therapeutic range" could cause drug toxicity.

## Volume of Distribution

The distribution characteristics of a drug are quantified by the *apparent volume of distribution*, which is abbreviated $V_D$. The apparent volume of distribution is defined as the volume required to contain the dose if it was distributed equally at the concentration in the plasma. Of course, drugs are not distributed equally throughout the body at the concentration in the plasma. Some drugs are stored in the peripheral tissues, and only a fraction of the total drug is in the plasma. These drugs have a large $V_D$; for example, the $V_D$ of fluoxetine (Prozac) is 2520 L in a 70-kg man, which is physically impossible since 2520 L of water weighs 2520 kg. Because fluoxetine is lipophilic and distributes to the peripheral compartment, leaving only a fraction of the dose in the plasma, the plasma concentration from a 40-mg dose averages approximately 30 ng/mL (1 nanogram = 1000 micrograms). If it is assumed that the dose is equally distributed at 30 ng/mL, it would *apparently* require 2520 L, or 36 L/kg, to contain the dose. Although the apparent volume of distribution is an abstraction rather than an actual volume, $V_D$ can be used to characterize the distribution of a drug according

to the values in Table 2–3. $V_D$ is also useful in pharmacokinetic calculations and in computing loading doses (see App. 2–1, Calculating Loading Doses).

## METABOLISM

Metabolism and excretion are the two processes by which drugs are eliminated from the body. Metabolism, also called *biotransformation*, is the elimination of a drug through enzymatic alteration of the chemical structure of the drug molecule to form a metabolite. The drug is eliminated from the body by conversion to a new chemical entity that is more water-soluble and more readily excreted from the body. The resulting metabolites may be active or inactive. Active metabolites retain the ability to interact with the target receptor and cause therapeutic and adverse effects of the parent drug. Some medicinals, called *prodrugs*, are not active in the form administered but are activated by metabolism in the intestinal wall or during the first pass through the liver. It is even possible for a metabolite to be more toxic than the parent drug. For example, one of the intermediary metabolites of acetaminophen (Tylenol) can cause liver necrosis if it is present in the high concentrations that occur in overdose or hepatic impairment. Although the major organ of me-

## TABLE 2–3.  INTERPRETATION OF VOLUME OF DISTRIBUTION

| If $V_d$ is approximately . . . | | | Examples | |
|---|---|---|---|---|
| L/kg | L/70 kg | Drug Distributes to . . . | Drug | $V_D$, L/kg |
| 0.6 | 40 | Total body water | Enalapril (Vasotec) | 0.6 |
| | | | Erythromycin | 0.8 |
| | | | Lithium | 0.8 |
| | | | Nifedipine (Procardia) | 0.8 |
| | | | Theophylline | 0.5 |
| 0.2 | 15 | Extracellular fluid | Amoxicillin | 0.2 |
| | | | Gentamicin | 0.2 |
| | | | Cephalexin (Keflex) | 0.2 |
| 0.04 | 3 | Plasma | Chlorpropamide (Diabinese) | 0.04 |
| | | | Warfarin | 0.13 |
| | | | Furosemide (Lasix) | 0.05 |
| >0.7 | >46 | Sequestered in peripheral tissues | Acetaminophen | 1.0 |
| | | | Diazepam (Valium) | 1.1 |
| | | | Digoxin | 6.2 |
| | | | Fluoxetine (Prozac) | 36 |

tabolism is the liver, drugs undergo metabolism in many different organs. Physiologic mechanisms that determine the liver metabolism of drugs are (1) amount of liver blood flow and (2) enzyme activity.

## Liver Blood Flow

Since the liver is the major organ of metabolism, liver blood flow is critical to drug elimination, because it determines the exposure of drugs to hepatic enzymes. Drugs designated as high hepatic extraction drugs (see Table 2–6 in the section on drug clearance below) are particularly sensitive to changes in liver blood flow and can accumulate to toxic concentrations if liver blood flow is impaired.

## Enzyme Activity

Although there are numerous specific enzyme reactions that metabolize drugs, two broad categories have been identified. *Phase I*, or nonsynthetic, reactions involve the addition or unmasking of a polar group on the drug molecule. *Phase II*, or conjugation, reactions entail joining of the drug molecule to a polar molecule. Two common conjugation reactions are *glucuronidation*, bonding the drug to a glucose molecule, and *acetylation*, bonding the drug molecule to an acetate molecule. Although the terms suggest that a Phase I reaction always precedes a Phase II reaction, drugs can undergo only Phase II metabolism or only Phase I metabolism, or can undergo both processes in any order. Drugs often have multiple pathways for metabolism and several active or inactive metabolites.

An important group of enzyme systems for metabolizing drugs and endogenous lipophilic substances such as steroidal hormones is the *cytochrome P-450 enzymes*, which have also been called the *mixed-function oxidases* or the *microsomal enzymes*. Cytochrome, like hemoglobin, is a hemoprotein. Eleven isozyme families of cytochrome P-450 have been identified, designated by "CYP" to indicate human cytochrome P-450, followed by the Arabic number to designate the P-450 family, followed by a capital letter to designate the subfamily, followed by a second Arabic number to designate the particular gene encoding the isozyme (Table 2–4). The cytochrome P-450 enzymes catalyze primarily Phase I reactions. A notable characteristic of these enzyme systems is their responsiveness to

environmental chemicals. Some chemicals increase the density and activity of cytochrome P-450 enzymes, a process called *induction*. Other chemicals can decrease the amount and activity of the cytochrome P-450 enzymes, which is referred to as enzyme *inhibition*. Induction and inhibition are the mechanism for important interactions of drugs with foods, environmental pollutants, and other drugs.

## Factors That Alter Metabolism

Metabolism is the most individual of pharmacokinetic processes, varying among individuals and within the same individual over time. Genetic inheritance is the major source of individual difference in drug metabolism. For example, in some racial groups, 5–20% of the population may lack one of the isozymes of cytochrome P-450, utilizing different pathways to metabolize drugs usually processed by that isozyme (Nemeroff, DeVane & Pollock, 1996). In the United States about half of the population are slow acetylators, more prone to develop certain adverse effects with drugs that are metabolized by acetylation, such as isoniazid (INH) and procainamide (Pronestyl). Very little of the genetic basis of drug metabolism has been adequately studied, so this important source of variation in drug response remains poorly understood.

Developmental and environmental factors also have profound effects on drug metabolism. The very young and the very old have less effective hepatic metabolism than young adults, but children actually have accelerated elimination of some drugs metabolized by cytochrome P-450. Since the constituents of cytochrome P-450 and other drug-metabolizing enzymes are iron, proteins, and vitamin cofactors, nutritional deficiency can impair drug metabolism. Thyroid function can speed or slow drug metabolism, and correction of hyperthyroid or hypothyroid states will alter dose requirements for many drugs. Diseases like cirrhosis and hepatitis decrease both the hepatic blood flow and enzyme activity, resulting in decreased drug elimination. Although patients with abnormal values on liver function tests often have impairment of drug metabolism, it is not possible to adjust dosages of metabolized drugs based upon laboratory tests of liver function. The clinician must rely on an assay of plasma concentration of the drug or evaluation of the clinical response to titrate dosages of hepatically eliminated drugs.

**TABLE 2–4. CYTOCHROME P-450 ISOZYMES, SUBSTRATES, INDUCERS, AND INHIBITORS**

| Isozyme | Substrates | Inducers | Inhibitors |
|---|---|---|---|
| CYP1A2 | Acetaminophen (Tylenol)<br>Caffeine<br>Clozapine (Clozaril)<br>Imipramine (Tofranil)<br>Tacrine (Cognex)<br>Theophylline<br>R-warfarin (Coumadin) | Charbroiled foods<br>Cigarette smoke<br>Cruciferous vegetables<br>Phenytoin (Dilantin)<br>Rifampin | Cimetidine (Tagamet)<br>Ciprofloxacin (Cipro)<br>Diltiazem (Cardizem)<br>Enoxacin (Penetrex)<br>Erythromycin<br>Fluvoxamine (Luvox)<br>Mexiletine (Mexitil)<br>Norfloxacin (Noroxin)<br>Tacrine (Cognex) |
| CYP2C9 | Amitriptyline (Elavil)<br>Diclofenac (Voltaren)<br>Ibuprofen (Motrin)<br>Imipramine (Tofranil)<br>S-warfarin (Coumadin) | | Cimetidine (Tagamet)<br>Disulfiram (Antabuse)<br>Fluconazole (Diflucan)<br>Fluvastatin (Lescol)<br>Metronidazole (Flagyl)<br>Trimethoprim-sulfamethoxazole<br>   (Bactrim, Septra) |
| CYP2C19 | Diazepam (Valium)<br>Imipramine (Tofranil)<br>Naproxen (Anaprox)<br>Omeprazole (Prilosec)<br>Phenytoin (Dilantin)<br>Propranolol (Inderal)<br>Tolbutamide (Orinase) | | Felbamate (Felbatol)<br>Fluoxetine (Prozac)<br>Fluvoxamine (Luvox)<br>Omeprazole (Prilosec) |
| CYP2D6 | Amitriptyline (Elavil)<br>Bupropion (Wellbutrin)<br>Clomipramine (Anafranil)<br>Codeine<br>Desipramine (Norpramin)<br>Dextromethorphan<br>Fluoxetine (Prozac)<br>Haloperidol (Haldol)<br>Imipramine (Tofranil)<br>Metoprolol (Lopressor)<br>Nortriptyline (Aventyl)<br>Paroxetine (Paxil)<br>Pentazocine (Talwin)<br>Propranolol (Inderal)<br>Risperidone (Risperdal)<br>Thioridazine (Mellaril)<br>Type 1c antiarrhythmics (eg,<br>   encainide, flecainide, propafenone)<br>Venlafaxine (Effexor) | ?Dexamethasone<br>?Rifampin | Amiodarone<br>Fluoxetine (Prozac)<br>Haloperidol (Haldol)<br>Paroxetine (Paxil)<br>Quinidine<br>Ranitidine (Zantac)<br>Thioridazine (Mellaril)<br>Venlafaxine (Effexor) |
| CYP3A4<br>(also in<br>intestinal<br>mucosa) | Alprazolam (Xanax)<br>Astemizole (Hismanal)<br>Carbamazepine (Tegretol)<br>Cisapride (Propulsid)<br>Corticosteroids<br>Cyclosporine<br>Diazepam (Valium) | Carbamazepine<br>(Tegretol)<br>Corticosteroids<br>Phenobarbital<br>Phenytoin (Dilantin)<br>Rifampin | Cimetidine (Tagamet)<br>Clarithromycin (Biaxin)<br>Diltiazem (Cardizem)<br>Erythromycin<br>Fluconazole (Diflucan)<br>Fluoxetine (Prozac)<br>Miconazole (Monistat) |

(continues on next page)

**TABLE 2–4.** *continued from previous page*

| Isozyme | Substrates | Inducers | Inhibitors |
|---|---|---|---|
| CYP3A4 (also in intestinal mucosa) | Diltiazem (Cardizem) Felodipine (Plendil) Lidocaine Lovastatin (Mevacor) Midazolam (Versed) Nifedipine (Procardia) Quinidine Simvastatin (Zocor) Terfenadine (Seldane) Triazolam (Halcion) Verapamil (Isoptin, Calan) | | Nefazodone (Serzone) Omeprazole (Prilosec) Propoxyphene (Darvon) Quinidine Fluvoxamine (Luvox) Grapefruit juice Itraconazole (Sporanox) Ketoconazole (Nizoral) Mibefradil (Posicor) Protease inhibitors (e.g., indinavir, ritonavir) |

*Sources: Hansten (1996); Pepper (1997b).*

## Metabolism Drug Interactions

A growing list of chemicals, including drugs, foods, and pollutants, have been identified that can induce or inhibit cytochrome P-450 enzyme systems, and recent research has identified the specific isozymes involved for some interactions. Table 2–4 lists the isozyme, the substrates metabolized by the isozyme, the drugs that induce the isozyme, and the drugs that inhibit the isozyme. When a cytochrome P-450 isozyme is induced by a drug or chemical, the rate of metabolism of any substrate of that isozyme is increased, which lowers the serum concentration and results in decreased drug effect. For example, a cigarette smoker metabolizes theophylline more rapidly and needs a higher dosage to attain the therapeutic effect. Conversely, when an isozyme is inhibited by a drug, any substrate of that isozyme will be metabolized more slowly, accumulating in the plasma with the potential to cause toxicity. At high serum concentrations astemizole (Hismanal) and cisapride (Propulsid), which are metabolized by CYP3A4, causing potentially lethal cardiovascular adverse effects. Patients taking these agents and inhibitors of CYP3A4 such as erythromycin and ketoconazole (Nizoral) have developed lethal dysrhythmias. CYP3A4 is also located in intestinal mucosa where grapefruit juice may inhibit it during presystemic metabolism, increasing bioavailability and causing toxicity of diltiazem (Cardizem) and other CYP3A4 substrates (Hansten, 1996; Pepper, 1997b; Riesenman, 1995). Drugs such as cimetidine (Tagamet) and albuterol (Proventil) alter hepatic blood flow and affect metabolism of high hepatic extraction drugs.

## EXCRETION

Excretion involves the removal of drugs, active metabolites, or inactive metabolites from the body. Although drugs and metabolites are excreted through the sweat, saliva, and other secretions, renal elimination through the urine is the most common route of excretion. Biliary excretion is another common route of elimination. For drugs eliminated unchanged (that is, unmetabolized) or as active metabolites, decreased excretion results in accumulation of the drug and toxicity. The four physiologic processes that determine excretion are (1) glomerular filtration, (2) tubular secretion, (3) passive reabsorption, and (4) enterohepatic recirculation. The first three mechanisms, which are illustrated in Figure 2–10, are relevant to renal excretion, while enterohepatic recirculation involves biliary excretion.

## Glomerular Filtration

Molecules of drugs and metabolites in plasma that are not bound to plasma protein filter into the renal tubular filtrate at Bowman's capsule. Blood flow to the kidneys maintains filtration pressure, and decreased blood flow impairs drug excretion. Creatinine clearance is a valid laboratory indicator of glomerular filtration used to adjust dosages of renally excreted drugs. Molecules in the filtrate that are not reabsorbed will be excreted from the body in the urine.

## Tubular Secretion

Located in the walls of the tubule are protein carriers which actively transport substances into the renal tubules, even against a concentration gradi-

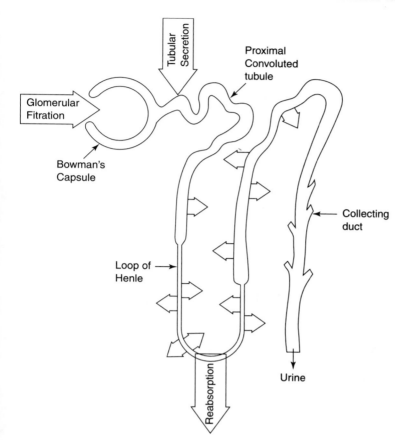

**Figure 2–10.** Processes of renal excretion. Drug molecules are excreted by glomerular filtration into the renal tubule and active tubular secretion by protein carriers in the proximal convoluted tubule. During passage through the nephron lipid soluble, nonionized drug molecules are reabsorbed, and remaining molecules are excreted in the urine.

ent. The tubules have two types of transport systems, one for acids and one for bases. Penicillin is transported by the acid transport system from the plasma into the proximal convoluted tubule by a carrier-mediated process called tubular secretion. This mechanism accounts for the very short half-life of penicillin of one-half hour.

## Passive Reabsorption

Drug molecules in the renal tubules can be reabsorbed by passive diffusion back into the body. Lipid-soluble, nonpolar, nonionized substances will be readily returned to the circulation. Because the pH of urine has wide variability, an acid or base may be nonionized and reabsorbed at one urine pH and ionized and eliminated at a different urine pH.

## Enterohepatic Recirculation

After Phase II metabolism, conjugates excreted into the bile come into contact with intestinal bacteria that can hydrolyze the bond between the drug and the conjugate, which restores the drug to its pharmacologically active, lipid-soluble form, which is then reabsorbed. Figure 2–11 illustrates how this recycling of the drug extends its duration of action. For example, estrogens undergo enterohepatic recirculation, so that a small amount of hormone has prolonged effects.

## Factors That Alter Excretion

The renal function of the very young (preterm infants and neonates) and the elderly is not as effective as other age groups, so dosages of drugs that are renally excreted unchanged or as active metabolites must be reduced for patients in these groups. Pregnancy can actually increase excretion secondary to the effects of increased blood volume on renal blood flow, so dosage increases of some drugs may be required to treat serious disorders during pregnancy (see Chap. 17). Renal disease and dehydration impair excretion of drugs. Drugs eliminated by biliary excretion can have impaired elimination in gallbladder disease.

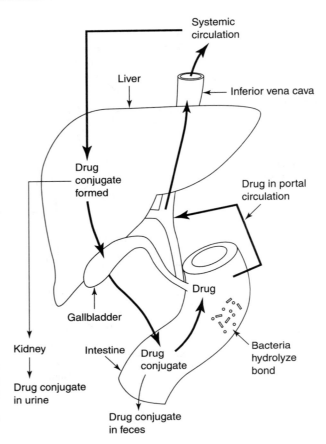

**Figure 2–11.** Enterohepatic recirculation. Drug molecules from the systemic circulation are conjugated in the liver and excreted via the bile into the intestines. Bacteria in the intestines enzymatically hydrolyze the bond of the drug conjugate, releasing drug in its lipid soluble form which is reabsorbed through the portal system to the systemic circulation. During each cycle, some hydrophilic drug conjugate is excreted with the urine or feces.

## Excretion Drug Interactions

Competition for protein carriers, ion trapping, and decreased renal blood flow are drug interactions that alter renal drug excretion. When probenecid (Benemid) is given concurrent with penicillin, the two substances compete for the protein carrier responsible for tubular secretion of penicillin in the nephron, prolonging the half-life of the penicillin and raising its peak serum concentration. This drug interaction has been used therapeutically; patients receiving tubularly secreted penicillins and cephalosporins are given probenecid (Benemid) to improve the antibiotic response. Competition for protein carriers also occurs between drugs and endogenous substances, such as the competition of uric acid with thiazide and loop diuretics for the same tubular secretion carrier. As a result, these diuretics raise serum uric acid and can trigger acute gout in genetically susceptible patients.

Acidic drugs are trapped in alkaline urine, and conversely alkaline drugs are trapped in acidic urine; both conditions promote excretion of the drugs. Treatment of poisoning often involves modification of urine pH so that the ionized drug is trapped in the urine and excreted. Overdose of the acid, phenobarbital, is managed with sodium bicarbonate infusion to alkalinize the urine. Amphetamine overdose is treated by acidification of the urine. Table 2–5 shows drugs that may have altered excretion due to ion trapping. For example, a patient on quinidine who uses megadose ascorbic acid therapy to treat a cold can develop recurrence of the arrhythmia because the basic drug will be ion-trapped in the acidic urine and excreted. Conversely, using sodium bicarbonate (baking soda) for gastric upset could trigger toxicity because the drug would be nonionized and reabsorbable in alkaline urine.

Decreased blood pressure reduces glomerular filtration, so antihypertensive drugs and other agents that decrease blood pressure impair elimination of drugs cleared by the kidneys.

## TABLE 2–5. DRUGS WITH ELIMINATION DEPENDENT ON URINE PH

| Elimination Increased by Acid Urine (Bases) | Elimination Increased by Alkaline Urine (Acids) |
|---|---|
| Amphetamines | Aspirin |
| Chloroquine (Aralen) | Acetazolamide (Diamox) |
| Ephedrine | Choline salicylate |
| Mexiletine (Mexitil) | (Arthropan) |
| Quinidine | Choline magnesium |
| Quinine | trisalicylate (Trilisate) |
| | Nitrofurantoin (Furadantin, |
| | Macrodantin) |
| | Phenobarbital |
| | Probenecid (Benemid) |
| | Salsalate (Disalcid) |

Nonsteroidal antiinflammatory agents also reduce renal blood flow and drug elimination by decreasing synthesis of prostaglandins. Prostaglandins are endogenous chemicals that dilate the renal artery and sustain renal blood flow, especially in conditions like congestive heart failure when compensatory mechanisms decrease renal blood flow.

Enterohepatic recirculation is interrupted when antibiotic therapy kills the bacteria that normally hydrolyze the bond in the drug conjugate, causing the plasma concentration of drugs that are normally recycled to decline. Women taking oral contraceptives are advised to use a backup contraception method for the remainder of the cycle after a course of broad-spectrum antibiotics. Similarly, women on hormone replacement therapy may experience return of hot flashes during antibiotic therapy.

## Drug Clearance

The measure of drug elimination by all routes of metabolism and excretion is clearance, which is defined as the rate of removal of a drug in proportion to plasma concentration. Clearance (CL) is reported as the volume of plasma cleared of the drug per unit of time. The clearances of some common drugs are shown in Table 2–6. If the plasma concentration of a hypothetical drug is 2 μ/mL and it is eliminated at 2 mg/h, the clearance would be 1 L/h or about 17 mL/min. (This is because 1000 mL or 1 L of plasma would be needed to contain 2 mg at a

concentration of 2 μg/mL.) Like volume of distribution, clearance is a useful abstraction, rather than a representation of absolute reality. That is, after 1 h there would not be 1 L of plasma somewhere in the patient's body with no drug and the remaining 2 L of plasma with 2 μg/mL of the drug. Rather, the overall plasma concentration would decline slightly, depending on how much drug stored in the peripheral compartment moved into the central compartment to replace the drug that was eliminated. The concept of clearance is useful in understanding the elimination characteristics of a drug and in pharmacokinetic calculations, particularly in the computation of maintenance dose (see App. 2–2, Calculating Maintenance Doses).

## HALF-LIFE

The elimination half-life of a drug is the amount of time required for half of the drug to be eliminated from the body. Figure 2–12 illustrates

## TABLE 2–6. EXAMPLES OF ROUTE AND RATE OF CLEARANCE OF COMMON DRUGS

| Drug Types | Clearance, L/h per kg* |
|---|---|
| **High Hepatic Extraction Drugs** | |
| Imipramine (Tofranil) | 0.9 |
| Labetalol (Normodyne, Trandate) | 1.50 |
| Lidocaine (Xylocaine) | 0.549 |
| Meperidine (Demerol) | 1.02 |
| Morphine | 3.286 |
| Propranolol | 0.72 |
| Verapamil (Isoptin, Calan) | 0.90 |
| **Other Drugs Eliminated by Liver** | |
| Acetaminophen | 0.3 |
| Carbamazepine (Tegretol) | 0.076 |
| Metronidazole (Flagyl) | 0.077 |
| Theophylline | 0.041 |
| **Drugs with Primarily Renal Elimination as Unchanged Drug** | |
| Ampicillin | 0.23[†] |
| Ciprofloxacin (Cipro) | 0.360[†] |
| Digoxin | 0.111 |
| Gentamicin | 0.077 |
| Vancomycin | 0.084 |

*Assuming normal renal and hepatic function.
[†]High clearance due to tubular secretion.

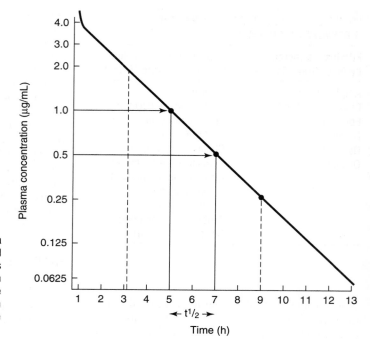

**Figure 2–12.** Elimination half-life. The plasma profile for intravenous administration plotted with concentration on a log scale demonstrates linear drug elimination with a constant fraction of the drug removed per period of time. For the hypothetical drug in this figure, the elimination half-life is 2 hours, the time required for the plasma concentration to decrease by half.

that elimination half-life is measured as the amount of time it takes for the plasma concentration to decline by 50%. Because the drug in the peripheral compartment and the drug in the plasma compartment are at equilibrium, changes in concentration of the drug in the plasma represent changes of the total amount in the body, regardless of whether the drug is primarily located in the blood or primarily sequestered in the peripheral tissues. Therefore, a drop in plasma concentration of 50% means that the amount of drug in the whole body has declined by 50%.

Half-life ($t_{1/2}$) is determined by the volume of distribution and clearance of a drug according to the following formula:

$$t_{\frac{1}{2}} = 0.7 \left[ \frac{V_D}{CL} \right]$$

Analysis of this formula reveals why it is important to consider both the volume of distribution and the clearance of a drug. Fluoxetine (Prozac) has a clearance of 0.58L/h per kilogram, which ranks it with the high hepatic extraction drugs, yet its half-life averages 53 h because it has an extraordinary volume of distribution of 36 L/kg. Even though any fluoxetine that passed through

the liver would be immediately metabolized, most of it is sequestered in peripheral tissues and is not subject to elimination.

The duration of drug action corresponds roughly with the half-life for many drugs, because the plasma concentration often falls below the minimum effective concentration after one half-life, but the effects of some drugs last well beyond one elimination half-life. Corticosteroids initiate a series of chemical reactions, but need to be present only for the initial reaction. Thus, the biologic half-life of corticosteroids far exceeds the elimination half-life. For drugs like the angiotensin-converting enzyme inhibitors, the peak drug level is so much greater than the minimum effective concentration that the plasma concentration exceeds the minimum effective concentration even after several half-lives have passed. A drug is largely eliminated from the body in about four half-lives, because half of the remaining drug is removed during each subsequent half-life:

| Number of Half-Lives | Percentage of Drug Eliminated |
|---|---|
| 1 | 50 |
| 2 | 75 |
| 3 | 87.5 |
| 4 | 93.75 |

## Dose-Dependent Kinetics

For most drugs a constant *proportion* of the drug is eliminated per unit of time, so that during each half-life 50% of the drug is eliminated. This is called *first-order kinetics*, which is how most drugs are eliminated. When there is not excess enzyme capacity for metabolism of a drug, the drug is removed at a constant *amount* per unit of time. This is called *dose-dependent* or *zero-order* kinetics. Common drugs with dose-dependent kinetics are aspirin, phenytoin (Dilantin), and ethanol. Aspirin has a half-life of 3–4 h and first-order kinetics at usual analgesic dosages (650 mg every 4 h). At antiarthritis dosages (4 g per day), the half-life of aspirin is 18 h and the drug is eliminated by dose-dependent kinetics. For drugs with dose-dependent kinetics, the clinician should titrate dosages in small increments, as well as monitor plasma concentration and clinical response frequently.

## STEADY STATE

In Figure 2–1 the plasma profile represented is for a single oral dose. Most drugs are given on a repetitive basis, with the repeat dose administered before the previous dose has been eliminated. Figure 2–13 illustrates that if a drug is repeatedly administered, a *steady state* occurs

after approximately four half-lives. A steady state occurs when absorption and elimination are equal and the average plasma concentration reaches a plateau. Regardless of whether the total daily dosage is administered as a single dosage, four times daily, ten times daily, or as a constant intravenous infusion, a steady state is approximated after four half-lives. With less frequent dosage, the plasma concentration fluctuates widely around the average concentration; that is, the peaks are higher and the troughs are lower than with more frequent dosing.

## CLINICAL IMPLICATIONS OF PHARMACOKINETICS

Rational pharmacotherapeutics requires thorough assessment and analysis of patient factors that may alter pharmacokinetics. Thinking in terms of how diseases and drugs alter the mechanisms of each of the pharmacokinetic processes, rather than trying to remember all the contraindications and precautions for each drug, is an effective outline for this analysis. One of the most important clinical implications of pharmacokinetics is the need for dosage reduction and meticulous patient monitoring when drug elimination is impaired. A drug excreted by the kidneys more than 30% unchanged or as an active metabolite will accumulate when there is

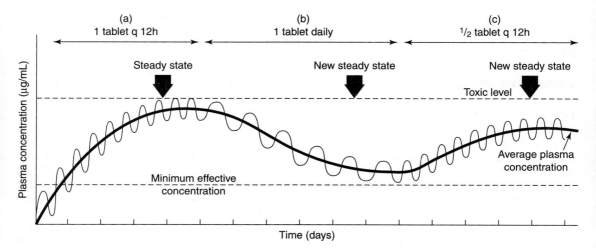

**Figure 2–13.** Steady state. (a) The average concentration of a drug plateaus after approximately four half-lives with repeated dosing. (b) Following a dosage change, it takes four half-lives for a new steady to occur. (c) Dividing a daily dosage into more frequent doses results in less extreme peak and trough values, which may control adverse effects at time of peak concentration or loss of therapeutic effect at trough levels.

renal impairment. For many drugs there are formulas and tables to guide the dosing of renally excreted drugs based upon creatinine clearance. Because there is no comparable laboratory test to guide dosage in hepatic impairment, it is prudent to start doses at one fourth to one third the usual starting dose and titrate slowly upward. Since dose adjustments should be made only after a steady state is approximated, the interval between increments during dose titration should be longer in both renal and hepatic impairment, which decrease clearance and cause prolonged half-life and extended time to a steady state. After the initial dosage is selected, plasma concentration is a useful measurement to use in dosage adjustment for drugs with a valid drug assay procedure (see App. 2–3, Adjusting Dosage Using Laboratory Drug Levels).

## PHARMACODYNAMIC PHASE

The pharmacodynamic phase has been characterized as what the drug does to the body to elicit the pharmacologic effect. The processes of pharmacodynamics are *drug-receptor binding* and *receptor-effector coupling*. Binding is the interaction of the drug with receptors, whereas coupling is how the interaction, directly or through a series of chemical and physiologic steps, evokes the therapeutic and adverse effects of the drug. Whereas the pharmacokinetic processes determine the concentration of a drug at the receptor, the pharmacodynamic processes determine the relationship between the concentration at the receptor and the nature and degree of the response.

## MECHANISMS OF ACTION

Drugs work by chemical, mechanical, general membrane, and receptor mechanisms. An example of a chemical mechanism is the acid-base interaction of antacids with gastric hydrochloric acid, or the inactivation of heparin (an acid) by protamine sulfate (a base). When bulk laxatives adsorb fluids and lipids in the gastrointestinal tract, the increased mass stimulates peristalsis through a mechanical action. General anesthetics do not interact with any specific receptor, but rather dissolve in the lipid layer of cell membranes in the central nervous system. This general membrane effect disrupts membrane function, resulting in loss of consciousness. How-

ever, most drugs elicit their pharmacologic responses through specific receptor interactions.

## DRUG-RECEPTOR BINDING

Drug-receptor interactions involve the reversible joining of a drug (D) and a receptor (R) to form a drug-receptor complex (DR), represented by the following equation for receptor binding:

$$D + R \Leftrightarrow DR$$

Because the bonds between drugs and receptors are usually electrostatic (weak chemical bonds), the interaction is reversible. Otherwise, drug effects would not terminate until new receptors were synthesized to replace those complexed with the drug.

### Dose-Response Relationships

Figure 2–14a illustrates the relationship between the dose of a drug and the response. As the dose is incremented, the response increases until all of the receptors are filled and the curve plateaus. Once the receptors are saturated, further dose increments do not increase the effect. Because pharmacokinetic factors affect the dose-response relationship, a more precise representation of pharmacodynamic processes is the concentration-response graph, which depicts the relationship between the concentration *at the receptor* and the response. Figure 2–14b demonstrates that plotting the concentration-response data on a log scale results in the more easily interpretable S-shaped curve.

   *Maximal efficacy* ($E_{max}$), the response attained when the receptors are saturated, is one important parameter of the concentration-response curve used to compare drugs. Another useful measure is the concentration or dose which elicits half of the maximal response ($EC_{50}$ or $ED_{50}$), which is the measure of drug *potency*. The meanings of *drug potency* and *drug efficacy* are often confused. Sales promotions often hype the potency of a product, which means only that each dose requires fewer milligrams than an equally effective dose of the comparison drug. For example, famotidine (Pepcid) is the most potent $H_2$ blocker, which means only that it takes 40 mg of famotidine to achieve the same effect as 300 mg of ranitidine (Zantac). It does not mean that famotidine is any more effective

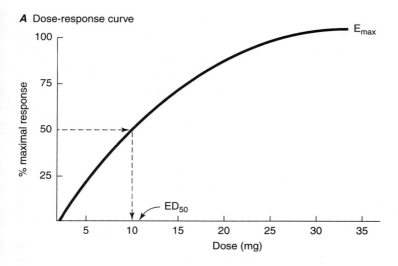

**A** Dose-response curve

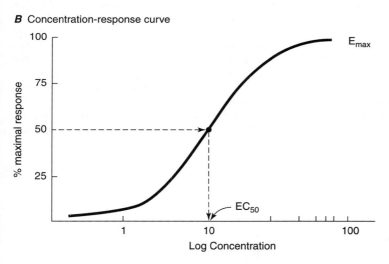

**B** Concentration-response curve

**Figure 2–14.** Dose-response and concentration-response relationships. **A.** Graph of dose-response relationship with dose on an arithmetic scale results in a hyperbolic curve. **B.** Graph of concentration response with concentration on a logarithmic scale results in the readily interpreted S-shaped curve. [$E_{max}$ is maximal efficacy; $ED_{50}$ is the dose that elicits 50% of the maximal response; $EC_{50}$ is the concentration at the receptor that elicits 50% of the maximal response.]

than ranitidine; that is, both drugs have the same $E_{max}$.

## Ligands

Any chemical which interacts with a receptor is referred to as a ligand. Substances that interact with receptors can be either exogenous drugs or endogenous chemicals naturally occurring in the body such as a hormones, neurotransmitters, peptides, or prostaglandins. The term *ligand* encompasses both endogenous substances and drugs. Classical receptors are regulatory proteins that mediate the actions of endogenous ligands. When drugs interact with classical

receptors, they may act either as agonists or as antagonists. *Agonists* bind to and activate the receptor, causing the change in function of the receptor that elicits the pharmacologic response. *Antagonists* also bind to the receptor, but do not alter their function. Rather, by occupying the receptor, antagonists prevent the endogenous ligand from binding to it, which is why antagonists are also called *blockers*. For example, terbutaline is an adrenergic agonist that interacts with beta$_2$ receptors on smooth muscle in the bronchi, eliciting bronchial dilation. This response is the same as occurs when the endogenous ligand norepinephrine interacts with these receptors. Propranolol is an antagonist that blocks beta₂ receptors, which prevents norepinephrine from binding to the beta₂ receptor and results in bronchial constriction due to the absence of adrenergic stimulation. Besides classical receptors, a frequent receptor site for drugs is on enzymes, large proteins that catalyze biochemical interactions. By binding to the enzyme a drug may change the shape of the enzyme or otherwise inhibit its interaction with the substrate. For example, clavulanic acid is an inhibitor of beta-lactamase, an enzyme produced by some penicillin-resistant bacteria. When clavulanic acid and amoxicillin are combined (Augmentin), beta-lactamase–producing strains of *Haemophilus influenzae, Moraxella cattarhalis*, gonococci, and other organisms are susceptible to the amoxicillin. The clavulanic acid inhibits the inactivation of the amoxicillin by the beta-lactamase, permitting the amoxicillin to impair bacterial cell wall synthesis and kill the organism.

***Receptors.*** Receptors are large protein molecules, such as lipoproteins, glycoproteins, or enzymes, which are often embedded in cell membranes with the ligand binding sites located on the outer surfaces of cells. It is important to distinguish receptor binding, which is pharma-

codynamic and related to the drug effect, from other kinds of protein binding with drugs, such as plasma protein binding and binding to protein carriers, which are pharmacokinetic and involve the disposition of the drug by the body. Proteins are ideal drug receptors since they have many reactive sites and regulatory functions in the body. In addition, due to the three-dimensional structure of proteins, consisting of folds, sheets, and helical shapes, interaction of the ligand with one part of the protein molecule can cause a change in the spatial conformation of a distal section of the molecule, bringing it into contact with another chemical, which activates the next step in the chain of events that results in drug response. Figure 2–15 illustrates the three-dimensionality of a receptor class that has been called serpentine, because the large molecular chain crosses the cell membrane several times. Ligands must be large enough molecules to bind to several reactive sites that make up the receptor, so drugs usually have a molecular weight between 100 and 1000, large enough to fit the receptor, but small enough for biotransport.

Most classical receptors are named for their endogenous ligand, although opiod receptors were labeled for drugs used centuries before the receptors were identified. The earliest receptors

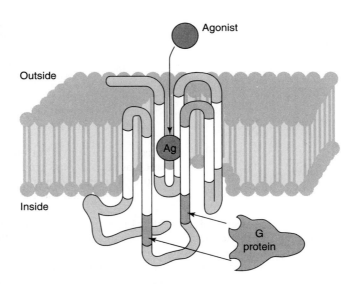

**Figure 2–15.** Serpentine receptor. The three dimensional structure of the receptor brings binding sites for the agonist (Ag) into proximity. Binding of the agonist causes conformational changes in the receptor molecule so that intracellular sites react with the G protein which triggers reactions leading to the clinical effect.

**Source:** Bourne & Roberts (1995).

to be characterized were the receptors for acetylcholine, called cholinergic receptors, and the receptors for norepinephrine, called adrenergic receptors. More recently, receptors have been identified for serotonin, gamma-aminobutyric acid (GABA), histamine, dopamine, opioids, adenosine, glycine, insulin, and numerous other hormones, neurotransmitters, and peptides. Receptor subtypes have been identified for most receptors. It is thought that the subtypes represent slight variants in the structure of the receptor protein, but subtypes may also have different coupling mechanisms. Because the receptor subtypes often mediate different effects, it has been possible to develop drugs for specific subtypes to target particular therapeutic responses or to avoid adverse effects. For example, once it was known that the histamine receptor involved in allergic responses ($H_1$ receptor) was distinct from the histamine receptor that controlled gastric acid secretion ($H_2$ receptor), pharmacologists were able to synthesize cimetidine (Tagamet) and other drugs that selectively block the $H_2$ receptor. Such "designer drugs" are now a common source of new drug products. Many receptor subtypes have been identified by a numeric subscript like the histamine receptors $H_1$, $H_2$, and $H_3$. Some receptor subtypes received Greek letter names, like the alpha- and beta-adrenergic receptors and mu, kappa, sigma, epsilon, and delta opioid receptors. Subdivisions of receptor subtypes have also been given subscript numbers, as in $beta_1$- and $beta_2$-adrenergic receptors. Cholinergic receptors are unique in that the major subtypes were named muscarinic and nicotinic by early pharmacologists who discovered that they could be distinguished by their response to plant extracts from a mushroom and the tobacco plant, respectively.

## STRUCTURE-ACTIVITY RELATIONSHIPS

The shape, size, electrical charge, and atomic composition of a drug determines whether it will bind to a receptor and whether it will be an agonist or an antagonist. The chemical structure also governs its receptor *affinity*, which is defined as propensity to bind to a receptor. Receptor affinity influences the concentration of a drug required at the receptor to elicit a desired response. The more avidly a drug binds to a receptor, the lower the concentration of drug required. This structure-activity relationship allows selectivity of drug molecules for specific receptors or receptor subtypes. For example, at low doses propranolol (Inderal) has affinity for both $beta_1$ and $beta_2$ subtypes of adrenergic receptors, but atenolol (Tenormin) has affinity for the $beta_1$ subtype only. Thus, at low doses only propanolol causes dyspnea. At higher doses, such as usual antihypertensive and antianginal dosages, selectivity is lost and both propranolol and atenolol cause dyspnea in susceptible patients. Thus, even when drugs are selective, that is, have low affinity for a receptor subtype, they will bind to the receptor when the concentration at the receptor is sufficiently high.

## Dissociation Constant

The dissociation content for the drug-binding equation presented above is called the equilibrium dissociation constant ($K_D$). $K_D$ is defined as the concentration of drug at which half of the receptors are occupied. $K_D$ is the measure of affinity of a drug for the receptor and reflects the potency of a drug. A low $K_D$ means that the drug has high affinity for the receptor.

## Stereoselectivity

Many drugs exhibit chirality; that is, they have paired forms with the same atomic composition existing in mirror-image spatial orientation, called enantiomers. Like the right and left hands of a human, the enantiomers are nonsuperimposable pairs, as illustrated in Figure 2–16. In pure solution one of the enantiomers rotates polarized light to the right (dextrorotary), whereas a pure solution of the other enantiomer will rotate polarized light to the left (levorotary). From this optical property is derived the convention of naming the pairs as the *d*- and *l*-enantiomers, such as *d*-propoxyphene (the analgesic Darvon). Other nomenclature uses the s- and r- or D- and L- prefixes, which are based on the absolute configuration of the atoms in the molecule independent of rotation of light, such as L-epinephrine. Because the shape of a ligand must be complementary to the receptor, two enantiomers might not fit the receptor equally well, just as a right and left hand do not fit equally well into the left glove. This is called stereoselectivity because one enantiomer has greater affinity for the receptor. Most of the activity of beta blockers is attributed to the *l*-isomers because they have greater affinity (lower $K_D$) for

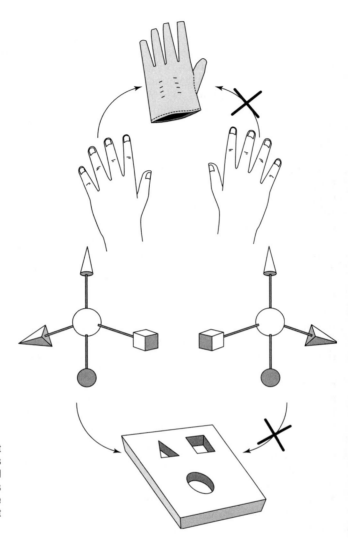

**Figure 2–16. Stereoselectivity.** The right and left human hands are nonsuperimposable mirror images and only the left hand fits well in the left glove. Chiral drugs are also nonsuperimposable mirror images with paired enantiomers. The enantiomer that fits the receptor best has more affinity and elicits the greatest response.

the receptors than the *d*-isomers. The alpha-beta blocker, labetalol (Normodyne, Trandate), is a chiral drug with an *l*-enantiomer that blocks beta receptors and a *d*-enantiomer that blocks the alpha receptors. For some enantiomers such as the intravenous anesthetic ketamine and methylphenidate (Ritalin), it has been hypothesized that one enantiomer causes the beneficial effect and the other enantiomer causes the adverse effects (Brocks & Jamali, 1995). The pharmacokinetics of enantiomers may differ, and enantiomer-specific drug interactions with warfarin (Coumadin) have been identified. Drug groups that include numerous agents with chiral properties are nonsteroidal antiinflammatory drugs, beta agonists, beta blockers, calcium channel blockers, warfarin, antiarrhythmics, psychotropics, and anesthetics. Over half of these chiral agents are currently marketed as the racemic mixture containing equal concentrations of the active enantiomer and the inactive (or actively toxic) enantiomer. For example, timolol and naproxen are supplied as the pure active enantiomers, while other beta-blockers and nonsteroidal antiinflammatory drugs are racemates. In the future, researchers, regulatory agencies, and manufacturers are expected to increase emphasis on evaluating the significance of chirality for each drug and modifying the products as necessary.

## RECEPTOR-EFFECTOR COUPLING

Coupling encompasses all the chemical and physiologic processes between the drug-receptor binding and the observed clinical effect. As the couplings on a train hold the railroad cars together, receptor-effector coupling is the aspect of pharmacodynamics that links the drug-receptor interaction to the reactions leading to the drug effect, represented by the unidirectional arrows in the equation below:

$$D + R \Leftrightarrow DR \to \to \to Effect$$

For example, when a patient receives digoxin for congestive heart failure, the clinician may monitor the clinical response using weight and lung sounds. The pharmacologic effects of digoxin are initiated when the digoxin binds to its receptor site on an enzyme in the cardiac muscle cell membrane called $Na^+$, $K^+$-ATPase. This enzyme, also known as the sodium pump, normally pumps $Na^+$ out of the cell in exchange for $K^+$. The binding of the digoxin to the enzyme decreases its effectiveness, causing accumulation of $Na^+$ inside the cell that is removed by another pump in exchange for $Ca^{2+}$. This increases the intracellular concentration of $Ca^{2+}$. The interaction of the contractile proteins actin and myosin in muscles is inhibited by a protein called troponin C. During the cardiac cycle, $Ca^{2+}$ is released intermittently and it interacts with troponin C to remove the inhibition of actin and myosin, resulting in the periodic muscle contraction of the myocardium. The increased $Ca^{2+}$ inside the cell when digoxin inhibits the sodium pump increases myosin-actin interaction, which is manifested as increased force of myocardial contraction. This improves both pulmonary circulation, resulting in disappearance of rales, and systemic circulation, which decreases edema and triggers weight loss. All these steps represent coupling of digoxin's clinical effects to its drug-receptor interaction.

## SIGNAL TRANSDUCTION

In recent years the first step in coupling, signaling, or signal transduction has been the focus of intense research. Signal transduction involves the molecular mechanisms whereby the binding of drug and receptor, which usually occurs extracellularly, is translated into intracellular messages that control cell function. These mechanisms provide an explanation for the action of some drugs that do not act at receptors such as metformin (Glucophage), and they may provide targets for the development of new drug classes. Figure 2–17 schematically represents the four signaling mechanisms that have been characterized for classical receptor systems: intracellular receptors, transmembranous enzymes, gated channels, and G protein–second messenger systems (Bourne & Roberts, 1995).

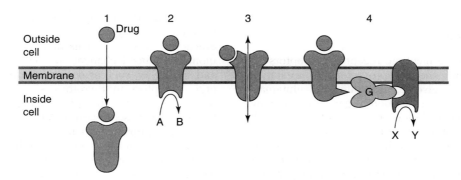

**Figure 2–17.** Signal transduction mechanisms. There are four known signal transduction mechanisms: **(1)** A lipid soluble ligand crosses the membrane and acts on an intracellular receptor, which may be an enzyme or regulator of gene transcription, **(2)** the ligand binds to the extracellular domain of a transmembranous protein, thereby activating an enzymatic activity of its cytoplasmic domain, **(3)** the ligand binds directly to and directly regulates the opening of an ion channel, and **(4)** the ligand binds to a cell surface receptor linked to an effector second messenger by a G protein.

**Source:** Bourne & Roberts (1995).

## INTRACELLULAR RECEPTORS

Ligands acting at intracellular receptors must be lipid-soluble to cross the cell membrane. The highly lipid soluble steroidal hormones (glucocorticoids, mineralocorticoids, and sex hormones) bind to receptors in the cytoplasm of the cell. The ligand-receptor complex migrates to the nucleus where it affects genetic transcription by binding to DNA sequences near the gene whose expression is stimulated. The onset of action of drugs working by this mechanism requires a lag period of 30 min to several hours for the synthesis of new proteins that produce the drug effects. This is why corticosteroid therapy is used to prevent rather than treat an asthmatic attack. Similarly, this mechanism is associated with long-lasting effects that persist until the new proteins stimulated by the drugs are metabolized. Other ligands known to work by directly affecting genetic transcription are thyroid hormone and vitamin D. Nitric oxide, an endogenous ligand with an intracellular enzyme, is probably involved in the pharmacodynamics of nitroglycerin and other nitrates.

## Transmembranous Enzymes

These transmembranous enzymes consist of a ligand-binding component on the outside of the cell and an enzyme on the cytoplasmic side of the membrane. When the extracellular component binds to the ligand, the protein receptor undergoes conformational change that activates the intracellular enzyme to catalyze a biochemical reaction. Insulin, growth factors, and atrial natriuretic factor are endogenous ligands with this signaling mechanism.

## Gated Channels

Acetylcholine nicotinic receptors, receptors for GABA, and the receptors for the excitatory amino acids glycine, aspartate, and glutamate are proteins that function as gates on ion channels through cell membranes. Binding of ligands to the receptors causes a conformational change that closes or opens the channel. For example, the antianxiety effects of diazepam (Valium) are attributed to binding with a receptor near the GABA receptor, resulting in increased affinity of GABA for its receptor. GABA binding opens chloride channels, and the influx of chloride into the cell inhibits neuronal depolarization. This mechanism occurs within milliseconds, so gated channels are often the signaling mechanism in the nervous system where information must be processed rapidly.

## G Proteins and Second Messengers

By binding to an extracellular receptor, a ligand can cause increased concentration of a chemical within the cell called the second messenger. The second messenger goes on to interact with intracellular constituents. Common second messengers are calcium ions, phosphoinositides, and cyclic adenosine 3',5'-monophosphate (cyclic AMP, or cAMP). These receptor systems usually have three components, the extracellular surface receptor, the G protein located on the internal surface of the membrane, and the second messenger. Interaction of the ligand with the surface receptor, which is commonly of the serpentine type, causes a conformational change in the receptor protein, bringing it into contact with the G protein. This activates an effector element, usually an enzyme or an ion channel, causing an increase in the concentration of the second messenger. For example, the G protein may activate the enzyme adenyl cyclase that catalyzes the conversion of intracellular ATP to cAMP, which goes on to stimulate protein kinases that initiate many intracellular reactions. G proteins with second messengers are the signaling mechanisms for muscarinic receptors for acetylcholine and alpha$_1$ and beta receptors for norepinephrine, serotonin receptors, and many peptide receptors.

## RESPONSE VARIABILITY

Some variability in response to drugs can be attributed to changes in the number and coupling efficacy of receptors. This may be due to hormonally induced changes in receptor number and sensitivity, such as occurs with beta-adrenergic receptors in thyrotoxicosis. In addition, drugs can induce receptor changes. Agonist therapy can cause *down-regulation* of the number of receptors, which manifests clinically as tolerance, increasing dose requirements to achieve the therapeutic response. The tolerance to beta$_2$-adrenergic agonist bronchodilators in asthma has been attributed to receptor down-regulation in which the receptors are taken into the cell by endocytosis and metabolized. Antagonist therapy can result in *up-regulation*, an increase in the number of receptors. Beta blockers must be tapered when they are discontinued, because abrupt withdrawal can cause rebound hypertension, angina, or even fatal myocardial infarction. The rebound is attributed to beta receptor up-regulation during therapy; with sudden discontinuation of the blocker, the increased number of receptors is suddenly accessible to endogenous norepinephrine.

## TYPES OF ANTAGONISTS

Receptor antagonists are classified as *competitive antagonists* and *irreversible antagonists*. Competitive or surmountable antagonism exists when additional agonist will overcome the receptor blockade. Opiod receptor blockade by naloxone (Narcan) is reversed if more opioid agonist, such as morphine, is administered. This blockade is called *competitive* because the agonist and antagonist molecules compete to occupy the receptors, and the ligand with the greatest affinity (lowest $K_D$ and greatest concentration at the receptor site) will dominate. Figure 2-18a shows that a competitive antagonist shifts the concentration-response curve to the right, requiring a greater dose of the agonist to get the maximal effect. *Irreversible antagonism* occurs if the addition of agonist does not overcome the blockade. Also called *noncompetitive antagonism*, it is thought to be due to binding of the antagonist by strong covalent chemical bonds or binding near the receptor, causing a conformational change in the receptor that prevents the agonist from binding to it. Figure 2-18a indicates that an irreversible antagonist decreases the maximal efficacy attainable from the agonist. An example of an irreversible antagonist is the alpha-adrenergic blocker phenoxybenzamine (Dibenzyline) used to treat pheochromocytoma, a hypertensive disease characterized by periodic release of large amounts of norepinephrine. If a competitive antagonist like prazosin (Minipress) is used in pheochromocytoma, it is displaced by norepinephrine when the hypertensive crisis occurs, but phenoxybenzamine is not displaced regardless of how much norepinephrine is released.

The term *antagonism*, which has specific meaning related to receptor antagonists, is also used generally for neutralization of the effects of one drug by another, regardless of mechanism. Even drugs that interact pharmacokinetically, such as drugs that prevent absorption of other drugs, are sometimes called antagonists. In addition to pharmacokinetic antagonism and receptor antagonism, drugs can counteract the effects of others drugs through *chemical antagonism* and *functional antagonism*. An example of chemical antagonism is the acid-base reaction that causes the reversal of heparin effects by protamine sulfate. Functional or physiologic antagonism involves the counteracting of one drug by another through a different receptor system on a different physiologic pathway. For example, bradycardia caused by the beta-adrenergic receptor blocker propranolol (Inderal) can be reversed by administering the cholinergic receptor blocker atropine. Propranolol decreases the heart rate by blocking receptors in the sympathetic nervous system, whereas atropine antagonizes the inhibitory action of the parasympathetic nervous system by blocking receptors for the vagus nerve.

## TYPES OF AGONISTS

Two types of agonists have been identified based on the maximum pharmacologic effect attained when all the receptors are occupied. Most drugs are *full agonists* that elicit the total capability of the receptor system when given in sufficient doses. As shown in Figure 2-18b, *partial agonists* do not elicit this maximal response, and have a lower $E_{max}$ even when the receptors are fully occupied. In fact, in the presence of a full agonist, a partial agonist functions as a competitive antagonist, reversing the agonist effects. Buprenorphine (Buprenex) is a partial agonist at the mu opioid receptors and cannot provide, even at maximal doses, as much analgesia as the full mu agonist morphine. Some drugs are *agonist-antagonists*, operating as agonists at one receptor subtype and antagonists at another subtype. The opioid nalbuphine (Nubain) is an agonist at kappa receptors and an antagonist at mu receptors. Agonist-antagonists also can reverse the effects of full agonists. Administered to a patient who has a full mu receptor agonist present, such as morphine, nalbuphine reverses the analgesic effects of the mu receptor. If the patient is physically dependent on morphine, nalbuphine will elicit withdrawal symptoms.

## PHARMACODYNAMIC DRUG INTERACTIONS

Many pharmacodynamic drug interactions involve antagonism by one of the mechanisms

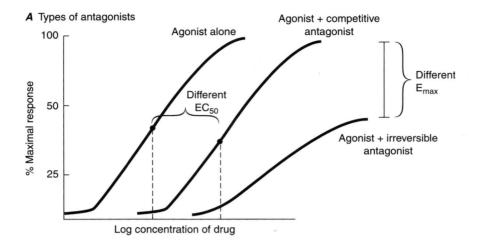

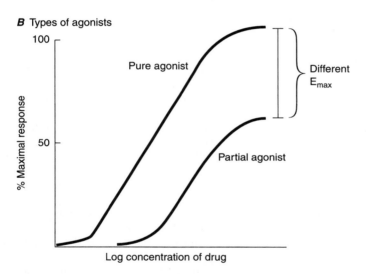

**Figure 2–18.** Concentration-response curves for various agonists and antagonist types. **A.** There are two types of receptor antagonists. Competitive antagonists do not affect the maximal efficacy ($E_{max}$) of an agonist, but do increase the dosage required to elicit a response of a particular magnitude ($EC_{50}$). Irreversible antagonists decrease maximal efficacy and cannot be reversed regardless of the amount of agonist added. **B.** Partial agonists do not elicit the magnitude of maximal effect ($E_{max}$) as do full agonists.

described above. Other important interactions are additive effects, in which the combination of two drugs increases the incidence or severity of a drug response. This can occur through the same receptor system, such as the combination of prazosin (Minipress) for high blood pressure and thioridazine (Mellaril) for schizophrenia. Both block alpha receptors, so they have additive hypotensive effects. Additive effects also can occur through separate physio-

logic and pharmacologic pathways. Both prazosin (Minipress) and the diuretic hydrochlorothiazide decrease blood pressure, but through entirely different mechanisms. Although the prescriber purposely can use drugs for their additive therapeutic benefits, many additive effects result in an adverse response. In both of the previous examples, the additive effects could lead to hypotension, syncope, and falls.

## ADVERSE DRUG EFFECTS

The nomenclature for adverse drug effects includes many overlapping and imprecise terms, such as iatrogenic disease, drug-induced disease, side effect, toxic effect, and idiosyncratic reaction. In 1986 Kellaway formulated the classification of adverse drug effects shown in Table 2–7 for use in helping patients to identify harmful and nuisance adverse effects. An important distinction in this classification is the differentiation of *unwanted pharmacologic effects*, which are predictable based upon the drug-receptor interactions, and pathologic reactions that are the unpredictable emergence of a disease condition unrelated to the activity of the drug at receptors, such as the development of anaphylaxis, cancer, or neutropenia. Often the pathologic mechanism is hypersensitivity, an antigen-antibody allergic reaction mediated by the immune system.

### TABLE 2–7. CLASSIFICATION OF ADVERSE DRUG EFFECTS

| Category | Mechanism | Examples Drug/Group | Adverse Effect |
|----------|-----------|---------------------|----------------|
| Excessive therapeutic effect | Same receptor/ same effector | Metoclopramide (Reglan) | Diarrhea |
| | | Anticoagulants | Bleeding |
| | | Thrombolytics | Bleeding |
| | | Antidiabetic agents | Hypoglycemia |
| | | Antihypertensives | Hypotension |
| | | Sedatives | Stupor/coma |
| Unwanted pharmacologic effect | Same receptor/ different effector | Opioids | Constipation |
| | | Haloperidol (Haldol) | Parkinsonism |
| | | Trihexyphenidyl (Artane) | Dry mouth |
| | | Terbutaline (Brethine) | Hyperglycemia |
| | | Nitroglycerin | Headache |
| | | Verapamil (Isoptin, Calan) | Constipation |
| | Different receptor/ different effector | Propranolol (Inderal) | Dyspnea |
| | | Chlorpheniramine (Chlor-Trimeton) | Drowsiness |
| | | Haloperidol (Haldol) | Dry mouth |
| | | Erythromycin | Diarrhea |
| | | Penicillin | Seizures |
| | | Thioridazine (Mellaril) | Hypotension |
| | | ACE inhibitors | Nonproductive cough |
| Pathological reactions | Hypersensitivity | Captopril (Capoten) | Neutropenia |
| | | Penicillin | Anaphylaxis |
| | | Sulfonamides | Stevens-Johnson Syndrome |
| | Teratogenesis | Lithium | Cardiovascular defects |
| | | Warfarin (Coumadin) | Hypoplastic nasal bridge, chondrodysplasia |
| | Carcinogenesis | Chemotherapeutic agents | Various cancers |
| | | Glucocorticoids | Various cancers |
| | Other, unknown | Acetaminophen (Tylenol) | Nephritis |
| | | HMG CoA reductase inhibitors | Rhabdomyolysis |
| Superinfection | Inhibits normal flora | Tetracycline | Vaginal candidiasis |
| | | Broad-spectrum antibiotics | Pseudomembranous colitis |
| Drug interaction | Pharmacokinetic | Erythromycin + cisapride (Propulsid) | Dysrhythmia |
| | Pharmacodynamic | Opioid + Antihistamine | Somnolence |

## CLINICAL IMPLICATIONS OF PHARMACODYNAMICS

The understanding of pharmacodynamic properties plays a major role in the selection of a drug to treat a disease or symptom. To ignore this consideration is prescribing by rote, putting patients at risk for inappropriate or harmful therapy. The pharmacodynamics of adverse drug effects also merits attention, since appropriate prevention, management, and patient education derives from a thorough understanding of the mechanisms of the adverse effects. Too often patient education about adverse effects is merely a list of potential effects, but unless patients are taught how to detect the effects and what to do if an effect occurs, their ability to participate in self-care is limited. Not all adverse effects need to be reported to the clinician in a midnight call, but evaluation of many adverse effects should not be deferred until the next visit. Based upon the classification of adverse effects in Table 2–7, excessive therapeutic effects, pathological reactions, superinfection, and drug interaction require consultation with the prescriber or health care provider within hours to days of when they are first detected. Most unwanted pharmacologic effects are transient and can be managed by the patient, but if the effect is severe, bothersome, or continuous, it should be reported to a health care professional. Since these effects are predictable based upon the pharmacodynamics of the drug, the clinician can provide anticipatory counseling on how to avoid the effect and how to minimize its impact on comfort and functional status if it occurs.

Prevention and management of adverse effects will vary depending upon the type of adverse effect. The two most common types are excessive therapeutic effects and unwanted pharmacologic effects. Excessive therapeutic effects occur when the adverse and therapeutic responses are produced at the same receptor on the same effector, such as postural hypotension caused by the antihypertensive prazosin (Minipress). Pharmacologic options for prevention or management of excessive therapeutic effects are minimizing the dose, which could compromise the therapeutic response; choosing a drug from a different drug group; or prescribing multidrug therapy to minimize the dose of each agent, such as adding a diuretic to another antihypertensive. Replacing the drug with nonpharmacologic therapy could be considered, depending upon severity and sequelae of the condition. Using a drug to treat an adverse effect of another drug is usually contraindicated, but nonpharmacologic interventions such as teaching the patient with postural hypotension to change position slowly and keep well-hydrated may render the adverse effects tolerable.

There are two types of unwanted pharmacologic effects. The first occurs when the therapeutic and adverse effects involve the same receptor subtype on different effector organs, such as hyperglycemia from oral albuterol (Proventil) for asthma. Any of the options listed for managing an excessive therapeutic effect may be beneficial, but consideration should also be given to prescribing the medication via a route that maximizes the drug concentration at the site of the receptors for the therapeutic effect, such as administering albuterol by inhalation. The second mechanism of unwanted pharmacologic effects involves different receptors on different organs for the therapeutic and adverse effects, which can be avoided by prescribing a more selective drug in the same drug group. For example, if a nonselective beta blocker such as propranolol (Inderal) causes dyspnea, a cardioselective agent like atenolol (Tenormin) could be tried, or any of the strategies proposed above for other mechanisms of adverse effects could also be used.

## CONCLUSION

Three phases of drug action—pharmaceutics, pharmacokinetics, and pharmacodynamics—mediate variability in drug response. By understanding the processes and mechanisms for each phase, the prescriber is able to select optimal drug therapy for each patient's unique response patterns. One of the greatest challenges of pharmacotherapeutics is keeping up with the rapid advances in the field of pharmacology; it has been proposed that the half-life of pharmacology knowledge is less than 5 years. Understanding of the underlying principles of pharmaceutics, pharmacokinetics, and pharmacodynamics also allows the clinician to adapt to this rapidly changing environment and to critically appraise the therapeutic significance of the new developments.

## REFERENCES

*Ad Hoc* Subcommittee of the Liaison Committee of the World Health Organization and the International Society of Hypertension. (1997). Effects of calcium antagonists on the risks of coronary heart disease, cancer, and bleeding. *Journal of Hypertension, 15,* 106–115.

Bourne, H. R., & Roberts, J. M. (1995). Drug receptors and pharmacodynamics. In B. G. Katzung (Ed.), *Basic and clinical pharmacology* (6th ed.). Norwalk, CT: Appleton & Lange.

Brocks, D. R., & Jamali, F. (1995). Stereochemical aspects of pharmacotherapy. *Pharmacotherapy, 15,* 551–564.

Furberg, C. D. & Psaty, B. M. (1996). Calcium antagonists: Not appropriate as first line antihypertensive therapy. *American Journal of Hypertension, 9,* 122–125.

Hansten, P. D. (1996). Substrates and inhibitors for selected cytochrome P450 isozymes. *Drug Interactions Newsletter,* 905–906.

Kellaway, G. (1986). The patient. In W. H. W. Inman (Ed.), *Monitoring for drug safety* (2nd ed.) (pp. 637–649). Boston: MTP Press.

Nemeroff, C. B., DeVane, C. L., & Pollock, B. G. (1996). Newer antidepressants and the cytochrome P450 system. *American Journal of Psychiatry, 153,* 311–320.

Pepper, G. A. (1997*a*). Calcium channel blocker controversy. *Clinical Letter for Nurse Practitioners, 1* (4), 8.

Pepper, G. A. (1997*b*). The perils of P450. *Clinical Letter for Nurse Practitioners, 1* (1), 7–8.

Riesenman, C. (1995). Antidepressant drug interactions and the cytochrome P450 system: A critical appraisal. *Pharmacotherapy, 15* (6 Pt 2), 84S–99S.

# APPENDIX 2–1

## CALCULATING LOADING DOSES

Because the danger of exceeding toxic levels is substantial, loading doses are reserved for urgent situations when it is critical to attain steady-state plasma concentrations immediately. Usually loading doses are given by intravenous bolus and followed by an intravenous infusion to maintain the desired plasma concentration, but a loading dose can be given orally as a single dose or divided into several doses given at intervals of several hours to allow the drug to distribute between doses. Digoxin is sometimes "loaded" in hospitalized patients using this divided oral dose method. Since the function of a loading dose is to fill up the distribution volume in a single dose, rather than over the four half-lives usually required to approximate the steady state, the key parameters required to compute the loading dose are volume of distribution ($V_D$) and the desired plasma concentration ($C_p$). If the drug is given orally, bioavailability ($F$) must also be considered. All three parameters can be found in standard references. The formula for computing loading dose is:

$$\text{Loading dose} = \frac{V_D \times C_p}{F}$$

*Example:* To compute the loading dose of theophylline for a 50-kg adolescent female, the clinician must first determine the target plasma concentration ($C_p$). The therapeutic range for theophylline is 10–20 µg/mL. Because it is prudent to begin in the lower end of the therapeutic range, the $C_p$ selected is 10 µg/mL. The $V_D$ reported in standard references must be adjusted for the weight of the patient. From Table 2–3 the $V_D$ of theophylline is 0.5 L/kg or 25 L for this 50-kg patient. Since the bioavailability of theophylline is 0.96, it is virtually 1.0, which is used in the calculation. The loading dose of 250 mg was calculated as follows:

$$\text{Loading dose} = \frac{25\,\text{L} \times [10\,\mu\text{g/mL}]}{1.0}$$

$$= 25,000\,\text{mL} \times 10\,\mu\text{g/mL}$$

$$= 250,000\,\mu g = 250\,\text{mg}$$

# APPENDIX 2–2

## CALCULATING MAINTENANCE DOSES

The dose of a drug prescribed is generally based upon the usual dosage recommended by the manufacturer, modified by clinical considerations such as patient weight. For drugs with nar- row therapeutic ranges that are followed by laboratory drug assays (blood levels), computation of maintenance dose individualizes the dosage for a desired plasma concentration. The goal of maintenance dosing is to replace the drug that is eliminated during each dosing interval, so that the target plasma concentration is sustained. Therefore, the critical parameters in calculating maintenance dose are the clearance (CL) and the desired therapeutic concentration ($C_p$). Since maintenance doses are usually given orally, bioavailability ($F$) and dosing interval ($\tau$ or tau) are considered. The formula for calculation of maintenance dose is:

$$\text{Maintenance dose} = \frac{C_L \times C_p}{F} \times \tau$$

*Example:* The clinician wants to compute the maintenance dose of theophylline required to sustain a plasma concentration of 12 μg/mL for a 50-kg adolescent using an immediate-release dosage form administered three times daily. The target $C_p$ was historically determined from patient responses to various plasma concentra-

tions of theophylline. CL may be computed from individualized pharmacokinetic studies or obtained from standard references. The dosing interval ($\tau$) is 8 h, based upon the usual frequency of dosing with the preparation selected. Bioavailability ($F$) of 0.96 is used for illustration, although it is so close to 1.0 that it might be omitted from the calculation. The CL of 0.04 L/h per kg from Table 2–6 adjusted for the patient's weight is 2.0 L/h. The maintenance dose of 200 mg t.i.d. was computed as follows:

$$\begin{aligned}
\text{Maintenance dose} &= \frac{2\,\text{L/h} \times 12\ \mu\text{g/mL}}{0.96} \times 8\text{h} \\[6pt]
&= \frac{2000\,\text{mL/h} \times 12\ \mu\text{g/mL}}{0.96} \times 8\text{h} \\[6pt]
&= \frac{24{,}000\ \mu\text{g/h}}{0.96} \times 8\text{h} \\[6pt]
&= 200{,}000\ \mu\text{g/dose} \\[6pt]
&= 200\ \text{mg t.i.d.}
\end{aligned}$$

## APPENDIX 2–3

## ADJUSTING DOSAGE USING LABORATORY DRUG LEVELS

Even if a maintenance dose was calculated for a particular patient using values from standardized tables, the measured plasma concentration might not equal the target plasma concentration. Patients vary widely from the average values in standardized tables in actual absorption, liver function, and renal function. The dose ($D_2$) required to attain a desired plasma concentration for a particular patient can be computed from the current dose ($D_1$), the current plasma concentration ($C_1$), and the desired plasma concentration ($C_2$) using the following formula:

$$\frac{D_1}{D_2} = \frac{C_1}{C_2}$$

*Example:* The plasma concentration for a 14-year-old girl taking theophylline 200 mg t.i.d. is

10 μg/mL. She is experiencing dyspnea and wheezing and her past history indicates plasma theophylline concentrations of 14 μg/mL are required for disease control. The new dose of theophylline of 280 mg t.i.d. was computed as follows:

$$\frac{200\,\text{mg}}{D_2} = \frac{10\ \mu\text{g/mL}}{14\ \mu\text{g/mL}}$$

$$\frac{200{,}000\,\text{mg}}{D_2} = \frac{10\ \mu\text{g/mL}}{14\ \mu\text{g/mL}}$$

$$D_2 = 280\ \text{mg}$$

If the dose is raised to 280 mg and the target plasma concentration is not attained, the clinician should check to see that the blood samples for drug assay are collected at the proper time to ensure appropriate values.

# 3

# PHARMACOTHERAPEUTIC IMPACT OF RENAL OR HEPATIC DYSFUNCTION

*Thomas J. Comstock*

## GENERAL CONSIDERATIONS

Dosage regimen design for patients with renal and/or hepatic impairment requires knowledge of the pharmacokinetic characteristics of a drug as well as the physiologic changes that occur as a result of the decreased organ function. Pharmacokinetic changes that accompany organ dysfunction usually are manifested as decreased elimination, such as decreased metabolism by the liver and decreased excretion by the kidneys, but also may be manifested as changes in absorption and distribution.

Overall drug elimination from the body can be considered as the sum of elimination by two primary pathways, such that the total rate of elimination from the body is equal to renal plus nonrenal elimination, where nonrenal elimination is predominantly hepatic metabolism.

As a general rule, when a drug is eliminated more than 30% by an organ system, then impairment of that organ system may necessitate changes in the dosage regimen in order to avoid excessive accumulation of the drug and subsequent toxicity. The degree of organ impairment and the fraction of the drug that normally is eliminated by that route determine the amount of change in a dosage regimen. Drugs with a narrow therapeutic range, for example, digoxin 1–2 µg/L or phenytoin 10–20 mg/L, will require more individualization of the regimen and closer monitoring compared to those with a wider therapeutic range, such as many analgesic compounds.

Although drug elimination is an important consideration, changes in absorption and distribution of drugs also may occur with organ dysfunction. This chapter will focus on the pharmacokinetic alterations that occur with drugs administered to patients with liver or kidney disease and the actions the clinician should take to optimize the dosage regimen in order to obtain the desired clinical outcome and avoid unnecessary toxicity.

## ASSESSMENT OF ORGAN FUNCTION

Adjustment of dosage regimens is dependent on some knowledge of organ function. Whereas renal function can be estimated using several clinical tools, hepatic function is not easily quantified. Despite this limitation, an understanding of the processes involved in drug elimination by the liver is useful as a guide to clinical decision making.

### HEPATIC FUNCTION

The levels of the hepatic enzymes aspartate aminotransferase (AST) and alanine aminotransferase (ALT), commonly referred to as "liver function tests," are not useful as quantitative measures of hepatic drug metabolism. These enzymes are increased under conditions of hepatic inflammation, such as acute hepatitis, but do not reflect drug elimination capability. Drug clearance by the liver is complex and related to hepatic blood flow, plasma protein binding of a drug, and intrinsic hepatic clearance. A drug is delivered to the liver via the portal vein (~1050 mL/min) and hepatic artery (~350 mL/min) and is present within the blood in equilibrium between the protein-bound and unbound states. The primary driving force for hepatic blood flow is cardiac output, which may be significantly reduced during heart failure. As a drug flows through the liver, the unbound drug is able to move into the hepatocyte, where it may undergo metabolism and/or biliary excretion. Formed metabolites then are able to reenter the systemic circulation or be excreted in the bile. The fraction of a drug that is removed, or cleared, as it passes through the liver is the hepatic extraction ratio (E), and has a range in value from 0–1. The pharmacokinetic parameter that best describes drug elimination is clearance. As discussed in Chap. 2, clearance is the volume of plasma that is cleared totally of a drug per unit time. For example, the clearance of theophylline in a nonsmoking adult is 40 mL/min. Clearance of a drug by an individual organ is the product of the flow through the organ and the extraction ratio of the drug. For drugs with a high extraction ratio, the hepatic clearance approaches hepatic blood flow, and any change in hepatic blood flow will have a proportionate effect on hepatic elimination of the drug.

Drugs eliminated by hepatic metabolism can be considered as high-, middle-, or low extraction drugs based on the fraction of the drug that is removed as blood flows through the liver. High extraction drugs are characterized by E > 0.7, middle as 0.3 < E < 0.7, and low as E < 0.3. Whereas hepatic blood flow is the primary determinant for the removal of high extraction ratio drugs, elimination of low extraction ratio drugs is dependent on plasma protein binding and intrinsic clearance. Intrinsic clearance refers to the ability of the liver (hepatocytes) to eliminate the drug without the restrictions of blood flow or protein binding. Generally, this refers to the ability of the liver to metabolize the drug. Drugs in this category are susceptible to drug interactions from drugs such as cimetidine that compete for metabolizing enzymes or to induction of enzymes by drugs such as rifampin and phenobarbital, resulting in an increased elimination of other drugs and subtherapeutic

plasma concentrations. Examples of high and low extraction drugs are included in Table 3–1.

Drug metabolizing enzymes of the liver are categorized broadly as being responsible for Phase I reactions (synthetic) or Phase II reactions (conjugation). Phase I reactions consist of oxidation, reduction, hydrolysis, and others, and may result in formation of an "active" metabolite, such as the demethylation of codeine to form morphine. A large group of enzymes responsible for many of the Phase I oxidative reactions is the cytochrome P-450 system (sometimes referred to as microsomal enzymes). This set of enzymes can be subdivided into approximately 20 different isozymes, such as CYP2D6 and CYP3A4. Each isozyme is responsible for a different metabolic pathway. The presence and quantity of these isozymes is genetically determined, which in part accounts for variability in pharmacokinetics among individuals. As a result of these oxidative pathways metabolites then may be further metabolized to other species or eliminated in the urine. Metabolism of a drug by Phase II or conjugation reactions (such as glucuronidation, sulfation, or acetylation) results in larger, more polar compounds, which are subsequently eliminated either in the urine or through the biliary system into the gastrointestinal tract (GIT). Active metabolites also may result from this process as well, such as the formation of N-acetylprocainamide from the acetylation of procainamide. Elimination of some glucuronide conjugates into the GIT may undergo hydrolysis by β-glucuronidase with subsequent reabsorption of the parent compound, a process known as enterohepatic recycling (Rowland & Tozer, 1995).

The numerous metabolic pathways through which drug elimination occurs in the liver have precluded identification of a single test to quantitate hepatic metabolic function. Furthermore,

## TABLE 3–1. EXAMPLES OF HIGH AND LOW HEPATIC EXTRACTION DRUGS

| High Extraction | Low Extraction |
| --- | --- |
| Propranolol | Theophylline |
| Lidocaine | Warfarin |
| Verapamil | Phenytoin |
| Meperidine | Ibuprofen |
| Morphine | Procainamide |
| Nitroglycerin | Phenobarbital |

hepatic blood flow and plasma protein binding are also determinants of hepatic drug clearance. Attempts have been made to use markers representative of the various drug elimination pathways through the liver, including antipyrine and aminopyrine for Phase I metabolism, lorazepam for Phase II metabolism, and indocyanine green (ICG) for hepatic blood flow. These markers have been shown to distinguish between patients with hepatic cirrhosis and normal subjects, but have not been proven effective for quantitation of hepatic function within these extremes. The tests are potential research tools but have limited use in the clinic.

More appropriate clinical tools to assess hepatic drug metabolism include a combination of the serum albumin and bilirubin concentrations as well as the prothrombin time. Individually, abnormal tests are not indicative of hepatic dysfunction, but when taken together may reflect severe hepatic disease such as cirrhosis. For example, several conditions may lead to hypoalbuminemia, including not only cirrhosis, but also malabsorption, malnutrition, and nephrotic syndrome. An albumin value of <2.5 g/dL is consistent with hepatic cirrhosis since it reflects the decreased synthetic capacity of the liver. Likewise, a prolonged prothrombin time > 15 s in a patient not receiving warfarin may suggest severe hepatic disease, reflecting decreased synthesis of clotting factors and other synthetic activity within the liver. Elevation of the bilirubin concentration is suggestive of an inability to excrete bilirubin and thus hepatobiliary disease. Together, abnormalities in these markers point toward severe hepatic dysfunction and should be considered as a sign of decreased drug elimination by the liver. A scoring system for cirrhosis, which includes these tests as well as other clinical signs, has been used as a semi-quantitative assessment of hepatic function, and is shown in Table 3–2 (Pugh, Murray-Lyon, Dawson, Pietroni, & Williams, 1973).

## RENAL FUNCTION

Each kidney normally consists of approximately 1 million nephrons, the functional unit. Excretion of a drug through the nephron is achieved through the net combination of filtration, secretion, and reabsorption. Filtration is accomplished at the glomerulus and allows for the passive movement of protein-free plasma from the glomerulus into the proximal tubule. The concentration of solute in the early proximal tubule is similar to the unbound concentration in the plasma. Secretion occurs by an active transport process whereby drug is carried from the peritubular capillary circulation, across the tubular cell, and into the tubular lumen. Reabsorption of drug generally occurs as a passive process in the collecting tubule, moving from the tubule into the circulation. Factors such as urine flow and pH of the urine may influence tubular reabsorption. Increased urine flow will decrease reabsorption, and an increase in urine pH for weak acids (eg, salicylate) or decreased pH for weak bases (eg, amphetamine) will decrease reabsorption by trapping the ionized form of the drug in the lumen, resulting in increased urinary excretion.

Measurement of kidney function is based on the premise that filtration, secretion, and reabsorption all change in parallel when there is a loss of functional nephrons. This concept is known as *Bricker's intact nephron hypothesis*, which states that net kidney function is proportional to the number of functional nephrons. Based on this, measurement of the glomerular filtration rate (GFR) provides an assessment of overall function.

## TABLE 3–2. PUGH'S CRITERIA FOR THE ASSESSMENT OF HEPATIC CIRRHOSIS

| Criterion | 1 point | 2 points | 3 points |
|---|---|---|---|
| Encephalopathy (grade) | None | 1 or 2 | 3 or 4 |
| Ascites | Absent | Slight | Moderate |
| Bilirubin (mg/dL) | 1–2 | 2–3 | >3 |
| Albumin (g/dL) | >3.5 | 2.8–3.5 | <2.8 |
| Prothrombin time (s > control) | 1–4 | 4–10 | >10 |

Scoring system: 5–6 total points = mild dysfunction; 7–9 = moderate dysfunction; > 9 = severe dysfunction
*Source: Pugh (1973).*

Approximately 20% of cardiac output perfuses the kidney, at 1200 mL/min. Renal plasma flow is therefore about 625 mL/min, after correcting the renal blood flow for hematocrit. The filtration fraction of plasma across the glomerulus is 20%, and the resultant glomerular filtration rate is about 125 mL/min in individuals with normal kidney function. Determination of the GFR can be accomplished by measuring the renal clearance of a solute that is freely filtered across the glomerulus, is not protein-bound, and does not undergo tubular secretion or reabsorption. The "gold standard" test for measurement of GFR is inulin clearance, but it has limited use in the clinical setting. A more common marker for GFR is creatinine, an endogenous product of muscle metabolism. Creatinine is also not bound to plasma proteins, is freely filtered across the glomerulus, and is not reabsorbed. Unlike inulin, approximately 10% of the elimination of creatinine by the kidneys is due to tubular secretion in subjects with normal kidney function. As renal function declines, the fraction of creatinine that is secreted increases to about 50%, so that the creatinine clearance overestimates GFR in patients with reduced kidney function. Despite this limitation, it is the most useful clinical marker for renal function and drug elimination by the kidneys (Comstock, 1997). Urea, or the blood urea nitrogen (BUN) concentration, has also been suggested as a marker of renal function. Although it also is freely filtered at the glomerulus, and is not protein-bound, it does undergo substantial reabsorption, particularly under conditions of decreased effective circulating volume, such as volume depletion, congestive heart failure, ascites, or nephrotic syndrome. Urea is an ineffective osmole and is able to freely cross cell membranes. It follows water, and the above conditions all result in increased water reabsorption from the proximal tubule. The subsequent decrease in urea excretion, and elevated BUN are not a reflection of kidney function or GFR. Creatinine does not undergo appreciable reabsorption, which accounts for the elevated BUN:creatinine ratio under these conditions.

Creatinine clearance can be determined by direct measurement of the creatinine excretion rate or estimated using population-based equations. Measurement of creatinine clearance requires collection of a timed urine sample, usually 24 h, although shorter collection times may be used (2–4 h) and are as accurate as 24-h collections. Ideally, a midpoint serum creatinine concentration is measured, although it is more convenient to collect the sample at the end of the timed interval, as long as the patient has stable kidney function. Calculation of the measured creatinine clearance is as follows:

$$CL_{cr}, mL/min = (V_{urine} \times C_{urine})/(C_{serum} \times time)$$

where:

$V_{urine}$ = total volume of the urine collection
$C_{urine}$ = concentration of creatinine in the urine sample
$C_{serum}$ = concentration of creatinine in the serum sample
time = duration of the urine collection

For example, a 55-year-old man (70 kg), who is instructed to collect his urine for 24 h, returns to the clinic with his container with 1360 mL of urine. The concentration of creatinine in the urine is reported to be 92 mg/dL, and his plasma creatinine concentration is 1.4 mg/dL. His creatinine clearance is:

$$CL_{cr} = \frac{1360\,mL \times 92\,mg/dL}{1.4\,mg/dL \times 1440\,min} = 62\,mL/min$$

It often is inconvenient to perform a measured creatinine clearance, and inaccurate collections can lead to falsely low measures of kidney function (for instance, if all of the urine is not collected). Often it is more convenient to estimate kidney function. The Cockcroft–Gault estimation method for creatinine clearance was described initially in 1976 and has served as a useful tool to estimate kidney function in adult patients:

$$CL_{cr}(male), mL/min = \frac{(140 - age)\,IBW}{72(S_{cr})}$$

$$CL_{cr}(female) = CL_{cr}(male) \times 0.85$$

where:

$S_{cr}$ = serum creatine concentration (mg/dL)
IBW = ideal body weight, kg
IBW(male) = 50 kg + 2.3 kg for every 1 in > 5 ft in height
IBW(female) = 45.5 kg + 2.3 kg for every 1 in > 5 ft in height

This method provides the individualized creatinine clearance. A normalized clearance based on 72 kg is:

$$CL_{cr}(male), mL/min/72\ kg =$$
$$(140 - age, years)/S_{cr}$$
$$CL_{cr}(female) = CL_{cr}(male) \times 0.85$$

For the previous example, the creatinine clearance is estimated as:

$$CL_{cr} = \frac{140 - 55}{1.4} = 61\ mL/min/72\ kg$$

The measured and estimated creatinine clearances are not always similar, and consideration must be given to factors that will alter the plasma creatinine concentration since it is the primary measured determinant of the estimated creatinine clearance.

Patients with very low body mass or those with spinal cord injuries are not good candidates for estimation of creatinine clearance since the creatinine production rate is very low and the creatinine clearance is falsely elevated. Furthermore, false elevations of the serum creatinine concentration may occur with exercise or some medications, such as cimetidine or trimethoprim, and may falsely lower the estimate of kidney function. The blood sample for measurement of creatinine should be not be obtained following the ingestion of a meat meal, as the creatinine in the meat will be absorbed and falsely elevate the patient's creatinine concentration. Preferably, the sample should be obtained in the morning before a meal is ingested. These conditions and others are listed in Table 3–3.

Estimation of kidney function in pediatric patients can be accomplished after considering developmental changes in renal function following birth. Renal function rapidly approaches normal values, corrected for body size, within the first year of life and can be estimated according to Schwartz, Feld, & Langford (1984), as follows:

$$CL_{cr}\ mL/min\ per\ 1.73\ m^2 =$$
$$(0.45 \times height, cm)/S_{cr}$$

For patients in the range of 1–12 years, the following equation by Schwartz, Haycock, Edelman, & Spitzer (1976) should be used:

$$CL_{cr}\ mL/min\ per\ 1.73\ m^2 =$$
$$(0.55 \times height, cm)/S_{cr}$$

## DOSING ISSUES—HEPATIC IMPAIRMENT

Whereas it is difficult to quantify hepatic metabolic function because of the vast array of factors influencing drug elimination and the multiple metabolic pathways, certain pharmacokinetic changes may be anticipated based on drug characteristics in patients with hepatic cirrhosis (Brouwer, Dukes, & Powell, 1992). The half-life $(t_{1/2})$ for elimination of a drug is determined by both the clearance (CL) of the drug from the body and its volume of distribution $(V_D)$. A decreased clearance or an increased $V_D$ results in a prolonged elimination half-life. The relationship between these parameters is $t_{1/2} = (0.693 \times V_D)/CL$. When the clearance of a drug is reduced in hepatic failure and the volume of distribution is increased, such as for a protein-bound, high extraction drug such as lidocaine, there will be pronounced effects on the elimination half-life and caution must be exercised in patients with severe hepatic disease.

| TABLE 3–3.  COMMON FACTORS INTERFERING WITH THE INTERPRETATION OF CREATININE CLEARANCE AS A MEASURE OF KIDNEY FUNCTION | |
|---|---|
| **Elevation of Serum Creatinine** | **Mechanism** |
| Acetoacetate | Analytical interference |
| Ascorbic acid | Analytical interference |
| Cephalosporins | Analytical interference |
| 5-Flucytosine | Analytical interference |
| Exercise | Increased production |
| Diet (meat ingestion) | Absorption |
| Drugs (cimetidine, trimethoprim, probenecid) | Decreased tubular secretion |

Drug absorption following oral administration involves disintegration (for solid dosage forms), dissolution, and absorption. The absorption process involves passage of drug molecules through the wall of the GIT and into the portal circulation where they are then delivered to the liver before entry into the systemic circulation. Both the GIT and liver are capable of drug metabolism during the absorption process, and the bioavailability of the absorbed drug is dependent on the fraction that escapes metabolism. For a high E drug, bioavailability is very low, and a relatively large oral dose must be administered in order to achieve adequate plasma concentrations, such as for propranolol. Lidocaine administered orally results in subtherapeutic concentrations of lidocaine and toxic concentrations of an active metabolite, thus precluding the oral administration of lidocaine to achieve systemic effects. Hepatic cirrhosis results in a significant reduction in effective hepatic blood flow as well as metabolic activity, resulting in as much as a twofold increase in absorption of high E drugs, necessitating dose reduction.

Volume of distribution is determined by the physiologic compartments for drug distribution, ie, extracellular and intracellular spaces, and protein binding of the drug in both the plasma and tissue compartments. Significant changes in the physiologic volume of distribution are not likely to occur in patients with hepatic disease, unless the drug has a small volume of distribution, such as is the case for the aminoglycoside antibiotics, which are limited to the extracellular space. For these drugs, in the presence of severe ascites, the $V_D$ may increase by as much as 50%. Most changes in the $V_D$ of patients with hepatic disease, however, are attributed to hypoalbuminemia. Decreased plasma protein binding as a result of fewer available binding sites will lead to the increased unbound drug moving into the extravascular space, thus resulting in an increased $V_D$. These changes are only significant for highly protein bound drugs (>90%). The impact of $V_D$ changes on the elimination parameters of a drug depend on whether it is characterized as a low or high E compound. The low E drug will show an increased $V_D$, and the net effect on elimination will depend on whether the drug is eliminated by Phase I or Phase II enzymes. Phase I–eliminated drugs will most likely show a reduced clearance, and therefore a significantly prolonged elimination half-life, when combined with the increased $V_D$. Phase II–eliminated drugs may show a minimal

effect on half-life since the hepatic clearance may actually increase because more of the drug is available for metabolism, and Phase II processes tend to be spared from the effects of cirrhosis. Highly protein bound drugs that are also high E compounds will show an increased $V_D$ and decreased hepatic clearance, and therefore a significantly prolonged elimination half-life.

Altered hepatic clearance of drugs in patients with liver disease is dependent on the drug and its elimination characteristics. Low extraction drugs eliminated by Phase I processes will have a reduced hepatic clearance, whereas those eliminated by Phase II processes will retain near-normal clearance. High extraction drugs will show reduced clearance as a result of a decreased effective hepatic blood flow. These changes in elimination should be reflected in the dosage regimen for the patient.

## DOSING ISSUES—RENAL IMPAIRMENT

The new dosage regimen in the patient with reduced kidney function must take into consideration the changes in absorption and distribution as well as the expected changes in excretion. Factors to consider include concomitant drug therapy, organ dysfunction, and secondary effects of the disease (Lam, Banerji, Hatfield, & Talbert, 1997; Matzke & Frye, 1997).

### ABSORPTION

Although not well studied, altered absorption of drugs may occur in the patient with renal dysfunction. For the patient with end-stage renal disease (ESRD), numerous medications are often prescribed in order to manage secondary complications. Among these are calcium products for binding dietary phosphorus, iron supplements for the treatment of anemia, and multivitamin preparations. Absorption of fluoroquinolone antibiotics is significantly impaired when coadministered with these products, and digoxin bioavailability may be reduced when administered with antacids. These interactions may also occur in patients with normal kidney function. Generally, these interactions can be avoided by separating the administration of interacting drugs by at least 1 h, and 2 h if following a meal.

Another consideration with regard to absorption is the potential effect of renal failure and uremia on the function of other organs. For example, hepatic drug metabolism of high hepatic extraction drugs has been shown to be impaired in renal failure. As a result, the absorption of high extraction drugs may be expected to increase when administered to patients with end-stage renal disease. This has been demonstrated for propranolol and propoxyphene, where the absorption was increased by severalfold. This effect has not been observed with all high extraction compounds; the calcium antagonists show similar bioavailability in patients with normal and impaired renal function. Additional therapeutic monitoring is warranted when high hepatic extraction drugs are administered to patients with ESRD.

## DISTRIBUTION

Two potential changes in distribution may occur in patients with renal impairment, including volume and protein binding. Increased body water content is not likely to have a significant effect on drug distribution, although those patients receiving a drug with distribution limited to the extracellular volume (eg, aminoglycoside antibiotics) may show an increased volume of distribution for the drug.

A more important consideration is the change in protein binding that may occur in the patient with renal disease. These changes may be related to decreased albumin concentration and thus a reduced number of binding sites available for the drug molecule, competition from uremic toxins for the drug-binding site, or altered conformation of the albumin molecule that results in a decreased affinity for the drug. Each of these conditions may result in a decreased fraction of the drug that is bound to the albumin molecule and an increased amount of the drug available for distribution to the tissue and available for elimination (eg, metabolism). These changes in protein binding are only of concern for drugs bound more than 90% to plasma albumin. Changes in binding for drugs bound less than 90% generally do not result in significant changes in the free concentration of the drug to warrant concern. The best example of changes in protein binding in patients with kidney disease is phenytoin (Dilantin). In subjects with normal kidney function and serum albumin concentration, phenytoin is bound 90% to albumin. The usual therapeutic plasma concentration range is 10–20 mg/L based on the total plasma concentration; therefore, the unbound or free therapeutic concentration range is 1–2 mg/L. Patients with end-stage renal disease have a reduced plasma protein binding of 80%. Considering the goal of therapy is to have the same unbound concentration (the fraction available to interact with the receptor), the therapeutic total concentration range is then 5–10 mg/L since the 20% unbound will provide the same unbound concentration range, 1–2 mg/L. In patients with renal function between normal and end-stage there is an intermediate reduction in protein binding, and the total therapeutic plasma concentration range should be adjusted accordingly. Despite the change in the therapeutic range for phenytoin, the impact of these binding changes on the phenytoin dosage regimen is negligible. Although there is an increase in the volume of distribution of phenytoin, there is a proportionate increase in its hepatic clearance since more drug is available to the hepatocyte for metabolism.

Changes in tissue binding also may affect the volume of distribution for a drug. For example, digoxin is distributed mostly to the tissue compartment and has an apparent distribution volume of approximately 500 L. In patients with renal impairment, digoxin is displaced from tissue, binding sites and redistributes to the plasma compartment, resulting in a lowered volume of distribution. In ESRD it may be reduced to approximately 200 L. The impact of this change for the clinician is to administer a lower loading dose in order to avoid potentially toxic concentrations. The reduced maintenance dose necessary in patients with renal impairment is mostly a result of decreased renal elimination of digoxin, not changes in distribution.

## ELIMINATION

The most important changes in dosage regimens for patients with renal impairment are due to decreased renal elimination of a drug excreted by the kidneys. As a general rule, if a drug is eliminated more than 30% by the kidneys, then dosage regimen adjustment will usually be necessary in the patient with reduced kidney function. Dosage regimen adjustment for these drugs is based on several assumptions: drug excretion is proportional to kidney function; dose individualization is based on concentrations of the parent compound; and metabolites, which may accumulate with renal dysfunction, are not considered to be pharmacologically active. This is not always true; some compounds accumulate as active metabolites, such as normeperidine following meperidine (Demerol) administration, and N-acetylprocainamide following procainamide administration.

For drug elimination from the body, it is useful to consider renal and nonrenal processes. Generally, renal impairment will result in a proportionate decrease in the renal component of drug elimination. The greater the loss of kidney function, the more of an effect on overall drug elimination, resulting in prolongation of the elimination half-life. Figure 3–1 illustrates this general principle. The y-axis intercept is considered the fixed, or nonrenal, clearance and is independent of kidney function, whereas the line represents the renal clearance as a function of kidney function, generally assessed as creatinine clearance. This approach to modifying the dosage regiment for a drug in patients with renal impairment is often applied to drugs eliminated at least in part by the kidneys. Figure 3–2 illustrates the principle applied to the anticonvulsant gabapentin. Note the y-intercept is 0, indicating there is no nonrenal elimination of gabapentin, and all of the elimination is dependent on renal function. For gabapentin, dose adjustments are recommended at various degrees of kidney function, and guidelines are presented in the package insert. The process for dosage adjustment is (1) defining the goals of therapy, (2) assessment of kidney function, and (3) appropriate dose adjustment based on kidney function.

Consider the normal dosage regimen for a patient, expressed as a dose administered at a specified frequency, such as 200 mg every 12 h. At the steady state, this regimen will result in a plasma concentration within the therapeutic range. Unless there are pharmacodynamic changes or alterations in protein binding of the drug, the patient with renal disease should be expected to maintain the same therapeutic plasma concentration range. The new dosage regimen for the patient can be expressed using the patient-specific drug clearance obtained from its relationship to kidney function. Often the summary guidelines are available from the manufacturer of the drug product. Except for the circumstances described previously, the fraction of dose absorbed is usually unchanged in patients with renal failure.

Although this method for individualizing therapy in the patient with renal impairment is useful in determining a new dose rate for the patient, it does not specify whether the dose, dosing interval, or both variables should be changed. As a general guideline, the dosage should remain constant and the interval prolonged for antibiotics. This approach will maintain similar peak plasma concentrations, which may be necessary for antibacterial effect. It is also reasonable to prolong the interval when the normal dosage regimen is inconvenient, such as every 6 h. It would be beneficial to extend the dosing interval to every 12 or 24 h in order to improve the ease of the dosing schedule rather than reducing the dose.

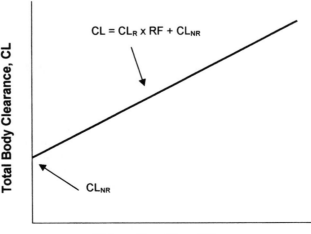

$$CL = CL_R \times RF + CL_{NR}$$

$CL_{NR}$

**Total Body Clearance, CL**

**Kidney Function, RF**

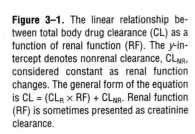

**Figure 3–1.** The linear relationship between total body drug clearance (CL) as a function of renal function (RF). The y-intercept denotes nonrenal clearance, $CL_{NR}$, considered constant as renal function changes. The general form of the equation is $CL = (CL_R \times RF) + CL_{NR}$. Renal function (RF) is sometimes presented as creatinine clearance.

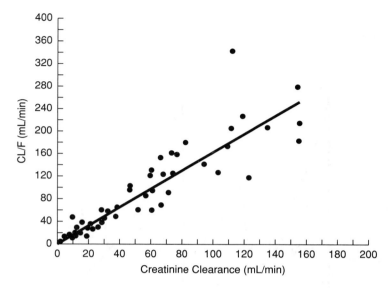

**Figure 3–2.** Relationship between gabapentin apparent oral clearance (CL/F) and creatinine clearance ($CL_{CR}$): $CL/F = (1.61 \times CL_{CR}) + 3.57$; Pearson correlation coefficient = 0.90 ($p < 0.05$). Bioavailability ($F$) of gabapentin is approximately 50% and independent of kidney function.

**Source:** Blum et al (1994).

On occasion, it may be necessary to maintain the dose for nonantibiotics and adjust the interval. This method is appropriate when the dosing interval is already at a convenient frequency, such as once per day, or there is a narrow therapeutic range and there is a need to minimize the peak-to-trough fluctuation in plasma concentrations. Figure 3–3 illustrates the resulting plasma concentration-versus-time profile when the dose, dosing interval, or both variables are modified in the process of individualizing therapy.

This approach to dosage regimen adjustment in patients with renal disease includes several assumptions such as stable kidney function, a linear relationship between drug clearance and renal function as assessed using the creatinine clearance, normal hepatic function, normal cardiovascular function, normal protein binding and volume of distribution, no changes in bioavailability, similar therapeutic plasma concentration ranges compared to normal subjects, and no active metabolites. Each of these factors should be considered when drugs are administered to patients with impaired renal function.

## DIALYSIS

Maintenance dialysis for patients with ESRD occurs primarily through either chronic hemodialysis (HD), three times weekly, or continuous ambulatory peritoneal dialysis (CAPD). During HD, the patient's blood is pumped through an artificial kidney that contains a semipermeable membrane across which the accumulated toxins in the blood diffuse into a dialysate solution on the opposing side. The rate of solute movement across the membrane depends on several variables, such as molecule size, plasma protein binding, membrane pore size, membrane thickness and surface area, and blood and dialysate flow rates. The amount of solute removed also depends on the length of the dialysis procedure, which is usually 3–4 h.

Drugs with a molecular weight of less than 500 and not bound to plasma proteins are removed from the plasma across conventional hemodialysis membranes (eg, cellulose acetate and cuprophane), but the total amount removed depends on how readily the drug moves from the tissue compartment into the plasma. Drugs with a much higher molecular weight, such as vancomycin (~1500) and erythropoietin (~35,000) are not able to cross the membrane. Drugs bound to plasma proteins, such as albumin or $\alpha_1$-acid glycoprotein, are functionally not able to cross the membrane due to the large size of the drug-protein complex (>65,000). The more a drug is bound to protein, the less likely it is that significant elimination will occur through dialysis. For example, phenytoin is bound 90% in patients with normal kidney function, and this is reduced to 80% in patients with end-stage renal disease. Although the free fraction is twice the normal value, most of the drug remains bound to albumin and is not removed by dialysis.

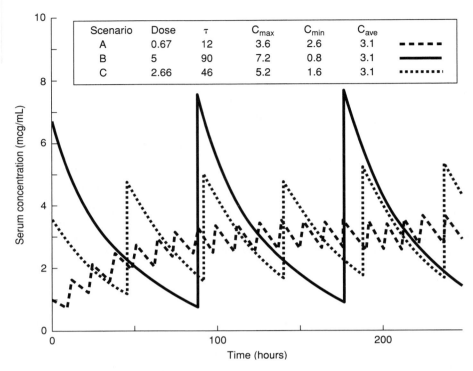

| Scenario | Dose | $\tau$ | $C_{max}$ | $C_{min}$ | $C_{ave}$ | |
|----------|------|--------|-----------|-----------|-----------|---|
| A | 0.67 | 12 | 3.6 | 2.6 | 3.1 | ----- |
| B | 5 | 90 | 7.2 | 0.8 | 3.1 | ───── |
| C | 2.66 | 46 | 5.2 | 1.6 | 3.1 | ········· |

**Figure 3–3.** Representation of the consequences of (**A**) altering the dose and maintaining the dosing interval; (**B**) changing the interval and maintaining the same dose; or (**C**) changing both the dose and interval. Note the peak-to-trough fluctuation with each scenario.

**Source:** Matzke & Frye (1997).

Newer membranes, commonly known as *high-flux* membranes, which have a larger pore size (eg, polysulfone, polyacrylonitrile, and polymethylmethacrylate), are able to permit the clearance of molecules up to 10,000 Da. For example, vancomycin supplementation must be administered to patients undergoing high-flux dialysis therapy, whereas conventional cellulose membranes often permitted a single dose of vancomycin to treat an infection because of its prolonged elimination half-life (DeSoi, Sahm, & Umans, 1992). These considerations are important when assessing the need for supplemental delivery of a drug following dialysis therapy. As a guideline, replacement dosing will be necessary when dialysis increases drug elimination by at least 30%.

Peritoneal dialysis is a slow, continuous dialysis, which usually consists of four exchanges of dialysate in the peritoneal cavity per day. Drug clearance is dependent on molecular size and protein binding, such that smaller and lesser-

bound drugs have a higher clearance. Since the dialysate flow is very low with CAPD, the net removal of most drugs is insignificant relative to clearance by other routes, and dose adjustments are generally not necessary. Patients undergoing CAPD occasionally develop peritonitis and require intraperitoneal administration of antibiotics. Absorption of drugs administered by the intraperitoneal route may vary from 50–90% and depends on the residence time in the peritoneal cavity. Larger molecules, such as proteins, are not as efficiently absorbed, but they may be absorbed sufficiently to meet systemic needs, such as for insulin in patients with diabetes mellitus (Taylor, Abdel-Rahman, Zimmerman, & Johnson, 1996).

## SUMMARY

Dosage regimen design must take into consideration the hepatic and renal functions of patients.

Significant changes in the elimination profile of a drug may occur in the patient with altered organ function, and an alternative choice of drug may be appropriate. Choosing a drug eliminated by hepatic metabolism will minimize the risk of excessive accumulation in the patient with renal dysfunction. Furthermore, the clinician must adjust the regimen for changes in absorption and distribution that may accompany organ disease. Multiple organ dysfunction will require additional monitoring and care to ensure that the risk of toxicity is minimized while achieving therapeutic goals. For patients with end-stage renal disease, maintenance dialysis regimens may also influence dosage regimen design, depending on the type of dialysis performed. Recognition that dialysis methods may vary greatly and affect drug elimination will minimize the risk of adverse effects in that population.

## REFERENCES

Blum, R. A., Comstock, T. J., Sica, D. A., Schultz, R.W., Keller, E., Reetze, P., Bockbader, H., Tuerck, D., Busch, J.A., Reece, P.A., & Sedman, A. J. (1994). Pharmacokinetics of gabapentin in subjects with various degrees of renal function. *Clinical Pharmacology and Therapeutics, 56,* 154–159.

Brouwer, K. L. R., Dukes, G. E., & Powell, J. R. (1992). Influence of liver function on drug disposition. In W. E. Evans, J. J. Schentag, & W. J. Jusko (Eds.), *Applied pharmacokinetics: Principles of therapeutic drug monitoring* (3rd ed.) (pp. 6/1–6/59). Vancouver, WA: Applied Therapeutics.

Cockcroft, D. W., & Gault, M. H. (1976). Prediction of creatinine clearance from serum creatinine. *Nephron, 16,* 31–41.

Comstock, T. J. (1997). Quantification of renal function. In J. T. DiPiro, R. L. Talbert, G. C. Yee, G. R. Matzke, B. G. Wells, & L. M. Posey (Eds.), *Pharmacotherapy: A pathophysiologic approach* (3rd ed). Stamford, CT: Appleton & Lange.

DeSoi, C. A., Sahm, D. F., & Umans, J. G. (1992). Vancomycin elimination during high-flux hemodialysis: Kinetic model and comparison of four membranes. *American Journal of Kidney Diseases, 20,* 354–360.

Lam, Y. W. F., Banerji, S., Hatfield, C., & Talbert, R. L. (1997). Principles of drug administration in renal insufficiency. *Clinical Pharmacokinetics, 32,* 30–57.

Matzke, G. R., & Frye, R. F. (1997). Drug therapy individualization for patients with renal insufficiency. In J. T. DiPiro, R. L. Talbert, G. C. Yee, G. R. Matzke, B. G. Wells, & L. M. Posey (Eds.), *Pharmacotherapy: A pathophysiologic approach* (3rd ed). Stamford, CT: Appleton & Lange.

Pugh, R. N., Murray-Lyon, I. M., Dawson, J. L., Pietroni, M. C. & Williams, R. (1973). Transection of the oesophagus for bleeding oesophageal varices. *British Journal of Surgery, 60,* 646–649.

Rowland, M., & Tozer, T. N. (Eds.). (1995). *Clinical pharmacokinetics: Concepts and applications* (3rd ed). Baltimore: Williams & Wilkins.

Schwartz, G. J., Feld, L. G. & Langford, D. J. (1984). A simple estimate of glomerular filtration rate in full-term infants during the first year of life. *Journal of Pediatrics, 104,* 849–854.

Schwartz, G. J., Haycock, G. B., Edelman, C. M. Jr., & Spitzer, A. (1976). A simple estimate of glomerular filtration rate in children derived from body length and plasma creatinine. *Pediatrics, 58,* 259–263.

Taylor, C. A., III, Abdel-Rahman, E., Zimmerman, S. W., & Johnson, C. A. (1996). Clinical pharmacokinetics during continuous ambulatory peritoneal dialysis. *Clinical Pharmacokinetics, 31,* 293–308.

# GENERAL ISSUES

**II**

# 4

# SAFETY IN PHARMACOTHERAPY

*Lea Ann Hansen*

Every therapeutic process is more than picking a drug "recipe" from a book for a given diagnosis. After a pharmacotherapeutic regimen has been implemented, proper monitoring is critical to a successful outcome for the patient. This step may, in fact, be more difficult to carry out than the initial diagnosis and therapy selection since very little information is available in texts or in scientific papers about the best way to follow up. Knowing how, what, and who to monitor comes from "experience"—yet it is this ability that distinguishes the astute clinician from others. Patient responses to a specific therapy are generally unpredictable. Sometimes, we can predetermine if a patient is more or less likely to have a good outcome, but it is rarely an exact science.

Even in settings where follow-up programs have been studied, there are wide-ranging results. Virgo, Vernava, Longo, McKirgan, and Johnson (1995) describe in detail the literature on follow up after potentially curative colorectal cancer treatment; the points raised in the article and accompanying editorial (Loprinzi, 1995) can be extrapolated to any disorder. Bottom line, they found that even though different strategies can vary in cost by as much as $800 million for a national cohort of patients, there are few data to support better outcomes for the more intensive programs.

When developing a monitoring plan for an individual patient, it is important to have a logical, comprehensive strategy to use even if it may seem cumbersome at first. Later, your "experience" will streamline the process. One such strategy, with examples, follows:

1. Outline all of the parameters that could be used to monitor efficacy. The decision to actually use any or all of these parameters will be a later step. How can you determine if the medication is working? The patient's symptoms (pain, shortness of breath) related to the disease state should lessen and possibly resolve. A physical finding (blood pressure, edema), laboratory test (urinalysis, CBC), or radiological test (chest x-ray) used for diagnosis should normalize with proper therapy. If additional sequelae of the disease that were not present in the patient initially (suicidal thoughts in a depressed patient) represent worsening of the illness, how would you detect them? Familiarize yourself with the usual course of events in treating the condition.

2. Consider all the parameters that can be used to monitor side effects of treatment. Many drug references can provide you with an extensive list of possible side effects. How can they be detected? Ask your patients to report symptoms (call you if they have bleeding or bruising) or question them about specific possibilities at a later time. Consider an additional physical exam or laboratory test to detect frequently reported problems (transaminase levels for hepatic toxicity).

3. Decide which of these parameters you will actually monitor. Many facets of this decision relate primarily to the need to detect either poor efficacy or development of toxicity, ie, consequences of an undetected problem. Availability

59

of testing and feasibility contribute to the decision. Not all references will provide adequate information to determine the relative importance of each issue. Be aware of situations that could cause mortality or severe morbidity. For example, for a patient on allopurinol, a seemingly simple rash can progress into Stevens-Johnson syndrome, a potentially fatal condition. Although such an occurrence is rare, evaluation for rash should be part of the monitoring plan. Also consider the frequency of occurrence for a certain problem; if a problem occurs in more than 1% of patients, it is likely to be encountered at some point in a busy practice. If it occurs in 10% of patients or more, specific procedures to handle the problem should be in place.

4. Decide how frequently each parameter will be monitored. Obviously, it is not feasible to monitor every parameter all the time, so the interval must coincide with how quickly a patient's status is likely to change (eg, a few days for a minor bacterial infection compared to a few weeks to months for hyperlipidemia), feasibility (a reliable patient with a high level of interest in his or her health can be taught self-monitoring), and economics of the testing. Structured telephone follow-up is a useful tool that is probably not implemented as frequently as it could be. One study assessed the impact of doubling the time interval between face-to-face interactions and substituting three telephone calls for the omitted clinic visit. The group receiving the telephone calls had decreased total clinic visits, less need for medication, fewer hospital admissions, and fewer hospital days than did the group with routine follow-up. The subset of the population whose health was poor or fair, especially, used fewer health care resources when telephone interaction was used (Wasson et al, 1992).

The ability to change the overall outcome by detecting a problem should also be considered. For example, a patient on the most aggressive triple therapy for HIV has few additional options if it is ineffective. The most important focus for the monitoring plan is, therefore, to detect toxicity. Documentation of efficacy in this example can be somewhat less stringent, although the financial costs of monitoring may be justified if the cost of unrecognized ineffective therapy is high.

Documentation in the medical record should include the therapy plan with the specific drug(s) and doses, in addition to the monitoring plan described above. Mechanisms should be used to facilitate collection of that data. Patient self-reports should be logged. Laboratory values are frequently written on a flowsheet. Other types of data can be brought to the same level of prominence by documenting them in a similar manner: for example, pain ratings and bowel movement frequency in a patient on opioid analgesics, number of nitroglycerin tablets used for angina, or number of hours of sleep obtained by an insomniac.

## COMPLIANCE WITH PHARMACOTHERAPEUTIC REGIMEN

The best drug therapy available will not help the patient if it is does not reach the site of action in the body. Incorrect use of medications is common in patients of all ages. Originally this behavior was described as "noncompliance." This term has more recently been replaced by "nonadherence," implying more patient involvement in determining the course of treatment. Since the majority of research uses the term noncompliance, it will be used here.

Noncompliance can lead to increased overall yearly expenditures (health care costs and indirect costs) of $25–100 billion. Noncompliers are also more likely to die, as in the beta blocker heart attack trial (2.6 times higher mortality in 1 year) (Coons et al, 1994). Most formal studies of compliance use an assessment of the proportion of a prescribed regimen used by the patient. Simple measures such as pill counts or patient diaries can be inaccurate and can potentially overestimate compliance rates. Studies frequently fail to consider inappropriately administered medication as a type of noncompliance.

Obviously, an informed patient is more likely to make correct decisions about treatment. Patient education issues are discussed in the next section. Besides knowledge deficit, other factors that can lead to suboptimal compliance include:

- Drug side effects
- Complexity of the regimen
- Adaptation to the lifestyle change
- Age greater than 75 years
- Female sex
- Living alone
- Lack of a support system

Socioeconomic status has not been consistently predictive (Coons et al, 1994). Previous experience leads patients to their own unique appraisal of the situation and the importance of the treatment, although belief in the importance of health does not always translate into compliant behavior (Wierenga & Hewitt, 1994). Previous success with behavioral change seems to be a strong predictor of future success with health habit changes (Rakowski, Wells, Lasater, & Carelton, 1991). Adapting the medication to the patient's lifestyle may be more effective than vice versa. Patients with serious illnesses, such as myocardial infarction, may be less compliant if they are highly prone to psychological distress (Rose, Conn, & Rodeman, 1994). Anxiety management may promote adherence as much as education.

Elderly patients may have impairments that hinder their ability to take medication, such as decreased vision, decreased physical functioning, or cognitive impairment. Atkin, Finnegan, Ogle, and Shenfield (1994) found that of 120 elderly patients admitted to a hospital who were well enough to give consent, 63% were unable to open at least one of seven types of medication containers. A screw-top bottle could be opened by 92.7% and a flip-top by 85.8%. A childproof container could only be opened by 43.4%. Even 7-day medication organizers, promoted to assist compliance, caused difficulty for 24%. Seventy-two percent could not break a scored tablet. Men were significantly less likely than women to have difficulties in opening containers.

## TEACHING AND COUNSELING

Initially, a patient educational program should include an assessment of the patient's willingness to learn, any barriers to learning, and specific learning needs. A patient may understand the basic issues of treatment but develop a more negative attitude toward it if a situation arises that he or she feels incapable of handling (eg, a missed dose of medication). Simple written medication leaflets in conjunction with oral counseling are preferred by patients, especially by middle-aged adults (Harvey & Plumridge, 1991). Low-literacy patients may react to a complicated learning situation by withdrawing while indicating the material was understood even if it was not (Hussey, 1991).

Sophisticated training programs have been shown to increase knowledge and compliance. A program such as Medication Management Module for Schizophrenic Patients (Eckman,

Liberman, Phipps, and Blair, 1990) consists of sessions held 3 h per week for 15–20 weeks. The program has specific educational objectives, goal setting, redundancy of information, multimedia instructional techniques, checking for assimilation of material presented, modeling, use of positive reinforcement and shaping techniques, role playing, coaching and active prompting of correct responses, homework assignments, and immediate positive or corrective feedback. This program increased the patients' ability to utilize certain medication-related skills from 40–50% and their compliance from 67–82%. Unfortunately, an assessment of health care resource utilization after completion of this extensive intervention was not reported.

In elderly hospitalized patients with a diagnosis of congestive heart failure, a review to consolidate medications into a two or three times daily regimen and intensive multidisciplinary education, including charts detailing drug regimens and patient self-monitoring techniques, reduced readmission rates during the following 90 days from 45.7% in the control group to 33.3%. Hospital days during this interval were reduced by 1.4 days per patient, but neither of these differences was statistically significant due to the small sample size (Rich et al, 1993).

Dividing educational material into understandable pieces is important, but it is very difficult in many health care systems to identify which person is responsible for education in every setting. It is important that each subsequent educator be aware of previous activity. Otherwise, useless repetition of basic information and omission of the more difficult material can result. Therefore, educational programs are incomplete unless content, patient comprehension, and ongoing needs are documented in the medical record.

## MISUSE OF MEDICATIONS

When a medication is not used as prescribed or is used at a different dosage, it is being misused (Finch, 1993). Usually this is unintentional. Education or a strengthened support system may be needed. Instances of intentional misuse should not always be considered abuse; for example, lack of understanding may lead a person to use leftover antibiotics for a new symptom.

Over-the-counter medications or herbal therapies can also be misused, often without the knowledge of the health care provider. Patients may not consider that such medications might be dangerous and disregard the label directions. Fung, Weintraub, and Bowen (1995) reported a case of a 69-year-old woman who was admitted to the intensive care unit with symptoms resembling a stroke. Only after intubation and discussions of withdrawing medical therapy had taken place was it discovered that the patient's magnesium level was 6.65 mmol/L (normal, 0.80–1.20 mmol/L). After fluid diuresis, the patient recovered and admitted to taking two large bottles of magnesium-containing antacids per day for chronic GI complaints. A similar but milder presentation had resulted in a hospital admission just 4 months earlier.

Another type of misuse of medications is the prescribing of "unnecessary" medications. A study by Lindley, Tully, Paramsothy, and Tallis (1992) suggests that 6.3% of all hospital admissions are related to adverse effects from medications. About half of these are due to inappropriate prescriptions, including use of contraindicated and unnecessary medications plus those that interacted with previous therapy. This supports the adage that "a drug that is not indicated is contraindicated." Lindley et al also found that the drug-related admission rate was significantly higher for inappropriate drugs compared to appropriate drugs (5.1% vs. 1.1%). Willcox, Himmelstein, and Woolhandler (1994) found that 23.5% of a cohort of 6171 elderly patients were taking a medication that had been previously deemed inappropriate by a panel of geriatrics experts and of those, 20.4% were taking two or more. Critical evaluation of all components of a medication profile should be a regular part of patient care. It can be difficult to obtain a complete medication history when multiple prescribers are involved. Problematic drug use has been well documented in nursing homes as well (Beers, Fingold, & Ouslander, 1992).

## ABUSE OF DRUGS

Abuse refers to drug use outside the normally accepted standard for that drug such that negative consequences occur. Data from the mid-1980s estimated that 15% of the U.S. population over 12 years of age had used a prescription medication for nonmedical reasons (Britton, Lobeck, and Kelly, 1994). Health professionals have a responsibility to detect substance abuse and intervene when it is suspected. However, this responsibility, coupled with fear that patients may be deceptive or that regulatory authorities may take action, can cause excessive vigilance. Prescribers must recognize the difference between addiction and physical dependence with its associated withdrawal symptoms. The latter can occur with appropriate therapy.

Waldrop and Mandry (1995) surveyed the perceptions of health professionals at an urban teaching hospital about opioid dependence among patients in pain. Staff physicians had the lowest percentage of perceived dependency (4% of all patients, 8% of sickle cell anemia patients). Resident physicians believed 9% of all patients and 17% of sickle cell patients were dependent. Nurses' ratings were 7% and 13% for the two groups. All these values are higher than any incidence of dependence documented in the literature: generally less than 1%. This example implies that unnecessary withholding of therapy for legitimate problems could occur, potentially a greater overall harm than allowing a few abusers to have access to medications.

Many categories of drugs have abuse potential. Agents acting on the central nervous system are most prominent, but others, such as anabolic steroids or thyroid medications, have been used outside of medical indications. An excellent review by Finch (1993), outlines characteristics of patients who are potent medication abusers, including:

- Previous substance abuse (assess this in every patient)
- Changes in functional status or personal relationships
- Early requests for refills (because a prescription was allegedly lost or stolen)
- Missed clinic appointments, with subsequent after-hours calls for prescription renewals
- Forgery of prescriptions
- Strong preference for a particular drug ("allergic" to others, "nothing" else works)
- Solicitation of prescriptions from multiple prescribers

Some health care systems have established multidisciplinary committees to identify and intervene when medication abuse is suspected (Britton et al, 1994). Actions that can be taken include limitations on quantity dispensed, requiring that the patient sign a receipt for a specific quantity of drug at each refill, restricting the prescription of the abused drug to one provider, or referral to a substance abuse treatment program.

# REFERENCES

Atkin, R. A., Finnegan, T. P., Ogle, S. J., & Shenfield, G. M. (1994). Functional ability of patients to manage medication packaging: A survey of geriatric inpatients. *Age and Ageing, 23,* 113–116.

Beers, M. H., Fingold, S. F., & Ouslander, J. G. (1992). A computerized system for identifying and informing physicians about problematic drug use in nursing homes. *Journal of Medical Systems, 16,* 237–245.

Britton, M. L., Lobeck, F. G., & Kelly, M. W. (1994). Multidisciplinary committee on the abuse of prescription medications. *American Journal of Hospital Pharmacy, 51,* 85–88.

Coons, S. T., Sheahan, S. L., Martin, S. S., Hendricks, J., Robbins, C. A., & Johnson, J. A. (1994). Predictors of medication noncompliance in a sample of older adults. *Clinical Therapeutics, 16,* 110–117.

Eckman, T. A., Liberman, R. P., Phipps, C. C., & Blair, K. E. (1990). Teaching medication management skills to schizophrenic patients. *Journal of Clinical Psychopharmacology, 10,* 33–38.

Finch, J. (1993). Prescription drug abuse. *Primary Care, 20,* 231–238.

Fung, M. C., Weintraub, M., & Bowen, D. L. (1995). Hypermagnesemia: Elderly over-the-counter drug users at risk. *Archives of Family Medicine, 4,* 718–723.

Harvey, J. L., & Plumridge, R. J. (1991). Comparative attitudes to verbal and written medication information among hospital outpatients. *Annals of Pharmacotherapy, 25,* 925–928.

Hussey, L. C. (1991). Overcoming the clinical barriers of low literacy and medication noncompliance among the elderly. *Journal of Gerontology Nursing, 17,* 27–29.

Lindley, C. M., Tully, M. P., Paramsothy, V., & Tallis, R. C. (1992). Inappropriate medication is a major cause of adverse drug reactions in elderly patients. *Age and Ageing, 21,* 294–300.

Loprinzi, C. L. (1995). Follow-up testing for curatively treated cancer survivors; what to do? *JAMA, 273,* 1877–1878.

Rakowski, W., Wells, B. L., Lasater, T. M., & Carelton, R. A. (1991). Correlates of expected success at health habit change and its role as a predictor in health behavior research. *American Journal of Preventive Medicine, 7,* 89–94.

Rich, M. W., Vinson, J. M., Sperry, J. C., Shah, A. S., Spinner, L. R., Chung, M. K., & Davila-Roman, V. (1993). Prevention of readmission in elderly patients with congestive heart failure. *Journal of General Internal Medicine, 8,* 585–590.

Rose, S. K., Conn, V. S., & Rodeman, B. J. (1994). Anxiety and self-care following myocardial infarction. *Issues in Mental Health Nursing, 15,* 433–444.

Virgo, K. S., Vernava, A. M., Longo, W. E., McKirgan, L. W., & Johnson, F. E. (1995). Cost of patient follow-up after potentially curative colorectal cancer treatment. *JAMA, 273,* 1837–1841.

Waldrop, R. D., & Mandry, C. (1995). Health professional perceptions of opioid dependence among patients with pain. *American Journal of Emergency Medicine, 13,* 529–531.

Wasson, J., Gaudette, C., Whaley, E., Sauvigne, A., Baribeau, P., & Welch, H. G. (1992). Telephone care as a substitute for routine clinic follow-up. *JAMA, 267,* 1788–1793.

Wierenga, M. E., & Hewitt, J. B. (1994). Facilitating diabetes self-management. *The Diabetes Educator, 20,* 138–142.

Willcox, S. M., Himmelstein, D. U., & Woolhandler, S. (1994). Inappropriate drug prescribing for the community-dwelling elderly. *JAMA, 272,* 292–296.

# 5

# PSYCHOLOGICAL, SOCIOLOGICAL, AND CULTURAL FACTORS

*Jeanette F. Kissinger and Kathleen J. Sawin*

A 36-year-old white male presents at an ambulatory clinic complaining of "pain in my left hand." The hand is edematous, with erythematous induration extending 4 in. above the wrist. The client came to the clinic because the pain was interfering with driving his truck. Examination revealed two small healed abrasions on the dorsal side of the hand. When queried about the healed wounds, he stated that he had been punctured and cut on barbed wire the previous week and had been treated at this clinic. His past records at the clinic documented the treatment given at the time of the initial injury and showed that he was given a prescription for Augmentin. When asked if he had taken the Augmentin, he said he had not. When asked why, he stated, "I lost the prescription in my truck." He had been on a delivery to Chicago and had just returned from that run. He had not sought any other medical or over-the-counter (OTC) treatment for his hand, and stated that the swelling and redness began 2 days prior. Told of the seriousness of the resulting cellulitis, he was given the appropriate treatment—all now at greater expense, monetarily and physically, to the patient as well as at a higher total cost of health care.

As health care providers we must ask ourselves: Did he understand the health risk if he did not take the prescribed medication? Did he know that a phone call would have replaced the lost prescription, if it was lost? Did he understand he was at risk (susceptible) for complications? Was there a financial/insurance *or any*

*other* reason for not following through and getting the prescription filled? Did he believe in preventive measures, or did he believe you can treat the problem when it occurs? Did his health orientation (seek help when it hurts or interferes with your occupation) or family tradition prevent him from taking the Augmentin?

When we prescribe a drug, we need to factor in the characteristics of the drug or drug schedule (see Chap. 4 in this book on safety), of the person we wish to take the medication, and of the provider/patient relationship associated with the likelihood of the drug actually being taken. If health care providers wish to achieve positive health outcomes from the therapies and medications they prescribe, they must consider all influences on the clients' medication-taking behavior and adherence (compliance) to the prescribed regime.

Rubel and Carro (1992) state that the major barrier to successful health outcomes from the treatment of tuberculosis (TB) today is the lack of adherence to the prescribed medications. An extensive qualitative study (Robertson, 1992) found that patients evaluate their prescribed medical regimes before deciding on a course of action, and these evaluations are based on their own beliefs, values, and knowledge. Arakelian (1992) concludes that health care professionals and patients disagree on the definition of compliance. Subjects felt they were compliant if they were feeling well, heard their doctors' comments that they were doing fine, and in some instances were checking their own blood pressure or sugar levels. For some, treatment regimes were found to be more problematic than illness.

Health care professionals who assume that the prescribed drug regimen is the patient's only approach and treatment and that compliance is static need to examine their own beliefs. The literature uses both *adherence* and *compliance* synonymously. Many find that *compliance* conveys a negative connotation. *Adherence* implies a collaborative relationship in which the client and health care provider come to an agreement regarding the desired outcome and the treatment to achieve it. (Adherence is the preferred term of the authors, but both terms are used here to reflect current usage.) In many cases, patient input in the decision is critical (Biley, 1992) and avoiding that step may decrease the likelihood of an effective use of prescribed drugs. It is not the intent of the authors to discuss the entire range of factors that influence adherence, so this chapter focuses on beliefs, culture, religion, traditions, world views, and relevant psychosocial theories.

## DEMOGRAPHICS OF THE HEALTH CARE CONSUMER

### AGE AND SEX

Dramatic changes are occurring in the age pyramid—and, thus, the "market profile" of health care consumers—due in part to the baby boom, the increasing growth of the 65+ age group, and females outliving males by more than 7 years. Thomas (1993) finds that not only are women the major decision makers regarding consumption of health care, they use health services more frequently than men, particularly during childbearing and their senior years. As the population ages, the health care system will overwhelmingly be dominated by women. Why is this important? Their needs are different, most research has been done on men, and women constitute a large percentage of the workforce. All these facts contribute to the reality that the health care provider desiring positive health outcomes must approach prescribing therapies to women in a more collaborative manner. The increased aging of the population has necessitated further differentiations in what constitutes "old." The active 60s, the declining 70s, and the frail 80s not only have different health needs but also have different views of who should control

their health behavior and how the health problem should be fixed (Thomas, 1993).

## RACIAL AND ETHNIC DIVERSITY

When the census was taken in both 1980 and 1990, respondents were asked to indicate their ancestry. It was interpreted that the responses would indicate the ethnic group the person identified with and still had some strong attachment with regardless of how many generations they were removed from it. Over 80% of the respondents reported a single ancestry. Others reported double or triple ancestry. Among the white population, English, German, and Irish were the most often cited ethnic groups. French and Italian came next, followed by Scottish, Polish, and Mexican at slightly lesser rates. The five states with the largest European ancestry groups are California, New York, Minnesota, Illinois, and Pennsylvania (Henwood, 1994). The assimilation of the European immigrants is such that they share many of the "American" values and norms concerning health care and health behavior. However, diversity does exist in many health traditions and beliefs.

During the 1980s and continuing at a slower rate in the 1990s, a third of the U.S. population growth was due to immigration, most of it from Asia. The Asian population in the United States has doubled from 1980 to 1990. Asians, Hispanics, and African-Americans, although still minorities, are increasing faster than non-Hispanic whites. Their influence on society is increasing commensurate with their numbers. It is projected that by the year 2000, three states— California, Texas, and Florida—will have a "minority majority" (Henwood, 1994).

African-Americans constitute 12% of the U.S. population, increasing one-and-a-half times faster than the overall population. Consequently, this segment of the population has a higher proportion of children and lower proportion of elderly than the total population.

Nine percent of the population is Hispanic, which increased 53% in the 1980s. This ethnic group, as with the Asians, continues to grow much faster than the African-American population because of the combined effects of immigration and fertility (Thomas, 1993).

Considering all these trends, nearly one fourth of the U.S. population and nearly half of the nation's children in the 1990s are racial or ethnic minorities. The immigrant pool will continue to diversify. The Immigration Act of 1990 had this as an intent and also ensures a continuous flow of immigrants into the United States. Unlike the typical European immigrant who shared many of the norms and values of middle America, these new immigrants have different attitudes towards the health care system and different patterns of health behavior and health traditions. Their intent is also different: they come to the United States to work and then retire in their original homeland. They tend to stay within their own ethnic group and often manage to neither need nor desire to learn English or interact outside their enclave.

## EDUCATION

Current trends point to a huge divergence of educational levels. If this trend continues, in the early part of the new century, patients will be either highly educated or close to functionally illiterate. This will have a great bearing on whether patients understand directions for their therapy. On the other hand, those who are well educated will demand to collaborate in the process of decision making regarding their treatment. Knowledge has been consistently shown to be necessary for informed patients but not sufficient to predict health behavior (Bradley, 1995; Conway, Pond, Hamnett, & Watson 1996; Montgomery, 1996). Intervention programs based on knowledge alone have not been successful in behavior change. However, behaviors, including medication use, have been changed with interventions that integrate knowledge with experiences, that change expectations, that encourage confidence in performing behaviors, and that enhance skills necessary for behavior change (assertiveness, communication skill, psychomotor skill) (J. B. Jemmott, L. S. Jemmott, & Fong, 1992; L. S. Jemmott & J. B. Jemmott, 1991). Clinicians cannot expect prescriptive behavior to change just because they have "taught" the patient new knowledge.

## SELECTED CULTURAL FACTORS INFLUENCING MEDICATION-TAKING BEHAVIOR

Belief categories related to health/illness, culture, religion, traditions, and world view are not distinct. There is overlap among all these factors

given the holism of people and the process of socialization. *Culture*, as defined by *The American Heritage Dictionary*, is "the aggregate of socially transmitted beliefs, traditions, behavior patterns, skills, and all other products of human work and convictions characteristic of a community or population" (Morris, 1993). All the factors listed above are included in the broad term *culture*. Ethnicity is not a synonym; it is subsumed under the umbrella term. Culture is used here to refer to specific socialization effects for the particular ethnic group addressed.

The groups discussed here are the white ethnic (German Americans, Irish Americans, Italian Americans, and Polish Americans) and the minority ethnic (Asian-Americans, Hispanic Americans, African-Americans, and Native Americans). The authors can attempt here only to address those ethnic groups of the U.S. population that constitute the largest percentages.

## WHITE ETHNIC GROUPS

- *German Americans: Beliefs*: Health is the ability to enjoy life and have energy to do things; illness is caused by stress, environmental changes, drafts, and germs, but also can be punishment or caused by an "evil eye." *Culture*: Strong family ties; everything in life has a purpose; the year is measured by the church calendar. *Religion/tradition*: Holy days are celebrated with festivities and take precedence over other commitments. *World view*: Emphasis is on the past and present, but also on plan for future.

- *Irish Americans: Beliefs*: Flesh is weak; ignore bodily complaints. *Culture*: Strong extended family ties; high alcohol use; problem expressing love and affection; male dominance. *Religion*: Strong faith in God, and the Catholic church's saints. *Tradition*: Celebrate saints' days with festivities and alcohol. *World view*: Past, present, and future oriented.

- *Polish Americans: Beliefs*: Health is when you are feeling OK; keep healthy by being pure; walk and exercise; be happy and put faith in God; illness is because of a poor diet and perhaps an "evil eye." *Culture*: Use folk medicine and faith healers. *Religion*: Strong faith in God and the Mother of God. *Traditions*: Wear scapulars for protection; celebrate saints' days and have special rituals, ie, blessing of the throats, to protect health; honor relics of the saints; make novenas and pilgrimages. *World view*: major focus on past and present.

• *Italian Americans: Beliefs*: Health is being able to take advantage of the present; illness is caused by drafts, contamination, suppression of emotions, stress, grief, fear, anxiety, "evil eye," and "curses." *Culture*: Male is the head of household, while female is the heart; rely on family to provide continuity in life and for coping; avoid talk of sex or menstrual cycle; expect immediate treatment for illness; report symptoms very dramatically; expect explanations of illness and treatment to be given in great detail. *Religion*: Strong faith in God; death is God's will and should not be discussed. *Tradition*: Most celebrations center around family; rituals to avoid "evil eye" and undo "curses." *World view*: Focus on present and future; internal locus of control—belief that they can effect the outcome of a situation by their actions.

Some general commonalties of the white ethnic group are: time is money; the future is valued more than the present; small talk and personal space are valued.

## MINORITY ETHNIC GROUPS

• *Asian-Americans: Beliefs*: Illness is due to poor working conditions, poverty, crowding, imbalance of yin and yang; cannot treat a "hot" illness with a "hot" herb or "hot" medication; there are seven pulses that are used for diagnosis, using three fingers; 100 conditions can be diagnosed by the color and texture of the tongue; many diagnostic tests are not needed and need not be so painful; blood is the source of life and cannot be regenerated; immunizations and x-rays are acceptable. *Culture*: Value silence; avoid confrontation; self-expression should be repressed; loyalty of the young to the old; accept without questioning; family is multigenerational and is the chief social network; father is the main decision maker; male is valued more than female; the body is a gift; believe in prevention of illness; the health care system's task is to prevent illness; should not have to pay when one is ill; best to die with body intact. *Religion*: Evil is removed by purification; rituals are used to prevent illness and restore balance in yin and yang. *Tradition*: Use both Western and Oriental healing; use medicinal herbs and folk healers; fortune tellers can tell of the event that caused the illness; family takes care of the disabled. *World view*: major focus is on the present; communication is largely nondirect; use strong self-control to avoid an incident that would bring shame.

• *Hispanic Americans: Beliefs*: Health is a gift from God as a reward for good behavior—it is the result of good luck; illness is an imbalance of hot/cold or wet/dry—a punishment; if the four body humors are disrupted, you will have a disease; malaise, fatigue, or a headache are caused by a "bad eye" (an unwanted condition resulting from the look/gaze of an individual thought to possess special powers). The solution is to find the person who gave the bad eye and have him care for the ill person; illness is also caused by a "soul loss" (a depressed emotional state). *Culture*: "Envidia"—Belief that one's success may provoke the envy of friends, thus the potential of illness from a "bad eye"; father is the decision maker; traditional gender and family roles, but women are the primary healers; men are considered "macho"; strong effort to retain cultural identity. *Religion*: Demonstratively religious; have shrines in homes; wear medals and amulets and pray to prevent illness. *Tradition*: Use teas, herbs, spices, and folk healers; will not take a hot medication to treat a hot condition; make a pilgrimage, visit shrines, offer medals, candles, and make promises to God to be cured from a severe illness; hold big celebrations for holidays, birthdays, and other family or religious occasions; parental assistance, physical and financial, continues to the children long after they have become adults. *World view*: Focus is on the present; time is relative—day, afternoon, or night—with a wider frame of reference; there is a lack of focus on clock time, ie., being on time for appointments, taking medications, etc.; have an external locus of control (believe that their actions will not influence the outcome of situations); in communication, eye contact is important.

• *African-Americans: Beliefs*: Health is a gift from God; trouble and pain are God's will; do not view illness as a burden; illness is a natural occurrence because of disharmony caused by demons, sin, and evil spirits; the cure is to get rid of the evil by voodoo, herbs, roots, and laxatives. *Culture*: Female is the dominant family force; grandmother is the major decision maker; elderly are held in high esteem; strong bonds in the extended family; nonrelatives often live in same household; the health care system is not considered for prevention. *Religion*: Reliance on the healing power of religion; social network; trust the advice of the preacher. *Traditions*: Use healers and folk medicine for most problems, ie, prevent colds by taking cod liver oil, use sulfur and molasses as a spring tonic, wear copper or silver bracelets to protect (harm will occur if they are removed); use of alcohol (greatest health problem). *World view*: In communication, eye contact is important but is not synonymous with attention; have a closer personal space; present oriented, but those with a strong religious belief are future oriented as well; time is flexible; a person with status is expected to arrive late.

- *Native Americans: Beliefs*: Health is equanimity with nature and the universe; disregard germ theory; illness has a mythical component associated with evil spirits; cure is to rid the body of the evil spirits; they are not to be blamed for their illness, since the cause is external. *Culture*: Treat body with regard; believe in self-control; witches have power to interact with the evil spirits and can bring illness and misery on those who chafe them; lineage is from mother; close relationship with nature; are true ecologists. *Religion*: Intertwined with their relationship with nature; give libation to the god of the earth, offer prayer sticks, and dance to the god of the wind, etc.; healer and medicine man are wise in the ways of the land and nature and have the ability to know supernatural effects. *Traditions*: Wear or carry amulets, etc., to guard against the power of witches; use herbs and rituals; follow advice of the medicine person; consult with singers and healers; are hesitant to use Western medicine because of conflicting perceptions of what the illness is, what the cause is, and how it should be treated; use of alcohol (greatest health problem). *World view*: Present time orientation; patterns of their social life are not bound by clock time, but by patterns in nature and need; the locus of control is both external (victim when ill) and internal (believe they have the power to control themselves); in communication, nonverbal cues are very important; it is proper to avoid eye contact when speaking and using a soft and low voice conveys respect; direct questions are considered an intrusion on privacy; the pointing of an object at another is considered an insult and a threat.

## SELECTED PSYCHOSOCIAL FACTORS INFLUENCING MEDICATION-TAKING BEHAVIOR

Five of the most useful models or concepts worth considering when exploring medication use are discussed briefly below.

## THE HEALTH BELIEF MODEL

The health belief model (HBM) was originated by social scientists in the 1950s who wondered

why people did not use free chest screening for TB. The model has been revised and focused on a wide variety of health behaviors. The central concepts of the current version are susceptibility, seriousness, benefits, barriers, and cues to action. To act, individuals have to see themselves as susceptible to a condition, see the condition as serious, see benefits to the behavior undertaken to prevent or treat the condition, see few barriers to performing these behaviors, and be prompted to act by cues in the environment. A literature review indicates the majority of studies support barriers and susceptibility as the major predictors of health behavior (Hand & Bradley, 1996).

However, it is important to look at patterns. Barriers, such as time, transportation, schedules, financial cost, change in habits—real or perceived—are the most important variable to explore when patients are not able to follow the prescribed treatment or drug regime. For example, Marlenga (1995) found that even though dairy farmers knew they were susceptible to sun-mediated cancer and it was a serious problem, they did not use protective sunscreen because of barriers. In addition, Patel & Spaeth (1995) found barriers a significant predictor to eyedrop use for glaucoma. Similarly, barriers were cited as reasons for not using inhalers (Hand & Bradley, 1996).

Benefits, on the other hand, are useful to understand why people do follow through with prescribed behavior (French, Kurczynski, Weaver, & Pituch, 1992). Patients took antipsychotic medication if they saw benefits of the medication, and saw the condition as severe and themselves as susceptible (Budd, Hughes, & Smith, 1996). Bond, Aiken, and Somerville (1992) looked at medication and other behaviors in adolescents with diabetes. They conceptualized threat as a combination of susceptibility and severity, and created a variable that operationalized benefits minus costs (barriers). The most successful metabolic control was achieved with a low perceived threat and high perceived benefits minus costs.

A series of studies (Champion, 1985, 1987, 1988; Champion & Miller, 1996; Miller & Champion, 1996) explores predictors of self–breast-examination behavior and mammogram use in women. Although the same variables were predictive of the target behavior in this population, there was variance by individual. Thus the intervention designed by Champion (1994, 1995) and Champion &

Huster (1995) allowed for individual targeting of the individual's health belief profile. This individually negotiated intervention was successful in establishing long-term increases in target behavior. Providers need to explore the issues of threat and benefit/barrier ratio when discussing drugs with patients. Questions that assess barriers and susceptibility might be routinely assessed when the clinician gives a prescription. Asking, "Is there anything that will make it hard for you to get this prescription filled today?" could be a first-line screening question for all prescriptions. If the clinician feels the patient does not see himself or herself at risk, say, "I think you are at high risk for this to develop into a bigger problem and I want you to take this medicine for 7 days. What do you think about that?" In working with patients who have chronic illness, all four variables may need to be explored so that the clinician can determine which of the concepts is most important to the individual patient being seen. Interventions can then be targeted to individual patterns.

## THE THEORY OF PLANNED BEHAVIOR

In the 1970s two social scientists (Ajzen & Fishbein, 1980; Fishbein & Ajzen, 1975) advocated three constructs to explain why persons did or did not participate in health behavior. The three constructs of the theory of reasoned action are: (1) individuals' attitude toward the behavior; (2) their "subjective norm," or perception of what those important to them thought about the behavior; and (3) their intention to perform the behavior. In this model, behavioral intention is the only variable directly related to the behavior itself.

Overall evidence for the predictive utility of the model was found as long as attitude was measured specifically (Jemmott & Jemmott, 1991; Morrison, Gilmore, & Baker, 1995; Pender, 1996). That is, attitude towards a specific medication regime would need to be measured. Overall attitude toward taking medication would not be helpful in predicting hypertension medication use, or attitudes toward hypertension medications would not be helpful in predicting birth control medication use.

The theory of planned behavior is an extension of the theory of reasoned action (Ajzen, 1988, 1991). The dimension added was "perceived behavioral control," which is proposed to affect behavior directly and indirectly through intentions. Perceived behavioral control has been conceived as perceived ease or difficulty engaging in behavior and is viewed as a reflection of past experiences and anticipated impediments or obstacles (Ajzen, 1988). The concept has been seen by the author as somewhat similar to Bandura's self-efficacy (Ajzen, 1991). However, the conceptual definition of ease/difficulty of engaging in the behavior cannot be equated with the conceptual definition of self-efficacy and may in fact be closer to the conceptual definition of the benefit/barriers concept of the HBM. The support for this added variable is mixed (Wambach, 1997 & Pellino, 1997).

In addition, several researchers have identified three variables which moderate the model's effectiveness: the measure of intention employed, the type of behavior, and the presence of a choice among alternatives. Modification to account for goal intentions, choice situations, and differences between intention and estimation measures has been proposed (Sheppard, Hartwick, & Warshaw, 1988).

## SELF-EFFICACY

More recently, several theorists have tested the addition of the self-efficacy variable developed by Bandura (1986) to both the health-belief model and the theory of reasoned action. In social cognition theory, it is not only the specific value attitude toward the behavior (ie, good idea vs. bad idea) that is thought to be predictive but the specific belief that the subject can perform the behavior change needed. An increasingly complex body of literature supports the effect of self-efficacy on the development of outcome behavior. The majority of this literature is in health promotion activities, such as smoking cessation and exercise behavior. The "lessons learned" indicate that self-efficacy is often a powerful predictor of behavior if measured specifically.

A growing number of studies have evaluated self-efficacy in medication-taking behavior. Their findings parallel the literature on health promotion behaviors. Measured specifically, self-efficacy predicted medication-taking behaviors for persons with epilepsy, diabetes, and AIDS. It is important to ask the client, "What do you think the likelihood is that you can take this medication three times a day [or however prescribed]?"

## VALUE OF THE PROVIDER/PATIENT RELATIONSHIP

The patient/provider relationship is another variable scientists are recently suggesting we add to these models of behavior. Several studies suggest that the provider has a powerful impact on health behavior (Elliot, 1994; Paskett, Carter, Chu, & White, 1990; Rosenberg, Burnhill, Waugh, Grimes, & Hillard, 1995; Somkin, 1993). The impact may be cumulative or inconsistent, but when studies addressing contraceptive use, mammogram use, or inhaler use are analyzed using multivariate techniques, provider relationship is a frequent predictor (Hand & Bradley, 1996; Rosenberg et al, 1995). Specifically, provider recommendation for a test (Champion, 1996; Van Essen, Kuyvenhoven, & de Melker, 1997) or a change in behavior (smoking) is frequently predictive even when other predictors are accounted for. The provider needs to realize the power of the relationship and use it: "Will you try this for me for 2 weeks to see if it is useful? You will need to take the medication every day for 2 weeks for us to evaluate its use. Do you think you can do that for me?" However, part of the relationship with the provider may be the attitude that all regimes are not appropriate for all patients and a willingness on the provider's part to explore options. The provider might say, "We have two choices: an injection or a 10-day course of antibiotics. Since you choose the 10-day course, can we count on you to complete that treatment? Is that something you can do for us?"

## INTEGRATION OF MODELS PREDICTING MEDICATION-TAKING BEHAVIOR

Several studies have indicated that integrating variables from a variety of models increases precision. Results of Champion's work indicate that the predisposing variables of seriousness, benefits, health motivation, control, knowledge of breast cancer and mammography guidelines, socioeconomic status, age, physician recommendation for mammography, and prior breast symptoms were significantly related to having had recent mammography (Champion, 1996). In addition, the predictor variables suggested by Ajzen and Fishbein (1980), plus gender and the specific measure of condom use self-efficacy, were predictive of intentions to use condoms 3 months later (Jemmott & Jemmott, 1992; Morrison, Gillmore, & Baker, 1995). The tradi-

tional theory of reasoned action worked well to predict condom use intentions and behavior. Support was also found for inclusion of gender and self-efficacy, but not behavior in the prediction of intention to use condoms, but not behavior (Morrison, Gillmore, & Baker, 1995). Other studies have found that interventions provided by creditable providers, which address knowledge, attitude, and skills, can have a long-term impact on health behavior (J. B. Jemmott, L. S. Jemmott, & Fong, 1992, L. S. Jemmott & J. B. Jemmott, 1991).

Recently, Pender (1996) has revised her model combining the predictive variables of other theories. The expectancy-value theory (the basis of the health belief model and the theory of reasoned action) and social cognitive theory (renamed from social learning theory, and the basis of self-efficacy) are articulated as the theoretical underpinnings of this model. The model also includes individual characteristics and experiences, such as previous experience with the behavior, since past behavior is repeatedly shown to be the best predictor of future behavior. For components of the model, see Figure 5–1. Pender reports that the model explains health-promoting lifestyles such as exercise, fitness and cardiac rehabilitation program participation, and hearing protection programs. She recommends that researchers testing this revised model develop rigorous measures of behavior-specific variables if they do not already exist.

One particularly intriguing study suggests an important relationship to be tested in clinical practice. With a large sample in a experimental study, pretreatment perceptions of barriers were found to be predictive of short-term behavior change. After the treatment was initiated, self-efficacy was found to be predictive of long-term success. In getting patients to adopt an important drug regime, combating barriers may be critical for short-term prescriptions. However, once the treatment is initiated and the initial barriers are overcome, building self-efficacy for a program of long-term pharmacotherapy may be crucial. As the patient overcomes these barriers and builds new behaviors, continuing to reinforce the patient's confidence may prove to be a powerful force in increasing self-efficacy (Mudde, Kok, & Strecher, 1995). This may indeed be a part of the behavior of providers that patients have reacted to and report as a "positive relationship" with the provider. This finding also supports the need for the clinician to be familiar with the most recent

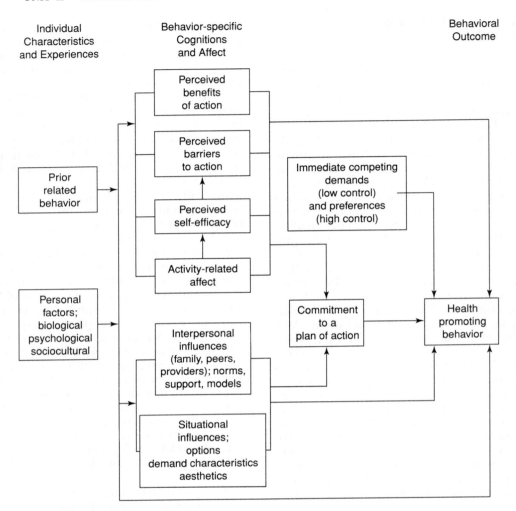

**Figure 5-1.** Pender Model.

theory impacting medication-taking behavior, discussed in the next section (Prochaska, Velicier, Rossi, & Goldstein, 1994).

## THE TRANSTHEORETICAL MODEL OF BEHAVIOR CHANGE

Usually in chronic illness, when we begin, modify, or increase the medications prescribed, we are asking patients to make a fundamental change in their behavior for the long term. Thus, understanding not only factors associated with behavior but also stages of behavior change becomes very important. Currently, the dominant theory in the literature explaining the process is

the *transtheoretical model of behavior change*. Prochaska et al. (1994) used their work with smoking cessation to identify the stages of change that a person goes through, whether the person is adopting a new behavior or quitting a health-threatening behavior. This model has five stages

1. *Precontemplation:* A person is not thinking about adopting a particular behavior.
2. *Contemplation:* A person is seriously thinking about adopting a particular behavior.
3. *Planning or preparation:* A person who has tried to change a behavior is seriously thinking about engaging in the contemplated change (making small or sporadic changes).

4. *Action:* This phase covers the first period during which the person has made the behavior change consistently.

5. *Maintenance:* This period begins 6 months after action has started and continues indefinitely.

Each stage gives health care providers unique opportunities for influence. The movement between each stage is a balance of pros and cons discussed as variables in the previous theories. Minor changes in the balance of pros and cons are predicted as the force that moves a person from one stage to another. This work suggests different interventions to use at various stages to maximize change. Consciousness raising and self-reevaluation are more important in the early stages and behavioral processes—such as reinforcement, counterconditioning, support from providers/significant others, and stimulus control—are more important for understanding and predicting transition from preparation to action and from action to maintenance. Thus, the provider using data such as lab results or a log of weekly blood pressure readings could raise a patient's consciousness that change is needed, and positive outcome data—such as hemoglobin $A_{IC}$ (used to monitor long-term control of blood glucose level), serum levels, and decrease in bothersome symptoms—could reinforce changed medication-taking behavior. It is particularly important for the clinician to assess the patient's willingness to maintain the medication regime when immediate clinical results are not evident.

The transtheoretical model of behavior change is congruent with the findings of the previously cited study that identified barriers as the critical variable in initiating the behavior and self-efficacy as the critical variable in maintaining behavior change. Indeed, Champion (Champion & Huster, 1995) in her ongoing study of mammography behavior has found that salient beliefs for health behavior vary over the stages of behavior change. Women compliant with mammography guidelines had significantly higher scores on seriousness, benefits, health motivation, and control, as well as significantly lower scores on barriers. In addition, scores on susceptibility, seriousness, benefits, barriers, and health motivation were significantly different across stages of mammography-seeking behavior change (precontemplation, contemplation, and action/maintenance). The health provider may need to combine several interventions to impact medication behavior change depending on the stage of behavior change.

In complex situations, such as taking medication for chronic illness or monitoring efficacy of drug treatment with measures of peak flow, remember that change takes time to establish. The provider's own expectations may be as follows: (1) The patient needs to start this medication or treatment program immediately (after all, I've known about this medication for a long time and am convinced it is the best course of action) or (2) relapses are avoidable. For the patient, however, changing his or her life to integrate this medication into it is a new idea, and one she or he might have to consider before adopting. In addition, relapses or inappropriate cessation of medication for limited or prolonged periods occur frequently. Marlatt and Gordon (1985) indicate that relapses are most common in times of negative emotional states (anger, frustration, depression, boredom), social situations (negative situations such as conflict with other significant persons), or physical craving (for food or substances). Persons attempting to establish long-term therapeutic use of prescriptive medications are at high risk for relapse. Relapse prevention might include maximizing intention with contracts, assessing barriers, *and* making a plan to deal with them, increasing skills necessary to perform the behavior, assessing social support and making a plan to optimize it if there is a deficit, or creating interventions that maximize a person's sense of confidence in the targeted behavior.

Simons studied interventions used by nurses which they believed to be effective in enhancing patient adherence to a prescribed regime. Thirty-eight nurses reviewed interventions and five interventions met the stringent criteria of the intervention content validity used. Nurses reported that behavior modification, coping enhancement, mutual goal setting, patient contracting and self-modification were interventions appropriate to impact client behavior. The researchers identified multiple activities used in each of these intervention categories (Simons, 1992).

## DISCUSSION

The Review of the Literature reveals in many instances that the patient sees the health care provider as a consultant who gives advice that can be acted upon, adapted, or ignored. The patient evaluates the regime based on the variables discussed in this chapter. In the past the health care provider assumed that his or her advice would automatically be followed. Today, the health care provider needs to explore all the variables that a patient uses to evaluate the plan. It is apparent that not all health care consumers share the beliefs, norms, and expectations of the health care provider. Perhaps that is the most important piece of adherence: the realization that the provider community has a culture (broad term) all its own. We expect patients to tell us their symptoms and to take our prescriptions with minimal questioning, follow them, and pay for the service. We expect them to value preventive care as much as we do. We expect them to complete their therapy because we explained how important it was. However, the beliefs, perceptions, values, and traditions vary among ethnic groups. A patient who is present oriented may hear the advice for exercise or take away the medications to prevent an infection, but never do them or take them because he or she does not believe that's the health care providers' task; or the patient may only be able to focus on here and now, and does not value the future as much as the present. The perception of time by someone who is present oriented may not be ruled by the clock but by social activities or physical need. Telling this person or the parent to take or give the medication three times a day may not hold any meaning. Those who have an external locus of control may not follow through on the prescribed activities—warm soaks, stretching exercises, etc.—because they do not really believe that their actions will affect the outcome. They may need a significant other to remind and prod them to adhere.

Roles in the family are important, and their significance varies among ethnic groups. If the patient is not the major decision maker regarding health by virtue of his or her role in the family, the person who is (grandmother, father, nonrelative) needs to understand the regime and its importance to achieve adherence.

The literature has shown that respect is an important factor in adherence. We may think we are being respectful, but if we are talking in a medium voice and saying, "What did you say?" to a Native American, it is interpreted as disrespectful. If we avoid eye contact while taking notes or writing prescriptions in the presence of the patient, this may be considered disrespect by a majority of patients. If a negative comment is made regarding the use of folk medicine or a healer the patient has already consulted, the patient may disregard all that is prescribed. The external-locus-of-control belief that health is a matter of luck and mostly controlled by external forces in nature is the basis of folk medicine. Violating a person's personal space while doing a routine exam may be offensive to the patient and cause nonadherence to the prescriptive regime.

If a patient's concept of time is flexible and based on social life and need rather than a clock, giving him or her an appointment for 10:00 A.M. on Monday may hold no meaning except that it is in the morning. It may be more expeditious for this patient to be followed at a walk-in clinic (Giger and Davidhizar, 1991). The same applies to taking medications three or four times a day.

With cultural information in mind, the health care provider needs to assess specific attitudes regarding medication-taking behavior. Although each of the frameworks can be useful to the provider, the evidence suggests barriers, self-efficacy, and stages of behavior change have the most pragmatic value. The health care provider may gain further guidance through the emerging evidence that to affect medication-taking behavior, strategies need to be stage-specific.

## IMPLICATIONS FOR PRACTICE

Based on the variation in the ethnic groups, individual belief patterns, and patient/provider relationships, how can health care providers optimize medication-taking behavior, enhancing the possibility of a positive health outcome? The following are some suggestions, by no means inclusive:

1. When patients present for care, ask them how you can help them; what is it they want to happen (goal)?
2. When possible, relate their actions to the symptoms or the problem, ie, moving furniture 2 days ago to musculoskeletal pain, or a high-sodium/high-fat breakfast at the local Shoney's buffet to ankle edema and elevated blood pressure.
3. Ask them what they think caused their symptoms.
4. Ask them if they have used any home remedies, broader than OTC treatment, or consulted any-

one else for their problem. This will give you an idea of how strongly they follow the traditions of their ethnic group.

5. When there are several equally effective options for treatment, give the patient the choice, ie, IM injection or 10 days of medication.

6. When the treatment is collaboratively decided upon, explain it thoroughly, using terms at the level of the patient's knowledge. The collaborative decision may be made with the family's major decision maker, if possible. If the patient has an external locus of control, it is important to know if he or she believes the treatment will take care of the problem. It is recognized that many patients will say, "You're the doc, what do you think?"

7. Ask if any family, ethnic, or religious belief would make them uneasy in following the prescribed therapy, ie, no hot medications for hot illnesses; does not believe in prevention, so stops therapy when symptoms disappear; using certain appliances on the Sabbath (Baldonado, 1996).

8. Ask patients to tell you how they will fit the therapy into their lifestyle, ie, children cannot take medicine at school; a diabetic works the night shift. Guide patients in problem-solving, but let them come up with the solution. Let them own the problem and the solution.

When developing a long-term medication regime, all of the above, especially the barriers addressed in items 7 and 8, need to be considered, in addition to the following:

9. What possible reinforcement does this plan need to support long-term success?

10. What projected stress or changes would put the plan in jeopardy? What substitute strategies can be developed to support the plan?

11. If relapse is imminent, what plans are there for immediate access to health care personnel? Is the patient agreeable to a contract that specifies no modification of medication regime without contacting the provider?

The following considerations are applicable for both short- and long-term medication regimes:

12. Assess the patients' beliefs regarding seriousness, susceptibility, benefits, and barriers to the course of action. Design an explanation of the medication needed that is congruent with the your assessment of the patients' beliefs in these areas.

13. Get a commitment from the patients to follow through on the plan. Have them verbalize whether they think they will be able to carry out the plan. If it is a smoking cessation contract, have them sign the discharge slip, ie, "I will decrease the cigarettes smoked by one each day this week." The literature shows that a commitment on the part of patients results in better adherence.

14. Consider including the following in your instructions: "If anything comes up that makes you consider changing this plan or stopping the medication, will you contact me to discuss it before you change the plan if possible, but at least as soon as you can?"

The above suggestions are certainly not inclusive. Health care providers need to ask themselves this bottom-line question, "What do I need to know about these clients to help them effectively use pharmacological and other therapies to achieve the desired positive health outcomes?" The issues discussed in this chapter such as culture, norms, beliefs, theories, and patient/provider relationships provide a framework to make these decisions.

## REFERENCES

Ajzen, I. (1988). *Attitudes, personality and behavior*. Chicago: Dorsey Press.

Ajzen, I. (1991). The theory of planned behavior. *Organizational Behavior and Human Decision Processes, 50*, 179–211.

Ajzen, I., & Fishbein, M. (1980). *Understanding Attitudes and Predicting Social Behavior*, Englewood Cliffs, NJ: Prentice-Hall, Inc.

Arakelian, M. (1992). Review of the meaning of compliance. *Nursing Scan in Research, 5*(5), 1–2.

Baldonado, A. A. (1996). Transcending the barriers of cultural diversity in health care. *Journal of Cultural Diversity, 3*(1), 20–22.

Bandura, A. (1986). *Social foundations of thought and action: A social cognitive theory*. Englewood Cliffs, NJ: Prentice Hall.

Biley, F. (1992). Some detriments that effect patient participation in decision-making about nursing care. *Journal of Advanced Nursing, 17*(4), 414–421.

Bond, G. G., Aiken, L. S., & Somerville, S. C. (1992). The health belief model and adolescents with insulin-dependent diabetes mellitus. *Health Psychology, 11*(3), 190–198.

Bradley, C. (1995). Health beliefs and knowledge of patients and doctors in clinical practice and research. *Patient Education and Counseling, 26*(1–3), 99–106.

Budd, R. J., Hughes, I. C., & Smith, J. A. (1996). Health beliefs and compliance with antipsychotic medication. *British Journal of Clinical Psychology, 35*(Pt 3), 393–397.

Champion, V. L. (1985). Use of the health belief model in determining frequency of breast self-examination. *Research in Nursing & Health, 8*(4), 373–379.

Champion, V. L. (1987). The relationship of breast self-examination to health belief model variables. *Research in Nursing & Health, 10*(6), 375–382.

Champion, V. L. (1988). Attitudinal variables related to intention, frequency and proficiency of breast self-examination in women 35 and over. *Research in Nursing & Health, 11*(5), 283–291.

Champion, V. L. (1994). Strategies to increase mammography utilization. *Medical Care, 32*(2), 118–129.

Champion, V. L. (1995). Results of a nurse-delivered intervention on proficiency and nodule detection with breast self-examination. *Oncology Nursing Forum, 22*(5), 819–824.

Champion, V. L., & Huster, G. (1995). Effect of interventions on stage of mammography adoption. *Journal of Behavioral Medicine, 18*(2), 169–187.

Champion, V., & Miller, A. M. (1996). Recent mammography in women aged 35 and older: Predisposing variables. *Health Care of Women International, 17*(3), 233–245.

Conway, S. P., Pond, M. N., Hamnett, T., & Watson, A. (1996). Compliance with treatment in adult patients with cystic fibrosis. *Thorax, 51*(1), 29–33.

Devine, E. C., & Reifschneider, E. (1995). A meta-analysis of the effects of psychoeducational care in adults with hypertension. *Nursing Research, 44*(4), 237–248.

Elliot, W. J. (1994). Compliance strategies. *Current Opinion in Nephrology & Hypertension, 3*(3), 271–278.

Fishbein, M., & Ajzen, I. (1975). *Belief, attitude, intention, and behavior: An introduction to theory and research.* Boston: Addison-Wesley.

French, B., Kurczynski, T., Weaver, M., & Pituch, M. (1992). Evaluation of the Health Belief Model and decision making regarding amniocentesis in women of advanced maternal age. *Health Education Quarterly, 19*(2), 177–186.

Giger, J. N., & Davidhizar, R. E. (1991). *Transcultural Nursing.* Baltimore: Mosby.

Hand, C. H., & Bradley, C. (1996). Health beliefs of adults with asthma: Toward an understanding of the difference between symptomatic and preventive use of inhaler treatment. *Journal of Asthma, 33*(5), 331–338.

Henwood, D. (1994). *The state of the U.S.A. atlas: The changing face of American life in maps and graphics.* New York: Simon & Schuster.

Jemmott, J. B., Jemmott, L. S., & Fong, G. T. (1992). Reductions in HIV risk-associated sexual behaviors among Black male adolescents: Effects of an AIDS prevention intervention. *American Journal of Public Health, 82*(3), 372–377.

Jemmott, L. S., & Jemmott, J. B. (1991). Applying the theory of reasoned action to AIDS risk behavior: Condom use among Black women. *Nursing Research, 40*(4), 228–234.

Jemmott, L. S., & Jemmott, J. B. (1992). Increasing condom-use intentions among sexually active Black adolescent women. *Nursing Research 41*(5), 273–279.

Marlatt, G. A., & Gordon, J. R. (1985). *Relapse prevention: Maintenance strategies in the treatment of addictive behaviors.* New York: Guilford Press.

Marlenga, B. (1995). The health beliefs and skin cancer prevention practices of Wisconsin dairy farmers. *Oncology Nursing Forum, 22*(4), 681–686.

Miller, A. M., & Champion, V. L. (1996). Mammography in older women: One-time and three-year adherence to guidelines. *Nursing Research, 45*(4), 239–245.

Montgomery, A. J. (1996). AIDS education: Knowledge, sexual attitudes and sexual behavioral responses of selected college students. *ABNF Journal, 7*(2), 57–60.

Morris, W. (Ed.). (1993). *The American Heritage dictionary.* Boston: American Heritage and Houghton Mifflin.

Morrison, D. M., Gillmore, M. R., & Baker, S. A. (1995). Determinants of condom use among high-risk heterosexual adults: A test of the theory of reasoned action. *Journal of Applied Social Psychology, 25*(8), 651–676.

Mudde, A. N., Kok, G., & Strecher, V. J. (1995). Self-efficacy as a predictor for the cessation of smoking: Methodological issues and implications for smoking cessation programs. *Psychology & Health, 10*(5), 353–367.

Pasket, E. D., Carter, W. B., Chu, J. E., & White, E. (1990). Compliance behavior in women with abnormal pap smears: Developing and testing a decision model. *Medical Care, 28*(7), 643–656.

Patel, S. C., & Spaeth, G. L. (1995). Compliance in patients with eyedrops for glaucoma. *Ophthalmic Surgery, 26*(3), 233–236.

Pellino, T. A. (1997). Relationships between patient attitudes, subjective norms, perceived control, and analgesic use following elective orthopedic surgery. *Research in Nursing and Health, 20,* 97–105.

Pender, N. J. (1996). *Health promotion in nursing practice*. Stamford, CT: Appleton & Lange.

Prochaska, J. O., Velicier, W. E., Rossi, J. S., & Goldstein, M. G. (1994). Stages of change and decisional balance for 12 problem behaviors. *Health Psychology, 13*(1), 39–46.

Robertson, M. (1992). The meaning of compliance: Patient perspective. *Qualitative Health Research, 2*(1), 7–26.

Rosenberg, M. J., Burnhill, M. S., Waugh, M. S., Grimes, D. A., & Hillard, P. J. (1995). Compliance and oral contraceptives: A review. *Contraception, 52*(3), 137–141.

Rubel, A. J., & Carro, L. C. (1992). Social and cultural factors in successful control of TB. *Public Health Reports, 107*(6), 626–636.

Sheppard, B. H., Hartwick, J., & Warshaw, P. R. (1988). The theory of reasoned action: A meta-analysis of past research with recommendations for modifications and future research. *Journal of Consumer Research, 15*(3), 325–343.

Simons, M. R. (1992). Interventions related to compliance. *Nursing Clinics of North America, 27* (2), 477–494.

Somkin, C. P. (1993). Improving the effectiveness of breast self-examination in the early detection of breast cancer: A selective review of the literature. *Nurse Practitioner Forum, 4*(2), 76–84.

Thomas, R. (1993). *Health care consumers in the 1990s*. New York: American Demographics Books.

Van Essen, G. A., Kuyvenhoven, M. M., & de Melker, R. A. (1997). Why do healthy elderly people fail to comply with influenza vaccinations? *Age and Aging, 26*(4), 275–297.

Wambach, K. A. (1997). Breastfeeding intention and outcome: A test of the theory of planned behavior. *Research in Nursing & Health, 20*, 51–59.

## ADDITIONAL RESOURCES

Douglas, J. H. (1993). Issues in transcultural nursing highlighted in three international conferences. *Journal of Transcultural Nursing, 5*(1), 34.

Matsumoto, D., Pun, K. K., Nakstani, M., Kadowaki, D., Weissman, M., McCarter, L., Fletcher, D., & Takeuchi, S. (1995). Cultural differences in attitudes, values, and beliefs about osteoporosis in first and second generation Japanese-American women. *Women & Health, 23*(4), 39–56.

Spector, R. (1991). *Cultural diversity in health and illness*. Stamford, CT: Appleton & Lange.

# 6

## REGULATORY CONTROL OF DRUGS

*Gene White*

## THE FEDERAL FOOD, DRUG, AND COSMETIC ACT

The law that specifically defines the term "drug" and provides the legal basis for regulating the development, manufacture, marketing, and distribution of drugs in the United States is the Federal Food, Drug and Cosmetic Act (FDCA) that was enacted in 1938. The FDCA prohibits adulterated or misbranded drugs from being introduced into interstate commerce, or becoming adulterated or misbranded while in interstate commerce, or the receipt of such drugs after shipment in interstate commerce. Likewise, the Act provides that all drugs marketed after 1938 must prove that they are safe and effective for the conditions for which they are recommended before receiving the Food and Drug Administration's approval for marketing. After getting approval, manufacturers must establish a system for receiving information regarding the use of such drugs and report to the Food and Drug Administration (FDA) any adverse information that may call into question the drug's safety and effectiveness.

The Durham-Humphrey Amendment to the FDCA divides drugs into two categories. If the FDA determines that adequate directions for the safe and effective use of the drug by a layman for the conditions recommended cannot be written, then the drug must be dispensed only pursuant to a valid prescription. Therefore, the drug's immediate container must bear the label "Caution: Federal Law Prohibits Dispensing Without a Prescription." The drug is then called *a legend drug*. If the FDA determines that such directions can be written, a prescription is not needed to purchase the drug. It is then referred to as an *over-the-counter drug*.

Persons regulated by the provisions of this law could be subjected to strict liability or liability without fault. This means that a person could be criminally convicted even though the violation was done unintentionally or without knowledge that the event had occurred. Those placing themselves under the provisions of this law should take it very seriously.

## FEDERAL CONTROLLED SUBSTANCE ACT

In the late 1960s America found itself in the middle of a growing drug abuse problem. While illicit drugs were a large part of the problem, so were legal drugs. Some legend drugs that could only be legally dispensed pursuant to a prescription were being diverted for illegal use. It was determined that certain drugs needed to be under stricter regulation than that imposed by the FDCA. Therefore, in 1970 Congress enacted the Federal Controlled Substance Act (CSA).

The CSA places certain drugs into one of five schedules by using the following three criteria:

- Does the drug have a currently accepted medical use in the United States?

- Does the drug have a potential for abuse?
- What is the severity of dependence of the drug, both psychologically and physiologically?

The five schedules are designated as C-I, C-II, C-III, C-IV, and C-V, with the severity of controls decreasing as the numbers get larger. See Table 6–1 for a description of the schedules. In general, drugs in schedules C-II, C-III and C-IV are legend drugs and require a prescription before they can be legally dispensed. Some preparations in Schedule C-V require a prescription. However, there are preparations in Schedule C-V that have acceptable directions for use and

### TABLE 6–1. DESCRIPTION OF DRUG SCHEDULES

C-I    The only schedule of drugs that do not have a recognized medical use in the United States and therefore cannot be legally marketed. These drugs may be used for research purposes.

C-II    Drugs that have a currently accepted medical use in the United States and a high abuse potential, with severe psychological or physiological dependence. Examples: Morphine, Demerol, Cocaine, Codeine, Methadone, Amphetamine, Ritalin and the fast acting barbiturates (amo-, pento-, and secobarbital).

C-III    Drugs that have a currently accepted medical use in the United States and an abuse potential below that of C-I and C-II. Abuse of these drugs may lead to moderate or low physical dependence or high psychological dependence. Examples: certain codeine products such as Empirin No. 3, Tylenol No. 4, Paregoric, Anabolic Steroids, and certain barbiturates in combination with other active medicinal ingredients.

C-IV    The same as C-III except a lower abuse potential. Overuse of these drugs causes only a limited physical or psychological dependence. Examples: Chloral Hydrate, phenobarbital, and certain tranquilizers such as Librium and Valium.

C-V    The same as C-IV except there is a lower potential for abuse and less physical and psychological dependence than C-IV. Examples: preparations containing a limited quantity of a narcotic drug in combination with a non-narcotic active medicinal ingredient and used for anti-cough purposes. Also diphenoxylate in combination with atropine sulfate for antidiarrheal purposes.

may be obtained without a prescription. These preparations may be sold over-the-counter in limited quantities within 48 hours to any one person. The pharmacist is required to keep a bound book showing the name of the C-V preparation, the quantity sold, the name and address of the purchaser, the date of the purchase, and the pharmacist's initials.

The appropriate schedule of controlled substances can usually be determined by reading the manufacturer's label attached to the immediate container of the drug. The schedule number will be shown in the upper right hand corner inside a C that is at least twice as large as any other printing on the label, or it will appear as background print over the entire label with other label requirements superimposed. All other legend drugs that are not in one of the five schedules are usually referred to as non-controlled legend drugs. However, there are several states that have given these non-controlled legend drugs the designation of C-VI drugs.

## PRESCRIPTIONS

### ELEMENTS OF A PRESCRIPTION

Before a pharmacist can legally dispense a legend drug, it must be authorized by a valid prescription. It is the pharmacist's responsibility to be certain that the required tangible and intangible characteristics are present to constitute such a prescription.

Tangible (physical) Characteristics:

1. Patient's full name and address.
2. Prescriber's full name and address.
3. Prescriber's DEA number if a controlled substance is prescribed.
4. Drug name.
5. Drug strength and dosage form, if appropriate.
6. Quantity to be dispensed.
7. Directions for use.
8. Refill instructions, if applicable.
9. Substitution rights.
10. Signed and dated by the prescriber on the day issued.

Intangible (nonphysical) Characteristics:

Federal regulations written pursuant to the CSA provide the following: "A prescription for a controlled substance to be effective must be issued *for a legitimate medical purpose* by an individual practitioner *acting within the usual course of his professional practice*. The responsibility for the proper prescribing and dispensing of controlled substances is upon the prescribing practitioner, but a corresponding responsibility rests with the pharmacist who fills the prescription." Code of Federal Regulations.

If the pharmacist knows or should have known that the prescribed controlled drug will not be used for legitimate medical purposes, such as maintaining a patient's addiction to drugs or prescribing a central nervous system stimulant to assist a driver in sleep deprivation for extended periods of time, then the prescription is not a valid authorization to dispense medication. Likewise, if a dentist prescribes an antibiotic to treat a gunshot wound or a physician prescribes a tranquilizer to calm down a neighbor's hyperactive cat, the prescriber would not be acting within the usual course of his professional practice and the prescription would be invalid. Most states, either by statute or regulation, have applied these intangible characteristics to non-controlled, legend drugs.

## WHO MAY PRESCRIBE LEGEND DRUGS

The FDCA provides that legend drugs can be dispensed only upon the written or oral prescription of *a practitioner licensed by law* to administer such drugs. In general, it is state law that determines who can become a practitioner licensed by law to administer such drugs. This normally covers Medical Doctors (M.D.), Dentists (D.D.S.), Osteopaths (D.O.), Podiatrists (D.P.M.), and Veterinarians (D.V.M.). States have now begun to grant limited prescriptive authority to other health practitioners such as Nurse Practitioners, Physician Assistants, Optometrists, and Pharmacists. Among those states that have enacted such laws, the terms and conditions of the prescriptive authority vary greatly.

## FILLING PRESCRIPTIONS

The general rule for C-II drugs is that the pharmacist must have a written prescription before the medication can be legally dispensed. There is an exception in an emergency situation if the proper procedure is followed. In this case, an emergency situation is defined as one in which:

1. The patient's health will be adversely affected without the medication.
2. No other medication will work.
3. The prescriber cannot reasonably be expected to get the pharmacist a prescription.

The pharmacist may then accept an oral prescription for a C-II drug and reduce it to writing showing all of the information needed except the prescriber's signature. An amount of drug sufficient to get a patient through the emergency situation up to a maximum three-day supply may be dispensed. If the pharmacist does not recognize the prescriber or has any reason to doubt the authenticity of the prescriber, the pharmacist must make a reasonable effort to determine that the oral order came from a bona fide practitioner. Within 72 hours from giving the oral order, the prescriber must send the pharmacist a written prescription for the medication already dispensed (postmarked within 72 hours). The written prescription must contain the phrase, "Authorization for emergency dispensing" and bear the date of the oral order. The written prescription from the prescriber must be attached to the order prepared by the pharmacist and kept on file. If the written order is not received (postmarked) from the prescriber within 72 hours, the pharmacist is required to report the prescriber to the Drug Enforcement Agency. Should the pharmacist fail to report the prescriber, then the statutory authority allowing the pharmacist to dispense a C-II drug on oral order is revoked and the pharmacist has illegally distributed a C-II drug.

Prescriptions for C-II drugs may not be refilled. It is permissible to partially fill a C-II prescription in several instances:

1. If the pharmacist does not have the full quantity prescribed; then the prescription may be partially filled. The remaining portion must be dispensed within 72 hours of the partial filling or it cannot be dispensed and the prescriber must be notified.
2. C-II prescriptions for patients in long-term care facilities (LTCF) may be partially filled in the following manner. The prescriber may write for up to a maximum 60-day supply of a C-II drug. The pharmacist may partially fill the prescription until the total quantity prescribed is dispensed or up to 60 days from the date of issuance, which ever comes first.
3. A prescription for a C-II drug may be partially filled for an ambulatory patient with a medical diagnosis documenting a terminal illness. The practitioner must classify the patient as termi-

nally ill and the pharmacist must verify and record such notation on the prescription. The prescription may be partially filled for a maximum of 60 days from the date of issuance or until the total quantity of medication prescribed is dispensed, which ever comes first.

Prescriptions for C-III or C-IV drugs may be received from the prescriber either orally or in writing. If received orally they must be promptly reduced to writing and show all of the necessary information except the prescriber's signature. If so authorized by the prescriber, C-III and C-IV prescriptions may be refilled up to five times or within six months from the date of issuance, whichever comes first. After this six month period, these prescriptions may not be filled or refilled.

Prescriptions for noncontrolled legend drugs may also be received either in writing or orally and promptly reduced to writing. These prescriptions may be refilled as authorized by the prescriber on the face of the original prescription. The length of time in which these prescriptions can be filled or refilled varies among the states, but is usually around two years from the date of issuance.

## FILING OF PRESCRIPTIONS

The CSA provides three methods for filing the hard prescription copy in a pharmacy:

1. Prescriptions may be kept in three separate files. One file for the C-II prescriptions, one for C-III, C-IV, and C-V prescriptions, and another file for noncontrolled legend prescriptions.
2. The file for C-II prescriptions and a separate file for C-III, C-IV, C-V and noncontrolled legend prescriptions.
3. One file for C-II, C-III, C-IV, C-V prescriptions and a separate file for noncontrolled legend prescriptions.

When C-III, C-IV and C-V prescriptions are mixed with any other prescriptions, they must be marked with a red C at least one inch high in the lower right hand corner of the prescriptions. Some states require that C-II prescriptions always be filed by themselves and therefore only allow methods 1 and 2.

## REFILL INFORMATION

When a prescription is refilled the pharmacist must note, on the hard copy of the prescription or in a computer, the date of the refill, the amount dispensed if different from the quantity prescribed, and the pharmacist's initials. Most pharmacies maintain electronic records of prescriptions and quantities dispensed and refilled. Rules on how to maintain these records will vary depending on the state.

## DISPENSING GUIDELINES

The Poison Prevention Act is a federal law that requires that prescription medication be dispensed in child resistant containers unless it comes under one of the following exemptions.

1. The prescriber may request that the medication be dispensed in a container that is not child resistant. Such a request could cover all of the medication prescribed by the practitioner for one patient at a time, but not for all of the practitioner's patients at once.
2. The patient may request that their medication be dispensed in a non-childproof container. While the patient can give a blanket consent that all of their medication be dispensed in non-childproof containers, the pharmacist is required to check with the patient verbally each time medication is dispensed. While federal law does not require that the patient's consent be obtained in writing, it would certainly be prudent for the pharmacist to do so. Some state statutes provide immunity from civil liability when the pharmacist obtains a signed consent form from the patient.
3. Drugs dispensed to institutionalized patients may be packaged in non-childproof containers to be administered by institutional personnel.

Some O-T-C products such as Aspirin, Methyl Salicylate, Ibuprofen, and Methyl Alcohol are required to be in childproof containers. The manufacturer is allowed to select one size of this product other than the most popular size, and package it in a non-childproof container. This is done for the convenience of the elderly and handicapped, and the package must bear a label stating that "This package is for households without young children."

## REGISTRATION AND BIENNIAL INVENTORY

The CSA requires all pharmacies or pharmacists to register with the DEA every three years as a class 3 registrant. This registration allows pharmacists legally to possess and dispense schedule C-II through C-V drugs. Every pharmacy or pharmacist registrant must conduct a complete and accurate inventory of all controlled substances every two years. This inventory must be signed and dated by the pharmacist conducting the inventory. While not required by law, many pharmacists prefer to keep a perpetual inventory of controlled substances in order to detect shortages quickly. A complete and accurate record of all controlled substances received and dispensed or otherwise disposed of must be kept.

## REFERENCES

Code of Federal Regulations. 21 CFR Sect. 1306.04 (1991), 71.

Fink, J. & Simonsmeier, L. Laws governing pharmacy. *Facts & Figures Digest* (27th ed.). 890–934.

Pharmacy Law Digest. St. Louis: Facts and Comparisons. Supplemented annually.

# 7

# PHARMACOTHERAPY RESOURCES FOR THE PROVIDER

*Geneva Briggs*

All health care practitioners need up-to-date, easy-to-use, and easy-to-find resources to answer questions about medications in everyday practice. Ideally, the information should be unbiased and cover more than might be available on an FDA label, if necessary. This chapter addresses the various options and resources currently available to help you find the medication information you need. Because computerized resources change rapidly, any specific products mentioned may have evolved or no longer be available. The examples of each kind of product discussed here should pique your interest in the range and depth of resources you can turn to for help in your practice.

## PRINTED RESOURCES

Books and journals in printed and bound formats have been and still remain the primary resources for medication information. Although computerized information has exploded and has the advantage of being more current, not everyone has access to a computer or to either CD-ROM disk versions of texts and journals or to the Internet at their workplaces. Printed materials are widely available, are less costly, and allow the user to choose different versions so the information is most useful for a particular situation or practice. Their major disadvantage is the time lag between the date of writing and publication. Textbooks and handbooks are out of date as soon as they are

published because new medications and new research information about the use of both older and new medications are being released as the books are in production. Even materials updated yearly may not contain the very newest medications. The most current *printed text* information can be found in two resources:

- *Drug Facts and Comparisons:* Can be obtained in either a hardcover book updated yearly or in a loose-leaf format that is available as a subscription service and updated monthly.
- *American Hospital Formulary Service (AHFS) Drug Information:* Published yearly with new information sent quarterly in a softcover format.

The majority of written resources come in five major formats: textbooks, journals, newsletters, resource books, and handbooks (Shaughnessy, Slawson, & Bennett, 1994). Examples of all the formats are cited in Table 7–1. Textbooks often contain more information than the practitioner may want to read to find a quick answer to a simple question. And due to the publication time lag, newer medications and new uses for medications will not be addressed. Pharmacotherapy textbooks are valuable for an overall perspective on the treatment of a disease or condition with medications, but the user should ensure that he or she is using the most recent edition of a text for the most current information (Knott & Scott, 1994).

Journals provide the most recent information on medications, but the sheer number of journals can be daunting and can cause information

## TABLE 7–1. PRINTED AND COMPUTERIZED PHARMACOTHERAPY RESOURCES

| Pharmacotherapy Resource | Publisher | Description/Comments | Frequency of Publication and/or Updates |
|---|---|---|---|
| **Textbooks** | | | |
| Pharmacotherapy: A Pathophysiologic Approach | Appleton & Lange PO Box 120041 Stamford, CT 06912-0041 880-423-1359 | Comprehensive text on pharmacotherapeutics | Most recent edition: 1997 |
| Applied Therapeutics: The Clinical Use of Drugs | Applied Therapeutics, Inc. PO Box 5077 Vancouver, WA 98668-5077 360-253-7123 | Comprehensive text on pharmacotherapeutics; presents information in case-study format | Most recent edition: 1995 |
| Basic and Clinical Pharmacology | Appleton & Lange | Complete, yet concise pharmacology text; focuses on not only the basic mechanisms of drug action but also the clinical use of drugs and monitoring of therapeutic and adverse effects | Most recent edition: 1995 |
| **Reference Books** | | | |
| AHFS Drug Information | American Society of Health System Pharmacists 7272 Wisconsin Avenue Bethesda MD 20814 301-657-3000 | Extensive drug monographs; includes non-FDA-approved indications and doses | Yearly with quarterly updates |
| Drug Facts and Comparisons | Facts and Comparisons 111 West Port Plaza, Suite 423 St. Louis, MO 63146-9811 314-878-2515 | Easy-to-use information on administration, brand and generic identification, and available dosage forms; lists inactive ingredients such as alcohol and sugar and orphan drugs | Yearly with monthly updates |
| Drug Interaction Facts | Facts and Comparisons | Clinical significance, mechanisms, and management of drug-drug and drug-food interactions | Quarterly updates |
| Drug Interactions and Updates Quarterly | Applied Therapeutics, Inc. | Clinical significance, mechanisms, and management of drug-drug and drug-food interactions | Quarterly updates |
| Evaluations of Drug Interactions | PDS Publishing Co. 2388 Schuetz Road, Suite A-56 St. Louis, MO 63146 | Clinical significance, mechanisms, and management of drug-drug interactions | Bimonthly updates |
| Handbook of Nonprescription Drugs | American Pharmaceutical Association 2215 Constitution Avenue, NW Washington, DC 20037-2985 800-878-0729 | Although named as a handbook, this is really a hybrid textbook and medication resource, covers disease processes that | Every 3 years; most recent: 1996 |

*continues on next page*

**TABLE 7–1.** *continued*

| Pharmacotherapy Resource | Publisher | Description/Comments | Frequency of Publication and/or Updates |
|---|---|---|---|
| | | are treated with OTC products, such as sunburn or poison ivy; information about selected OTC medications | |
| Drugs in Pregnancy and Lactation | Williams and Wilkins PO Box 1496 Baltimore, MD 21203 800-638-0672 | Covers fetal and neonatal (breast-feeding) risks of maternal drug ingestion | Periodically; most recent edition: 1994 |
| Physician's Desk Reference | Medical Economics Data PO Box 430 Montvale, NJ 07645-1742 800-232-7379 | Contains FDA-approved package insert labeling, inactive ingredients, pictures of some products, manufacturers' addresses and phone numbers, not comprehensive | Yearly: biannual supplements for additional cost |
| Physician's Desk Reference—OTC | Medical Economics Data | Monographs and pictures for OTC medications | Yearly |
| Physician's Drug Reference—Generics | Medical Economics Data | Average wholesale prices, common off-label uses, class monographs, indications and therapeutic/pharmacologic category indexes, visual and imprint code identifications; drug information center, poison control center, and manufacturer listings | Yearly |
| Martindale: The Extra Pharmacopoeia | Drug Intelligence Publications 1241 Broadway Hamilton, IL 62341 | Good for identifying foreign medications; British publication | Every 5–6 years; most recent edition: 1993 |
| Drugs Available Abroad. A Guide to Therapeutic Drugs Available and Approved Outside the U.S. | Gale Research Inc. 645 Griswold Street, #835 Detroit, MI 48226-4006 800-877-4253 | Lists drugs available in other countries | Periodically; most recent edition: 1990 |
| USP DI, Volume I, Drug Information for the Health Care Professional | United States Pharmacopeial-Convention, Inc. 12601 Twinbrook Parkway Rockville, MD 20852 800-227-8772 | Drug monographs; adverse effects organized by severity; orphan drug products | Yearly with monthly updates |
| Drug Evaluations Annual | American Medical Association 800-621-8335 | Organized by therapeutic indication; thus, individual drugs may be discussed in more than one location; referenced | Yearly |

*continues on next page*

**TABLE 7–1.** *continued from previous page*

| Pharmacotherapy Resource | Publisher | Description/Comments | Frequency of Publication and/or Updates |
|---|---|---|---|
| **Handbooks** | | | |
| Quick Look Drug Book | Lexi-Comp Inc. 1100 Terex Road Hudson, OH 44236-3771 800-837-LEXI | Very brief monographs that include brand name, synonym, therapeutic category, use, usual dose, dosage forms | Yearly |
| Geriatric Dosage Handbook | Lexi-Comp Inc. | Brief monographs; dosage adjustments for patients with renal and hepatic failure | Yearly |
| Pediatric Dosage Handbook | Lexi-Comp Inc. | Brief monographs with pediatric dosing information | Yearly |
| Pocket Version—Drug Facts and Comparisons | Facts and Comparisons | Condensed version of Drug Facts and Comparisons; monographs have similar layout | Yearly |
| Pocket Guide to Evaluations of Drug Interactions | American Pharmaceutical Association | Condensed version of Evaluations of Drug Interactions; cross-referenced to the larger version | Most recent edition: 1996 |
| **Miscellaneous Handbooks** | | | |
| Nonprescription Products: Lists for Patients with Special Needs | American Pharmaceutical Association | Lists products free from potentially irritating substances such as alcohol, fragrance, lactose, sucrose, caffeine, dye, gluten, purine, and sulfite | Most recent edition: 1996 |
| Red Book | Medical Economics Data | Average wholesale prices, manufacturers' addresses and phone numbers, and drug information center and poison control center numbers | Yearly with monthly average wholesale price updates |
| **Newsletters** | | | |
| The Medical Sciences Bulletin | Pharmaceutical Information Associates Ltd. 2761 Trenton Road Levittown, PA 19056 (215) 949-0490 | Reviews new advances in clinical pharmacology; referenced | Monthly |
| Prescriber's Letter | Therapeutic Research Center P.O. Box 8190 Stockton, CA 95208 209-472-2440 | Up-to-date information on drug interactions and new medication uses gleaned from current primary literature; referenced | Monthly |

*continues on next page*

**TABLE 7–1.** *continued*

| Pharmacotherapy Resource | Publisher | Description/Comments | Frequency of Publication and/or Updates |
|---|---|---|---|
| The Medical Letter | The Medical Letter, Inc. 1000 Main Street New Rochelle, NY 10801 | Reviews of new medications, drug classes, new indications; referenced and unbiased | Monthly |
| Drug Newsletter | Facts and Comparisons | Lists newly approved medications and updates to indications and dosage forms; reviews recently reported drug interactions, primary literature, and investigational drugs | Monthly |
| Journal Watch | Journal Watch PO Box 9685 Waltham, MA 02254 800-843-6356 | Reviews current primary literature; referenced | Bimonthly |
| **Software—Drug Interactions** | | | |
| Drug Master Plus | Rapha Group Software 314-521-0808 | Drug-drug interaction screening; diskette | 3 times per year |
| RxTriage | Camdat 359 Northgate Drive Warrendale, PA 15086 800-875-8355 | Drug-drug and drug-food interaction screening, duplicate therapy screening, decision support; diskette | Quarterly |
| **CD-ROMs[a]** | | | |
| Drug Information Fulltext | American Society of Health System Pharmacists | Contains full text of AHFS Drug Information plus extra information and Handbook on Injectable Drugs; allows searching of database; network version is available | Yearly |
| Drug Facts and Comparisons | Facts and Comparisons | Contains same information as loose-leaf version | Yearly |
| DrugDex | Micromedex, Inc. 600 Grant Denver, CO 80203 800-525-9083 | Contains drug monographs and drug consults; referenced | Quarterly |
| MEDLINE Clinical Collection | National Library of Medicine/ Dialog OnDisc Dialog Information Services, Inc. 3460 Hillview Ave Palo Alto CA 94304 415-858-3785 | Includes 5 years of references and abstracts from 150 journals specializing in clinical medicine | Quarterly |
| MEDLINE (Standard) | National Library of Medicine/ Silver Platter Information 1750 Bridgeway–Suite B207 Sausalito, CA 94965 800-874-1130 | Full Medline database which indexes worldwide literature on medicine and the biosciences | Monthly |

*continues on next page*

**TABLE 7–1.** *continued from previous page*

| Pharmacotherapy Resource | Publisher | Description/Comments | Frequency of Publication and/or Updates |
|---|---|---|---|
| International Pharmaceutical Abstracts (IPA) | American Society of Health System Pharmacists | Abstracts from 600 world-wide pharmaceutical, medical, and health care journals since 1970 | Quarterly |
| Meyler's Side Effects of Drugs (SEDBASE) | Excerpta Medica/Silver Platter Information | Drug side effects, reactions, toxicity, and interactions; referenced | Semiannually |
| STAT!-Ref | Teton Data Systems 235 East Broadway Jackson, WY 83001 800-755-STAT | Full text and tables of major general references, eg, The Medical Letter, Hansten's Drug Interactions, AMA Drug Evaluations, USP-DI, and more | Quarterly |
| USP-DI | United States Pharmacopeia/ Micromedex, Inc. | Drug monographs; adverse effects organized by severity; orphan drug products | Quarterly |
| Clinical Pharmacology | Gold Standard Multimedia, Inc. 235 S. Main Street, Suite 206 Gainesville, FL 32601-6585 800-375-0943 | Over 2000 drug monographs; can maintain patient profiles, generate reports, write prescriptions, check for drug interactions; color pictures of drug products | Quarterly |
| Ask Rx | Camdat | Contains monograph information from USP DI Drug Information for the Health Care Professional on over 6000 medications; can search by side effect, screen patient profile for drug interactions; customizable patient printouts in English and Spanish | Quarterly |
| Drug Interaction Facts | Facts and Comparisons | Can obtain information on interactions by single drug or multiple drugs (up to 20) and by severity | Quarterly |

[a] Several of the CD-ROM products will screen for drug interactions.

*Sources: Baker, Smith, and Abate (1994); Cohen and Insel (1996); Day (1993); Mazza (1994); Neill (1996); Price and Goldwire (1994); Richards (1996); Troncale (1996).*

overload for the average practitioner. Newsletters summarize the latest developments in a particular field for a particular health care practitioner. Their targeted information can keep one abreast of significant findings of either current studies, which may or may not include medications (for example, *Journal Watch*, published by the New England Medical Association), or on medication issues (see *The Medical Letter*, published by *The Medical Letter, Inc.*).

Resource books contain medication information only, typically in monograph form. Monographs are detailed descriptions of drugs containing generic and brand names, indications, pharmacology, mechanisms of action, contraindications, precautions, adverse effects, drug interactions, dosage, administration, dosage forms, and patient information (Price & Goldwire, 1994). *Drug Facts and Comparisons, Drug Evaluations Annual*, and *AHFS Drug Information* cover most medications marketed in the United States and contain FDA and non-FDA approved indications and dosing guidelines. *Drug Evaluations Annual* is organized as both a text and a resource book. Since *The Physician's Desk Reference* (PDR) contains FDA-approved package insert information about medications that a manufacturer chooses to pay to have published, it is not comprehensive (Cohen & Insel, 1996). Specialty resource books concentrate on a single area or topic, such as drug interactions, adverse effects of medications, or medication use in pregnancy. A *current* drug interactions resource book is a necessity for any health care practitioner who prescribes, dispenses, or administers medications because new drug interactions are constantly being discovered. Practitioners who work with children and child-bearing-age women should have references on pediatric dosing and medications in pregnancy and lactation. Handbooks usually contain only selected information about a few medications or limited information about multiple medications and are common for specialty areas such as geriatrics or pediatrics. Handbooks can be useful for a practitioner in a specialty area if the specific medications usually used are covered in sufficient detail. Handbooks also tend to be smaller and more portable.

## COMPUTER-BASED RESOURCES

In recent years the number of computer-based resources available has exploded. Many handbooks and reference books are available in both a printed and computer version (diskette or compact disk). The current compact disk read-only memory (CD-ROM) has storage capacity of over 600 megabytes of information (Baker, Smith, & Abate, 1994; Millman & Lee, 1995). This is equivalent to 250,000 to 300,000 pages of text and more than 400 floppy disks. Because CDs can hold so much information, the CD version of a reference may contain such extras as pictures, graphs, or tables not found in the printed version.

For primary literature information, MEDLINE, covering over 3700 international journals, is the most comprehensive database of citations for articles in medicine and bioscience. Many different CD-ROM products have evolved from the database: You can obtain the complete database from 1966 to the present, or only the most recent citations (3–5 years), or only citations from clinical journals. MEDLINE is also available from different on-line sources, discussed later.

Before making a significant investment in computer-based resource materials, the user should consider a few key points: computer accessibility, computer requirements, computer literacy of the end user, costs compared to the printed version if available, the frequency of upgrades and the associated costs, and the format of information obtained. A computer needs to be accessible at the time resource use is desired, and the user needs to be able to find the desired information quickly and efficiently. Consider the computer requirements for the program; given the space consumption and requirements of some programs, additional memory or a faster compact disk player may be needed. Some programs require multiple CD players or are cost-prohibitive for most single users; these versions are primarily intended for institution use and purchase. The information format in a program is also important. Some databases—*International Pharmaceutical Abstracts*, for example—are only bibliographic, providing only the citation and/or abstract of an article, whereas others contain the full text from an article. Consider how often a program is updated, if at all, and the costs of any updates or upgrades.

Carefully evaluate any software or compact disk program before buying to see that it meets identified needs. Many companies will allow a demonstration or trial period with their products. Look beyond the "bells and whistles" of a program to assess its true benefit to your practice.

## ON-LINE RESOURCES

On-line resources can connect you with many CD-ROM and printed materials, often for free. Connection to an on-line resource is usually through a personal computer or mainframe computer workstations. On-line resources are available in several ways: access to large databases in remote locations through direct computer connection (university library), through a commercial on-line service (not specifically medically related), or electronic bulletin boards sponsored by professional organizations or schools. On-line resources can conveniently answer questions quickly if you are computer literate and hardware is available for immediate use. Before committing to an on-line service, consider the amount of time you will likely use the service, its billing plan, and the format and quality of information obtained. Some services have an hourly use charge and are accessed through a long-distance telephone call, an additional charge. Also consider what additional computer equipment may be necessary to access an on-line service (i.e., modem or communications software).

Commercial on-line services such as CompuServe, Prodigy, and America Online offer access to the Internet and have medically related discussion groups in which health professionals and nonprofessionals can participate. Consider answers to pharmacotherapy questions obtained from discussion groups of unknown reliability. Such groups might, in fact, be good resources for obtaining leads to information or finding out how someone else dealt with a particularly difficult patient or situation. Directing patients to computer discussion groups may help them deal with and understand their illnesses.

Internet-based technology has changed the way biomedical information is distributed. The result has been widespread availability of clinical, research, and educational resources through personal computers (Lowe, Lomas, & Polonkey, 1996; Kramer & Cath, 1996; Potts, 1996). Table 7–2 lists some World Wide Web sites that contain or can assist practitioners in finding medication-related information on the Internet. Many additional professional organizations, government agencies, and pharmaceutical companies are developing their own Web sites, so be sure to browse to see what is new in your specialty.

## PATIENT MEDICATION INFORMATION

Medication information resources for patients also come in printed and computer formats (see Table 7–3). Sometimes the patient information segment is part of a larger information database such as DrugDex. The same issues discussed previously should be considered when choosing a patient education resource. Additionally, consider the reading level of the information provided, customizability, and availability in multiple languages if applicable to a practice setting.

The printed output of a computer program, for example, might not be legible for an elderly patient needing a larger-print format.

## OTHER RESOURCES

Other sources of medication information that warrant discussion include pharmaceutical companies, drug information centers, and poison control centers.

Pharmaceutical companies provide medication information through two primary sources—manufacturer's sales representatives (MSRs) and in-house drug information centers. A pharmaceutical company is obviously a good source for basic product information (Shaughnessy et al, 1994). Under current FDA regulations, the MSR can provide a health professional with information on FDA-approved and unapproved uses of a product (Wechsler, 1997). Additional information about nonapproved uses can be given to a health professional by a pharmaceutical company's in-house drug information center. The in-house drug information centers only provide information about an individual company's products, but may be able to assist your quest for information on various uses, adverse effects, and drug interactions with their products. One problem with obtaining information from a pharmaceutical company is that the information has the potential to be biased (Shaughnessy et al, 1994). And obtaining answers from manufacturer's in-house drug information centers can take 1–14 days (Price & Goldwire, 1994). A list of pharmaceutical companies' addresses and phone numbers is available in both the PDR and the RedBook.

Drug information centers, usually affiliated with a university and/or large medical center, sometimes can be a valuable resource for answering difficult questions. Unfortunately, not all centers take calls from the outside community. If you have access to a drug information center, consider the following prior to calling: Is there a fee for the service? Have all other resources been exhausted? How fast can the center respond with an answer? Usually a center will want to know what resources have already been used to avoid duplication.

Most communities have access to a poison control center through a toll-free number. The centers assist both the general public with information and health professionals treating a potential poison ingestion. The number of the local center should be available in the telephone book

## TABLE 7–2. WEB SITES FOR PHARMACOTHERAPY INFORMATION

| Site Name | Site Address | Comments |
|---|---|---|
| MedPulse | http://www.medscape.com/ | Offers peer-reviewed, practice-oriented information; full-text articles; MEDLINE; updated daily, free, but health care provider must register |
| RxList | http://www.rxlist.com/ | Drug monograph database |
| HELIX | http://www.helix.com/ | Drug databases, on-line forums with other health professionals, association information, continuing education, and MEDLINE; free, but health care provider must register |
| PharmInfoNet | http://www.pharminfo.com/pin_hp.html | Drug-related research bulletins and links to other web sites; DrugDB—a database of hundreds of widely prescribed and newly approved medications; DrugFAQs—frequently asked questions about medications; DrugPR—press releases from pharmaceutical companies |
| HyperDOC | http://www.nlm.nih.gov/ | National Library of Medicine (NLM) home page; over 40 databases, PREMEDLINE (in-process citations and abstracts before entered in MEDLINE; updated weekly; have not gone through NLM quality control); MEDLINE; charge to use most databases and must open account to use |
| FDA | http://www.fda.gov/ | Information from FDA on drugs, medical devices, foods, biologics, toxicology, and cosmetics |
| World Health Organization | http://www.who.ch/ | Statistical information, weekly epidemiologic record, world health report, and vaccination information for world travel |
| National Institutes of Health (NIH) | http://www.nih.gov/ | NIH research news, grants and contracts, and health information |
| Centers for Disease Control (CDC) | http://www.cdc.gov/ | Disease outbreaks, CDC recommendations, and vaccination information for world travel |

Sources: Kramer and Cath (1996); Lowe, Lomas, and Polonkey (1996); Potts (1996).

under emergency numbers. Before calling, have the following information available: age of the patient, substance ingested or clues to the ingestion, amount ingested, time of ingestion, and patient signs and symptoms.

## SUGGESTED MINIMUM PHARMACOTHERAPY LIBRARY

Below is a suggested minimum pharmacotherapy library:

- Pharmacotherapy reference text (most recent edition)
- Updated drug information resource program or book
- Updated drug interaction screening program or book
- Newsletter subscription for area of practice interest
- Handbook for area of practice interest
- Access to very current information or obscure information that may not be in any of these resources—through an on-line service, drug information center, or both

## TABLE 7–3. PATIENT EDUCATION RESOURCES

| Pharmacotherapy Resource | Publisher | Description/Comments | Frequency of Publication and/or Updates |
|---|---|---|---|
| **Books** | | | |
| USP DI, Volume II, Advice for the Patient | United States Pharmacopeial Convention, Inc. 12601 Twinbrook Parkway Rockville, MD 20852 800-227-8772 | Patient information on same products as in USP-DI, Volume I, Drug Information for the Health Professional | Yearly with monthly updates |
| Patient Drug Facts | Facts and Comparisons 111 West Port Plaza Suite 423 St. Louis, MO 63146-9811 800-223-0554 | Patient information on same products as in Drug Facts and Comparisons; color pictures for product identification | Yearly with quarterly updates |
| The Medication Teaching Manual: The Guide to Patient Drug Information, 6th edition | American Society of Health System Pharmacists 7272 Wisconsin Avenue Bethesda MD 20814 301-657-3000 | One-page patient information sheets on over 500 medications; easy to read; available in Spanish | Periodically |
| **Software** | | | |
| MedTeach | American Society of Health System Pharmacists | Patient information sheets on over 500 medications; easy to read; available in Windows or MS-DOS versions; also available in Spanish; can customize printout | Quarterly (additional cost) |
| AskAdvice Patient Education Software | Camdat 359 Northgate Drive Warrendale, PA 15086 800-875-8355 | Can be used with AskRx or standalone, patient medication information printouts can be customized; average reading level: post–high school | Quarterly |

Sources: Baker, Smith, and Abate (1994); Fox (1996); Price and Goldwire (1994).

## CONCLUSION

All health care providers who prescribe, dispense, or administer medications need current and easily accessible medication information. This chapter has given a brief overview of the available resources and suggested a minimum library to have available in practice.

## REFERENCES

Baker, D. E., Smith, G. H., & Abate, M. A. (1994). Selected topics in drug information access and practice: An update. *Annals of Pharmacotherapy,* 28, 1389–1394.

Cohen, J. S. & Insel, P. A. (1996). The Physicians' Desk Reference: Problems and possible improvements. *Archives of Internal Medicine,* 156, 1375–1380.

Day, R. P. (1993). Desktop drug information. *Annals of Internal Medicine,* 119, 936–938.

Fox, G. N. (1996). Ask Advice patient education software. *Journal of Family Practice,* 42, 626–627.

Knott, T. L. & Scott, U. K. (1994). New perspectives in information retrieval. *Clinical Reviews in Allergy,* 12, 201–210.

Kramer, J. M. & Cath, A. (1996). Medical resources and the internet: Making the connection. *Archives of Internal Medicine,* 156, 833–842.

Lowe, H. J., Lomas, E. C., & Polonkey, S. E. (1996). The World Wide Web: A review of an emerging internet-based technology for the distribution of biomedical information. *Journal of the American Medical Informatics Association, 3*, 1–14.

Mazza, J. J. (1994). A library for internists, VIII: Recommendations from the American College of Physicians. *Annals of Internal Medicine, 120*, 699–720.

Millman A. & Lee, N. (1995). CD ROMs, multimedia, and optical storage systems. *BMJ, 311*, 676–678.

Neill, R. A. (1996). Clinical pharmacology. *Journal of Family Practice, 42*, 88.

Potts, J. F. (1996). Winding your way through the Web. *Postgraduate Medicine, 100*, 35–42.

Price, K. O. & Goldwire, M. A. (1994). Drug information resources. *American Pharmacy, NS34*, 30–39.

Richards, J. W. (1996). PDR generics. *Journal of Family Practice, 42*, 419.

Shaughnessy, A. F., Slawson, D. C., & Bennett, J. H. (1994). Becoming an information master: A guidebook to the medical information jungle. *Journal of Family Practice, 39*, 489–499.

Troncale, J. A. (1996). Drug interaction facts on disk. *Journal of Family Practice, 42*, 626.

Wechsler, J. (1997). Final reform bill "modernizes" FDA, permits dissemination of off-label and economic data. *Formulary, 32*, 1254.

# 8

# ADVERSE DRUG EVENTS AND DRUG INTERACTIONS

*Geneva Briggs*

Responsible drug therapy requires knowing not only the efficacy of a particular drug in a particular disorder or disease state but also what combinations and conditions might actually aggravate a situation. It also requires knowing that unexpected reactions such as allergies may occur. This chapter covers both adverse drug events—those reactions or incidents that are not wished for—and drug interactions—some of which are indeed factored into the pharmacotherapy and some for which providers should be alert.

## ADVERSE DRUG EVENTS

An adverse drug event is an unwanted or undesirable occurrence resulting from the use of a medication. An adverse drug event, as defined in this chapter, includes adverse drug reactions resulting from allergy, intolerance, drug interaction, or unknown mechanism and medication misadventures (hospitalization, death, etc.) caused by use of a medication. *Adverse drug event* is a more inclusive term than *adverse drug reaction*, but the terms are sometimes used interchangeably.

Information about adverse drug events with medications is gathered from clinical trials, spontaneous reporting by health professionals and occasionally by consumers to manufacturers and government agencies, and published case reports. The full extent of adverse events

with medications is unknown because reporting of adverse drug events is a spontaneous, incomplete process. The majority of reports come from hospitals, yet the majority of drug use is in the outpatient setting. Minor gastrointestinal disturbances, rash, itching, drowsiness, insomnia, weakness, headache, tremulousness, muscle twitches, and fever account for up to 71% of reported reactions (Atkin & Shenfield, 1995). It is estimated that 2–11% of all hospitalizations are the result of adverse medication events (Atkin & Shenfield, 1995; Beard, 1992; Johnstone, Kirking, & Vison, 1995; Nelson & Talbert, 1996). When hospitalized, a patient has about a 1.5–44% chance of having an adverse drug event, with the chance of having a life-threatening adverse drug event estimated to be between 1.1–3% per hospitalized patient (Atkin & Shenfield, 1995). Many events do not result in hospitalizations but cause significant morbidity. The treatment of adverse drug events is costly to both the health care system and society. Drug-related morbidity and mortality has been estimated to cost $76.6 billion annually in the United States (Johnson & Bootman, 1995).

## WHAT IS AN ADVERSE DRUG REACTION?

Many definitions have evolved as to what constitutes an adverse drug reaction. The World Health Organization (WHO) defines an adverse drug reaction as any noxious, unintended, and undesired effect of a drug that occurs at a dose used in humans for prophylaxis, diagnosis, or therapy (Anonymous, 1975). The Food and Drug Administration (FDA) has broadened the definition of a reportable adverse drug reaction to include any adverse event associated with the use of a drug in humans, whether or not considered drug-related. These adverse events may occur in the course of the use of a drug product in professional practice; from drug overdose, whether accidental or intentional; from drug abuse; from drug withdrawal; and from any significant failure of expected pharmacological action (Department of Health and Human Services, 1985).

## CLASSIFICATION

Adverse drug reactions are categorized into two groups: predictable and unpredictable. *Predictable reactions* are generally dose-dependent and related to the pharmacologic actions of the drug. These reactions include side effects, toxicity, drug interactions, and secondary effects related to pharmacologic properties but not the primary therapeutic properties (ie, sedation from antihistaminic activity of a tricyclic antidepressant). *Unpredictable reactions* are usually dose-independent, are not always related to the pharmacologic actions of the drug, and are related to the individual's immunologic response or genetic differences (Rieder, 1994). Examples of unpredictable reactions include drug intolerance (exaggerated pharmacologic or toxic effects in vulnerable subsets of patients) and idiosyncratic, anaphylactoid, and allergic (immunologically mediated) reactions.

To evaluate whether a reaction is due to a medication, consider the temporal relationship of medication administration to the reaction, previous reports of the same or similar reaction, patient history of a similar reaction or reaction to a similar class of medication, and resolution of the reaction upon discontinuation of the substance (Kando, Yonker, & Cole, 1995). Also consider alternative causes for the reaction, presence of toxic drug concentrations, any positive dose-response relationship, and recurrence of the reaction when the drug is reintroduced (Kando et al, 1995). Rechallenge is seldom possible or ethical, but if attempted, discontinuation of the drug should be five times the elimination half-life before reintroduction to ensure that the drug has been eliminated com-

pletely from the body. Also, the reaction should have completely resolved symptomatically, and any abnormal laboratory values should be normalized (Girard, 1987). Most cases of rechallenge are by accident, which is why documentation of reactions is very important for prevention. Based on all these issues, reactions can be classified as definitely, probably, possibly, or indistinguishably caused by the suspected agent (Atkin & Shenfield, 1995).

A reaction can be considered mild if symptomatic treatment or dosage alteration is necessary but a change in medication is not required. Moderate reactions do require a change in medication. A severe reaction is defined as one that is unexpected or untoward or results in permanent disability or death (Kando et al, 1995).

### Predictable Reactions

Predictable reactions usually are related to the pharmacologic properties of a medication. Several characteristics are risk factors for predictable reactions (Kando et al, 1995):

- Advanced age
- Female gender
- History of a previous adverse event
- Multiple medications
- Duration of hospital stay
- Liver disease
- Renal disease

In addition to being at higher risk for reactions, women appear to have higher rates of gastrointestinal reactions than men (Kando et al, 1995).

### Unpredictable Reactions

Unpredictable reactions include *anaphylactoid, allergic,* and *idiosyncratic* reactions. There are no predictive factors for anaphylactoid and idiosyncratic reactions. Some factors do impact the risk of developing allergic reactions, such as age, gender, genetics, associated illnesses, drug-related factors such as route of administration, and previous drug administration. Young children have a lower risk of allergic reactions because of limited prior exposure to medications. Women have higher rates of cutaneous reactions (Bigby, Jick, Jick, & Arndt, 1986). Patients with atopic dermatitis, allergic rhinitis, and asthma tend to have more severe allergic reactions than patients without these conditions (Van Arsdel, 1991).

Genetic ability to metabolize drugs also can affect the rate of allergic reactions. Patients who are slow acetylators, for example, are more likely to develop drug-induced lupus when treated with procainamide or hydralazine (Beringer & Middleton, 1993). Concomitant illnesses such as infectious mononucleosis, lymphocytic leukemia, and gout are associated with higher incidences of macropapular rashes with ampicillin (Van Arsdel, 1991). AIDS patients have higher incidences of cutaneous reactions with sulfonamides and amoxicillin-clavulanate (Van Arsdel, 1991).

Dose, frequency of exposure, and route of administration affect the frequency of some allergic reactions. Some allergic reactions only occur with high doses, whereas others require intermittent exposure to a drug for a reaction to develop. Topical administration is most sensitizing followed by intramuscular, intravenous, and then oral (Van Arsdel, 1991). A history of an allergic reaction to a drug or chemically similar drug is the most reliable risk factor for development of a subsequent reaction (Beringer & Middleton, 1993).

## REPORTING ADVERSE EVENTS

Reporting adverse drug events is a professional and legal obligation, so appropriate information on medication-related problems is communicated to the broader medical community. Within the United States, the FDA has primary responsibility for collecting, analyzing, and disseminating information on adverse drug events. The individual manufacturer has responsibility to collect pre- and postmarketing information on its products. Postmarketing surveillance is important for several reasons. A medication is studied in limited numbers of patients prior to marketing, so reactions that occur rarely (ie, 1 in 100,000 exposures) are often not detected. Dose-dependent reactions are usually discovered in premarketing studies, but idiosyncratic reactions may not be. Also, medications are not necessarily studied in patients with multiple diseases, complicating factors, or complicated medication regimens. Reactions are detected once a product reaches the general market and is given to complicated patients. Additionally, most drug interactions are not discovered until after a medication is marketed and given to many patients because the inclusion criteria of premarketing studies usually limit the number of concomitant medications a study subject is receiving.

Lack of knowledge of all the risks associated with a new medication is attributable to deficiencies in the premarketing process, referred to as "the Five Toos" (Sills, 1986):

- *Too few patients to detect rare events:* Thirty thousand people would have to take a medication to detect an adverse drug reaction that occurs in 1 in 10,000 exposures (McCloskey, 1996).
- *Too simple:* Patients who take multiple medications or have complicated medical conditions are excluded from clinical trials.
- *Too median-aged:* Most trials do not represent the very young and old.
- *Too narrow:* Indications for a newly approved drug are narrow based on premarketing clinical trials, but once marketed the drug may be used for other related but untested indications.
- *Too brief:* Most clinical trials are short; some adverse drug events may not appear for years.

Appropriate reporting often depends on where one is practicing. Hospitals and some other organized medical systems usually have an organization-specific process for reporting adverse drug events. An adverse drug event reporting system is mandated by the Joint Commission on Accreditation of Hospital Organizations (JCAHO). In these types of settings, reporting should follow the organizational process. The end result of health system reporting should be dissemination of the information within the organization and to the appropriate reporting body (ie, FDA).

In a solo practice or clinic setting without a structured reporting system, reports should be filed directly with the FDA through the MedWatch program. The MedWatch program was initiated in 1993 to simplify and consolidate reporting of serious adverse drug events and medical device problems. Events are reported on the MedWatch form (Fig. 8–1). The form can be mailed, faxed, or sent by modem to the FDA. Reactions to vaccines are reported on a different form (Vaccine Adverse Event Reporting System—VAERS), shown in Figure 8–2. The phone number for MedWatch is 800-FDA-1088; for VAERS it is 800-822-7967.

To get the most useful information, the FDA requests that only serious adverse events be reported through MedWatch. To be considered a *serious event*, the patient outcome is death, life-threatening, hospitalization (initial or prolonged), disability (significant, persistent, or permanent), or a congenital anomaly, or inter-

**Figure 8–1.** Sample form: MedWatch.

# ADVICE ABOUT VOLUNTARY REPORTING

**Report experiences with:**
- medications (drugs or biologics)
- medical devices (including in-vitro diagnostics)
- special nutritional products (dietary supplements, medical foods, infant formulas)
- other products regulated by FDA

**Report SERIOUS adverse events. An event is serious when the patient outcome is:**
- death
- life-threatening (real risk of dying)
- hospitalization (initial or prolonged)
- disability (significant, persistent or permanent)
- congenital anomaly
- required intervention to prevent permanent impairment or damage

**Report even if:**
- you're not certain the product caused the event
- you don't have all the details

**Report product problems** – quality, performance or safety concerns such as:
- suspected contamination
- questionable stability
- defective components
- poor packaging or labeling

**How to report:**
- just fill in the sections that apply to your report
- use section C for all products except medical devices
- attach additional blank pages if needed
- use a separate form for each patient
- report either to FDA or the manufacturer (or both)

**Important numbers:**
- 1-800-FDA-0178    to FAX report
- 1-800-FDA-7737    to report by modem
- 1-800-FDA-1088    for more information or to report quality problems
- 1-800-822-7967    for a VAERS form for vaccines

**If your report involves a serious adverse event with a device** and it occurred in a facility outside a doctor's office, that facility may be legally required to report to FDA and/or the manufacturer. Please notify the person in that facility who would handle such reporting.

**Confidentiality:** The patient's identity is held in strict confidence by FDA and protected to the fullest extent of the law. The reporter's identity may be shared with the manufacturer unless requested otherwise. However, FDA will not disclose the reporter's identity in response to a request from the public, pursuant to the Freedom of Information Act.

---

The public reporting burden for this collection of information has been estimated to average 30 minutes per response, including the time for reviewing instructions, searching existing data sources, gathering and maintaining the data needed, and completing and reviewing the collection of information. Send your comments regarding this burden estimate or any other aspect of this collection of information, including suggestions for reducing this burden to:

Reports Clearance Officer, PHS
Hubert H. Humphrey Building,
Room 721-B
200 Independence Avenue, S.W.
Washington, DC 20201
ATTN: PRA

and to:
Office of Management and Budget
Paperwork Reduction Project
(0910-0230)
Washington, DC 20503

Please do NOT return this form to either of these addresses.

FDA Form 3500-back    **Please Use Address Provided Below – Just Fold In Thirds, Tape and Mail**

- - - - - - - - - - - - - - - - - - - - - - - - - - - - - - - - - - - - - - - - - - - - - - - - - - - - - - - - - - - - - - - - - - - - - - - - - - - - - - - -

**Department of
Health and Human Services**
Public Health Service
Food and Drug Administration
Rockville, MD  20857

**Official Business**
Penalty for Private Use $300

NO POSTAGE
NECESSARY
IF MAILED
IN THE
UNITED STATES
OR APO/FPO

| **BUSINESS REPLY MAIL** |
| FIRST CLASS MAIL   PERMIT NO. 946  ROCKVILLE, MD |
| *POSTAGE WILL BE PAID BY FOOD AND DRUG ADMINISTRATION* |

MED**W**ATCH
**The FDA Medical Products Reporting Program
Food and Drug Administration
5600 Fishers Lane
Rockville, MD  20852-9787**

**Figure 8–1.** (*continued*)

vention is required to prevent permanent impairment or damage. Serious events that occur from medications (prescription or over-the-counter drugs or biologics), medical devices, nutritional products (dietary supplements, infant formulas), homeopathic remedies, or health food store products should all be reported. The actions the FDA can take on reported adverse drug reactions include labeling changes, letters to health professionals, requirement of further study by the manufacturer, or withdrawal of a drug from the market.

**VACCINE ADVERSE EVENT REPORTING SYSTEM**
24 Hour Toll-free information line 1-800-822-7967
P.O. Box 1100, Rockville, MD 20849-1100
**VAERS**
PATIENT IDENTITY KEPT CONFIDENTIAL

**For CDC/FDA Use Only**

VAERS Number _____

Date Received_____

| Patient Name: | Vaccine administered by (Name): | Form completed by (Name): |
|---|---|---|
| Last          First          M.I. | Responsible Physician _____ Facility Name/Address | Relation      ☐ Vaccine Provider    ☐ Patient/Parent to Patient   ☐ Manufacturer      ☐ Other |
| Address | | Address (if different from patient or provider) |
| City          State          Zip | City          State          Zip | City          State          Zip |
| Telephone no. (_____)_____ | Telephone no. (_____)_____ | Telephone no. (_____)_____ |

| 1. State | 2. County where administered | 3. Date of birth   /   /   mm   dd   yy | 4. Patient age | 5. Sex  ☐ M ☐ F | 6. Date form completed   /   /   mm   dd   yy |
|---|---|---|---|---|---|

| 7. Describe adverse event(s) (symptoms, signs, time course) and treatment, if any | 8. Check all appropriate: |
|---|---|
| | ☐ Patient died     (date ___/___/___)  ☐ Life threatening illness mm  dd  yy  ☐ Required emergency room/doctor visit  ☐ Required hospitalization (_____days)  ☐ Resulted in prolongation of hospitalization  ☐ Resulted in permanent disability  ☐ None of the above |

| 9. Patient recovered  ☐ YES  ☐ NO  ☐ UNKNOWN | 10. Date of vaccination   /   /   mm   dd   yy  Time_____ AM PM | 11. Adverse event onset   /   /   mm   dd   yy  Time_____ AM PM |
|---|---|---|
| 12. Relevant diagnostic tests/laboratory data | | |

13. Enter all vaccines given on date listed in no. 10

| | Vaccine (type) | Manufacturer | Lot number | Route/Site | No. Previous doses |
|---|---|---|---|---|---|
| a. | | | | | |
| b. | | | | | |
| c. | | | | | |
| d. | | | | | |

14. Any other vaccinations within 4 weeks prior to the date listed in no. 10

| | Vaccine (type) | Manufacturer | Lot number | Route/Site | No. Previous doses | Date given |
|---|---|---|---|---|---|---|
| a. | | | | | | |
| b. | | | | | | |

| 15. Vaccinated at:  ☐ Private doctor's office/hospital    ☐ Military clinic/hospital  ☐ Public health clinic/hospital    ☐ Other/unknown | 16. Vaccine purchased with:  ☐ Private funds  ☐ Military funds  ☐ Public funds  ☐ Other /unknown | 17. Other medications |
|---|---|---|
| 18. Illness at time of vaccination (specify) | 19. Pre-existing physician-diagnosed allergies, birth defects, medical conditions (specify) | |

| 20. Have you reported this adverse event previously?    ☐ No    ☐ To health department    ☐ To doctor    ☐ To manufacturer | **Only for children 5 and under** |
|---|---|
| | 22. Birth weight _____ lb. _____ oz. | 23. No. of brothers and sisters |

| 21. Adverse event following prior vaccination (check all applicable, specify) | **Only for reports submitted by manufacturer/immunization project** |
|---|---|

| | Adverse Event | Onset Age | Type Vaccine | Dose no. in series | 24. Mfr. / imm. proj. report no. | 25. Date received by mfr. / imm. proj. |
|---|---|---|---|---|---|---|
| ☐ In patient | | | | | | |
| ☐ In brother or sister | | | | | 26. 15 day report?  ☐ Yes ☐ No | 27. Report type  ☐ Initial ☐ Follow-Up |

Health care providers and manufacturers are required by law (42 USC 300aa-25) to report reactions to vaccines listed in the Table of Reportable Events Following Immunization. Reports for reactions to other vaccines are voluntary except when required as a condition of immunization grant awards.

Form VAERS -1

**Figure 8–2.** Sample form: Vaccine Adverse Event Reporting System (VAERS).

"Fold in thirds, tape & mail - DO NOT STAPLE FORM"

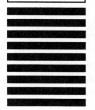

NO POSTAGE
NECESSARY
IF MAILED
IN THE
UNITED STATES
OR APO/FPO

## BUSINESS REPLY MAIL
FIRST-CLASS MAIL   PERMIT NO. 1895   ROCKVILLE, MD

*POSTAGE WILL BE PAID BY ADDRESSEE*

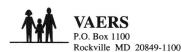

**VAERS**
P.O. Box 1100
Rockville MD  20849-1100

## DIRECTIONS FOR COMPLETING FORM
(Additional pages may be attached if more space is needed.)

### GENERAL

- Use a separate form for each patient. Complete the form to the best of your abilities. Items 3, 4, 7, 8, 10, 11, and 13 are considered essential and should be completed whenever possible. Parents/Guardians may need to consult the facility where the vaccine was administered for some of the information (such as manufacturer, lot number or laboratory data.)
- Refer to the Reportable Events Table (RET) for events mandated for reporting by law. Reporting for other serious events felt to be related but not on the RET is encouraged.
- Health care providers other than the vaccine administrator (VA) treating a patient for a suspected adverse event should notify the VA and provide the information about the adverse event to allow the VA to complete the form to meet the VA's legal responsibility.
- These data will be used to increase understanding of adverse events following vaccination and will become part of CDC Privacy Act System 09-20-0136, "Epidemiologic Studies and Surveillance of Disease Problems". Information identifying the person who received the vaccine or that person's legal representative will not be made available to the public, but may be available to the vaccinee or legal representative.
- Postage will be paid by addressee. Forms may be photocopied (must be front & back on same sheet).

### SPECIFIC INSTRUCTIONS

Form Completed By:  To be used by parents/guardians, vaccine manufacturers/distributors, vaccine administrators, and/or the person completing the form on behalf of the patient or the health professional who administered the vaccine.

Item 7:   Describe the suspected adverse event. Such things as temperature, local and general signs and symptoms, time course, duration of symptoms diagnosis, treatment and recovery should be noted.

Item 9:   Check "YES" if the patient's health condition is the same as it was prior to the vaccine, "NO" if the patient has not returned to the pre-vaccination state of health, or "UNKNOWN" if the patient's condition is not known.

Item 10:   Give dates and times as specifically as you can remember. If you do not know the exact time, please
and 11:   indicate "AM" or "PM" when possible if this information is known. If more than one adverse event, give the onset date and time for the most serious event.

Item 12:   Include "negative" or "normal" results of any relevant tests performed as well as abnormal findings.

Item 13:   List ONLY those vaccines given on the day listed in Item 10.

Item 14:   List any other vaccines that the patient received within 4 weeks prior to the date listed in Item 10.

Item 16:   This section refers to how the person who gave the vaccine purchased it, not to the patient's insurance.

Item 17:   List any prescription or non-prescription medications the patient was taking when the vaccine(s) was given.

Item 18:   List any short term illnesses the patient had on the date the vaccine(s) was given (i.e., cold, flu, ear infection).

Item 19:   List any pre-existing physician-diagnosed allergies, birth defects, medical conditions (including developmental and/or neurologic disorders) for the patient.

Item 21:   List any suspected adverse events the patient, or the patient's brothers or sisters, may have had to previous vaccinations. If more than one brother or sister, or if the patient has reacted to more than one prior vaccine, use additional pages to explain completely. For the onset age of a patient, provide the age in months if less than two years old.

Item 26:   This space is for manufacturers' use only.

**Figure 8–2.** (*continued*)

## PREVENTION

It is estimated that 30–80% of all adverse drug events are preventable (Nelson & Talbert, 1996; Pearson et al, 1994; Schumock & Thornton, 1992). Although not all adverse drug events can be prevented, many can be avoided. Some simple things can be done to prevent or avoid reactions: appropriate dosing of medications based on gender, age, and concomitant medications and conditions; avoidance of drug interactions when possible; and labeling of patient records with prior reactions. To prevent future reactions, any adverse drug reaction should be documented in detail in the patient's record. Patients should also be educated to communicate any reactions they have had to all health care providers. Patients who have had serious reactions, such as anaphylaxis or angioedema, should be told how to obtain bracelets or necklaces to wear that identify the problem medication and reaction. Prescribers should have knowledge of the drugs they prescribe, select them objectively, provide the patient with risk-versus-benefit information to enable the patient to make an informed decision as to whether to accept the therapy or not, and warn about unwanted reactions and interactions (Day, 1995).

## DRUG INTERACTIONS

Medications can interact with other medications, disease states, food, or the social habits of the patient. Such interactions frequently occur, but most are not clinically significant. Although usually thought of in a negative sense, interactions can be positive in nature and intentionally used to benefit the patient. This section will discuss the different types of interactions and give some common, significant examples for each type.

## DRUG-DRUG INTERACTIONS

Drug-drug interactions can be classified as pharmacokinetic or pharmacodynamic. The drug whose action is altered by an interaction is termed the *object drug*, and the drug that alters the action is the *precipitant drug*.

*Pharmacokinetic interactions* include positive and negative effects on drug absorption, distribution, metabolism, and excretion (see Chap. 2 for explanation of these terms). Gastrointestinal absorption can be affected by drug binding in the GI tract, altered GI motility, altered intestinal flora, and altered gastrointestinal pH (Benjamin & Buckman, 1996). Absorptive interactions can affect both the rate and extent of absorption. The most important interactions usually affect the overall extent of absorption (Hansten & Horn, 1996b). Sucralfate forming insoluble complexes with ciprofloxacin is an example of a binding interaction (Garrelts et al, 1990). Anticholinergics, which slow GI motility, and metoclopramide, which increases GI motility, can affect the rate of absorption of many medications, but changes in GI motility rarely affect the overall extent of absorption significantly (Hansten & Horn, 1996b). $H_2$ antagonists may markedly reduce absorption of drugs that require an acidic medium to dissolve adequately, such as ketoconazole (Lelawongs et al, 1988).

*Distribution interactions* occur when drugs compete for binding sites on plasma proteins or tissues. When this happens, the free or unbound serum concentration of one or both drugs may increase, which may result temporarily in increased drug response. Protein-binding interactions are usually important when the displaced drug is highly bound, has a limited body distribution, is slowly eliminated, and has a low therapeutic index (Benjamin & Buckman, 1996). The enhanced pharmacologic effects of such a displaced drug usually only occur for a few days because more unbound drug is available for elimination by the liver and kidneys. For example, warfarin is a highly protein bound drug susceptible to protein-binding drug-drug interactions. Chloral hydrate is one drug that can displace warfarin from protein-binding sites, resulting in an increase in hypoprothrombinemic effect that could last for up to a week (Hansten & Horn, 1996b). With continued combination therapy, the total plasma concentration of warfarin declines and the free warfarin concentration returns to preinteraction levels.

Liver metabolism can be increased by enzyme induction or decreased by enzyme inhibition (Hansten & Horn, 1996b). The onset of induction usually is gradual over 1–2 weeks. Dissipation of the reaction once the inducing agent is removed may take longer than 2 weeks. Some examples of liver enzyme inducers include barbiturates, carbamazepine, rifampin, and phenytoin (Lee, 1996). Enzyme inhibition usually occurs rapidly (within one or more doses of the inhibitor). An exception is erythromycin, whose effect may be delayed by several days. Enzyme inhibitors include cimetidine, erythromycin, isoniazid, ketoconazole, and fluoxetine (and other selective serotonin reuptake inhibitors) (Lee, 1996).

Renal elimination of drugs can be altered by many mechanisms, including alteration of urinary pH affecting passive tubular secretion, active tubular secretion, and glomerular filtration (nephrotoxicity) (Hansten & Horn, 1996b). Probenicid competes with penicillin to reduce active tubular secretion and renal clearance of the penicillin (Hansten & Horn, 1996b). The penicillin-probenicid interaction has been used to enhance the effect of the penicillin. An example of nephrotoxicity causing a drug-drug interaction is when a digitalized patient treated with gentamicin develops aminoglycoside-induced renal failure, which leads to digoxin toxicity.

A *pharmacodynamic interaction* occurs when a drug affects the outcome or toxicity of another drug without any change in the second drug's serum concentration. Pharmacodynamic effects of drugs can be additive or antagonistic. Pharmacodynamic interactions can be therapeutic (eg, combinations of antihypertensives), can result in adverse effects (eg, multiple anticholinergic drugs), or can result in negation of therapeutic effect [eg, nonsteroidal antiinflammatory drugs (NSAID) blunting the antihypertensive effect of clonidine]. These types of interactions occur commonly, but when anticipated, do not usually cause serious difficulties.

Table 8–1 lists selected important drug interactions. The reader is cautioned to always consult an updated drug interactions text and the package labeling for drug products prior to prescribing, dispensing, or administering any medication.

## DRUG–DISEASE INTERACTIONS

Drug-disease interactions can occur when a medication adversely or positively impacts a disease. Drug-disease interactions are usually thought of in a negative sense because a positive impact on a disease would be viewed as a therapeutic effect of the medication. Medications can affect diseases in various ways, such as when hydrochlorothiazide increases glucose and impairs glycemic control in the diabetic (White & Campbell, 1995). Clinicians should be aware of the important drug-disease interactions for the diseases commonly seen in their patients. The

reader is referred to Unit III for discussion of specific drug-disease interactions.

## DRUG–FOOD INTERACTIONS

Interaction between drugs and food does not always get the attention it deserves. Since the frequency of ingestion of food with medications is far greater than the frequency of ingestion of two or more medications together, these interactions need to be considered. Nutrients may positively or negatively affect the bioavailability and ultimate efficacy of oral medications through many mechanisms. Negative effects to consider are binding with the medication to form nonabsorbable complexes and reduced absorption due to delayed gastric emptying, destruction by gastric acid, or altered ionization status of the medication (Chiesara, Borghini, & Marabini, 1995). Positive effects include increased absorption in the presence of certain types of food such as fat. Table 8–2 lists selected clinically significant drug-food interactions.

## DRUG–SOCIAL HABIT INTERACTIONS

Social habits, such as smoking tobacco or marijuana and alcohol consumption, can interact with medications. Nicotine and polycyclic hydrocarbons from tobacco induce liver enzyme metabolism (Schein, 1995). Since cigarette smoke increases the metabolism of theophylline, tacrine, flecainide, propranolol, diazepam, chlordiazepoxide, and propoxyphene, smokers may require larger dosages (Schein, 1995). There appears to be a relation between cigarettes smoked per day and the magnitude of many smoking-drug interactions. Heavy smokers (>25 cigarettes/day) are more likely to manifest interactions with drugs (Hansten & Horn, 1996a). Smoking may pharmacodynamically increase the risk of adverse events in patients with cardiovascular or peptic ulcer disease and in women on oral contraceptives (Schein, 1995). Diabetics who smoke may require one third the insulin of nonsmokers. This appears to be due to increased catecholamine and corticosteroid release caused by smoking and to reduced subcutaneous insulin absorption due to smoking-induced vasoconstriction (Hansten & Horn, 1996a).

Delta-9-tetrahydrocannabinol (THC), cannabidiol, and other cannabinoids found in marijuana can inhibit or increase metabolism of some drugs (Hansten & Horn, 1993a). Duration

**TABLE 8–1. SELECTED CLINICALLY SIGNIFICANT DRUG-DRUG INTERACTIONS**

| Object Drug | Interacting Drug | Mechanism/Management |
|---|---|---|
| Terfenadine | Erythromycin, clarithromycin, ketoconazole | Erythromycin, clarithromycin, and ketoconazole inhibit the metabolism of terfenadine. Excessive serum concentrations of terfenadine may cause cardiac arrhythmias. Avoid concomitant use. |
| Quinolone antibiotics | Sucralfate | Sucralfate can significantly reduce absorption of quinolone antibiotics. If concomitant use is necessary, give the quinolone several hours before the sucralfate. |
| Monoamine oxidase inhibitors (MAOIs) | Meperidine | Meperidine blocks the neuronal uptake of serotonin, and MAOIs inhibit central nervous system (CNS) metabolism of serotonin. The combination of meperidine and MAOIs results in accumulation of CNS serotonin, leading to agitation, blood pressure increase, hyperpyrexia, and convulsions. |
| | Tricyclic antidepressants, selective serotonin reuptake inhibitors | Combination can result in excessive CNS serotonin, resulting in agitation, blood pressure increase, hyperpyrexia, and convulsions. |
| Lithium | Nonsteroidal antiinflammatory drugs (NSAIDs) | NSAIDs inhibit the renal clearance of lithium, resulting in increased serum lithium concentrations and potential toxicity. Lithium concentrations and patient symptoms should be monitored closely when NSAID therapy is initiated or discontinued. |
| | Thiazide diuretics | Thiazide diuretics increase serum lithium concentrations and potential toxicity. Concomitant use should be undertaken with caution. Lithium concentrations and patient symptoms should be monitored closely when thiazide therapy is initiated or discontinued. |
| Warfarin | Trimethoprim/sulfamethoxazole (Bactrim, Co-Trimoxazole) | Trimethoprim/sulfamethoxazole combinations inhibit the metabolism of warfarin and compete with warfarin for plasma protein-binding sites. These two factors result in increased hypoprothrombinemic response to warfarin. Warfarin dosage adjustment is necessary when the combination is used. |
| | Amiodarone | Amiodarone inhibits the metabolism of warfarin, resulting in excessive anticoagulation unless warfarin dosage is adjusted. |
| Theophylline | Erythromycin | Erythromycin can inhibit the metabolism of theophylline, resulting in increased serum concentrations of theophylline. If a combination is necessary, reduce the theophylline dose during erythromycin therapy. |
| Potassium-sparing diuretics, potassium supplements | Angiotensin-converting enzyme inhibitors | Angiotensin-converting enzyme inhibitors tend to increase serum potassium. Concurrent use of potassium supplements or potassium-sparing diuretics can result in hyperkalemia. |
| Cisapride | Azoles (ketoconazole, miconazole, itraconazole), terfenadine | Azole antifungals and terfenadine inhibit the metabolism of cisapride, causing increased cisapride concentrations and possible toxicity, including arrhythmias. |

*Sources: Benjamin and Buckman (1996); Finley, Warner, and Peabody (1995); Quinn and Day (1995); Sporer (1995); Thompson and Oster (1996); Wells, Holbrook, and Crowther (1994) and Anastasio, Cornell, and Menscer (1997).*

## TABLE 8–2.  CLINICALLY SIGNIFICANT DRUG-NUTRIENT INTERACTIONS

| Medication | Interaction | Mechanism/Management |
|---|---|---|
| **Decreased Absorption/Bioavailability** | | |
| Alendronate | Food and any liquids other than water | Must be taken with 6–8 oz of plain water 30 min before meal |
| Erythromycin base and stearate | Food reduces absorption | May be due primarily to effects of food on gastric acidity; space 2 h apart |
| Penicillin G | Food, especially milk, and metal ions reduce absorption | May be due to binding; space 2 h apart |
| Tetracycline | Dairy products (calcium), iron | Chelation can decrease absorption by >50%; take tetracyclines 1 h before or 2 h after food |
| Fluoroquinolones (ciprofloxacin, ofloxacin, lomefloxacin, enoxacin) | Iron, calcium, copper, magnesium, manganese, zinc | Binding can decrease absorption significantly; space 2 h apart or temporarily discontinue cation-containing products if possible |
| Etidronate (Didronel) | Milk, iron, calcium, aluminum | Binding; separate by 2 h |
| Didanosine | Food | Acid-labile drug that should be taken under fasting conditions because food stimulates acid secretion |
| Zidovudine | Food | Reduced bioavailability; take on empty stomach |
| Captopril | Food | Unknown mechanism; on empty stomach or at same time each day |
| Azithromycin | Food | Food reduces absorption significantly; space 2 h apart |
| Sucralfate | Food | Sucralfate binds with proteins in food; space 2 h apart |
| Theophylline timed-release (Theo-Dur Sprinkle, Theo-24, Uniphyl) | Food | Rate of absorption can be affected, causing high theophylline concentrations; avoid taking with high-fat foods or take 1 h before eating |
| Fat-soluble vitamins | Mineral oil (used as a laxative) | By acting as a physical barrier, mineral oil prevents absorption of vitamins A, D, E, and K |
| Digoxin | High-fiber food, fiber laxatives | Digoxin binds to the fiber |
| Iron, folic acid, vitamin A, essential fatty acids | Cholestyramine, colestipol | Bile acid sequestrants can bind listed nutrients and prevent absorption |
| Enteral feedings | Phenytoin suspension, carbamazepine suspension, warfarin | Binding to components in the enteral formulation decreases absorption |
| **Increased Absorption/Bioavailability** | | |
| Atovaquone | High-fat food | Enhances absorption |
| Calcium channel blockers (felodipine, nifedipine) | Grapefruit juice | Flavonoid glycosides present in grapefruit juice inhibit the metabolism of these agents by the cytochrome P-450 (CYP1A2 and CYP3A4) enzymes in the liver |
| Cyclosporine | Grapefruit juice | Inhibition of the hepatic and extrahepatic cytochrome P-4503A metabolism results in higher serum levels of cyclosporine |

*continues on next page*

**TABLE 8–2.** *continued from previous page*

| Medication | Interaction | Mechanism/Management |
|---|---|---|
| Griseofulvin | Fatty food | Serum levels are double those of fasting state |
| Lovastatin | Food | Increased absorption |
| Nitrofurantoin | Food or milk | Increased absorption by 200–400%, most likely because of delayed gastric emptying, allowing increased time for dissolution |
| **Pharmacodynamic Interactions** | | |
| Warfarin | Food high in vitamin K | Exogenous vitamin K antagonizes the anticoagulant effect of warfarin |
| MAOI (phenelzine, tranylcypromine) | Tyramine-containing foods and beverages | Combination can result in hypertensive crisis and death due to tyramine buildup |
| **Others** | | |
| Antineoplastic agents | Food | Antineoplastics suppress appetite, resulting in decreased food intake and nutritional deficiency |
| Iron, folic acid, vitamin A, essential fatty acids | Cholestyramine, colestipol | Bile acid sequestrants can bind listed nutrients and prevent absorption |
| Enteral feedings | Phenytoin suspension, carbamazepine suspension, warfarin | Binding to components in the enteral formulation decreases absorption |

Sources: *Chiesora, Borghini, and Marabini (1995); D'Arcy (1995); Kirk (1995); and Yamreudeewong, Hennan, Fazio, Lower, and Cassidy (1995).*

of marijuana smoking affects the direction of the interaction. Inhibition of metabolism occurs within hours of use, while induction requires 10–14 days of regular use to occur. The potency of the marijuana, additional smoking of cigarettes, and concurrent alcohol consumption can also impact the interaction of marijuana with medications. For instance, marijuana increases the metabolism of theophylline (Hansten & Horn, 1993a; Yamamoto, Wantanabe, Narimatusu, & Yoshimura, 1995). Pharmacodynamic interactions also occur with marijuana. Anticholinergic agents (including tricyclic antidepressants) can produce additive increases in the heart rate, whereas propranolol tends to attenuate marijuana-induced tachycardia. Excessive marijuana use can impair glucose control in diabetics by an unknown mechanism. Combined use of alcohol with marijuana may result in additive perceptual, cognitive, and motor impairment.

Alcohol interacts with numerous medications (Hansten & Horn, 1993b). The combination of disulfiram with as little as 15 mL of alcohol can cause a disulfiram reaction (nausea, vomiting, headache, cutaneous flushing, vasodilation, respiratory difficulties, tachycardia, confusion, drowsiness, hypotension, shock, and even death).

The combination of alcohol and metronidazole or oral sulfonylureas (primarily chlorpropamide) can cause a mild disulfiram-like reaction. Alcohol, even in limited daily quantities, potentiates the hepatotoxicity of acetaminophen (Zimmerman & Maddrey, 1995). Cases of fatal hepatotoxicity have been reported with usual doses of acetaminophen (3–4 g/day) and limited alcohol intake in the presence of illness and reduced nutrition intake. Hepatic metabolism of drugs is modified by ethanol intake (Lieber, 1995). Acute binges inhibit the microsomal oxidative enzyme systems, impairing metabolism of barbiturates, chloral hydrate, tolbutamide, and warfarin. Chronic ethanol ingestion stimulates the microsomal enzymes of the liver and thus accelerates metabolism of the same drugs that acute binge drinking inhibits. Patients with alcoholic liver disease will have impaired liver metabolism (Morgan & McLean, 1995).

The effects of alcohol are additive with the pharmacodynamic effects of central nervous system depressants, including antihistamines, opiates, barbiturates, benzodiazepines, antipsychotics, and antidepressants. Alcohol can increase the gastric mucosal damage from aspirin and other NSAIDs. Additive hypoglycemic effects occur when acute alcohol intake is combined with insulin and oral hypoglycemics.

## CLINICAL OUTCOME

The outcome of a drug interaction is dependent on several factors: sequence of drug administration, duration of therapy with the combination, dose of the two drugs, other drugs taken by the patient, and the therapeutic index of the object drug (Hansten & Horn, 1996b). Adverse effects from a drug interaction are situational and may require a combination of factors to be present or occur at the same time. For example, a patient stabilized on cimetidine who is started on warfarin would not experience a problem unless the cimetidine dose was changed or the drug discontinued. Conversely, a patient on warfarin who is started on cimetidine without a decrease in warfarin dose may have a significant increase in prothrombin time due to metabolic inhibition of warfarin by the cimetidine.

## AVOIDING DRUG INTERACTIONS

When deciding whether an interaction from a drug combination is possible, current drug interaction texts should be consulted (see Chap. 7 for information on resources). When new drugs come to market, the adverse effects problem described earlier occurs in a similar manner with drug interactions. Drug interaction studies are sometimes conducted premarketing with the most likely interacting drugs (eg, a new drug is metabolized by a particular liver enzyme system; a study with known inhibitors of this system would be conducted) (Kuhlmann, 1994; Slaughter & Edwards, 1995). Unfortunately, the drug interaction studies are likely to have been conducted with healthy volunteers, which does not always reflect what will occur in patients. Also with new drugs, only drug-drug and possibly drug-disease interactions may be known prior to marketing. Drug-nutrient and drug–social habit interactions may not be discovered until a drug is in wide use.

Avoiding drug interactions begins with identifying patients at risk (ie, the patient is receiving warfarin, which is known to have significant interactions). Patients receiving medications with known interactions should be (1) educated about what medications and/or nonprescription medications to avoid and (2) warned always to notify any health care practitioner that they are taking potentially problematic medication. Patient records should also contain a warning. Once a pa-

tient is identified as being at risk for a drug interaction, appropriate precautions should be taken to minimize adverse consequences. Management strategies will depend on the type of interaction:

- Some combinations are absolutely contraindicated: monoamine oxidase (MAO) inhibitors and selective serotonin reuptake inhibitors (SSRI).
- Alternatives should be used with other combinations: theophylline and erythromycin—use a different antibiotic.
- Most absorption interactions can be easily managed by appropriate spacing of medications: separate antacid from ciprofloxacin by 2 h.
- Other interactions may require monitoring, although the drug combination does not need to be avoided: an antihypertensive and TCA (tricyclic antidepressant)—both can cause orthostatic hypotension, but this can be monitored.

## REFERENCES

Anastasio, G. D., Cornell, K. O., & Menscer, D. (1997). Drug Interactions: Keeping it straight. *American Family Physician, 56,* 883–895.

Anonymous. (1975). *Requirements for adverse reaction reporting.* Geneva: World Health Organization.

Atkin, P. A., & Shenfield, G. M. (1995). Medication-related adverse reactions and the elderly: A literature review. *Adverse Drug Reactions and Toxicological Reviews, 14,* 175–191.

Beard, K. (1992). Adverse drug reactions as a cause of hospital admission in the aged. *Drugs and Aging, 2,* 356–367.

Benjamin, D. M., & Buckman, R. W. (1996). Minimizing the risk of adverse drug interactions. *Female Patient, 21,* 47–61.

Beringer, P. M. & Middleton, R. K. (1993). Anaphylaxis and drug allergies. In L. E. Young & M. A. Koda-Kimble (Eds.), *Applied therapeutics.* Vancouver, WA: Applied Therapeutics, Inc.

Bigby, M., Jick, S., Jick, H., & Arndt, K. (1986). Drug-induced cutaneous reactions. A report from the Boston Collaborative Drug Surveillance Program on 15,438 consecutive inpatients, 1975 to 1982. *JAMA, 256,* 3358–3363.

Chiesara, E., Borghini, R., & Marabini, L. (1995). Dietary fibre and drug interactions. *European Journal of Clinical Nutrition, 49,* S123–S128.

D'Arcy, P. F. (1995). Nutrient-drug interactions. *Adverse Drug Reactions and Toxicological Reviews, 14,* 233–254.

Day, A. T. (1995). Adverse drug reactions and medical negligence. *Adverse Drug Reaction Bulletin, 172,* 651–654.

Department of Health and Human Services. (1985). New drug and antibiotic regulation: Section 314.80, post marketing reporting of adverse drug experiences. *Federal Register, 50*, 7500–7501.

Finley, P. R., Warner, M. D., & Peabody, C. A. (1995). Clinical relevance of drug interactions with lithium. *Clinical Pharmacokinetics, 29*, 172–191.

Garrelts, J. D., Godley, P. J., Peterie, J. D., Gerlach, E. H., Yakshe, C. C. (1990). Sucralfate significantly reduces ciprofloxacin concentrations in serum. *Antimicrobial Agents and Chemotherapy, 34*, 931–933.

Girard, M. (1987). Conclusiveness of rechallenge in the interpretation of adverse drug reactions. *British Journal of Clinical Pharmacology, 23*, 73–79.

Hansten, P. D., & Horn, J. R. (1996a). Cigarette smoking and drug interactions. *Drug Interactions Newsletter, 16*, 943–946.

Hansten, P. D., & Horn, J. R. (1996b). Drug interactions. *Drug Interactions Newsletter, 16*, 893–904.

Hansten, P. D., & Horn, J. R. (1993a). Effects of marijuana smoking on drug actions. *Drug Interactions Newsletter, 13*, 107–109.

Hansten, P. D., & Horn, J. R. (1993b). Ethanol drug interactions. *Drug Interactions Newsletter, 13*, 525–538.

Johnson, J. A., & Bootman, J. L. (1995). Drug-related morbidity and mortality. A cost-of-illness model. *Archives of Internal Medicine, 155*, 1949–1956.

Johnstone, D. M., Kirking, D. M., & Vison, B. E. (1995). Comparison of adverse drug reactions detected by pharmacy and medical records departments. *American Journal of Health-System Pharmacy, 52*, 297–301.

Kando, J. C., Yonker, K. A., & Cole, J. O. (1995). Gender as a risk factor for adverse events to medications. *Drugs, 50*(1), 1–6.

Kirk, J. K. (1995). Significant drug-nutrient interactions. *American Family Physician, 51*, 1175–1182.

Kuhlmann, J. (1994). Drug interaction studies during drug development: Which, when, how? *International Journal of Clinical Pharmacology and Therapeutics, 32*, 305–311.

Lee, M. (1996). Drugs and the elderly: Do you know the risks? *American Journal of Nursing, 96*, 25–31.

Lelawongs, P., Barone, J. A., Colaizzi, J. L., Hsuan, A. T., Mechlinski, W., Lejendre, R., & Guarnieri, J. (1988). Effect of food and gastric acidity on absorption of orally administered ketoconazole. *Clinical Pharmacy, 7*, 228.

Lieber, C. S. (1995). Medical disorders of alcoholism. *New England Journal of Medicine, 333*, 1058–1065.

McCloskey, B. A. (1996). Improving adverse drug reaction reporting in the community setting. *Medical Interface, May*, 85–87.

Morgan, D. J., & McLean, A. J. (1995). Clinical pharmacokinetic and pharmacodynamic considerations in patients with liver disease. An update. *Clinical Pharmacokinetics, 29*, 370–391.

Nelson, K. M., & Talbert, R. L. (1996). Drug-related hospital admissions. *Pharmacotherapy, 16*, 701–707.

Pearson, T. F., Pittman, D. G., Longley, J. M., Grapes, Z. T., Vigliotti, D. J., & Mullis, S. R. (1994). Factors associated with preventable adverse drug reactions. *American Journal of Hospital Pharmacy, 51*, 2268–2272.

Quinn, D. I., & Day, R. O. (1995). Drug interactions of clinical importance. An updated guide. *Drug Safety, 12*, 393–452.

Rieder, M. J. (1994). Mechanisms of unpredictable adverse drug reactions. *Drug Safety, 11*, 196–212.

Schein, J. R. (1995). Cigarette smoking and clinically significant drug interactions. *Annals of Pharmacotherapy, 29*, 1139–1148.

Schumock, G. T., & Thornton, J. P. (1992). Focusing on the preventability of adverse drug reactions. *Hospital Pharmacy, 27:*538.

Sills, J. M., Tanner, L. A., Milstien, J. B. (1986). Food and Drug Administration monitoring of adverse drug reactions. *American Journal of Hospital Pharmacy, 43*, 2764–2770.

Slaughter, R. L., & Edwards, D. J. (1995). Recent advances: The cytochrome P450 enzymes. *Annals of Pharmacotherapy, 29*, 619–624.

Sporer, K. A. (1995). The serotonin syndrome. Implicated drugs, pathophysiology and management. *Drug Safety, 13*, 94–104.

Thompson, D., & Oster, G. (1996). Use of terfenadine and contraindicated drugs. *JAMA, 275*, 1339–1341.

Van Arsdel, P. P., Jr. (1991). Classification and risk factors for drug allergy. *Immunology and Allergy Clinics of North America, 11*, 475–480.

Wells, P. S., Holbrook, A. M., & Crowther, N. R. (1994). Interactions of warfarin with drugs and food. *Annals of Internal Medicine, 121*, 676–683.

White, J. R., & Campbell, R. K. (1995). Drug/drug and drug/disease interactions and diabetes. *Diabetes Education, 21*, 283, 285–286.

Yamamoto, I., Wantanabe, K., Narimatusu, S., & Yoshimura, H. (1995). Recent advances in the metabolism of cannabinoids. *International Journal of Biochemistry and Cell Biology, 27*, 741–746.

Yamreudeewong, W., Hennann, N. E., Fazio, A. Lower, D. L., & Cassidy, T. G. (1995). Drug-food interactions in clinical practice. *Journal of Family Practice, 40*, 376–384.

Zimmerman, H. J., & Maddrey, W. C. (1995). Acetaminophen (paracetamol) hepatotoxicity with regular intake of alcohol: Analysis of instances of therapeutic misadventure. *Hepatology, 22*, 767–773.

# 9

# EVALUATING PATIENT SELF-CARE AND OVER-THE-COUNTER DRUGS

*Karen D. Rich*

## THE MEDICATION SELF-CARE MOVEMENT

Over the past decade, individuals increasingly have looked first to self-care management when confronted with changes in health. It is estimated that self-care, without physician intervention, accounts for the management of 70–95% of all illnesses (Vuckovic & Nichter, 1997). This growing trend in attitudes and beliefs has been referred to as the "self-care movement" (Holt & Hall, 1993). Coons (1990) defines self-care as "any activity initiated or performed by an individual to regain, maintain, or improve his or her health (or the health of family members and friends)." Numerous other labels have been attached to these activities including: symptom-motivated health-related activities, self-diagnosis, decision making regarding one's own health, and taking action to prevent, detect, treat, or rehabilitate health problems (Green, 1990; Holt & Hall, 1993; Segall, 1990; Sorofman, Tripp-Reimer, Lauer, & Martin, 1990) All these statements identify the patient as an active participant, if not the driver, in the health care system.

Self-care encompasses a wide variety of therapeutic modalities. These modalities range from doing nothing to changing activity level or dietary considerations; to using avoidance behaviors (ie, avoiding stress or alcohol), homemade preparations (ie, baths or salves) or appliances (ie, thermometers or heating pads), herbal or folk remedies, biofeedback or relaxation techniques, or nonprescription medications; to borrowing prescription medications from another individual or using leftovers from a previous illness (Segall, 1990; Stoller, Forster, & Portugal, 1993). Many of the factors contributing to the growing popularity of the self-care movement are listed in Table 9–1.

Most research on self-care has focused on prescription medication use, because of the difficulties in obtaining solid data on patient over-the-counter (OTC) medication use: (1) with unlimited access to nonprescription drugs, accurate data gathering is problematic; (2) it is hard to clearly assess morbidity from OTC drug use; and (3) sorting out the risk-to-benefit ratios of OTC medication use is complex due to the large variability in the way people use OTC drugs (Vickery, 1985).

## CONSUMER SOPHISTICATION AND EDUCATION

Individuals are becoming more educated regarding medical issues, partly because of increased media coverage of medical topics (Newton, Pray, & Popovich, 1994). An estimated 300,000 OTC products are available in the United States (Nonprescription Drug Manufacturers Association, 1996a), often in nonpharmacy venues (ie, grocery stores, gas stations, or convenience stores). This may leave the patient with the impression that OTC drugs are not "real" medications because no prescription is

## TABLE 9–1. FACTORS INFLUENCING THE TREND TOWARD SELF-CARE

- Rising costs of medical care
- Increased individual responsibility
- Rising education level in the general population
- Lack of available medical services
- Skepticism of medical care
- Desire to exercise self-control
- Desire to avoid contact with health professionals or lack of relationship with health provider
- Medication availability
- Impatience with illness due to loss of productivity
- Pharmaceutical advertising

Adapted from: Coons (1990) and Vuckovic and Nichter (1997).

required to obtain them (Henry, 1994) and they are so easily obtained.

Asking very specific questions regarding OTC drug use is important during the patient history and medication interview, something some health care practitioners may forget. At times this information can be key in diagnosing and resolving potential OTC drug-induced problems (Davies, Fattah, & Clee, 1994). Unless health care professionals inquire about OTC drug use routinely, most experiences they will have with patient self-directed OTC medication use will be when something negative happens (Vickery, 1985). This in turn may lead providers to doubt their patients' abilities to make self-care decisions and, thus, to not embrace the concept of patient self-care.

This lack of trust in patient decision-making capabilities has been challenged by several consumer surveys in recent years. In a compilation of 13 national consumer studies conducted by independent researchers over the past 15 years, the Nonprescription Drug Manufacturers Association (NDMA, 1996*b*) reports increased consumer sophistication. As evidence for this, the NDMA asserts that "Americans know when to take OTC medicines, how much to take, when to stop and when to seek professional help" (NDMA, 1996*a*). Specifically, the surveys reported that 93% of consumers read label directions prior to using a medication, that 80% of consumers always or often find OTC labels easy to understand, and that the majority of consumers use OTC drugs at doses well below the suggested maximum and well within the specified duration of treatment.

In clinical practice, practitioners are bound to find large variations in patient sophistication and health-related education. This patient-specific information should guide the clinician in working with the patient to identify the appropriate level of self-care versus health professional assistance needed. Table 9–2 lists the most common problems consumers report self-treating.

## DEMOGRAPHICS OF OTC DRUG USE

Since the elderly population is often associated with polypharmacy, several studies have evaluated the OTC medication practices of the elderly (Chrischilles et al, 1992; Conn, 1991; Delafuente, Meuleman, Conlin, Hoffman, & Lowenthal, 1992; Hershman, Simonoff, Frishman, Paston, & Aronson, 1995; Stoller et al, 1993). Conflicting results have emerged when trying to determine predictors for OTC drug use. The traditional prescription drug models do not accurately reflect nonprescription drug use in the elderly. One large study of prescription and nonprescription drug use in adults 65 years of age or older identified several significant factors in nonprescription drug use (Fillenbaum et al, 1993), namely, female sex, urban residence, younger age, more education, and poor self-rated and medical status. Another large study by Chrischilles et al (1992) of community-dwelling elderly individuals found similar results. Nonprescription drug use was positively correlated with female gender, former smokers, physical impairment, depressive symptoms, and poor self-perceived health status. In contrast, a cross-sectional study of community-dwelling elderly found the only predictors of

## TABLE 9–2. TOP 10 PROBLEMS CONSUMERS ARE LIKELY TO TREAT WITH OTC DRUGS

- Headache
- Athlete's foot
- Lip problems
- Common cold
- Chronic dandruff
- Premenstrual symptoms
- Menstrual symptoms
- Upset stomach
- Painful, dry skin
- Sinus problems

**Source:** Nonprescription Drug Manufacturers Association (1996*a*). Used with permission.

nonprescription drug use were an increased number of symptoms in the previous month, higher income, and living alone (Conn, 1991). Still another study found no correlation between gender or perceived health status and OTC drug use in the elderly (Hershman et al, 1995). Categories of OTC drug use most commonly reported by the elderly included vitamins and minerals, analgesics and antiinflammatories, laxatives, and antacids (Delafuente et al, 1992; Hershman et al, 1995).

A 1990 study by Green of self-care behaviors in college-age students found that the most common self-care modality used for minor illnesses was rest (32.8%), followed by self-medication (28.9%) and then physician visits (14.4%) A U.S. population-based survey of OTC drug use by more than 8,000 preschool-age children was conducted by Kogan, Pappas, Yu, and Kotelchuck (1994). During the survey, 70% of mothers who identified their children as being ill during the previous 30 days reported giving their children OTC medications. Overall, 53.7% of 3-year-olds in this study had received an OTC medication in the past 30 days.

## ACCESSIBILITY AND ADVERTISING

Accessibility and effective marketing are key motivators in encouraging patient self-care with OTC medications. Because nonprescription drugs are not bound by the same constraints as prescription medications, it is relatively easy for patients to obtain OTC drugs. It has been estimated that consumers can purchase nonprescription drugs from about ten times more locations than prescription drugs (Palumbo, 1991), since they are widely available at grocery stores, gas stations, convenience stores, and other nonpharmacy locations.

Another factor contributing to the use of OTC drugs by patients is the powerful effect of advertising by manufacturers. Advertisements for prescription drugs try to convince patients to visit their physicians or primary caregivers and request a specific drug. However, there is no guarantee that the practitioner will choose to prescribe that drug. Advertisements of OTC drugs, however, bypass the health care provider and must persuade only the patient to purchase the drug (Gossel, 1991, Palumbo, 1991). Advertising costs may account for up to 40% of the purchase price of some OTC products, especially if the therapeutic category has a variety of competitive products from which the patient may select (Smith, 1996).

Negative advertising has become more widely used to persuade consumers to purchase one product over another as the therapeutic categories become inundated with choices. Advertisers try to focus on a competitor's side-effect profile and enhance consumer fear of a product. One example of this was the 1996 television ad campaigns by the makers of Tylenol and Advil (Holt, 1996). McNeil Consumer Products—makers of Tylenol—emphasized the risks hypertensive or peptic ulcer disease patients may be subject to when taking Advil, while Whitehall-Robins—makers of Advil—focused on the alcohol warning label on Tylenol and potential liver failure as reasons for choosing Advil over Tylenol.

## OTC DRUG USE AND HEALTH CARE COSTS

Probably the greatest driving force behind the promotion of self-care and OTC drug use is the desire to lower health care costs. Data from independent researchers indicates that OTC drugs accounted for less than 2% of total U.S. health care expenditures during 1995. Approximately $16 billion was spent on nonprescription drugs out of the estimated $1 trillion spent on health care (NDMA, 1996a). After the switch of 0.5% hydrocortisone from prescription to nonprescription status in 1979, an estimated $600 million was saved by U.S. patients (Temin, 1983). The implied cost savings of OTC drug use come from a combination of fewer practitioner office visits, reduced prescription expenses, less time lost from work (time spent at practitioner office visits or picking up prescriptions), less travel, and an increased number of OTC drug users (Andersson, 1995; Gossel, 1991; Holt & Hall, 1993) A typical nonprescription medication can be purchased for an average of $4, while a physician visit adds an average of $40 plus a prescription medication of around $25 (NDMA, 1996a). The NDMA projects that by the year 2000, $34 billion will be saved because of increased OTC drug use (Smith, 1996).

## OTC DRUG USE AND HEALTH CARE PLANS

Insurance coverage, or lack thereof, is an increasingly important determinant in patient access to health care. Patients without adequate insurance coverage or access to health care for other reasons may choose to self-treat with OTC drugs out of necessity. Additionally, encouragement of OTC drug use may benefit patients participating in health care plans with capitated prescription reimbursement. This is particularly true for patients with chronic conditions, where it is likely that the maximum limit will be reached during a coverage period.

On the other hand, most health care plans do not cover OTC medications. Patients with prescription drug insurance coverage may be reluctant to purchase OTC medications if the after-insurance cost of the prescription medication is lower than the price of an OTC drug (Snyder, 1996b). In one study, patients with the most comprehensive Medicare coverage were 10–15% more likely to select a prescription drug over OTC alternatives (Stuart & Grana, 1995). The same principle applies to patients receiving Medicaid. Patients may be reluctant to purchase an OTC drug that may cost more than the average copayment (Snyder, 1996a). A 1995 study by Gurwitz, McLaughlin, & Fish showed significant cost savings to an HMO due to the prescription-to-OTC switch of vaginal antifungal products. This cost savings was attributed to fewer physician visits and a reduction in medication costs for the HMO. However, one question raised by this study concerns the true economic benefits to the patients when the cost of the medication is shifted to the patient from the HMO. Ensuring that the patient does not pay more for the OTC drug than he or she would for a prescription copayment will be key to encouraging increased use of OTC drugs in the future (Muirhead, 1995).

# REGULATION OF OTC DRUGS

## FOOD AND DRUG ADMINISTRATION APPROVAL PROCESS

The 1938 Federal Food, Drug and Cosmetic (FD&C) Act was the first legislation to require that manufacturers prove the safety of their products for humans (references used in this section were Gilbertson, 1993; Gossel, 1991). The act required that products be cleared through a new drug application (NDA) prior to marketing. The act also required proper labeling and instructions for use. This legislation had been under consideration for several years, but was finally enacted after the deaths of more than

100 people due to the use of the toxic solvent ethylene glycol in a newly formulated sulfanilamide elixir (U.S. Food and Drug Administration, 1977).

Several amendments were made to the 1938 FD&C Act. The 1951 Durham-Humphrey Amendment [*Federal Food, Drug and Cosmetic Act*, Section 503(b), 21 USC 353(b)] provided criteria for drugs that must be limited to prescription-only use, for separating prescription and nonprescription drugs into two distinct classes, and for requiring adequate labeling instructions. The 1962 Kefauver-Harris Amendment (*Federal Food, Drug and Cosmetic Act*, Section 505, 21 USC 355.32) was key in requiring manufacturers to prove effectiveness for intended uses as well as the safety of drugs prior to approval. It also required review of all drugs approved between 1938–1962 to ensure they met the efficacy standards set by the amendment. A review of prescription medications was conducted in the 1960s by a procedure called the Drug Efficacy Study Implementation (DESI). Near the end of that review, it was determined that nonprescription medications also needed extensive review. Due to the massive number of OTC products available (approximately 300,000), the FDA decided to evaluate OTC products by active ingredient (approximately 700), subdivided by therapeutic category; see Table 9–3. This review is formally known as the OTC drug review and was begun in 1972.

# THE OTC DRUG REVIEW

The OTC drug review is a three-phase process: (1) advisory panel review, (2) tentative final monograph publication, and (3) final monograph publication. The results of each phase are published in the *Federal Register*. Phases 2 and 3 are still ongoing. The ultimate goal of this rule-making process is to establish standards for active ingredients (as opposed to new drug applications, which evaluate final dosage forms) and labeling OTC products in each therapeutic category.

## Phase I

This phase lasted about one decade and involved over 300 individuals who served on advisory panels. The advisory panels classified active ingredients into one of three categories upon review:

## TABLE 9–3.  PRODUCT CATEGORIES BY WHICH THE FDA IS REVIEWING OTC DRUG INGREDIENTS

Acne
Anorectal
Antacid
Anthelmintic
Anticaries
Antidiarrheal
Antiemetic
Antiflatulent
Antifungal
   Diaper rash[a]
Antimicrobials
  Alcohol (topical)
  Antibiotics, first aid
  Antiseptics (topical)
  Diaper rash[a]
  Mercurials
Antiperspirant
Aphrodisiac
Benign prostatic hypertrophy
Boil ointments
Camphorated oil
Cholecystokinetic
Corn/callus removers
Cough/cold/allergy
  bronchodilator/antiasthmatic
    combinations
  Anticholinergic
  Antihistamine
  Antitussive
  Bronchodilator
  Expectorant
  Nasal decongestant
Dandruff/seborrhea/psoriasis
Daytime sedative
Deodorants (int.)
Digestive aids
Exocrine pancreatic insufficiency
External analgesic
  Astringents (wet dressings)[b]
  Diaper rash[a]
  Fever blister/cold sore (external)[b]
  Insect bites and stings
  Male genital desensitizers
  Poison (ivy/oak/sumac)
    treatment/prevention[b]

Fever blister/cold sore (internal)
Hair grower/loss
Hexachlorophene
Hormone (topical)
Hypo/hyperphosphatemia
Ingrown toenail relief
Insect repellents (internal)
Internal analgesic
   Leg muscle cramps
Laxative
Menstrual products
Nailbiting/thumbsucking deterrents
Nighttime sleep-aid
Ophthalmic products
Oral health care
Oral mucosal injury
Overindulgence remedies
   Ingredients intended to minimize or prevent
   inebriation
Pediculicides
Poison treatment
  Antidotes—toxic ingestion
  Emetics
Relief of oral discomfort
Salicylanilides (TBS)
Skin bleaching
Skin protectant
  Astringents (wet dressings)[b]
  Diaper rash[a]
  Fever blister/cold sore (external)[b]
  Insect bites and stings[b]
  Poison (ivy/oak/sumac) treatment/prevention[b]
Smoking deterrent
Stimulant
Stomach acidifier
Sunscreen
Sweet spirits of nitre
Topical otic (earwax)
Topical otic (swimmer's ear)
Vaginal contraceptive
Vaginal drug products
Vitamin/mineral
Wart remover
Weight control

[a]See also antimicrobials, external analgesics, and skin protectants.
[b]See also skin protectants.
*Source: Gilbertson (1993).*

- *Category I:* Generally recognized as safe and effective (GRASE) for the claimed therapeutic indication.
- *Category II:* Not generally recognized as safe and effective (NRASE) or having unacceptable indications.
- *Category III:* Insufficient data available to permit final classification.

The panels also recommended labeling instructions. In the end, the review panels summarized their recommendations and submitted 58 reports to the Food and Drug Administration (FDA). These were published in the *Federal Register* to give notice of proposed rulemaking and to invite public comment.

## Phase II

The second phase, tentative final monograph publication, is where the FDA reviews the recommendations from the review panels, public comment, or newly available data and then publishes a proposed rule in the *Federal Register*. Once again, time is allowed for public comments, hearings, or objections.

## Phase III

The last phase, final monograph publication, is the point at which the FDA publishes its final rule after considering all new information since the tentative final monograph. The final rule is then published in the *Code of Federal Regulations*. Usually the rule is considered to be in effect 1 year after publication in the *Federal Register*. At this point, all manufacturers must comply with regulations. New OTC products do not require submission of an NDA if they meet the regulations of the final monograph for that particular active ingredient.

## Impact of the Review

The OTC drug review has had a significant impact on the availability of some active ingredients. All in all, the OTC drug review examined 722 active ingredients. Counting multiple therapeutic claims for some ingredients, a total of 1454 ingredients promoted for specific uses were evaluated. Of the 1454 ingredients, the FDA first banned 233 substances as active ingredients across 19 different therapeutic classes as of May 7, 1991 (*Clinical Pharmacy*, 1991). In 1993 the FDA removed an additional 415 substances across seven different therapeutic classes (Gilbertson, 1993).

## PRESCRIPTION-TO-OTC STATUS RECLASSIFICATION

The OTC drug review has been responsible for the reclassification of over 40 prescription drugs to OTC status since the review began. The 1951 Durham-Humphrey Amendment defined three different criteria limiting drugs to prescription-only use [*Federal Food, Drug and Cosmetic Act*, Section 503(b), 21 USC 353(b)]:

- Habit-forming agents (listed specifically in the act)
- Drugs not safe for use except under the supervision of a licensed practitioner because of toxicity or other collateral measures necessary to use
- NDA which limits drug to prescription-only use

Currently, the second criteria probably has the most impact as agents are brought forward for potential reclassification. The criteria the FDA relies upon when considering a drug for prescription-to-OTC status switch include a high margin of safety (low potential for toxicity, low potential for misuse or abuse, low risk-to-benefit ratio), consideration of whether the condition is self-diagnosable and self-treatable, and adequate labeling (directions, warnings, ability of patient to comprehend instructions). There are currently four different mechanisms by which a drug may be reclassified as an OTC drug (see as shown in Figure 9–1). The most common mechanism by which drugs are reclassified currently is through filing a supplemental NDA (mechanism 3).

- *Mechanism 1:* Filing a new NDA for a currently prescription-only drug
- *Mechanism 2:* "Switch regulation": filing a petition to exempt a prescription drug from prescription requirements
- *Mechanism 3:* Filing a supplemental NDA for OTC status for a drug currently restricted to prescription-only use
- *Mechanism 4:* OTC drug review process

Many parties benefit from reclassification of prescription drugs to OTC status. Manufacturers benefit when a patent expiration is pending since reclassifying an agent to OTC status extends the life of the drug. Consumers benefit from a wider selection of agents to assist them in self-care as well as the potential cost savings for reasons discussed previously. This is especially true for the new classes of drugs recently making the prescription-to-OTC switch (ie, $H_2$ antagonists and vaginal yeast preparations). And practitioners can spend less time treating less se-

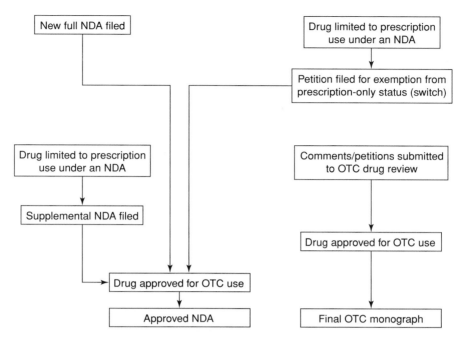

**Figure 9–1.** Mechanisms for reclassifying prescription drugs to OTC

**Source:** Gilbertson (1993).

rious patient care problems, and devote more time to serious problems. Table 9–4 lists the drugs switched from prescription to OTC status since 1975.

One market research firm predicts that future growth in the OTC market will be largely due to prescription-to-OTC status switches. Growth will develop from the actual switches as well as extension lines around that product (Snyder, 1995). As the OTC market grows, consideration of potential problems associated with OTC medication use must be considered.

## POTENTIAL PROBLEMS WITH OTC DRUG USE

### IMPROPER USE

Though OTC drug use has many positive aspects, most notably reduction in health care costs and ease of access and availability to the patient, there are also potential drawbacks. Of greatest concern is that patients will use the drugs improperly or for improper indications. Improper drug use may potentially harm the

patient, cause a delay in the patient seeking treatment for a serious underlying condition, or interact adversely with other drugs or substances the patient is taking. The potential for harm is especially worrisome for the patient who perceives OTC medications as completely safe and without any potential for side effects or harm because of their nonprescription status. Although OTC medications are reviewed rigorously to ensure a high safety margin, even OTC medications can have severe side effects if used improperly (Cetaruk & Aaron, 1994). Rebound headache caused by chronic, improper OTC analgesic use is one example of the consequences of improper use (Elkind, 1991).

### LACK OF COUNSELING

A consumer survey in 1995 by the consulting firm Kline & Co. reported that 60% of individuals surveyed reported relying on professional advice to select an OTC product (Griffle, 1995). Although this indicates that a majority of patients request assistance in the selection of OTC drugs, there is still a large percentage who

## TABLE 9–4. INGREDIENTS AND DOSAGES TRANSFERRED FROM RX-TO-OTC STATUS BY THE FOOD AND DRUG ADMINISTRATION SINCE 1975

| Ingredient | Adult Dosage | Product Category | Date of OTC Approval | Product Examples |
|---|---|---|---|---|
| 1. Brompheniramine maleate | 4 mg/4–6 h (oral) | Antihistamine | September 9, 1976 | Dimetane (A. H. Robins) |
| 2. Chlorpheniramine maleate | 4 mg/4–6 h (oral) | Antihistamine | September 9, 1976 | Allerest (Pharmacraft), Chlor-Trimeton (Schering), Contac (SmithKline), Sudafed Plus (Warner-Lambert) |
| 3. Oxymetazoline hydrochloride | 0.05% aqueous solution (topical) | Nasal decongestant | September 9, 1976 | Afrin (Schering), Duration (Plough), Dristan Long Lasting (Whitehall), Neo-Synephrine 12 Hour (Bayer) |
| 4. Pseudoephedrine hydrochloride | 60 mg/4 or 4–6 h (oral) 240 mg max/24 h | Nasal decongestant | September 9, 1976 | Sudafed (Warner-Lambert), Neo-Synephrinol (Bayer) |
| 5. Pseudoephedrine sulfate | 60 mg/4 or 4–6 h (oral) | Nasal decongestant | September 9, 1976 | Afrinol (Schering), Chlor-Trimeton (Schering) |
| 6. Xylometazoline hydrochloride | 0.01% aqueous solution (topical) | Nasal decongestant | September 9, 1976 | Orrivin (Ciba) |
| 7. Doxylamine succinate (NDA) | 25-mg single dose only (oral) | Sleep aid | October 18, 1978 | Unisom (Pfizer) |
| 8. Hydrocortisone | 0.25–0.50% (topical) | Antipruritic (antiitch) | December 4, 1979+ | Cortaid (Upjohn), Lanacort (Combe) |
| 9. Hydrocortisone acetate | 0.25–0.50% (topical) | Antipruritic (antiitch) | December 4, 1979+[a] | Bactine (Miles), Caldecort (Pharmacraft) |
| 10. Acidulated phosphate fluoride rinse | 0.02% fluoride in aqueous solution | Dental rinse | March 28, 1980 | |
| 11. Sodium fluoride rinse | 0.05% aqueous solution (topical) | Dental rinse | March 28, 1980 | Flourigard (Colgate-Palmolive) |
| 12. Stannous fluoride gel | 0.4% gel (topical) | Anticaries gel | March 28, 1980 | Gelkam Gel (Colgate-Palmolive) |
| 13. Stannous fluoride rinse | 0.1% aqueous solution (topical) | Dental rinse | March 28, 1980 | Stan Care (Block) |
| 14. Ephedrine sulfate | 0.1–1.25% (topical) | Anorectal/vasoconstrictor | May 27, 1980 | Pazo Ointment (Bristol-Myers) |
| 15. Epinephrine hydrochloride | 0.005–0.01% (topical) | Anorectal/vasoconstrictor | May 27, 1980 | |
| 16. Phenylephrine hydrochloride | 0.25% (topical) | Anorectal/vasoconstrictor | May 27, 1980 | |
| 17. Chlorpheniramine maleate (NDA) | 12 mg/12 h (oral timed-release) | Antihistamine | July 23, 1981 | Triaminic 12 (Sandoz) |
| 18. Phenylpropanolamine hydrochloride (NDA) | 75 mg/12 h (oral timed-release) | Nasal decongestant | July 23, 1981 | Triaminic 12 (Sandoz) |

| # | Drug | Dosage | Category | Approval Date | Product (Company) |
|---|------|--------|----------|---------------|-------------------|
| 19. | Diphenhydramine hydrochloride (NDA) | 25 mg/4 h (oral) | Antitussive | August 7, 1981 | Benylin (Parke-Davis) |
| 20. | Haloprogin | 1.0% (topical) | Antifungal | March 23, 1982 | Micatin (Ortho) |
| 21. | Miconazole nitrate | 2.0% (topical) | Antifungal | March 23, 1982 | Micatin (Ortho) |
| 22. | Diphenhydramine hydrochloride | 50-mg single dose only (oral) | Sleep aid | April 23, 1982 | Sominex 2 (Beecham), Sleep-eze 3 (Whitehall) |
| 23. | Diphenhydramine monocitrate | 76-mg single dose only (oral) | Sleep aid | April 23, 1982 | Excedrin PM (Bristol-Myers) |
| 24. | Dyclonine hydrochloride | 0.05–0.1% solution or suspension, 1–3 mg as lozenge | Oral anesthetic | May 25, 1982 | Sucrets Maximum Strength (SmithKline) |
| 25. | Dexbrompheniramine maleate (NDA) | 6 mg/12 h (oral timed-release) | Antihistamine | September 3, 1982 | Drixoral (Schering) |
| 26. | Pseudoephedrine sulfate (NDA) | 120 mg/12 h (oral timed-release) | Nasal decongestant | September 3, 1982 | Afrinol Repetabs (Schering) |
| 27. | Triprolidine hydrochloride | 2.5 mg/4–6 h | Antihistamine | November 26, 1982 | Actifed Capsules (Warner-Lambert), Actidil Syrup and Capsules (Warner-Lambert) |
| 28. | Tioconazole (NDA) | 1% cream | Antifungal | February 18, 1983 | TZ-3 (Pfizer) |
| 29. | Ibuprofen (NDA) | 200 mg/4–6 h (oral) | Internal analgesic/antipyretic | May 18, 1984 | Advil (Whitehall), Nuprin (Bristol-Myers) |
| 30. | Dexbrompheniramine maleate | 2 mg/4–6 h (oral) | Antihistamine | January 15, 1985 | Drixoral (Schering) |
| 31. | Diphenhydramine hydrochloride | 25–50 mg/4–6 h (oral) | Antihistamine | January 15, 1985 | Benadryl 25 (Warner-Lambert) |
| 32. | Pseudoephedrine hydrochloride (NDA) | 120 mg/12 h (oral timed-release) | Nasal decongestant | June 17, 1985 | Actifed (Warner-Lambert) |
| 33. | Triprolidine hydrochloride (NDA) | 5 mg/12 h | Antihistamine | June 17, 1985 | Actifed 12-hour Capsules (Warner-Lambert) |
| 34. | Oxymetazoline hydrochloride (NDA) | 0.025% solution/drops (topical) | Ocular vasoconstrictor | May 30, 1986 | Ocuclear (Schering) |
| 35. | Pyrantel pamoate | 11 mg/kg of body weight; maximum dose 1 g (oral) | Anthelmintic | August 1, 1986 | Antiminth (Pfizer) |
| 36. | Povidone iodine sponge (NDA) | 10% (new dosage form) | Antimicrobial | January 7, 1987 | E-Z Scrub 241 (Deseret) |
| 37. | Diphenhydramine hydrochloride | 25–50 mg/4–6 h (oral) | Antiemetic | April 30, 1987 | |
| 38. | Dexbrompheniramine maleate (NDA) | 3 mg/6–8 h (oral) | Antihistamine | May 22, 1987 | Drixoral Plus (Schering) |

*continues on next page*

**TABLE 9-4.** *continued from previous page*

| Ingredient | Adult Dosage | Product Category | Date of OTC Approval | Product Examples |
|---|---|---|---|---|
| 39. Chlophedianol hydrochloride | 25 mg/6–8 h (oral) | Antitussive | August 12, 1987 | Nyquil (Procter & Gamble) |
| 40. Doxylamine succinate | 7.5–12.5 mg/4–6 h (oral) | Antihistamine | August 24, 1987 | |
| 41. Loperamide (NDA) | 4 mg, then 2mg, 8 mg/day (oral) | Antidiarrheal | March 3, 1988 | Imodium A-D (Johnson & Johnson) |
| 42. Hydrogenated soybean oil and lecithin | 12.4 g powder in 2–3 oz water 20 min before gall bladder x-rays | Cholecystokinetic | February 28, 1989 | Liposperse (Merck) |
| 43. Clotrimazole (NDA) | 1% lotion and cream/2 times daily | Antifungal | October 23, 1989 | Lotrimin AF (Schering) |
| 44. Permethrin (NDA) | 1% cream rinse | Pediculicide (head lice) | May 5, 1990 | Nix (Warner-Lambert) |
| 45. Clotrimazole (NDA) | 1% cream and 100-mg inserts | Anticandidal | November 30, 1990 | Gyne-Lotrimin (Schering), Mycelex-7 (Miles) |
| 46. Miconazole nitrate | 2.0% cream and 100-mg inserts | Anticandidal | March 13, 1991 | Monistat 7 (Ortho) |
| 47. Hydrocortisone | Above 0.50–1.0% | Antipruritic (antiitch) | August 30, 1991[a] | |
| 48. Hydrocortisone acetate | Above 0.50%–1.0% | Antipruritic (antiitch) | August 30, 1991[a] | |
| 49. Clemastine fumarate (NDA) | 1.34 mg/12 h | Antihistamine | August 21, 1992 | Tavist-1 (Sandoz Consumer) |
| 50. Clemastine fumarate [in combination with phenylpropanolamine HCl (NDA)] | 1.34 mg/12 h | Antihistamine/decongestant | August 21, 1992 | Tavist-D (Sandoz Consumer) |
| 51. Dexchlorpheniramine maleate | 2 mg/4–6 h (oral) | Antihistamine | December 9, 1992 | |
| 52. Naproxen sodium (NDA) | 200 mg/4–6 h (oral) | Internal analgesic/antipyretic | January 11, 1994 | Aleve (Procter & Gamble) |
| 53. Pheniramine maleate with naphazoline HCl (NDA) | 0.3%; 0.025% in solution | Ophthalmic antihistamine/decongestant | June 8, 1994 | Naphcon A (Alcon), Opcon A (Bausch & Lomb), Ocuhist (Akorn) |
| 54. Antazoline phosphate with naphazoline HCl (NDA) | 0.5%; 0.05% in solution | Ophthalmic antihistamine/decongestant | July 11, 1994 | Vasocon A (Ciba) |
| 55. Famotidine (NDA) | 10 mg, up to 20mg/day | Acid reducer | April 28, 1995 | Pepcid AC (J&J Merck) |
| 56. Ibuprofen suspension 100mg/5mL for pediatric use (NDA) | 7.5 mg/kg up to 4 times a day | Internal analgesic/antipyretic | June 16, 1995 | Children's Motrin (McNeil Consumer) |
| 57. Cimetidine (NDA) | 200 mg up to twice per day | Acid reducer | June 19, 1995 | Tagamet HB (SmithKline) |

| | Drug | Dosage/Form | Indication | Date | Brand (Manufacturer) |
|---|---|---|---|---|---|
| 58. | Ketoprofen (NDA) | 12.5 mg/4–6 h | Internal analgesic | October 16, 1995 | Orudis KT (Whitehall-Robins), Actron (Bayer) |
| 59. | Ranitidine (NDA) | 75 mg up to twice per day | Acid reducer | December 19, 1995 | Zantac 75 (Warner Wellcome) |
| 60. | Butoconazole nitrate (NDA) | 2.0% cream and applicators (3 days) | Anticandidal | December 26, 1995 | Femstat 3 (Procter & Gamble) |
| 61. | Minoxidil (NDA) | 2.0% topical solution | Hair grower | February 9, 1996 | Rogaine (Pharmacia & Upjohn) |
| 62. | Nicotine polacrilex (NDA) | 2-mg and 4-mg gum | Smoking cessation | February 9, 1996 | Nicorette (SmithKline Beecham) |
| 63. | Nizatidine (NDA) | 75 mg up to twice daily | Acid reducer | May 9, 1996 | AXID AR (Whitehall-Robins Healthcare) |
| 64. | Miconazole nitrate (NDA) | 2.0% cream and 200-mg inserts | Anticandidal | April 16, 1996 | Monistat 3 (Ortho) |
| 65. | Nicotine transdermal system (NDA) | 15-mg patch | Smoking cessation | July 3, 1996 | Nicotrol (McNeil Consumer) |
| 66. | Clotrimazole (NDA)[b] | 1% cream and 200-mg inserts | Anticandidal | July 29, 1996 | Gyne-Lotrimin 3 (Schering-Plough) |
| 67. | Nicotine transdermal system (NDA) | 21-, 14-, and 7-mg patch | Smoking cessation | August 2, 1996 | Nicoderm CQ (SmithKline Beecham) |
| 68. | Bentoquatam (NDA)[b] | 5% lotion | Poison ivy protection | August 26, 1996 | Ivy Block (EnviroDerm) |
| 69. | Cromolyn sodium | 4% nasal solution | Allergy prevention and treatment | January 6, 1997 | Nasalcrom (McNeil Consumer) |
| 70. | Tioconazole | 6.5% vaginal ointment | Anticandidal | February 11, 1997 | Vagistat-1 (Bristol-Myers Squibb) |

[a]FDA approval for OTC marketing is on an interim basis pending adoption of a Final Monograph.
[b]New OTC NDA–Not previously Rx.
NDA = new drug application.
Source: Nonprescription Drug Manufacturers Association, February 1997. Used with permission.

do not consult a health care professional about the use of OTC medications. For those patients who may rely solely on the manufacturer (via package labeling) for information about proper use, the necessary instructions may not be adequately communicated, as one study showed when reviewing manufacturer instructions to patients for use of OTC eyedrops (Kabongo, 1993). Given their training and availability, pharmacists make ideal candidates for OTC medication consultation. Unfortunately, such counseling on OTC medications may not take place since the drugs are often physically separated from the prescription drug dispensing area and are available in a variety of nonpharmacy venues. One study asserts that pharmacy consultations regarding OTC drugs may influence patient decision making. In this study, a pharmacy consultant was available for patients in the OTC drug aisles. Forty percent of patients changed their minds about drug selection after the interaction; 25.4% of patients purchased a different item than originally intended; 1.3% were referred to a physician; and 13.4% decided not to purchase any OTC medication after consultation (Nichol, McCombs, Johnson, Spacapan, & Sclar, 1992). Although the limitations of the study do not allow for direct attribution of the changes in patient decisions to the pharmacy consultant interaction, the study does make a strong argument for the potential for significant patient benefit from increased access to pharmacists when making OTC drug purchases.

## LABELING CONCERNS

The FDA requires label instructions to be "stated in terms that are likely to be read and understood by the average consumer, including those of low comprehension under customary conditions of purchase and use" [*Federal Food, Drug and Cosmetic Act*, Section 502(c), 21 USC 352(c)]. The NDMA compilation of nationwide surveys by independent research firms suggests that patients read labels at the time of purchase or before first use over 90% of the time (NDMA, 1996*b*). In addition, 87–90% of patients reportedly understand the information on the label. However, a 1992 study by Holt and colleagues questioned the validity of the latter assertion. Over 300 patients were given a survey form with examples of different label instructions and asked to explain how they would take

the medications. No verbal instructions or explanations were given in order to simulate circumstances under which many patients obtain nonprescription drugs. High variability in patient response was found to such simple instructions as "Take 1 tablet 3 times daily" or "Take 1 tablet twice daily," particularly with regard to hourly spacing throughout the day. This example illustrates the risk health professionals run by thinking that patients will necessarily interpret instructions the way the health care provider intends them. Functional reading ability does not necessarily guarantee comprehension or understanding (Palumbo, 1991). Verbal counseling in addition to written counseling is needed in many cases for proper patient understanding.

Product line extensions introduce another hazard in OTC use recommendations by health practitioners. Expanding a product line capitalizes on the popularity of a particular product by using the same name in new products (ie, Tylenol P.M. or Robitussin-DM). However, the new products do not always contain the main ingredient found in the original product. Patients and health care practitioners may inadvertently select an inappropriate agent for the patient because of this practice (Newton et al, 1994; Rupp & Parker, 1993). Table 9–5 illustrates this point with one OTC product line. Several suggestions have been made to decrease OTC selection confusion, such as that manufacturers limit product line extensions unless a specific patient need will be satisfied, restrict the use of brand names to products containing the active ingredients, and adopt a standard nomenclature for suffixes used in product line extensions (Rupp et al, 1993). The FDA has been evaluating the "user friendliness" of patient labeling for both readability and ease of comprehension (Rosendahl, 1995). Increased flexibility in wording and uniform, easier-to-read label formats are expected changes in the future.

## DELAY IN OBTAINING NEEDED TREATMENT

Delaying needed treatment because of OTC drug use can be a real concern, particularly with some health conditions. Reports of severe illness and detrimental effects of delays in treatment by physicians have ranged from untreated pelvic inflammatory disease caused by use of OTC vaginal yeast infection products (Kabongo, 1993) to a perforated eardrum being treated with OTC

## TABLE 9–5. ROBITUSSIN PRODUCTS

| Product | Active Ingredients |
| --- | --- |
| Robitussin | Guaifenesin 100 mg/5 mL |
| Robitussin-CF | Guaifenesin 100 mg/5 mL<br>Phenylpropanolamine HC 12.5 mg/5 mL<br>Dextromethorphan hB 10 mg/5 mL |
| Robitussin-DM | Guaifenesin 100 mg/5 mL<br>Dextromethorphan Hbr 10 mg/5 mL |
| Robitussin Night Relief | Pseudoephedrine Hcl 10 mg/5 mL<br>Pyrilamine maleate 8.3 mg/5 mL<br>Dextromethorphan Hbr 5 mg/5 mL |
| Robitussin-PE | Guaifenesin 100 mg/5 mL<br>Pseudoephedrine Hcl 30 mg/5 mL |
| Robitussin Pediatric | Dextromethorphan 7.5 mg/5 mL |
| Robitussin Pediatric Cough & Cold | Dextromethorphan 7.5 mg/5 mL<br>Pseudoephedrine HCl 15 mg/5 mL |

*Source: Drug Facts & Comparisons (1997).*

earwax drops (Bennet & McFarlane, 1992). In one survey of 138 physician members of a practice group composed of family physicians, obstetricians, and gynecologists, 24% indicated that reclassification of vaginal yeast infection preparations to OTC status was a positive change, 19% indicated the reclassification was a negative change, and 57% reported no impact of the reclassification on their practices. However, only 8.2% of the physicians estimated that none of their patients had delayed treatment for a bacterial or viral infection during the preceding year because of OTC yeast product use. Each of the remaining physicians reported anywhere from 1 to more than 11 occasions during the preceding year when patients had delayed treatment for a nonyeast infection because of OTC use of vaginal preparations (Tylor & Lipsky, 1994). This illustrates the difficulty a patient may have in properly self-diagnosing some problems, especially when symptoms may be nonspecific or, as in this case, when the patients could not differentiate between types of vaginitis (Schaff, Perez-Stable, & Borchardt, 1990). Pharmacists have also reported concern over patients misdiagnosing themselves. One pharmacist reported experience with elderly patients diagnosing themselves as having an ulcer and trying to purchase an OTC $H_2$ antagonist when their chief complaint on questioning was chest pain (Slezak, 1996).

## GUIDELINES FOR APPROPRIATE USE OF OTC DRUGS

OTC medications are appropriate for many conditions, including to treat symptoms of minor, self-limiting illnesses; to prevent a disease or disorder (ie, aspirin to prevent stroke); to manage chronic conditions [ie, nonsteroidal antiinflammatory drugs (NSAIDs) for arthritis]; or to cure certain conditions (ie, vaginal yeast infections) (Holt & Hall, 1993). OTC medications can also significantly reduce health care costs. Self-care measures, particularly nonprescription drug use, should be recognized as an important part of the overall health status of the patient by both health care providers and patients alike. A thorough history of OTC drug use should be obtained during the patient visit. Utilizing a review-of-systems approach has been advocated to help prompt patients to divulge information regarding OTC drug use (Holden, 1992; Ponte, 1990).

Patients may pay significantly more for a brand name product because of advertisement costs (Smith, 1996). With many generic versions of most OTC products available, practitioners can help reduce patient costs by suggesting an equivalent generic product in place of a branded one or recommend that the patient consult with the pharmacist when selecting a product.

Although the FDA is currently examining labeling practices, do not assume that the patient will receive adequate instructions on OTC drug use simply by reading the label. It is important to counsel patients on the appropriate use of OTC medications as well as prescription medications. According to a 1992 study by Holt et al, patients seemed to best interpret the correct responses to instructions that were given with specific hourly intervals (ie, "every 12 hours" instead of "twice a day"). Although the profession of pharmacy has placed greater emphasis in recent years on increasing patient counseling both for prescription and OTC medications, the wide access of OTC medications to the patient may preclude a pharmacist-patient interaction. Thus, the health care provider needs to counsel the patient on recommended OTC use at the time of the visit. To maximize the benefits of OTC use and decrease the likelihood of adverse events, the following should be emphasized in the counseling process:

- Reason for self-treatment
- Description of drug or treatment
- Proper administration of drug or treatment
- Potential side effects and precautions
- Normal response time and what to do if the desired response does not occur

As with all other facets of health care, the practitioner must use discretion in the recommendation of OTC drugs based upon the perceived level of patient sophistication and education and the seriousness of the condition being treated.

## REFERENCES

Andersson, F. (1995). Why is the pharmaceutical industry investing increasing amounts in health economic evaluations? *International Journal of Technology Assessment in Health Care, 11*(4), 750–761.

Bennett, J. D., & McFarlane, H. W. (1992). Unsuspected factors in 'self-limiting' ailments. *British Journal of Clinical Practice, 46*(3), 210–211.

Cetaruk, E. W., & Aaron, C. K. (1994). Hazards of nonprescription medications. *Emergency Medicine Clinics of North America, 12*(2), 483–510.

Chrischilles, E. A., Foley, D. J., Wallace, R. B., Lemke, J. H., Semia, T. P., Hanlon, J. T., Glynn, R. J., Ostfeld, A. M., & Guralnik, J. M. (1992). Use of medications by persons 65 and over: Data from the established populations for epidemiologic studies of the elderly. *Journal of Gerontology, 47*(5), M137–144.

*Clinical Pharmacy* (1991), *10*, 88, 93.

Conn, V. S. (1991). Older adults: Factors that predict the use of over-the-counter medication. *Journal of Advanced Nursing, 16*, 1190–1196.

Coons, S. J. (1990). The pharmacist's role in promoting and supporting self-care. *Holistic Nursing Practice, 4*(2), 37–44.

Davies, P., Fattah, H., & Clee, M. D. (1994). Undisclosed self-medication—a clinical pitfall. *British Journal of Clinical Practice, 48*(6), 333.

Delafuente, J. C., Meuleman, J. R., Conlin, M., Hoffman, N. B., & Lowenthal, D. T. (1992). Drug use among functionally active, aged, ambulatory people. *Annals of Pharmacotherapy, 26*, 179–183.

*Drug Facts & Comparisons* (1997). St. Louis: Facts & Comparisons.

Elkind, A. H. (1991). Drug abuse and headache. *Medical Clinics of North America, 75*(3), 717–732.

Fillenbaum, G. G., Hanlon, J. T., Corder, E. H., Ziqubu-Page, T., Wall, W. E., & Brock, D. (1993). Prescription and nonprescription drug use among black and white community-residing elderly. *American Journal of Public Health, 83*(11), 1577–1582.

Gilbertson, W. E. (1993). FDA's review of OTC drugs. In T. R. Covington, L. C. Lawson, & L. L. Young. (Eds.), *Handbook of nonprescription drugs* (10th ed). Washington, DC: American Pharmaceutical Association.

Gossel, T. A. (1991). Implications of the reclassification of drugs from prescription-only to over-the-counter status. *Clinical Therapeutics, 13*(2), 200–215.

Green, K. E. (1990). Common illnesses and self-care. *Journal of Community Health, 15*(5), 329–338.

Griffle, K. G. (1995). Opinions. *Drug Topics 139*(18), 52–53.

Gurwitz J. H., McLaughlin, T. J., & Fish, L. S. (1995). The effect of an Rx-to-OTC switch on medication prescribing patterns and utilization of physician services: The case of vaginal antifungal products. *Health Services Research, 30*(5), 672–685.

Henry, J. A. (1994). Hazards of self-medication. *British Journal of Clinical Practice, 48*(6), 285.

Hershman, D. L., Simonoff, P. A., Frishman, W. H., Paston, F., & Aronson, M. K. (1995). Drug utilization in the old old and how it relates to self-perceived health and all-cause mortality: Results from the Bronx aging study. *Journal of the American Geriatric Society, 43*, 356–360.

Holden, M. D. (1992). Over-the-counter medications: Do you know what your patients are taking? *Postgraduate Medicine, 91*(8), 191–194, 199–200.

Holt, C. (1996) Tylenol vs. Advil. *American Druggist, 213*(4), 19.

Holt, G. A., Dorcheus, L., Hall, E. L., Beck, D., Ellis, E., & Hough, J. (1992). Patient interpretation of label instructions. *American Pharmacy, NS32,* 58–62.

Holt, G. A., & Hall, E. L. (1993). The self-care movement. In T. R. Covington, L. C. Lawson, & L. L. Young (Eds.). *Handbook of nonprescription drugs,* (10th ed.). Washington, DC: American Pharmaceutical Association.

Kabongo, M. L. (1993). Problems with over-the-counter vaginal preparations. *American Family Physician, 48*(4), 579.

Kogan M. D., Pappas G., Yu S. M., & Kotelchuck, M. (1994). Over-the-counter medication use among US preschool-age children. *JAMA 272*(13), 1025–1030.

Muirhead, G. (1995). Coverage for OTCs? *Drug Topics, 139*(16), 38.

Newton, G. D., Pray, W. S., & Popovich, N. G. (1994). New OTCs: A selected review. *American Pharmacy, NS34*(2), 31–38, 40.

Nichol, M. B., McCombs, J. S., Johnson, K. A., Spacapan, S., & Sclar, D. A. (1992). The effects of consultation on over-the-counter medication purchasing decisions. *Medical Care, 30*(11), 989–1003.

Nonprescription Drug Manufacturers Association. (1996a). OTC Facts and Figures. *NDMA Fact Sheets*, May.

Nonprescription Drug Manufacturers Association. (1996b). American consumers support self-medication and practice it responsibly. *NDMA Fact Sheets*, April.

Nonprescription Drug Manufacturers Association. (1997). Ingredients and dosages transferred from Rx- to OTC-status by the Food and Drug Administration since 1975. *NDMA Fact Sheets*, April.

Palumbo, F. B. (1991). The impact of the Rx to OTC switch on practicing pharmacists. *American Pharmacy, NS31*(4), 41–44.

Ponte, C. D. (1990). What nonprescription medications are you taking, Mrs. Jones? *Drug Intelligence and Clinical Pharmacy: The Annals of Pharmacotherapy, 24*:1118.

Rosendahl, I. (1995). OTC labeling. *Drug Topics, 139*(14), 47.

Rupp, M. T., & Parker, J. M. (1993). Drug names; When marketing and safety collide. *American Pharmacy, NS33,* 39–42.

Schaff, V. M., Perez-Stable, E. J., & Borchardt, K. (1990). The limited value of symptoms and signs in the diagnosis of vaginal yeast infections. *Archives of Internal Medicine, 150,* 1929–1933.

Segall, A. (1990). A community survey of self-medication activities. *Medical Care, 28*(4), 301–310.

Slezak, M. (1996). Steering patient switches. *American Druggist, 213*(7):32–35.

Smith, M. C. (1996). Pharmacists and nonprescription medication: Paradox and prospect. *Drug Topics, 140*(2), 78–85.

Snyder, K. (1995). Rising tide: New wave of Rx-to-OTC switches coming. *Drug Topics, 139*(19), 76.

Snyder, K. (1996a). A better deal? Will Medicaid reimburse for Rx-to-OTC switches? *Drug Topics, 140*(6), 41.

Snyder, K. (1996b). PBM encouraging OTC use to counter medication costs. *Drug Topics, 140*(3), 72.

Sorofman, B., Tripp-Reimer, T., Lauer, G. M., & Martin, M. E. (1990). Symptom self-care. *Holistic Nursing Practice, 4*(2), 45–55.

Stoller, E. P., Forster, L. E., & Portugal, S. (1993). Self-care responses to symptoms by older people: A health diary study of illness behavior. *Medical Care, 31*(1), 24–42.

Stuart, B., & Grana, J. (1995). Are prescribed and over-the-counter medicines economic substitutes? *Medical Care, 33*(5), 487–501.

Temin, P. (1983). Costs and benefits in switching drugs from Rx to OTC. *Journal of Health Economics, 2,* 187–205.

Tylor, C. A., & Lipsky M. S. (1994). Physicians' perceptions of the impact of the reclassification of vaginal antifungal agents. *Journal of Family Practice, 38*(2), 157–160.

U.S. Food and Drug Administration. (1977). Safety and effectiveness of over-the-counter drugs: The FDA's OTC drug review. *Pediatrics, 59,* 309–311.

Vickery, D. M. (1985). A medical perspective. *Drug Information Journal, 19,* 155–158.

Vuckovic, N., & Nichter M. (1997). Changing patterns of pharmaceutical practice in the United States. *Social Science and Medicine, 44*(9), 1285–1302.

# 10

# HERBAL THERAPIES FOR COMMON HEALTH PROBLEMS

*Ellis Quinn Youngkin and Debra S. Israel*

In the nineteenth and prior centuries, herbal remedies for a wide variety of complaints were commonly found on pharmacy shelves. Then, in the twentieth century, such preparations took a back seat to prescription medicines, many of which had as their bases the very same herbs that had lost favor as the new century evolved. Now herbs (botanicals used to treat disease conditions, often chronic) and phytomedicinals (galenicals made by extracting herbs with various solvents) are back in a big way, conservatively estimated at $1.5 billion in the retail market in the United States (Tyler & Foster, 1996). Alternative therapies as a whole are so popular that approximately 33% of all American adults are using them annually (Campion, 1993). The Office of Alternative Medicine was established in 1992 by the National Institutes of Health (NIH) at the instruction of Congress to support research in the field (Marwick, 1992). As the country enters a new millennium, the herbs that were touted for their wonders hundreds, and even thousands, of years ago will continue to be in wide use, only they will have the advantage of modern scientific evaluation behind their use.

The safety and effectiveness of selected herbal therapies must be of concern to health care providers who are asked daily about such remedies by their patients. Thousands of people are planning to take or are already taking herbal preparations, and providers must be knowledgeable about their use. A survey of family practice patients indicated that half had used or were using alternative therapies, and only 53% had told their physician (Elder, Gillcrist, & Minz, 1997). Patients used the nontraditional therapies because they believed they would work. Physician factors like acceptance, open-mindedness, nonjudgmental attitudes, acknowledging the need for the person to be in control of their own care, the limits of traditional medicine, and "narrow-mindedness" were mentioned in the discussion of whether the patients told their physicians or not about the use of alternative therapies. A 1994 Robert Wood Johnson Foundation National Access to Care Survey found that nearly 25 million Americans (almost 10% of the sample of 3,450) saw a professional for one of four alternative therapies: acupuncture, therapeutic massage, relaxation techniques, and chiropractic therapies (Paramore, 1997). Although herbal therapies were not mentioned, it is reasonable to assume that their use by the public is as or more wide-spread. For the provider to simply say, "There are no quality-controlled standards for production, or no double-blind, placebo-controlled clinical trials, so don't use them," to a patient is short-sighted and akin to telling the sexually active teen to "Just say no." People are going to use herbal remedies, so being informed is imperative. A better and more realistic provider approach is to know the answers to the questions in the following paragraph.

Which herbal therapies are effective and safe for common problems such as constipation, headache, dysmenorrhea, or head cold? What is the scientific support in the literature and where does it come from? What is the best dosage to use and for how long? In what form should the therapy be provided? Additionally, other questions to ask the patient are suggested by Tyler and Foster (1996): Has the patient used the product before and what happened? Are there any allergies to plant materials? Who is using or planning to use the product (the patient or someone else in the household, such as a child)? Does the patient understand the importance of closely following label instructions for use? Is the patient taking any other prescription or non-prescription medications (that could interact negatively with the herbal therapy)? Most importantly for women, are they pregnant or breast-feeding?

Some herbal preparations can be harmful. For example, the Food and Drug Administration (FDA) advised that ma huang (ephedrine) and kola nut nutritional products used together may be harmful (Youngkin & Israel, 1996). Over 100 reports of deaths or serious health problems, such as heart attack, irregular heart beat, seizure, stroke, and psychosis, were reported in 1994 from combining ephedrine and the kola nut, which contains caffeine (Hurley, 1995). Other serious diseases have been reported from herbal use, including hepatitis from an herbal medicine used for weight loss (Larrey et al, 1992).

Thus, health care providers must carefully determine what herbal preparations their patients are taking, how much, and by what route, and what conventional drugs the patients are taking that may interact negatively with these herbal ingested substances in light of illness and/or symptoms. This chapter will provide the practitioner with some background information on selected acceptable herbal therapies for some commonly encountered complaints in primary care, as well as some general information.

## SAFETY, EFFECTIVENESS, REGULATION, AND DANGERS

Over 1400 herbs are sold commercially, most as dietary supplements, and only nine are said to be safe and effective by the FDA (V. E. Tyler, personal communication to D. Israel, 1996). For the FDA to classify a substance as safe and effective, sufficient information has to be submitted for adequate evaluation (Tyler & Foster, 1996). That the FDA has not classified an herb

as safe and effective does not mean the herbal preparation is automatically unsafe or ineffective; it means that a lack of data exists for Category I placement. Nevertheless, in 1994, the Dietary Supplement Health and Education Act ruled that herbs could be labeled with information on their effects in the body but must contain a disclaimer that the product has not received FDA review and is not intended for use as a drug but as a dietary supplement (Hurley, 1995). It is understandable why companies are not willing to invest huge sums to gain clinical evidence of safety and effectiveness since most herbs are not patentable (Tyler & Foster, 1996).

In other countries, especially in Europe and Great Britain, herbal therapies have been used longer, and research has been conducted for years so that herbal preparations are frequently considered for treatment along with conventional medicines (Tyler, 1994). Although studies may not have been the tightly controlled trials U.S. researchers respect most, there have been respectable studies in which providers can have some comfort for suggesting or supporting an herbal therapy. Germany has a very successful system to investigate herbal therapies through the Federal Health Agency–appointed Commission E (Tyler & Foster, 1996). This commission has been studying the safety and efficacy of herbs since 1978, and it has published hundreds of monographs on herbs. Risk-benefit ratios for the safety and effectiveness of studied herbs offer significant insights for providers who need to help patients make informed decisions. Asian practitioners, especially the Chinese, have used herbs for thousands of years for every condition imaginable. A wealth of scientific data exists from these countries.

Since there are no government oversights or industry standards for the quality of herbal preparations available in America, the consumer does not know what she or he is getting (Youngkin & Israel, 1996). One cannot be sure exactly what part of the plant is being used (flowers, stem, root, seeds, fruit, or other), what other substances have been added (adulterants), or how concentrated the particular product is. Tyler (1994) warns that active, expensive plant parts are more likely to be adulterated, and some products may not contain any of the advertised active ingredient at all (Tyler & Foster, 1996). *Consumers are advised to buy preparations marketed by a reputable firm that states a standardized dose on the package.* Tyler (March 1997) advises carefully reading labels to note quantity per dose, storage instructions, and active ingredients, as well as buying from sources where stock turnovers are at least every 3 to 6 months.

The regulation of teas falls in a "gray" area of regulation between food and drugs, according to the FDA (Snider, 1991). Herbal teas are not regulated since they are considered foods. Care is especially important in the use of imported teas or ones grown at home since the concentration may be very high, and thus dangerous, if consumed in excess (Youngkin & Israel, 1996).

Other areas of concern include the danger of homegrown plants being mistakenly identified as safe herbs, but actually not being herbs at all, leading to poisonings (Youngkin & Israel, 1996). Also, some imported herbal preparations are laced with undeclared drugs and toxic substances that may be particularly dangerous to people looking for treatments for chronic conditions that have not responded to conventional medicines (Napier, 1994). In addition, prolonged use of products thought to be generally safe may lead to toxicity; long-term testing data are simply not available (Tyler & Foster, 1996). Some products are advertised for certain outcomes but are useless except for placebo effect. Weight-loss herbal products are one category of preparations that do nothing more than cause fluid loss from a laxative or diuretic effect. Of concern are products that tout a combined weight-loss and energy-boost effect. These may have multiple herbs in them that in combination may be harmful, such as ephedrine and kola nut.

Miller (1996), a gerontological nurse specialist, advises patients to be sure they have no medical condition that might need treatment before taking nonprescription remedies; discuss such remedies with their provider; use products that contain just one ingredient; check warnings on labels and seek help if any untoward symptoms occur; understand that safety standards are not required of such products; and consider that if it sounds too good to be true, it most likely is not true.

Many herbal preparations are mixtures of herbs, necessitating that the consumer be knowledgeable about a wide variety of herbs in order to separate information about each component for safety. The references at the end of this chapter provide some excellent resources to buy and keep on hand to evaluate herbal preparations. Many lay resources are not based on science, and although they may have accurate information, in many no or few references are given to help the consumer feel confident about safe and effective use.

Lastly, for ultimate safety, no herbal therapies should be used by pregnant women, nursing mothers, or infants and young children until definitive data exist to prove safety (Tyler & Foster, 1996).

## DOSAGE FORMS OF HERBAL THERAPIES

Herbs are prepared in different ways to get the most effective active ingredients from the specific herb. For instance, if some herbs are dried, such as St. John's Wort or feverfew, properties are lost (Keville, 1996). For other herbs that contain a lot of water, like calendula or comfrey, drying is the best method of preparation. Table 10–1 gives an overview of various preparations of herbs for use internally or externally. Bissett (1994) has edited a large handbook of herbs that is a helpful reference of pictures of the plants and the dried herbs, as well as scientific phytopharmaceutical information.

## COMMON CONDITIONS AND HERBAL REMEDIES

Selected conditions commonly encountered in primary health care are presented in alphabetical order in this section. One or more herbal remedies that have scientific support for use and appropriate dose and form are given. *Any signs or symptoms of adverse effects that the patient develops require stopping the herbal therapy immediately and calling the health care provider or going to an emergency room if serious.* Providers are reminded that herbs are drugs, despite patients' common misconception that they are "natural" and, therefore, "safe." As drugs, allergic responses and untoward effects can occur. Table 10–2 provides definitions of terms commonly used to describe herbal actions. Table 10–3 provides the common and scientific names of a selection of commonly used herbs.

### ANXIETY AND STRESS

#### St. John's Wort

This herb comes from the dried flowering tops of a member of the St. John's wort family that grows in Europe, Asia, Africa, North America,

## TABLE 10–1. DELIVERY FORMS OF HERBS AND PHYTOMEDICINALS

- *Infusions (teas)*: Herbs steeped in hot water; plant materials are in a coarsely comminuted form unless commercially cut extra fine for quick tea. Infusions can be cold; used for fragrant herbs that lose their essential oils if heated.
- *Decoctions*: Generally, roots and bark simmered gently for longer periods to produce the tea.
- *Poultices*: Fresh plants pounded, blended, or chewed into a sticky paste form, spread on an injury, and wrapped with a bandage. Another type of poultice is made from powder mixed with water to form the paste for external use.
- *Capsules or tablets*: Finely powdered herbs for oral ingestion; they release the active ingredient in the stomach. They may be enteric-coated to protect from inactivation in the stomach if the herb is damaged by acid.
- *Syrups*: Tinctures, liquid extracts, glycerites, or teas.
- *Extracts or galenicals*: Liquid or solid phytomedicinals that can be standardized more readily because the herb is extracted with solvents.
- *Tinctures*: Concentrated liquid herbal extracts diluted by adding to water or juice; alcohol is the solvent used for extracting the herb.
- *Vinegars*: Prepared like tinctures but with an infusion of herb into vinegar, not alcohol; herbal vinegars are not strong enough for medicinal use.
- *Body oils*: Made from herbs for massage or for external remedies, such as for sore muscles.
- *Skin salves*: Thickened herbal oils that adhere to the skin.
- *Compresses*: Can be hot or cold if the cloth is soaked in an herbal liquid preparation such as tea, diluted tincture, oil, or water.
- *Herbal bath*: Generally, a relaxation method, but herbal therapies can be combined with other therapies, such as aromatherapy, to accomplish a medicinal goal such as stimulation of circulation or muscle relaxation. Small baths for feet or hands can be prepared from teas or oils.
- *Glycerites*: Syrupy liquids made with glycerin without alcohol as an alternative to more potent tinctures.

*Sources:* Keville (1996) and Tyler and Foster (1996).

and Australia (Leung & Foster, 1995). It contains a number of components including naphthodianthrone pigments, flavonoids, flavonols, and a volatile oil. It has anxiolytic, antidepressant, and antiinflammatory properties, but its most important activity is said to be as a treatment for mild or moderate depression (Harrer & Sommer, 1994). It is thought to function as a monoamine oxidase inhibitor (MAO), increasing serotonin levels and feelings of well-being (St. John's wort, 1997). It was found superior to placebo in treating depression in eight clinical trials, and equal to standard antidepressants in three trials, with fewer side effects from the herbal therapy (Fugh-Berman, 1996). A review of controlled clinical trials with depressed patients taking hypericum extracts found positive results in most of the 12 placebo-controlled trials (Voltz, 1997). In examining the three published studies that compared hypericum with synthetic antidepressants, the herbal extract was associated with improvement in depressed symptoms, but the review found that comparators had not been dosed adequately. The authors found no trials with severely depressed

patients, and urged more studies since most were methodologically flawed. An earlier meta-analysis had concluded, after reviewing results from 23 randomized trials, 15 of which were placebo-controlled, and 8 of which compared hypericum with another drug, that hypericum extracts were more effective than placebo for treating mild to moderately severe depressive disorders. Again further studies were advised. In one study, hypericum extract, 900 mg daily over 4 weeks, was found effective in treating people with seasonal affective disorder (SAD) (Kasper, 1997). Total score of the Hamilton Depression Rating Scale was reduced significantly for the people given hypericum. Added bright light therapy did not significantly improve results from no added bright light therapy.

Research is ongoing to evaluate the antiviral properties of an herbal component, hypericin. It has broad-spectrum viricidal abilities (Bricklin, 1996). Precautions with St. John's wort include the possibility of photodermatitis. People with light skin are advised to not expose skin to direct sunlight when taking this herb or to use sunscreen (Hebel, 1996; Leung & Foster, 1995).

## TABLE 10–2.  COMMONLY USED DEFINITIONS OF HERBAL TERMS

| | |
|---|---|
| Abortifacient | Induces expulsion of fetus |
| Adaptogen | Strengthens organs or entire organism (synonym for *tonic*) |
| Alterative | Produces gradual favorable change in body |
| Analgesic | Relieves pain |
| Antacid | Neutralizes acids |
| Antiabortive | Helps inhibit abortion process |
| Antiasthmatic | Relieves asthma symptoms |
| Antibiotic | Inhibits or destroys microorganisms |
| Anticatarrhal | Counters mucus formation |
| Antihydrotic | Reduces or suppresses perspiration |
| Antiseptic | Helps inhibit bacterial growth on skin |
| Antispasmodic | Relieves spasms or cramps |
| Aphrodisiac | Increases sexual desire or potency |
| Astringent | Contracts organic tissue; reduces secretions |
| Calmative | Sedates or tranquilizes |
| Carminative | Induces expulsion of gas from intestines |
| Cholagogue | Stimulates release and secretion of bile from gallbladder |
| Demulcent | Soothes irritated tissue, especially mucous membranes |
| Diaphoretic | Promotes perspiration |
| Diuretic | Increases expulsion of urine |
| Emetic | Induces vomiting |
| Emmenagogue | Promotes menstrual flow |
| Emollient | Used externally; softens and soothes |
| Expectorant | Promotes discharge of mucus from respiratory passages |
| Febrifuge | Helps body reduce fevers (also known as *antipyretic*) |
| Galactogogue | Increases secretion of milk |
| Hemostatic | Stops bleeding |
| Laxative | Promotes bowel movements (also called *purgative*) |
| Mucilaginous | Characterized by a gummy or gelatinous consistency |
| Nervine | Calms nervous tension |
| Rubefacient | When applied to skin, causes local irritation that increases circulation, which relieves internal pains |
| Sialogogue | Stimulates secretion of saliva |
| Stimulant | Excites or quickens activity of physiologic processes |
| Stomachic | Strengthens or tones stomach |
| Tonic | Strengthens organs or entire organism (synonym for *adaptogen*) |

*Sources:* Hoffman (1991) and Tierra (1990).

Special care must be taken if the person is also taking another drug that causes photosensitivity, like tetracycline (Bricklin, 1996a). Some nausea has been reported (Bloomfield, Nordfors, & McWilliams, 1997). It is not currently known if this herb is associated with the same warnings as MAOs, such as avoiding foods high in tyramine or tryptophan (since a hypertensive crisis may result) or avoiding concomitant antidepressant therapy (since serious adverse effects may occur). Caution in using this herb is recommended. Patients should never stop a prescribed antidepressant to take St. John's wort without provider approval and close monitoring, nor should the patient add St. John's wort to an already prescribed antidepressant.

## TABLE 10-3. COMMON, SCIENTIFIC, AND/OR OTHER NAMES OF SELECTED HERBS

Aloe vera:   *Aloe barbadensis*, Barbados aloe, Curacao aloe

Angelica:   *Angelica archangelica*, garden angelica, European angelica

Bearberry:   *Arctostaphylos uva ursi*, uva-ursi, Ericaceae

Black cohosh:   *Cimicifuga racemosa*, black snake root, rattleweed, rattleroot, squawroot

Caffeine:   Contained in *Coffea arabic L.* or other *Coffea* (coffee); *Camellia sinensis (L.)* O. Kuntze (tea); *Cola nitida* (kola or cola); *Theobroma cacao* L. (Cocoa); *Paullinia cupana* H.B.K. (cuarana paste); *Ilex paraguariensis* St.Hil. (mate)

Caigua:   *Cyclanthera pedata*, wild cucumber, achojcha

Capsicum:   *Capsicum spp.*, cayenne pepper, chile pepper, red pepper

Chamomile:   *Matricaria recutia, Chamaemelum nobile*, German or Hungarian chamomile

Chaste tree berry:   *Vitex agnus-castus*, chaste tree, chaste berry, Vitex

Cranberry:   *Vaccinium macrocarpon*, cranberry juice

Echinacea:   *Echinacea angustifolia, E. purpurae, E. pallida*, Sampson root

Elder:   *Sambuccua canadensis nigra*, elderberry

Eleuthero:   *Eleutherococcus senticosus*, Siberian ginseng

Ephedra:   *Ephedra sinica*, ma huang, Ephedraceae

Evening primrose oil:   *Oenothera biennis*, black currant, borage seed oil

Feverfew:   *Tanacetum parthenium*, Chrysanthemum parthenium

Garlic:   *Allium sativum L.*, clove garlic

Ginger:   *Zingiber officinale Rosc.*, African ginger, black ginger, race ginger, gingerroot

Ginkgo biloba:   *Ginkgo biloba L.*, ginkgo tree

Ginseng:   *Panax ginseng* (Oriental), *Panax quinquefolius* (American), Asiatic ginseng, wonder-of-world (Chinese ginseng), five-fingers, five-leafed ginseng (American ginseng)

Goldenrod:   *Solidago virgaurea L.* (American), *S. serotina, S. Canadensis L.*

Hawthorn:   *Crataegus laevigata* (Pior) DC., *C. oxyacantha auct., C. monogyna Jacq.*, May bush, May tree, thorn-apple tree, whitehorn

Horehound:   *Marrubium vulgare L.*, marrubium

Kava:   *Piper methysticum*

Licorice:   *Glycyrrhiza glabra L.* (European), *G. uralensis Fisch.* (Chinese), licorice root, sweet licorice, sweet wood

Melissa:   *Melissa officinalis L.*, lemon balm

Nettle:   *Urtica diocia*, common nettle, stinging nettle, great stinging nettle

Peppermint:   *Menthax piperita L.*, mint

Plantago seed/husk:   *Plantago psyllium L.* (Spanish); *P. indica L.* (French); *P. ovata* Forskal (Blond Psyllium or Indian Plantago seed)

Pygeum:   *Pygeum africanum*

St. John's wort:   *Hypericum perforatum L.*, amber, goatweed, Johnswort, Klamath weed

Saw palmetto:   *Serenoa epens, Sabal serrulata*

Senna:   *Senna alexandrina, Cassia acutifolia, C. angustifolia*

Slippery elm:   *Ulmus rubra Muhl., U. fulva*

Tea tree oil:   *Melaleuca alternifolia*, tea tree

Valerian:   *Valeriana officinalis L.*, valerian

Witch hazel:   *Hamamelis virginiana L., H. vernalis Sarg.*

*Sources:* Mindell (1992), Tierra (1990), Tyler (1994), Tyler and Foster (1996), and Youngkin and Israel (1996).

**Advised Dosage.** 2–4 g of herb, generally in capsule form. This is calculated to contain 0.2–1.0 mg hypericin, the flavonoid known to have antidepressant action (Harrer & Sommer, 1994; Hyperici herba, 1989). One article advises taking no more than 300 mg at one time and no more than 900 mg daily (Bricklin, 1996a). The 300 mg dose of St. John's wort one to three times daily is cited in the lay as well as professional literature (Bloomfield, Nordfors, & McWilliams, 1997; The natural mood booster, December 1997). Dr. Tyler suggests pouring a cup of boiling water over 1 to 2 teaspoons (2 to 4 grams) of the herb, steep for 10 minutes and drink (Foltz-Gray, 1997). One to 2 cups daily for six weeks is advised to lead to improved feelings.

## Valerian

Some individuals use valerian to relieve anxiety and tension. However, this herb can act as a stimulant in some people, causing anxiety (see Insomnia section, this chapter for more information on valerian). Use valerian with caution for anxiety.

## Kava

This herb comes from the underground root of the kava plant (a pepper plant, *Piper methysticum*) and is also called kava-kava or ava (Norton & Ruze, 1994; Tyler, October 1997). *Piper methysticum*, the scientific name, means intoxicating pepper. Used as a ceremonial drink for thousands of years by Pacific Islanders (Fiji, Polynesia, Melanesia, Micronesia) to create a feeling of relaxation, kava was approved by the German Commission E in 1990 to relieve stress, anxiety, and restlessness (Keville, 1996; Norton & Ruze, 1994; Tyler, October 1997). Ingested as a beverage, kava creates an intoxicated state of tranquility. Active ingredients are chemical compounds called pyrones, known to relax in 30 to 120 minutes by effects on the central nervous system (Tyler, October 1997). Clinical studies have demonstrated a decrease in feelings of anxiety (Keville, 1996). Related symptoms were relieved in menopausal women who felt increased well-being. Other research has demonstrated brain wave effects from kava in some types of anxiety similar to effects of benzodiazepines, but without lessened alertness or addition. Improved memory, alertness, and vigilance are reported. Side effects include mild, reversible gastrointestinal upsets and allergic skin reactions. Taking Kava longer than three months may lead to a yel-

low discoloration of the skin, nails, and hair; visual disturbances; balance disturbances; and allergic skin reactions (scaliness) (Keville, 1996; Tyler, October 1997). The scaly (ichthyosiform) eruption is known as kava dermopathy, and may interfere with cholesterol metabolism (Norton & Ruze, 1994). This herb should not be used in pregnancy, lactation, or if depressed. It has potential for abuse because it is potent, thus future controls may be needed (Tyler, October 1997). An interaction between kava and alprazolam leading to coma has been reported (Almeida & Grimsley, 1997).

**Advised Dosage.** Seek a product standardized to contain 30% kavalactones (pyrones). Tyler (October 1997) states that in a 150 mg capsule, there are approximately 50 mg of kavalactones. One capsule may be taken twice a day, but he advises starting at a low dose.

## BREAST TENDERNESS

### Chaste Tree Berry

See *Premenstrual Symptoms*.

### Evening Primrose Oil

See *Muscle/Joint Pain and Inflammation*.

## BRONCHIAL ASTHMA

### Ephedra

The aboveground (aerial) parts are used of the species, found in warm, dry areas of Asia, the Americas, and Europe (Tyler & Foster, 1996). It is commonly called *ma huang*, and the stem contains the active ingredients, primarily an alkaloid mixture of ephedrine and pseudoephedrine. Ephedra has been used to treat bronchial asthma for at least 5000 years, producing bronchodilation, vasoconstriction, and decreased bronchial edema (Hebel, 1996; Tyler, 1994). However, ephedra can be very dangerous, producing nervousness, insomnia, and palpitations when used to excess (Tyler, 1994). Other side effects noted include skin flushing, vomiting, and possible toxic psychosis (Hebel, 1996). People with heart conditions, hypertension, diabetes, or thyroid disease must not use it. The FDA is expected to regulate its use since reports of toxicity are increasing. Some states restrict sales since it is used in the manufacture of illegal methamphetamine and methcathinone

(Tyler, 1994). It must not be used with kola nut since it may cause serious problems.

Advised Dosage. 2 g steeped in 240 mL boiling water for 10 min and drunk as a tea. This is equivalent to 15–30 mg of ephedrine (Tyler, 1994).

## COLDS AND FLU

### Echinacea

This herb comes from aerial (aboveground) parts and/or roots of the purple coneflower, a member of the aster family found naturally in the midwestern United States (Tyler & Foster, 1996). Active ingredients vary with the source of the herb, but include a number of acids, essential oils, alkylamides, polysaccharides, and other constituents. It is used orally as a prophylaxis against cold and flu symptoms, for treatment of *Candida albicans* infections, and for its immunostimulating actions (Bauer & Wagner, 1991; Braunig, Dorn, & Knick, 1992; Bricklin, 1996b; Foster, 1991c). According to Dr. Adriane Fugh-Berman, formerly with the Office of Alternative Medicine of NIH, it may be used as complementary treatment with antibiotic therapy for serious infection. In a review of 26 clinical trials, 30 of 34 groups studied were said to have positive results with immunostimulation (Fugh-Berman, 1996). Some 32 well-done studies are reported by Tyler to give support for use of this herb to ward off a fully developed cold (Foltz-Gray, November 1997). The herb can be used topically in ointment for wound healing, eczema, burns, psoriasis, herpes simplex, and other skin irritations (Leung & Foster, 1995; Echinaceae purpureae herba, 1989), but is contraindicated in tuberculosis, leukosis, multiple sclerosis, collagenosis, HIV infections, lupus, and other autoimmune diseases since the immune system is already over-stimulated and partly to blame for these illnesses (Bricklin, 1996b; Echinaceae purpureae herba, 1989). No side effects have been reported with the use of this herb (Hebel, 1996). Some people are allergic to plants in the daisy family, and echinacea can cause a reaction in these individuals (Foltz-Gray, November 1997).

Advised Dosage. 6–9 mL daily of the expressed fresh juice of *Echinacea purpurea* for up to 8 weeks; immunostimulation declines after that time (Echinaceae purpureae herba, 1989). If the *Echinacea pallida* root is used, the daily dosage, usually administered in a tincture (1:5) prepared with 50% ethanol, is equal to 900 mg (Echinaceae pallidae radix, 1992). If the *Echinacea angustifolia* root is taken, the dosage is 1 g of capsules, tablets, or tincture t.i.d. (Bradley, 1992). Fugh-Berman (1996) reports that more information is needed to clarify recommended dosages, preparations, and circumstances. Tyler advises taking echinacea as a tablet or capsule at the first sign of a cold or sore throat. It should be taken as directed on the packaging for up to one week; longer is not beneficial. He chooses tablet or capsule form since these tend to be standardized, which the liquid is not (Foltz-Gray, November 1997).

### Elder

Berries of the elderberry tree have long been used as a folk remedy for the flu, colds, and neuralgia (Keville, 1996; Mindell, 1992). Keville (1996) reported that research in Israel found that compounds in the berries could stop invasion of healthy cells in the laboratory by the flu virus. In a flu epidemic, Israelis gave a syrup of the berries to kibbutz members; they recovered more quickly than those who used standard treatments. Publication of research results is pending from the Israeli studies (Arnot, 1996). Elder is said to enhance the immune system as well as stop cold and flu viruses. Flowers from the elder plant may have diuretic and laxative properties, but these effects are not well established. The Centers for Disease Control reported several cases of nausea, vomiting, weakness, numbness, and stupor occurring in persons attending a picnic in 1984, all of whom ingested elderberry juice. Stems and leaves should not be used in making juice since extracts of these plant parts may contain cyanide (Hebel, 1996).

Advised Dosage. 1 tablespoon syrup or one lozenge q.i.d.; available as Sambucol in the United States.

### Horehound

See *Coughs*.

## CONSTIPATION

### Plantago Seed and Husk

This herb is also called psyllium or plantain, and comes from cleaned, dried, ripened seeds grown in Europe, India, and Pakistan; seeds and seed husks contain insoluble (80%) and soluble (20%) fiber (Tyler & Foster, 1996). The components act as a bulk laxative as the seed coats swell, increasing intestinal volume and stimulation, and the mucilage from the seeds provides lubrication and increased transit time (European Scientific Cooperative, 1992; Plantaginis ovatae testa, 1990). There is also evidence that plantago seed lowers cholesterol and low-density lipoprotein (LDI) levels (Plantaginis ovatae testa, 1990; Sprecher et al, 1993). Rarely, allergic reactions occur with use. Plantago seed should not be used in people with diabetes mellitus or GI obstructions.

*Advised Dosage.* 7.5 g with 150 mL water for each 5 g of drug taken 30 to 60 min after a meal or after taking other medications (Plantaginis ovatae testa, 1990; Tyler, Brady, & Robbers, 1988). The average daily dose is 4–20 g.

## Senna

The preparation is made from dried leaflets of Alexandria and Tinnevelly senna, from the Middle East and Asia primarily, that act as a cathartic (Leung & Foster, 1995; Tyler, 1994; Tyler, Brady, & Robbers, 1988). Senna can cause cramps, and chronic abuse causes potassium loss, electrolyte and fluid imbalance, and reduced effectiveness of other drugs such as cardiac glycosides. It can cause a potential for toxicity of such drugs, and its use is contraindicated in pregnancy or lactation.

*Advised Dosage.* 2 g or as directed on labeling (Sennae folium, 1993; Tyler, Brady, & Robbers, 1988). Use of this herb beyond 1–2 weeks is not recommended unless the patient is under the supervision of a health care practitioner (Tyler & Foster, 1996).

## COUGH

### Horehound

Horehound comes from the dried aerial flowering parts of a member of the mint family found in Europe and the United States (Tyler & Foster, 1996). The leaves contain a volatile oil and other active ingredients, especially marrubiinic acid, which has a strong choleretic activity (Tyler, 1994). German health authorities have approved the herb for coughs, colds, as a digestive aid, and

as an appetite stimulant (Marrubii herba, 1990). The FDA has said it is ineffective as a cough suppressant and expectorant. This herb may produce a hypoglycemic effect although this has not been well established (Hebel, 1996). Overall, horehound is considered safe.

*Advised Dosage.* 2 g dried cut herb steeped in 240 mL of boiling water with daily intake of 0.75–1 L of the infusion. Horehound-flavored candy is sold as a cough suppressant (Tyler, 1994).

### Licorice

Licorice is reputed to calm coughs and have expectorant qualities. The extract is used in lozenges, candies, and teas (Tyler, 1994). However, in the U.S., most licorice candy is flavored with anise oil and contains no real licorice. Tyler advises looking for Lakerol, a combination of licorice and menthol, on the label (Foltz-Gray, November 1997). See Gastric Ulcers in this chapter for more information on licorice.

## DEPRESSION

### St. John's Wort

See *Anxiety and Stress.*

## DYSMENORRHEA

### Black Cohosh

Black cohosh comes from the dried rhizome and roots of a member of the buttercup family native to North America (Tyler & Foster, 1996). The main active components are glycosides and isoflavones. Black cohosh is used in Europe, primarily Germany, to treat neurovisceral and psychic problems associated with menopause, premenstrual complaints, dysmenorrhea, and uterine spasms (Bradley, 1992; Cimicifugae racemosae rhizoma, 1989). Possible side effects are GI disturbances. Additive hypotensive effects may be seen if black cohosh is used along with antihypertensive medications (Hebel, 1996). Use in pregnancy and lactation is contraindicated.

*Advised Dosage.* A daily dosage of a decoction or tincture made from dried rhizome corresponding to 40–200 mg may be used for not longer than 6 months according to German authorities (Bradley, 1992).

## FATIGUE

### Eleuthero

Eleuthero is the dried root of a shrubby member of the ginseng family found in Asia; it is marketed as "Siberian ginseng" in the United States in preparations that use the roots, stem, and leaves of the plant (Tyler & Foster, 1996). It is not a true ginseng herb. The herb's active compounds are numerous eleutherosides. Alcohol extracts are said to have assistive activities in such conditions as hyperthermia and gastric ulcers. Russian clinical studies are the basis for German Commission E approval for use in fatigue, concentration, debility, and reduced work ability (Bradley, 1992; Farnsworth et al, 1985; Foster, 1991h; Eleutherococci radix, 1991). Rare side effects such as drowsiness have been reported, and it should be used with caution in patients with hypertension (Eleutherococci radix, 1991). Patients who are febrile or who have had a myocardial infarction should not use this herb (Hebel, 1996).

Advised Dosage. 2–3 g of powdered or cut root in a decoction daily. A 33% ethanol root extract was used in the Russian studies with dosages of 2–16 mL one to three times a day for up to 60-day courses with 2–3 weeks rest between as many as five courses in a year (Eleutherococci radix, 1991; Farnsworth et al, 1985).

### Ginseng

See *Memory, Concentration, and Alertness Problems.*

## FLATULENCE

### Chamomile

This popular herb comes from the dried flower heads of the German chamomile; Roman chamomile, grown mainly in Great Britain, is different chemically from the German variety (Tyler & Foster, 1996). An essential oil in the German variety has well over 100 components. The dried flower heads and the volatile oil have antiinflammatory, antispasmodic, and antimicrobial actions. Chamomile is used for GI

spasms, inflammatory diseases, and as an antiflatulent (European Scientific Cooperative, 1990; Foster, 1991b). Persons allergic to ragweed, asters, or chrysanthemums should use it with caution (Tyler, 1993, 1994) since contact dermatitis and hypersensitivity reactions have occurred. The primary concern, though rare (five reported cases in nearly 100 years), is anaphylactic shock in the event of allergic reaction (Tyler, 1994).

Advised Dosage. For GI problems, 3 g of dried flower heads steeped in 150 mL of hot water for 10 min three to four times daily (between meals) (Tyler & Foster, 1996). Another source recommends 2 teaspoonsful of chamomile leaves in one cup of boiling water, covered and steeped for 15 minutes (Foltz-Gray, November 1997).

## GASTRIC ULCERS

### Licorice

The preparation is made from the dried rhizome and roots from European, Chinese, or other varieties of licorice (Tyler & Foster, 1996). One important component for quality is glycyrrhizin, which is many times sweeter than sugar and is converted to an acid compound with hydrolysis. Licorice increases prostaglandins E and $F_{2\alpha}$ in the stomach, providing a protective gastric mucosal effect and healing of ulcers (Tyler, 1994). Many studies show licorice and its compounds to be effective for ulcer treatment (Fugh-Berman, 1996). Antacids, cimetidene, and deglycyrrhizinated licorice were compared in 500 confirmed ulcer patients; all healed equally well (Kassir, 1985). See the section on Cough earlier in this chapter for other uses of licorice.

The main concern with use of licorice is that along with its beneficial gastric effects comes an increase in glucocorticoids, sodium retention, potassium excretion, and elevation in blood pressure. Farese, Biglieri, Shackleton, Irony, and Gomez-Fontes (1991) discussed the literature on these potential dangers. Licorice use must be carefully controlled and monitored because of these maleffects. Inappropriate dosing or long-term use (>4–6 weeks) can be dangerous (Tyler, 1994; Tyler & Foster, 1996). If licorice is used with a thiazide diuretic, increased potassium may be lost and an increase in digitalis glycoside sensitivity results. One study of healthy volunteers found decreases in potassium and RAA axis values from modest amounts of licorice daily for less than a week (Epstein, Espiner, Donal, & Hughes, 1977). One journal article reported hypertension, enlargement of the heart, and pulmonary edema in a man who overate licorice candy (Chamberlain & Abolnik, 1997). Contraindications for use include liver cirrhosis, cholestatic liver diseases, hypertonia, hypo-kalemia, and pregnancy and lactation.

Advised Dosage. For gastric or duodenal ulcers, 5–15 g of finely cut or powdered root per day (contains 200–600 mg of glycyrrhizin) in infusions not to exceed 4–6 weeks (Liquiritiae radix, 1990). As a tea, for cough, Tyler advises one to two teaspoons of licorice-root powder (Foltz-Gray, 1997). For digestive problems, he advises preparing by adding a half cup boiling water to a teaspoonful of the herb, simmer for 5 minutes, cool, strain, and drink up to three times daily.

### Slippery Elm

See *Sore Throat and Laryngitis*.

## GASTRITIS AND COLITIS

### Slippery Elm

See *Sore Throat and Laryngitis*.

## HAY FEVER

### Nettle

See *Prostate Enlargement (Benign)* for a description of the herb and its primary use. The freeze-dried herb in capsules has been found to be helpful for sneezing and itching of hayfever (Bricklin, 1996b). Nettle and a placebo were used to treat 69 hayfever patients in Oregon. Of the nettle group 58% had moderate to excellent relief in a week versus only 37% of the placebo group. More research is indicated.

Advised Dosage. One capsule a day for several days (begin low to see if there is an allergy to the nettle). If there is no allergy, increase to one to capsules, t.i.d. If no relief is observed with up to six capsules after 1–2 weeks, stop the herb. *Do not eat uncooked plants; they may be poisonous.* Also, the bristly hairs of the plant can act like little needles to inject the substance under the skin, causing irritation (Bricklin, 1996b). Mild

gastrointestinal side effects are reported (Tyler, December 1997).

## HEADACHES

### Caffeine

A number of plants contain caffeine, such as coffee (dried ripe seeds from the madder family), tea leaves and buds, kola (dried cotyledon from the cola family), cocoa or cacao (roasted seed of the cocoa family), guarana (crushed seeds from a member of the soapberry family), and mate or yerba mate (dried leaves of a member of the holly family) (Tyler & Foster, 1996). The active ingredient is caffeine or trimethylxanthine (Tyler, Brady, & Robbers, 1988). Actions are as central nervous system (CNS) stimulants, and they are used to decrease drowsiness. If combined with analgesics, the action of the analgesic is potentiated up to 40%. If combined with ergot alkaloids, it offers some migraine headache relief. In beverages, caffeine has a short-lived, weak diuretic effect (Tyler, 1994). People with conditions such as hypertension should not use caffeine.

Advised Dosage. 100–200 mg of caffeine per day (Tyler, 1994); 250 mg equals approximately two cups of brewed coffee.

### Feverfew

Feverfew comes from the dried leaves of a member of the aster family, native to Europe, and is grown as an ornamental flower in the United States (Tyler & Foster, 1996). The main active chemical components are sesquiterpenes, primarily parthenolide. Parthenolide is believed to stop serotonin effects on blood vessels (Foltz-Gray, November 1997). The minimal standard for parthenolide in Canada is 0.2% to ensure efficacy, and the two published clinical trials used a comparable amount (Awang et al, 1991; Heptinstall et al, 1992). Feverfew is used for prevention and treatment of migraine headache to decrease the frequency, severity, duration, and associated nausea (Awang et al, 1991; Bradley, 1992; Foster, 1991d; Fugh-Berman, 1996; Heptinstall et al, 1992; Johnson, Kadam, Hylands, & Hylands, 1985). Other uses include fevers, menstrual problems, and other painful problems (Awang, 1989; Tyler & Foster, 1996). Side effects may include gastric discomfort, mouth ulcers, loss of taste, and dermatitis (Fugh-Berman, 1996; Hebel, 1996). Swelling of the mouth, lips, or tongue may occur if fresh leaves are eaten, but is less likely if capsules are taken (Fugh-Berman, 1996). Patients taking feverfew chronically should be cautioned about abruptly stopping the herb since a "postfeverfew syndrome" has been described (poor sleep patterns, anxiety, muscle and joint stiffness, and rebound of migraine symptoms) (Hebel, 1996).

Advised Dosage. 125 mg with a minimum parthenolide content of 0.2% a day in a tablet or capsule (Tyler, 1994). British researchers found that those individuals with regular migraines who used feverfew for 4 months had 24% fewer headaches than those who were not taking the herb (Foltz-Gray, November 1997).

## HEMORRHOIDS

### Plantago Seeds and Husk

See *Constipation*.

### Witch Hazel

Witch hazel comes from twigs and leaves of a botanical native to North America, cultivated in Europe, and made commercially in the United States as a distilled extract (Tyler & Foster, 1996). Hydroalcohol extracts are used in Europe (Tyler, 1994). The tannins in witch hazel are believed to cause the astringent effect, but this effect is due to added alcohol in the commercially available steam distillate that does not contain tannins. Witch hazel is used as an antiinflammatory and astringent for hemorrhoids and skin and mucous membrane injuries (Hamamelidis folium et cortex, 1990; Tyler, 1994). This herbal preparation has no precautions. It is applied topically as needed.

## HYPERLIPIDEMIA

### Garlic

Dried or fresh bulbs from the lily family, garlic has been cultivated for 5000 years worldwide (Tyler & Foster, 1996). Garlic is an allium, and its active ingredients are a volatile oil containing many sulfur compounds. The most important of these is allicin, which when self-condensed into ajoene has antiplatelet aggregation and antibac-

terial activity. Allicin is produced when an amino acid derivative that contains sulfur, alliin, in the intact cells of garlic is released with crushing of the cells. Contact with an enzyme in neighboring cells, allinase, yields alliin, a very potent, odoriferous antibiotic (Tyler, 1994). In addition, garlic has antifungal, antiinflammatory, hypotensive, and antioxidant effects, with cholesterol- and triglyceride-lowering activities (Foster, 1991e; Phelps & Harris, 1993). Numerous clinical studies have supported its lowering of cholesterol and triglycerides, as well as some lowering of blood pressure. The equivalent of one-half to one clove of garlic daily is effective in lowering serum cholesterol about 9%, according to clinical trials (Warshafsky, Kamer, & Sivak, 1993). Other studies show an effect ranging from 1 to 20% (Fugh-Berman, 1996). Twelve weeks of use lowered diastolic blood pressure 13 points in one double-blind trial of patients with mild hypertension (Auer et al, 1990). Silagy and Neil (1994) reviewed trial results for effect on blood pressure and concluded that a garlic powder preparation has some clinical use in mild hypertension, but suggested the need for more rigorous studies. Garlic rarely may cause an allergic reaction; the most common side effect is GI discomfort. Onion, another allium, has platelet-clumping prevention properties, as well as lipid-lowering properties (Fugh-Berman, 1996). Prevention of stomach and colon cancer is attributed to alliums, thought to be due to antibacterial properties (Johnson & Vaughn, 1969).

Advised Dosage. 400–1200 mg of dried powder or 2–5 g of fresh bulbs. The daily dosage is equal to 4–12 mg of alliin (2–5 mg of allicin) (Allii sativi bulbus, 1988; Bradley, 1992).

## INSOMNIA

### Hawthorn

The preparation is made from the dried leaves with flowers and/or fruits from the rose family grown in the wild or cultivated in Europe and China (Tyler & Foster, 1996). Active ingredients are procyanidins and flavonoids. The flowering tops are used for sleep-inducing preparations (European Scientific Cooperative, 1992). Hawthorn is used in Europe for treatment of diminished cardiac performance (stages I and II), mild/ stable angina pectoris, mild dysrhythmia, and other heart conditions not requiring digitalis

(Tyler & Foster, 1996). If it is used for cardiac reasons, the patient should have medical supervision (Tyler, 1994). Low doses of hawthorn appear to be safe, but higher doses may cause hypotension (Hebel, 1996).

**Advised Dosage.** 3–4 g of the dried herb given in 1-g doses in an infusion (European Scientific Cooperative, 1992).

## Valerian

Valerian is derived from the dried or fresh root of a member of the valerian family and is produced in Belgium, France, Russia, and China (Leung & Foster, 1995). The root and its essential oil contain more than 120 chemical components, some of which offer sedative and antispasmodic activity (Tyler & Foster, 1996). It is used as a sleep aid that is particularly helpful when the person is excited or nervous (European Scientific Cooperative, 1992). Most of the literature on valerian is from Germany, but there have been two double-blind trials in English that found its use promotes sleep (Leathwood, Chauffard, Herck, & Munoz-Box, 1982; Lindahl & Lindwall, 1989). Valerian is generally thought to have low toxicity, but some adverse effects have been reported. Four cases of hepatotoxicity have been linked to valerian usage (MacGregor, Abernathy, Dahabra, Cobden, & Hayes, 1991). In addition, headaches, excitability, uneasiness, and cardiac changes have been reported in controlled clinical trials (Hebel, 1996).

**Advised Dosage.** 2–3 g taken one to three times per day or an equivalent regimen (Tyler & Foster, 1996). Bricklin (1996a) advises one or two cups of valerian tea before bedtime, prepared from a teaspoon of the dried root, as a reasonable dose. Also, 200–300 mg of the extract containing 0.8% valerenic acid is another suggested dose. Bricklin warns that this herb has a bad odor.

## IRRITABLE BOWEL SYNDROME

### Chamomile

See *Flatulence*.

### Peppermint

Peppermint comes from the dried leaves and flowering tops of a mint family member grown in Europe, Egypt, and the United States (Tyler & Foster, 1996). Its essential oil is the active ingredient. In Europe, enteric-coated capsules of the oil are used to treat distention, recurrent colicky abdominal pain, and varied bowel habits (Leung & Foster, 1995). Few to no side effects have been reported (Foster, 1991g). Peppermint is felt to be safe for normal persons, but if used in excess it can cause heartburn and esophageal sphincter relaxation. It should be avoided in children and infants because it may cause laryngeal and bronchial spasms (Tyler, 1994).

**Advised Dosage.** Hot infusions daily of 1.5–3 g of dried leaf (Menthae piperitae folium, 1985), made by pouring 160 mL of boiling water on 1–1.5 g of the herb and steeped up to 10 min taken three to four times daily (Tyler, 1994). If enteric-coated peppermint oil in capsules are used, 0.2–0.4 mL is the usual dose, and up to three doses daily may be taken (Menthae piperitae aeatheroleum, 1990).

### Plantago Seed and Husk

See *Constipation*.

## MEMORY, CONCENTRATION, AND ALERTNESS PROBLEMS

### Ginkgo Biloba

The extract comes from the dried leaves of the *Ginkgo biloba* (maidenhair tree) of the ginkgo family (only surviving member of this family or genus of plants), which contain flavones, biflavonoids, and organic acids (Tyler & Foster, 1996; Kleijnen & Knipschild, 1992). More than 250 pharmacologic and clinical studies have been published, most on a specific standardized leaf extract from which possibly toxic ginkgoic acid is removed (Foster, 1991f). Ginkgo increases vasodilation and peripheral blood flow, and offers protection against hypoxia. Gingko biloba, like aspirin, can prevent clot formation (Is gingko biloba, January 1998). It is used for varicose problems; postthrombotic syndrome; chronic cerebral vascular insufficiency; short-term memory loss; cognitive disorders due to depression, dementia, tinnitus, and vertigo; and obliterative arterial disease of the lower extremities (Fugh-Berman, 1996; Tyler & Foster, 1996). It may be helpful for intermittent claudication (Is gingko biloba, January 1998). A review of clinical trials of this drug indicates that it is an appropriate therapy for symptoms for which the extracts are indicated, but further double-blinded research is advised (Kleijnen & Knipschild, 1992). One study of 60 men with impotence indicated it may improve blood flow in 8 weeks, with regained potency in 6 months, but this was not a trial controlled with a placebo (Sikora et al, 1989). Kleijnen and Knipschild (1992) reviewed 40 trials on ginkgo and cerebral insufficiency, concluding that positive effects exist, but stated more studies were needed. In a 52-week, randomized, double-blind, placebo-controlled, parallel group, multicenter study, researchers found that Egb 761, the extract of ginkgo biloba used in Europe for cognitive symptoms disorders, was associated with modestly improved (statistically significant) cognitive performance and social functioning in patients suffering from mildly to severely demented Alzheimer disease or multi-infarct dementia (LeBars, Katz, Berman, Itil, Freedman, & Schatzberg, 1997). The use of the extract was safe in this study. The highly refined extract used was significantly different from gingko products available over-the-counter in the United States. There is not strong data currently to indicate if ginkgo biloba would improve mental alertness in healthy people. European studies are said to be small and flawed, leaving many unanswered questions (Is gingko biloba, 1998). Ginkgo may cause minor reversible gastric disturbances, and rarely, headache, dizziness, and vertigo (Warburton, 1988). Two cases of bleeding after long-term use have been reported (Is gingko biloba, 1998). It may interact with aspirin or other anticoagulant drugs. It is not advised in pregnancy or lactation.

Advised Dosage. 120–160 mg of standardized leaf extract daily (Warburton, 1988). In capsules, 40 mg of the standardized leaf is advised three times a day.

## Ginseng

Ginseng comes from the dried roots of Asian or American ginseng, members of the ginseng family cultivated extensively in Asia and the United States (Foster, 1991a). Asian ginseng is the focus of most research. Much used in China, American ginseng is greatly prized there, but it is used for different purposes from the Asian variety (Fugh-Berman, 1996). The Siberian variety, with different properties and actions, is not

the same genus as the Asian and American varieties. The primary active ingredients are saponins, including ginsenosides. Ginseng has been used for thousands of years for a variety of problems. It is classified as an adaptogen that assists with various stress resistances through shorter reaction times, increased alertness, better concentration and grasp of abstract concepts, and better visual and motor coordination (Ng & Yeung, 1986; Shibata et al, 1985). The German Commission E approves its use for fatigue, loss of concentration, diminished work capacity, and as an aid during convalescence (Ginseng radix, 1991). People in Korea who consumed red and white ginseng extract or powder (not fresh) had lower overall cancer rates (Yun & Choi, 1995).

Ginseng is believed generally safe, but excessive consumption over a long time is said to cause hypertension, jitteriness, nervousness, and skin rash (Ginseng side effects?, 1996; Tyler, 1994). Rarely, insomnia and diarrhea have been described, although there is a recent report of possible ginseng-associated Stevens-Johnson syndrome (Dega, Laporte, Frances, Herson, & Chosidow, 1996) although this may have been due to impurities in the product (Faleni & Soldati, 1996). It should be noted that some women taking ginseng may complain of abnormal spotting and bleeding from the uterus, leading to the belief that ginseng has estrogenic activities (Fugh-Berman, 1996). Dr. Varro Tyler says that pure ginseng has no estrogenic effect, but the product could contain other added components, unknown to the consumer. This is seen especially with Chinese preparations (Ginseng side effects?, 1996). Women with abnormal bleeding should see their providers immediately. Providers should be aware that ginseng products may contain as much as 34% alcohol, and most do contain some alcohol. U.S. Customs has been requested by the Bureau of Alcohol, Tobacco and Firearms of the Treasury Department to seek to recall ginseng products containing alcohol.

Advised Dosage. 1–2 g of fresh root in appropriate forms daily (Ginsing radix, 1991). Fresh Korean ginseng is more easily obtained from ethnic markets and herbal pharmacies and can be used for tea. Look for "standardized" on the label for more reliable products if buying capsules or extract (Ginseng side effects?, 1996). Chewing a quarter-sized chunk of fresh root will provide the daily dosage as well as provide assurance of freshness without adulteration.

## MENOPAUSAL SYMPTOMS

### Black Cohosh

See *Dysmenorrhea*.

### Chaste Tree Berry

See *Premenstrual Symptoms*.

## MOUTH ULCERS

### Chamomile

See *Flatulence*.

## MUSCLE/JOINT PAIN AND INFLAMMATION

### Capsicum

This herb is also called cayenne, red pepper, or chili pepper; it comes from the dried ripe fruit of members of *Solanaceae* family (Tyler, 1994). It is FDA-approved for topical analgesia (Tyler, 1993, 1994). The active ingredient is capsaicin. When applied topically, capsaicin decreases arthritic joint pain (Fugh-Berman, 1996). In one double-blind, controlled study, tenderness and pain of osteoarthritis was decreased by 40%; however, no beneficial effects on rheumatoid arthritis were found (McCarthy & McCarty, 1992). Capsaicin is useful for fibromyalgia, herpes zoster pain and itching after the shingles have resolved, and cluster headache pain. Postmastectomy pain syndrome was found to respond significantly better than placebo to capsaicin. Capsaicin may also be safe and effective for treatment of diabetic neuropathy. It causes substance P, a neuropeptide that mediates pain impulse transmission from the peripheral nerves to the spinal cord, to be depleted (Tyler, 1994). This effect takes several weeks to occur. Hands must be thoroughly washed after application of these products to prevent transfer to eyes and mucous membranes. If the cream gets in eyes or on sensitive skin, it will cause burning. No sound evidence of capsicum improving blood vessel elasticity and lowering blood pressure has been found (Ask Dr. Tyler, May 1997). The FDA has approved 0.075% capsaicin in a cream base for over the counter (OTC) sale.

**Advised Dosage.** Application topically four to five times a day for at least 4 weeks.

### Evening Primrose (Black Currant, Borage Seed) Oil

Evening Primrose Oil (EPO) comes from seeds of the evening primrose, a member of the primrose family, native to eastern North America, but naturalized widely elsewhere (Tyler & Foster, 1996). Black currant and borage seeds are used similarly. The primary active component is a fixed oil containing *cis*-linoleic acid and *cis*-gamma-linolenic acid (GLA) (Leung & Foster, 1995). GLA from converted linoleic acid in the body is believed from studies to be hindered by aging, high cholesterol, high saturated fat and transfatty acid intake, viral infections, stress, high alcohol intake, diabetes mellitus, premenstrual syndrome (PMS), and eczema (Horrobin, 1990). Thus, supplemental GLA is thought to be helpful in these conditions (Briggs, 1986; Horrobin, 1990). Other studies of the use of EPO for eczema indicate that it may be an important therapy for reducing itching, scaling, and severity in this condition with adults and children (Fugh-Berman, 1996; Lovell, Burton, & Horrobin, 1981; Schalin-Karrila, Mattila, Jansen, & Uotila, 1987). EPO has been found to be as effective as bromocriptine for breast pain (Gately, Miers, Mansel, & Hughes, 1992) and helpful in pain reduction for rheumatoid arthritis (Belch et al, 1988). In one double-blind study comparing EPO and olive oil for rheumatoid arthritis patients, EPO improved morning stiffness at 3 months; olive oil improved pain on the articular index at 6 months, an unexpected effect (Brzeski, Madhok, & Capell, 1991). EPO preparations are considered safe; headache, nausea, and diarrhea have been the reported side effects.

**Advised Dosage.** For atopic eczema, four 250-mg capsules b.i.d.; for GLA supplementation, 600–6000 mg per day (Horrobin, 1990). Mindell (1992) advises 250-mg capsules up to three times daily for PMS symptoms, to be started 2–3 days before symptoms usually begin.

### Willow Bark

This herb is derived from the dried bark from the branches of a number of species of willow native to Europe, with most naturalized to North America (Tyler & Foster, 1996). The active ingredients are phenolic glycosides (predominately salicylates and tremulacin), flavonoids, tannins, and other components. It is used as an antiinflammatory, analgesic, antipyretic, and astringent to treat arthritis, colds, flu, headache, and gout (Bradley, 1992). In the body, salicylic acid is formed but has no effect on platelet function. Pain reduction is from antiprostaglandin activity (Bradley, 1992; Tyler, 1994). Such a large amount (0.75–5 L) of willow bark tea would have to be drunk to obtain a therapeutic effect that too much tannin for safe levels would also be consumed. So consumers will have to wait until this herb is available in the United States in a standardized, phytomedicinal form, as it now is in Europe. Consumers may use aspirin or other antiinflammatory medicines as alternatives to willow bark therapy.

## NAUSEA AND MOTION SICKNESS

### Ginger

The preparation comes from the dried or fresh rhizome of *Zingiber officinale Roscoe* (Tyler, 1994), and it acts as a carminative, an antiemetic, a cholagogue, and a positive inotropic. Studies in humans provide conflicting results. Germany allows labeling for dyspepsia and motion sickness. However, Fugh-Berman (1996) says that more research is needed to determine its effectiveness in combatting motion sickness. In controlled studies, it was found to be effective for preventing nausea and vomiting postoperatively (Bone, Wilkinson, Young, McNeil, & Charlton, 1990); it also helped with dizziness in another small study (Grontved & Hentzer, 1986). It is better than Dramamine in motion sickness induced in laboratory settings, but not necessarily helpful in the real situation. In one double-blind, crossover trial of pregnant women with morning sickness, ginger was preferred over placebo by 70% for decreasing nausea and vomiting (Fischer-Rasmussen, Kjaer, Dahl, & Asping, 1990). However, Stewart, Wood, Wood, & Mims (1991) found no anti-motion-sickness activity with powdered ginger or significant gastric function alteration. Tyler (1998) reports that 1 gram of ginger reduced motion sickness symptoms better than 100 mg of Dramamine in a 1982 study, and that similar studies have supported such results. He states that shogaol and gingeol compounds are most likely responsible for the anti-nausea action, acting directly on the stomach

and not the central nervous system. Therefore, people don't complain of drowsiness or mouth dryness. Tyler further indicates that ginger may be useful to relieve gas, indigestion, menstrual cramps, and even have a role in preventing cancer, but more controlled studies are needed. In advised dosages for motion sickness, it causes no side effects or toxic reactions. It is not advised for postoperative nausea since it may prolong bleeding time and cause immunologic changes. Tyler and Foster (1996) state that it is contraindicated in pregnancy and for gallstone pain.

**Advised Dosage.**  For motion sickness, two 500-mg capsules PO, 30 min apart 20 to 25 minutes before travel followed by one or two capsules prn every 3 to 4 h (Bradley, 1992; Tyler, 1994; Tyler, 1998). Additionally, a tea from 2 teaspoons of powdered ginger (from spice rack) or made from ½ to 1 teaspoon grated fresh ginger may be used (Tyler, 1998). A piece of candied ginger 1 inch square and ¼ inch thick equal to about 1 gram of ginger can be obtained from Asian food stores. Canada Dry and Schweppes contain the real ginger and 12 ounces is needed for a therapeutic dose.

## OBESITY

A number of herbal fiber products, laxatives, diuretics, and proposed "herbal weight loss remedies" have received recent attention since serious complications associated with two popular prescription medications for weight loss resulted in discontinuation of use. Some of the herbal therapies are not recommended, some can be dangerous if abused, and some have real application if used safely. See Chapter 32 for further discussion of herbal therapies in the management of obesity.

## PREMENSTRUAL SYMPTOMS

### Black Cohosh

See *Dysmenorrhea.*

### Chaste Tree Berry

This herb comes from fruits from a member of the verbena family, which grows as shrubs or trees in West Asia and southwestern Europe (Tyler & Foster, 1996). The primary active ingredients are flavonoids, but the fruits also contain an essential oil and glycosides (Gorler, Oehlke, & Soicke, 1985). There is evidence that this herb inhibits the secretion of prolactin by the pituitary gland. Used for thousands of years for menstrual problems, this herb has been approved by the German Commission E for PMS, mastalgia, menopausal symptoms, and other menstrual disorders (Agni casti fructus, 1992). It may cause GI side effects occasionally, and itching and rash rarely. Chaste tree berry possibly may interfere with dopamine-receptor antagonists, and it is contraindicated in pregnancy. Long-term effects are not known.

**Advised Dosage.** The average daily dose of alcoholic extracts or tinctures of pulverized fruits provides the equivalent of 20 mg of crude fruit or 30–40 mg of fruits in decoction (Agni casti fructus, 1992).

## Evening Primrose Oil

See *Muscle/Joint Pain and Inflammation.*

## PROSTATE ENLARGEMENT (BENIGN)

### Nettle

This herb comes from aboveground plant leaves and root parts of the stinging nettle, a member of family Uricaceae (Tyler, 1994). Clinical studies support the use of the root to treat benign prostatic hypertrophy (BPH); the active ingredients are not identified, but there are many compounds in this herb. The most recent hypothesis is that a lectin compound and polysaccharides are responsible for the therapeutic activity. It is believed that the herb decreases testosterone synthesis. In two of ten studies, scientific rigor was met, and urine output increased significantly in those two studies, although no change in flow or ability to totally empty the bladder occurred (Tyler, December 1997). Tyler believes saw palmetto and pygeum to be better choices for treatment of BPH. In Germany, nettle is an approved treatment for early prostate adenoma and BPH (Tyler, 1994). Local rash and irritation and mild GI disturbances are side effects (Tyler, 1993, 1994). No contraindications are known. The dried leaves also have the ability to increase urine flow (Tyler, 1994), but the active ingredients have not been identified. See *Hayfever* for other uses.

**Advised Dosage.** For BPH, 4–6 g daily as tea; for urinary flow enhancement, 4 g (three to four teaspoonsful of the botanical in 150 mL of boiling water). One cup three to four times a day with additional water (Tyler, 1994).

### Saw Palmetto

This herb is developed from the dried fruits from a member of palm family growing in the wild in Georgia and Florida (Tyler & Foster, 1996). The fruits contain an essential oil and a fixed oil with free fatty acids and neutral substances. Although not specifically identified, the antiandrogenic parts are in the fruit's acidic lipophilic fractions (Leung & Foster, 1995; Tyler, 1994). This herb is used in Europe for BPH; the active ingredient reduces testosterone and dihydrotestosterone by 40% in tissue samples. German studies have proved its effectiveness for stages 1 and 2 of BPH (Braeckman, 1994; Sabal fructus, 1991; Tyler, 1994). One double-blind French study found that it improved nocturia significantly, also decreasing residual urine and increasing flow rate (Champault, Patel, & Bonnard, 1984). Saw palmetto may prove to be a more useful way to inhibit the same enzyme inhibited by finasteride in prostate enlargement treatment without the impotence or loss of libido side effect some men report (Fugh-Berman, 1996). Tyler (December 1997, p. 70) calls it the "most promising" herbal therapy for BPH, pointing out that it is effective, has few side effects, and is inexpensive. Fifteen studies have been completed, more than half had high research methodologies, and most found statistically significant positive effects with saw palmetto use. No contraindications are known. Rarely, gastric upset is reported.

**Advised Dosage.** 320 mg of a lipophilic fruit extract (two 80-mg capsules, b.i.d.) (Bricklin, 1995a; Tyler & Foster, 1996).

### Pygeum

This herb, pygeum africanum, comes from an evergreen tree, prunus africana, found in southern and central Africa (Keville, 1996; Tyler, December 1997). Tyler states that the pygeum is the next best treatment for BPH after saw palmetto. Almost fifty percent of twenty-six European studies on the extract were scientifically sound and found that pygeum was associated with significant BPH system improvement.

However, German Commission E has not studied this herb, so safety, side effects, and efficacy statements have not been provided. Over the twenty years of studies, long-term administration indicated that the herb was tolerated satisfactorily.

Advised Dosage. 100 to 200 mg daily of a lipid extract of the bark, but be aware of the lack of German Commission E examination of this herb (Tyler, December 1997).

## SKIN PROBLEMS

### Aloe Vera

Aloe vera is a mucilaginous gel that comes from the center of the leaf of the aloe vera, a lily family member (Tyler & Foster, 1996). The juice of the aloe plant leaf is used as a cathartic. The active ingredients in the gel include polysaccharides. The gel is used for first-degree burns and minor skin irritations for its antiinflammatory, emollient, pain-lessening, and wound-healing features (Heggers, Pelley, & Robson, 1993). The fresh gel is applied topically as needed, and it is considered safe. Aloe, as a topical agent for wound healing, has been found to significantly increase wound contraction (Heggars, Kucuk-celebi, Listengarten, et al., 1996). The researchers speculated that aloe increases collagen activity and improves the breaking strength of the resulting scar. Tyler (1994) reported that the internal form of aloe, a potent stimulant laxative, is made up of several species of dried latex, is used in Europe but little in the United States, and is quite different in composition from the gel. Mindell (1992) advises one capsule up to three times daily or one tablespoon of the juice or gel up to three times daily for digestive disorders. He cautions against use in pregnancy, by children, or by the elderly.

### Evening Primrose Oil

See *Muscle/Joint Pain and Inflammation*.

### Melissa

The preparation is developed from leaves of lemon balm, a member of the mint family (Tyler & Foster, 1996). The ingredients are a volatile oil, a tannin, flavonoids, and other compounds (Leung & Foster, 1995). It is used as a calmative, antispasmolytic, and carminative, and for sleep inducement and GI symptoms (Leung & Foster, 1995). Melissa also has antibacterial and antiviral effects (antiviral effects against herpes simplex types I and 2) (Tyler, 1994). The cream containing 1% of the dried extract of lemon balm must be begun at the first sign of infection; it works best in days 1 and 2 of treatment (Wobling & Leonhardt, 1994). No side effects are reported.

Advised Dosage. For skin infections, primarily herpetic, see above; applied topically as needed.

### Tea Tree Oil

A steam-distilled volatile oil made from the leaves of a shrub or small tree, this is a member of the Myrtacea family found in swampy or wet areas in Australia (Tyler & Foster, 1996). The oil contains terpene hydrocarbons and other components and is bacteriostatic and germicidal if it contains high levels of terpinen-4-ol; it is used to treat a variety of lesions and injuries (boils, abcesses, cuts, sores, abrasions, suppurant wounds, athlete's foot, and acne vulgaris). Some people may be sensitive to the oil and develop a skin irritation or allergy, but it is generally not toxic (Tyler, 1994).

Advised Dosage. Topical application; concentration is 0.4–100% depending on the reason for use and area for treatment (Tyler, 1994). Can be applied to washed, dried areas with a cotton swab.

### Other

Many studies of traditional Chinese medicinal plant decoctions used for atopic eczema have been published, but it is not possible from the literature to identify specific plants. One such example is a study by Sheehan and Atherton (1992) that found superior improvement to placebo in 47 children treated with such a compound. The expectation is that wider use of such therapies will be forthcoming.

## SORE THROAT AND LARYNGITIS

### Slippery Elm

The preparation comes from the dried inner bark of a member of the elm family found in eastern North America (Tyler & Foster, 1996).

The inner bark contains mucilage, starch, and tannins. Its action is as a mucilaginous demulcent, emollient, and nutrient to soothe irritated mucous membranes. Slippery elm also will relieve gastritis, colitis, and gastric or duodenal ulcers (Bradley, 1992). As a soothing demulcent for sore throats, slippery elm has received FDA approval. It is safe, and no precautions are advised.

Advised Dosage. 0.5–2 g powdered bark steeped in 10 parts hot water (5–20 mL) taken as needed. Commercially prepared tablets and troches may be purchased (Bradley, 1992).

## URINARY INFECTION/INFLAMMATION

### Bearberry

Bearberry is made from the dried leaves of a plant that grows in cold regions of the Northern Hemisphere (Tyler & Foster, 1996). It contains phenolic glycosides with antiseptic action, plus other components like flavonoids and tannins. Bearberry has minimal diuretic action; it is primarily an antibacterial for urinary tract infections (UTIs). It must be given with alkaline fluids to release active ingredients, so a high-alkaline diet is required (milk, tomatoes, potatoes, fruits, fruit juices) or 6–8 g sodium bicarbonate daily may be taken (Tyler, 1994). Bearberry may cause nausea and vomiting in a few persons.

Advised Dosage. 10 g of dried cut or powdered herb macerated overnight in 150 mL of cold water is the daily dose. This corresponds to 400–700 mg arbutin. One week or less of use is advised (Uvae ursi folium, 1984).

### Cranberry

The juice or extract of the American cranberry is used to treat UTIs. The therapeutic ingredients are fructose and an unidentified compound (Tyler, 1994). In the 1920s, cranberry was recognized as having a bacteriostatic effect; now, action is thought to be due to prevention of adhesion of bacteria to mucosal cells (Sobota, 1984). If it is given to incontinent persons, it decreases pH and degradation of bacteria, thus decreasing the ammonia odor (Lawrence Review, 1994). Avorn et al (1994) found that cranberry juice reduced the frequency of bacteriuria in a

study of over a hundred elderly women. Non-adhesion properties were found only in plants of the *Vaccinium* genus (family, Ericaceae) in a study looking at seven juices. Blueberry and cranberry juices are the only ones in this family considered safe for use (Ofek et al, 1991). No precautions are indicated, although ingestion of large amounts (more than 3–4 L/day) may result in gastrointestinal disturbances, including diarrhea (Hebel, 1996). It is useful for prophylaxis with diaphragm users, women who have coitally related UTIs, and elderly women (Fugh-Berman, 1996).

Advised Dosage. For prevention of UTIs, 90 mL of juice daily; for treatment of UTIs, 360–960 mL daily. Available in capsules containing dried cranberry and extract; six capsules are equivalent to 90 mL of cranberry juice cocktail where one third of the cocktail is cranberry juice (Tyler, 1994).

### Goldenrod

The preparation is from the dried flowering aboveground (aerial) parts of European or American species of the aster family (Tyler & Foster, 1996). Active ingredients include saponins, diterpenes, tannins, flavonoids, and other components. It is used to prevent or treat urinary calculi and kidney stones. It should be avoided if the user is allergic to aster family members, and is contraindicated in impaired cardiac or kidney function.

Advised Dosage. 3–5 g of herb steeped in 240 mL of boiling water for infusion. Daily dosage is generally 6–12 g (Solidaginis virgaureae herba, 1990; Tyler, 1994).

## OTHER PREPARATIONS ON THE HORIZON OR BEING STUDIED

### Caigua

Caigua is a dried vegetable from Central and South America, better known as wild cucumber or, in some countries, as achojcha (Bricklin, 1996b). Its scientific name is *Cyclanthera pedata*. Scientists are studying caigua for its cholesterol-lowering ability. In one small study of 24 postmenopausal women, it lowered total cholesterol 22%, lowered LDL cholesterol 33%, and raised HDL cholesterol 33% (Bricklin, 1996b).

It is used in soups and stews, stuffed in peppers, and steamed alone. Its high fiber content may be the reason for its exciting effects. It is not yet available in the United States.

## Lavender

Found in flowers from a member of the mint family, lavender contains an essential oil used for centuries as a fragrance in perfumes, soaps, and sachets, as well as an aromatherapy for relaxation, anxiety-stress-depression relief, upset stomachs, and headaches (Mindell, 1992). In a recently reported study in Great Britain, 1% essential oil of lavender was used in a lubricating oil for massage in an intensive care unit by nurses (Dunn, Sleep, & Collett, 1995). Mood improvement and anxiety reduction were found. Lavender may also exert a hypoglycemic action and appears to relieve perineal discomfort postpartum. It can also act as an insect repellant. Few data are available on toxicity, but there are several recent reports of contact dermatitis reactions to lavender oil and fragrance (Hebel, 1996).

## REFERENCES

Agni casti fructus (Kenuschlammfruchte). Bundes-anzeiger. 1985 Mar 5; replaced 1992 Dec 2. Monograph reported in Tyler and Foster, 1996.

Allii sativi bulbus (Knoblauchzwiebel). Bundesanzeiger. 1988 July 6. Monograph reported in Tyler and Foster, 1996.

Almeida, J. C. & Grimsley, E. W. (1997). Coma from the health food store: Interaction between kava and alprazolam. *Annals of Internal Medicine*, 125(11), 940–941.

Arnot, B. (1996, February). Health check: Can a berry fight the flu? *Good Housekeeping*, 58.

Ask Dr. Tyler. (May 1997). *Prevention*, 82–83.

Auer, W., Eiber, A., Hertkorn, E. et al. (1990). Hypertension and hyperlipdiaemia: Garlic helps in mild cases. *British Journal of Clinical Practice* (Suppl. 69), 3–6.

Avorn, J., Monane, M., Gurwitz, J.H., Glynn, R., Choodnovskiy, I., & Lipsitz, L. (1994). Reduction of bacteriuria and pyuria after ingestion of cranberry juice. *JAMA*, 271(10), 751–754.

Awang, D. V. C. (1989). Herbal medicine: Feverfew. *Canadian Pharmaceutical Journal*, 122, 266–270.

Awang, D. V. C., et al. (1991). Parthenolide content of feverfew (*Tanacetum parthenium*) assessed by HPLC and $^1$H-NMR spectroscopy. *Journal of Natural Products*, 54, 1516–1521.

Bauer, R., & Wagner, H. (1991). *Echinacea* species as potential immunostimulatory drugs. In H. Wagner & N. R. Farnsworth (Eds), *Economic and medicinal plant research, Vol. 5* (pp. 253–320). Orlando, FL: Academic Press.

Belch, J. J. F., Ansell, D., Madhok, R., et al. (1988). Effects of altering dietary essential fatty acids on requirements for non-steroidal anti-inflammatory drugs in patients with rheumatoid arthritis. *Annals of Rheumatic Disease*, 47(2), 96–104.

Bisset, N. B. (1994). *Herbal drugs and phytopharmaceuticals: A handbook for practice on a scientific basis*. Boca Raton, FL: CRC Press.

Bloomfield, H. H., Nordfors, M., & McWilliams, P. (1997). *Hypericum & depression*. Los Angeles: Prelude Press.

Bone, M. E., Wilkinson, D. J., Young, J. R., McNeil, M. B., & Charlton, M. B. (1990). Ginger root: A new antiemetic. The effect of ginger root on postoperative nausea and vomiting after major gynecological surgery. *Anaesthesia*, 45, 669–671.

Bradley, P. R. (Ed). (1992). *British herbal compendium*. Vol. I. Bournemouth, Dorset, England: British Herbal Medicine Association.

Braeckman, J. (1994). The extract of *Serenoa repens* in the treatment of benign prostatic hyperplasia: A multicenter open study. *Current Therapeutic Research*, 55, 776–785.

Braunig, B., Dorn, M., & Knick, E. (1992). Echinaceae purpureae radix. *Zeitschrift Phytother*, 13, 7–13.

Bricklin, M (1995a, August). The herbs for the prostate. *Prevention*, 19, 20.

Bricklin, M. (1995b, July). Herbs that turn back the clock. *Prevention*, 19–21.

Bricklin, M. (1996a, January). Herbs that ease the mind. *Prevention*, 15, 16, 18.

Bricklin, M. (1996b, August). Healing plants around the world. *Prevention*, 21–22.

Bricklin, M. (1996c, October). Two hot herbal healers. *Prevention*, 23–25.

Briggs, C. J. (1986). Evening primrose. *Canadian Pharmaceutical Journal*, 119, 248–254.

Brzeski, M., Madhok, R., & Capell, H. A. (1991). Evening primrose oil in patients with rheumatoid arthritis and side effects of non-steroidal anti-inflammatory drugs. *British Journal of Rheumatology*, 30, 370–372.

Campion, E. W. (1993). Why unconventional medicine? *New England Journal of Medicine, 328*, 282–283.

Capsaicin Study Group (1991). Treatment of painful diabetic neuropathy with topical capsaicin. *Archives of Internal Medicine*, 151, 2225–2229.

Chamberlain, J. J. & Abolnik, I. Z. (1997). Pulmonary edema following a licorice binge. *Western Journal of Medicine*, 167(3), 184–185.

Champault, B., Patel, J. C., & Bonnard, A. M. (1984). A double-blind trial of an extract of plant *Serenoa repens* in benign prostatic hyperplasia. *British Journal of Clinical Pharmacology, 18,* 461–462.

Cimicifugae racemosae rhizoma (Cimicifugawurzelstock). Bundesanzeiger. 1989 Mar 2. Monograph reported in Tyler and Foster, 1996.

Dega, H. Laporte, J. L., Frances, C., Herson, S., & Chosidow, O. (1996). Ginseng as a cause for Stevens-Johnson syndrome? [letter]. *Lancet,* 347:1134

Dunn, C., Sleep, J., & Collett, D. (1995). Sensing an improvement: An experimental study to evaluate the use of aromatherapy, massage and periods of rest in an intensive care unit. *Journal of Advanced Nursing, 211*(1), 34–40.

Echinaceae pallidae radix (blassfarbene Kegelblumenwurzel). Bundesanzeiger. 1992 Aug 29. Monograph reported in Tyler and Foster, 1996.

Echinaceae purpureae herba (Purpursonnenhutkraut). Bundesanzeiger. 1989 Aug 29. Monograph reported in Tyler and Foster, 1996.

Elder, N. C., Gillcrist, A., & Minz, R. (1997). Use of alternative health care by family practice patients. *Archives of Family Medicine, 6*(2), 181–184.

Eleuterococci radix (Eleutherococcus - senticosus - Wurzel). Bundesanzeiger. 1991 Jan 17. Monograph reported in Tyler and Foster, 1996.

Epstein, M. T., Espiner, E. A., Donal, R. A., & Hughes, H. (1977). Effect of eating licorice on the renin-angiotensin-aldosterone axis in normal subjects. *British Medical Journal, 1,* 488–490.

European Scientific Cooperative for Phytotherapy (ESCOP). (1990). *Proposal for European monographs* (Vol. 1). Bevrijdingslaan, The Netherlands: ESCOP Secretariat. Reported in Tyler and Foster, 1996.

European Scientific Cooperative for Phytotherapy (ESCOP). (1992). *Proposal for European monographs* (Vol. 2). Bevrijdingslaan, The Netherlands: ESCOP Secretariat. Reported in Tyler and Foster, 1996.

Faleni, R., & Soldati, F. (1996). Ginseng as cause of Stevens-Johnson Syndrome? [letter; comment]. *Lancet, 348*(9022), 267.

Farese, R. V., Biglieri, E. G., Shackleton, C. H. L., Irony, I., & Gomez-Fontes, R. (1991). Licorice-induced hypermineralcorticoidism. *New England Journal of Medicine, 325*(17):1223–1227.

Farnsworth, N. R., et al. (1985). Siberian ginseng (*Eleutherococcus senticosus*): Current status as an adaptogen. In H. Wagner, H. Hikino, & N. R. Farnsworth (Eds), *Economic and medicinal plant research,* (Vol. 1) (pp. 155–215). Orlando, FL: Academic Press. Reported in Tyler and Foster, 1996.

Fischer-Rasmussen, W., Kjaer, S. K., Dahl, C., & Asping, U. (1990). Ginger treatment of hyperemesis gravidarum. *European Journal of Obstetrics, Gynecology, and Reproductive Biology, 38,* 19–24.

Foltz-Gray, D. (November 1997). Move over aspirin. *Prevention,* 97–103, 180.

Foster, S. (1991a). Asian ginseng: *Panax ginseng* (Botanical Series 309) (pp. 1–8). Austin, TX: American Botanical Council.

Foster, S. (1991b). Chamomile: *Matricaria recutita* and *Chamaemelum nobile* (Botanical Series 307) (pp. 1–7). Austin, TX: American Botanical Council.

Foster, S. (1991c). *Echinacea: The purple cone flowers* (Botanical Series 301) (pp. 1–7). Austin, TX: American Botanical Council.

Foster, S. (1991d). Feverfew: *Tanacetum parthenium* (Botanical Series 310) (pp. 1–8). Austin, TX: American Botanical Council.

Foster, S. (1991e). Garlic: *Allium sativum* (Botanical Series 311) (pp. 1–7). Austin, TX: American Botanical Council.

Foster, S. (1991f). Ginkgo: *Ginkgo biloba* (Botanical Series 304) (pp. 1–7). Austin, TX: American Botanical Council.

Foster, S. (1991g). Peppermint: *Menthax piperita* (Botanical Series 306) (pp. 1–7). Austin TX: American Botanical Council.

Foster, S. (1991h). Siberian ginseng: *Eleutherococcus senticosus* (Botanical Series 302) (pp. 1–7). Austin, TX: American Botanical Council.

Fugh-Berman, A. (1996). *Alternative medicine: What works. A comprehensive, easy-to-read review of the scientific evidence, pro and con.* Berkeley, CA: Odouson Press.

Gately, C. A., Miers, M., Mansel, R. E., & Hughes, L. E. (1992). Drug treatments for mastalgia: 17 years experience in the Cardiff mastalgia clinic. *Journal of the Royal Society of Medicine, 85,* 12–15.

Ginseng radix (Ginsengwurzel). Bundesanzeiger. 1991 Jan 17. Monograph reported in Tyler and Foster, 1996.

Ginseng side effects? (1996, October). Mailbag. *Prevention,* 10, 13.

Gorler, K., Oehlke, D., & Soicke, H. (1985). Iridoidführung von Vitex agnuscastus. *Planta Medica, 51,* 530–531. Reported in Tyler and Foster, 1996.

Grontved, A., & Hentzer, E. (1986). Vertigo-reducing effect of ginger root: A controlled clinical study. *Journal of Oto-Rhino-Laryngology and Its Related Specialties, 48,* 282–286.

Hamamelidis folium et cortx (Hamamelisblatten undrende). Bundesanzeiger. 1985 Aug 21; revised 1990 March 13. Monograph reported in Tyler and Foster, 1996.

Harrer, G., & Sommer, H. (1994). Treatment of mild/moderate depression with hypericium. *Phytomedicine*, *1*, 3–8.

Hebel, S. K. (Ed.). (1996). *The Lawrence review of national products*. St. Louis: Facts and Comparisons.

Heggers, J. P., Kucukcelebi, A., Listengarten, D., Stabenau, J., Ko, F., Broemeling, L. D., Robson, M. C., & Winters, W. D. (1996). Beneficial effect of aloe on wound healing in an excisional wound model. *Journal of Alternative Complementary Medicine*, *2*(2), 271–277.

Heggers, J. P., Pelley, R. P., & Robson, M. C. (1993). Beneficial effects of aloe in wound healing. *Phytother Res* [Spring special issue] 7, 548–552.

Heptinstall, S., Awang, D. V., Dawson, B. A., (1992). Parthenolide content and bioactivity of feverfew (*Tanacetum parthenium*(L.) Schultz-Bip.): Estimation of commercial and authenticated feverfew products. *Journal of Pharmacy and Pharmacology*, *44*, 391–395.

Hoffman, D. (1991). *The new holistic herbalist* (3rd ed.) New York: Element.

Horrobin, D. F. (1990). Gamma linolenic acid, an intermediate in essential fatty acid metabolism with potential as an ethical pharmaceutical and as a food. *Review of Contemporary Pharmacotherapy*, *1*(1), 1–41.

Hurley, D. (1995, May). Pharmacists need to increase knowledge of herbal remedies as use skyrockets. *Pharmacy Practice News*, 24–25.

Hyperici herba (Johanniskraut). Bundesanzeiger. 1984 Dec 5; rev 1989 Mar 2. Monograph reported in Tyler and Foster (1996).

Is gingko biloba a memory booster? (January 1998). University of California at Berkeley. *Wellness Letter*, *14*(3), 1–2.

Johnson, E. S., Kadam, N. P., Hylands, D. M., & Hylands, P. J. (1985). Efficacy of feverfew as prophylactic treatment of migraine. *British Medical Journal*, *291*, 569–573.

Johnson, M. G., & Vaughan, R. H. (1969). Death of *Salmonella gypinmurium* and *Escherichia coli* in the presence of freshly reconstituted dehydrated garlic and onion. *Applied Microbiology*, *17*(6), 903–905.

Kasper, S. (1997). Treatment of seasonal affective disorder (SAD) with hypericum extract. *Pharmacopsychiatry*, *30* Supplement 2, 89–93.

Kassir, Z. A. (1985). Endoscopic controlled trial of four drug regimens in the treatment of chronic duodenal ulcers. *Irish Medical Journal*, *78*, 153–156.

Keville, K. (1996). *Herbs for health and healing*. Emmaus, PA: Rodale Press.

Kleijnen, J., & Knipschild, P. (1992). *Ginkgo biloba. Lancet*, *340*, 1136–1139.

Larrey, C., Vial, T., Pauwies, A., Biour, M., David, M., Michel, H. (1992). Hepatotoxicity after gremander (*Teucrium chamaedrys*) administration: Another instance of herbal medicine hepatotoxicity. *Annals of Internal Medicine*, *117*, 129–132.

Lawrence Review of National Products. (1994 July). Reported in Tyler and Foster, 1996.

Leathwood, P. D., Chauffard, F., Herck, E., & Munoz-Box, R. (1982). Aqueous extract of valerian root (*Valeriana officianlis* L.) improves sleep quality in man. *Pharmacology, Biochemistry and Behavior*, *17*, 65–71.

LeBars, P. L., Katz, M. M., Berman, N., Itil, T. M., Freedman, A. M., & Schatzberg, A. F. (1997). A placebo-controlled, double-blind, randomized trial of an extract of Ginkgo biloba for dementia. North American Egb Study Group, *Journal of the American Medical Association*, *278*(16), 1327–1332.

Leung, A. Y. & Foster, S. (1995). *Encyclopedia of common natural ingredients used in foods, drugs, and cosmetics* (2nd ed.). New York: Wiley.

Lindahl, O., & Lindwall, L. (1989). Double blind study of a valerian preparation. *Pharmacology, Biochemistry and Behavior*, *32*, 1065–1066.

Linde, K., Ramirez, G., Mulrow, C. D., Pauls, A., Weidenhammer, W., & Melchart, D. (1996). St. John's wort for depression—an overview and meta-analysis of randomised clinical trials. *British Medical Journal* *313*(7052), 253–258.

Liquiritiae radix (Sussholzwurzel). Bundesanzeiger. 1985 May 15; revised 1990 March 13. Monograph reported in Tyler and Foster, 1996.

Lovell, C. R., Burton, J. L., & Horrobin, D. F. (1981). Treatment of atopic eczema with evening primrose oil. *Lancet*, *1*(8214), 278.

MacGregor, F., Abernathy, V., Dahabra, S., Cobden, I. & Hayes, P. (1991). Hepatotoxicity of herbal remedies. *British Medical Journal*, 299:1156–1159.

Marrubii herba (Andornkraut). Bundsanzeiger. 1990 Feb 1. Monograph reported in Tyler and Foster, 1996.

Marwick, C. (1992). Congress wants alternative therapies studied; NIH responds with programs. *JAMA*, *268*, 957–958.

McCarthy, G. M., & McCarty, D. J. (1992). Effects of topical capsaicin in the therapy of painful osteoarthritis of the hands. *Journal of Rheumatology*, *19*, 604–607.

Menthae piperitae aetheroleum (Pfefferminzblätter). Bundesanzeiger. 1990 Mar 13. Monograph reported in Tyler and Foster, 1996.

Menthae piperitae folium (Pfefferminzblätter). Bundesanzeiger. 1985 Nov 30; rev 1990 Mar 13. Monograph reported in Tyler and Foster, 1996.

Miller, C. A. (1996). Alternative healing products: Herbal and homeopathic remedies. *Geriatric Nursing, 17*(3), 145–146.

Mindell, E. (1992). *Earl Mindell's herb bible*. New York: Fireside.

Napier, K. (1994, March). Unproven medical treatments lure elderly. *FDA Consumer*.

Ng, T. B., & Yeung, H. W. (1986). Scientific basis of the therapeutic effects of ginseng. In R. P. Steiner (Ed.), *Folk medicine, the art and the science* (pp. 139–152). Washington, DC: American Chemical Society.

Norton, S. A., & Ruze, P. (1994). Kava dermopathy. *Journal of the American Academy of Dermatology, 31*(1), 89–97.

Ofek, I., Goldhar, J., Zafriri, D., et al. (1991). Anti-*Escherichia coli* adhesion activity of cranberry and blueberry juices. *New England Journal of Medicine, 324*(22), 1599.

Paramore, L. C. (1997). Use of alternative therapies: Estimates from the 1994 Robert Wood Johnson Foundation National Access to Care Survey. *Journal of Pain Symptoms Management, 13*(2), 83–89.

Phelps, S., & Harris, W. S. (1993). Garlic supplementation and lipoprotein oxidation susceptibility. *Lipids, 28*(5), 475–477.

Plantaginis ovatae testa (Indische Flohsamenschalen); Plantaginis ovatae semn (Indische Flohsamen). Bundesanzeiger. 1990 Feb 1. Monograph in Tyler and Foster, 1996.

Sabal fructus (Sagepalmenfrüchte). Bundesanzeiger. 1989 Mar 2; revised 1990 Feb 1; 1991 Jan 17. Monograph reported in Tyler and Foster, 1996.

St. John's Wort. (August 1997). *Women's Health Watch, IV*(12), 5.

Schalin-Karrila, M., Mattila, L., Jansen, C. T., & Uotila, P. (1987). Evening primrose oil in the treatment of atopic exzema: Effect on clinical status, plasma phospholipid fatty acids, and circulation blood prostaglandins. *British Journal of Dermatology, 117*, 11–19.

Sennae folium (Sennesblatter). Bundesanzeiger. 1989 Mar 2; revised 1990 Feb 1; 1991 Jan 17. Monograph reported in Tyler and Foster, 1996.

Sheehan, M. P., & Atherton, D. J. (1992). A controlled trial of traditional Chinese medicine plants in widespread, non-exudative atopic eczema. *British Journal of Dermatology, 126*, 179–184.

Shibata, S., et al. (1985). Chemistry and pharmacology of *Panax*. In H. Wagner, H. Hikino, & N. R. Farnsworth (Eds.), *Economic and medicinal plant research* (Vol. 1) (pp. 217–284). Orlando, FL: Academic Press. Reported in Tyler and Foster, 1996.

Sikora, R., Sohn, M., Deutz, F-J., et al. (1989). *Ginkgo biloba* extract in the therapy of erectile dysfunction [abstract]. *Journal of Urology, 141*:188A.

Silagy, C. A., & Neil, H. A. W. (1994). A meta-analysis of the effect of garlic on blood pressure. *Journal of Hypertension, 12*, 463–468.

Sobota, A. E. (1984). Inhibition of bacterial adherence by cranberry juice: Potential use for the treatment of urinary tract infections. *Journal of Urology, 131*, 1013–1016.

Solidaginis virgaureae herba (Echtes Goldrutenkraut). Bundesanzeiger. 1987 Oct 15; revised 1990 Mar 13. Monograph reported in Tyler and Foster, 1996.

Snider, S. (1991). Herbal teas and toxicity. *FDA Consumer*. Rockville, MD: DHHS Publication No. 92-1185.

Sprecher, D. L., Harris, B. V., Goldberg, A. C., et al. (1993). Efficacy of psyllium in reducing serum cholesterol levels in hypercholesterolemic patients on high- or low-fat diets. *Annals of Internal Medicine, 119*, 545–554.

Stewart, J. J., Wood, M. J., Wood, C. D., & Mims, M. E. (1991). Effects of ginger on motion sickness susceptibility and gastric function. *Pharmacology, 42*, 111–120.

The natural mood booster. (December 2, 1997). *Prevention's Guide: Healing Herbs*, 8.

Tierra, M. (1990). *The way of herbs*. New York: Pocketbooks.

Tyler, V. E. (1993). *The honest herbal: A sensible guide to the use of herbs and related remedies* (3rd ed.). New York: Pharmaceutical Products Press.

Tyler, V. E. (1994). *Herbs of choice: The therapeutic use of phytomedicinals*. New York: Pharmaceutical Products Press.

Tyler, V. E. (March 1997). Herbal medicine 101. *Prevention*, 72–76.

Tyler, V. E. (October 1997). Nature's stress buster. *Prevention*, 90–95.

Tyler, V. E. (December 1997). Promising herbs for prostate problems. *Prevention*, 69–72.

Tyler, V. E. (February 1998). Spotlight on ginger. *Prevention*, 82–85.

Tyler, V. E., Brady, L. R., & Robbers, J. E. (1988). *Pharmacognosy* (9th ed.). Philadelphia, PA: Lea & Febiger.

Tyler, V. E., & Foster, S. (1996). Herbs and phytomedicinal products. In *Handbook of nonprescription drugs* (pp. 695–711). Washington, DC: American Pharmaceutical Association.

Uvae ursi folium (Barentraubenblatter). Bundesanzeiger. 1984 Dec 5. Monograph reported in
Tyler and Foster, 1996.

Voltz, H. P. (1997). Controlled clinical trials of hypericum extracts in depressed patients—an overview.
*Pharmacopsychiatry, 30* Supplement 2, 72–76.

Warburton, D. M. (1988). Clinical psychopharmacology
of *Ginkgo biloba* extract. In E. W. Funfgeld (Ed.),
*Rokan (Ginkgo biloba): Recent results in pharma-
cology and clinic* (pp. 327–345). Berlin: Springer-
Verlag. Reported in Tyler and Foster, 1996.

Warshafsky, S., Kamer, R. S., & Sivak, S. L. (1993).
Effect of garlic on total serum cholesterol: A meta-
analysis. *Annals of Internal Medicine, 119,* 599–605.

Watson, C. P. N., & Evans, R. J. (1992). The postmastectomy pain syndrome and topical capsaicin:
A randomized trial. *Pain, 51,* 375–379.

Wobling, R. H., & Leonhardt, K. (1994). Local therapy of herpes simplex with dried extract from
*Melissa officinalis. Phytomedicine, 1,* 25–31.

Youngkin, E. Q., & Israel, D. (1996). A review and
critique of common herbal alternative therapies.
*Nurse Practitioner, 21*(10), 39–62.

Yun, T-K., & Choi, S. Y. (1995). Preventive effect
of ginseng intake against various human cancers:
A case-control study on 1987 pairs. *Cancer
Epidemiology, Biomarkers, and Prevention, 4*(4),
401–408.

# 11

## IMMUNIZATIONS

*Debra K. Hearington*

Vaccination attempts to protect humans from disease have been reported since the sixth century, although the first written reports are from the eleventh century (Plotkin & Plotkin, 1994). The twentieth century has seen the practice develop and flourish, and the incidence of many diseases that once caused significant morbidity and mortality has dramatically declined. One such disease, smallpox, was declared eradicated from the world in 1980 (World Health Organization [WHO], 1980). Polio has been eradicated from the United States and Europe. Others, including measles in the Western Hemisphere and polio worldwide, probably will be eradicated within the next few years.

This chapter will briefly discuss vaccine-controllable diseases, immunization schedules, and vaccines in development. The reader should refer to Plotkin & Mortimer (1994), the most current edition of the Department of Health and Human Services (DHHS) publication *Epidemiology & Prevention of Vaccine-Preventable Diseases*, and the Centers for Disease Control (CDC) publications, *Morbidity and Mortality Weekly Report* (MMWR), for more information.

## SELECTED PRINCIPLES OF IMMUNITY

Vaccines confer active immunity to disease. *Active immunity* occurs following exposure and recovery from an infection in certain diseases. For example, recovery from chicken pox, *vari-* *cella* infection, confers active immunity to chicken pox so that individuals rarely suffer from that disease a second time. Active immunity also occurs following inoculation, ingestion, or inhalation of an altered form of an infectious organism or product of the organism (eg, toxin) that has been modified to induce immunity but not produce disease (Sell, 1996). Conferring lifelong immunity to diseases against which immunizations are effective may require more than one dose of the vaccine. *Passive immunity* occurs when immune products are transferred from one living being to another.

Passive immunity is temporary, usually lasting several weeks to months. Newborn infants have immunity to specific infectious agents because antibodies have been transferred from the mother in utero. This immunity generally lasts 3–4 months (Sell, 1996). Humoral antibodies may also be transferred in human immunoglobulin and immunoglobulins from the serum of immunized animals. Pooled human immune globulin is useful in treating exposures to hepatitis A and measles, and specific human immune globulin may be given for exposures to hepatitis B, pertussis, rabies, tetanus, vaccinia (cowpox), and infection with varicella-zoster (Sell, 1996). Specific equine immune globulin may be given after bites by snakes and black widow spiders, and exposure to diphtheria and botulism toxins (Sell, 1996). Immune globulins must be given immediately following exposure to the infecting organisms, and in some cases, must be repeated.

Once a large proportion of a population of people are immunized, other unimmunized people are indirectly protected because transmission of the infectious agent may be interrupted. This concept is called *herd immunity* (Hinman & Orenstein, 1994). Herd immunity is an important factor in the eradication of diseases against which immunizations are effective.

## CHILDHOOD IMMUNIZATIONS

Immunization against diseases known to cause significant morbidity and mortality in the population is begun in infancy. Those diseases are pertussis, poliomyelitis, and meningitis caused by *Haemophilus* influenza type B (HIB), diphtheria, tetanus, rubeola, mumps, hepatitis B, and chicken pox. Rubeola causes severe damage to fetuses, and the population is immunized to protect the unborn. Immunizations begun in infancy have been successful in protecting children from illnesses often fatal in the first year of life, such as pertussis and meningitis caused by *Haemophilus* influenza type B. Certain immunizations cannot be given in the first year of life because of limited efficacy or because of the high risk of an allergic reaction to a vaccine component, such as egg protein. Those immunizations include varicella and measles-mumps-rubella (MMR).

See the recommended childhood immunization schedule (Fig. 11–1) for the timing of childhood immunizations.

## POLIOMYELITIS

The poliovirus is an enterovirus, with three serotypes, that replicates in the oropharynx and the intestinal tract. Often, the infection (viremia) following is asymptomatic. However, the infection may result in apparently minor illness with no sequelae or minor illness followed by severe illness—aseptic meningitis or paralytic poliomyelitis. Mild illness is characterized by fever, sore throat, headache, and/or gastrointestinal symptoms. Nonparalytic poliomyelitis is characterized by the appearance of meningitis symptoms 1–2 days following the onset of mild illness, and occurs in 1–2% of patients. Recovery is usually complete; however, in a small percentage of cases, mild muscle weakness or paralysis occurs. Paralytic poliomyelitis is characterized by sudden onset of muscle weakness and aches in the back and/or extremities and progresses to flaccid paralysis and loss of deep tendon reflexes. Paralytic poliomyelitis may occur with or without prodromal symptoms, and happens in less than 2% of all poliovirus infections. Paralysis generally does not progress after the temperature returns to normal, and recovery occurs gradually over several months. Some patients experience residual muscle weakness or paralysis for the rest of their lives. The death rate from paralytic poliomyelits is 2–10% of cases (CDC, 1997f; Committee on Infectious Diseases, 1998; DHHS, 1996; Melnick, 1994).

A postpolio syndrome occurs in 25–40% of persons 30–40 years following paralytic poliomyelitis. They experience muscle pain and may have an exacerbation of existing weakness or develop new weakness or paralysis (CDC, 1997f). Those who develop postpolio syndrome were infected in the 1940s and 1950s when wild poliovirus was circulating (CDC, 1997f; Melnick, 1994).

The virus is transmitted by direct fecal-oral contact and indirectly by contaminated sewage and water, and contact with infectious saliva or feces (CDC, 1997f). Humans are the only reservoir, which is an advantage in the eradication effort. The Western Hemisphere was certified to be free of indigenous wild poliovirus in September, 1994, because there is no evidence of any polio infection caused by circulating wild virus in this part of the world (Hull, Ward, Hull, Milstien & deQuadros, 1994). The World Health Assembly adopted the goal of global eradication by the year 2000, which now appears feasible (CDC, 1997f).

There are two vaccines currently available: oral polio vaccine (OPV) and inactivated polio vaccine (IPV). An inactivated, injectable vaccine was introduced in the United States in 1955 and was less potent than the most recent injectible IPV licensed for use in 1987. When the trivalent OPV, a live attenuated vaccine, became available in the early 1960s, use of IPV declined for all except immunocompromised persons (CDC, 1997f).

No adverse reactions to IPV have been documented, but a hypersensitivity reaction may occur in those sensitive to streptomycin, polymyxin B, and neomycin. There is a small risk of paralysis following administration of OPV (CDC, 1997f). The condition known as vaccine-associated paralytic poliomyelitis (VAPP) carries a risk of 1 case in 2.4 million doses of OPV administered and 1 case per 750,000 first doses ad-

Vaccines [1] are listed under the routinely recommended ages. ⌐Bars⌐ indicate range of acceptable ages for vaccination. Catch-up immunization should be done during any visit when feasible. ⟨Shaded ovals⟩ indicate vaccines to be assessed and given if necessary during the early adolescent visit.

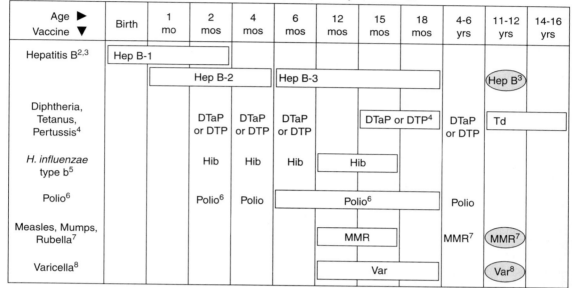

| Age ▶<br>Vaccine ▼ | Birth | 1<br>mo | 2<br>mos | 4<br>mos | 6<br>mos | 12<br>mos | 15<br>mos | 18<br>mos | 4-6<br>yrs | 11-12<br>yrs | 14-16<br>yrs |
|---|---|---|---|---|---|---|---|---|---|---|---|
| Hepatitis B[2,3] | Hep B-1 | | | | | | | | | | |
| | | | Hep B-2 | | Hep B-3 | | | | | (Hep B[3]) | |
| Diphtheria,<br>Tetanus,<br>Pertussis[4] | | | DTaP<br>or DTP | DTaP<br>or DTP | DTaP<br>or DTP | | DTaP or DTP[4] | | DTaP<br>or DTP | Td | |
| H. influenzae<br>type b[5] | | | Hib | Hib | Hib | Hib | | | | | |
| Polio[6] | | | Polio[6] | Polio | | Polio[6] | | | Polio | | |
| Measles, Mumps,<br>Rubella[7] | | | | | | MMR | | | MMR[7] | (MMR[7]) | |
| Varicella[8] | | | | | | Var | | | | (Var[8]) | |

Approved by the Advisory Committee on Immunization Practices (ACIP), the American Academy of Pediatrics (AAP), and the American Academy of Family Physicians (AAFP).

[1]  This schedule indicates the recommended age for routine administration of currently licensed childhood vaccines. Combination vaccines may be used whenever any components of the combination are indicated and its other components are not contraindicated. Providers should consult the manufacturers' package inserts for detailed recommendations.

[2]  *Infants born to HBsAg-negative mothers* should receive 2.5 µg of Merck vaccine (Recombivax HB®) or 10 µg of SmithKline Beecham (SB) vaccine (Engerix-B®). The 2nd dose should be administered at least 1 mo after the 1st dose. The 3rd dose should be given at least 2 mos after the second, but not before 6 mos of age.
*Infants born to HBsAg-positive mothers* should receive 0.5 mL hepatitis B immune globulin (HBIG) within 12 hrs of birth, and either 5 µg of Merck vaccine (Recombivax HB®) or 10 µg of SB vaccine (Engerix-B®) at a separate site. The 2nd dose is recommended at 1–2 mos of age and the 3rd dose at 6 mos of age.
*Infants born to mothers whose HBsAg status is unknown* should receive either 5 µg of Merck vaccine (Recombivax HB®) or 10 µg of SB vaccine (Engerix-B®) within 12 hrs of birth. The 2nd dose of vaccine is recommended at 1–2 mo of age and the 3rd dose at 6 mos of age. Blood should be drawn at the time of delivery to determine the mother's HBsAg status; if it is positive, the infant should receive HBIG as soon as possible (no later than 1 wk of age). The dosage and timing of subsequent vaccine doses should be based upon the mother's HBsAg status.

[3]  Children and adolescents who have not been vaccinated against hepatitis B in infancy may begin the series during any childhood visit. Those who have not previously received 3 doses of hepatitis B vaccine should initiate or complete the series during the 11–12 year-old visit, and unvaccinated older adolescents should be vaccinated whenever possible. The 2nd dose should be administered at least 1 mo after the 1st dose, and the 3rd dose should be administered at least 4 mos after the 1st dose, and at least 2 mos after the 2nd dose.

[4]  DTaP (diphtheria and tetanus toxoids and acellular pertussis vaccine) is the preferred vaccine for all doses in the vaccination series, including completion of the series in children who have received 1 or more doses of whole-cell DTP vaccine. Whole-cell DTP is an acceptable alternative to DTaP. The 4th dose (DTP or DTaP) may be administered as early as 12 mos of age, provided 6 mos have elapsed since the 3rd dose and if the child is unlikely to return at age 15–18 mos. Td (tetanus and diphtheria toxoids) is recommended at 11–12 years of age if at least 5 years have elapsed since the last dose of DTP, DTaP or DT. Subsequent routine Td boosters are recommended every 10 years.

[5]  Three *H. influenzae* type b (Hib) conjugate vaccines are licensed for infant use. If PRP-OMP (PedvaxHIB® [Merck]) is administered at 2 and 4 mos of age, a dose at 6 mos is not required.

[6]  Two poliovirus vaccines are currently licensed in the US: inactivated poliovirus vaccine (IPV) and oral poliovirus vaccine (OPV). The following schedules are all acceptable by the ACIP, the AAP, and the AAFP, and parents and providers may choose among them:
  1. 2 doses of IPV followed by 2 doses of OPV
  2. 4 doses of IPV
  3. 4 doses of OPV
The ACIP recommends 2 doses of IPV at 2 and 4 mos of age followed by 2 doses of OPV at 12–18 mos and 4–6 years of age. *IPV is the only poliovirus vaccine recommended for immunocompromised persons and their household contacts.*

[7]  The 2nd dose of MMR is recommended routinely at 4–6 yrs of age but may be administered during any visit, provided at least 1 mo has elapsed since receipt of the 1st dose and that both doses are administered beginning at or after 12 mos of age. Those who have not previously received the second dose should complete the schedule no later than the 11 to 12-year visit.

[8]  Susceptible children may receive varicella vaccine (Var) at any visit after the first birthday, and those who lack a reliable history of chickenpox should be immunized during the 11–12 year-old visit. Susceptible children 13 years of age or older should receive 2 doses, at least 1 month apart.

**Figure 11–1.** Recommended childhood immunization schedule: United States, January–December 1998.

ministered (CDC, 1997f). VAPP occurs because persons vaccinated with OPV excrete live virus in their stools for up to 6 weeks following immunization, which may cause infection in susceptible (unimmunized and immunocompromised) persons. Since there are no more cases of wild poliovirus infection and an inactivated vaccine is available, the risk of VAPP occurring because of the oral vaccine is considered

unacceptable. Therefore, the Advisory Committee on Immunization Practices (ACIP), the American Academy of Pediatrics (AAP), and the American Academy of Family Physicians (AAFP) have approved a sequential schedule of administering polio vaccines to children. The schedule appears in Fig. 11–1.

Providers may elect to follow a sequential schedule, give IPV alone, or give OPV alone.

The footnotes to the schedule (Fig. 11–1) will guide the provider in administering the correct number of doses depending upon the vaccine chosen. Immunocompromised individuals, including those receiving immunosuppressive therapy in any form and those with acquired or congenital immunodeficiency illnesses, should receive only IPV. Children and other healthy persons needing polio vaccine, who live with immunocompromised people, should also receive only IPV.

There is some controversy regarding the recommended switch to an IPV/OPV sequential schedule or to IPV alone. Some believe that switching to IPV alone is unnecessary because polio will be eliminated altogether in 5–8 years, making vaccination unnecessary. Also, the cost of IPV is higher and compliance may be affected because infants get several immunization shots in the first year of life (Peters, 1997). A concern about an IPV-only schedule is the risk of inadequate gastrointestinal (GI) immunity, although the IPV does confer some GI immunity. These concerns were addressed by the ACIP in recommending the sequential schedule. The sequential schedule calls for two doses of IPV before the age of 6 months and two doses of OPV, one given at 12–18 months and the other at 4–6 years. All these options should be discussed with the person receiving the vaccine or the parents or legal guardians of a minor receiving the vaccine. When administering the vaccine to a child incompletely or never immunized, the ACIP recommends using OPV, except in the contraindicated situations mentioned above. The child should receive three doses at 4-week intervals, and the fourth dose at 4–6 years of age. It is not recommended that adults 18 years and older residing in the United States be routinely immunized due to their low risk for exposure to polioviruses and some degree of immunity from childhood immunization. The CDC recommends vaccination for adults in the following circumstances: the adult is traveling to areas where poliomyelitis is endemic or epidemic; the adult is a member of a community or specific population group with disease caused by wild polioviruses; the adult is a laboratory worker who handles specimens that may contain polioviruses; the adult is a health care worker who may have contact with persons excreting wild polioviruses; or the adult has never been vaccinated and has children who will be receiving OPV. IPV only is recommended for adults who have never been vaccinated because of the higher risk of VAPP in adults. In this case, two doses of IPV should be administered at intervals of 4–8 weeks, with a third dose 6–12 months after the second. Adults who received primary immunization with OPV or IPV and are in the above risk categories may receive either OPV or IPV for their subsequent immunization. The CDC recommends that vaccination in pregnancy be avoided even though adverse effects of IPV or OPV on pregnant women or fetuses have not been documented. However, should a pregnant woman require immediate protection, she should be immunized according to the recommended schedule for adults (CDC, 1997f, pp. 16–17).

For more information on the above information or immunization of people not covered in the above information, contact the CDC at 1-800-CDC-SHOT (1-800-232-7468).

## PERTUSSIS

Pertussis, also known as whooping cough, is a disease characterized by severe, paroxysmal coughing spasms leading to cyanosis and vomiting. Complications include subconjunctival hemorrhages, epistaxis, facial edema, ulceration of the lingual frenulum, pneumonia, pneumothorax, dehydration, otitis media, hernias, rectal prolapse, encephalitis with seizures, and malnutrition (DHHS, 1996, p. 59; Mortimer, 1994b, pp. 91–92). The disease, caused by *Bordetella pertussis*, a gram-negative bacillus, initially appears to be a mild upper respiratory infection with low-grade fever and an occasional cough that increasingly becomes more spasmodic and paroxysmal (Mortimer, 1994b, p. 91). The disease is spread through close contact (respiratory route) and lasts 2–6 weeks. Erythromycin is the drug of choice, but generally it is not effective unless administered early (Wright, Edwards, Decker, & Zeldin, 1995). DHHS recommends that erythromycin or trimethoprim-sulfamethoxazole be given prophylactically to household and close contacts of the infected person for 14 days, regardless of age and vaccination history, to minimize or prevent transmission. In addition, close contacts under age 7 who have not completed the four-dose primary series should complete the series as soon as possible, and anyone who completed the series but has not received a pertussis-containing vaccine within 3 years of exposure should receive a booster dose (DHHS, 1996, p. 60).

Studies have shown that adults may now be the primary source of *Bordetella pertussis* transmission to children and other susceptible adults (DHHS, 1996; Edwards et al, 1993; Herwaldt, 1991; Nelson, 1978; Nennig, 1996; Schmitt et al, 1996; Wright et al, 1995). The disease also has been recognized in adolescents with chronic cough (Cromer et al, 1993, DHHS, 1996). This is thought to be due to declining immunity in adolescents and adults and the presence of *Bordetella pertussis* in the community (Cromer et al, 1993; Wright et al, 1995). This trend has led to the recommendation that adults be given booster doses of acellular pertussis vaccine to reduce transmission to other adults and children (Edwards et al, 1993; Nennig et al, 1996).

Two forms of pertussis vaccine are available: whole-cell preparations and acellular preparations. Severe adverse reactions including high fever (>40.5°C or 105°F); persistent, inconsolable crying for longer than 3 hours; seizures, with and without fever; a hypotonic, hyporesponsive episode; and encephalopathy have been reported following administration of whole-cell preparations (CDC, 1997e; DHHS, 1996; Mortimer, 1994b, p. 113). They occur infrequently, and based on studies that showed a possible causal relationship between whole-cell pertussis vaccine and severe neurologic reactions and studies that did not demonstrate such a relationship, practitioners are somewhat divided on the issue of giving whole-cell pertussis vaccines. However, it has been documented that more adverse reactions, including severe local reactions, are reported following whole-cell pertussis vaccine than acellular pertussis vaccine (CDC, 1997e; Decker et al, 1995). This, combined with studies demonstrating equal, if not better, efficacy of acellular pertussis vaccines, has led to the recent ACIP recommendation to immunize infants and children with acellular pertussis vaccine (CDC, 1997e).

Pertussis vaccine, either whole-cell or acellular, is available combined with diphtheria and tetanus vaccines. A preparation of whole-cell pertussis vaccine combined with diphtheria, tetanus, and *Haemophilus* influenza type B (HIB) vaccines also is available. Other combination preparations of acellular pertussis and other vaccines are in research and development at the present time. See Fig. 11–1 for the schedule for administering pertussis vaccine to children.

# DIPHTHERIA

Toxigenic strains of *Corynebacterium diphtheriae*, a gram-positive bacillus, cause diphtheria, which usually is transmitted by close person-to-person contact (respiratory spread) and rarely by direct contact with skin lesions or materials contaminated with the discharge of skin lesions. The disease may involve any mucous membrane, and sites of infection include the nose, tonsils, and throat, larynx, conjunctiva, skin, and genitalia. A membrane forms that is white in the nose and bluish-white progressing to greyish-green and black if bleeding has occured in the mouth and throat. The membrane adheres to the tissue, and extensive membrane formation in the throat or larynx (depending on the site of disease) may lead to airway obstruction. Symptoms depend on the site of involvement, but include low-grade fever, mucopurulent nasal discharge (may be blood-tinged), sore throat, anorexia, hoarseness, and barking cough with laryngeal involvement; in severe disease, prostration, stupor, coma, and lymphadenopathy and marked edema in the neck are present. Cutaneous involvement is manifested by ulcers with clearly demarcated edges and membrane or a scaling rash, although any chronic skin lesion may contain *C. diphtheriae* (DHHS, 1996, pp. 36–37). Complications include myocarditis, neuritis, palatal, ocular, and diaphragmatic paralysis; and death (DHHS, 1996, pp. 37–38; Mortimer, 1994a).

Treatment is with both diphtheria antitoxin and antibiotics—erythromycin PO or IM or procaine penicillin G IM, and the infected person should be isolated. The person is not contagious after 48 h of antibiotic administration. Diphtheria antitoxin is available in the United States only through an investigational drug protocol through the CDC (CDC, 1997a). Contacts should be given a diphtheria toxoid booster and IM benzathine penicillin G or oral erythromycin (DHHS, 1996, p. 42). Having the infection does not appear to result in lifelong immunity; therefore, booster doses should be given at the appropriate intervals, even with a history of diphtheria illness.

Reporting of nontoxigenic strains of *C. diphtheriae* is no longer required, and contacts do not need to be investigated. All cases caused by toxigenic strains are reportable.

Diphtheria toxoid is available in combination with tetanus toxoid and/or pertussis vaccine, and effectiveness is estimated to be 97% after the primary series is completed (three doses in adults and four doses in infants, spaced at the recommended intervals). Adults require a diphtheria toxoid booster every 10 years to boost waning immunity (DHHS, 1996, p. 42). Multiple boosters at less than 10-year intervals should not be given as Arthus-type hypersensitivity reactions may occur. Anaphylaxis is rare. Mild illness and immunosuppression are not contraindications to receiving diphtheria toxoid vaccine.

See Fig. 11–1 for the recommended schedule in children.

## TETANUS

Tetanus is not a communicable illness, but one that is often fatal. Therefore, protection by immunization is extremely important. It is caused by an exotoxin produced by *Clostridium tetani*, a gram-positive rod, and results in skeletal muscle spasm and rigidity first involving the jaw and neck. Humans and animals harbor the organism, which is found in the intestines and feces, and can also be found in soil, street dust, and manure. Spores may also be found on the skin and in contaminated heroin (DHHS, 1996, p. 47). The organism enters at wound sites and the spores germinate, producing toxins that are disseminated through the circulatory and lymphatic systems. Tetanus may be local, where muscle contraction and spasm is limited to the area of injury. Localized tetanus is unusual in humans, but it may occur and precede the development of generalized tetanus (Wassilak, Orenstein, & Sutter, 1994, p. 58). Cephalic tetanus is rare and may occur with otitis media when the organism is present in middle ear fluid or following head injuries. Neonatal tetanus may occur following infection of the unhealed umbilical stump. The most common form is generalized tetanus, beginning with jaw muscle rigidity (lockjaw) followed by neck stiffness and spasm of the facial muscles in some cases. Difficulty in swallowing, abdominal muscle rigidity, spasms of other muscles, fever, sweating, increased blood pressure, and periodic tachycardia also occur. Complications include laryngospasm, fractures, coma, pulmonary embolism, aspiration pneumonia, and death (DHHS, 1996, pp. 48–49; Wassilak et al, 1994, p. 58).

Treatment includes administration of human tetanus immune globulin (TIG) at diagnosis; ad-ministration of procaine penicillin, aqueous crystalline penicillin G, or metronidazole; and administration of agents to relieve muscle spasm, in addition to other supportive therapy (Wassilak et al, 1994, pp. 60–61). Infection does not produce immunity, so those with a history of tetanus disease need to be immunized with tetanus toxoid according to the appropriate schedule for age and previous vaccination history.

Tetanus toxoid is combined with diphtheria toxoid and/or pertussis vaccine. Following the primary series, immunity generally lasts 10 years. Therefore, persons should receive booster doses every 10 years following the primary series. A repeat dose of tetanus toxoid should be given when "dirty" wound injuries occur more than 5 years after a tetanus booster. When the injured are unsure of the date of last tetanus booster, a booster should be given. In the case of an injured person who has had two doses or less of tetanus toxoid, or who is uncertain of a prior history of tetanus immunization, tetanus immune globulin should be given in addition to the immunization (DHHS, 1996, pp. 55). Pregnancy, immunosuppression, or presence of minor illness is not a contraindication to tetanus immunization.

Local reactions, erythema, induration, and pain at the injection site are common. An abscess at the injection site may also occur, and local reactions are generally self-limited.

See Fig. 11–1 for the recommended immunization schedule.

## MEASLES

The measles virus belongs to the Paramyxoviridae family, genus *Morbillivirus*. Infection with this virus causes illness that begins with fever, upper respiratory symptoms, and conjunctivitis. Koplik's spots appear on the buccal mucosa 1–2 days preceding the development of a red, maculopapular rash beginning at the hairline and proceeding downward. The lesions are discrete but may become confluent on the upper body and face, and initially they blanch with pressure. The rash then fades in the order it progressed, and desquamation may occur over severely involved areas. Other symptoms include malaise, anorexia, diarrhea, and generalized lymphadenopathy. Complications include diarrhea, otitis media, pneumonia, encephalitis, hepatitis, appendicitis, pericarditis, myocarditis, thrombocytopenia, laryngotracheobronchitis, ileocolitis, glomerulonephritis, hypocalcemia, and Stevens-Johnsons syndrome. Subacute sclerosing panencephalitis (SSPE) is a rare, severe complication of measles infection and may occur years after infection (1 month to 27 years). SSPE is a degenerative disease of the central nervous system resulting in behavioral and personality changes, seizures, coma, and death (Markowitz & Katz, 1994, p. 229). Measles in pregnancy may result in spontaneous abortion or premature birth, although there is no evidence that infection in the first trimester causes birth defects (unlike rubella) (DHHS, 1996, pp. 85–88; Markowitz & Katz, 1994).

Treatment is primarily supportive, although high doses of vitamin A seem to reduce morbidity and mortality in developing countries. No other forms of therapy for measles or SSPE have been shown to be effective (Markowitz & Katz, 1994). Immune globulin may be administered prophylactically to susceptible persons in whom the vaccine is contraindicated following exposure to the measles virus. Susceptible persons include children under 1 year of age, pregnant women, immunocompromised persons, and others with a contraindication to administration of a live vaccine (Markowitz & Katz, 1994).

Periodic measles outbreaks have occurred since the onset of mass immunization programs; however, the number of reported cases began declining in 1992 (DHHS, 1996, p. 96). There was a slight increase in 1994, from 312 confirmed cases in 1993 to 961 cases in 1994. The outbreaks were noted to be primarily among people in groups that oppose vaccination. In 1995, the number of cases dropped to 309, the lowest since national surveillance began (CDC, 1997c). Increasingly, the cases reported in the United States have been imported, and they often lead to an outbreak among children and adults who have not had a second measles vaccination. The data suggest that wild-type virus transmission in the United States has been interrupted numerous times, which favors the goal of eradication (CDC, 1997c).

A live attenuated vaccine for measles is available alone or in combination with mumps and rubella vaccines. The recommended schedule has been changed several times, but it is now known that two doses are required to establish and maintain long-term immunity. The vaccine is ineffective in infants under 1 year of age because the presence of maternal antibody inhibits the immune response to the vaccine (CDC, 1997c). Children should receive the first dose at 12–15 months of age and a repeat dose at school entry. For those who are already in school and who have not received the second dose, the booster dose should be given at entry to middle or high school. College students should receive a second dose of measles vaccine if they have not previously had one or if they have no evidence of immunity. Health care workers and international travelers also need to get the vaccine if they have not been immunized with two doses of measles vaccine after the first birthday or they have no evidence of immunity (DHHS, 1996, pp. 97–98).

The vaccine contains a small quantity of egg protein because it is grown in chick culture; therefore, caution must be used in immunizing those with a history of severe hypersensitivity reactions to eggs. Extreme caution should also be used when immunizing those with a history of severe reactions to neomycin. Mild illness is not a contraindication to vaccination with measles vaccine. Pregnancy and immunosuppression are contraindications, although measles vaccine may be given to persons with HIV infection. In persons who have received blood products recently, measles vaccine should be delayed. Contact the CDC for information on when to immunize those who have received blood products (DHHS, 1996, pp. 99–100).

Adverse events following vaccination with live measles vaccine include fever, rash, and thrombocytopenia. The fever and rash occur 5–12 days postvaccination and occur because of replication of the measles vaccine virus. Fifteen percent or less experience fever; 5% or less experience rash (DHHS, 1996, p. 99).

## RUBELLA

Rubella is a generally mild, exanthematous disease caused by the rubella virus, a togavirus (genus *Rubivirus*). The disease is characterized by a maculopapular, erythematous rash beginning on the face and neck and progressing downward. In young children there is often no prodrome, but the prodrome in older children and adults consists of low-grade fever, malaise, mild conjunctivitis, upper respiratory symptoms, and lymphadenopathy. The rash may be pruritic, is fainter than the measles rash, and does not coalesce (DHHS, 1996, p. 112). Arthralgia and arthritis occur in up to 70% of adult women and may last as long as 1 month. Complications include chronic arthritis, encephalitis, orchitis, neuritis, panencephalitis, and hemorrhages caused by thrombocytopenia. Congenital infection results in birth defects (up to 85% of infants infected in the first trimester of pregnancy), and the primary goal of immunization against rubella is to protect the unborn fetus. Congenital rubella syndrome can affect all organ systems, and damage occurs when infection is present in the first 20 weeks of pregnancy. After that, defects from rubella infection are rare (DHHS, 1996, p. 114; S.L. Plotkin, 1994).

*In recent years, more than one half of cases of congenital rubella syndrome occurred because of missed opportunities for vaccination in the mothers* (CDC, 1997i, p. 353).

Treatment is supportive. Ordinary immune serum globulin and hyperimmune globulin have been used in an attempt to prevent fetal infection in pregnant women exposed to rubella, but this has not been shown to be effective (DHHS, 1996, p. 119; S.L. Plotkin, 1994). A rubella vaccine is available singly and mixed with mumps and measles vaccines, and confers lifelong immunity. Adverse events following immunization include fever, lymphadenopathy, arthralgia, and occasionally, rash and acute arthritis. Rubella vaccine should not be administered to persons with moderate to severe illness (minor illness is not a contraindication), immunosuppressed persons, pregnant women, and persons with a recent history of receiving antibody-containing blood products. HIV infection is not a contraindication to immunization. Women who receive rubella vaccine should avoid pregnancy for 3 months. A vaccine virus has been isolated from the pharynx of vaccinees, and while they are not contagious to others, breast-feeding mothers may infect their infants. Those infants may develop a mild illness with rash, without serious effects. Therefore, breast-feeding is not a contraindication to rubella immunization (DHHS, 1996, p. 121).

## MUMPS

The mumps virus is a paramyxovirus that is spread by respiratory droplets. Following replication in the nasopharynx and lymph nodes, the virus spreads to multiple tissues and glands, including the meninges, salivary glands, testes, ovaries, and pancreas. The most common manifestation is parotitis (inflammation of the salivary glands), which may be unilateral or bilateral. Thirty to forty percent of infected persons experience parotitis. A prodrome of myalgia, anorexia, malaise, headache, and low-grade fever may occur. Mumps may present as a lower respiratory infection in young children. Mumps infections may be asymptomatic in up to 20% of cases. Complications include meningoencephalitis (adults are at greater risk), orchitis, oophoritis, myocarditis, deafness, nephritis, pancreatitis, mastitis, arthropathy, and fetal death. Death may also result from mumps infection (Cochi, Wharton, & Plotkin, 1994; DHHS, 1996, pp. 102–104). Mumps disease confers lifelong immunity.

Treatment is supportive. Postexposure prophylaxis with mumps immune globulin or immune globulin (IG) has not been shown to be effective.

Vaccination with live virus mumps vaccine is estimated to be 95% efficacious, and immunity is presumed to be lifelong (DHHS, 1996, p. 106). Adverse reactions to mumps vaccine are rare but include parotitis, low-grade fever, rash, pruritus, and purpura. Mumps vaccine is available singly, with rubella vaccine, and with measles and rubella vaccines.

Contraindications to vaccination include a history of severe allergy to eggs and neomycin, persons with moderate to severe illness, immunosuppressed persons, pregnant women, and those recently transfused with antibody-containing blood products. Women should not become pregnant for 3 months after receiving the vaccine. Protocols have been developed for immunizing those with egg allergy. Persons with HIV may receive the vaccine (DHHS, 1996, pp. 107–108).

## *HAEMOPHILUS* INFLUENZA TYPE B

*Haemophilus influenzae*, a gram-negative coccobacillus, causes many types of infection in children under 5 years of age. The most common are meningitis, epiglottitis, pneumonia, arthritis, cellulitis, otitis media, and bronchitis. Otitis media and bronchitis may also be caused by nontypable strains of *H. influenzae*. Osteomyelitis and pericarditis also may occur. Most infections require hospitalization and treatment with antibiotics—chloramphenicol, cefotaxime, or ceftriaxone. Ampicillin-resistant strains are common in the United States; therefore, ampicillin should not be used to treat infections thought to be caused by HIB. Transmission is thought to be by respiratory droplet spread. Household contacts may be pro-phylaxed with rifampin to prevent disease spread and eliminate the carrier state (DHHS, 1996, p. 145–147; Ward, Lieberman, & Gochi, 1994).

Immunization against HIB was first recom-mended in 1985 for all children at 24 months of age (Ward et al, 1994). With further vaccine de-velopment, immunization is now recommended beginning at 2 months of age. Several HIB vac-cines are available singly or in combination with diphtheria, tetanus, and whole-cell pertussis vaccines. Health care personnel administering the vaccine should be sure to review the package insert of the vaccine to be sure the HIB vaccine chosen is appropriate for the age of the child being immunized.

Adverse events following HIB vaccination in-clude swelling, redness, and pain at the injection site. Fever and irritability are infrequent. Previous anaphylactic reaction to HIB vaccine is a contraindication to receiving further doses. Minor illness is not a contraindication to vacci-nation.

## VARICELLA

Chickenpox is a common childhood disease, caused by the varicella-zoster virus, a her-pesvirus. The virus is transmitted by respiratory droplets and is highly contagious. Viral replica-tion occurs and can be transmitted to others be-fore the characteristic skin rash appears. The rash may be preceded by a prodrome of malaise, headache, decreased appetite, and low-grade fever. Macular lesions then appear, beginning on the trunk and face and spreading to extremi-ties. The lesions progress from macules to papules to vesicles, which may then be scratched open and ooze fluid. The vesicles eventually scab over. Lesions erupt in crops gen-erally over a 3-day period and are present in var-ious stages of progression all over the body at the same time. The disease is contagious from 48 h prior to eruption of the lesions until all le-sions have scabbed over. The disease is trans-mitted by the respiratory droplet route and by direct contact with skin lesions.

Chickenpox is relatively benign in most healthy children, but severe complications can occur. Adults, children under 1 year, and im-munocompromised children tend to have more serious disease and a higher rate of complica-tions and death (DHHS, 1996, pp. 187–188;

Takahashi & Gershon, 1994). The most common complication of varicella infection is secondary bacterial infection of skin lesions. Other com-mon complications include pneumonia, dehy-dration, and involvement of the central nervous system, including aseptic meningitis, encephali-tis, and cerebellar involvement. Reye's syndrome has been reported in cases of children who took aspirin during the acute illness. More rarely, ap-pendicitis, transverse myelitis, thrombocytope-nia, hemorrhagic varicella, purpura fulminans, glomerulonephritis, arthritis, myocarditis, clini-cal hepatitis, orchitis, uveitis, iritis, and Guillain-Barré syndrome have been reported.

Uncomplicated cases of chickenpox are man-aged primarily with supportive therapies; anti-histamines and oatmeal baths provide some relief for itching. If fever is present, acet-aminophen may be prescribed. As with any acute illness, increased fluid intake is important.

Complicated cases and chickenpox in high-risk cases are managed according to the compli-cations that appear. Therapy is directed at the specific symptoms that appear (for example, an-tibiotics for secondary bacterial infections and intravenous fluids for dehydration). Acyclovir is used orally or intravenously in higher-risk cases, such as immunocompromised clients and adults. Informed clients may request acyclovir, thinking that it will reduce the severity of illness. It has been shown to reduce numbers of lesions and number of days of fever, but not the course of the illness in otherwise healthy children (Balfour et al, 1990). Acyclovir should be given within 24 h of the onset of rash.

Varicella-zoster immune globulin (VZIG) is effective against chickenpox; however, it must be given within 96 h of exposure to be effective in preventing or modifying clinical varicella. Administration of VZIG should be considered for susceptible, unvaccinated children and adults, including immunocompromised persons, pregnant women, newborns whose mothers de-veloped clinical disease 5 days before to 2 days after delivery, and preterm infants with postna-tal exposure. VZIG is given intramuscularly, never intravenously.

Varivax, a live attenuated vaccine, is available and is recommended for routine vaccination of all children at 12–18 months of age, and by the thirteenth birthday for children never vaccinated with no history of actual disease. After age 13, varicella infections tend to be more severe, and two doses of vaccine are required to insure ade-quate immunity (DHHS, 1996, p. 193). When two doses are given, they should be separated by 4–8 weeks. If more than 8 weeks have passed, the second vaccine may still be administered without starting the series over. Breakthrough disease may occur in some vaccinated individuals, although the disease is mild with fewer lesions and no fever in most cases. If a patient does develop significant rash (greater than 100 lesions) and fever following vaccine administration, it could be due to wild-virus vaccine from a recent exposure. Clinicians should consider this probability in addition to considering the possibility of infection caused by the vaccine virus (Feder, La Russa, Steinberg, & Gershon, 1997).

Contraindications to varicella vaccine include previous history of severe allergic reaction to a vaccine component (the vaccine contains trace amounts of neomycin and gelatin) or following a previous dose of vaccine, moderate or severe illness, immunosuppression, HIV infection, and a history of receiving antibody-containing blood products in the previous 5 months (DHHS, 1996, p. 198). The risk of varicella to the developing fetus is very low; however, in the absence of reliable data on varicella vaccination in pregnancy, pregnant women should not be immunized (DHHS, 1996, p.198; Takahashi & Gershon, 1994). However, should a pregnant woman be inadvertently vaccinated, the clinician should report the case to the Varicella Vaccination in Pregnancy Registry established by the CDC and the varicella vaccine manufacturer. The registry collects data on maternal-fetal outcomes following varicella vaccination in pregnancy. The phone number is 1-800-986-8999 (DHHS, 1996, p. 198).

Controversy has surrounded the recommendation of routine varicella vaccination of children and reportedly one third of physicians surveyed by the Merck Company are not recommending the vaccine (Watson & Haupt, 1997). Issues cited involve adding another injection to the childhood immunization schedule, especially for a disease that is relatively benign in healthy children; questions regarding the duration of immunity following vaccination; waning immunity among immunized children leading to the risk of varicella infection in adulthood; transmission of the virus from the vaccine itself; questions of increased risk of varicella-zoster in adults; and safety, efficacy, and storage issues (Watson & Haupt, 1997). Twenty-year studies in Japan and 10-year studies in the United States have indicated persistent immunity. This could be due to two factors: vaccine

efficacy and/or persistent immunity secondary to natural "boosters" by continuing wild-virus circulation (Asano et al, 1994; Kuter et al, 1991; Watson et al, 1994; Watson et al, 1993). Long-term follow-up studies are continuing, but if questions persist and if the evidence indicates, a recommendation to repeat the dose in adolescence may be made (Plotkin, 1996). Breakthrough disease following immunization, another concern, is generally mild and occurs at a very low rate, 110–150 cases in 11,000 children vaccinated since 1981 (Watson & Haupt, 1997). When a rash develops following vaccination, the transmission of the virus to household contacts is approximately 17%. In those cases, the household contacts had direct contact with the vaccinee's rash. There is no documentation of airborne spread (Watson & Haupt, 1997).

Studies have shown the risk of varicella-zoster to be decreased in persons who have received the varicella vaccine, rather than increased as some have feared. During varicella virus infection, the virus descends from skin lesions to the dorsal root ganglia, entering a latent phase. Zoster occurs when the virus reactivates (Plotkin, 1996). Since some skin lesions may appear following varicella immunization, the virus may migrate to the dorsal root ganglia, leading to the potential for zoster infection; however, fewer ganglia would be infected than in the case of wild-virus infection. Also, the incidence of rash following immunization is low, less than 6% overall, so the long-term effect of the varicella vaccine may be a decrease in the incidence of zoster (Plotkin, 1996, Watson & Haupt, 1997). All cases of zoster reported to date (8 in more than 9000 vaccinated children and 1 case in more than 1500 adolescents and adults vaccinated) have been mild and not associated with complications, such as postherpetic neuralgia. The rate reported in children is four to five times less than occurs in zoster following natural varicella infection (DHHS, 1996, p. 197).

The most compelling argument for widespread childhood vaccination is the effect of immunization on wild-virus transmission. If the majority of children are vaccinated, adults will have decreased exposure to wild virus. The net effect will be to decrease the incidence of disease in children and adults. The incidence will be further decreased if present recommendations to immunize susceptible adults and children over age 13 are followed (Plotkin, 1996).

The most common complications following immunization are injection-site complaints (pain, redness, and swelling) and fever. Less common are rash at the site and generalized rash (Watson & Haupt, 1997).

## HEPATITIS B

The hepatitis B virus (HBV) is a hepadnavirus that can cause acute and/or chronic infection. The mortality rate of acute fulminant hepatitis, which occurs in 1–2% of those with acute hepatitis, is 63–93%. Chronic disease occurs in approximately 10% of acute hepatitis cases. Infants are much more likely to become HBV carriers after acquiring HBV infection from their mothers at birth (90%) than adults with acute hepatitis leading to the chronic carrier state (6–10%). Thirty percent to 50% of HBV-infected children become carriers. Twenty-five percent of carriers develop chronic active hepatitis, which often leads to cirrhosis, and the rate of liver cancer in persons with chronic infection is 12 to 300 times that of noncarriers. Dialysis patients and persons with certain immunodeficiency diseases (eg, HIV) develop the chronic carrier state following acute hepatitis at a higher rate than previously healthy persons (DHHS, 1996, pp. 127–128; Krugman & Stevens, 1994).

HBV infection occurs more frequently in Pacific Islanders, Alaskan natives, persons receiving multiple transfusions of blood and blood products, persons engaging in high-risk behaviors (multiple sexual partners, intravenous drug abusers), and immigrants from other countries with high rates of hepatitis B infection (Africa, Asia, parts of the Middle East, and the Amazon Basin, in particular) (AAP Committee on Infectious Diseases, 1992; DHHS, 1996, p. 131; Krugman & Stevens, 1994). Four percent of cases occur secondary to household contact with a chronic carrier, and 2% of cases occur in health care workers. Twenty-five percent of cases have no identifiable risk factors (DHHS, 1996, p. 132). The incidence in the United States peaked in 1985 with approximately 70 cases per 100,000 population; the rate was approximately 40 cases per 100,000 in 1992 (DHHS, 1996, p. 132).

Acute hepatitis B is transmitted by parenteral or mucosal exposure to blood and blood products, contaminated needles and syringes, tattooing, hemodialysis, oral surgery, semen, intimate sexual contact, and perinatally. Hepatitis B may be transmitted through contact between broken skin and contaminated blood and saliva (bites).

It does not appear to be transmitted by kissing or by contact with body fluids with a lower concentration of HBV, such as tears, sweat, urine, stool, or respiratory droplets. Also, touching contaminated surfaces and then touching skin lesions or mucous membranes may be a source of infection (DHHS, 1996, p. 130).

Acute hepatitis B infection may be subclinical and virtually asymptomatic. The incubation period is from 6 weeks to 6 months postexposure. The prodromal phase is characterized by fever, headache, malaise, anorexia, nausea and vomiting, right upper quadrant pain, myalgia, arthralgia, arthritis and skin rashes, and dark urine. Diarrhea or constipation may occur. One to 2 days later, jaundice appears and the person develops hepatomegaly with tenderness and light or grey stools. This phase generally lasts 1–3 weeks. The convalescent phase lasts for weeks or months, and although jaundice, anorexia, and other symptoms disappear, malaise and fatigue may persist. Most cases result in complete recovery and immunity from reinfection (a function of anti-HBs antibody); however, chronic infection may also result. Complications of acute hepatitis B are fulminant hepatitis and chronic infection (DHHS, 1996, pp. 127–128; Krugman & Stevens, 1994).

Treatment is supportive. Interferon-α is used to treat chronic hepatitis B infection, with a success rate of 25–50% (DHHS, 1996, p. 129). Clearly, prevention is the best option.

Two recombinant hepatitis B vaccines are available in the United States, Recombivax HB and Engerix-B. Both are safe and effective. Initially, immunization was recommended for high-risk groups but was unsuccessful because of the underidentification of risk and lack of preventive health care in identified high-risk groups. The present strategy for hepatitis B prevention recommended by the DHHS is fourfold: prenatal testing of all pregnant women for HbsAg, routine vaccination of all newborn infants, vaccination of certain adolescents, and vaccination of adults at high risk of infection. Prenatal testing of pregnant women will identify infants who need immunoprophylaxis for hepatitis B and household contacts who need vaccination (DHHS, 1996, p. 134). All intimate and household contacts with carriers should also be immunized.

Since national recommendations were made, many states have mandated the practice and the rates of infant immunization with hepatitis B vaccine have increased. However, barriers still exist, such as the number of shots needed to complete the series, cost, resistance among providers, and the belief among parents that their child is not at risk (Woodruff et al, 1996). However, the benefits have been documented: HBV transmission among Native American children in Alaska has been interrupted because of the infant immunization program, and preliminary studies indicate a decreased liver cancer rate among vaccines in Japan (AAP Committee on Infectious Diseases, 1992; Cheng-Liang Lee & Ying-Chin Ko, 1997).

The present recommended schedule for infant immunization is a three-shot series with injections given at birth, 1–2 months, and 6–18 months of age or at 1–2 months, 4 months, and 6–18 months of age. The best time for giving preterm infants their first hepatitis B immunization has not been determined, but at least one study has shown immunization at hospital discharge with the series completed at the appropriate intervals to yield a response-to-immunization rate of 90%. Nonresponders in that study had higher birth weights and gestational ages and gained less weight before vaccine initiation than responders, but after a fourth dose, they responded with seroconversion (Kim et al, 1997). Other previous studies had shown suboptimal response rates that seemed to be somewhat dependent on weight at vaccine initiation, which led to an AAP recommendation to delay immunization in preterm infants until hospital discharge or 2 months of age (Kim et al, 1997). Kim et al (1997) suggest that based on the present data, preterm infants receive anti-HBs serologies following immunization to determine seroconversion status and the need for a fourth shot. Infants (term and preterm) born to HbsAg-positive mothers need to receive immunoprophylaxis with hepatitis B immune globulin and hepatitis B vaccine at birth or as soon as possible thereafter (DHHS, 1996, p. 136).

A combination vaccine of hepatitis B and *Haemophilus* influenza type B vaccines has been approved recently for use in children. It may be given at 2, 4, and 12–15 months of age (Clinician Reviews, 1997). Combinations of hepatitis B and other vaccines are also in development (AAP Committee on Infectious Diseases, 1992).

The recommended vaccine schedule for children and adults is a three-shot series, given at time 0, 1 month later and then 2–12 months later. Dialysis patients and immunocompromised patients may require a fourth dose. Postvaccination testing for immunity may be useful in those groups and for persons at occupational risk for exposure to hepatitis B (DHHS, 1996, p. 140).

Postvaccination testing may also be useful in persons who are more likely to be nonresponders: aged over 40 years, male, obese, a smoker, those who suffer from chronic illness, those who received hepatitis B vaccine in the buttock, those who received incorrect doses of vaccine, and/or those who were not vaccinated according to the recommended intervals (DHHS, 1996, p. 140).

The vaccine is always given intramuscularly, and the dose varies according to the vaccine selected. That information is available on the package insert supplied with the vaccine. Hepatitis B vaccine may be safely given at the same time as diphtheria, tetanus and pertussis (DTP), diphtheria, tetanus, acellular pertussis (DtaP), HIB, polio, and MMR vaccines (AAP Committee on Infectious Diseases, 1992).

For unimmunized persons exposed to hepatitis B, hepatitis B immune globulin should be given and hepatitis B vaccination initiated. HBIG should always be given as close as possible to the time of exposure, eg, immediately after birth or a needlestick. When sexual contact is involved, HBIG should be given within 14 days of the last sexual contact. Household contacts of someone just diagnosed with hepatitis B should be prophylaxed if they are unimmunized infants or contacts that have had identifiable blood exposure such as with shared toothbrushes and razors (DHHS, 1996, p. 141).

Pregnancy and immunosuppression are not contraindications to vaccination since the vaccine is made of noninfectious HbsAg particles. Data regarding the effects of hepatitis B immunization on the developing fetus are not available, but the risk of severe disease in the mother and chronic infection in the infant is great if the mother acquires hepatitis B in pregnancy. The only known contraindication is that of previous severe allergic reaction to hepatitis B vaccine or a component of the vaccine (DHHS, 1996, p. 143; Krugman & Stevens, 1994).

Adverse events are rare, but include pain at the injection site, fatigue, headache, irritability, and low-grade fever.

## ELECTIVE IMMUNIZATIONS FOR SELECTED INFECTIOUS DISEASES

### INFLUENZA

Influenza viruses (Orthomyxoviridae family) are highly contagious and cause serious and sometimes fatal illness, primarily in persons over age

65. There are three known basic antigen types—A, B, and C. Type A has three hemagglutinin subtypes (H1, H2, and H3) and two neuraminidase subtypes (N1 and N2). Influenza A causes moderate to severe illness in all age groups and can infect animals as well as humans. Influenza B, which is more stable antigenically than type A, causes milder disease and affects only humans, primarily children. Type C only affects humans, and most cases are subclinical. Type A demonstrates high antigenic variability (type B to a lesser extent), which leads to epidemics of new variants of influenza viruses each year. The mortality rate from influenza and related complications is high—an influenza A pandemic in 1918–1919 caused an estimated 20 million deaths and in nine U.S. epidemics from 1972–1973 to 1991–1992, more than 20,000 deaths occured in each season. In each of four of those epidemics, more than 40,000 deaths occurred; more than 90% of those deaths were among persons over age 65 (CDC, 1997g; Maassab, Shaw, & Heilman, 1994).

Influenza is manifested by sudden onset of fever, myalgia, sore throat, and nonproductive cough. Rhinorrhea, headache, chest burning, intestinal symptoms, and ocular symptoms may also occur. Influenza viruses A, B, and C are not the cause of the viral intestinal illnesses characterized by fever, vomiting, diarrhea, and myalgia that most refer to as the "flu" or the "intestinal flu." Various other infectious agents are involved in those illnesses. The health care provider needs to clearly communicate to clients the difference between the two types of illnesses, and the prevention and treatment of each.

Complications of influenza include secondary bacterial pneumonia (most common complication) and primary influenza viral pneumonia, which is less common but carries a high fatality rate. Myocarditis and worsening of chronic pulmonary diseases are also complications. Reye's syndrome may occur in children and may be associated with type B influenza (DHHS, 1996, pp. 161–162).

Treatment is supportive; there is no known cure. The antivirals amantadine hydrochloride and rimantadine hydrochloride are available for treatment within 48 h of the onset of symptoms. They are not curative, but may reduce the duration of fever and other symptoms. When used prophylactically, they are 70–90% effective in warding off infection; however, they are only effective against influenza type A. Rimantadine generally causes fewer side effects in the elderly than amantadine (DHHS, 1996, p. 172).

Inactivated whole-virus and split-virus vaccines are available in the U.S. The split-virus vaccine, also labeled as *subvirion* or *purified-surface-antigen* vaccine, has a lower potential for causing febrile reactions and therefore should be used for children less than 12 years of age. Adults may be given either the split-virus or whole-virus vaccine. Each year the vaccine is reformulated according to the strains that are thought to be likely to circulate in the upcoming year. The vaccine contains three strains, usually two type A and one type B, and is only good for the year for which it is formulated. For example, the vaccine for the 1997–1998 "flu season" contained A/Bayern/07/95-like (H1N1), A/Wuhan/359/95-like (H3N2), and B/Beijing/184/93-like hemagglutinin antigens. U.S. manufacturers used antigenically equivalent strains for the above antigens—A/Johannesburg/82/96 (H1N1), A/Nanchang/933/95 (H3N2), and B/Harbin/07/94 (CDC, 1997j). The strains are identified by virus type, A or B; geographic origin, eg, Johannesburg; strain number, eg, 82; year of isolation, eg, 96; and virus subtype, eg, H1N1 (CDC, 1997j; DHHS, 1996, p. 160). The vaccine should be given only in the year for which it is developed; otherwise, the vaccine will not confer adequate protection. The vaccine is 90% effective in healthy young adults when the vaccine strain is similar to the circulating strain. Efficacy in the elderly has been estimated to be 40–60%; however, it is 50–60% effective in preventing hospitalization and 80% effective in preventing death in immunized elderly who develop clinical illness (DHHS, 1996, p. 166). A nasal inhalation influenza immunization is now being used in clinical trials, and FDA approval is expected by the fall of 1999.

Persons targeted for immunization include persons aged 65 or older; persons over 6 months of age with chronic illnesses such as asthma, emphysema, cardiovascular disease, HIV disease, and immunosuppression; residents of long-term care facilities; and persons aged 6 months to 18 years receiving chronic aspirin therapy. Pregnant women should be immunized, preferably after the first trimester, unless high-risk conditions are present and the influenza season will begin during the first trimester. Because no major systemic effects are associated with the vaccine, the vaccine is not a live-virus vaccine, and data on more than 2000 pregnancies have not shown adverse fetal effects, it is thought to be safe during pregnancy. In addition, persons who have contact with the above high-risk populations, such as health care workers, caretakers, and household contacts, should receive influenza immunizations. Foreign travelers should also be immunized, since influenza viruses are present worldwide and may occur at different times of the year. Travelers may contact the CDC or local health department for information regarding influenza activity in the country or countries of interest (DHHS, 1996, p. 168).

The influenza vaccine should be administered from October through mid-November, but may be given as early as September and at any time during the influenza season. October through mid-November is the optimal time because the influenza season usually peaks between late December and early March, and antibody levels in some vaccinated persons may begin to decline within a few months of vaccine administration. Therefore, the vaccine should be given 4–6 weeks prior to the date of anticipated outbreak (CDC, 1997g). One dose of the vaccine is sufficient; however, previously unvaccinated (against influenza) children aged 9 years or less should be given two doses 1 month apart to ensure adequate antibody response. The second dose should be given prior to December, if possible (CDC, 1997g).

Adverse effects are few, but include pain, redness, and induration at the injection site. Mild systemic effects, such as fever, malaise, and myalgia, have also been reported. Immediate hypersensitivity reactions are rare.

Contraindications to vaccination with influenza virus are severe egg allergy and allergy to other vaccine components, primarily thimerosal. The Murphy and Strunk (1985) protocol for influenza vaccination may be considered for those with severe egg allergy and medical conditions that place them at high risk for complications of influenza. Intradermal skin tests may be performed first to determine egg protein sensitivity. Those with negative skin tests results may receive the vaccine. Those with positive skin tests results may be immunized with small doses of diluted and then undiluted vaccine in 15-min intervals. Emergency equipment for immediate resuscitation in case of anaphylactic reaction must be available (Murphy & Strunk, 1985).

## PNEUMOCOCCAL DISEASE

*Streptococcus pneumoniae*, also called pneumococcus, causes pneumococcal disease, most commonly manifested as pneumonia, bacteremia, and/or meningitis. It also causes 30–60% of episodes of acute otitis media in children. Pneumococcus is the most common cause of nursing home–acquired pneumonia, and it accounts for 50% of hospital-acquired pneumonia and up to 36% of community-acquired pneumonia (CDC, 1997d; DHHS, 1996, p. 176). Children under 2 years of age and persons 65 years of age and older are at higher risk for developing pneumococcal infection. The elderly have a higher complication and fatality rate following pneumococcal infection than do previously healthy children and adults. Pneumococcal meningitis is seen more often in blacks, and pneumococcal disease occurs more often in males than females (CDC, 1997h; DHHS, 1996, p. 179)

Symptoms of pneumococcal pneumonia include sudden onset of fever and shaking chills, with cough, pleuritic chest pain, malaise, weakness, tachycardia, tachypnea, and dyspnea developing shortly thereafter. Sputum is mucopurulent and rusty in color. Symptoms of pneumococcal meningitis are similar to other forms of bacterial meningitis—fever, headache, lethargy, nausea, vomiting, nuchal rigidity, and irritability. Cranial nerve signs, seizures, and coma may follow. Pneumococcus is transmitted by droplets and by "autoinoculation" from the upper respiratory tract (DHHS, 1996, p. 179).

Pneumococcal infections are treated with penicillin (drug of choice) or cephalosporins for penicillin-allergic people. Erythromycin may be prescribed for pneumonia and ceftriaxone or chloramphenicol (not the drug of choice) for meningitis. However, penicillin-resistant strains are emerging, and resistance to other antibiotics is also rising in the United States and in other parts of the world (CDC, 1997h; Lepow, 1994, p. 504).

Two 23-valent polysaccharide pneumococcal vaccines are available in the United States, Pneumovax 23 and Pnu Immune 23. Eighty-five to ninety percent of the serotypes causing invasive pneumococcal disease in children and adults in the United States are represented in the 23-valent vaccines. Although studies have yielded inconsistent results regarding efficacy in preventing pneumonia, the 23-valent vaccines have been shown to be 60–70% effective in preventing invasive disease (CDC, 1997h; DHHS, 1996, p. 181). Eighty percent or more of healthy young adults receiving the vaccine develop an antigen-specific antibody response; although how this response correlates with protection against disease hasn't been shown (CDC, 1997h). The vaccine generates poor antibody response to most of the serotypes in children less than 2 years of age. Children aged 2–5 years may have inconsistent responses to some of the common pediatric serotypes (CDC, 1997h); however, a study of a 5-valent pneumococcal vaccine given in three doses to children younger than 2 years with and without HIV infection demonstrated the vaccines to be safe and immunogenic for all children receiving the vaccine (King et al, 1997). This is very important because 80% of childhood pneumococcal disease occurs in this age group (DHHS, 1996, p. 181). Antibody response to the 23-valent vaccine also is poor or absent in immunocompromised individuals over age 2. More study involving repeated doses of vaccine in cases likely to be unresponsive to a single dose needs to be done.

The Advisory Committee on Immunization Practices (ACIP) of CDC recommends that the vaccine be given to all persons aged 65 years and over, persons aged 2 years and over with chronic illness, persons aged 2 years and over with functional or anatomic asplenia, persons aged 2 years and over living in environments in which the risk for disease is high, and immunocompromised persons aged 2 years and over at high risk for developing infection (CDC, 1997h). Risk factors in otherwise immunocompetent individuals include chronic cardiovascular diseases, chronic pulmonary diseases, chronic liver diseases, diabetes mellitus, persons with functional or anatomic asplenia, and children with sickle cell disease. Asthma is not associated with increased risk for pneumococcal disease unless it occurs with other chronic pulmonary disease or long-term systemic corticosteroid use (CDC, 1997h).

Serotype-specific antibody levels decline 5–10 years following vaccination and decrease more rapidly in some groups than others. How this affects protection against disease is unknown (CDC, 1997h). One study demonstrated that protection may last for at least 9 years following initial vaccination (Butler et al, 1993), but more studies are needed. At the present time, ACIP recommends revaccination for those 2 years or older at greatest risk for serious pneumococcal infection "and for those who are likely to have a rapid decline in pneumococcal antibody levels, provided that 5 years have elapsed since receipt of the first dose of pneumococcal vaccine" (CDC, 1997h). Children aged 10 and younger considered to be at highest risk for severe pneumococcal disease should be revaccinated after 3 years. Persons 65 years old and older should be revaccinated if they received the first dose before age 65 and 5 years or more have passed since the first dose. Those at highest risk for rapid antibody decline after initial vaccination are those with functional or anatomic asplenia, nephrotic syndrome, renal failure, renal transplantation, leukemia, lymphoma, Hodgkin's disease, multiple myeloma, generalized malignancy, other conditions associated with immunosuppression, and those receiving immunosuppressive chemotherapy, including long-term systemic corticosteroids. If vaccination status is unknown, those in the above categories should receive the pneumococcal vaccine (CDC, 1997h).

Local reactions such as redness, pain, and swelling are the most common adverse reactions to vaccine. Very few experience fever, muscle aches, and severe local reactions. Severe allergic reactions are very rare—about 5 in every 1 million doses (DHHS, 1996, p. 182).

A history of severe allergic reaction to a previous dose of pneumococcal vaccine or a vaccine component (phenol or thimerosal in pneumococcal vaccines) and moderate to severe illness are contraindications to vaccination. Pregnant women should not be given pneumococcal vaccine since the safety of pneumococcal vaccine in pregnancy has not been evaluated. Ideally, women at high risk for pneumococcal disease should be vaccinated before pregnancy (DHHS, 1996, p. 183).

## HEPATITIS A

Hepatitis A is a hepatovirus (Picornaviridae family) that generally causes mild disease in those infected. Infected children under age 5 are usually asymptomatic; those acquiring the disease after puberty usually exhibit clinical symptoms. The incubation period is about 1 month with a range of 15–45 days. Symptoms include sudden onset of fever (usually low-grade), malaise, nausea, headache, myalgia, and arthralgia. The disease is transmitted by contaminated food and water and is more common in countries with poor sanitation. Diagnosis depends upon laboratory testing to differentiate hepatitis A from other forms of viral hepatitis. Hepatitis A disease can be prolonged over several months, but never develops into chronic liver disease. Recovery from hepatitis A confers life-long immunity. Treatment is supportive.

Passive immunization with standard, pooled human immune globulins is available and is about 85% effective; however, the duration of immunity is only 2–5 months depending upon the dose given. An inactive hepatitis A vaccine is now available for active immunization of those at risk for hepatitis A disease and for travelers. The vaccine is approximately 90% effective in adults following a single dose of the vaccine; however, immunity may wane after 1 year. Therefore, a booster shot 6 months after the first shot is recommended for adults, primarily those who are frequent travelers and/or those planning to stay abroad for extended periods. The recommended schedule for children aged 2–17 calls for a primary dose with a booster dose 6–18 months later. Immunity is thought to last for 10 years following a booster dose (Clinician Reviews, 1996; Jilg, Deinhart, & Hilleman, 1994; Nettleman, 1993).

It is unknown if the hepatitis A vaccine is harmful to a fetus; however, because it is an inactivated virus, the risk is thought to be low. The provider should evaluate the risk-benefit profile based on the individual client's situation. The vaccine may be safely given to immunocompromised persons because it is inactivated (CDC, 1996, p. 20).

Side effects include soreness at the injection site, headache, and malaise in adults and soreness or induration at the injection site, feeding problems, and headache in children. No serious adverse reactions have been reported (CDC, 1996, p. 19).

## MENINGOCOCCAL DISEASE

Meningococcal disease is caused by *Neisseria meningitidis*, a gram-negative bacillus. It primarily manifests as meningitis and meningococcemia, although myocarditis, endocarditis, pericarditis, conjunctivitis, pharyngitis, urethritis, and cervicitis may also be seen. Meningococcemia begins with sudden onset of fever, malaise, myalgia, headache, and often vomiting and diarrhea. A maculopapular rash occurs in most cases, and it progresses to a petechial rash. Meningococcal septicemia may lead to hypotension, disseminated intravascular coagulation (DIC), and death. In cases of meningococcal meningitis, meningeal signs, vomiting, headache, and petechial rash are common (Lepow, 1994). The mortality rate for meningococcal meningitis is 13% and 11.5% for meningococcal septicemia (CDC, 1997b). *N. meningitidis* is transmitted by the respiratory system; carriers are asymptomatic.

The antibiotic of choice in managing meningococcal disease is aqueous penicillin G. Ceftriaxone also is highly effective; chloramphenicol and cefotaxime are other antibiotics that can be successfully used. Small doses of dexamethasone may be given in meningitis cases before antibiotic therapy is initiated and continued for 14 days to reduce the chance of deafness and to alleviate other central nervous system symptoms. Supportive therapy to manage shock and DIC may also be necessary (Lepow, 1994). Close contacts of persons with meningococcal disease should be prophylaxed as soon as possible after onset of disease in the primary patient with oral rifampin or intramuscular ceftriaxone. Ciprofloxacin is an acceptable alternative for prophylaxis in nonpregnant, nonlactating adults. Both rifampin and ciprofloxacin are contraindicated in pregnancy; ceftriaxone is not. Children should not be given ciprofloxacin unless no alternative is available (CDC, 1997b).

Persons with underlying medical conditions, immunosuppressed persons, persons with immunocompromising disease, and persons with asplenia are at increased risk for meningococcal disease. The disease used to be common in military recruits, but the rates have decreased dramatically due to immunization of all military recruits (CDC, 1997b). The rates of meningococcal disease are highest in children 3–12 months of age (CDC, 1997b).

A quadrivalent polysaccharide vaccine, Menomune, is available in the United States and should be administered to those considered to be at high risk for disease, especially those with functional or anatomic asplenia and those with terminal complement component deficiency diseases. This vaccine contains the four serogroups known to cause meningococcal disease in humans—A, C, Y, and W-135. Serogroups B and C account for most of the meningococcal disease in the United States, although the proportion of cases caused by Y strains is increasing (CDC, 1997b).

The vaccine is ineffective in children under 2 years of age, but may be given to children as young as 3 months of age in cases where the child is at high risk for infection. If given to infants and young children, two doses 3 months apart should be administered. Antibody levels in adults have been shown to decline in 2–3 years; therefore, revaccination may be considered if necessary within 3–5 years. The vaccine may be given in pregnancy.

Vaccines have been developed to target serogroups A and C, and serogroup B alone.

New vaccines for serogroups A and C have yet to be evaluated. Serogroup B vaccines have been evaluated, and efficacy is estimated to be 57–83% in older children and adults. However, efficacy is poor in children under 4, who have the highest rate of disease. None of the serogroup B vaccines are licensed for use in the United States (CDC, 1977b).

## RABIES

Clinical rabies is rare in the United States, primarily because of the routine vaccination of dogs and cats. However, infected wild animals such as skunks, raccoons, bats, and foxes constitute a continuing source of human risk. Bites or scratches from those animals and infected, unvaccinated domesticated animals may transmit the rabies virus to humans, causing encephalitis and death in most cases. By 1994, there were only five known cases of survival from rabies infection, three of whom suffered long-term sequelae (Plotkin & Koprowski, 1994, p. 651). Children are at high risk due to their animal-friendly behavior, although all age groups are equally at risk of contracting the disease with exposure. Raccoons are the primary reservoirs of rabies in the mid-Atlantic and southeastern states, skunks in the north and south central states and California, the gray fox in Arizona and Texas, the coyote in Texas, and the arctic fox and red fox in Alaska and upper New York state. Dogs along the U.S.-Mexico border are also likely to be infected (Phelps, 1997). Rodents, such as squirrels, hamsters, and guinea pigs, and lagomorphs (hares and rabbits) are generally not a source of infection, but groundhogs may be a source of infection (Phelps, 1997).

Corneal transplantation was a source of infection in six cases. Two cases were acquired from airborne exposure in the laboratory, and two were acquired from airborne exposure in bat-infested caves (Phelps, 1997). The clinician should ask about these potential sources of infection when attempting to rule out rabies disease.

Rabies has an incubation period of 20–90 days (range 4 days to 19 years) and initial clinical manifestations are relatively nonspecific (Phelps, 1997). If the initial injury is in the head or face, the incubation period is shorter. The initial symptoms in humans include headache, malaise, anorexia, fatigue, fever, and pain or paresthesia at the site of exposure (Phelps, 1997; Plotkin & Koprowski, 1994). Anxiety, apprehen-

sion, irritability, insomnia, and depression also may occur. Following the prodrome, hyperactivity, disorientation, hallucinations, seizures, bizarre behavior, nuchal stiffness, and paralysis develop and may occur intermittently and be associated with stimulation. Hydrophobia occurs in most cases. Other manifestations that may appear are hyperventilation, muscle fasciculations, and hypersalivation (Phelps, 1997; Plotkin & Koprowski, 1994). In some cases, the patient may not exhibit the hyperactivity and other irritable CNS signs. Instead, paralysis appears and the disease progresses to stupor and coma (Phelps, 1997). The course of illness is rapid, less than 2 weeks. Death may occur suddenly after cardiac and respiratory arrest, or more gradually following the development of coma and use of intensive life support (Phelps, 1997; Plotkin & Koprowski, 1994).

Preexposure prophylaxis with three intramuscular doses of 1 mL of human diploid cell vaccine (HDCV) or rabies vaccine adsorbed (RVA) on days 0, 7, and 21 or 28 or three intradermal doses of 0.1 mL of HDCV on days 0, 7, and 28 may be initiated in persons at high risk for exposure. Those persons include anyone who works with domestic or wild animals such as veterinarians, animal handlers, animal control workers, and wildlife workers; spelunkers who are exposed to bat-infested caves; those who handle live rabies virus in laboratories, and travelers to countries where rabies is endemic in dogs (CDC, 1991, pp. 11–12; Phelps, 1997). If the person must also take antimalarials before traveling to a rabies-enzootic area, the intradermal HDCV therapy should be initiated at least 1 month prior to traveling, or the intramuscular route used, because chloroquine phosphate (and perhaps other antimalarials) interferes with the antibody response to intradermal HDCV (CDC, 1991, p. 12). Booster doses must be given if exposure to rabid animals occurs or if immunity has waned as determined by serologic tests of antibody levels (CDC, 1991, pp. 12–13; Phelps, 1997).

Postexposure treatment is available and must be initiated as soon as possible following exposure. The challenge is to identify the exposure and match clinical symptoms with the possible cause, because in some cases no known exposure can be documented. Then the risk that the animal was infected must be considered. In two cases identified by Phelps (1997), a bite or scratch apparently did not occur. In one case, a bat was found in a child's bedroom, and in another, a man opened the mouth of a dead bat to examine the teeth. Once a bite or scratch has occured and the risk for infection is determined to be high, the wound should be washed thoroughly with soap and water. Human rabies immune globulin (HRIG) should be administered immediately, one-half dose directly in the wound and the remainder injected intramuscularly in the gluteal area. Human diploid cell vaccine (HCDC) must also be administered intramuscularly in the deltoid or anterior thigh in small children (never in the buttocks in any client) on days 0, 3, 7, 14, and 28 (CDC, 1991, p. 7; Phelps, 1997). Protocols for intradermal injection have been developed and also are effective, as well as less expensive. Treatment may be delayed for up to 48 h while awaiting laboratory test results (if the animal causing the injury was caught), when the risk of infection is determined to be low as in the case of a dog bite when the vaccination status of the dog is unknown (Phelps, 1997). However, when in doubt, treat. Treatment may be halted if laboratory tests show the animal was not infected with rabies.

When a person has been previously treated with HDCV, either as preexposure or postexposure prophylaxis, a two-dose schedule may be followed with HDCV given on days 0 and 3, without HRIG (CDC, 1991, p. 7). If other rabies vaccines were used for previous vaccination and antibody response has been documented, the two-dose schedule with HDCV may be followed. If antibody response has not been documented, the full postexposure schedule with HDCV and HRIG must be followed (Plotkin & Koprowski, 1994).

Pain, redness, swelling, and itching at the injection site are the most common reactions seen. Systemic reactions, such as headache, nausea, muscle aches, dizziness, and abdominal pain may also occur. Immune-complex-like reactions, including itching, arthralgia, arthritis, allergic edema, nausea, vomiting, malaise, and fever may occur after booster doses. Guillain-Barré-like illness has been reported in three cases, it resolved without sequelae (Phelps, 1997). If an allergic reaction to HDCV is observed, an alternative vaccine such as RVA may be given since it has a different tissue origin. Prophylactic antihistamines may be used for those with a history of severe allergies, and epinephrine should be available if needed when those persons are vaccinated. Those receiving steroids or other immunosuppressive medications should have antibody levels checked following vaccination.

Pregnancy is not a contraindication to rabies vaccination (Plotkin & Koprowski, 1994).

Contact the local or state health department or the rabies section of the Centers for Disease Control (404-639-1050 or 1075) for more information and advice on diagnosis and treatment.

## TUBERCULOSIS

Tuberculosis (TB) disease, caused by *Mycobacterium tuberculosis*, accounts for most death and disease in the world. It causes serious illness in those who develop active disease. Many are asymptomatic at the onset of infection and develop symptoms from months to years after primary infection with *M. tuberculosis*. This is referred to as reactivation, postprimary, adult-type, or reinfection tuberculosis. Initially, symptoms are mild and include mild cough, night sweats, malaise, weight loss, fatigue, irritability, and low-grade fever. The disease may ultimately progress to severe pulmonary disease, disseminated tuberculosis, and/or tuberculous meningitis leading to death if untreated. Early detection often is difficult because in both of those manifestations of TB, tuberculin skin tests may be negative and chest radiographs may be normal (Starke & Connelly, 1994).

In Europe and the United States, improving sanitation, living conditions, and socioeconomic conditions led to the decline in deaths from tuberculosis. Conditions that favor transmission of the disease are crowded living and working conditions, war, famine, and population displacement (as in refugee situations). There is also an association between the development of tuberculosis and infection with human immunodeficiency virus (HIV).

Treatment is available with antibiotics; however, drug-resistant strains of *M. tuberculosis* are proliferating, especially among the population infected with HIV. While the available vaccine, bacille Calmette-Guérin (BCG), has never been used in the United States, its use may be considered now because of the rapid development of drug resistance. Unfortunately, studies regarding the efficacy of the BCG vaccine have yielded widely varying results, probably because of the nature of tuberculosis disease and the lack of reliable serological markers for immunity to mycobacteria. The effects on tuberculous disease of nontuberculous mycobacteria, which are prevalent in the environment, are unknown. Their immunologic effects on humans may contribute in some way to the prevention and control of tuberculosis (Starke & Connelly, 1994). Studies done in areas in which the prevalence of environmental mycobacteria is low have yielded high vaccine efficacy rates. Conversely, studies done in areas of high mycobacteria prevalence have yielded the lowest efficacy rates (Starke & Connelly, 1994).

The primary method of controlling tuberculosis disease spread in the United States is by skin-testing children at 12 months of age, school entry (age 4 or 5), and other significant events such as college entry or at the time of employment in certain companies; aggressive investigation of known case contacts; and prophylactically treating those with positive skin tests and/or chest radiographs without clinical evidence of disease. BCG vaccine is recommended only in cases where the risk of transmission of TB from intimate and prolonged exposure is high and the noninfected person cannot be removed from the environment, and in groups with high TB infection rates. BCG vaccine causes local reactions, including scarring and lymphadenitis. It should not be given to immunocompromised individuals, those with HIV infection, or those who are pregnant. More research into the use of BCG in HIV-infected persons and into the development of new, more effective tuberculosis vaccines is needed if we hope to more adequately protect people from and eliminate tuberculosis disease (Starke & Connelly, 1994).

See Chapter 22 for more information on diagnosing and treating tuberculosis.

## TRAVELER'S IMMUNIZATIONS

Persons traveling abroad are at risk of contracting selected diseases based on the prevalence of those diseases in the country of destination. Persons traveling to developing countries are at increased risk of common diseases generally not seen in the more developed countries with appropriate sanitation and food and water controls. This section will briefly review some of the diseases for which a traveler may be at risk and available vaccines for prevention.

### DISEASES ASSOCIATED WITH CONTAMINATED FOOD AND WATER

Cholera, hepatitis A, typhoid fever, and traveler's diarrhea are all associated with ingestion of contaminated food and water and are more preva-

lent among travelers to developing countries than the developed world. Primary emphasis is placed on prevention by cautioning travelers to avoid eating raw vegetables and fruits and raw or partially cooked shellfish, fish, and meat and to avoid drinking tap water and unpasteurized milk. Ice should be avoided, but beverages made from boiled water are safe. Bottled carbonated beverages are safe; however, the lips of bottles with metal caps may be a source of contamination. Boiling water is the most reliable way to purify it, but using iodine and portable water purifiers is also effective (Nettleman, 1993, 1996).

The majority of persons contracting *cholera* are asymptomatic or experience mild diarrhea for a few days. The cholera vaccine efficacy is approximately 50%, and two doses must be given 1 month apart. Immunity lasts 6 months or less. Because of the inadequate effectiveness of the vaccine, vaccine side effects, and the very low risk of contracting cholera, vaccination is no longer recommended (Nettleman, 1993, 1996).

The *hepatitis A* vaccine is safe and efficacious for many years when given in two doses, as noted previously. All travelers to developing countries, especially those who will not be staying in tourist areas, who will be eating in local restaurants, and/or who will stay for an extended period of time, should get the vaccine. Immune globulin is approximately 85% effective in preventing hepatitis A infection when given within 2 months prior to the exposure, and it is another option for travelers. If travel is to occur within 1 month of receiving the first hepatitis A vaccine, the traveler should also receive immune globulin (Nettleman, 1993, 1996).

An inactivated parenteral vaccine and a live attenuated oral vaccine are available for protection against *typhoid fever*; however, neither is 100% effective. Therefore, as with cholera, prevention of exposure is of utmost importance. Studies have shown the efficacy of parenteral typhoid vaccine to be 51–77% and 67% or better with oral vaccine. The parenteral vaccine is given in two doses, 4 weeks apart. The oral vaccine is given in four doses, 1 dose every other day. Booster doses are needed every 3 years for the parenteral vaccine and every 5 years for the oral vaccine, although long-term follow-up data on the oral vaccine are lacking. There is a high incidence of adverse effects with the parenteral vaccine; fewer adverse effects are seen with the oral vaccine. The oral vaccine should not be given to immunocompromised persons and children under 6 years of age; the parenteral vaccine may be given to immunocompromised persons and children over 6 months of age. Safe use of either vaccine in pregnancy has not been established (Nettleman, 1996; Woodruff, Pavia, & Blake, 1991).

*Traveler's diarrhea* can be caused by a variety of bacteria, most commonly enterotoxigenic *Escherichia coli, Salmonella, Shigella*, and *Campylobacter*. There are no available vaccines for prevention; however, the traveler should have antibiotics available in case diarrhea develops. Adults may take fluoroquinolones or trimethoprim-sulfamethoxazole to treat the diarrhea. Short-term travelers may wish to take daily ciprofloxacin to prevent diarrhea. Antimotility agents, such as Pepto-Bismol, loperamide, or diphenoxylate hydrochloride, may also be used. If bloody diarrhea, severe abdominal pain, or high fever is present, the traveler should not take antimotility agents and should seek medical attention (Nettleman, 1993, 1996).

## MALARIA, JAPANESE ENCEPHALITIS, AND YELLOW FEVER

*Malaria* is transmitted by the female *Anopheles* mosquito, *Japanese encephalitis* by the *Culex* mosquito, and yellow fever by the *Aedes* mosquito. Travelers to areas where the above diseases are endemic should take the appropriate precautions to minimize exposure, such as using insect repellants, protective clothing, and mosquito netting. Chloroquine may be taken to reduce the likelihood of acquiring malaria. In areas of chloroquine resistance, mefloquine may be taken; however, it should not be taken by those also taking antiarrhythmics or beta blockers. When these drugs cannot be taken, or when the traveler is going to an area of mefloquine resistance, daily doxycycline may be taken. For travel to areas of chloroquine and mefloquine resistance, or when mefloquine cannot be taken, travelers may take a treatment supply of pyrimethamine-sulfadoxine (Fansidar) with them in case symptoms of illness develop. Primaquine should be given prophylactically to travelers who have had extended stays and significant mosquito exposure in areas where *Plasmodium vivax* or *P. ovale* malaria is endemic. Primaquine is usually taken during the last 2 weeks of chloroquine chemoprophylaxis (Nettleman, 1996; Sears & Sack, 1995).

Contact the local or state health department or the CDC for the most current information on areas where malaria is present, and whether the malarial strains are known to be resistant to chloroquine or mefloquine.

An inactivated-virus vaccine is available to protect against *Japanese encephalitis*, prevalent in much of Asia. It should be given to travelers expecting to stay in endemic areas during the seasons in which disease transmission is most likely (May through October) for longer than 1 month. The vaccine is given in three doses (Nettleman, 1993, 1996).

*Yellow fever* occurs in South America and Africa. Travelers to areas with known infected mosquito populations should receive the live attenuated vaccine. Some countries require proof of yellow fever vaccination before they will allow travelers to enter. The CDC licenses official vaccination centers where the traveler may receive the vaccine and the International Certificate of Vaccination documenting vaccination against yellow fever (Nettleman, 1996).

## MENINGOCOCCAL DISEASE

Travelers to areas where meningococcal disease is prevalent should receive the available polysaccharide capsular vaccine. Meningococcal disease is endemic in sub-Saharan Africa and epidemics have been reported in Brazil, Kenya, Tanzania, and Saudi Arabia. Outbreaks also have occurred in New Delhi and Nepal. Immunization is recommended for travelers to Burundi and northern India (Sears & Sack, 1995). The type B serotype causes most of the cases of meningococcal disease in the United States and was the cause of the outbreak in Brazil. Types A and C predominate in other countries. The vaccine is effective against types A, C, Y, and W135. No vaccine against type B is available (Nettleman, 1993). See the section on elective immunizations for selected infectious diseases for more information about meningococcal disease.

## PLAGUE

The average traveler is at very low risk of acquiring human plague (transmitted by fleas on rodents); however, those who will be working or living in close contact with rodents should be immunized (Nettleman, 1996; Sears & Sack, 1995).

## POLIOMYELITIS

Because poliomyelitis still exists in developing countries, the CDC recommends that travelers to those countries be immunized. If more than 10 years have passed since the primary series was completed, a booster dose of OPV or IPV may be given. In adults who were never immunized, IPV should be given according to the appropriate primary series schedule (CDC, 1997f). See the section on childhood immunizations for more information about polio vaccines.

Travelers should be sure their "routine" immunizations are up-to-date, including diphtheria/tetanus and rubeola. Influenza and pneumococcal vaccines should be administered to those at risk for those infections (see the section on elective immunizations for selected infectious diseases). Travelers should also be aware of diseases endemic in the countries of destination and precautions that should be taken to avoid exposures. Insect-borne diseases, such as dengue fever, leishmaniasis, filariasis, and Lyme disease, have no available vaccines for protection, therefore, precautions with repellants, appropriate clothing, and netting should be taken. Also, schistosomiasis may be contracted by wading or swimming in fresh water so travelers should swim only in chlorinated pools and salt water, upstream from sewage dumps (Nettleman, 1996; Sears & Sack, 1995).

Health care providers should refer questions regarding recommendations for vaccination and precautions for travelers to foreign countries to local or state health departments or the CDC. Additionally, when travelers return from foreign countries with unidentified illness or when illness defying diagnosis presents in patients who have traveled to other countries, health care providers should consult with experts in travel medicine and/or infectious diseases and the CDC. Many diseases may appear months to years after exposure, and others are difficult to diagnose because they are uncommon in the United States. Prompt consultation and referral, if necessary, are crucial to ensure appropriate treatment and to prevent complications.

For current information regarding requirements and recommendations for travelers, call the CDC at 404-332-4559. This service is available 24 hours a day, 7 days a week.

## DECISION MAKING REGARDING IMMUNIZATIONS

Special consideration must be given to children, immunocompromised persons, the elderly, and pregnant and lactating women. In addition, those not immunized in childhood according to the routine schedule require special consideration in getting "caught up." Timing and administration of multiple vaccines must also be considered, as well as efficacy when antibody-containing blood products have been administered prior to immunization. Figure 11–2 lists a catch-up schedule for childhood vaccines, and Figure 11–3 is a recommended schedule for adult vaccines. Whenever a question arises about specific circumstances, such as whether or not to give a vaccine after an individual has received blood products, when the next dose of a vaccine should be given or if the series needs to be started over, and dosing information, the provider should refer to the package inserts or call the state or local health department or the Centers for Disease Control.

Risks and benefits of vaccine administration must be carefully considered when administering elective vaccines. Most of the more commonly given vaccines yield more benefits than risks, and therefore should be administered to those at risk for the diseases prevented by the vaccine. The risk-benefit profile is one of the reasons why sequential IPV/OPV schedules are now recommended for childhood polio immunization.

The provider should take advantage of every opportunity to immunize. Numerous reports of outbreaks of certain illnesses note that there were missed opportunities to immunize those who were ultimately stricken with disease. Some opportunities are missed because the provider is concentrating on other aspects of care and may not focus on the need for immunization if the client does not ask. Others are missed because providers may elect not to immunize if the client has a mild illness. Some of the barriers to immunization of children (and adults, in some cases) include the cost of vaccines, the access to care, the number of vaccine injections that must be given at each visit, and the number of visits required to ensure adequate immunization. *The provider should review the client's immunization status at every preventive health care visit or every sick visit if the client does not make and/or keep appointments for primary, preventive care visits.* This is especially true for the elderly, who are at high risk for acquiring influenza and pneumococcal disease, among others. Adults over age 50 are also at risk for tetanus and diphtheria as immunity wanes. Sixty-seven percent of cases of tetanus reported

Legend: ■ Children < 24 months of age   ▨ Children > 24 months of age

| | Time 0 | 1 MONTH INTERVAL | 1 MONTH INTERVAL | 1 MONTH INTERVAL | 1 MONTH INTERVAL | 1 MONTH INTERVAL | 1 MONTH INTERVAL | 1 MONTH INTERVAL | 1 MONTH INTERVAL | 1 MONTH INTERVAL | AGE 4-6 YEARS | BOOSTERS |
|---|---|---|---|---|---|---|---|---|---|---|---|---|
| HEPATITIS B | #1 | #2 | | | | #3 at least 2 months after #2 | #3 at least 4 months after #2 | | | | | |
| | #1 | #2 | | | | | | | | | | |
| DIPTHERIA, TETANUS & PERTUSSIS (DTP or DTaP)[1] | #1 | | #2 | | #3 | | | | | #4* 6 months after dose #3 and/or age 4-6 years | | Q 10 years |
| | #1 | | #2 | | #3 | | | | | #4 | #5 | Age 11-12 & then Q 10 yrs |
| H. INFLUENZAE TYPE B[2] | 1 Dose | | | | | | | | | | | |
| | #1 | | #2 | | #3 | | | | | | | #4 15-18 mos. of age |
| POLIO[3] | IPV or OPV #1 | | IPV or OPV #2 | | | IPV or OPV #3 6-12 months after #2 | | | | | IPV or OPV #4 | |
| | IPV or OPV #1 | | IPV or OPV #2 | | | IPV or OPV #3 6-12 months after #2 | | | | | IPV or OPV #4 | |
| MEASLES, MUMPS, RUBELLA[4] | #1 | | | | | | | | | | #2** or #2 at 11-12 yrs | #2** or #2 at 11-12 yrs |
| | #1 | | | | | | | | | | #2 | |
| VARICELLA[5] | #1 | #2*** | | | | | | | | | | At 11-12 yrs[5] |
| | #1 | | | | | | | | | | | |
| INFLUENZA[6] | #1 | | #2 | | | | | | | | | Yearly |
| | #1 | | #2 | | | | | | | | | Yearly |
| HEPATITIS A[7] | #1 | | | | | | #2 6-18 months later | | | | | |
| PNEUMOCOCCAL[8] | #1 | | | | | | | | | | | 3-5 Years |
| MENINGOCOCCAL[9] | #1 | | | #2 | | | | | | | | 3-5 Years |

1. May use DT in children ≥ 6. Use Td for children ≥ 11. If DTP used for children < 4 yrs, use DTaP for 4-6 yrs of age booster. *If #4 dose is given at ≤ 18 mos of age, a 5th dose is given at 4-6 yrs of age.

2. One dose may be given to children ≥ 15 mos. Children ≥ age 5 yrs do not need to be immunized against HIB. **Not required if PRP-OMP is used for 1st 2 vaccinations.

3. Sequential IPV/OPV recommended for children (IPV for doses 1 & 2 & OPV for doses 3 & 4); however, IPV only or OPV only schedules may be used. * If dose #3 of IPV or OPV is given after 4 yrs of age, a 4th dose is not needed.

4. MMR dose 1 may not be given prior to 12 mos of age. **#2 dose may be given 1 mo after 1st dose as long as both doses are given after 12 mos of age.

5. Varicella may be given at or after 12 mos of age. Unvaccinated children without history of disease should be vaccinated at age 11-12 yrs. ***Persons age 13 and over should receive 2 doses at least 1 month apart.

6. In children age 9 yrs or less not previously vaccinated against influenza, a 2nd dose 1 mo later (preferably before December) should be given.

7. Should not be given to children less than 2 yrs of age (see text for indications).

8. Should be given to children aged 2 yrs and over at high risk for pneumococcal disease (see text)

9. Ineffective in children < age 2 yrs, but may be given to children age 3 mos or older, with a 2nd dose 3 mos later. In children over age 2, 1 dose is needed with a booster 3-5 yrs later if necessary. See text for indications.

**Figure 11–2.** "Catch-up" immunization schedule for children and adults not previously immunized according to the routine childhood schedule.

| | Time 0 | 1 MONTH INTERVAL | 1 MONTH INTERVAL | 1 MONTH INTERVAL | 1 MONTH INTERVAL | 1 MONTH INTERVAL | 1 MONTH INTERVAL | 1 MONTH INTERVAL | 1 YEAR INTERVAL | 5 YEAR INTERVAL | 10 YEAR INTERVAL | 10 YEAR INTERVAL |
|---|---|---|---|---|---|---|---|---|---|---|---|---|
| HEPATITIS B [1] | #1 | #2 | | | | #3 | | | | | | |
| ADULT TETANUS DIPTHERIA TOXOID (Td) | #1 | | #2 | | | | | | #3 6-12 months later | | | Repeat Q 10 years + |
| POLIO [2] (E-IPV) | #1 | #2 | | | | | #3 6-12 months after #2 | | | | | |
| MMR [3] | #1 | #2 | | | | | | | | | | |
| VARICELLA [4] | #1 | #2 | | | | | | | | | | |
| HEPATITIS A | #1 | | | | #2 | | | | | | | |
| INFLUENZA [5] | YEARLY | | | | | | | | YEARLY | | | |
| PNEUMOCOCCAL [6] | | | | | | | | | | 5 YEAR INTERVAL | | |
| MENINGOCOCCAL [7] | | | | | | | | | | 3-5 YEARS | | |

+  In case of injury and ≥ 5 years have elapsed since previous tetanus booster, repeat booster.

1  Dialysis and immunocompromised patients may require 4th dose (see text).

2  E-IPV only should be given to previously vaccinated adults. Previously vaccinated adults who completed the primary series with OPV, may be given an OPV or E-IPV booster in adulthood if necessary (see text).

3  With questionable past immunization history against any or all components, entering college, military or health care work, history or receiving killed measles vaccine between 1963-1967, women of childbearing age, international travel and/or questionable documentation of immunity to measles, mumps, and rubella diseases, MMR is the vaccine of choice.

4  May be given in adults with no documentation of previous varicella disease or immunity.

5  Must be given annually in October through November.

6  For persons with chronic illness, those living in institutions (including nursing homes and rehabilitation facilities), persons ≥ age 65, and all others at risk including immunocompromised persons. A booster dose may be given after 5 years and SHOULD be given to those ≥ 65 years of age who received their 1st dose prior to age 65.

7  For persons considered at high risk for contracting meningococcal disease (see text).

**Figure 11-3.** Immunization schedule for adults, including those not immunized in childhood.

in the United States each year are among adults over age 50, and studies have shown that up to 40% of adults have inadequate levels of antitoxin antibodies. Additionally, up to 60% of adults lack a protective level of antibodies against diphtheria (Clinical Guidelines, 1997). Every effort should be made to see that adults and children are adequately immunized. See Fig. 11–3 for an adult immunization schedule.

Providers also should assist clients to seek immunizations at reduced or no cost by referring them to sites that offer immunizations required by law to those who are unable to pay, as in the case of the local health department. Elective immunizations may also be obtained at reduced cost at local health departments in most cases. Providers should also strive to educate clients on the importance and necessity of information. Many people have forgotten, or simply do not know, how severe certain diseases are, and therefore they may not be as motivated to be adequately immunized. It is very important that parents understand the necessity of child immunizations at the appropriate time. It often is helpful to review the schedule and the rationale for immunization with them. Pointing out that most of the injections are given in the first 15–18 months of life, and that "catching up" an older child is frightening and painful because of the number of injections required at such frequent intervals, may gain the reticent parent's compliance with an immunization schedule.

## REPORTING OF ADVERSE EVENTS AND THE NATIONAL VACCINE INJURY COMPENSATION PROGRAM

The Department of Health and Human Services established the Vaccine Adverse Event Reporting System (VAERS) in 1990 to comply with conditions specified in the National Childhood Vaccine Injury Act of 1986. Prior to that time, the CDC and the FDA monitored reports of adverse events. Adverse effects after administration of vaccines purchased with public money were reported to the CDC, and adverse effects of vaccines purchased with private money were reported to the FDA. The agencies worked together to create VAERS. Those responsible for vaccine administration are required to report anaphylaxis, encephalitis, residual seizure disorders, paralytic poliomyelitis, and acute complications or sequelae of these events

to VAERS. Additionally, providers are encouraged to report any clinically significant adverse event following administration of U.S. licensed vaccines in case those events may later be causally associated with vaccine administration. Copies of forms for reporting adverse events are mailed to physicians in the United States likely to administer vaccines and state health departments that, in turn, distribute forms to public health clinics. Vaccine manufacturers also report to VAERS (Chen et al, 1994).

The VAERS 24-hour phone number is 800-822-7967. Callers may receive assistance in completing the forms, obtaining additional reporting forms, and answering questions about VAERS (Chen et al, 1994).

The Vaccine Injury Compensation Program (VICP) was established as a result of the National Childhood Vaccine Injury Act of 1986 and went into effect in October 1988. Claims for injuries or death resulting from DTP, DtaP, diphtheria/tetanus (DT), tetanus toxoid (TT), tetanus/diphtheria (Td), MMR or individual component vaccines, IPV, and OPV may be made. For more information on this program, write or call the program:

National Vaccine Injury Compensation Program
Health Resources and Services Administration
Parklawn Building, Room 8-05
5600 Fishers Lane
Rockville, MD 20857
Telephone 301-443-6593

Persons needing specific information on how to file a claim may call 800-338-2382 toll-free.

## NEW HORIZONS

Vaccines for many diseases are in the process of research and development. Such diseases include hepatitis C and E, cytomegalovirus, rotavirus, and HIV. Adenovirus vaccines are used in military recruits, but are not available for general use. Improvements are sought in vaccines currently used, such as for pertussis and meningococcus, to increase efficacy and decrease adverse events. Additionally, many different combination vaccines are in development so that the number of immunizations given in a routine childhood visit may be decreased. New technologies will expand the scope of traditional vaccination from prevention of disease to changing the physiology of disease and for immunological treatment of disease. Diseases and conditions that would ultimately be affected include allergy, infertility, cancer, and AIDS (Ellis, 1994).

Human rotavirus causes severe diarrhea, abdominal cramping and vomiting, leading to dehydration and death if untreated. It is a leading cause of death in children in developing countries (approximately 1 million children per year). In the United States, approximately 100,000 children are hospitalized and 125 die annually. Treatment is directed at managing hydration status until the disease resolves. There is no cure. A vaccine, shown to reduce severe diarrheal illness and resultant dehydration in several clinical trials, was approved by the FDA on December 12, 1997, and routine vaccination of full-term infants has been recommended by the CDC's Advisory Committee on Immunization Practices (Getting rid, 1998). The vaccine, RotaShield, marketed by Wyeth-Lederle, should be given in 3 oral doses at 2, 4 and 6 months of age (CDC panel, 1998).

## PROGRAMS FOR IMPROVING IMMUNIZATION RATES

Many local, regional, state, and national programs have been developed to address the continuing problem of underimmunization of preschool children. The president of the United States initiated the Childhood Immunization Program in 1993 to "(1) eliminate indigenous cases of 6 vaccine-preventable diseases (i.e., diphtheria, HIB disease [among children aged less than 5 years], measles, poliomyelitis, rubella, and tetanus [among children aged less than 15 years]) by 1996; (2) increase vaccination coverage levels to at least 90% among 2-year-old children by 1996 for each of the vaccinations recommended routinely for children (for hepatitis B, the objective is set for 1998); and (3) establish a vaccination-delivery system that maintains and further improves high coverage levels." (CDC, 1994). Activities to meet those goals include efforts to improve quality and quantity of vaccination delivery services, increase community participation and education, reduce vaccine cost for parents by implementing the Vaccines for Children program (begun October 1, 1994), improve surveillance for coverage and disease, form and strengthen partnerships, and improve vaccines (CDC, 1994). The

"National Infant Immunization Week" was established in 1993, and each year materials are sent to health care providers and related professional organizations and to various community organizations and leaders across the country to facilitate activities to increase public awareness.

Contact your local or state health department for information on programs to improve immunization rates in your area.

## SUMMARY

Tremendous progress has been made in vaccine development in the last 40 years. However, many diseases for which vaccines are available are still prevalent even thought they are now, for the most part, preventable. It is important to remember that although no vaccine is 100% safe or 100% effective, immunizing the population is successful in achieving herd immunity and controlling or eliminating disease. Smallpox has been declared eradicated from the world; polio is soon to follow and then, with continued diligent immunization efforts, perhaps measles. Hepatitis B immunization may be instrumental in decreasing the numbers of people with hepatocarcinoma (Cheng-Liang Lee & Ying-Chin Ko, 1997).

The provider must convey to clients the importance of receiving all necessary immunizations on time and when circumstances necessitating immunization arise, such as traveling or when at high risk for contracting a vaccine-preventable illness. The provider should also be able to explain to clients what the diseases look like to facilitate understanding of why the vaccines are so important. Third, providers must take advantage of every opportunity to immunize their clients. Many cases of vaccine-preventable diseases occur in cases in which opportunities to vaccinate were missed by providers.

New vaccines are in development; some are improvements of existing vaccines, some are combinations of existing vaccines, some are new forms of vaccines, such as the new influenza nasal inhalation vaccine preparation, and others are being developed for diseases for which there are no current vaccines. Up-to-date information is available from the Centers for Disease Control via the World Wide Web: www.cdc.gov/nip/home.html. To find out the location of immunization clinics in your area and answers to commonly asked questions, call 1-800-232-2522. See Chapter 37 for immunization issues specific to children and HIV infection.

## REFERENCES

American Academy of Pediatrics Committee on Infectious Diseases. (1992). Universal hepatitis B immunization. *Pediatrics, 89,* 795–800.

Asano, Y., Suga, S., Yoshikawa, T., Kobayashi, I., Yasaki, T., Shibata, M., Tsuzuki, K., & Ito, S. (1994). Twenty year follow-up of protective immunity of the Oka strain live varicella vaccine. *Pediatrics, 94*(4, Pt 1), 524–526.

Balfour, H. H., Jr., Kelly, J. M., Suarez, C. S., Heussner, R. C., Englund, J. R., Crane, D. D., McGuirt, P. V., Clemmen, A. F., & Aeppli, D. M. (1990). Acyclovir treatment of varicella in otherwise healthy children. *Journal of Pediatrics, 116*(4), 633–639.

Butler, J. C., Breiman, R. F., Campbell, J. F., Lipman, H. B., Broome, C. V., & Facklam, R. R. (1993). Pneumococcal polysaccharide vaccine efficacy: An evaluation of current recommendations. *JAMA, 270,* 1826–1831.

CDC panel calls for use of rotavirus vaccine. (1998). *Newstand@thrive.*

Centers for Disease Control. (1991, March 22). Rabies prevention—United States, 1991: Recommendations of the Advisory Committee on Immunization Practices (ACIP). *MMWR, 40*(#RR-3).

Centers for Disease Control. (1994, February 4). Reported vaccine-preventable diseases—United States, 1993, and the Childhood Immunization Initiative. *MMWR, 43*(4), 57–60.

Centers for Disease Control. (1996, December 27). Prevention of hepatitis A through active or passive immunization: Recommendations of the Advisory Committee on Immunization Practices (ACIP). *MMWR, 45*(#RR-15).

Centers for Disease Control. (1997a, May 2). Availability of diphtheria antitoxin through an investigational new drug protocol. *MMWR, 46*(17), 380.

Centers for Disease Control. (1997b, February 14). Control and prevention of meningococcal disease: Recommendations of the Advisory Committee on Immunization Practices (ACIP). *MMWR, 46*(#RR-5).

Centers for Disease Control. (1997c, June 13). Measles eradication: Recommendations from a meeting cosponsored by the World Health Organization, the Pan American Health Organization, and CDC. *MMWR, 46*(#RR-11).

Centers for Disease Control. (1997d, January 24). Outbreaks of pneumococcal pneumonia among unvaccinated residents in chronic-care facilities—Massachusetts, October 1995, Oklahoma, February 1996, and Maryland, May–June 1996. *MMWR, 46*(3), 60–62.

Centers for Disease Control. (1997e, March 28). Pertussis vaccination: Use of acellular pertussis vaccines among infants and young children. *MMWR, 46*(#RR-7).

Centers for Disease Control. (1997f, January 24). Poliomyelitis prevention in the United States: Introduction of a sequential vaccination schedule of inactivated poliovirus vaccine followed by oral poliovirus vaccine. *MMWR, 46*(#RR-3).

Centers for Disease Control. (1997g, April 25). Prevention and control of influenza: Recommendations of the Advisory Committee on Immunization Practices (ACIP). *MMWR, 46*(#RR-9).

Centers for Disease Control. (1997h, April 4). Prevention of pneumococcal disease: Recommendations of the Advisory Committee on Immunization Practices (ACIP). *MMWR, 46*(#RR-8).

Centers for Disease Control. (1997i, April 25). Rubella and congenital rubella syndrome—United States, 1994–1997. *MMWR, 46*(16), 350–354.

Centers for Disease Control. (1997j, April 18). Update: Influenza activity—United States and worldwide, 1996–97 season, and composition of the 1997–98 influenza vaccine. *MMWR, 46*(#15).

Chen, R. T., Rastogi, S. C., Mullen, J. R., Hayes, S. W., Cochi, S. L., Donlon, J. A., & Wassilak, S. G. (1994). The Vaccine Adverse Event Reporting System (VAERS). *Vaccine, 12,* 542–550.

Cheng-Liang Lee & Ying-Chin Ko. (1997). Hepatitis B vaccination and hepatocellular carcinoma in Taiwan. *Pediatrics, 99,* 351–353.

Clinical Guidelines. (1997). Tetanus and diphtheria immunization/prophylaxis in adults and older adults. *The Nurse Practitioner, 22*(3), 116–120.

Clinician Reviews. (1996). New vaccine for hepatitis A prevention. *Clinician Reviews, 6*(5), 32.

Clinician Reviews. (1997). Infant and adolescent immunizations: New guidelines reflect latest policy changes. *Clinician Reviews, 7*(2), 67–77.

Cochi, S. L., Wharton, M., & Plotkin, S. A. (1994). Mumps vaccine. In S. A. Plotkin & E. A. Mortimer, Jr., *Vaccines* (2nd ed.). Philadelphia: W. B. Saunders.

Committee on Infectious Disease. (1998). Recommended childhood immunization schedule—United States, January–December 1998. *Pediatrics 101*(1), 154–157.

Cromer, B. A., Goydos, J., Hackell, J., Mezzatesta, J., Dekker, C., & Mortimer, E. A. (1993). Unrecognized pertussis infection in adolescents. *American Journal of Diseases of Children, 147,* 575–577.

Decker, M. D., Edwards, K. M., Steinhoff, M. C., Rennels, M. B., Pichichero, M. E., Englund, J. A., Anderson, E. L., Deloria, M. A., & Reed, G. F. (1995). Comparison of 13 acellular pertussis vaccines: Adverse reactions. *Pediatrics, 96*(3), 557–566.

Department of Health and Human Services. (1996). Epidemiology and prevention of vaccine-preventable diseases (3rd ed.). Washington, DC: DHHS.

Edwards, K. M., Decker, M. D., Graham, B. S., Mezzatesta, J., Scott, J., & Hackell, J. (1993). Adult immunization with acellular pertussis vaccine. *JAMA, 269*, 53–56.

Ellis, R. W. (1994). New technologies for making vaccines. In S. A. Plotkin & E. A. Mortimer, Jr., *Vaccines* (2nd ed.). Philadelphia: W. B. Saunders.

Feder, H. M., LaRussa, P., Steinberg, S., & Gershon, A. (1997). Clinical varicella following varicella vaccination: Don't be fooled. *Pediatrics, 99*, 897–899.

Getting rid of rotavirus. (1998). *Environmental Health Perspectives, 106*(3).

Herwaldt, L. (1991). Pertussis in adults: What physicians need to know. *Archives of Internal Medicine, 151*, 1510–1512.

Hinman, A. R., & Orenstein, W. A. (1994). Public health considerations. In S. A. Plotkin & E. A. Mortimer, Jr., *Vaccines* (2nd ed.). Philadelphia: W. B. Saunders.

Hull, H. F., Ward, N. A., Hull, B. P., Milstien, J. B., & deQuadros, C. (1994). Paralytic poliomyelitis: Seasoned strategies, disappearing disease. *Lancet, 343*, 1331–1337.

Jilg, W., Deinhardt, F., & Hilleman, M. R. (1994). Hepatitis A vaccine. In S. A. Plotkin & E. A. Mortimer, Jr., *Vaccines* (2nd ed.). Philadelphia: W. B. Saunders.

Kim, S. C., Chung, E. K., Hodinka, R. L., DeMaio, J., West, D. J., Jawad, A. F., & Watson, B. (1997). Immunogenicity of hepatitis B vaccine in preterm infants. *Pediatrics, 99*, 534–536.

King, J. C., Vink, P. E., Farley, J. J., Smilie, M., Parks, M., & Lichenstein, R. (1997). Safety and immunogenicity of three doses of a five-valent pneumococcal conjugate vaccine in children younger than two years with and without human immunodeficiency virus infection. *Pediatrics, 99*, 575–580.

Krugman, S., & Stevens, C. E. (1994). Hepatitis B vaccine. In S. A. Plotkin & E. A. Mortimer, Jr., *Vaccines* (2nd ed.). Philadelphia: W. B. Saunders.

Kuter, B. J., Weibal, R. E., Guess, H. A., Matthews, H., Morton, D. H., Neff, B. J., Provost, P. J., Watson, B. A., Starr, S. E., & Plotkin, S. A. (1991). Oka/Merck varicella vaccine in healthy children: Final report of a two-year efficacy study and seven-year follow-up studies. *Vaccine, 9*, 643–647.

Lepow, M. L. (1994). Meningococcal vaccines. In S. A. Plotkin & E. A. Mortimer, Jr., *Vaccines* (2nd ed.). Philadelphia: W. B. Saunders.

Maassab, H. F., Shaw, M. W., & Heilman, C. A. (1994). Live influenza virus vaccine. In S. A. Plotkin & E. A. Mortimer, Jr., *Vaccines* (2nd ed.). Philadelphia: W. B. Saunders.

Markowitz, L. E., & Katz, S. L. (1994). Measles vaccine. In S. A. Plotkin & E. A. Mortimer, Jr., *Vaccines* (2nd ed.). Philadelphia: W. B. Saunders.

Melnick, J. L. (1994). Live attenuated poliovirus vaccines. In S. A. Plotkin & E. A. Mortimer, Jr., *Vaccines* (2nd ed.). Philadelphia: W. B. Saunders.

Mortimer, E. A., Jr. (1994a). Diphtheria toxoid. In S. A. Plotkin & Mortimer, E. A., Jr., *Vaccines* (2nd ed.). Philadelphia: W. B. Saunders.

Mortimer, E. A., Jr. (1994b). Pertussis vaccine. In S. A. Plotkin & E. A. Mortimer, Jr., *Vaccines* (2nd ed.). Philadelphia: W. B. Saunders

Murphy, K. R., & Strunk, R. C. (1985). Safe administration of influenza vaccine in asthmatic children hypersensitive to egg proteins. *Journal of Pediatrics, 106*, 931–933.

Nelson, J. D. (1978). The changing epidemiology of pertussis in young infants: The role of adults as reservoirs of infection. *American Journal of Diseases of Children, 132*:371–373.

Nennig, M. E., Shinefield, H. R., Edwards, K. M., Black, S. B., & Fireman, B. H. (1996). Prevalence and incidence of adult pertussis in an urban population. *JAMA, 275*, 1672–1674.

Nettleman, M. D. (1993). *Emporiatrics: An introduction to travel medicine*. College of Medicine, University of Iowa, Iowa City, IA.

Nettleman, M. D. (1996). Preparing the international traveler. *Gastroenterology Clinics of North America, 25*, 451–469.

Peters, S. (1997, February). The state of pediatric immunizations today. *ADVANCE for Nurse Practitioners*. 43–49.

Phelps, R. (1997). Rabies: Confronting the continuing threat. *Contemporary pediatrics, 14*(7), 136–150.

Plotkin, S. A. (1996). Commentary: Varicella vaccine. *Pediatrics, 97*, 251–253.

Plotkin, S. A., & Koprowski, H. (1994). Rabies vaccine. In S. A. Plotkin & E. A. Mortimer, Jr., *Vaccines* (2nd ed.). Philadelphia: W. B. Saunders.

Plotkin, S. A., & Mortimer, E. A., Jr. (1994). *Vaccines* (2nd ed.). Philadelphia: W. B. Saunders.

Plotkin, S. L. (1994). Rubella vaccine. In S. A. Plotkin & E. A. Mortimer, Jr., *Vaccines* (2nd ed.). Philadelphia: W. B. Saunders.

Plotkin, S. L., & Plotkin, S. A. (1994). A short history of vaccination. In S. A. Plotkin & E. A. Mortimer, Jr., *Vaccines* (2nd ed.). Philadelphia: W. B. Saunders.

Schmitt, H.-J., Wirsing von König, C. H., Neiss, A., Bogaerts, H., Bock, H. L., Schulte-Wissermann, H., Gahr, M., Schult, R., Folkens, J. U., Rauh, W., & Clemens, R. (1996). Efficacy of acellular pertussis vaccine in early childhood after household exposure. *JAMA, 275*(1), 37–41.

Sears, S. D., & Sack, D. A. (1995). Medical advice for the international traveler. In L. R. Barker, J. R. Burton, & P. D. Zieve (Eds.), *Principles of ambulatory medicine* (4th ed.). Baltimore: Williams & Wilkins.

Sell, S. (1996). *Immunology, immunopathology, and immunity* (5th ed.). Stamford, CT: Appleton & Lange.

Starke, J. R., & Connelly, K. K. (1994). Bacille Calmette-Guerin vaccine. In S. A. Plotkin & E. A. Mortimer, Jr., *Vaccines* (2nd ed.). Philadelphia: W. B. Saunders.

Takahashi, M., & Gershon, A. A. (1994). Varicella vaccine. In S. A. Plotkin & E. A. Mortimer, Jr., *Vaccines* (2nd ed.). Philadelphia: W. B. Saunders.

Ward, J., Lieberman, J. M., & Cochi, S. L. (1994). *Haemophilus influenzae* vaccines. In S. A. Plotkin & E. A. Mortimer, Jr., *Vaccines* (2nd ed.). Philadelphia: W. B. Saunders.

Wassilak, S. G. F., Orenstein, W. A., & Sutter, R. W. (1994). Tetanus toxoid. In S. A. Plotkin & E. A. Mortimer, Jr., *Vaccines* (2nd ed.). Philadelphia: W. B. Saunders.

Watson, B., Gupta, R., Randall, T., & Starr, S. (1994). Persistence of cell-mediated and humoral immune responses in healthy children immunized with the live attenuated varicella vaccine. *Journal of Infectious Diseases, 169*, 197.

Watson, B., & Haupt, R. M. (1997). Varicella vaccine: Removing the roadlocks. *Contemporary Pediatrics, 14*(5), 166–181.

Watson, B., Pierey, S., Plotkin, S. A., et al. (1993). Modified chickenpox in children immunized with the Oka/Merck varicella vaccine. *Pediatrics, 91*:17.

Woodruff, B. A., Pavia, A. T., & Blake, P. A. (1991). A new look at typhoid vaccination: Information for the practicing physician. *JAMA, 265*, 756–759.

Woodruff, B. A., Stevenson, J., Yusuf, H., Kwong, S. L., Todoroff, K. P., Hadler, J. L., Connecticut Hepatitis B Project Group, Hoyt M. A., & Mahoney, F. J. (1996). Progress toward integrating hepatitis B vaccine into routine infant immunization schedules in the United States, 1991 through 1994. *Pediatrics, 97*, 798–803.

World Health Organization (1980, May 2). Smallpox declared eradicated. *MMWR.*

Wright, S. W., Edwards, K. M., Decker, M. D., & Zeldin, M. H. (1995). Pertussis infection in adults with persistent cough. *JAMA, 273*, 1044–1046.

# III

# SPECIAL ISSUES AND PATIENT POPULATIONS

# 12

## PEDIATRIC ISSUES

*Katharine A. Gracely-Kilgore*

Several factors influence the choice and administration of medications to pediatric and adolescent patients. These factors include the pharmacokinetics and physiologic differences of childhood, the developmental stage of the child, practical needs of the child and family, safety issues, and pediatric patients' response to pain. Since the focus of this book is on ambulatory care, this chapter will not address IV or emergency drugs.

## USE OF DRUGS IN CHILDREN— HISTORICAL PERSPECTIVE AND CURRENT CONTROVERSIES

Up until the period following World War II children were simply given smaller adult doses with no relation to weight or age (Lucey, 1992). Then a "series of therapeutic disasters" from 1950 to 1970 (Lucey, 1992, p. xiii), helped awaken pediatric providers to the dangers of haphazard medication administration and the need for more careful and precise dosing.

- In the early 1950s, it was discovered that delivering a high percentage of oxygen for long periods of time to premature infants caused retinopathy of prematurity and possible subsequent blindness (Phelps, 1993).
- In the 1960s, several neonates died when given chloramphenicol because their natural low levels of the liver enzyme glucuronyl transferase were

unable to conjugate the drug (Howry, Bindler, & Tso, 1981; Nahata, 1993). The infants developed hypotension, hypoxemia, and eventually shock and death, and had an ashen gray color, thus the name "Gray-baby" syndrome (Smith, 1992).

- In the 1970s, it was reported that premature babies who were repeatedly bathed in 3% hexachlorophene (Phisohex) suffered vacuolar encephalopathy of the brainstem (Ghadially & Shear, 1992).

The Food and Drug Administration (FDA) is the agency that oversees the safety and efficacy of drugs used in the United States. In 1962, amendments were made to the regulations that ensured that medications used in infants and children were to be tested in infants and children before being approved (Yaffe & Aranda, 1992). Before this time, there were no assurances that pediatric drugs had been tested in the pediatric population.

As of 1992, less than 25% of the drugs available in the United States had been shown to be safe and effective for children (Yaffe & Aranda, 1992). The other drugs available for use in pediatrics may be safe, but they have not had sufficient testing to support their safety and efficacy, and are therefore not FDA-approved (*Handbook of Pediatric Drug Therapy*, 1990; Yaffe & Aranda, 1992). Lack of testing may be a function of, as in the case of ranitidine and omeprazole, "a lack of interest by pharmaceutical companies to pursue clinical trials to get additional indications for a potential market that is much smaller than the adult population" (Karjoo & Kane, 1995, p. 270). The term *therapeutic orphan* (Yaffe & Aranda, 1992, p. 5) refers to the situation in which a pediatric patient is deprived of the use of a drug because it has only been approved for use in adults. However, some providers may choose to use an unapproved drug for a patient if they feel that the benefits outweigh the risks, as in the case of using ciprofloxacin for patients with cystic fibrosis (Buck, 1992). This "off label" drug use is controversial (Wilson, Kearns, Murphy, & Yaffe, 1994). There is the potential for the health care provider to be caught in a situation where a drug unapproved by the FDA might be considered. For legal reasons, the provider is strongly encouraged to only use FDA-approved drugs.

A recent controversy is the recommendation of the American Academy of Pediatrics for mandatory labeling by pharmaceutical companies of the inactive ingredients contained in prescription and over-the-counter medications. Oral medications are not required to have inactive ingredients listed, yet some of them can cause adverse reactions in children, including seizures, headaches, bronchospasm, diarrhea, and allergic reactions. There are more than 773 of these ingredients and they can include sweeteners, dyes, coloring agents, and preservatives. Also, fragrances and flavoring agents are not required to be listed.

## PHARMACOKINETICS: PEDIATRIC VARIATIONS

Physiologically, children's and adolescents' bodily systems develop at different rates, with some systems maturing much sooner than others. The ways that drugs are absorbed, distributed, metabolized, and excreted varies with the maturity of various body systems (see Table 12–1). Conversely, some medications may affect the development process itself and the results will not be readily apparent for many years (Yaffe & Aranda, 1992).

This section will address these four pharmacokinetic areas by age, following FDA groupings. The FDA categorized children into groups according to age because it was felt that some age-dependent factors may affect the safety and efficacy of drugs used in children (Yaffe & Aranda, 1992). The FDA groups referred to in this chapter are: neonate (birth to 1 month), infant-toddler (1 month to 2 years), child (2 years

to onset of puberty), and adolescent (onset of adolescence to adult life) (Yaffe & Aranda, 1992). The discussion will not include premature infants because of the specialized nature of the care of this population.

## NEONATE

### Absorption

The skin of neonates has a thinner dermis, epidermis, and stratum corneum layers (Bindler & Howry, 1991; *Handbook of Pediatric Drug Therapy*, 1990), thus resulting in greater permeability. Neonates' large skin surface in relation to body weight (Blumer & Reed, 1992; *Handbook of Pediatric Drug Therapy*, 1990) causes systemic availability to be 2.7 times that of adults (Blumer & Reed, 1992). Because of these factors, the weakest strength of any medication must be ordered and used sparingly. Hexachlorophene, salicylic acids, rubbing alcohol, phenol (*Handbook of Pediatric Drug Therapy*, 1990), lindane (see Drug Table 806), and strong steroids (see Drug Table 807) are to be avoided, and the health care provider and the caregivers must be cautious with the use of over-the-counter (OTC) preparations (Cetta, Lambert, & Ros, 1991). Fluorinated steroids should never be applied to the face at any age. Inflamed, burned, or denuded skin (Blumer & Reed, 1992) or skin covered with disposable diapers or occlusive dressings (Pagliaro, 1995) absorbs medication to a greater degree (Blumer & Reed, 1992; Pagliaro, 1995). Therefore, when treating severe diaper rash, medications need to be applied sparingly.

Drugs can easily pass into the nasolacrimal duct of the eye, thus causing increased systemic absorption, especially of anticholenergics (Pagliaro, 1995). One or two drops of any medication is sufficient. If necessary to impede absorption, the caregiver can practice nasolacrimal obstruction (NLO), which is gentle external pressure at the inner canthus to close the drainage system. Increased production of tears causes decreased absorption (Pagliaro, 1995), so the caregiver must not give eyedrops if the neonate is crying. For treating a blocked tear duct, with its increased tearing, ointment may be preferred, or an alternate route may need to be chosen.

A major factor in drug absorption is the gastrointestinal (GI) tract. A variable and prolonged gastric emptying time, prolonged transit time and peristalsis (Blumer & Reed, 1992; *Handbook of Pediatric Drug Therapy*, 1990), and greater small

**TABLE 12–1. PEDIATRIC PHARMACOKINETIC DIFFERENCES AS COMPARED TO ADULTS**

| | Neonate | Infant | Child |
|---|---|---|---|
| **Absorption** | | | |
| Gastric acidity | Achlorhydria at 10–30 days after birth | Reaches adult levels at 1–2 years | |
| Gastric emptying time | Prolonged 6 to 8 h; irregular peristalsis | Reaches adult levels at 6–8 months; irregular peristalsis | Same as adult |
| GI motility intestinal transit time | Highly variable; influenced by the presence/absence of food | | |
| Pancreatic enzyme activity | Decreased | Full activity capacity dependent on specific enzyme | |
| GI surface area | More sensitive to chemicals that may cause more nausea, vomiting, and diarrhea | | |
| Dietary components | Acidic/alkaline foods will alter gastric pH | | |
| Skin permeability | Thinner stratum corneum; more surface area/body weight | Thinner stratum corneum | |
| **Distribution** | | | |
| Total body water | Increased | | Same as adult |
| Albumin | Lower, concentrations (3.0–4.0 g/dL); lower binding affinity | Plasma proteins reach adult levels by 1 year | |
| Blood-brain barrier | More permeable | Similar to adult | |
| Fat composition | Lower than adult (15–20% of TBW); lipid-soluble drugs stored to a lesser degree | 21–26% TBW | Adolescent boys lose fat (12% of TBW); adolescent girls accumulate fat (25% of TBW) |
| **Metabolism** | | | |
| Liver | Some hepatic enzymes reduced; most metabolize drugs at a rate several times lower than adult | | Most enzyme systems mature by 2–4 years of age |
| **Excretion** | | | |
| Renal blood flow | Reduced | 9 months reaches adult levels | |
| Glomerular filtration | Decreased | 9 months reaches adult levels | |
| Tubular function | Decreased | >9 months reaches adult levels | Decrease in renal tubular clearance with the onset of adolescence |

Source: Used with permission of Nurse Practitioner (1997), 22(3), 18.
TBW = total body weight.

intestinal surface all contribute to increased absorption of oral medications and the potential for overdose if too large a dose is given (Sagraves, 1995). Medications given via the lower rectum have greater systemic absorption (Kauffman, 1992), so the health care provider must be cautious of overdosage. However, suppositories are erratically absorbed, especially if feces are present (Kauffman, 1992), so other routes are preferred over the rectal.

Other considerations in this age group include the fact that infants are nose breathers until 3 months of age, so drops should be instilled to one side of the nose at a time. Also, tooth discoloration has been associated with the use of ciprofloxacin (Lumbiagannon, Pengsaa, & Sookpranee, 1991). The neonate has many immature body systems, so the health care provider must be alert to the risk of toxicity with the use of **any** drug because of increased absorption and must monitor the patient carefully.

## Distribution

Peripheral circulation is poorly developed, and vasoconstriction occurs in response to cold, causing decreased absorption (Bindler & Howry, 1991). A decreased muscle mass (25% of body weight versus 40% in adults) provides a smaller area for absorption of intramuscular medications (Bindler & Howry, 1991), so intramuscular or subcutaneous routes are not the best choices for the neonate. The oral route is preferred unless the infant is very ill, in which case medication is given intravenously.

Immature myelinization of the central nervous system (CNS) until age 2 years (Bindler & Howry, 1991; Lehne, Moore, Crosby, & Hamilton, 1990) enables drugs to pass the blood-brain barrier more easily (Lehne et al, 1990). Encephalopathy is more commonly seen as a toxic side effect (Bindler & Howry, 1991). The risk of CNS depression is great in the neonate (Lehne et al, 1990), so one must monitor the patient carefully if CNS drugs such as phenobarbital are prescribed (see Drug Table 308.1).

## Metabolism

The liver affects drug metabolism in neonates and infants because of their immature enzyme systems. There is variability in this impact since enzyme systems mature at different rates (Skaer, 1991). Most drugs are metabolized slower in neonates, but in some there may be an increased metabolism. Most enzyme systems mature between 2–4 years of age. Fewer total plasma proteins (Sagraves, 1995) and less albumin (Niederhauser, 1997), along with the lower binding affinity of albumin, allow for more free drug to be available for absorption (Sagraves, 1995), especially phenobarbital, phenytoin, and salicylates (Nahata, 1993). Also, maternal hormones and a large amount of free and fatty acids bind with plasma proteins, thus restricting the binding of drugs with plasma proteins (Bindler & Howry, 1991). Drugs such as sulfonamide antibiotics can compete with albumin-binding sites (see Drug Table 102.9; 102.10) and can cause increased risk of kernicterus in the neonate (Barone, 1996; Skaer, 1991).

## Excretion

Due to the smaller number of tubular cells, shorter tubules, and decreased renal flow in neonates (Bindler & Howry, 1991), their glomerular filtration rate is decreased (Behrman & Vaughan, 1987; Merenstein & Gardner, 1989; Reed & Besunder, 1989). This results in drugs having a longer half-life and increased absorption, especially digoxin, penicillins, aminoglycosides, salicylates and thiazide diuretics (see Drug Tables 102.6, 207, 208.4, 307) (Niederhauser, 1997). Dosage intervals of drugs, especially those mentioned above, may have to be increased (Wink, 1991).

## INFANTS

## Absorption

The GI emptying time reaches adult levels at 6 to 8 months (Blumer & Reed, 1992), and greater small intestine surface area (Kauffman, 1992), increases absorption of oral medications. Because body surface area doubles by 1 year of age (Kauffman, 1992), topical agents are still greatly absorbed. As an example, Maswoswe, Egbunike, Stewart, et al (1994) discuss a 6-month-old child with an itchy rash associated with varicella who died from diphenhydramine toxicity (see Drug Table 705) from application of Caladryl to its entire body for several days. Because of increased absorption, transdermal patches are not FDA-approved for pediatric patients (Pagliaro, 1995). Certain drugs are contraindicated at this age. Oil-based nasal sprays can cause aspiration and lipid pneumonia (Pagliaro, 1995), and accurate dosages of opioid drugs can cause respiratory depression in children under 1 year of age (Kauffman, 1992).

## Distribution

Muscle mass is decreased, and although most immunizations and their booster doses are given intramuscularly during infancy and childhood, the oral route is preferred for ill young children.

Acutely ill children may need intravenous medication.

## Metabolism

As the neonate matures into infancy, "Both hepatic and renal function not only equals, but in some cases exceeds normal adult function between one year and puberty." (Kauffman, 1992, p. 213).

## Excretion

By 9 months of age most excretion functions have reached adult levels (Niederhauser, 1997).

## CHILD

### Absorption

For the child, maturing systems are still vulnerable. Fluoroquinolones have been found to be toxic to cartilage (see Drug Table 102.4) (Todd, 1995) and are therefore not recommended for children under the age of 12 years. Tetracycline has been found to cause tooth staining in children under 8 years of age. Acetaminophen can lead to liver toxicity if overdosed (Kiebler & Mowry, 1994). A shorter GI transit time in the young child decreases absorption of sustained-release drugs (Pederson & Moller-Peterson, 1984; Rogers, Kalisker, Weiner, & Szafler, 1985), so drugs such as Ritalin-SR or Theolair-SR should not be used. Gastric emptying time exceeds or equals adult levels (Kauffman, 1992), which results in increased absorption (Green & Mirkin, 1984; Kearns & Reed, 1989), especially of liquid medications (Kauffman, 1992).

### Distribution

By childhood most distribution functions reach adult levels.

## ADOLESCENT

### Absorption

Inflammatory bowel disease (Yaffe & Aranda, 1992) or any condition associated with diarrhea and/or vomiting, such as an eating disorder or viral gastroenteritis, can cause decreased absorption of oral medications, including oral contraceptives. With oral contraceptives, the use of a back-up method of birth control must be reinforced during an acute illness. For a chronic condition, a different method of birth control, such as medroxyprogesterone (Depo-Provera), may need to be chosen (see Drug Table 603.6).

## DEVELOPMENTAL STAGES AND ADMINISTERING MEDICATIONS

When administering medications, or more likely, when counseling caregivers on how to administer medications, the health care provider always must consider the developmental level of the child. For example, the approach to giving medications to toddlers is very different from the approach to school-aged children. The reader is referred to Erik Erikson's and Jean Piaget's theories of child development for background information.

### NEONATE

Since separation from parents is one of the biggest fears of neonates, it is recommended that caregivers hold the neonates securely when administering any medication. And even though it may seem silly, caregivers should also tell the neonates that they are getting medicine to make them feel better. In this way the caregivers will be in the habit of explaining the reason for the medication to the children, and this matter-of-fact explanation to children will help increase compliance when children are older. It is sometimes difficult to open neonates' eyes, so drops must be applied quickly. When giving oral medications, it is best to put the medicine in a nipple or special device, so the infants can suck the medicine. Do not put it in a bottle of formula or other liquids, because the infants may not finish the bottle or refuse it because of the taste and therefore not get the full dose. The caregiver also can give very small amounts of the medicine slowly to the inside of the cheek with an oral syringe. The neonates' taste has not developed, so the medicine should not be spit out, and the infants will take the medicine better if they are hungry (Bindler & Howry, 1991). To help encourage neonates or infants to swallow, the caregiver can stroke the throat or blow a puff or air into the face, which is called the *Santmyer swallow reflex* (Pagliaro, 1995). Masks are used to deliver nebulizer treatments for lung conditions. Rectal suppositories are sometimes given to neonates, eg, glycerin suppositories for constipation. The suppositories should never be cut because the medication is not evenly dispersed (Pagliaro, 1995).

## INFANT

Administration of eye medication is seen as frightening and as an intrusion to infants (Pagliaro, 1995). Infants and toddlers do not like nose sprays because of the tickling sensation, taste, and difficulty in breathing, and they feel that it is an invasion of their bodies (Pagliaro, 1995). Therefore, they should be told what to expect, that it will last only a short time, and that they can have a drink of their favorite liquid after accepting the spray; infants should be held gently during the administration.

Giving oral medications can be a "challenge." Infants under 3 months can turn away from oral medications, and when the sense of taste develops they can spit out a medication that they do not like. To help disguise medication, mix it with small amounts of certain soft foods, such as applesauce, yogurt, or pudding, unless the medication becomes unstable in these foods (Chater, 1993). Stranger anxiety develops around 9 months, so let the caregivers give the medication. If strangers must do it, they can play games such as peek-a-boo with the infants first to gain their trust before administering medications. Infants also can reach for and grasp the medication cup, and crawl away if not held.

## TODDLER

Certain characteristics are unique to toddlers. The first is negativism. Toddlers' favorite word is "NO," so expect that as an answer to any question you ask. Do not ask them if they are ready to take their medication; state that it is time for their medication. Only give choices for those things that you want as the result: which cup to use, the choice of Band-Aid or sticker, which arm to use first, etc. Do not get into a power struggle; set limits and do what you have to do quickly, especially with procedures or injections. Tell toddlers JUST before giving medication or an injection that you are going to give it. Do not discuss what will happen in the future; they are concerned with the present (Pagliaro, 1995). Ignore negative behavior and praise positive behavior.

Toddlers like routine and having things done in the same way (Wong, 1993a). It gives them a sense of control and security. They may want the same cup or the same drink after taking medicine, or insist upon taking the medicine a certain way. Place a desired sticker where the children tell you to.

Toddlers are egocentric. They see illness, medication, and painful procedures as being their fault and a form of punishment (Dixon, 1992). Reinforce that they are not at fault. To help them gain a sense of control, let them play with the equipment, such as a mask, beforehand if possible, and definitely afterwards. Let them hold the cup if you know they are going to take the medication. Let them give it to a doll or stuffed animal first, if that will help them cooperate. Give short and simple explanations. "This medicine is to help your ear infection go away so you can get better," is sufficient. Let the caregivers help hold the children if they wish to. Praise the children for cooperating and cuddle them afterwards. Allow for outlet of aggression in a play situation (Pagliaro, 1995), especially after an unpleasant procedure, such as an injection.

If toddlers absolutely refuse oral medication, another route may have to be chosen (Pagliaro, 1995). However, an effective method of administering oral medication to a resisting child is to place the oral syringe diagonally across the tongue while delivering the medication into the inside of the cheek (Bindler & Howry, 1991). Toddlers should never be told that medication is candy (Chater, 1993; Pagliaro, 1995).

Rectal medication is to be avoided because of the possible negative feelings associated with toilet training (*Handbook of Pediatric Drug Therapy*, 1990) as well as fear of body entry.

## PRESCHOOLER

Preschoolers are more cooperative than toddlers. They like to help (Pagliaro, 1995). Let them hold or play with the equipment; this gives them a sense of control. Children will usually take medication willingly if given a simple, truthful explanation: "This will help you get better." If expected to take a medication, they usually will cooperate (Pagliaro, 1995). Reinforce their cooperation by praising positive behaviors.

Other characteristics of preschoolers are animism and magical thinking (Dixon, 1992; Wong, 1993a). When explaining things, choose words carefully. They see things in a concrete sense. Objects in their world seem to be alive. "Germs in your throat" may seem to them to be unseen alive objects. They also think that all their blood will come out after receiving an injection, and that a Band-Aid will stop the blood loss. It helps to show the site and show that there is no blood loss. They will understand better if a procedure is demonstrated on a doll or stuffed animal and/or with a drawing (Pagliaro, 1995).

Their time concept is limited (Wong, 1993b). Explain each time a medication is given why they must take it (Pagliaro, 1995). Also, associate times for medication with events in their life: lunch, dinner, and bedtime (Pagaliaro, 1995).

When prescribing oral medications, order liquids unless the child can tolerate chewable tablets. The taste of the medication may need to be disguised. Do not call the medication candy. The caregiver may need to give medication to an imaginary friend first before giving it to the child. For inhalation medications, metered-dose inhalers (MDIs) are the vehicle of choice. Spacers improve drug delivery (the mist goes to the lungs, not to the back of the mouth and throat) and spacers also let the child see and hear the delivery. Four-year-olds can use InspirEase. They can see it go in and out, and it will make a noise if inhaled and exhaled too fast. See Chapter 22.

## SCHOOL-AGER

School-agers want to feel a sense of accomplishment (Selekman, 1993). If possible, let them help, eg, by shaking the bottle of medication (Martin, 1992). Let them decide which liquid to take with the medication or whether to have a tablet, capsule, chewable tablet, or liquid. They can assume some responsibility in remembering to take their medication. They agree even when not understanding (Pagliaro, 1995), so explain carefully and ask them to explain the information to you. Use drawings to explain how the body works, the need to take medication, and how medications work. Reassure them that medication is not punishment. Use the word "medication," not "drug" (Martin, 1992). They are learning about drug abuse in school and that drugs are bad.

Five- or six-year-olds may be able to take a tablet or a capsule, depending upon the size. The health care provider must be certain of the children's ability to swallow tablets before ordering them. Chewable tablets are a good choice at this age, since they do not require refrigeration. Some chewable tablets have a tart taste and may be refused. Tablets can be crushed, and some capsules can be opened and put in food.

## ADOLESCENT

Adolescents may alternate between cooperation and negativism. They should be encouraged to take part in the decision making regarding their medication (Khunti, 1996). They are able to give themselves medication, but may not always remember or want to. Having a chart to mark the dose taken instead of constant verbal questions or reminders is a better way to keep track of medications taken. Once-a-day dosing is best; twice-a-day dosing is also good.

Adolescents want to be treated like adults, but may still need to be treated like children. They may not ask for help in administering eye- or eardrops. They should be able to tolerate tablets, but may still prefer liquids. Most older adolescents have abstract thinking and can understand reasons for illness and the necessity of needing medication. *Truthfully* explain the facts to adolescents. Communicate with them in an honest, understanding, and nonjudgmental way so the adolescents will feel comfortable in talking with the provider and disclose needed information. Ask what other drugs they are taking, over-the-counter as well as illicit (Hein, 1992). Adolescents may use alcohol or illegal drugs that can interact with prescription drugs (Hein, 1992).

Adolescents do not like to feel different. With a chronic illness, they may feel different, and refuse to take their medication. A support group or meeting or talking on the phone with just one other person with the same illness may help alleviate this feeling of alienation or isolation. Also, pointing out some of their favorite celebrities with the same condition may help. The health care provider should explain things in such a way as to make compliance "cool."

Adolescents are concerned with the present. They will want an "instant" cure for acne, and may be frustrated with the slow progress of treatment.

Female adolescents may need vaginal medication for the first time. Explain how it works and use a diagram to show how it is inserted. Be sensitive to their feelings and embarrassment or lack of embarrassment.

## TABLE 12–2. PRACTICAL TIPS: DOSES OF COMMON ANTIBIOTICS FOR CHILDREN

| Drug | Weight, lb | Dosage | Youngest Age Medication Safely Given |
|---|---|---|---|
| Amoxicillin; 40 mg/kg/d; q 8 h | | 125 mg/5 cc | |
| | 6 | 1/4 tsp | Neonate |
| | 10 | 1/2 tsp | |
| | 16 | 3/4 tsp | |
| | 20 | 1 tsp | |
| | | 250 mg/5 cc | |
| | 26 | 3/4 tsp | |
| | 40 | 1 tsp | |
| Amoxicillin/clavulanate potassium (Augmentin); 40 mg/kg/d; q 12 h | | 400 mg/5 cc | |
| | 11 | 1/4 tsp | Neonate |
| | 22 | 1/2 tsp | |
| | 33 | 4/5 tsp | |
| | 44 | 1 tsp | |
| | 55 | 1 1/3 tsp | |
| | 66 | 1 2/3 tsp | |
| | 77 | 2 tsp | |
| Azithromycin (Zithromax); 10 mg/kg; 5 mg/kg/d; q 24 h | | 100 mg/5 cc | |
| | 22 | 1 tsp on day one 1/2 tsp next 4 days | 6 months |
| | | 200 mg/5 cc | |
| | 44 | 1 tsp on day one 1/2 tsp next 4 days | |
| | 66 | 1 1/2 tsp on day one 3/4 tsp next 4 days | |
| Cefaclor (Ceclor); 40 mg/kg/d; q 12 h | | 375 mg/5 cc | |
| | 20 | 1/2 tsp | 1 month |
| | 40 | 1 tsp | |
| Cefadroxil (Duricef); 30 mg/kg/d; q 12 h | | 250 mg/5 cc | |
| | 10 | 1/4 tsp | 1 month |
| | 20 | 1/2 tsp | |
| | 30 | 3/4 tsp | |
| | 40 | 1 tsp | |
| | 50 | 1 1/4 tsp | |
| | 60 | 1 1/2 tsp | |
| Cefixime (Suprax); 8 mg/kg/d; q 24 h | 14 | 1/2 tsp | 6 months |
| | 21 | 3/4 tsp | |
| | 28 | 1 tsp | |
| | 35 | 1 1/4 tsp | |
| | 42 | 1 1/2 tsp | |
| | 49 | 1 3/4 tsp | |
| | 56 | 2 tsp | |

*continues on next page*

TABLE 12–2. *continued*

| Drug | Weight, lb | Dosage | Youngest Age Medication Safely Given |
|---|---|---|---|
| Cefpodoxine proxetil (Vantin); 10 mg/kg/d; q 12 h | | 50 mg/5 cc | 5 months |
| | 14 | 1/2 tsp | |
| | 18 | 3/4 tsp | |
| | | 100 mg/5 cc | |
| | 25 | 1/2 tsp | 5 months |
| | 36 | 3/4 tsp | |
| | 49 | 1 tsp | |
| Cefprozil (Cefzil); 30 mg/kg/d; q 12 h | | 125 mg/5 cc | |
| | 10 | 1/2 tsp | 6 months |
| | 15 | 3/4 tsp | |
| | | 250 mg/5 cc | |
| | 20 | 1/2 tsp | |
| | 30 | 3/4 tsp | |
| | 40 | 1 tsp | |
| Ceftibutin (Cedax); 9 mg/kg/d; q 24 h | 11 | 1/2 tsp | 6 months |
| | 22 | 1 tsp | |
| | 33 | 1 1/2 tsp | |
| | 44 | 2 tsp | |
| Cefuroxime axetil (Ceftin); 30 mg/kg/d; q 12 h | | 125 mg/5 cc | 3 months |
| | 9 | 1/2 tsp | |
| | 13 | 3/4 tsp | |
| | 18 | 1 tsp | |
| | 22 | 1 1/4 tsp | |
| | 26 | 1 1/2 tsp | |
| | 33 | 1 3/4 tsp | |
| | 37 | 2 tsp | |
| Clarithromycin (Biaxin); 15 mg/kg/d; q 12 h | | 125 mg/5 cc | 6 months |
| | 20 | 1/2 tsp | |
| | 37 | 1 tsp | |
| | | 250 mg/5 cc | |
| | 55 | 3/4 tsp | |
| | 73 | 1 tsp | |
| Erythromycin; 30–50 mg/kg/d; q 6 h | | 200 mg/5 cc | |
| | 15 | 1/4 tsp | Neonate |
| | 25 | 1/2 tsp | |
| | 50 | 1 tsp | |
| | 100 | 1 1/2 tsp | |
| | >100 | 2 tsp | |
| Erythromycin ethylsuccinate (50 mg/kg/d); Acetyl sulfisoxazole (150 mg/kg/d) (Pediazole) q 6 h | 18 | 1/2 tsp | 2 months |
| | 35 | 1 tsp | |
| | 53 | 1 1/2 tsp | |
| | >100 | 2 tsp | |
| Bicillin L-A (Penallin G Benzathine) | Neonate | 50,000 units/kg | Neonate |
| | <2 years | 300,000 units | |
| | >2 years; <60 lb | 600,000 units | |
| | >60 lb | 1,200,000 units | |

*continues on next page*

**TABLE 12–2.** *continued from previous page*

| Drug | Weight, lb | Dosage | Youngest Age Medication Safely Given |
|---|---|---|---|
| Loracarbef (Lorabid); | | 200 mg/5 cc | 6 months |
| 30 mg/kg/d; q 12 h | 15 | 1/2 tsp | |
| | 29 | 1 tsp | |
| | 44 | 1 1/2 tsp | |
| | 57 | 2 tsp | |
| Penicillin V Potassium | 18 | 1/2 tsp of 125 mg/5 cc | Neonate |
| (Pen-Vee K); 25–50 mg/kg/d; | 35 | 1 tsp of 125 mg/5 cc | |
| q 6 h | >35 | 1 tsp of 250 mg/5 cc | |
| Trimethoprim (8 mg/kg/d); | 22 | 1 tsp | 2 months |
| Sulfamethoxazole | 44 | 2 tsp | |
| (Co-Trimoxazole) | 66 | 3 tsp | |
| (40 mg/kg/d) (Bactrim, | 88 | 4 tsp | |
| Septra) q 12 h | | | |

*Adapted from Barone (1996), Gennrich & Chan (1996), and Physician's Desk Reference (1997), & tables produced by manufacturers of medications.*

**TABLE 12–3. PRACTICAL TIPS: PEDIATRIC DOSES OF COMMON OVER-THE-COUNTER MEDICATIONS**

| Drug | Weight/Age | Dosage | Youngest Age Medication Safely Given |
|---|---|---|---|
| Acetaminophen (Tylenol); | 11 lb | 1/4 tsp of 160 mg/5 cc (0.4 mL of 80 mg/mL) | Neonate |
| 10 mg/kg/dose; q 4 h | 17 lb | 1/2 tsp of 160 mg/5 cc (0.8 mL of 80 mg/mL) | |
| | | 160 mg/5 cc | |
| | 23 lb | 3/4 tsp | |
| | 35 lb | 1 tsp | |
| | 47 lb | 1 1/2 tsp | |
| | 59 lb | 2 tsp | |
| | 71 lb | 2 1/2 tsp | |
| | 95 lb | 3 tsp | |
| | >95 lb | 4 tsp | |
| Chlorpheniramine | | 2 mg/5 cc | |
| (Chlor-Trimeton); | 3 months–2 years | 1/4 tsp | 3 months |
| 1–2 mg/dose; q.i.d. | 2–6 years | 1/2 tsp | |
| | 6–12 years | 1 tsp | |
| | >12 years | 2 tsp | |
| Guaifenesin (Robitussin), q.i.d. | | 100 mg/5 cc | |
| 12 mg/kg/day | 3 months–2 years | 1/4 tsp | 3 months |
| | 2–6 years | 1/2 tsp | |
| | 6–12 years | 1 tsp | |
| | >12 years | 2 tsp | |

*continues on next page*

**TABLE 12–3.** *continued*

| Drug | Weight/Age | Dosage | Youngest Age Medication Safely Given |
|---|---|---|---|
| Ibuprofen (Advil, Motrin); | | 100 mg/5 cc | |
| 5 mg/kg/dose; q 6–8 h | 17 lb | 1/4 tsp | 6 months |
| For temp > 102.5, double | 23 lb | 1/2 tsp | |
| the dose | 35 lb | 3/4 tsp | |
| | 47 lb | 1 tsp | |
| | 59 lb | 1 1/4 tsp | |
| | 71 lb | 1 1/2 tsp | |
| | 95 lb | 2 tsp | |
| Pseudoephedrine (Sudafed); | | 30 mg/5 cc | |
| 4 mg/kg/d; q.i.d. | 3 months–2 years | 1/4 tsp | 3 months |
| | 2 years–6 years | 1/2 tsp | |
| | 6 years–12 years | 1 tsp | |
| | >12 years | 2 tsp | |
| Pseudoephedrine | | 7.5 mg/0.8 mL | |
| (PediaCare); q.i.d. | 11 lb | 0.4 mL | 3 months |
| | 17 lb | 0.8 mL | |
| | 23 lb | 1.2 mL | |
| | 35 lb | 1.6 mL | |
| **Combinations** | | | |
| Dimetapp; q.i.d.[a] | 6–11 months | 1/4 tsp | 6 months |
| | 1–6 years | 1/2 tsp | |
| | 6–12 years | 1 tsp | |
| | >12 years | 2 tsp | |
| Triaminic (all products); q.i.d.[b] | 3 months–2 years | 1/4 tsp | 3 months |
| | 2–6 years | 1/2 tsp | |
| | 6–12 years | 1 tsp | |
| | >12 years | 2 tsp | |

[a] Contains brompheniramine maleate and phenylpropanolamine HCl.
[b] Ingredients differ; may include pseudoephedrine, phenylpropanolamine HCl, chlorpheniramine maleate, dextromethorphan HBr, acetaminophen, or guaifenesin.
*Adapted from Barone (1996), Gennrich & Chan (1996), and Physician's Desk Reference (1997), & tables produced by manufacturers of medications.*

Adolescents may be modest if needing an injection in the hip. They may still be afraid of needles (Schichor et al, 1994). Adolescents may need reminders or charts to rotate sites for insulin injections.

## PRACTICAL TIPS FOR PRESCRIBING MEDICATIONS

When prescribing medications, there are only two acceptable methods for calculating doses. These are milligrams of drug per kilogram of body weight (mg/kg) and milligrams of drug per square meter of body surface (mg/m$^2$). The surface area is a relationship between the height and weight and is the most accurate. However, not all drug doses are calculated by the body surface area formula by the manufacturers; most have been calculated in milligrams per kilogram. If there are questions regarding pediatric dosing, the American Academy of Pediatrics indicates that the manufacturer's packets are the official source of medication dosages (American Academy of Pediatrics Committee on Drugs, 1978).

Easy reference tables now are produced by drug companies for their products. They list age, weight and dose, and may also state the size of the container to order. If tables do not exist, providers are encouraged to create their own tables of frequently used medications. Several examples of some of the most common antibiotic drugs are included in Table 12-2 and common over-the-counter medications in Table 12-3. Although some providers are weighing children in kilograms, the prevalent practice is to weigh in pounds. Thus the practice guides (see Table 12-2) in this chapter will cite pounds, not kilograms.

The provider's choice of medication needs to reflect understanding of ease of dosing, cost, potential to develop resistancy, as well as caregiver/patient preference. For example, many providers may consider using second and third generation broad spectrum antibiotics for the treatment of otitis media. Several studies support that either 1) a once-a-day dosing (Mandel, Casselbrant, Kurs-Lasky, & Bluestone, 1996) or 2) a loading dose followed by a shorter course (Khurana, 1996) of a broad spectrum antibiotic, can achieve outcomes equivalent to the traditional 10-day course of oral antibiotic in terms of cure, relapse, and comfort. In addition, the recent use of ceftriaxone (Rocephin) as a one-time intramuscular injection has also been found to be equally effective as the traditional 10-day course (Barnett, et al, 1997; Bauchner, Adams, Barnett, & Klein, 1996; Chamberlain, 1994; Green & Rothrock, 1993). In one of these studies (Bauchner et al, 1996), parents overwhelmingly indicated a preference for a one-time injection for their child's next case of otitis media. However, for the provider the choice of medication is difficult. It is not clear which choice puts the patient at the greater risk of developing resistant organisms, the use of broad spectrum antibiotic or the incomplete use of a 10-day traditional narrow spectrum medication. Clearly more data is needed to answer this question.

Currently high risk populations, such as persons who are homeless, or migrant workers (see Chapter 15), or some emergency room patients, might be candidates for the one-time intramuscular medication for specific bacterial infections (Varsano et al, 1997). Other special circumstances, particularly in cases where the ability to tolerate or absorb oral drugs is compromised, or in children unable to take oral medication, might also lead the provider to consider using an injection (Varsano et al, 1997). Yet if one is assured that the caregiver will be able to administer the complete course of medication, the narrowest spectrum antibiotic is still preferred, taking into account the cost and caregiver preference for frequency of administration. Parents not in a high risk group who request one-time injection need to have information about the risk of developing resistant organisms discussed with them in a respectful manner.

There are many practical tips for writing prescriptions, teaching, and safety that have been generated from providers experienced in pediatric care that may be helpful to those less familiar with this population. Tips for medication writing are summarized in Table 12–4, teaching tips for parents and families in Table 12–5, and safety issues in Table 12–6.

## PAIN IN CHILDREN AND ADOLESCENTS

Pain from injections and blood tests seems to be expected in pediatrics. Sometimes adults become immune to the reactions of children and adolescents to painful procedures. On the other hand, some adults have not forgotten their experience as children and are still afraid of needles as adults.

In pediatrics, painful procedures are caused by vaccinations, other injections, and the taking of blood through a fingertip or vein. To help the child cope, for the neonate and small infant, it is best to cuddle them after the injection. Beginning at 8–12 months, infants associate pain with the needle and syringe, so the health care provider must keep the syringe out of sight just until time to give the injection (Bindler & Howry, 1991). Toddlers should be told that the injection will hurt, but only for a short time. They need to be held securely, and be given the injection quickly. For older infants and children, providers can try diversionary measures: blowing when receiving the injection, closing eyes, wriggling toes, counting to 10 (Pagliaro, 1995), tapping another part of the body, and looking the other way. McCaffery and Beebe (1989) have advocated pinching and grasping the deltoid muscle when giving an injection there, ice massage, use of hot and cold, imagery, singing, listening to music, tapping a rhythm, rhythmic massage, and slow rhythmic breathing.

A newer method of pain relief is the use of EMLA cream which contains 2.5% lidocaine and 2.5% prilocaine (Farrington, 1993; Goede &

## TABLE 12–4. PRACTICAL TIPS: PRESCRIPTION WRITING

1. Always get a **weight** at **every** pediatric visit. A child can lose weight easily with an illness. Even if the infant or child was seen 3 days ago, today's weight is critical to calculate correct medication dosage.
2. **Do not go above the recommended adult doses** when ordering for adolescents. If drugs were ordered by milligram per kilogram, too high a dose would be ordered.
3. As a rule, **start** with the **smallest dose** or the **weakest strength**, especially if treating a neonate. For example, topical gel preparations, such as tretinoin for acne, are stronger than lotions or creams.
4. "**Round up**" the dose if it falls between the given choices **unless it is a toxic drug or has severe side effects**, since compliance is not usually 100%.
5. With **acetaminophen** products, **calculate** the dose by **weight**, not age.
6. It has been difficult to dose patients **under 2 years of age** for OTC preparations. If a schedule does not exist, a provider can use the milligram per kilogram value of at least one of the ingredients to calculate the dose needed if there is a compelling reason to use a specific medication and no other practical options exist. See Table 12–2.
7. In **writing a prescription**, be very explicit in your terminology. It is best to write out numbers. State "chewable" tabs if that is what is desired. State "suspension," especially for Cortisporin otic opthalmic medication. Be consistent in writing "tsp," "cc," or "ml," and tell the caregiver the term that you are writing. If you write "5 mL," tell the caregiver to give "5 mL," not "one teaspoon." This also helps remind them to use a measuring device and not a household teaspoon. Write a zero preceding decimals (Burg & Bourret, 1994), but not after. Print or type if your handwriting is not legible (Burg & Bourret, 1994). Order the exact amount needed. If more is given, the caregiver may be tempted to use more than is needed, or use the remainder for another sick child.
8. You may write the reason for the antibiotic on the prescription. For example: "for ear infection" (J.M. Shalf, Personal Communication, July 15, 1996).
9. An example of a written prescription:
   Amoxicillin susp 125 mg/5 cc
   150 cc
   5 cc PO t.i.d. × 10 days for ear infection
   No refills
10. If medication needs to be sent to **school** or **day care**, write on prescription for two bottles and have the pharmacist split the amounts according to the number of days needed. Some school systems require a special form that includes the name of the medication, dosage, and time and duration to be given.
11. **New schedules** are frequently introduced. Review the literature on the proposed change and/or consult with collaborating physicians and/or pharmacists for efficacy or side effects of proposed changes (Bauchner, Adams, Barnett, & Klein, 1996; Chamberlain, Boenning, Waisman, Ochsenschlanger, & Klein, 1994; Goldfarb & Medendorp, 1994; Johnson, Schuh, Koren, & Jaffe, 1996; Rowe & Klassen, 1996). For example, cefpodoxime proxetil can now be given once a day and amoxicillin/clavulanate potassium has been changed to twice a day.

---

Betcher, 1994). It must be applied to intact skin 1 to 2 hours before the procedure, depending upon the depth of penetration desired, with the maximum depth of approximately 5 mm being achieved at 2 hours (Farrington, 1993). Although numerous studies have shown that EMLA reduces pain associated with venipuncture, lumbar punctures, or intravenous insertion, the data on its use to reduce injection pain is scarce and conflicting. Three studies (Morris et al, 1994; Raveh et al, 1995; Taddio et al, 1994) support the ability of EMLA to reduce pain of injections. Only one of these studies (Taddio et al, 1994) involved children. In contrast, a Danish study found EMLA did not reduce pain in

MMR immunizations in older children (Hansen & Sorensen, 1993). The provider needs to monitor future research developments to determine the advisability of EMLA use for immunizations in children.

Several studies have explored the use of diversionary methods in a clinical setting and two studies found that having children blow was the easiest and most effective (French, Painter, & Coury, 1994; Geldmaker, 1994). Children can blow against a mobile, a pinwheel, or imaginary birthday candles. For older children, it is best to explain that they will experience pain for a short time, but the pain will end. Be sensitive to their psychological level; they may respond at a more

## TABLE 12–5. PRACTICAL TIPS: TEACHING

1. Always **explain** the name of the medication (brand and generic), the class of drug, what it is for, why it was cho-sen, and any side effects (Martin, 1992; Wink, 1991). This will help to increase compliance by increasing the care-giver's or patient's understanding.
2. If ordering an **extended-release** tablet or capsule, teach the caregiver or the patient the terms associated with these drugs: CR (controlled-release or continuous-release), Dur(duration), LA(long-acting), SA(sustained-action), SR(sustained-release or slow-release), TD(time-delay), XR(extended-release), EC(enteric-coated), and En-tab or Entab (enteric tablet) (Pagliaro, 1995, p. 19). Reinforce the idea of **not crushing or opening** these tablets or cap-sules (Pagliaro, 1995; Sagraves, 1995).
3. Give **verbal and written** instructions reinforcing any special instructions about medications, eg, decreasing doses of prednisone or when to stop a medication if different from the usual time period.
4. Reinforce the idea of **proper storage**. Most antibiotics need refrigeration, and caregivers and patients need to be reminded of this. If traveling, order a medication that does not need to be refrigerated, such as cefixime, cefurox-ime axetil, or trimethoprim-sulfamethoxazole or chewable if available (see Drug Tables 102.2, 102.3 & 102.10).
6. Have the caregivers or patient read back to you any instructions you have given them. By having them read the in-structions back to you, you screen for understanding and reading level. Having written instructions is helpful, be-cause listening and retention are decreased when someone is distracted by worry about a sick child, or a crying baby or other children in the room. The health care provider can give preprinted instructions with appropriate blanks to be filled in for various situations or alternate forms of instruction, such as audio- or videotape, if the pa-tient's or the caregiver's vision and/or reading is not optimal. Copies of written instructions can be placed in the chart to facilitate communication. Check for understanding of key information by stressing important items.

## TABLE 12–6. PRACTICAL TIPS: SAFETY ISSUES

1. Reinforce using a **measuring device** for giving medications, not the household teaspoon (Martin, 1992), which can hold anywhere from 2.5 to 9.7 cc (Pagliaro, 1995).
2. Advise patients to drink plenty of **fluids** when taking pills (Martin, 1992) and to only take one pill at a time if more than one is ordered (Pagliaro, 1995).
3. **Avoid liquid oil formulations** such as **castor oil or mineral oil** in infants/toddlers due to the risk of aspiration and lipid pneumonia (Pagliaro, 1995).
4. Aminoglycoside eardrops should **not** be instilled if there is a risk of eardrum perforation; hearing loss or deaf-ness can occur. (Livingstone & Livingstone, 1989b). Auralgon eardrops are also contraindicated if the eardrum is perforated (Barone, 1996) (see Drug Table 402-2).
5. Beware of "compounding pharmacists," those who make their own drugs or change already manufactured ones (Perrin, 1996).
6. Granting refills on a prescription depends upon many factors. If one would like to see a patient back, it is best not to write prescriptions with refills. Certain medications should never have refills (controlled substances and usually antibiotics). It is permissible to order refills on medicines that might be necessary in an emergency situation, for example, albuterol for asthmatics. It is also a good idea not to order refills until you know the patient better.
7. Caregivers should understand **drops** versus dropperfuls. Several medications for neonates and infants are or-dered in drops, and overdoses have occurred because the caregiver mistakenly gave dropperfuls instead of drops (Rudy, 1992). Many caregivers also use one dropper, for example, one that comes with acetaminophen drops, for different medications. They need to be taught to use only the dropper that comes with the medication. It is a good idea to have samples of different medication droppers available so parents can be shown the one that belongs with the medication ordered (Pagliaro, 1995).
8. **Reinforce follow-up**. Caregivers should know to call or return to the clinic if there is no improvement in 48 h with antibiotics, or whenever deemed necessary. Caregivers may tend to give more of a medication if they see no improvement. You as the health care provider also need to see how the child is reacting to the medication. A phone call from you in a few days can be very helpful.

*continues on next page*

**TABLE 12–6.** *continued*

9. **Always explain allergic symptoms and the possibility of an allergic reaction with any medication ordered.** Allergic symptoms in children can include rash, hives, vomiting, diarrhea, anaphylaxis, or any other unusual symptoms (Cochran, 1991). Neomycin is a common allergen and is contained in Cortisporin otic suspension and Neosporin (see Drug Tables 402.1 & 805). Caregivers may not realize that a certain medication is in a certain class. They may only know the brand name. That is why you should state the brand name as well as the class when giving a prescription. For example, "I'm ordering amoxicillin, which is a penicillin. Is your child allergic to penicillin?" **Always ask more than once about allergies.** Caregivers may forget in their anxiety about their child.

10. **Allergies should be displayed in a prominent place in the chart.**

11. Check with African-American patients about their ability to take **acetaminophen, aspirin**, or **sulfa**. Glucose-6-phosphate dehydrogenase (G6PD) deficient patients will have a hemolytic anemic reaction if given these drugs (Barone, 1996) (see Drug Tables 301, 307, 102.9, 102.10).

12. **Be explicit in charting** any medications given, including dosage, frequency, and duration. Ask at each visit the current medications, along with the dose given, including OTCs.

13. **Storage** of medications at home should be in a safe place, not in the bathroom, but in a locked box on a high shelf. Medication in the refrigerator should be on a high shelf, and in a box that is difficult to open. When visiting relatives, caregivers should remind them to keep their medications out of the reach of children, especially purses, where many people keep medicines. Most medications for the elderly do not have child-resistant packaging (Rodgers, 1996).

14. Reinforce **not sharing** medications or putting them in other unlabeled containers, especially when sending a child to camp (Lishner & Busch, 1994).

15. Have **Syrup of Ipecac** at home in case of accidental poisoning. Have the **poison control phone number** handy and always call poison control before giving the Ipecac.

16. Advise caregivers to check labels for **additives** such as alcohol, sugars, sodium (Pagliaro, 1995), food dyes, and preservatives (Sagraves, 1995).

17. Use the **clinical rule of thumb** to double-check doses chosen. The average 12-year-old gets 100% of the adult dose, a 6-year-old gets approximately one half of the adult dose, and a 2–3-year-old gets approximately one quarter of the adult dose. If these approximations do not match calculated doses, check your calculations.

---

immature level than their chronological age. An analgesic can be given for the pain if necessary. The reader is referred to the literature for more detailed information about pain.

## SUMMARY

Prescribing and administering medications to children can be challenging but not insurmountable. Important information as well as practical guidelines have been highlighted in this chapter. The provider should consult Chapter 5 for further considerations helpful in working with families. In addition issues for pediatric rehabilitation are addressed in Chapter 14.

The author would like to express her thanks to the following for their input to this chapter. Jerome M. Shalf, MD, Christie Lessels, RN, MS, CFNP, David Ballowe, and Janet Younger, Ph.D., CPNP, for her review of an earlier draft of this manuscript.

## REFERENCES

American Academy of Pediatrics Committe on Drugs (1978). Unapproved uses of approved drugs: The physician, the packaging insert, and the PDR. *Pediatrics,* 62 (2), 262–264.

Barnett, E. D., Teele, D. W., Klein, J. O., Cabral, H. J., & Kharasch, S. J. (1997). Comparison of ceftriaxone and trimethoprim-sulfamethoxazole (sulfamethoxozole) for acute otitis media. *Pediatrics* 99(1):23–28.

Barone, M. A., (Ed). (1996). *The Harriet Lane handbook* (14th ed.). (pp. 475, 487, 499–504, 600, 641). St. Louis: Mosby.

Bauchner, H., Adams, W., Barnett, E., & Klein, J. (1996). Therapy for acute otitis media. *Archives of Pediatric and Adolescent Medicine, 150,* 396–399.

Behrman, R. E., & Vaughan, V. C. (1987). *Nelson's textbook of pediatrics* (13th ed.) (pp. 231–237). Philadelphia: WB Saunders. Cited in Wink (1991).

Bindler, R. M., & Howry, L. B. (1991). *Pediatric drugs and nursing implications* (pp. 1–45). Norwalk, CT: Appleton & Lange.

Blumor, J. L., & Reed, M. D. (1992). Principles of neonatal pharmacology. In S. J. Yaffe & J. V. Aranda (Eds.), *Pediatric pharmacology: Therapeutic principles in practice* (2nd ed.) (pp. 164–177). Philadelphia: W. B. Saunders.

Buck, G. (1992). Fluoroquinolone antibiotics. *Pediatric Nursing, 18,* 168, 173.

Burg, F. D., & Bourrett, J. A. (1994). *Current pediatric drugs.* Philadelphia: W. B. Saunders.

Cetta, F., Lambert, G. H., & Ros, S. P. (1991). Newborn chemical exposure from over-the-counter skin care products. *Clinical Pediatrics, 30,* 286–289.

Chamberlain, J. M., Boenning, D. A., Waisman, Y., Ochsenschlager, D. W., & Klein, B. L. (1994, November). Single-dose ceftriaxone versus 10 days of cefaclor for otitis media. *Clinical Pediatrics,* 642–646.

Chater, R. W. (1993). Pediatric dosing: Tips for tots. *American Pharmacy, NS33,* 55–56.

Cochran, F. B. (1991). Hypersensitivity to carbamazepine mimicking infection. *Clinical Pediatrics, 30,* 95–96.

Dixon, S. D. (1992). Two years: Learning the rules—Language and cognition. In S. D. Dixon & M. T. Stein, *Encounters with children: Pediatric behavior and development* (p. 248). St. Louis: Mosby–Year Book.

Farrington, E. (1993). Lidocaine 2.5%/prilocaine 2.5% EMLA cream. *Pediatric Nursing, 19,* 484–486, 488.

French, G. M., Painter, E. C., & Coury, D. L. (1994). Blowing away shot pain, a technique for pain management during immunization. *Pediatrics 93* (3), 384–388.

Geldmaker, B. (1994). *Pediatric Pain Interviews* (Video). Richmond, Virginia Commonwealth University.

Gennrich, J. L. & Chan, P. D. (1996). *Pediatric Drug Reference* (pp. 12, 23, 33, 38, 40, 53, 55, 62). Fountain Valley, CA: Current Clinical Strategies Publishing.

Ghadially, R., & Shear, N. H. (1992). Topical therapy and percutaneous absorption. In S. J. Yaffe & J. V. Aranda (Eds.), *Pediatric pharmacology: Therapeutic principles in practice* (2nd ed.) (pp. 72–77). Philadelphia: W. B. Saunders.

Goldfarb, J., & Medendorp, S. (1994, November). New therapies for otitis media. *Clinical Pediatrics,* 647–648.

Goode, I. A. & Betcher, D. L. (1994). EMLA. *Journal of Pediatric Oncology Nursing 11,* 38–41.

Green, S. M. & Rothrock, S. G. (1993). Single-dose intramuscular ceftriaxone for acute otitis media in children. *Pediatrics, 91* (1), 23–30.

Green, T. P., & Mirkin, B. L. (1984). *Clinical pharmacokinetics: Pediatric considerations.* In L. Z. Benet, N. Massoud, & J. G. Gambertoglio, (Eds.), *Pharmacokinetic basis for drug treatment* (pp. 269–282). New York: Raven Press. Cited in Kauffman (1992).

Handbook of pediatric drug therapy. (1990). Springhouse, PA: Springhouse (pp. 1–7).

Hansen, B. W., & Sorensen, P. V. (1993). The EMLA cream versus placebo in MMR vaccination of older children in general practice. *Ugeskr Laeger,* 155(29):2263–2265.

Hein, K. (1992). Drug therapeutics in the adolescent. In S. J. Yaffe & J. V. Aranda (Eds.), *Pediatric pharmacology: Therapeutic principles in practice* (2nd ed.) (pp. 220–233). Philadelphia: W. B. Saunders.

Johnson, D. W., Schuh, S., Koren, G., & Jaffe, D. M. (1996). Outpatient treatment of croup with nebulized dexamethasone. *Archives of Pediatric and Adolescent Medicine, 150,* 349–355.

Karjoo, M., & Kane, R. (1995). Omeprazole treatment of children with peptic esophagitis refractory to ranitidine therapy. *Archives of Pediatric and Adolescent Medicine, 149,* 267–271.

Kauffman, R. E. (1992). Drug therapeutics in the infant and child. In S. J. Yaffe & J. V. Aranda (Eds.), *Pediatric pharmacology: Therapeutic principles in practice* (2nd ed.) (pp. 212–219). Philadelphia: W. B. Saunders.

Kearns, G. L., & Reed, M. D. (1989). Clinical pharmacokinetics in infants and children: A reappraisal. *Clinical Pharmacokinetics, 17,* 29–67. Cited in Kauffman (1992).

Khunti, K. (1996, February). Issues in adolescent asthma: Compliance. *Maternal and Child Health,* 36–38.

Khurana, C. M. (1996). A multicenter, randomized, open label comparison of azithromycin and amoxicillin/clavulanate in acute otitis media among children attending day care or school. *Pediatric Infectious Disease Journal, 15* (9 suppl), S24–S29.

Kiebler, B., & Mowry, J. B. (1994). Acetaminophen's potential for morbidity and mortality. *Pediatric Nursing, 20,* 491–494.

Lehne, R. A., Moore, L. A., Crosby, L. J., & Hamilton, D. B. (1990). *Pharmacology for nursing care* (pp. 29–84). Philadelphia: W. B. Saunders. Cited in Wink (1991).

Lishner, K., & Busch, K. (1994). Safe delivery of medications to children in summer camps. *Pediatric Nursing, 20,* 249–253.

Livingstone, C., & Livingstone, D. (1989). Drug delivery. Part 6: Formulations for the eye, nose, and ear. *The Pharmaceutical Journal, 242,* 688–689. Cited in Pagliaro, A. M. (1995).

Lucey, J. F. (1992). Forward to the second edition. In S. J. Yaffe & J. V. Aranda (Eds.), *Pediatric pharmacology: Therapeutic principles in practice* (2nd ed). Philadelphia: W. B. Saunders.

Lumbiagannon, P., Pengsaa, K., & Sookpranee, T. (1991). Ciprofloxacin in neonates and its possible adverse effect on teeth. *Pediatric Infectious Disease Journal, 10*, 619–620. Cited in Buck (1992).

Martin, S. (1992). Catering to pediatric patients. *American Pharmacy, NS32*, 47–50.

Maswoswe, J. J., Egbunike, I., Stewart, K. R., et al. (1994). Suspected fatal diphenhydramine toxicity by application to the skin of an infant with varicella. *Hospital Pharmacy, 29*, 26, 28–30, 53. Cited in Pagliaro (1995).

McCaffery, M., & Beebe, A. (1989). *Pain: Clinical manual for nursing practice* (pp. 133, 143, 146, 155, 173, 176, 177, 213). St. Louis: C. V. Mosby.

Merenstein, G. B., & Gardner, S. L. (1989). Handbook of neonatal intensive care (2nd ed.) (pp. 141–159). St. Louis: C. V. Mosby. Cited in Wink (1991).

Morris, K. P., Hughes, C., Hardy, S. P., Matthews, J. N., & Coulthard, M. G. (1994). Pain after subcutaneous injection of recombinant human erythropoietin: does Emla cream help? *Nephrology Dialysis and Transplant, 9*(9):1299–1301.

Nahata, M. C. (1993, August). Therapeutic considerations in pediatric patients. *Pharmacy and Therapeutics*, 752–762.

Niederhauser, V. P. (1997). Prescribing for children: Issues in pediatric pharmacology. *Nurse Practitioner, 22* (3), 16–30.

Pagliaro, A. M. (1995). Administering drugs to infants, children, and adolescents. In L. A. Pagliaro & A. M. Pagliaro (Eds.), Problems in pediatric drug therapy (3rd ed.) (pp. 3–101). Hamilton, IL: Drug Intelligence Publications.

Pederson, S., & Moller-Petersen, J. (1984). Erratic absorption of a slow-release theophylline sprinkle product. *Pediatrics, 74*, 534–538. Cited in Kauffman (1992).

Perrin, J. H. (1996). Pediatrician and compounding pharmacist: A dangerous liaison. *Archives of Pediatric and Adolescent Medicine, 150*, 224–226.

Phelps, D. L. (1993). Retinopathy of prematurity. *Pediatric Clinics of North America, 40*, 705–714.

*Physician's Desk Reference* (50th ed.) (1997). (pp. 406–412, 747–751, 1067–1070, 1443–1445, 1476–1472, 1513–1516, 1557, 2043–2046, 2112–2115, 2257, 2258, 2340–2342, 2480, 2484). Montvale, N.J.: Medical Economics.

Raveh, T., Weinberg, A., Sibirsky, O., et al. (1995). Efficacy of the topical anesthetic cream, EMLA, in alleviating both needle insertion and injection pain. *Annals of Plastic Surgery, 35*(6), 576–579.

Reed, M. D., & Besunder, J. B. (1989, October). Developmental pharmacology: Ontogenic basis of drug disposition. *Pediatric Clinics of North America, 36*, 1053–1074. Cited in Wink (1991).

Rodgers, G. B. (1996). The safety effects of child-resistant packaging for oral prescription drugs. *JAMA, 275*, 1661–1665.

Rogers, R. J., Kalisker, A., Weiner, M. B., & Szafler, S. (1985). Inconsistent absorption from a sustained-release theophylline preparation during continuous therapy in asthmatic children. *Journal of Pediatrics, 106*, 496–501. Cited in Kauffman (1992).

Rowe, P. C., & Klassen, T. P. (1996). Corticosteroids for croup. *Archives of Pediatric and Adolescent Medicine, 150*, 344–346.

Rudy, C. (1992). A drop or a dropper: The risk of overdose. *Journal of Pediatric Health Care, 6*, 40, 51–52.

Sagraves, R. (1995, November/December). Pediatric dosing information for health care providers. *Journal of Pediatric Health Care*, 272–277.

Schichor, A., Bernstein, B., Weinerman, H., Fitzgerald, J., Yordan, E., & Schechter, N. (1994). Lidocaine as a diluent for ceftriaxone in the treatment of gonorrhea. *Archives of Pediatric and Adolescent Medicine, 148*, 72–75.

Selekman, J. (1993). Health promotion of the school-age child and family. In D. L. Wong, *Whaley & Wong's essentials of pediatric nursing* (4th ed.) (p. 425). St. Louis: C. V. Mosby.

Simon, R. E. (1996). Ibuprofen suspension: Pediatric antipyretic. *Pediatric Nursing, 22*, 118–120.

Skaer, T. L. (1991). Dosing considerations in the pediatric patient. *Clinical Therapeutics, 13*, 526–544.

Smith, A. L. (1992). Chloramphenicol. In S. J. Yaffe & J. V. Aranda (Eds.), *Pediatric pharmacology: Therapeutic principles in practice* (2nd ed.) (pp. 276–286). Philadelphia: W. B. Saunders.

Taddio, A., Nulman, I., Goldbach, M., Ipp, M., & Koren, G. J. (1994). Use of lidocaine-prilocaine cream for vaccination pain in infants. *Journal of Pediatrics 124*(4):643–648.

Todd, J. K. (1995). Antimicrobial therapy of pediatric infections. In W. W. Hay, Jr., J. R. Groothuis, A. R. Hayward, & M. J. Levin (Eds.), *Current pediatric diagnosis and treatment* (12th ed.) (pp. 1012–1016). Norwalk, CT: Appleton & Lange.

Varsano, I., Volvitz, B., Horev, Z., Robinson, J., Laks, Y., Rosenbaum, I., Cohen, A., Eilam, N., Jaber, L., Fuchs, C., & Amir, J. (1997). Intramuscular ceftriaxone compared with oral amoxicillin-clavulante for treatment of acute otitis media in children. *European Journal of Pediatrics 156*(11), 858–863.

Wilson, J. T., Kearns, G. L., Murphy, D., and Yaffe, S. J. (1994). Paediatric Labeling Requirements. *Clinical Pharmacokinetics, 26,* 308–325.

Wink, D. M. (1991). Giving infants and children drugs: Precision + caution = safety. *Maternal Child Nursing, 16,* 317–321.

Wong, D. L. (1993a). Health promotion of the toddler and family. In D. L. Wong, *Whaley & Wong's essentials of pediatric nursing* (4th ed.) (pp. 345, 347). St. Louis: C. V. Mosby.

Wong, D. L. (1993b). Health promotion of the preschooler and family. In D. L. Wong, *Whaley & Wong's essentials of pediatric nursing* (4th ed.) (p. 369). St. Louis: C. V. Mosby.

Yaffe, S. J., & Aranda, J. V. (1992). Introduction and historical perspective. In S. J. Yaffe & J. V. Aranda (Eds.), *Pediatric pharmacology: Therapeutic principles in practice* (2nd ed.) (pp. 3–9). Philadelphia: W. B. Saunders.

# 13

## GERIATRIC ISSUES

*Geneva Briggs*

Much of current U.S. healthcare practice is concerned with the needs of the older adult. As the vanguard of the "baby boomer" generation now advances from middle into old age, that demographic bulge is going to require even more attention and resources. At this time, the elderly—those over 65 years of age—consume 35% of prescription and 40% of nonprescription medications (Piraino, 1995). Age-related changes, the increased number of chronic diseases, and health care professionals' varying levels of knowledge and skill contribute to some of the significant issues in geriatric pharmacotherapy: adverse drug events, excessive and inappropriate medications, and nonadherence (Seppala & Sourander, 1995; Willcox, Himmelstein, & Woolhandler, 1994). The goals of pharmacotherapy for the elderly client should include obtaining maximal benefit with minimal harm.

The following discusses age-related changes in medication handling and response. Most of the research on this subject has been conducted in the young-old (55–65 years) and not the middle-old (65–85) or the old-old (>85). Because no one ages at the same rate, it is best to individualize your approach with each patient.

## PHARMACOKINETIC CHANGES WITH AGING

The four phases of pharmacokinetics are absorption, distribution, metabolism, and excretion. The effects of aging on those phases are summarized in Table 13–1. In brief, although there are changes in drug absorption with aging, none of these are clinically significant or affect how medications are given to the elderly (Schenker & Bay, 1994). Conditions common to the elderly—achlorhydria, malabsorption, constipation, or diarrhea—can reduce drug absorption (Lee, 1996). Drug distribution is altered in the elderly because of changes in body composition. These changes include a decrease in lean body mass, increased body fat, and decreased total body water (Piraino, 1995). The increase in body fat can lead to excess storage of fat-soluble drugs, such as diazepam, a long-acting benzodiazepine. Water-soluble drugs, such as aminoglycosides and alcohol, can reach higher serum levels in the elderly due to reduced total body water (Schenker & Bay, 1994).

With aging there can be a decline in plasma albumin levels (Cooper & Gardner, 1989). Since many drugs are bound to serum albumin, this change can mean an increase in unbound drug in the system and, potentially, an increase in adverse effects (Lee, 1996). Alterations in protein binding affect the initial dose used, but not necessarily the maintenance dose because clearance of a drug from the body is also affected by the free fraction of the drug (Wallace & Verbeeck, 1987). Steady-state effects of maintenance regimens are not altered by protein-binding changes alone. Changes in protein binding are important for drugs that are highly bound to albumin, such as phenytoin and salicylates.

## TABLE 13–1. PHARMACOKINETIC PHASES AND CHANGES WITH AGING

| Pharmacokinetic Parameter | Physiologic Change with Aging |
|---|---|
| Absorption | Increased gastric pH |
| | Increased GI transit time |
| | Decreased blood flow to muscles |
| | Decreased skin hydration |
| | Increase in keratinized cells |
| Distribution | Decreased lean body mass |
| | Decreased total body water |
| | Increased total body fat |
| | Decreased albumin levels |
| Renal elimination | Decreased glomerular filtration rate |
| | Decreased secretion |
| Metabolism | Decreased liver mass and volume |
| | Decreased liver blood flow |
| | Diminished enzyme activity |

*Sources: Katzung (1992), Piraino (1995), and Stein (1994).*

With aging there is a decrease in liver mass, volume, and blood flow (Vestal et al, 1975; Woodhouse & Wynne, 1988). These declines are important because the liver is a major route of drug elimination. Liver metabolic activity declines 1% per year after the age of 40 (Vestal et al, 1975). Liver metabolism can be divided into two broad phases: oxidative (phase I) and conjugative (phase II). Phase I metabolism is impaired the most in the elderly (Schenker & Bay, 1994). A group of drugs that undergo significant phase I metabolism are the long-acting benzodiazepines, such as diazepam, flurazepam, and chlordiazepoxide. The elimination half-life of the long-acting benzodiazepines is significantly prolonged in the elderly versus a younger population. The half-life of diazepam in an elderly person is 82 h versus 37 h in a younger person (Ray, Griffen, & Downey, 1989). Aging does not appear to affect phase II metabolism.

Kidney function declines in two thirds of the population at a rate of 1% per year beginning in the fourth to fifth decade of life (Lindeman, 1992). This decline affects pharmacotherapy significantly because the kidney is also a major organ for drug elimination. The decreased glomerular filtration rate leads to the prolongation of the half-life of renally eliminated drugs and can lead to accumulation of these drugs within the body.

Most dosage adjustments in the elderly are due to decreases in renal function (Lindeman, 1992).

Age-related changes in renal function are not necessarily reflected in an increase in serum creatinine because of the concurrent decrease in muscle mass (Smythe, Hoffman, Kizy, & Smuchowski, 1994). Renal function can be estimated using numerous equations, some of which are more accurate than others. Although not necessarily the most accurate, the Cockcroft-Gault equation is the most commonly used because it is easy to calculate (Cockcroft & Gault, 1976; Smythe et al, 1994):

$$CrCl\ (mL/min) = \frac{(140 - age)(wt)}{72 \times (SCr)} \times 0.85\ (for\ women)$$

CrCl = creatinine clearance
SCr = serum creatinine in mg/dL
wt = kgs

## PHARMACODYNAMIC CHANGES WITH AGING

Pharmacodynamics is the study of what a drug does to the body. When a change in body response occurs with a drug, finding the cause is difficult and may include such reasons as: altered pharmacokinetics, diminished homeostatic responses, or true changes in receptor interaction (Katzung, 1992). The elderly are known to have a decreased response to beta-adrenergic receptor stimulators and blockers (Vestal, Wood, & Shand, 1979). Whether this change is due to aging, disease, or both is unknown, and this change is probably not clinically significant. Studies have also supported the commonly held belief that the elderly have an increased sensitivity to benzodiazepines, narcotic analgesics, warfarin, metoclopramide, and alcohol even when pharmacokinetic changes are taken into account (Katzung, 1992).

## ALTERATIONS IN HOMEOSTATIC MECHANISMS THAT AFFECT MEDICATIONS

With aging, homeostatic mechanism changes alter an elderly patient's response to medications. One well-described change is a decrease in baroreceptor sensitivity (Ray, Griffen, Shaffner, Bargh, & Melton, 1987). This can cause orthostatic changes alone, and is compounded by medications that lower blood pressure, such as antihypertensives, antipsychotics, and levodopa. Orthostatic hypotension can result in falls and subsequent hip fractures and head injuries.

The elderly are also sensitive to the anticholinergic effects of many medications (Sunderland et al, 1987). With aging, a cholinergic deficit in the brain may occur that is thought to account for the benign forgetfulness the elderly may experience (Sunderland et al, 1987). The primary medication classes with anticholinergic properties are tricyclic antidepressants, antipsychotics, and antihistamines. Beyond the usual adverse effects of dry mouth, constipation, and urinary retention, these medications can cause confusion in the elderly (Sunderland et al, 1987). Patients with dementia are especially prone to the adverse effects of such drugs.

The use of flurazepam, diazepam, chlordiazepoxide, amitriptyline, doxepin, imipramine, thioridazine, or haloperidol significantly increases an older person's risk of having a hip fracture or an automobile accident (Ray et al, 1987; Ray et al, 1989). The reason for this increased risk is not known, but it may be due to alterations in pharmacokinetics (benzodiazepines), changes in homeostatic mechanisms (tricyclic antidepressants and antipsychotics), or changes in pharmacodynamics that have not been identified.

## MEDICATION ISSUES

### POLYPHARMACY

The elderly take more prescription and nonprescription medications than the average population (Lee, 1996). Studies indicate the elderly take a range of 2.5–5.3 prescription and 0–4 over-the-counter medications daily (Baum, Kennedy, & Forbes, 1984; Nolan & O'Malley, 1988). Because of the complexity of medication regimens, concerns about compliance, and costs of medications, try to streamline your patient's medication regimen. Reasons to target the regimens of the elderly include the high rate of medication use; changes in pharmacokinetics, pharmacodynamics, and homeostatic mechanisms; the high rate of adverse drug events in this age group; and the often limited incomes of the elderly (Colley & Lucas, 1993).

## ADVERSE DRUG EVENTS

The over-65 population is prone to adverse drug events because of alterations in the body's handling of medications and the number of medications they take, but probably not age itself (Atkin & Shenfield, 1995). It is estimated that 10–31% of hospital admissions and 7% of hospital readmissions among the elderly are due to adverse drug events (Beard, 1992; Bero, Lipton, and Bird, 1991). An adverse event is thought to occur during 5–10% of all hospital admissions irrespective of a patient's age (Col, Fanale, & Kronholn 1990). In addition, the elderly do not tolerate or recover from adverse events as well as younger people (Atkin & Shenfield, 1995). Diseases can present atypically in the elderly and confusion, falls, or incontinence may actually be the result of an adverse drug event. Be extra vigilant when starting an elderly person on a new medication, both to identify new problems that may occur and to ensure new problems are not dismissed by the patient or practitioner as simply part of the aging process.

## ADHERENCE

Adherence is a problem in all age groups, not just the elderly. Fifty percent of all patients are estimated to be nonadherent with medications (Col et al, 1990). The elderly are especially at risk since (Salzman, 1995):

- They take increased numbers of medications.
- They may have acquired disabilities that make taking or remembering medications difficult (stroke, arthritic changes, dementia).
- They may have limited incomes to pay for costly medications.
- They possibly may be illiterate or have trouble seeing to read.

Health care providers should be particularly alert for adherence problems. Some strategies for improving adherence are medication and disease education, written information to supplement verbal education, and devices such as pillboxes or non-child-resistant tops. Be conscious of patients' hearing deficits that can impair their understanding of verbal instructions.

## TOXICITY/POISONINGS

Accidental poisoning in the elderly accounted for 25% of calls to a state poison control center in one study (Kroner, Scott, Waring, & Zanga, 1993). The elderly are more likely to require hospitalization and to die from poisonings. The most frequently implicated drugs in fatal poisonings in the elderly are analgesics, cardiovascular medications, theophylline, and antidepressants (Haselberger & Kroner, 1995). Remind patients about dosages, proper storage, and what to do when doses are missed. Advise them to read the label each time and take medications in a well-lit area. This simple recommendation will prevent them from accidentally taking the wrong medication or ingesting a nonmedicinal substance. For patients with visual impairment, strategies such as specific medication bottle placement for easier and safer use are necessary. All medications should be kept out of reach of children *and* confused adults.

## STEPS TO HEALTHY PRESCRIBING

To summarize all the issues highlighted in this chapter, the following are suggested steps for healthy prescribing of medications for the elderly (Beers & Ouslander, 1989; Piraino, 1995; Stein, 1994). These tips are not only helpful for the elderly, but make good sense for any patient.

1. Take a careful medication history (prescription, over-the-counter, homeopathic, etc.).

2. Have patients bring all items they regularly take to visits for review.

3. Prescribe only for a specific and rational indication.

4. Consider the patient's overall condition, including mental status, quality of life, and nutritional status, before prescribing.

5. Define the goal of therapy.

6. Begin with lowest available dose and increase doses slowly.

7. Use the fewest drugs and simplest regimen possible.

8. Talk with the patient and/or caregivers about the treatment plan.

## TABLE 13–2.  MEDICATIONS TO AVOID OR USE WITH CAUTION IN THE ELDERLY

**Avoid because of excessive side effects**
Amitriptyline (Elavil)
Atropine
Barbiturates
Belladonna alkaloids
Carisoprodol (Soma)
Chlordiazepoxide (Librium)
Chlorpropamide (Diabinese)
Chlorzoxazone (Paraflex)
Clidinium
Cyclobenzaprine (Flexeril)
Diazepam (Valium)
Dicyclomine (Bentyl)
Diphenhydramine (Benadryl)
Doxepin (Sinequan)
Flurazepam (Dalmane)
Hyoscamine (Levsin)
Indomethacin (Indocin)
Meperidine
Meprobamate (Miltown, Equanil)
Metaxalone (Skelaxin)
Methyldopa
Methocarbamol (Robaxin)
Oxybutynin (Ditropan)
Pentazocine (Talwin)
Phenylbutazone
Propantheline (Pro-Banthine)
Propoxyphene (Darvon)
Propranolol
Reserpine
Ticlopidine (Ticlid)
Trimethobenzamide (Tigan)

**Avoid because of questionable efficacy**
Dipyridamole (Persantine)
Ergoloid mesylate (Hydergine)
Isoxsuprine (Vasodilan)

**Use with caution but at appropriate geriatric doses**
Alprazolam (Xanax)
Cimetidine (Tagamet)
Digoxin
Haloperidol (Haldol)
Hydrochlorothiazide
Lorazepam (Ativan)
Ranitidine (Zantac)
Oxazepam (Serax)
Temazepam (Restoril)
Thioridazine (Mellaril)
Triazolam (Halcion)

*Sources: Beers (1997), Beers et al (1991), Lee (1996), and Piraino (1995).*

9. Reinforce verbal education with written materials (at the appropriate educational level and in large type).

10. Consider the cost of medications to patients.

11. Periodically review and "weed out" outdated or no longer needed medications.

12. Have the patient maintain a medication list to show to all health care providers.

13. Alert the patient and caregivers about potential adverse effects and have them monitor for these.

14. Maintain a high index of suspicion regarding adverse events and drug interactions.

15. Exercise caution with newly marketed medications; the effects in the elderly may not be known.

16. Avoid problem medications or use with extreme caution (see Table 13-2).

## REFERENCES

Atkin, P. A., & Shenfield, G. M. (1995). Medication-related adverse reactions and the elderly: A literature review. *Adverse Drug Reactions and Toxicology Reviews, 14,* 175–191.

Baum, C., Kennedy, D. L., & Forbes, M. B. (1984). Drug use in the United States in 1981. *JAMA, 241,* 1293–1295.

Beard, K. (1992). Adverse reactions as a cause of hospital admission in the aged. *Drugs and Aging, 2,* 356–367.

Beers, M. H. (1997). Explicit criteria for determining potentially inappropriate medication use by the elderly. An update. *Archives of Internal Medicine, 157,* 1531–1536.

Beers, M. H., & Ouslander, J. G. (1989). Risk factors in geriatric drug prescribing. A practical guide to avoiding problems. *Drugs, 37,* 105–112.

Beers, M. H., Ouslander, J. G., Rollingher, I., Reuben, D. B., Brooks, J., & Beck, J. C. (1991). Explicit criteria for determining inappropriate medication use in nursing home residents. *Archives of Internal Medicine, 151,* 1825–1832.

Bero, L. A., Lipton, H. L., & Bird, J. A. (1991). Characterization of geriatric drug-related hospital readmissions. *Medical Care, 29,* 989–1003.

Cockcroft, D. W., & Gault, M. H. (1976). Prediction of creatinine clearance from serum creatinine. *Nephron, 16,* 31–41.

Col, N., Fanale, J. E., & Kronholm, P. (1990). The role of medication noncompliance and adverse drug reactions in hospitalizations of the elderly. *Archives of Internal Medicine, 150,* 841–845.

Colley, C. A., & Lucas, L. M. (1993). Polypharmacy: The cure becomes the disease. *Journal of General Internal Medicine, 8,* 278–283.

Cooper, J. K., & Gardner, C. (1989). Effect of aging on serum albumin. *Journal of the American Geriatrics Society, 37,* 1039–1042.

Haselberger, M. B., & Kroner, B. A. (1995). Drug poisoning in older patients. Preventative and management strategies. *Drugs and Aging, 7,* 292–297.

Katzung, B. G. (1992). Special aspects of geriatric pharmacology. In B. G. Katzung (Ed.), *Basic and clinical pharmacology* (5th ed.). Norwalk, CT: Appleton & Lange.

Kroner, B. A., Scott, R. B., Waring, E. R., & Zanga, J. R. (1993). Poisoning in the elderly: Characterization of exposures reported to a poison control center. *Journal of the American Geriatrics Society, 41,* 842–846.

Lee, M. (1996). Drugs and the elderly: Do you know the risks? *American Journal of Nursing, 96,* 25–31.

Lindeman, R. D. (1992). Changes in renal function with aging: Implications for treatment. *Drugs and Aging, 2,* 423–431.

Nolan, L., & O'Malley, K. (1988). Prescribing for the elderly, II: Prescribing patterns: Differences due to age. *Journal of the American Geriatrics Society, 36,* 142–149.

Piraino, A. J. (1995, June 15). Managing medication in the elderly. *Hospital Practice,* 59–64.

Ray, W. A., Griffen, W. R., & Downey, W. (1989). Benzodiazepines of long and short half-life and the risk of hip fractures. *JAMA, 262,* 3303–3307.

Ray, W. A., Griffen, M. R., Schaffner, W., Bargh, D. K., & Melton, L. J. (1987). Psychotropic drug use and the risk of hip fracture. *New England Journal of Medicine, 316,* 363–369.

Salzman, C. (1995). Medication compliance in the elderly. *Journal of Clinical Psychiatry, 56* (Suppl. 1), 18–22.

Schenker, S., & Bay, M. (1994). Drug disposition and hepatotoxicity in the elderly. *Journal of Clinical Gastroenterology, 18,* 232–237.

Seppala, M., & Sourander, L. (1995). A practical guide to prescribing in nursing homes. Avoiding the pitfalls. *Drugs and Aging, 6,* 426–435.

Smythe, M., Hoffman, J., Kizy, K., & Smuchowski, C. (1994). Estimating creatinine clearance in elderly patients with low serum creatinine concentrations. *American Journal of Hospital Pharmacy, 51,* 198–204.

Stein, B. E. (1994). Avoiding drug reactions: Seven steps to writing safe prescriptions. *Geriatrics, 49,* 28–36.

Sunderland, T., Tariot, P. N., Cohen, R. M., Weingartner, H., Mueller, E. A., & Murphy, D. L. (1987). Anticholinergic sensitivity in patients with dementia of the Alzheimer type and age-matched controls: A dose-response study. *Archives of General Psychiatry, 44*, 418–426.

Vestal, R. E., Norris, A. H., Tobin, J. D., Cohen, B. H., Shock, N. W., & Andres, R. (1975). Antipyrine metabolism in man: Influence of age, alcohol, caffeine and smoking. *Clinical Pharmacology and Therapeutics, 18*, 425–432.

Vestal, R. E., Wood, A. J., & Shand, D. G. (1979). Reduced B-adrenoceptor sensitivity in the elderly. *Clinical Pharmacology and Therapeutics, 26*, 181–186.

Wallace, S. M., & Verbeeck, R. K. (1987). Plasma protein binding of drugs in the elderly. *Clinical Pharmacokinetics, 12*, 41–72.

Willcox, A. M., Himmelstein, D. U., & Woolhandler, S. (1994). Inappropriate drug prescribing for the community-dwelling elderly. *JAMA, 272*, 292–296.

Woodhouse, K. W., & Wynne, H. A. (1988). Age-related changes in liver size and hepatic blood flow: The influence on drug metabolism in the elderly. *Clinical Pharmacokinetics, 15*, 287–296.

# 14

# INDIVIDUALS WITH DISABILITIES

*Stephanie G. Metzger*

A holistic approach to pharmacotherapeutic interventions will ensure that individuals with disabilities are not treated only as a medical condition. Health care and health maintenance issues for individuals with disabilities provide a unique challenge and opportunity for primary health care providers. Although it is essential to have a firm understanding of each diagnosis, the physical, cognitive, and emotional considerations of the individual cannot be lost within the diagnosis. The conceptual issues that arise are globally explored in this chapter, and implications for the pediatric population are included. Specific health issues and common health problems for individuals with disabilities are also reviewed. Since the scope of pharmacotherapy management for this population is broad, this chapter focuses on the information needed by the generalist primary care provider. The provider must also be aware of the individual's functional abilities in order to make effective pharmacotherapy choices.

Legislative reform during the last decades has helped to equalize life opportunities for individuals with disabilities. The Americans with Disabilities Act (ADA) of 1990 encompasses civil rights protection so that no individual with a disability can be discriminated against in opportunities for employment, public services, public accommodations, or health care. Unfortunately, social prejudices and misconceptions continue to make life needlessly difficult for such individuals (Blumberg, 1992). Society

has not completely realized that challenged individuals strive for the same roles in life fulfillment, relationships, and meaningful employment as their nondisabled peers. The health care provider must be sensitive to each unique individual to obtain complete, accurate information on which to base pharmacotherapeutic options. All too often, the level of disability is determined not by physical or cognitive limitations but by the attitude of health care workers and architectural barriers within health care settings (Krotoski, Nosek, & Turk, 1996).

## PRIMARY HEALTH CARE ISSUES AND PHARMACOTHERAPY

The Chinese culture uses two symbols to illustrate crisis, one meaning danger and one meaning opportunity. An opportunity exists in the primary care setting to provide comprehensive care in an atmosphere of normalcy for individuals with disabilities. The primary care needed involves health maintenance and anticipatory guidance, managing common conditions associated with the disability and monitoring specialized pharmacotherapeutic treatment related to the disability. The control of health care delivery rests with each individual, and physiologic management is enhanced by integrating treatment into routine (Nosek, 1992). Individuals with disabilities, their families, and their support systems have the same developmental needs and tasks all of us have. Active participation in life experiences is critical to the attainment of developmental milestones.

Primary care providers generally do not initiate major drug therapies for individuals with disabilities. However, the provider is often responsible for monitoring the efficacy and side effects of any special pharmacotherapy and therefore should be aware of possible interactions with commonly prescribed medications. Effective primary care for individuals with disabilities mandates interdisciplinary collaboration. It is essential that each team member coordinate his or her specialties to address the unique needs of each individual with a disability. For the pediatric population, a family-centered approach that fosters communication and collaboration between the family and the team is stressed. This approach also is useful with the adult population.

The primary care provider may serve as a consultant to the individual with a disability to help with decision making. Recognize and appreciate that the individual or family members may be more knowledgeable than you are about specific issues relating to the disability. In an atmosphere of teamwork, this does not have to be an uncomfortable position for you. For example, asking an individual who has recurrent urinary tract infections to collaborate regarding self-catheterization will foster communication and empower the individual. The provider and the individual must synchronize to ensure complete and unbiased information about treatment, interventions, and outcomes.

To promote health in individuals with a disability, primary health care needs must be addressed. Pharmacotherapeutic treatment and routine health care management, coupled with medical and psychosocial anticipatory guidance, must not be fragmented by the health care delivery system. The provider should collaborate with subspecialists to address any unique complexities. Each disability, whether congenital or acquired, has its own trajectory and uses rehabilitation services at various points along the health care continuum. Rehabilitation, which is a custom-designed, educational problem-solving process, helps the individual minimize the effects of the disability and promotes functional outcomes. The primary care provider does not abdicate care but works with subspecialists to enhance organization and problem solving to achieve effective symptom management and to monitor treatment modalities. The provider may

not be an expert on the individual's disability but may be an expert on the individual (Blumberg, 1992). This allows you to give maximal support and advocacy, which is essential if the individual is not to be lost within a sea of subspecialists and pharmacotherapeutic interventions.

Primary health care for children with disabilities involves developmental assessment, health maintenance screening, and immunization procedures that may be neglected or overlooked. Caring for a child with a disability involves caring for the entire family. Families often may feel that they struggle for control over the care of their child and must be recognized as experts (Mausner, 1995). Families of disabled children have 24-hour daily responsibility for the coordination and care of their child; involvement with the health care team fluctuates. Since each family is unique, their perception of the disability is more important than the severity of the disability or the intensity of the caregiver demands. Whether a child has a congenital or acquired disability, family expectations are altered. All families grieve for the loss of their perfect child and make life adjustments that tend to characterize their disabled child as an asset or as a liability (Stallard & Dickinson, 1994). Families of disabled children question emancipation and the ability to master self-care skills. Cognitive abilities and the social implications of being disabled often leave children poorly prepared for adulthood and unable to make the transition to independence. Primary care providers may find themselves ill-prepared to help an adult attain independence, especially when community supports are sparse. Interdisciplinary collaboration with rehabilitation specialists is necessary from the onset of the disability to promote self-care activities and independence (Briskin & Liptak, 1995; O'Sullivan, Mahoney, & Robinson, 1992).

The age of onset of the disability shapes life experiences and self-definition. A progressive disability such as multiple sclerosis requires periodic self-concept adjustments as the symptoms determine functional abilities. A sudden disability means that stages of grief and acceptance will be influenced by developmental stage. For example, a 14-year-old person with a disability has a different adolescent experience than an adult who acquires a disability and has experienced adolescence as a nondisabled individual. Family and social support systems, financial resources, and access to the health care system combined with individual personality influence functional outcomes regardless of disability or the developmental age when the disability is acquired (Patterson & Blum, 1996).

# SPECIFIC ISSUES IN PHARMACOTHERAPY

## COGNITIVE ISSUES

The goal of the provider is for the individual to adhere to the pharmacotherapeutic plan. Deviation from the prescribed treatment plan may be intentional or not. Detailed assessment of cognitive and functional abilities may be necessary to determine reasons for noncompliance. Assessment of cognitive ability is essential since pharmacotherapeutic interventions require such abilities and strategies. For example, an individual who sustained a brain injury through trauma or cerebral vascular accident may recover functional self-care abilities but have long-term memory storage and retrieval deficits. Prescribing a medication with the least number of daily dosages may help ensure that the medication is taken.

Bear in mind that there is a clear distinction between traumatic and nontraumatic spinal cord injury. Traumatic spinal cord injury usually does not hinder cognitive abilities, unless accompanied by brain injury. Congenital spinal cord injury often has a central nervous system component and possibly associated decreased cognitive capabilities. An individual with a spinal cord injury may require either cognitive considerations or adaptations in packaging, or both. Individuals with impaired cognition, for whatever the reason, will benefit from the least number of medications possible, with the fewest dosage requirements. Individuals with epilepsy, for example, may have memory problems and, without specific memory strategies, be unable to maintain a pharmacotherapeutic schedule. Dose schedules can be modified to coincide with physical cues such as setting a watch alarm, meal times, or the availability of a support person for administration. Daily or weekly medication containers may be helpful in an environment free of children. Color-coded bottles, charts, and calendars—along with written dosage schedules and instructions for what to do in case of a missed dose—can ensure that pharmacotherapeutic treatment is successful. Remember to update written instructions even for minor changes.

# SEXUALITY ISSUES

All humans are sexual beings, although individuals with a disability are often viewed as less than whole and assumed to be asexual or devoid of feelings and desires. Try to get a clear understanding of the medical aspects of the disability and its relation to sexuality prior to initiating pharmacotherapeutic intervention. Individuals with a disability may be homosexual or heterosexual; however expressed, it is important to recognize sexual preference and to include partners in sexual counseling. The literature has few studies relating to female sexuality, since it is falsely assumed that females are less interested or are passive participants in sexual activities (Nosek, Rintala, Young, et al, 1996). For example, research on female sexuality after a spinal cord injury is scarce compared with male sexuality research, due in part to the traditional asexual myth as well as the greater number of males with spinal cord injury (Sipski & Alexander, 1992). Research interest has centered on pregnancy and complications of pregnancy in spinal-cord-injured females, bracketing women's sexuality with the act of childbearing (Charlifue, Gerhart, Menter, Whiteneck, & Manley, 1992).

Acquired neurologic injury—such as a traumatic brain or spinal cord injury or a cerebral vascular accident—often results not only in physical disabilities but also influences sexuality. Injuries may cause impairment to motor and sensory areas, limiting mobility or balance and changing or depleting sensory areas. For example, aphasia may limit speech, thereby decreasing communication, and apraxia may limit voluntary movements. Neurologic injury may change emotions, affect, social response, perception, and cognition. Timing sexual activity to coincide with peak concentrations of analgesic or antispasmodic medications may enhance sexual function. The serum level of sex hormones may be altered by tricyclic antidepressants, such as imipramine, and medications such as calcium channel blockers may produce sexual dysfunction. When assessing sexual concerns, it is important to remember that difficulty in sexual expression and activity may be caused by physical factors, such as mobility or genital function, or environmental or situational factors, as well as pharmacotherapeutic interventions.

Development of a sexual identity is different for individuals who have been disabled from birth compared to those who become disabled as adults (Nosek, Rintala, Young, et al, 1996). Children and adolescents with a disability may not have the opportunity to understand their bodies, changes within them, and how to appropriately channel emerging sexual feelings. Parents of children with disabilities can be so devoted to the physical management of their child and the accompanying dependency issues that sexuality is denied. Parents may also view their disabled child as a child for life or question lifespan and therefore not foster attainment of a sexual identity. Providers can help parents to develop a specific plan for sexuality education based on functional ability, not chronological age. Children with disabilities are sexually maltreated at a rate 1.7 times higher than their nondisabled peers, and education is the most effective protection from such abuse (American Academy of Pediatrics, 1996). Feelings of sexual inadequacy and undesirability may foster vulnerability to sexual exploitation, and primary care providers must use careful assessment techniques to detect possible abuse or exploitation (Nosek, 1995).

## WOMEN'S HEALTH ISSUES

Physical inaccessibility is often the reason cited by women with disabilities for delay or avoidance of gynecological care. There is also a dearth of health care providers—generalists or specialists—who are willing to help and are knowledgeable in gynecological care for women with disabilities. Research has shown that in a barrier-free environment, health care providers can positively influence the maintenance of women's health. This environment allows women to learn about reproductive health as well as preventive health measures, such as breast self-examination (Nosek, Young, Rintala, et al, 1995). Women with disabilities not only face health care issues related to their disability but also specific issues related to sensuality and sexuality.

Pelvic examinations are an integral part of women's health care. A physically accessible examination table must lower to 19 inches to allow for independent transfer and have arm support for safe and comfortable positioning. Women with decreased range of motion and spasticity may require adaptations of the gynecological examination. Spasticity is often exacerbated by examination positioning, which may trigger ad-

ductor spasms. Use the knee-chest position or side-lying position to decrease positional spasticity. Warming the speculum or reversing the speculum to use a handle-up position may also decrease spasticity. If a Pap smear is not indicated, Xylocaine gel may be applied to the speculum to decrease the potential for spinal-cord-induced autonomic dysreflexia as well as spasticity. The examination should be scheduled to coincide with the maximum concentration of antispasmodic medication. Women who use intrathecal Lioresal for control of severe spasticity may require a bolus of medication to be delivered prior to examination. Both spasticity and spinal cord injury will be discussed later in this chapter.

Contraceptive options for women with disabilities involve discussion and consideration of many factors. Although safe sex is paramount, the risk of pregnancy and the risks associated with the contraceptive method must be considered. Latex allergies, mobility issues, manual dexterity, and cognitive issues factor into the choices offered. For example, the physiological risks of thrombosis associated with oral contraceptives, impaired sensation for use of the IUD, and dexterity issues related to barrier methods must be openly discussed and evaluated in women with spinal cord injury. Norplant, which does not employ estrogen, may provide an option for women with motoric issues who are not physiologically at risk for hormonal contraception. Depo-Provera may be an option if time and transportation are available for quarterly administration. Contraceptive issues must be approached with the same level of comfort and commitment used with all activities of daily living.

Pregnancy, labor and delivery, and parenting are lifestyle choices for women with disabilities that may require routine health care considerations or complex interventions. Health issues such as neurogenic bowel and bladder, skin management, and thrombosis may be intensified with pregnancy and labor and delivery. Women with disabilities may also need referral to specialists for issues related to fertility. No matter what the level of the intervention, the primary care provider will be involved with a team of specialists to ensure maximal health. For a comprehensive discussion of health care for women with disabilities, refer to Sawin (1998).

# NEUROGENIC BOWEL AND BLADDER ISSUES

The ability to maintain continence is a survival instinct present in wild animals as well as children and adults. Neurogenic bowel and bladder are common health maintenance issues for individuals with a disability that often become a silent secondary disability, limiting both social and sexual opportunities. These issues can be assessed by the primary care provider to initiate treatment or referred to an advanced practice nurse or rehabilitation specialist if complex interventions and management are required.

Urinary incontinence may be the result of a spinal cord injury, multiple sclerosis, cerebral vascular accident, or spinal dysraphism. It causes embarrassment, decreases therapy and mobility options, causes skin breakdown and urinary tract infection, and may be the deciding factor between social functioning and long-term care (Linsenmeyer, 1991). Before initiating pharmacotherapeutic management, the reason for the incontinence must be established. The mnemonic DIAPPERS—D(delirium), I(infection), A(atrophic vaginitis), P(pharmaceuticals), P(psychosocial), E(endocrine), R(reduced mobility), and S(stool impaction) (Resnick & Yalla, 1985)—may help assess the reversible causes of incontinence. Reversible causes must be corrected before pharmacotherapeutic treatment is given. A neurogenic bladder may result in an inability to store urine, an inability to empty urine, or both. Urodynamic evaluation guides pharmacotherapeutic treatment and is necessary to determine if the neurogenic bladder is due to causes within the bladder, such as coordination of bladder contraction and bladder pressure, or to causes related to the bladder outlet or the external sphincter.

Although various pathophysiologies may contribute to a neurogenic bladder, the goal of treatment is to prevent upper urinary tract deterioration and to provide socially acceptable continence (Decter & Bauer, 1993). The general principles of urinary management are the same for both the pediatric and adult populations, and continence is sought through catheterization and pharmacotherapeutic agents. However, psychosocial factors and compliance vary among age groups. The young child will be dependent on parental intervention and possibly uninterested in management, whereas the adolescent may be very socially motivated to become continent. Clean intermittent catheterization is the treatment of choice to preserve upper urinary

tract function in the presence of a neurogenic bladder. Latex-free catheters are used, and the individual is taught the technique based on cognitive ability, dexterity, and mobility. Depending on cognitive ability, a child as young as 6 can begin to participate in catheterization by naming the supplies and may be independent between the ages of 8 and 12 (Peterson, Rauen, Brown, & Cole, 1994). Similarly, an individual with a high-level spinal cord injury may direct an attendant in this procedure. Those who are unable to perform urethral catheterization may need to be evaluated for surgical options, such as to create an abdominal reservoir that can be self-catheterized. It is important to realize that a urine culture from an individual who is self-catheterizing may contain flora and fauna suggestive of a urinary tract infection. However, if the individual is asymptomatic, without fever, pain, or altered urinary pattern, antibiotic treatment is not initiated as the flora and fauna are due to colonization, not active infection. Instead, fluids are increased along with the maintenance of a strict catheterization procedure and schedule. Only when symptoms of an infection are present is treatment initiated with culture-sensitive antibiotics (Decter & Bauer, 1993).

Pharmacotherapeutic treatment is initiated based on the prominent cause of the neurogenic bladder as determined by the urodynamic evaluation. Anticholinergic agents are frequently used to relax the smooth muscle of the bladder. Oxybutynin is the first-line drug of choice to decrease intravesicular pressure and increase bladder capacity. It may be instilled intravesically if the anticholinergic side effects produced by oral administration are intolerable. If oxubutynin fails, a favorable response may result from a trial with propantheline and dicyclomine, both anticholinergic medications with differing sites of action. Imipramine, a tricyclic antidepressant, is used in the treatment of neurogenic bladder to suppress bladder contractions and increase bladder capacity. Alpha blockers such as phenylpropanolamine or ephedrine also may be employed to improve urinary storage.

The ability to maintain bowel continence is based on rectal compliance and capacity and the autonomic and somatic nervous system's ability to coordinate defecation. Treating neurogenic bowel is based on maintaining a regular emptying pattern that does not allow stool to accumulate, thereby minimizing the complications of constipation and diarrhea. Constipation may lead to impaction when hardened fecal material obstructs the rectum. Paradoxical diarrhea or frequent watery stools may be a result of constipation, causing a dilated colon. Diarrhea may be interchanged with stool accumulation. Constipation may also exacerbate the symptoms of neurogenic bladder by decreasing bladder capacity.

A bowel training program prevents constipation and diarrhea by complete elimination of formed or semiformed stools. Elements of a bowel program may include adequate fluid intake, adequate dietary fiber, exercise to increase peristalsis, medications or techniques to stimulate evacuation, and timed evacuation. A reasonable goal is to have a pattern of regular soft stools at least every 2 days and to have no more than one bowel accident per month. The time involved in a bowel program should be between 30 and 45 minutes (King, Currie, & Wright, 1994). The ability to maintain continence is not voluntary, and factors such as medical condition and pharmacotherapeutic treatment, functional ability to participate in a bowel training program, financial resources, diet, lifestyle, and emotional desire for continence must all be evaluated. Every bowel program is customized, and the establishment of a successful bowel training program is labor-intensive for the individual as well as the provider and may take weeks to months to establish.

Pharmacotherapeutic interventions are based on the two distinct issues of stool motility through oral medication and stool evacuation through mechanical intervention. Colace, lactulose, and mineral oil are used for softening the stool. Lactulose, a nonabsorbable sugar, is often used for infants and young children. Bulking the stool through preparations such as psyllium (Metamucil) allows stool passage by changing consistency. Colonic motility may be stimulated through the use of senna or bisacodyl. Stool evacuation techniques include digital stimulation, suppositories, and enemas. Digital stimulation and suppositories trigger the colon to empty. Suppositories may be mild, such as glycerin, or may provide contact irritation, such as bisacodyl. Enemas also trigger evacuation of stool and may be used as part of a routine bowel program or may be used to relieve constipation. Enemas vary in amount of expansion used from very small, such as Therevac and Babylax enemas, to Fleet and bisacodyl enemas. Specialists in the treatment of neurogenic bowel also use preparations and techniques such as the Magic Bullet suppository, enema continence catheter, and biofeedback.

## MOBILITY ISSUES

Immobilization is a major consideration for some individuals with disabilities. The multisystem involvement of immobility causes metabolic and regulatory alterations. Nutritional recommendations as well as pharmacotherapeutic interventions must be considered, since obesity severely limits functional ability.

Medications that increase appetite or require food intake to decrease gastrointestinal distress may not be the most efficacious. Metabolic changes due to immobilization include loss of body protein and expansion of extracellular water volume, which alters drug kinetics. For example, gentamicin clearance is increased, which requires an increased dosage to maintain therapeutic levels. Cardiac complications are prevalent since a sedentary lifestyle lowers levels of high-density lipoprotein cholesterol. Orthostatic hypotension may be problematic, and sodium and fluid intake must be monitored since supplementary sodium chloride tablets may be necessary.

Since alpha-adrenergic blockers such as phenoxybenzamine potentiate orthostatic hypotension, they may not be the best choice for individuals with a spinal cord injury. A spinal cord injury also results in increased calcium excretion due to bone reabsorption of the paralyzed portion of the body. Kidneys unable to excrete all the increased calcium can lead to hypercalcuria and hypercalcemia. Hypercalcemia may cause nausea, vomiting, dehydration, lethargy, polydypsia, and polyuria. As part of the differential consideration, obtain a serum calcium level. Limiting oral calcium intake and vitamin D intake may decrease gastrointestinal absorption. Long-term control involves corticosteroids and oral phosphates. Increased calcium reabsorption also places the individual at risk for osteoporosis and urinary tract calculi.

Immobility and the lack of muscular pumping allow blood to pool in the calf, placing the individual at risk for deep venous thrombosis and of the complication of pulmonary embolism. The overall incidence of deep venous thrombosis in this adult population is 16.3%, with the highest incidence occurring in the first 2 weeks after injury, although deep venous thrombosis can occur beyond this time frame (Green et al, 1994). Note also that acute subclinical pulmonary embolism may be present in as many as 14% of individuals with spinal cord injury (Weingarden & Belen, 1992). The incidence of venous thrombosis in the pediatric population is poorly documented, and risk assessment is based on Tanner stage of physical maturity. Prophylactic treatment is questioned in the prepubertal population, but if diagnosed, treatment is recommended to decrease the risk of a pulmonary embolism (Radecki & Gaebler-Spira, 1994).

Prophylaxis management of deep venous thrombosis is beyond the scope of this chapter, and there is debate over the safety and efficacy of various prophylactic approaches. However, individuals with a spinal cord injury may be maintained on anticoagulation therapy for up to 6 months with various dosing and laboratory evaluation schedules monitored by the primary care provider. Remember too that the presence of a device to prevent blood clots from traveling, such as a Greenfield filter, does not exclude venous thrombosis from differential considerations. Clinical signs and diagnosis may be complicated by the alteration in, or absence of, sensation owing to changes in the neurologic system. Therefore, all complaints of pleuritic chest pain require a diagnostic evaluation.

## HETEROTOPIC OSSIFICATION

Heterotopic ossification is the abnormal formation of new bone in periarticular soft tissue areas of individuals who have sustained such traumatic injuries as a spinal cord injury, brain injury, or burns. Heterotopic ossification has been reported in 16–53% of individuals with spinal cord injury, most commonly between months 1 and 4 and rarely after month 12 postinjury (Hinck, 1994). Presenting findings are swelling, heat, loss of range of motion, and possibly fever. For individuals with a spinal cord injury, the hip is the most common site, followed by the knee, shoulder, and elbow. Differential considerations include deep vein thrombosis, cellulitis, joint sepsis, tumor, and fracture (Banovac, Gonzales, Wade, & Bowker, 1993). Roentgenograms may be negative during the early weeks because of insufficient ossification, and a triple-phase bone scan will be necessary for diagnosis. Laboratory evaluation will reveal an increase in the serum alkaline phosphatase level during the acute phase.

Early diagnosis and treatment of heterotopic ossification are essential to preserve function. Aggressive and regular passive range of motion is the treatment modality of choice. In the adult population, disodium etidronate may be used to attempt to limit or prevent the extent of ossification by inhibiting bone matrix mineralization. Although the ideal treatment length has not been established, the overall goal is to use the lowest effective dose for the shortest duration. An initial dosage of 5 mg/kg per day may be used for up to 6 months, with severe instances requiring dosages of 10 mg/kg per day for up to 3 months. Dosage above 20 mg/kg per day is contraindicated. Pharmacologic research on the prophylactic use of disodium etidronate is being undertaken (Dunn, Fitton, & Sorkin, 1994). Disodium etidronate is used cautiously in the pediatric population because of possible interference with bone metabolism in the developing skeleton (Molnar & Perrin, 1992).

## AUTONOMIC DYSREFLEXIA

Autonomic dysreflexia is a life-threatening phenomenon of elevated blood pressure caused by reflex activity of the sympathetic and parasympathetic nervous systems when a spinal cord lesion is above the sympathetic splanchnic outflow. Individuals with a spinal cord injury proximal to thoracic level 6 are at risk for a sudden uninhibited sympathetic response causing hypertension. The sudden paroxysmal hypertension may elevate systolic pressure as high as 200 mm Hg and diastolic pressure as high as 100 mm Hg. At any point, an increase in the baseline pressure of 20 mm Hg is considered autonomic dysreflexia. This condition may be constant, subside within 3 years of the spinal cord injury, or may be subject to remissions and exacerbations.

Autonomic dysreflexia can be triggered by noxious events to the body below the level of the spinal cord injury. Symptoms include a sudden onset of headache, hypertension, sweating, nasal congestion, and piloerection. Immediate removal of the noxious stimuli is essential. If this treatment is not effective, pharmacotherapy intervention is imperative. See Table 14–1. Prevention of noxious stimuli is accomplished through bowel, bladder, and skin management programs. Although the symptoms of mild autonomic dysreflexia are uncomfortable, severe hypertension associated with dysreflexia may lead to cerebral hemorrhage. Close monitoring is mandatory. Severe hypertension is an emergency, and immediate pharmacotherapy must be initiated. Associated hemodynamic changes also place the

**TABLE 14–1.  AUTONOMIC DYSREFLEXIA: CAUSES, SYMPTOMS, AND TREATMENTS**

| Symptoms | Causes | Interventions | Medication | Prevention |
|---|---|---|---|---|
| Hypertension<br>Headache<br>Flushing **above**<br>  lesion<br>Sweating **above**<br>  lesion<br>Pallor **below**<br>  lesion<br>Nasal congestion<br>Blurred vision<br>Dilated pupils<br>Bradycardia<br>Increased spasticity | | Monitor heart rate<br>Monitor blood pressure<br>Raise head of bed<br>Lower legs<br>Remove tight<br>  clothes<br>Remove equipment | *Sublingual*<br>Nifedipine<br><br>*PO*<br>Dibenzyline<br>Minipress<br>  Procardia<br><br>*IV*<br>Hydralazine<br>Hyperstat<br>Nipride | Educate family,<br>  caregivers,<br>  coworkers, and<br>  professional<br>  colleagues |
| **Bladder** | | | | |
| | Blocked/<br>  kinked catheter | Catheterize with<br>  Pontocaine<br>Drain slowly<br>Irrigate Foley<br>  catheter<br>Unkink tubing<br>Empty bag | | Establish and maintain effective<br>  bladder program |
| **Bowel** | | | | |
| | Impaction<br>Distention<br>Digital stimulation<br>Suppository<br>Enema<br>Hemorrhoids | Rectal exam and<br>  disimpaction with<br>  Xylocaine gel | | Establish and maintain effective<br>  bowel program |
| **Integumentary** | | | | |
| | Lesion<br>Pressure<br>Ingrown toenail<br>Positioning<br>Tight clothing<br>Tight straps on equipment<br>↑/↓ temperature<br>Sunburn | Topical anesthetic<br>  to skin lesion | | Establish and maintain effective skin<br>  monitoring program |
| **External or painful stimuli** | | | | |
| | Medical instrumentation<br>Sexual activity<br>Labor and delivery<br>Menstruation<br>Fracture<br>Infection<br>Urinary tract infection<br>Renal calculi<br>Epididymitis | | | Use anesthetic<br>  agents before<br>  procedures and<br>  painful conditions<br>Prompt treatment<br>  of symptomatic<br>  infections |

individual at risk for heart failure. Older individuals with spinal cord injury are at the greatest risk for such life-threatening consequences.

## SPASTICITY

Spasticity is one of the most common health problems for individuals with a disability and is often associated with cerebral palsy, traumatic brain injury, spinal cord injury, and multiple sclerosis. Spasticity is easy to recognize, complex to characterize, and difficult to treat. It is characterized as an abnormally increased and prolonged muscle contraction in response to rapid movements or rapid changes in position. Spasticity is often recognized by hyperactive deep tendon reflexes; Babinski's sign; increased resistance to passive movement; clonus, flexor, or extensor spasms; and abnormal voluntary movements. The amount and degree of spasticity fluctuate, and therefore multiple clinical assessments are necessary.

Evaluating spasticity revolves around the question of whether it interferes with functional ability. Ask the individual to demonstrate the functional activity affected by spasticity. Spasticity alters the ability to make smooth voluntary movements. Sitting or transferring may be affected, or it can alter cosmesis, cause skin breakdown or pain, disturb sleep, or interrupt sexual function. Conversely, spasticity may have a salubrious affect by providing muscle tone useful in gait, promoting limb repositioning, and improving circulation, thereby decreasing the risk of deep venous thrombosis (Young, 1994).

When an individual who is neurologically stable exhibits increased spasticity, precipitating factors must be evaluated. Any noxious physical stimuli—a urinary tract infection or kidney stone, pressure sore, acute infectious process or bowel or bladder distension—or psychological stimuli—such as stress—may exacerbate spasticity. Management of spasticity begins with physical and rehabilitative therapy to eliminate nociceptive stimuli. There are several pharmacotherapeutic agents available to treat spasticity. The frequency of doses and adverse effects may make control of severe spasticity difficult. If the agent improves the symptoms but fails to improve functional abilities, it is unlikely that another agent will be beneficial. The goals of treatment are to diminish spasticity without causing voluntary muscle weakness, to maintain the positive effects of spasticity, and to limit sedation caused by the medication. No standard pharmacotherapeutic intervention can be recommended since spasticity may be either spinal or cerebral in origin, and the site of origination guides pharmacotherapeutic treatment decisions. Flexor spasms in a complete spinal cord injury differ from severe spasticity associated with multiple sclerosis, which is markedly different from spastic diplegia in children with cerebral palsy (Schapiro, 1994).

The primary care provider may begin treatment of spasticity or is more often involved in the monitoring of treatment initiated by a specialist. Medications must be closely monitored since abrupt withdrawal by the individual or the provider may yield potentially serious consequences. General muscle relaxants such as methocarbamol are not effective in the treatment of spasticity and should not be initiated. Lioresal, a gamma-aminobutyric acid agonist, is the first-line pharmacotherapeutic treatment of choice and is more beneficial in spinal cord injury and multiple sclerosis than in cerebrally originated spasticity. Lioresal has a wide dose range and experts in the treatment of spasticity may far exceed the maximum recommended dose range of 80 mg per day. Adverse effects of drowsiness, weakness, fatigue, confusion, and headache are common and usually dissipate within several days of initiation. These effects can be reduced by starting with a low dose and increasing dosage at a 7-day interval instead of the usual 4-day interval. Lioresal may decrease seizure threshold, a consideration for individuals with epilepsy. It may also have an additive central nervous system depressant effect if used with other depressants. A withdrawal syndrome that may include psychosis, hallucinations, or seizures as well as rebound spasticity is likely if Lioresal is abruptly discontinued without slowly weaning the dose (Fromm, 1994).

Both clonazepam and diazepam may be useful as combination therapy with Lioresal and are often used to decrease nocturnal spasms. Sedative effects may be problematic for daytime use. Diazepam is used for spasticity that originates in the spinal cord and also has some efficacy in individuals with cerebral palsy. The side effects of decreased cognitive ability and motor control often render diazepam an unacceptable choice. True physiologic addiction may take place, and abrupt withdrawal can include seizures. A paradoxical reaction of insomnia, anxiety, hostility, hallucinations, and increased spasticity has been reported with long-term use.

Clonidine has shown marked improvement in spasticity, particularly after a cerebral vascular accident (Sandford, Spengler, & Sawasky, 1992). However, such side effects as hypotension and constipation may be unacceptable in individuals with spinal cord injury. Clonidine may induce bradycardia that dissipates when the medication is discontinued (Rosenblum, 1993).

Dantrolene may be effective in treating spinal cord spasticity and spasticity with a cerebral origin, but it has fallen out of favor since other pharmacotherapeutic options are available. Hepatotoxicity is a concern, and it should not be used in individuals with severe hepatic disease. Before initiating therapy, baseline liver function tests must be obtained and then monitored at routine intervals. A clinically apparent response to treatment may not be noticed until 1 week after dose adjustment. If a response is not seen within 2 weeks at a maximum dosage level, discontinue use because of the hepatic risks. The adverse effect of weakness makes dantrolene an unacceptable choice for individuals with multiple sclerosis.

The oral agents used to treat spasticity have sedating properties, and the dose required to adequately decrease severe spasticity may impair cognition and functional abilities (Segatore & Miller, 1994). Referrals may be necessary for treatment options aside from or in conjunction with oral pharmacotherapeutic agents. Experts in the management of spasticity may use botulinum toxin injections into the neuromuscular junction to weaken spastic muscles. Dosage is dependent on the desired effect. For example, the dose required for precise control of a fine motor muscle is lower than the dose to control painful spasms in a nonfunctional limb. The average duration of response to injection is 2–6 months depending on the dose and the size and activity of the muscle (Gooch & Sandell, 1996). Ablative surgery, the selective dorsal root rhizotomy, may be used for severe spasticity. Ideal candidates for this procedure are between the ages of 2 and 6 years, and an extensive rehabilitation program is required afterward.

For severe spasticity, a new treatment uses intraspinal drug therapy to precisely deliver the antispasmodic agent directly to the receptors within the spinal cord. A surgically implanted, externally programmable pump is used to deliver intrathecal Lioresal. Intraspinal drug therapy has resulted in improvement in functional abilities as well as lifestyle activities such as sleep, bladder management, and relief of dis-

comfort (Savoy & Gianino, 1993). Such practical issues as cost, surgical risk, refilling intervals, individual commitment, and available expertise must be considered prior to pump implantation (Teddy, 1995).

## LATEX ALLERGY

Awareness of latex sensitivity and allergy has increased over the past decade. This is due in part to a 1991 recall of latex enema tips by the Food and Drug Administration (FDA) as well as the establishment of universal precautions that require repeated exposure to latex for health care providers. Latex is a natural material found in the milky sap of the *Hevea brasiliensis* plant, the rubber tree. Individuals at risk for developing an allergy are those who are repeatedly exposed to products containing latex, such as health care providers and individuals with spina bifida, spinal cord injury, or congenital genitourinary tract anomalies, as well as those undergoing multiple surgeries. Identify at-risk individuals and treat an allergic reaction promptly.

During an allergy history, explore allergies to tropical fruit, chestnuts, and avocados that have all been associated with latex sensitivity (Lavaud et al, 1992). A history of an allergic reaction to a glove or balloon is also crucial. Individuals with spina bifida have an 18–40% incidence of latex sensitivity (Food and Drug Administration, 1991). Leger and Meeropol (1992) compared latex allergy in individuals with spina bifida to individuals with neuromuscular and orthopedic conditions and found that 20% of individuals with spina bifida had latex allergy as compared to 1.1% of those with the other disorders. They also found that the spinal cord injury population had a lower incidence of latex allergy as compared to the spina bifida population. This higher incidence is thought to be due to exposure to latex from birth in individuals with spina bifida (Vogel, Schrader, & Lubicky, 1995). It can be extrapolated that individuals with congenital genitourinary anomalies will also have a higher incidence of latex allergy due to exposure from birth. The second largest risk group is health care workers, with estimates ranging from 2.6% to 16.9%. More than 1,000 episodes of anaphylaxis and 15 deaths were reported to the FDA (Wood, 1997).

Symptoms of a local allergic response to latex include watery eyes, itching, sneezing, and hives, whereas a systemic reaction results in anaphylaxis. Reactions occur when latex touches the skin or mucous membranes or enters the bloodstream (Hamann, 1993). Sensitivity may become so great that opening a package of latex gloves can trigger a reaction due to the airborne particles. Definitive evidence for latex allergy is difficult because each test—the skin prick, intradermal, or radioallergosorbent—measures only the amount of the reaction at that particular point in time (Brown, 1994). A "latex alert" should be used as a safeguard for those who are in a high-risk group but who have not had any symptoms of an allergic reaction. The identification of "latex allergy" is for individuals who have displayed latex sensitivity either locally or systemically and who must have a latex-free environment. All children at risk of latex allergy must be identified, particularly before undergoing surgical procedures (Wood, 1997). A medic alert bracelet and autoinjectable epinephrine are essential for high-risk individuals (Romanczuk, 1993).

It is both difficult and time-consuming to know all the products that contain latex since there are no current labeling requirements. An individual with a latex sensitivity or allergy is at greatest risk from gloves, catheters, balloons, balls (Koosh and tennis), condoms, dental dams, nipples, pacifiers, tape, chux, rubber bands, and Band-Aids. The Spina Bifida Association maintains a current list updated twice a year that can be obtained by calling 1-800-621-3141. Latex allergy must be considered when injecting medications in the office or in the hospital. Do not draw up medications into a syringe through the rubber cap on a medication vial or inject medications into latex ports on intravenous tubing.

At-risk individuals require preassessment by anesthesia, and dental and surgical procedures should be scheduled for the first case in the morning in a latex-free environment. Same-day procedures are not appropriate because of intensive postoperative monitoring requirements. Patients with a history of latex allergy are treated 24 hours preoperatively and postoperatively with IV or oral diphenhydramine and methylprednisolone 1 mg/kg per dose and cimetidine 5 mg/kg per dose every 6 h. Individuals at high risk are treated every 12 h preoperatively with oral diphenhydramine 1 mg/kg per dose, followed by prednisone 0.5 mg/kg per dose every 12 h. In the case of anaphylaxis, treatment includes the above medications as well as epinephrine and airway support (Kwittken et al, 1992).

## PRESCRIPTIVE CONSIDERATIONS

A unique issue for individuals with disabilities is the appropriate use of nonpharmacologic prescriptions. Individuals with disabilities see many specialists and use specialized equipment and therapy resources to maximize their functional abilities. Technological advances offer a myriad of options and therapies that must be wisely assessed by the primary care provider. The goals for therapeutic interventions as well as the health/dollar benefits should be known before providing the prescription.

Equipment ranges from the simple—a reacher or bath seat—to the complex—orthotic intervention for ambulation or powered mobility. The prescribing provider must really understand what models, brands, and vendors are most appropriate for the individual and the disability. For example, a standard, prefabricated orthosis may be prescribed when a hinged, custom-made orthosis would allow for more dorsiflexion and improve functional gait. If the funding for the prefabricated orthosis is used, there may not be funding options for the customized orthosis. Similarly, prescribing a child's wheelchair that cannot be adjusted as the child grows or ordering a nonadjustable axle plate that does not allow the wheels to be moved to the most optimal pushing position is disastrous. A team approach allows the provider, individual, therapists, rehabilitation specialist, and reimbursement source to coordinate and prescribe proper fitting and functioning assistive devices and therapies to increase functional abilities. A suboptimal choice is a major negative outcome; therefore, a standard prescription for therapeutic equipment or a blanket request for therapy does not exist.

In addition, unique teaching needs for medication or equipment must be considered in this population. Evaluate the learning needs of your patients and alter education as appropriate. For example, individuals with visual impairments may need a special system devised for safety and instructions that are accessible in an audiotape. The practitioner will need to know if patients have access to a Kerzler reader and would prefer written instructions. If learning disabilities are an issue, a multiple approach, such as visual and auditory, might be optimal for complex regimes.

## SUMMARY

Primary care for individuals with a disability is the crux of health maintenance. The unique complexities presented by the disability allow the provider to address issues related to pharmacotherapeutic intervention, routine health care, common health conditions, and health issues related to the disability. The primary care provider does not abdicate care, but can both provide care and guide and direct care provided by subspecialists. Pharmacotherapeutic interventions must be customized for the disability and the combined effects on the body systems. A holistic view of the individual by the primary care provider forms the basis of collaboration and partnership, which is essential to maximize health. All too often, it is forgotten that an individual with a disability is an ordinary person who does ordinary things in extraordinary ways.

## REFERENCES

American Academy of Pediatrics. (1996). Sexuality education of children and adolescents with developmental disabilities. *Pediatrics, 97*(2), 275–278.

Banovac, K., Gonzales, F., Wade, N. & Bowker, J. J. (1993). Intravenous disodium etidronate therapy in spinal cord injury patients with heterotopic ossification. *Paraplegia, 31*(10), 660–666.

Blumberg, L. (1992). Don't put disabled children on display. *Contemporary Pediatrics, 9*, 61–70.

Briskin, H., & Liptak, G. S. (1995). Helping families with children with developmental disabilities. *Pediatric Annals, 24*(5), 262–266.

Brown, J. P. (1994). Latex allergy requires attention in orthopaedic nursing. *Orthopedic Nursing, 13*(1), 7–11.

Charlifue, S. W., Gerhart, K. A., Menter, R. R., Whiteneck, G. G., & Manley, M. S. (1992). Sexual issues of women with spinal cord injuries. *Paraplegia, 30*, 192–199.

Decter, R. M., & Bauer, S. B. (1993). Urologic management of spinal cord injury in children. *Urologic Clinic of North America, 20* (3), 475–483.

Dunn, C. J., Fitton, A., & Sorkin, E. M. (1994). Etidronic acid. A review of its pharmacological properties and therapeutic efficacy in resorptive bone disease. *Drugs and Aging, 5*(6), 446–474.

Food and Drug Administration. (1991). Medical alert: Allergic reactions to latex-containing medical devices. MDA91-1, 1–2.

Fromm, G. H. (1994). Balofen as an adjuvant analgesic. *Journal of Pain and Symptom Management, 9*(8), 500–509.

Gooch, J. L., & Sandell, T. V. (1996). Botulinum toxin for spasticity and athetosis in children with cerebral palsy. *Archives of Physical Medicine and Rehabilitation, 77*(5), 508–511.

Green, D., Chen, D., Chmiel, J. S., Olsen, N. K., Berkowitz, M., Novick, A., Alleva, J., Steinberg, D., Nussbaum, S., & Tolotta, M. (1994). Prevention of thromboembolism in spinal cord injury; Role of low molecular weight heparin. *Archives of Physical Medicine and Rehabilitation, 75*, 290–292.

Hamann, C. P. (1993). Natural rubber latex protein sensitivity in review. *American Journal of Contact Dermatitis, 4*(1), 4–21.

Hinck, S. M. (1994). Heterotopic ossification: A review of symptoms and treatment. *Rehabilitation Nursing, 19*(3), 169–173.

King, J. C., Currie, D. M., & Wright, E. (1994). Bowel training in spina bifida: Importance of education, patient compliance, age, and anal reflexes. *Archives of Physical Medicine and Rehabilitation, 75*, 243–247.

Krotoski, D. M., Nosek, M. A., & Turk, M. A. (1996). Women with physical disabilities. In D. M. Krotoski, M. A. Nosek, & M. A. Turk, (Eds.), *Women with physical disabilities.* Baltimore: Paul H. Brookes Publishing.

Kwittken, P. L., Becker, J., Oyefara, B., Danziger, R., Pawlowski, N. A., & Sweinberg, S. (1992). Latex hypersensitivity reactions despite prophylaxis. *Allergy Proceedings, 13*(3), 123–127.

Lavaud, F., Cossart, C., Reiter, V., Bernard, J., Deltour, G., & Holmquist, I. (1992). Latex allergy in patients with allergy to fruit. *Lancet, 339*: 492–493.

Leger, R., & Meeropol, E. (1992). Children at risk: Latex allergy and spina bifida. *Journal of Pediatric Nursing, 7* (6), 371–376.

Linsenmeyer, T. A. (1991). Neuro-urologic rehabilitation via pharmacologic agents. *Neurorehabilitation, 1*: 22–32.

Mausner, S. (1995). Families helping families: An innovative approach to the provision of respite care for families of children with complex medical needs. *Social Work in Health Care, 21*(1), 95–106.

Molnar, G. E., & Perrin, J. C. S. (1992). Head injury. In G. E. Molnar (Ed.), *Pediatric rehabilitation* (2nd ed.). Baltimore: Williams & Wilkins.

Nosek, M. A. (1992). Primary care issues for women with severe physical disabilities. *Journal of Women's Health, 1*(4), 245–248.

Nosek, M. A. (1995). Sexual abuse of women with physical disabilities. *Physical Medicine and Rehabilitation, 9*(2), 487–502.

Nosek, M. A., Rintala, D. H., Young, M. E., Howland, C. A., Foley, C. C., Rossi, D., & Chanpong, G. (1996). Sexual functioning among women with physical disabilities. *Archives of Physical Medicine and Rehabilitation, 77*, 107–115.

Nosek, M. A. Young, M. E., Rintala, D. H., Howland, C. A., Foley, C. C., & Bennet, J. J. (1995). Barriers to reproductive health maintenance among women with physical disabilities. *Journal of Women's Health, 4*(5), 505–518.

O'Sullivan, P., Mahoney, G., & Robinson, C. (1992). Perceptions of pediatrician's helpfulness: A national study of mothers of young disabled children. *Developmental Medicine and Child Neurology, 34*(12), 1064–1071.

Patterson, J., & Blum, R. W. (1996). Risk and resilience among children and youth with disabilities. *Archives of Pedriatics and Adolescent Medicine, 150*(7), 692–698.

Peterson, P. M., Rauen, K. K., Brown, J., & Cole, J. (1994). Spina bifida: The transition into adulthood begins in infancy. *Rehabilitation Nursing, 19*(4), 229–238.

Radecki, R. T., & Gaebler-Spira, D. (1994). Deep vein thrombosis in the disabled pediatric population. *Archives of Physical Medicine and Rehabilitation, 75*, 248–250.

Resnick, N. M., & Yalla, S. V. (1985). Current concepts: Management of urinary incontinence in the elderly. *New England Journal of Medicine, 313*(13), 800–805.

Romanczuk, A. (1993). Latex use with infants and children: It can cause problems. *MCN, 18*, 208–212.

Rosenblum, D. (1993). Clonidine-induced bradycardia in patients with spinal cord injury. *Archives of Physical Medicine and Rehabilitation, 74*(11), 1206–1207.

Sandford, P. R., Spengler, S. E., & Sawasky, K. B. (1992). Clonidine in the treatment of brainstem spasticity. Case report. *American Journal of Physical Medicine and Rehabilitation, 71*(5), 301–303.

Savoy, S. M., & Gianino, J. M. (1993). Intrathecal baclofen infusion: An innovative approach for controlling spinal spasticity. *Rehabilitation Nursing, 18*(2), 105–113.

Sawin, K. J. (1998). Health care concerns for women with physical disability and chronic illness. In E. Youngkin & M. Davis (Eds.), *Women's health: A primary care clinician's guide* (2nd ed.). Stamford, CT: Appleton & Lange.

Schapiro, R. T. (1994). Symptom management in multiple sclerosis. *Annals of Neurology, 36*, S123–129.

Segatore, M., & Miller, M. (1994). The pharmacotherapy of spinal spasticity: A decade of progress I. Theoretical aspects. *Spinal Cord Injury Nursing, 1*(3), 66–69.

Sipski, M. L., & Alexander, C. J. (1992). Sexual function and dysfunction after spinal cord injury. *Physical Medicine and Rehabilitation Clinics of North America, 3*(4), 811–828.

Stallard, P., & Dickinson, F. (1994). Groups for parents of pre-school children with severe disabilities. *Child Care Health, and Development, 20*(3), 197–207.

Teddy, P. J. (1995). Implants for spasticity. *Baillieres Clinical Neurology, 4*(1), 95–114.

Vogel, L. C., Schrader, T., & Lubicky, J. P. (1995). Latex allergy in children and adolescents with spinal cord injuries. *Journal of Pediatric Orthopedics, 15*, 517–520.

Weingarden, S. I., & Belen, J. G. (1992). Clonidine transdermal system for treatment of spasticity in spinal cord injury. *Archives of Physical Medicine and Rehabilitation, 73*, 876–877.

Wood, R. A. (1997). Anaphylaxis in children. *Patient Care*, 161–179.

Young, R. R. (1994). Spasticity: A review. *Neurology, 44*(11), S12–20.

# 15

## MIGRANT AND HOMELESS POPULATIONS

*Sandra L. Graves*

The provision of quality primary care to migrant workers and homeless clients poses significant challenges. Since lifestyle and environmental issues compound their situations, the pharmacotherapeutic considerations in the care of these two vulnerable populations are addressed in this chapter within the context of those variables. Pediatric implications for migrants and the homeless also are included.

## THE MIGRANT FARM WORKERS POPULATION

The size of the population of migrant farm workers and their dependents is currently estimated to be slightly more than 4 million people (Go & Baker, 1995). However, this is most likely an underestimation because of their transient nature and because of the number of workers who migrate in and out of the United States (Rust, 1990). Three major streams of migrant workers exist: (1) the West Coast stream heading north from southern California to northern California, Oregon, and Washington; (2) the Central stream traveling up the Mississippi Valley to Ohio, Michigan, Indiana, and Illinois from Texas and Arizona; and (3) the East Coast stream moving from southern Florida up the East Coast to Maryland, Delaware, New Jersey, New York, and New England (Go & Baker, 1995; Mobed, Gold, & Schenker, 1992). The streams are comprised primarily of individuals who are from Mexico, Puerto Rico, Jamaica, Haiti, and Central America but includes Native Americans and African-Americans (Mobed, Gold, & Schenker, 1992). For the purposes of this chapter, migrant farm workers are defined as those individuals who "migrate to obtain temporary agricultural employment" as distinguished from seasonal farm workers who "are seasonally employed in agriculture within one local area" (Martin, Gordon, & Kupersmidt, 1995).

## COMMON HEALTH PROBLEMS OF MIGRANT WORKERS

Significant gaps in information exist concerning the health status of the migrant worker populations. Rust (1990) completed a retrospective literature review on the health of migrant workers and found limited documentation on either the more common causes of infection or the incidence, prevalence, or risk factors for cancer, heart disease, or stroke. Go and Baker (1995) studied Eastern Shore migrant workers in Maryland and found that their most common health problems were (in decreasing order of frequency for adults) dental, dermatologic infections, hypertension, diabetes mellitus, and gynecologic/family planning needs. The significant occupational health problems of this documented group include accidents, pesticide-associated illnesses, musculoskeletal and soft tissue injuries, and degenerative joint diseases (Go & Baker,

1995; Mobed, Gold & Schenker, 1992). In addition, there is a significant risk of communicable diseases, including tuberculosis, because of crowded and unsanitary living conditions.

Major health problems of migrant workers' children aged 5 through 15 were found to be communicable diseases, such as pediculosis and upper respiratory infections, ear/eye/nose/throat problems, dental problems, anemia, and injuries (Go & Baker, 1995). A study by Martin, Gordon, and Kupersmidt (1995) also found that children of migrant and seasonal farm workers were exposed to extreme levels of violence: Fifty-two percent of the children surveyed had been exposed to the results of some type of violence. Of these children exposed to violence, forty-six percent witnessed someone being beaten, mugged, shot at, and/or murdered; and nineteen percent had been victims of violence themselves. This exposure to violence, compounded by the issues of poverty and a transient lifestyle, may be reflected in these children's higher risk for emotional and behavioral problems.

## LIFESTYLE FACTORS THAT CONTRIBUTE TO DISEASE

The barriers that exist in the delivery of health care to migrant workers and their families include limited access to health care facilities, a lack of health care insurance, language and cultural barriers, varied definitions of health and illness, and lower educational levels (Poss & Meeks, 1994). In addition, the housing and working conditions of this group significantly impact on their health status, both in terms of transmission of communicable diseases as well as in the healing process. Crowded living conditions are often compounded by inadequate facilities for personal hygiene, providing an excellent environment for exposure to communicable diseases. Also, because of the transient nature of their lives, treatment for selected communicable diseases may be incomplete, adding to their risk of infection.

With regard to family support systems, Poss and Meeks (1994) noted that Hispanic men tended to bring their families with them, whereas the Jamaican and African-American migrant workers tended to travel alone. This cultural pattern has significant implications for practice in terms of the resource needs of the population as well as the support systems in place for care of the ill.

## THE HOMELESS POPULATION

Documentation of the extent of the homeless population varies significantly depending on the definition used and on whether one uses government statistics or statistics from advocates for the homeless (Link et al, 1994). According to Gelberg (1992), between 250,000 and 3 million people are estimated to be homeless. There is consensus, however, that the number of people who are homeless grew significantly during the 1980s. Approximately one quarter to one third of those individuals are women and children, who are the fastest growing component of the homeless population (Wood, 1992; Wright, 1991). It is important to keep in mind that the factors that frequently lead a person to homelessness, such as substance abuse, mental illness, or domestic violence, significantly influence their general health status and greatly impact their utilization of health care resources (Usatine, Gelberg, Smith, & Lesser, 1994). In addition, because of their lifestyle, access to medications and compliance with a plan of care become much more difficult.

## COMMON HEALTH PROBLEMS OF THE HOMELESS

The homeless have higher prevalence rates of physical morbidity and mortality as compared to the general population. They also have a poorer perception of their individual health status than the general population (Gelberg, 1992). Their most common health problems have been well documented in the literature. The most common acute presenting problems include upper respiratory infections; trauma; skin conditions, both minor and serious; back, joint, and fracture pain; and respiratory problems (Carter, Green, Green, & Dufour, 1994; Scholler-Jaquish, 1996; Usatine, Gelberg, Smith, & Lesser, 1994).

Thirty to forty percent of this population also suffer from one or more chronic health conditions. These include: hypertension, diabetes mellitus, peripheral vascular disease, chronic obstructive pulmonary disease, heart disease, and seizures. Typically, compared to the general population, these individuals have had these conditions for an extended length of time, and they have left them untreated, therefore, the conditions are of greater severity (Carter, et al,

1994; Fleischman & Farnham, 1992; Scholler-Jaquish, 1996; Usatine et al, 1994).

Communicable diseases such as tuberculosis (TB) are of significant concern in this population. The association among poverty, over-crowding, and tuberculosis has been historically well documented. Given overcrowded poorly ventilated shelter conditions, and the percentage of homeless who have substance abuse problems or mental illness, the increase in tuberculosis cases during the 1980s should have been expected (Brudney, 1993). Recent research (Barnes et al, 1996) also indicates that primary tuberculosis caused most of the tuberculosis cases reported in an urban Los Angeles setting. It was concluded that greater resources were needed for case finding, for the use of ultraviolet lights and other environmental controls, and for prompt assessment and treatment of individuals with a recent infection. Multiple-drug-resistant TB (MDR-TB) was not common until 1987 and continues to occur most frequently in HIV-infected individuals (Jo, 1993). HIV infection is a major risk factor for the development of TB.

Homeless people are at greater risk for HIV because of their increased high-risk behaviors, including intravenous drug usage and sexual contact with persons who have been exposed to HIV (Allen et al, 1994). In 1989, when the Centers for Disease Control and Prevention collaborated with several state and local health departments, survey data reflected elevated HIV seroprevalence rates and HIV risk behaviors among homeless adults and runaway youths (Allen et al, 1994).

Substance abuse and chronic mental illness are significant health problems in this population. Depending on the definition used, the prevalence of mental illness ranges from 16–91% (Gelberg, 1992). Usatine, Gelberg, Smith, and Lesser (1994) found that at least 33% of the homeless have severe mental illnesses, including schizophrenia, major depressive disorders and bipolar affective disorders. These conditions can, in fact, precipitate homelessness and tend to worsen with life on the street.

As previously noted, the demographics of the homeless population have changed in recent years. Once considered predominately male, the homeless population has seen a significant increase in the number of women and children. Women frequently report significant histories of violence both in terms of their families of origin and in their previous or current relationships.

Mental health concerns and substance abuse are frequently cited as problems. In addition, an increased frequency of gynecologic and genitourinary problems is seen. These women usually prioritize the health needs of their children over their own and do not seek care until their condition has progressed (Hatton, 1997; Hodnicki & Horner, 1993; Norton & Ridenour, 1995).

Limited documentation exists regarding the specific health problems and concerns of homeless women who are pregnant. Common concerns for pregnant women such as urinary frequency, a change in vaginal discharge, morning sickness, fatigue, and a unhealthy diet are much more difficult to deal with in a shelter or homeless environment. An increased risk of infections, such as urinary tract infections, as well as an increased risk of mental health problems, such as depression, has been documented (Killion, 1995).

Children are the most vulnerable members of the homeless population. Wright (1991) noted that although the illnesses that homeless children exhibit are quite common in the general pediatric population, the consequences of these diseases are significantly different. Several studies comparing the health of homeless children with housed children of lower socioeconomic means showed an increased frequency of serous otitis and of communicable diseases such as pediculosis and scabies, as well as a significantly higher rate of injuries (Murata, Mace, Strehlow, & Shuler, 1992). Minor upper respiratory infections, followed by minor skin problems, ear disorders, gastrointestinal problems, trauma, eye disorders, and lice infestations were the most common presenting complaints in Wright's review of the literature regarding the most common health problems of homeless children (Wright, 1991). With regard to chronic conditions, anemia, asthma, and recurrent otitis media are quite common and often go untreated (Redlener & Karich, 1994). Developmental delays, learning difficulties, and mental health problems, including depression, also are increasingly common (Kemsley & Hunter, 1993; Redlener & Karich, 1994; Wood, Valdez, Hayashi, & Shen, 1990; Wright, 1991).

## LIFESTYLE FACTORS THAT CONTRIBUTE TO DISEASE

Life on the streets focuses on survival. Homelessness puts these individuals at a significantly higher exposure risk for infection and other health-related problems. Their primary concerns revolve around the need for shelter and food; taking care of one's health needs and seeking health care is not seen as a high priority. Time is cyclical and present-oriented, rather than linear or future-oriented, for most of these individuals ie, determined by the time of day that the meals are served or the shelters open (Gelberg, 1992).

Shelters are too often overcrowded and unsanitary. Beds are not always available so individuals may be forced to sleep on the floor or in chairs. The situation may be compounded by poor hygiene regimens, exposing them to an increased risk of communicable diseases (Usatine et al, 1994). As Brickner et al (1993, p. 151) note, "The physical deterioration that results from trauma, inadequate nourishment, exposure, and the inability to remain clean creates a bodily environment that allows infection to occur more easily."

The nutritional status of homeless individuals significantly impacts their health status. Their diet is often high in calories, starches, and salt and limited in fruits and vegetables. Modified diets are frequently not possible in an environment that relies heavily on donations.

Access to health care means overcoming financial, transportation, physical, and psychological barriers. The homeless often rely on low visibility as a mechanism for survival. Contact with the traditional delivery system can also be very threatening for the care providers as well as for those who are homeless as some providers are very uncomfortable in working with clients whom they perceive as not utilizing the system appropriately or whom they believe to be "undesirable." (Gelberg, 1992).

## MEDICATION AND TREATMENT CONSIDERATIONS FOR MIGRANT WORKERS AND THE HOMELESS

Significant similarities exist between migrants and the homeless concerning medication and treatment considerations. Both populations perceive barriers between them and the services actually available to them, and neither are frequently able to comply fully with the management plan. Given the presenting complaints most commonly seen in a primary care setting, the clinician is confronted with significant is-

sues. (Table 15–1 highlights selected issues for the clinician who provides care to these populations). The client may present with a more advanced stage of illness. For migrants, this could reflect the varied cultural interpretation of the significance of the illness or injury. They may be hesitant to seek care given the possible impact on their employment. In general, the homeless do not seek care until there is little alternative because of the multiple barriers to care that exist (Brickner et al, 1993; Usatine et al, 1994).

Clinic location and appointment schedules are very important. Utilization of a clinic will depend on clinic hours being coordinated with other services that the populations utilize and limited waiting times.

These clients may also confront significant attitudinal barriers on the part of the health care provider or resource used. The practitioner must have both the interest and the skill to address the complex needs of the migrant or homeless client. The need for specialty referral or hospitalization may be "overlooked" even if required. Translation resources are often quite limited, making the investigation of the presenting complaint, the delineation of the differential diagnosis, and the development of the management plan flawed. The homeless population rarely trusts the traditional health care delivery system so development of nonthreatening relationships is essential.

Medication should be given to both the homeless and migrant workers rather than using prescriptions because of problems in their getting a prescription filled. Also consider the storage requirements of any medications. Nyamathi and Shuler (1989) completed a retrospective study of the factors affecting medication compliance of 61 homeless males sheltered at the Union Rescue Mission in Los Angeles. The study examined those factors that positively or negatively impacted the compliance with the medication regime as well as those that impacted perception of health. The most common reasons negatively affecting compliance with medication usage included the lack of privacy, lack of a storage area, the increased risk of medication being stolen, and the difficulty in obtaining medication. Refrigeration is frequently not available. Pills often are ground to powder while being carried. Consider also providing only enough medication to cover the individual until the next visit, as loss or sale of medication is quite common. Once-a-day dosing is the best option when possible (Brickner et al, 1993).

**TABLE 15–1. CONSIDERATIONS IN CHOOSING MEDICATION FOR MIGRANT AND HOMELESS POPULATIONS**

| Consideration | Action | Example* |
|---|---|---|
| Stage of illness—clients seek care when in more advanced stage. | Treat more aggressively with more broad-spectrum antibiotic. | Treat pneumonia with a cephalosporin if it is available in clinic. |
| Clinic location and structure; appointment schedule and hours | If client lives a distance from clinic or cannot return to clinic, treat more aggressively. | Treat child with borderline otitis media with whatever acceptable antibiotic is available in the clinic. If once-a-day medication (ie, Cipro) is available, use it. |
| Lack of acceptance in community or lack of translators | Avoid problematic community settings. If a pharmacy is known to treat migrant or homeless people with disrespect, find other alternatives. Develop a list of well-respected volunteers for translation and transportation, and to assist with community relations issues. | Women who have a yeast infection could be treated by over-the-counter Monistat. Clinic either provides the medicine or finds escort to the pharmacy to facilitate optimum outcome. |
| Difficulty in filling prescriptions | Provide medication rather than prescription. | Provide worker with low back pain with nonsteroidal antiinflammatory in appropriate doses with gastric-sparing teaching information. |
| Difficulty with multiple doses and medications requiring storage | Treat when possible with as few doses per day as available. If practical, give daily dose to patient at homeless shelter. | Give once-a-day medication to child with acute otitis media if clinic samples or voucher if program exists. First-line choice of medication is determined more by what's available, the budget of the clinic, and community resources. Although amoxicillin may be the drug of choice in noncomplicated situations, Cipro or another daily medication should be used if available. A recently approved single injection of ceftriaxone would be another available option. |
| Viral infection—increased risk of the development of a secondary bacterial infection. | Treat more aggressively. | Lower respiratory infections that may be viral need antibiotic treatment due to multiple risk factors. |

*These are clinical examples which reflect the chapter references and the clinical experiences of the author/editors.

Decisions regarding antibiotics for treatment of acute infections must include consideration of the cost of medication, the frequency of dosing, and the patient's ability to understand the use of the drug. For migrant workers particularly, considerations also include the worker's time in the fields, access there to food and water, and the risk of side effects related to sun exposure. Bear in mind that with some viral conditions there is great risk of a secondary bacterial infection. Since monitoring conditions and modifying lifestyle in terms of increased fluids and rest are difficult at best, antibiotics are often more frequently prescribed. The following clinical situation highlights some of the challenges faced by the clinician.

Anthony was a 37-year-old Caucasian male who presented at the clinic complaining of the "flu." He had noted nasal congestion and an intermittent productive cough for approximately 4 days. He described the sputum as white. He had not felt well but did not believe he had a fever. He was a one-pack-per-day smoker. He was sleeping at one of the temporary shelter sites and had been working the day labor pool. His physical exam was normal although an intermittent cough was noted. A chest x-ray was not easily available. The decision was made to use an oral antibiotic, as well as to administer a PPD (purified protein derivative).

Dermatologic conditions pose a real challenge with regard to pharmacotherapeutic intervention for the migrant population. Depending on the etiology of the condition, ongoing exposure to the irritant is a given. The availability of medication and the frequency of the dosage is a struggle. Adequate hygiene and appropriate dressing or protection from the elements may not be feasible.

As previously noted, the prevalence of untreated or undertreated chronic illness in both populations is quite high. Therefore, it is important to assess for chronic conditions whenever the client makes contact with the delivery system. The treatment of chronic conditions in both populations frequently does not reflect textbook standards because those guidelines are unrealistic.

Diabetes mellitus and hypertension are examples of this point. Treatment of these diseases requires continuity of care, monitoring, and lifestyle modifications to manage the conditions. The American Diabetic Association guidelines for diagnosis and treatment of diabetes requires monitoring of blood sugars and a stable living situation. As noted by Fleischman & Farnham (1992) and by Usatine et al (1994) attempting to control a diabetic homeless person is a dangerous goal since there is significant instability in eating and activity patterns. Syringes, alcohol swabs, and medication may be subject to theft or sale. Learning to inject oneself, monitoring one's condition, etc., require frequent visits and the development of a trusting relationship. Therefore, the goal is often moderate control of blood glucose without hypoglycemia, using oral hypoglycemics as much as possible.

With regard to hypertension, as noted by the Fifth Report of the Joint National Committee on Detection, Evaluation, and Treatment of High Blood Pressure (U.S. Department of Health and Human Services, 1993), recommen-dations for follow-up of an elevated initial set of blood pressure measurements range from immediate intervention to confirming an elevation within 2 months, depending on the initial reading. In the homeless population, there is an increased frequency of hypertension in younger individuals, and it is therefore wise to check blood pressure on all adults. Of course, several blood pressure readings at more frequent intervals is optimal for a more accurate assessment. Decisions about when to implement drug therapy must be carefully individualized in light of the increased risk of noncompliance, limited follow-up, and difficulty in modifying lifestyle in terms of diet, stress, and substance abuse. The choice of a drug should reflect the following considerations: once-a-day dosing if possible, limited need for laboratory monitoring (use a potassium-sparing diuretic when possible), and choice of a drug with no rebound phenomenon (Brickner et al, 1993; Fleischman & Farnham, 1992). Drugs worth considering for initial therapy include potassium-sparing diuretics and beta blockers. However, one must consider the fact that beta blockers are somewhat less effective in the African-American population and should be avoided in individuals with a history of asthma or chronic obstructive pulmonary disease (COPD). The following example highlights some of the challenges faced by the clinician in treatment of individuals with hypertension.

Alanzo is a 42-year-old Hispanic male who lives in one of the area's migrant camps. He was seen one week ago for a tooth abscess and at that time his blood pressure reading was 160/100 in his right arm and 162/98 in his left arm. When questioned about a history of hypertension, Alanzo noted that "a while back" someone had told him his blood pressure was high, but he had not filled the prescription. He did not remember if a cardiac evaluation had been completed. He denied a past medical history of asthma, diabetes mellitus, or COPD. He did not know a great deal about his family history but noted that his mother had a history of high blood pressure. He was a one-pack-per-day smoker. His alcohol intake varied. His blood pressure on repeat exam was 164/102 right arm, and 162/100 left arm. A physical examination and standard laboratory testing were completed. The client was started on a beta blocker and was asked to return to the clinic in 1 week.

To treat tuberculosis, the current guidelines (Centers for Disease Control, 1992) emphasize the value of *directly observed therapy*. (For a full discussion of tuberculosis, see Chapter 22.) Outpatient therapy should include isoniazid and rifampin, in addition to pyrazinamide and ethambutol for the first 2 months. Therapy should be modified based on the results of the drug susceptibility tests obtained on the positive cultures of the client. To achieve directly observed therapy with these transient groups, it is important to be able to provide housing and other supports; use incentives such as money, food coupons, and/or gifts; and develop a trusting relationship between the staff worker administering the therapy and the client to ensure completion of treatment (Jo, 1993).

## CONTINUITY OF CARE ISSUES

Given the nature of both populations, continuity of care poses significant challenges. The foundation of any therapeutic health provider–client relationship is openness and trust; however, the amount of time it takes to establish even limited levels can be quite lengthy. The transient nature of both populations, combined with rotational clinic staffing, often prohibits this.

Documentation can be very difficult since individuals may have limited knowledge of the specific details of their past medical histories. Obtaining copies of records takes time, and the client often does not remember the specific community or setting where a service was provided. The client may be hesitant to provide such historical information given a basic lack of trust in the traditional medical system. It is useful to provide the client with a copy of the records if you know or suspect the person is leaving the community.

## COMMUNITY RESOURCE IMPLICATIONS

Accessing the appropriate level of care and the appropriate medication for migrant workers or their families or those who are homeless poses significant challenges to the primary care provider. Since these groups tend to use the existing health care delivery system as a last resort, early intervention is generally not possible. The clients may also have one or more unmonitored, uncontrolled chronic illnesses. Substance abuse

or mental illness often compounds the difficulties in the provision of services. Further, these individuals struggle to prioritize health care needs with other basic needs for food, shelter, and clothing. Providing health care services in community settings where other basic services are available can decrease barriers to access (Gelberg, Gallagher, Anderson, & Koegel, 1997).

Accessing medication for these mostly uninsured groups can be time-consuming and frustrating. Advocacy groups, faith communities, and other community-based groups often devote immense time and effort to coordinating resources for medications. Provider networking within their communities is critical to the effective treatment of these vulnerable populations.

## REFERENCES

Allen, D. M., Lehman, J. S., Green, T. A., Lindegren, M. L., Onorato, I. M., Forrester, W., & the Field Services Branch. (1994). HIV infection among homeless adults and runaway youth, United States, 1989–1992. *AIDS, 8*, 1593–1598.

Barnes, P. F., El-Hajj, H., Preston-Martin, S., Cave, M. D., Jones, B. E., Otaya, M., Pogoda, J., & Eisenach, K. D. (1996). Transmission of tuberculosis among the urban homeless. *JAMA, 275*(4), 305–307.

Brickner, P. W., McAdam, J. M., Torres, R. A., Vicic, W. J., Conanan, B. A., Detrano, T., Piantieri, O., Scanlan, B., & Scharer, L. K. (1993). Providing health services for the homeless: A stitch in time. *Bulletin of the New York Academy of Medicine, 70*(3), 146–170.

Brudney, K. (1993). Homelessness and TB: A study in failure. *Journal of Law and Medical Ethics, 21*(3–4), 360–367.

Carter, K. F., Green, R. D., Green, L., & Dufour, L. T. (1994). Health needs of homeless clients accessing nursing care at a free clinic. *Journal of Community Health Nursing 11*(3), 139–147.

Centers for Disease Control (1992, April 17). *Prevention and control of tuberculosis in U.S. communities with at-risk minority populations and prevention and control of tuberculosis among homeless persons.* Recommendations of the Advisory Council for the Elimination of Tuberculosis. *MMWR, 14*, 1–23.

Fleischman, S., & Farnham, T. (1992). Chronic disease in the homeless. In D. Wood (Ed.), *Delivering health care to homeless persons.* New York: Springer.

Gelberg, L. (1992). Health of the homeless: Definition of problem. In D. Wood (Ed.),

*Delivering health care to homeless persons*. New York: Springer.

Gelberg, L., Gallagher, T. C., Anderson, R. M., & Koegel, P. (1997). Competing priorities as a barrier to medical care among homeless adults in Los Angeles. *American Journal of Public Health, 87*(2), 217–220.

Go, V., & Baker, T. (1995). Health problems of Maryland's migrant farm laborers. *Maryland Medical Journal, 44*(8), 605–608.

Hatton, D. C. (1997). Managing health problems among homeless women with children in a transitional shelter. *Image—The Journal of Nursing Scholarship, 29*(1), 33–37.

Hodnicki, D. R., & Horner, S. D. (1993). Homeless mothers' caring for children in a shelter. *Issues in Mental Health Nursing, 14*, 349–356.

Jo, H. S. (1993). Assessment and management of persons coinfected with tuberculosis and human immunodeficiency virus. *Nurse Practitioner, 18*(11), 42–49.

Kemsley, M., & Hunter, J. K. (1993). Homeless children and families: Clinical and research issues. *Issues in Comprehensive Pediatric Nursing, 16*(2), 99–108.

Killion, C. M. (1995). Special health care needs of homeless pregnant women. *Advances in Nursing Science, 18*(2), 44–56.

Link, B. G., Susser, E., Stueve, A., Phelan, J., Moore, R. E., & Struening, E. (1994). Lifetime and five-year prevalence of homelessness in the United States. *American Journal of Public Health, 84*(12), 1907–1912.

Martin, S. L., Gordon, T. E., & Kupersmidt, J. B. (1995). Survey of exposure to violence among the children of migrant and seasonal farm workers. *Public Health Reports, 110*(3), 268–276.

Mobed, K., Gold, E. B., & Schenker, M. B. (1992). Occupational health problems among migrant and seasonal farm workers. *Western Journal of Medicine, 157*, 367–373.

Murata, J., Mace, J. P., Strehlow, A., & Shuler, P. (1992). Disease patterns in homeless children:

A comparison with national data. *Journal of Pediatric Nursing, 7*(3), 196–204.

Norton, D., & Ridenour, N. (1995). Homeless women and children: The challenge of health promotion. *Nurse Practitioner Forum, 6*(1), 29–33.

Nyamathi, A., & Shuler, P. (1989). Factors affecting prescribed medication compliance of the urban homeless adult. *Nurse Practitioner, 14*(8), 47–54.

Poss, J. E., & Meeks, B. H. (1994). Meeting the health care needs of migrant farmworkers: The experience of the Niagara County migrant clinic. *Journal of Community Health Nursing, 11*(4), 219–228.

Redlener, I., & Karich, K. M. (1994). The homeless child health care inventory: Assessing the efficacy of linkages to primary care. *Bulletin of the New York Academy of Medicine, 71*(1), 37–48.

Rust, G. S. (1990). Health status of migrant farmworkers: A literature review and commentary. *American Journal of Public Health, 80*(10), 1213–1217.

Scholler-Jaquish, A. (1996). RN to BSN students in a walk-in health clinic for the homeless. *N & HC: Perspectives on Community, 17*(3), 119–123.

U.S. Department of Health and Human Services (1993). *The Fifth Report of the Joint National Committee on Detection, Evaluation, and Treatment of High Blood Pressure*. Washington, DC: National Institutes of Health.

Usatine, R. P., Gelberg, L., Smith, M. H. & Lesser, J. (1994). Health care for the homeless: A family medicine perspective. *American Family Physician, 49*(1), 139–146.

Wood, D. (1992). The evaluation and managment of homeless families and children. In D. Wood (Ed.), *Delivering health care to homeless persons*. New York: Springer.

Wood, D. L., Valdez, R. B., Hayashi, T., & Shen, A. (1990). Health of homeless children and housed, poor children. *Pediatrics, 86*(6), 858–866.

Wright, J. (1991). Children in and of the streets health. Social policy and the homeless young. *American Journal of Diseases of Children, 145*, 516–519.

# 16

# INDIVIDUALS WITH CHRONIC PAIN

*Cynthia J. Simonson and Lori W. Lush*

Each year, millions of Americans seek medical assistance for the relief of intolerable pain. Pain is often the symptom that motivates a patient to call his or her primary care practitioner. Pain researchers estimate that at any given time one tenth to one third of the population experiences chronic pain (Burckhardt, 1994). Despite the widespread prevalence of pain and the abundance of analgesic therapies, pain is generally undertreated and often ranks low on the medical treatment priority list. In an effort to establish better treatment of pain, the Agency for Health Care Policy and Research (AHCPR) of the Public Health Service developed evidence-based guidelines for the treatment of acute pain, cancer pain, and acute low back pain. These AHCPR guidelines are cited throughout this chapter and are excellent additions to the primary care practitioner's resource library.

This chapter includes subsections describing the four types of pain, the use of pain assessment tools, various nonpharmacologic analgesic interventions, and the pharmacologic treatments used in managing pain. A chronic pain treatment guideline is also presented. Although many of the concepts described can be used in the treatment of most other painful conditions, this chapter focuses primarily on the management of patients with chronic pain.

## PAIN TYPES

### ACUTE VERSUS CHRONIC PAIN

Pain can be classified as either acute or chronic, depending on its onset and duration. Acute pain has an easily defined onset and is transient, occurring only between the time of tissue injury and tissue recovery. Acute pain serves a major medical function by alerting patients and clinicians that tissue damage may exist (Bushnell & Justins, 1993). For a thorough review of the management of acute pain, please refer to the AHCPR Acute Pain Management Guideline (Acute Pain Management Guideline Panel, 1992).

Although acute pain is a symptom of another medical condition, chronic pain is a syndrome in its own right (Bushnell & Justins, 1993). Chronic pain persists or recurs over an extended period of time and interferes with the patient's functioning. Clinicians may not be able to explain the origin of a chronic pain, and thus patients may be told that the pain is "in their head." Unlike acute pain, chronic pain serves no useful medical function (Burckhardt, 1994). The personality changes that can occur in patients experiencing chronic pain include feelings of helplessness, hopelessness, and meaninglessness (Bushnell & Justins, 1993). Patients become increasingly depressed and dysfunctional, and may suffer a diminished quality of life (Burckhardt, 1994).

Unlike acute pain, the goals of treating chronic pain are not to eliminate the pain completely, but to teach the patient coping mechanisms, increase the patient's level of functioning, and attempt to reduce pain to its most tolerable level (Rowlingson, 1992). This can be a challenging process involving numerous trials of different pharmacologic and nonpharmacologic interventions (Portenoy, 1996).

## NOCICEPTIVE VERSUS NEUROPATHIC PAIN

Pain also can be classified by its source; it is either nociceptive or neuropathic. Nociceptive pain is the result of stimulation of pain receptors, called nociceptors, located throughout the body (Portenoy, 1996). Nociceptive pain can be further subdivided into somatic and visceral pain. Somatic nociceptive pain originates from the skin or skin structures and is dull and aching in quality. This type of pain is well localized to a specific area of the body. Tendinitis, post surgical pain, and musculoskeletal pain are examples of somatic nociceptive pain. Visceral nociceptive pain originates from the internal organs as a result of infiltration, compression, or stretching of these tissues. Visceral nociceptive pain is difficult to localize and is often referred to sites distant from the site of origin. Myocardial infarction pain, referred to the arm and shoulder, is a classic example of visceral nociceptive pain (Caraceni, 1996). Nociceptive pain of either subgroup responds well to nonsteroidal antiinflammatory agents and opioids alone or in combination (Barenholtz & Bellamy, 1995).

Neuropathic pain originates from compression or injury to a peripheral nerve fiber or the central nervous system. Patients describe this type of pain as shooting, electrical, or burning in nature. Postherpetic neuralgia, trigeminal neuralgia, and diabetic neuropathy are examples of neuropathic pain syndromes. In general, neuropathic pain is less responsive to commonly used analgesic medication classes. Adjunct analgesics including antidepressants, anticonvulsants, and antiarrhythmics may be required in the treatment of this type of pain (Barenholtz & Bellamy, 1995).

Although the four previously mentioned pain types are distinct, all may be present in a patient simultaneously. This is particularly true in patients with cancer pain or geriatric patients with multiple health problems. To provide maximal pain relief, combinations of interventions may be necessary, particularly when different pain types coexist (Bushnell & Justins, 1993).

## PAIN ASSESSMENT

Pain is a subjective experience with both physical and psychologic elements. The expression of pain may or may not be related directly to the presence or degree of physical injury. Its expression is influenced by psychosocial, cultural, genetic, biochemical, and religious factors. Since pain is experiential, the best way to assess pain is to listen to and believe the patient. The AHCPR Cancer Pain Management Guideline recommends the following assessment guidelines:

- Health professionals should ask about pain and believe the patient's report.
- The initial evaluation of pain should include a detailed history, including an assessment of pain intensity and characteristics, a physical assessment emphasizing the neurologic examination, and a psychosocial assessment.
- Pain should be assessed with easily administered rating scales and should document the efficacy of management plans.
- Changes in pain patterns or the development of new pain should trigger a diagnostic evaluation and modification of the treatment plan.

## NONPHARMACOLOGIC ANALGESIC THERAPIES

Many nonpharmacologic analgesic treatments are available and can be very useful in the treatment of chronic pain. The AHCPR Cancer Pain Management Guidelines recommend that because of the many misconceptions about pain and its treatment, education for patients and their families should be a part of all management strategies. Information should be given about the ability to effectively control pain, and myths about opioids should be corrected. It is also recommended that psychosocial interventions be included early in the course of pain management, but that they not be used as substitutes for analgesics. Information about support groups, community resources, and spiritual support should be included. Patients should be encouraged to report the occurrence of new pain to their health care practitioner before seeking palliation from modalities such as acupuncture, massage therapy, and healing touch therapy.

Nonpharmacologic therapies can be divided into two groups: counterirritation or psychological methods (Twycross, 1994). Counterirritation includes treatments such as massage, chemicals applied to the skin, cold, heat, transcutaneous electrical nerve stimulation (TENS), vibration, and acupuncture (Twycross, 1994; McCaffery, 1989; Rhiner et al, 1993, Smith et al, 1990). Psychological methods include distraction, imagery, meditation, relaxation, art or music therapy, hypnosis, biofeedback, cognitive-behavioral therapy, and psychodynamic therapies (Twycross, 1994; McCaffery, 1989; Rhiner, 1993; Smith, 1990; & Loscalzo, 1996). A third category called energies could be added and would include treatments such as healing touch therapy. (Wytias, 1994; Malkin, 1994; Krieger, 1990).

These nonpharmacologic treatments sometimes can be adequate alone. They are most often used in conjunction with analgesics and other nonpharmacologic treatments. Not all patients find these treatments beneficial, but they almost always should be given a trial.

## PHARMACOLOGIC ANALGESIC THERAPIES

### ASPIRIN, SALICYLATES, AND NONSTEROIDAL ANTIINFLAMMATORY DRUGS

Nonsteroidal antiinflammatory drugs (NSAIDs) are among the most frequently prescribed analgesic medications (Brooks & Day, 1991). NSAIDs inhibit the enzyme cyclooxygenase to prevent prostaglandin and thromboxane synthesis. Prostaglandins sensitize nociceptors and decrease the pain threshold to pain mediators such as bradykinin, substance P, and histamine (Paice & Citari, 1997). By suppressing the actions of prostaglandins, NSAIDs produce analgesia and have antiinflammatory properties (Levy & Smith, 1989).

NSAIDs are generally used for the treatment of mild to moderate pain (Management, 1994). They are considered first-line therapy in most rheumatic disorders (Willkens, 1992). NSAIDs

are commonly used in combination with other analgesic medications, such as opioids. Combining opioids and NSAIDs produces greater pain relief than when either modality is used alone. In addition, NSAIDs have an opiate-sparing effect that allows lower doses of opioids to be used (Acute Pain Management, 1992).

Over 20 NSAIDs are commercially available. Many are now available in less costly over-the-counter or generic forms (see Drug Table 306). Thus far, no study has shown one NSAID to be more efficacious than another (Willkens, 1992). However, there is a significant interpatient variability in response (American Pain Society [APS], 1992). If an NSAID of one structural class is not effective at maximally tolerable doses, a trial of a second NSAID of a different structural class may be beneficial (APS, 1992; Levy, 1996) (see Drug Table 306). A patient may need therapeutic trials with several NSAIDs before one is found that is effective and tolerable (Levy & Smith, 1989).

Adverse effects produced by NSAIDs can be grouped into two categories: those mediated through inhibition of prostaglandin synthesis and those considered idiosyncratic (Willkens, 1992). In addition to their role in pain and inflammation, prostaglandins perform many protective functions throughout the body (Kenny, 1992). In the gastrointestinal tract, prostaglandins protect the gastric mucosa by increasing mucous production and inhibiting gastric acid output (Willkens, 1992). Vasodilatory prostaglandins protect the kidneys by ensuring renal blood flow and regulating fluid and electrolyte excretion (Brooks & Day, 1991). Thromboxane $A_2$ and prostaglandin endoperoxidases are involved in platelet aggregation (Kenny, 1992). By inhibiting the synthesis of these prostaglandins, use of NSAIDs can lead to gastrointestinal upset and ulceration, compromised renal function, and platelet inhibition. Bronchospasm may also occur with the use of NSAIDs because of the inhibition of bronchodilating leukotrienes (Willkens, 1992).

Dermatitis, central nervous system effects, hepatitis, acute interstitial nephritis, and hepatotoxicity are a few of the idiosyncratic reactions that have been reported by patients receiving NSAIDs (Willkens, 1992). The incidence of allergic reactions to NSAIDs is small. However, 5–10% of adult asthmatics are aspirin-sensitive (Kenny, 1992). Aspirin-sensitive patients should also avoid NSAIDs due to the possibility of cross-reactions (APS, 1992).

Although all NSAIDs produce similar adverse effects, there are slight differences in the severity of these reactions (Levy & Smith, 1989). Ibuprofen and nonacetylated salicylates produce fewer gastrointestinal adverse effects than aspirin (Management, 1994; Levy, 1996). With regard to platelet inhibition, aspirin irreversibly binds thromboxane synthetase and affects platelet aggregation for the life of the platelet (ie, 4–7 days) (Management of Cancer Pain, 1994; Levy, 1996), whereas NSAIDs transiently inhibit platelet aggregation and nonacetylated salicylates have little or no antiplatelet effect (APS, 1992; Management, 1994; Levy, 1996). Studies suggest sulindac and piroxicam are more renal-sparing and piroxicam and meclofenamate produce fewer hepatic effects (Levy & Smith, 1989).

There are also differences among NSAIDs in their pharmacokinetic profiles. Piroxicam and oxaprozin have long half-lives that allow once-daily dosing (see Drug Table 306). In patients who have trouble remembering to take their medications, choosing an agent with a long half-life can help to increase medication compliance (Levy & Smith, 1989). However, NSAIDs with long half-lives have a greater incidence of gastrointestinal injury due to constant prostaglandin suppression. Choosing an NSAID with a shorter half-life (eg, ibuprofen) may be more appropriate in high-risk patients (Pitner, Wiley, & Pennypacker, 1994).

NSAIDs have a ceiling effect. Each NSAID has a maximum dose beyond which there is no additional analgesic benefit (APS, 1992) (see Drug Table 306). Within the dosing range, the dose required to produce analgesia is generally smaller than that needed for the NSAIDs' antiinflammatory effects (Levy & Smith, 1989).

NSAIDs are an integral part of the management of mild to moderate pain and should be used unless there is a contraindication (APS, 1992). Efficacy being equal, over-the-counter availability, generic availability, cost, adverse effect profiles, and pharmacokinetic differences become the primary determinants in drug selection.

## ACETAMINOPHEN

Acetaminophen is widely used for the relief of mild to moderate pain (Bushnel & Justins, 1993). According to the AHCPR Guidelines, acetaminophen is the safest most effective treatment for acute low back pain (Acute Low Back, 1994). Acetaminophen works centrally, through inhibition of the cyclooxygenase enzyme (Bushnel & Justins, 1993). The analgesic potency of acetaminophen, aspirin and NSAIDs is comparable (Management, 1994). However, unlike aspirin and the NSAIDs, acetaminophen has no antiinflammatory properties (Bushnell & Justins, 1993).

Acetaminophen produces very few adverse reactions (see Drug Table 301). Unlike aspirin and the NSAIDs, it does not cause gastrointestinal adverse effects and does not affect platelet function (APS, 1992; Bushnell & Justins 1993; Levy, 1996). Acetaminophen may be used in aspirin-sensitive patients (Hillier, 1990). Because of the association between aspirin and Reye's syndrome, acetaminophen is the analgesic and antipyretic of choice in children (Bushnel & Justins, 1993). The most serious adverse effect of acetaminophen is dose-related hepatotoxicity. Acetaminophen undergoes a saturable metabolic process. Beyond the saturation point, an alternative hepatotoxic metabolite is formed (Bushnell & Justins, 1993). To avoid hepatotoxicity, the manufacturer recommends limiting the maximum daily acetaminophen dose to 4 g (Paice & Citari, 1997; Levy, 1996). Patients with chronic alcoholism or liver disease are more susceptible to hepatotoxicity and may experience liver damage at lower acetaminophen doses (APS, 1992).

Acetaminophen is available over-the-counter in a variety of generic formulations. It is available in both oral and rectal preparations (see Drug Table 301). Because of its attractive adverse effect profile, relatively low cost, and comparable analgesic efficacy, acetaminophen is an acceptable first-line treatment for many painful conditions (Hillier, 1990).

## OPIOIDS

Opioids are used in the treatment of moderate to severe pain (Acute Pain Management, 1992). Opioids are commonly used in the postoperative and malignant pain settings. Although the routine use of opioids in nonmalignant pain is controversial, opioids are an acceptable alternative for other analgesic interventions that have been ineffective (Barenholtz & Bellamy, 1995).

Opioids produce their pharmacologic and adverse effects through binding to opioid receptors throughout the central nervous system and peripheral tissues (Acute Pain Management, 1992). There are three types of opioid receptors: mu, kappa, and delta. The mu receptor is considered the prototypical opioid receptor (Acute Pain Management, 1992; Cherny, 1996). When stimulated, the mu receptor produces analgesia, miosis, euphoria, reduced gastrointestinal motility, respiratory depression, urinary retention, sedation, nausea, tolerance, and physical dependence (Acute Pain Management, 1992; Cherny, 1996). Kappa receptor stimulation produces analgesia, dysphoria, psychotomimetic effects, miosis, and respiratory depression. Stimulation of the delta opioid receptor produces analgesia without respiratory depression (Cherny, 1996).

Opioids are classified as controlled substances by the Food and Drug Administration (FDA). As such, there is a known potential for abuse. When prescribing, monitoring, and counseling patients about opioid therapy, it is important to differentiate between the terms tolerance, physical dependence, and psychological dependence (Management, 1994). Tolerance and physical dependence are normal physiologic changes that occur in most patients who receive opioids for more than 1 month (APS, 1992). Tolerance is defined as the need for a higher dose, after repeated administration, to maintain the same effect (Cherny & Foley, 1996). Physical dependence occurs when the body becomes accustomed to receiving opioids. If the opioids are withdrawn, the body will exhibit withdrawal symptoms within 6–72 h. To avoid opioid withdrawal, the dose of opioids should be slowly tapered (25% reduction in dose every other day) upon drug discontinuation (APS, 1992). Psychological dependence, or addiction, indicates that the patient is taking the medication for reasons other than its intended use. This occurrence is not a characteristic of the drug class alone, but is a combined effect of biochemical, societal, and psychological factors affecting the patient (APS, 1992).

Opioids are classified by their ability to stimulate or block opioid receptors (Acute Pain Management, 1992). Pure agonists include morphine, codeine, dihydrocodeine, hydrocodone, oxycodone propoxyphene, hydromorphone, methadone, meperidine, oxymorphone, levorphanol, and fentanyl. These medications exert their action primarily by stimulation of the mu opioid receptor. Unlike NSAIDs, pure opioid agonists do not have a ceiling effect; additional analgesia may be obtained by increasing the opioid dose (Management, 1994).

Buprenorphine is the only commercially available partial agonist. It is a partial agonist at the mu opioid receptor, but an antagonist at the kappa receptor (Cherny, 1996). Compared to the pure agonists, buprenorphine is less effective and has an analgesic ceiling effect (Management, 1994). If given to a patient receiving high doses of a pure opioid agonist, withdrawal symptoms may occur (APS, 1992). This is due to buprenorphine's relatively lower analgesic potency and its displacement of the pure agonist at the opioid receptor sites (Cherny, 1996).

Mixed agonist-antagonists include pentazocine, butorphanol, dezocine, and nalbuphine (Foley, 1982). These agents are agonists at the kappa receptor and weak antagonists at the mu receptor (Cherny, 1996). Patients who are opioid-tolerant should not be given a mixed agonist-antagonist. The mu antagonism of the mixed agents risks opioid withdrawal symptoms (Management, 1994). Similar to partial agonists, mixed agonist-antagonists have an analgesic ceiling effect (Acute Pain Management, 1992). Because of their primary kappa receptor stimulation, these agents are known to produce psychotomimetic effects (Cherny, 1996). The role of these agents in the treatment of severe pain and chronic pain is limited (Foley, 1982).

Naloxone and naltrexone are opioid antagonists. All opioid receptor types are blocked by these agents. The primary role of the opioid antagonists is to displace opioid agonists from their receptor sites to reverse opioid-induced adverse effects (Cherny, 1996).

Opioids can also be grouped by the severity of pain in which they are used. Codeine, dihydrocodeine, hydrocodone, and propoxyphene are less potent and are used in the treatment of moderate pain (Cherny & Foley, 1996). Although a few of these agents are available as single-entity preparations, most are combined with aspirin or acetaminophen. The acetaminophen content in the combination products limits the ability to escalate the dose (APS, 1992). These agents are short-acting and must be dosed frequently (ie, every 2–4 h) (Cherny, 1996).

Opioids used for severe pain can be grouped by their duration of action. Morphine, oxycodone, oxymorphone, hydromorphone, meperidine, and fentanyl are short-acting agents (Cherny, 1996). Morphine is the prototypical opioid. It is used as a standard of comparison for all other opioids (Bushnell & Justins, 1993).

Morphine is available in many formulations and is the most cost-effective opioid choice (Rowlingson, 1992; Management, 1994). Hydromorphone is more potent than morphine. Because of its high solubility and potency, hydromorphone is often used for subcutaneous administration of relatively high opioid doses (APS, 1992). Meperidine is considerably less potent than morphine and is converted to a neurotoxic metabolite. This agent has no role in the treatment of chronic pain (APS, 1992). Of the short-acting opioids, morphine (MS Contin, Kadian, Oramorph SR), oxycodone (OxyContin), and fentanyl (Duragesic Patches) are formulated in sustained-release preparations to increase patient convenience and to provide a constant level of pain relief (Cherny, 1996).

Methadone and levorphanol are potent, long-acting, pure opioid agonists. Methadone is used in the prevention of opioid withdrawal for patients that are physically dependent on opioids. When used in this capacity, methadone is usually given once daily. Patients receiving methadone for analgesic purposes may require dosing every 4–8 h. These medications are not considered first-line agents because of the difficulty in rapidly titrating to an effective dose (Cherny, 1996).

Methadone, however, is considered a second choice drug in the management of cancer pain. Methadone has a number of unique characteristics including excellent oral and rectal absorption, no known active metabolites, high potency, low cost, and longer administration intervals, as well as an incomplete cross-tolerance with respect to other mu-opioid receptor agonist drugs (Ripamonti, 1997). However, its use is limited by the remarkably long and unpredictable half-life, large inter-individual variations in pharmacokinetics, the potential for delayed side effects, and the limited knowledge of correct administration intervals and the equianalgesic ratio with other opioids when administered chronically (Ripamonti, 1997). Serious adverse effects can be avoided if the initial titration is done on an as needed basis. When a steady state of pain control with tolerable side effects has been reached, an around-the-clock schedule can be established based on the 24h dose needed for good pain control (Cherny & Foley, 1996).

Adverse effects that may occur with the use of opioid medications include nausea and vomiting, sedation, constipation, urinary retention, pruritus, and respiratory depression (Management, 1994). Nausea, vomiting, and sedation occur early in therapy or immediately after a dosage increase. Tolerance develops quickly to these effects (Cherny, 1996). Patients who have a history of experiencing opioid-induced nausea and vomiting may require scheduled antiemetics for the first several days of opioid therapy until tolerance occurs (Management, 1994). If sedation is problematic, smaller, more frequent doses may be used (Cherny, 1996). Stimulant medications, such as caffeine and methylphenidate, have been administered to counteract sedation in cancer pain patients receiving high doses of opioids, (APS, 1992; Cherny, 1996).

Constipation is the most frequently reported adverse effect with the chronic use of opioids (Cherny & Foley, 1996). Unlike other opioid-induced adverse effects, tolerance does not develop to constipation (Cherny, 1996). Patients should be given a stimulant laxative (senna, bisacodyl, or phenolphthalein) and possibly a stool softener (docusate) on a routine basis (Cherny, 1996). Osmotic laxatives (lactulose, magnesium citrate) or bowel preparations, such as Golytely, may be needed intermittently. Oral naloxone can be given for refractory constipation. Naloxone is not well absorbed by the oral route; therefore, the risk of precipitating opioid withdrawal is small. If patients experience nausea, early satiety, and bloating, these may be signs of delayed gastric emptying and the use of metoclopramide or cisapride may be helpful (Cherny & Foley, 1996).

Urinary retention and pruritus are more commonly seen when opioids are administered by the epidural or intrathecal route. Bear in mind that antidepressants also cause urinary retention and may be a contributing factor when opioids and antidepressants are combined (Management, 1994). Pruritus may also be treated with antihistamines (APS, 1992).

The most serious and most feared opioid-induced adverse reaction is respiratory depression. Clinically significant respiratory depression is rare when opioids are given to patients who are experiencing acute pain (Bushnell & Justins, 1993). Patients receiving opioids chronically rarely experience this effect since tolerance develops to respiratory depression (APS, 1992). Signs of central nervous system depression accompany respiratory depression and include somnolence, unarousability, mental confusion, and slowed respiratory rate. Since its use will precipitate withdrawal in the opioid-dependent patient, naloxone should be reserved for potentially life-threatening situations (Cherny, 1996).

When naloxone is required, the dose should be titrated slowly to response (0.4 mg diluted with 10 mL saline given intravenously in 0.5-cc increments every 2 min) (APS, 1992).

Opioids may be administered by many routes of administration, including subcutaneous, intramuscular, intravenous, epidural, intrathecal, oral, buccal, sublingual, transnasal, transdermal, rectal, and by inhalation (Acute Pain Management, 1992; Bushnell & Justins, 1993; Cherny, 1996). Patients who are unable to take oral medications to reach a tolerable dose orally have many available options. The least invasive, most cost-effective method should be tried before moving to more invasive techniques. In general, the oral route of administration is preferred because of its convenience and lower cost (Acute Pain Management, 1992). Intramuscular injections should be avoided; they are painful and the medication is erratically absorbed from the site of administration (Management, 1994).

Fortunately, unlike other analgesic classes, opioids have well-accepted equianalgesic doses, which allows the clinician to convert between agents and between routes of administration. Most opioids require a dosage increase when converting from the parenteral to the oral route. Close monitoring after an opioid conversion or dosage change is required to evaluate the need for further dosage adjustments (Hillier, 1990).

A method commonly used after titrating to a relatively stable opioid dose is to prescribe one long-acting agent and one "as needed" short-acting agent. The long-acting opioid (sustained-release morphine, oxycodone, methadone, or levorphanol) should be used on a scheduled basis, with "as needed" short-acting medications prescribed for pain that is not relieved by the scheduled dose (APS, 1992). The "as needed" or breakthrough dose should be approximately 15–50% of the total daily scheduled medication dose. Patients who routinely require frequent breakthrough doses within a dosing interval (eg, more than two doses in 4 h or more than six doses in 24 h) need an increase in their scheduled medication. The goal of this technique is to maintain a constant level of pain relief with the scheduled medication, while only occasionally requiring the breakthrough medication (Cherny, 1996).

## ANTIDEPRESSANTS

Tricyclic antidepressants are the drugs of choice for many patients with chronic pain, particularly those in whom commonly used analgesic agents have proven ineffective (Burckhardt, 1994). Antidepressants have been used in a variety of chronic pain conditions including cancer pain, tension and migraine headache, postherpetic neuralgia, diabetic neuropathy, arthritis, and low back pain (Egbunike & Chaffee, 1990). Although antidepressants have been used in treating many painful conditions, they are most effective in treating burning neuropathic pain states (McQuay, 1988).

The precise mechanism of the analgesic action of antidepressants is not understood. Initially, antidepressants were thought to provide analgesia simply by relieving depression. Subsequent studies found antidepressants produced analgesia in nondepressed patients, demonstrating that antidepressants possess an analgesic activity independent of their antidepressant action (Burckhardt, 1994). Antidepressants are believed to produce analgesia by inhibiting the reuptake of serotonin and norepinephrine, neurotransmitters involved in the descending inhibitory pain pathway (McQuay, 1988).

Antidepressants are considered "dirty" drugs in that they interact with or affect many receptors and neurotransmitters in the body. Although these interactions produce the desired pharmacologic effects, they also lead to many adverse effects (Kehoe & Jacisin, 1992).

Many antidepressants are marketed today. The first-generation, older agents have cyclic structures. Cyclic antidepressants are categorized as either tertiary or secondary amines. In general, compounds with tertiary amine structures (eg, amitriptyline, imipramine, and doxepin) possess more serotonergic activity than noradrenergic activity. Conversely, secondary amines (eg, nortriptyline, desipramine, and protriptyline) preferentially affect norepinephrine to a greater extent than serotonin (Magni, 1991).

Second-generation, newer antidepressants (eg, trazodone, nefazodone, bupropion, and the selective serotonin reuptake inhibitors, such as fluoxetine, paroxetine, sertraline, and fluvoxamine) are structurally unrelated to the cyclic antidepressants and are more selective in the receptors and neurotransmitters they affect. These agents have not been used as extensively in the treatment of pain as the cyclic antidepressants. There is a theory that the "dirtier" antidepressant medications are more effective analgesics (Magni, 1991). This appears to be true since the second-generation antidepressants appear less effective than the cyclic compounds (McQuay, 1988).

Adverse effects caused by antidepressants include anticholinergic, cardiovascular, and central nervous system effects (American Psychiatric Association [APA], 1993). In general, tertiary amines appear to produce more adverse effects than secondary amines, and the second-generation antidepressants are better tolerated (Preskorn, 1994).

Anticholinergic adverse effects are the most common and also the most bothersome produced by this medication class. These include blurred vision, constipation, urinary retention, and dry mouth. Sugarless gum or candy may help relieve dry mouth. Pharmacologic interventions, including pilocarpine eye drops (blurred vision), hydration and bulk laxatives (constipation), and bethanechol (urinary retention) may be required to counteract these effects (APA, 1993).

Antidepressants affect the cardiovascular system through several mechanisms: alpha receptor blockade, blockade of norepinephrine reuptake, and through an antiarrhythmic effect similar to the type I antiarrhythmic medication quinidine (APA, 1993). Orthostatic hypotension caused by alpha receptor blockade can be a significant problem, occurring in approximately 20% of patients (Kehoe & Jacisin, 1992). Less orthostasis has been reported with the use of nortriptyline (APA, 1993).

Because of their interactions with histamine receptors, certain antidepressants (eg, amitriptyline, imipramine, doxepin, and trazodone) can cause central nervous system sedation. This "adverse reaction" may be beneficial in the patient with pain and insomnia. Conversely, the selective serotonin reuptake inhibitor fluoxetine produces central nervous system stimulation and may lead to insomnia (Kehoe & Jacisin, 1992).

Seizures are one of the more serious central nervous system adverse effects seen in patients receiving antidepressants. Antidepressants lower the seizure threshold. Patients at risk for experiencing seizures (ie, patients with epilepsy or head injuries, patients who receive concomitant seizure-threshold–reducing medications such as phenothiazines, substance abusers, or patients who experience withdrawal from alcohol or sedatives/hypnotics) should be monitored closely (Kehoe & Jacisin, 1992).

Other adverse reactions produced by antidepressants include weight changes and sexual dysfunction. Weight gain may occur with tricyclic antidepressants, whereas weight loss is more common with fluoxetine and other selective serotonin reuptake inhibitors. Sexual dysfunction has been reported with all antidepressant classes (APA, 1993).

Amitriptyline has been the most widely studied antidepressant for its analgesic properties (APS, 1992). Because of this, it should be considered the first-line agent (Management, 1994). However, because it is a tertiary amine with many adverse reactions, certain patient populations (eg, patients with benign prostatic hypertrophy, narrow-angle glaucoma, significant cardiovascular problems, and the elderly) may not be able to tolerate amitriptyline's adverse effect profile. These patients may require a secondary amine cyclic antidepressant or a second-generation antidepressant with fewer adverse effects (APS, 1992; Barenholtz & Bellamy, 1995).

Doses of antidepressants for pain management are lower than those used for depression (APS, 1992). Small doses should be started initially (ie, 10–25 mg of amitriptyline or doxepin) and then increased in small increments (10–25 mg) at 2–4-day intervals to an effective dose (approximately 75–150 mg) (Management, 1994). When used for their analgesic properties, most antidepressants should be given as a single bedtime dose, taking advantage of the sedating properties while minimizing bothersome anticholinergic properties that peak during sleep (APS, 1992). Often, early morning oversedation will subside in the first weeks of treatment (APA, 1993). Be cognizant of the potential for nocturnal orthostatic hypotension, especially in elderly patients, when the entire daily dose is given at bedtime (APS, 1992).

The onset of analgesic action is variable, occurring from a few days to several weeks after therapy is initiated (McQuay, 1988). Therapeutic analgesic serum concentrations have not been established (Barenholtz & Bellamy, 1995). If a patient is being evaluated for therapeutic failure, a drug level may be drawn to rule out noncompliance or bioavailability problems (Kehoe & Jacisin, 1992). If a patient has a therapeutic failure with an antidepressant of one structural class, a medication in another class may be tried (APA, 1993).

Matching the medication to the patient is somewhat of a challenge because of the many intolerable adverse effects of these medications. Antidepressants used as analgesic adjuvants generally are not completely effective and are rarely used as single drug therapy (Barenholtz & Bellamy, 1995). However, antidepressants have an alternative mechanism of action that when combined with other analgesic medication classes, may provide additional pain relief.

## ANTICONVULSANTS

Anticonvulsants are used in the treatment of many neuropathic pain syndromes (Barenholtz & Bellamy, 1995). Overall, these agents are more effective in treating neuropathic pain that is shooting or electrical in quality (Bushnel & Justins, 1993). In this setting, the two most commonly used anticonvulsants are carbamazepine and phenytoin (Portenoy, 1996). Valproic acid and clonazepam have also been studied as analgesic adjuvants (Management, 1994). Among these medications, only carbamazepine has FDA labeling for the treatment of a painful condition, trigeminal neuralgia (Barenholtz & Bellamy, 1995).

Anticonvulsants are believed to exert their analgesic activity by inhibiting aberrant nerve firing, leading to neural membrane stabilization. However, the specific mechanism by which each anticonvulsant provides membrane stabilization differs (McQuay, 1988). Carbamazepine is more effective than phenytoin and should be considered the drug of choice (Barenholtz & Bellamy, 1995).

The recommended starting dose of carbamazepine is 100 mg twice daily. Due to rate-limiting sedation, the dose must be gradually increased to effect. A dose range of 200–1600 mg daily is generally effective. Carbamazepine induces its own metabolism. After a few weeks of therapy, an increase in carbamazepine dosage may be required because of increased drug clearance (Barenholtz & Bellamy, 1995).

If phenytoin is used, the initial dose is 300 mg of the sustained-release preparation, given once daily (Barenholtz & Bellamy, 1995). Phenytoin undergoes Michaelis-Menten nonlinear pharmacokinetics. Upon reaching its metabolism saturable point, small dosage increases will lead to large increases in drug concentration and possibly toxicity (Graves, 1993). Symptoms that occur at a concentration near the upper limit or above the therapeutic range include nystagmus, slurred speech, ataxia, and confusion (Barenholtz & Bellamy, 1995). To avoid toxicity, small incremental dosage adjustments of phenytoin are required, especially when nearing the upper limit of the therapeutic range (Graves, 1993).

Analgesia should begin to occur within the first few days of therapy. After several months of use, the patient should be weaned from the anticonvulsant medication. If pain recurs, the medication can be reinstituted (Barenholtz & Bellamy, 1995).

In rare instances, carbamazepine and phenytoin have caused hepatic dysfunction, neutropenia, and thrombocytopenia. Liver function tests and complete blood counts should be monitored at baseline and intermittently for the first few months of therapy (Barenholtz & Bellamy, 1995). Patients should be instructed to contact their primary care practitioner or pharmacist if they experience fever, sore throat, flu-like symptoms, bruising, or jaundice. Since chronic use of phenytoin can lead to gingival hyperplasia, patients receiving phenytoin should be encouraged to use good oral hygiene (Barenholtz & Bellamy, 1995).

A relationship between concentration and analgesic effect has not been clearly established for the anticonvulsants. Generally, the same therapeutic range used for management of seizures has been used in the treatment of pain. When these medications are used as analgesic adjuvants, drug concentrations are rarely used to monitor therapy. As with the antidepressants, drug concentrations should be used to avoid toxicities and to monitor compliance (Barenholtz & Bellamy, 1995).

## ANTIARRHYTHMICS

The antiarrhythmic agents mexiletine and lidocaine are used in the management of severe neuropathic pain (Management, 1994). Lidocaine and mexiletine block sodium channels to inhibit aberrant nerve firing. Because these agents selectively inhibit hyperactive neurons, healthy neuronal discharge is unaffected (Barenholtz & Bellamy, 1995). Mexiletine can be initiated at an oral dose of 150 mg daily for 7 days. If tolerated, it is increased to 150 mg t.i.d. If relief is inadequate, the dose can be titrated every 5–7 days to a maximum of 1200 mg per day (on a b.i.d. to t.i.d. schedule) (Paice & Citari, 1997; Portenoy, 1994). Gastrointestinal side effects and tremor are dose-related adverse effects. To lessen gastrointestinal upset, patients may take mexiletine with food. As with the anticonvulsants and antidepressants, a concentration-response relationship for analgesia has not been established and routine drug concentration sampling is not indicated (Barenholtz & Bellamy, 1995).

## CORTICOSTEROIDS

Corticosteroids have antiinflammatory properties that make them useful in the management of many painful conditions. Corticosteroids exert their antiinflammatory properties through inhibiting leukotriene and prostaglandin synthesis. The most common use of corticosteroids is in the treatment of nerve compression pain in patients with cancer (Bushnell & Justins, 1993).

## GENERAL TREATMENT GUIDELINES

The following points describe strategies used in the management of patients with chronic pain.

- Always believe your patient's report of pain and communicate that belief (Management, 1994).
- Keep the regimen as simple and as cost-effective as possible.
- Use the oral route of administration whenever possible because of its convenience and lower cost (Acute Pain Management, 1992).
- Individualize the analgesic regimen for each patient (Management, 1994).
- Maximize the dose of each medication before declaring it a therapeutic failure.
- Analgesic medication should be given on a scheduled basis. It is easier to prevent pain than to control pain of a higher intensity (Acute Pain Management, 1992).
- For patients with chronic, nonmalignant pain, maximize all other therapies before opting for an opioid (Barenholtz & Bellamy, 1995).
- For mild pain, patients should receive either acetaminophen, aspirin, or an NSAID (Management, 1994).
- For moderate pain, or if mild pain persists or increases, a pure opioid analgesic used to treat moderate pain (eg, codeine or hydrocodone) should be added to the previous step (Management, 1994).
- For severe pain, or if moderate pain persists or increases, the dosage of the opioid should be increased or the patient should be converted to a more potent opioid agonist (eg, morphine or oxycodone) (Management, 1994).

- An analgesic adjuvant (eg, antidepressant or anticonvulsant) can be used at any point in therapy, if appropriate (Management, 1994).

## REFERENCES

Acute Low Back Problems in Adults Clinical Practice Guideline Panel. (1994). *Acute Low Back Problems in Adults. Clinical Practice Guideline.* AHCPR Pub. No. 95-0643. Rockville, MD: Agency for Health Care Policy and Research, Public Health Service, U.S. Department of Health and Human Services.

Acute Pain Management Guideline Panel. (1992, February) *Acute pain management: Operative or medical procedures and trauma. Clinical practice guideline.* AHCPR Pub. No. 92-0032. Rockville, MD: Agency for Health Care Policy and Research, Public Health Service, U.S. Department of Health and Human Services.

American Pain Society. (1992). *Principles of analgesic use in the treatment of acute pain and cancer pain* (3rd ed). Skokie, IL: American Pain Society.

American Psychiatric Association. (1993). Practice guideline for major depressive disorder in adults. *American Journal of Psychiatry, 150* (Suppl. 4), 1–26.

Barenholtz, H. A., & Bellamy C. D. (1995). Atypical analgesics and pain. *U.S. Pharmacist 20,* 54–69.

Brooks, P. M., & Day, R. O. (1991). Nonsteroidal anti-inflammatory drugs—Differences and similarities. *New England Journal of Medicine, 324,* 1716–1725.

Burckhardt, C. S. (1994). Chronic pain. *Clinics in Podiatric Medicine and Surgery, 11,* 135–145.

Bushnell, T. G., & Justins D. M. (1993). Choosing the right analgesic. *Drugs, 46,* 394–408.

Caraceni, A. (1996). Clinicopathologic correlates of common cancer pain syndromes. *Hematology/Oncology Clinics of North America: Pain and Palliative Care, 10*(1), 57–77.

Cherny, N. I. (1996). Opioid analgesics. *Drugs, 51,* 713–737.

Cherny, N. I., & Foley, K. M. (1996). Nonopioid and opioid analgesic pharmacotherapy of cancer pain. *Hematology/Oncology Clinics of North America: Pain and Palliative Care, 10*(1), 79–102.

Egbunike, I. G., & Chaffee, B. J. (1990). Antidepressants in the management of chronic pain syndrome. *Pharmacotherapy, 10,* 262–270.

Foley, K. M. (1982). The practical use of narcotic analgesics. *Medical Clinics of North America, 66,* 1091–1104.

Graves, N. M. (1993). Pharmacokinetics and interactions of antiepileptic drugs. American Journal of Hospital Pharmacy, 50(Suppl. 5), S23–S29.

Hillier, R. (1990) Control of pain in terminal cancer. *British Medical Bulletin, 46*, 279–291.

Kehoe, W. A., & Jacisin, J. J. (1992). Selecting and monitoring antidepressant medications. *American Journal of Pain Management, 2*, 17–26.

Kenny, G. N. (1992). Potential renal, haematological and allergic adverse effects associated with non-steroidal anti-inflammatory drugs. *Drugs, 44*, 31–37.

Krieger, D. (1990). Therapeutic touch: Two decades of research, teaching and clinical practice. *Imprint, 37*(3), 83, 86–88.

Levy, M. H. (1996). Pharmacologic treatment of cancer pain. *The New England Journal of Medicine, 335*, 1124–1132.

Levy, R. A., & Smith D. L. (1989). Clinical differences among nonsteroidal anti-inflammatory drugs: Implications for therapeutic substitution in ambulatory patients. *Annals of Pharmacotherapy, 23*, 76–83.

Loscalzo, M. (1996). Psychological approaches to the management of pain in patients with advanced cancer. *Hematology/Oncology Clinics of North America: Pain and Palliative Care, 10*(1), 139–155.

Magni, G. (1991). The use of antidepressants in the treatment of chronic pain. *Drugs 42*, 730–748.

Malkin, K. (1994). Use of massage in clinical practice. *British Journal of Nursing, 3*(6), 292–294.

Management of Cancer Pain Guideline Panel. (1994, March). *Management of cancer pain. Clinical practice guidelines*. AHCPR Publication No. 94-0592. Rockville, MD. Agency for Healthcare Policy and Research, U.S. Department of Health and Human Services, Public Health Service.

McCaffery, M., & Beebe, A. (1989). *Pain: Clinical manual for nursing practice*. St. Louis: The CV Mosby Co.

McQuay, H. J. (1988). Pharmacological treatment of neuralgic and neuropathic pain. *Cancer Surveys, 7*, 141–159.

Paice, J. A., & Citari, A. A. (1997). Cancer pain management: New therapies. *Oncology Nursing Updates 4*,(2), 2–10.

Pitner, J. K., Wiley, M. K., & Pennypacker, L. (1994). Prevention of NSAID-induced gastropathy in the elderly. *Consultant Pharmacist, 9*, 568–579.

Portenoy, R. K. (1996). Adjuvant analgesic agents. *Hematology/Oncology Clinics of North America: Pain and Palliative Care, 10*(1), 103–119.

Preskorn, S. H. (1994). Antidepressant drug selection: Criteria and options. *Journal of Clinical Psychiatry, 55*, (9; Suppl. A), 6–22.

Rhiner, M., Ferrell, B. R., Grant, M. M. (1993). A structured nondrug intervention program for cancer pain. *Cancer Practice, 1*(2):137–143.

Ripamonti, C., Zecca, E., Bruera, E. (1997). An update on the clinical use of methadone for cancer pain. *Pain, 70*, 109–115.

Rowlingson, J. C. (1992). *Management of chronic pain*. Philadelphia: Lippincott, 199–211.

Smith, I. W., Airey, S., Salmond, S. W. (1990). Nontechnologic strategies for coping with chronic low back pain. *Ortho Nursing, 9*(4):26–34.

Spross, J. A. (1994). Pain, suffering, and spiritual well-being: Assessment and interventions. *Quality of Life: A Nursing Challenge, 2*(3):71–79.

Twycross R. (1994). *Pain Relief in Advanced Cancer*. New York: Churchill Livingstone, 527–552.

Willkens, R. F. (1992). The selection of a nonsteroidal anti-inflammatory drug. Is there a difference? *Journal of Rheumatology, 19* (Suppl. 36), 9–12.

Wytias, C. A. (1994). Therapeutic touch in primary care. *Nurse Practitioner Forum, 5*(2), 91–96.

# 17

# PREGNANCY AND LACTATION

*Laurie A. Buchwald*

The fact that pregnancy is a natural event does not preclude the need for occasional medication use. Whether an over-the-counter preparation or a prescription drug is used, most women will find it necessary to take some kind of medication during a 40-week gestation. The same is true for the woman who is lactating. One study revealed that 44–92% of women use at least one medication during pregnancy, with an average use of 3.0–5.5 medications per woman (Artal, Lee, & Martin, 1993). Given this, providers who care for pregnant and lactating women must have an understanding of the changes that occur in maternal physiology and pharmacokinetics. This chapter addresses these changes as well as highlights positive pharmacotherapeutics during the preconception period and drug management of common illnesses and discomforts during pregnancy and lactation.

## PHYSIOLOGIC CHANGES DURING PREGNANCY

Pregnancy induces a number of physiologic changes (see Table 17–1). The tone and motility of the gastrointestinal (GI) tract—including the stomach, the small bowel, and the colon—are decreased. This is most likely due to the smooth muscle relaxing effects of progesterone (Cruikshank, Wigton, & Hays, 1996). Although the literature is unclear as to whether this decrease in GI motility results in delayed gastric emptying, it is likely that it does occur (Baer & Williams,

1996). Estrogen and progesterone levels rise, as do the levels of triglycerides, cholesterol, and phospholipids, resulting in an increased competition for protein-binding sites. "With fewer binding sites, a larger percentage of drug remains free to move to receptor sites or across the placenta" (Baer & Williams, 1996, p. 174). The liver does not enlarge, and there is no significant increase in hepatic blood flow (Murray & Seger, 1994). Total body water increases by as much as 8 L, and total body fat and weight are also significantly increased (Hedstrom & Martens, 1993). Maternal cardiac output increases by 30–50% during pregnancy, and plasma volume also increases by 50% (Cruikshank, Wigton, & Hays, 1996). The glomerular filtration rate is 50% higher than in the nonpregnant woman, and causes a decrease in blood-urea-nitrogen (BUN) and creatinine levels.

Changes also occur in the respiratory, integumentary, skeletal, and endocrine systems, but it is beyond the scope of this chapter to review those changes that do not significantly affect drug response during pregnancy.

## CHANGES IN PHARMACOKINETICS DURING PREGNANCY

The properties of pharmacokinetics are discussed in Chap. 2. The following is a review of those properties that are affected by the changes in maternal physiology.

**TABLE 17–1. MATERNAL PHYSIOLOGIC CHANGES AFFECTING PHARMACOKINETICS**

- Increase in total body water: approximately 8 L
- Increase in total body fat and weight gain: 3–4 kg
- Decreased tone and motility of the GI tract
- Increased glomerular filtration rate: 50%
- Increased cardiac output: 30–50%
- Increased blood volume: 50%
- Increased plasma protein production
- Decreased plasma albumin concentration
- Increased competition for plasma protein binding sites

*Adapted from Baer and Williams (1996), Forney (1996), and Murray and Seger (1994).*

## ABSORPTION

The absorption of medications during pregnancy may be affected by several factors. The decrease in GI tone and motility may cause the drug to remain in the stomach longer, leading to increased absorption. Nausea and vomiting, symptoms commonly experienced by women in the first trimester, often alter the eating habits of pregnant women and may ultimately reduce the amount of drug available for absorption (Forney, 1996).

## DISTRIBUTION

Of the four kinetic properties, distribution is affected most by maternal physiologic changes. The increase in plasma volume results in an increased volume for distribution and can lead to a prolonged drug elimination half-life (Murray & Seger, 1994). Decreased albumin levels result in a limited number of receptor or binding sites. Hormones, which are strongly protein-bound, compete for the available sites, leaving fewer sites available for binding drugs. Ultimately, this results in a wide distribution of free, unbound drug in the body (Forney, 1996). A 3–4-kilogram increase in body fat means that drugs distributed to fatty tissues remain in the body longer (Murray & Seger, 1994).

## BIOTRANSFORMATION

The liver is the primary site for metabolism of drugs. Since blood flow through the liver is relatively unchanged during pregnancy, this property of kinetics is essentially unaffected.

## EXCRETION

The elimination of drugs from the body through the kidneys is the most important route of excretion. Renal blood flow increases by 25–50%, and glomerular filtration increases by 50% (Forney, 1996). As a consequence, those drugs that have substantial renal excretion have increased rates of clearance (Murray & Seger, 1994).

## PLACENTAL TRANSFER

Medications that cross through the placenta must pass through the syncytiotrophoblast, the stroma of the intervillous space, and the fetal capillary wall (Cunningham et al, 1997). This histological barrier is not an actual physical barrier, and throughout pregnancy, a wide range of substances pass to the fetus. Most medications cross the placenta by simple diffusion, but movement also occurs by active transport and pinocytosis, a mechanism by which minute particles may be engulfed and carried across the cell. Cohen (1992) notes that several factors affect placental drug transfer and drug effects on the fetus. Lipid solubility is one such factor. Drugs that are lipid-soluble tend to diffuse readily across the placenta and enter the fetal circulation. Molecular weight and size also affect the rate and amount of drug transferred across the placenta. Drugs with molecular weights of 250–500 d can cross the placenta easily (Cohen, 1992). Most drugs used therapeutically have molecular weights lower than 600 d and, therefore, cross the placenta without difficulty (Murray & Seger, 1994). Protein binding must also be considered. The binding of drugs to maternal plasma proteins causes transfer to be slow. In essence, medications that have a small molecular size and are non-protein-bound, nonionized, and lipophilic readily cross the placenta and may negatively impact the developing fetus.

## GUIDELINES FOR MEDICATION USE IN PREGNANCY

The Food and Drug Administration (FDA) has developed a drug classification system designed to guide providers as they choose medications for their pregnant clients (see Table 17–2). Risk factors have been assigned to all drugs based on

## TABLE 17-2. FOOD AND DRUG ADMINISTRATION PREGNANCY RISK CLASSIFICATION

**Category A**
Controlled studies in women fail to demonstrate a risk to the fetus in the first trimester (nor is there evidence of a risk in later trimesters), and the possibility appears remote.

**Category B**
Either animal reproduction studies have not demonstrated a fetal risk (there are no controlled studies in pregnant women) or animal reproduction studies have shown an adverse effect (other than a decrease in fertility) that was not confirmed in controlled studies in women in the first trimester (and there is no evidence of a risk in later trimesters).

**Category C**
Either studies in animals have revealed adverse effect on the fetus (teratogenic or embryocidal effects or other) and there are no controlled studies in women, or studies in women and animals are not available. Drugs should be given only if the potential benefit justifies the potential risk to the fetus.

**Category D**
There is positive evidence of human fetal risk, but the benefits from use in pregnant women may be acceptable despite the risk (eg, if the drug is needed in a life-threatening situation or for a serious disease for which safer drugs cannot be used or are ineffective). An appropriate statement should be included in the "warnings" section of the labeling.

**Category X**
Studies in animals or human beings have demonstrated fetal abnormalities or there is evidence of fetal risk based on human experience, or both, and the risk of the drug in the pregnant women clearly outweighs any possible benefit. The drug is contraindicated in women who are or may become pregnant. An appropriate statement must be included in the "contraindications" section of the labeling.

*Adapted from Baer and Williams (1996) and Briggs, Freeman, and Yaffe (1994).*

the level of risk that the drug poses to the developing fetus. One of the problems with developing this classification system is that controlled drug trials to determine safety, efficacy, and pharmacokinetic alterations in pregnancy are rare. Because of the lack of data, many agents are given a category C designation. This category includes a statement that the drug should be given only if potential benefits justify potential risks to the fetus. Barron, Lindheimer, and Davison (1995) caution the provider not to view category C drugs as safe, and to remember that adverse fetal effects may occur.

## DRUG TERATOGENESIS

A teratogen is any substance, agent, or process capable of causing abnormal development (Sever & Mortensen, 1996). Conover (1994) describes four variables that must be considered when assessing the teratogenic effects of an agent: (1) the characteristics of the agent, (2) the timing of the exposure, (3) the dosage and

chronicity of the exposure, and (4) fetal susceptibility. Concurrent exposure to other agents, individual maternal metabolism, and route of administration also must be evaluated (Kochenour, 1994). The "classic" teratogenic period is between day 31 and day 71 after the first day of the last menstrual period. Niebyl (1996) notes that drugs administered early in this classic period will affect the organs developing at that time, such as the heart or neural tube. The ear and palate are forming at the end of the teratogenetic period and may be affected by drugs administered during that time. Although providers must proceed with caution, it should be remembered that most agents present less than a 1 percent risk for malformations (Conover, 1994). Table 17-3 lists some medications suspected or proven to be teratogens.

## DRUG THERAPY DURING LACTATION

The past two decades have seen a significant increase in the number of women who breast-

## TABLE 17–3. KNOWN OR SUSPECTED TERATOGENS/ SIGNIFICANT ADVERSE EFFECTS ON THE FETUS[a]

| | |
|---|---|
| Angiotensin-converting enzyme (ACE) inhibitors (D) | Diethylstilbestrol (X) |
| Accutane (X) | Disulfuram (C) |
| Alcohol | Estrogens (X) |
| Aminopterin (X) | Etretinate (X) |
| Aminoglycosides | Haloperidol (C) |
| Antidepressants | Hydroflumethiazide (D) |
| Busulfan (D) | Isotretinoin (X) |
| Carbamazepine (C) | Lithium (D) |
| Chlorambucil (D) | Methimazole (D) |
| Chloramphenicol (C) | Methotrexate (D) |
| Chlordiazepoxide (D) | Penicillamine (D) |
| Chlorpropamide (D) | Phencyclidine (X) |
| Clomiphene (X) | Phenytoin (D) |
| Clomipramine (C) | Propylthiouracil (D) |
| Cocaine (C) | Radioactive iodine |
| Cortisone (D) | Tetracycline (D) |
| Coumarins (D) | Thalidomide |
| Cyclophosphamide (D) | Thioguanine (D) |
| Cytarabine (D) | Trimethadione (D) |
| Danazol (X) | Vaccines, eg, MMR (X), Varicella (X) |
| Dextroamphetamine (C) | Valproic acid (D) |
| Diazepam (D) | Warfarin (D) |

[a] FDA pregnancy designation in parentheses.
*Adapted from Cohen (1992), Cunningham et al (1997), Reeder, Martin, and Koniak-Griffin (1997), Remich (1998), and Sherwen, Scoloveno, and Weingarten (1995).*

feed. Considering this, clinicians must understand how drugs are excreted into breast milk.

## THE TRANSMISSION OF DRUGS THROUGH BREAST MILK

O'Dea (1992) notes three general concepts regarding drug transfer in breast milk. First, drug ingestion by a breast-feeding infant is usually less than 1–2 percent of the total maternal dose. Second, those drugs that have wide distribution throughout the body usually have a low concentration in breast milk. Third, only the free or unbound portion of the drug is available for diffusion into breast milk.

A drug must first be absorbed into the maternal circulation for it to be excreted into the

breast milk. Many of the same factors that influence placental transfer of drugs also influence drug excretion into breast milk (see Table 17–4). Most drug molecules pass into breast milk by passive diffusion, but some are moved by pinocytosis, facilitated diffusion, and active transport (Forney, 1996). The ease of movement of a drug into maternal circulation is influenced by such factors as small molecular size, high lipid solubility, and whether it is nonprotein bound and nonionized (Murray and Segar, 1994).

## CLASSIFICATION OF DRUGS USED DURING LACTATION

The Committee on Drugs of the American Academy of Pediatrics (AAP) has reviewed drugs in lactation and categorized them as follows:

1. Contraindicated (see Table 17–5A)
2. Requires temporary cessation of breast-feeding
3. Effects unknown but may be of concern
4. Use with caution
5. Usually compatible (Silberstein, 1993, p. 535).

The committee recommends that the following questions and options be considered when prescribing drug therapy to lactating women:

1. Is the drug therapy really necessary?
2. Use the safest drug.

## TABLE 17–4. FACTORS INFLUENCING DRUG TRANSFER THROUGH BREAST MILK

- Absorption of drug by the mother's body: half-life, absorption rate, route of administration
- Movement of drug from maternal plasma to breast milk
- Molecular size and weight: smaller size = greater transfer
- pH of the drug: nonionized drugs = greater transfer
- Lipid solubility: increased solubility = greater transfer
- Protein binding: non-protein-bound = greater transfer
- Drug distribution: wide distribution = low concentration

*Adapted from Akridge (1998), Murray and Segar (1994), and O'Dea (1992).*

## TABLE 17–5A. DRUGS THAT ARE CONTRAINDICATED DURING LACTATION

| | |
|---|---|
| Alcohol | Iodine |
| Aminoglycosides | Lithium |
| Amphetamines | Marijuana |
| Bromocriptine | Methotrexate |
| Chronic aspirin use | Minor tranquilizers |
| Cocaine | Narcotics |
| Chloramphenicol | Nicotine/tobacco |
| Cimetidine | Phencyclidine (PCP) |
| Cyclophosphamide | Phenindione |
| Cyclosporine | Quinolones |
| Doxorubicin | Tetracycline |
| Ergotamine | Thiouracil |
| Gold salts | Vancomycin |
| Heroin | |

*Adapted from Akridge (1998), Eisenstat and Carlson (1995), Murray and Seger (1994), O'Dea (1992), and Sherwen, Scoloveno, and Weingarten (1995).*

3. If there is a possibility that a drug may present a risk to the infant, consider measuring the blood level in the nursing infant.

4. Drug exposure to the nursing infant may be minimized by having the mother take the medication just after completing a breast-feeding and/or just before the infant is due a lengthy sleep period (Committee on Drugs, 1994, p. 137).

Drugs usually considered compatible with lactation are shown in Table 17-5B.

## PRECONCEPTION CARE

The concept of identifying and reducing a woman's reproductive risks before conception is known as *preconception care*. The components of preconception care as outlined by Jack and Culpepper (1991) include risk assessment, health promotion, and medical intervention. Risk assessment allows the health care provider to determine if the woman is engaging in any high-risk behaviors such as tobacco, alcohol, or illicit drug use. This is also the time to identify existing medical conditions. Health promotion offers the opportunity to teach the woman healthy lifestyle behaviors and to avoid teratogens. Interventions during the preconception period include changing medications if necessary, referrals to high-risk clinics or substance

abuse treatment centers, and making sure that immunizations are current. The goal of preconception care is to maximize the health of the woman and to give prospective parents the opportunity to make lifestyle adjustments to improve their chances of a successful outcome in pregnancy (Bailey, 1998).

## SCREENING FOR SUBSTANCE USE AND ABUSE

Tobacco, alcohol, illicit drugs, and caffeine can adversely affect pregnancy. Substance abuse occurs in approximately 10% of all pregnancies (Cunningham et al, 1997). One factor to consider when assessing for substance abuse is that illicit drug users seldom abuse only one drug. Specific questions should be asked about each substance to obtain an accurate history. Another factor to consider is that many illegal substances contain impurities and contaminants. These impurities have adverse effects on both the mother and the fetus (Cunningham et al, 1997). Providers should be aware of the various screening tools available to aid in the assessment of substance abuse.

### Alcohol

The use of alcohol during pregnancy has been implicated in mental-retardation, intrauterine fetal demise, growth retardation, low birth

## TABLE 17–5B. DRUGS THAT ARE USUALLY COMPATIBLE DURING LACTATION

| | |
|---|---|
| Acetaminophen | Minoxidil |
| Amoxicillin | Oral contraceptives |
| Azithromycin | Penicillins |
| Beta adrenergic agonists | Piroxicam |
| Cephalosporins | Procainamide |
| Cisplatin | Propranolol |
| Cromolyn | Suprafen |
| Dicloxacillin | Terbutaline |
| Diltiazem | Theophylline |
| Erythromycin | Ticarcillin |
| Ibuprofen | Tolmetin |
| Ipratropium (Altrovent) | Trimethoprim-sulfa- |
| Labetalol |    methoxazole |
| Methimazole | Valproic acid |
| Metronidazole | Verapamil |
| Mexilitine | |

*Adapted from Akridge (1998) and Eisenstat and Carlson (1995).*

weight, central nervous system abnormalities, behavioral deficits, spontaneous abortions, and abruptio placentae (Cefalo & Moos, 1995). What is arresting about this is that all of these conditions—known to have been caused by alcohol use—are preventable. Fetal alcohol syndrome (FAS) is the most common environmental cause of mental retardation in developed countries (Sokol & Martier, 1996). The research is unclear as to whether alcohol use in any amount is safe, but as little as 1 oz of alcohol per day has been implicated (Remich, 1998). Assess each patient for the use of alcohol. Counsel her about the known detrimental effects of alcohol, and encourage her to stop using it during the preconception period and pregnancy. Refer the patient to an appropriate program if she is unable to limit her intake on her own.

## Tobacco

Associations have been found among smoking and infertility, spontaneous abortions, ectopic pregnancies, placental complications (abruptio placentae, placenta previa), low birth weight, preterm birth, lags in developmental milestones, and infant mortality (Cefalo & Moos, 1995; Remich, 1998). Providers should encourage women who smoke to reduce or quit the habit by providing appropriate education and literature, support, and referrals to smoking cessation programs if necessary.

## Illicit Drugs

Illicit drug use during pregnancy has been correlated with fetal addiction, prematurity, low birth weight, placental abruption, stillbirth, and behavioral and learning disabilities (Cefalo & Moos, 1995; Niebyl, 1996; Remich, 1998). Commonly abused drugs include cocaine, heroin, marijuana, and methamphetamines. As noted previously, polydrug use is frequent, and women who abuse illicit drugs often use alcohol and nicotine as well (Cohen & Keith, 1994). All patients, regardless of socioeconomic background, should be evaluated for illicit drug use. Those with identified problems should be referred to a substance abuse treatment program. Although it is important to emphasize the detrimental side effects of substance abuse of any kind, doing so in a guilt-provoking manner will not encourage women to stop. In fact, this approach will only serve to alienate substance-abusing patients.

## Caffeine

Animal studies have found a relationship between caffeine and malformations, but studies with humans have not found evidence of teratogenic effects (Cunningham et al, 1997). When counseling women on caffeine use in the preconceptual period and pregnancy, tell them that it may increase diuresis, worsen mood swings, increase fetal or newborn heartbeat irregularities, and increase spontaneous abortion risk (Remich, 1998). During lactation, caffeine is not contraindicated (Johnson, 1996).

## GUIDELINES FOR MEDICATION USE IN THE PRECONCEPTION PERIOD

The following general guidelines for preconception counseling regarding medication use should be considered:

- It is impossible to state with complete assurance that any medication used during pregnancy is completely safe, but there are relatively few drugs that are definitely known to be teratogenic in humans.
- All medications, including over-the-counter remedies, should be reviewed and assessed for their risk-to-benefit ratio.
- Many variables interact to determine the effect of a drug on the developing fetus.
- Category X drugs should be avoided for all women likely to become pregnant, and, when possible, avoid category D drugs as well (or use the lowest possible dose).
- Women who require medication for their own health needs should be made aware that although the general rule is to avoid medications, drug therapies are beneficial to pregnancy outcome in some circumstances, and, in those cases, the safest choice is to take the prescribed medication (Cefalo & Moos, 1995).

## POSITIVE PHARMACOTHERAPEUTICS DURING THE PRECONCEPTION PERIOD

### Vitamins and Minerals

Vitamins are not produced in the body and must be supplied by the diet. In the United States, it is rare to find women who have a vitamin deficiency because so many foods are enriched or fortified. A well-balanced diet can provide most of the nutrients for optimal maternal and fetal health, except for iron and folic acid. Several studies, including the Medical Research Council and the Budapest trial, have shown conclusively that a woman's risk for having a pregnancy affected by neural tube defects can be substantially reduced by taking folic acid periconceptually (Daly, Kirke, Molloy, Weir, & Scott, 1995). This research has prompted the Centers for Disease Control (CDC) to recommend that all women of reproductive age take 0.4 mg of folic acid per day.

## Prenatal Vitamin

A prenatal vitamin is generally prescribed for all pregnant women. The dosage of vitamins in most prenatal supplements reflects the increased recommended daily allowance (RDA) for pregnancy (Cefalo & Moos, 1995). Each tablet should contain at least (Remich, 1998, p. 485):

30 mg of elemental iron

15 mg of zinc

2 mg of copper

250 mg of calcium (not as calcium phosphate)

2 mg of vitamin $B_6$

0.8–1.0 mg of folic acid

50 mg of vitamin C

200 I.U. of vitamin D

Administration: One tablet by mouth each day.

Side effects: Constipation, nausea, GI upset.

Client education: Take the tablet on an empty stomach with a drink that is high in vitamin C (avoid taking with coffee, tea, or milk)

FDA designation: Category A.

## Iron Supplement

The recommended intake of elemental iron to prevent iron deficiency anemia (IDA) is 30–60 mg per day (the amount generally found in one prenatal vitamin). See Table 17–6. The recommended amount of elemental iron needed to treat IDA is 120 mg per day.

Administration: One tablet by mouth one to three times a day depending on the level of IDA.

Side effects: Constipation, GI upset

Client education: Take on an empty stomach with a drink high in vitamin C (avoid taking with coffee, tea, or milk)

FDA designation: Category A

### TABLE 17–6. PERCENTAGE OF ELEMENTAL IRON IN COMMON IRON PREPARATIONS

| Preparation (325 mg) | Percentage of Elemental Iron (%) | Elemental Iron, (mg) |
|---|---|---|
| Ferrous Sulfate | 29 | 60–65 |
| Ferrous Gluconate | 12 | 37–39 |
| Ferrous Fumarate | 33 | 107 |

Adapted from Samuels (1996) and Star et al (1990).

## IMMUNIZATIONS DURING PREGNANCY AND LACTATION

The preconception period is the time to determine if all childhood immunizations have been given and to ensure that immunity has been conferred. Immunizations are generally not performed in pregnant women, but several, as noted in Table 17–7, can be administered for the same indications as in nonpregnant women (Reilly & Clemenson, 1993). In 1997, the Centers for Disease Control recommended that all women in their second and third trimesters of pregnancy be offered the influenza vaccine. The decision to immunize should be made only after the risk of disease has been weighed against the risk of vaccination.

### RUBELLA

A resurgence of rubella infection occurred between 1988 and 1991, and the greatest incidence affected individuals over the age of 15 years (Cefalo & Moos, 1995). The major cause of this resurgence was the failure to im-

### TABLE 17–7. SUMMARY OF RECOMMENDATIONS FOR IMMUNIZATIONS DURING PREGNANCY

| Usual Indications | High Risk Only | Contraindicated |
|---|---|---|
| Rabies | Hepatitis B | Measles |
| Pneumococcus | Poliomyelitis | Mumps |
| Tetanus-Diptheria | | Rubella |
| Influenza | | Varicella |

Adapted from Cunningham et al (1997), Reeder, Martin, and Koniak-Griffin (1997), Reilly and Clemenson (1993), Remich (1998).

munize children. For this reason, a second measles-mumps-rubella (MMR) vaccine was added to the immunization schedule. Women of reproductive age are at risk for being nonimmune to rubella, and in fact, 6–11% remain seronegative for the rubella antibody (Remich, 1998). When a pregnant woman contracts this highly contagious disease, there is a 50% chance that the fetus will become infected. Congenital rubella syndrome may lead to a wide variety of manifestations, including growth retardation, cataracts, deafness, congenital heart defects, and organomegaly (Shandera & Tierney, 1992). All women of reproductive age should have documented evidence of immunity to rubella. If a woman is seronegative prior to pregnancy, she should be given the rubella vaccine and counseled to wait 3 months before becoming pregnant. Cefalo and Moos (1995) note that the teratogenic risk is negligible should conception occur within 3 months of receiving the vaccination. However, if a woman is found to be seronegative during prenatal testing, she should not be given the vaccine and should be cautioned to avoid anyone with a rash or viral illness (Remich, 1998).

## HEPATITIS B VIRUS

Hepatitis B infection is a major cause of acute hepatitis and its more serious sequelae: chronic hepatitis, cirrhosis, and hepatocellular carcinoma (Cunningham et al, 1997). Transfer of the infection from the hepatitis B-positive mother to the fetus is thought to be by ingestion of infected material during delivery or exposure subsequent to birth. Transplacental transmission is uncommon. Of 18,000 infants born to mothers who test positive for hepatitis B, 4000 will become chronically infected (Cunningham et al, 1997). Hepatitis B is transferred from mother to infant in 75% of cases in which the mother contracted the disease in the third trimester but will be transferred in only 10% of the cases when the virus is contracted during the first trimester (Reilly & Clemenson, 1993). Infection can usually be prevented by the administration of hepatitis B immune globulin soon after birth, followed promptly by the hepatitis B vaccine (Cunningham et al, 1997). All women should be screened for hepatitis B during the prenatal period. Women with risk factors and a negative surface antigen should receive hepatitis B vaccination, which is not contraindicated in preg-

nancy (Reilly & Clemenson, 1993; Remich, 1998).

## VARICELLA

Pregnant women should not receive the vaccination; and nonpregnant women should not become pregnant for 3 months after vaccination (Remich, 1998).

# DRUG MANAGEMENT OF COMMON DISCOMFORTS IN PREGNANCY AND LACTATION

This section addresses the pharmacotherapeutic management of the discomforts that commonly accompany pregnancy. The more serious illnesses such as migraine headaches, pyelonephritis, or hyperemesis gravidarum are not addressed. Refer to other sources for discussions of more complicated illnesses during pregnancy, and for nonmedication management of common discomforts. The health care provider is encouraged to try conservative measures first where appropriate before resorting to the use of medications.

## TENSION HEADACHE

### Diagnosis

More common than migraine, the tension headache is a frequent complaint during pregnancy. The pain often starts in the back of the neck and head, and progresses to feeling a tight "rubberband" pressure around the head. The pain is often bilateral, dull, and steady. The headache may begin in the morning, but will usually worsen throughout the day. Photophobia and gastrointestinal distress are uncommon.

### Drug Management

Acetaminophen is the preferred medication for headache pain during pregnancy, as there is no evidence of teratogenic effect. Aspirin and ibuprofen may increase the bleeding time and have undesired harmful effects on the pregnancy, especially during the third trimester (Feller & Franko-Filpasic, 1993; Silberstein, 1993). Acetaminophen is excreted into breast milk in small concentrations only and is considered compatible with breast-feeding (Briggs,

Freeman, & Yaffe, 1994). Although ibuprofen is generally not recommended during pregnancy, it does not enter breast milk in significant quantities, and does not pose a significant risk during lactation. See Table 17–8.

## URINARY TRACT INFECTION

Pregnancy increases a woman's risk for developing urinary tract infections (UTIs). Several physiologic changes occur that promote these infections, including increased glomerular filtration rate and urinary volume, loss of ureteral tone leading to urinary stasis, and changes in the chemical composition of the urine (Lucas & Cunningham, 1993).

### Diagnosis

*Asymptomatic bacteriuria* occurs in 4–12% of pregnant women and is diagnosed when a culture shows 100,000 colonies of one type of bacteria per milliliter of urine (Duff, 1993; Reilly & Clemenson, 1993). The significance of asymptomatic bacteriuria is in its potential to cause pyelonephritis, which develops in up to one third of pregnant women with untreated bacteriuria (Lucas & Cunningham, 1993). The majority of upper UTIs occur as a result of undiagnosed or untreated lower UTIs.

*Acute cystitis* affects 1–3% of pregnant women, and is diagnosed when the urinalysis shows white cells and bacteria. Nitrites and red blood cells may also be present. Often, the client is symptomatic for dysuria, frequency, hesitancy, and urgency. *Escherichia coli* accounts for 80–90% of UTIs in obstetric clients. *Klebsiella, Enterobacter, Proteus, Enterococcus faecalis,* and group B streptococcus account for most of the rest of the cases (Lucas & Cunningham, 1993).

### Drug Management

Clients with asymptomatic bacteriuria and acute cystitis are best treated with a short course of antibiotics: A 3-day course may be as effective as a 7–10-day course (Duff, 1993; Duff, 1996). However, providers often err on the side of overtreatment in that a 1-week course of therapy is usually given (Lucas & Cunningham, 1993). Several authors recommend that 10–14-day therapies be reserved for recurrent infections only (Duff, 1993; Duff, 1996; Lucas & Cunningham, 1993; Vercaigne & Zhanel, 1994), whereas others note that less than a 10-day treatment has not been proven effective in pregnant women (Abbott, 1994; Artal, Lee, & Martin, 1993; Reilly & Clemenson, 1993). Considering the discrepancy in recommendations, a protocol developed in consultation with an obstetrician, outlining appropriate therapy guidelines, is recommended.

When possible, antibiotic selection should be made based on sensitivity testing. Should treatment be initiated empirically, sulfisoxasole or nitrofurantoin macrocrystals are excellent choices because most uropathogens are susceptible to them (Duff, 1993). Briggs, Freeman, and Yaffe (1994) cite a 1985–1992 study that suggested an association between the combination trimethoprim-sulfamethoxazole and congenital defects. This has led some to believe that this combination antibiotic (ie, Bactrim, Septra) should be avoided during the first trimester, whereas others believe it should not be used at all during pregnancy. However, this combination drug has been widely used, and there have been no reports of increased fetal abnormalities (Hodgman, 1994). Nitrofurantoin should be avoided near term because of the theoretical risk of hemolytic anemia in the newborn (Artal, Lee, & Martin, 1993; Briggs, Freeman, & Yaffe, 1994). The use of sulfonamides near term should also be avoided because of the risk of fetal kernicterus (Artal, Lee, & Martin, 1993). It is thought that the sulfa drugs displace bilirubin and allow for an increase in unconjugated bilirubin which is deposited in fetal brain tissue (Hedstrom & Martens, 1993). The AAP recommends that exposure to sulfonamides via breast milk should be avoided in the ill, stressed, or premature infant, and in infants with hyperbilirubinemia or G6PD deficiency (Murray & Seger, 1994). See Table 17–9.

---

**TABLE 17–8. MEDICATIONS FOR TENSION HEADACHES**

| Drug | FDA Designation | AAP Category |
|------|-----------------|--------------|
| Acetaminophen | B | Compatible |
| Aspirin | C | Use with caution |
| Ibuprofen* | B (D during third trimester) | Compatible |

*not recommended for use during pregnancy.
FDA and AAP designations from Briggs, Freeman, and Yaffe (1994).

## TABLE 17–9. MEDICATIONS FOR URINARY TRACT INFECTIONS

| Drug/Dosage | FDA Designation | AAP Category |
|---|---|---|
| Sulfisoxazole: 2 g, then 1 g, q.i.d. | B | Compatible |
| Sulfamethoxazole-Trimethoprim DS: 800 mg then 160 mg b.i.d. | C | Compatible |
| Nitrofurantoin monohydrate/macrocrystals: One b.i.d. | B | Compatible |
| Ampicillin: 250 mg q.i.d. | B | No category[a] |
| Amoxicillin: 250 mg t.i.d. | B | Compatible |
| Cephalexin: 250 mg q.i.d. | B | No category[a] |

[a] Ampicillin and cephalexin are not assigned a category, but both are excreted into breast milk in low concentrations.
*Adapted from Duff (1993) and Reilly and Clemenson (1993).*

## NAUSEA AND VOMITING

Many women experience nausea and vomiting during the first trimester of pregnancy. Nausea develops in approximately 85% of women by 16 weeks of pregnancy, and 65 percent experience vomiting (Abbott, 1994). Although the etiology of nausea and vomiting is unclear, the high levels of circulating pregnancy-related hormones have been implicated (Abbott, 1994; Cunningham et al, 1997). Emotional and dietary factors may also contribute to the increased incidence of nausea and vomiting.

### Drug Management

After ensuring that more serious conditions such as hyperemesis gravidarum have been ruled out, nonpharmacologic measures should be attempted first to alleviate the nausea and vomiting. If dietary and lifestyle changes have proven ineffective, initiation of the medications listed in Table 17–10 may hasten the resolution of the problem. As necessary, consult with the collaborating physician, and then initiate promethazine (Phenergan) by mouth or rectal suppository. The medication should be used cautiously, at the lowest possible dose, and in conjunction with more conservative measures (Hollander, 1994).

## INDIGESTION/HEARTBURN

Pregnancy causes relaxation of the lower esophageal sphincter and decreased peristalsis and motility. These changes in the GI tract often cause reflux indigestion and esophagitis in the pregnant woman. Dietary and lifestyle changes should be the first interventions recommended. If these suggestions are unsuccessful in relieving the indigestion, the following medications may be recommended.

### Drug Management

The FDA and AAP have not provided classifications for antacid preparations, but they are generally considered safe in pregnancy (Artal, Lee, & Marten, 1993). Eisenstat and Carlson (1995) suggest the following, however:

- Aluminum hydroxide may increase the risk of fetal malformations in the first trimester, but is safe during the rest of pregnancy.
- Calcium carbonate is safe in the first semester, but may increase the risk of fetal hypomagnesemia in mid and later pregnancy.
- Magnesium compounds safety is unknown in early pregnancy and may increase the risk of fetal hypomagnesemia in the last trimesters.

The use of sodium bicarbonate should be avoided by pregnant women since sodium retention is common and may lead to edema as the result of ingestion of excessive amounts (Cunningham et al, 1997). $H_2$ blockers should only be used for those patients who do not respond to therapy, and only after consultation

## TABLE 17–10. MEDICATIONS FOR NAUSEA AND VOMITING

| Drug | FDA Designation | AAP Category |
|---|---|---|
| Vitamin $B_6$ (pyridoxine); 50 mg t.i.d. or q.i.d. | A | Compatible |
| Doxylamine | B | Data not available |
| Meclizine | B | Data not available |
| Cyclizine | B | Data not available |
| Phenergan (promethazine) | C | No category |

with a specialist. Calcium carbonate, one to two tablets every hour as needed, is useful for hyperacidity as well as providing a source of calcium (Remich, 1998).

## CONSTIPATION

The slowing of the GI tract in pregnancy, compounded by the addition of iron in the prenatal vitamin, often leads to constipation. The expanding uterus may also act as a mechanical obstacle to normal bowel evacuation (Hollander, 1994). Forty percent of women complain of constipation at some time during pregnancy, with 20% doing so in the third trimester (Cunningham et al, 1997).

### Drug Management

If the initiation of dietary and lifestyle interventions does not alleviate the constipation, then the clinician may recommend bulk-forming laxatives or stool-softening agents. Cathartics should not be used in pregnancy, particularly when the woman is high risk for preterm labor (Remich, 1998). The woman should avoid nonabsorbable oil preparations such as mineral oil because they may interfere with the absorption of lipid-soluble vitamins (Cunningham et al, 1997). See Table 17–11.

## UPPER RESPIRATORY INFECTIONS AND ALLERGIC RHINITIS

Pregnancy does not predispose women to upper respiratory infections (URIs), but the symptoms of a URI may be exaggerated by the normal vascular congestion that many experience. Rhinitis affects 20% of pregnant women and is thought to occur because of the increase in estrogen production (Lekas, 1992). URI symptoms may include rhinorrhea, rhinitis, cough, and sore throat. The challenge for the provider will be to determine whether the URI is viral or bacterial in origin, or if the symptoms may be associated with seasonal allergies.

### Drug Management

Recommend conservative, nonpharmacologic measures first, but know which medications are safe for the patient to use (see Table 17–12). Pseudoephedrine, a sympathomimetic, is the decongestant of choice in pregnancy (Murray & Seger, 1994) and can be used to alleviate the symptoms of allergic disorders or URIs. The best treatment for cough is increased intake of water, but dextromethorphan (an antitussive) and guaifenesin (an expectorant) may be used should the cough be refractive to fluids. Antihistamines, such as diphenhydramine, chlorpheniramine, and brompheniramine, are helpful in relieving allergy symptoms (rhinorrhea, itchy and watery eyes, postnasal drip). Neither the Collaborative Perinatal Project nor the Boston Collaborative Drug Surveillance Program identified any significant difference in frequency of congenital anomalies among children of mothers who took any of these "cold" medicines (Murray & Seger, 1994). New prescription antihistamines such as Claritan and Zyrtec are category B, and can be used to treat the symptoms of allergic rhinitis. These drugs

## TABLE 17–11. MEDICATIONS FOR CONSTIPATION

| Drug | FDA Designation | AAP Category |
|------|-----------------|--------------|
| Docusate sodium | C | No category |
| Metamucil | B | No category |

## TABLE 17–12. MEDICATIONS FOR URIS AND ALLERGIC RHINITIS

| "Cold" Medications | FDA Designation | AAP Category |
|--------------------|-----------------|--------------|
| Pseudoephedrine | C | Compatible |
| Dextromethorphan | C | No known category |
| Guaifenesin | C | No known category |

| Allergic Rhinitis | FDA Designation | AAP Category |
|-------------------|-----------------|--------------|
| Claritin | B | |
| Allegra | B | Category C |
| Zyrtec | B | |
| Diphenhydramine | C | No category[a] |
| Chlopheniramine | B | No data available |
| Brompheniramine | C | Compatible |

[a] The drug manufacturer considers the drug to be contraindicated in breast-feeding because of the increased sensitivity of newborns or premature infants to antihistamines.

are not recommended for use in the treatment of URIs.

## PHARYNGITIS/SINUSITIS/OTITIS MEDIA

Should the URI symptoms lead you to diagnose a bacterial infection, the appropriate antibiotic must be selected. Knowing the latest recommendations for diagnosing and treating bacterial infections is mandatory. For the pregnant woman, the antibiotic must also be effective against the maternal infection and cause no harm to the developing fetus (Hedstrom & Martens, 1993).

### Drug Management

In general, it is safe to prescribe penicillins and cephalosporins during pregnancy, turning to erythromycin as an alternative when an allergy to penicillin exists (see Table 17–13) (Murray & Seger, 1994). No reports of animal or human teratogenicity have been associated with the use of penicillins or cephalosporins. The same is true of erythromycin. The drugs are excreted into breast milk in low concentrations, and there have been no reports of adverse effects in the nursing infant (Murray & Seger, 1994). *Tetracyclines should never be used during pregnancy*.

## VAGINITIS

Vaginal infections are a routine complaint during pregnancy. The most frequent infections are bacterial vaginosis (BV), *Trichomonas vaginalis*, and vulvovaginal candidiasis (VVC).

### Bacterial Vaginosis

BV is responsible for approximately 45% of vaginal infections and has been associated with preterm delivery, premature rupture of membranes, intraamnionic infection, and postpartum infection (Duff, 1993; Wendel & Wendel, 1993). BV results from an overgrowth of anaerobic bacteria. Clients may complain of vaginal discharge, odor, and mild lower abdominal discomfort, or they may be asymptomatic. The presence of homogeneous discharge, vaginal pH of greater than 4.5, positive amine "whiff" test, and clue cells support the diagnosis of BV (Reilly & Clemenson, 1993).

Drug Management.  Metronidazole is the treatment of choice for BV, yet studies conflict regarding the possibility of teratogenesis (Murray & Seger, 1994). The drug is mutagenic in bacteria and carcinogenic in rodents, yet these properties have never been shown in humans (Briggs, Freeman, & Yaffe, 1994). Some providers do use metronidazole during the first trimester of pregnancy, as it is a category B drug. As yet, there is no definitive support for this and the CDC continues to recommend waiting until the second trimester before using it. The CDC (1997) recommends metronidazole 250 mg p.o. t.i.d. for 7 days. Clindamycin 300 mg p.o. b.i.d. for 7 days or metronidazole 2 g p.o. in a single dose are alternatives. Metronidazole gel, 0.75%,

### TABLE 17–13.  MEDICATIONS FOR BACTERIAL INFECTIONS

| Infection | Antibiotic | FDA Designation | AAP Category |
|---|---|---|---|
| Pharyngitis | Penicillin V | B | Compatible |
| | Amoxicillin | B | No category[a] |
| | Erythromycin | B | Compatible |
| Sinusitis or otitis media | Ampicillin | B | No category[a] |
| | Amoxicillin | B | No category[a] |
| | Bactrim | C | Compatible |
| | Cefuroxime | B | No category[a] |
| Otitis media | (Same as listed for sinusitis) | | |

[a] These antibiotics are excreted into the breast milk in low concentrations; adverse effects are rare, but three potential problems exist for the nursing infant: modification of bowel flora, direct effects on the infant (allergic response/sensitization), and interference with interpretation of culture results (Briggs, Freeman, & Yaffe, 1994).

one applicator-full per vagina b.i.d. for 5 days is also suggested as an alternative. Clindamycin vaginal cream should not be used; it has been implicated in increased preterm births. Clindamycin, as an alternative drug, may safely be used in pregnancy. Partners do not need to be treated, although some recommend doing so if the woman presents with recurrent infections after taking all of the prescribed medication (Bennett, 1994). See Table 17–14.

## Trichomonas Vaginalis

*Trichomonas* is identified in 20% of women during prenatal examinations, and has been found to be associated with an increased incidence of premature rupture of membranes near term, but not with preterm labor and delivery (Reilly & Clemenson, 1993; Wendel & Wendel, 1993). Women complain of yellow-green, foul-smelling, frothy discharge, and not uncommonly, of intermittent vaginal spotting and dyspareunia. The diagnosis is made by the identification of motile trichomonads on microscopic examination, although they may be present only 60% of the time.

**Drug Management.**   Metronidazole is the only trichomonacidal drug available in the United States, and it is quite effective in eradicating *T. vaginalis* (Wendel & Wendel, 1993). Initial treatment should be a single dose of 2 g for both partners, with 375 mg or 500 mg given b.i.d. should initial treatment fail (Schaffer, 1998; Wendel & Wendel, 1993). Metronidazole should not be given during the first trimester. Please refer to the discussion regarding metronidazole in the BV section.

## Vulvovaginal Candidiasis

VVC accounts for 20–30% of vaginal infections in pregnant women. The *Candida* species are considered to be part of the normal vaginal flora, and symptoms of infection are thought to develop when an overgrowth of these organisms occurs (Duff, 1993). Symptoms include vaginal and vulvar pruritis and irritation, and a white, curd-like discharge. The wet mount reveals hyphae, pseudohyphae, and budding yeast.

**Drug Management.**   Oral agents, designated as category C, are not recommended in pregnancy; topical agents are the only therapies that should be used (Schaffer, 1998). Table 17–14 lists several topical agents of proven value in the treatment of VVC. Candidiasis is not considered to be sexually transmitted, and therefore, the partner does not need to be treated.

## SEXUALLY TRANSMITTED DISEASES

Sexually transmitted diseases (STDs), of which there are many, are common during pregnancy. Some STDs are uncomplicated and easily treated; others are associated with preterm labor, premature rupture of membranes, chorioamnionitis, and postpartum endometritis. Potential infections in the neonate include sepsis, conjunctivitis, and pneumonitis. Risk factors for STDs include low socioeconomic status, urban status, multiple sexual partners, illicit drug use, and youth. Since it is neither possible nor appropriate to assume which woman will have an STD, most providers choose to screen all prenatal patients for gonorrhea, chlamydia, hepatitis B, and syphilis. All women should be counseled and a consent form signed prior to being tested for HIV. It is recommended that the most current copy of the *CDC Treatment Guidelines* for STDs be available. For a more in-

## TABLE 17–14.   MEDICATIONS FOR VAGINITIS

| Drug | FDA Designation | AAP Category |
|---|---|---|
| **Bacterial Vaginosis and Trichomonas Vaginalis** | | |
| Metronidazole | B[a] | Use with caution[b] |
| Clindamycin | B | Compatible |
| **Vulvovaginal Candidiasis** | | |
| Miconazole (Monistat) | C[c] | No data available |
| Clotrimazole (Gyne-Lotrimin) | B | No data available |
| Terconazole (Terazol-7) | C[c] | No data available |
| Butoconazole (Femstat) | C[c] | No data available |

[a] The CDC considers this drug to be contraindicated during the first trimester (Briggs, Freeman, & Yaffe, 1994).
[b] The AAP recommends discontinuing breast-feeding for 12–14 h to allow for the excretion of the drug, after a single 2-g dose (Briggs, Freeman, & Yaffe, 1994).
[c] Used topically, no association has been found between this drug and congenital malformations (Briggs, Freeman, & Yaffe, 1994).

## TABLE 17–15. MEDICATIONS FOR UNCOMPLICATED STDS IN PREGNANCY

| STD | Drug | FDA Designation | AAP Category |
|---|---|---|---|
| Gonorrhea | Ceftriaxone 125 mg IM (or alternate cephalosporin)[a] plus | B | Compatible |
| | Erythromycin 500 mg q.i.d. × 7 days[b] | B | Compatible |
| Chlamydia | Erythromycin 500 mg q.i.d. × 7 days*[b] or erythromycin 250 mg × 14 days | B | Compatible |
| Syphilis (primary, secondary, and early latent of less than 1 year's duration) | Penicillin G[c] benzathine 2.4 million u IM × 1 | B | No category |
| Syphilis (late latent) | Penicillin G benzathine 7.2 million u divided in three doses of 2.4 million u IM, at 1-week intervals | B | No category |
| HPV (human papillomavirus) | Cryotherapy with trichloracetic acid (TCA) 80–90%; repeat weekly if necessary up to 3–4 weeks, then refer.<br>• Lesions have a tendency to proliferate during pregnancy<br>• Podophyllin, imiquimod, podofilox are contra-indicated during pregnancy | N/A | N/A |
| HSV (herpes simplex virus) | Acyclovir, Famciclovir, Valacyclovir[d] | | |
| Pediculosis pubis | Permethrin 1% lotion applied to affected areas and washed off after 10 min or pyrethrins with piperonyl butoxide applied to affected areas and washed off after 10 min; repeat 1 week as needed; *lindane should not be used* | B | |
| Scabies | Permethrin 5% lotion applied to all areas of the body from the neck down; wash off after 8–14 h; *lindane should not be used* | B | |

[a] Cephalosporin-intolerant women should be treated with one dose of spectinomycin 2 gm I.M.
[b] Amoxicillin 500 mg t.i.d. × 7 days may be used if erythromycin cannot be tolerated.
[c] Women who are allergic to penicillin should be treated with penicillin after desensitization, as there are no proven alternatives. Referral to an obstetrican for desensitization is indicated.
[d] The safety of Acyclovir, Famciclovir, and Valacyclovir in pregnancy has not been established. See the current CDC Treatment Guidelines for a discussion of use in pregnancy.
*Adapted from Morbidity and Mortality, 1998.*

depth discussion of STDs, refer to Chapter 36. Table 17–15 provides medication managment for uncomplicated STDs in pregnancy. More complex disorders should be managed in consultation with, or referred to, an obstetrician or infectious disease specialist.

## REFERENCES

Abbott, J. (1994). Medical illness during pregnancy. *The Pregnant Patient, 12*(1), 115–127.

Akridge, K. M. (1998). Postpartum and lactation. In E. Q. Youngkin & M. S. Davis (Eds.), *Women's health: A primary care clinical guide* (pp. 639–701). 2nd ed. Stamford, CT: Appleton & Lange.

Artal, R., Lee, R. V., & Martin, J. N. (1993). When the pregnant patient gets sick. *Patient Care 27*(6), 89–107.

Baer, C. L., & Williams, B. R. (1996). *Clinical pharmacology and nursing.* Springhouse.

Bailey, C. W. (1998). Assessing health during pregnancy. In E. Q. Youngkin & M. S. Davis (Eds.), *Women's health: A primary care clinical guide* (pp. 441–476). 2nd ed. Stamford, CT: Appleton & Lange.

Barron, W. M., Lindheimer, M. D., & Davison, J. M. (Eds.). (1995). *Medical disorders in pregnancy.* St. Louis: Mosby–Year Book.

Bennett, E. C. (1994). Vaginitis and sexually transmitted diseases. In E. Q. Youngkin & M. S. Davis (Eds.), *Women's health: A primary care clinical guide* (pp. 203–240). Norwalk, CT: Appleton & Lange.

Briggs, G. G., Freeman, R. K., & Yaffe, S. J. (1994). *Drugs in pregnancy and lactation*. Baltimore: Williams & Wilkins.

Cefalo, R. C., & Moos, M. K. (1995). *Preconceptional health care: A practical guide*. St. Louis: Mosby–Year Book.

Cohen, M. S. (1992). Special aspects of perinatal and pediatric pharmacology. In B. G. Katzung (Ed.), *Basic and clinical pharmacology* (pp. 853–861). Norwalk, CT: Appleton & Lange.

Cohen, L. S., & Keith, L. G. (1994). Drug abuse in pregnancy. In F. P. Zuspan & E. J. Quilligan (Eds.), *Current therapy in obstetrics and gynecology* (pp. 241–242). Philadelphia: W. B. Saunders.

Committee on Drugs (1994). The transfer of drugs and other chemicals into human milk. *Pediatrics, 93*(1), 137–142.

Conover, E. (1994). Hazardous exposures during pregnancy. *Journal of Obstetric, Gynecologic and Neonatal Nursing, 23*(6), 524–532.

Cruikshank, D. P., Wigton, T. R., & Hays, P. M. (1996). Maternal physiology in pregnancy. In S. G. Gabbe, J. R. Niebyl, & J. L. Simpson (Eds.), *Obstetrics: Normal and problem pregnancies* (pp. 91–110). New York: Churchill Livingstone.

Cunningham, F. G., MacDonald, P. C., Gant, N. F., Leveno, K. J., Gilstrap, L. C., Hankins, G. D. V., & Clark, S. L. (1997). *Williams obstetrics* (19th ed.). Stamford, CT: Appleton & Lange.

Daly, L. E., Kirke, P. N., Molloy, A., Weir, D. G., & Scott, J. M. (1995). Folate levels and neural tube defects. *The Journal of the American Medical Association, 274*(21), 1698–1702.

Duff, P. (1993). Antibiotic selection for infections in obstetric patients. *Seminars in Perinatology, 17*(6), 367–378.

Duff, P. (1996). Maternal and perinatal infections. In S. G. Gabbe, J. R. Niebyl, & J. L. Simpson (Eds.), *Obstetrics: Normal and problem pregnancies* (pp. 1193–1246). New York: Churchill Livingstone.

Eisenstat, S. A., & Carlson, K. J. (1995). Use of medication in pregnancy and lactation. In K. J. Carlson & S. A. Eisenstat. *Primary care of women*. St. Louis: Mosby.

Feller, C. M., & Franko-Filipasic, K. J. (1993). Headaches during pregnancy: Diagnosis and management. *Journal of Perinatal and Neonatal Nursing, 7*(1), 1–10.

Forney, S. L. (1996). Drug therapy in childbearing and breastfeeding clients. In N. L. Pinnell (Ed.), *Nursing pharmacology* (pp. 100–109). Philadelphia: W. B. Saunders.

Hedstrom, S. & Martens, M. G. (1993). Antibiotics in pregnancy. *Clinical Obstetrics and Gynecology, 36*(4), 886–892.

Hodgman, D. E. (1994). Management of urinary tract infections in pregnancy. *The Journal of Perinatal and Neonatal Nursing, 8*(1), 1–11.

Hollander, D. (1994). Gastrointestinal problems in pregnancy. In F. P. Zuspan & E. J. Quilligan (Eds.), *Current therapy in obstetrics and gynecology* (pp. 248–251). Philadelphia: W. B. Saunders.

Jack, B. W., & Culpepper, L. (1991). Preconception care. *Journal of Family Practice, 32*(3), 306–313.

Johnson, C. A. (1996). Breastfeeding. In C. A. Johnson, B. E. Johnsen, J. L. Murray, & B. S. Apgar (Eds.). *Women's health care handbook*. Philadelphia: Hanley & Belfus, 323–339.

Kochenour, N. (1994). Medications in early pregnancy. In J. T. Queenan (Ed.), *Management of high-risk pregnancy* (pp. 36–42). Boston: Blackwell Scientific.

Lekas, M. D. (1992). Rhinitis during pregnancy and rhinitis medicamentosa. *Otolaryngology: Head and Neck Surgery, 107*(6), 845–849.

Lucas, M. J., & Cunningham, F. G. (1993). Urinary infection in pregnancy. *Clinical Obstetrics and Gynecology, 36*(4), 855–867.

Morbidity and Mortality Weekly Report. (1998, January 23). *1998 Guidelines for treatment of sexually transmitted diseases, 47*(No. RR-1), Atlanta, GA: U.S. Department of Health and Human Services, PHS, Centers for Disease Control and Prevention.

Murray, L., & Seger, D. (1994). Drug therapy during pregnancy and lactation. *Emergency Medicine Clinics of North America, 12*(1), 129–149.

Niebyl, J. R. (1996). Drugs in pregnancy and lactation. In S. G. Gabbe, J. R. Niebyl, & J. L. Simpson (Eds.), *Obstetrics: Normal and problem pregnancies* (pp. 249–277). New York: Churchill Livingstone.

O'Dea, R. F. (1992). Medication use in the breastfeeding mother. *NAACOG's Clinical Issues, 3*(4), 598–604.

Reeder, S. J., Martin, L. L., & Koniak-Griffin, D. (1997). *Maternity nursing: Family, newborn, and women's health care*. Philadelphia: Lippincott.

Reilly, K., & Clemenson, N. (1993). Infections complicating pregnancy. *Primary Care, 20*(3), 665–684.

Remich, M. (1998). Promoting a healthy pregnancy. In E. Q. Youngkin & M. S. Davis (Eds.), *Women's health: A primary care clinical guide* (pp. 447–531). 2nd ed. Stamford, CT: Appleton & Lange.

Samuels, P. (1996). Hematologic complications of pregnancy. In S. G. Gabbe, J. R. Niebyl, & J. L. Simpson (Eds), *Obstetrics: Normal & problem pregnancies* (pp. 1083–1100). New York: Churchill Livingstone.

Schaffer, S. D. (1998). Vaginitis and sexually transmitted diseases. In E. Q. Youngkin & M. S. Davis (Eds.). *Women's health: A primary care clinical guide*, 2nd ed (pp. 265–299). Stamford, CT: Appleton & Lange.

Sever, L. E., & Mortensen, M. E. (1996). Teratology and the epidemiology of birth defects: Occupational and environmental perspectives. In S. G. Gabbe, J. R. Niebyl, & J. L. Simpson (Eds.), *Obstetrics: Normal and problem pregnancies* (pp. 185–213). New York: Churchill Livingstone.

Shandera, W., & Tierney, L. (1992). Infectious diseases: Viral and rickettsial. In S. A. Schroeder, L. M. Tierney, S. J. McPhee, M. A. Papadakis, and M. A. Krupp (Eds.), *Current medical diagnosis and treatment* (pp. 1009–1036). Norwalk, CT: Appleton & Lange.

Sherwen, L. N., Scoloveno, M. A., & Weingarten, C. T. (1995). *Nursing care of the childbearing family*. Norwalk, CT: Appleton & Lange.

Silberstein, S. D. (1993). Headaches and women: Treatment of the pregnant and lactating migraineur. *Headache, 33,* 533–540.

Sokol, R. J., & Martier, S. (1996). High risk pregnancy: Alcohol. *Contemporary OB/GYN, 12,* 19–23.

Star, W. L., Shannon, M. T., Sammons, L. N., Lommel, L. L., & Gutierrez, Y. (1990). *Ambulatory obstetrics: Protocols for nurse practioners/nurse midwives*. San Francisco: The Regents, University of California.

Vercaigne, L. M., & Zhanel, G. G. (1994). Recommended treatment for urinary tract infection in pregnancy. *Annals of Pharmacotherapy, 28,* 248–250.

Wendel, P. J., & Wendel, G. D., Jr. (1993). Sexually transmitted diseases in pregnancy. *Seminars in Perinatology, 17*(6), 443–451.

# 18

# CONTRACEPTIVES

*Catherine Berardelli and Vivien E. James*

This chapter, which explores the full spectrum of contraceptive alternatives available to patients today, would have been otherwise impossible to write had it not been for the undaunting activist work of women such as Margaret Sanger (Caufield, 1998; Lynaugh, 1991; Ruffing-Rahal, 1986). A women's rights activist, pioneer in family planning, and a nurse (Schuster, 1993), Sanger braved governmental condemnation and imprisonment in order to answer the pleas of women in her care to "Please tell me the secret . . ." (Lynaugh, 1991, p. 124) of preventing unwanted pregnancies. It was Margaret Sanger who, among other contributions, introduced the diaphragm in the United States and fought for women's reproductive rights through her early work in the family planning movement. It is our hope that this chapter will assist clinicians in providing thoughtful, sensitive, thorough information to patients, enabling them to be informed decision makers about their own reproductive health.

Contraception, or fertility control, has been defined as the deliberate management of conception or childbirth. This control and management may be achieved using a variety of devices, chemicals, surgical procedures, fertility awareness methods, and postcoital methods. Thus, choosing a contraceptive method is an important decision involving the ability to anticipate and plan for the occurrence of sexual intercourse. It has been reported, however (Hanson, 1996, p. 31), that approximately "60% of all pregnancies in the United States are unintended," suggesting that planning

has either been ineffective or nonexistent. Norris (1988, p. 135) has suggested that one's "ability to anticipate and prepare for intercourse is contingent on the ability to think about sexual intercourse, contraception, and the negative impact on one's life of an unplanned pregnancy." This notion has important implications for clinicians in practice, especially as it relates to patient education. The clinician's mission is to assist patients in choosing contraceptive methods best fitting their personal lifestyles while taking into consideration the feelings and attitudes of the patient and the patient's partner. To that end, this chapter will discuss all currently available forms of contraception and also provide information about methods on the horizon. A compilation of perfect use and typical use failure rates from various contraceptive methods is provided in Table 18–1.

## FACTORS AFFECTING REPRODUCTIVE CHOICE

The reproductive life span of a woman may encompass 40 or more years, and for men the production of sperm is continuous throughout life. Therefore, it is natural to expect that a variety of contraceptive methods may be used. As family planning needs change, it is necessary for sexual partners to acquire accurate information about the factors that may affect their contraceptive needs in order to more accurately reevaluate their pregnancy prevention choices.

**TABLE 18–1. PERCENTAGE OF ACCIDENTAL PREGNANCY DURING FIRST YEAR OF USE ASSOCIATED WITH CONTRACEPTION METHODS**

| Method | Perfect Use Failure Rate % | Typical Use Failure Rate % |
|---|---|---|
| No method | 85 | 85 |
| Withdrawal | 14.7 | 27.8 |
| Periodic abstinence | | 20 |
| Spermicide alone | 6 | 21 |
| Cervical cap with spermicide | 11.5 | 18 |
| Diaphragm with spermicide | 6 | 18 |
| Condom | | |
| Male | 3 | 12 |
| Female | 5 | 21 |
| IUD | | |
| Progesterone T | 1.5 | 2 |
| Copper T | 0.6 | 0.8 |
| Oral contraceptives | | 3 |
| Combined | 0.1 | |
| Progestin only | 0.5 | |
| Depo-Provera | 0.3 | 0.3 |
| Norplant | 0.09 | 0.09 |

*Adapted from "Choice of Contraceptives" (1995) and Hatcher et al (1994).*

Caufield (1998) enumerates a number of factors influencing the selection of birth control methods. These factors, listed in Table 18–2, mandate the existence of a true collaborative effort between the patient and health care provider to determine the method that best fits into the tapestry of people's reproductive lives.

## SEXUAL HISTORY TAKING

Developing the skills necessary to complete a thorough sexual history enhances the clinician's ability to effectively counsel patients regarding their choice of contraceptive method. Alexander (1996) notes that sexual history taking is a skill requiring the clinician to become comfortable with sexual language, including the straightforward jargon with which the patient may be more familiar. In addition, clinicians need to be skilled in a wide variety of therapeutic communication techniques to facilitate information gathering. The single most important therapeutic communication technique at the clinician's disposal is that of attentive, active listening.

Empowering the patient to provide information that may feel embarrassing and uncomfortable to them requires a private place for taking a sexual history. This is essential so that the sharing of intimate information can be done in relative comfort and safety. In addition, a warm greeting and a genuinely respectful attitude will help initiate rapport at the outset of the interview. It also is important that the patient be fully aware of the nature of the interview, the type of information being requested, and the purpose for which the information is being obtained. Table 18–3 includes a listing of skills and techniques that often help in gathering sensitive information from patients.

## SEXUALLY TRANSMITTED DISEASE RISK RELATED TO CONTRACEPTIVE CHOICES

Both men and women bear responsibility for making contraceptive decisions and seeking birth control methods reflecting their reproductive needs. Consideration must also be given to how effective each method is in preventing sexually transmitted diseases (STDs). As part of the clinician's sexual history taking, and within the context of contraceptive decision making, a full assessment regarding the patient's risk of contracting STDs should be conducted.

**TABLE 18–2. FACTORS INFLUENCING SELECTION OF BIRTH CONTROL METHODS**

| | |
|---|---|
| Age and maturity | Stage of reproductive life |
| Relationship status | Health history |
| Cultural and religious beliefs | Presence of physical/ mental limitation |
| Motivation/degree of cooperation | Individual locus of control |
| Comfort with one's own body | Monogamous versus multiple sexual partners |
| Cost and effectiveness of method | Method safety/convenience |
| Previous method experience | Noncontraceptive benefits |
| Frequency of intercourse | Access to health care |

*Source: Caufield (1998).*

## TABLE 18–3. TECHNIQUES IN SENSITIVE INFORMATION GATHERING

- Patient modesty and privacy is of paramount importance
- Assure patient confidentiality
- Clearly state what information can and cannot be held in confidence
- Develop attentive listening skills
- Ask questions in nonjudgmental manner
- Ask questions about specific behaviors instead of lifestyle issues
- Never assume sexual orientation
- Use open-ended questions
- Allow time, including periods of silence, for patients to elaborate
- Pay attention to verbal and nonverbal cues
- Never prejudge

*Adapted from Alexander (1996) and Caufield (1998).*

Even though abstinence is the one best method for both preventing pregnancy and STDs, it is simply not a viable contraceptive alternative for many. Therefore, when counseling a patient about contraception, it is important to discuss disease transmission and risk reduction strategies as well. In using data from a comprehensive literature review conducted by Cates and Stone in 1992, O'Connell (1996, p. 476) states, "[A woman] has a much higher risk of contracting an infection than of becoming pregnant. Even on the day a woman's risk of pregnancy is highest, the day before ovulation, the risk of contracting gonorrhea from an infected man is four times greater than the risk of pregnancy." Youngkin (1995, p. 743) poignantly notes that "sexually transmitted diseases are like a huge runaway train . . . an estimated 12 million new STD cases occur yearly in the United States." Thus, in addition to discussing the effectiveness in preventing pregnancy and the safety, cost, and convenience of a particular contraceptive method, clinicians must also discuss the method's protection effectiveness against contracting STDs.

## BARRIER METHODS

Barrier methods have been providing a mechanical barricade to advancing sperm since the seventeenth century (Hatcher et al, 1994), and they provide effective protection from pregnancy and STDs if they are used correctly and consistently. These methods include male and female condoms, diaphragms, cervical caps, and spermicides including vaginal contraceptive films. The mechanism of action, effectiveness, advantages, disadvantages, and patient education requirements of each are discussed below.

## MALE CONDOMS

Historians have identified several uses for the condom throughout history (Himes, 1963). Egyptian men in 1350 B.C. are said to have worn them as decorative covers for their penises, and in the 1560s Fallopius, an Italian anatomist, described a protective linen sheath used to cover the penis during intercourse. However, it was not until the 1700s when penile sheaths made from animal intestines were given the name *condom* and were used to protect men from "venereal disease and numerous bastard offspring" (Hatcher et al, 1994, p. 146).

Condoms currently on the market are made from latex rubber, polyurethane, and the nonsynthetic intestinal tissue of certain animals. They come in a wide variety of colors, shapes, sizes, textures, and thicknesses (Caufield, 1998; Hatcher et al, 1994), preventing pregnancy by blocking sperm from entering the vagina and cervix. Some contain spermicidal lubrication, most commonly nonoxynol-9, which is used to immobilize and kill sperm following ejaculation.

Latex condoms help prevent transmission of STDs, including herpes virus, hepatitis B, and HIV, by preventing direct contact with body fluids. Current research has shown the nonsynthetic condom to be more porous than the latex condom, thereby lessening its effectiveness in preventing the transmission of STDs (Cates & Stone, 1992). Individuals with latex allergies now have the option of using a polyurethane condom that is nonallergenic, stronger than the latex condom, and more effective in controlling the transmission of STDs than those condoms made of animal intestine ("Choice of Contraceptives," 1995). A nonallergenic condom made of latex-free natural rubber is being tested. This condom, made from a synthetic thermoplastic elastomer, is made from FDA-approved material for synthetic nonallergenic gloves (Caufield, 1998).

Effectiveness is directly related to consistent and correct usage (Caufield, 1998; Hatcher et al,

1994; Potter, 1996). Current statistics measure pregnancy prevention effectiveness in terms of failure rate for typical versus perfect use. O'Connell (1996) notes that for women between the ages of 15 and 44, failure rates vary between 18.5% (typical use) and 9.8% (perfect use). Caufield (1998), Hatcher et al (1994), and Potter (1996) suggest that failure rates vary between 12% (typical use) and 3% (perfect use). Failure rates increase dramatically if patients use petroleum-based lubricants. Advantages and disadvantages of condoms are provided in Table 18–4.

Condom users should be cautioned regarding the use of mineral oil or petroleum-based lotions or lubricants. "Choice of Contraceptives" (1995) highlights a study conducted by Voeller et al in 1989 that notes a barrier strength reduction of 90% when latex condoms are used in conjunction with oil-based lubricants and lotions. They suggest the use of water-soluble lubricants.

Patient education needs to stress the importance of checking the expiration date on condoms prior to use and that they can only be used once. In addition, patients need to understand that condoms must be placed on the penis before contact with perineal area, they need to be rolled all the way on, and they should be held tight when removing to avoid spillage. It is advisable to use a second method, such as spermicide, to enhance effectiveness.

## FEMALE CONDOMS

In 1993, the FDA approved the Reality female condom for distribution in the United States in response to increased demand for an easily reversible, easily accessible, woman-controlled method of contraception that also addressed concerns regarding the increase of STDs among women (Boston Women's Health Collective, 1992). Made of thin polyurethane approximately 17 cm long with one closed and one open flexible end, the female condom completely shields the vagina and cervix and partially covers the perineal area. When properly inserted, the condom prevents sperm from entering the vagina and cervix and provides a protective barrier against most STDs, including HIV (Caufield, 1998).

The effectiveness of female condoms in preventing unwanted pregnancy varies from a 21% failure rate with typical use to a 5% failure rate with perfect use. Its effectiveness is similar to those of the diaphragm and cervical cap in the United States (Caufield, 1998). The manufacturer currently suggests that the Reality condom can be left in place for up to 8 h. Patients should be aware that the Reality condom can be used only once and then must be discarded. Table 18–5 lists the advantages and disadvantages of female condoms.

Proper insertion technique is an important teaching consideration. The inner ring of the closed end should be squeezed together and inserted until the ring is past the pubic bone, com-

**TABLE 18–4. ADVANTAGES AND DISADVANTAGES OF CONDOMS**

| Advantages | Disadvantages |
|---|---|
| • Easily accessible (no prescription needed)<br>• Cost-effective<br>• Significant STD protection (latex or polyurethane)<br>• Male participation in contraception<br>• Enhances erection<br>• Can be used during lactation | • Allergic reaction to latex or lubrication<br>• Slippage/breakage<br>• Unwillingness of male partner to use<br>• Interferes with sexual spontaneity<br>• Decreased pleasure and/or sensation<br>• Skin condoms ineffective protection against STDs including HIV<br>• Heat may weaken rubber condoms |

*Adapted from Caufield (1998) and Hatcher et al. (1994).*

**TABLE 18–5. ADVANTAGES AND DISADVANTAGES OF FEMALE CONDOMS**

| Advantages | Disadvantages |
|---|---|
| • Easily accessible<br>• Easily reversible<br>• Requires no prescription<br>• Protective against STDs and HIV<br>• Can be used during lactation<br>• Can be inserted well before intercourse<br>• Can be removed immediately after intercourse | • Three times as costly as male condoms<br>• Can only be used once<br>• Cumbersome to insert<br>• Slippage can occur<br>• May be esthetically unpleasing (noise with use, ring dangles outside vagina) |

*Adapted from Boston Women's Health Collective (1992), Caufield (1998), and Hatcher et al. (1994).*

pletely covering the cervix. It is important to check to make sure the pouch has not become twisted during insertion since this would make penile insertion very difficult. The pouch should then extend along the vagina and on to the perineum.

## DIAPHRAGM

Used since the late 1800s in Europe, the diaphragm gained acceptance in the United States during the 1920s. It is a dome-shaped cup with a flexible spring-like rim made of heavy latex rubber, which when combined with a spermicidal cream or jelly, provides both a mechanical barrier to shield the cervix and a chemical to kill sperm. To be effective, the diaphragm must be inserted into the vagina prior to intercourse so that the posterior rim rests in the posterior fornix and the anterior rim fits snugly behind the pubic bone (Caufield, 1998; Hatcher et al, 1994). It must remain in this position for at least 6 h after intercourse but should not be worn longer than 24 h because of the possible increased risk of developing toxic shock syndrome.

Diaphragms are available in four styles and a range of sizes indicating the cup size in millimeters (see Table 18–6). To ensure effectiveness with proper usage, any diaphragm must be properly sized and fitted.

Proper fitting of a diaphragm requires a vaginal examination. An estimate of the diagonal length of the vaginal canal from the posterior vaginal fornix to the symphysis pubis provides the measurement necessary for determining the appropriately sized diaphragm. This estimated measurement is accomplished by inserting the middle and index fingers into the vagina until the middle finger touches the posterior vaginal wall. Mark the point on the clinician's hand that touches the symphysis pubis, and then select a diaphragm diameter corresponding to the length between the middle finger and the point where contact was made with the symphysis pubis. When inserted, the diaphragm should fit snugly against the pubic bone, should completely cover the cervix, and should touch the lateral vaginal walls. Movement by the patient, such as walking, sitting, or squatting, should not displace the diaphragm and should not cause discomfort. Table 18–7 lists the advantages and disadvantages of diaphragms.

Women with chronic urinary tract infections, a history of toxic shock syndrome, a severely displaced uterus or vaginal cystocele, scoliosis, or spina bifida should be counseled to use another form of birth control.

Once the diaphragm has been fitted, the patient will need to practice insertion and removal. Teaching should include timing of diaphragm insertion (within 6 h before intercourse) and

### TABLE 18–6. COMPARISON OF DIAPHRAGMS

| Diaphragm Type | Sizing | Special Considerations |
|---|---|---|
| Coil spring rim | Koromex (latex): 50–95 mm<br>Ortho coil (latex): 50–95 mm<br>Ramses (gum rubber): 50–95 mm | Has sturdy rim with firm spring strength; well suited for woman with average vaginal musculature and average pubic arch depth |
| Arcing spring rim | Koroflex (latex): 60–95mm<br>Ortho All-Flex (latex): 55–95 mm<br>Ramses Bendex (gum rubber): 65–95 mm | Sturdy rim with firm arching spring strength eases insertion; well suited for most women; can be retained in presence of rectocele or cystocele and in women with relaxed muscle tone |
| Flat spring rim | Ortho-White (latex): 55–95 mm | Thin gentle spring strength especially useful in women with firm musculature, in women with a shallow notch behind the pubic bone, or in nulliparous women; can be inserted with plastic introducer |
| Wide seal rim | Milex Wide-Seal (latex: 60–95 mm; comes in either arcing or spring coil | Flexible flange on inside rim of dome keeps spermicide in place and enhances seal between rim and vaginal wall |

*Adapted from Caufield (1998); Hatcher et al. (1994).*

## TABLE 18–7. ADVANTAGES AND DISADVANTAGES OF DIAPHRAGMS

| Advantages | Disadvantages |
| --- | --- |
| • Cost-effective | • Requires accurate fitting |
| • Can be used 1–2 years with proper care | • Initial cost for fitting may be high |
| • Good method for women needing contraception on irregular basis | • May interfere with sexual spontaneity |
| • Easily reversible | • Increased incidence of UTIs, especially with arcing spring |
| • Can use during lactation | • Allergic reactions to latex/rubber or spermicide |
| • Provides some protection against STDs | • Takes time to learn insertion and removal |
| • Does not require partner involvement | • Requires refitting for loss or gain of weight or after pregnancy, abortion, or miscarriage |
| • Protects against cervical neoplasia | |

Adapted from Boston Women's Health Collective (1992) and Caufield (1998).

how to check for proper placement (the patient should be able to feel the outline of the cervix through the soft rubber cup, and the rim of the diaphragm should fit snugly behind the pubic bone). Like condoms, diaphragms react to petroleum-based products, producing a birth control product that is ineffective due to destruction of the rubber. Therefore, if lubricants are being used, the patient should be warned to use only water-soluble products (Boston Women's Health Collective, 1992; Hatcher et al, 1994).

## CERVICAL CAP

This barrier method, resembling a small version of a diaphragm with a deep cup, is made of soft rubber (Caufield, 1998) and is meant to fit snugly over the cervix, creating a seal between the soft flexible rim and the outer edge of the cervix. It provides a barrier against advancing sperm, and when spermicide is put inside the dome prior to insertion, the chemical aids in killing sperm, thereby achieving dual pregnancy and some STD prevention.

Approved for distribution by the FDA in 1988, the Prentif cavity rim cervical cap, currently the only one approved by the FDA, maintains effec-

tiveness ratings similar to the diaphragm: 6% failure rate with perfect use and 18% failure rate with typical use (Boston Women's Health Collective, 1992). Like the diaphragm, the cervical cap must be fitted by a properly trained health care provider and manifests similar advantages and disadvantages. It provides continuous protection for up to 48 h and may be left in place without adding additional spermicide for no more than 48 h.

Women with cervical erosion or laceration should not be fitted with a cervical cap, and women with a long or irregularly shaped cervix may be unable to wear the cervical cap. Other contraindications for use include allergy to latex or rubber. Having a history of abnormal Pap tests or cervical cancer may be a contraindication to use; however, no studies looking specifically at cervical cap use in women with these problems have been conducted to date (Caufield, 1998).

It is important for a woman to understand how much spermicide to use in conjunction with the cervical cap: enough to fill about one third of the cap, which is then spread around the inside of the cap without applying any to the rim. Too much spermicide can cause a break in the suction of the cap to the cervix (Boston Women's Health Collective, 1992; Caufield, 1998). To prevent odors, the cervical cap can be soaked for approximately 20 min in a solution of one cup of water to one tablespoon of either cider vinegar or lemon juice. The cap should then be thoroughly rinsed and dried before use.

Other barrier methods, such as the FemCap, a silicone rubber cap, and the Lea's shield, an oval silicone rubber "one-size-fits-all" device (Caufield, 1998), are currently being tested, but have not been approved for distribution in the United States by the FDA.

## SPERMICIDE

Distributed as foams, jellies, creams, suppositories, and films spermicide must be inserted into the vagina prior to intercourse and works by immobilizing and killing sperm (Caufield, 1998). When used as the sole protective device, a spermicide provides protection for one episode of sexual intercourse and is effective for approximately 1 h after insertion. The most common active spermicidal ingredients are nonoxynol-9 and octoxynol. Both are equally effective in preventing pregnancy; the failure rate with typical use is 21% versus 6% with perfect use ("Choice of Contraceptives," 1995).

New spermicides are in development. Clinical trials are currently underway to determine the safety of a spermicide employing benzalkonium chloride. In addition, other types, designed to dissolve more quickly but remain stable in warm to hot climates, are being developed. A new nonoxynol-9 agent, named Advantage 24, is being marketed. This gel adheres to the vaginal walls to provide spermicidal activity for up to 24 h (Caufield, 1998). Another product, sulphated polymers, being studied inhibits viral entry into mucosal cells by an electrostatic layer that, in theory, puts a positive charge around infected material (Female-controlled methods, 1996).

Caufield (1998) highlights in vitro studies demonstrating the lethal effect of nonoxynol-9 on organisms causing most of the common STDs, including chlamydia, gonorrhea, genital herpes, and syphilis. In addition, several clinical studies have shown significant protection against gonorrhea and chlamydia for women using spermicidal products containing nonoxynol-9 (Hatcher et al, 1994; Youngkin, 1995). Conflicting results have been found in human studies on HIV transmission (Caufield, 1998). Advantages and disadvantages of spermicides are provided in Table 18–8. Some concern exists about the possible harmful effects of high-dose, high frequency application with nonoxynol-9 products. The biodetergent characteristic of the spermacide may create micro-ulcerations, more points of entry for pathogenic organisms, and enhance STD transmission (Female-controlled methods, 1996).

Timing is everything when using spermicides. Spermicides that come in the form of foams, jellies, or creams should be applied no more than 15 min before vagina-to-penis contact is anticipated. If the patient chooses suppositories or vaginal contraceptive film, she needs to follow package instructions and wait the appropriate amount of time before intercourse to allow the adequate dispersement of the spermicide. No matter what type of spermicide is used, patients need to be cautioned about the need to reapply the spermicide prior to each episode of intercourse in order to maintain effectiveness of the method. Patients should be advised to keep a supply on hand and to make sure they check the expiration date before use. In addition, use of a second method, such as one of the barrier methods, is recommended to enhance effectiveness. Finally, should irritation or burning occur with use, the patient is advised to discontinue use (Boston Women's Health Collective, 1992; Caufield, 1998; Hatcher et al, 1994).

## INTRAUTERINE DEVICES

A popular form of contraceptive protection during the 1960s and 1970s, being used by as many as 10% of "contracepting women in the United States," (Hatcher et al, 1994, p. 347), the intrauterine device (IUD) declined in popularity during the early 1980s. Currently IUDs are used by only about 2% of the population at risk for pregnancy. The decrease in popularity of the IUD is commonly attributed to the high incidence of pelvic infections and septic abortions brought about by the use of one particular type of IUD, the Dalkon shield (Knutson, 1997).

Currently, only two IUDs are commercially available in the United States, the Progestasert and the ParaGard Copper T380A. Both are T-shaped and made of plastic with strings attached to aid in removal ("Choice of Contraceptives," 1995). The Progestasert has been on the market continuously since 1976 and contains 38 mg of progesterone in a delivery system releasing 65 $\mu$g daily (Knutson, 1997). This product must be replaced yearly and has been found to decrease menstrual flow and cramping as a result of the slow release of progesterone.

The ParaGard Copper T380A, a copper-bearing IUD containing barium sulphate to fa-

### TABLE 18–8. ADVANTAGES AND DISADVANTAGES OF SPERMICIDES

| Advantages | Disadvantages |
|---|---|
| • Widely available without prescription or examination | • May interfere with spontaneity |
| • Cost-effective | • Must be on hand at or near time of intercourse |
| • Easily available as a backup method | • Skin irritation of vulva or penis related to allergy |
| • Can reduce STI transmission | • Inability to learn correct insertion technique |
| • Completely reversible | • Abnormal vaginal anatomy interfering with placement |
| • Can provide lubrication during intercourse | |

*Adapted from Caufield (1998) and Hatcher et al (1994).*

cilitate x-ray visibility, has been on the market since 1988. This T-shaped polyurethane device has a very fine copper wire wound around it and a white polyethylene string attached to the end to facilitate removal (Caufield, 1998). As of 1994, the FDA increased the length of continuous use for this IUD from 8 to 10 years (Knutson, 1997).

The mechanism of action for IUDs, although not proven, appears to be multidimensional and affects three primary areas: fertilization, implantation, and the endometrium (Caufield, 1998). Studies have shown that the presence of the IUD appears to create an inflammatory response that is toxic to ova and interferes with sperm survival by rendering them immobile. In addition to being toxic, this inflammatory response appears to markedly increase the ova's speed of transport through the fallopian tube, thereby decreasing the possibility of fertilization (Caufield, 1998; Hatcher et al, 1994; Knutson, 1997). Secondly, the increase of prostaglandin, as part of the inflammatory response, appears to prevent ova implantation on the endometrial lining and leads to destruction of the blastocyte (Caufield, 1998). Lastly, the endometrium appears to be affected by an IUD in two ways. ParaGard Copper T380A appears to interfere with the uptake of estrogen by the uterine mucosa, and the Progestasert's daily release of progesterone produces an atrophic endometrium with long-term use (Caufield, 1998).

Knutson (1997, p. 23) notes that effectiveness differs slightly depending on which IUD is used. For typical use, ". . . the copper-bearing IUD has a failure rate of 0.8% and the progesterone-bearing IUD has a failure rate of 2.0%. Perfect use rates are 0.6% and 1.5%, respectively." Caufield (1998) notes effectiveness can be influenced by the size and shape of the IUD, as well as by the rate of expulsion and the age and parity of the woman.

All potential IUD users must be carefully screened for contraindications prior to insertion of the device. The suggested patient profile is a woman without a history of pelvic inflammatory disease or ectopic pregnancy, who is in a mutually monogamous relationship, has had one full-term pregnancy, and desires reversible, long-term contraception (Caufield, 1998). Table 18–9 enumerates the manufacturer-specific contraindications to IUD use.

After a thorough health history is taken, the physical examination should include a bimanual pelvic examination with particular attention to the size, shape, consistency, and position of

## TABLE 18–9. CONTRAINDICATIONS TO IUD USE

| Progestasert | ParaGard T380A |
|---|---|
| • History of pelvic surgery that may be associated with increased risk of ectopic pregnancy | • Known allergy to copper |
| | • Diagnosed Wilson's disease |
| | • Untreated cervicitis or vaginitis |
| • Presence or history of STDs | • Conditions associated with increased susceptibility to infections, eg, AIDS, leukemia, chronic steroid therapy |
| • Untreated cervicitis or vaginitis | • Previously inserted IUD not removed |
| • Conditions associated with increased susceptibility to infection, eg, AIDS, leukemia, chronic steroid therapy, diabetes, history of endocarditis | |
| • Incomplete involution after abortion or birth | |

### General Contraindications
• History of pelvic inflammatory disease
• Intravenous drug abuse
• Non-mutually monogamous relationship
• Genital bleeding of unknown etiology
• Pregnancy or suspected pregnancy
• Abnormality of uterus resulting in distortion of uterine cavity
• Genital actinomycosis

*Adapted from Caufield (1998) and prescribing information for ParaGard Copper T380A (Ortho) and Progestasert (ALZA).*

uterus. In addition the following laboratory studies should be completed: a Pap smear, STD screen, vaginal wet mount, hematocrit, and pregnancy test in absence of menses or in cases of irregular menses (Knutson, 1997). Thorough counseling regarding the advantages and disadvantages of the method should be included during the preinsertion visit. Time during this preinsertion visit should be sufficient to clarify information and obtain a prior written consent. Any preexisting condition such as anemia or vaginal infection should be treated prior to insertion of the IUD.

Knutson (1997) highlights the current controversy regarding the relative merits of prophylactic antibiotic use at the time of IUD insertion. Some clinicians prescribe either 200 mg of doxycycline, administered 1 h prior to insertion, or 500 mg of erythromycin, administered 1 h prior and 6 h following insertion, to decrease the chance of uterine infection following insertion. However, a randomized controlled clinical trial, conducted by Walsh and colleagues in 1994, found no statistically significant difference between a group given prophylactic antibiotic therapy prior to insertion and a group given a placebo prior to insertion. And, as Knutson (1997, p. 31) clearly admonishes, "The bottom line defense from infection is scrupulous aseptic technique for insertion. Do not be tempted to rely on prophylactic antibiotics as a substitute for sterile technique." Advantages and disadvantages of the IUD are listed in Table 18–10.

An IUD may be inserted at any time during the menstrual cycle as long as the woman is not pregnant. Caufield (1998) suggests that midcycle insertion, when the cervix is softer, may cause less discomfort. Hatcher et al (1994) note an increased incidence of IUD expulsion and higher infection rate when IUDs are inserted during menses. All phases of IUD insertion require the practitioner to use a slow, steady, and gentle movement. It will be necessary to redetermine uterine position with bimanual examination prior to insertion. Methods of insertion vary slightly with the type of IUD; therefore, the health care provider should always read and follow the manufacturer's instructions for insertion.

Patient education should include a thorough explanation of what to expect during and after IUD insertion. Women should be instructed how and when to check for the IUD string, how to recognize the signs and symptoms of infection, and how to monitor for danger signs using the acronym PAINS: P = period, late or with abnormal spotting or bleeding; A = abdominal pain and/or pain with intercourse; I = infection symptoms or exposure; N = not feeling well, ie, experiencing fever, chills, or pelvic pain; S = string is either missing or shorter or longer than normal (Caufield, 1998).

## STERILIZATION

Hatcher et al (1994, p. 379) write, ". . . voluntary surgical contraception . . . has become one of the most widely used methods of family planning in the world . . ." and go on to note that ". . . nearly 14 million women rely on sterilization as their contraceptive method: 9.6 million rely on female sterilization, and 4.1 million on vasectomy."

Defined as the surgical interruption or closure of pathways for sperm or ova, this method of contraception is considered permanent. However, surgical procedures have been developed to successfully reverse this contraceptive method. In addition, the FDA approved the Filshie clip (Filshie clip recommended, 1996; News alert for family, 1996) for distribution in the United States. The device, made of silicone-rubber–lined titanium, is designed to occlude the fallopian tube by compression with less tissue destruction than other clips or rings currently on the market. Amy Pollack, M.D., president of Access to Safe and Voluntary Contraception International (News alert for family, 1996, p. 130), notes that minimal tissue damage offers a better chance of method reversal, which may be "an important point for many women who may choose the method early in their contracepting years."

Caufield (1998), Hatcher et al (1994), and Potter (1996) identify voluntary surgical sterilization as a highly effective method of birth control with failure rates noted to be as low as 0.1% during the first year. However, Peterson (1996) suggests that relying on first-year failure rate statistics is misleading. He reports the results of a Centers for Disease Control (CDC) 10-year study looking at female contraception. The results of this study indicated a much higher failure rate over time. Table 18–11 reveals the differing statistical information.

Peterson (1996, p. 5) cautions clinicians not to generalize the findings because "it is an aver-

## TABLE 18–10. ADVANTAGES AND DISADVANTAGES OF IUDS

| Advantages | Disadvantages |
| --- | --- |
| • Requires no continuing action, once inserted | • Insertion requires trained health provider |
| • Allows for sexual spontaneity | • Must regularly check for presence of IUD string |
| • Continuously effective | |
| • Cost-effective, once inserted | • May increase risk for pelvic infections |
| • Progesterone IUD may decrease menstrual flow and dysmenorrhea | • Does not decrease risk of contracting STDs |
| • Can be used during lactation | • May cause increased dysmenorrhea and menstrual flow |

*Adapted from Caufield (1998) and Knutson (1997).*

## TABLE 18–11. STERILIZATION FAILURE RATES

| Author | Female Sterilization Failure Rates | Male Sterilization Failure Rates |
|---|---|---|
| Caufield (1998) | 1.9% overall cumulative rate over 10 years | 0.1% first year lowest expected<br>0.15% first year typical expected |
| Hatcher et al (1994) | 0.4% first year lowest expected<br>0.4% first year typical expected | 0.1% first year lowest expected<br>0.15% first year typical expected |
| Potter (1996) | 0.1% first year lowest expected<br>0.15% first year typical expected | Not reported |
| CDC, CREST Study: Peterson (1996) | 1.9% overall cumulative rate over 10 years | Not studied |
| Filshie clip (Contraception Report, 1996) | 0.1% first year cumulative rate<br>0.7% 2-year cumulative rate | Not studied |

*Adapted from Caufield (1998), Hatcher et al (1994), and Peterson (1996).*

age of widely differing rates for specific methods." It is important, however, for clinicians to incorporate the U.S. Collaborative Review of Sterilization (CREST) study findings in their presterilization counseling sessions so the patient and her partner can make the best choice based on full comprehension of current information.

As part of the 10-year CDC study, the CREST study (Peterson, 1996) also found that approximately 6% of the women in the study consulted a health care provider regarding the possibility of reversal at some point during the 5 years following their sterilization procedure. The study found that women under 30 made up the largest percentage of women seeking information about reversal. Other factors influencing possible regret included changes in marital status, death of a child, socioeconomic status, and whether the sterilization was performed in conjunction with cesarean section (Peterson, 1996). Wilcox, Chu, and Peterson (1990) have identified the following characteristics that make patients ideal candidates for tubal reanastomosis: (1) younger than 43, (2) documented ovulation, (3) of average weight for height, (4) at least 4 cm of healthy tubal tissue remaining.

As with all other forms of fertility control, voluntary surgical sterilization is a personal decision best made after reviewing all the options and carefully weighing the risks and benefits. Seven areas to be included when providing presterilization counseling to patients are outlined in Table 18–12 (Pollack, 1996). Advantages and

## TABLE 18–12. PRESTERILIZATION COUNSELING GUIDELINES

- Stress the permanency of the method
- Include both partners and discuss both male and female procedures
- Provide full discussion of all fertility control options
- Provide information about failure rates, both 1-year and cumulative
- Reinforce risk reduction activities related to sexually transmitted infections
- Be aware of factors that may lead to poststerilization regret
- Provide full complement of information on all patient-appropriate surgical procedures

*Adapted from Knutson (1997) and Pollack (1996).*

disadvantages of sterilization are discussed in Table 18–13.

## FERTILITY AWARENESS METHODS

There are a variety of techniques women can use to determine fertile from infertile periods during the menstrual cycle (Northrup, 1995). These fertility awareness methods (FAMs) help women determine their fertile period by learning to "read" the expected physiological changes caused by hormonal fluctuations occurring during the normal menstrual cycle (Caufield, 1998; Hatcher et al, 1994; Northrup, 1995; Planned Parenthood Federation of America [PPFA] 1992).

Women who become attuned to and learn to recognize the measurable body changes that occur around the time of ovulation can use this information to effectively manage their fertility over time without the need to rely on other devices. A FAM's main mechanism of action as a contraceptive method, avoidance of unprotected intercourse during the woman's fertile period, is based on the following factors: (1) an ova is usually released each cycle; (2) the ova is released 14 days before menstruation; (3) the ova lives for approximately 24 h; and (4) sperm may live for 5 days in a woman's body. Therefore, women may be fertile for as long as 5 days before ovulation, because of sperm life, and for up to 3 days after ovulation, because of ova life.

### TABLE 18–13. ADVANTAGES AND DISADVANTAGES OF STERILIZATION

| Advantages | Disadvantages |
|---|---|
| • Provides permanent fertility control | • Inherent risks of any surgical procedure |
| • Highly effective, convenient, one-time decision | • Difficult to reverse |
| | • Cost initially high |
| • Long term: low cost, low risk | • Vasectomy not immediately effective |
| • Certain techniques can be done immediately after abortion or childbirth | • Not protective against HIV/AIDS or other STDs |
| • Considered immediately effective | |

*Adapted from Knutson (1997) and Peterson (1996).*

The two most common FAMs include monitoring a woman's basal body temperature (BBT) on a daily basis and checking cervical mucus changes daily. Using the two methods together, called the *symptothermal method*, provides important confirmatory information for patients who choose this method of fertility control.

A woman's basal body temperature, the lowest temperature reached by the body of a healthy person during waking hours, fluctuates with the ovulatory cycle as much as $0.8°F$ (Northrup, 1995). Using this method requires a thermometer that measures in tenths of a degree and a BBT chart. BBT should be taken daily before rising, eating, or drinking and charted to observe ovulatory patterns over time.

Ovulation occurs at a point in the menstrual cycle at which progesterone levels increase as a result of the surge in luteinizing hormone. Concomitantly, there is a rise in the BBT of $0.4°–0.8°F$. This temperature increase continues until menstruation, at which point there will be a return to preovulation BBT. If conception has occurred, the BBT will remain elevated.

Over the course of several months, patterns should emerge providing valuable information as to fertile and infertile periods, enabling the patient to predict the end of the fertile period and the beginning of the luteal (nonfertile) phase (Caufield, 1998). If using this method alone, women should be counseled to refrain from unprotected intercourse from day 4 of the menstrual cycle until after BBT has been elevated for 3 days (PPFA, 1992), unless pregnancy is desired.

Determining ovulatory patterns by observing changes in the cervical mucus was first developed in the early 1960s by Billings (Boston Women's Health Collective, 1992), who sought a method of contraceptive protection in compliance with the teachings of the Catholic Church.

Secreted by the exocrine glands lining the cervical canal, cervical mucus changes character in response to hormonal changes throughout the menstrual cycle (Caufield, 1998). In order to determine the time of ovulation, a patient is instructed to assess the vaginal area for level of wetness or dryness on a daily basis and also to note changes in color and consistency of the mucus. It is normal for women to experience several days of dryness immediately following menstruation. Then there will be a period when the mucus will appear milky white, translucent yellow, or clear and slightly sticky. Corresponding to a peak in estrogen, which occurs immediately before ovulation, the amount of mucus increases and it becomes clear and slippery to touch, similar in consistency to egg whites (PPFA, 1992). Mucus with this consistency facilitates the movement of sperm toward the awaiting ova.

After ovulation has occurred, the amount of mucus decreases, and it returns to a milky white, sticky consistency. Before ovulation, dry days when no cervical fluid is present are the days considered safe (Caufield, 1998). A daily record should be kept noting the cervical mucus changes.

The symptothermal method combines the BBT and cervical mucus methods along with noting other physiological changes such as breast tenderness, change in libido, and mittelshmerz. Experts contend that combining FAMs offers patients the highest degree of effectiveness in pregnancy protection versus using each method independently. The failure rate with perfect use ranges between 1% and 3%. Some experts add an optional sign of fertility: the position of the cervix and its openness. The cervix is usually deeper/higher in the vagina, softer, open, and wet close to ovulation (Caufield, 1998). Advantages and disadvantages of FAMs are listed in Table 18–14.

Preparation for using this method of fertility control and understanding how to accurately interpret the charts requires thorough and ongoing education. Table 18–15 describes the content areas essential for FAMs. These should be incorporated into the teaching plan for patients choosing to use FAMs.

### TABLE 18–15. ESSENTIAL CONTENT AREAS IN PREPARATION FOR USING FAMs

- Normal menstrual cycle
- Mechanics of the method
- Required equipment
- Method selection
- Charting the data
- Determining fertile period
- Alternative sexual activity during fertile periods

Sources: Northrup (1995) and PPFA (1992).

## COITUS INTERRUPTUS (WITHDRAWAL)

This method of fertility control has been used throughout history and was "a natural response to the discovery that ejaculation into the vagina caused pregnancy" (Hatcher et al, 1994, p. 341). It involves having the man remove his penis from the vagina and perineal area before ejaculation in an effort to keep sperm and ova separate. Although few statistical data exist to accurately determine effectiveness, most contraceptive experts suggest that the failure rate with perfect use in the first year is about 4% and 19% with typical use (Caufield, 1998; Hatcher et al, 1994). Advantages and disadvantages of coitus interruptus are listed in Table 18–16.

## ORAL CONTRACEPTIVES

Oral contraceptives (OCs) are the most popular method of birth control and are used by more than 13 million women in the United States (Hatcher et al, 1994). This popularity is due to

### TABLE 18–14. ADVANTAGES AND DISADVANTAGES OF FERTILITY AWARENESS METHODS

| Advantages | Disadvantages |
| --- | --- |
| • Increases user knowledge of reproductive cycle<br>• Acceptable to most religious groups<br>• Actively involves both partners<br>• No side effects<br>• Cost-effective<br>• Provides information about potential fertility problems | • Does not provide protection against HIV/AIDS or other STDs<br>• Mandates cooperation between partners<br>• Not reliable if cycle is irregular, lactating, or perimenopausal<br>• Perceived lack of sexual spontaneity |

Adapted from Northrup (1995) and PPFA (1992).

### TABLE 18–16. ADVANTAGES AND DISADVANTAGES OF COITUS INTERRUPTUS

| Advantages | Disadvantages |
| --- | --- |
| • Does not cost anything<br>• Involves no artificial devices or chemicals<br>• Can be used during lactation<br>• It is always available | • Requires control on the part of the man<br>• Not protective against STDs, HIV/AIDS<br>• Diminished sexual pleasure<br>• Premature ejaculation |

Sources: Boston Women's Health Collective (1992), Caufield (1998), and Hatcher et al (1994).

several factors including high efficacy, simplicity of use, rapid reversal in effects after discontinuation, and menstrual cycle benefits (Dickey, 1993). After oral contraceptives were synthesized in the 1950s, many formulation changes were made in the hopes of ameliorating potential complications and adverse effects (Weisberg, 1995). These changes include a reduction in the doses of estrogen and progestin, timing of the progestin in the cycle, and newly available third-generation progestins that differ in pharmacologic activity from other progestins.

The first pill marketed, Enovid 10, contained constant doses of both estrogen and progestin; however, doses were much higher than those used today and resulted in an increased risk of thromboembolism. Today, doses of estrogen and progestin are 5 and 25 times lower, respectively, than those used in the initial formulations. Sequential formulations were introduced in the 1960s, but are no longer marketed. These pills contained estrogen given during the first 2 weeks; then progestin was added during the third week of the cycle. Sequential OCs were shown to be less effective and associated with an increased risk of endometrial cancer (Bucci & Carson, 1997).

## CURRENT FORMULATIONS

The majority of women taking OCs receive combination pills, a mixture of synthetic estrogen and one of several progestins. Combination pills are marketed as fixed, biphasic, or triphasic OCs depending on whether or not the hormone dose varies throughout the 21-day cycle. Most OCs contain a "fixed" amount of estrogen and progestin in each pill; therefore, every pill in the 21-day active-pill cycle is the same. Biphasic OCs, introduced in 1982, are composed of two pill strengths. Estrogen remains constant throughout the cycle; however, the progestin dose is lower during the first 10 days of the cycle. Triphasic OCs were developed to decrease the total monthly dose of progestin, potentially leading to a reduction in adverse effects. These pills also are advertised as more closely resembling menstrual cycle hormonal changes (Baird & Glasier, 1993). Clinical advantages of biphasic and triphasic formulations have not yet been elucidated (Baird & Glasier, 1993). Recently, an estrophasic pill, Estrostep, has been approved by the FDA. This OC contains three strengths that vary in estrogen content, gradually increas-

ing the dose throughout the cycle and resulting in lower monthly estrogen doses. Progestin-only pills are known as "minipills" and are primarily used in women who have contraindications to estrogen or do not tolerate combination pills. Minipills will be discussed in more detail in the section on progestin-only contraceptives. Table 18–17 lists selected OCs with their respective formulation types. Nearly ten new OC formulations are in some phase of study for FDA approval and are expected to be marketed in the coming months (New medicines, 1997).

## MECHANISM OF ACTION AND EFFICACY

As previously discussed, OCs are comprised of estrogen and progestin or progestin only (minipills). OCs prevent pregnancy by a variety of mechanisms and have a wide range of effects, resulting in a myriad of potential symptoms. Estrogenic effects that prevent conception include: (1) inhibition of ovulation by suppression of follicle-stimulating hormone (FSH) and luteinizing hormone (LH), which occurs because the pituitary gland "thinks" a woman is already pregnant; and therefore, hormones which would normally stimulate the ovary are not released; (2) inhibition of implantation with high doses of estrogen alters uterine secretions and endometrial cellular structure; (3) acceleration of ovum transport; and (4) degeneration of the corpus luteum (luteolysis), which prevents normal implantation and placental attachment. Progestins are thought to (1) inhibit ovulation by suppression of LH; (2) produce thick cervical mucus, which hampers sperm transport; (3) inhibit the enzymes that allow sperm to penetrate the ovum (capacitation); (4) slow ovum transport; and (5) inhibit implantation due to atrophic changes in the endometrium.

As a result of these varied mechanisms, OCs are an extremely effective method of birth control with perfect use failure rate within the first year of 0.5% and 0.1% for progestin-only and combined OCs, respectively. With typical use, it is estimated 3% of women will become pregnant within the first year of use with either progestin-only or combination OCs (Hatcher et al, 1994).

## COMPONENTS AND BIOLOGICAL ACTIVITY OF ORAL CONTRACEPTIVES

In the United States, OCs contain one of either two synthetic estrogens, ethinyl estradiol or mes-

**TABLE 18–17. SELECTED ORAL CONTRACEPTIVE FORMULATIONS**

| Formulation | Drug | Estrogen | Amount, μg | Progestin | Amount, mg |
|---|---|---|---|---|---|
| Fixed | Ovral | Ethinyl estradiol | 50 | Norgestrel | 0.5 |
| (mono-phasic) | Ovcon 50 | Ethinyl estradiol | 50 | Norethindrone | 1.0 |
| | Demulen 50 | Ethinyl estradiol | 50 | Ethynodiol diacetate | 1.0 |
| | Genora/Norethin/ | Mestranol | 50 | Norethindrone | 1.0 |
| | Norinyl/Ortho-Novum 1/50 | Ethinyl estradiol | 30 | Norgestrel | 0.3 |
| | Lo/Ovral | Ethinyl estradiol | 30 | Desogestrel | 0.15 |
| | Desogen/Ortho-Cept | Ethinyl estradiol | 35 | Norethindrone | 0.4 |
| | Ovcon 35 | Ethinyl estradiol | 30 | Levonorgestrel | 0.15 |
| | Levlen/Nordette/ Min-Ovral | Ethinyl estradiol | 35 | Norgestimate | 0.25 |
| | Ortho-Cyclen | Ethinyl estradiol | 35 | Norethindrone | 0.5 |
| | Brevicon/Modicon/ | Ethinyl estradiol | 35 | Norethindrone | 1.0 |
| | Nelova 0.5/35 | Ethinyl estradiol | 30 | Norethindrone acetate | 1.5 |
| | Genora/Nelova/ Norethin/Norinyl/ Ortho-Novum 1/35 | Ethinyl estradiol | 35 | Ethynodiol diacetate | 1.0 |
| | Loestrin 1.5/30 | Ethinyl estradiol | 30 | Norethindrone acetate | 1.5 |
| | Demulen 1/35 | Ethinyl estradiol | 35 | Ethynodiol diacetate | 1.0 |
| Biphasic | Ortho-Novum 10/11 | Ethinyl estradiol | 35 | Norethindrone | 0.5, 1.0 |
| Triphasic | Ortho-Novum 7/7/7 | Ethinyl estradiol | 35 | Norethindrone | 0.5, 0.75, 1.0 |
| | Tri-Levlen/Triphasil | Ethinyl estradiol | 30/40/30 | Levonorgestrel | 0.05, 0.075, 0.125 |
| | Tri-Norinyl | Ethinyl estradiol | 35 | Norethindrone | 0.5, 1.0 |
| | Tri-Cyclen | Ethinyl estradiol | 35 | Norgestimate | 0.180, 0.215, 0.250 |
| Estrophasic | Estrostep | Ethinyl estradiol | 20/30/35 | Norethindrone | 1.0 |
| Minipill | Ovrette | None | — | Norgestrel | 0.075 |
| | Micronor/Nor Q.D. | None | — | Norethindrone | 0.35 |

*Sources: Bucci and Carson (1997) and Estrostep package insert.*

tranol. These compounds differ from one another in terms of potency. Mestranol is an inactive form of estrogen that must be converted by the liver to the pharmacologically active form of estrogen, ethinyl estradiol. It is thought that mestranol is approximately 67% as potent as ethinyl estradiol. Therefore, Ortho-Novum 1/50, which contains 50 μg of mestranol, has roughly the same estrogenic effects as Ortho-Novum 1/35, which contains 35 μg of ethinyl estradiol (Dickey, 1993; Hatcher et al, 1994). Both mestranol and ethinyl estradiol only produce estrogenic activity.

In contrast, the eight progestins currently available in the United States for use in OC for-

mulations differ in progestational, androgenic, estrogenic, and endometrial (prevalence of spotting and breakthrough bleeding) activity. These progestins, along with their respective biological activities, are listed in Table 18–18. Estrogenic effects occur with certain progestins secondary to their metabolism to estrogenic substances. Additionally, antiestrogenic effects may be present. Androgenic effects are due to the structural similarity between progestins and testosterone. Norgestimate, desogestrel, and gestodene (an investigational progestin in the United States) are considered third-generation progestins and, when compared with levonorgestrel, are associ-

## TABLE 18–18. BIOLOGIC ACTIVITY OF ORAL CONTRACEPTIVE PROGESTINS

| Progestin | Progestational Activity | Estrogenic Activity | Androgenic Activity |
|---|---|---|---|
| Norethindrone | + | + | + |
| Norethindrone acetate | + | + | + |
| Ethynodiol diacetate | ++ | + | + |
| Norethynodrel | + | +++ | 0 |
| Levonorgestrel | +++ | 0 | ++++ |
| Norgestrel | +++ | 0 | ++++ |
| Desogestel | +++ | 0 | +++ |
| Norgestimate | + | 0 | ++ |
| Gestodene | ++++ | 0 | ++ |

*Adapted from Bucci and Carson (1997), Dickey (1993), and Drug Interaction Facts on Disk (1995).*

ated with reduced androgenic effects. Moreover, estrogenic effects do not occur with several progestins, including norgestimate, desogestrel, gestodene, and levonorgestrel. Interestingly, levonorgestrel has higher androgenic activity than norethindrone. It would be desirable to clinically compare the third-generation progestins and norethindrone since norethindrone is associated with less androgenicity than levonorgestrel. Unfortunately, properly controlled clinical trials comparing norethindrone, norgestimate, and desogestrel are rare; therefore, determining the actual clinical relevance of these purported improvements in lower androgenicity and progestational selectivity remains unknown (Bucci & Carson, 1997; Chapdelaine & Desmarais, 1989; Chez, 1989; Coenen, Thomas, Borm, Hollanders, & Rolland, 1996; Corson, 1995, Darney, 1995; James, 1993; Kafrissen, 1992; Phillips, Hahn, & McGuire, 1992; Speroff & DeCherney, 1993; Stone, 1995).

Since progestins vary in their propensity for causing estrogenic, progestational, androgenic, and endometrial activity, understanding the differences between the progestins is essential for selecting appropriate OCs and managing adverse effects. Pharmacological differences between OCs result from the type of progestin used and the estrogen and progestin dose in the formulation. For example, Ortho-Novum 7/7/7, containing norethindrone and ethinyl estradiol 35 µg, has greater estrogenic activity than Tri-Cyclen, containing norgestimate and the same dose of ethinyl estradiol, because of the added estrogenic effect from norethindrone being converted, in vivo, to estrogen. Table 18–19 compares the

relative pharmacologic effects of selected OCs. Using information from this table will allow the practitioner, in a logical, systematic manner, to choose the most appropriate OC and switch OCs if adverse effects develop. Table 18–20 describes potential adverse effects associated with each type of activity.

## MANAGING ADVERSE EFFECTS

As discussed previously, adverse effects from OCs may be classified by the type of activity responsible for them (Table 18–20). In most cases, management involves switching patients to an OC with a different estrogenic, progestational, androgenic, or endometrial activity level, depending on which adverse effect is present (see Table 18–19 for pharmacologic activity of respective OCs).

In addition to pharmacologic activity, the time framework in which the adverse effect develops is important to management. Adverse effects from OCs may be worst in the first several months, constant over time, worse over time, or worse after pill discontinuation (Dickey, 1993; Hatcher et al, 1994). By determining when the adverse effect occurred and if it is worse upon starting OCs, it may be possible to continue therapy for at least 3 months instead of switching pills. Side effects that normally dissipate after the first 3 months include nausea, dizziness, cyclic weight gain, edema, breast fullness and tenderness, and breakthrough bleeding. Conversely, some side effects such as acne, depression, and decreased libido may be constant

## TABLE 18–19. ACTIVITY OF SELECTED ORAL CONTRACEPTIVES[a]

| Oral Contraceptive | Endometrial Activity[b] | Estrogenic Activity | Progestational Activity | Androgenic Activity |
|---|---|---|---|---|
| **50-µg Estrogen** | | | | |
| Ovral | 4.5 | ++++ | ++++ | +++ |
| Ortho-Novum 1/50 | 10.6 | +++ | ++ | ++ |
| Ovcon 50 | 11.9 | ++++ | +++ | ++ |
| Demulen 50 | 13.9 | ++ | ++++ | ++ |
| Norlestrin 1/50 | 13.9 | +++ | +++ | +++ |
| **Sub-50-µg estrogen (monophasic)** | | | | |
| Lo-Ovral | 9.6 | ++ | ++ | ++ |
| Desogen/Ortho-Cept | 9.9 | ++ | ++++ | + |
| Ovcon 35 | 11.0 | ++++ | + | + |
| Levlen/Nordette | 14.0 | ++ | ++ | ++ |
| Ortho-Cyclen | 14.3 | +++ | + | + |
| Brevicon 0.5/35 | 14.6 | ++++ | + | + |
| Ortho-Novum 1/35 | 14.7 | +++ | +++ | ++ |
| Loestrin 1.5/30 | 25.2 | + | +++++ | +++ |
| Loestrin 1/20 | 29.7 | + | +++ | +++ |
| Demulen 1/35 | 37.4 | + | ++++ | ++ |
| **Sub-50-µg estrogen (multiphasic)** | | | | |
| Ortho-Novum 10/11 | 19.6 | ++++ | ++ | ++ |
| Ortho-Novum 7/7/7 | 12.2 | ++++ | ++ | ++ |
| Tri-Norinyl | 14.7 | ++++ | ++ | ++ |
| Tri-Levlen/Triphasil | 15.1 | ++ | + | ++ |
| Tri-Cyclen | 17.5 | +++ | + | ++ |
| **Progestin-only** | | | | |
| Ovrette | 34.9 | 0 | + | + |
| Micronor/Nor-QD | 42.3 | 0 | + | + |

[a]OCs cannot be precisely compared because activity rates are from different noncomparative studies in distinct patient populations.
[b]Percentage of spotting and breakthrough bleeding.
*Adapted from Bucci and Carson (1997) and Dickey (1993).*

over time. Table 18–21 reviews management strategies for commonly occurring OC adverse effects.

Rarely, serious side effects may occur with OCs and patients should be instructed to contact their provider if the following warning signs (ACHES) develop: A = abdominal pain (severe); C = chest pain (severe), shortness of breath, or coughing up blood; H = headaches; E = eye problems such as blurred vision, flashing lights, or blindness; and S = severe leg pain (calf or thigh). These signs may signal gallbladder disease; hepatic adenoma; a blood clot in the lungs or myocardial infarction; stroke, hypertension, or migraines; other temporary vascular problems; or a blood clot in the legs.

## BENEFITS, RISKS, AND UNCERTAINTIES ASSOCIATED WITH OCS

In the majority of cases, OCs are a safe and reliable method of birth control for women under 50 who do not smoke. Surprisingly, women who use combination OCs are at a lower risk for development of endometrial and ovarian cancer. OCs may also benefit women at risk for pelvic inflammatory disease and ectopic pregnancies

**TABLE 18–20.  SELECTED ADVERSE EFFECTS ASSOCIATED WITH HORMONAL ACTIVITY**

| System | Estrogen Excess | Progestin Excess | Androgen Excess | Estrogen Deficiency | Progestin Deficiency |
|---|---|---|---|---|---|
| General | Chloasma<br>Chronic nasal<br>  pharyngitis<br>Allergic rhinitis | Appetite<br>  increase<br>Depression<br>Fatigue<br>Hypoglycemia<br>  symptoms<br>Libido decrease<br>Neurodermatits<br>Weight gain<br>  (noncyclic) | Acne<br>Cholestatic<br>  jaundice<br>Hirsutism<br>Libido increase<br>Oily skin and<br>  scalp<br>Rash and<br>  pruritus<br>Edema | Nervousness<br>Vasomotor<br>  symptoms | N/A |
| Cardiovascular | Capillary fragility<br>CVA<br>DVT<br>Telangiectasias<br>Thromboembolic<br>  disease | Hypertension<br>Leg vein<br>  dilation | N/A | N/A | N/A |
| Reproductive | Breast cystic<br>  changes<br>Dysmenorrhea<br>Hypermenorrhea<br>Increase in breast<br>  size | Cervicitis<br>Flow length<br>  decrease<br>Moniliasis | N/A | Absence of<br>  withdrawal<br>  bleeding<br>Bleeding and<br>  spotting<br>  during pill<br>  days 1–9<br>Continuous<br>  bleeding and<br>  spotting<br>Flow decrease<br>Vaginitis<br>  (atrophic) | Breakthrough<br>  bleeding and<br>  spotting during<br>  pill days 10–21<br>Delayed with-<br>  drawal bleeding<br>Dysmenorrhea<br>Heavy flow and<br>  clots |
| Premenstrual | Bloating<br>Dizziness, syncope<br>Edema<br>Headache (cyclic)<br>Irritability<br>Leg cramps<br>Nausea, vomiting<br>Visual changes<br>  (cyclic)<br>Weight gain (cyclic) | N/A | N/A | N/A | Bloating<br>Dizziness, syncope<br>Edema<br>Headache (cyclic)<br>Irritability<br>Leg cramps<br>Nausea, vomiting<br>Visual changes<br>  (cyclic)<br>Weight gain (cyclic) |

N/A = not applicable.
*Adapted from Bucci and Carson (1997), Dickey (1993), and Hatcher et al (1994).*

and those who have ovarian cysts, benign breast disease, severe dysmenorrhea, iron deficiency anemia, endometriosis, hirsutism, and acne (Baird & Glasier, 1993; Dickey, 1993; Hatcher et al, 1994; Mango, Ricci, Manna, Miggiano, & Serna, 1996). Recent evidence suggests OCs also may prevent pelvic inflammatory disease caused by chlamydial infection, which was previously thought not to be affected by OC use (Spinillo et al, 1996).

**TABLE 18–21. MANAGEMENT STRATEGIES FOR COMMONLY OCCURRING ADVERSE EFFECTS**

| Adverse Effect | Causal Factors | Management Strategies |
|---|---|---|
| **Menstrual Disorders** | | |
| Absence of withdrawal menses | • Insufficient estrogen to develop endometrium and vessels<br>• Most common in women taking low-dose estrogen OCs<br>• May appear after OCs have been taken for several months | • Rule out pregnancy<br>• Continue same OC without menses<br>• Switch to OC with same amount estrogen but increased endometrial activity<br>• Switch to OC with larger estrogen dose (up to 50 μg ethinyl estradiol) |
| Dysmenorrhea | • Rare in anovulatory cycles unless there is passage of blood clots<br>• Endometriosis | • Switch to OC with more progestin/androgen activity and less estrogen activity<br>• Use an NSAID |
| Heavy menstruation | • Insufficient progestin activity or excess estrogen activity | • Rule out pathological causes<br>• Switch to OC with more progestin/androgen activity or less estrogen activity |
| Breakthrough bleeding (BTB) and spotting | • Early BTB: insufficient estrogen activity, associated with failure to menstruate during off days<br>• Late BTB: insufficient progestin activity<br>• Most common with low-dose OCs<br>• Most common reason for discontinuation | • Rule out pathological condition or pregnancy<br>• Allow three cycles for patient to adjust to OC<br>• Switch to OC with more endometrial activity |
| **Sensory-Nervous System** | | |
| Dizziness | • Associated with fluid retention<br>• Usually disappears after third cycle | • Switch to OC with less estrogen activity |
| Headache | • May be due to estrogen<br>• Usually associated with fluid retention or vascular spasm | • Switch to OC with less estrogen activity<br>• May have to discontinue OC if headache persists |
| Depression | • May be due to progestin<br>• Characterized by apathy, listlessness, feelings of dejection, anorexia, insomnia, and restlessness | • Switch to OC with less progestin activity<br>• Consider discontinuing OC if depression occurs in patients with history of depression<br>• Vitamin $B_6$ (pyridoxine) may be used |
| **Other Side Effects** | | |
| Acne and Hirsutism | • Associated with androgenic activity | • Switch to OC with the estrogen activity<br>• Switch to OC with less androgen activity |
| Nausea and Vomiting | • Associated with estrogen dose<br>• Most severe with initial cycles | • Take with food or at bedtime<br>• Switch to OC with less estrogen activity |
| Weight Change | • Associated with both estrogen and progestin depending if cyclic or non-cyclic weight gain. | • Switch to OC with less progestin and less androgen if appetite increases hypoglycemic symptoms<br>• Switch to OC with less estrogen activity if cyclic weight gain in breast, hips and thighs |

Sources: Dickey (1993) and Hatcher et al (1994).

Although many benefits have been documented with OCs, caution should be exercised when deciding to use OCs in certain women because of the potential for exacerbation of a variety of conditions. Table 18–22 lists absolute and relative contraindications to OC use.

## CARDIOVASCULAR COMPLICATIONS AND METABOLIC CHANGES

With the availability of new third-generation progestins and the reduction in dosage of estrogen in combination OCs, the risks for cardiovascular disease, including effects on lipid metabolism, hypertension, glucose tolerance, venous thromboembolism, myocardial infarction, and stroke, have been reduced compared with the increased risk for cardiovascular disease associated with older OC formulations. The Oxford Family Planning Association Contraceptive Study published in 1977 demonstrated an increase in the risk of death from cardiovascular disease of 4.7-fold in women taking OCs containing 50 μg of estrogen (Vessey, McPherson, & Johnson, 1997). No evidence suggests that OCs containing low doses of estrogen place women at an increased risk for developing cardiovascular disease, although certain patient-specific characteristics may place a woman at an increased risk.

### TABLE 18–22. CONTRAINDICATIONS TO OC USE

| Absolute | Relative |
|---|---|
| • Cardiovascular: thrombophlebitis, thromboembolic disorders, cerebral vascular disease | • Migraine headaches |
| | • Hypertension |
| | • Uterine leiomyoma |
| | • Gestational diabetes |
| | • Elective surgery |
| • Liver function markedly impaired | • Epilepsy: anticonvulsants may decrease efficacy of OCs |
| • Breast cancer: known or suspected | |
| • Vaginal bleeding: undiagnosed, abnormal | • Obstructive jaundice in pregnancy |
| • Pregnancy: known or suspected | • Sickle cell disease or sickle cell–hemoglobin C disease |
| • Smokers over 35 years | • Systemic lupus erythematosus |
| | • Diabetes mellitus |
| | • Gallbladder disease |

Source: Hatcher et al (1994).

## Hypertension

Hypertension is a relative contraindication to OC use even if a woman's blood pressure is well controlled on antihypertensive medications (Narkiewicz et al, 1995). Both estrogen and progestin may cause mild elevations in blood pressure in approximately 5% of normotensive women and 9–16% of hypertensive women. Monitoring blood pressure in women taking OCs is recommended, and if it is elevated, switching to an OC with a lower progestational activity or discontinuing therapy should result in a normalization of blood pressure within 3 months. Women are more likely to develop hypertension with increasing age, longer duration of OC use, and family history of hypertension. However, hypertension may occur in women without risk factors and at any time while receiving OCs (Baird & Glasier, 1993; Bucci & Carson, 1997; Dickey, 1993).

## Lipid Metabolism

OCs may alter lipid metabolism. Estrogen has beneficial effects on the lipid profile, and partially for this reason, it is given to postmenopausal women to reduce the risk of cardiovascular disease. Conversely, progestins, especially those with appreciable androgenic activity, may raise LDL-cholesterol and lower HDL-cholesterol. Differences among OC formulations in the propensity to affect the lipid profile have been demonstrated in various clinical studies. Some studies suggest that third-generation progestin formulations containing desogestrel, gestodene, and norgestimate have resulted in beneficial effects on the lipid profile, raising HDL-cholesterol and reducing LDL-cholesterol, and suggest a potential cardioprotective effect with long-term use (Baird & Glasier, 1993; Brill et al, 1996; Godsland et al, 1990; Kauppinen-Makelin, Kyusi, Ylikarkala, & Tikkanen, 1992; Krauss & Burkman, 1992; Lobo, Skinner, Lippman, & Cirillo, 1996; Speroff & De Cherney, 1993). Regardless of the lipid profile changes resulting from OCs, the detrimental cardiovascular effects (stroke, venous thromboembolism, and myocardial infarction) demonstrated with OC use are thought to be caused by the thrombogenic properties of OCs. Therefore, lipid alterations produced by OCs are not thought to be clinically significant (Baird & Glasier, 1993).

## Glucose Intolerance

Most women without diabetes do not experience glucose intolerance while taking low-dose OCs, although high-dose older OC formulations have resulted in increased glucose levels, increased plasma insulin levels, and decreased glucose tolerance. The new progestins, norgestimate and desogestrel, are not thought to alter glucose metabolism. If an OC is prescribed to a woman who has a history of glucose intolerance, it would be advisable to choose one containing a third-generation progestin to minimize adverse carbohydrate effects, and to monitor glucose tolerance on a periodic basis (Hatcher et al, 1994). Please refer to the special populations section in this chapter for information on the use of OCs in women with diabetes.

## Venous Thromboembolism and Pulmonary Embolism

Venous thromboembolism and pulmonary embolism are rare, yet serious, complications of OCs and for this reason OCs should not be used in women with a history of deep venous thrombosis (DVT). The estrogen component of OCs has been shown to increase the hepatic synthesis of selected vitamin K–dependent clotting factors and fibrinogen, decrease the activity of antithrombin III and protein S (endogenous inhibitors of clotting), and increase platelet aggregation. These effects lead to an increased propensity for thrombosis, especially in women who smoke. The incidence of venous thromboembolism was reported in early studies to be 3 to 11 times higher in women who used OCs compared to nonusers. More recent studies with second-generation progestins indicate the relative risk for venous thromboembolism to be 2.8 in users compared with nonusers (Alving & Comp, 1992; Baird & Glasier, 1993; Bucci & Carson, 1997; Hatcher et al, 1994). In 1995, controversy surrounding desogestrel- and gestodene-containing OCs and the potential increase in relative risk for venous thromboembolism prompted a "Dear Doctor" letter to be sent to physicians in the United Kingdom. This warning was based on data from four large observational studies (Farley, Meirik, Chang, Marmot, & Poulter, 1995; Jick et al, 1995; Poulter, Chang, Farley, Meirik, & Marmot, 1995; Spitzer et al, 1996) suggesting that desogestrel and gestodene OCs resulted in an approximate twofold increase in the risk of venous thromboembolism compared with

OCs containing other progestins. Appropriate interpretation of these studies is important. Although an increased relative risk with desogestrel and gestodene OCs was found, the risk is still less than that associated with older, high-dose pills and with pregnancy. Additionally, the relative risk, even though significantly greater, still represents a small actual increase in frequency. For example, if the baseline risk for DVT within a population is 1 in 10,000 women per year, a second-generation OC would have a risk of 3.6 in 10,000, and desogestrel or gestodene OCs would have a risk of about 5 in 10,000 women per year. Therefore, using second-generation OCs would prevent 2 DVTs per 10,000 women per year. Moreover, these observational studies were not randomized, and bias could have influenced the results (Grimes, 1996; Koster, Small, Rosendaal, & Helmerhorst, 1995; Lewis, Heinemann, et al, 1996; Lidegaard & Milsom, 1996). In conclusion, taking a careful family and personal history for increased risk of venous thromboembolism is highly recommended. Risk factors for venous thromboembolism include hereditary thrombophilia, lupus anticoagulant, malignancy, immobility or trauma, obesity, and varicose veins (Mills et al, 1996). It may be advisable for women who have risks for venous thromboembolism not to be initially started on a desogestrel- or gestodene-containing OC and, if started, to obtain a signed informed consent. If a woman is currently receiving a third-generation OC and has risk factors for venous thromboembolism, the woman should be advised to switch to an OC that does not contain desogestrel or gestodene or use another contraceptive method (Grimes, 1996; Mills et al, 1996).

## Myocardial Infarction

In addition to an increased risk for venous thromboembolism, women who receive OCs have a greater relative risk for myocardial infarction (MI), primarily if other cardiovascular risks are present. The risk of MI increases with advancing age and cigarette smoking. Women who smoke and are over 35 years old are at an increased risk for MI and other cardiovascular conditions such as stroke and venous thromboembolism. For this reason, OCs should not be used in women older than 35 years of age who smoke. New data indicate OCs with less than 50 μg of estrogen may be used in healthy, nonsmoking women up to 50 years old (Bucci & Carson, 1997; Dickey, 1993; Hatcher et al, 1994).

Risk for MI also may vary depending on the type of progestin in the OC formulation. A recent study (Lewis, Spitzer, et al, 1996) reported that third-generation progestins are associated with a reduction in MI risk or with no difference in risk compared to second-generation OCs. Women taking OCs containing less than 50 μg of estrogen and a second-generation progestin had a significantly increased odds ratio of acute MI of 3.1 compared to nonusers of OC. In those women receiving third-generation OCs the odds ratio was 1.1, indicating no increase in MI risk compared to women not receiving OCs. The risk of MI with second-generation OCs is still considered low when compared to results of studies published in the 1970s with higher-dose OCs. Therefore, the excess risk of venous thrombo-embolism reported in other studies may be weighed against the reduction in MI risk with the third-generation progestin OCs (Lewis, Spitzer, et al, 1996)

### Stroke

Another complication associated with OCs is stroke, either thrombotic (ischemic) or hemorrhagic. Early data with higher-dose pills suggested the risk of stroke was five times greater in pill users versus nonusers, with even greater risk in those women who smoked (Bucci & Carson, 1997; Lidegaard, 1993). A recent study (World Health Organization [WHO] Collaborative Study, 1996a) demonstrated that the risk of hemorrhagic stroke was not increased in younger women and was only slightly increased in older women when receiving currently prescribed low-dose OCs. Another study examining the risk of thrombotic and hemorrhagic stroke has also concluded that new, low-dose OCs do not place healthy women of childbearing age at any greater risk for stroke (Buring, 1996; Petitti et al, 1996). Women with diabetes and hypertension generally were not given OCs in this study. Another study (WHO Collaborative Study, 1996b) evaluated ischemic stroke and combined oral contraceptives and found the incidence of ischemic stroke to be low in women of reproductive age. Furthermore, the risk can be reduced if users are younger and do not smoke or have a history of hypertension.

### NEOPLASTIC EFFECTS

The association between OC use and breast cancer has been evaluated in many epidemiologic reports (Hawley, Nuevo, DeNeef, & Carter, 1993; Herbst & Berek, 1993; McGonigle & Huggins, 1991). Recently a meta-analysis (Collaborative Group, 1996) using data from 54 epidemiologic studies, including a total of 53,297 women with breast cancer and 100,239 women without breast cancer, was conducted. This meta-analysis concluded that in women currently taking OCs and within 10 years of discontinuing OCs, there was a small increase in the risk of contracting breast cancer. Current OC users had a 24% greater risk of breast cancer compared to nonusers. The risk was greater in higher-dose OCs and decreased progressively after OC discontinuation. If diagnosed, breast cancer in OC users was less clinically advanced than breast cancer diagnosed in non-OC users. Moreover, a slightly decreased risk of breast cancer was found in those women who had stopped using OCs for more than 10 years. It is unclear whether these findings were due to earlier diagnosis of breast cancer, to biological hormonal effects, or to a combination of these factors.

The effect of OCs on cervical cancer remains unclear because of the many variables other than OC use that may influence the risk of cervical cancer. These variables include number of sexual partners and age at first coitus, exposure to human papillomavirus, use of barrier contraceptives, and smoking. Because the risk of cervical cancer is unknown, periodic cervical screening should be performed.

As briefly discussed earlier, women who use combination OCs are at a lower risk for development of endometrial and ovarian cancer. Epidemiologic evidence indicates that combination OC users, compared to nonusers, have a 40% and 50% lower likelihood of developing ovarian and endometrial cancer, respectively, after 2 years of use. Moreover, this protection appears to endure for at least 15 years after OCs have been discontinued. This decreased risk is thought to involve the maintenance of regular withdrawal bleeding (Baird & Glasier, 1993; Centers for Disease Control, 1987a, 1987b; Schlesselman, 1989).

Although extremely rare, an increase in hepatocellular adenomas has been associated with OC use. These benign tumors, occurring in 1.3 per million women between 31–44 years of age using OCs, may lead to rupturing of the liver capsule and death. Ongoing, severe abdominal pain is a sign of this complication (Hatcher et al, 1994).

## DRUG INTERACTIONS

Obtaining an accurate medication history is essential to ensure that drug interactions do not go unnoticed or compromise patient care. Medication history taking may be complicated in OC users because many women do not consider the pill to be a "drug"; therefore, they may not disclose taking OCs when asked about current medications. Additionally, multiple physicians may be involved, one prescribing the OC and another prescribing a potentially interacting medication. Many medications have the potential to reduce the efficacy of OCs, thereby putting a woman at risk for pregnancy. Breakthrough bleeding may be a sign that a drug interaction has occurred (Dickey, 1993). Mechanisms by which drugs may interact with OCs include interference with gastrointestinal absorption, alteration in gastrointestinal bacterial flora, and pharmacokinetic changes. Additionally, OCs may interfere with other medications or exacerbate various disease states, thereby reducing the effectiveness of drug therapy. Table 18–23 provides information on drug interactions with oral contraceptives along with management strategies.

In addition to medications altering the serum concentration of OCs, grapefruit juice and vitamin C may increase the bioavailability of ethinyl estradiol. The clinical importance of this interaction has not yet been demonstrated; however, if estrogen concentrations are elevated significantly, a woman may be at risk for cardiovascular complications (Bucci & Carson, 1997; Weber et al, 1996).

## CHOOSING AN ORAL CONTRACEPTIVE AND INITIATING THERAPY

Before deciding to place a woman on an OC, the clinician needs to address several issues such as contraindications, drug interactions, patient lifestyle, compliance, acceptance, toleration, and cost. According to an economic study on contraception, the most cost-effective forms of contraception are the copper-T IUD, vasectomy, and injectable and implantable contraceptives. Oral contraceptives cost approximately $1800 over 5 years, but save almost $12,000 in costs related to prevented pregnancies (Trussell et al, 1995). Additionally, advantages and disadvantages of OCs should be discussed with patients.

Once it has been determined to use an OC, many formulations are available, each with differences in potential side effects and tolerability. Since high-dose OCs are associated with increased risks, typically OCs with less than 50 µg of ethinyl estradiol are selected. Patients may have inherent sensitivities to the estrogenic, progestational, androgenic, or endometrial effects of OCs. If a woman appears more sensitive to a certain type of activity, initial OC selection should minimize this effect. For example, a woman who is more sensitive to estrogenic effects may have a history of migraine, severe nausea, vomiting, or hypertension during pregnancy; large or fibrocystic breasts; and heavy menses. An OC with lower estrogenic activity would be an appropriate choice for this patient. A woman would be considered to be progestin-sensitive if she has a history of toxemia, excessive weight gain, tiredness, or varicose veins during pregnancy; depression; and excessive premenstrual edema. Androgen sensitivity is associated with irregular heavy menses, acne, hirsutism, and oily skin. An OC with high progestational activity and low androgenic activity would be appropriate in this setting. Tables 18–19 and 18–20 also may be used to guide a practitioner in OC selection (Dickey, 1993; Hatcher et al, 1994).

Before a woman is placed on an OC, a complete medical history and physical examination should be conducted and repeated at least once a year while using OCs. The physical examination may be deferred by the physician if requested by the patient. The physical examination should include blood pressure, breasts, abdomen, and pelvic organs. Cervical cytology and any pertinent laboratory tests should also be checked.

## PATIENT INSTRUCTIONS AND COMPLIANCE ISSUES

Although the annual failure rate is 0.1% with perfect OC use, typical users have an annual failure rate averaging 3%, and higher failure rates may occur in certain populations. The primary reason for this discrepancy between perfect and typical failure rates is lack of compliance. As many as one half of women discontinue OCs within the first year of use, primarily due to fear of potential side effects and actual side effects such as breakthrough bleeding. Those OC users who discontinue therapy may not adopt alternate means of birth control, placing them-

**TABLE 18–23. SELECTED DRUG INTERACTIONS WITH COMBINED ORAL CONTRACEPTIVES AND MANAGEMENT STRATEGIES**

| Drug Class | Generic Name (Trade) | Effect | Patient Management |
|---|---|---|---|
| **Drugs Which May Reduce Effectiveness of Oral Contraceptives** | | | |
| Antibiotics | Erythromycin<br>Griseofulvin<br>Penicillins<br>Rifampin<br>Tetracycline | Antibiotics may eliminate GI bacteria, thereby disturbing the enterohepatic circulation of estrogen, which results in lower serum estrogen concentrations. GI transport may increase or diarrhea may also decrease absorption of estrogen. Griseofulvin or rifampin may increase estrogen metabolism | Use alternative method of contraception during the treatment course and for at least 1 week after discontinuing the antibiotic (1 month for rifampin). |
| Antivirals | Ritonavir (Norvir)<br>Nevirapine (Viramune) | Ritonavir may lower estrogen levels by about 40%; nevirapine may lower serum levels of OCs | Use alternative method of contraception. |
| Anticonvulsants (including barbiturates) | Carbamazepine (Tegretol)<br>Felbamate (Felbatol)<br>Phenobarbital<br>Phenytoin (Dilantin)<br>Primidone (Mysoline) | Induction of liver microsomal enzymes (increases metabolism), leading to decreased OC effect | Use alternative method of contraception or consider a higher-dose product (50 μg ethinyl estradiol; monitor for signs of estrogenic side effects). Valproic acid does not appear to interact with OCs. |
| Antidiabetic agents | Troglitazone (Rezulin) | May lower the serum concentration of OCs by 30% | Use alternative method of contraception or another medication to treat type II diabetes mellitus. |
| **Effect of Oral Contraceptive on Other Drugs or Disease States** | | | |
| Anticoagulants | Warfarin (Coumadin) | OCs increase vitamin-K–dependent clotting factors, decrease efficacy of anticoagulant | Do not use OCs in patients who require anticoagulation. |
| Antidiabetic agents | Insulin; oral hypoglycemics | High-dose OCs may impair glucose tolerance | Use low-dose estrogen and progestin OC or alternative method. |
| Antihypertensives | | OCs may increase blood pressure | Use alternative method in patients with hypertension or switch to low-dose OC. |
| Beta blockers | Acebutolol (Sectral)<br>Metoprolol (Lopressor)<br>Propranolol (Inderal) | OCs lower metabolism of some beta blockers, thereby increasing their effects | Increase dose of beta blocker if needed; monitor cardiovascular status. |
| Bronchodilators | Theophylline | Increase effect of theophylline | Use with caution. |
| Corticosteroids | Prednisone | OCs raise serum levels | May need to lower dose of steroid. |
| Tricyclic antidepressants | Amitriptyline (Elavil) and others | OCs may increase the metabolism of tricyclic antidepressants (TCAs), thereby increasing their effects | Monitor for TCA toxicity and lower dose if necessary. |
| Antibiotics | Troandomycin | Increase risk of cholestasis | Use alternative method of contraception. |

*Adapted from Dickey (1993), Drug Interaction Facts on Disk (1995), Hatcher et al (1994), Pharmacist's Letter (1997), and Norvir, Rezulin, and Viramune package inserts.*

selves at an additional risk for pregnancy. Providing adequate counseling is crucial in improving compliance and enhancing OC effectiveness (Filshie clip, 1996; Grimes, 1996, Rosenberg, Burnhill, Waugh, Grimes, & Hillar, 1995; Rosenberg, Waugh, & Meehan, 1995). Table 18–24 provides counseling suggestions for providers to use with their patients in the hopes of improving patient compliance.

Specific directions for taking OCs should be discussed and provided to patients in writing along with the package insert and product information required for estrogen products. Patients should be instructed to read all directions and take the pill at approximately the same time every day, which promotes compliance and consistent plasma concentrations. There are 21-day and 28-day pill packs, each containing 21 "active" pills. The 28-day pill packs contain seven placebo pills taken during the last week. Taking a pill daily with no off days may be easier for some women to remember. OCs are started on the first day of menses or on the first Sunday after the onset of menses. If menses begin on Sunday, the women should start taking the OC that same Sunday. Initiating OCs on Sunday will usually avoid menses during the weekend. Those patients starting OC on the first day of menses will not require any backup contracep-

tive method; however, Sunday starters need to use an alternate contraception method as a backup for 7 days (until the next Sunday). The patient's next menses will begin during the seven placebo tablets if using a 28-day pill pack. If using a 21-day pill pack, the patient should be instructed to start the next pack 1 week after finishing the last, even if she is still menstruating (Hatcher et al, 1994).

Missing scheduled pills is a common occurrence in both adolescents and older women. One study revealed that adolescents miss an average of three pills per month. Another report determined that 30% of women between 18–30 years of age miss one or more pills per month (Rosenberg, Burnhill, Waugh et al, 1995; Rosenberg, Waugh, & Meehan, 1995). In addition to providing patient education to improve compliance and reduce the incidence of missing pills, it is equally important to make sure patients understand what to do if an active pill or pills have been missed. If an inactive pill has been missed, the patient should be instructed to throw away the missed pills and start the next pill pack on the regularly scheduled day. Since these are placebo tablets, missing one of the last seven pills in a 28-day OC pack will not put a woman at risk for pregnancy. Data suggest that the most critical times to miss pills are directly prior to or after the 7-day hor-

## TABLE 18–24.  SUGGESTIONS FOR IMPROVING COMPLIANCE

| Recommendation | Comment |
|---|---|
| Three things all women should know before starting OCs | 1. How to take the OC.<br>2. What to do if they miss a pill or pills.<br>3. Common, transient, and serious side effects. |
| Dispel OC misinformation | Also discuss health benefits from OCs. |
| Instructions | Verbal and written instructions given to all patients, discussed point by point; each follow-up visit should offer another copy of instructions. If questions arise at a later point, make sure the patient knows how to get additional information. |
| Demonstrate use of pill pack | All users, especially first-time users. Compliance enhanced with 28-day pack. |
| Time of day to take OC | Help select specific time; may want to briefly discuss daily schedule to identify optimal time; taking after dinner or with a bedtime snack may cause nausea. |
| Extra refills | Include extra cycle in prescription for missed pills or lost packets. |
| Missed pills procedure | Discuss backup method. |
| STDs | Discuss prevention of STDs. Provide condom and discuss proper use. |
| Follow-up visits; inquire about problems | A nonjudgmental approach to uncover and solve problems with taking pills. Ask what was done if a pill was missed. |
| Repeated compliance problems | Counsel women about using another method if OC user has repeated difficulty remembering to take OC. |

Adapted from Oral contraception (1994) and Rosenberg, Burnhill, Waugh, et al (1995).

mone-free period (Potter, 1994). Table 18–25 provides guidelines for missed "active" pills. Other reasons to use an alternate form of contraception in addition to missed pills include diarrhea, vomiting, and administration of interacting drugs that might reduce the effectiveness of OCs. Diarrhea or vomiting may reduce the amount of estrogen and progestin absorbed. Table 18–23 provides a list of drugs that may reduce the efficacy of OCs. A backup method should be used in these situations for the remainder of the cycle. OCs do not protect against STDs, including HIV. For this reason, consistently and correctly using latex or polyurethane condoms is highly recommended. Some practitioners recommend using an alternate method during the first pill pack, although FDA guidelines state a backup method is only required for the first 7 days in those patients starting on Sunday (Anonymous, 1994; Bucci & Carson, 1997; Filshie clip, 1996; Hatcher et al, 1994).

Return to fertility may be delayed after OCs have been discontinued. Some practitioners suggest that women wait two to three normal menstrual periods before becoming pregnant to allow for reestablishment of ovulation and menses. No increase in birth defects has been shown in women who conceived in the month after OC discontinuation (Bucci & Carson, 1997).

## PROGESTIN-ONLY CONTRACEPTIVES

### The "Minipill"

The minipill is a progestin-only pill that delivers the same dose of progestin every day (see Table 18–17 for a list of minipill OCs). Minipills are prescribed to a minority of women. They are not used as frequently as combination OCs because of decreased efficacy and a propensity for untoward side effects such as breakthrough bleeding or spotting. However, in certain patients, minipills may offer advantages over combination OCs. Reasons to choose a minipill include: a contraindication to the estrogen component of combined OC (ie, thromboembolism); risk for estrogen-related side effects such as hyperten-

## TABLE 18–25. GUIDELINES FOR MISSED "ACTIVE" PILLS

| Pills Missed | Time in Cycle | Patient Interactions |
|---|---|---|
| 1 | Anytime | • Take pill as soon as you remember. Take the next pill at your regular time (you may take 2 pills in one day).<br>• Backup method of contraception is not necessary |
| 2 | First 2 weeks | • Take 2 pills on the day you remember and 2 pills the next day.<br>• Then take 1 pill a day until you finish the pack.<br>• You MAY BECOME PREGNANT if you have intercourse in the 7 days after you miss pills. You MUST use another contraceptive method for those 7 days. |
| 2 | Third week | • Day 1 starter: Throw out the pill pack and start a new pack that same day.<br>• Sunday starter: Keep taking 1 pill every day until Sunday; on Sunday, throw out pill pack and start a new pack that same day.<br>• It is expected that you will not have a period this month. However, if you miss your period 2 months in a row, call your doctor or clinic because you may be pregnant.<br>• You MAY BECOME PREGNANT if you have intercourse in the 7 days after you miss pills. You MUST use another contraceptive method for those 7 days. |
| 3 | Anytime | • Day 1 starter: Throw out the pill pack and start a new pack that same day.<br>• Sunday starter: Keep taking 1 pill every day until Sunday; on Sunday, throw out pill pack and start a new pack that same day.<br>• It is expected that you will not have a period this month. However, if you miss your period 2 months in a row, call your doctor or clinic because you may be pregnant.<br>• You MAY BECOME PREGNANT if you have intercourse in the 7 days after you miss pills. You MUST use another contraceptive method for those 7 days. |

Sources: Oral contraception (1994), Hatcher et al (1994), Potter (1994), and the Ortho-Novum package insert.

sion, headache, and varicose veins; previous patient experiences of intolerable side effects from estrogen in combination OC; smokers older than 35 years of age; and breast-feeding mothers. Estrogen suppresses lactation, and since this effect is not present with progestin-only OCs, the minipill is an excellent choice for a breast-feeding mother. Starting on the first day of menses, patients take the minipill every day without a 7-day pill-free interval. A backup method of contraception is not necessary during the initial cycle because effects on cervical mucus appear immediately; however, it may be prudent to use an alternate method during this time because of the potential to forget pills or take them late during the initial cycle. Table 18–26 provides additional information on progestin-only pills (Bucci & Carson, 1997, Caufield, 1998; Hatcher et al, 1994).

## Long-Acting Progestin Contraceptives

Medroxyprogesterone Acetate. Depot-medroxy progesterone acetate (DMPA) (Depo-Provera) inhibits ovulation by suppression of FSH and LH levels and by eliminating the LH surge. Additionally, DMPA produces an atrophic endometrium and thick cervical mucus, decreasing sperm penetration. DMPA is administered as a 150-mg deep IM injection given in the gluteal, deltoid, or quadricep muscle within 5 days after the onset of menstrual bleeding and repeated every 3 months. Initially, administration during the first few days of the menstrual cycle ensures an immediate contraceptive effect, improves efficacy, and avoids administration in pregnancy. There are two commercial strengths of DMPA, 100- and 400-mg/mL suspensions; however the 400-mg/mL suspension should not be used as a contraceptive method because of inconsistent bioavailability and decreased efficacy. Prior to injection, the vial should be shaken to produce an even dispersion of the suspension. Massaging the injection site is not recommended because this is associated with higher initial serum levels but lower levels after 90 days. Although DMPA should be administered every 3 months, there is a 2-week "grace period" in which the patient may be late in receiving the next injection yet still be pro-

## TABLE 18–26.  PROGESTIN-ONLY PILLS (MINIPILLS)

| | |
|---|---|
| Mechanism | • Inhibit ovulation by suppression of LH.<br>• Produce thick cervical mucus, which hampers sperm transport.<br>• Inhibit the enzymes that allow sperm to penetrate the ovum (capacitation).<br>• Slow ovum transport.<br>• Inhibit implantation due to atrophic changes in the endometrium. |
| Effectiveness | • Low failure rate: 0.5% per year.<br>• Typical failure rate: 3% per year. |
| Major adverse effects | • Menstrual cycle disturbance. |
| Advantages | • No adverse effects related to estrogen.<br>• Safer than combined OCs.<br>• Nursing mothers: Does not reduce lactation.<br>• May use in women who cannot receive estrogen (refer to estrogen contraindications) or in women who are experiencing intolerable adverse effects from estrogen. However, according to FDA requirements, package insert information for minipills lists contraindications related to estrogen. |
| Disadvantages | • May be less effective than combined OC. Compliance with minipills is essential.<br>• Timing is critical to ensure effectiveness. Must be taken no more than 27 hours between doses.<br>• Slightly higher risk for ectopic pregnancy and functional ovarian cyst. |
| Precautions | • A backup contraceptive method during the initial 7–28 days on minipills should be used.<br>• If a minipill is taken over 3 h late, another contraceptive method should be used for 48 h.<br>• If a minipill is missed, a backup method should be used until the woman restarts or until her next period. |

*Sources: Bucci and Carson (1997), Caufield (1998), Dickey (1993), and Hatcher et al (1994).*

tected from becoming pregnant (Bucci & Carson, 1997; Hatcher et al, 1994; Hickey & Fraser, 1995).

Advantages and disadvantages of DMPA are listed in Table 18–27. Irregular, unpredictable spotting, heavy bleeding, and, after the first several injections, amenorrhea, are the most frequent side effects from DMPA. Before starting therapy, these unpredictable changes should be discussed with patients (Nelson, 1996). Fertility may be delayed after discontinuation of DMPA for up to 24 months. After 15 and 24 months from the last injection, 75% and 95% of women conceive, respectively. Therefore, if a woman is planning on conceiving within the next year, DMPA is not an appropriate method. Bone density may be negatively affected by DMPA use. One study, involving 30 women treated with DMPA for at least 5 years, 30 premenopausal women, and 30 postmenopausal women, concluded that DMPA users had significantly lower bone mineral density in comparison to premenopausal nonusers. The DMPA group did have higher bone mineral density than the postmenopausal group (Hickey & Fraser, 1995). Another study evaluating the effect of DMPA on bone density found that bone turnover was increased (Naessen, Olsson, & Gudmundson, 1995). These effects appear to be reversible, and the clinical significance of bone density changes remains unknown.

Other adverse effects include weight gain (1–4 kg per year on average depending on the study), depression, headache, abdominal bloating, asthenia, dizziness, nervousness, mild elevations in serum triglycerides, decreases in HDL-cholesterol, and increases in LDL-cholesterol and total cholesterol (Bucci & Carson, 1997; Frederiksen, 1996; Hatcher et al, 1994; Hickey & Fraser, 1995; Sangi-Haghpeyka, Poindexter, Bateman, & Ditmore, 1996; Westhoff, 1995, 1996). One study evaluating the use of DMPA in an urban setting noted a low continuation rate at 1 year of 28.6%. Patients discontinued therapy because of intolerable side effects and changes in their menstrual cycle (Sangi-Haghpeykar et al, 1996).

DMPA had been used in other countries for several decades prior to approval for use in the United States by the FDA in 1993. The reason for this delay was concern over the potential for an increased risk for breast cancer, documented in studies on beagle dogs given prolonged exposure to high-dose DMPA. Subsequently, two large, retrospective case-controlled studies have evaluated the risk for breast cancer in women treated with DMPA (Paul, Skegg, & Spears, 1989; WHO Collaborative Study, 1991). In DMPA users, the overall risk of breast cancer is no higher than in nonusers; however, the risk in certain populations is higher. One study found a slight increase in risk in the first 4 years of use

## TABLE 18–27. ADVANTAGES AND DISADVANTAGES OF DEPOT MEDROXYPROGESTERONE ACETATE (DMPA)

| Advantages | Disadvantages |
|---|---|
| • Safe, effective, reversible method<br>• Long-acting<br>• Does not require medical personnel to remove (unlike Norplant)<br>• Simple to administer<br>• Privacy maintained<br>• Patient memory only required for follow-up injections every 3 months (does not need to remember daily or with intercourse)<br>• May give to patients for whom estrogen is contra-indicated<br>• Drug interactions not reported with use<br>• Will not suppress lactation<br>• Reduces iron-deficiency anemia, sickle cell anemia; may decrease number and severity of sickle crises<br>• Considered immediately effective | • Menstrual disturbance: occurs in the majority of women with irregular unpredictable spotting or continuous heavy bleeding (uncommon); amenorrhea after 1 year of use develops in 33–50% of women; primary reason for discontinuation<br>• Delayed fertility<br>• Risk of osteoporosis: decreased bone mineral density<br>• Weight gain<br>• Depression<br>• Breast cancer risk: may enhance the growth of pre-existing tumors |

Sources: Bucci and Carson (1997), Hatcher et al (1994), and Hickey and Fraser (1995).

(WHO Collaborative Study, 1991). The risk did not increase over time. Another study showed that women under 35 years of age at diagnosis who had ever received DMPA were at elevated risk. Women between ages 25–34 were observed to have a relative risk of 2.0, and those who had been given DMPA for more than 2 years before age 25 had an even higher relative risk of 4.6 (Paul et al, 1989). Findings from these studies suggest that DMPA may enhance the growth of preexisting tumors, and the risk for breast cancer appears to be similar to the risk found with oral contraceptives (Kaunitz, 1996).

The effect of DMPA on other types of reproductive cancers has also been studied. DMPA is associated with a reduction of 80% in endometrial cancer. Ovarian and cervical cancers appear to be unaffected by the use of DMPA (Hickey & Fraser, 1995; Kaunitz, 1996; Thomas, Ray, & WHO (1995).

Levonorgestrel Implant.    In December 1990, the Food and Drug Administration approved the long-acting levonorgestrel implant (Norplant). Levonorgestrel is the synthetic progestin contained in the six flexible, nonbiodegradable, hollow silastic (silicon rubber) tubes that are inserted under the skin of the upper arm. The progestin slowly diffuses into systemic circulation for 5 years, and serum levels of levonorgestrel gradually decline over this time. The level of progestin is lower than that found in combination OCs. The mechanism of action for Norplant includes ovulation inhibition and thickening of cervical mucus and is similar to the mechanism of Depo-Provera.

Because heavier women have a larger volume of distribution with lower serum concentration of levonorgestrel, leading to an increased risk of pregnancy, the earlier "hard" tubing Norplant systems were not recommended to be used in women weighing more than 154 pounds. However, new "soft" tubing systems are now available, and pregnancy rates are lower with a risk of becoming pregnant over the 5 years of 1%, regardless of weight. Insertion is recommended during the first 7 days of the menstrual cycle to ensure ovulation is inhibited. If insertion is delayed past this time, a backup method of contraception is recommended (Brache, Alvarez, Faundes, Cochon, & Theverin, 1996; Hatasaka, 1995).

Norplant has side effects that are similar to other progestin-only contraceptive methods. The most common adverse effect is irregular

menstrual bleeding, occurring during the first year in about 60–70% of women (Biswas et al., 1996). Table 18–28 shows selected common adverse effects that may occur in women using Norplant. Other side effects include headache, nausea, dizziness, depression, acne, weight gain, and hirsutism (Hatasaka, 1995).

Drug interactions with phenytoin, phenobarbital, carbamazepine, primidone, and rifampin may occur due to the increase in hepatic metabolism of levonorgestrel. Unlike DMPA, fertility returns quickly, within 1 month after removal of the implant. Before deciding to insert Norplant, it is important to consider absolute and relative contraindications to use. Absolute contraindications are: genital bleeding of unknown cause, pregnancy, acute liver disease, thromboembolic disease, breast cancer, or liver tumors. Relative contraindications include: drugs which interact with Norplant, mental depression, breast-feeding in women less than 6 weeks postpartum, severe acne, chronic disease, hypercholesterolemia, smoking, ectopic pregnancy history, hypertension, diabetes mellitus, gallbladder disease, cardiovascular disease, and severe vascular headaches.

Continuation rates for Norplant range from 76–95% after 1 year of use. Patient counseling plays an important role in maintaining patient satisfaction and improving long-term use of this method (Hatasaka, 1995; Haugen, Evans, & Kim, 1996). Several removal techniques exist

### TABLE 18–28.  SELECTED COMMON ADVERSE EFFECTS FROM NORPLANT

| Adverse Effect | Incidence, % |
|---|---|
| Many bleeding days or prolonged bleeding | 27.6 |
| Spotting | 17.1 |
| Amenorrhea | 9.4 |
| Irregular bleeding | 7.6 |
| Frequent bleeding onsets | 7 |
| Removal difficulties | 6.2 |
| Scanty bleeding | 5.2 |
| Breast discharge | ≥5 |
| Cervicitis | ≥5 |
| Musculoskeletal pain | ≥5 |
| Abdominal discomfort | ≥5 |
| Leukorrhea | ≥5 |
| Vaginitis | ≥5 |
| Pain or itching near implant site | 3.7 |

Source: Norplant package insert.

and have been published elsewhere (Hatasaka, 1995). Once removed, the effects of Norplant are terminated quickly.

## CONTRACEPTIVES IN SPECIAL PATIENT POPULATIONS

Women with either insulin dependent or non-insulin-dependent diabetes mellitus can be prescribed progestin-only OCs or low-dose OCs if serious vascular complications are not present and if they are followed closely by their provider. Before starting therapy, weight, blood pressure, glucose control, and fasting lipids should be evaluated and checked every 3–4 months thereafter. Microalbuminuria should also be determined. Depo-Provera and Norplant may be used in diabetic women; however, these contraceptives have been shown in some studies to result in statistically, but not clinically, significant negative effects on glucose tolerance and lipid levels (Betschart, 1996; Kjos, 1996; Womack & Beal, 1996).

Women with epilepsy are usually treated with anticonvulsants such as phenobarbitol, carbamazepine, phenytoin, and ethambutol, which may lower serum concentrations of OCs, thereby increasing risk for pregnancy. High-dose (ie, 50 μg of ethinyl estradiol) OCs may be used in these situations, but poor cycle control and lack of reliability are possibilities. Therefore, other contraceptive methods are recommended (Weisberg, 1995).

Women with disabilities have special needs related to fertility management. Moreover, in many cases contraception information is not provided to women who have disabilities. Spinal cord injury patients, because of decreased mobility, are at an increased risk for deep vein thrombosis; therefore, estrogen-containing OCs augment this potential risk. Women with spinal cord injuries may still become pregnant and may give birth without complications. Hormonal therapy may affect the course of multiple sclerosis, and OCs are contraindicated in women who are paralyzed or who have restricted mobility. There are conflicting data regarding the use of OCs in women with cystic fibrosis. Bronchial mucus may become scant, and endocervical polyps may develop. However, one small study found that pulmonary function and respiratory symptoms were not affected in young women treated with OCs (Sawin, 1998).

## EMERGENCY CONTRACEPTION

Emergency (postcoital) contraception (EC) "is still a well-kept secret in the U.S." (Hanson, 1996), and only approximately 10% of physicians inform patients about its availability. In Europe, prepackaged "morning-after pills" have been available since the early 1980s. The term *morning-after pill* is deceiving since EC may be given the same night or up to 3 days after unprotected intercourse. Because of the lack of public awareness regarding EC and the high rate of unplanned pregnancies (60% of all pregnancies), there has been a recent movement from the family planning community to publicize EC regimens.

EC is not effective if implantation has already occurred, and, for this reason, regimens should be given as soon as possible and within the first 72 h after unprotected intercourse. EC works by several mechanisms including: production of impenetrable cervical mucus, pituitary hormone secretion suppression, ovulation inhibition, corpus luteum disruption, luteal phase shortening, endometrial hormonal receptor suppression, endometrial development modification, and tubal transport time alteration (Hanson, 1996).

Several EC regimens exist. One of the most frequently used EC regimens is two Ovral (ethinyl estradiol 50 μg and norgestrel 0.5 mg) tablets administered within 72 h of unprotected intercourse followed by two tablets 12 h later. OCs containing levonorgestrel and ethinyl estradiol may also be used (Lo/Ovral: ethinyl estradiol 30 μg, norgestrel 0.3 mg; Nordette: ethinyl estradiol 30 μg, levonorgestrel 0.15 mg); however, because the dose of hormones is lower, four tablets are taken immediately followed by four more tablets 12 h later. The copper IUD may also be inserted within 5–7 days after unprotected intercourse except in cases of rape or STDs. If combination OCs are administered appropriately, EC is effective, with a failure rate of less than 2% (Hanson, 1996).

EC may result in several side effects because of the increased hormonal exposure. Nausea and/or vomiting occur in 30–50% and 15–20% of patients, respectively. Some clinicians advocate prescribing an antiemetic medication to be taken concurrently. If a patient vomits within 1 hour after taking the dose, repeating the dose would be recommended. Other side effects include headache, dizziness, breast tenderness, fluid retention, and menstrual irregularity (Bucci & Carson, 1997; Hanson, 1996). To date, studies evaluating contraindications to EC hormonal regimens have not been conducted. Since many of the contraindications to OCs stem from the potential complications with long-term use, these contraindications should not pertain to EC regimens because they are used for a short time period (ACOG Practice Patterns, 1996).

In conclusion, EC is inexpensive, effective, and safe. Millions of pregnancies that are unwanted could be potentially averted if EC were available to and used by more women. Unfortunately, many women and providers remain unaware about EC methods. Additionally, manufacturers in the United States do not market a specific EC method; rather, routine OCs are administered in different regimens. Furthermore, reluctance on the part of the women or providers may exist because of misunderstandings. EC is not an abortifacient; rather, it prevents pregnancy from occurring (Anonymous, 1995). An EC hotline toll-free service is available 24 hours a day (1-800-584-9911). Additionally, Internet users may obtain EC and other contraceptive information from the Planned Parenthood Web site (http://www.ppfa.org/ppfa/contraception/choices).

## FUTURE CONTRACEPTIVES

Currently, no perfect contraceptive method exists. The methods described in the preceding sections vary in efficacy, adverse effects, and other characteristics. Future contraceptive methods should be acceptable, effective, easy to use, free of long- and short-term adverse effects, affordable, suitable for different times of the reproductive cycle, and suitable in different age groups. Several new contraceptive methods are being investigated and include: one-rod and two-rod implants, biodegradable implants, biodegradable norethindrone pellets, transdermal contraceptives, vaginal rings, vaginal sponges, vaginal shields, female condoms, testosterone injections, calcium channel blockers, and vaccines. In addition to its use as an abortifacient, mifepristone appears to inhibit implantation; thus, it may be used in the future as an emergency contraceptive method (Bonn, 1996; Coutinho, 1996; Dao, Vanage, Marshall, Bardin, & Koide, 1996; Griffin & Farley, 1996; Habenicht & Stock, 1996; Kekkonen,

Heikinheimo, Mandelin & Lahteenmaki 1996; Sivin et al, 1997).

## REFERENCES

ACOG Practice Patterns. (1996). Emergency oral contraception. Washington, D.C.: ACOG.

Alexander, L. (1996). Taking a sexual history to help patients prevent STDs. *Contraception Report, 7,* 12–14.

Alving, B., & Comp, P. (1992). Recent advances in understanding clotting and evaluating patients with recurrent thrombosis. *American Journal of Obstetrics and Gynecology, 167,* 1184–1191.

Anonymous. (1994). Oral contraceptive compliance: Strategies for ensuring correct and continued use of the pill. *Contraceptive Technology Update, 15,* 3–7.

Anonymous. (1995). Consensus statement on emergency contraception. *Contraception, 52,* 211–213.

Baird, D., & Glasier, A. (1993). Hormonal contraception. *New England Journal of Medicine, 328,* 1543–1549.

Betschart, J. (1996). Oral contraception and adolescent women with insulin-dependent diabetes mellitus: Risks, benefits, and implications for practice. *Diabetes Educator, 22,* 374–378.

Biswas, A., Leong, W., Ratnam, S., O.A.S. (1996). Menstrual bleeding patterns in Norplant-2 implant users. *Contraception, 54,* 91–95.

Bonn D. (1996). What prospects for hormonal contraceptives for men? *Lancet, 347,* 316.

Boston Women's Health Collective. (1992). *The new our bodies, ourselves* (25th anniversary ed:). New York: Simon & Schuster.

Brache, V., Alvarez, F., Faundes, A., Cochon, L., & Theverin, F. (1996). Effect of preovulatory insertion of Norplant over luteinizing hormone secretion and follicular development. *Fertility and Sterility, 65,* 1110–1114.

Brill, K., Then, A., Beisiegel, U., Jene, A., Wunsch, C., & Leidenberger, F. (1996). Investigation of the influence of two low-dose monophasic oral contraceptives containing 20 µg ethinylestradiol/75 mg gestodene, on lipid metabolism in an open randomized trial. *Contraception, 54,* 291–297.

Bucci, K., & Carson, D. (1997). *Contraception.* In J.T. Dipero (Ed.), *Pharmacotherapy: A pathophysiologic approach* (3rd ed.). Stamford, CT: Appleton & Lange.

Buring, J. (1996). Low-dose oral contraceptives and stroke. *New England Journal of Medicine, 335,* 54.

Cates, W., & Stone, K. (1992). Family planning, sexually transmitted diseases and contraceptive choice. A literature update, part I. *Family Planning Perspectives, 24*, 75–84.

Caufield, K. A. (1998). Controlling fertility. In E. Q. Youngkin & M. S. Davis (Eds.), *Women's health: A primary care clinical guide* (2nd ed.). Stamford, CT: Appleton & Lange.

Centers for Disease Control, National Institute of Child Health and Human Development. (1987a). Combination oral contraceptive use and the risk of endometrial cancer. *JAMA, 257*, 796–800.

Centers for Disease Control, National Institute of Child Health and Human Development. (1987b). The reduction in risk of ovarian cancer associated with oral-contraceptive use: The cancer and steroid hormone study. *New England Journal of Medicine, 316*, 650–655.

Chapdelaine, A., & Desmarais, J. (1989). Clinical evidence of the minimal androgenic activity of norgestimate. *International Journal of Fertility, 34*, 347–352.

Chez, R. A. (1989). Clinical aspects of three new progestogens: Desogestrel, gestodene, and norgestimate. *American Journal of Obstetrics and Gynecology, 160*, 1296–1300.

Choice of contraceptives. (1995). *The Medical Letter, 37*, 9–12.

Coenen, C., Thomas, C., Borm, G., Hollanders, J., & Rolland, R. (1996). Changes in androgens during treatment with four low-dose contraceptives. *Contraception, 53*, 171–176.

Collaborative Group on Hormonal Factors in Breast Cancer. (1996). Breast cancer and hormonal contraceptives: Further results. *Contraception, 54*, 1S–106S.

Corson, S. (1995). Norgestimate. *Clinical Obstetrics and Gynecology, 38*, 841–848.

Coutinho, E. M., Athayde, C., Barbosa, I., et al. (1996). Results of a user satisfaction study carried out in women using Uniplant Contraceptive Implant. *Contraception, 54*, 313–317.

Dao, B., Vanage, G., Marshall, A., Bardin, C., & Koide, S. (1996). Anti-implantation activity of antiestrogens and mifepristone. *Contraception, 54*, 253–258.

Darney, P. (1995). The androgencity of progestins. *American Journal of Medicine, 98* (SIA), 104A–110A.

Dickey, R. (1993). *Managing contraceptive pill patients* (7th ed.). Durant, OK: Essential Medical Information Systems, Inc.

Drug Interaction Facts on Disk. (1995). St. Louis, MO: Facts and Comparisons, Inc..

Farley, T., Meirik, O., Chang, C., Marmot, M., & Poulter, N. (1995). WHO Collaborative Study of Cardiovascular Disease and Steroid Hormone Contraception. Effect of different progestagens in low oestrogen oral contraceptives on venous thromboembolic disease. *Lancet, 346*, 1582–1588.

Female-controlled methods are key to AIDS prevention. (1996). *Contraceptive Technology Update, 17*(11), 135–137.

Filshie clip recommended for approval for use in the United States. (1996). *The Contraception Report, VII*(3), 12–14.

Frederiksen, M. (1996). Depot medroxyprogesterone acetate contraception in women with medical problems. *Journal of Reproductive Medicine, 41* (Suppl.), 414–418.

Godsland, I., Crook, D., Simpson, R., et al. (1990). The effects of different formulations of oral contraceptive agents on lipid and carbohydrate metabolism. *New England Journal of Medicine, 323*, 1375–1381.

Griffin, P., & Farley, T. (1996). Hormonal contraception for men. *Lancet, 347*, 830–831.

Grimes, D. (1996). Risk of venous thromboembolism with third-generation OCs. *Contraception Report, 7*, 3–15.

Habenicht, U., & Stock, G. (1996). Development of new immunocontraceptives—industrial perspective. *American Journal of Reproductive Immunology, 35*, 517–522.

Hanson, V. (1996, June). Facing facts on emergency postcoital contraception. *Contemporary Obstetrics and Gynecology, 31*, 34, 41–42, 45–46, 48, 52.

Hatasaka H. (1995). Implantable levonorgestrel contraception: 4 years of experience with Norplant. *Clinical Obstetrics and Gynecology, 38*, 859–871.

*Hatcher, R., Trussell, J., Stewart, F., Stewart, G., Kowal, D., Guest, F., Cates, W., & Policar, M. (1994). *Contraceptive technology* (16th rev. ed.). New York: Irvington.

Haugen, M., Evans, C., & Kim, M. (1996). Patient satisfaction with a levonorgestrel-releasing contraceptive implant. Reasons for and patterns of removal. *Journal of Reproductive Medicine, 41*, 849–854.

Hawley, W., Nuovo, J., DeNeef, C., & Carter, P. (1993). Do oral contraceptive agents affect the risk of breast cancer? A meta-analysis of the case-control reports. *Journal of the American Board of Family Practice, 6*, 123–135.

Herbst, A., & Berek, J. (1993). Impact of contraception on gynecologic cancers. *American Journal of Obstetrics and Gynecology, 168*, 1980–1985.

---

*The 1998 edition of *Contraceptive Technology*, a book frequently cited in this chapter, was not yet available at the time of this writing. The reader is advised to refer to the 17th edition for updated information.

Hickey, M., & Fraser, I. (1995). The contraceptive use of depot medroxyprogesterone acetate. *Clinical Obstetrics and Gynecology, 38,* 849–858.

Himes, N. (1963). *Medical history of contraception.* New York: Gamut Press.

James, V. (1993). Just say no? A contraceptive update. *Pharmacy Perspectives in Ambulatory Care, 5,* 12–20.

Jick, H., Jick, S., Gurewich, V., et al (1995). Risk of idiopathic cardiovascular death and nonfatal venous thromboembolism in women using oral contraceptives with differing progestagen components. *Lancet, 346,* 1589–1593.

Kafrissen, M. (1992). A norgestimate-containing oral contraceptive: Review of clinical studies. *American Journal of Obstetrics and Gynecology, 167,* 1196–1202.

Kaunitz, A. (1996). Depot medroxyprogesterone acetate contraception and the risk of breast and gynecologic cancer. *Journal of Reproductive Medicine* 41, (Suppl.) 419–427.

Kauppinen-Makelin, R., Kyusi, T., Ylikarkala, O., & Tikkanen, M. (1992). Contraceptives containing desogestrel or levonorgestrel have different effects on serum lipoproteins and post-heparin plasma lipase activities. *Clinical Endocrinology, 36,* 203–209.

Kekkonen, R., Heikinheimo, O., Mandelin, E., & Lahteenmaki, P. (1996). Pharmacokinetics of mifepristone after low oral doses. *Contraception.* 54, 229–234.

Kjos, S. (1996). Contraception in diabetic women. *Obstetrics and Gynecology Clinics of North America, 23,* 243–257.

Knutson, C. (1997). A new generation of IUD use: Taking a fresh look at an old contraceptive. *Advance for Nurse Practitioners, 5,* 22–24, 27, 31.

Koster, T., Small, R., Rosendaal, F., & Helmerhorst, F. (1995). Oral contraceptives and venous thromboembolism: A quantitative discussion of the uncertainties. *Journal of International Medicine, 238,* 31–37.

Krauss, R., & Burkman, R. (1992). The metabolic impact of oral contraceptives. *American Journal of Obstetrics and Gynecology, 167,* 1177–1184.

Lewis, M., Heinemann, L., MacRae, K., et al. (1996). The increased risk of venous thromboembolism and the use of third generation progestagens: Role of bias in observational research. *Contraception,* 54, 5–3.

Lewis, M., Spitzer, W., Heinemann, L., et al. (1996). Third generation oral contraceptives and risk of myocardial infarction: An international case-control study. *British Medical Journal, 312,* 88–90.

Lidegaard, O. (1993). Oral contraception and risk of a cerebral thromboembolic attack: Results of a case-control study. *British Medical Journal, 306,* 956–963.

Lidegaard, O., & Milsom, I. (1996). Oral contraceptives and thrombotic diseases: Impact of new epidemiological studies. *Contraception, 53,* 135–139.

Lobo, R., Skinner, J., Lippman, J., & Cirillo, S. (1996). Plasma lipids and desogestrel and ethinyl estradiol: A meta-analysis. *Fertilization and Sterilization, 65,* 1100–1109.

Lynaugh, J. (1991). The death of Sadie Sachs. *Nursing Research, 40,* 124–125.

Mango, D., Ricci, S., Manna, P., Miggiano, G., & Serna, G. (1996). Clinical and hormonal effects of ethinylestradiol combined with gestodene and desogestrel in young women with acne vulgaris. *Contraception, 53,* 163–170.

McGonigle, K. F., & Huggins, G. R. (1991). *Fertilization and Sterilization, 56,* 799–819.

Mills, A., Wilkinson, C., Bromham, D., Elias, J., et al. (1996). Guidelines for prescribing combined oral contraceptives. *British Medical Journal, 312,* 121–122.

Naessen, T., Olsson, S., & Gudmundson, J. (1995). Differential effects on bone density of progestogen-only methods for contraception in premenopausal women. *Contraception, 52,* 35–39.

Narkiewicz, K., Graniero, G., D-Este, D., Mattarie, M., Zonzin, P., & Palatini, P. (1995). Ambulatory blood pressure in mild hypertensive women taking oral contraceptives: A case-control study. *American Journal of Hypertension, 8,* 249–253.

Nelson, A. (1996). Counseling issues and management of side effects for women using depot medroxyprogesterone acetate contraception. *Journal of Reproductive Medicine, 41,* (Suppl.) 391–400.

New medicines in development for women. (1997). *America's Pharmaceutical Research Companies.* Washington, D.C.: PhRMA.

News alert for family planners: Filshie clip finally available in the United States. (1996). *Contraceptive Technology Update, 17,* 129–131.

Norris, A. (1988). Cognitive analysis of contraceptive behavior. *Image: Journal of Nursing Scholarship, 20,* 135–140.

Northrup, C. (1995). *Health Wisdom for Women,* 2:3–5.

O'Connell, M. (1996). The effect of birth control methods on sexually transmitted disease/HIV risk. *Journal of Obstetric, Gynecologic, and Neonatal Nursing, 25,* 476–480.

Oral contraception compliance: Strategies for ensuring correct and continued use of the pill. (1994). *The Contraception Report, V,* 13–17.

Paul, C., Skegg, D., & Spears, G. (1989). Depot medroxyprogesterone (Depo-Provera) and risk of breast cancer. *British Medical Journal, 299,* 759–762.

Peterson, H. (1996). Update on female sterilization: Failure rates, counseling issues, and post-sterilization regret. *Contraception Report, VII,* 4–11.

Petitti, D., Sidney, S., Bernstein, A., Wolf, S., Quesenberry, C., & Ziel, H. (1996). Stroke in users of low-dose oral contraceptives. *New England Journal of Medicine, 335,* 8–15.

Pharmacist's Letter. (1997). *13,* 5.

Phillips, A., Hahn, D., & McGuire, J. (1992). Preclinical evaluation of norgestimate, a progestin with minimal androgenic activity. *American Journal of Obstetrics and Gynecology, 167,* 191–196.

Planned Parenthood Federation of America. (1992). *Facts about fertility awareness methods (FAM).* New York: PPFA.

Pollack, A. (1996). Guidelines for pre-sterilization counseling. *The Contraception Report, VII(3),* 12–14.

Potter, L. (1994, November). Will the new OC instructions increase compliance? *Advance for Nurse Practitioner,* 11–13.

Potter, L. (1996). How effective are contraceptives? The determination and measurement of pregnancy rates. *Obstetrics and Gynecology, 88* (Suppl. 3), 13S–23S.

Poulter, N., Chang, C., Farley, T., Meirik, O., & Marmot, M. (1995). WHO Collaborative Study of Cardiovascular Disease and Steroid Hormone Contraception. Venous thromboembolic disease and combined oral contraceptives: Results of international multicentre case-control study. *Lancet, 346,* 1575–1582.

Rosenberg, M., Burnhill, M., Waugh, M., Grimes, D., & Hillar, P. (1995). Compliance and oral contraceptives: A review. *Contraception, 52,* 137–141.

Rosenberg, M., Waugh, M., Meehan, T. (1995). Use and misuse of oral contraceptives: Risk indicators for poor pill taking and discontinuation. *Contraception, 51,* 283–288.

Ruffing-Rahal, M. (1986). Margaret Sanger: Nurse and feminist. *Nursing Outlook, 34,* 246–249.

Sangi-Haghpeykar, H., Poindexter, A., Bateman, L., & Ditmore, J. (1996). Experiences of injectable contraceptive users in an urban setting. *Obstetrics and Gynecology, 88,* 227–233.

Sawin, K. (1998). Issues for women with physical disability and chronic illness. In E. Q. Youngkin & M. S. Davis (Eds.), *Women's health: A primary care clinical guide* (2nd ed.). Stamford, CT: Appleton & Lange.

Schlesselman, J. (1989). Cancer of the breast and reproductive tract in relation to use of oral contraceptives. *Contraception, 40,* 1–38.

Schuster, E. A. (1993). Greening the curriculum. *Journal of Nursing Education, 32(8),* 381–383.

Sivin, I., Viegas, O., Campodonico, I., et al. (1997). Clinical performance of a new two-rod levonorgestrel contraceptive implant: A three-year randomized study with Norplant implants as controls. *Contraception, 55,* 73–80.

Speroff, L., DeCherney, A. (1993). Advisory Board for the New Progestins. Evaluation of a new generation of oral contraceptives. *Obstetrics and Gynecology, 81,* 1034–1047.

Spinillo, A., Gorini, G., Piazzi, G., Baltaro, F., Monaco, A., & Zara, F. (1996). The impact of oral contraception on chlamydial infection among patients with pelvic inflammatory disease. *Contraception, 54,* 163–168.

Spitzer, W., Lewis, M., Heinemann, L., et al. (1996). Third generation oral contraceptives and risk of venous thromboembolic disorders: An international case-control study. *British Medical Journal, 312,* 83–88.

Stone, S. (1995). Desogestrel. *Clinical Obstetrics Gynecology, 38,* 821–828.

Thomas, D., Ray, R., and the WHO Collaborative Study of Neoplasia and Steroid Contraceptives. (1995). Depot-medroxyprogesterone acetate (DMPA) and risk of invasive adenocarcinomas and adenosquamous carcinomas of the uterine cervix. *Contraception, 52,* 307–312.

Trussell, J., Leveque, J. A., Koenig, J. D., et al. (1995). The economic value of contraception: A comparison of 15 methods. *American Journal of Public Health, 85,* 494–503.

Vessey, M., McPherson, K., & Johnson, B. (1997). Mortality among women participating in the Oxford Family Planning Association Contraceptive Study. *Lancet, 2,* 727–731.

Walsh, T., Bernstein, G., Grimes, D. (1994). Effect of prophylactic antibiotics on morbidity associated with IUD insertion: Results of a randomized controlled trial. *Contraception, 50,* 319–327.

Weber, A., Jager, R., Borner, A., et al. (1996). Can grapefruit juice influence ethinylestradiol bioavailability? *Contraception, 53,* 41–47.

Weisberg, E. (1995). Prescribing oral contraceptives. *Drugs, 49,* 224–231.

Westhoff, C. (1996). Depot medroxyprogesterone acetate contraception metabolic parameters and mood changes. *Journal of Reproductive Medicine, 41* (suppl.), 401–406.

Westhoff, C., Wieland, D., & Tiezzi, L., (1995). Depression in users of depot-medroxyprogesterone acetate. *Contraception, 51,* 351–354.

WHO Collaborative Study of Neoplasia and Steroid Contraceptives. (1991). Breast cancer and depot-medroxyprogesterone acetate: A multinational study. *Lancet, 338,* 833–838.

WHO Collaborative Study of Cardiovascular Disease and Steroid Hormone Contraception. (1996a). Haemorrhagic stroke, overall stroke risk, and combined oral contraceptives: Results of an international, multicentre, case-control study. *Lancet, 348,* 505–510.

WHO Collaborative Study of Cardiovascular Disease and Steroid Hormone Contraception. (1996b). Ischaemic stroke and combined oral contraceptives: Results of an international, multicentre, case-control study. *Lancet, 348,* 498–505.

Wilcox, L., Chu, S., Peterson, H. (1990). Characteristics of women who considered or obtained tubal reanastomosis: Results from a prospective study of tubal sterilization. *Obstetrics and Gynecology, 75,* 661–665.

Womack, J., & Beal, M. (1996). Use of Norplant in women with or at-risk for noninsulin-dependent diabetes. *Journal of Nurse-Midwifery, 41,* 285–296.

Youngkin, E. (1995). Sexually transmitted diseases: Current and emerging concerns. *Journal of Obstetric, Gynecologic, and Neonatal Nursing, 24,* 743–758.

# 19

# MENOPAUSE AND HORMONAL REPLACEMENT THERAPY

*Susan Rawlins and Robert L. Martin*

Menopause is not a disease; rather it is an anticipated developmental achievement of women. Occurring between the ages of 45 and 55 in most women, it is the culmination of a variety of universally occurring physiologic events. Understanding these menopausal physiologic events allows the provider to anticipate and support the woman during the varied presentations of normal menopause.

Menopause, by commonly accepted definition, is the last episode of menstrual bleeding experienced by a woman and is therefore a retrospective assessment (Hargrove & Eisenberg, 1995). The climacteric or perimenopause is the time of transition surrounding the actual menopause. During the early climacteric period of natural menopause, most women experience abnormal ovarian follicular function with anovulation, alternating periods of hyperestrogenism and hypoestrogenism, decreased serum progesterone, and increased serum gonadotrophins (Santoro, Brown, Adel, & Skurnick, 1996). Testosterone levels also decline, but in natural menopause the decline is very gradual. The anovulatory cycles produce irregular, unpredictable vaginal bleeding for several years before amenorrhea eventually develops. Vasomotor instability and alterations in mood, memory, and sexual functioning accompany the changes in the menstrual cycle in some women. Over the course of several years, the low serum estrogen levels lead to progressive urogenital atrophy, rapid demineralization of the bones, and

unfavorable lipoprotein changes. Although the function of androgens in women is not completely understood, low serum testosterone levels, especially after bilateral salpingo-oophorectomy, have been associated with decreased libido (Pearce, Hawton, & Blake, 1995). The hormonal milieu of the climacteric places perimenopausal women at increased risk for endometrial cancer (Santoro et al, 1996). Although most women experience at least a few symptoms related to their changing hormonal profile, only a small minority find these symptoms truly problematic (Porter, Penney, Russell, Russell, & Templeton, 1996).

Pharmacologic management of the climacteric is not directed toward curing this natural condition; the goal is relief of distressing symptoms and prevention of long-term morbidity and premature mortality. During the early years of this century, most women died shortly before or soon after menopause, so the physiologic consequences of menopause were of little concern. Due to improvements in public health and medical science, most women today successfully achieve menopause and many can expect to live more than 30 years thereafter (Hargrove & Eisenberg, 1995). The consequences of menopause are now a concern of all women and society as well, for long life without good health is a burden, not a blessing. This chapter addresses the pharmacologic interventions that can improve health and well-being by preventing or delaying the onset of common conditions associated with menopause as well as other conditions common to aging women. The conditions include: perimenopausal anovulatory bleeding, vasomotor instability, urogenital atrophy, impaired memory, altered psychological functioning, osteoporosis, coronary heart disease, colorectal cancer, and stroke.

The anovulatory cycles that occur during perimenopause result in unpredictable vaginal bleeding that can be quite distressing to most women. This problem is amenable to hormone therapy. The alterations in psychological functioning that occur in some women during the climacteric can have their roots in many areas other than hormonal decline. However, poor sleep—a common problem of perimenopausal women—may be directly related to hormonal and vasomotor changes. Changes in libido, also, may be multifactoral in cause, but one influencing factor may be hormonal declines in estrogen and testosterone. Such conditions as rheumatoid arthritis and autoimmune disease may receive some protective effect from hormonal replacement therapy (HRT); more studies are needed to confirm this (Sowers & La Pietra, 1995). A discussion of the potential risks associated with hormone replacement therapy is presented later in the chapter. These risks vary from life-threatening, such as breast and endometrial cancer, to nuisance problems, like breast tenderness and unpredictable uterine bleeding.

## CONDITIONS ASSOCIATED WITH MENOPAUSE

### DYSFUNCTIONAL UTERINE BLEEDING

Menstrual cycle changes begin early in the climacteric in response to altered ovarian function. The progression through this transition is marked by alternating ovulatory and anovulatory cycles with resulting excess estrogen and inadequate progesterone. This hormonal milieu produces the unpredictable vaginal bleeding that affects many perimenopausal women and predisposes them to develop endometrial hyperplasia. Management of this problem includes low-dose oral contraceptives and combination hormone replacement therapy (Santoro et al, 1996).

### VASOMOTOR INSTABILITY

Vasomotor instability, commonly called a *hot flash* or *flush*, is the most common and one

of the more distressing experiences women undergo during the transition through menopause (Kwawukume, Ghosh, & Wilson, 1993; Sagraves, 1995). In the North American Menopause Society Survey, 80% of women reported menopausal symptoms, with 72% experiencing hot flashes, 50% experiencing irregular bleeding or emotional changes, and approximately 30% reporting sexual relationship changes. Although hot flashes are common, only 20–45% seek medical intervention for this problem (Wich & Carnes, 1995). The menopausal hot flash results from instability in the thermoregulatory centers of the brain in response to the decline in estrogen. This condition, although almost universal in its occurrence, has great variation in presentation between women and in the same woman over time (von Muhlen, Kritz-Silverstein, & Barrett-Conner, 1995). The period of vasomotor instability lasts from 1–2 years in most women who experience it, and up to 15 years or more in some (Rosenberg, Kroll, & Vandromme, 1996). Thin women, especially those who smoke cigarettes, are more likely to experience hot flashes than heavier women and nonsmokers (Schwingl, Hulka, & Harlow, 1994). The hot flash is usually one of the first signs of approaching menopause and is often the reason many women seek health care (Hargrove & Eisenberg, 1995).

## PSYCHOLOGICAL AND COGNITIVE FUNCTIONING

Pathologic mood disorders do not increase in general in women experiencing natural menopause. When menopausal women in the general population are studied, only a minority have true clinical depression (Avis, 1997), although there may be a transitory increase in depressive symptoms during the perimenopause transition, especially if the transition is prolonged (Avis, Brambilla, McKinlay, & Vass, 1994). Many women report positive feelings about menopause and, even with symptoms, they do not find the menopausal experience to be a distressful life event (von Muhlen et al, 1995).

In contrast, women who seek medical care for menopausal symptoms report increased rates of emotional instability and decreased cognitive functioning as well as general feelings of psychological distress (Schmidt et al, 1996; Sherwin, 1994). Some women appear to experience a mild dysphoric disorder during the perimenopausal phase that includes symptoms of depression, irritability, fatigue, insomnia, and forgetfulness. For some, the dysphoric mood and cognitive decline are thought to be secondary to sleep disruption caused by the physical symptoms of menopause, such as hot flashes (Asplund & Aberg, 1995; Wich & Carnes, 1995). These psychological symptoms are less well studied than the physical manifestations of menopause, but they appear to improve with estrogen therapy. True depression seems to be more common in women with previous episodes of depression or in women who have experienced other psychological dysfunctions associated with the hormonal fluctuations of reproduction, such as postpartum depression or premenstrual syndrome (Avis et al, 1994; Pearlstein, 1995). The etiology of these symptoms is multifactorial, with important influences from sociocultural factors as well as changes in the neurochemistry of the brain (Dennerstein, 1996; Sherwin, 1994).

Cognitive functioning declines with aging. Estrogen replacement therapy has been shown to improve short-term verbal memory in healthy menopausal women (Sherwin, 1994). In addition, through improved cerebral vascular blood flow, as well as other mechanisms, estrogen may prevent cognitive decline and dementia in elderly women as well as improve cognitive functioning in demented women (Fillit, 1995). Menopausal estrogen therapy may delay the onset and possibly prevent the development of Alzheimer's disease in elderly women (Paginini-Hill, 1996; Tang et al, 1996).

It is important to emphasize that not all menopausal women have an increased risk of major depression and estrogen is not appropriate therapy for those women who are clinically depressed. However, estrogen has been shown to elevate mood in nondepressed, mildly dysphoric women (Dennerstein, 1996; Pearlstein, 1995).

## UROGENITAL ATROPHY

The genital and urinary tracts arise from a common embryonic precursor cell line and both contain abundant estrogen receptors (Klutke & Bergman, 1995). After several years of diminished estrogen, the urogenital tract begins to atrophy (Fantl, 1994; Klute & Bergman, 1995). The vulvar epithelium thins, and the collagen and adipose tissue supporting structures diminish (Hammond, 1996). The vagina shortens, loses elasticity, and thins from eight to ten cell layers to three to four cell layers (Bachmann, 1995). Vaginal secretions decrease in volume and become more alkaline with a corresponding change in vaginal flora (Nilsson, Risberg, & Heimer, 1995). The urethra and trigone of the bladder also atrophy with estrogen loss (Bachmann, 1995). These alterations of the physiology of the urogenital tract increase the likelihood of trauma, infection, and pain (Hammond, 1996). Not surprisingly, menopausal women experience dyspareunia, cystitis, stress, and urge incontinence (Bachmann, 1995). Many women accept incontinence as a consequence of aging and do not report this condition unless specifically asked by their provider. Urinary incontinence may affect up to 35% of women aged 60 and older. Incontinence leads to psychosocial deterioration and isolation for many of these women (Rosenberg et al, 1996). Good vaginal health, an essential component of high-level wellness in women, is enhanced by estrogen replacement.

## SEXUALITY

In spite of the physical changes of the vulva and vagina, most women continue to be sexually active throughout their lives and place great value on this aspect of their relationships. Of those who report not being sexually active, the most common reason for lack of sexual activity is the absence of a functional partner (Lindgren, Berg, Hammer, & Zuccon, 1993). When questioned, approximately one third to one half of menopausal women report problems in one or more areas of sexual functioning (Sherwin, 1994). These problems include decreased libido, arousal, and orgasm. One contributing factor to a decline in sexual functioning may be the disruption of the rapid eye movement (REM) phase of sleep, which commonly occurs during menopause. Both men and women experience nocturnal genital congestion during REM sleep, which helps maintain the ability to mount a sexual response (Graziottin, 1996). Serum androgen levels are lower in menopausal women than in reproductive-aged women. The addition of testosterone to estrogen replacement therapy may increase libido and sexual enjoyment in some women (Sherwin, 1994). The risks of androgen therapy are discussed later in the chapter.

## OSTEOPOROSIS

Osteoporosis currently effects 26 million women and is characterized by decreased bone mass and compromised structural integrity of the skeleton (Anonymous, 1991). It has been reported that the more than 1.5 million osteoporotic fractures occurring each year contribute approximately $10 billion to the cost of health care in the United States (Barrett-Connor, 1995). Women experience accelerated bone loss during the first few years of menopause and are at increased risk for developing osteoporosis. Although there is no consensus concerning treatment of established osteoporosis after the first fracture, primary prevention of osteoporosis is an achievable goal for most women (Chapuy & Meunier, 1995).

## CARDIOVASCULAR DISEASE

Cardiovascular disease is discussed in detail in Chapter 20. It is the leading cause of death in women, and increased risk of cardiovascular disease has been linked to the loss of estrogen that accompanies menopause (National Center for Health Statistics, 1993). As women enter the climacteric, they experience changes in serum lipoproteins, including increased cholesterol and LDL-C that increase their risk for heart disease (Matthews, Wing, Kuller, Meilahn, & Plantinga, 1994). Although the lipoprotein changes are important in the development of cardiovascular disease, there are many other contributing factors. Estrogen replacement therapy prevents death from heart disease by promoting a favorable lipoprotein profile as well as improving blood vessel endothelial function, increasing coronary blood flow, and acting as an antioxidant (Guetta & Cannon, 1996; Lip, Beevers, & Zarifis, 1995; Schwartz, Freeman, & Frishman, 1995). Cardiovascular risk factors can be viewed as nonmodifiable (advancing age, race, and family history) or modifiable (lifestyle, cholesterol levels, and management of concomitant disease). To prevent cardiovascular disease, interventions should be directed to the modifiable risk factors, such as low-fat diet, exercise, smoking cessation, maintenance of appropriate weight and cholesterol levels, and controlling hypertension and diabetes (Arnstein, Buselli, & Rankin, 1996).

## SPECIFIC CONSIDERATIONS FOR PHARMACOTHERAPY

### WHEN DRUG THERAPY IS NEEDED

Although the inherent risks of hormone replacement are acknowledged, there is developing consensus that many, if not most, postmenopausal women will benefit from hormone replacement therapy in terms of both longer life and better quality of life (Cooper & Whitehead, 1995; Ettinger, Friedman, Bush, & Quesenberry, 1996; Limouzin-Lamothe, Mairon, Joyce, & Le Gal, 1994; Writing Group for the PEPI Trial, 1995). Emphasis on treatment has shifted from relief of short-term symptoms affecting quality of life to primary prevention of long-term, life-threatening conditions. It is well established that estrogen has a marked benefit on the reduction of hot flashes and prevention/reversal of urogenital atrophy (Derman, Dawood, & Stone, 1995; Klutke & Bergman, 1995; Wiklund et al, 1992). In addition, many women, especially those who have had surgically induced menopause, report increased feelings of well-being while taking estrogen replacement, with improvements in sleep patterns, memory, and satisfaction with sexual functioning (Asplund & Aberg, 1995; Derman et al, 1995; Graziottin, 1996; Limouzin-Lamothe, et al, 1994; Myers, 1995; Pearce et al, 1995; Schiffman, Sattely-Miller, Suggs, & Graham, 1995). Estrogen is not an appropriate treatment for major depression, but may benefit women with mild perimenopausal dysphoric disorders (Pearlstein, 1995). Estrogen therapy is a cornerstone in the prevention of osteoporosis with documented decreases in fracture rates and maintenance of bone density. These benefits are most apparent if estrogen is begun soon after menopause, before significant loss of bone has occurred (Cauley et al, 1995; Chapuy & Meunier, 1995; Lindsay, 1996; Marcus et al, 1994; Slemenda, Longcope, Peacock, Sui, & Johnston, 1996; Watts et al, 1995) but also may benefit older postmenopausal women as well as those with established osteoporosis (Kohrt & Birge, 1995). Estrogen exerts both a direct and indirect effect on cardiovascular risk. Women develop a lipoprotein profile that is associated with increased risk of cardiovascular disease as they reach menopause. Estrogen has a direct effect on the cardiovascular system through improvement in clotting factors, endothelial function, vasodilatation, and waist-to-hip fat distribution. Estrogen replacement is known to restore a more favorable lipoprotein profile, which indirectly improves the cardiovascular system (Lichtman, 1996a; Lip et al, 1995; Writing Group, 1995). There is also increasing evidence for a role for estrogen in the prevention and the delay of the onset of Alzheimer's disease (Brinton, 1997; Paganini-Hill, 1996), colorectal cancer (Calle & Thun, 1997), and stroke (Corson, 1995).

## SHORT-TERM AND LONG-TERM GOALS OF PHARMACOTHERAPY

Short-term goals of pharmacotherapy include the relief of vasomotor symptoms, control of anovulatory uterine bleeding, improvement in psychological and cognitive functioning, and overall improvement in perceived quality of life by decreasing the frequency and severity of symptoms of the climacteric. Long-term therapy is designed to protect women from osteoporosis and cardiovascular disease without increasing the incidence of other causes of mortality or morbidity. As more data are acquired, estrogen replacement may be recommended for delaying or preventing Alzheimer's disease and colon cancer (Fillit, 1995; Paganini-Hill, 1996). Other areas of research are: examining hormone therapy and tooth loss, cardiovascular events after balloon angioplasty, fecal incontinence, and balance.

## NONPHARMACOLOGIC THERAPY FOR CONTROL OF MENOPAUSAL SYMPTOMS

1. *Hot flashes:* (The following are not as effective as HRT, and offer no protection for bones or heart). Lichtman (1996b) provides an excellent review of nonpharmacologic therapy for hot flashes.
   - Cool ambient room temperatures, especially at night while sleeping
   - Biofeedback training
   - Personal dietary triggers (if known) for avoidance
   - Vitamin E (400 mg PO daily)
   - Aerobic exercise
   - Layering clothing
2. *Vaginal dryness*
   - *Lubricant use:* Over-the-counter moisturizers such as Replens or Gyne-Moistrin can

increase vaginal comfort (Scharbo-DeHaan, 1996).
   - *Sexual intercourse:* Although formal studies are lacking, sexual intercourse encourages genital vascular congestion and may improve vaginal moisture and suppleness (Lichtman, 1996b; Scharbo-DeHaan, 1996).
   - *Masturbation:* Autoerotic activities have been recommended by some authors to improve vaginal lubrication (Lichtman, 1996b).
3. *Urinary incontinence:* These therapies are effective in some women, but do not reverse urogenital atrophy. For a general review of incontinence therapy, see Nygaard, 1996.
   - *Kegal exercises:* Kegals improve pelvic floor muscle tone and involve alternating contraction and relaxation of the pubococcygeus muscle. Women should begin with ten alternating 3-s contractions and relaxations per day and gradually increase to 10-s contractions and relaxations 80–150 times per day (Walsh Scura & Whipple, 1997).
   - *Bladder retraining:* Patients gradually increase the time between voiding by 15 min weekly until they are voiding every 3–4 h (Walsh Scura & Whipple, 1997).
   - *Diuretics avoidance:* Incontinence therapy is enhanced if prescribed drugs, and dietary compounds, that induce diuresis can be avoided (Hurt, 1996).
   - *Surgical intervention:* For a review of surgical interventions, see Mostwin, Genadry, Sanders, and Yang, 1996.
4. *Osteoporosis prevention:* (these therapies are more effective when combined with HRT).
   - *Weight-bearing exercise:* A recommended regimen is 50–60 min/day at least three times per week.
   - Calcium intake of 1500 mg/day (not on estrogen) or 1000 mg/day (on estrogen) (Berga, 1996).
   - Vitamin D 400–800 IU/day or at least 15 min of direct sunlight daily (Lichtman, 1996b).
   - *Variable-resistance weight training*: One successful regimen is 20-min sessions, three times per week (Notelovitz et al, 1997).
   - Avoid smoking and refrain from taking more than two drinks each of caffeine or alcohol per day (Ettinger et al, 1996).
5. *Cardiovascular disease:*
   - Low-fat diet.
   - *Aerobic exercise* (with provider approval): Sedentary menopausal women should be en-

couraged to begin a variety of self-directed, moderate-intensity activities with the goal of achieving 30 min of moderate-intensity activity most days of the week ("Counseling to Promote Physical Activity," 1997).

## TIME FRAME FOR INITIATING PHARMACOTHERAPY

Pharmacotherapy should be initiated when a woman expresses a desire for symptomatic relief and has no contraindications. Therapy should be directed toward controlling the presenting complaint, for example, hot flashes, vaginal dryness, or irregular menstrual cycles. In an asymptomatic woman, therapy should be initiated shortly after the menopause (within 6 months of the last menstrual period) to have the maximal effect on preventing osteoporosis (Cauley et al, 1995). Begin estrogen therapy early in the menopause to prevent the accelerated bone loss that occurs during the first 6–8 years after menopause. Prevention of bone loss is critical, because rebuilding bone that has been lost is not very successful with the pharmacologic methods available today (Chapuy & Meunier, 1995; Vedi, Croucher, Garrahan, & Compston, 1996). For osteoporosis protection, estrogen therapy should be continued for at least 10 years and probably for life (Cauley et al, 1995). Eiken, Nielson, & Kolthoff (1997) found a significant difference in the incidence of fractures in women on HRT over an 8-year period compared to the placebo group. Additionally, women who discontinued HRT developed decreased bone densities at rates similar to the women taking placebo. The optimal time to start and the duration of estrogen for cardioprotection is unknown, but cardioprotective benefits are provided with osteoporosis regimes. Additionally, atherosclerotic changes begin shortly after menopause, so it seems reasonable that hormone therapy should be initiated as soon after menopause as possible. See Table 19–1 for an overview of the drug classes used for the pharmacologic management of the climacteric.

## HISTORY AND PHYSICAL EXAMINATION PRIOR TO THERAPY

Before initiating therapy, a thorough history and complete physical examination are required. The history should focus on identifying any contraindications for hormone use as well as risk fac-

### TABLE 19–1. OVERVIEW OF DRUG CLASSES FOR PHARMACOLOGICAL MANAGEMENT OF THE CLIMACTERIC

Combination oral contraceptives
Estrogens
  Natural estrogens
    Conjugated equine estrogens
    Esterified estrogens
    Micronized estrogens
    Estropipate
  Synthetic estrogens
    Diethylstilbestrol
    Ethinyl estradiol
    Quinesterol
Progestins
  Natural progesterone
  Progesterone derivatives
    Medroxyprogestrone acetate
    Megace
  19-nortestosterone derivatives
    Norethindrone
    Norethindrone acetate
Androgens
  Natural testosterone
  Dehydroepiandrosterone
  Synthetic testosterone
Estrogen–androgen combinations
Estrogen–progestin combinations
Bone resorption inhibitors
  Alendronate sodium
  Calcitonin
Calcium supplements
  Calcium carbonate
  Calcium citrate
  Calcium lactate
  Calcium gluconate
Selective estrogen receptor modulators

tors for heart disease (Table 19–2), breast cancer (Table 19–3), and osteoporosis (Table 19–4).

In addition, determine the woman's perception of the need for and risks of hormone replacement so that these issues can be addressed during counseling. Any current herbal or alternative therapies she may be using must be identified as they can have an additive effect with estrogen. A complete physical examination with special emphasis on breast and pelvic findings should be conducted.

The contraindications to the use of the estrogen in combination oral contraceptive pills are

## TABLE 19–2.  RISK FACTORS FOR HEART DISEASE

Obesity
Hypertension
Diabetes mellitus
Cigarette smoking
Sedentary lifestyle
Estrogen deficiency
Increased blood viscosity

*Adapted from Gorodeski and Utian, 1994.*

## TABLE 19–4.  RISK FACTORS FOR OSTEOPOROSIS

Caucasian or Asian Race
Family history
Low body mass index
Early menopause
Oligomennorhea/amenorrhea
Early childbearing
Smoking
Alcohol intake
High caffeine intake

*Adapted from Lichtman, 1996a.*

discussed in Chapter 18. Contraindications to the low doses of estrogen used in menopausal hormone replacement therapy are similar but not identical. The accepted contraindications are: (1) undiagnosed abnormal vaginal bleeding (2) active liver disease (3) current or recent thrombophlebitis or thromboembolic disease (4) breast cancer, and (5) endometrial cancer (Josse, 1996). In addition to the absolute contraindications listed above, other conditions are considered relative contraindications and require careful consideration of the benefits and risks before initiation of and careful, frequent monitoring while using therapies that include estrogen. These conditions are: (1) migraine headaches (2) history of thromboembolism, (3) familial hypertriglyceridemia, (4) uterine leiomyomas, (5) endometriosis (6) gall bladder disease, (6) strong family history of breast cancer, and (7) chronic hepatic dysfunction (Josse, 1996).

Once abnormal vaginal bleeding has been diagnosed and treated, estrogen may be initiated. Although a general consensus has not been achieved, some physicians will consider hormone replacement therapy for long-term survivors of breast and endometrial cancer (Chapman et al,

## TABLE 19–3.  RISK FACTORS FOR BREAST CANCER

Female gender
Increasing age
Personal history of breast cancer
Family history of breast cancer
Atypical hyperplasia on breast biopsy
Early menarche < age 12
Late menopause > age 50
Nulliparity
First full-term pregnancy after age 30

*Adapted from American Cancer Society, 1997b.*

1996; DiSaia, 1996; Theriault, 1996) as well as for women with resolved thromboembolic disease or liver disease (Shoupe & Mishell, 1994). Although controversial, consideration may be given to a nonoral form of estrogen for women with elevated triglycerides (>500 mg/dL) or gall bladder dysfunction (McGowan, 1996; Van Erpecum, Van Berge Henegouwen, Verschoor, Stoelwinder, & Willokens, 1991). Continuous combined hormone therapy may help control migraine headaches in those women whose headaches are induced by cyclic changes in hormones (Byyny & Speroff, 1996, p. 145).

Common conditions that are not contraindications for estrogen replacement are cervical cancer, diabetes, hypertension, or cardiovascular disease, including stroke (Shoupe & Mishell, 1994). It is notable that the Postmenopausal Estrogen/Progestin Interventions (PEPI) trial (Writing Group, 1995) found no change and possibly a decrease in blood pressure with women on hormone therapy. Women with risk factors for osteoporosis, cardiovascular disease, or colorectal cancer could reap the most benefits from hormone replacement therapy.

### Laboratory Tests

For many women, the age of onset and characteristic symptoms and physical findings allow the diagnosis of menopause without laboratory confirmation. In other women, laboratory data may provide critical information to help the clinician select the appropriate treatment. The following laboratory tests can be used to identify problems associated with the climacteric.

### Gonadotropin Measurements

If the diagnosis of menopause cannot be made with confidence from the history and physical examination findings, measurement of gonado-tropins may help establish the diagnosis. Elevated levels of gonadotropins (FSH > 30 IU/L and LH > 40 IU/L) indicate menopausal status (Byyny & Speroff, 1996). Because FSH increases before and to a greater extent than LH, it is the preferred measurement and it is seldom necessary to measure LH. Many women, during the early transition years, will be symptomatic and have normal gonadotropins. After eliminating pathologic causes of symptoms, a symptomatic woman with normal gonadotropins can be started on a trial of hormone replacement or low-dose oral contraceptives (Santoro et al, 1996).

## Mammography

The American Cancer Society recommends that all low-risk women obtain mammograms annually beginning at the age of 40 regardless of menopausal status or estrogen therapy (American Cancer Society, 1997a). Because estrogen may play a role in tumor progression in some breast cancers, mammograms should be obtained before initiating estrogen therapy and annually thereafter.

## Endometrial Biopsy

For any woman experiencing abnormal vaginal bleeding, a biopsy should be obtained to rule out endometrial cancer before initiating hormone therapy (Hargrove & Eisenberg, 1995). The slender cannula biopsy instruments make this an atraumatic office procedure for most women.

## Bone Density Measurements

For women with increased risk factors for osteoporosis or for those who do not choose to take estrogen, a measurement of bone density will monitor bone integrity and help predict fracture risk (Chung & Maroulis, 1996; Hargrove & Eisenberg, 1995). The most precision is obtained with dual energy x-ray absorptimetry (DEXA), but cost-effective screening can be obtained with single-photon absorptiometry (SPA) of the radius or calcaneus (Byyny & Speroff, 1996, p. 439).

## CLIENT INFORMATION

All perimenopausal women need to be counseled on how to achieve and maintain a healthy life-style. Older women tend to be given unacceptably low rates of clinical preventative services (Bergman-Evans & Walker, 1996). Counseling should include information on nutrition, exercise, sexual health, rest and recreation, stress reduction, immunizations, dental health, smoking cessation, alcohol and drug use/abuse, and injury and violence prevention (American College of Obstetricians and Gynecologists [ACOG], 1995). In addition to the general counseling, women need specific information about the risks and benefits of any treatment regimen selected.

## Oral Contraceptives

Perimenopausal women started on low doses of oral contraceptives (OCs) need to be reassured of the safety of this treatment modality in this age group. Women should be informed of the reduced risk of ovarian and endometrial cancer associated with OC use (Hulka & Brinton, 1995; Rosenberg et al, 1994). Women should be counseled that if hot flashes occur during the placebo pills, an evaluation is needed to determine the appropriateness of switching to hormone replacement therapy.

## Hormone Replacement Therapy

Women beginning hormone replacement therapy should be informed about the benefits and risks as well as prepared for the expected side effects with thorough and appropriate counseling. Each woman must decide if the benefits of therapy outweigh the combination of risks (genetic and biologic) and inconvenient side effects (environmental, lifestyle, and personal characteristics) that accompany estrogen replacement. A thorough history will identify the particular symptoms and risks an individual woman may face as she ages that can be relieved by HRT.

Hormone Replacement Therapy Risks. As with most pharmacologic interventions, hormone replacement is not risk-free. The most serious risks associated with hormone replacement include the development or promotion of reproductive tract cancers. Breast cancer is known to be estrogen-dependent in many women and is a concern of women taking exogenous estrogen. A multitude of studies have investigated the impact of estrogen replacement on the development of breast cancer with varying and often conflicting results (Theriault, 1996). All women in this age group have an increased risk of breast cancer, and the effect of hormone replacement on that risk is not absolutely known. Speroff (1996, 1997) suggests that the very nature of the data being so inconsistent indicates that if there is an increased risk, it may be small or the effect of a more pronounced impact in certain subgroups of women. The results of the randomized study of HRT effects by the Women's Health Initiative are due in 2005 and will shed much needed light on this issue.

Scientific evidence regarding the effect of hormone therapy on the development of ovarian cancer is also noted for conflicting results. Although one study (Rodriguez et al, 1995) found an increased risk of fatal ovarian cancer with ≥11 years of estrogen use, no consistent evidence of increased risk was found in the pooled analysis of 12 case-controlled studies of ovarian cancer risks (Whitemore, Harris, Itnyre, & the Collaborative Ovarian Cancer Group, 1992). In addition, an analysis of cancer incidence and deaths in 22,597 Swedish women using hormone replacement therapy showed no elevation of risk for a multitude of cancer sites including ovarian cancer (Persson, Yuen, Bergkvist, & Schairer, 1996). Further studies are needed to delineate the impact of postmenopausal estrogen on the development of ovarian cancer.

Other risks associated with menopausal hormone replacement therapy include an increase in asthma (Troisi, Speizer, Willett, Trichopoulos, & Rosner, 1995) and an increased risk of gallbladder disease requiring surgery (Grodstein, Colditz, & Stampfer, 1994).

In addition, it is well documented that there is an increased risk of endometrial hyperplasia and cancer in women with a uterus who take estrogen alone (Persson et al, 1996; Writing Group, 1995). Most, but not all, of the endometrial cancer experienced by women during estrogen replacement therapy tends to be well differentiated with an excellent cure rate (Woodruff & Pickar, 1994). The risk for endometrial cancer can be significantly reduced but not totally eliminated by adding a progestin to the estrogen replacement in women who have a uterus (McGonigle et al, 1994; Writing Group, 1995).

Hormone Replacement Side Effects. A woman should be given anticipatory guidance to prepare her for the most common nuisance side effects. Make her a partner in establishing the appropriate therapy. She needs to monitor and report side effects to allow optimal titration of the dosage. Unpredictable bleeding for the first 4–6 months of therapy is common. Nuisance side effects involve both the estrogen and progestin components of HRT. The estrogen component has been associated with complaints of nausea, edema, breast tenderness, contact lens intolerance, headache, and aggravation of porphyria. The progestin component can create premenstrual syndrome symptoms, such as fatigue, depression, edema, breast tenderness, insomnia, or chloasma (Wich & Carnes, 1995).

### Bone Resorption Inhibitors

Alendronate sodium, a third-generation bisphosphonate, has been shown to improve bone density in the hip and spine and decrease fracture rates (Chesnut et al, 1995; Liberman et al, 1995). It is currently approved for use in patients with osteoporosis, but studies are in progress for preventive use. The usual starting dose of alendronate is 10 mg/day. Strongly counsel the patient:

1. To take the drug in the morning at least 30 min before any food, drink, or other medication and with a large (6 to 8 oz) glass of water.
2. Not to lie down for at least 30 min after taking the medication.
3. To contact her health care provider if heartburn or difficulty swallowing develops, since this may herald esophageal ulcerations.

Calcium interferes with the absorption of alendronate and should be taken at least 30 min after the morning dose (Chung & Maroulis, 1996.)

Calcitonin also inhibits bone resorption. In short-term studies, it is effective in decreasing spinal bone loss associated with early menopause (Reginster et al, 1995). In addition, in one small study, calcitonin plus 500 mg of elemental calcium reduced osteoporotic fractures (Rico, Revilla, Hernandez, Villa, & Alvarez de Buergo, 1995). One unique aspect of calcitonin is that it has an analgesic effect and relieves pain associated with vertebral fractures (Notelovitz, 1997).

## OUTCOMES MANAGEMENT

### SELECTION OF THE APPROPRIATE AGENT

Pharmacologic management of the climacteric is an art as well as a science. You must balance the personal preferences and characteristics of the individual with the known medical risks and benefits of any drug intervention. The most difficult management decisions usually occur during the perimenopausal period. After thorough evaluation and consideration of the contraindications to each therapy, the clinician has the pharmacologic options for management discussed below.

## Oral Contraceptives

During the perimenopausal years (ages 40–50), women will often present with unpredictable anovulatory vaginal bleeding, hot flashes, or both. Low-dose oral contraceptives are ideal first-line drugs for this group of women. They prevent pregnancy; induce regular, predictable menstrual bleeding; and reduce the risk of ovarian and endometrial cancer while providing the estrogen to maintain bone health and prevent hot flashes (Grimes & Economy, 1995; Shaaban, 1996; Trossarelli et al, 1995). The woman who is having anovulatory bleeding but not having hot flashes also is a candidate for low-dose OCs once endometrial cancer has been ruled out. Because even low dose OC's have higher doses of estrogen than needed by menopausal women, the clinician should switch her from OCs to hormone replacement therapy when:

- she has hot flashes on the placebo pills
- her serum FSH (measured after the placebo pills and before starting the active pills) is >30 IU/L
- her FSH/LH ratio is >1
- her estradiol ($E_2$) level is <20 pg/mL (Creinin, 1996).

## Progestin

If the perimenopausal woman with irregular anovulatory bleeding prefers to not take OCs, cyclic withdrawal to oral progestin is an appropriate alternative therapy. Medroxyprogesterone acetate (MPA) 10 mg daily for the first 10 days of the month will prevent endometrial hyperplasia (Byyny & Speroff, 1996, p. 110). Estrogen should be started when the woman fails to have withdrawal bleeding from the progestin.

## Hormone Replacement

There are many treatment options appropriate for the average menopausal woman. For the woman with a uterus, estrogen is used for symp-tom control, osteoporosis prevention, and cardiovascular disease prevention, and a progestin is added to decrease the risk of endometrial cancer. For the woman without a uterus, oral estrogen alone will control symptoms and provide the anticipated long-term benefits. Under special circumstances, a progestin is appropriate for women who have had a hysterectomy, for example, those with a history of endometriosis or those with elevated triglycerides (Byyny & Speroff, 1996, pp. 195, 202). In the United States, the most thoroughly studied oral estrogen is conjugated equine estrogen (CEE) Premarin, which contains ten different estrogenic compounds (Ansbacher, 1996). Esterified estrogens (Estratab), micronized estradiol (Estrace), and transdermal estrogens (Estraderm, Climara, and Vivelle) are not identical compounds to conjugated estrogens, but in small-scale, short-term studies, they have demonstrated similar benefits in menopausal women (Gordon et al, 1995). Conjugated estrogen 0.625 mg is the lowest effective dose known to prevent osteoporosis. This dose also will control hot flashes in the average menopausal woman. For the young, surgically menopausal woman, a higher initial dose may be required to control hot flashes. With higher doses of estrogen, a higher dose of progestin may be needed for endometrial protection (Nand, Webster, & Wren, 1995). Over time, the dose should be titrated downward until symptoms are controlled by the 0.625-mg dose. Older women started on estrogen after years of extremely low endogenous estrogen may need very low starting doses to prevent unacceptable side effects, and their dose titrated upward to the goal dose of 0.625 mg daily (Lichtman, 1996b). A recent study reported in *The Harvard Woman's Health Watch* (Low-dose estrogen, 1996) found that 0.3 mg/day of estrogen replacement therapy given to women with a uterus may preserve the bone mineral density without increasing the risk of hyperplasia compared to those given a placebo. All the women in this study also took 1000 mg of calcium.

Transdermal estrogen systems are available for nonoral delivery of hormones. The 0.05-mg patch is the usual starting dose and is thought to be approximately equivalent to 0.625 mg of oral conjugated estrogen. The transdermal patch offers very stable serum levels of estradiol and may control symptoms in women who are sensitive to the fluctuations in serum levels of estrogen that occur during oral therapy. Some women may prefer a nonoral estrogen. Transdermal estrogen, especially in conjunction with oral MPA, may not produce the favorable changes in cholesterol, LDL-C, and HDL-C seen with oral preparations (Lemay, Dodin, Cedrin, & T-Lemay, 1995). Long-term, prospective, randomized, and well-controlled studies are needed to demonstrate the benefits of transdermal estrogen for osteoporosis prevention and cardiovascular protection. Injectable estrogen is not appropriate for menopausal hormone replacement.

Once the agent and starting dose have been selected, a regimen must be chosen. There is no one "right" way to prescribe hormone replacement; rather, appropriate options should be tailored to the particular woman's symptoms, needs, and preferences. Adherence to therapy depends heavily on the client's thorough understanding of the short-term and long-term benefits and preparation for the anticipated side effects. Women who have undergone a hysterectomy should be prescribed estrogen alone, in doses sufficient to control symptoms, but at least equivalent to 0.625 mg of conjugated equine estrogen. Women who have retained their uteruses are at increased risk for developing endometrial hyperplasia if they take estrogen alone. For these women, a progestin is added to the regimen to inhibit endometrial growth (Writing Group, 1995). Currently the most commonly prescribed progestins for menopausal hormone replacement are medroxyprogesterone acetate (MPA) or norethindrone (NET). The PEPI trials reported excellent lipid and endometrial results using micronized progesterone. This preparation under the brand name Prometrium is available in 25 countries worldwide. Solvay Pharmaceuticals, Inc. has acquired the license for marketing Prometrium in the United States and Canada. U.S. release is pending at this time. Currently, micronized progesterone is available only from compounding pharmacies. Prempro (daily combination of CEE 0.625 mg and MPA 2.5 mg continuously) and Premphase (daily CEE 0.625 mg with MPA 5 mg added the last 14 days) are prepackaged blister packs that simplify dosing. This may improve patient compliance.

Two treatment regimens for women with a uterus are: continuous estrogen with cyclic progestin and continuous daily estrogen and progestin. The estrogen with cyclic progestin regimen produces withdrawal bleeding in almost all women (Writing Group, 1995). Continuous estrogen/progestin regimes are ac-companied by unpredictable vaginal bleeding in 60–70% of woman for the first few months (Nand, Webster, & Wren, 1995; Bachman, Timmons & Abernethy, 1996). For most women, this bleeding usually subsides by about 6 months and amenorrhea ensues. For a few unfortunate women, bleeding will continue indefinitely. Although both regimens relieve menopausal symptoms, compliance may be better with continuous combined therapy (Doren, Reuther, Minne, & Schneider, 1995). Any continued bleeding after 6 months or increase in amount, duration, or frequency of bleeding requires evaluation.

Early in menopause, the endometrium remains exquisitely sensitive to estrogen, and women on continuous estrogen/progestin regimes may experience significant breakthrough bleeding. In addition, women who are experiencing unpredictable heavy bleeding during the perimenopause may have substantial breakthrough bleeding on continuous estrogen/progestin therapy (Corson, 1995). After counseling about the expected bleeding patterns, it is appropriate for the woman to choose her replacement regimen.

Start-up problems should be anticipated, and women should be prepared for breast tenderness, vaginal bleeding, and the inconvenience of daily dosing. Frequent contact between women and their providers will facilitate improved treatment adherence. Problems can be identified, and changes in dosages or drugs, can be initiated before the woman becomes discouraged and electively discontinues treatment. A suggested follow-up schedule is: (1) telephone contact during the first month of treatment, (2) an office visit every 3 months until a suitable dose and regimen have been established, and (3) yearly visits thereafter. Annual physical examination and laboratory studies are required for continued hormone therapy.

## SELECTIVE ESTROGEN RECEPTOR MODULATORS (SERMS)

The new class of drugs gaining notice and favor for the prevention of osteoporosis is selective estrogen receptor modulators or SERMs. The anticipated belief is that SERMs, also called "designer estrogens" and "estrogen antagonists," can provide all or most of the benefits of estrogen replacement therapy without the dangers (Drug offers estrogen, 1997; HRT: An option,

1997). SERMs are similar to estrogen in that they attach to receptors within cells; yet unlike estrogen, they do not signal cell growth and division as seen in breast or endometrial cancer (Bryant & Dere, 1998; Hol, Cox, Bryant, & Draper, 1997; Mitlak & Cohen, 1997).

The first widely-used SERM, tamoxifene, is a breast cancer treatment that acts to lock out the estrogen effect from the breast cells, thus reducing their ability to live and grow (HRT: An option, 1997). In addition, serum cholesterol reduction and bone density are maintained. However, with tamoxifene, the endometrial effect is not antagonized and endometrial cancer risk is increased.

A newer SERM, raloxifene, is a benzothiophene, and is proving not only to block estrogen receptors in both the breast and the endometrium (antagonist action), but it increases bone mass and lowers cholesterol (agonist action) (Bryant & Dere, 1998; Drug offers estrogen, 1997). Edward Lukin of the Mayo Clinic in Rochester, reported findings of a study of 143 postmenopausal women with osteoporosis and a history of fracture at the American Society for Bone and Mineral Research in the Fall of 1997 (Drug offers estrogen, 1997). Raloxifene increased bone mass in the women receiving it. A worldwide study of 12,000 women offers preliminary results of raloxifene increasing bone density and lowering total cholesterol, LDL cholesterol, and fibrinogen, as well as causing no breast tenderness or bloating (HRT: An option, 1997). However, hot flashes have been exacerbated in some women and HDL cholesterol did not increase as it does with estrogen therapy.

In the months to come, pharmaceutical companies will be marketing or investigating more than 35 new products (patches, pills, and devices) for osteoporosis prevention, menopausal symptoms and hormonal therapy (New Medicines, 1997). Among these will be a wave of SERMs aimed at postmenopausal prevention of osteoporosis. Readers are urged to keep abreast of current drug therapies and supporting scientific evidence for use as these drugs and devices come on the market.

## Bone Resorption Inhibitors

For those who cannot or will not take estrogen, prescribe alendronate or calcitonin for postmenopausal women with osteopenia or established osteoporosis (Chesnut et al, 1995; Hodsman, Adachi, & Olszynski, 1996, Liberman et al, 1995; Reginster et al, 1995; Rico et al, 1995). Calcium supplementation of at least 1000 mg day should be used in conjunction with either drug. Alendronate may be the better choice for increasing bone mass and decreasing fracture risk (Notelovitz, 1997).

## Calcium Supplementation

Because intake of adequate calcium is vital to maintaining bone mass regardless of whether hormonal or nonhormonal therapies are chosen, try to ensure that appropriate dietary and supplemental sources of calcium are taken by menopausal women. All adult women and menopausal women on estrogen therapy should obtain 1 g of elemental calcium daily either through diet or a combination of diet and supplementation. Menopausal women not taking estrogen require 1.5 g of elemental calcium (Berga, 1996). Daily calcium intake of greater than 2 gs/day should be avoided. Several formulations of calcium are available for supplementation: calcium carbonate contains the highest proportion of elemental calcium by weight, but calcium chelates such as citrate may be more effective for promoting bone formation (Chung & Maroulis, 1996).

Excess dietary calcium may induce unfavorable calcium-mineral interactions, particularly with iron, zinc, and magnesium. Since calcium inhibits iron absorption, encourage women with low dietary iron intake to consume their calcium between or after meals. A zinc deficiency could develop in women with low levels of dietary zinc on high-calcium diets, so zinc may need to be supplemented. Finally, excess calcium can cause magnesium deficiency in special circumstances such as diabetes or alcoholism. To prevent magnesium deficiency, 100 mg of magnesium for every 500 mg of calcium is recommended for these situations. Most cases of calcium-induced mineral deficiency occur with calcium intake of greater than 2 g/day (Whiting, Wood, & Kim, 1997).

## MONITORING FOR EFFICACY

Efficacy is demonstrated by resolution of presenting symptoms and continued adherence to the treatment regimen. When a woman has multiple symptoms, it is not unusual for one or more symptoms to be relieved but not all. For example, hot flashes may be controlled, but genital atrophy continues. If the woman is otherwise asymptomatic and is on at least 0.625 mg of CEE or the equivalent, supplementation with vaginal estrogen (vaginal cream or a silastic ring) is preferred to increasing the dose of oral estrogen. Some women experience decreased sexual desire and increased sexual dysfunction that is unresponsive to estrogen replacement alone. After several months of estrogen trial, if decreased libido continues to be a problem, a trial of an estrogen/androgen combination therapy can be tried. It is important to note that the oral estrogen/androgen combination prevents the favorable changes in lipoproteins seen with estrogen alone and careful monitoring is advisable (Watts et al, 1995). Although protection from osteoporosis has been demonstrated, it is not known whether this regimen provides protection against cardiovascular disease. A progestin should still be used for endometrial protection with estrogen/androgen combination therapy.

Relief of symptoms provides more information on therapy efficacy than laboratory tests, but laboratory studies are available.

1. *Vaginal cytology:* The maturation index supplies information about local tissue response to estrogen. Adequate estrogen therapy produces abundant superficial cells, whereas a high percentage of parabasal cells indicates low estrogen.

2. *Bone density measurements:* Women who are at high risk for osteoporosis or who had evidence of decreased bone mass prior to estrogen therapy should have a periodic measurement of bone density (Corson, 1995).

3. *Serum estrogen levels:* In women who continue to be symptomatic on 1.25 mg of CEE or equivalent doses of other estrogens, including nonoral routes, measuring serum estradiol will differentiate estrogen deficiency from other causes of symptoms. Serum estradiol levels of 40–100 pg/mL are adequate for menopausal symptom control. Because conjugated equine estrogens are compounds with many estrogenic substances, monitoring estradiol is more effective when estradiol-containing compounds are used (Corson, 1995). With adequate serum estradiol levels and continuing symptoms, a thorough search must be made for other causes.

## MONITORING FOR TOXICITY

The greatest risks of estrogen therapy are the increased risk of endometrial cancer, possible increased risk of breast cancer, possible increased risk of ovarian cancer, possible increased risk of asthma, and an increased risk of gallbladder disease. Monitoring for these risks involves cooperation between provider and patient. Any unexpected abnormal vaginal bleeding must be evaluated by endometrial biopsy. With cyclic administration of a progestin, bleeding is expected to occur during the last few days of progestin or the week after the progestin is stopped. A high index of suspicion is indicated and a biopsy should be performed if heavy bleeding occurs at any time, if bleeding persists over time, or if bleeding occurs at unexpected times. Vaginal probe sonography can be used to evaluate endometrial status. If the endometrium measures <5 mm in double-wall thickness, endometrial cancer is very unlikely (Hargrove & Eisenberg, 1995). Endometrial biopsy is recommended when the endometrial thickness is ≥5 mm. The woman should be informed of the need to return for evaluation if any of the above bleeding patterns occur.

Although the relationship of HRT and the development of breast cancer remains unclear, surviving breast cancer in the long term is improved with early detection and treatment. Therefore, women should be taught and encouraged to perform monthly breast self-examinations and providers must carefully evaluate each woman annually for suspicious changes in the breast. Diagnostic mammograms and biopsies should be performed as needed, and screening mammograms should be done annually.

Women taking HRT should be counseled to return for evaluation of any unusual abdominal pain. Gallbladder disease should be considered and investigated when appropriate symptoms are present in women who are taking HRT.

Estrogen/androgen combination therapy is not associated with the favorable changes in lipoproteins seen with estrogen alone and should be used with caution in women with elevated blood lipids or other cardiovascular disease risks (Speroff, 1996; Watts et al, 1995).

## FOLLOW-UP

The duration of hormone replacement therapy for optimal disease prevention and health promotion is unknown. For control of hot flashes, hormone replacement is needed for only a few months to a few years; for prevention of urogenital atrophy, osteoporosis, and cardiovascular disease, a minimum of 10 years and possibly lifelong therapy is necessary.

A woman on HRT should have a thorough history, with emphasis on identifying annoying side effects, reviewing the risks and benefits of the current therapy, and completing a physical examination annually. In addition, a generally healthy lifestyle should be encouraged, involving regular exercise, a low-fat, high-fiber diet, and adequate calcium intake as well as avoiding smoking and excessive alcohol and caffeine.

There is much to learn about the optimal management of women's health during the midlife years. In the coming years, the results of the National Institutes of Health Women's Health Initiative Study will provide more concrete information about the clinical outcomes of long-term hormone replacement therapy. Another study in progress, the Hormone Estrogen/Progestin Replacement Study, may provide information about the effect of hormone replacement on women with preexisting heart disease. With the results of these and future studies, a more desirable hormone replacement regime may be developed that creates fewer side effects and risks for women and accrues greater benefits.

## REFERENCES

American Cancer Society. (1997a). American Cancer Society workshop on guidelines for breast cancer detection. Chicago, March 7–9, 1997 [Internet: http://www.cancer.org/mammog.html].

American Cancer Society. (1997b). What are the risk factors for breast cancer? [Internet: http://www.cancer.org/brrisk.html].

American College of Obstetricians and Gynecologists. (1995, August). *Health maintenance for perimenopausal women*. ACOG Technical Bulletin, No. 210 Washington, DC: ACOG.

Anonymous. (1991). Consensus development conference: Osteoporosis. *American Journal of Medicine, 90*, 107–110.

Ansbacher, R. (1996). Estrogens: Conjugated and esterified therapeutic substitution. *Female Patient, 21*, 12–15.

Arnstein, P. M., Buselli, E. F., & Rankin, S. H. (1996). Women and heart attacks: Prevention, diagnosis, and care. *Nurse Practitioner, 21*(5), 57–71.

Asplund, R., & Aberg, H. E. (1995). Body mass index and sleep in women aged 40 to 64 years. *Maturitas, 22*(1), 1–8.

Avis, N. E. (1997). Hormones and mood among menopausal women. *Menopausal Medicine, 5*(1), 5–9.

Avis, N. E., Brambilla, D., McKinlay, S. M., & Vass, K. (1994). A longitudinal analysis of the association between menopause and depression: Results from the Massachusetts women's health study. *Annals of Epidemiology, 4*, 214–220.

Bachmann, G. A. (1995). Influence of menopause on sexuality. *International Journal of Fertility and Menopausal Studies, 40*(Suppl. 1), 16–22.

Bachmann, G. A., Timmons, M. C., & Abernethy, W. D. (1996). Breakthrough bleeding patterns in two continuous combined estrogen/progestogen hormone replacement therapies, one of which included androgens. *Journal of Women's Health, 5*(3), 205–212.

Barrett-Connor, E. (1995). The economic and human costs of osteoporotic fracture. *American Journal of Medicine, 98*(2A), 35–85.

Berga, S. L. (1996). Ways of optimizing calcium intake: The NIH's new guidelines call for different amounts of calcium at various stages of life to promote long-term bone health. *Contemporary Ob/Gyn, 41*(6), 84–91.

Bergman-Evans, B., & Walker, S. N. (1996). The prevalence of clinical preventive services utilization by older women. *Nurse Practitioner, 21*(4), 88–106.

Brinton, R. D (1997). Estrogen replacement therapy and Alzheimer's disease. *Menopausal Medicine, 5*(1), 5–9.

Bryant, Y. U. & Dere, W. H. (1998). Selective estrogen receptor modulators: An alternative to hormone replacement therapy. *Proceedings of Society of Experimental Biology & Medicine, 217*(1), 45–52.

Byyny, R. L., & Speroff, L. (1996). *A clinical guide for the care of older women. Primary and preventive care* (2nd ed.) (pp. 79–141, 143–160, 161–226, 425–452). Baltimore: Williams & Wilkins.

Calle, E. E., & Thun, M. (1997). The epidemiology of the effects of estrogen and aspirin on colorectal cancer. *Menopausal Medicine, 5*(1), 9–12.

Cauley, J. A., Seeley, D. G., Ensrud, K., Ettinger, B., Black, D., & Cummings, S. R. (1995). Estrogen replacement therapy and fractures in older women. *Annals of Internal Medicine, 122*(1), 9–16.

Chapman, J. A., DiSaia, P. J., Osann, K., Roth, P. D., Gillotte, D. L., & Berman, M. L. (1996). Estrogen replacement in surgical stage I and II endometrial cancer survivors. *American Journal of Obstetrics and Gynecology, 175*(5), 1195–1200.

Chapuy, M. C., & Meunier, P. J. (1995). Prevention and treatment of osteoporosis. *Aging: Clinical and Experimental Research, 7*(4), 164–173.

Chesnut, C. H., III, McClung, M. R., Ensrud, K. E., Bell, N. H., Genant, H. K., Harris, S. T., Singer,

F. R., Stock, J. L., Yood, R. A., Delmas, P. D., Kher, U., Pryor-Tillotson, S., & Santora, A. C., II. (1995). Alendronate treatment of the postmenopausal osteoporotic woman: Effect of multiple dosages on bone mass and bone remodeling. *American Journal of Medicine, 99*, 144–152.

Chung, P. H., & Maroulis, G. B. (1996). Osteoporosis: An update on prevention and treatment. *Female Patient, 21*, 39–50.

Cooper, A., & Whitehead, M. (1995). Menopause: Refining benefits and risks of hormone replacement therapy. *Current Opinion in Obstetrics and Gynecology 7*(3), 214–219.

Corson, S. L. (1995). A practical guide to prescribing estrogen replacement therapy. *International Journal of Fertility and Menopausal Studies, 40*(5), 229–247.

Counseling to promote physical activity. (1997). *Primary Care Update Ob/Gyns, 4*(3), 97–105.

Creinin, M. (1996). Laboratory criteria for menopause in women using oral contraceptives. *Fertility and Sterility, 66*(1), 101–104.

Dennerstein, L. (1996). Well-being, symptoms and the menopausal transition. *Maturitas, 23*(2), 147–157.

Derman, R. J., Dawood, M. Y., & Stone, S. (1995). Quality of life during sequential hormone replacement therapy: A placebo-controlled study. *International Journal of Fertility and Menopausal Studies, 40*(2), 73–78.

DiSaia, P. (1996). Hormone replacement therapy in breast cancer patients. *Contemporary Ob/Gyn*, 67–84.

Doren, M., Reuther, G., Minne, H. W., & Schneider, H. P. G. (1995). Superior compliance and efficacy of continuous combined oral estrogen-progestogen replacement therapy in postmenopausal women. *American Journal of Obstetrics and Gynecology, 173*(5), 1446–1451.

Drug offers estrogen benefits, not side effects. (September 12, 1997). *Sun-Sentinel*, 4A.

Eiken, P., Nielson, S. P., & Kolthoff, N. (1997). Effects on bone mass after eight years of hormonal replacement therapy. *British Journal of Obstetrics and Gynaecology, 104*(6), 702–707.

Ettinger, B., Friedman, G. D., Bush, T., & Quesenberry, C. P., Jr. (1996). Reduced mortality associated with long-term postmenopausal estrogen therapy. *Obstetrics and Gynecology, 87*(1), 6–12.

Fantl, J. A. (1994). The lower urinary tract in women—effect of aging and menopause on continence. *Experimental Gerontology, 29*(3–4), 417–422.

Fillit, H. (1995). Future therapeutic developments of estrogen use. *Journal of Clinical Pharmacology, 35*(Suppl. 9), 25S–28S.

Gordon, S. F., Thompson, K. A., Ruoff, G. E., Imig, J. R., Lane, P. J., Schwenker, C. E., & the Transdermal Estradiol Patch Study Group. (1995). Efficacy and safety of a seven-day, transdermal estradiol drug-delivery system: Comparison with conjugated estrogens and placebo. *International Journal of Fertility and Menopausal Studies, 40*(3), 126–134.

Gorodeski, G. L., & Utian, W. H. (1994). Epidemiology and risk factors of cardiovascular disease in postmenopausal women. In R. Lobo (Ed.), *Treatment of the post-menopausal woman: Basic and clinical aspects* (pp. 199–222). New York: Raven Press.

Graziottin, A. (1996). HRT: The woman's perspective. *International Journal of Gynaecology and Obstetrics, 52*(Suppl. 1), S11–16.

Grimes, D. A., & Economy, K. E. (1995). Primary prevention of gynecologic cancers. *American Journal of Obstetrics and Gynecology, 172*(1), 227–235.

Grodstein, F., Colditz, G. A., & Stampfer, M. J. (1994). Post menopausal hormone use and cholecystectomy in a large prospective study. *Obstetrics and Gynecology, 83*, 5–11.

Guetta, V., & Cannon, R. O., III. (1996). Cardiovascular effects of estrogen and lipid-lowering therapies in postmenopausal women. *Circulation, 93*, 1928–1937.

Hammond, C. B. (1996). Menopause and hormone replacement therapy: An overview. *Obstetrics and Gynecology, 87*(Suppl. 2), 2S–15S.

Hargrove, J. T., & Eisenberg, E. (1995). Menopause. *Medical Clinics of North America, 79*(6), 1337–1356.

Hodsman, A., Adachi, J., & Olszynski, W. (1996). Prevention and management of osteoporosis: Consensus statements from the Scientific Advisory Board of the Osteoporosis Society of Canada. 6. *Canadian Medical Association Journal, 155*(7), 945–948.

Hol, T., Cox, M. B., Bryant, H. U., & Draper, M. W. (1997). Selective estrogen receptor modulators and postmenopausal women's health. *Journal of Women's Health, 6*(5), 523–531.

HRT: An option for the future. (August 1997). *Harvard Women's Health Watch, IV*(12), 1.

Hulka, B. S., & Brinton, L. A. (1995). Hormones and breast and endometrial cancers: Preventive strategies and future research. *Environmental Health Perspectives 103*(Suppl. 8), 185–189.

Hurt, W. G. (1996). Urinary incontinence in older women. *Menopausal Medicine, 4*(3), 1–4.

Josse, R. G. (1996). Effects of ovarian hormone therapy on skeletal and extraskeletal tissues in women. *Canadian Medical Association Journal, 155*(7), 929–934.

Klutke, J. J., & Bergman, A. (1995). Hormonal influence on the urinary tract. *Urology Clinics of North America, 22*(3), 629–639.

Kohrt, W. M., & Birge, S. J., Jr. (1995). Differential effects of estrogen treatment on bone mineral density of the spine, hip, wrist and total body in late postmenopausal women. *Osteoporosis International, 5*(3), 150–155.

Kwawukume, E. Y., Ghosh, T. S., & Wilson, J. B. (1993). Menopausal age of Ghanaian women. *International Journal of Gynaecology and Obstetrics, 40*(2), 151–155.

Lemay, A., Dodin, S., Cedrin, I., & T-Lemay, L. (1995). Phasic serum lipid excursions occur during cyclical oral conjugated oestrogens but not during transdermal oestradiol sequentially combined with oral medroxyprogesterone acetate. *Clinical Endocrinology, 42*(4), 341–351.

Liberman, U. A., Weiss, S. R., Broll, J., Minne, H. W., Quan, H., Bell, N. H., Rodriguez-Portales, J., Downs, R. W., Jr., Dequeker, J., Favus, M., Seeman, E., Recker, R. R., Capizzi, T., Santora, A. C., II, Lombardi, A., Shah, R. V., Hirsch, L. J., Laurence, J., & Karpf, D. B. (1995). Effect of oral alendronate on bone mineral density and the incidence of fractures in postmenopausal osteoporosis. *New England Journal of Medicine, 333*(22), 1437–1443.

Lichtman, R. (1996a). Perimenopausal and postmenopausal hormone replacement therapy–Part 1: An update of the literature on benefits and risks. *Journal of Nurse-Midwifery, 41*(1), 3–28.

Lichtman, R. (1996b). Perimenopausal and postmenopausal hormone replacement therapy–Part 2: Hormonal regimens and complementary and alternative therapies. *Journal of Nurse-Midwifery, 41*(3), 195–210.

Limouzin-Lamothe, M. A., Mairon, N., Joyce, C. R., & Le Gal, M. (1994). Quality of life after the menopause: Influence of hormonal replacement therapy. *American Journal of Obstetrics and Gynecology, 170*(2), 618–624.

Lindgren, R., Berg, G., Hammar, M., & Zuccon, E. (1993). Hormonal replacement therapy and sexuality in a population of Swedish postmenopausal women. *Acta Obstetrica et Gynecologica Scandinavica 72*, 292–297.

Lindsay, R. (1996). The menopause and osteoporosis. *Obstetrics and Gynecology, 87*(Suppl. 2), 16S–19S.

Lip, G. Y., Beevers, G., & Zarifis, J. (1995). Hormone replacement therapy and cardiovascular risk: The cardiovascular physicians' viewpoint. *Journal of Internal Medicine, 238*(5), 389–399.

Low-dose estrogen for HRT. (1996, December). *Harvard Women's Health Watch, IV*(4), 7.

Marcus, R., Greendale, G., Blunt, B. A., Bush, T. L., Sherman, S., Sherwin, R., Wahner, H., & Wells, B. (1994). Correlates of bone mineral density in the post menopausal estrogen/progestin interventions trial. *Journal of Bone and Mineral Research, 9*(9), 1467–1476.

Matthews, K. A., Wing, R. R., Kuller, L. H., Meilahn, E. N., & Plantinga, P. (1994). Influence of the perimenopause on cardiovascular risk factors and symptoms of middle-aged healthy women. *Archives of Internal Medicine, 154*, 2349–2355.

McGonigle, K., Karlan, B., Barbuto, D., Leuchter, R., Lagasse, L., & Judd, H. (1994). Development of endometrial cancer in women on estrogen and progestin hormone replacement therapy. *Gynecologic Oncology, 55*, 126–132.

McGowan, M. P. (1996). Managing dyslipidemias in the postmenopausal woman. *Menopausal Medicine, 4*(3), 5–8.

Mitlak, B. H., & Cohen, F. J. (1997). In search of optimal long-term female hormone replacement: The potential of selective estrogen receptor modulators. *Hormone Research, 48*(4), 155–163.

Mostwin, J. L., Genadry, R., Sanders, R., & Yang, A. (1996). Anatomic goals in the correction of female stress urinary incontinence. *Journal of Endourology, 10*(3), 207–212.

Myers, L. S. (1995). Methodological review and meta-analysis of sexuality and menopause research. *Neuroscience and Biobehavioral Reviews, 19*(2), 331–341.

Nand, S. L., Webster, M. A., & Wren, B. G. (1995). Continuous combined piperazine oestrone sulphate and medroxyprogesterone acetate hormone replacement therapy: A study of bleeding pattern, endometrial response, serum lipid and bone density changes. *Australian and New Zealand Journal of Obstetrics and Gynaecology, 35*(1), 92–96.

National Center for Health Statistics. (1993). *Vital statistics of the United States, 1989, Vol. II, Mortality, Part A* (DHHS Publication No. PHS 93-1101). Washington, DC: U.S. Government Printing Office.

New medicines in development for women. (10/97). *America's Pharmaceutical Research Companies*, PhRMA, Washington, D.C.

Nilsson, K., Risberg, B., & Heimer, G. (1995). The vaginal epithelium in the postmenopause—cytology, histology and pH as methods of assessment. *Maturitas, 21*(1), 51–56.

Notelovitz, M. (1997). Osteoporosis: Alternatives for keeping bones strong. *Contemporary Nurse Practitioner, 2*(1), 7–19.

Nygaard, I. E. (1996). Nonoperative management of urinary incontinence. *Current Opinions in Obstetrics and Gynecology, 8*(5), 347–350.

Paganini-Hill, A. (1996). Oestrogen replacement therapy and Alzheimer's disease. *British Journal of Obstetrics and Gynaecology, 103*(S13), 80–86.

Pearce, J., Hawton, K., & Blake, F. (1995). Psychological and sexual symptoms associated with the menopause and the effects of hormone replacement therapy. *British Journal of Psychiatry, 167*(2), 163–173.

Pearlstein, T. B. (1995). Hormones and depression: What are the facts about premenstrual syndrome, menopause, and hormone replacement therapy? *American Journal of Obstetrics and Gynecology, 173*, 646–653.

Persson, I., Yuen, J., Bergkvist, L., & Schairer, C. (1996). Cancer incidence and mortality in women receiving estrogen and estrogen-progestin replacement therapy—Long-term follow-up of a Swedish cohort. *International Journal of Cancer, 67*(3), 327–332.

Porter, M., Penney, G. C., Russell, D., Russell, E., & Templeton, A. (1996). A population based survey of women's experience of the menopause. *British Journal of Obstetrics and Gynaecology, 103*(10), 1025–1028.

Reginster, J. Y., Deroisy, R., Lecart, M. P., Sarlet, N., Zegels, B., Jupsin, I., de Longueville, M., & Franchimont, P. (1995). A double-blind, placebo-controlled, dose-finding trial of intermittent nasal salmon calcitonin for prevention of post-menopausal lumbar spine bone loss. *American Journal of Medicine, 98*(5), 452–458.

Rico, H., Revilla, M., Hernandez, E. R., Villa, L. F., & Alvarez de Buergo, M. (1995). Total and regional bone mineral content and fracture rate in postmenopausal osteoporosis treated with salmon calcitonin: A prospective study. *Calcified Tissue International, 56*(3), 181–185.

Rodriguez, C., Calle, E. E., Coates, R. J., Miracle-McMahill, H. L., Thun, M. J., & Heth, C. W., Jr. (1995). Estrogen replacement therapy and fetal ovarian cancer. *American Journal of Epidemiology, 141*(9), 828–835.

Rosenberg, L., Palmer, J. R., Zauber, A. G., Warshauer, M. E., Lewis, J. L., Jr., Strom, B. L., Harlap, S., & Shapiro, S. (1994). A case-control study of oral contraceptive use and invasive epithelial ovarian cancer. *American Journal of Epidemiology, 139*(7), 654–661.

Rosenberg, S., Kroll, M., & Vandromme, J. (1996). Decision factors influencing hormone replacement therapy. *British Journal of Obstetrics and Gynaecology, 103*(Suppl. 13), 92–98.

Sagraves, R. (1995). Estrogen therapy for post-menopausal symptoms and prevention of osteoporosis. *Journal of Clinical Pharmacy and Therapeutics, 35*(Suppl. 9), 2S–10S.

Santoro, N., Brown, J. R., Adel, T., & Skurnick, J. H. (1996). Characterization of reproductive hormonal dynamics in the perimenopause. *Journal of Clinical Endocrinology and Metabolism, 81*(4), 1495–1501.

Scharbo-DeHaan, M. (1996, December). Hormone replacement therapy. *Nurse Practitioner*, 1–15.

Schiffman, S. S., Sattely-Miller, E. A., Suggs, M. S., & Graham, B. G. (1995). The effect of pleasant odors and hormone status on mood of women at midlife. *Brain Research Bulletin, 36*(1), 19–29.

Schmidt, R., Fazekas, F., Reinhart, B., Kapeller, P., Fazekas, G., Offenbacher, H., Eber, B., Schumacher, M., & Freidl, W. (1996). Estrogen replacement therapy in older women: A neuropsychological and brain MRI study. *Journal of the American Geriatrics Society, 44*(11), 1307–1313.

Schwartz, J., Freeman, R., & Frishman, W. (1995). Clinical pharmacology of estrogens: Cardiovascular actions and cardioprotective benefits of replacement therapy in postmenopausal women. *Journal of Clinical Pharmacology, 35*, 314–329.

Schwingl, P. J., Hulka, G. S., & Harlow, S. D. (1994). Risk factors for menopausal hot flashes. *Obstetrics and Gynecology, 84*(1), 29–34.

Shaaban, M. (1996). The perimenopause and contraception. *Maturitas, 23*(2), 181–192.

Sherwin, B. B. (1994). Sex hormones and psychological functioning in postmenopausal women. *Experimental Gerontology, 29*(3–4), 423–430.

Shoupe, D., & Mishell, D., Jr. (1994). Contraindications to hormone replacement in treatment of the postmenopausal woman. In R. Lobo (Ed.), *Treatment of the post-menopausal woman: Basic and clinical aspects* (pp. 415–418). New York: Raven Press.

Slemenda, C., Longcope, C., Peacock, M., Sui, S., & Johnston, C. C. (1996). Sex steroids, bone mass, and bone loss. A prospective study of pre-, peri-, and postmenopausal women. *Journal of Clinical Investigation, 97*(1), 14–21.

Sowers, M. R., & La Pietra, M. T. (1995). Menopause: Its epidemiology and potential association with chronic diseases. *Epidemiologic Reviews, 17*(2), 287–302.

Speroff, L. (1996). Postmenopausal hormone therapy and breast cancer. *Obstetrics and Gynecology, 87*(Suppl. 2), 445–545.

Speroff, L. (1997). Postmenopausal hormone therapy and breast cancer. An Internal Medicine Special Report. Sponsored by the Oregon Health Sciences University and produced by *Contemporary OB/GYN*.

Tang, M-X., Jacobs, D., Stern, Y., Marder, K., Schofield, P., Gurland, B., Andrews, H., & Mayeux, R. (1996). Effect of oestrogen during menopause on risk and age at onset of Alzheimer's disease. *Lancet, 348*, 429–432.

Theriault, R. L. (1996). Hormone replacement therapy and breast cancer: An overview. *British Journal of Obstetrics and Gynaecology, 103*(Suppl. 13), 87–91.

Troisi, R. J., Speizer, F. E., Willett, W. C., Trichopoulos, D., & Rosner, B. (1995). Menopause, postmenopausal estrogen preparations, and the risk of adult-onset asthma: A prospective cohort study. *American Journal of Respiratory and Critical Care Medicine, 152,* 1183–1188.

Trossarelli, G., Gennarelli, G., Benedetto, C., deAloysio, D., Mauloni, M., Fanizza, G., & Covelli, A. (1995). Climacteric symptoms and control of the cycle in women aged 35 years and older taking an oral contraceptive with 0 150mg desogestrel and 0.020mg ethinylestradiol. *Contraception. 51,* 13–18.

Van Erpecum, K. J., Van Berge Henegouwen, G. P., Verschoor, L., Stoelwinder, B., & Willekens, F. L. (1991). Different hepatobiliary effects of oral and transdermal estradiol in postmenopausal women. *Gastroenterology, 100*(2), 482–488.

Vedi, S., Croucher, P. I., Garrahan, N. J., & Compston, J. E. (1996). Effects of hormone replacement therapy on cancellous bone microstructure in postmenopausal women. *Bone, 19*(1), 69–72.

von Muhlen, D. G., Kritz-Silverstein, D., & Barrett-Connor, E. (1995). A community-based study of menopause symptoms and estrogen replacement in older women. *Maturitas, 22*(2), 71–78.

Walsh Scura, K., & Whipple, B. (1997). How to provide better care for the postmenopausal woman. *American Journal of Nursing, 97*(4), 36–43.

Watts, N. B., Notelovitz, M., Timmons, M. C., Addison, W. A., Wiita, B., & Downey, L. J. (1995). Comparison of oral estrogens and estrogens plus androgen on bone mineral density, menopausal symptoms, and lipid-lipoprotein profiles in surgical menopause. *Obstetrics and Gynecology, 85*(4), 529–537.

Whitemore, A. S., Harris, R., Itnyre, J., & the Collaborative Ovarian Cancer Group. (1992). Characteristics relating to ovarian cancer risk: Collaborative analysis of twelve U.S. case controlled studies. II. Invasive epithelial ovarian cancers in white women. *American Journal of Epidemiology, 136,* 1184.

Whiting, S. J., Wood, R., & Kim, K. (1997). Calcium supplementation. *Journal of the American Academy of Nurse Practitioners, 9*(4), 187–192.

Wich, B. K., & Carnes, M. (1995). Menopause and the aging female reproductive system. *Endocrinology and Metabolism Clinics of North America, 24*(2), 273–295.

Wiklund, I., Berg, G., Hammar, M., Karlberg, J., Lindgren, R., & Sandin, K. (1992). Long-term effect of transdermal hormonal therapy on aspects of quality of life in postmenopausal women. *Maturitas, 14*(3), 225–236.

Woodruff, J., & Pickar, J. (1994). Incidence of endometrial hyperplasia in post-menopausal women taking conjugated estrogens (Premarin) with medroxyprogesterone acetate or conjugated estrogen alone. *American Journal of Obstetrics and Gynecology, 170,* 1213–1223.

Writing Group for the PEPI Trial. (1995). Effects of estrogen or estrogen/progestin regimes on heart disease risk factors in postmenopausal women. The Postmenopausal Estrogen/Progestin Interventions (PEPI) trial. *JAMA, 273*(3), 199–208.

# IV

## Pharmacotherapy for Common Primary Care Disorders

# 20

# CARDIOVASCULAR DISORDERS

*Judith Bunnell Sellers and Mary L. Brubaker*

Cardiovascular disease represents the greatest health problem in the United States. It is estimated that as many as 50 million Americans have high blood pressure. Although death rates from coronary heart disease and hypertension are decreasing (American Heart Association Monograph, 1995), cardiovascular problems still remain the most common cause of death and disability.

Great strides have been made in the early detection and treatment of cardiovascular disorders. Treatments include lifestyle modifications along with pharmacologic management. Recently prevention and patient education have undergone scrutiny as the practitioner strives to improve overall patient outcome rather than focus on clinical endpoints. However, management plans that include satisfaction, evaluation, and compliance for a patient group with differing motivations, genetics, cultural factors, and unique responses to treatment present a great challenge.

There are few cookbook techniques available to the practitioner that help develop logical treatment plans and evaluation of current regimens. Nor are there guidelines that help deal with the myriad of new medications, each with advantages and disadvantages. During 1997, there were a variety of agents undergoing different phases of testing. There were 22 new treatments in the pipeline for stroke, 18 agents for myocardial infarction, 17 for congestive heart failure, 12 for angina, 10 for hypertension, 9 for peripheral vascular diseases, 7 for hyperlipide-

mia, 5 for arrhythmia and coronary artery disease, and 3 for atherosclerosis.

Despite the obstacles, the practitioner can help patients begin their own education and treatment, and together, they can improve quality of life while reducing the cost to our society.

This chapter will discuss the diagnosis and treatment of hypertension, congestive heart failure, arrhythmias including atrial fibrillation, peripheral vascular conditions, coronary artery disease, ischemic heart disease and angina, mitral valve prolapse, and hyperlipidemia.

## HYPERTENSION

### BLOOD PRESSURE REGULATION

Under normal conditions, blood pressure (BP) is regulated by a complex system of neurohumoral and renal feedback loops. These feedback loops control cardiac output and total peripheral resistance. When the balance between cardiac output (CO) and total peripheral resistance (TPR) is disturbed, changes in blood pressure occur (BP = CO × TPR).

Cardiac output is the heart rate (HR) times the stroke volume (SV). Heart rate and stroke volume have sympathetic and parasympathetic control mechanisms. Stroke volume is also determined by cardiac contractility, preload, and afterload. Peripheral resistance is determined by venous and arterial forces and opposition to

309

the forces. Peripheral resistance is, therefore, the vascular reactivity—vasodilatation and vasoconstriction in response to various neural and humoral impulses. Of importance in the humoral regulation is the renin-angiotensin-aldosterone (RAA) system.

Renin is released by the juxtaglomerular cells of the kidney. Renin changes angiotensinogen from the liver into angiotensin I, an inactive decapeptide. Angiotensin I is converted to angiotensin II by the angiotensin-converting enzyme (ACE). Angiotensin II, a powerful vasoconstrictor, increases peripheral resistance, thereby increasing blood pressure. Angiotensin II also stimulates the secretion of aldosterone from the adrenal cortex, which in turn promotes sodium and water retention in the kidney. Again, under *normal* conditions, this system is activated when arterial blood pressure drops, thereby increasing blood pressure by increasing cardiac output and peripheral resistance.

## ETIOLOGY

The etiology of essential hypertension remains a mystery. Blood pressure normally increases in response to both internal and external forces. Continued elevation of blood pressure results in thickening of the arteries and arterioles from constant vasoconstriction and the high force exerted in the vessels. As the blood pressure continues to be elevated, hypertrophy and hyperplasia in the blood vessels occur and arterioles become permanently narrowed.

Early in the development of hypertension, it is thought that cardiac output increases. Although not proven, the increase in cardiac output may be accompanied by or may stimulate peripheral resistance. The hemodynamic theory postulates that there is an increase in retention of sodium and water that increases cardiac output. As the extracellular fluid volume increases, the regulatory mechanisms compensate by stimulating vasoconstriction. Blood volume remains high, total peripheral resistance continues to increase, and hypertension results (Haak, Richardson, Davey, & Parker-Cohen, 1994; Massie, 1996b).

In the early stages, there is no damage to blood vessels. If the condition is recognized and the cardiac output is decreased, the arterioles return to the normal tone. However, in some susceptible individuals the cardiac output may decrease, but the vascular tone does not return

to normal. In this case, blood pressure remains high and vascular damage starts.

A second theory regarding the mechanisms that promote hypertension lays the blame on a defect in the autoregulatory mechanisms that determine vasoconstriction and vasodilatation. As with the hemodynamic theory, there is an increase in cardiac output. The autoregulatory mechanisms react by causing vasoconstriction. The kidneys respond by increasing the excretion of sodium and water, and the cardiac output and blood volume return to normal; however, the autoregulatory mechanisms do not return the vascular system tone to normal. Rather, it is thought that the autoregulatory system establishes a new blood pressure baseline that is hypertensive and that it works to maintain (Haak et al, 1994; Naftilan & Dzau, 1990).

A third theoretical approach to the etiology of hypertension involves sodium. Sodium and the accompanying water retention seem to be the stimulus for the increased cardiac output that the other theories identify as the beginning of hypertension. There may be two mechanisms causing this phenomenon. First, there may be an inherited defect in the kidney for sodium excretion. An intake of sodium of more than 50 mEq/day places a strain on the kidney and activates the defect.

The second possible mechanism may be an inability of the sodium-potassium pump to work properly. Normally, the sodium-potassium pump moves sodium and potassium across the cell membrane. It is possible that a hormone may inhibit sodium release from the cells. Intracellular sodium increases as does intracellular calcium. Intracellular calcium enhances contractility, particularly of the smooth muscles of the vascular tree. The resulting vasoconstriction and increased peripheral resistance lead to hypertension (Haak et al, 1994). In long-standing hypertension, patients have normal or decreased cardiac output and hypertension is maintained through peripheral resistance (Naftilan & Dzau, 1990).

In light of the above theories, there are four factors that are important for determining the best treatment:

1. At first, *cardiac output increases* possibly because of sodium and water retention caused by either an inherited defect and moderate to high sodium intake or a defect in the sodium-potassium pump.

2. *Peripheral resistance increases* possibly because of a response to increased cardiac output, a re-

sponse to inappropriate autoregulation, or a response to increased calcium in the cells.

3. *Renin and angiotensin activation* causes vasoconstriction, sympathetic activation, and aldosterone secretion, which in turn promotes retention of sodium and loss of potassium.

4. *Peripheral resistance increases* with normal or low CO, which maintains high blood pressure in long-standing hypertension.

Isolated systolic hypertension (ISH) is an important type of hypertension that was once thought insignificant. Elevations in systolic hypertension are due to either increased cardiac output or peripheral resistance, or both. ISH is often associated with aortic valvular insufficiency, arteriovascular (AV) fistulas, thyrotoxicosis, and Paget's disease. The cause is a rigidity of the aorta and is most common among the elderly. As the aorta becomes less responsive, total peripheral vascular resistance increases, and cardiac output increases to maintain systemic circulation. ISH is associated with a high risk for cardiovascular morbidity and mortality and therefore requires treatment (Joint National Committee, 1997; Langer, Criqui, & Barrett-Connor, 1993; Massie, 1996b; Sagie, Larson, & Levy, 1993; Systolic Hypertension in the Elderly Program Cooperative Research Group, 1993).

Pseudohypertension, common among the elderly, is the result of a decrease in arterial compliance and sclerosis of the large arteries. The elderly may demonstrate symptoms of low blood pressure and have no end-organ changes even though BP readings are consistently high. Osler's maneuver is sometimes recommended to rule out pseudohypertension. The Osler maneuver is considered positive when the radial artery is still palpable even though the blood pressure cuff is inflated enough to occlude the artery. In this case, the high blood pressure is the result of a rigid brachial artery. Although this maneuver continues to be recommended, it may not be effective (Hla, Samsa, & Stoneking, 1991; Tsapatsaris, Napolitana, & Rothchild, 1991).

## SPECIFIC CONSIDERATIONS FOR PHARMACOTHERAPY

### When Drug Therapy Is Needed

Early recognition and treatment of hypertension has long been considered important in the prevention of end-organ failure. Consequences of untreated or inadequately treated hypertension include:

- *Cardiovascular complications,* such as left ventricular hypertrophy with heart failure, coronary artery disease, myocardial infarction, and sudden death
- *Peripheral vascular complications,* such as intermittent claudication and gangrene
- *Renal complications,* such as parenchymal damage, nephrosclerosis, renal arteriosclerosis, renal insufficiency, and renal failure
- *Cerebrovascular complications,* such as transient ischemia, cerebrovascular accident (CVA), cerebral thrombosis, aneurysm, and hemorrhage
- *Retinal complications,* such as retinal vascular sclerosis, exudation, and hemorrhage

### Short- and Long-Term Goals of Pharmacotherapy

The primary goal of pharmacotherapy is to return the blood pressure to normal levels using the least expensive, least complex form of therapy. At the same time, therapy should avoid or reverse hyperlipidemia, glucose intolerance, and left ventricular hypertrophy. Maintaining the blood pressure within a normal range will decrease morbidity and mortality and promote quality of life.

### Nonpharmacologic Therapy

Treatment of mild and moderate hypertension has been proven to reduce morbidity and mortality (Massie, 1996b; Naftilan & Dzau, 1990; National High Blood Pressure Working Group, 1993; Sadowski, & Redeker, 1996). Blood pressure must be considered in the context of total risk factors since attempts to reduce blood pressure without working to alter total risk frequently meets with failure. Lifestyle interventions are initiated prior to or in conjunction with pharmacologic therapy and are a lifelong process of change.

Recommended changes that have been shown effective in some individuals include smoking cessation, weight reduction if appropriate, dietary sodium restriction to less than 2.3 g/day, relaxation techniques, decrease or elimination of caffeine, and discontinuance of certain pressure drugs (oral contraceptives, adrenal steroids, sodium-containing antacids, nonsteroidal anti-inflammatory drugs [NSAIDs], and some antidepressants). Other possibly effective nonpharmacologic treatments include potassium, calcium, and magnesium supplements, alcohol restriction, regular aerobic activity, and a vegetarian and/or low-saturated-fat diet (Massie, 1996b; Naftilan & Dzau, 1990; Sadowski & Redeker, 1996).

Lifestyle change is always approached gradually with all age groups, particularly the elderly. Research in elders 60–85 years of age has found a combined program of decreased sodium intake, loss of weight (as appropriate), and increased physical activity to significantly decrease blood pressure by the end of a 6-month period (JNC VI, 1997). An exercise program starting slowly and increasing to 30 min three to five times a week will result in less muscle strain and use of NSAIDs. The exercise program will help a reasonable weight reduction program. An increase in fiber and fruit will help decrease calories and increase potassium and calcium. The increase in fiber also will help decrease constipation. The effectiveness of any program for the elderly will not be demonstrated for 3–6 months (JNC VI, 1997; National High Blood Pressure Education Program, 1993; Applegate, Miller, & Elam, 1992; Sagie et al, 1993).

## Time Frame for Initiating Pharmacotherapy

If lifestyle modifications have not lowered blood pressure to the desired range, the practitioner must decide whether to begin pharmacologic interventions. The Joint National Committee (JNC VI) guidelines direct the practitioner to individualize the patient's drug therapy, giving consideration to the severity of blood pressure elevation, target organ damage, and the presence of other conditions and risk factors. The practitioner should also include in the decision-making process such factors as the cost of medication, metabolic and subjective side effects, and drug-drug interactions.

Although controversy still exists, treatment of ISH decreases the risk of a stroke by three times. Treatment should be initiated at systolic blood pressures of 160 or greater even though the diastolic pressure is less than 90 (Systolic Hypertension in the Elderly Program [SHEP] Cooperative Research Group, 1991).

The JNC VI report makes recommendations on a therapeutic approach based on diastolic blood pressure (JNC VI, 1997) (See Table 20–1).

## Overview of Drug Classes for Treatment

The treatment of hypertension includes drugs from a variety of classes which can be used as monotherapy or in combination. See Drug Table 205.

## Assessment Needed Prior to Therapy

The goals of the assessment are to determine if the person really has hypertension, to search for secondary (treatable) causes, to assess end-organ damage, to identify risk factors, and to assess comorbidity. When diagnosing the severity of hypertension, risk factors and end-organ disease must be taken into consideration so that the most appropriate therapeutic measures are taken.

## TABLE 20–1. THERAPEUTIC APPROACH USING BLOOD PRESSURE, RISK FACTORS, AND TARGET ORGAN DISEASE/CARDIOVASCULAR DISEASE

| Average blood pressure mmHg | No risk factors, no target organ damage, no clinical cardiovascular disease | One risk factor, not including DM, no target organ damage, no clinical cardiovascular disease | Target organ damage, clinical cardiovascular disease and/or DM with or without other risk factors |
|---|---|---|---|
| 130–139/85–89 | Lifestyle modification | Lifestyle modification | Drug therapy for those with heart failure, renal insufficiency, or diabetes |
| 140–159/90–99 Stage I | Lifestyle modification up to 12 mo | Lifestyle modification up to 6 mo | Drug therapy |
| ≥160/≥100 Stage 2 and 3 | Drug therapy | Drug therapy | Drug therapy |

Adapted from JNC VI (1997).

**Determination of hypertension.** The established criteria for hypertension come from the JNC. Hypertension is not diagnosed on the basis of a single blood pressure reading. It is generally defined as sustained elevation of systolic and/or diastolic blood pressure. In general, a high blood pressure reading at three different visits constitutes hypertension. The immediacy of confirmation of the elevated blood pressure and treatment are dependent on the blood pressure level. Table 20–2 indicates levels and stages of hypertension (JNC VI, 1997).

**Clinical assessment.** The history-taking part of the examination should include the following:

- Age, sex, race, and family history.
- Hypertensive history including severity, duration, symptoms, precipitating events, comorbid factors, and prior treatment and response to treatment.
- Symptoms of transient ischemic attack (TIA), CVA, coronary artery disease (CAD), angina, premature ventricular contraction (PVC), and congestive heart failure (CHF).
- Symptoms of periodic headaches, palpitations, perspiration (pheochromocytoma), muscular weakness, cramps, polyuria (primary aldosteronism), intermittent claudication, and headaches (coarctation of the aorta, PVC).
- Risk/lifestyle factors including family history, smoking, alcohol use, stress, obesity, diabetes, lack of exercise, and high sodium intake.
- Medications including oral contraceptives, steroids, thyroid hormone, cocaine, licorice, and OTC medications such as cold medications, diet pills, and nasal sprays. NSAIDs are linked to the development of hypertension as well as having an adverse effect on the action of antihypertensive medications (JNC VI, 1997; Tsapatsaris et al, 1991).

### TABLE 20–2. DIASTOLIC AND SYSTOLIC LEVELS AND STAGES OF HYPERTENSION

| Category of Severity | Blood Pressure (mmHg) | |
| --- | --- | --- |
| | *Systolic* | *Diastolic* |
| Optimal | <120 | <80 |
| Normal | <130 | <85 |
| High Normal | 130–139 | 85–89 |
| Hypertension | | |
| Stage 1 | 140–159 | 90–99 |
| Stage 2 | 160–179 | 100–109 |
| Stage 3 | ≥180 | ≥110 |

The physical examination should include the following:

- Vital signs and weight. Check BP in both arms, and check postural hypotension.
- Funduscopic evaluation of arteriosclerotic and hypertensive changes (AV nicking, arteriolar narrowing, exudates, papilledema).
- Neck: distended veins, bruits, or thyroid enlargement.
- Cardiac and chest: evidence of hypertrophy and heart failure, valvular disease, murmurs, or gallops.
- Abdominal: masses and bruits, especially over renal arteries.
- Peripheral arteries: palpate and auscultate for bruits.
- Neurologic evaluation.
- Evidence of gout, thyroid disorder, or Cushing's syndrome.

Laboratory studies help determine risk factors, end-organ failure and secondary etiology and should include:

- CBC
- Urinalysis
- Serum sodium, potassium, calcium, uric acid, and glucose to screen for secondary hypertension from hyperparathyroidism, hyperaldosteronism, renal insufficiency, diabetes, gout, or nephrosclerosis
- Lipids
- Serum creatinine and creatinine clearance
- Electrocardiogram, chest x-ray, and echo cardiogram

The following are additional clues that may identify the physiologic mechanism involved in hypertension and therefore the most appropriate treatment regimen.

1. Edema, weight gain, chronic renal failure = *increased extracellular volume.*
2. Decreased weight, orthostatic hypotension, diuretic effect creating an increase in BUN = *decreased extracellular volume.*
3. Narrow pulse pressure, high diastolic pressure, cold extremities = *increased vascular resistance.*
4. Wide pulse pressure, orthostatic hypotension, warm extremities = *decreased vascular resistance.*
5. Tachycardia, wide pulse pressure = *increased cardiac output.*
6. Increased BUN, $S_3$ gallop = *decreased cardiac output.*

**The elderly and hypertension.** The pathophysiology of hypertension in the elderly is different from that found in younger individuals. The elderly generally have:

- Lower plasma volumes
- Decreased aortic compliance
- Decreased plasma-renin activity
- Decreased aldosterone levels
- Reduced baroreceptor sensitivity
- Decreased renal clearance
- Higher likelihood of salt sensitivity

Cardiac function in the older person changes. Maintaining cardiac output becomes a function of increased left ventricular volume and increased stroke volume. However, the older person with hypertension actually has a decreased cardiac output. The predominant vascular abnormality is the reduced arterial distensibility due to rigidity of the vessels (Sadowski & Redeker, 1996).

## Patient/Caregiver Information

Although most lifestyle changes promote health and well-being, the outcome for treatment of hypertension remains equivocal. Pharmacologic therapy has proved effective in reducing morbidity and mortality in large populations. Patient compliance in the treatment of hypertension represents a major key to success.

Patients should be educated on the reduced effect of their antihypertensive therapy caused by various over-the-counter preparations such as NSAIDs and ibuprofen and diet aids that contain phenylpropanolamine or ephedra (herbal fen-phen). Some patients will experience an increase in blood pressure with oral nasal decongestants such as pseudoephedrine.

## OUTCOMES MANAGEMENT

### Selecting an Appropriate Agent

The JNC VI (1997) guidelines direct the practitioner to individualize each patient's drug therapy, giving consideration to the severity of blood pressure elevation, target organ damage, and the presence of other conditions and risk factors. In addition to these, consideration must be given to cost, the ease in following the treatment regimen, the potential for drug-drug interactions, and the profile of side effects including sexual, psychological, and cognitive functions.

Initiation of pharmacotherapy has been guided by the step-care approach, and yet individualization and consideration of coexisting conditions may enhance clinical as well as patient compliance and desired outcomes. The variety of agents permits tailoring of the therapy to the individuals and the physiologic mechanism of their hypertension. Whatever therapy is chosen, the blood pressure should be decreased slowly over 2–6 months (McVeigh et al, 1995).

The JNC VI treatment algorithm recommends diuretics and beta blockers as the preferred agents for uncomplicated hypertension since they lower morbidity and mortality. ACE inhibitors, calcium channel blockers, alpha receptor blockers, alpha and beta blockers, and angiotensin II antagonists are also acceptable as monotherapy. About 50–60% of patients with mild hypertension will respond to any agent used as monotherapy. The guidelines continue with recommendations if the response from the initial agent is inadequate. The practitioner either can increase the drug dose, substitute another agent, or add a second agent from a different drug class. If with moderate doses of monotherapy, the BP is higher than desired, the practitioner may wish to try another agent particularly if the patient is experiencing adverse effects. If the moderate doses of monotherapy have lowered the BP but not yet to the desired level, a patient with Stage 1 HTN may need to try another agent, whereas a patient with Stage 2 would benefit from the addition of a second agent from a different class. If a second drug, primarily a diuretic, is added to any other antihypertensive agent, then about 80% of patients will respond (McVeigh, Flack, & Grimm, 1995). If the response is again inadequate, continue to add agents from another drug class or refer to a hypertension specialist.

It is important also to consider contraindications or coexisting conditions when deciding upon an agent of choice. A goal could be to treat these patients with hypertension and a coexisting condition with monotherapy.

The JNC VI report gives information on drug therapy that might be considered when there are compelling indications or there may be a favorable effect on a comorbid condition. Below is a list of drug therapy for these situations. (JNC VI, 1997).

- Compelling Indications
  - Diabetes mellitus (type 1) with proteinuria: ACE I
  - Heart failure: ACE I, diuretics

- ISH (older patients): diuretics (preferred), calcium antagonists (long-acting dihydropyridine)
- MI: beta blockers (non-intrinsic sympathomimetic activity), ACE I (with systolic dysfunction)

- Favorable Effects on Comorbid Conditions
  - Angina pectoris: beta blockers, calcium channel blockers
  - Atrial tachycardia and fibrillation: beta blockers, calcium antagonists (non-dihydropyridines)
  - Cyclosporine-induced hypertension (caution with the dose of cyclosporine): calcium antagonists
  - Diabetes mellitus (type 1 and 2) with proteinuria: ACE I (preferred), calcium antagonists
  - Diabetes mellitus (type 2): low dose diuretics
  - Dyslipidemia: alpha blockers
  - Essential tremor: beta blockers (non-cardioselective)
  - Heart failure: carvedilol, losartan potassium
  - Hyperthyroidism: beta blockers
  - Migraine: beta-blockers (non-cardioselective), calcium antagonists (non-dihydropyridine)
  - Myocardial infarction: diltiazem, verapamil
  - Osteoporosis: thiazides
  - Preoperative hypertension: beta blockers
  - Prostatism (BPH): alpha blockers
  - Renal insufficiency (caution in renovascular hypertension and creatinine level ≥ 3 mg/dL): ACE I

- Situations in which drug therapy may have an unfavorable effect on comorbid conditions
  - Bronchospastic disease: beta blockers
  - Depression: beta blockers, central alpha antagonists, reserpine
  - Diabetes mellitus (type 1 and 2): beta blockers, high dose diuretics
  - Dyslipidemia: beta blockers (non-intrinsic sympathomimetic activity), diuretics (high dose)
  - Gout: diuretics
  - Second or third degree heart block: beta blockers, calcium antagonists (non-dihydropyridine)
  - Heart failure: beta blockers (except carvedilol), calcium antagonists (except amlodipine, felodipine)
  - Liver disease: labetalol, methyldopa
  - Peripheral vascular disease: beta blockers
  - Pregnancy: ACE I, angiotensin II receptor blockers
  - Renal insufficiency: potassium sparing agents
  - Renovascular disease: ACE I, angiotensin II receptor blockers

Additional information that may be helpful is the work of Materson et al (1993), Materson & Reda (1994), and Carter et al (1994). These researchers evaluated the effectiveness of monotherapy in controlling blood pressure in young and elderly Caucasians and African-Americans. A high percentage of young Caucasians will respond to beta blockers, ACE inhibitors, calcium channel blockers, prazosin, and clonidine. Diuretics were least effective. In elderly Caucasians, all of the above including diuretics are effective. Young African-Americans responded to calcium channel blockers, whereas elderly African-Americans showed responsiveness to diuretics, calcium channel blockers, and clonidine. Materson (Tobian et al, 1994) personalized this data into an algorithm to help him choose beginning and subsequent antihypertensive therapy. It is presented below.

In mild to moderate hypertension:

- Young African-American: calcium channel blocker
- Young Caucasian: ACE inhibitor or beta blocker
- Older African-American: calcium channel blocker, or diuretic
- Older Caucasian: calcium channel blocker, or diuretic; ACE inhibitor, or beta blocker

If the initial response with the lowest possible dose is inadequate, then either increase the dose, change to an alternative drug, add a thiazide diuretic, or add a second drug at a low dose.

If adding a second drug, consider the following combinations:

- Thiazide diuretics with any of the nondiuretic drugs
- ACE inhibitor plus a calcium channel blocker
- Alpha blocker plus a beta blocker
- ACE inhibitor plus an alpha blocker (monitor for hypotension)

In severe hypertension begin with diltiazem and a dihydropyridine calcium channel blocker (edema is an adverse effect).

In resistant hypertension determine if the patient is taking and absorbing the drug(s). Add an adequate dose of a diuretic or add a loop diuretic, especially if there is renal failure.

Recent studies have demonstrated the benefit of treating isolated systolic hypertension. The final results from the Systolic Hypertension in the Elderly Program (SHEP) published in 1991 concluded that low-dose chlorthalidone as a first-step medication could reduce the incidence of total stroke by 36% along with a 32% decrease in major cardiovascular events. Atenolol at 25 mg/day or reserpine at 0.05 mg/day are used if the systolic blood pressure was not reached with first-step drug therapy. The results of this study assisted the members of the JNC V to make their recommendations for thiazide diuretics and beta blockers as first choice in the treatment of hypertension (Tobian et al, 1994). Kostis, Davis, and Cutler (1997) performed an analysis on the data from the SHEP study to determine if heart failure, which is often preceded by ISH, was reduced by a diuretic-based antihypertensive stepped-care treatment. They concluded that a low-dose chlorthalidone regimen produced an 80% risk reduction in patients with a prior myocardial infarction and exerted a strong protective effect in preventing heart failure.

Other large studies such as the Multiple Risk Factor Intervention Trial and the European Working Party on Hypertension in the Elderly Trial evaluated the incidence of morbidity and mortality in patients with either or both elevations of systolic and diastolic blood pressure (Lapalio, 1995). The Swedish Trial in Old Patients with Hypertension (STOP-Hypertension) evaluated the benefits of treating hypertension in older patients (70–84 years). Patients included in the study had systolic blood pressure of 180–230 mm Hg with a diastolic pressure of at least 90 mm Hg, or a diastolic pressure of 105–120 mm Hg irrespective of systolic pressure. The authors concluded that treatment of hypertension in patients, both men and women, in this age range resulted in reduction in cardiovascular morbidity and mortality (Dahlof et al, 1991). The drug therapy used in this study included atenolol 50 mg and hydrochlorothiazide 25 mg plus amiloride 2.5 mg, metoprolol 100 mg, or pindolol 5 mg. All the medications were given once a day.

These studies focused on the use of diuretics and/or beta blockers in the treatment of hypertension. As such, they were the only pharmacotherapy that could be shown to reduce morbidity and mortality. The Systolic Hypertension in Europe (SYST-EUR) trial group presented their findings on the results of starting with the dihydropyridine calcium antagonist nitrendipine in a stepwise antihypertensive regimen. Enalaril and/or hydrochlorothiazide were added if the sitting systolic blood pressure remained above 150 mm Hg. The group reported 42% fewer strokes and 26% fewer cardiac endpoints

(CHF, MI) when compared with placebo recipients.

It is important to remember that elderly patients are more susceptible to developing orthostatic hypotension resulting from antihypertensive treatment. There also is some degree of autonomic dysfunction in the elderly, so treatment should not be aggressive. Initiating pharmacotherapy with half the usual recommended dose and increasing slowly should help prevent incidences of cerebral or cardiac hypoperfusion.

The results of the Antihypertensive and Lipid Lowering Heart Attack Prevention Trial (ALL-HAT) are expected in the year 2002. This prospective study of 40,000 patients over 55 years of age is comparing various classes of antihypertensive and should provide additional insight to choosing antihypertensive therapy (Gavras, Manolis, & Gavras, 1997).

## Monitoring for Efficacy and Toxicity

*Diuretics.* Diuretics are considered first-line therapy for the treatment of hypertension in patients without cautionary/contradictory comorbid conditions. When not used as monotherapy, diuretics are often used to augment the initial therapy of calcium channel blockers, ACE inhibitors, or beta blockers. The pharmacodynamics of thiazide diuretics are inhibition of sodium and water reabsorption and arterial vasodilation. The initial drop in blood pressure is from a decreased cardiac output that is later followed by a reduction in peripheral resistance (Tackett, 1995).

The thiazide diuretic hydrochlorothiazide (HCTZ) is the most widely prescribed. In the past, HCTZ was often used as monotherapy and at much larger doses per day. Patients experienced such adverse events as hyperglycemia and hyperlipidemia. A lowering of the dose to 12.5–25 mg/day reduces the likelihood of these adverse events while decreasing the systolic blood pressure in the range of 15–20 mm Hg and diastolic blood pressure 8–15 mm Hg (Materson & Reda, 1994; Neaton et al, 1993). The more potent loop diuretics (furosemide, butamide) have the disadvantage of requiring more frequent dosing but are advantageous in patients with creatinine clearances of <30 mL/min. The loop diuretic torsemide has the unique pharmacokinetic property of a longer half-life and can be prescribed once a day (Gavras et al, 1997). The potassium-sparing diuretics should be used in patients who develop hypokalemia while on low-dose thiazide treatment and are unable to take potassium supplements or express a desire to avoid multiple drug regimens.

**Beta blockers.** There are data to support beta blockers' ability to reduce morbidity and mortality, making them first-line therapy according to the JNC VI guidelines (JNC, 1997; Sever et al, 1993). Beta blockers have been shown to be an effective single-drug therapy in young and middle-aged patients, as well as in patients with coronary artery disease. Beta blockers decrease the rate, myocardial contractility, and conduction velocity of the heart, resulting in a decreased cardiac output. In addition, inhibition of renin release and a reduction of sympathetic nervous system activity centrally contribute to the antihypertensive effect. Beta blockers can produce a significant reduction in left ventricular hypertrophy that is not possible with the use of diuretics (Tackett, 1995).

The agents do vary in their cardioselectivity (atenolol, betaxolol, bisoprolol, metoprolol), intrinsic sympathomimetic activity ([ISA]-acebutolol, cartelol, penbutolol, pindolol), penetration of the blood brain barrier (lipid solubility—propranolol, timolol, metoprolol), and additional alpha blockade (labetalol).

The nonselective beta blockers without ISA are associated with the adverse events of hyperglycemia and hyperlipidemia. However, these changes may be temporary and the exact clinical significance is minimal. The patient should be monitored for the occurrence. Other adverse events to consider when prescribing beta blockers include a tendency to cause peripheral vasoconstriction, have a negative inotropic and chronotropic action on the heart, bronchoconstriction, and accentuation of insulin resistance. Beta blockers may be counterproductive in patients who must lose weight or increase exercise. A paradoxical increase in BP in volume-dependent patients may occur. On the other hand, beta blockers are well suited in treating hypertension in patients who also have angina, arrhythmias, or migraines. Beta blockers without ISA are indicated in patients following myocardial infarction since they have been shown to prevent the recurrence of infarction and sudden death.

Like most antihypertensive therapy, doses of beta blockers are started at the low end of the range and increased or augmented with another agent such as a diuretic to achieve outcome.

Longer dosing intervals can successfully treat hypertension (HTN) and should assist in patient compliance.

**Alpha blockers.** The alpha$_1$ blockers (prazosin, doxazosin, terazosin) can lower blood pressure along with reducing cholesterol, improving glucose tolerance, and increasing insulin sensitivity. These agents will not induce reflex increases in cardiac output and renin release. They have proven useful in the coexisting conditions of peripheral vascular disease, benign prostatic hypertrophy, CHF, asthma, and impotence. Although these are very beneficial aspects, the adverse events of hypotension and tachyphylaxis limit the usefulness of these agents.

It is important to advise patients about first-dose or reinstituted-dose orthostatic hypotension and reflex tachycardia. Educate patients to take the first dose, or one that is missed after one or two doses, at bedtime or at a time when they can recline for a few hours.

**Alpha$_2$ agonists.** The two currently prescribed agents are clonidine and reserpine. Clonidine may be effective in patients with severe HTN or renin-dependent disease. Although clonidine lowers BP without reflex tachycardia or metabolic changes in the patient, it does cause CNS sedation, partial tachyphylaxis, and interference with sexual function. Rebound hypertension may occur in some individuals with the discontinuation of clonidine. Concomitant administration with a beta blocker or in the presence of peripheral neuropathy may enhance the alpha activity, leading to a paradoxical increase in BP.

The SHEP study (1993) evaluated the use of reserpine in the treatment of ISH. Reserpine in doses limited to 0.25 mg per day was found to be cost-effective and have minimal adverse events and a long duration of action. Depression was avoided at the lower dosage range. The long duration of action requires at least 3 weeks of treatment before assessing the effect.

**ACE inhibitors.** The cardioprotective and renoprotective effects of ACE inhibitors make these agents useful in patients with reduced left ventricular function (CHF) and proteinuria (Lebovitz et al, 1994). ACE inhibition causes suppression of the vasoconstrictor angiotensin II and potentiation of the vasodilator bradykinin. The suppression of angiotensin II results in suppression of aldosterone secretion. Together there is decreased vasoconstriction, sodium and water retention, along with vasodilation via bradykinin. Bradykinin also enhances insulin sensitivity. ACE inhibitors appear consistently and effectively to decrease left ventricular mass in hypertensive patients.

An estimation of the renin state of a patient should be attempted to avoid profound hypotension with the initiation of the ACE inhibitor. High-renin states occur in patients with dehydration, reduced salt intake, renovascular hypertension, CHF, liver disease, or diuretic-therapy-induced volume contraction. To reduce the chance of hypotension, begin at lower doses (one half normal or at the bottom of dosage range) and titrate slowly to the desired outcome. The ACE inhibitors have a slow onset and a long duration of action, allowing for once-a-day dosing. Assessment of activity should be 3–4 weeks after initiating therapy.

Patients may mistake allergy-like symptoms of cough for chronic allergies or sinusitis. There is no way to predict the occurrence of renal insufficiency caused by ACE inhibitors in patients. The patient's serum creatinine should be followed for several weeks to monitor for onset.

Because of the blockade of aldosterone, the patient is susceptible to hyperkalemia. The practitioner will need to routinely monitor for this possibility with initiation of therapy and dosage adjustments. The patient should be educated on the avoidance of potassium-containing supplements or salt substitutes.

Suspect noncompliance, NSAID use, or excessive salt intake whenever there is an increase in the patient's blood pressure. The teratogenic effects of ACE inhibitors precludes the use of these agents during pregnancy.

**Calcium channel blockers.** Calcium channel blockers are numerous but may be divided into two groups: L-type and T-type. The L-type divides into two subgroups. The first subgroup contains verapamil and diltiazem. The second group contains nifedipine and the other dihydropyridines. Overall, the L-type channels are found in the plasma membrane, sinoatrial node, and atrioventricular node. By blocking the voltage-dependent L-type channels, these calcium channel blockers contribute to pacemaker activity, regulate AV conduction, vasodilate coronary and peripheral arteries, and, in some cases, have a negative inotropic effect on the heart. The second subgroup (nifedipine and other dihydropyridines) has a greater vasodilatory effect,

whereas diltiazem and verapamil (first subgroup) affect the heart rate and contractility to a greater degree.

Concerns for using nifedipine include cardiac ischemia, proteinuria, glucose intolerance, and the development of peripheral edema. Psaty et al (1995) suggested that patients with no pre-existing cardiac disease appear to be at higher risk for coronary events when using short-acting calcium channel blockers. Additional studies with other short-acting dihydropyridines also suggest the possibility of harm (Psaty et al, 1997). It is important to remember that the short-acting dihydropyridines do not carry an indication for the treatment of chronic hypertension. Verapamil and diltiazem benefit patients with LV dysfunction, reduce diabetic proteinuria, and have an additive effect with diuretics. The L-type calcium channel blockers are effective in elderly, African-American, and salt-sensitive patients. The efficacy of the medication does not depend on salt restriction.

The T-type calcium channel blockers belong to the tetralol class. Currently the only available agent is mibefradil dihydrochloride. Although this agent binds to receptor sites on L-type channels, it triggers the closure of T-type channels as well. What we know about the T-type channels is that they are not essential for cardiac excitation, but play a role in activating smooth muscle contraction. They respond to lower levels of voltage stimulation and are transient in nature. The T-type channels are present in sinus node, vascular smooth muscle, and neuroendocrine cells. Finally, the T-type channels do not appear in great numbers in the normal myocardial cells, which suggests that blockade is not likely to have a negative impact on cardiac contraction. Thus, the proposed value of the T-type calcium channel blocker is a beneficial reduction in heart rate with little or no negative inotropic effect. Mibefradil is about 250 times more potent at increasing coronary blood flow than decreasing myocardial contractility. It is also more potent at inducing coronary vasodilation than at suppressing AV conduction or sinus rate. As of this writing (June 1998) mibefradil has been taken off the market because of bad drug interactions.

**Vasodilators.** The direct-acting vasodilators hydralazine and minoxidil are considered second- or even third-line agents because of the side effects of reflex tachycardia and water and sodium retention. Consequently, a diuretic, beta blocker, or alpha agonist should be prescribed concurrently. In turn, vasodilators may improve the efficacy of beta-blocker and diuretic therapy.

Minoxidil is also considered a potassium channel opener (Barber et al, 1994). Through this mechanism, minoxidil acts as an indirect calcium channel antagonist. When the potassium channels are opened, the influx of calcium is inhibited.

***Angiotensin II inhibitors.*** The newest additions to the antihypertensive lineup are the angiotensin II inhibitors (losartan, valsartan). These agents block the effects of angiotensin II, with no effect on the metabolic pathway of bradykinin. Without angiotensin II there is limited vasoconstriction and secretion of aldosterone. With no disruption of the normal inactivation of bradykinin, there is less incidence of cough and allergic reactions.

There are two types of angiotensin II receptors: $AT_1$ and $AT_2$. At this time only the functions of the $AT_1$ type are known and manipulated pharmacologically. The $AT_1$ receptors are found on vascular endothelium and are responsible for vasoconstriction, stimulation of thirst, and sodium reabsorption. These receptors are involved in vascular and myocardial restructuring and remodeling. The $AT_2$ receptors are found in the adrenal medulla and the uterus and in fetal tissues (Weir, 1996).

In summary, there are several approaches to the treatment of hypertension and a plethora of agents. The future will bring the JNC VI, more large studies, and even more new agents along with commercial combination products. Look for combinations of ACE inhibitors and calcium channel blockers to join the combinations of ACE inhibitors and diuretics, and beta blockers and diuretics to simplify treatment regimens in pursuit of patient compliance.

## Follow-up Recommendations

The goal of therapy is to maintain the blood pressure within normal limits and prevent end-organ failure. If the treatment is appropriate treatment and blood pressure becomes stable, management becomes relatively routine. The provider should consider consultation with a physician for any patient with a stage III or IV hypertension.

A follow-up physical examination will include funduscopic examination, symptoms of dizziness or syncope, heart size, heart sounds, symptoms of shortness of breath, palpitations, chest pain, lung sounds, peripheral pulses, bruits, temperature, and sensation. Diagnostic studies should include creatinine, lipids, blood sugar, electrolytes, and an EKG. Other diagnostic procedures should be conducted as indicated by the history and physical.

The JNC VI summarizes the recommended follow-up time frame based on the classification (Table 20–3).

With unstable blood pressure:

1. Refer to a physician and then follow frequently. This may be three times a week or more depending on the severity of the BP readings and the need for ongoing education and monitoring of effects of medications. Unstable blood pressure is best followed in consultation with a cardiologist or physician.

2. During follow-up visits, try to ascertain the degree of compliance with nonpharmacologic and pharmacologic treatments. Lack of compliance continues to be a major problem in management of hypertension.

3. Assess the number and degree of side effects of medications.

4. Continue to assess other medications, especially over-the-counter medications the patient may be taking.

5. Continue patient education.

With stable blood pressure:

1. Recheck every 3–6 months. The frequency depends on needs of the patient for education, ongoing monitoring, and compliance. Telephone follow-up or more frequent visits may improve compliance with treatment plan.

2. Always assess signs and symptoms of adverse reactions to medication(s), compliance with the treatment plan, and effectiveness of therapy.

3. Conduct an annual physical examination with focus on risk factors and end-organ involvement.

4. Consult a physician when there are signs and symptoms of additional cardiovascular problems or a change in response to the medication.

## HEART FAILURE

Heart failure, a complication of heart disease, is a common diagnosis in the inpatient setting, particularly for people 65 and older. Heart failure is

## TABLE 20–3.  RECOMMENDED FOLLOW-UP TIME FRAME FOR HYPERTENSION

| Blood Pressure (mm Hg) | | |
| Systolic | Diastolic | Recommended Follow-up |
| --- | --- | --- |
| <130 | 85 | Recheck in 2 yrs |
| 130–139 | 85–89 | Recheck in 1 year |
| 140–159 | 90–99 | Confirm within 2 mo |
| 160–179 | 100–109 | Evaluate→care within 1 mo |
| ≥180 | ≥110 | Immediate care or within 1 week depending on clinical situation |

*Adapted from JNC VI (1997).*

associated with limitation of activity and decrease in quality of life. Limitation of activity varies from minimal limitation to inability to carry out any physical activity. One-year survival after the diagnosis varies from 57% for men and 64% for women. However, the 5-year survival drops to 25% for men and 38% for women. The more severe the disease, the lower the 1- and 5-year survival rates. The death rate for heart failure in 1990 was almost 38,000. Also, the people with a diagnosis of heart failure have a higher likelihood of succumbing to a sudden cardiac death than the overall population (Konstam et al, 1994).

## DEFINITION

Heart failure occurs when the myocardium is unable to pump enough blood to meet the metabolic demands of the body. Heart failure is a problem of volume overload and poor tissue perfusion. The result is a constellation of symptoms that limit functional abilities. Heart failure can be either a systolic or diastolic dysfunction.

## PATHOPHYSIOLOGY

The problem inherent in heart failure is the ineffective functioning of the myocardium due to systolic and/or diastolic dysfunction. The myocardium loses muscle mass often because of ischemia. Decreased muscle mass leads to dilated cardiomyopathy, resulting in a decrease in cardiac output and therefore ineffective tissue perfusion. The result of myocardial changes is an alteration in myocardial contractility, preload, afterload, and heart rate. Decreased contractility and increased preload and afterload increase pressure in the associated cardiac chamber. As the pressure increases, the myocardial fibers lengthen. Ventricular dilatation and elevation of diastolic pressure results. Hemodynamically, when the heart is unable to meet the demands of the body and is considered in failure, two factors account for the clinical presentation: decreased cardiac output and elevation of ventricular diastolic pressures.

In an attempt to compensate for the loss of myocardial effectiveness, the body sets into motion a complex system of neurohormonal mechanisms. These reflexes attempt to restore blood pressure through increasing peripheral resistance, altering the left ventricular function, and increasing sodium and water retention. The heart rate is increased with sympathetic stimulation. This may lead to arrhythmias and additional ischemia. Although compensatory and protective mechanisms take place, in someone with heart failure they act to increase cardiac afterload, which in turn continues to decrease cardiac performance and increase volume overload (Fig. 20–1).

In the early stages of heart failure, the compensatory mechanisms may be successful in

- increased capillary pressure – – ➤ pulmonary or systemic edema
- decreased cardiac output – – ➤ neurohormonal responses: decreased renal blood flow – – ➤ activation of renin-angiotensin-aldosterone system – – ➤ sodium and water retention – – ➤ increased peripheral resistance and left ventricular afterload, and increased preload
- increased sympathetic activity – – ➤ stimulation of myocardial contractility, heart rate, venous tone – – ➤ increase in preload, tachycardia, ischemic attacks, increased pulmonary edema
- increased peripheral resistance – – ➤ reduction in renal blood flow, left ventricular afterload
- increased arginine vasopressin – – ➤ vasoconstriction, inhibits water excretion

**Figure 20–1.** The compensatory mechanisms in heart failure (from Haak et al, 1994; Kloner & Dzau, 1990; Kradjan, 1993; Massie, 1996a).

maintaining the needs of the body. As failure of the myocardium progresses, however, the physiologic needs of the body are not met and the clinical symptoms become apparent.

## TYPES OF HEART FAILURE

Heart failure is frequently classified by the predominant mechanism of failure. With the new pharmacotherapy for heart failure, the most important and accurate classification is diastolic and systolic dysfunction. Heart failure is also classified as failure of the right side or left side and low output or high output. However, most patients with heart failure have a combined left ventricular systolic dysfunction and diastolic dysfunction, and management is determined by the patient's functional level.

### Systolic Dysfunction

The most common form of heart failure is left ventricular systolic dysfunction. The mechnisms of systolic dysfunction are decreased cardiac output → decreased ejection fraction → increased left ventricular end-diastolic pressure → increased ventricular preload → decreased contractile force → decreased blood pressure → compensatory responses.

The etiology is coronary artery disease, myocardial infarction, chronic hypertension, and valvular abnormalities.

Symptoms include dyspnea on exertion, fatigue, weakness, orthopnea, peripheral edema, and chronic cough. The patient also may complain of restlessness, insomnia, nocturia, anorexia, memory loss, and confusion (Dracup, 1996; Haak et al, 1994; Kloner & Dzau, 1990; Kradjan, 1993; Massie, 1996a).

### Diastolic Dysfunction

The mechanisms of diastolic dysfunction are reduced ventricular compliance (ventricles rigid and unable to relax enough to accept all blood) → increased ventricular diastolic pressure → increased atrial pressures → increased pressure in pulmonary and systemic venous systems. Normal ventricular function and ejection fraction are indicative of diastolic dysfunction.

The etiology is left ventricular hypertrophy due to hypertension, hypertrophic or restrictive cardiomyopathy, diabetes, and pericardial disease.

Many of the same symptoms of left ventricular systolic dysfunction apply, particularly dyspnea and peripheral edema (Dracup, 1996; Haak et al, 1994; Kloner & Dzau, 1990; Kradjan, 1993).

Possible symptoms of right heart failure include peripheral edema, ascites, weakness, mental confusion, hepatic congestion, right upper quadrant abdominal pain, anorexia, constipation, bloating, nausea, vomiting, splenomegaly, jugular venous distension (JVD), and hepatojugular reflux (HJR).

Possible symptoms of left heart failure include dyspnea, orthopnea, paroxysmal nocturnal dyspnea, inability to exercise, weakness, fatigue, nocturia, mental confusion, cough, hemoptysis, basilar crackles, pleural effusions, pulmonary edema, $S_3$ heart sound.

## SPECIFIC CONSIDERATIONS FOR PHARMACOTHERAPY

### When Drug Therapy Is Needed

Heart disease is a progressive chronic condition that may severely limit functional abilities. Prevention is a major factor. Management of hypertension and other cardiovascular diseases as well as diabetes may decrease the incidence of heart failure. Evaluation for a drug-induced cause is important. Once it is determined that there is no other etiology for the presentation of congestive heart failure, the practitioner will need to initiate pharmacotherapy. The choice of agents and the aggressiveness of treatment will be based on the patient's signs and symptoms. Untreated CHF can progress to further disability, more hospitalizations, and decreased quality of life.

### Short- and Long-Term Goals of Pharmacotherapy

The goals of therapy are to control the symptoms of CHF so that the patient may continue with as many activities of daily living as possible, and to reduce mortality. Short-term therapy is directed at decreasing fluid congestion in the periphery and lungs while assisting the heart's contractility. By breaking the vicious cycle of CHF, long-term pharmacotherapy can be directed towards maintaining cardiac function while slowing the progression of the disease.

Quality-of-life considerations may vary depending on the severity of the disease. If the patient has mild symptoms, then survival is primary followed by exercise capacity and then symptom management. With moderate symptoms, the patient may desire more exercise capacity, with survival followed by symptom control. The patient with severe symptoms may express control of symptoms as primary, followed by exercise capacity and lastly, survival.

## Nonpharmacologic Therapy

Nonpharmacologic treatment involves lifestyle modifications, particularly diet and activity. Dietary changes include a moderate (2-g) sodium restriction. This usually is achieved by teaching the patient to add no salt during cooking or at the table. Sodium restriction is often difficult for patients to follow, and a more severe restriction results in noncompliance (Massie, 1996a). The American Heart Association has many helpful publications for patients and families, including a cookbook that uses alternate spices to improve flavor.

Because of the depressant effect of alcohol, it is recommended that it be either eliminated or restricted to one drink a day. Caffeine should be limited because of the stimulatory effect on the heart. Finally, fluid intake needs to be assessed and limited when necessary (Dracup, 1996; Kloner & Dzau, 1990; Massie, 1996a).

When heart failure symptoms are severe, resting the heart through a decrease in activity may facilitate recompensation of the myocardium. Activity restriction during the acute phase is needed to reduce symptoms. Limited activity along with pharmacologic therapy may promote copious diuresis. A semireclined position promotes increased renal profusion, leading to increased diuresis. However, after the acute phase, patients are encouraged to begin an exercise program. In most cases, an exercise program that emphasizes a gradual increase in activity is beneficial in reducing symptoms and improving endurance.

## Time Frame for Initiating Pharmacotherapy

Pharmacotherapy should be initiated along with lifestyle modifications. The type of pharmacotherapy for CHF will depend on the presenting symptomology of the patient. Hospitalization and aggressive treatment will be necessary for patients who present in acute or severe failure. Additional treatments will be based upon

resolution of acute symptoms and the desired functional level.

See Drug Tables 205.1, 205.7, 207, 208.

## Assessment Prior to Therapy

The history and physical examination concentrate on the signs and symptoms of heart failure, which relate to the alteration in function of the heart. Left-sided heart failure is the most common and involves systolic left ventricular dysfunction. The most helpful classification is according to functional limitations (see Table 20–4).

Using the functional classification, a patient may present without any symptoms; therefore, it is important to perform a complete history and physical examination. Because systolic and diastolic heart failure frequently occur together, the assessment needs to include information on both manifestations of the disease (Dracup, 1996; Kloner & Dzau, 1990; Kradjan, 1993; Massie, 1996a).

### Areas of focus

HISTORY.  Previous medical history includes hypertension, myocardial infarction, congenital heart problems, untreated streptococcal infection, and coronary artery disease. Symptoms include onset and severity, ability to perform activities of daily living including instrumental activities, usual exercise, and changes in ability, sleep patterns, and mental status.

RESPIRATORY.  Commonly, the patient will complain of shortness of breath with exertion. As the syndrome progresses, the symptoms increase.

---

### TABLE 20–4. NEW YORK HEART ASSOCIATION CLASSIFICATION OF HEART FAILURE

- Class I: No limitation on activity. No fatigue, dyspnea, or palpitations with physical activity.

- Class II: Slight limitation on activity. Comfortable at rest but fatigue, palpitations, and dyspnea with ordinary physical activity.

- Class III: Marked limitation of activity. Comfortable at rest but fatigue, palpitations, and dyspnea, during ordinary physical activity.

- Class IV: Unable to carry out any physical activity without discomfort. Fatigue, palpitations, and dyspnea at rest.

Be sure to ascertain symptoms of a nonproductive cough, often worse when lying down. Patients may be comfortable at rest but have dyspnea when changing clothes or during assessment of gait and balance. Observe the patient during conversation. Note the ability to complete sentences without distress. Inquire about the number of pillows or if able to sleep lying down.

**GASTROINTESTINAL.**   Assess appetite, nausea, vomiting, and pain.

**PAIN.**   Check for angina, chest pain, right upper quadrant pain caused by right heart failure and the resultant congestion in the liver, loss of appetite, nausea, and peripheral edema.

**URINARY.**   Assess for nocturia.

**PRECIPITATING EVENTS AND CONDITIONS.**   Assess for previous myocardial infarction, hypertension, use of NSAIDs (sodium-retaining), pulmonary embolism, infection, anemia and use of beta blockers and other negative inotropic drugs.

**WEIGHT.**   With severe heart failure, weight loss with cachexia may be apparent. Weight gain over a short period of time is indicative of fluid overload.

**COLOR.**   Assess for cyanosis.

**VITAL SIGNS.**   Check for tachycardia, hypotension, and decreased pulse pressure.

**NECK.**   Check height of pulsations of jugular veins, jugular distention, and carotid pulses. Evaluate pulse pressure, the presence of atrial stenosis, and hepatojugular reflux. Thyroid examination is important. Hyperthyroidism and hypothyroidism represent two treatable causes of heart failure.

**LUNGS.**   Check for crackles at the bases, dullness to percussion (pulmonary effusion), expiratory wheezes, and rhonchi.

**HEART.**   Check enlargement of the heart, downward and lateral displacement of the point of maximal impulse (PMI) and diffuse PMI, parasternal lift, diminished first heart sound, $S_3$ gallop (heard just after $S_2$) that may start in the left ventricle, and a fourth heart sound that may be heard. Murmurs could indicate valvular disease or dilated ventricles.

**ABDOMEN.**   Hepatic enlargement, tender or nontender, may occur with right-sided failure. Pressure on the liver may produce a positive hepatojugular reflux. Also assess ascites and upper right quadrant tenderness.

**EXTREMITIES.**   Pitting edema of the legs may be in the lower legs and extend to the thighs and abdomen. Assess temperature and color of extremities.

**LABORATORY.**   A CBC should be done to check for anemia, one sign in high-output cardiac failure. With severe heart failure, polycythemia may occur.

**CHEMICAL PROFILE.**   Azotemia, low sedimentation rate, respiratory alkalosis, elevated liver enzymes, and elevated bilirubin and BUN may occur. Do a thyroid profile and check thiamine level if high output is suspected.

**URINALYSIS.**   Proteinuria and high specific gravity may be present.

**ELECTROCARDIOGRAM.**   This helps define possible etiologies such as secondary arrhythmias, valvular disease, myocardial infarction, coronary artery disease, and ventricular hypertrophy. A stress test electrocardiogram is indicated if ischemia is suspected.

**ECHOCARDIOGRAM.**   The echocardiogram is preferred and justified because it helps differentiate between systolic and diastolic dysfunction. An ejection fraction of less than 40% indicates systolic dysfunction. The normal ventricular function and ejection fraction are indicative of diastolic dysfunction. The echocardiogram also reveals the size and function of the ventricles and atria and is able to detect valvular problems, old myocardial infarctions, and other possible etiologies of heart failure.

**CHEST X-RAY.**   Examine the x-ray for the size and shape of the heart. Typically, the chest x-ray shows cardiomegaly. Interstitial edema, alveolar fluid, dilation of the veins of the upper lobe, and perivascular edema may indicate pulmonary venous hypertension. The chest x-ray may also show pleural effusion, common with heart failure.

## Patient/Caregiver Information

It is important that the patient and the patient's family be informed and understand the diagnosis, including the prognosis, and symptoms of worsening heart failure and actions to take in the event these symptoms occur. Information should be provided on activity and dietary recommendations. The effects of medications, dosing, side effects, and mechanisms to enhance compliance should be discussed.

## OUTCOMES MANAGEMENT

### Selecting an Appropriate Agent

In the ambulatory setting, treatment may be initiated with diuretics to reduce volume overload. Additional treatments can be added to reduce symptoms, improve functional status (ACE inhibitors, digoxin), and reduce mortality (ACE inhibitors, isosorbide dinitrate/hydralazine).

The Agency for Health Care Policy and Research (AHCPR) has developed an algorithm for the pharmacotherapeutic management of congestive heart failure based on the severity of dyspnea on exertion (DOE), volume overload, and the presence of hypertension or concomitant angina (Konstam et al, 1994):

Begin by determining the severity of DOE.

Mild:
 Presence of volume overload?
  No: Initiate and titrate ACE inhibitor.
  Yes: Initiate diuretic; initiate and titrate ACE inhibitor.
 Symptoms resolved?
  No: Add diuretic.
  Yes: Monitor.
 Symptoms resolved?
  No: Add digoxin.°
  Yes: Monitor.
 Symptoms resolved?
  No: Persistent volume overload?°°
   Yes: Aggressive diuretic therapy.
   No: Persistent dyspnea?
    Yes: Hydralazine and/or nitrates.
    No: Persistent hypertension?
     Yes: Direct vasodilator or alpha blocker.
     No: Concomitant angina?
      Yes: Nitrates and aspirin.

Moderate:
 Initiate diuretic; initiate and titrate ACE inhibitor.
 Symptoms resolved?
  Yes: Monitor.
  No: Begin at ° above and proceed.
Severe:
 Initiate diuretic, ACE inhibitor, and digoxin.
 Symptoms resolved?
  Yes: Monitor.
  No: Begin at °° above and proceed.

### Monitoring for Efficacy and Toxicity

*Diuretics.* Diuretics (thiazides, potassium-sparing, and loop) are the drugs of choice for reducing the symptoms of volume overload and the accompanying pulmonary and/or peripheral edema. To date, diuretics have not been shown to decrease the mortality of CHF. Diuretics, through their reduction of atrial and ventricular diastolic pressure, may inhibit the progression of ventricular hypertrophy. However, in patients without signs and symptoms of volume overload, diuretics may be harmful because of induction of neurohormonal activation (Cohn, 1996).

Thiazide diuretics (hydrochlorothiazide, indapamide, metolazone), whose site of action is the early distal convoluted tubule, can manage mild volume overload. Thiazide diuretics become less effective when the glomerular filtration rate is less than 30 mL/min.

Loop diuretics (furosemide, bumetanide, torsemide) remove a greater percentage of sodium and water and are favored when volume overload is more severe. Loop diuretics act in the ascending limb of the loop of Henle, induce a prostaglandin-mediated increase in renal blood flow, and maintain their activity in renal impairment. Loop diuretics maintain their effectiveness as glomerular filtration rates decrease, but are reduced with concurrent administration of nonsteroidal antiinflammatory drugs (Brater, 1985; Ellison, 1991).

Among the three loop diuretics, torsemide has several unique features (White & Chow, 1997). Torsemide produces less potassium loss because of less action at the proximal convoluted tubule. Its bioavailability is similar to bumetanide but greater than furosemide. Torsemide's half-life is longer than the other two and permits true once-a-day dosing. About 25% of torsemide is excreted unchanged in the urine; for bumetanide this fraction is 50% and for furosemide 50–80%. Torsemide does not interact with cimetidine and warfarin. A helpful dosage equivalence scale is 10–20 mg of torsemide = 1 mg of bumetanide = 40 mg of furosemide.

The effectiveness of diuretics can be assessed by the following:

- Increase in exercise tolerance
- Decrease in pulmonary congestion and rales
- Weight loss
- Less edema (using these first four parameters, the practitioner and the patient may develop criteria for self-adjustment of diuretic pharmacotherapy to maintain desired weight)
- Less neck vein distention (more aggressive diuretic pharmacotherapy may be needed if the patient has an elevated pressure in the internal jugular vein or evidence of hepatojugular reflux)
- Disappearance of $S_3$ gallop

If the activity of the loop diuretic diminishes, the addition of a thiazide diuretic (metolazone or hydrochlorothiazide) provides a synergistic effect. The rationale is that the loop diuretic is increasing the delivery of sodium to the distal convoluted tubule, resulting in an increased amount removed by the thiazide diuretic. The possibility of an edematous gastrointestinal tract may be the cause of decreased efficacy since there is diminished rate of absorption, with lowered peak concentrations (Brater, 1985).

It should be noted that diuretics can increase the activity of renin, thus decreasing their efficacy. With chronic use, the patient needs to be monitored for the onset of hypokalemia, hyponatremia, hypomagnesemia, hypochloremic alkalosis, hyperglycemia, and hyperuricemia. Hypokalemia occurs in 10–36% of patients receiving diuretics. There is an average decrease of between 0.5 and 0.7 mmol/L of serum potassium with long-term use of diuretics. The decrease is dose-related and more likely to occur in patients who have unrestricted sodium intake. Hypokalemia should be treated with potassium replacements to decrease the likelihood of hypochloremic alkalosis and persistent hypokalemia. Hypokalemia can also exacerbate digitalis intoxication in patients receiving digoxin.

Alternatively, potassium-sparing diuretics (amiloride, spironolactone, triamterene) may be used to minimize potassium loss with diuresis since they are more potent natriuretic agents. Their site of action is the late distal convoluted tubule and collecting ducts. It is important to monitor closely the serum potassium level whenever these agents are used in treatment. This is especially important in patients receiving

potassium supplements (don't forget about the potassium salts used by patients vs. table salt) or an ACE inhibitor (which reserves potassium at the kidney). Serum magnesium needs to be evaluated in patients with refractory hypokalemia.

If the patient becomes fatigued or hypotensive or has azotemia in the presence of a normal jugular venous pressure, excessive diuresis is the likely cause. The dose of the agent should be reduced or discontinued. In patients with diastolic dysfunction, diuretics need to be used cautiously to avoid volume depletion, orthostatic hypotension, and aggravation of the CHF.

***ACE inhibitors.*** ACE inhibitors reduce preload and afterload by arterial and venous dilation. The pharmacodynamics of these agents involve inhibition of angiotensin II (afterload reduction) and the resultant inhibition of aldosterone secretion (preload reduction). In addition, ACE inhibitors prevent the breakdown of the vasodilator bradykinin. Because of the evidence demonstrating increased survival, these agents are considered first-line therapy, versus digoxin, for mild to moderate CHF and especially in patients with symptomatic CHF associated with reduced systolic ejection or left ventricular remodeling (Cohn, 1996; Pfeffer et al, 1992; SOLVD Investigators, 1991). Current ACE inhibitors indicated to treat CHF are captopril, enalapril, fosinopril, lisinopril, quinapril, and ramipril. The others (benazepril, moexipril, trandolapril) have not been studied yet in the treatment of CHF. There are differences among these agents in regards to their pharmacokinetics; however, the outcome is comparable. Captopril and lisinopril are not prodrugs and therefore do not need to be converted by the liver to an active form. Fosinopril is 50% fecally and 50% renally eliminated (as is trandolapril for HTN), whereas the others are 90% renally eliminated. Ramipril and quinapril are not removed by hemodialysis as are the others, except lisinopril, which is unknown.

The desired response to ACE inhibitors requires several weeks of administration. This time period probably is due to the adjustment needed by the body's various hormonal responses. The plasma renin activity is not indicative of the long-term success of these medications (Packer et al, 1993). Doses need to be started low and can be adjusted upwards about every 2–3 days, though weekly is more realistic, until symptomatic relief occurs. The target doses are captopril 50 mg t.i.d., enalapril 10 mg b.i.d., lisinopril 20 mg daily, and quinapril 20–40 mg/day, unless the patient develops intolerable side effects.

Special attention should be given to the patient's fluid and sodium status before initiating an ACE inhibitor in order to prevent hypotension and renal insufficiency. If the patient is on diuretic therapy or has recently had an increase in his or her dose, the starting doses of ACE inhibitors should be reduced (captopril 6.25–12.5 mg t.i.d., enalapril 2.5 mg one or two times per day, lisinopril 5 mg/day, and quinapril 5 mg/day) to help prevent hypotension. A reduction in diuretic doses or an increase in sodium intake should minimize the chance of renal insufficiency. A helpful parameter is if the serum sodium concentration is less than 135 mmol/L, the patient probably will have a high level of plasma renin activity and thus increased sensitivity to the ACE inhibitors (Cohn, 1996).

Retention of potassium is another possible adverse effect. Although hyperkalemia rarely develops, other sources of potassium (diet, salt substitutes, potassium supplements) should be discussed with the patient.

Other patient complaints include rash, dysgeusia, reflex tachycardia, hypotension, and a dry, hacking cough. Up to 40% of the population get a cough independent of ACE inhibitor therapy, although the incidence is greater when an ACE inhibitor is prescribed.

**Cardiac glycosides: digoxin.** Digoxin has a positive inotropic and a negative dromotropic effect on the heart. The pharmacodynamics of digoxin include inhibition of NaK-ATPase, increased vagal tone, and some evidence of blunting of excessive neurohumoral activation. The net effects are an increase in cardiac index, a decrease in systemic vascular resistance and pulmonary capillary wedge pressure (PCWP), and little change in arterial blood pressure.

In recent years the therapeutic efficacy of digoxin has been disputed for patients with heart failure and normal sinus rhythm. However, the withdrawal of digoxin can have an adverse effect (Cohn, 1996). In the Digitalis Investigation Group (DIG) study it was noted there was no significant effect of digoxin on mortality, as with ACE inhibitors or hydralazine-isosorbide dinitrate, but there was a reduction in the hospitalization rate and improvement in patient symptoms (Young, 1996). Digoxin should be used in patients along with diuretics and either an ACE

inhibitor or hydralazine-isosorbide dinitrate early in the course of the disease.

Special pharmacokinetic considerations of digoxin include its large volume of distribution and predominantly renal elimination. Because of a significant distribution phase, serum levels should be collected at least 6–12 h after the oral dose, but ideally just before the next dose. Therapeutic serum levels are generally in the range of 0.8–2.0 ng/mL.

A serum level must be evaluated in conjunction with any adverse signs and symptoms the patient may exhibit since there is not a good correlation between serum levels and the presence of signs and symptoms of toxicity. The half-life of digoxin normally is 1.5 h in a patient with normal renal function, but is extended to 5 days in anuric patients.

Most patients with heart failure and normal sinus rhythm can be started on digoxin without the need for loading doses. Doses range from 0.125–0.5 mg/day. If a patient needs an earlier onset of therapy than 6–10 days, loading doses should be given. Doses are based on ideal body weight in the range of 10–20 µg/kg. A common administration schedule is to give one half of the calculated dose initially, then one fourth every 6–8 h for the two remaining doses. Table 20–5 presents daily doses of digoxin based on corrected creatinine clearance (140 − [age/serum

### TABLE 20–5. DAILY DIGOXIN DOSE

| Digoxin Dose (mg/day) | Corrected Creatinine Clearance (mL/min/70 kg) | Weight (kg) |
|---|---|---|
| 0.125 | 10 | 50–80 |
| 0.125 | 20 | 50–70 |
| 0.125 | 30 | 50–60 |
| 0.125 | 40–50 | 50 |
| 0.25 | 10 | 90–100 |
| 0.25 | 20 | 80–100 |
| 0.25 | 30 | 70–100 |
| 0.25 | 40–50 | 60–100 |
| 0.25 | 60–70 | 50–90 |
| 0.25 | 80–90 | 50–80 |
| 0.25 | 100 | 50–70 |
| 0.375 | 60–70 | 100 |
| 0.375 | 80–90 | 90–100 |
| 0.375 | 100 | 80–100 |

Adapted from Young (1996).

creatinine concentration in mg/dL] × 0.85 if female) and body weight (in kg) as used in the DIG study (Young, 1996).

Adverse effects may be either noncardiac (nausea, vomiting) or cardiac (dysrhythmias). Additionally, hypokalemia, hypomagnesemia, and hypercalcemia will predispose the patient to cardiac manifestations.

**Vasodilators.** If dyspnea persists, a vasodilator (hydralazine and/or nitrates) should be added to the diuretic, ACE inhibitor, and digoxin regime. It has been shown that an ACE inhibitor or the combination of hydralazine and isosorbide dinitrate can decrease mortality (Cohn et al, 1986; Cohn et al, 1991; CONSENSUS Trial Study Group, 1987; SOLVD Investigators, 1991). Based on this, if an ACE inhibitor used as initial therapy is not tolerated, hydralazine and isosorbide dinitrate should be initiated because of evidence of reducing mortality and improving ejection fractions. In clinical trials the daily dose of 300 mg of hydralazine and 160 mg of isosorbide dinitrate was desired but not always achieved because of headaches in some patients (Cohn, 1996).

Vasodilators exert their effect either by a direct vasodilation as with hydralazine or by activation of guanylate cyclase to increase cyclic guanosine monophosphate (GMP). Nitrates reduce preload, whereas hydralazine reduces afterload.

Isosorbide dinitrate is administered routinely every 6 h. The practitioner may be concerned that the tolerance that develops with nitroglycerin may also extend to isosorbide dinitrate. To date the literature is equivocal in CHF patients, but this does not appear to be a problem compared to treatment of patients with angina (Leier et al, 1983; Packer, 1990). If it develops in a CHF patient, nitrate intervals of 8–12 h may be necessary.

Hydralazine doses often are higher in patients with CHF versus hypertension (300 mg/day). Adverse effects often limit the usefulness of the hydralazine and isosorbide dinitrate regime.

Vasodilators not recommended in CHF include alpha-adrenergic blockers such as prazosin (Cohn et al, 1986), minoxidil, an arterial vasodilator (Franciosa et al, 1984), and calcium channel blockers (Elkayam et al, 1990; Goldstein et al, 1991; Multicenter Diltiazem Postinfarction Trial Research Group, 1988). Calcium channel

blockers may be of value in patients with pure diastolic dysfunction.

**Beta blockers.** Recent evidence suggests that in stable CHF patients, low doses of a beta blocker (metoprolol 6.25 mg bid), with gradual titration over 4–6 weeks to higher doses, can be beneficial. This is based on the neurohormonal model of heart failure in which activation of the sympathetic nervous system and the renin-angiotensin-aldosterone system contributes to the hemodynamic and clinical abnormalities. Currently, beta blockers may be useful in patients with idiopathic dilated cardiomyopathy. Dosing guidelines for successful outcomes include:

1. Start slowly titrating the dose every 1–4 weeks.
2. Improvements may not be seen for 3–12 months.
3. Effectiveness may be greater in patients with high adrenergic activity, resting tachycardia, and depressed left ventricular function.
4. Nonselective agents with peripheral vasodilating properties may be better because of an increase in beta$_2$ and alpha$_1$ receptors from continual adrenergic stimulation.

Two currently available agents are metoprolol and carvedilol. Metoprolol is a selective beta blocker with peripheral vasodilatory effects. Carvedilol is a nonselective beta blocker with vasodilating action via alpha-adrenergic blockade. Carvedilol also has calcium channel blocking activity at high doses. Although this action does not provide additional benefits in blood pressure reduction, it may be responsible for local vascular bed vasodilation. The cardioprotective effect of carvedilol may be due to its antioxidant properties. Carvedilol prevents the generation of oxygen free radicals and the oxidation of LDL and uptake into coronary vasculature (Chen & Chow, 1997). Carvedilol carries an FDA indication for the treatment of mild or moderate heart failure of ischemic or cardiomyopathic origin when used in combination with digoxin, diuretics, and ACE inhibitors. When carvedilol was compared to placebo in patients with chronic heart failure, the risk of death and hospitalization for cardiovascular causes was reduced by 65% when used in combination with digoxin, diuretics, and an ACE inhibitor (Packer et al, 1996).

The investigational agent bucindolol is a nonselective beta blocker without intrinsic sympathomimetic or alpha$_1$ receptor activity. It is a direct vasodilator and may have some coronary vasodilation properties. The net result is an improvement in left ventricular function and submaximum exercise duration.

***Other agents.*** Several inotropes have been investigated for their use in CHF. They include enoximone (Uretsky et al, 1990), imazodan (Goldberg et al, 1991), xamaterol (Xamaterol in Severe Heart Failure Study Group, 1990), flosequinan ("Flosequinan for Heart Failure," 1993), and vesnarione (Feldman et al, 1993). The agents have mechanisms of phosphodiesterase inhibition, beta-adrenergic agonism, arterial and venous dilating properties, and augmentation of cardiac contractility. To date none of these agents have been proven to be more effective than current treatments. Flosequinan, a quinolone, did reach the market but was removed because of excess mortality.

The calcium channel blockers felodipine and amlodipine have been studied in the treatment of CHF. These two agents have an action more restricted to the vascular walls and may augment vasodilation induced by ACE inhibitors (Cohn, 1996). More recently it has been proposed that in CHF the cells are programmed for cell death by tissue necrosis factor alpha and interleukin-6, leading to decreased myocardial contractility. The beneficial effects of amlodipine may be the result of its inhibition of interleukin-6.

The angiotensin II type 1 receptor blockers may also prove useful in the treatment of CHF. Their action is similar to that of the ACE inhibitors, but they do not interfere with the metabolism of bradykinin. As such, there should be less potential to induce cough. Another advantage may be the local inhibition of angiotensin II effects when compared to the ACE inhibitors. However, the effect of angiotensin II receptor blockers on mortality is unknown. These agents should be reserved for patients who cannot tolerate the ACE-inhibitor-induced cough or the side effects of hydralazine–isosorbide dinitrate therapy (White & Chow, 1997).

### Follow-up Recommendations

There is no standard frequency of follow-up. After the initial diagnosis and treatment and once the patient is stabilized, visits to the provider may be as frequent as every 2–3 weeks or every 3–6 months. Patient education and evaluation of effectiveness of therapy are needed during early stages.

Each visit includes the patient's perception of symptoms discussed previously as well as vital signs and heart and lung sounds. Always reevaluate using the New York Heart Association classification (Table 20–4).

Closely follow electrolytes, chest x-rays, and electrocardiograms, as well as renal (BUN and creatinine) and liver function tests.

If diuretics are being used, observe for signs of excessive diuresis: weight change, orthostatic hypotension, dry mouth, thirst, weakness, oliguria, nausea, vomiting, dizziness, confusion, falls, cramps, restlessness, and drowsiness.

If ACE inhibitors are part of the regimen, check for cough, rash, swelling of the face, eye, lips, or tongue, sore throat, fever, hypotension, dehydration, vomiting, diarrhea, potassium level, and renal function.

Monitor steady-state blood levels of digitalis just prior to next dose or in the presence of signs of toxicity (confusion, nausea, vomiting, dizziness, arrhythmias, headaches, visual disturbances, weakness).

Always ask about other medications including over-the-counter medications, especially NSAIDs, since these agents promote sodium and water retention and decrease renal function in the elderly.

## ARRHYTHMIAS

Arrhythmia, or dysrhythmia, is a disturbance in cardiac rhythm. The conduction system of the heart begins in the sinoatrial (SA) node of the heart. The SA impulse activates the atria and AV node. The AV node transmits the impulse across the septum to the bundle of His in the ventricles. The impulse then moves through the ventricles by way of the right and left bundle branches and the Purkinje system. Disturbances in rate and rhythm are due to disturbances in this electrophysiologic system and are most frequently caused by reentry problems or disturbances in automaticity (Graboys, 1990; Haak et al, 1994; Waldo & Witt, 1993).

Some definitions of the mechanisms of arrhythmias follow (Graboys, 1990; Haak et al, 1994; Waldo & Witt, 1993):

- *Impulse conduction:* Impulse conduction is altered at the SA or AV node, in the ventricular conduction system, or within the atria or ventricles. It is associated with the development of reentry circuits.

- *Reentry:* When the normal pathway for depolarization is blocked, the impulse seeks another route. The alternate pathway is unidirectional and causes a delay in depolarization and impulse conduction. This delay causes another impulse to be initiated at the original site. Reentry circuits may be at the SA or AV nodes or may be alternate pathways that circumvent either node. Reentry mechanisms may be the most important in arrhythmias.
- *Automaticity:* The capacity of special cells in the cardiac muscle to automatically generate depolarization is known as automaticity. Spontaneous depolarization or pacemaker activity normally occurs in the SA and AV nodes as well as the bundle of His. However, the SA node works at a faster rate and usually prevents the slower pacemakers in the AV node and Purkinje system from firing unless it is dysfunctional.
- *Abnormal impulse formations* are arrhythmias caused by problems with automaticity. As described, the SA node is the normal pacemaker. Ectopic pacemakers (nonnormal pacemakers) are outside the SA node. Abnormal rhythms occur when the ectopic pacemaker cells reach threshold before the SA node discharges the impulse, thus initiating a beat before the SA node. The ectopic pacemaker continues to generate impulses after repolarization.

Pharmacotherapy for arrhythmias is organized according to electrophysiological effects. Therefore, to understand pharmacotherapy for arrhythmias, it is important to examine the electrophysiologic properties of the cardiac muscle and to define commonly used terms.

- *Depolarization:* Change in the voltage at the cell membrane caused by the initiation of the action potential; electrical activation of cells. Allows movement of sodium, calcium, and potassium across the cell membrane.
- *Repolarization:* Deactivation of the electrical activity at the cell membrane. The depolarization and repolarization can be described in phases (Table 20–6).
- *Action potential:* The first step in contraction is when the cardiac cells are excited, changing the distribution of ions at the cell membrane. Ions move through channels into the myocardial cells. The movement of ions causes changes in membrane voltage. Channels in each cell allow the action potential to move through cells, causing depolarization of the cell.
- *Resting membrane potential:* Describes the voltage difference at the cell membrane. The resting membrane potential indicates a higher negative

**TABLE 20–6. PHASES OF DEPOLARIZATION AND REPOLARIZATION**

- Phase 0: Depolarization and rapid movement of calcium or sodium into the cell; referred to as upstroke
- Phase 1: Early repolarization; slow influx of calcium into the cell
- Phase 2: Plateau; continuation of repolarization with slow influx of sodium and calcium into the cells
- Phase 3: Repolarization; potassium moves outside cell; repolarization but not quite resting
- Phase 4: Return to resting potential via the sodium/potassium ATPase pump with magnesium serving as a catalytic enzyme

charge outside the cell membrane and is noted as $-60--80$ mV (millivolts) depending on the location. This value is an important determinant of the speed of impulse conduction. At the SA node (pacer) the resting membrane potential is less negative. Therefore, it is able to be receptive to new impulses sooner than other cardiac cells with a more negative resting membrane potential. Resting potential in the cardiac cells is the time of repolarization.

- *Fast channel:* Rapid conduction of impulses. The channel opens, allowing the rapid influx of sodium or calcium ions into the cell depending on the cardiac tissue. The movement of sodium into the cell causes depolarization of the cell.
- *Slow channel:* After the rapid influx of sodium, the channel allows the slow influx of calcium. Conduction of impulses at this time is slow.
- *Action potential duration* (APD): Time from the beginning of the action potential to the return of the resting potential; phases 0–4.
- *Refractory period:* Time from the start of depolarization through contraction.
- *Effective refractory period* (ERP): Time from the beginning of the action potential to the beginning of repolarization when no new action potential can be initiated. It is the time needed to open the sodium and calcium channels; phases 0–3.5.
- *Relative refractory period:* Short time from the end of the ERP to the end of repolarization when the membrane potential is beginning to be negative; able to depolarize but a stronger than usual stimulus is needed.

There are many cardiac arrhythmias. The usual classifications are supraventricular, ventricular, and conduction arrhythmias (see Table 20–7).

## TABLE 20-7. CARDIAC ARRHYTHMIAS

| Arrhythmia | Description/Etiology | Signs/Symptoms |
| --- | --- | --- |
| **Supraventricular: Originate in the SA node, atria, AV node, and bundle of HIS** | | |
| Sinus arrhythmia | Variable filling times, oxygen demand, and arterial pressure. Common in young adults and varies with respirations. | Variable rate. P waves have 1:1 ratio, and may have regular irregularity. QRS complex for every P wave. |
| Sinus bradycardia | Increased vagal influence on SA node or sign of organic disease. Increases preload and decreases arterial pressure. Etiology: hyperkalemia, digoxin toxicity. | Heart rate <50. Elderly: weakness, confusion, falls. |
| Sinus tachycardia | SA node increases impulse formation. Increases myocardial demand. Decreased filling times, decreased arterial pressure. Etiology: fever, exercise, emotion, pain, anemia, heart failure, shock, thyroid disease, drugs, alcohol. | Heart rate >100 with regular rhythm. Onset and ending usually gradual. Number of beats per minute may vary with changes in position, holding the breath, or medication. |
| Premature beats: atrial | Ectopic formation of beats occurring before SA node impulse or before reentry circuit started. May have decreased filling time and/or decreased arterial pressure. Etiology: hypercalcemia, electrolyte disturbances, hypoxia. | P wave not normal for patient. Ventricular contraction premature. Common in adults, frequently in normal hearts. |
| Paroxysmal supraventricular tachycardia | Most common form of paroxysmal tachycardia. Decreased filling time and decreased arterial pressure; increased myocardial oxygen demand. Reentry circuit involving the SA or AV node or accessory pathway is most common mechanism. Etiology: digitalis toxicity, AV block. | Occurs in young adults with normal hearts. Attacks have sudden onset and ending. May last hours. Heart rate 140-220/min, regular rhythm. Often asymptomatic with exception of knowing heart is racing. May have mild chest pain and/or shortness of breath. ECG: P:QRS complex variable. |
| Atrial fibrillation | Rapid disorganized depolarization originating in ectopic sites in the atria. Atrial contraction ineffective. Decreased filling time, blocked impulses at the AV node creating irregular ventricular contraction. Etiology: *Cardiac:* valvular disease, cardiomyopathy, MI, hypertension, CAD, pericarditis, cardiac surgery: *Pulmonary:* pneumonia, COPD, pulmonary embolus; *Endocrine:* thyroid disease, pheochromocytoma: *Medications:* theophylline, beta-adrenergic agonists, amphetamines, alcohol. | Atrial heart rate 400-600/min. Heart rate 80-180, pulse irregular, pulse deficit (difference between apical and palpable pulse) high with high ventricular rate. May be accompanied by lightheadedness, fatigue, problems with exercise and endurance, angina, dyspnea, fainting. Chronic common condition; incidence increases with age. ECG: P wave not clear, QRS complex irregularly irregular and narrow, P-R interval variable. |
| Atrial flutter | Impulses form ectopically in atria; only every second, third, or fourth impulse is transmitted through AV node. Reentry mechanism involved. Decreased filling time. Etiology: COPD, CAD, CHF, atrial septal defect, rheumatic heart disease, AV block. Associated with atrial fibrillation. | Atrial heart rate 250-350/min. Variable P:QRS complex, QRS complex narrow. |

*continues on next page*

**TABLE 20–7.** *continued*

| Arrhythmia | Description/Etiology | Signs/Symptoms |
|---|---|---|
| **Ventricular: Originate below the bundle of HIS; generally have wide QRS complex and elevated T wave** | | |
| Premature beats: ventricular | Ectopic origination of beats that override the SA node. Decreased cardiac output due to lack of atrial filling for that beat. May have bigeminy (every second beat premature) or trigeminy (every third beat premature). Etiology: if frequent occurrence, hypo- or hyperkalemia, hypoxia, hypercalcemia, hyperthyroidism, heart disease, increased incidence with aging, mitral prolapse. | Wide QRS complex, no P wave before complex. Patient may complain of "skipped" beat sensation. Exercise returns heart to normal rhythm. Asymptomatic when no other cardiac disease. With heart disease, associated with sudden death. |
| Ventricular tachycardia | Three or more consecutive premature ventricular beats. Mechanism is most often reentry, but may also have ectopic origin. Decreased cardiac output, increased oxygen demand on myocardium. Etiology: most common complication of MI or dilated cardiomyopathy, mitral prolapse, myocarditis. Most will have diagnosed or detectable heart disease. | Ventricular rate of 160–240/min. May be irregular or regular. No change with carotid sinus pressure. May be sustained or nonsustained (lasts less than 30 s). Symptoms vary from asymptomatic to syncope and/or symptoms of poor cerebral perfusion. P wave absent. |
| Ventricular fibrillation | Ectopic pacemaker activity throughout the heart results in individual portions beating independently. No obvious electrical cycle, no cardiac output. Etiology: acute MI, hyperkalemia, acidosis, severe ischemia. | No P wave, no QRS complex. Not compatible with life. |
| **Conduction: Originate between the SA node and atrium, in the AV node itself, and/or in the ventricles; classification is above the ventricles, below the bundle of HIS, or in the ventricles** | | |
| Sick sinus syndrome | Group of arrhythmias resulting from dysfunction of the SA node. It can be a generalized disorder of the heart with the SA node abnormality only one part. In elderly, SA node and conduction system have patchy fibrosis. Presentation on ECG resembles sinoatrial exit block, sinus arrest, chronic sinus bradycardia or both supraventricular tachycardias and bradycardias (tachybrady). Etiology: most frequently associated with medications especially digitalis, calcium channel blockers, beta blockers, sympatholytic agents, or antiarrhythmics. Also occurs with sarcoidosis, amyloidosis, and cardiomyopathy. | Most asymptomatic. Patients may experience syncope, dizziness, and confusion resulting in falls in the elderly. Patients may complain of palpitations. Rhythm changes from one arrhythmia to another; isometric exercises do not produce a significant change in heart rate. |
| Atrioventricular blocks | Three types defined as first-, second-, or third- (also called complete block) degree blocks. | ECG: nodal block, QRS complex usually narrow; infranodal block, QRS complex wide. |

*continues on next page*

**TABLE 20–7.** *continued from previous page*

| Arrhythmia | Description/Etiology | Signs/Symptoms |
|---|---|---|
| First-degree block | All AV impulses transmitted. Etiology: digitalis, calcium channel blockers, organic disease, ischemia, infarction, fibrosis, inflammatory processes, hypo- or hyperkalemia. | ECG: PR interval <0.20; asymptomatic. |
| Second-degree block | Mobitz type I and II: intermittent blocked beats, associated with decreased cardiac output and increased preload for the next beat. Mobitz type I usually AV node; type II usually bundle of His. Etiology (both): hypokalemia, altered AV node cell metabolism, CAD, MI, hypoxia, increased preload, valvular surgery, valvular disease, diabetes. Mobitz type I, digoxin toxicity, beta blockers; type II, antiarrhythmics, tricyclic antidepressants. | Mobitz type I: PR interval gradually lengthens, RR interval shortens before blocked beat. QRS complex drops as PR interval lengthens. Mobitz type II: abrupt onset with no preceding lengthening of AV conduction time. P:QRS complex may vary. |
| Third-degree (complete) block | Lesion below bundle of His, associated with both left and right bundle branch block. No transmission of atrial impulses through the AV node. Slow heart rate sustained by ectopic ventricular pacemaker. Etiology: hypokalemia, MI (especially inferior wall), abnormal cell metabolism below the bundle of His. | Wide QRS complex. P waves independent of QRS. Ventricular heart rate <50/min. Rate not increased with exercise. $S_1$ heart sound changes intensity, pulse pressure wide, varying systolic blood pressure, cannon venous neck pulsations. Symptoms include weakness and dyspnea; more severe when ventricle unable to increase stroke volume. |
| Atrioventricular dissociation | Ventricular pacemaker sends impulses faster than sinus rate. When AV node is in refractory period, it is unable to transmit impulses from the atria. Etiology: arrhythmias, third-degree block. | P waves independent of QRS but do not necessarily indicate an AV block. AV dissociation may not be third-degree block. |
| Ventricular block | Impulses blocked at any point and may involve either right, left, or both branches. RBBB more common than LBBB since the left bundle has dual blood supply. At risk for development of complete block. Etiology: cardiac disease including CAD, inflammatory heart disease, postcardiac surgery, cardiomyopathies, post MI. | ECG able to differentiate between types of blocks. May have syncope and symptoms of bradycardia. |

*Supraventricular section of table adapted from Friedman (1990), Graboys (1990), and Massie (1996a). Ventricular section adapted from Friedman (1990) and Graboys (1990). Conduction section adapted from Friedman (1990).*

## SPECIFIC CONSIDERATIONS FOR PHARMACOTHERAPY

### When Drug Therapy Is Needed

There are many types of arrhythmias, ranging from common, to asymptomatic, to life-threatening. Antiarrhythmic pharmacotherapy has not been proved completely effective, and many medications have side effects that are more harmful than the arrhythmia. Therefore, the value of using pharmacotherapy is evaluated by the potential mortality or morbidity of the arrhythmia and the associated side effects of the medications. Treatment of arrhythmias is most often based on the history and symptoms of the patient, potential side effects of medications, and provider comfort with a particular agent.

## Short- and Long-Term Goals of Pharmacotherapy

Pharmacotherapy and the associated short- and long-term goals are dependent on the condition being treated and the underlying disease state. Pharmacotherapy is often used in symptomatic patients until a pacemaker or permanent correction of the arrhythmia is possible. These types of arrhythmias include bradycardia and second- and third-degree heart blocks. Drugs may be used in conjunction with permanent pacing such as with acute ventricular block or an MI with ventricular block. Finally, pacing may be instituted followed by pharmacotherapy.

As with any disease state, the goals of therapy are to prevent mortality and morbidity, prevent complications, and promote quality of life. Pharmacologic therapy is used to restore the rate and force of contraction, change thresholds, change refractory periods, decrease myocardial demand, prevent reentry, and alter repolarization and depolarization. The goals include:

1. *Prevention of sudden death.* Sudden cardiac death is most often associated with ventricular fibrillation. Prior to fibrillation, the patient usually demonstrates ventricular tachycardia, complete heart block, or sinus node arrest. Correction of the arrhythmia and underlying disease, using pharmacotherapy as well as other interventions, is crucial for the prevention of sudden death.
2. *Correction of life-threatening arrhythmias.* Ventricular standstill, tachycardia, fibrillation, and premature beats may be precursors of sudden death. Acute paroxysmal supraventricular tachycardia in the presence of heart disease requires termination of the attack as well as prevention of future attacks. Aggressive treatment with pharmacotherapy and mechanical interventions is essential.
3. *Prevention of complications.* The elderly, in particular, may experience syncope associated with an arrhythmia, increasing their chance of falling. The falls may result in hip, wrist, and other fractures. These in turn limit functional abilities and decrease quality of life. Arrhythmias with a higher incidence of syncope include AV block, automaticity problems as found with sick sinus syndrome, ventricular and supraventricular tachycardia, and heart disease. Atrial fibrillation and paroxysmal supraventricular tachycardia are highly correlated with

thromboembolitic stroke (Aronow, Ahn, & Gutstein, 1996; Aronow, Ahn, Mercando, Epstein, & Gutstein, 1996) as well as other embolic problems. Because of the strong association with CVA, converting the rhythm to normal sinus rhythm is essential. Treatment includes anticoagulants and aspirin plus medications to control the ventricular rate.

## Nonpharmacologic Therapy

Some arrhythmias respond to nonpharmacologic interventions. Treatment begins with identification of the cause and treatment of any reversible conditions.

- *Atrial premature beats:* May disappear if heart rate is increased.
- *Paroxysmal supraventricular tachycardia:* The Valsalva maneuver, lowering the head below the body, stretching the arms and trunk, coughing, or holding the breath are methods that the patient can use to try to terminate the attack. Carotid sinus pressure over one carotid sinus and then the other is often successful in interrupting an attack. However, this should be performed only by professionals, in patients without a bruit or history of transient ischemic attacks. An ECG or auscultation should be used to monitor the heart rate during the procedure.
- *Symptomatic bradycardia, Moritz II AV block, or complete heart block:* Require a permanent pacemaker.

## Time Frame for Initiating Pharmacotherapy

Initiation of pharmacotherapy is based on the patient's tolerance of the arrhythmia and whether any correctable cause is identified. Factors that must be considered in evaluating the patient's ability to tolerate the arrhythmia include the heart rate, duration of the arrhythmia, and any underlying cardiac disease and its severity. Arrhythmias that should be treated and are responsive to pharmacotherapy include atrial fibrillation or flutter, paroxysmal supraventricular tachycardia, automatic atrial tachycardias, and ventricular tachycardia.

See Drug Table 202.

## Assessment Needed Prior to Therapy

### History and physical examination
- *Symptoms:* Inquire about onset and duration of symptoms such as dizziness, syncope, lightheadedness, fatigue, confusion, and falls in the elderly population and palpitations or sensations

of skipped beats or a racing heart. Inquire about chest pain, angina, shortness of breath, and dyspnea.

- *Risk factors:* Explore coronary artery disease (CAD), previous myocardial infarction, cardiac surgery, inflammatory heart disease, cardiomyopathies, valvular disease, hypertension, previous CVA, alcohol or drug abuse, and rheumatic heart disease.
- *Medication history:* Review medications, including OTC and herbal, for anticholinergic and sympathomimetic effects. Examples to consider include digoxin, beta blockers, calcium channel blockers, antiarrhythmic medications, tricyclic antidepressants, antipsychotics, cold remedies, and diet aids.
- *Physical examination of the heart:* Always auscultate heart sounds and observe the rate, rhythm, pulse deficit, pattern (such as regularity of irregular heart rate), variations in first heart sound, intensity of heart sounds, response to exercise, and changes in heart sounds with position or respirations. Examine for orthostatic hypotension.

### Diagnostic testing

- *Electrocardiogram:* This is best done when the patient is experiencing a symptom; therefore, ambulatory monitoring is important for diagnosing arrhythmia. If symptoms accompany exercise or stress, an exercise ECG is useful. Frequent syncope may require inpatient monitoring.

- *Electrophysiologic testing:* An intracardiac ECG with programmed atrial and/or ventricular stimulation is good for complex arrhythmias. It is used after the initial ECG and ambulatory ECG prove inconclusive to evaluate the effectiveness of pharmacotherapy in people with life-threatening arrhythmias or accessory pathway arrhythmias, as a differential diagnostic tool for ventricular or supraventricular arrhythmias, and for evaluation of pacing devices.
- *Laboratory:* CBC, chemical profile, especially of electrolytes and blood sugar, thyroid profile, and digoxin level (if appropriate).

## Patient/Caregiver Information

Educate the patient regarding the role of stress, lack of sleep, chocolate, and alcohol in increasing vulnerability of the heart to electrophysiologic induction of atrial flutter and fibrillation. If the patient also is taking digoxin therapy, the heart rate during exercise should be kept below 140–150 beats per minute.

Patients should be aware that the resting heart rate may be elevated during time of illness.

## OUTCOMES MANAGEMENT

### Selecting an Appropriate Agent and Monitoring for Efficacy and Toxicity

*Atrial fibrillation or flutter.* Pharmacotherapeutic management of symptomatic patients is first directed at restoring and maintaining the sinus rhythm or controlling the ventricular rate, and then to preventing thromboembolism. Heart rate control is a requirement for all patients. Direct-current cardioversion (DCC) is the most widely used and successful treatment in the restoration of sinus rhythm. Drug therapies to control ventricular rate include digoxin, calcium channel blockers such as verapamil and diltiazem, and beta blockers. Anticoagulants such as warfarin and aspirin are prescribed to reduce the risk of a thromboembolic event. The type I antiarrhythmics (quinidine, procainamide, flecainide) and type III antiarrhythmics (amiodarone, sotalol) are often prescribed in an attempt to sustain sinus rhythm.

In managing a patient with atrial fibrillation or flutter (Bauman, Parker, & McCollam, 1995), the practitioner needs to evaluate the onset or duration of the arrhythmia and the severity of symptoms. The treatment algorithms differ for atrial fibrillation onset of less than 48 h or greater than 48 h and then if either acute (<12 months) or chronic (>12 months).

If atrial fibrillation onset is less than 48 hours, therapy is as follows (Golzari, Cebul, & Bahler, 1996):

Step 1. Control ventricular rate, consider antithrombotic therapy, and observe for spontaneous conversion

Step 2. Prompt electrical or pharmacologic conversion

Step 3. Need for antiarrhythmic therapy—yes, if unstable hemodynamics or frequent recurrences; no, if stable hemodynamics, infrequent recurrences, or first episode

The duration of the atrial fibrillation is the best predictor of the success of either electrical or pharmacologic conversion and the probability of maintaining sinus rhythm. Often about 50% of the patients with new-onset atrial fibrillation of short duration will spontaneously convert to sinus rhythm within 24–48 h (Prystowsky et al,

1996). If atrial fibrillation has been present for longer than 1 year, restoring sinus rhythm is more difficult. Occasionally long-standing atrial fibrillation will spontaneously convert and appears to be a result of left atrial fibrosis.

DCC has a success rate of greater than 80% in restoring sinus rhythm. However, there are adverse effects associated with cardioversion. These include embolic events, hypotension, pulmonary edema, depressed left ventricular contractility, and arrhythmias. Even so, cardioversion is an effective treatment modality.

If atrial fibrillation has been present for longer than 48 h, use the following algorithm (Golzari et al, 1996):

Step 1. Control ventricular rate and start antithrombotic therapy (heparin and/or warfarin or aspirin)
Step 2. Duration of atrial fibrillation <1 year Warfarin therapy for 3–4 weeks or determine by transesophageal echocardiography the presence of intracardiac thrombi—if none present, proceed to cardioversion.
　　　Cardioversion or pharmacologic conversion
　　　　　Need for antiarrhythmic therapy— yes, unstable hemodynamics or frequent recurrences; no, stable hemodynamics, infrequent recurrences, or first episode
　　　　　Continue warfarin 1–2 months and monitor for recurrences
　　Duration of atrial fibrillation >1 year Chronic antithrombotic therapy; ensure control of ventricular rate (this approach can also be considered for duration <1 year instead of cardioverting the patient)

Drugs that may be useful in pharmacologic conversion include quinidine, procainamide, and the new agents amiodarone, propafanone, flecainide, and sotalol. The adverse effects of quinidine make it a less useful agent now with the newer agents and the widespread use of cardioversion (Flaker et al, 1992). Intravenous procainamide is the treatment of choice for patients with Wolff-Parkinson-White syndrome who have a preexcited ventricular response during atrial fibrillation as long as they are hemodynamically stable. Digoxin will not convert patients out of atrial fibrillation to sinus rhythm. The electrophysiologic effects of digoxin are to

shorten the atrial refractory period, which can increase the chance of initiating and perpetuating this arrhythmia.

The type IC agents flecainide and propafanone have been successful in converting atrial fibrillation to sinus rhythm in patients with recent onset. If the arrhythmia is of less than 7 days duration, flecainide 200 mg or propafanone 600 mg as a single dose has shown similar efficacy in conversion to sinus rhythm (Golzari et al, 1996). Flecainide should be avoided in the post–myocardial infarction setting because of increased mortality. Both of these agents via their pharmacodynamics allow more atrial impulses to be conducted through the AV node, which may result in a faster ventricular rate. Propafanone may prove to be of value in treating paroxysmal atrial fibrillation; however, the hematologic adverse effects have limited its widespread use in this setting.

Sotalol has both type II (beta-blocker) and type III (cardiac action potential duration prolongation) properties. The efficacy of this agent has yet to be well established. Current studies suggest conversion to sinus rhythm with sotalol is no better than a placebo and less than quinidine (Golzari et al, 1996) in maintaining sinus rhythm in more than 50% of the patients (Prystowsky et al, 1996).

Amiodarone may have the greatest potential for converting and maintaining sinus rhythm even with its slow onset. Almost two thirds of patients remained in sinus rhythm for up to 1 year while receiving amiodarone (Prystowsky et al, 1996). A low dose of 200 mg of amiodarone per day is often successful in maintaining sinus rhythm while minimizing the adverse effects seen in 75% of the patients when ≥400 mg per day is prescribed (Gosselink et al, 1992; Lacy et al, 1997). Amiodarone's place in treatment may be in symptomatic patients with drug-refractory, recurrent atrial fibrillation. Also, amiodarone appears to have the lowest proarrhythmic effect of all the above-mentioned agents.

Even with the use of antiarrhythmics, reversion to atrial fibrillation within 1 year occurs in almost half of the patients. This reflects the limited efficacy of these drugs and the high incidence of treatment cessation caused by adverse effects.

Concomitant ventricular rate control therapy can be accomplished with the use of digoxin, a calcium channel blocker (verapamil, diltiazem), or a beta blocker. In patients with severe symptoms these medications may be administered intravenously, whereas in the less symptomatic patients they may be given orally to control the ventricular rate.

By enhancing vagus nerve activity on the heart, digoxin decreases conduction through the AV node with a slowing of the ventricular response. The adequacy of the dose can be judged by a ventricular rate goal of 70–90 beats per minute. Remember that digoxin does not convert patients out of atrial fibrillation and cannot adequately control the ventricular response during exercise. Digoxin, either alone or in combination with other agents, works best in the management of atrial fibrillation in patients who are minimally symptomatic (mild palpitations) and/or who have congestive heart failure related to impaired systolic ventricular function. In the latter, beta blockers and calcium channel blockers are undesirable because of their negative inotropic effects.

Daily maintenance doses of digoxin range from 0.125–0.375 mg. Patients with impaired renal function will need their dosage adjusted accordingly (refer to the section on congestive heart failure). Measurement of serum levels will help in determining patient compliance and to rule out digoxin toxicity. However, the patient should be evaluated for symptoms of digoxin toxicity such as nausea, vomiting, weakness, and visual disturbances since there is not always a correlation between serum level and toxicity. A therapeutic serum level of digoxin is 0.8–2.0 µg/mL. Blood sampling should occur at steady state (7–14 days depending on renal function) and at least 6–8 h after the dose or just before the next scheduled dose. The practitioner should also monitor potassium and magnesium serum levels and maintain electrolytes within normal levels to reduce the incidence of digoxin toxicity.

To assist digoxin in the control of the acute and long-term ventricular rate, especially during exercise-related increases, propranolol, verapamil, or others of these drug categories may be added. Propranolol, a beta blocker, is a type II antiarrhythmic that decreases conduction through the AV node, prolonging the PR interval. It also has a direct slowing effect on the sinus rate. The calcium channel blocker verapamil is a type III antiarrhythmic that slows calcium flux across the slow channels of vascular smooth muscle and cardiac cells. Verapamil depresses the AV node and has a negative

chronotropic effect on the SA node. Diltiazem, also a calcium channel blocker, has a similar effect but to a lesser degree. Neither of the calcium channel blockers will convert patients to a sinus rhythm. A benefit of verapamil and diltiazem is that their effect on rate control is not diminished during exercise or stress. A limitation to the use of beta blockers or calcium channel blockers is coexisting CHF. Calcium channel blockers may inhibit the nonrenal clearance of digoxin.

Although evidence for long-term antiarrhythmics is unclear, recent studies reveal the value of antithrombotic therapy in patients with atrial fibrillation to prevent stroke either prior to cardioversion or with chronic atrial fibrillation (Laupacia, Albers, Dunn, & Feinberg, 1992; Stroke Prevention in Atrial Fibrillation Investigators, 1991). The patient most likely to benefit is one who is over 60 years of age; has valvular, ischemic, or hypertensive heart disease; has respiratory or systemic disease; and has no contraindications to warfarin therapy. In patients with no identified risk factors, atrial fibrillation alone, or who are noncompliant, the use of 325 mg of aspirin per day should be considered (Stroke Prevention in Atrial Fibrillation Investigators, 1994). Dosing warfarin to achieve international normalizing ratio (INR) values of 2.0–3.0 is recommended (see Table 20–8).

### TABLE 20–8. ANTICOAGULATION RECOMMENDATIONS FOR PATIENTS WITH ATRIAL FIBRILLATION

| Age | Risk Factors[a] Present | |
|-----|------|---|
| <65 | None | ASA 325 mg/day or no therapy |
| <65 | Yes | Warfarin INR 2–3 or ASA 325 mg/day in patients with significant bleeding risk factors |
| 65–75 | None | |
| 65–75 | Yes | Warfarin INR 2–3 or ASA 325 mg/day in patients with significant bleeding risk factors |
| >75 | | |

[a] Risk factors are hypertension, previous stroke or TIA, heart failure, diabetes mellitus, coronary artery disease, mitral valve disease, prosthetic heart valve, and thyrotoxicosis.

Some simple suggestions for initiating warfarin therapy are presented in Table 20–9 (Hulisz, 1997; Wittkowsky, 1995).

Two other initiating regimens are:

1. 10 mg daily for 3 days; however, this regimen was designed to reach a prothrombin time of 1.5–2.0 times baseline (Carter et al, 1987; Sawyer et al, 1985).

2. 4–5 mg daily; this is the average dose for the population as a whole; however, the time necessary to reach a desired INR is prolonged.

Future dose alterations can be adjusted based on the following algorithm:

| INR of 2.0 to 3.0 | Adjustment |
|---|---|
| <2.0 | Increase by 5–15% |
| 3.1–3.5 | Decrease by 5–15% |
| 3.6–4.0 | Hold 0–1 doses; decrease by 10–15% |
| >4.0 | Hold 0–2 doses; decrease by 10–15% |
| INR of 2.5 to 3.0 | Adjustment |
| <2.5 | Increase by 5–15% |
| 3.6–4.0 | Decrease by 5–15% |
| 4.1–4.5 | Hold 0–1 doses; decrease by 10–15% |
| >4.5 | Hold 0–2 doses; decrease by 10–15% |

Chronic atrial fibrillation or flutter greater than 12 months is managed by blocking the AV node as in acute scenarios. However, DCC is not attempted unless the patient has severe symptoms. In both situations, long-term anticoagulation is warranted.

***Paroxysmal supraventricular tachycardia.*** The treatment of PSVT is governed by the severity of symptoms and/or width of the ARS complex and possible arrhythmias. In patients with severe symptoms, DCC is the primary treatment. If the patient is experiencing mild symptoms, pharmacotherapy is directed by the width of the QRS complex. When the QRS complex is narrow and regular, suggesting AV node reentrant tachycardia, the treatments consist of verapamil, diltiazem, or adenosine. If the QRS complex is wide and regular, suggesting VT, the treatment is adenosine or procainamide. Finally, if the QRS complex is wide and irregular, suggesting AF with an accessory pathway, procainamide is the treatment of choice (Bauman et al, 1995).

Continued therapy will be necessary if patients have frequent or severe symptoms. Trials of agents such as verapamil, digoxin, quinidine, procainamide, beta blockers, flecainide, propafanone, or amiodarone can be done to determine the best therapy. Electrophysiologic stud-

## TABLE 20–9.  INITIATING WARFARIN DOSE USING BASELINE PT INR

| Day | INR | Warfarin Dose (mg) | OR | INR | Warfarin Dose (mg) |
|---|---|---|---|---|---|
| 1 | <1.4 | 10 | | <1.5 | 10 (5 mg if <50 kg) |
| 2 | <1.8 | 10 | | <1.6 | 10 |
| | 1.8 | 10 | | 1.6–2.0 | 5 |
| | >1.8 | 5 | | 2.1–3.0 | 2.5 |
| | | | | >3.0 | 0 |
| 3 | <2.0 | 10 | | <2.0 | 10 |
| | 2.0–2.1 | 5 | | 2.0–2.5 | 5 |
| | 2.2–2.3 | 4.5 | | | |
| | 2.4–2.5 | 4 | | | |
| | 2.6–2.7 | 3.5 | | 2.6–3.5 | 2.5 |
| | 2.8–2.9 | 3.0 | | | |
| | 3.0–3.1 | 2.5 | | | |
| | 3.2–3.3 | 2.0 | | | |
| | 3.4 | 1.5 | | | |
| | 3.5 | 1.0 | | | |
| | 3.6–4.0 | 0.5 | | >3.5 | 0 |
| | >4.0 | None | | | |

*Adapted from Hulisz (1997) and Wittkowsky (1995).*

ies along with therapy may be helpful in determining the origin and direction of reentry (Desanctis & Ruskin, 1993).

### Ventricular arrhythmias.

Because of the life-threatening nature of many of the ventricular arrhythmias, a cardiology consultation or referral is recommended. Therapy is probably best initiated by the cardiologist with maintenance and follow-up care, in many instances, by the primary care provider.

#### VENTRICULAR PREMATURE BEATS.

In patients without appreciable heart disease, pharmacotherapy may be warranted if the palpitations significantly interfere with the patient's life. If this is the situation, propranolol, a beta blocker, has been successful.

In patients with heart disease, the decision to use pharmacotherapy is not as apparent. The results of the cardiac arrhythmia suppression trial (CAST) studies indicate that while ectopy was suppressed, the risk of death was increased (Echt et al, 1991). Currently, patients who are post–myocardial infarction with complex ventricular ectopy remain at risk for death, and therapies besides beta blockers designed to reduce this risk need further evaluation. Low-dose amiodarone is under investigation as a possible alternative agent (Ceremuzynski et al, 1992).

#### VENTRICULAR TACHYCARDIA.

VT is often precipitated by electrolyte disturbances, ischemia, organic heart disease, or drug toxicity. As such, initial management should be directed toward detection and correction of the condition.

In acute episodes of VT in which the patient is severely symptomatic, DCC should be performed. Again, the possibility of an underlying cause such as myocardial infarction should be investigated.

Intravenous lidocaine (with hospitalization) may be necessary in patients with transient VT as seen in acute myocardial ischemia or digoxin toxicity. Once the underlying cause is identified and treated, further antiarrhythmic therapy is unlikely.

Advanced cardiac life support (ACLS) guidelines should be used in the management of a patient with asymptomatic or mild symptoms associated with an acute episode of VT (Emergency Cardiac Care Committee, 1992).

Management of chronic, recurrent sustained VT is important since these patients are at risk

for sudden death and should be directed by an experienced practitioner or cardiologist. An electrophysiologic study performed in the hospital can assist in the selection of effective pharmacotherapy and the possible role of pacemaker therapy in patients not responsive to drug therapy (Desanctis & Ruskin, 1993).

Drug therapy can be selected from all four types of antiarrhythmics. Quinidine, procainamide, and disopyramide (type Ia) are effective in suppressing sustained ventricular arrhythmias; however, their side-effect profiles make them less acceptable to the patient. The major side effects associated with quinidine are gastrointestinal problems such as diarrhea, cramps, and nausea. Procainamide therapy is often terminated in patients who develop a positive antinuclear antibody titer or a positive lupus erythematosus preparation. Disopyramide has anticholinergic side effects of blurred vision, dry mouth, and urinary retention in males that reduce patient compliance.

Mexiletine and tocainide (type Ib) are effective in suppressing sustained ventricular arrhythmias when combined with a beta blocker or another agent like quinidine or procainamide. Flecainide (type Ic) must be monitored for potential cardiac toxicity, including proarrhythmic effects, in patients with advanced heart disease and left ventricular dysfunction.

Propafanone is a mixed agent with type Ic, weak beta-blocking action and, at higher doses, some calcium channel blocking action. This agent is also associated with a significant incidence of proarrhythmic effects and several side effects that likely would affect patient compliance. These include nausea, vomiting, constipation, dizziness, rash, and a bitter metallic taste.

Moricizine has weak type Ic properties with moderate activity in sustained ventricular arrhythmias. Sotalol is a nonselective beta blocker with type III antiarrhythmic properties. When doses exceed 320 mg per day, the incidence of torsade de pointes increases because of the prolongation of the QT interval.

Amiodarone, also a type III agent, can be used in patients with life-threatening ventricular arrhythmias. However the practitioner must be aware of the significant incidence of adverse reactions and drug interactions.

The treatment of sustained ventricular arrhythmias is best handled by an experienced practitioner or cardiologist. Electrophysiologic studies, surgical excision of the focus, and implantable automatic cardioverter defibrillators may be necessary in patients who are unable to tolerate drug therapy or who are resistant to pharmacologic management.

## Follow-up Recommendations

Follow-up is based on the problem, etiology, symptoms, possible complications, and medications. Unfortunately, because there are many types of arrhythmias that may or may not be associated with symptoms and may or may not be life-threatening, prescribed times for follow-up vary.

However, when initiating pharmacotherapy, the pharmacodynamics of the medication may help identify the frequency of visits. During the initial treatment phase, visits every day may be appropriate to observe for adverse reactions. Keep the following suggestions in mind for the follow-up:

1. *History and physical examination:* Always auscultate heart sounds, and check vital signs, including orthostatic hypotension. Inquire about nausea and other GI disturbances, symptoms of CNS disturbance, palpitations, and shortness of breath or wheezing.
2. *ECG:* Observe for new arrhythmias, heart block, and left ventricular function.
3. *Laboratory:* Appropriate tests are determined by the common side effects of the medications prescribed. Included are thyroid function, electrolytes, renal function, liver function, and CBC.
4. If the patient is placed on an anticoagulant for atrial fibrillation, obtain a prothrombin time reported as an INR to eliminate laboratory variation.

## PERIPHERAL VASCULAR DISEASE

Peripheral vascular disease (PVD) encompasses multiple conditions affecting the circulation to and from the extremities. In order to understand and manage PVD, it is important to understand atherosclerosis (see the section on coronary heart disease).

Arterial insufficiency is commonly caused by atherosclerosis. This section covers arterial insufficiency and specific conditions that are responsive to some form of nonsurgical therapy. Differences between occlusive problems of the aorta and iliac arteries (conservative care), the lower leg and foot, thromboangiitis obliterans,

and Raynaud's phenomenon are presented. Table 20-10 summarizes occlusive and venous PVD processes and signs and symptoms.

## SPECIFIC CONSIDERATIONS FOR PHARMACOTHERAPY

### When Drug Therapy Is Needed

Many arterial aneurysms and occlusive diseases require surgical intervention. Conditions such as aneurysm, aortic dissection, occlusion of major arteries, and other acute manifestations of arterial disease may either be treated with or without medications until surgical intervention. In most cases, medication in combination with nonpharmacologic therapy is needed to promote the optimal level of function and quality of life.

### Short- and Long-Term Goals of Pharmacotherapy

When treating the peripheral vascular disorders of occlusive PVD or Raynaud's phenomenon, the goal is symptom relief. Pharmacotherapy is directed at relief of the symptoms of intermittent claudication and nocturnal leg cramps. Ideally, the long-term goals of therapy are to slow the progression of the disease, which should improve blood flow and relieve pain. With improved blood flow, ulcerations and progression to gangrene may be prevented. If the symptom of severe pain persists, then a pain care plan should be initiated.

### Nonpharmacologic Therapy

Any patient with peripheral vascular disease, independent of the primary location of the disease process, must be encouraged to make specific lifestyle changes.

Smoking cessation is essential. Counseling should include education on the effects of smoking specific to the patient's circulation problem and how symptoms are exacerbated. If the patient is a future surgical candidate, the surgeon may require smoking cessation prior to surgery to improve and maintain outcomes.

Walking daily promotes the development of collateral circulation and improves function. If the patient experiences intermittent claudication, instruct him or her to stop for about 3 min, but resume walking for the allotted time (Ernst & Fialka, 1993).

## TABLE 20–10. PERIPHERAL VASCULAR DISEASE

| Occlusive Disease | Process | Signs/Symptoms |
| --- | --- | --- |
| Aorta/iliac arteries | Aorta: starts distal to bifurcation. Iliac: starts proximal to bifurcation. Atherosclerosis that eventually occludes one or both iliac arteries and aorta just below renal arteries. | Intermittent claudication in calf muscles, thighs, and buttocks. Pain is usually bilateral. Leg weakness, especially when walking. Impotence in men common. Pulses: femoral pulses absent or weak. Distal pulses often absent. Bruit: possibly aorta or over iliac or femoral arteries. Skin: atrophic changes. Color and temperature changes not necessarily apparent unless distal arteries involved. |
| Femoral/popliteal arteries | Occlusion of superficial arteries in area of knee and thigh. Atherosclerosis starts in distal part of superficial femoral artery and may extend to popliteal artery. The superficial femoral artery slowly becomes completely occluded. | Intermittent claudication in calf and foot. Atrophic changes of lower leg: hair loss, thin skin, loss of subcutaneous tissue and muscle mass. Dependent rubor, blanching of skin with elevation of extremity, foot cool to touch. Pulses: absence of popliteal and pedal. |
| Lower leg/foot | Atherosclerotic changes in tibial and common peroneal arteries; pedal arteries most common. | Development of collateral circulation may create a stable or slowly progressive disease process. Symptoms may be minimal to severe. Intermittent claudication. Aching and fatigue during exercise or exertion, usually first in calf muscles. With progression of disease, pain may be constant or walking a minimal distance will cause cramping. May have pain at rest, especially at night. Pulses: pedal absent. Skin: dependent rubor, cool to touch, hairless, atrophic. |
| Thromboangiitis obliterans (Buerger's disease) | Affects both arteries and veins. Inflammatory as well as thrombic processes involved. The inflammatory process is intermittent with characteristic exacerbations and remissions. Process occurs in segments with exacerbations producing occlusions in new areas. Thrombic process occurs in distal arteries, usually in lower extremities in the foot and lower leg, but also in fingers. | Most common in men <40 who smoke. History of frequent episodes of superficial thrombophlebitis in different areas of extremity with resulting small tender bands along superficial veins. Intermittent claudication, rest pain, numbness, tingling, burning, or other changes in sensation. Affected part: cold and pale or rubor that may be pronounced with dependent position and may not change color when elevated; asymmetric changes in toes; possible ulcerations around nail beds. Pulses: dorsalis pedis, posterior tibial, ulnar, or radial may be diminished or absent. |

*continues on next page*

**TABLE 20–10.** *continued*

| Occlusive Disease | Process | Signs/Symptoms |
|---|---|---|
| Raynaud's disease | Digital arteries involved. Etiology unknown: probably due to sympathetic nervous system abnormality. Arteries sensitive to vasospastic stimuli causing paroxysmal digital cyanosis. Progressive. Raynaud's phenomenon: same process but associated with disorders such as rheumatoid arthritis, systemic lupus erythematosis, and other connective tissue disease, and in conjunction with thromboangiitis obliterans and thoracic outlet syndrome. | Most common in women ages 15–45. Attacks are paroxysmal, bilateral and are usually precipitated by cold. They typically start with pallor or cyanosis of one or two fingertips followed by rubor and sometimes pain, throbbing, sensory changes, and edema. Warming creates termination of attack. Raynaud's phenomenon: unilateral, nonprogressive. |

| Venous Disease | Process | Signs/Symptoms |
|---|---|---|
| Varicose veins | Superficial veins, usually of lower extremities, become dilated, elongated, and tortuous. Etiology: may be inherited, fundamental weakness in walls, or valvular incompetence. | May be asymptomatic. Usual: dull, aching, heavy feeling or easy fatigue from standing. Vessels dilated, tortuous, visible beneath skin in leg and thigh. Skin: may have brown discoloration and thinning above ankle. |
| Thrombophlebitis (general) | Occlusion of vein, either partial or complete, accompanied by inflammation. Results in platelet aggregation on the vein wall followed by thrombus formation. Trauma to wall of vein most frequent cause. From beginning of process to inflammatory changes is 7–10 days. Fibroblasts attack the thrombus, causing scarring of the vessel and valvular destruction. | |
| Thrombophlebitis (specific) Deep vein | Usually starts in calf but may be in pelvis. Process extends up popliteal and femoral veins. Etiology: post surgical, oral contraceptives especially in women who smoke and are over 30, hypercoagulability as seen in some cancers. | May be asymptomatic until embolus occurs. Frequently complain of aching, tightness or pain in calf. Most noticeable when walking. Signs not always present: swelling of calf, fever, tachycardia, positive Homan's sign (leg pain with dorsiflexion of foot) |
| Superficial | Most common site in saphenous vein of legs, but may be in any superficial vein. Unknown etiology or post trauma; early sign of cancer of the pancreas, associated with other cancers. | Tenderness, erythema and edema along vein, warm to touch, fever. Changes linear rather than circular. |
| Chronic insufficiency | Result of inadequate venous return over a period of time. Blood pools in lower legs; circulation sluggish to the point that waste products not removed. Etiology: usually due to deep vein thrombophlebitis and the resulting destruction of walls and valves of vessels. Also may be due to trauma, neoplastic obstruction in pelvic veins or varicose veins. | Skin: hyperpigmentation of lower legs especially the skin over the feet and ankles, shiny, thin. Edema of the leg. Itching, discomfort in legs when standing. Stasis dermatitis and recurrent ulcer formation common. |

Protection of the involved extremity(ies) prevents accidental injury that could result in major complications. With circulation compromised, normal healing processes are slow to nonexistent. Generally, the involved extremity should be kept warm and not exposed to either cold or hot temperatures. Keep the extremity clean and moisturized but not moist.

Varicose veins are usually managed with nonpharmacologic treatment or surgery. Varicose veins with minimal symptomatology are frequently managed with elastic stockings if the patient does not want surgery. The medium or heavy stockings give support to the veins of the lower leg and should be worn during times when the patient is standing. However, the patient should avoid standing for long periods of time or wearing constrictive clothing. When the stockings are not worn, elevation of the legs is recommended. Using stockings and elevation of the extremities, in addition to managing symptoms, may also prevent progress of the condition.

Specific conditions requiring a cardiology or surgical consult include: aortic abdominal aneurysm, popliteal and femoral aneurysm, aortic dissection, occlusive disease, arterial thrombus or embolism, varicose veins (depending on the extent of the condition), and thromboangiitis obliterans.

## Time Frame for Initiating Pharmacotherapy

Pharmacotherapy should be initiated simultaneously with exercise and lifestyle modifications in patients who remain symptomatic.

See Drug Tables 205.4, 205.6, 205.7, 206.

## Assessment Needed Prior to Therapy

### History and physical examination

- *Medical:* Check chronic conditions associated with atherosclerosis, neoplasms, previous surgical procedures, diabetes, liver, kidney disease, and trauma.

- *Social:* Assess occupational history, smoking habits, and alcohol use.

- *Symptoms:* Check pain location, quality, duration, aggravating factors, relief measures (what and effectiveness), and frequency (including pain at rest); presence of intermittent claudication; ability to walk before symptoms: two blocks (mild arterial occlusion); less than one block (moderate to severe occlusion); and discomfort when standing. Skin symptoms include changes in skin color, temperature, texture, and hair and

presence of numbness, tingling, and burning sensations. Check heart sounds, murmurs, arrhythmias, vital signs, bruits, and BP both arms (observe difference). Check pulses, temperature and color of extremities, atrophic changes, ulcerations, and dermatitis. Color changes with dependent positioning. In the abdomen check bruits, pain, and organomegaly.

- *Diagnostic studies:*
  Electrocardiogram: for aortic aneurysm or aortic dissection.
  Ultrasound: for abdominal aneurysm or peripheral artery aneurysm.
  Arteriogram: for thromboangiitis obliterans.
  Aortography: for occluded aorta or iliac arteries.
  X-ray: for chest if an embolism is suspected, for lower leg and foot to identify calcification from occlusion of peripheral arteries.
  Ascending contrast venogram: for accurate diagnosis of deep vein thrombophlebitis (expensive and uncomfortable).
  Doppler ultrasound: for deep vein thrombosis.

- *Laboratory:* CBC and chemical profile will assist in differential diagnosis of hypercoagulation, pancreatic disease, liver disorders, and infectious processes (Haak et al, 1994; Hobbs, 1991; Lally, 1992; Tierney, 1996; Wilt, 1992).

## Patient/Caregiver Information

Patients should be advised to stop smoking and keep walking (Housley, 1988). Graduated pressure elastic stockings should be worn when standing and legs should be elevated whenever possible. Constrictive clothing around the legs, such as tight socks, stockings, or garters, should be avoided. Although elastic stockings are the nonpharmacologic treatment of choice, they are made of thick, heavy material and are difficult to get on. Therefore, patients often do not wear the stockings as regularly as necessary for full benefit. Teaching the importance of pressure to prevent symptoms and additional problems plus techniques to assist in dressing may promote compliance with treatment strategies.

## OUTCOMES MANAGEMENT

### Selecting an Appropriate Agent

Treatment begins by minimizing risk factors and controlling coexisting conditions such as diabetes, hypertension, and smoking. Managing hyperlipoproteinemia can slow the progression of the disease (see the section on treatment of hyperlipidemias for additional information).

## Monitoring for Efficacy and Toxicity

### Intermittent claudication

PENTOXIFYLLINE.   Pentoxifylline has several mechanisms that have proven beneficial in the treatment of intermittent claudication (IC) and is approved by the FDA. Overall, pentoxifylline reduces blood viscosity and improves blood flow. This is accomplished by increasing red blood cell deformability, while decreasing platelet adhesiveness and blood fibrinogen. Pentoxifylline may be more effective when used early in the disease state when the patient presents with moderately severe ischemia without rest pain, ischemic ulcers, or severe claudication (Ernst, Kollar, & Resch, 1992).

The efficacy of pentoxifylline is measured by the time it takes before pain begins upon exertion. Improvement may take 2–3 weeks, but at least 8 weeks is needed to evaluate efficacy.

ANTIPLATELET AGENTS.   Aspirin with or without dipyridamole and ticlopidine has been evaluated in the treatment of PVD (Bevan et al, 1992). Aspirin alone has little effect (Hess et al, 1985), whereas the combination of aspirin with dipyridamole may decrease disease progression. However, aspirin's value as an antithrombotic must be considered as a part of a treatment regimen. Ticlopidine studies showed mixed results. Improvement in pain-free walking time and ulcer healing were demonstrated in some small, early studies, whereas a large 5-year study showed no significant improvement (Balsano et al, 1989; Katsumura et al, 1982).

CALCIUM CHANNEL BLOCKERS.   Interest in using calcium channel blockers in IC stems from their vasodilatory effects and their potential antiatherosclerosis effect (Fleckenstein-Grun, Thimm, Czirifuzs, & Matyas, 1994; Frey & Just, 1994). It is the latter that is intriguing since slowing the progression of atherosclerosis is a cornerstone of treatment. However, the evidence on the safety of calcium channel blockers is inconclusive so they should be used with caution.

VASODILATORS.   The vasodilators, including isosorbide dinitrate, have been used in treatment, yet currently are not recommended in the treatment of IC and occlusive PVD (Berkow, 1992b). Vasodilators often "steal" blood flow from the diseased vessels since the vasodilatory action is less than that on nondiseased vessels. The concomitant drop in blood pressure contributes to further diminished blood flow through these vessels (Coffman, 1988).

BETA BLOCKERS.   Beta blockers are often prescribed for patients with coronary artery disease and hypertension. Concern surrounds the use of these agents if the patient also has concomitant PVD. Studies are equivocal, showing no difference, a worsening of symptoms, and an improvement in symptoms (Ingram et al, 1982; Smith & Warren, 1982; Hiatt, Stoll, & Nies, 1985; Roberts et al, 1987). In theory, beta blockers inhibit $beta_2$-induced vasodilation during exercise. This, coupled with reduced systemic blood flow through stenotic arteries or collateral vessels, suggests these agents would be detrimental. At this time beta blockers should be used cautiously in patients with intermittent claudication. Begin with low doses and titrate slowly while monitoring for increased PVD symptoms (Heintzen & Strauer, 1994).

INVESTIGATIONAL AGENTS.   Several antiplatelet drugs are currently being evaluated for their use in PVD. These include prostaglandin $E_1$ and $I_2$, which are potent vasodilators and inhibitors of platelet aggregation (Grant & Goa, 1992). Presently these agents are only available as intravenous infusions. Others in clinical evaluation are picotamide, trapidil, and cilostazol (Balsano & Violi, 1993).

Defibrotide, a calcium channel blocker, has been shown to improve symptoms and treadmill exercise time in approximately half the patients. It has been demonstrated that defibrotide increases tissue plasminogen activator production and release, $PGI_2$ formation, and inhibition of platelet activation (Ulutin, 1988). L-carnitine, an amino acid which improves muscle metabolism, improved walking distance in studies that supplied 2 g twice a day for 3 weeks (Brevetti et al, 1988).

ACE inhibitors may be an alternative in patients with hypertension and IC. These agents may preserve collateral blood flow.

### Raynaud's phenomenon

CALCIUM CHANNEL BLOCKERS.   Nifedipine is the drug of choice for patients with Raynaud's disease who continue to experience symptoms after nonpharmacologic management is implemented. The peripheral vasodilating effects of this calcium channel blocker may be able to prevent the vascular response caused by cold exposure and alpha$_2$-receptor-mediated activity. Although nifedipine doses of 10–30 mg three times a day have been shown to be beneficial, objective changes in blood flow do not correlate well with the response (Coffman, 1991). Other calcium channel blockers have variable benefits. Doses of 30–120 mg three times a day of diltiazem showed benefit but not to the extent of nifedipine. Diltiazem may be preferred in patients who do not tolerate the side effects of nifedipine (Coffman, 1989). Verapamil, with fewer peripheral vasodilating properties, showed no subjective or objective benefit. The remainder of the calcium channel blockers (nicardipine, isradipine, felodipine, and amlodipine) have reportedly shown some benefit in patients but not conclusively (Leppert et al, 1989; Rupp et al, 1987).

**ALPHA$_1$-ADRENERGIC ANTAGONISTS.** Prazosin at doses of 1 mg three times a day has shown moderate benefit in a majority of patients (Wollersheim et al, 1986, 1988). Compliance may be an issue since this agent has significant side effects, especially if the dose is increased. Older agents, such as reserpine, guanethidine, methyldopa, phentolamine, and phenoxybenzamine should be avoided because of significant side effects. Dosage recommendations continue to be made in the literature for reserpine 0.125–1.0 mg/day, guanethidine 10–50 mg/day, and phenoxybenzamide 10 mg q.i.d. (Hancock, 1996a). Research continues on a superior agent, but to date none have exceeded nifedipine's action. When applied to the hands, nitroglycerin ointment resulted in fewer and less severe attacks (Coffman, 1991; Roath, 1989); however, the side effects may decrease usefulness. Other medications that have or are being evaluated include niacin, serotonin receptor antagonists, ACE inhibitors, and thymoxamine, an alpha$_1$ antagonist (Challenor et al, 1991; Coffman et al, 1989; Cooke & Nicolaides, 1990).

**Nocturnal leg muscle cramps.** With the FDA's removal of quinine from over-the-counter distribution and the deletion of leg cramps as an indication for use, the mainstay of treatment is nonpharmacologic. However, if the practitioner believes the benefit of quinine therapy exceeds the risks, careful monitoring of the patient is necessary. In addition, the dose should not exceed the prescribed amount of 200–300 mg taken at bedtime with an additional dose taken earlier in the evening if necessary. The patient may find it helpful to keep a diary of the number and extent of leg cramps during therapy.

### Follow-up Recommendations

Appropriate follow-up of patients is dependent on severity of condition and treatment regimen.

- For arterial disease, follow-up should include investigation of new symptoms and monitoring of blood pressure, pulses, and bruits. Providers must be alert to symptoms of any atherosclerotic or arteriosclerotic conditions.
- For venous disease, always check pulses, color, temperature, and atrophic changes in the skin. Observe and treat stasis ulcers.
- Monitor PTT if the patient is on anticoagulant therapy.
- Question the patient about exercise and smoking and alcohol use.
- Continue education about dietary modifications and protection of the involved part.
- Question the patient about new medications, including over-the-counter medications and birth control pills.

## CORONARY HEART DISEASE

Coronary heart disease includes coronary artery disease (CAD) and ischemic heart disease. The underlying problem is the deprivation of oxygen to the heart muscle caused by atherosclerosis of the coronary arteries. As the coronary arteries become occluded, the decreased blood supply injures cells with ischemia as a result. Angina pectoris is the result of myocardial ischemia.

### CORONARY ARTERY DISEASE

The development of ischemic heart disease begins with CAD. A major factor in the development of CAD is atherosclerosis. It is likely that atherosclerosis is associated with hyperlipidemia and the accumulation of LDL cholesterol.

#### Atherosclerosis

Atherosclerosis, a form of arteriosclerosis, is a chronic abnormal thickening and hardening of the arteries. This condition is due to deposits of fat in the form of cholesterol and fibrin in the arterial wall.

Although the exact mechanism is unknown, changes occur within the arterial wall. The vascular smooth muscle cells move close to the basement membrane. It is thought the cells secrete enzymes that attack the basement membrane, allowing the formation of atherosclerotic lesions. Atherosclerotic lesions are classified as a fatty streak, fibrous plaque, or complicated lesion. A fatty streak lesion is a smooth muscle cell filled with lipid material and appears flat and yellow. Fatty streaks are found in the aorta of children less than 1 year of age. The lesion does not cause narrowing or obstruction, may be reversible, and appears regardless of gender, race or environment (Haak et al, 1994; Brown, 1993). Fatty streak lesions may give rise to fibrous plaque lesions (Schwartz, 1992).

Fibrous plaque lesions indicate advancing atherosclerotic processes. The lesion is a smooth muscle cell that is full of lipid material and encircled with a matrix of collagen, elastic fibers, and mucoprotein. The white, elevated lesion begins the occlusive process by invading the walls of the artery and then protruding into the artery lumen. The fibrous plaque is most often found where arteries bifurcate or curve or in areas of narrowing (Brown & Kloner, 1990; Haak et al, 1994; O'Keefe, 1995).

Complicated lesions are calcified fibrous plaques. As the lesions grow and become hard, there is ulceration or disintegration of the lining of the artery. The complicated, advanced lesions are the most frequent cause of occlusion of the artery (Haak et al, 1994; O'Keefe, 1995).

Collateral circulation develops in response to the decreasing blood supply. Because the atherosclerotic process is slow, new arteries may form around the area of potential occlusion, thereby minimizing the symptoms experienced. However, the collateral vessels also develop atherosclerotic plaques and in turn become occluded. Symptoms may not appear for 40–50 years after the beginning of the disease process.

Neither arteriosclerosis nor atherosclerosis is isolated in a single vessel nor unique to a single disease. The major arteries are most frequently affected. The manifestations of atherosclerosis are dependent on the extent of the pathologic process, the number of vessels involved, location of the involved vessels, age, genetic predisposition, physiologic status, and other risk factors. Symptoms are not noted by the individual until about 60% of the vessel is occluded (Haak et al, 1994). In addition to the narrowing and occlusion, arteries may lose structural components of the vessel wall, leading to aneurysms.

## Additional Risk Factors

In addition to atherosclerosis and hyperlipidemia, the development of CAD is associated with (Haak et al, 1994):

- *Hypertension:* Continuous pressure on the walls of the arteries causes damage to the walls and either precipitates or exacerbates the process of atherosclerosis.
- *Cigarette smoking:* The mechanism is unknown, but the release of epinephrine and norepinephrine caused by nicotine increases BP by an increase in heart rate and peripheral vascular resistance. The catecholamines may also release fatty acids, resulting in higher LDL cholesterol. Other possible mechanisms include an increase in adhesiveness of the platelets, causing increased clot formation in the arteries, or hypoxemia, which may result in atherosclerosis caused by increased permeability of the arterial walls.
- *Diabetes mellitus:* This condition is associated with hyperlipidemia, hypertension, and obesity.
- *Genetic factors:* CAD is more likely to occur if there is a familial history of a myocardial event, especially before the age of 50. This genetic predisposition is usually associated with hyperlipidemia and occurs more often in men than women.
- *Hypoestrogenemia:* Women with low estrogen levels are more at risk for the development of CAD than women with normal estrogen levels. However, oral contraceptives (OCs) are associated with increased triglyceride and total cholesterol levels, increased platelet aggregability, and altered prothrombin and clotting factors, leading to possible MI in premenopausal women. Although OCs were once thought contraindicated for women 35–50, they have been found safe for nonsmoking women. Present data do not indicate an increased risk of CAD and years taking OCs. The relationship between estrogen and CAD continues to be investigated.
- *Lifestyle/personality:* A sedentary lifestyle and Type A personality have been associated with a high incidence of coronary heart disease; however, research has not verified this relationship.

## Myocardial Ischemia

Myocardial ischemia begins with inadequate blood flow to supply the needs of the myocardium. The first signs occur when the demand for oxygen increases, such as during exercise, increased systolic blood pressure, stress, hyperthyroidism, and anemia. An ischemic attack occurs when a major artery is narrowed by 50%.

If the attack lasts up to 20 minutes, the cells lose their ability to contract and therefore decrease the function of the myocardium. Deprived of oxygen, the cells are unable to use glucose through aerobic metabolism and turn to anaerobic metabolism. The result is an accumulation of lactic acid.

Clinically, the individual will have symptoms of chest pain (angina pectoris), arrhythmias, and electrical abnormalities on an ECG.

Angina pectoris is the most common presenting symptom of myocardial ischemia. The patient presents with precordial chest pain that is transient and frequently associated with exertion or stress. See Table 20–11 for a listing of the types of angina.

Angina has been classified by the Canadian Cardiovascular Society according to severity during activity, which may be helpful for the provider and patient in assessment of the problem (see Table 20–12).

## SPECIFIC CONSIDERATIONS FOR PHARMACOTHERAPY

### When Drug Therapy Is Needed

Pharmacotherapy is directed at reducing myocardial oxygen consumption, improving coronary artery blood flow, slowing the progression of the disease process, and preventing morbidity and mortality associated with CHD. The initiation of drug therapy should be considered in any patient who experiences symptoms. Drug therapy should be used in conjunction with lifestyle modifications. In addition, early recognition and treatment of hyperlipidemia, hypertension, and diabetes mellitus is important.

### Short- and Long-Term Goals of Pharmacotherapy

The long-term goal is to ensure that the supply of oxygen and nutrients to the myocardium equals the demand. Therefore, the immediate goal of pharmacotherapy is the prevention of angina and restoration of cardiovascular function. Long-term drug therapy is directed at reducing the risk of further cardiovascular or cerebral incidents.

### Nonpharmacologic Therapy

Prevention through diet, exercise, and smoking cessation, as discussed in the sections on hypertension and hyperlipidemia, is applicable to the treatment of CHD. Early detection and treatment of diabetes and hypertension will help decrease the progress of atherosclerosis and the development of CAD.

### Time Frame for Initiating Pharmacotherapy

The initiation of pharmacotherapy should be individualized and based on the history and physical examination, as well as any presenting signs and symptoms of angina (see the assessment

## TABLE 20–11. TYPES OF ANGINA PECTORIS

| Type of Angina | Description |
| --- | --- |
| Stable angina | Exertional, classic angina. Discomfort is predictable, precipitating factors known, and the pattern of discomfort the same for each episode. Usually brought on by exertion and relieved with rest (Brown & Kloner, 1990; Haak et al, 1994). |
| Unstable angina | Between stable angina and a myocardial infarction. It is also known as preinfarction angina and acute coronary insufficiency. Onset and characteristics of pain differ for each episode. There is an increasing frequency, duration, and severity of attacks. May occur at rest (Haak et al, 1994; Massie, 1996a; O'Keefe, 1995). |
| Prinzmetal angina | Variant angina. Discomfort occurs at rest and is unpredictable. It is associated with vasospasms of coronary arteries. When pain occurs during sleep, it is associated with REM sleep. It may have a transient ST elevation (Brown & Kloner, 1990; Haak et al, 1994). |
| Syndrome X | Typical presentation of angina but no evidence of coronary artery disease or spasm. Myocardial ischemia due to disease of coronary microcirculation (Brown & Kloner, 1990; Haak et al, 1994; Massie, 1996a). |

*Adapted from Abrams (1991) and Massie (1996a).*

## TABLE 20–12. CANADIAN CARDIOVASCULAR SOCIETY CLASSIFICATION SYSTEM

- Class I: No limits to normal activity, but angina occurs with prolonged exertion
- Class II: Slight limitation on normal activity; angina with walking >2 blocks
- Class III: Marked limitation in normal activity; angina with walking <2 blocks
- Class IV: Severe limitation in normal activity; angina with little activity or at rest

---

section for differential diagnosis). If the patient is experiencing angina, determination of the type and classification will direct the course of action:

1. If the patient meets the definition of unstable angina, hospitalization or a cardiology consult is required.

2. In the patient with chronic stable, severe angina pectoris, the presenting circumstances will direct whether the patient can be treated in the outpatient setting or require hospitalization. If the patient is experiencing more than five episodes of chest pain daily with minimal exertion, hospital evaluation is recommended.

3. In the patient with chronic stable, mild angina pectoris, an outpatient evaluation and initiation of pharmacotherapy when indicated is recommended.

See Drug Tables 205.5, 205.6, 205.7, 206.

## Assessment Needed Prior to Therapy

*History.*  The practitioner should cover the following items with the patient (Arnstein, Buselli, & Rankin, 1996; Brown & Kloner, 1990; Massie, 1996a; O'Keefe, 1995):

- *What precipitates discomfort:* Cover activities that bring on discomfort such as walking up stairs or hills, or other forms of exercise or exertion; past infectious disease with fever; and stress, anxiety, meals, cold air, or smoking. Ask the patient the number of times a week, day, or month the discomfort occurs.

- *Description of discomfort:* This is usually described as discomfort, pressure, heaviness, or even burning or squeezing and may radiate to the left neck, jaw, or epigastrium. Discomfort typically moves from the sternum, to the left shoulder, to the upper arm, and down the fore-

arm to the wrist and fourth and fifth fingers. Radiation of pain may also be to the right in the same pattern, but this is not as frequent as the left. Discomfort lasts 15 s or up to 15 min. Characteristically, the pain is relieved by rest. Pain that can be pointed to with one finger is usually not angina. Levine's sign is the patient describing discomfort using a fist over the sternum. Angina during sleep may be due to increased venous return in the supine position.

- *Measures tried and measures effective in relieving pain:* Angina is suspected if relief of pain occurs within ½–2 min of taking nitroglycerin. Angina is also suspected if nitroglycerin is taken prior to anticipated exertion and no discomfort occurs with the exertion. Relief of esophageal spasm, however, may also occur with nitroglycerine. Relief when leaning forward is more indicative of pericarditis than angina. Discomfort lasting only a few seconds is not usually angina.

- *Risk factors:* Cigarette smoking or a family history of hyperlipidemia, hypertension, heart attacks, and diabetes puts the patient at risk. Additional factors include catecholamines, oral contraceptives, age and gender.

- *Any previous diagnostic tests.*

### Differential diagnosis

- *Neuromuscular origin:* Pain is increased with inspiration and herpes rash; pain occurs with palpation.

- *Gastrointestinal origin:* esophageal involvement, peptic ulcer disease, or gastritis, or gallbladder disease. Pain is usually not related to exertion. Food may decrease or make pain worse. Pain may be relieved with antacids. Pain is often in lower chest.

- *Psychogenic origin:* Pain not related to exertion; hyperventilation present.

- *Pulmonary origin:* Dyspnea, cough, and pleuritic pain of sudden onset, sharp, and exacerbated by inspiration; may or may not be associated with exertion or signs of right ventricular failure. May mimic angina.

- *Cardiovascular origin:* Complete assessment of discomfort is necessary to differentiate types of angina or sharp pain; pain is worse in supine position or pain that is sharp or tearing, often in the back, indicative of pericarditis or dissecting aortic aneurysm.

### Physical examination.

*Physical examination.*  Because of the multiple causes of chest pain, the physical examination is not always conclusive. Therefore, the examination must include many different areas of assessment.

*Cardiovascular examination.*  Elevated systolic and diastolic blood pressure; heart sounds show gallop, apical systolic murmur, $S_4$ heart sound, and arrhythmias, which are typical during an attack. Vital signs, heart sounds, presence of bruits, quality of pulses, and heart size are important parameters for examination.

*Chest and respiratory examination.*  Breath sounds, friction rubs, and signs of hyperinflation are evident with percussion. Perform palpation of anterior ribs, especially at intercostal junctions.

*Spinal examination.*  Palpation of the cervical or thoracic spine may produce severe pain similar to angina. Pain usually occurs on the outer arm and thumb rather than fourth and fifth fingers.

*Abdominal examination.*  Check for epigastric tenderness and right upper quadrant pain.

*Funduscopic examination.*  Examine for changes associated with hypertension or atherosclerosis.

*Laboratory examination.*  Any patient suspected of having CAD needs additional studies to both diagnose CHD and rule out other causes of chest pain (Abrams, 1991; Massie, 1996a).

*Hematologic examination.*  Obtain CBC, chemical profile including lipids, and thyroid profile. Make sure diabetes, hyperlipidemia, anemia, polycythemia, and thyroid abnormalities are not causative factors.

*Other tests.*  Myocardial ischemia is associated with electrical changes. However, the ECG may be normal or may show an old myocardial infarction, ST or T changes, conduction defects, or left ventricular abnormalities. Ischemia may be noted with depressed ST segments, T wave inversion, or ST elevation. These changes occur during an attack. An exercise ECG is the most helpful and noninvasive test. ST depression or chest pain is precipitated by exercise. Exercise testing is indicated for confirmation of angina, to determine the activity limitation and its severity, to assess the prognosis of those with diagnosed CHD, and to evaluate therapeutic response. Ambulatory ECG monitoring may detect silent ischemia. Possible additional tests are stress thallium, coronary angiography, and echocardiogram.

## Patient/Caregiver Information

The most important information for a patient with CHD is recognition of symptoms requiring emergency care. The patient should be instructed to have available sublingual nitroglycerin tablets and to use them when experiencing chest pain. The tablets may or may not produce a stinging sensation under the tongue, but additional doses at 5-min intervals should be based on the continuation of chest pain. The patient should keep the nitroglycerin tablets in the original container and replace them approximately every 6 months if the container is opened or if tablets are exposed to excessive environmental or body heat.

The patient should be instructed about those activities that may precipitate angina. These include activity that places strain on the thoracic or upper extremity muscles such as lifting, walking uphill, and physical activity. The patient may also experience angina without exertion such as following meals or exposure to cold, upon awakening, after strong emotions, and following carbon monoxide inhalation. If sexual intercourse causes discomfort, it should be avoided; patients need to be assured that without discomfort it is perfectly safe. If the patient knows that such an activity will result in chest pain, then the patient can use sublingual nitroglycerin prior to that activity.

## OUTCOMES MANAGEMENT

### Selecting an Appropriate Agent

Selection of drug therapy is made on an individualized basis. The degree and type of angina will direct the need for monotherapy or a combination of nitrates, beta blockers, calcium channel blockers, and/or aspirin (Hutter, 1996).

### Monitoring for Efficacy and Toxicity

*Nitrates.*  Nitrates are effective in treating all forms of angina. The site of action is the peripheral vascular tree, especially the venous and coronary blood vessels. Nitrates can dilate severely atherosclerotic vessels as well. The vasodilation lowers blood pressure, which in turn reduces myocardial wall tension, a major determinant of myocardial oxygen need. This results in a more favorable balance of myocardial oxygen supply and demand.

The sublingual dosage form is effective in treating acute episodes of angina, whereas the long-acting preparations are effective in preventing the development of angina. Monotherapy with sublingual nitroglycerin can be given in patients with less severe and occasional anginal attacks (less than one per day). The dose of sublingual nitroglycerin that decreases blood pressure by 10 mm Hg or heart rate by 10 beats per minute provides an optimum hemodynamic effect (Raehl & Nolan, 1995). The patient will often experience the adverse effects of dizziness, lightheadedness, and headache, but these can be reduced by teaching the patient to sit while taking the nitroglycerin. Headache pain can be managed with acetaminophen. Pain relief should begin in 3–5 min and lasts approximately 30 min. The patient should repeat the dose every 5 min for a total of three doses if pain is not relieved. If the patient is still experiencing angina after three doses or if the patient must repeat the dose every 30–60 min, he or she should be instructed to seek emergency care.

Longer-acting preparations should be considered in patients experiencing more severe and frequent anginal attacks. A variety of dosage forms (ointment, patches, tablets, capsules) are available. Nitrate tolerance can develop with all these forms of nitrates. Therefore, a nitrate-free period of a minimum of 8–12 h each day is necessary to maintain efficacy (Talbert, 1997). Eight hours appears to be sufficient for nitroglycerin, while isosorbide may need 12 h of nitrate-free time (Berkow, 1992a). The nitrate-free period depends on the time of day the patient experiences the least number of anginal attacks (Parker et al, 1983, 1987). When an oral preparation such as isosorbide dinitrate is prescribed, the last dose of the day should not be later than 5:00 P.M. if taking three times a day. If taking twice a day, the doses should be at 7:00 A.M. and 2:00 P.M.

**Beta blockers.**    If the patient continues to experience angina during the nitrate-free period, then a beta blocker or calcium channel blocker can be given. By blocking the beta$_1$ receptors in the heart, beta blockers decrease heart rate, blood pressure, and contractility, with the net effect of reducing myocardial oxygen demand and increasing exercise tolerance. Beta blockers are useful as monotherapy treatment of chronic exertional stable angina or in combination with nitrates and calcium channel blockers. Beta

blockers and nitrates can work in a complementary fashion. The beta blockers can block the reflex tachycardia induced by nitrate therapy, and the nitrates can reduce the left ventricular volume created by the beta blockers. Beta blockers can reduce the risk of postmyocardial reinfarction (Raehl & Nolan, 1995). Careful consideration must be given to using those beta blockers with intrinsic sympathomimetic activity (ISA) and the resultant cardiovascular effects.

Dosing of beta blockers is titrated upward until the resting heart rate is 50–60 beats per minute. When the patient exercises, the maximal heart rate is either limited to 100 beats per minute or no more than 20 beats per minute or 10% over resting heart rate. Most beta blockers are effective in the treatment of angina when dosed no more than twice a day.

Adverse effects of beta blockers are numerous and are an extension of their pharmacodynamics. Beta blockers can produce additional cardiovascular changes of heart failure, bradycardia, heart block, hypotension, and peripheral vasoconstriction with intermittent claudication. Those beta blockers that are not cardioselective or lose this selectivity at higher doses can cause bronchospasm and alteration in glucose metabolism. The lipophilic beta blockers can cause CNS problems such as fatigue and depression.

Patients need to be educated about not abruptly stopping their beta blocker therapy since a buildup of catecholamines can result in an increased load on the heart to the point of myocardial infarction (Olsson et al, 1984). This is especially critical in patients with severe atherosclerosis or unstable angina (Raehl & Nolan, 1995). When a beta blocker needs to be discontinued, a downward reduction in the dose is required. There is no set rate for this reduction, but two alternatives are (1) to reduce the dose by half every 3–4 days, decrease the frequency to daily every 3–4 days, and hold at daily for 3–4 days before stopping (Raehl & Nolan, 1995); or (2) decrease the dose over 2 days while using the patient's heart rate as a guideline (Talbert, 1997).

**Calcium channel blockers.**    The calcium channel blockers are divided into four types. Type I consists of verapamil and diltiazem. The dihydropyridine derivatives, which include nifedipine, amlodipine, felodipine, isradipine, and nicardipine, are type II. The type III agents include cinnarizine and flunarizine, but these are currently not available. These agents have no effect on the calcium movement in the myocardium but rather vasodilate the peripheral smooth muscle. Type IV calcium channel blockers include bepridil. This agent blocks both the fast sodium and the slow calcium channels of the heart. Bepridil has been approved for the treatment of chronic stable angina as second-line therapy after the traditional agents have been tried and have failed. The reason for the reservation in the use of this agent is its quinidine-like effect and the possibility of causing agranulocytosis.

The type II agents are preferred because of their vascular selectivity, peripheral and coronary, when compared to the type I agents verapamil and diltiazem, and their minimal activity on myocardial conduction and contractility. Of the type II agents, nicardipine has the most vaso-selectivity followed by nifedipine, isradipine, and amlodipine with slightly less. Felodipine has the least vasoselectivity of this group. Not all of these agents have a FDA-approved indication (refer to Drug Table 205.6).

Calcium channel blockers can be added to nitrates and/or beta blockers (cautiously with verapamil or diltiazem) for additional benefit in patients remaining symptomatic. A calcium channel blocker is especially beneficial in patients with coexisting hypertension. Calcium channel blocker adverse events of concern are heart block, left ventricle dysfunction, bradycardia, and hypotension.

A new class of calcium channel blockers is now available. Mibefradil is a nondihydropyridine calcium channel blocker with elements of phenylethylamino and benzothiazepin structures. The premise for mibefradil is that it is a selective T-channel calcium blocker, whereas the current calcium channel blockers are L-channel calcium blockers. The difference in the blockade of L and T channels is that the L channel remains open for a long time following membrane depolarization, whereas the time the T channel is open is shorter or transient. Clinically, this translates into the following actions of mibefradil: it increases coronary blood flow about 250 times more than its decrease in myocardial contractility (verapamil's action is essentially equal); it lowers blood pressure and slightly reduces heart rate; it does not stimulate the neurohormonal system; it is not involved in cardiac excitation and therefore does not generate an action potential upstroke; it participates in the pacemaker activity of the sinoatrial node; and it plays a role in activating smooth muscle contraction (Gums, 1997).

**Aspirin.** Because of aspirin's ability to bind irreversibly to platelets and inhibit their aggregation, it has been suggested that the use of a single dose of aspirin each day may prevent the genesis of unstable angina or myocardial infarction. The daily dose of 80–325 mg may be given prophylactically in patients with coronary artery disease (Berkow, 1992a).

The following summarizes the pharmacotherapy care plans for each type of angina:

- *Stable angina:* Begin with nitroglycerin SL monotherapy in patients with less frequent angina. If the anginal attacks increase in frequency and severity, then the addition of a long-acting nitrate and/or beta blocker therapy is indicated. Beta blockers are preferred in patients who have had a myocardial infarction. Nitrates are the alternative when beta blockers are contraindicated, or a long-acting nitrate and a beta blocker can be considered for their synergistic activity as well as the fact that each offsets the adverse effects of the other. The nitrate will have to be dosed to avoid the development of tolerance. If the patient continues to be symptomatic, then maximizing the doses of the current agents is indicated until they are effective or until side effects prevent further escalation of the dose. Alternatively, additional drug therapy such as a calcium channel blocker can be started. Aspirin therapy (325 mg/day—enteric-coated in patients experiencing gastrointestinal irritation) should be given to patients who have a history of myocardial infarction. If the patient is intolerant to aspirin, then ticlopidine can be given. All therapy is titrated to the desired hemodynamic effect while minimizing the incidence of side effects.

- *Unstable angina:* If a patient presents to an ambulatory clinic with symptoms of unstable angina, initiate treatment with sublingual nitroglycerin and aspirin and then refer either to a cardiologist if low risk (new onset, <20 min in length, no pain at rest, normal or unchanged ECG) or transfer to an emergency room.

- *Variant angina:* Nitrates and calcium channel blockers appear to be effective in the treatment of variant (Prinzmetal's or vasospastic) angina. Sublingual nitroglycerin can provide symptomatic relief and should be encouraged. The cardioselective calcium channel blockers amlodipine, nicardipine, and nifedipine can reduce morbidity and mortality.

- *Syndrome X:* Syndrome X is also known as microvascular ischemia. There appears to be an imbalance between the inherent vasoconstrictor and vasodilator responses of the vessel. It is thought that there may be a link between this type of ischemia and mental stress.

No drug therapy is especially effective in the treatment of syndrome X. The calcium channel blockers and nitrates may provide some benefit but are not always successful. Although the beta blockers are less effective and may actually aggravate the condition through unopposed alpha stimulation, they may be able to block the norepinephrine release caused by the stress. The current recommendation is to use SL nitroglycerin for acute pain relief along with a calcium channel blocker while avoiding environmental and dietary stimulants.

## Follow-up Recommendations

Frequency of monitoring depends on the individual and the severity of the CHD. Consultation with a cardiologist is important to establish a treatment plan. Patients at high risk should be seen as frequently as every 2 weeks.

If a patient has unstable angina, hospitalization is necessary. When it is deemed safe to treat on an outpatient basis, follow-up within 72 h is generally essential. During follow-up, an ECG, evaluation of vital signs, another physical examination including heart sounds, and a hematocrit level should be done.

Education is important for anyone with angina and should cover the following items:

1. When to seek medical intervention for changes in pain frequency, intensity, and duration.
2. Importance of following the medical regimen.
3. Importance of smoking cessation and positive reinforcement for successes.
4. Exercise plan.
5. Diet.
6. Activities including driving, sexual relations, and exertion.
7. Use of nitroglycerin. Use when angina present, and repeat twice every 5 min if needed. If there is still no relief, seek medical intervention.
8. Stress reduction techniques.

Frequency of follow-up is individualized according to patient symptoms and the need for professional supportive management. At each follow-up visit:

1. Evaluate exercise, diet, smoking cessation, and stress reduction.
2. Discuss the medical regimen and the patient's ability to comply with the program.
3. Discuss medications and explore possible side effects.
4. The use of an ECG for monitoring is controversial. If the patient is having an asymptomatic MI (silent), the management strategies are the same as previously stated. If there is an acute MI, the ECG is indicated by the symptoms.
5. Do a blood chemistry and CBC.
6. Do a prothrombin time with INR if the patient is taking warfarin.
7. Monitor vital signs and heart and lung sounds.
8. Assess for development of additional risk factors, and inquire about any additional medications including over-the-counter drugs.

## MITRAL VALVE PROLAPSE

Mitral valve prolapse, also called floppy mitral valve, is a very common abnormality, particularly in young women. Although it was once thought to be the result of rheumatic heart disease, research indicates that it is likely of genetic origin and associated with other congenital connective tissue abnormalities such as Marfan's syndrome or simply an isolated abnormality. Abnormal volume regulation, autonomic nervous system function, and neuroendocrine function may accompany mitral valve prolapse.

Mitral valve prolapse is present when the anterior and posterior leaflets (cusps) of the mitral valve bulge or balloon into the atrium during systole. The abnormal function is due to thickened, enlarged, scalloped, and sometimes elongated leaflets. Mitral regurgitation, the most common physical finding, occurs when the abnormality is sufficient to allow blood to leak into the atrium.

Although the condition is common, symptoms are either nonexistent or vague. Most patients have no limit on physical function and frequently are more troubled psychologically by the diagnosis. Symptoms include nonspecific chest pain, palpitations, light-headedness, syncope, fatigue (particularly in the morning), lethargy, weakness, panic attacks, and anxiety. The variety of symptoms and the number seem unrelated to the extent of the prolapse. However, palpitations, chest pain, syncope, fatigue, and dyspnea are associated with altered autonomic function. The condition is usually nonprogressive. Complications occur if there is significant mitral regurgitation or secondary disease states. If there is progressive mitral regurgitation, it is usually due to dilatation of the mitral annulus or rupture of the chordal structures (Fortuin, 1996).

## SPECIFIC CONSIDERATIONS FOR PHARMACOTHERAPY

### When Drug Therapy Is Needed

Pharmacotherapy for mitral valve prolapse may be indicated for the following medical reasons: (1) preventing recurrence of rheumatic fever, (2) preventing infective endocarditis, (3) preventing thromboembolism, and (4) managing atrial arrhythmias.

Although the incidence of bacterial endocarditis is not positively known, the best medical treatment when infection occurs still has a 3–40% mortality rate (Chenoweth & Burket, 1997). Therefore, prophylactic antibiotic coverage is warranted in patients who have mitral valve prolapse. However, the American Heart Association recommends antibiotics in patients with regurgitation and not in the absence of regurgitation. Individuals who have a mitral valve prolapse associated with thickening and/or redundancy of the valve leaflets may be at increased risk for bacterial endocarditis, particularly men ≥45 years of age.

The AHA (Dajani et al, 1997) recommends antibiotic prophylaxis for the following cardiac conditions and medical procedures:

- Cardiac conditions (high risk):
  Prosthetic cardiac valves, including bioprosthetic and hemograft valves

  Previous infective endocarditis

  Complex cyanotic congenital heart disease including single ventrical states, transposition of the great arteries, and tetralogy of Fallot

  Surgically constructed pulmonary shunts or conduits

- Cardiac conditions (moderate risk):
  Most other congenital cardiac malformations, including patent ductus arteriosus, ventricular septal defect, and coarctation of the aorta

  Rheumatic and other acquired valvular dysfunctions, even after surgical repair

  Mitral valve prolapse with valvular regurgitation and/or thickened leaflets

  Hypertrophic cardiomyopathy

  Medical procedures:

  Dental procedures known to induce gingival or mucosal bleeding, including routine professional cleaning

Tonsillectomy and/or adenoidectomy

Surgical operations that involve intestinal or respiratory mucosa

Bronchoscopy with a rigid bronchoscope

Sclerotherapy for esophageal varices

Esophageal dilation

Endoscopic retrograde cholangiography with biliary obstruction

Biliary tract surgery

Urethral dilation or cystoscopy

Urinary tract surgery, including prostate surgery

### Short- and Long-Term Goals of Pharmacotherapy

The immediate benefit of prophylactic antibiotics is the prevention of bacterial endocarditis in susceptible individuals since bacterial endocarditis is associated with significant mortality and long-term morbidity. The use of pharmacotherapy in the prevention of thromboembolism or management of atrial arrhythmias needs to be individualized based on the overall status of the patient.

### Nonpharmacologic Therapy

Most patients are asymptomatic and do not require treatment. Complications usually occur after age 50, at which point surgery may be indicated. There generally is no restriction on activity. Vigorous exercise and sports are only restricted if there is another associated abnormality or if there is a decrease in intravascular volume associated with the prolapse and the person may experience syncope with exercise.

Adequate salt intake is indicated in patients with associated intravascular volume depletion, any abnormal renin-aldosterone response to volume depletion, or alterations in the autonomic nervous system (the patient has symptoms of chest pain, palpitations, fatigue, dyspnea, anxiety, or panic attacks).

Avoid caffeine, alcohol, and cigarettes if palpitations are present. (Carabello, 1991, 1993; Massie, 1996a).

### Time Frame for Initiating Pharmacotherapy

For prophylactic antibiotics to have a beneficial effect, serum and tissue levels must have reached peak levels prior to the dental or surgical procedure. All of the oral antibiotic regimens are given 1 hour prior to the procedure. When designed to prevent thromboembolism, therapy should be started in patients with documented systemic embolism or chronic or paroxysmal atrial fibrillation. Management of atrial arrhythmias may be necessary when paroxysms are frequent or reversion to normal sinus rhythm cannot be attained (Hancock, 1996b).

See Drug Tables 102, 202.

## Assessment Needed Prior to Therapy

*History.* Because many patients often are asymptomatic and any symptoms are vague and may not indicate a problem of cardiovascular origin, the history may be inconclusive. Inquire about functional limitations. Younger patients may experience palpitations, effort intolerance, or light-headedness due to hyperresponsiveness to an endogenous sympathetic stimulus (Fortuin, 1996). Inquire about any family history of valvular disease or disorders of connective tissue.

*Physical examination.* Cardiac auscultation will be the key to diagnosis because valvular disease causes murmurs. Listen for the characteristic midsystolic click. Clicks may be multiple and may be followed by a midsystolic murmur or a late systolic crescendo murmur. The click and/or murmur may vary from one examination to another, from one position to another, and with temperature, respirations, and time of day. Multiple clicks are possible and may indicate a higher degree of prolapse and regurgitation. Auscultate in the standing position because the abnormal sounds are accentuated when standing. A pansystolic murmur may indicate significant mitral regurgitation possibly caused by a ruptured chordae tendineae.

In checking the skeletal system, observe for long arms (longer than usual for height) and thoracic narrowing or other chest wall abnormalities (typical of Marfan's syndrome).

*Diagnostic measures.* The ECG may be normal. The chest x-ray will be normal. The echocardiogram is the most useful test to confirm physical findings and will also evaluate other valves. It should not be used as a routine screen since most mitral valve prolapses are benign.

## Patient/Caregiver Information

Any patient with mitral valve prolapse will need to take precautions prior to dental and surgical procedures (outlined in the previous section).

Written instructions should include the types of procedures and the importance of informing the provider of the presence of mitral valve prolapse.

Regular exercise and activities usually should be encouraged. If the patient experiences syncope with exercise or if there is another limiting factor, exercise should not be vigorous and competitive sports limited.

## OUTCOMES MANAGEMENT

### Selecting an Appropriate Agent

The American Heart Association (Dajani et al, 1997) recommends the following prophylaxis regimens for the prevention of infective endocarditis:

*Dental, upper respiratory tract, or esophageal procedures*
- Routine
  Amoxicillin:
    Adults: 2 g PO 1 h before procedure
    Children: 50 mg/kg PO 1 h before procedure
- Penicillin-allergic patients
  Clindamycin:
    Adults: 600 mg PO 1 h before procedure
    Children: 20 mg/kg 1 h before procedure

  OR

  Cephalexin or cefadroxil:
    Adults: 2 g PO 1 h before procedure
    Children: 50 mg/kg PO 1 h before procedure

  OR

  Azithromycin/clarithromycin:
    Adults: 500 mg PO 1 h before procedure
    Children: 15 mg/kg PO 1 h before procedure
- Patients unable to take oral medications
  Ampicillin:
    Adults: 2 g IM or IV 30 min before procedure
    Children: 50 mg/kg IM or IV 30 min before procedure
- Penicillin-allergic patients unable to take oral medications
  Clindamycin:
    Adults: 600 mg IV 30 min before procedure
    Children: 20 mg/kg IV 30 min before procedure

  OR

  Cefazolin:
    Adults: 1 g IM or IV 30 min before procedure
    Children: 25 mg/kg IM or IV 30 min before procedure

## Genitourinary/gastrointestinal procedures (excluding esophageal procedures)

- High-risk patients

  Adults: Ampicillin 2 g IV or IM plus gentamicin 1.5 mg/kg (maximum 120 mg) IV 30 min before procedure; amoxicillin 1 g PO or ampicillin 1 g IV 6 h after initial dose

  Children: Ampicillin 50 mg/kg IM or IV (maximum 2 g) plus gentamicin 1.5 mg/kg 30 min before procedure; 6 h later, ampicillin 25 mg/kg IV or IM or amoxicillin 25 mg/kg PO

- High-risk penicillin-allergic patients

  Adults: Vancomycin 1 g IV over 1–2 h plus gentamicin 1.5 mg/kg (maximum 120 mg) IV or IM; complete injection/infusion 30 min before procedure

  Children: Vancomycin 20 mg/kg IV over 1–2 h plus gentamicin 1.5 mg/kg IV or IM; complete injection/infusion 30 min before procedure

- Moderate-risk patients

  Adults: Amoxicillin 2 g PO 1 h before procedure or ampicillin 2 g IM or IV 30 min before procedure

  Children: Amoxicillin 50 mg/kg PO 1 h before procedure or ampicillin 50 mg/kg IM or IV 30 min before procedure

- Moderate-risk penicillin-allergic patients

  Adults: Vancomycin 1 g IV over 1–2 h; complete infusion 30 min before procedure

  Children: Vancomycin 20 mg/kg IV over 1–2 h; complete infusion 30 min before procedure

  NOTE: Total pediatric dose should not exceed adult dose.

Warfarin pharmacotherapy should be prescribed whenever the patient has had a previous episode of embolism or atrial fibrillation of paroxysmal or chronic nature and either rheumatic mitral valve disease, mitral annular calcification, or mitral valve prolapse. Warfarin should be dosed to achieve an INR of 2.0–3.0 (warfarin dosing algorithms are presented in the section on arrhythmias). Patients who have experienced a transient ischemic attack (TIA) of unknown etiology are candidates for 325 mg/day of aspirin therapy or ticlopidine 250 mg twice a day. If the TIAs continue, long-term anticoagulation with warfarin should be prescribed. In patients in whom warfarin is not tolerated, aspirin doses of 975 mg/day or ticlopidine 250 mg b.i.d. can be prescribed (Hancock, 1996b).

The most common arrhythmia is atrial fibrillation. The atrial fibrillation may be paroxysmal or become chronic and as such is often permanent. During paroxysmal episodes, countershock or quinidine therapy may cause reversion to normal sinus rhythm. Long-term therapy with antiarrhythmic agents such as quinidine and disopyramide may help maintain sinus rhythm, whereas many patients may have permanent fibrillation (Hancock, 1996b).

## Monitoring for Efficacy and Toxicity

Refer to the anti-infective agents in Drug Table 102 for a description of pharmacodynamics and pharmacokinetics and symptoms of toxicity and adverse reaction.

## Follow-up Recommendations

1. Repeat echocardiograms yearly if the patient has mitral systolic murmurs, increased left ventricular size, or thickening of the leaflets (cusps) because these complications are most common. Echocardiograms are indicated as the person ages since clinically significant regurgitation occurs with age.

2. Yearly visits include a complete history of symptoms associated with mitral valve prolapse and cardiac auscultation to detect additional clicks or new murmurs.

3. With age, more complications may occur, especially in males over 50. History and physical examination should update information on the following conditions: TIA, stroke, CHF, syncope, and arrhythmias. (Carabello, 1993; Chapman, 1994; Fontana, 1991; Haak et al, 1994).

## HYPERLIPIDEMIA

To understand both coronary artery disease and peripheral vascular disease, it is important to understand lipids, lipid metabolism, and the relationship between lipids and atherosclerosis (see the section on coronary heart disease).

The blood lipids, carried on lipoproteins, are mainly cholesterol and triglyceride. Cholesterol, essential for the manufacture and repair of plasma proteins, is part of all cell membranes, bile salts, and steroid hormones. Cholesterol originates endogenously through synthesis in the liver or exogenously from the diet. Dietary cholesterol comes only from foods of animal origin. Cholesterol is carried in the blood by very low density (VLDL), low density (LDL), and high density (HDL) lipoproteins.

Triglycerides are the main component of VLDLs. Triglycerides, derived from dietary fat, are needed to transfer food energy into cells. The majority of triglycerides are stored in tissues as glycerol, fatty acids, and monoglyceroids. The liver is responsible for converting them back into triglycerides. Thus, triglycerides are considered stored energy.

The process of cholesterol synthesis and transport is complex. Density is synonymous with the amount of triglyceride. However, it is an inverse relationship. The higher the triglyceride level, the lower the density of the lipoprotein. The largest lipoproteins, VLDL, carry cholesterol to the tissues and contain the most triglyceride. The lipoproteins are gradually transformed into smaller and smaller particles: VLDL to ILDL (intermediate LDL) to LDL and HDL. The smaller the particle, the higher the density and the lower the triglyceride level. The VLDL and LDL cholesterol are thought to deposit on the arterial wall and be a determinant of atherosclerosis. Thus, a high triglyceride level should correspond to a high VLDL and LDL.

The large low-density lipoproteins are transformed into smaller higher-density lipoproteins by lipoprotein lipase. This enzyme is produced in muscles and capillaries of adipose tissue. The level increases during exercise, which also increases the amount of HDL. HDL plays a significant role in cholesterol and triglyceride metabolism. HDL carries the excess cholesterol back to the liver to be excreted and may prohibit the uptake of LDL by the cells.

LDL is considered a precursor to atherosclerosis. HDL is considered protective, but the exact mechanism is unknown. Studies are exploring a variety of etiologies and treatments for atherosclerosis. These include: (1) oxidized LDL particles are more atherogenic than nonoxidized particles; (2) the role of antioxidant vitamins C and E and beta carotene in preventing the oxidization of LDL; (3) the function of estrogen as an antioxidant; (4) the number or size of the VLDL and LDL particles; (5) genetic disorders; (6) the role of lipids in thrombus formation independent of atherosclerotic plaques; and (7) the role of Lp(a), an apolipoprotein in the development of atherosclerosis (Scanu, 1991).

In summary, cholesterol, in the form of VLDL, LDL, and HDL, has major implications for the development of heart disease, particularly coronary artery disease. Lowering total cholesterol, and particularly LDL, decreases the incidence of coronary heart disease, may slow the progression of atherosclerosis, and may even reverse atherosclerotic changes (Braunwald et al, 1994; W. S. Aronow et al, 1995, 1996; W. Aronow et al, 1996). Lowering LDL and raising HDL are significant in reducing risk factors in the development of coronary heart disease.

## SPECIFIC CONSIDERATIONS FOR PHARMACOTHERAPY

### When Drug Therapy Is Needed

Lifestyle modifications should be the first line of management although drug therapy may be the best option for patients. Practitioners are fully aware that treatment of hyperlipidemia can result in a reduced risk of coronary heart disease death and nonfatal MI. Lowering the LDL using whatever strategies that produce the best outcome is the goal. However, the dietary restrictions of decreasing fats may prove unpalatable for some. Others may be compliant with dietary and exercise measures, yet continue to have elevated lipid levels. The practitioner's role must include educating the patient and the patient's family about the importance of lowering LDL and increasing HDL levels.

### Short- and Long-term Goals of Pharmacotherapy

The long-term goal of therapy is to prevent the progression of the atherosclerotic process, thereby decreasing morbidity and mortality from coronary heart disease and arterial peripheral vascular diseases.

Short-term goals must be aimed at identification of populations at risk and primary prevention. Individuals with high cholesterol, high LDL, and low HDL, but with no indication of coronary heart disease, need to be treated to try to prevent onset of disease. In addition, individuals with manifestations of CHD need to begin treatment to prevent the progression of the atherosclerotic process.

The goal of therapy is to bring LDL and HDL to within normal limits as well as to lower total cholesterol to within normal limits. LDL should be reduced to as low as possible, and in patients with established coronary heart disease this means to less than 100 mg/dL. Although numerical goals are set, a 1% reduction in total cholesterol is associated with a 2–3% reduction in CHD, and any reduction in LDL is a positive step (W. Aronow et al, 1996; Davey Smith,

Song, & Sheldon, 1993; Gordon et al, 1989; Hebert, Gazaino, & Hennekens, 1995; Peto, Yusuf, & Collins, 1991). One additional factor to consider when developing a therapeutic plan is the ratio of cholesterol to HDL. Generally, the higher the cholesterol:HDL ratio, the higher the risk for development of atherosclerosis and coronary heart diseases. Therefore, it is important to decrease the ratio between total cholesterol and HDL.

## Nonpharmacologic Therapy

*Diet.* Dietary changes begin when LDL is over 130–190 mg/dL on one to two fasting measures and cholesterol is 200–300 mg/dL. Because the majority of cholesterol enters the system via the diet, dietary changes may decrease cholesterol and LDL. Dietary management is delineated as a Step I or a Step II diet. The Step I recommendation is to decrease the dietary fat intake to less than 30% of the total calories. In addition, daily saturated fat intake is to be less than 10% of the calories with no more than 300 mg of cholesterol. Polyunsaturated fats, once thought more acceptable, are now found to decrease HDL and are therefore also restricted. Olive oil and canola oil do not decrease HDL, and their use should be promoted (Browner, 1996; Ramsey, Yeo, & Jackson, 1991).

The Step II diet is more restrictive. It should be started in anyone with established coronary heart disease or when the Step I diet has less than desired benefit. In the Step II diet, fat is restricted to 20% of calories, limiting saturated fat to 7%, and 200 mg of cholesterol per day.

Fiber is also implicated in the reduction of cholesterol. Soluble fiber, as found in oat bran, broccoli, apples, beans, and grapefruit, has been found modestly effective in decreasing cholesterol. Psyllium powders are also a source of soluble fiber. Although soluble fiber may be useful as part of the dietary management of hyperlipidemia, it must be approached with caution. If oat bran is used in baked goods containing oils and eaten with butter, the value of the oat bran is lost. Also, psyllium and high-fiber foods cause abdominal bloating and flatus, which may decrease adherence to dietary changes.

Alcohol, in moderation, is slightly effective in raising the HDL level. However, it is important to advise patients about the detrimental effects of alcohol such as obesity and alcohol abuse.

*Exercise.* Exercise in conjunction with weight loss may decrease LDL and increase HDL (Browner, 1996; Stone, 1990).

## Time Frame for Initiating Pharmacotherapy

The decision to proceed to drug therapy and the desired goals are based on the National Cholesterol Education Program (NCEP) guidelines (Expert Panel on Detection, Evaluation, and Treatment of High Blood Cholesterol in Adults, 1993) (see Table 20–13).

In the authors' opinion, drug therapy should be considered for patients particularly if they have an LDL between 100 and 130 mg/dL and already have had a cardiovascular event. A cardiovascular event suggests that the LDL level for this patient is indeed a risk factor for them.

The decision to begin drug therapy in patients with hypertriglyceridemia is based on the NCEP guidelines (Expert Panel, 1993) (see Table 20–14).

See Drug Table 204.

## Assessment Needed Prior to Therapy

Patients with hyperlipidemia are asymptomatic until pathologic changes associated with high cholesterol and high LDL occur. Therefore, it is important to assess risk factors for cardiovascu-

## TABLE 20–13. DRUG THERAPY INITIATION ACCORDING TO LDL LEVELS

| For Individuals With | Add Drug Therapy If LDL Is | LDL Goals |
|---|---|---|
| No CHD and with <2 other risk factors | ≥190 mg/dL after ≥6 months of diet (consider shorter diet trial if LDL is ≥220 mg/dL) | <160 mg/dL |
| No CHD but with ≥2 other CHD risk factors | ≥160 mg/dL after ≥6 months of diet (consider shorter diet trial if LDL is ≥220 mg/dL) | <130 mg/dL |
| Definite CHD or other atherosclerotic disease | ≥130 mg/dL after 6–12 weeks of Step 2 diet | ≤100 mg/dL |

*Adapted from Expert Panel (1993).*

## TABLE 20-14. DRUG THERAPY INITIATION ACCORDING TO TRIGLYCERIDE LEVEL

| Category | Triglyceride Level | Treatment |
|----------|-------------------|-----------|
| Definite | >400 mg/dL | Diet plus drugs |
| Borderline | 200–399 mg/dL | Diet, drugs if other risk factors |
| Normal | <200 mg/dL | Diet |

*Adapted from Expert Panel (1993).*

lar disease (Browner, 1996; NCEP Adult Treatment Panel II, 1993; Woodhead, 1996).

### History

**GENETIC PREDISPOSITION.**   A family history of cardiovascular events is an important factor in hyperlipidemia and coronary heart disease.

**SMOKING.**   This is a definite risk factor in all cardiovascular problems. In addition, smoking cessation may raise the HDL level.

**DIET.**   Obesity and an excess of fats in the diet are major risk factors for coronary heart disease. Excess fat is related to low HDL as well as high LDL. A nutritional assessment is crucial to successful dietary intervention. When exploring dietary habits, always inquire as to amounts and frequency of intake of foods. The following MEDIC may be useful in assessment and teaching (Browner, 1996; Ramsey et al, 1991; Stone, 1990):

- M = meats: Be sure to identify kind of meat, amount, and frequency
- E = egg yolk: Identify the number of eggs per day or week and the type and number of baked goods.
- D = dairy products: Ask about milk, including number of glasses and fat content, as well as cheese. Be sure to ask about cheese in cooking.
- I = invisible fat: This includes fats such as those found in nondairy creamers and baked goods.
- C = cooking oils: This includes table fats and snacks. Be sure to inquire about the type of oil and snacks.

**EXERCISE.**   A sedentary lifestyle contributes to lower HDL. The patient should be asked about type, duration, and frequency of exercise.

**SECONDARY CAUSES.**   Other causes may be responsible for the hyperlipidemia and therefore should be assessed. Included are:

- Obesity
- Diabetes
- Hypothyroidism
- Nephrotic syndrome
- Renal insufficiency
- Obstructive liver disease
- Cushing's disease
- Medications such as estrogen, oral contraceptives, steroids, thiazide, and beta blockers without ISA

**Physical examination.**   Unless the individual has diagnosed heart disease, there are few physical findings related to hyperlipidemia. A complete physical examination may reveal cardiovascular disease. However, laboratory testing probably is the best screening and diagnostic technique available.

### Laboratory screening

**CHOLESTEROL LEVEL.**   Anyone with diagnosed symptomatic cardiovascular disease or risk factors should be screened for elevated lipids. Baseline levels should be established in patients at risk of coronary heart disease within the next 10 years. This would include men over 35 and women over 45. Because hyperlipidemia is common and asymptomatic, the acceptable standard of practice ranges from dietary changes to routine screening. Laboratory screening includes total cholesterol, LDL, HDL, and triglyceride levels. If LDL is high, obtain at least one or two levels with the patient fasting (Sox, 1993).

**HYPOTHYROID PROFILE.**   Hypothyroidism may cause hyperlipidemia.

**CBC AND CHEMICAL PROFILE.**   These tests identify liver function and kidney function, as well as screening for diabetes (Browner, 1996).

### Patient/Caregiver Information

Patient compliance is a definite factor. During the asymptomatic period, the patient may not be able to justify changes in diet and activity or the expense of antilipidemic medications. Education on lifestyle modification techniques to minimize the side effects of medication and utilization of allied health professionals such as dieticians and pharmacists to reinforce the information is critical for patient understanding and compliance. As with many chronic problems, a case manager may be helpful to assist the practitioner in coordination of resources to reinforce education.

## OUTCOMES MANAGEMENT

### Selecting an Appropriate Agent

Pharmacotherapy for hyperlipidemia involves matching the lipid disorder with the best agent. Other considerations include the existence of concomitant disease states. Several treatment algorithms are available to assist the practitioner along with the NCEP guidelines. The NCEP guidelines recognize bile acid sequestrates, nicotinic acid, and statins as the major drug categories in the treatment of hyperlipidemias (Expert Panel, 1993). A simple treatment algorithm consists of the following:

- *Hypercholesterolemia:* bile acid resins (BAR), niacin, or statins
- *Mixed hyperlipidemia:* niacin or statins; possibly fibric acids
- *Hypertriglyceridemia:* niacin or fibric acids

If the response is inadequate, then a second agent is added or an alternative agent is used.

A more complicated NCEP treatment algorithm is based on the type of lipid disorder and recommends either single-drug treatment or combination therapy (Expert Panel, 1993) (see Table 20–15).

### Monitoring for Efficacy and Toxicity

***Statins.*** The statins (atorvastatin, fluvastatin, lovastatin, pravastatin, simvastatin) are HMG-CoA reductase inhibitors. The inhibition of this enzyme reduces the biosynthesis of cholesterol. This results in lowered LDL and triglyceride (TG) levels and elevated HDL levels. The effects of the statins are dose-dependent (Bradford et al, 1991; Jones et al, 1991; Scandinavian Simvastatin Survival Study Group, 1994). A substantial effect is seen with low doses, and only small gains are seen as the dose is increased. Dosage adjustments can be made very 4 weeks with laboratory studies performed just prior to next possible adjustment. To improve the efficacy of all the statins except atorvastatin, the patient should take the dose in the evening. The serum levels of the statins coincide with the nighttime increase in cholesterol biosynthesis. Atorvastatin appears to have equal efficacy whether taken in the morning or evening.

Atorvastatin has a greater LDL cholesterol–lowering potential than the other agents at the lowest daily dose. Atorvastatin 10 mg has low-

## TABLE 20–15.  DRUG OF CHOICE: RECOMMENDATIONS FOR LIPID DISORDERS

| Lipid Disorder | Drug of Choice | Combination Therapy |
|---|---|---|
| Polygenic hypercholesterolemia with desirable TG and HDL | BAR, niacin, statin, estrogen (post-menopausal women) | BAR-niacin, BAR-statin, niacin-statin |
| Familial hypercholesterolemia with desirable TG and HDL | Statin, BAR, niacin | As above |
| Mixed hyperlipidemia in non-diabetics (including LDL and TG) | Niacin, statin, gemfibrozil | Niacin-statin, statin-gemfibrozil, niacin-BAR, niacin-gemfibrozil |
| Mixed hyperlipidemia in diabetics (including LDL and TG) | Statin, gemfibrozil | Statin-gemfibrozil, statin-BAR, gemfibrozil-BAR |
| Polygenic hypercholesterolemia with isolated low HDL | Niacin, statin, estrogen (postmenopausal) | Statin-niacin |

*Adapted from Expert Panel (1993).*

ered LDL cholesterol by 39% compared to lovastatin 20 mg at 24%, simvastatin 5 mg at 24%, pravastatin 10 mg at 22%, and fluvastatin 20 mg at 25%. At the upper dose per day, atorvastatin lowered LDL by 60% compared to 34–40% for the others and triglycerides by 37% compared to 11–24% for the others. The effect on HDL was very similar (Kellick et al, 1997). If switching to atorvastatin is considered, begin with 10 mg per day regardless of the dose of the current HMG-CoA reductase inhibitor.

The statins are shown to slow progression of atherosclerotic lesions, resulting in fewer CHD events along with a good safety profile (Brown et al, 1990). Although side effects are uncommon, patients may complain of GI symptoms and headache. Hepatotoxicity and myopathy are more serious side effects. Baseline LFTs should be performed and repeated every 6–8 weeks during the first year or if patient is symptomatic to screen for elevations in transaminase enzymes. Recently the FDA approved monitoring for simvastatin of baseline LFTs and then semiannually only for the first year of treatment or until 1 year after the last elevation in dose. Levels three times the upper normal limit may occur and appear to be dose-dependent (Bradford et al, 1991). However, LFTs return to normal when the statin is discontinued. Myopathy is suspected when a patient complains of muscle aches, soreness, or weakness and is confirmed when the CPK is greater than 10 times the upper limit of normal.

Patients should be educated on the need for lovastatin to be taken with the evening meal to increase bioavailability, whereas pravastatin, simvastatin, and fluvastatin should be taken at bedtime. Again, atorvastatin can be taken without regard to meals or time of day.

### Bile acid resins (sequestrates).

The two BARs are cholestyramine and colestipol. These medications are anion exchange agents that bind bile acids, interrupting the recycling of bile acids through the enterohepatic circulation. The hepatocytes are stimulated to convert cholesterol into bile acids. The reduced concentration of cholesterol stimulates LDL receptor synthesis, which leads to the removal of circulating LDL, and thus reduced blood levels. The BAR mechanism is synergistic with other medications of different actions.

The BARs have numerous gastrointestinal side effects, such as nausea, bloating, epigastric fullness, constipation, and flatulence, that may affect patient compliance. Patient education on the importance of increased fluid intake (not waiting for the thirst stimulus) and fiber intake are important. A technique of mixing the powder with pulpy juices and swallowing with minimal air intake may help reduce the GI problems.

Because the BARs are exchange resins, there is an increased chance for drugs and vitamins to bind if taken within 4 h of the resin. Therefore, such drugs as niacin, digoxin, warfarin, thyroxine, thiazide diuretics, beta blockers, and any other anionic drugs need to be taken 1 hour before or 4 hours after the resin.

### Niacin.

Niacin lowers all serum lipids when administered in high doses because it reduces the production of VLDL particles by the liver. This reduction of VLDL, and consequently LDL, is a result of inhibition of lipolysis with decreased free fatty acids in plasma, decreased hepatic esterification of TG, a possible direct effect on the hepatic production of apolipoprotein B, and a reduction in the synthesis of apolipoprotein A [Lp(A)].

Doses of 1200–1500 mg/day are necessary to reduce TG and raise HCL. Doses of niacin often are 2000–3000 mg/day to lower LDL levels (McKenney et al, 1994). Doses of niacin should be started low and titrated slowly. Begin with a dose of 200–250 mg per day in divided dosages, and then increase by 200–250 mg per day every 3–7 days. At the large amounts, the majority of patients will experience at least one of the side effects of vasodilation, flushing, itching or headache. A 325-mg aspirin tablet given 30 min prior to the morning dose of niacin can reduce the symptoms. It is thought the side effects are mediated through prostaglandins. To minimize any GI side effects, the niacin may be taken with food.

The greatest concern with the use of niacin is hepatoxicity. This side effect is almost exclusively associated with sustained-release products and appears to be dose-dependent at doses greater than 1500 mg/day. The use of a crystalline form of niacin is associated with a lower incidence of hepatoxicity. Liver function tests should be performed at baseline and then every 6–8 weeks the first year or whenever the patient is symptomatic. Of note, the sustained-release products are classified as dietary supplements, not as drugs under the watchful eye of the FDA. Many patients may already be taking a form of niacin on their own, and the possibility should be explored when taking a medication history.

***Fibric acids.***   The fibric acids, clofibrate, fenofibrate, and gemfibrozil, lower triglyceride levels by increasing the enzymatic action of lipoprotein lipase. Gemfibrozil has been the single agent available to treat elevated triglycerides for some time since clofibrate has been associated with increased mortality and fenofibrate was recently released.

The fibric acid derivatives share similar adverse effects of myalgias, elevated liver enzymes, and gastrointestinal distress and rashes. The one concerning side effect is an increase in gallstone formation because of the increased concentration of cholesterol in the bile caused by these drugs.

***Probucol.***   Probucol is an antioxidant and is of value in the prevention of atherosclerosis. Although it lowers LDL levels, it also decreases HDL levels more. The utility of this drug may be in its ability to cause regression of xanthomas in patients with severe hypercholesterolemia (Yamamoto et al, 1986).

***Estrogen replacement therapy.***   Estrogen replacement therapy (ERT) is considered as an alternative for treating lipid disorders in postmenopausal women who are at high risk with either elevated LDL or reduced HDL levels or as secondary prevention in women with known coronary artery disease. This suggestion is based on epidemiology data, not well-controlled studies (Barrett-Connor & Bush, 1991; Grady et al, 1992; Gruchow et al, 1988; Stampfer et al, 1991). There is little risk of using estrogen in patients without a uterus; however, the benefits in patients also requiring progestins is not as well known.

Other benefits of ERT include prevention of osteoporosis and urogenital atrophy.

In summary, statins provide the greatest LDL lowering and are the most likely to achieve LDL goals. They are the easiest for patients to take and maximize compliance. In comparison with BAR and niacin, the statins are the most cost-effective treatment.

A BAR should be used when additional LDL reduction is needed.

Niacin should be used for the management of TG elevations and possibly low HDL levels.

Gemfibrozil should be used when niacin is not indicated, as in patients with diabetes and lipid triad disorder.

## Follow-up Recommendations

It is important to individualize the plan of care. Motivation for long-term changes and medications may prove difficult for some patients. Follow-up must allow time to discuss compliance with the plan, modify medications, and consider relaxing some restrictions on diet.

General follow-up on each visit should include investigation of risk factors for the development of possible complications including coronary heart disease, cerebrovascular disease, and peripheral vascular disease. Weight, vital signs, and discussion about diet and the long-term plan must be part of each visit.

Laboratory measurements should include cholesterol and LDL levels in 4–6 weeks and then again at 3 months following the institution of dietary changes. If LDL is lowered to between 100 and 130 mg/dL with dietary changes, check in 3 months and then every year. When the patient is on medications as well as a diet, lipid profiles should be done 2–4 times a year.

Liver function tests should be performed every 6–8 weeks up to 1 year to monitor for hepatotoxicity associated with the statins and sustained-release niacin.

## REFERENCES

Abrams, J. (1991). Angina pectoris: Mechanisms, diagnosis, and therapy. *Cardiology Clinics, 9*(1), 1.

American Heart Association Monograph. (1995).

Applegate, W., Miller, S., & Elam, J. (1992). Nonpharmacologic intervention to reduce blood pressure in older patients with mild hypertension. *Archives of Internal Medicine, 152,* 1162–1166.

Arnstein, P., Buselli, E., & Rankin, S. (1996). Women and heart attacks: Prevention, diagnosis, and care. *Nurse Practitioner, 21*(5), 57–69.

Aronow, W., Ahn, C., & Gutstein, H. (1996). Prevalence of atrial fibrillation and association of atrial fibrillation with prior and new thromboembolic stroke in older patients. *Journal of the American Geriatrics Society, 44*(5), 521–523.

Aronow, W. S., Ahn, A. D., Mercando, S., Epstein, S., & Gutstein, H. (1996). Correlation of paroxysmal supraventricular tachycardia, atrial fibrillation, and sinus rhythm with incidences of new thromboembolic stroke in 1476 old-old patients. *Aging Clinical Experimental Research, 8*(1), 32–34.

Aronow, W. S., Ahn, A. D., Mercando, S., Epstein, S., Gutstein, H., & Schoenfeld, M. (1995). Association of silent myocardial ischemia with new atherothrombotic brain infarction in older patients with extracranial internal or common carotid arterial disease with and without previous atherothrombotic brain infarction. *Journal of the American Geriatrics Society, 43*(11), 1272–1274.

Balsano, F., Coccheri, S., Libbretti, A., et al. (1989). Ticlopidine in the treatment of intermittent claudication: A 21 month double-blind trial. *Journal of Laboratory and Clinical Medicine, 114,* 84–91.

Balsano, F., & Violi, F. (1993). Effect of picotamide on the clinical progression of peripheral vascular disease. A double-blind placebo-controlled study. The ADEP Group. *Circulation, 87,* 1563–1569.

Barber, D. A., Barber, C. H., Lee, C., et al. (1994). Angiotensin II receptor antagonist and potassium channel openers: Future cardiovascular therapy. *Pharmacy Times, 60,* 48–59.

Barrett-Connor, E., & Bush, T. L. (1991). Estrogen and coronary heart disease in women. *JAMA, 265,* 1861–1867.

Bauman, J. L., Parker, R. B., & McCollam, P. L. (1995). *Tachycardias. Pharmacotherapy self-assessment program* (2nd ed.). American College of Clinical Pharmacy, Kansas City, MO.

Berkow, R. (1992a). Myocardial ischemic disorders: Coronary artery disease. In R. Berkow & A. Fletcher (Eds.), *The Merck manual* (16th ed.) (pp. 498–507). Rahway, NJ: Merck.

Berkow, R. (1992b). Peripheral vascular disorders. In R. Berkow & A. Fletcher (Eds.), *The Merck manual* (16th ed.) (pp. 577–585). Rahway, NJ: Merck.

Bevan, E. G., Waller, P. C., Ramsay, L. E., et al. (1992). Pharmacological approaches to the treatment of intermittent claudication. *Drugs and Aging, 2,* 125–136.

Bradford, R. H., Shear, C. L., Chremos, A. N., et al. (1991). Expanded clinical evaluation of lovastatin (EXCEL) study results I: Efficacy in modifying plasma lipoproteins and adverse event profile in 8245 patients with moderate hypercholesterolemia. *Archives of Internal Medicine, 151,* 43–49.

Brater, D. C. (1985). Resistance to loop diuretics. Why it happens and what to do about it. *Drugs, 30,* 427–443.

Braunwald, E., Mark, D. B., Jones, R. H., et al. (1994). *Unstable angina: Diagnosis and management. Clinical practice guideline no. 10* (amended). AHCPR Publication no. 94-0602. Rockville, MD: Agency for Health Care Policy and Research and the National Heart, Lung, and Blood Institute, Public Health Service, U.S. Department of Health and Human Services.

Brevetti, G., Chiariello, M., Ferulano, G., et al. (1988). Increases in walking distance in patients with peripheral vascular disease treated with L-carnitine: A double-blind, crossover study. *Circulation, 77,* 767–773.

Brown, B. G. (1993). Lipid lowering and plaque regression: New insights into prevention of plaque disruption and clinical events in coronary disease. *Circulation, 87,* 1781.

Brown, E. J., & Kloner, R. (1990). Angina pectoris. In R. Kloner (Ed.), *The guide to cardiology* (2nd ed.) (pp. 173–198). New York: LeJacq Communications.

Brown, G., Albers, J. J., Fisher, L. D., et al. (1990). Regression of coronary artery disease as a result of intensive lipid-lowering therapy in men with high levels of apolipoprotein B. *New England Journal of Medicine, 323,* 1289–1298.

Browner, W. (1996). Lipid abnormalities. In L. Tierney, S. McPhee, & M. Papadakis (Eds.), *Current medical diagnosis and treatment* (35th ed.) (pp. 1069–1080). Stamford, CT: Appleton & Lange.

Carabello, B. (Ed.) (1991). Valvular heart disease. *Cardiology Clinics, 9*(2), 1.

Carabello, B. (1993). Mitral valve disease. *Current Problems in Cardiology, 18*(7), 423.

Carter, B. L., Frohlich, E. D., Elliott, W. J., et al. (1994). Selected factors that influence responses to antihypertensives. Choosing therapy for the uncomplicated patient. *Archives of Family Medicine, 3,* 528–536.

Carter, B. L., Taylor, J. W., Becker, A., et al. (1987). Evaluation of three dosage-prediction methods for initial in-hospital stabilization of warfarin therapy. *Clinical Pharmacy, 6,* 37.

Ceremuzynski, L., Kleczar, E., Drzeminska-Pakula, M., et al. (1992). Effect of amiodarone on mortality after myocardial infection: A double-blind, placebo-controlled, pilot study. *Journal of the American College of Cardiology, 20,* 1056–1062.

Challenor, V. F., Waller, D. G., Hayward, R. A., et al. (1991). Subjective and objective assessment of enalapril in primary Raynaud's phenomenon. *British Journal of Clinical Pharmacology, 31,* 477–480.

Chapman, D. (1994). The cumulative risks of prolapsing mitral valve. *Texas Heart Institute Journal 21*(4), 267–271.

Chen, B. P., & Chow, M. S. (1997). Focus on carvedilol: A novel beta adrenergic blocking agent for the treatment of congestive heart failure. *Formulary, 32*(8), 795–805.

Chenoweth, C. E., & Burket, J. S. (1997). Antimicrobial prophylaxis: Principles and practice. *Formulary, 32,* 692–713.

Coffman, J. D. (1988). New drug therapy in peripheral vascular disease. *Medical Clinics of North America, 72,* 259–263.

Coffman, J. D. (1989). *Raynaud's phenomenon.* New York: Oxford University Press.

Coffman, J. D. (1991). Raynaud's phenomenon: An update. *Hypertension, 17,* 593.

Coffman, J. D., Clement, D. L., Creager, M. A., et al. (1989). International study of ketanserin in Raynaud's phenomenon. *American Journal of Medicine, 87,* 264–268.

Cohn, J. N. (1996). The management of chronic heart failure. *New England Journal of Medicine, 335,* 490–498.

Cohn, J. N., Archibald, D. G., Ziesche, S., et al. (1986). Effect of vasodilator therapy on mortality in chronic congestive heart failure. Results of a Veterans Administration Cooperative Study. *New England Journal of Medicine, 314,* 1547–1552.

Cohn, J. N., Johnson, G., Ziesche, S., et al. (1991). A comparison of enalapril with hydralazine-isosorbide dinitrate in the treatment of chronic heart failure. *New England Journal of Medicine, 325,* 303–310.

CONSENSUS Trial Study Group. (1987). Effects of enalapril on mortality in severe congestive heart failure. Results of the Cooperative North Scandinavian Enalapril Survival Study (CONSENSUS). *New England Journal of Medicine, 316,* 1429–1435.

Cooke, E. D., & Nicolaides, A. N. (1990). Raynaud's syndrome. Thymoxamine, iloprost, and ACE inhibitors are among the effective treatments now available. *British Medical Journal, 300,* 553–555.

Dahlof, B., Lindholm, F. H., Hansson, L., et al. (1991). Morbidity and mortality in the Swedish trial in old patients with hypertension (STOP-Hypertension). *Lancet, 338,* 1281–1285.

Dajani, A. S., Taubert, K. A., Wilson, W., et al. (1997). Prevention of bacterial endocarditis: Recommendations by the American Heart Association. *JAMA, 277,* 1794–1801.

Davey Smith, G., Song, F., & Sheldon, T. (1993). Cholesterol lowering and mortality: The importance of considering initial level of risk. *British Medical Journal, 306,* 1363.

Desanctis, R. W., & Ruskin, J. N. (1993). Disturbances of cardiac rhythm and conduction. In D. Dale & D. Federman (Eds.), *Scientific American medicine* (1 Card VI, pp. 1–47). New York: Scientific American.

Dracup, K. (1996). Heart failure secondary to left ventricular systolic dysfunction. *Nurse Practitioner, 21*(9), 56–68.

Echt, D. S., Liebson, P. R., Mitchell, B., et al. (1991). Mortality and morbidity in patients receiving encainide, flecainide, or placebo. The cardiac arrhythmia suppression trial. *New England Journal of Medicine, 324,* 781–788.

Elkayam, U., Amin, J., Mehra, A., et al. (1990). A prospective, randomized, double-blind, crossover study to compare the efficacy and safety of chronic nifedipine therapy with that of isosorbide dinitrate and their combination in the treatment of chronic congestive heart failure. *Circulation, 82,* 1952–1961.

Ellison, D. H. (1991). The physiologic basis of diuretic synergism: Its role in treating diuretic resistance. *Annals of Internal Medicine, 114,* 886–894.

Emergency Cardiac Care Committee and Subcommittee, American Heart Association. (1992). Guidelines for cardiopulmonary resuscitation and emergency care. *JAMA, 268,* 2199–2241.

Ernst, E., & Fialka, V. (1993). A review of the clinical effectiveness of exercise therapy for intermittent claudication. *Archives of Internal Medicine, 153,* 2357.

Ernst, E., Kollar, L., & Resch, K. L. (1992). Does pentoxifylline prolong the walking distance in exercised claudicants? A placebo-controlled double-blind trial. *Angiology, 43,* 121–125.

Expert Panel on Detection, Evaluation, and Treatment of High Blood Cholesterol in Adults. (1993). Summary of the second report of the National Cholesterol Education Program (NCEP) expert panel on detection, evaluation, and treatment of high blood cholesterol in adults (Adult Treatment Panel II). *JAMA, 269,* 3015–3023.

Feldman, A., Bristow, M. R., Parmley, W. W., et al. (1993). Effects of vesnarinone on morbidity and mortality in patients with heart failure. Vesnarinone study group. *New England Journal of Medicine, 329,* 149–155.

Flaker, G. C., Blackshear, J. L., McBride, R., et al. (1992). Antiarrhythmic drug therapy and cardiac mortality in atrial fibrillation. *Journal of the American College of Cardiology, 20,* 527–532.

Fleckenstein-Grun, G., Thimm, F., Czirifuzs, A., & Matyas, S. (1994). Experimental vasoprotection by calcium antagonists against calcium-mediated arteriosclerotic alterations. *Journal of Cardiovascular Pharmacology, 24* (Suppl. 2), S75–S84.

Flosequinan for heart failure. (1993). *Medical Letter on Drugs and Therapeutics, 35,* 23–24.

Fontana, M. (1991). Mitral valve prolapse. *Current Problems in Cardiology 16*(5), 311.

Fortuin, N. J. (1996). Valvular heart disease. In J. D. Stobo, D. B. Hellmann, P. W. Landenson, et al. (Eds.), *The principles and practice of medicine* (23rd ed.) (pp. 59–67). Stamford, CT: Appleton & Lange.

Franciosa, J. A., Jordan, R. A., Wilen, M. W., et al. (1984). Minoxidil in patients with chronic left heart failure contrasting hemodynamic and clinical effects in a controlled trial. *Circulation, 70,* 63–68.

Frey, M., & Just, H. (1994). Role of calcium antagonists in progression of arteriosclerosis. Evidence from animal experiments and clinical experience. Part I. Preventive effects of calcium antagonists in animal experiments. *Basic Research in Cardiology, 89* (Suppl. 1), 161–176.

Friedman, P. (1990). Atrioventricular conduction disorders. In R. Kloner (Ed.), *The guide to cardiology* (2nd ed.) (pp. 317–325). New York: LeJacq Communications.

Frohlich, E. D. (1995). Continuing advances in hypertension: The joint national committee's fifth report. *American Journal of the Medical Sciences, 310,* S48–S52.

Gavras, I., Manolis, A., & Gavras, H. (1997). Drug therapy for hypertension. *American Family Physician, 55,* 1823–1834.

Goldberg, A. D., Nicklas, J., Goldstein, S., et al. (1991). Effectiveness of imazodan for treatment of chronic congestive heart failure. The Imazodan Research Group. *American Journal of Cardiology, 68,* 631–636.

Goldstein, R. E., Boccuzzi, S. J., Cruess, D., et al. (1991). Diltiazem increases late-onset congestive heart failure in postinfarction patients with early reduction in ejection. The Adverse Experience Committee; and the Multicenter diltiazem post infarction research group. *Circulation, 83,* 52–60.

Golzari, H., Cebul, R. D., & Bahler, R. C. (1996). Atrial fibrillation: Restoration and maintenance of sinus rhythm and indications for anticoagulation therapy. *Annals of Internal Medicine, 125,* 311–323.

Gordon, D. J., Probstfield, J. L., Garrison, R. J., et al. (1989). High-density lipoprotein cholesterol and cardiovascular disease: Four prospective American studies. *Circulation, 79,* 8–15.

Gosselink, A. T. M., Crijns, H. J. M., VanGelder, I. C., et al. (1992). Low-dose amiodarone for maintenance of sinus rhythm after cardioversion of atrial fibrillation or flutter. *JAMA, 267,* 3289–3292.

Graboys, T. (1990). Diagnosis and management of cardiac arrhythmias. In R. Kloner (Ed.), *The guide to cardiology* (2nd ed.) (pp. 301–315). New York: LeJacq Communications.

Grady, D., Rubin, S. M., Pettiti, D. B., et al. (1992). Hormone therapy to prevent disease and prolong life in postmenopausal women. *Annals of Internal Medicine, 117,* 1016–1037.

Grant, S. M., & Goa, K. L. (1992). Iloprost. A review of its pharmacodynamic and pharmacokinetic properties, and therapeutic potential in peripheral vascular disease, myocardial ischemia and extracorporeal circulation procedures. *Drugs, 43,* 889–924.

Gruchow, H. W., Anderson, A. J., Barboriak, J. J., et al. (1988). Postmenopausal use of estrogen and occlusion of arteries. *American Heart Journal, 115*(5), 954–963.

Gums, J. (1997). Cardiovascular disease therapy: Innovations in calcium channel blocker, an introduction to T-channel science. *Drug Topics* (Suppl.), 1–12.

Haak, S., Richardson, S., Davey, S., & Parker-Cohen, P. (1994). Alterations of cardiovascular function. In K. McCance & S. Huether, *Pathophysiology: The biologic basis for disease in adults and children* (2nd ed.) (pp. 1000–1084). St. Louis: C. V. Mosby.

Hancock, E. (1996a). Diseases of the aorta and large arteries. In D. Dale & D. Federman (Eds.), *Scientific American medicine* (1 Card XII 1–8). New York: Scientific American.

Hancock, E. (1996b). Valvular heart disease. In D. Dale & D. Federman (Eds.), *Scientific American medicine* (1 Card XI 1–16). New York: Scientific American.

Hebert, P., Gazaino, J., & Hennekens, C. (1995). An overview of trials of cholesterol lowering and risk of stroke. *Archives of Internal Medicine, 155,* 50.

Heintzen, M. P. & Strauer, B. E. (1994). Peripheral vascular effects of beta blockers. *European Heart Journal, 15* (Suppl. C), 2–7.

Hess, H., Mietaschk, A., Deichsel, G., et al. (1985). Drug induced inhibition of platelet function delays progression of peripheral occlusive arterial disease. A prospective double-blind arteriographically controlled trial. *Lancet, 1,* 415–419.

Hiatt, W. R., Stoll, S., & Nies, A. S. (1985). Effect of beta adrenergic blockade on the peripheral circulation in patients with peripheral vascular disease. *Circulation, 72,* 1226–1231.

Hla, K. M., Samsa, G., & Stoneking, H. (1991). Observer variability of Osler's maneuver in detection of pseudohypertension. *Journal of Clinical Epidemiology, 44,* 513–518.

Hobbs, J. T. (1991). ABC of vascular diseases: Varicose veins. *British Medical Journal, 303,* 918.

Housley, E. (1988). Treating claudication in five words. *British Medical Journal, 296,* 483.

Hulisz, D. T. (1997). Pharmacologic management of atrial fibrillation. *U.S. Pharmacist, 22,* 103–112.

Hutter, A. (1996). Ischemic heart disease: Angina pectoris. In D. Dale & D. Federman (Eds.), *Scientific American medicine* (1 Card IX 1–19). New York: Scientific American.

Ingram, D., House, A., Thompson, G., et al. (1982). Beta adrenergic blockade and peripheral vascular disease. *Medical Journal of Australia, 1,* 509–511.

Joint National Committee on Detection, Evaluation, and Treatment of High Blood Pressure. (1997). The sixth report of the joint national committee on detection, evaluation, and treatment of high blood pressure (JNC VI). *Archives of Internal Medicine, 157,* 2413–2446.

Jones, P. H., et al. (1991). Once daily pravastatin in patients with primary hypercholesterolemia: A dose response study. *Clinical Cardiology, 14,* 146–151.

Katsumura, T., Mishima, Y., Kamiya, K., et al. (1982). Therapeutic effect of ticlopidine, a new inhibitor of platelet aggregation, on chronic arterial occlusive disease, a double-blind study versus placebo. *Angiology, 33,* 357–367.

Kellick, K. A., Burns, K., McAndrew, E., et al. (1997). Focus on atorvastatin: An HMG-CoA reductase inhibitor for lowering both elevated LDL cholesterol and triglycerides in hypercholesterolemic patients. *Formulary, 32,* 352–363.

Kloner, R., & Dzau, V. (1990). Heart failure. In R. Kloner (Ed.), *The guide to cardiology* (2nd ed.) (pp. 359–381). New York: LeJacq Communications.

Konstam, M., Dracup, K., et al. (1994). *Heart failure: Evaluation and care of patients with left-ventricular systolic dysfunction. Clinical practice guideline no. 11.* AHCPR publication no. 94-0612. Rockville, MD: Agency for Health Care Policy and Research, Public Health Service, U.S. Department of Health and Human Services.

Kostis, J. B., Davis, B. R., & Cutler, J. (1997). Prevention of heart failure by antihypertensive drug treatment in older persons with isolated systolic hypertension. *JAMA, 278,* 212–216.

Kradjan, W. (1993). Congestive heart failure. In M. Koda-Kimble & L. Young (Eds.), *Applied therapeutics* (5th ed.). Vancouver, WA: Applied Therapeutics.

Lacy, C., Armstrong, L. L., Ingrim, N., et al. (1997). In *Drug information handbook* (4th ed.) (pp. 64–66). Ohio, Lexi-Comp.

Lally, E. V. (1992). Raynaud's phenomenon. *Current Opinion in Rheumatology, 4,* 825.

Langer, R., Criqui, M., & Barrett-Connor, E. (1993). Blood pressure change and survival after age 75. *Hypertension, 22,* 551–559.

Lapalio, L. R. (1995). Hypertension in the elderly. *American Family Physician, 52,* 1161–1165.

Laupacia, A., Albers, G., Dunn, M., & Feinberg, W. (1992). Antithrombotic therapy in atrial fibrillation. *Chest, 102,* 426S–433S.

Lebovitz, H., Wiegmann, T., Cnaan, A., et al. (1994). Renal protective effects of enalapril in hypertensive NIDDM: Role of baseline albuminuria. *Kidney International, 45,* S150–S155.

Leier, C. V., Huss, P., Magorien, R. D., et al. (1983). Improved exercise capacity and offering arterial and venous tolerance during chronic isosorbide dinitrate therapy for congestive heart failure. *Circulation, 67,* 817–822.

Leppert, J., Jonasson, T., Nilsson H., et al. (1989). The effects of isradipine, a new calcium channel antagonist, in patients with primary Raynaud's phenomenon: A single-blind dose-response study. *Cardiovascular Drugs and Therapy, 3,* 397–401.

Massie, B. (1996a). Heart. In L. Tierney, S. McPhee, & M. Papadakis (Eds.), *Current medical diagnosis and treatment* (35th ed.) (pp. 295–403). Stamford, CT: Appleton & Lange.

Massie, B. (1996b). Systemic hypertension. In L. Tierney, S. McPhee & M. Papadakis (Eds.), *Current medical diagnosis and treatment:* (35th ed.) Stamford, CT: Appleton & Lange. (pp. 384–402).

Materson, B. J., & Reda, D. J. (1994). Correction: Single-drug therapy for hypertension in men. *New England Journal of Medicine, 330,* 1689.

Materson, B. J., Reda, D. J., Cushman, W. C., et al. (1993). Single-drug therapy for hypertension in men: A comparison of six antihypertensive agents with placebo. The department of veteran affairs cooperative study group on antihypertensive agents. *New England Journal of Medicine, 328,* 914.

McKenney, J. M., Proctor, J. D., Harris, S., et al. (1994). A comparison of the efficacy and toxic effects of sustained- vs. immediate-release niacin in hypercholesterolemia patients. *JAMA, 271,* 672–677.

McVeigh, G. E., Flack, J., & Grimm, R. (1995). Goals of antihypertensive therapy. *Drugs, 49,* 161–175.

Multicenter Diltiazem Postinfarction Trial Research Group. (1988). The effect of diltiazem on mortality and reinfarction after myocardial infarction. *New England Journal of Medicine, 319,* 385–392.

Naftilan, A., & Dzau, V. (1990). Evaluation and management of hypertension. In R. Kloner (Ed.), *The guide to cardiology* (2nd ed.) (pp. 409–436). New York: LeJacq Communications.

National Cholesterol Education Program Adult Treatment Panel II. (1993). Summary of the second expert panel on detection, evaluation, and treatment of high blood cholesterol in adults. *JAMA, 269,* 3015.

National High Blood Pressure Education Program. (1993). National high blood pressure education program working group report on hypertension in the elderly. *Hypertension, 23,* 275.

National High Blood Pressure Education Program Working Group. (1993). National high blood pressure education program working group on primary prevention of hypertension. *Archives of Internal Medicine, 153,* 186.

National High Blood Pressure Education Program Coordinating Committee. (1990). The national high blood pressure education program working group report on ambulatory blood pressure monitoring. *Archives of Internal Medicine, 150,* 2270.

Neaton, J. D., Grimm, R. H., Jr., Prineas, R. J., et al. (1993). Treatment of mild hypertension study: Final results. *JAMA, 270,* 713.

O'Keefe, J. H. (1995). Insights into the pathogenesis and prevention of coronary artery disease. Treatment of mild hypertension study research group. *Mayo Clinic Proceedings, 70,* 69.

Olsson, G., Hjemdahl, P., Rehnqvist, N., et al. (1984). Rebound phenomena following gradual withdrawal of chronic metoprolol treatment in patients with ischemic heart disease. *American Heart Journal, 108,* 455.

Packer, M. (1990). Are nitrates effective in the treatment of chronic heart failure: Antagonist's viewpoint. *American Journal of Cardiology, 66,* 458–461.

Packer, M., Bristow, M. R., Cohn, J. N., et al. (1996). The effect of carvedilol on morbidity and mortality in patients with chronic heart failure. *New England Journal of Medicine, 334,* 1349–1355.

Packer, M., Narahara, K. A., Elkayam, U., et al. (1993). Double blind, placebo controlled study of the efficacy of flosequinan in patients with chronic heart failure. Principal investigators of the REFLECT Study. *Journal of the American College of Cardiology, 22,* 65.

Packer, M., Medina, N., Yushak, M., et al. (1985). Usefulness of plasma renin activity in predicting hemodynamic and clinical responses and survival during long-term converting enzyme inhibition in severe chronic heart failure. *British Heart Journal, 54,* 298–304.

Parker, J. O., Farrell, B., Lahey, K. A., et al. (1987). Effect of intervals between doses on the development of tolerance to isosorbide dinitrate. *New England Journal of Medicine, 316,* 1440–1444.

Parker, J. O., Fung, H. L., Ruggirello, D., et al. (1983). Tolerance to isosorbide dinitrate: Rate of development and reversal. *Circulation, 68,* 1074.

Pauly, R., Passanti, A., Crow, M., et al. (1992). Experimental models which mimic the differentiation and de-differentiation of vascular cells. *Circulation* (Supplement III), 68–73.

Peto, R., Yusuf, S., & Collins, R. (1991). Cholesterol-lowering trial results in their epidemiologic context. *Journal of the American College of Cardiology, 17*(III), 451.

Pfeffer, M. A., Braunwald, E., Moye, L. A., et al. (1992). Effect of captopril on mortality and morbidity in patients with left ventricular dysfunction after myocardial infarction. Results of the survival and ventricular enlargement trial. The SAVE investigators. *New England Journal of Medicine, 327,* 669–677.

Prystowsky, E. N., Benson, D. W., Fuster, V., et al. (1996). Management of patients with atrial fibrillation. A statement for healthcare professionals from the Subcommittee on Electrocardiograph and Electrophysiology, American Heart Association. *Circulation, 93,* 1262–1277.

Psaty, B. M., Heckbert, S. R., Koepsell, T. D., et al. (1995). The risk of myocardial infarction associated with antihypertensive drug therapies. *JAMA, 274,* 620–625.

Psaty, B. M., Smith, N. L., Siscovick, D. S., et al. (1997). Health outcomes associated with antihypertensive therapies used as first-line agents. A systematic review and meta-analysis. *JAMA, 277,* 739–745.

Raehl, C., & Nolan, P. (1995). Ischemic heart disease: Anginal syndromes. In M. Koda-Kimble & L. Young (Eds.), *Applied therapeutics: The clinical use of drugs* (6th ed.) (pp. 13-1–13-25). Vancouver, WA: Applied Therapeutics.

Ramsey, L., Yeo, W., & Jackson, P. (1991). Dietary reduction of serum cholesterol concentration: Time to think again. *British Medical Journal, 303,* 953.

Roath, S. (1989). Management of Raynaud's phenomenon. Focus on new treatments. *Drugs, 37,* 700–712.

Roberts, D. H., Tsao, Y., McLoughlin, G. A., et al. (1987). Placebo-controlled comparison of captopril, atenolol, labetalol, and pindolol in hypertension complicated by intermittent claudication. *Lancet, 2*(8560), 650–653.

Roffman, D. S. (1995). Heart failure. *U.S. Pharmacist* Feb 63–72.

Rupp, P. A. F., Mellinger, S., Kohler, J., et al. (1987). Nicardipine for the treatment of Raynaud's phenomena: A double-blind crossover trial of a new calcium entry blocker. *Journal of Rheumatology, 14,* 745–750.

Sadowski, A., & Redeker, N. (1996). The hypertensive elder. *Nurse Practitioner, 21*(5), 99–118.

Sagie, A., Larson, M., & Levy, D. (1993). The natural history of borderline isolated systolic hypertension. *New England Journal of Medicine, 29,* 1912–1917.

Sawyer, W. T., Poe, T. E., Canaday, B. R., et al. (1985). Multicenter evaluation of six methods for predicting warfarin maintenance dose requirements from initial response. *Clinical Pharmacy, 4,* 440.

Scandinavian Simvastatin Survival Study Group. (1994). Randomized trial of cholesterol lowering in 4444 patients with coronary heart disease: The Scandinavian Simvastatin Survival Study (4S). *Lancet, 344,* 1383.

Scanu, A. M. (1991). Update on lipoprotein (a). *Current Opinion in Lipidology, 2,* 253–258.

Schwartz, C. (1992). A modern view of atherogenesis. *American Journal of Cardiology, 71,* 9B.

Sever, P., Beevers, G., Bulpitt, C., et al. (1993). Management guidelines in essential hypertension: Report of the second working party of the British Hypertension Society. *British Medical Journal, 306,* 983.

Smith, R., & Warren, D. (1982). Effect of beta blocking drugs on peripheral blood flow in intermittent claudication. *Journal of Cardiovascular Pharmacology, 4,* 2–4.

SOLVD (Studies of Left Ventricular Dysfunction) Investigators. (1991). Effect of enalapril on survival in patients with reduced left ventricular ejection fractions and congestive heart failure. *New England Journal of Medicine, 325,* 293–302.

Sox, H. C. (1993). Screening for lipid disorders under health care systems reform. *New England Journal of Medicine, 328,* 1269.

Stampfer, M. J., Colditz, G. A., Willett, W. C., et al. (1991). Post-menopausal estrogen therapy and cardiovascular disease: Ten-year follow-up from the Nurses Health Study. *New England Journal of Medicine, 325,* 756–762.

Stanek, E., Moser, L., & Munger, M. (1995). *Heart failure.* Pharmacotherapy Self-Assessment Program (2nd ed.). American College of Clinical Pharmacy, Kansas, City, MO.

Stone, N. (1990). Clinical approach to hyperlipidemia. In R. Kloner (Ed.), *The guide to cardiology* (2nd ed.) (pp. 155–172). New York: LeJacq Communications.

Stroke Prevention in Atrial Fibrillation Investigators. (1991). Stroke prevention in atrial fibrillation: Final results. *Circulation, 84,* 527–539.

Stroke Prevention in Atrial Fibrillation Investigators. (1994). Warfarin versus aspirin for prevention of thromboembolism in atrial fibrillation: Stroke prevention in atrial fibrillation II study. *Lancet, 343,* 687–691.

Systolic Hypertension in the Elderly Program Cooperative Research Group. (1991). Prevention of stroke by antihypertensive drug treatment in older persons with isolated systolic hypertension. *JAMA, 265,* 3255–3264.

Systolic Hypertension in the Elderly Program Cooperative Research Group. (1993). Implications of the systolic hypertension in the elderly program. *Hypertension, 21,* 335–343.

Tackett, R. L. (1995). Update on hypertension. *Clinical Trends, 10,* 67–72.

Talbert, R. (1997). Ischemic heart disease. In J. T. Dipiro, R. L. Talbert, G. C. Yee, G. R. Matzke, B. G. Wells, & L. M. Posey (Eds.), *Pharmacotherapy: A pathophysiologic approach* (3rd ed.) (pp. 257–294). Stamford, CT: Appleton & Lange.

Tierney, L. (1996). Blood vessels & lymphatics. In L. Tierney, S. McPhee, & M. Papadakis (Eds.), *Current medical diagnosis and treatment* (35th ed.) (pp. 403–433). Stamford, CT: Appleton & Lange.

Tobian, L. Brunner, H. R., Cohn, J. N., et al. (1994). Modern strategies to prevent coronary sequelae and stroke in hypertensive patients differ from the JNC V consensus guidelines. *American Journal of Hypertension, 7,* 859–872.

Tsapatsaris, N., Napolitana, G., & Rothchild, J. (1991). Osler's maneuver in an outpatient clinical setting. *Archives of Internal Medicine, 151,* 2209–2211.

Ulutin, O. N. (1988). Clinical effectiveness of defibrotide in vaso-occlusive disorders and its mode of action. *Seminars in Thrombosis and Hemostasis, 14* (Suppl.), 58–63.

Uretsky, B. F., Jessup, M., Konstam, M. A., et al. (1990). Multicenter trial of oral enoximone in patients with moderate to moderately severe congestive heart failure: Lack of benefit compared to placebo. Enoximone multicenter trial group. *Circulation, 82,* 774.

Waldo, A. & Witt, A. (1993). Mechanisms of cardiac arrhythmias. *Lancet 341,* 1189.

Weber, M. A. (1993). Controversies in the diagnosis and treatment of hypertension: A persona review of JNC V. *American Journal of Cardiology, 72,* 3H–9H.

Weir, M. R. (1996). Angiotensin-II receptor antagonists: A new class of antihypertensive agents. *American Family Physician, 53,* 589–594.

White, C. M. & Chow, M. S. (1997). Pharmacologic management of congestive heart failure. *U.S. Pharmacist, 22,* 117–125.

Wilt, T. J. (1992). Current strategies in the diagnosis and management of lower extremity peripheral vascular disease. *Journal of General Internal Medicine, 7,* 87.

Wittkowsky, A. K. (1995). Thrombosis. In M. A. Koda-Kimble & L. Y. Young (Eds.), *Applied therapeutics: The clinical use of drugs* (6th ed.). Vancouver, WA: Applied Therapeutics.

Wollersheim, H., Thien, T., Fennis, J., et al. (1986). Double-blind, placebo-controlled stage of prazosin in Raynaud's phenomenon. *Clinical Pharmacology and Therapeutics, 40,* 219.

Wollersheim, H., Thien, T., et al. (1988). Dose response study of prazosin in Raynaud's phenomenon: Clinical effectiveness versus side effects. *Journal of Clinical Pharmacology, 28,* 1089–1093.

Woodhead, G. (1996). The management of cholesterol in coronary heart disease risk reduction. *Nurse Practitioner, 21*(9), 45–53.

Xamaterol in Severe Heart Failure Study Group. (1990). Xamaterol in severe heart failure. *Lancet, 336,* 1.

Yamamoto, A., Matsuzawa, Y., Yokoyama, S., et al. (1986). Effects of probucol on xanthomata regression in familial hypercholesterolemia. *American Journal of Cardiology, 57,* 29H–35H.

Young, J. B. (1996). Cahnera scientific meeting reports: Heart failure review. From the American College of Cardiology 46th Annual Scientific Meeting.

# 21

## UPPER RESPIRATORY DISORDERS

*Constance R. Uphold and Thomas E. Johns*

Many patients seen by primary care providers on a daily basis present with some form of upper respiratory disorder. Patient education can help prevent or reduce the severity of some of these disorders as well as ameliorate their condition during the course of the illness. These disorders collectively result in millions of hours lost from school or work and millions of dollars paid out for remedies good and ill-advised. Patient distress is real, whether the cause is a relatively benign common cold or a life-threatening attack of epiglottitis. Signs and symptoms can be difficult to differentiate initially—the patient has a runny nose, aches, fatigue, cough—from what cause? Meticulous history taking, a comprehensive physical examination, and/or diagnostic testing can help determine if these symptoms are indicative of allergic rhinitis, the common cold, sinusitis, pharyngitis, or croup, the subjects of this chapter.

## ALLERGIC RHINITIS

Allergic rhinitis is the most common nasal problem in the United States (Noble, Forbes, & Woodbridge, 1995) and ranks sixth as the most prevalent chronic illness (Consensus Conference Proceedings, 1995). Allergic rhinitis affects approximately 20% of all Americans (Bernstein, 1993) and accounts for over 11 million office visits annually (Consensus Conference Proceedings, 1995). Symptoms often lead to discomfort, absenteeism from school and work,

and expenditure of many dollars for health care services and medication (Nightingale, 1996).

Allergic rhinitis is an immunologically mediated condition stimulated by a type 1 antigen-antibody reaction (Noble et al, 1995). When an individual, often with a genetic predisposition to an allergy, is exposed to a specific antigen, allergen-specific IgE molecules are produced and then bind to mast cells in the respiratory epithelium. Reexposure to offending allergic stimuli results in degranulation of mast cells and basophils, which triggers the release of histamines, kinins, prostaglandins, and esterases, causing an immediate local vasodilation, mucosal edema, and increased mucous production. Four to eight hours later in persons with severe disease, a late-phase reaction with additional release of histamine and cellular infiltration of eosinophils, basophils, neutrophils, and mononuclear cells occurs. This late-phase reaction results in hyperresponsiveness to antigenic and nonantigenic stimuli and has been linked to the development of chronic disease (Swanson, 1996).

The most common form of allergic rhinitis has a seasonal pattern and is mainly associated with inhalant pollen allergens from trees, grass, and ragweed. The year-round, perennial type of allergic rhinitis is caused by dust mites, cockroaches, molds, and animal dander. In addition to these environmental sources, genetic factors play an important role. Persons with allergic rhinitis often have a positive family history of the condition (Bernstein, 1993).

A triad of nasal congestion, sneezing, and clear rhinorrhea is most characteristic of allergic rhinitis. Coughing, itching of the nose, throat, and eyes, complaints of postnasal drip, puffiness, and tearing of the eyes, and a sense of fullness in the ears may occur. The onset of symptoms is usually between the ages of 10–20 years, but may begin earlier in childhood (Bernstein, 1993; Smith, 1995). Chronic allergic rhinitis is a predisposing factor for the development and exacerbation of asthma, sinusitis, nasal polyposis, and otitis media (Consensus Conference Proceedings, 1995).

## SPECIFIC CONSIDERATIONS FOR PHARMACOTHERAPY

### When Drug Therapy Is Needed

When allergen avoidance is ineffective or impractical, drug therapy is indicated. Antihistamines, decongestants, nasal cromolyn, and/or nasal corticosteroids are all effective in reducing or preventing symptoms.

Antihistamines control symptoms of sneezing, rhinitis, pruritus, and conjunctivitis by blocking the effects of histamine on end organs (Smith, 1995). First-generation oral antihistamines are inexpensive and considered first-line therapy. Second-generation antihistamines such as astemizole, terfenadine, loratadine, and fexofenadine do not readily cross the blood-brain barrier, resulting in minimal sedation, and have minimal anticholinergic properties (Lockey et al, 1996). Cetirizine, considered a second-generation antihistamine, is an active metabolite of hydroxyzine and possesses mild sedative properties. With Food and Drug Administration (FDA) approval of fexofenadine and fexofenadine/pseudoephedrine, terfenadine and terfenadine/pseudoephedrine will be voluntarily withdrawn from the U.S. market by the manufacturer. Fexofenadine, the active metabolite of terfenadine, is devoid of significant cardiac adverse effects. It has been suggested that the risk-benefit ratio of terfenadine makes its use no longer acceptable. See Drug Table 705.

Levocabastine and azelastine are the first topical antihistamines. These topical agents are effective in reducing allergic symptoms, have a better safety profile, and are more beneficial in relieving nasal obstruction than oral antihistamines (Davies, Bagnall, McCabe, Calderon, & Wang, 1996; Krause, 1994).

Because antihistamines do not relieve nasal congestion, decongestants are sometimes required. Decongestants are sympathomimetics that cause vasoconstriction by stimulating alpha-adrenergic receptors in the nasal mucosa. Decongestants decrease tissue edema and nasal congestion, and they improve nasal airway patency and ventilation. Decongestants can be administered in oral or topical forms. Oral decongestants are often given in combination products with antihistamines to improve compliance, enhance effectiveness, and counterbalance the sedative effects of antihistamines. Topical decongestants are indicated for short-term use in patients with severe nasal congestion who need rapid relief. They may also be used prior to application of intranasal corticosteroids to reduce turbinate swelling and facilitate delivery and action of the steroid (Meltzer, 1995). See Drug Table 703.

Although the exact mechanism of action is unknown, topical corticosteroids reduce nasal vasodilation, edema, and inflammation (Noble et al, 1995; Swanson, 1996), but are ineffective in relieving ocular symptoms. Topical corticosteroids may be combined with antihistamines for enhanced effectiveness in reducing allergic reactions. Using corticosteroids topically can achieve high drug concentrations at receptor sites in the nasal mucosa with minimal risk of systemic effects (Mygind & Dahl, 1996). In contrast, systemic corticosteroids can cause numerous and possibly serious adverse reactions. Thus, oral corticosteroids are reserved for short-term therapy in patients with severe, debilitating rhinitis (Trevino & Gordon, 1993). See Drug Table 706.

Intranasal cromolyn sodium may also be effective in treating some patients with allergic rhinitis, particularly patients with high immunoglobulin E (IgE) levels. Cromolyn sodium interferes with the degranulation of sensitized mast cells (Smith, 1995) and is effective in relieving itching, sneezing, and rhinorrhea, but is less efficacious in treating nasal obstruction than other therapies (Horak, 1993). Nedocromil is a topical mast-cell stabilizer which is ten times more potent than cromolyn (Krause, 1994). Although nedocromil has a similar pharmacologic profile and possesses antiinflammatory activity, it is chemically unrelated to cromolyn sodium (Trevino & Gordon, 1993).

Intranasal ipratropium bromide has recently been approved by the FDA for symptomatic relief of rhinorrhea associated with allergic and nonallergic perennial rhinitis or symptomatic relief of rhinorrhea associated with the common cold in patients ≥12 years of age. Intranasal anticholinergics have an excellent safety profile and cause few side effects (Trevino & Gordon, 1993). Although these drugs reduce rhinorrhea, they have a minimal effect on nasal congestion (Consensus Conference Proceedings, 1995).

## Short-Term and Long-Term Goals of Pharmacotherapy

The short-term goal of pharmacotherapy is to eliminate, control, or reduce the symptoms arising from allergen triggers and inflammation while simultaneously minimizing the adverse side effects of therapy. The long-term goal is to prevent the onset of symptoms of allergic rhinitis and mimimize complications. Patients should be educated in the ways they can help themselves prevent and treat their own symptoms; see Table 21–1.

## Time Frame for Initiating Pharmacotherapy

Patients who have seasonal allergic rhinitis should begin pharmacological therapy 1–2 weeks before the anticipated season of sensitiv-

## TABLE 21–1. HOW PATIENTS CAN HELP THEMSELVES PREVENT AND TREAT ALLERGIC RHINITIS

### Prevention

*Control the Home Environment*

Frequent vacuuming, damp mopping, and dusting with damp cloth

Using air conditioning during summer months

Using dehumidifier in damp areas

Keeping doors and windows closed to decrease influx of pollen and mold

Eliminating carpets

Covering mattresses and pillows with bacteria-reducing cloth barriers

*Reduce other Allergens and Irritants*

Wearing protective mask when outside or mowing lawn

Wearing long-sleeve shirts and pants when gardening

Determining what triggers allergic reactions and avoiding offenders

Stopping smoking or avoiding second-hand smoke and other irritants

### Treatment

Exercising regularly

Using nasal saline sprays

ity and onset of symptoms. In contrast, perennial allergic rhinitis is treated year-round. Medications should be taken regularly rather than intermittently after symptoms have developed (Consensus Conference Proceedings, 1995). See Drug Table 705.

## Assessment Prior to Therapy

A *history* of onset, characteristics, duration, progression, and pattern of the symptoms should be obtained. Explore potential triggers such as exposure to animal dander, freshly cut grass, or dust mites, and ask about family history, other atopic diseases, and previous self-treatments (Uphold & Graham, 1994).

In the *physical examination*, inspect the eyes for signs typical of allergic rhinitis: tearing, lid swelling, periorbital edema, conjunctival injection, and darkening under the eyes (ie, allergic shiners). The nasal mucosa of patients with allergic rhinitis is pale and boggy, with a clear discharge. The pharynx should be observed for postnasal drip, tonsilar enlargement, and mild erythema (Smith, 1995). The lymph nodes, sinuses, nasal cavity, ears, and lungs should be carefully assessed to identify the following conditions which often coexist with allergic rhinitis: lymphoid hyperplasia, sinusitis, nasal polyps, otitis media, serous otitis media, and asthma (Consensus Conference Proceedings, 1995).

*Diagnostic testing* is needed when the patient's symptoms are severe and do not respond to allergen avoidance and medications or when immunotherapy is being considered. Skin testing is the gold standard of diagnostic testing (Noble et al, 1995). Nasal smears are not useful. Although a nasal smear that is positive for eosinophils is consistent with the diagnosis of allergic rhinitis, a positive smear may also be obtained in patients with nonallergic rhinitis eosinophilia syndrome (Noble et al, 1995). Radioallergosorbent testing is expensive and not as specific nor as sensitive as skin testing (Bernstein, 1993).

## Patient/Caregiver Information

Antihistamines have many side effects. Warn patients of the possibility of drowsiness and decreased ability to perform certain skills such as driving and use of machinery when taking sedating antihistamines. Inform patients that some antihistamines have strong anticholinergic properties, which may cause constipation and urinary retention (Smith, 1995). These untoward effects may be reduced by starting with low doses and gradually increasing the dosage over several days or advising the patient to take initial doses at bedtime (Noble et al, 1995). Remind patients to take antihistamines regularly to prevent symptoms and to allow the body time to adjust to unwanted sedation.

Patients should inform their health care provider that they are taking antihistamines. Sedating antihistamines can potentiate the effects of agents that cause central nervous system alterations such as alcohol, antianxiety agents, antipsychotics, and narcotic analgesics. First-generation antihistamines may have additive anticholinergic activity when administered concurrently with tricyclic antidepressants, antispasmodics, and antiparkinsonian medications (Ferguson, 1997).

Warn patients that terfenadine and astemizole should not be used in combination with certain medications such as fluconazole and ketoconazole or the macrolide antibiotics such as erythromycin and clarithromycin, which inhibit the metabolism of terfenadine and astemizole and may cause cardiac arrhythmias (Ament & Patterson, 1997; Krause, 1994). Caution patients not to exceed the recommended doses of medications, especially astemizole and terfenadine, due to potentially fatal cardiac arrhythmias (Smith, 1994). Teach patients to read drug labels before taking any over-the-counter medication since many cold products and sleep aids contain antihistamines. Astemizole and loratadine should be taken on an empty stomach (Noble et al, 1995).

Advise patients that intranasal decongestants may cause rebound congestion and should therefore be used for only 3 days. Teach patients that intranasal corticosteroids often have a delayed onset of activity and that symptoms may not improve for 1–2 weeks after starting therapy. Remind patients to take these drugs daily rather than sporadically or on an as-needed basis.

Because cromolyn nasal spray is ineffective in reducing allergic symptoms that are already present, advise patients that relief of symptoms may be delayed as long as 3–4 weeks when therapy is initiated. Addition of an antihistamine may be necessary until cromolyn reaches its full effect.

Intranasal medications must come in contact with the entire nasal mucosa to be effective. Therefore, nasal passages should be cleared prior to administering medications. Spray the

medication quickly and firmly into the nostril while keeping the head upright. Spray each nostril separately and wait at least 1 min before the second spray. If possible, avoid sneezing or blowing the nose for 5–10 min after using an intranasal inhaler. Cleanse the medicine canister device after each use to reduce the chance of contamination. Medications that are delivered intranasally may cause irritation and bleeding of the nasal mucosa, and in rare cases, nasal septal perforation. Therefore, intranasal medications should be sprayed away from the nasal septum (Smith, 1995; Swanson, 1996).

## OUTCOMES MANAGEMENT

### Selecting Appropriate Agents

*Antihistamines.* Antihistamines are classified into two groups: first-generation and second-generation antihistamines. First-generation antihistamines include agents such as diphenhydramine, hydroxyzine, chlorpheniramine, triprolidine, clemastine, and brompheniramine. Second-generation antihistamines include terfenadine, astemizole, loratadine, fexofenadine, and cetirizine. It should be emphasized that generally all antihistamines are equally effective (Hendeles, 1993a). Selection of an agent should be based more upon duration of action, side-effect profile, risk of drug interactions, and cost. Patient noncompliance may be the largest predictor of treatment failure. Antihistamine therapy for allergic rhinitis should be initiated with the least expensive first-generation antihistamine. The most commonly used agent is hydroxyzine. Hydroxyzine is similar in potency to cetirizine, yet less expensive because of generic availability (Hendeles, 1997). Chlorpheniramine is a suitable first-line alternative to hydroxyzine. Although sedation is an undesirable adverse effect of these agents, it may be minimized by slow dosage titration beginning with administration at bedtime only. After several days of bedtime dosing, a small morning dose may be added and increased based on symptom control and adverse effects. Tolerance to the sedative effects generally occurs after 1–2 weeks of continued dosing.

Because of the cost, second-generation antihistamines should be reserved for those patients unable to tolerate the traditional agents. These agents may be dosed once daily for enhanced patient compliance, with the exception of terfenadine and fexofenadine, which require twice-daily dosing for most patients (Nightingale, 1996). Caution should be applied when prescribing terfenadine or astemizole because these agents have been shown to induce torsades de pointes, a potentially fatal ventricular arrhythmia. Terfenadine and astemizole are metabolized hepatically by isoenzyme CYP3A4. Inhibitors of this enzyme (ie, erythromycin, clarithromycin, ketoconazole, HIV-1 protease inhibitors, fluconazole) have the potential to dramatically increase the serum concentration of terfenadine, astemizole, and desmethylastemizole, an active metabolite of astemizole. Loratadine is also metabolized by CYP3A4, but to date has not been associated with cardiovascular complications (Smith, 1994). In addition to avoiding the above drug interactions, patients should be counseled not to exceed 120 mg of terfenadine or 10 mg of astemizole daily. These agents are safe and effective when used at recommended doses in the absence of drug interactions. Decongestants may be added separately or in combined preparations with antihistamines to relieve nasal congestion not mediated by histamine receptors (Smith, 1994). See Drug Table 705.

*Decongestants.* Decongestants may be administered topically or orally to patients with nasal congestion as a symptom of allergic rhinitis. For short-term relief of nasal congestion or to enhance the delivery of an intranasal corticosteroid spray, topical phenylephrine, naphazoline, or oxymetazoline may be used for 3–5 days. Further use may be complicated by rebound congestion caused by rhinitis medicamentosa. Phenylpropanolamine and pseudoephedrine are the most effective oral decongestants available. Although phenylephrine is available in many over-the-counter products, its effectiveness has been questioned due to poor bioavailability and first-pass metabolism. Oral decongestants should be used with caution in patients with hypertension as they may cause elevations in blood pressure. Contraindications to decongestant use include severe hypertension, angle-closure glaucoma, and concurrent use of a monoamine oxidase inhibitor (Hendeles, 1993b). See Drug Table 703.

*Corticosteroids.* Intranasal corticosteroids are effective in controlling all symptoms of allergic rhinitis. Available products include beclomethasone, budesonide, flunisolide, fluticasone, triamcinolone, and dexamethasone. Dexamethasone should be avoided due to potentially significant systemic absorption, which may lead to adverse effects. Budesonide, fluticasone, triamcinolone, and possibly beclomethasone are effective if administered on a once-daily regimen. Budesonide, triamcinolone, and flunisolide contain solvents that may be irritating to the nasal mucosa of some patients. Aqueous formulations of beclomethasone, triamcinolone acetonide, and fluticasone are available and better tolerated. The relative cost of these agents varies, with triamcinolone and beclomethasone being the least expensive. Emphasis should be placed on regular use of these products versus on an as-needed basis. These agents should be added to antihistamine therapy as an adjunct to control nasal congestion or if antihistamine therapy fails to control symptoms (Badhwar & Druce, 1992; Mabry, 1992; Meltzer, 1995). See Drug Table 706.

*Cromolyn sodium, nedocromil, and ipratropium.* Cromolyn sodium and nedocromil are mast-cell stabilizers that may have utility in perennial allergic rhinitis if other therapies prove unsuccessful. They should be used to prevent symptoms from starting and not on an as-needed basis, for which they are generally ineffective. Mast-cell stabilizers should be reserved for those patients with chronic or severe symptoms. These agents are more costly compared to inhaled corticosteroids or antihistamines. Intranasal ipratropium may reduce rhinorrhea, but has no effect on nasal congestion. Its place in management of allergic rhinitis has yet to be defined (Badhwar & Druce, 1992).

## Monitoring for Efficacy

*Antihistamine.* Symptomatic relief begins to occur within several hours of administration but may take 2–4 weeks to reach its maximum effect. All antihistamines should be administered for 2–3 weeks prior to switching to an agent of another class.

*Decongestants.* An oral decongestant may be added if nasal congestion is not relieved by an antihistamine. Symptomatic improvement should occur within several hours of oral administration. Topical decongestants have a very rapid onset of action, usually relieving nasal congestion within minutes.

**Corticosteroids.** Most patients achieve moderate to significant symptomatic improvement within 2–4 weeks of initiating corticosteroid therapy provided it is used on a continuous and regular basis. A trial of 8 weeks may be necessary for assessing efficacy. Patients are generally initiated on the maximum recommended dose. If nasal symptoms are controlled, the dose may be gradually reduced to the lowest effective dose. Each new dose should be continued for at least 1 week before any subsequent changes are made (Hulisz & Fillwock, 1996).

**Cromolyn Sodium and Nedocromil.** The mast-cell stabilizers are used to prevent the symptoms of allergic rhinitis from initiating. The mast-cell stabilizers are expensive and require frequency of dosing, which can create compliance problems (Meltzer, 1995). Three to four weeks may be required before the beneficial effects of therapy are achieved (Hulisz & Fillwock, 1996).

## Monitoring for Toxicity

**Antihistamines.** The adverse-effect profile of first-generation antihistamines includes anticholinergic as well as histamine-blocking effects. Antagonism of central histamine receptors may result in sedation, dizziness, and paradoxical excitation in children and the elderly. Anticholinergic effects may include dry mouth, urinary retention, constipation, and blurred vision. Second-generation antihistamines are devoid of or have minimal sedative properties because of their reduced lipophilicity compared to first-generation agents. Cardiotoxicity has resulted from excessive serum concentrations of terfenadine and astemizole. This may result from doses above the recommended range, severe hepatic disease, or drug interactions (listed above). Cardiotoxicity has been reported, such as Q-T interval prolongation, atrioventricular heart block, and various ventricular arrhythmias, including torsades de pointes. Patients may experience unexplained dizziness, syncope, or blackout spells. Weight gain has also been reported with the second-generation antihistamines.

**Decongestants.** Adverse effects from decongestants result from central nervous system (CNS) stimulation caused by sympathomimetic effects. These include nervousness, restlessness, insomnia, tremor, dizziness, and headache. These adverse effects may counteract the sedative effects of antihistamine therapy. Tachycardia, palpita-

tions, and elevations of blood pressure have been known to occur.

**Corticosteroids.** Intranasal corticosteroids are generally well tolerated. Nasal stinging and burning may occur and are more common with beclomethasone and flunisolide because of propellants. Aqueous formulations of beclomethasone and fluticasone are available and better tolerated. Improper administration of these agents can result in rare complications such as hemorrhagic crusting, ulceration, and perforation. See Drug Table 706.

**Cromolyn Sodium and Nedocromil.** Adverse effects occur in less than 10% of patients (Meltzer, 1995). Common adverse effects associated with the use of intranasal mast-cell stabilizers include sneezing, nasal stinging and burning, and headaches.

## COMMON COLD

The common cold is the leading cause of acute morbidity as well as absenteeism from work and school. Children have approximately six to eight colds annually, whereas adults generally have two to four colds per year (Gwaltney, 1995a; Spector, 1995). Although colds are the most frequent reason for visiting health care providers, most colds can be effectively self-treated at home with over-the-counter medications (Bryant & Lombardi, 1993).

Common colds are caused by one of six different virus families. Rhinoviruses and coronaviruses are the most common viruses causing colds (Gwaltney, 1995a). In young children respiratory syncytial virus (RSV) is a common pathogen (Fireman, 1993). Viral invasion of the upper respiratory tract inflames all or part of the mucosal membranes from the nose to the bronchi. Transmission of the virus occurs through direct contact with infectious secretions on skin and environmental surfaces, brief transportation of large particles of respiratory secretions in the air, and airborne droplets (Gwaltney, 1995a).

Symptoms are usually self-limiting, lasting approximately 5–7 days. Patients typically complain of nasal discharge, congestion or obstruction, sneezing, coughing, postnasal discharge, sore throat, and hoarseness. Low-grade fever, malaise, and inflamed, watery conjunctivae may be present. Potential complications include otitis media, sinusitis, pneumonia, and exacerbation of chronic conditions such as asthma (Spector, 1995).

## SPECIFIC CONSIDERATIONS FOR PHARMACOTHERAPY

### When Drug Therapy Is Needed

Decongestants are useful agents for the relief of cold symptoms and are beneficial in preventing sinus and eustachian tube obstruction that may lead to sinusitis and otitis media. Decongestants cause vasoconstriction and reduce nasal secretions and congestion, thereby improving nasal airway patency and ventilation. Although topical decongestants are effective for short-term therapy and provide a rapid decrease in nasal airway resistance, they have the potential to produce rebound congestion if used for more than 3–5 days (Hendeles, 1993b). Oral decongestants are best when treatment is needed for more than 3–4 days (Bryant & Lombardi, 1993).

Cough suppressants such as codeine or dextromethorphan are beneficial when patients are unable to sleep or rest due to hacking, nonproductive coughs. However, suppression of a productive cough may lead to serious complications such as pneumonia because the body is unable to clear the lungs and airways of unwanted material (Hendeles, 1993a).

Antihistamines and expectorants are available in many over-the-counter medications. Antihistamines are not effective because nasal congestion in colds is not mediated by histamine receptors. Therefore, antihistamines have no role in the management of the common cold. Antihistamines have anticholinergic effects that dry mucous membranes, which may be beneficial; but antihistamines can also exacerbate symptoms and increase upper airway obstruction by impairing the flow of mucus (Spector, 1995). Expectorants are believed to thin sputum, increase the volume of phlegm, and stimulate the flow of mucus, but there is limited scientific evidence to support this view (Hendeles, 1993a). Water is the best expectorant and should be consumed liberally.

New pharmacologic therapies may prove beneficial in the management of common colds, such as intranasal ipratropium bromide (Doyle, Riker, & McBride, 1993; Hayden, Diamond, Wood, Korts, & Wecker, 1996), zinc gluconate lozenges (Mossad, Macknin, Medendorp, &

Mason, 1996), and vitamin C (Hemilia & Herman, 1996).

## Short-Term and Long-Term Goals of Pharmacotherapy

The goals are to relieve symptoms, reduce the risk of developing complications, and reduce the transmission of viral infection to others. Educate your patients in the ways they can help themselves prevent and treat their own symptoms; see Tables 21–1, 21–2.

## Time Frame for Initiating Pharmacotherapy

Pharmacotherapy is needed for comfort and should be initiated only when cold-related symptoms are intolerable. Topical decongestants should be used for no longer than 3–5 days. See Drug Tables 703–707.

## Assessment Prior to Therapy

Obtain a *history* of the course and characteristics of symptoms. Assess for complications by questioning the patient about fevers, headaches,

---

### TABLE 21–2. HOW PATIENTS CAN HELP THEMSELVES PREVENT AND TREAT UPPER RESPIRATORY INFECTIONS

**Prevention**
  Wash hands frequently to reduce spread of microorganisms
  Try to avoid people with colds or being in congested areas, especially during peak infectious seasons
  Cessation of smoking or avoidance of second-hand smoke and other irritants
  Avoidance of allergens and excessively dry heat

**Treatment**
  Humidification of air
  Increased fluid intake
  Rest
  Regular nasal hygiene with a saline irrigation
  Steam inhalation and warm compresses if patient has sinus pressure
  Elevating head of bed when sleeping to facilitate sinus drainage
  In younger children with nasal congestion, clearing the nose with bulb syringe
  Hard candy, lozenges, or warm saline gargles for sore throats

facial pain, severe sore throat, persistent cough, wheezing, and chest pain.

The *physical examination* should focus on the nose, pharynx, and lungs. In addition, the sinuses should be percussed and transilluminated. The ears should be examined, and lymph nodes should be palpated.

*Diagnostic testing* is not indicated unless complications are suspected (Uphold & Graham, 1994).

## Patient/Caregiver Information

Tactfully discuss the use and abuse of over-the-counter cold remedies. Explain that most colds are self-limited and resolve without any drug treatment. Emphasize that cold remedies are used to relieve symptoms and prevent complications rather than cure the infection. Teach patients to read labels on all medications bought for self-treatment. Most over-the-counter medications contain a combination of ingredients such as decongestants, antihistamines, analgesics, and expectorants that are usually ineffective in relieving symptoms and may cause adverse effects. If symptoms are intolerable, suggest the patient use a single-ingredient cold medicine containing a decongestant. Warn patients with diabetes, hypertension, glaucoma, and benign prostatic hypertrophy to use decongestants cautiously and only after consultation with their health care provider (Gadomski, 1994).

## OUTCOMES MANAGEMENT

### Selecting Appropriate Agents

*Decongestants.* Topical decongestants such as phenylephrine and oxymetazoline nasal sprays are currently recommended to relieve symptoms of nasal congestion and promote drainage of nasal secretions in patients with the common cold. They have a rapid onset on action and are devoid of drug–disease state interactions of oral decongestants. Oral decongestants are preferred if therapy continues longer than 3–5 days. Pseudoephedrine and phenylpropanolamine are suitable first-line agents and are present in many over-the-counter cough and cold preparations. Some authorities recommend use of name brand pseudoephedrine products. Bioequivalence is not uniform between slow-release pseudoephedrine preparations and immediate-

release products. Because of the age of this agent, it is exempt from regulation by the Food and Drug Administration (Hendeles, 1993b). Phenylephrine is not useful as an oral decongestant because of its extensive first-pass metabolism, resulting in poor bioavailability. Children typically do not respond to over-the-counter antihistamine-decongestant combinations and their routine use is not recommended (Smith & Feldman, 1993). See Drug Table 703.

*Antitussives.* Dextromethorphan and codeine may be helpful in suppressing a cough. A nonproductive cough should generally be suppressed only if it interferes with sleep. See Drug Table 704.

*Expectorants.* Maintaining an adequate fluid intake through the liberal consumption of water may prove to be the best expectorant. Guaifenesin, an ingredient in many over-the-counter cough and cold preparations, does not reduce cough frequency and provides no benefit as an expectorant. Symptomatic relief experienced by patients is probably reflecting the activity of other ingredients in combination products such as a decongestant or cough suppressant (Hendeles, 1993b). See Drug Table 707.

*Antipyretics/Analgesics.* Nonsteroidal antiinflammatory agents (NSAID) such as indomethacin, sulindac, and naproxen have documented effectiveness in reducing cough (Turner, 1997) and relieving headache and fever. Aspirin and acetaminophen are effective analgesics and antipyretics. Aspirin should not be used in children or adolescents because of the risk of Reye's syndrome.

*Anticholinergic Agents.* Numerous clinical trials have attempted to define the role of ipratropium bromide in the symptomatic relief of the common cold. It has demonstrated a reduction in nasal discharge, severity of rhinorrhea, and sneezing. (Hayden et al, 1996). Because of lack of comparative clinical trials between ipratropium bromide and oral decongestants and the increased cost associated with use of ipratropium bromide, routine first-line use of this agent is not recommended. It may prove useful in patients with disease-state contraindications to oral decongestants (ie, angle-closure glaucoma, severe hypertension).

***Vitamin C.*** The effectiveness of vitamin C in prevention and treatment of the common cold has elicited much debate and little hard fact. Data from clinical trials reveal conflicting information. Reviews of primary literature have noted a slight decrease in the duration and severity of symptoms (Hemila, 1994). At this time, no conclusions can be drawn. Well-designed clinical trials would prove useful in defining its role.

***Zinc Gluconate.*** Zinc gluconate lozenges have been studied to determine their effectiveness in the treatment of the common cold. When compared to placebo, patients receiving one lozenge every 2 hours while awake experienced significantly shorter time to complete resolution of symptoms and fewer days with coughing, headache, hoarseness, nasal congestion, nasal drainage, and sore throat. Fever, muscle ache, scratchy throat, and sneezing were unaffected by the zinc gluconate lozenges. Nausea and bad-taste reactions were more common in patients receiving zinc lozenges (Mossad et al, 1996). More recently, Jackson & Peterson (1997) completed a meta-analysis of published randomized clinical trials and found that there was little evidence for the effectiveness of zinc salt lozenges in reducing the duration of common colds.

## Monitoring for Efficacy

Resolution of symptoms is the goal of all treatment modalities. If decongestants are not effective in relieving symptoms, addition of intranasal ipratropium bromide may prove useful. Cough suppression with dextromethorphan or codeine may be beneficial. If symptoms such as cough persist for longer than 1 week or are accompanied by high fever, rash, or persistent headache, the patient should be reevaluated for complications.

## Monitoring for Toxicity

Refer to the Allergic Rhinitis section of this chapter for a detailed adverse-effect profile of decongestants and intranasal ipratropium bromide.

***Dextromethorphan.*** The potential for toxic effects of dextromethorphan is very low. Adverse effects are rare. Nausea, drowsiness, and dizziness have been reported. Signs of acute toxicity may include blurred vision, nystagmus, ataxia, and shallow respirations (Smith & Feldman, 1993).

***Codeine.*** With oral antitussive doses of codeine, the frequency of adverse effects is low, but they include nausea, vomiting, constipation, dizziness, sedation, and palpitations. Codeine may be habit-forming. Respiratory depression with oral antitussive doses of codeine seldom occurs. Patients with asthma or pulmonary emphysema should be monitored closely for signs of respiratory insufficiency (Smith & Feldman, 1993).

## INFLUENZA

Influenza is a viral infection that occurs in epidemics lasting about 5–6 weeks. Persons over 70 years of age are affected four times more than persons under 40 years of age. Influenza viruses are of three antigenic types: A, B, and C. Although all three types can cause infections in humans, only types A and B can cause severe illness. Influenza is highly contagious. Children are typically infected first and then transmit the virus to adults. The mode of transmission is through direct, person-to-person contact, large droplet infection, or objects contaminated with nasopharyngeal secretions (American Academy of Pediatrics, 1997).

Characteristic symptoms include abrupt onset of fever, myalgia, sore throat, and nonproductive cough. In contrast to other upper respiratory infections, persons with influenza often suffer severe malaise that may last for several days. Complications include pneumonia, myositis, and central nervous system conditions. Elderly persons and individuals with chronic health problems are at increased risk for complications. Individuals over age 65 account for approximately 90% of the influenza-associated deaths in the United States (U.S. Department of Health and Human Services [DHHS], 1996).

## SPECIFIC CONSIDERATIONS FOR PHARMACOTHERAPY

### When Drug Therapy Is Needed

In the United States, two approaches are available to minimize the deleterious effects of influenza: immunoprophylaxis with inactivated vaccine and therapy with an antiviral drug. See Chap. 11 for discussion of the influenza vaccine.

Amantadine is approved for prophylaxis and treatment of influenza A in adults and children over 1 year of age, whereas rimantadine is approved only for prophylaxis in children. The mechanism of action of these drugs is not completely known, but they are believed to interfere with the initial state of viral replication by either uncoating the virus or primary transcription of viral ribonucleic acid (Wintermeyer & Nahata, 1995). Pharmacotherapy with amantadine and rimantadine is particularly important for unvaccinated elderly patients or patients with underlying medical problems who are at increased risk for complicated influenza infection.

## Short-Term and Long-Term Goals of Pharmacotherapy

Goals of pharmacotherapy are to prevent influenza infections when used prophylactically and to reduce the duration and severity of symptoms in infected individuals. Patients should be advised that the best way to help themselves, once symptoms have begun, is to increase bed rest and fluid intake. See Table 21–2.

## Time Frame for Initiating Pharmacotherapy

For reduction of signs and symptoms, pharmacotherapy should be started within 48 hours of illness onset or as soon as possible after symptoms are recognized. Pharmacotherapy should be discontinued as soon as clinically warranted or approximately 24–48 h after the disappearance of signs and symptoms because of possible induction of antiviral resistance (U.S. DHHS, 1996). See Drug Table 106.

## Assessment Prior to Therapy

During the history taking, question the patient about onset, characteristics, and duration of symptoms. Specifically inquire about myalgias and malaise, which are characteristic of influenza but are not typical in other upper respiratory infections. Determine whether the patient had an annual influenza vaccine. To identify possible complications of influenza, questions regarding chest pain, hemoptysis, severe muscle pain, and central nervous system problems such as confusion should be asked. Explore whether household members or close contacts of the patient are experiencing similar symptoms.

Observe for general appearance of lassitude and distress. Particularly in elderly patients and young children, assess hydration status. Thoroughly examine sinuses, ears, nose, throat, and

chest. In severe cases, perform a complete abdominal and neurologic examination (Uphold & Graham, 1994).

*Diagnosis* can usually be made from epidemiologic data obtained from a local or state health department that confirms influenza infection in a particular region or community (U.S. DHHS, 1996).

## Patient/Caregiver Information

Remind the patient to watch for central nervous system adverse effects from the medications such as behavioral changes and agitation. Instruct the patient who is taking amantadine to be cautious of concurrent medications that affect the central nervous system (U.S. DHHS, 1996).

## OUTCOMES MANAGEMENT

### Selecting Appropriate Agents

Amantadine-resistant and rimantadine-resistant viruses have been identified and are cross-resistant; therefore, switching to the other agent is of no benefit. Either agent may be chosen as first-line therapy for treatment or prophylaxis in adults and prophylaxis in children. Only amantadine should be selected for treatment of type A influenza in children. In patients with mild to moderate renal insufficiency and the elderly with a history of CNS adverse effects from amantadine, rimantadine may be selected as initial therapy (U.S. DHHS, 1996).

### Monitoring for Efficacy

When used as prophylaxis, efficacy is determined by the presence or absence of type A influenza illness. Outcomes of treatment are based on resolution of signs and symptoms including fever, myalgia, sore throat, and cough. Patients should be monitored for signs of complications or advancing disease such as pneumonia, respiratory failure, exacerbation of congestive heart failure in elderly patients, or precipitation of a myocardial infarction (U.S. DHHS, 1996).

### Monitoring for Toxicity

Mild adverse effects such as nausea and anorexia occur with both amantadine and rimantadine and will usually subside with continued administration. More serious effects include behavioral changes, delirium, hallucinations, agitation, and seizures. Amantadine has been shown to have a higher incidence of central nervous system effects compared to rimantadine. These adverse effects of amantadine appear to be more common in patients with renal insufficiency, seizure disorders, and certain psychiatric disorders and in the elderly. Reducing the dose of amantadine may prevent or reduce these adverse effects. The dose of rimantadine should be reduced in patients with severe hepatic dysfunction (U.S. DHHS, 1996).

## SINUSITIS

Sinusitis remains one of the most common and difficult diseases to appropriately diagnose and treat despite recent advances (Willett, Carson, & Williams, 1994). Sinusitis is defined as an inflammation of the mucous membranes that line the paranasal sinuses (Yonkers, 1992). Typically, sinusitis is divided into three types based on duration of symptoms and extent of mucosal damage:

- *Acute sinusitis* has an abrupt onset with resolution of symptoms with therapy within 3 weeks.
- *Subacute sinusitis* has persistent purulent nasal discharge despite therapy but no permanent mucosal damage.
- *Chronic sinusitis* occurs with episodes of prolonged inflammation and or repeated or inadequately treated acute infections. Symptoms persist for longer than 3 months despite appropriate medical therapy, and there is often permanent damage to the mucosa (Fekete, 1993; Newman, Platts-Mills, Phillips, Hazen, & Gross, 1994; Willner, Lazar, Younis, & Beckford, 1994).

The pathogenesis of all types of sinusitis is similar. The main etiologic factor is obstruction of the osteomeatal unit, which leads to lower levels of oxygen within the sinuses, decreased clearance of foreign material, and mucous stasis resulting in infection. Any factor or condition that blocks the flow of secretions can lead to the development of sinusitis. For example, in acute sinusitis, upper respiratory infections are important predisposing factors (Schwartz, 1994; Wagenmann & Naclerio, 1992; Willett et al, 1994). Anatomical abnormalities such as a deviated nasal septum and nasal polyps are important antecedents to chronic sinusitis. Other less

common predisposing factors are extension of dental infections, barotrauma, neoplasm, trauma, and foreign bodies (Powell, 1993). Although allergies cause edema and swelling of nasal mucosa, research on the causative role of allergies in sinusitis is limited (Gwaltney, Jones, & Kennedy, 1997).

Pathogens involved in sinusitis depend on the duration of symptoms. In acute sinusitis, common pathogens are *Streptococcus pneumoniae*, *Haemophilus influenzae*, and *Moraxella catarrhalis* (Wald, 1992). Penicillin-resistant *S. pneumoniae* has been increasingly reported as a pathogen in upper respiratory infections such as sinusitis (Green & Wald, 1996). Anaerobic bacteria are of increased importance in sinusitis resulting from dental infections. In chronic or subacute sinusitis the infection is usually polymicrobial (Brook & Yocum, 1995). Previously, anaerobes such as alpha-hemolytic streptococcus, *Bacteroides* sp, *Veillonella* sp, and *Corynebacterium* sp were believed to predominate in chronic sinusitis (Stafford, 1993). Recent studies have demonstrated that anaerobes are not frequent pathogens. The most common aerobic organism involved in chronic sinusitis is *Staphylococcus* sp (Ramadan, 1995). Unusual pathogens such as *Chlamydia pneumoniae* and viruses may cause sinusitis in some patients.

Children with acute sinusitis tend to have subtle symptoms of cough, rhinorrhea, periorbital puffiness, fatigue, and malaise. Adults are more likely to have rhinorrhea, postnatal drip, headache, and facial pain (Arjmand & Lusk, 1995; Corren, 1993; Manning, 1993). In a recent study by Williams and Simel (1993), maxillary toothache, poor response to nasal decongestants, history of colored nasal discharge, purulent nasal secretion, and abnormal transillumination were the best predictors of acute sinusitis in adults. In patients of all ages, a diagnosis of sinusitis should be considered when signs and symptoms of an upper respiratory infection last longer than 7–10 days.

The signs and symptoms of subacute and chronic sinusitis are less specific than acute sinusitis. The hallmark of persistent sinusitis is a dull ache or pressure across the midface or headache (Godley, 1992). Other symptoms include nasal discharge, congestion, cough, postnasal drip, fetid breath, and fatigue (Schwartz, 1994). A daytime cough is a important predictor of chronic sinusitis in children (Wald, 1994).

All three types of sinusitis may exacerbate asthma or otitis media (Slavin, 1993; Willner et al, 1994). Without appropriate medical therapy, complications may develop and include extension of infection into the ocular orbit, meningitis, cavernous sinus thrombosis, subdural empyema, frontal osteomyelitis, and brain abscess (Corren, 1993; Fekete, 1993; Powell, 1993).

## SPECIFIC CONSIDERATIONS FOR PHARMACOTHERAPY

### When Drug Therapy Is Needed

Antibiotics are recommended for all types of sinusitis. In areas that have a low incidence of sinusitis due to beta-lactamase–producing strains of *H. influenzae* and *M. catarrhalis*, patients may be initially treated with an inexpensive, safe antibiotic such as amoxicillin. On the other hand, trimethoprim-sulfamethoxazole (TMP-SMX) is effective against beta-lactamase–producing organisms and thus may be used as first-line therapy; it is less effective against *S. pneumoniae*. Chronic sinusitis is treated with a longer course of therapy using broad-spectrum antibiotics (Willett et al, 1994).

Other pharmacological approaches should be used to correct the underlying obstruction of the osteomeatal unit. Irrigation of the nose with saline is effective in shrinking the edematous mucosa, improving mucociliary flow, and clearing nasal debris (Parsons & Wald, 1996). Topical decongestants may also reduce mucosal edema and promote sinus drainage but should be used for short periods of time because of the possibility of rebound mucosal congestion with extended use (Mabry, 1993). Oral decongestants serve the same function as topical agents, but they are less effective than topical agents. Oral decongestants have been recommended for treatment of both acute and chronic sinusitis (Godley, 1992; Mabry, 1993; Stafford, 1993). However, Yonkers (1992) states that oral decongestants probably lose their effectiveness after 5 days. Both types of decongestants may delay clearance of infected debris and decrease blood flow to the mucosa, which may impede the effectiveness of antimicrobial therapy. Mucolytics are often recommended to liquify secretions and facilitate evacuation of sinus contents (Mabry, 1993). Oral antihistamines and cromolyn sodium should be used only if the patient has allergies (Lewis, 1994).

Treatment of chronic sinusitis includes topical corticosteroid sprays to decrease inflammation and edema, decrease vascular permeability, and inhibit leukotriene release, as well as appropriate antibiotics (Stafford, 1993). Most experts do not recommend the use of topical steroids during acute sinusitis since they may reduce local immune reactions (Godley, 1992). Topical steroids also may be beneficial in the prophylaxis of recurrent acute sinusitis (Mabry, 1993). Systemic corticosteroids are usually reserved for patients who are unresponsive to topical steroids, patients with nasal polyps, or children with cystic fibrosis (Arjmand & Lusk, 1995; Zeiger, 1992).

### Short-Term and Long-Term Goals of Pharmacotherapy

Short-term goals of therapy include eradication of infection, reduction of tissue edema, and facilitation of sinus drainage. Long-term goals are maintenance of patency of the osteomeatal complex and prevention of recurrent infections and complications (Fekete, 1993; Schwartz, 1994). Patients should be educated to help themselves prevent and treat their symptoms; see Table 21–1.

### Time Frame for Initiating Pharmacotherapy

Sinusitis should be treated at the time of diagnosis to prevent life-threatening complications. Acute sinusitis is typically treated for 10 days in uncomplicated cases, whereas treatment of chronic sinusitis may extend 3–4 weeks. An alternative approach is to continue therapy for an additional 7 days after the patient becomes asymptomatic (Arjmand & Lusk, 1995; Gungor & Corey, 1997). Antibiotics may be beneficial in the management of recurrent sinusitis (Willner et al, 1994).

Medications to reduce obstruction in the osteomeatal unit, such as topical and oral decongestants, also should be initiated at the time of diagnosis. Topical corticosteroids, on the other hand, should be started in the later stages of subacute sinusitis or chronic sinusitis. See Drug Table 102.

### Assessment Prior to Therapy

The *history* should focus on identifying symptoms consistent with sinusitis such as purulent nasal discharge, headache that increases with bending, and a positive response to decongestants. Risk factors for developing sinusitis should be explored. Past medical history should include questions concerning previous episodes and treatments of sinusitis, ear infections, allergies, and asthma. Questions regarding high fevers, periorbital edema, severe headaches, and visual complaints should be included to explore the possibility of complications from sinusitis (Simon, 1995; Uphold & Graham, 1994).

The *physical examination* should focus on the nasal cavity. The frontal and maxillary sinuses should be transilluminated and percussed. The ears, pharynx, mouth, teeth, and chest should be examined for signs of infection. To assess for complications of sinusitis, look for periorbital swelling and perform a neurologic examination (Simon, 1995; Uphold & Graham, 1994).

The first episode of acute sinusitis is usually treated empirically with antibiotics. Sinus x-rays are indicated for recurrent acute sinusitis or patients whose condition indicates a need for early and accurate diagnosis. Radiographic x-rays reveal air-fluid level and opacification of the sinuses, which are helpful in diagnosing acute sinusitis (Arjmand & Lusk, 1995). However, sinus x-rays, particularly in children, are frequently misinterpreted and have been found to be misleading (Parsons, 1996). Computerized tomography (CT) has become the gold standard of radiographic study (Parsons, 1996), but CT is not cost-effective and should not be ordered routinely to diagnose acute sinusitis (Low et al, 1997). CT is usually reserved for management of recalcitrant cases and in patients needing surgical procedures (Willett et al, 1994).

The optimum way to confirm the diagnosis of maxillary and frontal sinusitis and identify the causative pathogen is to obtain sinus aspirates by antral puncture. However, that procedure is impractical in most primary care settings (Corren, 1993; Welch, 1993). Unfortunately, smears and cultures of nasal secretions, which can be easily collected, typically do not correlate with sinus pathogens because they are contaminated by flora of the nasopharynx (Yonkers, 1992).

### Patient/Caregiver Information

It is important to teach patients the proper use of nasal sprays (see patient information under Allergic Rhinitis). Education on strategies to prevent future bouts of sinusitis should be part of the management plan. For example, some patients should be taught to avoid certain environmental irritants and allergens. Patients with re-

current episodes of sinusitis should be instructed to begin decongestants at the first sign of sinusitis to facilitate sinus drainage and prevent mucus stasis, which often leads to infection (Simon, 1995).

## OUTCOMES MANAGEMENT

### Selecting Appropriate Agents

*Antimicrobial Treatment of Acute Sinusitis.* Antimicrobial selection for both adults and children is similar and should be based on the most likely pathogens involved. Inexpensive, safe antibiotics such as amoxicillin and TMP-SMX are good initial choices (Low et al, 1997). However, amoxicillin is not effective against beta-lactamase–producing strains of *H. influenzae* and *M. catarrhalis*, and TMP-SMX is less effective against *S. pneumoniae*. In geographic areas where a high percentage of beta-lactamase–producing pathogens are known, other agents such as amoxicillin-clavulanate, loracarbef, cefuroxime axetil, cefixime, and the macrolide antibiotics may be effective, but these agents are more costly. Sinusitis caused by penicillin-resistant *S. pneumoniae* is treated with high-dose amoxicillin (60–80 mg/kg per day) or high-dose beta-lactamase–stable antibiotics (Green & Wald, 1996). Treatment of acute sinusitis thought to originate from dental infection should include an agent such as amoxicillin-clavulanate that is effective against anaerobic organisms. Sinusitis in patients not responding to the above therapy may be due to *Chlamydia pneumoniae*. In this small percentage of patients (<10%), alternative therapy with a tetracycline, clarithromycin, or azithromycin should be initiated (Gwaltney, 1995c).

*Antimicrobial Treatment of Chronic Sinusitis.* Patients with chronic sinusitis are likely to have acute exacerbations of disease. Compared to acute sinusitis, acute infections associated with chronic sinusitis are more likely caused by gram-positive and gram-negative anaerobic bacteria (Wald, 1992). Therefore, antimicrobial selection should include coverage against these pathogens as well as the typical pathogens of acute disease. Single agents or combinations, such as amoxicillin-clavulanate, clindamycin, dicloxacillin-metronidazole, cefuroxime-metronidazole, or clarithromycin may be effective (Willet et al, 1994).

***Adjunctive Therapy for Acute and Chronic Sinusitis.***
Topical decongestants such as phenylephrine
nose drops and oxymetazoline nasal spray, as
well as oral decongestants such as pseudoephedrine, are recommended to improve maxillary ostial function. Because of rebound congestion and tolerance, decongestant nasal sprays
should be used only for 3 days. Topical corticosteroids such as beclomethasone dipropionate,
flunisolide, triamcinolone acetonide, and fluticasone may prove useful in the management of
chronic sinusitis, although no controlled clinical
trials have been conducted supporting their
benefit (Arjmand & Lusk, 1995; Gwaltney,
Jones, & Kennedy, 1997; Zieger, 1992).

## Monitoring for Efficacy

The efficacy of antimicrobial therapy is based on
resolution of signs and symptoms of the illness.
If symptoms do not begin to resolve within
5–7 days of initiating antimicrobial therapy, noncompliance, inappropriate drug selection, atypical pathogens, or resistant organisms must be
considered.

## Monitoring for Toxicity

Antimicrobial therapy with TMP-SMX has been
associated with rash, including Stevens-Johnson
syndrome, crystalluria, and photosensitivity. The
most frequently reported adverse effects of
penicillins or cephalosporins include rash and
urticaria. Amoxicillin-clavulanate has also been
associated with increased gastrointestinal com-
pliants, including diarrhea. Hypersensitivity reactions such as hives, laryngeal edema, and anaphylactic shock pose an immediate threat and
warrant medical attention. Gastrointestinal
complaints such as nausea, vomiting, and diarrhea are the most frequently reported adverse
effects of macrolide therapy.

# PHARYNGITIS

Pharyngitis (inflammation of the pharynx and
tonsils) is the fourth most common symptom
seen by health care providers (Centor & Meier,
1992). Although most patients who seek care
are concerned about streptococcal pharyngitis,
other etiologic agents are often involved.
Approximately 20–65% of all cases of pharyngitis result from noninfectious causes, such as
postnasal drip or irritation due to allergies,

smoking, or alcohol consumption (Pichichero,
1995). Viruses (ie, adenoviruses, Epstein-Barr
virus, herpesviruses, influenza viruses) are the
most frequent pathogens causing pharyngitis
(Gwaltney, 1995b). Bacteria such as *Mycoplasma pneumoniae* and *Chlamydia pneumoniae* may be important causes of sore throats in
adults. Other bacteria such as *Neisseria gonorrhoeae* and *Arcanobacterium haemolyticus* are
uncommon, sporadic etiologic agents associated
with pharyngeal infection (Pichichero, 1995).
*Corynebacterium diphtheriae* should be considered a likely pathogen only when the patient is
unimmunized. The most important pathogen to
identify is group A beta-hemolytic streptococci
(GABHS), also known as *S. pyogenes.*

Streptococcal pharyngitis occurs in approximately 30% of all children and 10% of all adults
complaining of sore throat. It is predominantly
an infection of school-aged children and is rare
in children younger than 3 years of age. The typical clinical course is short-lived with mild symptoms and signs of tonsillopharyngeal erythema,
enlarged anterior cervical nodes, and soft palate
petechiae (Ruppert, 1996). On the other hand,
some patients do experience severe throat pain,
headaches, chills, abdominal pain, high fever, an
edematous uvula, and a thick exudate covering
the pharynx and tonsils (Dajani et al, 1995).
Infections with certain strains of GABHS produce an erythrogenic toxin and result in scarlet
fever or scarlatina with a characteristic rash
(Gwaltney, 1995b; Uphold & Graham, 1994).
Other suppurative (ie, direct extension from the
pharyngeal infection) complications such as
peritonsillar abscess, cervical lymphadenitis,
mastoiditis, and sinusitis can occur.

Nonsuppurative complications that can arise
from immune responses to the acute infection
are a dangerous sequela of streptococcal
pharyngitis. Acute glomerulonephritis may appear 1–3 weeks postinfection and usually is not
prevented by appropriate antibiotic treatment.
In contrast, antibiotic treatment can prevent the
other significant nonsuppurative complication,
acute rheumatic fever. Although the incidence
of rheumatic fever is low in the United States,
since the mid-1980s there have been several
serious outbreaks (Blummer & Goldfarb, 1994).
Rheumatic fever involves inflammation of the
joints, heart, and subcutaneous tissue (Deeter,
Kalman, Rogan, & Chow, 1992). Jones devised
criteria for the diagnosis of acute rheumatic
fever, which were revised in 1984 and helpful in
clinical practice (Jones criteria, 1984).

# SPECIFIC CONSIDERATIONS FOR PHARMACOTHERAPY

## When Drug Therapy Is Needed

Although there are various etiologies of pharyngitis, health care providers especially want to identify and treat those patients with GABHS for a number of reasons:

1. Antibiotics can relieve symptomatic complaints rapidly. Even though many patients with streptococcal pharyngitis have mild, self-limited symptoms, others can develop severe pain, high fevers, and systemic complaints. Prompt treatment with antimicrobial therapy is recommended for patients who are acutely ill (Pichichero, 1995).

2. Prompt drug therapy can decrease the transmission of infection to others since patients are believed to be noninfectious after 24 h on antimicrobial therapy (Ruppert, 1996).

3. Drug therapy can reduce or prevent suppurative complications (Gwaltney, 1995b; Simon, 1995). Although antimicrobial therapy does not have a direct effect on the reduction of post-streptococcal glomerulonephritis, drug therapy may indirectly reduce the incidence of this non-suppurative complication by decreasing the communicability or spread of GABHS (Gerber & Markowitz, 1985).

Prevention of rheumatic heart disease is the most important reason for drug therapy (Peter, 1992). Acute rheumatic fever can lead to permanent cardiac valve damage (Alto & Gibson, 1992). Adequate antimicrobial treatment of GABHS can "virtually eliminate" the risk of developing acute rheumatic fever (American Academy of Pediatrics, 1997, p. 490).

Other drug therapies relieve the symptoms of pharyngitis. Acetaminophen or ibuprofen are helpful in reducing fevers and discomfort. Throat lozenges and topical anesthetic throat sprays may be beneficial for adults and older children (Ruppert, 1996).

## Short-Term and Long-Term Goals of Pharmacotherapy

The short-term goals of treatment for pharyngitis caused by GABHS are to resolve the infection, promptly relieve the symptomatic complaints, and prevent the transmission of the bacteria to others. The long-term goals of treatment are to prevent complications such as acute rheumatic fever. Patients should be instructed to increase fluid intake and use hard candy, cold drinks, or warm saline gargles to soothe throat pain. See Table 21–3 for additional information.

## Time Frame for Initiating Pharmacotherapy

Antimicrobial therapy should be started immediately in those patients with a positive rapid antigen test. Controversy exists as to initiation of antimicrobial treatment in those individuals with a negative rapid antigen test when a strong clinical suspicion of streptococcal pharyngitis

## TABLE 21–3. TREATMENT OF STREPTOCOCCAL PHARYNGITIS

| Agent | Dose | Mode | Duration |
|---|---|---|---|
| Penicillin G Benzathine | 600,000 U for patients ≤27 kg (60 lb); 1,200,000 U for patients >27 kg (60 lb) | Intramuscular | Once |
| Penicillin V | Children: 250 mg 2–3 times daily Adolescents and adults: 500 mg 2–3 times daily | Oral | 10 days |
| **For individuals allergic to penicillin** | | | |
| Erythromycin: | | | |
| Estolate | 20–40 mg/kg/day divided 2–3 times daily (maximum 1 g/day) | Oral | 10 days |
| Ethylsuccinate | 40 mg/kg/day divided 2–3 times daily (maximum 1 g/day) | Oral | 10 days |

*Source: Adapted from American Academy of Pediatrics (1997).*

still exists. Delaying therapy for as much as 9 days from the onset of symptoms does not increase the risk of rheumatic fever; therefore, not prescribing an antimicrobial until results of throat culture have been obtained (usually 24–48 h) is not unreasonable.

The *history* and *physical examination* should be aimed at determining whether the patient has streptococcal pharyngitis or another type of pharyngitis. For example, pharyngitis due to coxsackievirus is accompanied by lesions in the mouth and on the hands and feet. Patients with infectious mononucleosis have exudative pharyngitis as well as fever and fatigue (see Chap. 37 for further discussion of infectious mononucleosis). The severity of the pharyngitis and the risk the patient has for developing complications should also be assessed.

The physical assessment should focus on the skin, head, nose, throat, mouth, chest, and abdomen. For example, inspection and palpation of the skin can reveal circumoral flushing, Pastia's lines, and a fine pinpoint exanthem in patients who have scarlet fever. Examination of the head, nose, and mouth can identify signs suggestive of viral pharyngitis, such as a clear nasal discharge and mouth ulcers. Neck, chest and abdominal assessments can rule out signs of complications that may occur with lymphadenitis, pneumonia, and splenomegaly in infectious mononucleosis. Examining the pharynx is crucial in determining the likelihood of streptococcal pharyngitis and to rule out complications such as a peritonsillar abscess, which occurs with asymmetric tonsillar swelling (Ruppert, 1996; Uphold & Graham, 1994).

A throat culture is the *diagnostic test* of choice for patients complaining of sore throats. Rapid streptococcal tests may be used as an adjunct to throat cultures. Because specificity of these rapid tests is high, there is no need to perform a throat culture for confirmation of infection. However, the sensitivity of the rapid tests varies from 50–70%. Thus, a culture is needed when a patient has a negative rapid test and is suspected of having streptococcal pharyngitis (American Academy of Pediatrics, 1997; Bisno et al, 1997).

## Patient/Caregiver Information

Patients should be advised to take the full 10-day course of antibiotics even though they are likely to be asymptomatic within 24–48 h. If patients do not feel significantly better in 2–3 days,

they should return for further evaluation. Stress should be placed on informing the patient that the pharmacological treatment is aimed at resolving the acute infection as well as preventing the complications, particularly rheumatic fever. Side effects of medications and supportive home treatments should be discussed.

## OUTCOMES MANAGEMENT

### Selecting Appropriate Agents

Although numerous etiologies of pharyngitis have been described, antimicrobial treatment is aimed at eradication of GABHS from the pharynx to prevent rheumatic fever. Several factors should be considered when selecting the most appropriate antimicrobial treatment regimen. These factors include bacteriologic and clinical efficacy, compliance, cost, spectrum of activity, and potential side effects.

*Antimicrobial Treatment of Streptococcal Pharyngitis.* Although several classes of antimicrobial agents have been shown to eradicate group A streptococci from the pharynx, penicillin remains the drug of choice because of its proven efficacy and cost. The current recommended treatment for streptococcal pharyngitis consists of penicillin given as a 10-day, twice daily, oral regimen of penicillin V or a one-time dose of intramuscular penicillin G benzathine for patients expected to be noncompliant (American Academy of Pediatrics, 1997; Gerber, 1996; Shulman, 1996). See Table 21–3 for treatment options. Warm penicillin G benzathine to room temperature before administering to reduce the pain of intramuscular injection. Ampicillin and amoxicillin offer no clinical advantage and an increased cost over penicillin (American Academy of Pediatrics, 1997).

*Drug of Choice in Penicillin-allergic Patient.* Patients with immediate (anaphylactic-type) hypersensitivity to penicillin should receive erythromycin estolate or erythromycin ethylsuccinate for 10 days (American Academy of Pediatrics, 1997). Cephalosporins should be avoided as <20% of penicillin allergic patients can also be allergic to these agents (Gwaltney, 1995b).

*Alternative Antimicrobial Agents.* Antimicrobial agents including azithromycin, clarithromycin, cefadroxil, and cephalexin have been shown to effectively eradicate group A streptococci from the pharynx, although penicillin remains the only drug proven to prevent rheumatic fever (Gwaltney, 1995b; Shulman, 1996). Advantages of azithromycin include less gastrointestinal irritation compared to erythromycin and a convenient dosing regimen; a 5-day course of once-daily administration is currently indicated. Cephalosporins have been shown to have higher bacteriologic cure rates compared to penicillin, although the clinical significance of this finding warrants further investigation (Gwaltney, 1995b). A major disadvantage of the above agents is higher cost compared to penicillin or erythromycin.

***Drug of Choice for Patients whose Treatment Fails and Chronic Carriers of GABHS.*** In those patients who continue to harbor group A streptococci in the pharynx, a second course of antimicrobial should only be considered in symptomatic individuals or those who are asymptomatic with a previous history of rheumatic fever. Some studies suggest the presence of beta-lactamase–producing organisms in the upper respiratory tract may interfere with the activity of penicillin. Amoxicillin-clavulanate, clindamycin, or a combination of penicillin with rifampin given concurrently during the last 4 days of the regimen is recommended (Bisno et al, 1997; Gwaltney, 1995b).

Individuals who are chronic carriers of group A streptococci (positive throat culture without illness) are at low risk for development of rheumatic fever. However, when these individuals develop an acute upper respiratory tract infection, it may be difficult to distinguish infection from colonization. Therefore, a single course of antimicrobial therapy is indicated in this patient population (Gwaltney, 1995b).

***Drugs Not Indicated for Treatment of GABHS Pharyngitis.*** Agents not effective in the treatment of streptococcal pharyngitis include tetracyclines, trimethoprim-sulfamethoxazole, sulfonamides, and chloramphenicol (Gwaltney, 1995b).

## Monitoring for Efficacy

Signs and symptoms of streptococcal pharyngitis usually resolve several days after the initiation of antimicrobial therapy. Those patients who remain symptomatic or develop recurring symptoms and those who have had rheumatic fever and are at unusually high risk for recurrence should receive a throat culture 2–7 days after completion of the antimicrobial regimen (Dajani et al, 1995). Patients are considered noncontagious following 24 h of antimicrobial therapy.

## Monitoring for Toxicity

The most frequently reported adverse effects of penicillin or cephalosporins include rash and urticaria. Hypersensitivity reactions such as hives, laryngeal edema, and anaphylactic shock pose an immediate threat and warrant medical attention. Gastrointestinal complaints are the most frequently reported adverse effects of macrolide therapy.

## CROUP

Croup, or acute laryngotracheobronchitis, is a viral infection that produces inflammation and narrowing of the entire respiratory tract. The airway obstruction is greatest at the subglottic level. It is the most common cause of acute upper airway obstruction in children between the ages of 3 months and 6 years, with a peak occurrence in the second year of life. Croup is commonly caused by parainfluenza virus, although influenza, respiratory syncytial virus, rhinovirus, and *M. pneumoniae* may be causative pathogens (Hall, 1995).

Croup is characterized by fever, inspiratory stridor, hoarseness, and a barking cough that is worse at night. Children typically exhibit symptoms of the common cold one to several days before the onset of stridor. The symptoms usually resolve within 3–7 days, although the cough may last for a longer period (Hall, 1995).

Most children with croup have mild symptoms and are not brought in for medical attention. Of the children who present to the emergency department, approximately 20% have severe disease with cyanosis, hypoxemia, retractions, rales, and rapid respiratory rates and require hospitalization. Few children have respiratory failure that necessitates intubation (Fitzgerald et al, 1996; Pendergast, Jones, & Hartman, 1994).

Some children have repeated episodes of inspiratory stridor and are diagnosed with spasmodic croup. Spasmodic croup primarily occurs in children who have a history of atopy. Some believe this condition may be a hypersensitivity reaction to a past infection (Custer, 1993).

Other serious conditions have characteristic symptoms that resemble those of croup and must be included in the differential diagnosis. Epiglottitis and bacterial tracheitis require intensive therapy and hospitalization. In both cases the child appears toxic and is acutely ill (Doull, 1995).

## SPECIFIC CONSIDERATIONS FOR PHARMACOTHERAPY

### When Drug Therapy Is Needed

Currently, experts are debating whether children with mild symptoms should be treated with drugs and whether children with moderate to severe symptoms can be managed with these medications in outpatient settings.

Nebulized racemic epinephrine and nebulized L-epinephrine appear equally effective in reducing airway obstruction (Waisman et al, 1992). These agents stimulate alpha-adrenergic receptors, resulting in local vasoconstriction and a reduction in subglottic inflammation. Unfortunately, the action of these agents only lasts approximately 2 h, and children may have rebound mucosal vasodilatation and dyspnea.

Corticosteroids with their antiinflammatory effects improve the clinical course of croup in children (Klassen, Watters, Feldman, Sutcliffe, & Rowe, 1996). They may be given alone or in conjunction with or after nebulized epinephrine (Cruz, Stewart, & Rosenberg, 1995; Johnson, Schuh, Koren, & Jaffe, 1996; Klassen, Feldman, Watters, Sutcliffe, & Rowe, 1994; Ledwith, Shea, & Mauro, 1995). Although most authorities recommend that corticosteroids be reserved for children with severe symptoms, Rowe and Klassen (1996) conclude that strong evidence supports the routine use of nebulized budesonide or parenteral corticosteroids for the outpatient management of mild to moderate croup. Unfortunately, nebulized budesonide remains investigational and unavailable to the health care provider.

### Short-Term and Long-Term Goals of Pharmacotherapy

The goals are to reduce airway obstruction, shorten the course of disease, and prevent hospitalization and intubation. Caregivers should be educated to help treat their children's symptoms.

### Time Frame for Initiating Pharmacotherapy

The time frame for initiating pharmacotherapy is controversial. For children with moderate to severe symptoms of croup, most experts recommend that nebulized epinephrine be initiated immediately. Others (Cruz et al, 1995; Johnson et al, 1996) recommend that corticosteroids be used in conjunction with epinephrine or after epinephrine is administered.

It is even more controversial whether drugs should be initiated immediately for children with mild to moderate symptoms. Some experts (Klassen et al, 1996; Rowe & Klassen, 1996) recommend corticosteroids to prevent complications of croup if they are administered to all children, whereas others contend that croup is mainly a self-limited condition and children with mild to moderate symptoms should not receive epinephrine or corticosteroids (Hall, 1995).

See Drug Tables 601 and 701.

### Assessment Prior to Therapy

If a child is in respiratory distress, plan for immediate transfer to a hospital and quickly question parents regarding onset of symptoms, fluid intake, voiding, and level of alertness. For children with mild to moderate symptoms, take the time to gather a *history* of pattern, duration, characteristics, and severity of symptoms. Explore the presence of associated symptoms such as high fever and production of purulent sputum, which is more characteristic of bacterial tracheitis than croup (Gwaltney, 1995b). Inquire about immunization status to eliminate the likelihood of epiglottitis, since epiglottitis may be life-threatening, whereas croup is not.

During the *physical examination*, rapidly assess vital signs and respiratory status including respiratory rate, retractions, use of accessory muscles, nasal flaring, and cyanosis. Assess hydration status and decreased response to stimuli. Observe for signs of drooling and difficulty swallowing, which are characteristic of epiglottitis, an emergent problem requiring immediate transfer to a hospital. *Never attempt to examine the pharynx of a patient with signs and symptoms consistent with epiglottitis.* Perform a complete lung and heart examination (Uphold & Graham, 1994).

The *diagnosis* of croup is usually based on clinical presentation without diagnostic tests. If epiglottitis is suspected, a lateral inspiratory and expiratory chest x-ray and an anterior-posterior x-ray of the neck are recommended. If bacterial tracheitis is suspected, a culture of the sputum can confirm the diagnosis (Gwaltney, 1995b).

## Patient/Caregiver Information

Teach caregivers to carefully and frequently assess their child's hydration status, level of alertness, and respiratory rate. In particular, caution them that the effects of nebulized epinephrine are often short-lived and the child may have additional episodes of stridor and respiratory distress. Children treated with corticosteroids must be frequently monitored as well, even though the effects of these drugs are longer in duration. Since corticosteroids are only to be used for a short period of time, children should not experience adverse effects that occur with extended use of these agents. Ask the caregivers if the child has had exposure to varicella within the preceding 3 weeks or has received *Varicella* vaccine (Vari-vax) in the preceding 2 weeks. Fatalities have occurred when patients with varicella-zoster virus infection have ingested corticosteroids (Folland, 1997).

## OUTCOMES MANAGEMENT

Since croup is a predominately viral condition, antibiotics are only indicated in patients with fever for more than 5–7 days and showing deterioration of the condition. This is an attempt to manage bacterial superinfection.

## Selecting Appropriate Agents

*Epinephrine.* Nebulized racemic epinephrine has been used with success in the management of moderate to severe symptoms of croup. Local vasoconstriction and decreased subglottic inflammation account for its clinical benefit in relieving stridor. Rebound mucosal vasodilation and dyspnea may occur with discontinuance; therefore, close observation is necessary. Nebulized racemic epinephrine also has been shown to reduce the number of children requiring intubation for severe croup. Current recommendations are the administration of 0.5 mL of 2.25% racemic epinephrine hydrochloride in 3–5 mL of normal saline solution every 2 h (Custer, 1993). The levorotatory form of epinephrine (L-epinephrine) has been shown to be

equally effective compared to racemic epinephrine and is less expensive; it may be a suitable alternative (Waisman et al, 1992).

*Corticosteroids.* Corticosteroids have a longer duration of action than epinephrine. Therefore, corticosteroids are currently often used after nebulized epinephrine when treating children with moderate to severe symptoms of croup. A recent review of the literature yielded the following guidelines regarding the use of corticosteroids (Cruz et al, 1995; Johnson et al, 1996; Klassen et al, 1994; Rowe & Klassen, 1996):

- Patients with moderately severe to severe croup may benefit from oral or parenteral corticosteroids, or 2 mg of nebulized budesonide once available.
- Outpatients with mild to moderate croup may benefit from parenteral dexamethasone (0.6 mg/kg).
- Nebulized dexamethasone is not effective in improving clinical outcomes and is currently not recommended.

## Monitoring for Efficacy

A significant decrease in airway obstruction should occur 10–30 min after administering nebulized epinephrine and continue for 1–2 h. Frequent administration may be necessary because of this. Patients should be monitored for rebound congestion. Patients treated with epinephrine and corticosteroids should be monitored for up to 12 h prior to release.

## Monitoring for Toxicity

Toxicity from single doses of corticosteroids has not been reported in clinical trials. Racemic epinephrine given on a routine basis may result in tachycardia, restlessness, anxiety, and tremor.

## REFERENCES

Alto, W. A., & Gibson, R. (1992). Acute rheumatic fever: An update. *American Family Physician, 45,* 613–619.

Ament, P. W., & Patterson, A. (1997). Drug interactions with nonsedating antihistamines. *American Family Physician, 56,* 223–229.

American Academy of Pediatrics, Committee on Infectious Disease. (1997). *1997 Red book: Report of the Committee on Infectious Disease* (24th ed.). Elk Grove Village, IL: AAP.

Arjmand, E. M., & Lusk, R. P. (1995). Management of recurrent and chronic sinusitis in children. *American Journal of Otolaryngology, 16*, 367–382.

Badhwar, A. K., & Druce, H. M. (1992). Allergic rhinitis. *Medical Clinics of North America, 76*, 789–802.

Bernstein, J. A. (1993). Allergic rhinitis: Helping patients lead an unrestricted life. *Postgraduate Medicine, 93*, 124–132.

Bisno, A. L., Gerber, M. A., Gwaltney, J. M., Kaplan, E. L., & Schwartz, R. H. (1997). Diagnosis and management of Group A streptococcal pharyngitis: A practice guideline. *Clinical Infectious Diseases, 25*, 574–583.

Blummer J., & Goldfarb, J. (1994). Meta-analysis in the evaluation of treatment for streptococcal pharyngitis: A review. *Clinical Therapeutics, 16*, 605–620.

Brook, I., & Yocum, P. (1995). Antimicrobial management of chronic sinusitis in children. *Journal of Laryngology and Otology, 109*, 1159–1162.

Bryant, B. G., & Lombardi, T. P. (1993). Selecting OTC products for coughs and colds. *American Pharmacy, NS33 (1)*, 19–24.

Centor, R., & Meier, F. (1992). Sore throat. In L. Dornbrand, A. Hoole, & C. G Pickard (Eds.), *Manual of clinical problems in adult ambulatory care* (pp. 70–75). Boston: Little, Brown.

Consensus Conference Proceedings. (1995). *The chronic airway disease connection: Redefining rhinitis.* Los Angeles: UCLA School of Medicine, Office of Continuing Medical Education.

Corren, J. (1993, December). Making the clinical diagnosis of sinusitis. *Clinical Focus*, (Suppl.), 11–17.

Cruz, M. N., Stewart, G., & Rosenberg, N. (1995). Use of dexamethasone in the outpatient management of acute laryngotracheitis. *Pediatrics, 96*, 220–223.

Custer, J. R. (1993). Croup and related disorders. *Pediatrics in Review, 14*, 19–29.

Dajani, A. S., Ayoub E., Bierman, F. Z., Bismo, A. L., Dentry, F. W., Dureck, D. T., Ferrieri P., Freed, M., Gerber, M., Kaplan, E. L., Karchmer, A. W., Markowitz, M., Rahimbtoola, S. H., Shulman, S. T., Stollerman, G., Takahashi, M., Taranto, A., Taubert, K. A., & Wilson, W. (1993). Guidelines for the diagnosis of rheumatic fever: Jones criteria, updated 1992. *Circulation, 87*, 302–307.

Dajani, A. D., Taubert, K., Ferrieri, P., et al. (1995). Treatment of acute streptococcal pharyngitis and prevention of rheumatic fever. A statement for health professionals. *Pediatrics, 96*, 758–764.

Davies, R. J., Bagnall, A. C., McCabe, R. N., Calderon, M. A., & Wang, J. H. (1996).

Antihistamines: Topical vs oral administration. *Clinical and Experimental Allergy, 26, (Suppl. 3)*, 11–17.

Deeter, R. G., Kalman, D. L., Rogan, M. P., & Chow, S. (1992). Therapy for pharyngitis and tonsillitis caused by group A beta-hemolytic streptococci: A meta-analysis comparing the efficacy and safety of cefadroxil monohydrate versus oral penicillin V. *Clinical Therapeutics, 14*, 740–754.

Doull, I. (1995). Corticosteroids in the management of croup: Nebulised corticosteroids are the treatment of choice. *British Medical Journal, 311*, 1244.

Doyle, W. J., Riker, D. K., & McBride, T. P. (1993). Therapeutic effects of an anticholinergic-sympathomimetic combination in induced rhinovirus colds. *Annals of Otology, Rhinology and Laryngology, 102*, 521–527.

Fekete, T. (1993). Acute bacterial sinusitis: When sinus pain spells infection. *Family Practice Recertification, 15*(5), 27–34.

Ferguson, B. J. (1997). Allergic rhinitis: Options for pharmacotherapy and immunotherapy. *Postgraduate Medicine, 101*, 117–131.

Fireman, P. (1993). Pathophysiology and pharmacotherapy of common upper respiratory diseases. *Pharmacotherapy, 13*, 101S–109S.

Fitzgerald, D., Mellis, C., Johnson, M., Allen, H., Cooper, P., & Van Asperen, P. (1996). Nebulized budesonide is as effective as nebulized adrenaline in moderately severe croup. *Pediatrics, 97*, 722–725.

Folland, D. S. (1997). Treatment of croup: Sending home an improved child and relieved parents. *Postgraduate Medicine, 101*, 271–278.

Gadomski, A. (1994). Rational use of over-the-counter medications in young children. *JAMA, 171*, 1063–1064.

Gerber, M. A. (1996). Antibiotic resistance: Relationship to persistence of group A streptococci in the upper respiratory tract. *Pediatrics, 97*, 971–975.

Gerber, M. A., & Markowitz, M. (1985). Management of streptococcal pharyngitis reconsidered. *Pediatric Infectious Disease, 4*, 518.

Godley, F. A. (1992). Chronic sinusitis: An update. *American Family Physician, 45*, 2190–2199.

Green, M., & Wald, E. (1996). Emerging resistance to antibiotics: Impact on respiratory infections in the outpatient setting. *Annals of Allergy, Asthma, and Immunology, 77*, 167–175.

Gungor, A., & Corey, J. P. (1997). Pediatric sinusitis: A literature review with emphasis on the role of allergy. *Otolaryngology, Head & Neck Surgery, 116*, 4–15.

Gwaltney, J. M. (1995a). The common cold. In G. L. Mandell, J. E. Bennett, & R. Dolan (Eds.),

*Principles and practice of infectious diseases.* (4th ed.) (pp. 561–566). New York: Churchill Livingstone.

Gwaltney, J. M. (1995b). Pharyngitis. In G. L. Mandell, J. E. Bennett, and R. Dolin, (Eds.), *Principles and practice of infectious diseases.* (4th ed.) (pp. 566–572). New York: Churchill Livingstone.

Gwaltney, J. M. (1995c). Sinusitis. In G. L. Mandell, J. E. Bennett, & R. Dolan (Eds.), *Principles and practice of infectious diseases.* (4th ed.) (pp. 585–590). New York: Churchill Livingstone.

Gwaltney, J. M., Jones, J. G., & Kennedy, D. W. (1997). Medical management of sinusitis: Educational goals and management guidelines. *Annals of Otology, Rhinology, and Laryngology, 127* (suppl.), 22–30.

Hall, C. B. (1995). Acute laryngotracheobronchitis (croup). In G. L. Mandell, J. E. Bennett, and R. Dolin (Eds.), *Principles and practice of infectious diseases* (4th ed.) (pp. 573–579). New York: Churchill Livingstone.

Hayden, F. G., Diamond, L., Wood, P. B., Korts, D. C., & Wecker, M. T. (1996). Effectiveness and safety of intranasal ipratropium bromide in common colds: A randomized, double-blind, placebo-controlled trial. *Annals of Internal Medicine, 125,* 89–97.

Hemilia, H. (1994). Does vitamin C alleviate the symptoms of the common cold? A review of current evidence. *Scandinavian Journal of Infectious Diseases, 26,* 1–6.

Hemilia, H., & Herman, Z. S. (1996). Vitamin C and the common cold: A retrospective analysis of Chalmers' review. *Journal of the American College of Nutrition, 14,* 116–123.

Hendeles, L. (1993a). Efficacy and safety of antihistamines and expectorants in nonprescription cough and cold preparations. *Pharmacotherapy, 13,* 154–158.

Hendeles, L. (1993b). Selecting a decongestant. *Pharmacotherapy, 13,* 129S–134S.

Hendeles, L. (1997). Cetirizine: A new antihistamine with minimal sedation. *Pharmacotherapy, 15*(5), 967–968.

Horak, F. (1993). Seasonal allergic rhinitis: Newer treatment approaches. *Drugs, 45,* 518–527.

Hulisz, D. T., & Fillwock, L. D. (1996, July). Management of allergic rhinitis. *U.S. Pharmacist,* 49–60.

Jackson, J. L., & Peterson, C. (1997). A meta-analysis of zinc salt lozenges and the common cold. *Archives of Internal Medicine, 157,* 2373–2376.

Johnson, D. W., Schuh, S., Koren, G., & Jaffe, D. M. (1996). Outpatient treatment of croup with nebulized dexamethasone. *Archives of Pediatric and Adolescent Medicine, 150,* 349–355.

Jones criteria (revised, 1984) for guidance in the diagnosis of rheumatic fever. *Circulation, 69,* 204A–208A.

Klassen, T. P., Feldman, M. E., Watters, L. K., Sutcliffe, T., & Rowe, P. C. (1994). Nebulized budesonide for children with mild-to-moderate croup. *The New England Journal of Medicine, 331,* 285–289.

Klassen, T. P., Watters, L. K., Feldman, M. E., Sutcliffe, T., & Rowe, P. C. (1996). The efficacy of nebulized budesonide in dexamethasone-treated outpatients with croup. *Pediatrics, 97,* 463–466.

Krause, H. F. (1994). Therapeutic advances in the management of allergic rhinitis and urticaria. *Otolaryngology—Head and Neck Surgery, 111,* 364–372.

Ledwith, C. A., Shea, L. M., & Mauro, R. D. (1995). Safety and efficacy of nebulized racemic epinephrine in conjunction with oral dexamethasone and mist in the outpatient treatment of croup. *Annals of Emergency Medicine, 25,* 331–337.

Lewis, C. M. (1994). Protocol for acute and chronic sinusitis. *Journal of American College Health, 42,* 237–238.

Lockey, R. F., Wildlitz, M. D., Mitchell, D. Q., Lumry, W., Dockhorn, R., Woehler, T., & Grossman, J. (1996). Comparative study of cetirizine and terfenadine versus placebo in the symptomatic management of seasonal allergic rhinitis. *Annals of Allergy, Asthma, and Immunology, 76,* 448–454.

Low, D. E., et al. (1997). A practical guide for the diagnosis and treatment of acute sinusitis. *Canadian Medical Association Journal, 156* (6 suppl.), 51–53.

Mabry, R. L. (1992). Corticosteroids in the management of upper respiratory allergy: The emerging role of steroid nasal sprays. *Otolaryngology—Head and Neck Surgery, 107,* 855–860.

Mabry, R. L. (1993). Therapeutic agents in the medical management of sinusitis. *Otolaryngologic Clinics of North America, 26,* 561–570.

Manning, S. C. (1993). Pediatric sinusitis. *Otolaryngologic Clinics of North America, 26,* 623–638.

Meltzer, E. O. (1995). An overview of current pharmacotherapy in perennial rhinitis. *Journal of Allergy and Clinical Immunology, 95,* 1097–1110.

Mossad, S. B., Macknin, M. L., Medendorp, S. V., & Mason, P. (1996). Zinc gluconate lozenges for treating the common cold: A randomized, double-blind, placebo-controlled study. *Annals of Internal Medicine, 125,* 81–88.

Mygind, N., & Dahl, R. (1996). The rationale for use of topical corticosteroids in allergic rhinitis. *Clinical and Experimental Allergy, 26* (Suppl. 3), 2–10.

Newman, L. J., Platts-Mills, T. A. E., Phillips, D., Hazen, K. C., & Gross, C. W. (1994). Chronic sinusitis: Relationship of computed tomographic findings to allergy, asthma, and eosinophilia. *JAMA, 271*, 363–367.

Nightingale, C. H. (1996). Treating allergic rhinitis with second-generation antihistamines. *Pharmacotherapy, 16*(5), 905–914.

Noble, S. L., Forbes, R. C., & Woodbridge, H. B. (1995). Allergic rhinitis. *American Family Physician, 51*, 837–846.

Parsons, D. S. (1996). Chronic sinusitis: A medical or surgical disease? *Otolaryngologic Clinics of North America, 29*, 1–9.

Parsons, D. S., & Wald, E. R. (1996). Otitis media and sinusitis. *Otolaryngologic Clinics of North America, 29*, 11–25.

Pendergast, M., Jones, J. S., & Hartman, D. (1994). Racemic epinephrine in the treatment of laryngotracheitis: Can we identify children for outpatient therapy? *American Journal of Emergency Medicine, 12*, 613–616.

Peter, G. (1992). Streptococcal pharyngitis: Current therapy and criteria for evaluation of new agents. *Clinical Infectious Diseases, 14* (Suppl. 2), S218–S223.

Pichichero, M. E. (1995). Group A streptococcal tonsillopharyngitis: Cost-effective diagnosis and treatment. *Annals of Emergency Medicine, 25*, 390–403.

Powell, M. A. (1993). Question and answer: Adult sinusitis. *Journal of the American Academy of Nurse Practitioners, 5*, 179–180.

Ramadan, H. H. (1995). What is the bacteriology of chronic sinusitis? *American Journal of Otolaryngology, 16*, 303–306.

Rowe, P. C., & Klassen, T. P. (1996). Corticosteroids for croup: Reconciling town and gown. *Archives of Pediatric and Adolescent Medicine, 150*, 344–346.

Ruppert, S. D. (1996). Differential diagnosis of common causes of pediatric pharyngitis. *Nurse Practitioner, 21*(4), 38–48.

Schwartz, R. (1994). The diagnosis and management of sinusitis. *Nurse Practitioner, 19*(12), 58–63.

Shulman, S. T. (1996). Evaluation of penicillins, cephalosporins, and macrolides for therapy of streptococcal pharyngitis. *Pediatrics, 97*, 955–959.

Simon, H. B. (1995). Approach to the patient with sinusitis. In A. H. Goroll, L. A. May, & A. G. Mulley (Eds.), *Primary care medicine: Office evaluation and management of the adult patient.* Philadelphia: Lippincott.

Slavin, R. G. (1993, December). The pathophysiology of sinusitis. *Clinical Focus*, (Suppl.), 3–10.

Smith, L. J. (1995). Diagnosis and treatment of allergic rhinitis. *Nurse Practitioner, 20*(10), 58–66.

Smith, M. B. H., & Feldman, W. (1993). Over-the-counter cold medications: A critical review of clinical trials between 1950 and 1991. *JAMA, 269*(17), 2258–2263.

Smith, S. J. (1994). Cardiovascular toxicity of antihistamines. *Otolaryngology—Head and Neck Surgery, 111*, 348–354.

Spector, S. L. (1995). The common cold: Current therapy and natural history. *Journal of Allergy and Clinical Immunology, 95*, 1133–1138.

Stafford, C. T. (1993, December). Successful medical management of sinusitis. *Clinical Focus* (Suppl.), 18–24.

Swanson, K. A. (1996). Counseling patients about allergic rhinitis. *Journal of the American Pharmaceutical Association, NS36*, 300–307.

Trevino, R. J., & Gordon, B. R. (1993). Allergic rhinosinusitis: The total rhinologic disease. *Ear, Nose, and Throat Journal, 72*, 116–126.

Turner, R. B. (1997). Epidemiology, pathogenesis, and treatment of the common cold. *Annals of Allergy, Asthma, and Immunology, 78*, 531–537.

Uphold, C. R., & Graham, M. V. (1994). *Clinical guidelines in family practice.* Gainesville, FL: Barmarrae Books.

U.S. Department of Health and Human Services, Public Health Service, Centers for Disease Control and Prevention. (1996). Prevention and control of influenza: Recommendations of the Advisory Committee on Immunizations Practices. *Morbidity and Mortality Weekly Report, 45*(RR-5), 1–24.

Wagenmann, M., & Naclerio, R. M. (1992). Anatomic and physiologic considerations in sinusitis. *Journal of Allergy and Clinical Immunology, 3*, 419–423.

Waisman, Y., Klein, B. L., Boenning, D. A., Young, G. M., Chamberlain, J. M., O'Donnell, R., & Ochsenschlager, D. W. (1992). Prospective randomized double-blind study comparing L-epinephrine and racemic epinephrine aerosols in the treatment of laryngotracheitis (croup). *Pediatrics, 89*, 302–306.

Wald, E. R. (1992). Microbiology of acute and chronic sinusitis in children. *Journal of Allergy and Clinical Immunology, 3*, 452–456.

Wald, E. R. (1994). Chronic sinusitis in children. *Journal of Pediatrics, 127*, 339–347.

Welch, M. J. (1993). Topical nasal steroids for allergic rhinitis. *Western Journal of Medicine, 158*, 616–617.

Willett, L. R., Carson, J. L., & Williams, J. W. (1994). Current diagnosis and management of sinusitis. *Journal of General Internal Medicine, 9*, 38–45.

Williams, J. W., & Simel, D. L. (1993). Does this patient have sinusitis? Diagnosing acute sinusitis by history and physical examination. *JAMA, 270*, 1242–1246.

Willner, A., Lazar, R. H., Younis, R. T., & Beckford, N. S. (1994). Sinusitis in children: Current management. *Ear, Nose, and Throat Journal, 73,* 485–491.

Wintermeyer, S. M., & Nahata, M. C. (1995). Rimantadine: A clinical perspective. *Annals of Pharmacotherapy, 29,* 299–310.

Yonkers, A. J. (1992). Sinusitis—Inspecting the causes and treatment. *Ear, Nose, and Throat Journal, 71,* 258–262.

Zeiger, R. S. (1992). Prospects for ancillary treatment of sinusitis in the 1990s. *Journal of Allergy and Clinical Immunology, 3,* 478–495.

# 22

## LOWER RESPIRATORY DISORDERS

*Kathleen M. Tauer and Lauwana E. Hollis*

Lower respiratory tract infections have become a constant and increasingly prevalent part of primary care practice. The incidence of asthma across the life span has become commonplace even as pharmacotherapeutic modalities have made management easier. Pharmacotherapies have made advances in the management of cystic fibrosis, allowing these patients both longer and better-quality lives. Incidences of pneumonia are higher with a concomitant range of drugs available to treat the various types of the illness. And tuberculosis, once thought to be almost eliminated, is turning up with renewed regularity, even in new drug-resistant versions, especially among immune-suppressed patients. This chapter reviews causes and treatment options for asthma in adult, pediatric, and pregnant populations; bronchiolitis in children; chronic obstructive pulmonary disease (COPD); cystic fibrosis; pneumonia in adult, pediatric, and pregnant populations; and tuberculosis.

## ASTHMA

The incidence of asthma has risen significantly since the early 1980s, from approximately 6 million people then to the current estimate of 14–15 million people (Centers for Disease Control and Prevention [CDC], 1996a). Asthma affects approximately 4.8 million children in the United States today, making it one of the most common chronic diseases of childhood (CDC,

1996a). Hospitalization rates are the highest among African-Americans and children, with death rates from asthma highest among African-Americans aged 15–24 years (CDC, 1996a).

There are several theories as to why this significant increase in asthma is currently being seen:

1. Children are spending more time inside rather than outside, for whatever reason. The allergen particles indoors are smaller; house dust mites, animal proteins, fungi, and so on can more readily penetrate the lower airways, contributing to an allergic reaction and leading to an increase in inflammatory reaction and increased airway hyperresponsiveness (Martinez et al, 1995; Sporik, Holgate, Platts-Mills, & Cogswell, 1990).

2. Many children and adults have received antibiotics, vaccines, and other therapies to prevent and/or treat illnesses. When exposed to environmental insults, the T-lymphocyte cells that respond to infections and provide protective antibodies are poorly stimulated and do not respond appropriately. This may allow other T-lymphocyte cells that produce cytokines and inflammatory mediators to overreact and produce an intense response, leading in turn to allergic sensitization (Landau, 1996).

   Families with children in day care have been found to be less likely to have anyone in their household develop asthma (James, 1995).

3. There is increasing evidence that there may be a critical window in early infancy when sensiti-

zation to common environmental allergens may occur versus a tolerance to these agents. This may contribute to the development of atopy and/or asthma early on or later in life (Landau, 1996).

The current working definition of asthma developed by the National Heart, Lung and Blood Institute in its 1997 Expert Panel Report (National Asthma Education and Prevention Program [NAEPP], 1997) reads:

> Asthma is a chronic inflammatory disorder of the airways in which many cells and cellular elements play a role, in particular, mast cells, eosinophils, T-lymphocytes, macrophages, neutrophils, and epithelial cells. In susceptible individuals, this inflammation causes recurrent episodes of wheezing, breathlessness, chest tightness, and coughing, particularly at night or in the early morning. These episodes are usually associated with widespread but variable airflow obstruction that is often reversible either spontaneously or with treatment. The inflammation also causes an associated increase in the existing bronchial hyperresponsiveness to a variety of stimuli. (p. 2)

Recent data also indicate that subbasement membrane fibrosis can occur in some individuals that contributes to persistent abnormalities in lung function (Roche, 1991). Postmortem autopsy reports reveal that airway pathology involves both the large and small airways. Inflammatory changes, mucous plugging, and cellular debris are common. The airway smooth muscle undergoes hypertrophy characterized by new blood vessel formation, increased numbers of epithelial goblet cells, and alterations in the amount and composition of the extracellular airway matrix, especially in those with long-standing and severe asthma. This results in airway remodeling, which may make the asthma less responsive to treatment (Busse, 1993; Laitinen & Laitinen, 1994).

Variability between morning and evening peak expiratory flow (PEF) appears to reflect airway hyperresponsiveness and therefore may serve to measure asthma instability and severity (NAEPP, 1997). Airflow obstruction in asthma is recurrent and caused by a variety of changes (Howarth, Redington, & Montefort, 1993; Laitinen & Laitinen, 1994; NAEPP, 1997):

- Acute bronchospasms
- Airway edema
- Chronic mucous plug formation
- Airway remodeling

Preliminary data indicate that early intervention with antiinflammatory medications may modify the disease process. Inflammation is probably an early element of asthma as well as a late and persistent component (Agertoft & Pedersen, 1993; Laitinen & Laitenen, 1994).

Airway diameters change and enlarge as the infant grows to adulthood, with peak size occurring at 16–23 years of age (Burrows, 1987). After 30 years of age, the forced expiratory volume ($FEV_1$) declines normally at a steady rate of about 30 mL/year; an accelerated decline is seen in smokers (Burrows, 1987; Hanson & Midthun, 1992). In the person without lung obstruction few problems are noted, but in those with asthma and COPD the normal changes are compounded with already diminished airflow secondary to the disease process, thus changing the morbidity of the illness and making the quality of life poorer (Hanson & Midthun, 1992).

The NAEPP 1991 recommendations were organized around four components that are most effective for the management of asthma:

1. Use of objective measures of lung function to assess the severity of asthma and to monitor the course of therapy

2. Environmental control measures to avoid or eliminate factors that precipitate asthma symptoms or exacerbations

3. Comprehensive pharmacologic therapy for long-term management designed to reverse and prevent the airway inflammation characteristic of asthma as well as pharmacologic therapy to manage asthma exacerbations

4. Patient education that fosters a partnership among the patient, his or her family, and clinicians

The following sections discuss asthma assessment and monitoring; factors contributing to severity; pharmacologic therapy for daily management and acute exacerbations; and patient education for asthma in children, during pregnancy, and in adults based on the pathophysiology presented.

## ADULT ASTHMA

The onset of asthma usually occurs in childhood and adolescence, but increasingly asthma has its onset or recurrence in adults and the elderly. Many otherwise healthy adults often ignore and/or rationalize some of the common presenting symptoms of asthma, resulting in their asthma remaining undiagnosed for a long time. In older adults and the elderly, the classic asthma symptoms of cough, wheezing, chest tightness, and shortness of breath can mimic many other medical conditions: congestive heart failure, pulmonary embolism emphysema, chronic bronchitis, pneumonia, and/or tracheo-bronchial tumor (Braman, 1993). It has been estimated that about 50% of adults with asthma had their initial onset in childhood, followed by a period of remission and then a resurgence in midlife (Oswald et al, 1997).

In adult onset asthma, allergens can continue to play a role, but some patients have no family history or IgE antibodies to allergens. The mechanism of nonallergic asthma is not fully understood, although there is an inflammatory process that is similar but not identical to that of atopic asthma (Walker et al, 1992). Several other triggering factors can be gastroesophageal reflux, occupational pollutants, tobacco smoke, pollutants, and beta blockers (Chan-Yeung & Malo, 1994; Odeh, Oliven, & Bassan, 1991).

Asthma management in the adult can require aggressive daily pharmacotherapy primarily using inhaled steroids, long-acting beta$_2$ agonists, and now the new leukotriene antagonists. Older asthmatics usually require daily medications, whereas the younger asthmatic adult can often use a beta$_2$ agonist on an as-needed basis. Asthma also can be an unrelenting disease in the elderly and require oral systemic steroids (Braman, 1993).

In addition to the usual goals for the management of asthma in the adult, make sure that the daily asthma medications used do not exacerbate other coexisting medical conditions and lead to deleterious health effects.

## SPECIFIC CONSIDERATIONS FOR PHARMACOTHERAPY

### When Drug Therapy Is Needed

Because asthma is a chronic disease characterized by airway inflammation and bronchial hyperresponsiveness, daily medication is needed to control the symptoms, maintain normal activity levels, prevent recurrent exacerbations, optimize pharmacotherapy with minimal or no adverse effects, and prevent further irreversible lung changes (NAEPP, 1997).

Daily medications for those with mildly persistent to severe asthma has been shown to sig-

nificantly reduce and control symptoms so individuals can have fully normal functioning and healthy lives (Gianaris & Golish, 1994; NAEPP, 1997). Without adequate treatment of acute exacerbations and chronic symptoms, morbidity and mortality are increased, especially among African-Americans and Hispanics. The highest death rates for these groups are 3–5.5 times higher than for Caucasians (Carr, Zeitel, & Weiss, 1992). It is estimated that about 80% of asthma patients in the United States may be receiving suboptimal treatment for their asthma while asthma patients in Europe are more aggressively treated. In Sweden about 50% of asthma patients are now treated with inhaled steroids compared to about 15% of U.S. patients (Rachelefsky, 1995a). The NAEPP 1997 Expert Panel recommends more aggressive treatment for asthma patients of all ages. Their recommendations are as follows:

1. Identify factors that exacerbate asthma.
2. Monitor daily PEF with a symptom control record.
3. Write instructions on how to manage a decline in PEF.
4. Write instructions on managing an acute asthma exacerbation.
5. Intensive and extensive education should be given about asthma and its management.
6. Regular office visits with the health care provider can be combined with appropriate referral to a specialist.
7. Develop a partnership with the health care provider so that the decision making regarding asthma management is a joint effort between patient and provider.

### Short- and Long-Term Goals of Pharmacotherapy

The short-term goals of asthma pharmacotherapy are to recognize a decline in the PEF and/or change in the diurnal pattern of the PEF, institute early treatment that may prevent an acute asthma exacerbation, aggressively treat an acute asthma flare (decrease bronchospasms, increase bronchodilation, and reduce inflammation), and return the person to their previous level of functioning (NAEPP, 1997).

The long-term goals of asthma management are to control symptoms, prevent daily exacerbations, recognize and manage triggering factors that exacerbate asthma, control nocturnal symptoms, prevent EIB (exercise-induced broncho-spasms) through preventive medications, use daily medications regularly if necessary, decrease or ameliorate the long-term airway remodeling leading to irreversible lung changes, and reduce morbidity and mortality (NAEPP, 1997).

## Nonpharmacologic Therapy

- Assess and avoid triggering factors that can provoke an asthma flare.
- Exercise regularly.

## Time Frame for Initiating Pharmacotherapy

Once the diagnosis of asthma is established and the severity is determined, treatment must begin immediately with the appropriate agent(s). The goal is to resolve the symptoms as quickly as possible and restore normal lung function. In acute exacerbations the acute symptoms should resolve rapidly, but complete resolution of all symptoms may take several days to weeks, depending on the severity of the flare and other comorbid illnesses. Symptoms should continue to improve and not remain the same or decline.
    See Drug Table 701.2.

## Assessment Needed Prior to Therapy

See Tables 22–1, 22–2, and 22–3 for important history markers, physical examination findings, assessment parameters, and common diagnostic tests needed.

## Patient/Caregiver Information

All persons with asthma need to know how to use a peak flow meter and inhaler (see below).

1. Discuss the following with patients:
    - Patients need to have a complete health evaluation to find out if there are other health problems that could affect or be affected by asthma.
    - They need to be encouraged to discuss all symptoms and physical problems that make taking medication difficult.
2. In addition, patients need to understand that it is important for them to get help from a support group, family, friends, or a counselor when they feel stressed or depressed. Any life changes can increase the risk of having an asthma episode (NAEPP, 1997).

***How to use an inhaler.***    Inhalers can be used by all asthma patients who are 5 years of age and

## TABLE 22–1.  HISTORY AND PHYSICAL EXAMINATION FOR ASTHMA

### Pertinent Baseline History Markers
- Childhood symptoms
- Current symptoms suggestive of wheezing, shortness of breath, chest tightness, breathlessness during play or exercise
- Asthma diagnosed in childhood
- Symptom development
- Symptom description: seasonal pattern, limitation of ADL, sleep disturbance
- Hospitalizations for respiratory problems

- Current medications
- Associated health problems that could aggravate: nasal polyps, sinusitis, allergic rhinitis, eczema, gastroesophageal reflux disease (GERD), COPD, heart disease, hypertension, glaucoma, psychiatric problems
- Positive family history
- Occupation
- Hobbies, animals in the house

### Physical Examination and Possible Findings
- Eyes: lens cloudiness, glaucoma
- Nose: purulent rhinorrhea, polyps
- Sinuses: pain
- Throat: posterior pharyngeal hypertrophied lymphoid tissue
- Chest: change in shape

- Heart: murmurs, $S_3/S_4$
- Lungs: wheezing, rhonchi, prolonged expiratory phase, use of accessory muscles, decreased breath sounds
- Abdomen: hepatosplenomegaly
- Neurologic: mental confusion, change in cerebellar function, change in motor coordination from baseline

*Adapted from: Braman (1993), Martin (1996), NAEPP (1997), and Schaffer (1991).*

## TABLE 22–2. COMMON DIAGNOSTIC TESTS FOR ASTHMA AND THEIR POSSIBLE FINDINGS

| Diagnostic Tests | Possible Findings |
|---|---|
| Spirometry | Decreased $FEV_1$, FVC |
| Chest x-ray | Hyperinflation, rule out lung masses, cavities |
| Nasal smears | Eosinophils |
| Allergy tests | +/−[a] dust mites, animal dander, mold, pollen |

**Special Tests as Indicated**
Bronchoprovocation challenge
Sinus films
EKG
Other pulmonary tests
Liver function tests
Prothrombin time
Upper GI series

[a]+/− means finding may be either present or absent.
*Adapted from Braman (1993), NAEPP (1997), and Roncolli and Dempster (1996).*

older. Infants and young children will benefit most from a holding chamber and/or a face mask attached to the inhaler. These devices can also be useful to elderly patients.

### METERED DOSE INHALER WITHOUT A SPACER

1. Remove the cap and shake the inhaler.
2. Breathe out.
3. Put the mouthpiece in your mouth and at the start of a slow, deep inspiration, press the canister and continue to inhale deeply. Always hold the inhaler horizontal to the floor.
4. Hold your breath for 10–15 s.
5. Exhale into room air.
6. Wait 30–60 s and repeat steps 1 through 5.

Using a spacer is always preferred. It increases the amount of medication that is delivered to the lung and less is deposited on the tongue and in the back of the mouth. It also decreases the cough reflex, voice changes, and the risk of a yeast infection in the mouth. There are many models of spacers available, so ask your health care provider which one is right for you.
When using a spacer:

1. Remove the cap and shake the inhaler.

2. Put the inhaler either into the back of the spacer or insert only the canister into the appropriate holder in the spacer.
3. Breathe out.
4. Press on the canister, breathe in deeply and slowly.
5. Hold your breath for 10–15 s.
6. Exhale back into the spacer, inhale again without pressing the canister, and exhale into room air.
7. Wait 30–60 s and repeat steps 1 through 6.

If using a steroid inhaler, always rinse your mouth after using the inhaler.

### TURBUHALER

1. Unscrew and lift off the cover.
2. Hold the turbuhaler upright and twist the blue grip backwards and forwards twice if this is the first time the turbuhaler has been used. This "primes" the turbuhaler. For subsequent uses you need to twist the turbuhaler backwards and then forward only once.
3. DO NOT SHAKE THE TURBUHALER.
4. Breathe out, put the mouthpiece between your lips, and breathe in as deeply as possible.
5. Hold your breath for 10–15 s.
6. Exhale into room air.
7. DO NOT EXHALE back into the spacer.
8. Repeat steps 1 through 7 immediately after the first inhalation—you don't need to wait between inhalations.

If using a steroid inhaler, always rinse your mouth after using.

### AUTOHALER

1. Remove the protective cover from the canister by pulling down the lip on the back of the cover.
2. Hold the inhaler upright, push the lever up, and then shake the canister.
3. Breathe out. Hold the canister upright, put the mouthpiece in the mouth, and close the lips around it securely. Hold the canister so that the air vents at the bottom aren't blocked.
4. Inhale slowly and continue breathing when the inhaler "clicks."
5. Hold your breath for 10–15 s.
6. Exhale into room air.
7. Hold the canister upright and press the lever down. Wait 1 min between inhalations.

## TABLE 22–3. ASSESSMENT PARAMETERS FOR THE ADULT AND ELDERLY ON ASTHMA

| Medications | Disease State | Adverse Reactions in Asthma |
|---|---|---|
| Beta blockers[a] | Hypertension<br>Glaucoma | Can cause bronchospasms |
| Beta$_2$ agonist | CHF | Increases heart rate<br>Potentiates heart failure<br>Excess use (dose-dependent effect) can cause decrease in K+ and increase in QT interval on EKG<br>Beta$_2$ receptor function decreases with age |
| Systemic steroids | | Exacerbate TB, hypertension, peptic ulcer disease<br>Cause/aggravate/accelerate osteoporosis, DM, loss of attention span, myopathy, increased skin fragility, memory and mood swings |
| Methylxanthine[b,c]<br>(theophylline) | CHF, cirrhosis<br>Cholestasis<br>BPH<br>Peptic ulcer disease, GERD | Decreased clearance<br><br>Difficulty voiding<br>Relaxes the cardiac sphincter |
| NSAIDS/aspirin | Arthritis<br>Heart disease<br>Nasal polyps | Increased risk of bronchospasms, angioedema, urticaria |
| Nonallergic rhinitis<br>ACE inhibitors | Hypertension<br>CHF, diabetic nephropathy | Cough |

[a] Use of propanolol with zileuton can increase propanolol levels leading to increased beta$_2$ activity.
[b] Risk of seizures, cardiac arrhythmias, and death from methylxanthine toxicity increases with age; 16-fold greater risk of death.
[c] Erythromycin, cimetidine, allopurinal, ciprofloxacin, and zileuton increase methylxanthine levels; zafirlukast decreases theophylline levels.
*Adapted from: Braman (1993) and NAEPP (1997).*

8. After finishing, the lever must be pushed up ("on") before using the inhaler again. The inhaler won't operate if you don't follow these directions.

***How to use a peak flow meter.*** A peak flow meter is a device that measures how well air moves out of your lungs. When an asthma episode is occurring, the airways of the lung begin to narrow slowly. By taking your peak flow measurement daily, you can often detect early airway narrowing, sometimes hours or days before you have any asthma symptoms.

If medicine is started before symptoms, you may be able to halt an asthma flare quickly and before it becomes severe.

A peak flow meter is most important for patients who use daily asthma medication. Patients who are 4–5 years of age and older can usually use a peak flow meter accurately.

The following five steps are necessary in order to obtain an accurate peak flow:

1. Move the indicator (usually a small red tab) to the bottom of the scale.

2. Stand up.

3. Take a very deep breath.

4. Holding the peak flow meter horizontal to the floor, place the mouthpiece in your mouth and close your lips securely around it.

5. Blow into the meter as hard and fast as you can (for children, it is like blowing out birthday candles).

### OBTAINING THE RESULTS

1. Write down the number you get. If you cough or make a mistake, don't write that number down. Repeat it.

2. Repeat steps 1 through 5 one or two more times and write down the best of the three numbers.

3. FIND YOUR BEST PERSONAL PEAK FLOW NUMBER. Your best personal peak flow number is the highest peak flow you can obtain over a 2–3 week period when your asthma is under good control. Good control is when you feel good, can do your regular activitis, and have no asthma symptoms.

Your personal best peak flow number may be higher or lower than someone else who is your age, height, or sex. Everyone's asthma is different so you need to find your personal best number. Your asthma treatment plan will be based on your personal best number. To find your personal best peak flow number, take your peak flow:

1. Twice daily for 2–3 weeks.

2. In the morning when you wake up and between 12 noon and 2 P.M. The early afternoon may not be possible for everyone, so late afternoon or early evening is acceptable.

3. As per instructions by your health care provider.

## OUTCOMES MANAGEMENT

### Selecting an Appropriate Agent

The NAEPP (1997) has developed four categories to classify asthma severity: mild intermittent, mild persistent, moderate persistent, and severe persistent. Table 22–4 shows the clinical features associated with these asthma severity classification categories.

Two strategies are recommended for managing therapy in the newly diagnosed asthmatic patient and/or the poorly controlled asthmatic

## TABLE 22–4. CLASSIFICATION OF ASTHMA SEVERITY—CLINICAL FEATURES BEFORE TREATMENT[a]

| Step | Symptoms[b] | Nighttime Symptoms | Lung Function |
|---|---|---|---|
| Step 1: mild intermittent | Less than twice a week<br>Asymptomatic with normal PEF between exacerbations<br>Exacerbations brief (few hours to few days); intensity varies | Less than twice a month | $FEV_1$/PEF >80% of predicted<br>PEF variability <20% |
| Step 2: mild persistent | Daily symptoms<br>Exacerbations may affect activity | More than twice a month | $FEV_1$/PEF >80% of predicted<br>PEF variability 20–30% |
| Step 3: moderate persistent | Daily symptoms<br>Daily use of inhaled short-acting beta$_2$ agonist<br>Exacerbations affect activity<br>Exacerbations more than twice a week; may last days | More than once a week | $FEV_1$/PEF >60–80% of predicted<br>PEF variability >30% |
| Step 4: severe persistent | Continual symptoms<br>Limited physical activity<br>Frequent exacerbations | Frequent | $FEV_1$/PEF <60% of predicted<br>PEF variability |

[a] According to the Expert Panel Report II, the presence of one of the features of severity is sufficient to place a patient in that category. An individual should be assigned to the most severe grade in which any feature occurs. The characteristics noted in this table are general and may overlap because asthma is highly variable. Furthermore, an individual's classification may change over time.

[b] Patients at any level of severity can have mild, moderate, or severe exacerbations. Some patients with intermittent asthma experience severe and life-threatening exacerbations separated by long periods of normal lung function and no symptoms.

*Adapted from NAEPP (1997, p. 29).*

## TABLE 22–5. ASTHMA TREATMENT BY STEP[a]

| Long-Term Prevention | Quick Relief |
|---|---|
| **Step 1: Mild Intermittent Asthma** | |
| None needed | Short-acting bronchodilator, an *inhaled beta₂ agonist,* as needed. Use an inhaled beta₂ agonist or cromolyn before exercise or allergen exposure. Use if needed during a viral respiratory infection. If excessive use or not improving, call the health care provider. |
| **Step 2: Mild Persistent Asthma** | |
| Daily medication: Either *low-dose inhaled steroids, leukotriene modifiers, cromolyn,* or *nedocromil,* or sustained-release theophylline. If needed increase inhaled steroids or add long-acting bronchodilator (especially for nighttime symptoms): either long-acting inhaled beta₂ agonist, sustained-release theophylline, or long-acting oral beta₂ agonist. | *Bronchodilator* as needed for symptoms. If use exceeds three to four times a day on a regular basis, reassess asthma control. |
| **Step 3: Moderate Persistent Asthma** | |
| Daily medications: Either *medium-dose inhaled steroid or inhaled low-dose steroids and long-acting inhaled beta₂ agonist,* sustained-release theophylline, long-acting beta₂ agonist tablets, or leukotriene modifier (zafirlukast or zileuton). If needed: *Anti-inflammatory: medium- to high-dose inhaled steroids* in combination with the agents listed above and a *long-acting inhaled beta₂ agonist.* | Short-acting bronchodilator: *inhaled beta₂ agonist* as needed for symptoms. If use exceeds three to four times a day, asthma control should be reassessed. |
| **Step 4: Severe Persistent Asthma** | |
| Daily medications: *Anti-inflammatory: Inhaled high dose steroids and long-acting bronchodilator:* Either a *long-acting inhaled beta₂ agonist,* sustained-release theophylline, or long-acting beta₂ agonist tablets. | Short-acting bronchodilator: *inhaled beta₂ agonist* as needed. Daily use indicates the need for additional long-term control ther- |

[a] Preferred treatments are in italics.
*Adapted from NAEPP (1997).*

patient, both involving step therapy. The first strategy is to begin at a level consistent with the patient's disease and "step up" therapy to achieve control of the symptoms. The second strategy is to initiate therapy at a higher level than the patient's severity to achieve rapid control of symptoms. After control is achieved, "step down" therapy to a level consistent with the patient's disease (NAEPP, 1997). The NAEPP recommends the latter approach, which usually achieves control of symptoms with a short burst of oral corticosteroids.

***Step 1: mild intermittent asthma.*** The individuals in this category usually have EIB and can be symptomatic with viral respiratory infections and/or exposure to allergens. In the elderly who experience symptoms of EIB, bronchospasms

with a respiratory infection, or an allergen exposure, 50% resolve quickly with the standard treatment but the rest continue to have persistent symptoms (Braman, 1993). Table 22–5 lists the recommended treatment plan.

***Step 2: mild persistent asthma.*** Individuals in this category require daily medication. If the asthma is poorly controlled or symptoms at diagnosis are consistent with the criteria in this category, follow the treatment recommendations in Table 22–5.

Antiinflammatory medications diminish airway inflammation and airway hyperresponsiveness (Kerstjens et al, 1992; NAEPP, 1997; Robinson & Geddes, 1996). A good choice for an inhaled steroid is triamcinolone acetonide or beclomethasone. These inhaled steroids can be used two to four times a day, but if the frequency is problematic then consider flunisolide, which is used only twice a day. A spacer should be used with all inhalers. It increases medication deposition in the lung, decreases oropharyngeal deposition, and may help improve pulmonary function (NAEPP, 1997). The elderly may need an assistive device other than a spacer because of arthritis, musculoskeletal problems, and other factors that limit coordination. The VentEase is one such device. It is an adapter that facilitates activation of the MDI (metered dose inhaler) and bypasses deformities and coordination problems (Newman & Clarke, 1993).

In the younger and middle-aged adult, bronchodilators are very effective; the elderly have a decreased beta-adrenergic response in the airways (Braman, 1993). The cholinergic bronchoconstrictive reflexes are intact and do not diminish with age (Davis & Bayard, 1988; Kendall, Dean, Bradley, Gibson, & Warthington, 1982). Ipratropium bromide might be the preferred bronchodilator of choice for those over 60 years (Braman, 1993).

Many adults with asthma also have nocturnal symptoms. The use of a long-acting beta$_2$ agonist relieves nocturnal symptoms and improves overall asthma control, especially when used in conjunction with inhaled steroids. Those with nocturnal symptoms should have an evaluation to rule out other treatable problems that could be causing or aggravating the nighttime symptoms. The long-acting beta$_2$ agonist is helpful in the elderly patient, too, but these patients must be warned that this is not a rescue medication (DuBuske, 1994; NAEPP, 1997).

There is controversy regarding the use of sustained-release low-dose theophylline to control nocturnal symptoms. In NAEPP (1997) page 3-a3 states that "sustained release theophylline is an alternative but not preferred long-term-control medication." The health care provider in conjunction with the patient must make a decision whether to use theophylline after weighing the pros and cons. In the elderly, theophylline is not a safe drug to use because of concomitant diseases that may alter theophylline pharmacokinetics, multiple drug interactions, and often the inability to tolerate the medication (Braman, 1993).

In the elderly, obstructive lung disease, chronic bronchitis, and emphysema can coexist with asthma, making diagnosis difficult. Often a 2–3 week trial of oral systemic steroids can help determine the reversibility of the airflow obstruction and the extent of the therapeutic benefit of the steroids (Bousquet, Chanez, Vignola, & Michel, 1996; NAEPP, 1997).

Consider the step-up therapy if control deteriorates or the step-down therapy if control is maintained for several months.

***Step 3: moderate persistent asthma.*** If the asthma is poorly controlled or symptoms at diagnosis are consistent with criteria in this category, follow the treatment recommendations in Table 22–5 (Step 3). Improved asthma control has been noted with both a long-acting beta$_2$ agonist and a medium-dose inhaled steroid compared to doubling the dose of the current inhaled steroid (Woolcock, Lundbeck, Ringdal, & Jacques, 1996). Another option is to increase the potency of the medium-dose inhaled steroid. Fluticasone and budesonide are more potent than either triamcinolone or flunisolide on a per-puff basis, requires fewer inhalations, and may more effectively inhibit the inflammatory process in the airways (Barnes & Lee, 1992; Johnson, 1996; Okamoto, Noonan, DeBoisblanc, & Kellerman, 1996) (see Table 22-6).

Other therapeutic drugs are the leukotriene modifiers zileuton, zafirlukast, and montelukast. They are inhibitors of the metabolic pathway that activates the leukotrienes, which produce bronchoconstriction, airway inflammation, and bronchial hyperresponsiveness (Chanarin & Johnston, 1994; Henderson, 1994). Zileuton is a specific inhibitor of 5-lipoxygenase, thus inhibiting certain leukotrienes responsible for the effects of airway inflammation, edema, mucous secretion, and bronchoconstriction. Zileuton is currently being used as an adjunct therapy in asthma patients with moderate persistent to severe asthma. Zafirlukast is a selective leukotriene receptor antagonist of the components that cause anaphylaxis. Zafirlukast interferes with the development of airway edema, smooth muscle contraction, and altered cell activity associated with the inflammatory process in the lungs (*Drug facts and comparisons*, 1998; Wenzel & Kamada, 1996). Since the leukotrienes are relatively new in the treatment of asthma, there are no data that demonstrate their antiinflammatory effectiveness. Because asthma is a disease of airway inflammation, the leukotrienes are considered adjunct therapy only. The inhaled steroids still remain the first-line therapy. Zileuton, however, has demonstrated protection from an asthmatic response to cold dry air, exercise, and sensitivity to NSAIDS or aspirin (Israel et al, 1993).

Montelukast inhibits the physiologic activity at the cysteinyl leukotriene receptor (CYSLT). This leukoziluton inhibitor, similar to zileuton and zarfirlukast, interferes with airway inflammation. Montelukast is not considered monotherapy in the treatment of asthma. This drug

## TABLE 22–6. ESTIMATED COMPARATIVE DAILY DOSAGES FOR INHALED CORTICOSTEROIDS

| Drug | Low Dose | Medium Dose | High Dose |
|---|---|---|---|
| **Adults** | | | |
| Beclomethasone dipropionate | 168–504 μg | 504–840 μg | > 840 μg |
| 42 μg/puff | (4–12 puffs—42 μg) | (12–20 puffs—42 μg) | (>20 puffs–42 μg) |
| 84 μg/puff | (2–6 puffs—84 μg) | (6–10 puffs—84 μg) | (>10 puffs–84 μg) |
| Budesonide Turbuhaler | 200–400 μg | 400–600 μg | > 600 μg |
| 200 μg/dose | (1–2 inhalations) | (2–3 inhalations) | (>3 inhalations) |
| Flunisolide | 500–1,000 μg | 1,000–2,000 μg | > 2,000 μg |
| 250 μg/puff | (2–4 puffs) | (4–8 puffs) | (>8 puffs) |
| Fluticasone | 88–264 μg | 264–660 μg | > 660 μg |
| MDI: 44, 110, | (2–6 puffs—44 μg) or | (2–6 puffs—110 μg) | (>6 puffs—110 μg) or |
| 220 μg/puff | (2 puffs—110 μg) | | (>3 puffs—220 μg) |
| DPI: 50, 100, | (2–6 inhalations— | (3–6 inhalations— | (>6 inhalations— |
| 250 μg/dose | 50 μg) | 100 μg) | 100 μg) or |
| | | | (>2 inhalations— |
| | | | 250 μg) |
| Triamcinolone acetonide | 400–1,000 μg | 1,000–2,000 μg | > 2,000 μg |
| 100 μg/puff | (4–10 puffs) | (10–20 puffs) | (>20 puffs) |
| **Children** | | | |
| Beclomethasone dipropionate | 84–336 μg | 336–672 μg | >672 μg |
| 42 μg/puff | (2–8 puffs—42 μg) | (8–16 puffs—42 μg) | (>16 puffs—42 μg) |
| 84 μg/puff | (1–4 puffs—84 μg) | (4–8 puffs—84 μg) | (>8 puffs—84 μg) |
| Budesonide Turbuhaler | 100–200 μg | 200–400 μg | >400 μg |
| 200 μg/dose | | (1–2 inhalations— | (>2 inhalations— |
| | | 200 μg) | 200 μg) |
| Flunisolide | 500–750 μg | 1,000–1,250 μg | >1,250 μg |
| 250 μg/puff | (2–3 puffs) | (4–5 puffs) | (>5 puffs) |
| Fluticasone | 88–176 μg | 176–440 μg | >440 μg |
| MDI: 44, 110, | (2–4 puffs—44 μg) | (4–10 puffs—44 μg) or | (>4 puffs—110 μg) or |
| 220 μg/puff | | (2–4 puffs—110 μg) | (>2 puffs—220 μg) |
| DPI: 50, 100, | (2–4 inhalations— | (2–4 inhalations— | (>4 inhalations— |
| 250 μg/dose | 50 μg) | 100 μg) | 100 μg) or |
| | | | (>2 inhalations— |
| | | | 250 μg) |
| Triamcinolone acetonide | 400–800 μg | 800–1,200 μg | >1,200 μg |
| 100 μg/puff | (4–8 puffs) | (8–12 puffs) | (>12 puffs) |

NOTES:
- *The most important determinant of appropriate dosing is the clinician's judgment of the patient's response to therapy.* The clinician must monitor the patient's response on several clinical parameters and adjust the dose accordingly. The stepwise approach to therapy emphasizes that once control of asthma is achieved, the dose of medication should be carefully titrated to the minimum dose required to maintain control, thus reducing the potential for adverse effect.
- The reference point for the range in the dosages for children is data on the safety of inhaled corticosteroids in children, which, in general, suggest that the dose ranges are equivalent to beclomethasone dipropionate 200–400 μg/day (low dose), 400–800 μg/day (medium dose), and >800 μg/day (high dose).
- Some dosages may be outside package labeling.
- Metered-dose inhaler (MDI) dosages are expressed as the actuator dose (the amount of drug leaving the actuator and delivered to the patient), which is the labeling required in the United States. This is different from the dosage expressed as the valve dose (the amount of drug leaving the valve, all of which is not available to the patient), which is used in many European countries and in some of the scientific literature. Dry powder inhaler (DPI) doses (e.g., Turbuhaler) are expressed as the amount of drug in the inhaler following activation.

*Adapted from NAEPP (1997).*

has been approved for use in children aged 6 years and older (Singulair, 1998).

Early recognition of declining PEFs is important for immediate action to be initiated. It is imperative that elderly adults monitor PEF daily as their perception of bronchoconstriction is blunted, allowing deterioration for longer periods, which then necessitates hospitalization rather than outpatient treatment (Connolly, Crowley, Charan, Nielson, & Vestal, 1992). In the elderly with moderate persistent to severe asthma with frequent exacerbations and wheezing, it is unlikely that symptoms will improve over time. Almost all elderly with these symptoms will require chronic oral systemic steroids. Persistent airflow obstruction demonstrated by spirometry testing is common in this group (Braman, 1993; Braman & Davis, 1986). For the management of an acute asthma exacerbation, refer to Table 22–7.

Every effort should be made to determine the etiology of the flare and correct the problem. It is important at the follow-up visit that the health care provider review daily medications, inhaler technique, and changes in the home or work environment. Consultation with a pulmonary specialist is necessary.

**Step 4: severe persistent asthma.**  Severe persistent asthma requires collaboration with a pulmonary specialist. If the patient requires oral steroids, use the lowest dose for the shortest time possible. For the elderly needing oral steroids, monitor closely for adverse effects, especially if comorbid illnesses are present.

If the asthma is poorly controlled or symptoms at diagnosis are consistent with the criteria in this category, follow the recommendations in Table 22–5 (step 4).

## Monitoring for Efficacy

At each visit, ask the patient about any change in symptoms (cough with laughing, exercise, weather changes, environmental or work exposure), nocturnal symptoms, frequency of the beta$_2$ agonist use, PEF readings, changes in exercise tolerance, subjective symptoms, chest tightness, shortness of breath, wheezing, degrees of cough, and limitation of activities of daily living. The daily medications should be reviewed and inhaler use demonstrated to ensure correct technique and use of relief medications. The patient should be fully active with minimal

---

### TABLE 22–7. MANAGEMENT OF AN ACUTE ASTHMA EXACERBATION

**Initial Assessment**
History, physical examination (heart rate, respiratory rate, wheezing, decreased breath sounds, use of accessory muscles), PEF

| **Assess Severity** | |
|---|---|
| PEF: 50–80% of predicted or personal best | PEF <50% of predicted or personal best |

| **Initial Treatment** | |
|---|---|
| Inhaled short-acting beta$_2$ agonist: 2–4 puffs every 20 min three times or one nebulizer treatment | Inhaled short-acting agonist and an anticholinergic via nebulizer every 20 min or continuously for 1 h |

**Repeat Assessment**
Symptoms, physical examination, PEF

| **Good Response** | **Incomplete Response** | **Poor Response** |
|---|---|---|
| PEF >80% of predicted or personal best and increased from original PEF; no wheezing or shortness of breath; response to beta$_2$ agonist is sustained; continue beta$_2$ agonist q 3–4 h for 2–3 days; if on inhaled steroids, double dose for 7–10 days; +/– short burst of steroids, call clinician in 24 h. | PEF 50–80% of predicted or personal best and no change from original PEF; persistent wheezing and shortness of breath; continue beta$_2$ agonist; add oral steroids and taper; contact clinician immediately. | PEF <50% of predicted or personal best, marked wheezing and/or shortness of breath; repeat inhaled beta$_2$ agonist or nebulizer; add oral steroids and taper; if distress is increasing, severe, and/or unresponsive, send to the ER. |

*Adapted from NAEPP (1997).*

to no symptoms and feel that their asthma is not limiting his or her life. Elderly patients should be active and healthy and experience minimal symptoms secondary to their asthma and comorbid illnesses.

During the physical examination, check the following:

- Change from baseline
- Nose: purulent rhinorrhea
- Sinuses: pain
- Lungs: wheezing, crackles, rhonchi, decreased breath sounds, prolonged expiratory phase, respiratory rate
- Heart: murmurs, $S_3$ and/or $S_4$
- Skin: eczema
- Pulmonary function tests: $FEV_1$, FVC (if not available, use a PEF)

The examination may be more extensive but must be tailored to the patient's symptoms, age, other comorbid illnesses, state of health, frequency of beta$_2$ agonist use, exacerbations, and any visits to the emergency room or health care provider's office for asthma flares.

The laboratory tests are based on the history and physical examination. For an acute exacerbation, a WBC and chest x-ray may be required, but more lab tests are necessary if the patient is elderly and/or has a comorbid illness. If the patient is on theophylline, levels should be obtained periodically. In the elderly, theophylline levels should be checked more often, especially if a sudden onset of mental changes occurs. Numerous medications and other factors can interfere with theophylline metabolism. Theophylline levels should be checked if the following conditions exist: change in medication dosing, stopping or starting a medication that interferes with theophylline metabolism, a change in smoking frequency, and patients on zileuton or zafirlukast (Drug Facts and Comparisons, 1998). Levels should be drawn every 2–3 months, if the patient is elderly and/or taking medication that interferes with theophylline metabolism or the history or physical examination are suggestive of problems. An ALT/AST should be checked on patients at baseline if adding zileuton is considered. LFTs are checked once a month for 3 months and then yearly, unless symptoms develop consistent with liver dysfunction. If liver elevations do occur, they can remain unchanged, resolve, or progress with continued zileuton therapy (Costello, Meltzer, & Bleecker, 1994; Drug Facts and Comparisons, 1998). Elevated liver enzymes occur in approximately

3–4% of people on zileuton and usually occur within 3 months of starting the medication.

Prothrombin time is monitored in those patients taking zileuton or zafirlukast and warfarin. Zileuton and zafirlukast can interact with warfarin and cause a significant increase in prothrombin time (PT) and international normalized ratio (INR). PT and INR need to be monitored periodically (Drug Facts and Comparisons, 1998).

Montelukast has not been shown to inhibit the P-450 cytochrome. Therefore there are no clinically significant changes in the pharmacokinetics of theophylline, warfarin, terfenadine, or oral contraceptives with norethindrone/ethinyl estradiol or prednisone. It has been reported equally safe at the recommended dose for the elderly as well as younger adults but some elderly may experience greater sensitivity to this medicine than others taken for asthma.

The most common adverse reactions are headache, influenza-like symptoms, abdominal pain, cough, and approximately a 2% risk of an increased ALT level. It is recommended that a baseline LFT level be drawn. In patients with mild to moderate hepatic insufficiency, the metabolism of montelukast was decreased. Currently the developing drug company, Merck, does not recommend a dosage adjustment. However, appropriate clinical monitoring is warranted. At present, no safety data exist using montelukast in patients with severe hepatic insufficiency.

Montelukast is available in a 5-mg chewable tablet designed to be taken daily by children 6–14 years old and a 10-mg oral tablet for adolescents older than 15 years old and adults (Singulair, 1998).

## Monitoring for Toxicity

Patients should be questioned about any adverse reactions to their medications. Refer to Table 22–20 in the COPD section for the common toxicities and how to monitor them. In addition to the commonly discussed toxicities, the following adverse reactions need to be considered:

- *Beta$_2$ agonists:* Excessive use of inhaled beta$_2$ agonists must be discouraged, and the prescription for any beta$_2$ agonist should limit the adult from obtaining more than one inhaler per month.
- *Oral steroids:* Because women on oral steroids are at risk for trabecular bone loss they should be encouraged to participate in weight-bearing exercises to the best of their ability, eliminate smoking and alcohol, and maintain adequate calcium intake (Braman, 1993; NAEPP, 1997).

Daily elemental calcium intake of 1200–1500 mg and 400–800 units of vitamin D are essential. Avoid medications that can induce bone loss, ie, antacids with aluminum, tetracyclines, furosemide, anticonvulsants. It may be impossible to avoid using these medications, but if they are used close monitoring is required. If a patient is on long-term oral steroids, a bone densitometry evaluation is necessary because approximately 30% of bone is lost before there are changes on an x-ray (Braman, 1993; Spahn & Kamada, 1995). Cataracts can occur with oral prednisone use, even with a dose as low as 7.5 mg/day or greater. Annual eye examinations are advised. Inhaled steroids do not seem to cause the same risk of developing cataracts that oral steroids do (Kamada & Szefler, 1995; Toogood, 1993).

Suppression of the adrenal axis can be caused by oral steroids at doses of 7.5 mg/day or more of prednisone and in those who receive frequent "bursts" of high-dose steroids. Complete recovery of adrenal suppression from long-term use or frequent "bursts" can take from 6 months to 1 year (Spahn & Kamada, 1995).

- *Leukotriene modifiers:* The leukotriene modifiers zileuton and zafirlukast can have some adverse reactions. Zileuton can cause a transient rise in liver enzymes, bloating, abdominal discomfort or pain, and diarrhea. The abdominal complaints are usually dose-dependent and can be decreased by adjusting the medication dose to two or three times per day (Wenzel & Kamada, 1996). The efficacy of zileuton dosed at 3 times a day is very equivalent to 4 times a day; the efficacy decreases if dosed at 2 times a day but is still moderately effective (Wenzel & Kamada, 1996). Zileuton is metabolized by cytochrome P-450 so use caution when prescribing a medication that inhibits these enzymes. When taking zileuton, concurrent use causes an increase in propanolol, terfenadine, theophylline, and warfarin levels, and these should be monitored carefully. Zileuton has not been shown to decrease the effectiveness of prednisone, oral contraceptives, digoxin, or phenytoin. Zileuton is contraindicated in patients with active liver disease or ALT/AST levels more than three times normal. The elderly and those with renal impairment do not need a dose adjustment (Drug Facts and Comparisons, 1998). This drug is only indicated in patients 12 years and older.

Zafirlukast must be taken on an empty stomach and dosed one tablet twice a day. The most common side effects are headache and nausea. Mild to moderate respiratory infections are reported in patients older than 55 who are also using inhaled steroids (Drug Facts and Comparisons, 1998). Zafirlukast does not increase liver enzymes. In the elderly (>65 years) and those with hepatic impairment, there is an increase in the plasma levels of zafirlukast, and thus a dose adjustment may be necessary (Drug Facts and Comparisons, 1998).

## Follow-up Recommendations

Patients with mildly persistent to severe asthma who are stable can be seen every 6–12 months. The frequency of the office visits will depend on the patient's age, comorbid illness, medication use (especially theophylline and zileuton), and frequency of asthma flares and their severity. Spirometry should be done on all asthma patients once a year, and more often if there have been severe exacerbations. Other tests may be required, based on the patient's history, physical examination findings, and medication use.

## PEDIATRIC ASTHMA

Underdiagnosis of asthma in infants and children younger than 12 years is a frequent problem because many of the classic signs and symptoms seen in adolescents and adults may be absent in this age group. The diagnosis of asthma should always be considered if any of the following indicators are present (although these are not diagnostic by themselves, multiple indicators do increase the possibility of asthma):

- Wheezing in infants and young children who have a history of allergies is strongly associated with the development of asthma throughout childhood. However the absence of wheezing does not rule out asthma since many children with significant airflow variability and obstruction do not wheeze (Martinez et al, 1995; Roorda et al, 1993).
- Atopy is a strong predictor of asthma development in children. "Atopy is the genetic susceptibility to produce IgE directed toward common environmental allergens, including house-dust mites, animal proteins and fungi, etc." (Larsen, 1992, p. 1541). This production of IgE sensitizes mast cells and potentially other lung cells so that future exposure to specific antigens can activate these cells.
- Chronic cough triggered by exercise or viral infections. Can also be triggered by a constellation of nighttime factors: changes in body temperature, humidity levels, and recumbent position and decreases in cortisol and epinephrine levels and increase in endogenous PAF (platelet-activating factor), resulting in increased bronchoconstriction (Barnes & Lee, 1992; Martin, 1994; Martin, Cicutto, & Ballard, 1990).

- Symptoms occur or worsen when exposed to smoke, menses, changes in weather, airborne chemicals or dust, or strong emotions (NAEPP, 1997).

- Chest pain or stomachache with no other obvious etiology (Li & O'Connell, 1996).

- Chronic rhinitis and sinusitis (NAEPP, 1997).

## SPECIFIC CONSIDERATIONS FOR PHARMACOTHERAPY

### When Drug Therapy Is Needed

"Pharmacologic therapy is utilized to prevent and control the symptoms of asthma, reduce the frequency and severity of asthma exacerbations, and reverse airflow obstruction" (NAEPP, 1997, p. 3a–3). Because asthma is recognized as a chronic disorder with bronchial constriction that is at least partially reversible, chronic inflammation, and bronchial hyperresponsiveness, medications must be taken daily. The medications used for long-term control are antiinflammatory agents that attenuate inflammation by reducing the markers of inflammation in airway tissues and blocking mediator release in the early and late phases of antigen response and long-acting bronchodilators for control of nocturnal symptoms and exercise-induced bronchospasm (Charlesworth, 1996; NAEPP, 1997).

Immediate-relief medications, the short-acting bronchodilators, relax the airway smooth muscles and rapidly increase airflow, which reduces acute asthma exacerbations (NAEPP, 1997). There is mounting evidence that a significant number of children with asthma in childhood will have persistent symptoms in mid-adult life. A clinical review of a group of 286 children followed from age 7–35 years reveals that 70% of those with asthma have continued with intermittent wheezing and 90% of those with severe asthma have persistent symptoms. Abnormal lung function [decreased $FEV_1$ (forced expiratory volume) and $FEV_1/FVC$ (forced vital capacity)] was present in mid-life adults who had frequent and persistent asthma in childhood, although those with frequent wheezing had relatively minor lung abnormalities. Of those who wheezed with respiratory infections prior to age 7, none had any evidence of airway obstruction in mid-life (Oswald et al, 1997). Other studies done on children with wheezing and asthma suggest that absolute lung growth may be suboptimal, especially during adolescence, and that lung function may never return to normal even

though asthma becomes asymptomatic (Agertoft & Pedersen, 1993; Martinez et al, 1995). A number of other studies looked at childhood asthma and found similar results to Oswald's data; ie, all those with persistent wheezing and asthma had airflow obstruction in mid-life (Godden et al, 1994; Gold et al, 1994; Roorda et al, 1993). What the authors concluded was that aggressive early therapy with inhaled steroids in children with mild or mildly persistent asthma was not warranted, but such aggressive therapy was warranted in those with moderately persistent and severe asthma.

A Finnish study evaluated the use of inhaled budesonide among subjects that were divided into six groups based on the duration of their symptoms, ranging from less than 6 months to over 10 years. Inhaled budesonide use was evaluated after 3 months, and the most improvement was seen in the group with asthma present for 6 months or less. The subjects were reevaluated again 2 years after initiating treatment, with the least benefit seen in the group whose asthma was present for 10 years or more before treatment was initiated. These data suggest that early introduction of potent antiinflammatory agents could interrupt some of the irreversible component of the inflammatory process (Selroos, Pietinalho, Lofroos & Riska, 1995) (see Table 22–6). As more is learned regarding the pathophysiology of asthma, airway remodeling, and its long-term sequelae and more studies examine the aggressive and early use of inhaled steroids in children, the issue of when to initiate inhaled steroids in those with asthma may be resolved. However, aggressively treating children with moderately persistent or severe asthma with inhaled steroids may be prudent based on several studies that have been done showing less favorable long-term outcomes in those without inhaled steroids.

### Short- and Long-Term Goals of Pharmacotherapy

The short-term goals of treatment are to provide prompt relief of bronchoconstriction and the accompanying symptoms of chest tightness, wheezing, shortness of breath, and cough (Murphy & Kelly, 1996). Systemic steroids are also necessary in the treatment of moderately persistent and severe exacerbations to prevent progression, hurry recovery, and prevent a relapse during recovery (NAEPP, 1997).

The long-term goals of treatment are to prevent or reduce the severity and frequency of exacerbations, control the symptoms of asthma, reverse airflow obstruction, and perhaps reduce airway remodeling (Murphy & Kelly, 1996; NAEPP, 1997).

## Nonpharmacologic Therapy

The child's caregivers will need to control environmental factors that trigger an exacerbation. Relaxation techniques may also be useful (Rachelefsky, Fitzgerald, Page, & Santamaria, 1993).

## Time Frame for Initiating Pharmacotherapy

Early recognition of declining PEF is important, and immediate action is required. At diagnosis, medication(s) will be started, depending on the asthma classification designation. It is imperative that they begin immediately.

The following guidelines developed by the NAEPP (1997) utilizes a "stop light" approach to management. This makes it easier for children to know how to manage and intervene in their own asthma. Table 22–8 describes this plan. Patient education is vital along with clearly written management instructions for long-term care (NAEPP, 1997; Rachelefsky, 1995a).

## Assessment Needed Prior to Therapy

Refer to the section on asthma in adults. Only the differences in children will be discussed here. In young children less than 4–5 years, the medical history, physical examination, and empiric pharmacologic therapy may be the only diagnostic tools available to the clinician because the age of the child prohibits spirometry testing. In the older child, spirometry testing is an important diagnostic tool, especially if the symptoms are atypical. Refer to Table 22–9 for the history and physical examination. Refer to Table 22–10 for the diagnostic tests used in children.

## Patient/Caregiver Information

1. Discuss parent's anxiety regarding an asthma flare and review at each visit the clearly written instructions on "how to" manage a flare.
2. Role playing scenarios of an asthma flare at home and in school can help a parent gain more control and confidence in managing an asthma flare.
3. Teach all parents and children to use MDI, spacers, and peak flow meters.

---

### TABLE 22–8.  ASTHMA CONTROL PLAN: THE "STOP LIGHT" APPROACH

**Green Zone: All Clear**
80–100% of your personal best PEF[a] signals good control.
No asthma symptoms so continue taking your medications as usual. Able to do normal activities and sleep without symptoms.

**Yellow Zone: Caution**
50–80% of your personal best PEF signals caution.
Asthma symptoms may be mild to moderate and keep you from doing your usual activities.
Use an inhaled short-acting beta$_2$ agonist immediately either as a metered dose inhaler or nebulizer with cromolyn and follow the treatment regimen prescribed by your health care provider for managing your yellow zone.

**Red Zone: Medical Alert**
50% or less of your personal best signals a medical alert.
Asthma symptoms are serious.
You must use a short-acting inhaled beta$_2$ agonist immediately, either as a metered dose inhaler or nebulizer with cromolyn. Call your health care provider immediately and/or go directly to the ER.

---

[a] Normative standards are based on height, age, and sex for Caucasians. Differences exist for African-Americans, Native Americans, Hispanics, and Asians. Lung function varies across racial and ethnic populations so that the standards cannot be extrapolated to them. The most clinically useful standard then will be the child's personal best.
*Adapted from Coultas et al (1994), Marcus et al (1988), and NAEPP (1997).*

## TABLE 22–9. HISTORY AND PHYSICAL EXAMINATION OF CHILDREN WITH ASTHMA

### Pertinent History Markers

- Family history of asthma, allergies, eczema
- Classic symptoms of wheezing, shortness of breath, chest tightness, sputum production
- Precipitating factors that aggravate asthma-like symptoms: viral infections, exercise, environmental changes (cold air, weather changes, strong emotions, parent smoking)
- Pattern of symptoms: perennial, seasonal, episodic, continuous, or continuous with acute exacerbations
- History of frequent upper respiratory infections, chronic recurring rhinorrhea
- Effect of symptoms on activity level, schoolwork, sleep, and appetite
- Progression of symptoms
- Regular medications used, any relationship to exacerbations and medication use

### Physical Examination Needed and Possible Findings

- Vital signs: height and weight plotted on growth chart; may be <50% for age
- Skin: eczematous rash
- Eyes: vision, lens cloudiness
- Nose: rhinorrhea, allergic turbinates
- Oropharynx: posterior pharynx cobblestoning, mucus
- Heart: murmurs
- Lungs: wheezing, decreased breath sounds, use of accessory muscles
- Abdomen: tenderness

*Adapted from Luskin (1994), NAEPP (1997), and Shuttari (1995).*

4. The following needs to be discussed with parents of infants and young children:
   - It is important to keep all health care appointments, even if the infant is well.
   - It is important to act quickly with asthma symptoms.
   - Signs that indicate the need to seek immediate emergency care include:
     - Breathing rate increases to over 40 breaths/minute
     - Sucking or feeding stops
     - Skin between the infant's ribs is pulled in and tight
     - Chest gets bigger

- Coloring changes; blue fingers, nails, or lips; pale or red face
- Cry changes in quality
- Nostrils widen; grunting
- During an acute asthma episode parents should be warned NOT TO DO THE FOLLOWING:
  - Give large volumes of fluids; just give normal amounts.
  - Rebreath in a paper bag
  - Give OTC antihistamines and/or cold medicines
  - Breathe warm moist air from a shower (NAEPP, 1997)

## OUTCOMES MANAGEMENT

### Selecting an Appropriate Agent

Determining an agent to use in the pharmacologic management of pediatric asthma depends on severity and age. The same asthma classification categories developed by the NAEPP Expert Panel (NAEPP, 1997) are used for children as well as adults to make therapeutic decisions.

## TABLE 22–10. COMMON DIAGNOSTIC TESTS FOR CHILDREN WITH ASTHMA

| Diagnostic Tests | Possible Findings |
|---|---|
| Spirometry if the child is older than 4–5 years | Decreased $FEV_1$ and FVC |
| Bronchoprovocation challenge | $FEV_1$ after a beta$_2$ agonist challenge. If asthma, 12% improvement should be seen in $FEV_1$ |
| Nasal eosinophil smear | Positive |
| CBC | Eosinophilia |
| Skin testing | Usually positive for the common allergens; house-dust mites, fungi, animal protein (cat/dog hair) |
| Sweat test | Negative |
| Sinus x-ray | +/– sinusitis |
| Chest x-ray | +/– lung masses, infection, heart size, thoracic abnormalities |

+/– means finding may be either present or absent.
*Adapted from Luskin (1994) and NAEPP (1997).*

**Step 1: mild intermittent asthma.** Table 22–11 lists the long-term control and quick-relief medications for children less than 5 years of age. Patients in this category often experience symptoms with exercise (EIB), viral respiratory infections, and occasionally other triggering factors. A beta$_2$ inhaled agonist is the drug of choice, used on a prn basis for relief of symptoms; if pulmonary functions are normalized, then continued intermittent use is acceptable. If a beta$_2$ agonist is needed more than twice a week (except for exercise) and/or significant symptoms occur between exercise episodes, then the child should be reevaluated and/or moved to the next step of care. EIB can be present in healthy athletes without an asthma history (Natasi, Heinly, & Blaiss, 1995; Nixon, 1996; Rice, 1985). In all asthma patients, however EIB should be anticipated. EIB is a "bronchospastic event that is caused by a loss of heat, water or both from the lung during exercise because of hyperventilation of air that is cooler and drier than that of the respiratory tree" (McFadden & Gilbert, 1994, p. 1364). EIB usually occurs during or immediately after an activity, reaches its peak 5–10 min after stopping the activity and usually has resolved completely in another 20–60 min (Virant, 1991). In some, especially children, EIB may be the only precipitant of asthma. These children should be monitored regularly to ensure that

---

### TABLE 22–11. ASTHMA TREATMENT BY STEPS FOR CHILDREN

| Long-Term Control | Quick Relief |
|---|---|
| **Step 1: Mild Intermittent Asthma**<br>No daily medication needed. | Bronchodilator prn less than twice a week; inhaled short-acting beta$_2$ agonist by nebulizer or face mask and spacer/holding chamber (intensity of treatment depends on severity of exacerbation) or oral beta$_2$ agonist for symptom relief<br>With viral infections: beta$_2$ agonist two puffs q 4–6 h for 24 h and not to use more than every 6 weeks; can consider oral steroids if current exacerbation is severe or patient has a history of severe exacerbations. |
| **Step 2: Mild Persistent Asthma**<br>Daily anti-inflammatory medicine: either cromolyn (nebulized preferred) or MDI or nedocromil (MDI only) t.i.d. or q.i.d. (in infants and young children cromolyn is preferred) or low-dose inhaled steroids with spacer/holding chamber and face mask. | Bronchodilator as needed. |
| **Step 3: Moderate Persistent Asthma**<br>Daily anti-inflammatory medicines: either medium-dose inhaled steroids with spacer/holding chamber and face mask or (once control is established) medium-dose inhaled steroids and nedocromil; or medium-dose inhaled steroids and a long-acting bronchodilator (theophylline). | Bronchodilator as needed. |
| **Step 4: Severe Persistent Asthma**<br>Daily anti-inflammatory medicines: high-dose inhaled steroids with spacer/holding chamber and face mask; if needed, oral steroids 2 mg/kg per day and reduce to lowest effective dose or alternate-day dose that stabilizes symptoms. | Bronchodilator as needed. |

*Adapted from NAEPP (1997).*

they have no symptoms or reduction in their PEF in the absence of exercise. EIB can be a marker of inadequate asthma management (NAEPP, 1997). Recommended management strategies include:

- A beta₂ agonist metered dose inhaler (MDI) used approximately 20–30 min before exercise can be helpful for 2–3 h (deBenedictis, Martinati, Solinas, Tuteri, & Boner, 1996; NAEPP, 1997).

- In young children, albuterol liquid can be used at a dose of 0.15 mg/kg given approximately 1 h before exercise (Roncolli & Dempster, 1996).

- Cromolyn or nedocromil used 20–30 min before exercise can prevent EIB also (deBenedictis et al, 1996).

- A lengthy warm-up prior to exercise can be helpful and may preclude the need for medication or repeated medication.

- Long-term control of asthma symptoms with antiinflammatory medication will reduce airway responsiveness and is associated with a decrease in the frequency and severity of EIB (Barnes & Rederson, 1993; Spahn & Kamada, 1995; Vathenen, Knox, Wisniewski, & Tattersfield, 1991a).

**Step 2: mild persistent asthma.** The NAEPP Expert Panel recommends that children with persistent asthma—whether mild, moderate, or severe—receive daily long-term antiinflammatory medications. Table 22–11 (step 2) lists the long-term control and quick-relief medications used in children less than 5 years of age.

Cromolyn sodium, nedocromil, or *low-dose* inhaled steroids will provide the antiinflammatory relief needed. Many providers begin with cromolyn sodium or nedocromil because of the lower incidence of side effects; however, because of newer research, *serious* consideration should be given to using low-dose inhaled steroids (Johnson, 1996; Kamada et al, 1996).

In children younger than 5 years, a spacer/holding chamber and face mask is useful. It is anticipated that in 1998 the FDA will approve the use of a steroid solution that can be nebulized, which will make low-dose steroids more readily available to younger children (Pedersen, 1996).

For the management of an acute asthma exacerbation, refer to Table 22–7. For the differences in managing an acute asthma exacerbation in children, consider the following guidelines:

- In children, a nebulized mix of a short-acting beta₂ agonist (in doses of 0.1–0.15 mg/kg) and/or cromolyn (one ampule = 20mg) is routinely used. Some providers only use a short-acting beta₂ agonist (NAEPP, 1997).

- The nebulizer treatment is given every 20 min for three times, and then reassessment of the PEF is done. If there is improvement in the PEF, then continue the nebulizer treatment at the same dose every 3–4 h and carefully reassess regularly. The child should continue to take his or her regular medications in addition to the intensified nebulizer treatments (Murphy & Kelly, 1996).

- If the response to the nebulizer is good (PEF greater than or equal to 80% of personal best), then continue the treatments every 3–4 h until the improvement is sustained. Call the health care provider within 24 h (Murphy & Kelly, 1996; NAEPP, 1997).

- If the response is incomplete (PEF between 50–70%), then increase the nebulizer treatments to every 2 h and call the health care provider immediately for consultation. The provider may want the child to start oral steroids. The dose is 1–2 mg/kg of prednisone in two divided doses for 3–5 days (Lapin & Cloutier, 1995). A good response to the more frequent treatments should be noted within 12 h.

- If the nebulizer treatments must be increased to more than every 2 h, then the health care provider must be called immediately. Response to therapy must be carefully monitored (NAEPP, 1997).

- PEF should be measured regularly.

Assessment of the cause of the exacerbation should be undertaken. If no cause is found, then continue the medications as before; if a trigger is identified, then reduce, modify, or eliminate the agent. PEF should be measured once daily, preferably in the morning since the level is at its nadir then; however, if the child's asthma is not stable, PEFs can be checked twice daily, in the morning and evening (NAEPP, 1997).

**Step 3: moderate persistent asthma.** If symptoms persist despite the treatment measures instituted in Step 2, more aggressive therapy is required. As the severity of asthma increases, so does the potential for more side effects from the medications used. Consultation and/or referral to a pulmonary specialist is advisable. Table 22–11 (Step 3) lists the long-term control and quick-relief medications. Nocturnal asthma is often a feature of moderate or severe asthma and is probably related to diurnal variations in airway responsiveness (Jarjour, Gelfand, McGill, & Busse, 1996).

The use of low-dose sustained-release theophylline is controversial. Theophylline has been demonstrated to have only *modest* clinical effectiveness as a bronchodilator but at low doses has been shown to have some antiinflammatory properties (Barnes & Pauwels, 1994). It has been hypothesized that children younger than 7 years may have an increased sensitivity to theophylline and therefore increased side effects as well (Milgrom & Bender, 1995). Many children cannot tolerate the taste of theophylline and will vomit, and have subtle changes in memory, hand tremors, and anxiety (Bender, Lerner, & Poland, 1991). A comparison of standardized scholastic achievement test scores showed no differences between children taking theophylline and their sibling controls (Milgrom & Bender, 1995). With the advent of newer and less toxic drugs, theophylline is generally not used as a primary drug for asthma treatment. Many researchers do not recommend the use of theophylline for nocturnal asthma in children because of the potential toxicity profile, significant drug interactions, and the added expense of monitoring serum levels. A long-acting inhaled beta$_2$ agonist may be a better choice for nocturnal symptoms if the child is older than 12 years; if younger than 12 years, consider nebulized cromolyn (Clark, 1993; Niederhauser, 1997; Roncolli & Dempster, 1996).

***Step 4: severe persistent asthma.*** Consultation with and/or referral to a pulmonary specialist is highly recommended for children in this category. Table 22–11 (Step 4) lists the long-term control and quick-relief medications. Management of oral systemic steroids consists of:

- Giving the lowest possible daily dose or preferably an alternate-day dose
- Monitoring closely for steroid side effects
- When control is achieved, stepping down to minimal doses of oral steroids and then to inhaled high-dose steroids because they have fewer side effects than oral systemic steroids (Barnes & Redersen, 1993; Niederhauser, 1997).

Oral systemic prednisone is dosed at 1–2 mg/kg per day in two to three divided doses and then tapered slowly once the child is symptom-free and the PEF returns to the child's personal best (Drug Facts and Comparisons, 1998; Grant, Duggan, Santosham, & DeAngelis, 1996).

## Monitoring for Efficacy

Selection of a medication to use should be guided by the child's symptoms, severity of the asthma, safety profile of the medications, lowest effective daily dose, fewest number of medications on a daily basis, and reassessment of effectiveness and quality of daily life.

Each child must be taught to recognize symptom patterns that might indicate inadequate asthma control and maintain a symptom history record. He or she should check PEF once daily unless symptomatic and follow a detailed written action plan developed by the health care provider in the event of an exacerbation; this is a must for those with moderate to severe asthma and anyone with a history of severe exacerbations (NAEPP, 1997). The frequency of asthma exacerbations should be assessed at each visit. They may not be related to a triggering event but rather adherence to the treatment regimen, inhaler technique, side effects of the medications, incorrect level of medication usage for the activity, and an inappropriate diagnosis of the correct step classification and, therefore, incorrect pharmacotherapy (NAEPP, 1997). Each of these factors needs to be assessed regularly during office visits and after an acute asthma exacerbation. Quality of life should be periodically assessed for the child, which includes missed school days and disturbances in sleep and/or regular activities (NAEPP, 1997).

At each visit, assess the following changes from the baseline physical examination:

Skin: eczema, other rashes

Lungs: quality of breath sounds, change from last visit, wheezing, diminished breath sounds, respiratory rate, use of accessory muscles

Heart: murmurs, rate

PEF: FEV$_1$; if spirometry is used, then check FVC also

The rest of the examination depends on the complaint if it is other than respiratory and if this is a follow-up from an asthma exacerbation.

No consistent laboratory values are drawn unless the asthma exacerbation was secondary to pneumonia or the child is on long-term oral steroids. A blood glucose should be checked; consider a WBC with differential and other levels as appropriate.

## Monitoring for Toxicity

For a description of the most common adverse reactions to inhaled and oral beta$_2$ agonists, theophylline, and inhaled and oral steroids, refer to Table 22–20.

***Cromolyn/nedocromil.*** The most common side effects of using cromolyn or nedocromil are coughing and wheezing during nebulization, but they are less bothersome when used with a short-acting beta₂ agonist (Roncolli & Dempster, 1996). Serious adverse reactions are rarely reported with cromolyn sodium or nedocromil.

***Oral steroids.*** Children on oral systemic steroids have far more serious side effects than those on inhaled steroids, but the risks still exist, especially on the higher inhaled doses. The potential effect of high-dose inhaled steroids on growth is of concern, but childhood asthma does appear to be associated with delayed maturation and increased time of reduced growth prior to puberty. This delay, however, does not appear to affect the attainment of predicted final height (Allen, D. B., 1996). A meta-analysis recently done of the influence of inhaled beclomethasone on expected attainment of final adult height did not find any adverse effects regardless of dose, disease severity, or duration of asthma (Allen, Mullen, & Mullen, 1994). Doull, Freezer, & Holgate (1995) conducted an uncontrolled follow-up study of children over several years using inhaled budesonide at an average dose of 800 µg/day and found no adverse effect on long-term growth. The conclusion that might be drawn from these studies is that an inhaled steroid dose between 400–800 µg of budesonide or beclomethasone a day probably does not cause a negative effect on growth. Using a medium-dose inhaled steroid may have a potential but not predictable association with growth delay, while the higher-dose inhaled steroids potentially have the greatest risk for growth delay (Kamada & Szefler, 1995; Wolthers, 1996). Poorly controlled asthma can delay growth and has its own associated risks, balancing out the potential risks of inhaled steroids. Even high-dose inhaled steroids have significantly less potential for serious side effects than oral systemic steroids (NAEPP, 1997). With careful daily monitoring and a symptom control record, the number and severity of asthma flares in many children may be reduced. This can reduce the need for higher-dose inhaled steroids and/or oral systemic steroids. One study of children during steroid treatment found that they were more sad, irritable, tired, and argumentative and manifested both visual and verbal memory deficits while taking oral steroids, but not 24 or 48 h after discontinuing them (Bender et al, 1991). The development of cataracts is seen with oral systemic steroids, but no association has been seen during the use of inhaled steroids (Simons, Persaud, Gillespie, Cheang, & Schuckett, 1993). The development of cataracts from oral steroids is dose-dependent (>7.5 mg/day) and cumulative over time (Toogood, 1993). Adrenal suppression occurs on medium to high doses of oral steroids, but at low to medium doses of inhaled steroids there appears to be no significant effect (Duoll et al, 1995). A recent study done by Clark, Grove, Cargill, & Lipworth (1996), comparing fluticasone and budesonide at equivalent doses, found that fluticasone caused greater adrenal suppression than budesonide. This study might suggest that an inhaled steroid other than fluticasone should be the first choice.

## Follow-up Recommendations

Recommendations for monitoring children's asthma are:

1. Children with asthma should have regular health visits every 1–6 months, depending on the severity of the asthma, age of the child, and frequency of exacerbations.
2. At each office visit:
   (a) Assess PEF and ensure correct PEF and inhaler technique.
   (b) Review the symptom record and the daily PEF.
   (c) Review current medications and if symptoms have been controlled for the past 2–3 months, consider a step-down approach, decreasing the last medication added by 25% (NAEPP, 1997). Continue this step-down therapy until the lowest possible dose is achieved that is effective.
   (d) Most children with persistent asthma will always need a daily antiinflammatory to suppress underlying airway inflammation and will relapse if all antiinflammatory medications are withdrawn (Rachelefsky et al, 1993).
   (e) Reassess the written instructions for the home management of acute exacerbations and verbally review any questions regarding management concerns.
   (f) Discuss participation in sports and daily activities. Strongly encourage regular sports participation. A written plan should be given to the coach if the child participates on a sports team (NAEPP, 1997; Roncolli & Dempster, 1996).

3. A written management plan should be prepared for the school with the input of the child and parent and must include: rescue medications that must be readily available for the child to use during an acute asthma exacerbation and a plan for the child to self-administer these medications if old enough; factors in school that may trigger an asthma flare and ways to help the student avoid exposure; administration of long-term medications, when appropriate; and use of a short-acting beta$_2$ agonist or cromolyn to prevent EIB.

4. If the child is old enough, spirometry should be done every 6 to 12 months.

## ASTHMA IN PREGNANCY

With the increase in the incidence of asthma over the past 10 years in all age groups, there is a significant risk that asthma will be a complicating health problem of pregnancy. It is one of the most common pregnancy-related illnesses, affecting approximately 4% of all pregnancies (National Institutes of Health [NIH]/National Heart, Lung and Blood Institute [NHLBI], 1993). Asthma may occur either for the first time during a pregnancy or worsen during pregnancy. About one third of pregnant women with asthma have adverse health problems, one third will improve, and one third will remain stable (NIH/NHLBI, 1993). Those patients whose asthma worsens during the first trimester and continues to be difficult to control will usually follow the same course in subsequent pregnancies. In those women with severe asthma at the start of the pregnancy, severity peaks after 26 weeks of gestation (NIH/NHLBI, 1993).

Because of the potential risk of uncontrolled asthma adversely affecting both the mother and fetus, NIH's National Heart, Lung and Blood Institute issued an Executive Summary on the Management of Asthma during Pregnancy (1993) recommending aggressive therapy. The pharmacologic therapy must be just as aggressive as if the woman were not pregnant. All pregnant women with moderate or severe asthma and those with frequent and/or severe asthma flares, should be assessed and followed by consultations with a pulmonologist.

Throughout pregnancy there are hormonal and anatomic changes that alter the respiratory, cardiovascular, and circulatory systems. These changes alter the pregnant woman's normal breathing pattern, leading to hyperventilation and dyspnea, which decreases the $PCO_2$ but is compensated for by a rise in $PO_2$. Other changes are increased capillary engorgement in the mucous membranes, leading to an edematous and friable airway mucosa, and a decrease in TLV (total lung volume) and RV (residual volume); however, $FEV_1$ and respiratory rate remain the same (Elkus & Popovich, 1992; Johnson, Lawlor, & Weiner, 1994). With hyperventilation and mouth breathing, bronchospasms are more common because cool dry air may be delivered further down into the respiratory tree than usual (Schulman, Alderman, Ewig, & Bye, 1996). Dyspnea is prevalent in pregnant women, occurring in about 60–70% of all pregnancies, regardless of the presence of respiratory and/or cardiovascular illnesses (NIH/NHLBI, 1993).

In mild asthma, hypoxia is compensated for by hyperventilation, which keeps the $PO_2$ normal and the $PCO_2$ slightly decreased. As the airways become more constricted, ventilation-perfusion mismatching occurs. The result is arterial hypoxia. In severe obstruction, $PO_2$ continues to decrease while the $PCO_2$ rises to normal, signaling that the mother and especially the fetus are in the danger zone. Immediate treatment is required to prevent serious fetal and maternal complications (Pulmonary Disorders, 1997).

With asthma severity increased, the risks to the fetus include intrauterine growth retardation, increased perinatal mortality, preterm delivery, neonatal hypoxia, and low birth weight (NIH/NHLBI, 1993). The mother is at risk for preeclampsia, toxemia, hypertension, hyperemesis gravidarum, and vaginal hemorrhage (Kaliner, 1995). With respiratory status decline, consider the following as triggers for the asthma flare: allergies, sinusitis, gastroesophageal reflux disease (GERD), occupational exposure, and rarely, a pulmonary embolus (Kaliner & Lemanske, 1992).

## SPECIFIC CONSIDERATIONS FOR PHARMACOTHERAPY

### When Drug Therapy Is Needed

All pregnant women with asthma must be aggressively treated to control symptoms, prevent exacerbations, maintain normal pregnant lung function and activity levels, avoid or reduce the adverse effects from asthma therapy, and avoid complications of uncontrolled asthma flares to the fetus and the mother.

Since the majority of inhaled medications are safe to use during pregnancy, there is no rationale for withholding treatment. The use of antihistamines, OTC (over-the-counter) cold remedies, large volumes of fluid, steam, and breathing into a paper bag are *not* recommended. These home treatments delay the onset of immediate appropriate therapy and can increase the risk of hypoxia to the mother and fetus (NIH/NHLBI, 1993).

## Short- and Long-Term Goals of Pharmacotherapy

The short-term goals during an acute exacerbation are to dilate the bronchi, reverse the bronchospasms, and reduce airway inflammation. It is preferable to use only inhaled medications and not systemic steroids, but that may not be feasible. Because hypoxic complications to the fetus can occur rapidly, therapy must provide a quick response and sustain that improvement. If there is further deterioration, the exacerbation is severe, or the fetal kick count decreases, emergency help must be sought immediately (NIH/NHLBI, 1993).

The long-term goals are to prevent an asthma exacerbation, avoid environmental triggers (smoke, pollen, mold, animal protein, house dust-mites, etc.) to greatly reduce the risk of symptoms and need for additional medication, maintain the mother's normal lung function and

blood oxygenation to maintain the fetus's well-being and adequate oxygenation (NIH/NHLBI, 1993), and use the least amount of medication to maintain normal lung function but enough to control symptoms. The ultimate outcome is a well-oxygenated and healthy baby and mother.

### Nonpharmacologic Therapy

1. Check PEFs once daily, preferably at the same time.
2. Use a spacer every time an inhaler is used.
3. Avoid or reduce exposure to triggering factors at home and work.
4. Use fetal monitoring.
5. Measure $Po_2$ and $Pco_2$.
6. Exercise appropriately since exercise can improve vasomotor rhinitis of pregnancy.
7. If symptoms of allergic rhinitis, sinusitis, or gastroesophageal reflux disease (GERD) occur, initiate the necessary preventive management.

### Time Frame for Initiating Pharmacotherapy

Immediate recognition of declining PEF, quick early intervention, aggressive therapy, and slowly tapering the medications to the lowest effective dose are the goals. For the treatment of an acute asthma exacerbation, see Table 22–12.

---

### TABLE 22–12. MANAGEMENT OF ACUTE ASTHMA DURING PREGNANCY

**Assess Severity**

| | |
|---|---|
| PEF is 50–80% of personal best or predicted value; note symptoms suggestive of an asthma flare: cough, breathlessness, wheezing, chest tightness, and short of breath; the degree of symptoms correlates poorly with severity of exacerbation | PEF <50% of personal best or predicted value especially in third trimester; improvement not sustained; "kick" count decreases; proceed to emergency room immediately. |

↓

**Initiate Treatment**

Inhaled terbutaline two to four puffs q 20-min intervals for treatments or if unresponsive to terbutaline, use a single nebulizer treatment of albuterol

| Good Response | Incomplete Response | Poor Response |
|---|---|---|
| PEF >80% of personal best or predicted value; sustained response to beta$_2$ agonist for 4 h; continue beta$_2$ agonist q 3–4 h for 2–4 days; if on inhaled steroids, can double the dose for 7–10 days; contact the health care provider within 24 h | PEF 50–80% of personal best or predicted value; persistent chest tightness, shortness of breath, wheezing; continue beta$_2$ agonist; may need to begin oral prednisone, but call the clinician immediately for instructions and/or proceed to emergency room | PEF <50% of personal best or predicted value; proceed to emergency room immediately |

*Adapted from NAEPP (1997).*

In the pregnant woman if the asthma exacerbation becomes severe, deteriorates to become severe, or fetal kick count decreases, then intensive monitoring of the mother and fetus is critical. Medical treatment should be sought immediately to avoid further compromise.

## Assessment Needed Prior to Therapy

For complete history and physical examination findings, refer to Table 22–1. Additional history items address specific pregnancy-related experiences. A comprehensive asthma assessment in the pregnant woman includes: evaluation of fetal size, fetal heart rate, and fetal movement (see Table 22–13).

## Patient/Caregiver Information

1. Every patient should keep a daily PEF diary.
2. All patients need a written care plan for an acute exacerbation and it should be reviewed regularly.
3. All patients need a short-acting beta$_2$ agonist inhaler with a spacer and/or a nebulizer.
4. Pregnant women need to know:
   - Asthma symptoms will become worse for about one third of pregnant women.
   - Asthma symptoms may be the most severe between 29–36 weeks.
   - Uncontrolled asthma may affect the health of the baby. Not getting the baby oxygen, due to uncontrolled asthma, is a far greater risk than taking asthma medications.
   - Avoid the following during pregnancy: decongestants, some antibiotics such as tetracycline, live virus vaccines (killed are allowed),

allergy shots (do not begin but may be continued if initiated prior to pregnancy), and medicines such as brompheniramine, epinephrine, phenylephrine, and phenylpropanolamine.
5. All common asthma triggers need to be avoided.
6. Reassure patients that wheezing during labor and delivery is rare.
7. Breast-feeding is possible while taking asthma medications (NAEPP, 1997).

## OUTCOMES MANAGEMENT

### Selecting an Appropriate Agent

Consideration must be given to the safety of the drug used during pregnancy, utilizing the least amount of drug that will maintain control of symptoms, preventing an asthma exacerbation, and rapidly resolving an asthma flare in order to prevent maternal and fetal hypoxia. For an in-depth discussion on selecting an appropriate agent, refer to outcomes management in the adult asthma section.

***Bronchodilators.*** In the pregnant patient, the only bronchodilator that is a Category B and approved for use is terbutaline. Terbutaline should *only* be used as rescue medicine and management for EIB. Moderately persistent or severe asthma is often associated with nocturnal symptoms and will require treatment. The most often used drug, salmeterol, is a Category C drug. Symptom management, however, outweighs the risk of using this medication because of the greater risk of hypoxia to the fetus (Drug Facts and Comparisons, 1998). For further details refer to Drug Table 700.

***Inhaled steroids.*** Inhaled steroids will be necessary in all patients with mildly persistent (Step 2) to severe persistent asthma (Step 4). There are no contraindications to use in the pregnant woman, but consider trying a less potent steroid inhaler first. If the patient's asthma is not controlled using a less potent inhaled steroid, a more potent steroid inhaler and/or oral steroids will be required. With mild persistent asthma (Step 2), the woman can try cromolyn or nedocromil first and switch to a steroid inhaler if the asthma is not controlled.

For information on drugs to avoid, refer to outcomes management in the adult asthma section.

---

**TABLE 22–13. DIAGNOSTIC TESTS FOR THE PREGNANT WOMAN WITH ASTHMA**

Ultrasound at 12 to 20 weeks, depending on asthma severity

Sequential ultrasounds in second and third trimesters to evaluate fetal growth

Electronic fetal heart monitoring in third trimester to assess fetal well-being; more often if necessary

PEFs at each visit

Spirometry as baseline, but more often if repeat exacerbations

*Adapted from NIH/NHLBI (1993).*

## Monitoring for Efficacy

At each visit the clinician should obtain a symptom history suggestive of an asthma flare: cough (occurs at rest, upon laughing, with tobacco smoke or noxious fumes, etc.), shortness of breath, chest tightness, breathlessness, nighttime awakening with cough, change in exercise tolerance, wheezing, and any respiratory infections. Assess the frequency of use of the bronchodilator and if the patient is using the steroid inhaler or cromolyn/nedocromil correctly (Shaffer, 1991).

Physical examination findings should assess:

- *Lungs:* Same as for the adult but focus on lung sounds at bases and wheezing with forced expiration.
- *Heart:* Murmurs.

The remainder of the examination is appropriate for the number of weeks of pregnancy. Fetal monitoring should be used as appropriate for gestational age, severity of asthma, and frequency of severe asthma episodes. Pulmonary function studies should include $FEV_1$ and FVC.

At each visit assess the lungs and heart, changes in the patient's own baseline, the PEFs, and other tests as appropriate for patient's pregnancy and asthma condition.

No laboratory tests are done routinely for asthma follow-up unless an acute illness occurs or monitoring for a coexisting condition is necessary.

## Monitoring for Toxicity

A study of 180 pregnancies in which beta$_2$ agonists were used during the first trimester demonstrated no increased teratogenic risk to the fetus (Schatz et al, 1988). Beta$_2$ agonists can cause tremors and tachycardia, and frequent use can lead to tolerance and paradoxical worsening of symptoms. Occasional use is not harmful, but constant use can mask worsening disease and prevent prompt action that can correct impending fetal hypoxia.

The NIH/NHLBI Executive Summary Panel on the Management of Asthma in Pregnancy (1993) recommends beclomethasone, a less potent inhaled steroid and a Category C drug, as the initial choice for an inhaled steroid. The other inhaled steroids, flunisolide, budesonide, fluticasone, and triamcinolone acetonide, are also Category C drugs and should be second drug choices. However, if the pregnant woman is already on one of these steroid inhalers, she should continue the medication.

For complete information on the bronchodilators and steroid inhalers, refer to Drug Tables 701 and 702.

## Follow-up Recommendations

Asthma care should be incorporated as part of routine pregnancy care with special attention to:

- Symptom control
- Nocturnal symptoms
- Frequency of asthma flares, regardless of severity
- Frequency of beta$_2$ agonist use
- Daily medications
- Correct use of the spacer/inhaler
- PEF results
- Kick counts

The frequency of monitoring depends on the woman's pregnancy and asthma health; the more frequent and severe the exacerbations, the more frequent and intensive the monitoring.

## BRONCHIOLITIS

Bronchiolitis is one of the most common respiratory infections seen in infants and young toddlers. An inflammatory obstruction of the small airways (bronchioles), it is seen in children under the age of 2 years because airway resistance is mostly in the bronchioles at this age (Klassen et al, 1996). The most common etiology is viral, with respiratory syncytial virus (RSV) accounting for the majority of cases. Human parainfluenza and some adenoviruses have also been implicated (LaVia, Marks, & Stutman, 1992). This disease is self-limited in most healthy young infants and toddlers, but in those with comorbid illnesses—heart disease; BPD (bronchopulmonary dysplasia), and CF (cystic fibrosis)—and those who are premature, have had recent transplants, are immunosuppressed, or are on chemotherapy, the disease can be quite severe and requires more intensive health intervention (Fete & Noyes, 1996). Risk factors for developing RSV are listed in Table 22–14. All infants and toddlers with RSV risk factors need close follow-up and attention. Even many healthy infants and toddlers who develop RSV can become so severely ill that treatment in a pediatric intensive care unit is required.

## TABLE 22–14. RESPIRATORY SYNCYTIAL VIRUS RISK FACTORS

Infants of mothers who smoke

Males

Attendance at day care

Birth between April and September

Crowded living conditions

Bottle-feeding instead of breast-feeding

Age between 2–12 months; peak age is 6 months

*Adapted, with permission, from AAP (1998).*

RSV bronchiolitis is considered a risk factor for developing reactive airway disease and/or abnormal PFTs (pulmonary function tests) in later childhood. Bronchiolitis is manifested by symptoms of an upper respiratory infection; usually a low-grade fever is present, along with serous rhinorrhea and sneezing. It then progresses to a paroxysmal wheezy, bubbly cough, tachypnea, dyspnea, retractions, and irritability. If the respiratory distress continues, hypoxia and hypercarbia develop, leading to respiratory failure (LaVia et al, 1992). Rapid diagnosis is by immunofluorescence or enzyme-linked immunosorbent assay (ELISA) of RSV from the nasopharyngeal area (Fete & Noyes, 1996). The decision to treat as an outpatient versus an inpatient depends on age, severity of the symptoms, and other coexisting illnesses. The very young and preterm infant are at increased risk for apnea, whereas older infants and young toddlers are at risk for respiratory failure and/or dehydration (Klassen, 1997). The nurse practitioner or physician's assistant who first encounters the acutely ill infant or toddler with bronchiolitis will rarely manage the case alone, but in collaboration with the physician.

## SPECIFIC CONSIDERATIONS FOR PHARMACOTHERAPY

### When Drug Therapy Is Needed

The judicious use of a selected bronchodilator does seem to effectively improve oxygenation, lower respiratory and heart rates, and reduce airway resistance and stays in the hospital. The issues of how often to use a specific broncho-

dilator if the patient is admitted and if the bronchodilator retains its effectiveness if nebulized frequently have yet to be resolved (Klassen et al, 1996).

There is controversy regarding the effectiveness of glucocorticoids in the treatment of bronchiolitis. Research by Roosevelt et al (1996) and Klassen and colleagues (1996) found that there was no significant difference between those patients treated with or without glucocorticoids; thus, currently, treating bronchiolitis with glucocorticoids is not recommended. A study done by Reijonen, Kroppi, Kukka, and Remes (1996) demonstrated that early use of a nebulized antiinflammatory agent, either budesonide or cromolyn sodium, decreased the incidence of severe postbronchiolitis wheezing requiring hospitalization. Eighty-one percent of the children who received cromolyn sodium and 84% of those who received budesonide ceased wheezing after 2 months of treatment. The antiinflammatory agents were especially beneficial in children with atopy. The recommendation by Reijonen and colleagues (1996) is to continue the antiinflammatory agent for 2–4 months after inpatient treatment for bronchiolitis if the infant had atopy. Further research needs to be conducted to determine the best therapy to prevent postbronchiolitis reactive airway disease.

Recent studies have examined the use of respiratory syncytial virus immune globulin (RSVIG) to treat and prevent RSV in high-risk infants and toddlers. The studies demonstrated no difference in the duration of hospital stay, oxygen use, and need for mechanical ventilation between those treated with RSVIG and a placebo during an acute episode (Rodriguez et al, 1997). Currently RSVIG is only recommended to prevent RSV in high-risk children during the RSV season from early winter to late spring, but not to treat for acute illness.

Currently the American Academy of Pediatrics (AAP, 1998) recommends the use of aerosolized ribavirin *only* in the following children:

1. Those with heart disease, BPD, CF, or other chronic lung diseases, and those who have been immunocompromised (HIV), have had recent transplants, or are preterm infants

2. Those who are severely ill with $PaO_2 < 90\%$ and/or increased $PCO_2$

3. Those on mechanical ventilation

Aerosolized ribavirin has been shown to improve oxygenation and clinical scores and has been demonstrated to be safe and effective (AAP, 1998).

In infants and toddlers who are at increased risk for RSV, immunization for influenza is reasonable and prudent.

## Short- and Long-Term Goals of Pharmacotherapy

The short-term goals are to shorten the ER visit and to prevent and/or shorten the hospital stay.

The long-term goals are to (1) decrease mortality in high-risk infants and toddlers; (2) decrease the incidence of lower respiratory tract infections, RSV-associated hospitalizations, and intensive care stays; and (3) prevent postbronchiolitis reactive airway disease and abnormal PFTs in later childhood (Groothuis, Simoes, Hemming, & the Respiratory Syncytial Virus Immune Globulin Study Group, 1995).

## Nonpharmacologic Therapy

1. Give plenty of fluids for rehydration.
2. Use oxygen as needed.
3. Use mechanical ventilation as needed.

## Time Frame for Initiating Pharmacotherapy

Early diagnosis of RSV is essential to institute pharmacologic therapy if the infant or toddler meets the criteria established by the AAP (1998) for its use.

## Assessment Needed Prior to Therapy

A thorough history and physical examination with appropriate diagnostic tests is crucial. Refer to Tables 22–15 and 22–16 for the history, physical, and diagnostic information needs. Table 22–17 lists the possible criteria for hospitalization in an infant with comorbid problems.

## Patient/Caregiver Information

1. If the infant is managed as an outpatient, provide specific written instructions regarding changes to monitor, such as respiratory rate, ability to eat, playfulness, and lip color; worsening of other symptoms; and when to call the health care provider.
2. If using ribavirin, explain the rationale and duration of treatment and when to expect a clinical improvement.

---

### TABLE 22–15. HISTORY AND PHYSICAL EXAMINATION FOR BRONCHIOLITIS

**Pertinent History Markers**
- Birth history
- Medical problems in the nursery: any treatments, follow-up needed
- Health status since home from the hospital
- Respiratory infection history since birth, symptoms, treatment, any hospitalizations, diagnosis
- Current respiratory problem; beginning symptoms: rhinitis, coryza, +/– fever (normal to <100°), +/– earache; progression of symptoms: cough, feeding, and respiratory difficulties, vomiting, any home treatments
- Change in quality of eating and play
- Change in breathing pattern, +/– audible wheezing

**Physical Examination and Possible Findings**
- Vital signs: temperature normal to <100°
- Respirations: shallow, tachypnea
- Nose: purulent rhinorrhea, nasal flaring
- Lungs: thoracic-abdominal asynchrony, intercostal and substernal retractions, wheezing at end of a prolonged expiration
- Heart: increased rate
- Abdomen: hepatosplenomegaly

+/– means finding may be either present or absent.
*Adapted from Klassen (1997) and Panitch, Callahan, and Schidlow (1993).*

---

## OUTCOMES MANAGEMENT

### Selecting an Appropriate Agent

Supportive therapy is the mainstay of treatment for the healthy infant without risk factors who develops bronchiolitis. Usually rehydration and oxygen are all that is needed. If there is a moderately severe infection, it can be treated with a short hospital stay. Those with very mild disease and older than 6 weeks can be managed at home, with fluids, close monitoring, and frequent calls and visits to the health care provider. The use of aerosolized ribavirin in otherwise healthy infants and children is not warranted according to the AAP (1998).

Currently prophylactic RSVIG is only approved for high-risk children. The cost (about $1000 per IV treatment) is prohibitive for rou-

## TABLE 22–16. COMMON DIAGNOSTIC TESTS FOR BRONCHIOLITIS

| Diagnostic Test | Expected Findings |
| --- | --- |
| Chest x-ray | Hyperinflation common; 30% have scattered areas of consolidation |
| Pulse oximetry | >90%, unless severe respiratory distress; then may be <90% |
| RSV nasopharyngeal swab | Positive |
| CBC with differential | WBC with differential: normal or mildly elevated |

*Adapted from Klassen (1997).*

tine preventive treatment, but can be a cost saver when compared to a hospital stay, mechanical ventilation, and/or intensive care.

The bronchodilator most beneficial for RSV-infected infants or toddlers is racemic epinephrine. Nebulized racemic epinephrine has been shown to have greater effectiveness in decreasing the respiratory rate and pulmonary resistance than nebulized albuterol (Welliver, 1997). Clinical symptoms and oxygenation have been shown to be better using either racemic or subcutaneous epinephrine than albuterol (Menon, Sutcliffe, & Klassen, 1995).

Antibiotics, oral or intravenous glucocorticoids, and ribavirin have no place currently in the management of bronchiolitis. The research to date demonstrates that these treatment modalities are ineffective.

## Monitoring for Efficacy

Improvement in the high-risk infant or child receiving aerosolized ribavirin should be seen 36–48 h after initiating treatment. Recovery is usually complete within several days if no major complications occur. When using nebulized racemic epinephrine or subcutaneous epinephrine, improvement in the clinical scores has been seen in about 30 min and in oxygenation in 60 min, and the heart rate decreased in 90 min (Klassen, 1997). In those infants or toddlers treated as outpatients, improvement is noted within 48–72 h. The symptoms (respiratory rate, lip color, use of accessory muscles, ability to take fluids, etc.) should remain the same or improve but not worsen.

At each visit during the acute illness, check the following physical signs:

- Temperature: normal or elevated
- Respirations: rate, use of accessory muscles
- Lungs: wheezing, crackles, decreased breath sounds
- Heart: rate
- Abdomen: hepatosplenomegaly

Pulse oximetry should be checked if possible. If the infant or toddler looks toxic or the physical examination findings are deteriorating, then hospitalization is required. Other laboratory tests should be ordered as needed.

## Monitoring for Toxicity

Ribavirin has no known common side effects. A rare, less than 0.1% occurrence, is bronchospasm. Epinephrine, used in appropriate doses, lowers heart and respiratory rate rather than increases it because of better oxygenation and decreased work load of the heart, and it probably provides some dilating effect on the alveoli (Klassen, 1997).

## Follow-up Recommendations

In healthy infants and toddlers, a regular well-child visit can assess lungs, both at rest and after exercising, to ensure there is no wheezing. PFTs cannot be assessed in this age group. A good history from the parent may indicate any postbronchiolitic reactive airway problem.

In viral infections, bronchial hyperreactivity is common especially in boys and those with

## TABLE 22–17. CRITERIA FOR HOSPITALIZATION CONSIDERATION WITH BRONCHIOLITIS

**Selected Conditions**

BPD, CF, or other chronic lung diseases

Congenital heart disease

Prematurity

Underlying immunosuppressive diseases or therapy

Very young infant, less than 6 weeks

Severe illness: $Pao_2$ <90%; increased $CO_2$

Respiratory rate of 50 or greater/min

Unable to suck and breathe at same time (increased risk of dehydration, especially if young infant)

*Adapted, with permission, from AAP (1998).*

a family history of atopy and allergic disease. These patients must be treated with a bronchodilator during an acute exacerbation (Horst, 1994; Klassen, 1997). In those infants and toddlers with a comorbid illness, more frequent office visits are needed. The frequency is determined by age, complications while hospitalized, status after hospitalization, and nature of the comorbid illness. In preterm infants and those less than 2 months, there is about a 10% risk of apnea. These infants must be closely monitored and may need home apnea monitoring (Klassen, 1997).

## CHRONIC OBSTRUCTIVE PULMONARY DISEASE

Chronic obstructive pulmonary disease (COPD) is defined by the American Thoracic Society (ATS, 1995) as a disease state characterized by the presence of airflow obstruction due to chronic bronchitis or emphysema. COPD encompasses a spectrum of chronic respiratory diseases characterized by cough, sputum production, dyspnea, airflow limitation, and impaired gas exchange (Ferguson & Cherniack, 1993). The airflow obstruction of COPD is due to chronic bronchitis, emphysema, asthma, or some combination thereof (ATS, 1995). Table 22–18 shows some characteristics of chronic bronchitis and emphysema. Synonymous terms for COPD include chronic obstructive lung disease (COLD) and chronic obstructive airway disease (COAD).

COPD and allied conditions are the fourth leading cause of death in the United States (National Center for Health Statistics, 1997).

Smoking is the primary risk factor for COPD. Other risk factors include alpha$_1$ antitrypsin deficiency and occupational exposure to dust and fumes (Ferguson & Cherniack, 1993; Oxman et al, 1993; St. John, Gadek, & Pacht, 1993). Approximately 15% of smokers will go on to develop clinically significant COPD (ATS, 1995).

Healthy nonsmokers have an age-related decline in $FEV_1$ of about 30 mL/year starting in the mid-30s. This decline may accelerate to 75 mL/year in smokers (Hanson & Midthun, 1992). In a subset of susceptible smokers the decline in $FEV_1$ may reach 150 mL/year (ATS, 1995). Table 22–19 illustrates the COPD staging suggested by the ATS (1995).

## SPECIFIC CONSIDERATIONS FOR PHARMACOTHERAPY

### When Drug Therapy Is Needed

COPD patients need drug therapy to relieve acute and chronic symptoms and to improve their quality of life.

### Short- and Long-Term Goals of Pharmacotherapy

The short-term goals of pharmacotherapy are to treat infection, treat and control reversible symptoms (cough, bronchospasm), and to alleviate hypoxemia. The long-term goals of pharmacotherapy are to retard the progression of airflow limitation, minimize airflow limitation, prevent infection, reduce the need for hospitalization, and optimize functional capabilities (Ferguson & Cherniack, 1993; St. John et al, 1993).

### TABLE 22–18. SELECTED CHARACTERISTICS OF CHRONIC BRONCHITIS AND EMPHYSEMA

| Characteristic | Chronic Bronchitis | Emphysema |
|---|---|---|
| Age at diagnosis | ~50 years | ~60 years |
| Primary symptom | Cough | Dyspnea |
| Sputum | Copious, purulent | Scanty, mucoid |
| Chest x-ray changes | Peribronchial thickening, large heart | Flattened diaphragm, small heart |
| Hematocrit | 50–55% | 35–45% |
| Cor pulmonale | Common | Rare |
| Total lung capacity | Normal | Increased |
| Nickname | Blue Bloater | Pink Puffer |

*Adapted from Ingram (1994) and Williams (1995).*

**TABLE 22–19. SUGGESTED COPD STAGING**

| COPD Stage | Percentage of Predicted FEV$_1$ | Quality of Life Impact | Recommended Level of Care |
|---|---|---|---|
| Stage I (majority of patients) | >50 | Small | Primary care practitioner |
| Stage II | 35–49 | Moderate | Primary care with respiratory specialist |
| Stage III | <35 | Great | Respiratory specialist |

*Adapted from ATS (1995).*

## Nonpharmacologic Therapy

Nonpharmacologic treatment of COPD includes improvement and maintenance of adequate nutrition. Up to one quarter of outpatients with COPD and up to one half of inpatients with COPD may be malnourished (ATS, 1995). Nonpharmacologic treatment of COPD should also include some form of exercise training. There is no one form of exercise training suitable for every COPD patient. Exercise training needs to be individualized. Some form of activity such as walking, use of a treadmill, or stationary bicycling helps improve the patients' respiratory status and can help decrease dyspnea on exertion. Exercise training may also improve the patients' sense of well-being even if there is no objective improvement of pulmonary function (Carter, Coast, & Idell, 1992).

## Time Frame for Initiating Pharmacotherapy

COPD is a slowly progressive disease. Patients may have evidence of disease upon physical examination and pulmonary function tests long before they become subjectively symptomatic. Patients who are current smokers should be strongly encouraged to quit and offered specific smoking cessation therapy (drug and/or behavioral) at every clinician visit. Smoking cessation is the primary therapy to retard progression of airway disease.

Patients with COPD should begin treatment when their disease becomes symptomatic. It may take several days to several weeks for patients to optimally benefit from each step in pharmacotherapy.

## Assessment Needed Prior to Therapy

Baseline pulmonary function tests should be monitored for every patient and should include FEV$_1$ and FVC. Also the FEV$_1$:FVC ratio should be calculated. An FEV$_1$:FVC of $\approx$80% is considered normal, 60–75% is characteristic of mild obstruction, 50–60% is considered moderate obstruction, and <50% is considered severe obstruction (Williams, 1995). Pulmonary function tests may need to be performed over several visits to establish each patients' personal best.

Patients with underlying cardiovascular disease may need to avoid oral beta agonists and theophylline. If these agents are used, their benefits and risks need to be evaluated on a patient-by-patient basis. For sleep medications in COPD patients it is safer to use sedating antihistamines and chloral hydrate because they cause less respiratory depression than benzodiazepines. Sedating antidepressants (eg, amitriptylline, trazodone) may also improve sleep for those COPD patients with concomitant depression (ATS, 1995).

## Patient/Caregiver Information

Patients need to be as well educated as possible about their disease state and strongly encouraged to participate in their own care. It may take several days for patients to notice subjective improvement from their medication. For patients who are on regularly scheduled medication emphasize to the patient/caregiver that the medications need to be taken regularly even if they do not notice immediate benefit. Also periodically review the onset and duration of action and expected effects of the patient's medication regimen.

As with all medications, write down the patient's current medication regimen (including OTCs, alternative medications, and nutritional supplements) at each visit if changes are necessary and give a copy to the patient to carry with him or her. For example, suggest the patient carry a small notebook/calendar the size of a wallet or checkbook. The patient could also add notes and questions to this notebook.

Patients who smoke should be encouraged to quit at every clinician visit. Patients should be educated about the benefits of smoking cessation and that smoking cessation has been proven to slow the progression of COPD.

There are numerous drug interactions with theophylline. It is important to impress upon the patient the potential for interactions. Patients should check for interactions with theophylline whenever they start or discontinue any medication (prescription, OTC, or alternative therapies). It is also important to impress upon patients not to increase their dose of theophylline without consultation with their clinician.

Patients need to have their inhaler techniques reviewed periodically. Most patients benefit from a spacing device such as the Aerochamber.

## OUTCOMES MANAGEMENT

### Selecting an Appropriate Agent

Figure 22–1 shows a suggested treatment algorithm for the outpatient treatment of COPD (ATS, 1995; Ferguson & Cherniack, 1993; Friedman, 1995).

***Anticholinergics.*** Inhaled ipratropium bromide is the primary anticholinergic used in the treatment of COPD and is considered a first-line agent. It is available as both an oral multidose inhaler (MDI) and as a solution for nebulization. Because it is a water-soluble quaternary ammonium compound, it is poorly absorbed across the lung and therefore has minimal systemic toxicity. Ipratropium produces bronchodilation by inhibiting the vagal stimulation of the tracheobronchial tree (Skorodin, 1993). For patients who require the regular use of an inhaled anticholinergic and an inhaled beta$_2$-receptor agonist, a Combivent inhaler (ipratropium and albuterol) may be useful and aid in compliance.

***Beta$_2$-receptor agonists.*** There are numerous inhaled beta$_2$-receptor agonists available in the United States. They include albuterol, bitolterol, isoetharine, metaproterenol, pirbuterol, salmeterol, and terbutaline. Inhaled beta$_2$ agonists cause bronchodilation via relaxation of the smooth muscles of the bronchial tree. They also decrease airway resistance in those patients with reversible airway obstruction (*AHFS drug information*, 1997).

Inhaled beta$_2$ agonists can be used as first-line agents for COPD patients who cannot tolerate or receive no benefit from inhaled anticholinergics. Inhaled beta$_2$ agonists may also be used prn as a first-line agent for patients with mild COPD who do not have daily symptoms (ATS, 1995). They may also be used in conjunction with inhaled anticholinergics for an additive bronchodilatory effect.

The long-acting beta$_2$ agonist salmeterol was approved in 1998 for use in COPD. If long-acting inhaled beta$_2$ agonists are used, it is extremely important to educate the patient that their use is prophylactic and they are not effective for acute exacerbations. Patients using salmeterol may also use short-acting inhaled beta$_2$ agonists on an as-needed basis.

Oral beta$_2$ agonists available include albuterol, metaproterenol, and terbutaline. It is important to note that when administered orally, these agents also have some beta$_1$ activity and can therefore cause cardiac stimulation. Because of a greater risk of adverse effects, oral beta$_2$ agonists should be avoided unless a patient is unable to use inhaled forms or if inhaled forms result in suboptimal results (ATS, 1995; Ferguson & Cherniack, 1993; Skorodin, 1993).

***Theophylline.*** The theophyllines include aminophylline, dyphylline, oxtriphylline, and theophylline. For sake of simplicity only the term theophylline will be used. The use of theophylline in the management of COPD has fallen in and out of favor over the years, and its use is still controversial.

Fragoso and Miller (1993) state that theophylline has been shown to improve spirometry and dyspnea. Theophylline may also improve mucociliary clearance, respiratory muscle performance, cardiovascular function, central respiratory drive, gas exchange, and exercise capacity. Its main value is in improving respiratory muscle performance. Many pulmonologists regard theophylline as a third-line drug (Stauffer, 1995).

Patient dosing for theophylline needs to be individualized. Some patients may benefit from serum levels as low as 5–10 mg/L, but some patients may require serum levels in the range of 15–17 mg/L to show benefit (McKay, Howie, Thompson, Whiting, and Addis, 1993). It is important to assess the patient's response at each dosage. Since theophylline toxicity increases with increasing levels, it is important to monitor patients carefully and to educate patients re-

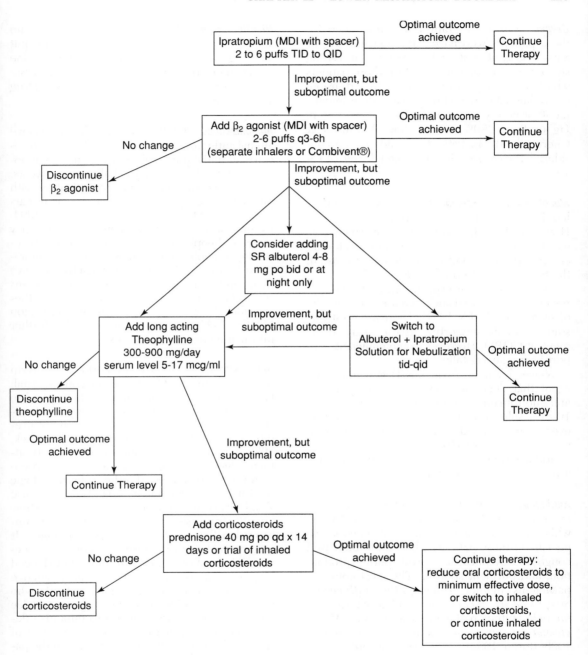

**Figure 22–1.** Algorithm for pharmacologic therapy in COPD.

Adapted from ATS (1995), Ferguson and Cherniak (1993), and Friedman (1995).

garding drug interactions and signs and symptoms of toxicity. Some patients may benefit from theophylline administered once daily in the evening to improve nocturnal bronchospasms (Stauffer, 1995).

In general, patients should be prescribed sustained-release forms of theophylline to maintain adequate blood levels, to minimize peak and trough differences, and to aid in patient compliance.

**Oxygen.** Oxygen therapy is recommended for those patients who have $PaO_2$ ≤55 mm Hg or $SaO_2$ ≤89% at rest, with exercise, or during sleep. It is also recommended for those patients who have evidence of pulmonary hypertension, cor pulmonale, mental or psychological impairment, or polycythemia and a $PaO_2$ of 56–59 mm Hg or $SaO_2$ ≤90% at any time (Ferguson & Cherniack, 1993). Patients should also be considered for oxygen therapy when flying (ATS, 1995).

**Mucolytics and expectorants.** Potassium iodide has historically been used as an expectorant. However, the risk of iodine toxicity usually outweighs the benefit of its use as an expectorant, and it is therefore not recommended for use in the treatment of COPD (*AHFS*, 1997).

Guaifenesin is an expectorant that increases respiratory tract fluid and decreases the viscosity of secretions (*AHFS*, 1997). There are no strong studies to date supporting its use in the treatment of COPD. However, some clinicians support its use anecdotally.

N-acetylcysteine (Mucomyst) is a mucolytic agent that decreases the viscosity of purulent and nonpurulent pulmonary secretions. A 10–20% solution can be inhaled via nebulization every 2–6 h if needed to aid in the removal of viscous secretions (*AHFS*, 1997).

Iodinated glycerol is no longer commercially available in the United States.

**Antibiotics.** Antibiotics are indicated in acute exacerbations of chronic bronchitis and COPD when there is evidence of bacterial infection, especially in those patients who exhibit increased cough and dyspnea, increased sputum production, and purulent sputum. The most common pathogens include *Haemophilus influenzae*, *Streptococcus pneumoniae*, and *Moraxella catarrhalis*. Other pathogens may include *Mycoplasma* sp. and *Chlamydia* sp. (Aboussouan, 1996; Rosen, 1992). Gram's stain of sputum may be helpful in identifying the type of organism. Antibiotic therapy should be directed at the most likely organisms. Refer to the pneumonia section of this chapter for a more detailed discussion of etiologic agents and preferred treatments. The duration of antibiotics should be 10–14 days with an assessment of efficacy within 5–7 days to determine if a change in therapy is needed (Rosen, 1992). COPD patients are at an increased risk of developing pneumonia.

**Nicotine replacement.** COPD patients who smoke should be strongly encouraged to quit smoking. Specific recommendations for nicotine replacement therapy and other smoking cessation strategies should be considered. See Drug Table 1003.

**Immunizations.** COPD patients should receive annual influenza vaccines. They should also receive an initial pneumococcal vaccine. Pneumococcal antibody titers may fall after several years, and it is recommended that revaccination with pneumococcal vaccine be evaluated every 6 years (Ferguson & Cherniack, 1993; Ingram, 1994; Rosen, 1992). Annual influenza vaccines may increase theophylline levels acutely. Patients receiving theophylline therapy should be monitored for theophylline toxicity when they receive their annual influenza vaccine. Some clinicians recommend decreasing the dose or holding theophylline for 24 h after vaccine administration (*AHFS*, 1997). Consult Chapter 11 for further information on immunizations.

**Corticosteroids.** The use of corticosteroids in the treatment of COPD remains controversial. Only a small percentage of patients respond to oral corticosteroids, and even fewer patients respond to inhaled steroids, but one cannot predict who will benefit (Ferguson & Cherniack, 1993; Gross, 1995). As indicated in the treatment algorithm (Fig. 22–1), a trial of corticosteroids is warranted if other pharmacologic treatments are less than optimal. Long-term use should be reserved for those patients who show benefit from steroids, as evidenced by improved airflow and/or exercise performance. It is important to distinguish between the objective benefit of oral corticosteroids as evidenced by pulmonary function tests and the subjective benefit that many patients feel. Patients who use inhaled steroids should use a spacing device and rinse the mouth after use to minimize deposition of drug in the mouth. Proper use of spacing devices should be reviewed with the patient periodically.

**Zileuton.** Zileuton is a 5-lipoxygenase inhibitor used in the treatment of asthma. To date there are no studies on its use in COPD. It may, however, be useful in those patients who have an asthmatic component to their COPD.

**Zafirlukast and montelukast.** Zafirlukast and montelukast are leukotriene receptor antagonists used in the treatment of asthma. To date there are no studies on their use in COPD. They may, however, be useful in those patients who have an asthmatic component to their COPD.

***Drugs to avoid.***    Patients who have an asthmatic component to their COPD should avoid non-selective beta blockers, including oral and ophthalmic products, because they may cause bronchoconstriction. Patients with severe COPD need to avoid benzodiazepines because of their respiratory depressant effects (ATS, 1995). Patients with underlying cardiovascular disease need to be cautious in their use of theophylline and oral beta$_2$ agonists.

## Monitoring for Efficacy

At each visit the clinician should question the patient regarding subjective symptoms such as cough (frequency and severity), sputum production (quality and quantity), dyspnea, and wheezing. The patient should also be questioned regarding the quality of sleep (ie, if they sleep well, better, or worse; need for inhalation therapy at night; several pillow orthopnea). Subjective assessment should include the patient's exercise tolerance (eg, the number of flights of stairs or city blocks they can handle).

A patient daily diary may be useful to record signs and symptoms and medication use. A chart may be useful to aid in consistency of reporting symptoms and to minimize the time it takes a patient to record symptoms (and therefore increase compliance). Keep in mind the age and visual acuity of the patient, and make the charts with big enough print and dark enough copies.

At each visit, assess the following changes from the baseline physical examination:

- Lung: breath sounds, crackles, rhonchi, rales, respiratory rate, use of accessory muscles, pursed lip breathing, shortness of breath (SOB) while speaking
- Cardiac: gallop, S$_3$ or S$_4$, distant heart sounds, JVD, six- and 12-min walking distance
- Pulmonary function tests: FEV$_1$, FVC

An alpha$_1$-antitrypsin level should be measured for those COPD patients who develop the disease at less than 50 years of age, when there is a family history of alpha$_1$-antitrypsin deficiency, or when emphysema occurs without a significant smoking history (Ingram, 1994). Arterial blood gas determinations are not usually

needed for stage I patients, but are indicated for stage II and stage III patients (ATS, 1995).

For patients taking theophylline, levels should be determined periodically. Initially, levels should be determined after a few days of therapy and after any change in dosage. There are numerous medications that interact with theophylline. Levels may need to be determined if a patient starts or stops any chronic medication. Smoking also influences theophylline metabolism. If a patient stops smoking, theophylline dosage may need to be adjusted. Patients requiring a single daily low dose of theophylline do not need frequent monitoring.

## Monitoring for Toxicity

Patients should be questioned regarding adverse effects of medications at each visit. Patients should be educated regarding common and serious side effects of their medication when it is initially prescribed. Patients should be advised to seek immediate care when serious adverse effects occur. Table 22–20 shows common toxicities and how to monitor them. FEV$_1$ and FVC should be monitored at each visit to determine if the patients' COPD is worsening.

## Follow-up Recommendations

Patients may need to be seen frequently when the effect of their chronic therapy is suboptimal (eg, once a week to once every 2 weeks) or if they are having an acute exacerbation of their illness (eg, acute bacterial or viral respiratory infection). Once patients are stable on their medication, they may be able to go several months between clinician visits. COPD is a chronic, progressive disease. Patients will need continuing care over their lifetime once the diagnosis of COPD is made.

# CYSTIC FIBROSIS

Cystic fibrosis (CF) is one of the most common genetically inherited diseases of Caucasians, occurring in 1 of 2500 live births. Because of better drug treatments and a coordinated team approach to care by major medical centers, the survival rate has increased to about 30 years. Approximately one third of CF survivors are currently over the age of 18 (Boucher, 1996). CF is

**TABLE 22–20. SELECTED ADVERSE REACTION MONITORING FOR DRUGS USED FOR COPD**

| Drug | Signs/Symptoms of Toxicity | Physical Examination Indicators of Toxicity | Laboratory Indicators of Toxicity |
|---|---|---|---|
| Inhaled ipratropium | Dry mouth, tachycardia, difficult urination | Tachycardia | |
| Inhaled beta$_2$ agonists | Tachycardia, tremors, nervousness, tolerance, paradoxical worsening | Tachycardia, tremors | |
| Oral beta$_2$ agonists | Tachycardia, tremors, nervousness, tolerance, paradoxical worsening | Hypertension, tachycardia, tremors | Hypokalemia |
| Theophylline | Nausea, vomiting, heartburn, nervousness, insomnia, tremors, seizure, tachycardia | Hypertension, tachycardia, tremors | Blood levels >20 mg/L, hypoglycemia |
| Oral corticosteroids | Symptoms of diabetes (polydipsia, polyphagia, polyuria), mental status changes | Hypertension, striae, skin thinning, purpura, cataracts, weight gain | Hypokalemia, hyperglycemia |
| Inhaled corticosteroids | Hoarseness, dysphonia, thrush | Thrush | |

Adapted from ATS (1995).

a result of a mutation of the gene on the long arm of chromosome 7 that encodes the CF transmembrane conductance regulator (CFTR) (Boucher, 1996). CFTR acts as a channel for chloride in the membranes of the airways and gut, which is one means of hydrating the airway and the intestinal tract. If the CFTR is defective, this may limit mucous hydration. Dehydrated airways lead to decreased mucociliary clearance, which encourages bacterial colonization and repeated infections (Puchelle, de Bentzmann, & Zahm, 1995). The most common etiologic agents of lung infections are *Staphylococcus aureus* and *H. influenzae* (later in the disease process, *Pseudomonas aeruginosa*) (Boucher, 1996). All body areas are probably affected by the lack of mucous hydration as well, ie, cervical glands, synovial cavities, bile ducts, etc. (Boucher, 1996).

The defective CFTR also leads to failure to secrete sodium bicarbonate (NaHCO$_3$) and water by the pancreatic ducts, causing retention of the enzymes in the pancreas, and ultimately destroying the pancreatic tissue. The secretions are thickened, and over time this leads to destruction of the beta cells resulting in diabetes, generally manifesting in the adolescent or young

adult (Puchelle et al, 1995). CF patients can secrete almost a normal volume of sweat into the sweat glands but cannot absorb the NaCl from that sweat. Thus, the definitive test for the diagnosis of CF still remains the sweat chloride test (Boucher, 1996).

Most CF patients present with the signs and symptoms of the disease in childhood, but a significant number are not diagnosed until their 20s (Boucher, 1996). The common presenting symptoms are (Matthews & Drotar, 1994):

- Failure to thrive/malnutrition
- Persistent respiratory problems, ie, persistent cough, chronic bronchitis, pulmonary infiltrates on x-ray, chronic purulent rhinorrhea, and sinusitis
- Malabsorption
- Family history of CF
- Meconium ileus

The most common complications that result from CF are (Boucher, 1996):

- Gallstones
- Diabetes

- Recurrent lung infections with eventual loss of lung function
- Delayed onset of puberty in both males and females
- Intestinal obstruction
- Pneumothorax
- Small volume hemoptysis
- Acute appendicitis

## SPECIFIC CONSIDERATIONS FOR PHARMACOTHERAPY

### When Drug Therapy Is Needed

Drug therapy is the mainstay for the CF patient to live a relatively comfortable and productive life and slow the progression of the disease. Infections should be treated rapidly and vigorously to restore the patient to the previous level of functioning. Without the appropriate nutrition, drug therapy, chest physiotherapy, and health care from a coordinated team, the CF patient's life would be limited to months rather than years.

### Short- and Long-Term Goals of Pharmacotherapy

The short-term goals are to treat any lung infections, resolve intestinal obstructions, and improve hydration and nutrition. The long-term goals include (Boucher, 1996; Mouton & Kerrebijn, 1990):

- Prevention of lung infections.
- Control the infection and restore the patient to his/her former state of well-being, if unable to eradicate.
- Promote mucociliary clearance and reduce the number of lung infections.
- Maintain normal absorption and nutrition through pancreatic enzyme replacement.
- Management of complications.
- Improve quality of life.

### Nonpharmacologic Therapy

Breathing exercises, chest physiotherapy, exercise training, and adequate hydration and nutrition are the main nonpharmacologic treatments available today.

Breathing exercises must be done once or twice daily and are always followed by chest phys-

iotherapy. To obtain the maximum benefit, the patient takes two deep breaths and exhales fully and forcefully so the mucus can be cleared. After exhaling, chest physiotherapy is performed. The sequence is repeated until mucus is expectorated (Mortenson, Falk, Groth, & Jensen, 1991).

Exercise tolerance and cardiopulmonary response to exercise are impaired in the CF patient. Exercise training has been shown to be beneficial by improving both aerobic fitness and cardiopulmonary efficiency (Nixon, 1996). Every CF patient should be evaluated through exercise testing so an individualized program can be initiated.

Adequate daily hydration and nutrition are crucial to overall pulmonary health. Research has demonstrated that undernutrition secondary to an energy imbalance is the result of three primary factors: (1) reduced energy intake because of dietary insufficiency and/or anorexia from respiratory disease, abdominal symptoms, and/or clinical depression; (2) increased energy loss secondary to maldigestion, and (3) increased energy expenditure from advanced lung disease (Durie & Pencharz, 1992). It is vital, therefore, to ensure that all CF patients regardless of duration of disease have a dietary consultation at every visit.

### Time Frame for Initiating Pharmacotherapy

Treatment should be initiated as soon as the diagnosis is established, whether the patient is 1 day old or 20 years old. The earlier the treatment is started, the better the short-term outcome will be. The long-term outcome is ultimately death, but the quality of life can be significantly improved with prompt treatment and frequent follow-up care by a CF medical health care team. Studies reveal that care delivered by a comprehensive CF team at a major medical center not only improves the quality of life but that CF patients experience fewer hospitalizations and more prompt and earlier recognition and treatment of infections. This improved quality of life is due to a more holistic approach because an entire team has the updated knowledge required to manage these patients (Boucher, 1996).

### Assessment Needed Prior to Therapy

The appropriate history and physical assessment as well as diagnostic test findings are described in Tables 22–21 and 22–22.

**TABLE 22–21.  SIGNIFICANT HISTORY AND PHYSICAL EXAMINATION NEEDED AND POSSIBLE FINDINGS FOR THE CF PATIENT**

| Pertinent History | Possible Findings |
|---|---|
| **Neonate** | |
| • First stool passed | Abdomen: may have distension<br>Rectal: possibly impacted stool |
| • Vomiting | |
| • Crying pattern | |
| **Infant/Toddler** | |
| • Failure to gain weight despite hunger and increased food | Height and weight plotted on chart |
| • May have foul-smelling, foamy, bulky stools | Abdomen: distention, tenderness |
| • Increased frequency but can be constipation (no BMs) | |
| • Wheezing, paroxysmal nonproductive cough | Lungs: wheezing, crackles, rhonchi |
| • Frequent respiratory infections | |
| | Heart: sound change |
| **School-Age/Adolescent** | |
| • Growth delay | Tanner stage: delay |
| • Delayed onset of puberty in girls and boys | |
| • Chronic respiratory problems: wheezing, productive cough, night cough, chest pain or hemoptysis, rhinorrhea | Lungs: wheezing, rhonchi, crackles<br>Chest: becoming barrel-shaped<br>Nails: clubbing |
| • Fatigue, change in energy level | |
| • Decrease in exercise tolerance | |
| • Purulent rhinorrhea | Nose: purulent rhinorrhea |
| • Stool pattern | Abdomen: tenderness, distention, hepatosplenomegaly |
| • Frequency of chest physiotherapy | |
| • Exercise plan adherence | |
| • Review daily diet, calorie intake, energy expenditure | |
| | Heart: sound changes |
| **Adults** | |
| • Symptom progression, especially at rest and night, more frequent and intractable pulmonary infections | Lungs: significant change in breath sounds, increased respiratory rate, shortness of breath |
| • Increasing hemoptysis, chest pain | Heart: sound changes, pulses |
| • Weight loss | Weight: every visit<br>Extremities: changes in sensations |

*Adapted from Boucher (1996), Bye et al (1994).*

## TABLE 22–22. PERTINENT DIAGNOSTIC TESTS FOR CYSTIC FIBROSIS

| Diagnostic Tests | Possible Findings |
| --- | --- |
| Sweat chloride | Positive |
| Flat plate of abdomen | Impacted stool, intussusception |
| Stool specimen | Positive for fat |
| Chest x-ray | Pneumonia or atelectasis |
| Liver function tests | Elevated; amylase low or absent |
| Sputum culture | S. aureus, H. influenzae, and/or Pseudomonas |
| Pulse oximetry | Decreased arterial $Po_2$ levels |
| Spirometry | Decreased $FEV_1$ and FVC |
| | Increased TLV and RLV |
| Blood glucose | Increased in prediabetic and diabetic state |
| WBC | Results depend on health state |
| **Special Tests** | |
| $B_{12}$ levels | |
| Levels of oto- and nephrotoxic drugs | Low, if enzyme replacement inadequate |
| Vitamin K levels | CF patients have altered pharmacokinetics |

*Adapted from Boucher (1996).*

## Patient/Caregiver Information

### Chest physiotherapy
1. All patients need written instructions regarding their chest physiotherapy.
2. The proper chest physiotherapy technique should be reviewed.

### Nutrition
1. Patients need to keep a diary of their food intake so it can be reviewed at each visit with a nutritionist.
2. Monitor weight regularly.
3. Teach patients to adjust enzyme replacement for special events, ie, birthday parties, holidays.
4. Teach patients to increase calories, fat, vitamins, and minerals during periods of rapid growth, ie, infancy and adolescence.

### General information
1. Directions for taking medications should be written, since most CF patients are on multiple drugs.
2. Patients should be cautioned to *never* stop taking the enzyme replacement, change brands, or adjust the dose themselves until first talking with their health care provider (Drug Facts and Comparisons, 1998).
3. Review the subtle signs of a respiratory infection so quick action can be initiated.
4. Encourage regular exercise.

## OUTCOMES MANAGEMENT

### Selecting an Appropriate Agent

The CF patient uses many therapeutic drugs. They include everything from bronchodilators to liquid food supplements.

***Bronchodilators.*** Bronchodilators available today include albuterol, pirbuterol, terbutaline, isoetharine, bitolterol, metaproterenol, and salmeterol. Inhaled beta₂ agonists cause dilation and relaxation of the smooth muscle in the airways, which decreases airway resistance in patients with reversible airway obstruction (Drug Facts and Comparisons, 1998).

In the CF patient, nebulization is the preferred administration route because it provides a mist that can help wet secretions (Frederiksen, Lanng, Koch, & Hoiby, 1996). Albuterol and metaproterenol are the only beta₂ agonists that can be nebulized. However, the safety of albuterol and metaproterenol in children <12 years and 6 years, respectively, has not been established. Even though safety for metaproterenol has been established for children >6 years, albuterol has been utilized most often and has the best safety record. It is the recommended beta₂ agonist of choice for nebulization. Pirbuterol, isoetharine, terbutaline, and bitolterol are not available to use in a nebulizer and safety has not been established in children <12 years (Drug Facts and Comparisons, 1998).

A beta$_2$ agonist is important in the treatment of CF. The first of the lung changes that occur in children is an increased RV/TLC (residual volume/total lung capacity), implying that the small airways are involved. As the disease progresses over years, there are reversible and nonreversible changes in FEV$_1$ and FVC in about 40–60% of patients. The reversible changes (airway relaxation can occur after constriction) might reflect either increased mucus in the lumen of the airway and/or airway reactivity, whereas the nonreversible changes (airways less flexible, more rigid, and damaged so relaxation is less possible) usually reflect chronic destruction and/or bronchiolitis (Boucher, 1996; Frederiksen et al, 1996).

Salmeterol, a long-acting bronchodilator, is not approved for use in children <12 years and has not been utilized in the CF population.

***Mucus liquifying agents.***    Dornase alfa is a purified solution of human recombinant DNA. CF patients accumulate very viscous and purulent mucus, making expectoration extremely difficult. This contributes to decreased pulmonary function and infection exacerbations (Puchelle et al, 1995). Dornase alfa hydrolyzes the DNA in the patient's lung sputum, making it less tenacious and sticky. Dornase alfa, 2.5 mg/ampule, is nebulized either in the morning or morning and evening. There are no safety data for children <5 yrs, but it is used because of its effectiveness (Sanchez & Guiraldes, 1995). The following precautions must be adhered to when using this medication (*AHFS*, 1997; Drug Facts and Comparisons, 1998):

1. Store in the refrigerator.
2. Do not mix or dilute with any other medication in the nebulizer because it can alter the property of dornase and cause a physiochemical change in the patient.
3. Use immediately after opening the ampule.

***Vitamins and pancreatic enzymes.***    It has been recognized that the degree of malnutrition correlates with the severity of the pulmonary disease and mortality (MacDonald, 1996). It is vital to aggressively prevent or treat a malnutrition state in order to promote the patient's well-being, allow catch-up growth, decrease lung infections, improve exercise tolerance, slow the deterioration of lung function, and perhaps prolong life. Dietary recommendations include: (1) a high-calorie diet, (2) liberal fat intake, and (3) vitamin

and mineral supplements. Nutrition and vitamin and mineral supplementation are revised based on the state of health, periods of growth, illnesses, antibiotic use, and advancing disease (Ramsey, Farrell, Pancharz, & The Consensus Committee, 1992).

CF patients, regardless of age, are prone to hyponatremic dehydration during periods of exercise, hot weather, and vomiting due to high losses of sodium sweat. These patients must be supplemented with sodium chloride, based on 1 mmol/kg per day (MacDonald, 1996).

Table 22–23 lists the recommendations for daily vitamins and energy supplementation for CF patients.

Pancreatic enzyme replacement is required for all CF patients with pancreatic deficiency. The supplements must be given with each milk feeding, meal, and snack. The guidelines in Table 22–24 can be used but must be individualized for each patient. There are no exact standards for dosing pancreatic enzyme replacement. The patient's health status must guide dosing. The most important dosing guideline to observe is: If more than 2000 units lipase/kg/meal or snack is required, then a consultation is imperative. Special consideration must be given to taking the pancreatic enzyme replacement correctly. The enteric-coated microcapsules *must not* be chewed, only swallowed. In the infant and toddler contents of the capsules can be sprinkled onto pureed fruit and fed. If the older child has difficulty swallowing the capsule, use the same technique (Drug Facts and Comparisons, 1998).

### Antibiotics

CHRONIC MEDICATIONS.    The principle behind using the antibiotic colistin M parenteral is that, inhaled by nebulization, colistin M seems to decrease the colony count of *Pseudomonas* in the lung. This may reduce hospitalizations and maintain lung function longer. Colistin M parenteral is nebulized in two divided doses of 20–300 mg/day (Hoiby, 1993). Ticarcillin powder, an antipseudomonal drug, is also nebulized to decrease the *Pseudomonas* colony count and preserve lung function (Sanchez & Guiraldes, 1995).

An aminoglycoside, tobramycin or gentamicin aerosolized, can also be used to decrease the *Pseudomonas* count since persistent bacterial eradication is not achievable. Tobramycin is given at a maximum dose of 600 mg two or three times daily and has been shown to be safe and effective. These inhaled aminoglycosides are

## TABLE 22–23.  DAILY VITAMIN AND ENERGY SUPPLEMENTS FOR CYSTIC FIBROSIS PATIENTS

| Vitamin and Energy Needs | Dosage/Day |
|---|---|
| **<2 Years** | |
| Vitamins A and D | Use any standard preparation, such as Poly-Vi-Sol; amount based on age |
| Energy[a] | 120–150% of daily requirements |
| **2–8 Years** | |
| Vitamin A | 5000 IU |
| Vitamin D | 400–800 IU; given in one multivitamin |
| Energy[a] | 120–150% |
| **8 Years to Adulthood** | |
| Vitamins A and D | One or two multivitamins |
| Energy | Averages about 130% or more |
| **Vitamin K[b]** | |
| <1 year | 2.5 mg/week or 2.5 mg twice a week if on antibiotics |
| >1 year | 5 mg twice a week; some recommend only for cholestatic liver disease or antibiotics, others regardless |
| **Vitamin E** | |
| 0–6 months | 25 IU |
| 6–12 months | 50–100 IU |
| 1–4 years | 100 IU |
| 4–10 years | 100–200 IU |
| >10 years | 200–400 IU |

[a] Must be individualized for each patient based on weight gain, nutritional status, and lung function declines. Energy requirements are increased as lung function declines.
[b] Antibiotic use may lead to decreased vitamin K production by intestinal flora; may need to double dose during this time. Amounts per age may vary by setting.
*Adapted from Green, Buchanan, and Weaver (1995) and Ramsey et al (1992).*

often used concurrently with oral or IV antibiotics during an acute lung infection (Smith & Ramsey, 1995; Webb, 1995).

***ACUTE MEDICATIONS.*** Antibiotics used for acute treatment of a lung infection are based on the most common organism and the sputum and/or blood cultures. The severity of the exacerbation will determine whether the treatment can be managed on an outpatient or inpatient basis. Usually two or three antibiotics are used, one inhaled and the other two either IV or oral. Since *Staphylococcus*, beta-lactamase-producing strains of *H. influenzae*, gram-negative bacteria, *M. catarrhalis*, and *Pseudomonas* are the most likely, coverage should be aimed at these organ-

## TABLE 22–24.  PANCREATIC ENZYME REPLACEMENT RECOMMENDATION FOR CYSTIC FIBROSIS

**Infants**
- 1000–2000 units lipase/120 mL of formula
- Increase as needed

**Children to Adults**
- 5000 units lipase/snack and meal
- Dosage should be increased in a stepwise manner
- If the requirement is >2000 units lipase/kg per meal and snack, then further investigation is imperative
- If the child has a larger than usual snack or meal, the child will need another one or two capsules

*Adapted from MacDonald (1996) and Ramsey et al (1992).*

isms. Other organisms such as *Proteus, Klebsiella,* or *Escherichia coli* cause a chronic low-grade infection rather than an acute infection. These organisms must always be considered in the diagnosis and treated (Boucher, 1996; Klein, 1991). Refer to the Antibiotic Drug Tables for more details.

Cephalosporins, especially the third generation, have more gram-negative coverage than the first or second generation and, therefore, are advantageous to use. The third-generation cephalosporins include ceftriaxone, cefotaxime, cefixime, cefpodoxime, ceftibuten, moxalactam (*AHFS,* 1997). The newer macrolides, penicillins, and trimethoprim-sulfamethoxazole can also be used. Table 22–25 lists the target organisms and the effective antibiotic.

### TABLE 22–25. ANTIBIOTICS EFFECTIVE AGAINST COMMON BACTERIA SEEN IN CYSTIC FIBROSIS PATIENTS

| Common Bacterial Organisms[b] | Effective Antibiotics |
|---|---|
| S. aureus | Penicillinase-resistant penicillin |
| | Usually hospitalized |
| Gram-negative bacteria | |
|  Proteus | Fluoroquinolones[c] |
|  Klebsiella | Amoxicillin/clavulanate or amoxicillin[d] |
|  E. coli | Third generation cephalosporins[d] |
| | TMP-SMX[d] |
| H. influenzae | TMP-SMX[d] |
| | Amoxicillin/clavulanate[d] |
| | 2nd & 3rd generation cephalosporins[d] |
| P. Aeruginosa | Antipseudomonal penicillin, other appropriate antibiotics[d] |
| | Inpatient treatment |

[a] Consultation with the health care team is imperative prior to treatment onset.
[b] Hospitalization may be required for patients with any of the common bacterial organisms
[c] Fluoroquinolones *only* indicated in CF children with *Pseudomonas* infections since increased risk of quinolone-induced cartilage toxicity; they have limited anaerobic activity (*Klein, 1991*).
[d] Depending on culture and sensitivities
Adapted from AHFS Drug Information (1997), Drug Facts and Comparisons (1998), and Musher (1998).

Because of the altered pharmacokinetics in the CF patient, the following principles must guide antibiotic prescription:

• Doses twice the normal doses are often needed.
• Renal clearance is increased.
• Treatment must be of sufficient duration to eradicate the organisms other than *Pseudomonas.* Persistent eradication of any of the bacteria seen in pulmonary infections in CF patients is not attainable. Complete eradication of *Pseudomonas* is not possible (Drug Facts and Comparisons, 1998; Webb, 1995).

**Steroids.** There is increasing evidence that a neutrophil-mediated inflammatory response may be involved in the early course of CF lung disease and may precede the onset of bacterial colonization (deBenedictis et al, 1996). Low-dose alternate-day oral steroids seem to be helpful. In children younger than school-age, the steroid (prednisone) dose is based on 1 mg/kg per day, whereas in the older child, the prednisone dose is usually 5–10 mg (deBenedictis et al, 1996). Data indicate that low-dose alternate-day prednisone does significantly delay linear growth after 24 months of therapy but causes fewer side effects than daily dosing (Rosenstein & Eigen, 1991). The $FEV_1$ improved, and serum IgG levels decreased. The FVC improved only in those patients colonized with *Pseudomonas.* The beneficial effects of prednisone were seen after 6 months of therapy but did not increase after that time. If no improvement is seen in pulmonary function tests after 6 months, the prednisone can be discontinued (Rosenstein & Eigen, 1991).

Inhaled steroids were used in two trials with conflicting results: one study indicated that there was no improvement in the PFTs, but a Danish study revealed there was improved pulmonary function in CF children (Frederiksen et al, 1996).

In high doses, the nonsteroidal antiinflammatory drug ibuprofen has been shown to have activity against neutrophils, including the inhibition of neutrophil migration. This decreases the progression of lung disease without significant toxicity (Konstans, Byrard, Hoppel, & Davis, 1995).

**$H_2$ blockers.** Inadequate neutralization of gastric acid can result in inactivation of the pancreatic lipase enzyme. It is theorized that the $H_2$

blockers could improve digestion and absorption when given as adjunctive therapy with the pancreatic enzyme replacement (Forstner & Durie, 1996). Any of the $H_2$ blockers, Pepcid, Zantac, Axid, or Tagamet, can be used effectively to enhance pancreatic enzyme absorption.

***Insulin.*** Both regular and intermediate-acting insulin may be required when the blood glucose reaches consistent levels higher than 180–200. The diabetes of CF tends to be mild. Ketoacidosis is rare, but there have been retinal, kidney, and other vascular complications noted. It has been discovered that in CF patients the onset of microvascular complications occurs 10 years after the onset of hyperglycemia (Hayes, O'Brien, O'Brien, Fitzgerald, & McKennon, 1995). Diabetic complications occur but have not been a significant issue since most CF patients died prior to the onset of major sequelae. With the increase in life expectancy, more serious complications will present new challenges to the health care provider (Hayes et al, 1995).

Tight glucose control is not recommended because ketoacidosis is rarely encountered and the blood glucose remains relatively stable. Decreased weight, body mass index (BMI), $FEV_1$, and FVC and an increase in the daily intake of pancreatic enzyme replacement can herald the onset of a prediabetic state. This change is insidious and affects overall health for years prior to diagnosis. It is important that attention is given to this constellation of changes so early intervention can be instituted. It has been shown that insulin therapy can improve lung function even in the prediabetic state (Hayes et al, 1995; Lanng, Thorsteinsson, Nerupo, & Koch, 1992).

***Liquid supplements.*** The CF patient often requires an extremely high daily calorie intake to maintain normal pulmonary and overall health. It can be difficult to consume the number of calories required, so liquid supplements can be used. They are calorie-dense without being overwhelmingly filling (Green, Buchanan, & Weaver, 1995). Both prescription and over-the-counter liquid supplements are equally effective.

***Drugs to avoid.*** Patients who have a reversible airway component to their pulmonary disease should avoid excessive beta$_2$ agonist use. Tolerance can develop and render the agonist minimally effective when needed, but time without the inhaler will render it effective again (*AHFS*, 1997).

## Monitoring for Efficacy

At each visit, the clinician needs to obtain a detailed history regarding the following: decreased appetite, weight loss or failure to gain weight, decrease in regular exercise tolerance pattern, fatigue, increased cough and/or night sweats, increase in respiratory rate, abdominal distention or discomfort, change in character of stools (bulky, greasy, foul-smelling), and personality changes (ie, irritability, signs of depression, anxiety, and eating disorders) (Pearson, Pumariega, & Seilheimer, 1991). Review the medication list with the patient, correct the mixing of the nebulizer solutions, check frequency of chest physiotherapy, note any subtle changes that the patient may have noticed, and review if any pancreatic enzymes needed to be adjusted. Fever and toxicity are rarely encountered in the CF patient, so careful assessment is important.

Possible physical examination findings to watch for include:

- Growth: height and weight, and head circumference in infants
- Tanner stage: age-appropriate
- Nose: purulent rhinorrhea
- Lungs: wheezing, crackles, rhonchi
- Heart: murmurs, $S_3$, $S_4$
- Abdomen: distention, tenderness, pain, hepatosplenomegaly
- Nails: clubbing
- Pulmonary function tests (declining levels can signal an acute pulmonary exacerbation): $FEV_1$, FVC, TLV, RV (Boucher, 1996)

The examination should be generally inclusive at each visit and even more detailed if a problem is detected during the history. It is important to be attuned to subtle changes, since 95% of CF patients die from complications of their lung infections (Boucher, 1996).

Laboratory data may need to be obtained, depending on the history, physical examination findings, and comorbid illnesses. These may include blood glucose, WBC with differential, stool for fat content, chest x-ray, LFTs, chemistry 18, blood gases, sputum cultures, and/or pulse oximetry.

## Monitoring for Toxicity

It is imperative that the patient and/or parents be questioned about any adverse reactions experienced. All the common adverse effects of each medication should be written down and re-

**TABLE 22–26. COMMON ADVERSE DRUG REACTIONS AND MONITORING IN CYSTIC FIBROSIS**

| Drug | Signs/Symptoms of Toxicity | Laboratory Indicators of Toxicity |
|------|----------------------------|-----------------------------------|
| Bronchodilator | Refer to Table 22–20 | |
| Dornase | None known | |
| Lipase | Abdominal pain or discomfort, change in stool pattern, hyper-uricemia | Increased fecal fat content, abnormal colonoscopy findings, decreased PFTs |
| Antibiotics | Maculopapular rash, diarrhea, nausea, vomiting | |
| Steroids | Refer to Table 22–20 | |
| H₂ blockers | Rare | |
| Insulin | None if the correct dose | |
| NSAIDs | Severe headaches, abdominal pain, substernal burning, photophobia, stiff neck, epigastric tenderness | Lumbar puncture, WBCs consistent with asceptic meningitis |

*Adapted from Drug Facts and Comparisons (1998).*

viewed when initially prescribed. Table 22–26 describes the common drug adverse reactions and ways to monitor them. It has been noted that CF patients do not develop gastric ulcers on either oral steroids or high-dose NSAIDs. It is speculated that the viscous stomach secretions may confer protection.

## Follow-up Recommendations

CF patients need to be seen by the health care team regularly because preventive care is crucial. The change from a chronic problem to an acute problem can be subtle. If the patient is seen regularly, every 6–8 weeks, and monitored frequently, any change in condition can be detected earlier. Intensive treatment can be initiated on an outpatient basis with fewer hospitalizations, less decline in function, and a more rapid return to activities of daily living. The tests that need to be performed will depend on the findings of the history and physical examination (Boucher, 1996).

# PNEUMONIA

## COMMUNITY-ACQUIRED PNEUMONIA IN ADULTS AND THE ELDERLY

Community-acquired pneumonia (CAP) is still one of the 10 leading causes of mortality among the elderly in the United States today and a major concern since the population is becoming increasingly older (Brown, 1993). Both the pneumococcal and influenza vaccines are readily available but are underutilized in this population. Pneumonia is more virulent in the elderly for a variety of reasons, including (Granton & Grossman, 1993; Mason & Nelson, 1996):

- Decrease in mucociliary clearance
- Decrease in lung recoil and chest wall compliance
- Impairment of cough reflex
- Decrease in production of antibodies to foreign antigens
- Impaired macrophage microbial response
- Impaired neutrophil migration
- Changes in the entire immune system (use of NSAIDs masks symptoms and reduces immune response)
- Nutritional deficits
- Environmental risk, which is highest if in a nursing home, followed by those with semiskilled care, and those at home

Perhaps an explanation of why CAP in the elderly may carry a higher mortality rate is the difficulty in establishing a diagnosis. The elderly rarely present with the "classic" pneumonia symptoms. Instead, they often present with mental status changes, new and/or increased falls, a worsening of their underlying illness, metabolic derangement, new incontinence, or failure to thrive (Granton & Grossman, 1993; Krieger, 1996). Unless the appropriate questions are asked or a family member is the historian, the pneumonia may be missed initially. When the pneumonia is finally diagnosed, the elderly person can be acutely ill, requiring hospitalization with a significantly greater risk of dying. The risk of severe pneumonia can be environment-related in the elderly. The frail, bedridden elderly in nursing homes or recently discharged from the hospital have the greatest risk of gram-negative and gram-positive organisms, such as *Pneumococcus, H. influenzae, Klebsiella, Staphylococcus,* gram-negative rods (GNR), and active tuberculosis. Atypical organisms that were once thought to be a rare cause of pneumonia in the elderly actually account for approximately 30% of the pneumonia cases today (Krieger, 1996). Consider mouth anaerobes if the elderly have teeth because anaerobic bacteria exist between teeth (Krieger, 1996).

Certain subgroups of adults, whether elderly or not, are at increased risk of pneumonia: smokers, alcohol abusers, users of immunosuppressive agents (NSAIDs and steroids, which the elderly tend to use regularly for the normal osteoarthritic pain), and those with cardiac/COPD/neoplastic/HIV/TB and neurologic disease (Leeper, 1996). In the young and middle-aged healthy nonsmoker and non-alcohol-abusing adult who develops pneumonia, the most likely etiology is a bacterial pneumonia (atypical and viral if during an epidemic). In persons with AIDS, however, *Pneumocystis carinii, S. pneumoniae,* and *H. influenzae* still remain the most common causes of pneumonia, but the clinician must always consider a broader differential. AIDS patients often have unusual causes of pneumonia such as fungal, *S. aureus, P. aeruginosa,* enteric gram-negative bacteria, and viral infections (Yu & Maurer, 1996). Always consider that active tuberculosis may also be the cause of the symptomatology. In the IVDA (intravenous drug abuser), besides *Klebsiella* and *H. influenzae,* consider rare fungi, anaerobes, and gram-negative and gram-positive bacteria, whereas in the alcoholic consider primarily *Klebsiella* and *Legionella* (Bartlett & Mundy, 1995; Bernstein & Locksley, 1997).

Table 22–27 summarizes the common pathogens and the clinical situations in which they are encountered.

The atypical pneumonias are the most common pneumonias that occur throughout the

## TABLE 22–27. CLINICAL SITUATIONS AND COMMON PATHOGENS IN COMMUNITY-ACQUIRED PNEUMONIA

| Clinical Situations | Pathogens |
|---|---|
| Alcoholism | a, b, c, e |
| COPD | a, b, f |
| Diabetes | a, h |
| Episodic | a, d |
| IVDA | a, c, e |
| Children, adolescents, young adults, populations living in close proximity | a, d |
| Chronic illness | a, e, h |
| Immunosuppressive state  NSAIDs  Steroids  Spleen dysfunction  HIV  Postinfluenza  Malignancies | a, b, c, e, h |
| Older adult men | c, e |
| Smokers | b, e |

Legend: a = *S. pneumonia*       e = *Legionella*
       b = *H. influenzae*       f = *M. catarrhalis*
       c = *Klebsiella*          g = TB
       d = *M.* or *C. pneumoniae*   h = GNR (gram-negative rods)
Adapted from Bernstein and Locksley (1997), Bozzoni et al (1995), Brown (1993), and Krieger (1996).

lifespan. They rarely occur before the age of 5 years, increase in frequency during school-age through young adults, and decline during middle age; however, they are an important pathogen in the elderly. The atypical pneumonias are usually self-limiting but can have significant extrapulmonary symptoms (Cunha & Ortega, 1996).

Table 22–28 lists the common atypical pneumonias and their clinical manifestations.

Other less common pneumonias to consider are coccidioidomycosis, histoplasmosis, tularemia, Q fever, *Chlamydia psittaci,* hantavirus, and hypersensitivity pneumonitis. These pneumonias should be suspected depending on whether the person has handled animals or birds or been exposed to fungal infections or where they have lived and traveled within the previous 6 weeks (Cunha & Ortega, 1996; Gales & McClain, 1997).

If an uncommon pneumonia or pneumonitis is suspected, a consultation or referral is war-

**TABLE 22–28.  COMMON ATYPICAL PNEUMONIAS AND CLINICAL MANIFESTATIONS**

| Atypical Pneumonia | Clinical Manifestations |
|---|---|
| *Mycoplasma pneumoniae* | Malaise, myalgias, arthralgias, low-grade fever +/– headache<br>Nonproductive cough, after several days +/– productive cough that persists<br>+/– OM, pharyngitis, tracheobronchitis<br>Extrapulmonary symptoms: cardiac, gastrointestinal, liver/spleen enlargement, elevation of LFTs; neurologic changes, hematologic abnormalities |
| *Chlamydia pneumoniae* | Biphasic course; erythematous, nonexudative pharyngitis with hoarseness first, then 1 week later cough begins; may be productive with bronchospasms and wheezing<br>+/– fever, cervical adenopathy<br>+/– eye involvement |
| *Legionella pneumophila* | Abrupt onset of myalgia, malaise, weakness, and headache; 24 h later fever, intermittent chills<br>Nonproductive cough; eventually 50% develop thin mucoid purulent, copious volume; hemoptysis in 30%<br>Diarrhea, nausea, vomiting, abdominal pain<br>Altered mental status |

+/– means finding may be either present or absent.
*Adapted from Bernstein and Locksley (1997), Cunha and Ortega (1996), and Prakash (1996).*

ranted. Very specific testing may be necessary, and several of these diseases can become chronic with significant sequelae and result in death.

## SPECIFIC CONSIDERATIONS FOR PHARMACOTHERAPY

### When Drug Therapy Is Needed

Because of the increased mortality of all pneumonias in the elderly, complicated usually by other comorbid illnesses, there is universal agreement that antibiotic therapy is the norm. In otherwise healthy nonelderly adults with bacterial or atypical pneumonia, treatment is warranted, but for the viral pneumonias without secondary infection supportive therapy is the accepted standard.

### Short- and Long-Term Goals of Pharmacotherapy

The short-term goals of treatment are to resolve the pneumonia, reduce the associated symp-

toms within 24–36 h, and reduce or prevent hospitalization.

The long-term goals are to reduce mortality; restore the person to the previous level of functioning; prevent recurrent episodes of pneumonia through adequate dental care, nutrition, hydration, and appropriate vaccination; and prevent or minimize an exacerbation of their comorbid illness during the acute pneumonia (File, Tan, & Plouffe, 1996; Musher, 1998).

### Nonpharmacologic Therapy

This can include the use of oxygen, plenty of hydration, and rest.

### Time Frame for Initiating Pharmacotherapy

Pneumonia must be treated as soon as possible in order to decrease the risk of mortality, especially in the elderly. The choice of treatment setting for the elderly with pneumonia is a decision based on the stability of comorbid illnesses, vital sign abnormalities, hypoxemia on room air, severe electrolyte and/or hematology abnormalities, low neutrophil count, and increased BUN and creatinine (Brown, 1993). In the nonhospitalized nonacute elderly, close follow-up is essential if the person lives alone. Usually the younger and middle-aged otherwise healthy adult can be safely treated as an outpatient.

### Assessment Needed Prior to Therapy

See Table 22–29 for baseline history information and physical examination criteria and Table 22–30 for findings specific to the common bacterial pneumonias.

Table 22–31 summarizes the common diagnostic tests to consider if the clinician suspects one of the community-acquired pneumonias.

### Patient/Caregiver Information

- Clear information must be given regarding signs and symptoms that indicate a worsening of the pneumonia.
- Review common side effects of the medication.
- In the elderly, supply written directions or when to call and/or a relative/neighbor/friend to check on them daily.

- Do a close follow-up, if the patient is elderly; otherwise follow up in 48–72 h.

## OUTCOMES MANAGEMENT

### Selecting an Appropriate Agent

Selection of an appropriate antibiotic depends on age and comorbid illnesses; other factors that can change the usual pathogen such as smoking, alcohol, and drug abuse; cost; broad-based coverage for the usual pathogens; and a single therapy if possible.

In 1993 the ATS formulated a set of guidelines that would treat community-acquired pneumonia using an empiric, not a syndrome-based, approach. The guiding principle behind this departure from the standard was to establish a diagnosis of pneumonia and a therapeutic plan employing an empiric regimen that takes into account the impact of age and comorbid illness on the risk for pneumonia. One of the most controversial decisions was to recommend that the sputum Gram's stain and culture not be used routinely as a diagnostic tool. There are multiple diagnostic tests to assist in identifying the offending pathogen, but there is *no one* test

### TABLE 22–29. HISTORY AND PHYSICAL EXAMINATION FOR BACTERIAL PNEUMONIAS

**History Information**
- Risk factors: alcohol, smoking, chronic lung disease, immunologic deficiency, IVDA, homelessness
- Nutrition
- Recent hospitalizations
- Recent pneumococcal/influenza vaccines
- Symptoms: initial onset of symptoms, progression of symptoms, self-treatment, worsening of other illnesses

- Daily medications: prescribed, OTC, and other self-medications
- Comorbid illnesses
- Living environment
- Immunosuppressive drugs; NSAIDs, and/or steroids
- Recent travel

**Physical Examination**
- Generally ill-appearing
- Vital signs:
  Increased respiratory rate, labored, use of accessory muscles
  Increased heart rate (increased 10–15 beats/min/temp degree)
- If heart rate is up significantly, need to consider CHF
- Hypotension in elderly
- Neck: JVD changes

- Skin: color, hydration
- Lips/teeth: cyanosis, cavities
- Lungs: dull percussion, + egophany, may/may not have consolidation or tactile fremitus, bronchial or tubular breath sounds, crackles; in elderly unable to breathe deeply, no crackles will be heard
- Abdomen: tenderness, hepatosplenomegaly
- Neurologic: changes in gait, balance, cerebral, cerebellar, CN I–XII

*Adapted from Austrian (1992), Brown (1993), Bartlett et al (1995), and Granton & Grossman (1993).*

## TABLE 22–30. HISTORY SPECIFIC TO THE COMMON BACTERIAL PNEUMONIAS

| | |
|---|---|
| Previous history of a URI | a, b |
| Fever: | |
|     Sudden onset of high fever | a, c |
|     Rare | d |
| Sudden shaking chills | a, c |
| Pleuritic chest pain | a, b, c |
| Productive cough: | |
|     Rusty-colored sputum | a |
|     Purulent sputum | b |
|     Thick, tenacious, purulent | c |
| Dyspnea | a, b, c, d |
| Pleuritic chest pain | a, b, c |
| Possibility of: | |
|     Vomiting/diarrhea | b, c |
|     Hypotension | b, d |
|     Mental confusion, asthenia | d |
|     Cyanosis, jaundice | c |
| Falls, new incontinence | d |
| Anorexia, failure to thrive | d |
| Worsening of comorbid illness | d |

Legend: a = *S. pneumoniae*; b = *H. influenzae*; c = *Klebsiella*; d = elderly.
*Adapted from Austrian (1992), Cunha and Ortega (1996), Moroney (1996), Granton and Grossman (1993), and Reilly (1993).*

available to make the diagnosis. Therefore, history becomes extremely important (Simon, 1995). There is considerable debate regarding this treatment approach, but these guidelines are to direct clinical practice only, so the clinician can still individualize treatment. Table 22–32 summarizes the ATS categories for the treatment of CAP.

***Adult without comorbid illness.*** In the young or middle-aged adult without comorbid illness the most common organisms causing infection are *S. pneumoniae, Mycoplasma pneumoniae, Chlamydia pneumoniae,* viruses, and, in smokers, *H. influenzae.* First-line therapy is erythromycin or the newer macrolides. The newer macrolides, azithromycin and clarithromycin, have the advantage of less frequent dosing and provide coverage for *H. influenzae.* Clarithromycin can cause considerable gastrointestinal side effects, but if it is taken with food, avoiding caffeine and spicy and greasy foods, most people can tolerate the medication. The medication leaves an "aluminum" or "tinny" taste in the mouth, but this can be decreased by having a small piece of

chocolate immediately after. Azithromycin can be taken on an empty stomach or with food without changing the bioavailability (Drug Facts and Comparisons, 1998).

Recently four new fluoroquinolones, levofloxacin, sparfloxacin, grepafloxacin, and trovafloxacin, have been approved for use in community-acquired pneumonia (CAP) and acute bacterial exacerbations of chronic bronchitis (ABECB). These drugs have enhanced activity against *S. pneumoniae*, including strains resistant to the beta-lactams and other antimicrobials. All have activity against *H. influenzae, M. pneumoniae, M. catarrhalis,* and *C. pneumoniae.*

These newer fluoroquinolones, like the older fluoroquinolones, increase the risk for photosensitivity as well as gastrointestinal disturbances. See Drug Table 102 for additional information. These newer fluoroquinolones all have the advantage of once-a-day dosing (Drug Facts and Comparisons, 1998; File, 1997).

Use of the older fluoroquinolones has been limited due to two problems: the rapid development of resistance for multiple bacteria and numerous drug interactions. The future of the newer fluoroquinolones may be in question as they potentially could be rendered ineffective (Musher, 1998).

Tetracycline is less often utilized because the need to avoid milk products at the time of administration, its phototoxicity, and gastrointestinal disturbances make taking this medication less than optimal. Because of these adverse side effects of tetracycline, compliance can be an issue, and the macrolides are therefore recommended instead (Bartlett & Mundy, 1995; Drug Facts and Comparisons, 1998; Fein, 1996).

*C. pneumoniae* is often unresponsive to erythromycin, so changing to azithromycin, clarithromycin, doxycycline, or a fluroquinolone is usually more effective. Treatment should be continued for 14–21 days whether treating *M.* or *C. pneumoniae.*

Many clinicians still use the penicillins and cephalosporins as their first-line drug therapy, but with increasing resistance to the penicillins from 10% to more than 30% in the United States, with high levels of resistance from 3–10% and even higher in other areas of the world, close follow-up is warranted to ensure that the pneumonia is resolving using penicillin (Pallares et al, 1995). Most of the strains have an intermediate resistance to the penicillins so many clinicians still treat uncomplicated pneumonias with higher

**TABLE 22–31. DIAGNOSTIC TESTS TO CONSIDER AND EXPECTED RESULTS FOR COMMUNITY-ACQUIRED PNEUMONIAS**

| Pneumonia | Chest x-ray | WBC with Differential | Chemistry 18 | Other Tests |
|---|---|---|---|---|
| *S. pneumoniae* | Homogeneous Usually LLL Can be bilateral | >12,000 with left shift (increased neutrophils and more immature white cells) | Changes based on age, comorbid illness | Sputum: rare to obtain without oral flora contamination; 50% positive |
| *H. influenzae* | Lobar/ bronchopneumonia | Usually increased | Usually normal | Sputum: depends on comorbid illnesses |
| *Klebsiella* | Lesion in URL +/− multiple lobes; lobar consolidation +/− necrotizing | Decreased in alcoholics secondary to folate deficiency/poor bone marrow function Others: 12,000–20,000 WBC | Usually normal | |
| *M. pneumoniae* | Patchy infiltrates in lower lobes | Normal–low; check if elderly | Normal but check if elderly/comorbid illness | |
| *C. pneumoniae* | Patchy bronchopneumonia | | | |
| *Legionella* | Diffuse patchy infiltrates and poorly defined nodular densities; bilateral infiltrates 50% | +/− abnormal | Low sodium Low serum phosphorus levels | |

+/− means finding could be either present or absent
*Adapted from Areno, San Pedro, and Campbell (1996), Bartlett and Mundy (1995), Cunha and Ortega (1996), and Moroney (1996).*

doses of penicillin. Resistance to the cephalosporins, erythromycin, and TMP/SMX is increasing as well so careful consideration to the antibiotic choice and closer follow-up is necessary (Schreiber & Jacobs, 1995).

***Adult with or without comorbid illness.*** For the adult older than 60 years with or without comorbid illness, the second- or third-generation cephalosporins, trimethoprim-sulfamethoxazole, or beta-lactam agents will generally provide coverage for the pathogens that are most prevalent in this age group: *S. pneumoniae*, *H. influenzae*, and the gram-negative bacteria.

The second-generation cephalosporins that can be used for treatment are cefaclor, loracarabef, and cefuroxime axetil; the third-generation cephalosporin cefpodoxime has a spectrum of action similar to the second-generation

cephalosporins. These agents have both gram-positive as well as gram-negative coverage, the most likely pathogens to cause pneumonia in the elderly. These cephalosporins are also beta-lactamase stable, which is important when treating *H. influenzae* and *Klebsiella* pneumonia since both organisms produce beta-lactamase and therefore render amoxicillin inactive (Drug Facts and Comparisons, 1998).

Trimethoprim-sulfamethoxazole (TMP-SMX) is also effective against *H. influenzae* and many other gram-negative organisms but fails to eradicate some gram-positive organisms. Amoxicillin-clavulanate potassium, with a beta-lactamase inhibitor, is effective against the most common gram-positive and gram-negative organisms usually seen in this age group. The older fluoroquinolones provide coverage for the common gram-negative and atypical organisms but are

**TABLE 22–32. LIKELY PATHOGENS CAUSING COMMUNITY-ACQUIRED PNEUMONIA AND EMPIRIC TREATMENT**

| No Comorbidity and <60 Years | With Comorbidity or >60 years |
|---|---|
| **Pathogens** | |
| S. pneumoniae | S. pneumoniae |
| M. pneumoniae | Viruses |
| Viruses | H. influenzae |
| C. pneumoniae | Gram-negative bacteria |
| H. influenzae | S. aureus |
| Consider tuberculosis, Legionella, or HIV in patients at risk | Consider Moraxella, tuberculosis, Legionella |
| | |
| **Empiric Treatment** | |
| Macrolides or tetracycline | • Second- or third-generation cephalosporins; trimethoprim-sulfamethoxazole<br>• Beta-lactam<br>• Beta-lactamase inhibitor with a macrolide if Legionella is documented |

Adapted from Areno et al (1996), Bartlett and Mundy (1995), Moroney (1996), and Niederman et al (1993).

equivocal for the common gram-positive organisms. However, the newer fluoroquinolones provide excellent coverage for gram-positive, *H. influenzae*, and atypical organisms. If *Legionella* is suspected, add a macrolide and hospitalize as the elderly have an increased morbidity and mortality (Bartlett & Mundy, 1995; Cassiere, Rodriguez, & Fein, 1996; Drug Facts and Comparisons, 1998; File et al, 1996; Moroney, 1996).

*The elderly patient.* The elderly patient in a long-term care facility usually has a comorbid illness, often with mental confusion, difficulty swallowing, dehydration, etc., which makes taking oral antibiotics almost impossible. This patient, if not critical, may respond well to ceftriaxone IM initially, and then switched to an oral second-generation cephalosporin or one of the newer fluoroquinolones when improvement is noted (Brown, 1993; Cassiere et al, 1996).

*Less common pneumonias.* Q fever and psittacosis, the less common pneumonias, can be treated on an outpatient basis with "cyclines" such as doxycycline, tetracycline, and minocycline. The other less common pneumonias need consultation and/or hospitalization because all can have serious sequelae (Relman & Schwartz, 1994).

Patients with HIV infections are usually treated as inpatients, but it depends on the organism, severity of the infection, positive or negative dissemination, status of the HIV infection, effectiveness of the protease inhibitors and the antibiotics, and other factors. These patients require the care of and consultation with infectious disease specialists (Yu & Maurer, 1996).

**Monitoring for Efficacy**

The usual course of treatment for the bacterial pneumonias is 10–14 days and for the atypical pneumonias 14–21 days; the course for the less common pneumonias depends on the etiologic agent (Bartlett & Mundy, 1995; Johnson & Cunha, 1993). Clinical signs and symptoms should be improving within 24–48 h; the maximum is 72 h unless deterioration occurs earlier. The WBC and fever should be normal or lower than at initial diagnosis within 48 h. The young patient and the patient without comorbid illness or other factors influencing pneumonia resolution will resolve symptoms the fastest. The history should be reviewed with each patient to ensure that the original positive history data related to the pneumonia symptoms are resolving. In the elderly, the neurologic examination and questions regarding improvement in behavioral changes will provide some of the best clues to the resolution of the pneumonia.

In slowly or nonresolving pneumonia always consider other factors that can influence the delay: the patient not taking the medication correctly; significant side effects so the patient discontinues the antibiotic; the antibiotic too expensive so the prescription never filled, etc.; as well as other coexisting problems (Mandell, 1996; Mittl et al, 1994).

The follow-up examination must include all the same systems that were examined at the baseline physical to make the diagnosis of pneumonia. In the young adult and those without comorbid illness, examine:

- Vital signs: respiratory rate, heart rate, BP
- Lungs: tactile fremitus, egophany, tubular breath sounds, crackles, rhonchi, use of accessory muscles

If there were any extrapulmonary symptoms, then recheck them.

In the elderly and those with comorbid illnesses, the physical exam must be more inclusive:

- Vital signs: respiratory rate, heart rate, B/P
- Skin: color, cyanosis
- Neck: JVD
- Heart: arrhythmias, murmurs, $S_3/S_4$
- Lungs: change in breath sounds from initial examination, tactile fremitus, egophany, crackles, rhonchi, wheezing (breath sounds can get worse in the elderly from baseline as rehydration recurs)
- Abdomen: hepatosplenomegaly, tenderness
- Neurologic: alertness, degree of confusion, balance, gait, CN I–XII, sensory, motor

Chest x-rays (CXRs) always lag behind clinical improvement so follow-up CXRs should not be repeated for at least 6–8 weeks after initiating treatment. CXRs often worsen once treatment is started, especially in the elderly, because dehydration can minimize the pulmonary infiltrates, but with rehydration the infiltrates are amplified (Cassiere et al, 1996). Legionella infections may require up to 20 weeks to clear radiographically, whereas *M. pneumoniae* usually clears within 2–4 weeks (Austrian, 1992; Fein, 1996). A study done by Mittl et al (1994) found that radiologic resolution was most influenced by age and the number of lobes involved. Multilobar pneumonia resolved more slowly than unilobar, and clearing decreased by 20% per decade. Most *S. pneumoniae* radiographically cleared by 12 weeks, whereas those with bacteremia still had some radiograph changes even at 3 months. Complete resolution did not occur until 18 weeks (Fein, 1994). Refer to Fig. 22–2 for the management of unresolved pneumonia.

In the elderly and those with renal impairment, a creatinine clearance calculation is necessary. Medication dosage is adjusted, depending on the degree of renal impairment: mild, moderate, or severe. If only serum creatinine is available, then convert to creatinine clearance using the following formula (PDR Generics, 1996)

$$\text{Males: } \frac{\text{Weight (kg)} \times (140 - \text{age})}{72 \times \text{serum creatinine}}$$

Females: $0.85 \times$ the value above

In those whose WBC with differential is >15,000, a repeat WBC should be redrawn at the follow-up visit. Other laboratory tests will be drawn as dictated by the history, physical, routine medications the patient is taking, potential interactions between the medications, and comorbid illnesses.

## Monitoring for Toxicity

The penicillins and cephalosporins can cause skin rashes and an anaphylactic reaction. Cefaclor can produce a serum-like sickness, but symptoms usually resolve 3–4 days after discontinuing the drug. These two categories of drugs rarely cause other major adverse side effects (*AHFS*, 1997).

Doxycycline and tetracycline, as with all the "cyclines," increase the risk of phototoxicity and erosive esophagitis, especially if taken at bedtime on an empty stomach. These are not the drugs of choice for an elderly patient, those with a history of a peptic or active ulcer, an adult who works outside, or someone with risk factors such as alcoholism and IV drug abuse (Drug Facts and Comparisons, 1998). Tetracycline must be taken 1 h before meals or 2 h after a meal without milk, which for some patients can be difficult.

Because the cephalosporins, fluoroquinolones, and penicillins are excreted through the kidney, a dose adjustment is usually necessary in the elderly and those with renal impairment (Conte, 1995). The fluoroquinolones can cause damage to growing cartilage and should not be used in anyone less than 18 years of age (Janwetz, 1995). The most frequent side effects, as with the majority of antibiotics, are gastrointestinal.

TMP-SMX, in susceptible individuals, can cause the following adverse reactions (Drug Facts and Comparisons, 1998):

- In sulfite-sensitive individuals this medication can trigger an asthma exacerbation.

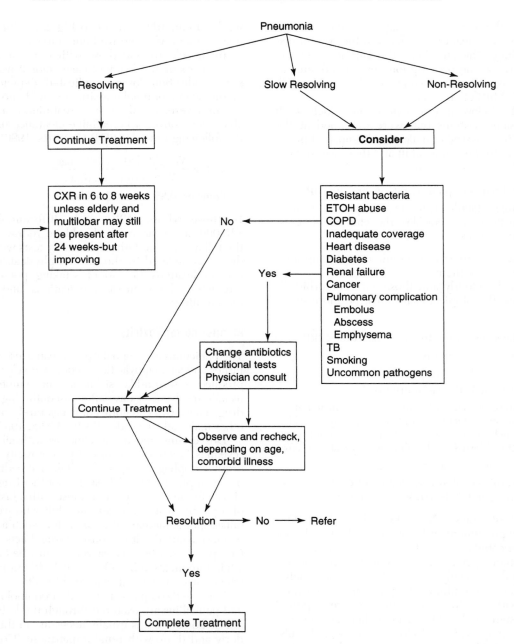

**Figure 22–2.** Algorithm for management of unresolved pneumonia.

Adapted from Fein (1996), Mittl et al (1994), and Moroney (1996).

- In patients with decreased renal function, a change in medication needs to be considered.
  - In patients with creatinine clearance less than 50 mL/min decrease the dose of sulfa.
  - DO NOT USE TMP-SMX if creatinine clearance is less than 15 mL/min.
- In patients with G6P deficiency, sulfa can cause hemolytic anemia.

For a complete listing of antibiotic side effects, refer to the Antibiotic Drug Tables.

## Follow-up Recommendations

The young or middle-aged adult with pneumonia can be followed up in the clinic within 48 h unless symptoms are worsening. At that visit the WBC and other laboratory values can be repeated based on original values and the patient's response to therapy. If the patient appears toxic at the follow-up visit or fails to respond to treatment, then consultation with the physician is necessary.

A CXR is repeated as described above. The older or elderly adult with pneumonia and/or comorbid illnesses should be followed up in 24 h, if not hospitalized, and then as often as necessary. The WBC and other appropriate tests are repeated based on the results of the original tests, comorbid illness, type and severity of pneumonia, the patient's response to therapy, and the patient's living environment (Fraser, 1993).

## PNEUMONIA IN CHILDREN AND ADOLESCENTS

Pneumonia occurs more commonly in the preschool-aged child and decreases in incidence in school-aged children and adolescents (Thompson, 1997). In developing countries though, pneumonia still remains a major health problem with a high incidence of mortality (Thompson, 1997). Pneumonia is caused by a variety of organisms: viral, bacterial, atypical, and other less common organisms. The principal organism will vary with the age of the child and season of the year, with males having a higher incidence of pneumonias (Prober, 1996). There is an increased incidence of pneumonia in children with altered local lung defenses and increased vulnerability. These are children with cystic fibrosis, prematurity, ciliary dyskinesia, and so on as well as those who live in homes with parents who smoke, with a lower socioeconomic environment, and with multiple children (Thompson, 1997).

Viral infections are the most common cause of pneumonia during the first several years of life, whereas atypical pneumonias are more common in the school-aged child and adolescent. Bacterial pneumonias are less common but do occur and tend to be more severe than those caused by nonbacterial infections (Prober, 1996).

## SPECIFIC CONSIDERATIONS FOR PHARMACOTHERAPY

### When Drug Therapy Is Needed

It is generally accepted that all bacterial pneumonias are treated with the appropriate antibiotics to prevent complications or metastatic

spread of the bacteria and empyema (Prober, 1996). Viral infections, however, are not treated with antibiotics; only supportive therapy is needed since the infection is self-limited and usually without complications. The most common viral organism is RSV, and it is only treated in certain circumstances. Refer to the section on Bronchiolitis for more details.

The atypical pneumonias, depending on severity, may be treated to shorten the course and prevent complications (Prakash, 1996).

### Short- and Long-Term Goals of Pharmacotherapy

The short-term goals of therapy are to resolve the infection and to recognize and intervene in early extrapulmonary symptoms. The long-term goals are to prevent recurrent episodes of pneumonia and complications (lung abscesses, bacteremia) especially if patients have associated comorbid illnesses such as cystic fibrosis, asthma, or prematurity (Prober, 1996).

### Nonpharmacologic Therapy

Stress increased fluids, rest, and adequate nutrition.

### Time Frame for Initiating Pharmacotherapy

Bacterial pneumonia should be treated at the time of diagnosis in order to prevent the condition from worsening and exacerbating a comorbid illness. A complete course of antibiotics for 2 weeks is required, but improvement should be noted in 24–36 h.

Viral pneumonias are managed with supportive care and if comorbid illnesses exist, close follow-up is necessary (Green, 1997).

Atypical pneumonias are treated depending on the age, severity, length of illness, and extrapulmonary manifestations. Once the diagnosis is established, treatment is begun immediately. Improvement should be seen in 36–72 h (Hammerschlag, 1996; Powell, 1996).

### Assessment Needed Prior to Therapy

Bacterial and viral pneumonias have great overlap in their signs and symptoms, so a careful history and physical exam can give valuable clues to the etiology of the pneumonia. Table 22–33 describes the history needed and potential examination findings in the child or adolescent with pneumonia. The above findings differ based on

## TABLE 22–33. HISTORY AND PHYSICAL EXAMINATION OF CHILDREN WITH PNEUMONIA

### Pertinent History Markers
- Age
- Season of year
- Past history: birth history and course in hospital, chronic illness, previous illness, hospitalizations, surgeries, frequent respiratory infections
- Onset of symptoms: rapid vs gradual
- Symptoms: laryngitis, malaise, chills, fever, tachypnea, chest pain, wheezing, body aches, cough (nonproductive/productive), headaches, vomiting, anorexia, abdominal pain, sore throat, hoarseness
- Progression of symptoms: Change in eating, playing, sleeping habits
- Others in family ill
- Daily medications, if any
- Where stays during day: day care, private, family
- Self-treatment
- Reason for visit

### Physical Examination and Possible Findings
- Vital signs:
  Temperature: increased in bacterial/viral infections (younger the child, higher the temperature), usually normal to low-grade in atypical pneumonia
  Respiratory/heart rate: increased in bacterial/viral pneumonia, usually normal in atypical
- Skin: maculopapular rashes
- Nose: nasal flaring, rhinorrhea
- Mouth: circumoral cyanosis
- Oropharynx: erythema of posterior pharynx
- Neck: cervical nodes, stiffness
- Lungs: intercostal, substernal, supraclavicular retractions, grunting, breath sounds on the opposite side may be exaggerated and tubular, inspiratory/expiratory wheezing, crackles, rhonchi, listen for nature of cough: staccato, dry, paroxysmal, productive
- Heart: murmurs
- Abdomen: distention, tenderness
- Neurologic: ability to arouse if lethargic

*Adapted from Irons (1994) and Schidlow and Callahan (1996).*

the pneumonia etiology and age of the patient. Table 22–34 summarizes common tests to diagnose pneumonia in children.

Concomitant disease states and contraindications include the following:

- Cystic fibrosis: The patient will need to be covered for *Pseudomonas* with two or three high-

dose antibiotics for at least 3–4 weeks. Monitor for drug interactions.
- Asthma: Theophylline has multidrug interactions that can decrease or increase theophylline clearance; zileuton interacts with terfenadine, causing prolongation of the QT complex.
- Heart disease: can cause more strain on the heart secondary to increased heart rate and mismatch in ventilation-perfusion quotient.

## Patient/Caregiver Information

1. Explain what signs and symptoms to monitor that would indicate a deterioration in the pneumonia.

2. Explain the common adverse effects of the antibiotics and how to minimize the symptoms.

3. Discuss important nonpharmacologic strategies.

4. Remind parents and patients to continue to give or take regular medications unless instructed otherwise.

5. For the older infant or toddler to age 12 years, follow the directions for taking Tylenol Elixir and Suspension liquid correctly. Take *only* every 4–6 h, *not to exceed* five doses in 24 h. *Use the special measuring cup provided only (no substitutions).* If needed for fever relief longer than 36–48 h, a call to the health care provider is necessary.

6. For young infants, follow the directions for taking Infant Tylenol Drops and Suspension Drops correctly. Dose exactly every 4–6 h, *not to exceed* four doses in 24 h. *Use the special measuring dropper only (no substitutions).* If fever persists longer than 36 h, call the health care provider. *Infant Tylenol Drops are more potent per dose than the Suspension so exact measuring is imperative.*

7. Children's ibuprofen oral suspension can be used. Follow the directions exactly. *Use the calibrated dosage cup only (no substitutions).* Dose every 6–8 h but *do not exceed* four doses in 24 h. If the fever lasts longer than 36 h, call the health care provider (Drug Facts and Comparisons, 1998; PDR Generics, 1996).

8. Refer to Chapter 12 for correct administration techniques for giving medications to children.

## OUTCOMES MANAGEMENT

### Selecting an Appropriate Agent

The most common cause of pneumonia in the newborn (birth to 1 month) age group is group B Streptococcus , *E. coli, C. trachomatis,* other

**TABLE 22–34. COMMON DIAGNOSTIC TESTS FOR CHILDREN WITH PNEUMONIA**

| Diagnostic Tests | Possible Findings |
|---|---|
| Chest x-ray | Nothing or patchy infiltrates, lobar consolidation, bilateral interstitial infiltrates, hyperinflation, pneumatoceles, effusions, nodular shadowing or enlargement of hilar lymph nodes (x-ray findings are variable depending on the type of pneumonia and from child to child) |
| WBC with differential | Usually >12,000 in bacterial pneumonia; normal/low in viral/atypical pneumonia |
| *Mycoplasma pneumoniae* PCR (polymerase chain reaction) | Positive |
| Viral specific-Ab tests | RSV, other viruses |

*Adapted from Prober (1996) and Schidlow and Callahan (1996).*

organisms like *S. aureus,* and gram-negative bacilli (Thompson, 1997). Group B streptococcal pneumonia generally appears within the first 6–12 h after birth and can progress to fulminant disease rapidly if not detected early (Schidlow & Callahan, 1996). Any newborn, 1 month or less, who is ill-appearing, symptomatic, and/or diagnosed with pneumonia must be hospitalized for a complete sepsis workup. These newborns are never treated as outpatients. The nurse practitioner or physician's assistant who examines an ill newborn will always seek consultation with the physician (Prober, 1996; Schidlow & Callahan, 1996).

The common offending organisms that cause pneumonia in the infancy and early childhood age group, in order of frequency, are (1) viruses, (2) *S. pneumoniae,* (3) *C. trachomatis,* (4) pertussis, and (5) *H. influenzae* in unimmunized children.

Table 22–35 reviews the organisms, history, clinical manifestations, and recommended treatment for infants and young children, and Table 22–36 summarizes these issues in children older than 5 and adolescents.

Febrile infants who experience difficulty eating, respiratory distress, and hypoxemia should be hospitalized, whereas afebrile infants without any of the previously mentioned symptoms, well-appearing, with no other associated illnesses, and having a parent who can monitor the infant closely can be treated as outpatients. The febrile infant should be hospitalized because the pneumonia course is more variable and complications more frequent.

When bacterial pneumonia is suspected, use ceftriaxone IM, a third-generation cephalosporin that covers both gram-negative and gram-positive organisms. When the infant or young child is able to tolerate oral fluids and the respiratory and heart rates approach normal, treatment can be changed to an oral antibiotic. The following preparations can be used: second- or third-generation cephalosporins, amoxicillin/clavulanic acid, or a macrolide (Klein, 1997; Prober, 1996).

Erythromycin provides coverage for *M.* or *C. pneumoniae* and *S. pneumoniae* but not for *H. influenzae* or the penicillin-resistant organisms of *Staphylococcus* (Drug Facts and Comparisons, 1998). Clarithromycin, available in suspension for children, is also effective against *S. pneumoniae, H. influenzae,* and *M.* and *C. pneumoniae.* The medication tastes badly, and most children will not take it. In children, azithromycin is equally as effective against the same organisms as clarithromycin, but easier to take: only one dose/day for 5 days in pill forms, so taste is not an issue. Azithromycin is available in a suspension but is not approved for treatment of pneumonia in children under 12 years (Drug Facts and Comparisons, 1998).

Erythromycin can abort or eliminate pertussis if it is started in the catarrhal phase but will not shorten the paroxysmal phase if started then. Relapse occurs if treatment in children is for less than 14 days. The dose is 40 mg/kg per day divided q.i.d. orally for 14 days. An alternate drug for the treatment of pertussis is TMP-SMX (trimethoprim-sulfamethoxazole) given in a dose of 5–10 mg/kg per day of TMP divided b.i.d. for 14 days (Drug Facts and Comparisons, 1998; Long, 1997; Niederhauser, 1997).

All the medications are given in either liquid or chewable preparations for the young infant, toddler, or preschooler. Dosages must be accu-

| TABLE 22–35. PNEUMONIAS IN INFANCY AND EARLY CHILDHOOD | | | |
|---|---|---|---|
| Organism | Significant History | Clinical Signs | Recommended Antibiotics |
| Respiratory syncytial virus | Refer to the section on bronchiolitis | | |
| Parainfluenza | Season of year, other illness in family or community<br><5 years of age<br>Gradual onset +/– fever, URI symptoms for several days, then +/– productive cough | Tachypnea<br>Tachycardia<br>Rarely fever, +/– rhonchi, rales, inspiratory/expiratory wheezing with prolonged expiratory phase | No treatment necessary unless secondary infection, rare in healthy children |
| S. pneumoniae<br>Infants: | Usually starts with a stuffy nose, decreased appetite, fretfulness for several days, then abrupt onset of high fever, restlessness, and respiratory distress<br>Infants may also have nausea, vomiting, diarrhea, +/– convulsions<br>Increased risk if HIV, sickle cell anemia, nephrotic syndrome, renal failure, splenectomy, transplant (for all ages) | Ill-appearing<br>Air hunger +/– cyanosis<br>Nasal flaring +/– retractions +/– grunting<br>+/– diminished breath sounds, fine crackles on affected side, but these findings are less common in infant/young child<br>Breath sounds on the opposite side may be enhanced and tubular<br>+/– abdominal distention secondary to increased air swallowing<br>+/– palpable liver secondary to downward displacement of the diaphragm; consider CHF<br>If lower lobe pneumonia, may be referred to abdomen, cause pain; if in upper lobes, can cause neck pain, nuchal rigidity | Usually hospitalized |

| | | | |
|---|---|---|---|
| Children: | Brief URI, develops shaking chills then high fever, restlessness, drowsiness, increased respirations, anxiety; can begin as dry hacky but productive sounding cough in the young child who rarely expectorates<br>Child may splint the affected side and/or lie on side with knees drawn up to chest | Tachypnea<br>Tachycardia<br>+/- circumoral cyanosis<br>Retractions, nasal flaring<br>Dullness to percussion, diminished tactile and vocal fremitus<br>Decreased breath sounds and fine crackles on affected side<br>Symptoms change as illness progresses; consolidation signs appear on days 2 to 3 and with resolution comes an increased productive cough of blood-tinged mucus | For outpatient treatment in children over 1 year of age:<br>ceftriaxone I.M.<br>macrolides<br>Augmentin/cephalosporins—if culture and sensitivities indicate |
| C. trachomatis | Occurs within the fourth to eleventh weeks of life but can occur later<br>Onset of nasopharyngitis, rhinitis is mucoid with some nasal obstruction being common<br>After a week, respiratory symptoms develop; 50% develop a paroxysmal staccato cough, separated by a brief inspiration—coughing spell does not result in cyanosis, emesis or an inspiratory whoop like pertussis<br>May have difficulty feeding and/or failure to thrive | Usually afebrile<br>Tachypnea (50–60/min)<br>General rales<br>Minimal expiratory wheezing, +/- prolonged expiratory phase<br>+/- conjunctivitis | Macrolides<br>azithromycin, clarithromycin, erythromycin |
| Pertussis | Usually <12 mos<br>Three stages of illness:<br>1. Often starts with coryza, conjunctivitis (1–2 weeks)<br>2. Followed by paroxysms of cough with post-tussive vomiting (2–4 weeks)<br>3. Convalescence (1–2 weeks) | Conjunctivitis<br>Low-grade fever<br>Leukocytosis especially in young children<br>Tachypnea | Treatment is only effective if begun in the catarrhal phase—treat with erythromycin 10 mg/kg q.i.d. × 14 days. Alternate treatment is 5–10 mg/kg of TMP b.i.d. for 14 days<br>Relapse occurs if treatment less than 14 days |

+/- = findings could be either present or absent.
*Adapted from Klein (1997), Prober (1996), Rubin and O'Hanley (1996), and Schidlow and Callahan (1996).*

## TABLE 22–36. PNEUMONIAS IN CHILDREN OLDER THAN 5 YEARS AND ADOLESCENTS

| Organism | History Information | Clinical Symptoms | Recommended Antibiotics |
|---|---|---|---|
| *M.* and *C. pneumoniae* | Wide array of presenting symptoms, but common is headache, abdominal pain, and vomiting<br>Onset is insidious; malaise, myalgias<br>Cough may begin as nonproductive and then progresses to productive cough with +/– chest pain that persists<br>In those with *C. pneumoniae,* usually starts with non-exudative pharyngitis and hoarseness, then 1 week later productive cough begins<br>May present as an exacerbation of a chronic illness, ie, asthma, undiagnosed reactive airway disease | +/– fever<br>+/– erythematous TMs<br>+/– sinus face pain<br>Scattered or localized crackles, tubular breath sounds over affected area, +/– wheezing<br>Paucity of clinical findings | Macrolides<br>  azithromycin<br>  clarithromycin<br>  erythromycin |
| *S. pneumoniae* | History and clinical manifestations as described in Table 22–35 | | Macrolides<br>  azithromycin<br>  clarithromycin<br>  erythromycin<br>Third generation cephalosporins<br>Augmentin (if cultures and sensitivities indicate |

Adapted from Klein (1997), Prakash (1996), Prober (1996), and Schidlow and Callahan (1996).

rate as the young infant or child varies in drug absorption, distribution, metabolism, and excretion (Niederhauser, 1997).

## Monitoring for Efficacy

The bacterial pneumonias tend to resolve rapidly after antibiotics are initiated. Improvement is noted within 24–48 h. The atypical pneumonias tend to resolve more slowly, but improvement should be noted after several days of antibiotics. In any child who remains symptomatic or whose symptoms resolve and then recur again, a reassessment is needed. In persistent symptoms always think cystic fibrosis, AIDS, foreign body, tracheobronchial anomalies, asthma or systemic disease (Schidlow & Callahan, 1996). Also when resolution is slow, consider the possibility that the medication is

given incorrectly or in an inaccurate dose or there is a change in the absorption of the medication (Niederhauser, 1997).

Chest x-ray resolution usually occurs in about 6–10 weeks after onset of antibiotics. If the chest x-ray fails to clear, then consider the above-cited medical conditions.

During the physical examination, look for:

- Vital signs: temperature, respiratory and heart rates
- Nose: flaring
- Lungs: wheezing, crackles, diminished breath sounds, rhonchi, use of accessory muscles
- Heart: murmurs

The physical examination is based on the patient's age, type of pneumonia, severity, and physical examination at diagnosis.

## Monitoring for Toxicity

The most common side effects are gastrointestinal and occasionally a rash. Diarrhea, if it occurs, can change the absorption rate of the medication. A change in medication may be necessary. Refer to Drug Table 102 for further information.

## Follow-up Recommendations

The young infant or child needs to be seen daily until the symptoms are resolved and improvement noted. If deterioration occurs, then the patient needs to be hospitalized and/or the diagnosis reconsidered. In the older child or adolescent with a bacterial pneumonia follow-up is recommended within 48 h. If symptoms are improving, repeat follow-up is at the clinician's judgment. In those who do not respond as expected, reconsider the diagnosis and other factors that could prevent resolution: other coexisting disease states, parental smoking, not giving the medication correctly, incorrect medication or resistant organism, etc. In those with an atypical pneumonia, follow up in 3–5 days unless deterioration occurs (Klein, 1997; Prober, 1996).

In any patient with a comorbid illness, follow-up must be daily and the patient examined by the consulting physician if not hospitalized.

## PNEUMONIA IN PREGNANCY

Pneumonia during pregnancy is an infrequent problem but has the potential to cause serious maternal and fetal distress. The fetus does not tolerate hypoxia, acidosis, fever, and tachycardia well, thus increasing the risk for preterm birth (Rodrigues & Niederman, 1992). Pneumonia is the most frequent cause of nonobstetric infection and the third leading cause of nonobstetric death (Rigby & Pastorek, 1996). The incidence of pneumonia and complications is increased in pregnant women with underlying lung disease (especially asthma), renal failure, chronic liver disease, diabetes, postsplenectomy, cigarette smoking, chronic alcohol abuse and illicit drug use, anemia, and HIV infection (Pulmonary Disorders, 1997; Rodrigues & Niederman, 1992).

The most common causative organisms are the same as for the nonpregnant woman: *M.* and *C. pneumoniae, S. pneumoniae,* and viruses. In pregnant women with HIV, coccidioidomycosis is the most common, but *P. carinii* can be the cause and is almost always fatal (McColgin,

Glee, & Brian, 1992). It is vital, therefore, to recognize the disease process and initiate prompt effective treatment, close observation, and follow-up. Pregnant women should be treated aggressively since an infectious pneumonitis can result in fetal complications and preterm labor (McColgin et al, 1992).

## SPECIFIC CONSIDERATIONS FOR PHARMACOTHERAPY

### When Drug Therapy Is Needed

In the preantibiotic era, maternal mortality was high. Fineland and Dublin's study done in 1939 showed a 32% mortality rate among 212 pregnant women with pneumonia. The studies done recently all demonstrated a significant decline in maternal and fetal morbidity and mortality with early diagnosis and appropriate antibiotic treatment (Macato, 1991). With the onset of antibiotic treatment, the incidence of preterm labor was also decreased (Madinger, Greenspoon, & Ellrodt, 1989).

Clearly there is unanimous agreement that all pregnant women must be treated with the appropriate antibiotic whenever pneumonia is diagnosed. Depending on the coexisting illness, severity of the pneumonia symptoms, and trimester, the pregnant woman may be hospitalized and treated with IV antibiotics. For the noncritical pregnant woman with pneumonia, outpatient treatment with intense follow-up is recommended.

### Short- and Long-Term Goals of Pharmacotherapy

The short-term goals of therapy are to direct the antibiotic therapy at the most likely organism(s), choose an antibiotic that is safe and effective during pregnancy, and resolve the pneumonia. The long-term goals of therapy are to prevent maternal and fetal complications through rapid diagnosis, aggressive treatment, and prevention of a recurrence.

### Nonpharmacologic Therapy

Urge hydration, rest, respiratory support, if needed, and cessation of smoking if warranted.

### Time Frame for Initiating Pharmacotherapy

A high index of suspicion should be maintained whenever an upper respiratory infection does not resolve within the usual time frame. An appropriate workup should be done and treatment begun immediately. Rapid improvement will be noted if there is no uncontrolled coexisting illness and/or an organism causing atypical pneumonia. Close follow-up is necessary.

## Assessment Needed Prior to Therapy

Refer to Table 22–29 for detailed history and physical examination findings for pneumonia in adults and the elderly. However, the additional history and physical findings in the pregnant woman may alert the clinician to a possible pneumonia; see Table 22–37. Additional tests are noted in Table 22–38.

There are no disease states where antibiotics cannot be used, but in certain diseases the antibiotics may have a Category C safety profile, cause oto- or neurotoxicity, and/or need dosage changes because of renal and liver disease, chemotherapy, alcohol or drug abuse, immunocompromise, and/or diabetes. If this occurs, consultation is necessary.

### TABLE 22–37. HISTORY AND PHYSICAL EXAMINATION FOR THE PREGNANT WOMAN WITH PNEUMONIA

**History Markers**
- Time of the year/area of the country: coccidioidomycosis occurs in drier months of the year and in endemic areas; Southwestern United States
- Other family members ill
- Nonspecific complaints: anorexia, headache, cough, and fever may be the initial symptoms for coccidioidomycosis
- Unresolved upper respiratory infection for 2 weeks or longer
- Smoking, alcohol, or illicit drug use
- Risk factors for HIV infection

**Physical Findings**
- Increased respiratory rate; may be earliest sign of infection
- Tachypnea
- Dry cough
- Change in pulse oximetry

*Adapted from NIH/NHLBI (1993) and Rodrigues & Niederman (1992).*

### TABLE 22–38. DIAGNOSTIC TESTS FOR THE PREGNANT PATIENT WITH PNEUMONIA

| | |
|---|---|
| Fetal ultrasound | 12–20 weeks, depending on severity and type of pneumonia |
| Sequential ultrasound | Done during the second and third trimester to evaluate fetal growth depending on type of pneumonia and its chronicity |
| Electronic fetal heart monitoring | Considered in third trimester to assess fetal well-being or if fetal problems suspected |

*Adapted from Rigby and Pastorek (1996) and Rodrigues and Niederman (1992).*

## Patient/Caregiver Information

- Alert the pregnant woman to signs and symptoms of upper respiratory infections that do not resolve.
- Discuss if the woman has increased rate of breathing, and then call the health care provider.
- Discuss smoking cessation and drug and alcohol avoidance.
- If the woman has a coexisting illness, manage carefully and if signs or symptoms flare, seek medical care immediately.

## OUTCOMES MANAGEMENT

### Selecting an Appropriate Agent

Antibiotics are the mainstay of treatment for community-acquired pneumonia, but which organism is most likely the causative agent depends on smoking status, age, and comorbid illnesses. Since community-acquired pneumonia is most frequently caused by *S. pneumoniae* and atypical and viral pathogens in the relatively healthy pregnant woman, treatment must be directed at providing coverage for these organisms. Selection of an agent to treat pneumonia during pregnancy necessitates consideration of drug hypersensitivity, safety during pregnancy, dose frequency, cost and other associated factors, chronic illnesses, and smoking and alcohol use. Table 22–39 lists the most common

**TABLE 22–39.  COMMON OFFENDING ORGANISMS AND ANTIBIOTIC THERAPY IN PREGNANT WOMEN WITH PNEUMONIA**

| Organism | Treatment Duration | Antibiotic |
|---|---|---|
| *S. pneumoniae* | Initial treatment for 14–21 days | Azithromycin,[a] erythromycin Penicillin,[b] amoxicillin[b] |
| | Treatment failure probably secondary to resistant organism; treat for 14 days, may need longer duration | Augmentin, first- and second-generation cephalosporin[c]: (cefaclor, cephalexin, cephradine, cefpodoxime proxetil, loracarbef), azithromycin |
| *H. influenzae* (smokers, ETOH abusers, immunocompromised) | Treat for 14–21 days | Second-generation cephalosporin |
| *M.* and *C. pneumoniae* | Treat for 10–14 days; some recommend 21 days | Erythromycin, azithromycin |
| Influenza A | Treatment for 5–7 days or 2 days after symptoms resolve | Amantidine[d] (possible hospitalization) |
| Varicella | | Acyclovir (usually hospitalized) |
| Coccidioidomycosis | | Hospitalize |
| *P. carinii* | | Hospitalize |

[a] Macrolides are the first-line drug therapy recommended by the ATS for treatment of CAP for patients <60 years without comorbid illness.
[b] 10 to >30% penicillin resistance.
[c] Increasing resistance to cephalosporins is 10 to 30%; second- and third-generation cephalosporins have more gram-negative coverage.
[d] Amantadine is a Category C drug; consultation is needed.
*Adapted from Bartlett and Mundy (1995), Drug Facts and Comparisons (1998), Fein (1996), and Levison (1998).*

pathogens and appropriate pharmacotherapy for pneumonia in pregnant women (Pulmonary Disorders, 1997).

**Antibiotics.**  For the pregnant woman, penicillin, amoxicillin, or azithromycin are safe drugs to use. Other excellent choices are the first- and second-generation cephalosporins, but the first-generation cephalosporins cephalexin and cephradine are inactivated by beta-lactamase-producing organisms. Several of the second-generation cephalosporins such as cefaclor are very stable in the presence of beta-lactamase enzymes, as is the third-generation cephalosporin cefpodoxime proxetil. Therefore, many organisms resistant to penicillins and some of the cephalosporins are susceptible to these second- and third-generation cephalosporins (Drug Facts and Comparisons, 1998). The pharmacokinetics of the cephalosporins change during pregnancy. They have (1) a shorter half-life, (2) lower serum levels, and (3) increased clearance (Drug Facts and Comparisons, 1998).

Amoxicillin/clavulanic acid will provide coverage for *S. pneumoniae* and *H. influenzae* but has more side effects than either azithromycin or the cephalosporins. Erythromycin can also be used but produces more side effects and at four-times-a-day dosing can be impractical. The estolate salt of erythromycin should be *avoided* during pregnancy as it can induce hepatotoxicity. The liver enzymes usually return to normal levels after discontinuing the drug (Briggs, Mahre, & Sibai, 1996). Clarithromycin, another newer macrolide, is a Category C drug and therefore *not approved* for use during pregnancy (Drug Facts and Comparisons, 1998). Unfortunately, resistance to the "mycins" is also increasing, and cross-resistance to all the agents in this group is usual (Schreiber & Jacobs, 1995).

**Antiviral agents.**  Influenza A is seen during epidemics and can cause pneumonia in pregnancy. Amantadine is the drug of choice for prophylaxis but is a Category C so a consultation is necessary. The drug must be given within 48 h of symptom onset, at a dose of 200 mg/day for 3–5 days or up to 48 h after symptoms resolve. This treatment can prevent or ameliorate the disease. Most of the complications of influenza are due to secondary bacterial infection, often *S. aureus*, *S. pneumoniae*, *H. influenzae*, and some gram-negative bacteria, which must be treated aggressively to prevent fulminant respiratory failure in the mother and fetal problems (Rodrigues & Niederman, 1992). During epidemics, amantadine as prophylaxis may be highly recommended for the pregnant woman who is at risk.

Varicella is a rare infection in pregnant women. It is estimated that about 95% of women of childbearing age have antibodies to varicella (Brunell, 1990). If the primary infection of varicella occurs during pregnancy, there seems to be an increased incidence and virulence of varicella pneumonia. This can lead to a more complicated infection and higher mortality rate, up to 35–40%, than in the nonpregnant state (Haake et al, 1990; Rodrigues & Niederman, 1992). If the varicella infection occurs in the first trimester, there is an increased risk of fetal malformations so these women should be hospitalized and treated with IV acyclovir (Broussard, Payne, & George, 1991). Table 22–40 lists the typical symptoms of varicella.

The chest examination can be unimpressive and correlates poorly with the severity of the varicella infection, showing diffuse changes with the maximum changes occurring at the height of the skin eruption (Rigby & Pastorek, 1996). Administration of varicella-zoster immunoglobulin (VZIG) can prevent or attenuate the varicella infections in exposed individuals if given within 96 h. Early recognition is imperative (Pulmonary Disorders, 1997).

In HIV-related infections, coccidioidomycosis is becoming an increasingly common infection both in the endemic and nonendemic areas. The areas where the spores may live are semiarid with hot dry summers, mild winters, and moderate rainfall (Rubin, 1996). The spores are hardy and can easily be transported outside the endemic area. An index of suspicion for this disease should be maintained if the pregnant woman presents with a suggestive history, recent travel to the Southwest, and/or signs of extrapulmonary manifestations. A coccidioidomycosis infection in the second and third trimester carries a high risk of mortality (Rigby & Pastorek, 1996). Approximately 35–50% who develop coccidioidomycosis have nonspecific complaints such as flu-like symptoms that appear 7–28 days after exposure and may also have eye, joint/muscle, skin, and pulmonary findings (Gales & McClain, 1997). The physical examination findings are often absent or very minimal with symptoms mimicking tuberculosis, cancer, pneumonia, and pleurisy (Gales & McClain, 1997). Pregnant women are usually at greater risk for dissemination of the coccidioidomycosis infection (Catanzaro, 1984). Because of the high mortality rate, early identification is imperative so that the pregnant woman can be hospitalized and treatment begun quickly.

*P. carinii* pneumonia (PCP) can also occur during pregnancy and requires a high index of suspicion in women who are at increased risk. This is a life-threatening illness and is characterized by a dry cough, fever, tachypnea, dyspnea, a decrease in arterial $Po_2$, and respiratory alkalosis (Rigby & Pastorek, 1996). These women must be referred immediately to a specialist in HIV treatment.

**Drugs to avoid.**    Any antibiotic that is a Category A or B is safe to use during pregnancy. The drugs that are in Category C are not considered first-line medications to use, but there are exceptions. The exceptions could include the case in which the drug is the only drug approved to treat severe infection and a chronic life-threatening infection, such as HIV, where toxic drugs are required. The nurse practitioner or physician's assistant in these cases would be collaborating with and transferring care to the physician specialist in the management of the pregnant woman and not directing the care alone (Drug Facts & Comparisons, 1998).

| TABLE 22–40.  COMMON SYMPTOMS OF VARICELLA | |
|---|---|
| **Signs and Symptoms of Varicella** | **Symptoms of Varicella Pneumonia** |
| • Persistent fevers, malaise | • Cough with dyspnea |
| • Myalgia occurs 2–5 days after onset of symptoms | • Tachypnea +/– pleuritic chest pain, hemoptysis |
| • Maculopapular/vesicular rash | • Hypoxemia |
| • Headaches | |

+/– means finding can be either present or absent.
*Adapted from Pulmonary Disorders (1997), Rigby and Pastorek (1996), and Yang and Rubin (1995).*

## Monitoring for Efficacy

The follow-up visit should be within 36–48 h after diagnosis. The pregnant woman needs to be questioned about symptom worsening or resolution, especially fever, cough, chest tightness, and dyspnea; associated nonpulmonary symptoms such as eye, skin, joint, and muscle problems; and smoking, alcohol, and illicit drug use.

Antibiotic therapy for atypical pneumonia is 10–21 days with relapses necessitating retreatment. Retreat with the second usual drug; ie, if erythromycin was used the first time, to retreat use azithromycin. Symptoms should begin to improve several days after initiating treatment. Refer to Table 22–28 for complete clinical manifestations of atypical pneumonia. A typical course of antibiotic therapy for bacterial pneumonia is 14–21 days. Improvement is seen in streptococcal pneumonia within 24–36 h after initiating treatment with the temperature, pulse, respiration, and pleuritic chest pain beginning to subside (Austrian, 1992). *H. influenzae* infection, if noninvasive, will respond to oral antibiotics rapidly, usually within 24–48 h. Antibiotics are given for 14–21 days as well. If the pregnant woman is not responding to the antibiotics as expected, reassess the diagnosis. Several causes should be considered:

- The organism is resistant to the antibiotic, especially penicillin- and/or macrolide-resistant.
- The patient is not taking the antibiotic or not taking it correctly.
- The diagnosis is incorrect.
- A comorbid illness or other associated factors, such as smoking, alcohol, or drug use, is influencing the disease course.

If all the causes have been taken into account, then most likely the organism is resistant and an antibiotic change is essential. Consider using augmentin, cefaclor, cefpodoxime, or azithromycin (Levison, 1998). Refer to Table 22–39 for a complete discussion of bacterial pneumonia treatment in this population.

Patients with varicella pneumonia and the HIV-related pneumonias are treated as inpatients so prompt recognition is important.

## Monitoring for Toxicity

Some antibiotics can cause gastrointestinal upset, pseudomembranous colitis, rash, and serum-like illnesses. If the gastrointestinal symptoms

are mild to moderate or an allergic reaction occurs, discontinuation of the drug is all that is usually needed. A change of antibiotics will be needed with attention to the cross-reactivity that can occur using either the penicillins or cephalosporins. Follow-up is needed to ensure that all allergic symptoms resolve and that the patient's pneumonia is resolving.

## Follow-up Recommendations

In the pregnant woman with pneumonia, close follow-up is necessary to ensure the safety of the woman and the fetus. Follow-up in the office should be within 36–48 h after diagnosis. The symptoms should be significantly better; temperature, pulse, and respiratory rate should be within the normal range or slightly elevated. The physical examination should indicate an improvement in the chest symptoms, unchanged fetal kick counts, and a normal WBC count. In many patients, the temperature may remain elevated for about 4 days. This does not indicate a change of antibiotics; however, if the temperature remains above normal for longer than 36–48 h, then a reevaluation is warranted. The chest x-ray is repeated in approximately 6–8 weeks if all symptoms have resolved or sooner if there is no response to the antibiotics (Austrian, 1992; NIH/NHLBI, 1993).

## TUBERCULOSIS

Tuberculosis (TB) is an infection caused by *Mycobacterium tuberculosis*. TB is spread primarily by airborne transmission via inhalation of aerosolized lung secretions (droplets) from the cough of an individual with active pulmonary tuberculosis disease. In immunocompetent patients, approximately 10% of those infected will go on to develop active TB disease at some point in their lifetime. The other 90% will have a latent infection without active disease and are considered noncontagious. It is important to distinguish the difference between TB infection and TB disease. Those with TB infection (positive purified protein derivative (PPD) but negative chest x-ray, and no disease symptoms) but without active disease do not transmit the mycobacterium. The primary site of infection of TB is the lung (approximately 85%), but infections can also occur throughout the body (U.S. Department of Health and Human Services [USDHHS], 1994).

The incidence of multiple-drug-resistant tuberculosis (MDR-TB) is on the rise. MDR-TB is defined as organisms that are resistant to both isoniazid and rifampin and may also be resistant to other medications as well. MDR-TB presents special problems because it is more difficult to treat and the duration of therapy is often longer than for nonresistant strains of TB.

There are certain populations considered at higher risk for contracting tuberculosis. They are listed in Table 22–41.

## SPECIFIC CONSIDERATIONS FOR PHARMACOTHERAPY

### When Drug Therapy Is Needed

The growth of *Mycobacterium tuberculosis* is very slow. It has a generation time of approximately 15–20 h. Most bacterial pathogens have a generation time of less than an hour. Hence twice-weekly or thrice-weekly therapy can be effective in selected situations.

Patients in high-risk groups (Table 22–41) and any others who have possibly been exposed to TB should be tested via the Mantoux skin test (PPD). A patient recently infected with TB will take from 2–10 weeks to develop a positive PPD. Hence close contacts of active TB cases who were initially PPD-negative should be retested 10 weeks after their last exposure to infectious TB.

Patients in the high-risk groups should be screened annually with a PPD. In those people who have not been tested for several years and who will be retested periodically, a two-step test should be done initially to distinguish boosted reactions and reactions due to new infection. The two-step test consists of an initial PPD and a second PPD within 1–3 weeks of the first. Those who have a negative reaction to the first step and a positive reaction to the second step are considered to have a boosted reaction from the first step and therefore do not have a new TB infection. People who are not at high risk for TB should not be routinely screened because of the risk of a false-positive PPD and inappropriate treatment (USDHHS, 1994). Criteria for a positive skin test are outlined in Table 22–42. Patients with a positive skin test should be fur-

---

### TABLE 22–41. PERSONS AT HIGH RISK FOR TUBERCULOSIS

- Foreign-born persons from high-prevalence countries (Asia, Africa, Oceania, Latin America)
- Low-income and medically underserved populations, including minorities at high risk (eg, African-Americans, Hispanics, Native Americans)
- Injecting drug users
- Alcoholics
- Persons with HIV infection
- Residents and personnel of correctional institutions, long-term care facilities, hospitals, and mental institutions
- The elderly
- Close contacts to infectious cases
- Migrant workers
- Persons with other medical risk factors, such as diabetes, malnutrition, postgastrectomy, end-stage renal disease, malignancies (leukemia, lymphoma), prolonged corticosteroid therapy
- Persons with chest x-ray demonstrating old fibrotic lesions

Note: Patients with HIV infection and TB infection may have a more than 100-fold greater risk for developing TB disease compared with those patients with TB infection alone.
*Adapted from ATS (1994) and USDHHS (1994).*

---

### TABLE 22–42. RECOMMENDED CRITERIA FOR TUBERCULIN POSITIVITY BY RISK GROUP

| Mantoux Test Induration Size | Group Considered to Be PPD-Positive |
|---|---|
| >5 mm | HIV-infected persons |
| | Injecting drug users with unknown HIV status |
| | Close contacts of a person with infectious TB |
| | Persons with chest x-ray suggestive of old, healed TB |
| >10 mm | Foreign-born persons from high-prevalence countries |
| | Low-income populations |
| | Injecting drug users known to be HIV-negative |
| | Correctional institution/nursing home staff/residents |
| | Mycobacterial lab employees |
| | Predisposing medical conditions |
| | Children younger than 4 years of age |
| >15 mm | No risk factors |

*Adapted from USDHHS (1994).*

ther evaluated for active TB disease versus TB infection. Those deemed to be infected without active disease should be evaluated for prophylactic therapy with isoniazid (INH). TB screening should always be carried out in consultation with the local health department (USDHHS, 1994).

## Short- and Long-Term Goals of Pharmacotherapy

The short-term goals of pharmacotherapy are to prevent progression to active disease in those who are infected and to prevent the spread of disease. Another goal of therapy is to provide the safest and most effective therapy in the shortest period of time. The long-term goals are to prevent development of drug-resistant TB and to prevent death from complications of TB.

## Nonpharmacologic Therapy

Contagious individuals must practice good hygiene until they become noninfectious. They must always cover their mouth when they cough, and cough into handkerchiefs or tissues, which should be properly disposed of. Most patients with active TB should be isolated until the sputum smear is negative, not just until some arbitrary deadline, such as 2 weeks of drug therapy, has passed. TB patients should also have their nutrition status assessed and be instructed on adequate nutritional guidelines.

## Time Frame for Initiating Pharmacotherapy

For patients with active tuberculosis, pharmacotherapy should be initiated immediately once the working diagnosis has been made so they can become noninfectious and minimize the spread of the disease.

Patients who are PPD converters without active disease are not considered infectious, and the decision to start or withhold therapy can be made over the course of several days. For patients who are recent PPD converters without active disease, the need for isoniazid prophylaxis should be individualized based on age, pregnancy status, and status of contact with an active disease case. For example, a patient who is 85 years old, has no other risk factors for disease, had a 10-mm PPD reaction, and has no contact with an active TB case does not need prophylaxis. In this case, the risk of INH-induced hepatitis outweighs the benefit of INH prophy-laxis. As another example, a 20-year-old patient who is 6 months pregnant,

has a 10-mm PPD reaction upon routine screening, and is not in contact with an active TB case does not need immediate INH prophylaxis. She should, however, be reevaluated for prophylaxis after delivery.

Treatment of TB infection and TB disease takes much longer than most other types of infectious disease. Therefore, it takes several months to achieve the goals of therapy.

## Assessment Needed Prior to Therapy

Patients with pulmonary TB usually have a cough and an abnormal chest x-ray, and they should be considered infectious (USDHHS, 1994). The primary clinician must promptly report all suspected or confirmed cases of TB to the health department so that appropriate contact investigation can be initiated (USDHHS, 1994). Patients should receive a complete history and physical exam prior to initiation of therapy. Special attention should be paid to the onset and duration of TB symptoms. Specific pulmonary TB symptoms include cough, chest pain, and hemoptysis. Systemic symptoms include fever, chills, night sweats, easy fatigability, loss of appetite, and weight loss.

The medical history should include questions related to the patients' history of TB exposure, infection, disease, and past treatment. If a patient is a contact of an active TB case, it may be very useful to obtain the culture and sensitivity results of the index case. The clinician may also contact the local health department for further information about TB treatment of the index case. If a patient received inadequate treatment or did not adhere to the treatment regimen, he or she may have a recurrence of TB that may be drug-resistant. It is therefore important to determine what drugs were used previously and for how long (Peloquin & Berning, 1994; USDHHS, 1994).

Diagnostic tests should include chest x-ray and sputum microscopic examination and culture. Abnormal chest x-rays may suggest TB, but they are not diagnostic. Chest x-rays may be used to rule out pulmonary TB in a patient with a positive PPD. Sputum smear samples should be examined under the microscope for acid-fast bacilli (AFB). The presence of AFB may also indicate the presence of mycobacteria other than *M. tuberculosis.* Many TB patients have negative AFB smears. A positive culture for *M. tuberculosis* confirms the diagnosis; however, TB may also be diagnosed and treated on the basis of clinical signs and symptoms without a positive culture.

A PPD test should be performed for all patients if it has not already been done. Up to 25% of patients with TB disease may have a negative PPD. More than 60% of patients with AIDs and TB disease may have a negative PPD. Patients who have recently been exposed to someone with TB disease and who have a negative initial PPD should have a second PPD placed 10 weeks after their last exposure to the infectious TB case (USDHHS, 1994).

For patients who will be receiving hepatotoxic medication(s) [eg, INH, pyrazinamide (PZA), rifampin (RIF)], baseline liver function tests should be measured. For those patients who will receive nephrotoxic agents, baseline BUN and serum creatinine should be determined.

Patients need to be assessed for any other chronic medical condition. Special attention should be paid to determining if the patient has chronic liver and/or renal disease.

Immunocompromised patients need to have therapy individualized and need to be monitored closely.

Patients with renal insufficiency should avoid the aminoglycosides if possible. Patients with renal insufficiency may also need to have doses of cycloserine, ethambutol, pyrazinamide, ciprofloxacin, and ofloxacin reduced. Patients who have neuropsychiatric disorders and who abuse alcohol need close supervision of TB therapy, preferably with directly observed therapy (DOT) (USDHHS, 1994).

### Patient/Caregiver Information

All patients and caregivers should be educated about tuberculosis in clear language. Educate them about the difference between TB infection and TB disease. They should also understand the modes of transmission and their drug regimens (dosing, frequency, adverse effects, and when to report adverse effects). Adherence to the medication regimen needs to be strongly emphasized, especially since patients will be on therapy for many months and may not feel sick. All information should be provided verbally as well as in writing and should be reviewed at each clinician visit.

### OUTCOMES MANAGEMENT

#### Selecting an Appropriate Agent

**Prophylaxis.** The primary drug for prophylactic therapy (TB infection) is INH. If a patient is in-

fected with MDR-TB, they should be referred to a TB specialist. Table 22–43 summarizes the criteria for those patients who should be considered for preventive therapy.

Regardless of skin test results, HIV-positive or suspected positive patients who are close contacts to infectious cases should be given prophylaxis if their risk of infection is deemed high and anergy is demonstrated (USDHHS, 1994).

Figure 22–3 offers an algorithm for TB management. A four-drug regimen—isoniazid, rifampin, pyrazinamide, and ethambutol (EMB) or streptomycin (SM)—should be initiated in patients for whom active TB cannot be initially ruled out. Once TB disease has been ruled out and the diagnosis of TB infection is made, the patient can continue therapy with an appropriate prophylactic regimen (USDHHS, 1994).

The standard prophylactic regimen for TB infection is daily INH. Twelve months of therapy reduces the risk of the development of TB disease by more than 90%. Six months of therapy reduces the risk by more than two thirds. Adults should receive at least 6 months of therapy, and children should receive at least 9 months of therapy. HIV-infected individuals should receive 12 months of therapy. For patients whose compliance is questionable twice weekly DOT at an INH dosage of 15 mg/kg is a reasonable alternative (USDHHS, 1994).

INH is contraindicated in those patients with drug allergy, history of INH-associated hepatic injury, history of severe adverse reactions to INH (eg, drug fever, rash, arthritis), and those patients with acute or unstable liver disease.

For patients who cannot tolerate INH or who are infected with INH-resistant TB, an alternative regimen is to give daily RIF in the usual doses and for the same duration as INH regimens. For patients who are likely to be infected with TB strains resistant to INH and RIF, observation without preventive therapy is recommended unless they are at very high risk for developing TB disease. Patients infected with INH- and RIF-resistant strains of TB and who are at high risk of developing TB disease should receive alternative prophylactic regimens consisting of at least two drugs to which the strain has been shown to be susceptible. For example, a 6-month regimen of daily EMB and PZA or PZA and a flouroquinolone (ofloxacin or ciprofloxacin) in the usual therapeutic doses can be given. In these cases a TB expert should be consulted (USDHHS, 1994). Peripheral neuropathy associated with INH therapy can be pre-

**TABLE 22–43. PATIENTS WHO SHOULD BE CONSIDERED FOR PREVENTIVE THERAPY**

| Age | ≥ 5 mm Increase in PPD Reaction | ≥ 10 mm Increase in PPD Reaction | ≥ 15 mm Increase in PPD Reaction |
|---|---|---|---|
| Regardless of age | Known HIV infection<br>Suspected HIV infection<br>Unknown HIV status and in-jecting drug user<br>Close contacts of infectious TB patients<br>Chest x-ray suggestive of previous TB with no or in-adequate treatment | Injecting drug users known to be HIV-negative<br>Predisposing medical condi-tions (see Table 22–41)<br>PPD converter from negative to positive within the past 2 years and <35 years old | PPD converter within the past 2 years and ≥35 years |
| <35 years of age | | Foreign-born from high-prevalence areas of the world<br>Medically underserved, low-income, populations<br>Residents of long-term-care facilities<br>Children <4 years old | |

*Adapted from USDHHS (1994).*

vented by daily administration of 10–50 mg of pyridoxine (vitamin B$_6$).

***Active disease.*** Five different treatment options for pulmonary TB (active TB disease) are illustrated in Fig. 22–4. The Centers for Disease Control and Prevention recommend an initial four-drug treatment regimen until culture and sensitivity results are available because of the emergence of MDR-TB across the country. The initial regimen should consist of INH, RIF, PZA, and ETH or SM unless specifically contraindicated. Any regimen consisting of twice-weekly or three-times-weekly therapy needs to be DOT.

Effective treatment of TB is accomplished through the use of multiple drugs. It is extremely important to avoid monotherapy and to avoid adding a single drug to a failing regimen. These mistakes contribute to the emergence of MDR-TB (Peloquin & Berning, 1994). If resistance to any of the first-line drugs is demonstrated or if the patient is still symptomatic and is smear- or culture-positive after 3 months of drug therapy, expert consultations should be sought (USDHHS, 1994).

If sputum cultures are still positive or if patients are still symptomatic after 2 months of therapy, the patient should be reevaluated for drug-resistant disease. While the drug sensitivity

patterns are being determined, the patient may be continued on the original regimen or it may be augmented by the addition of three drugs not given previously (USDHHS, 1994).

***Drug-resistant TB.*** When INH resistance is documented during the initial four-drug regimen (options 1, 2, 3, and 4 in Fig. 22–4), INH should be discontinued and the other three drugs should be continued for the full 6 months. Alternatively, TB resistant only to INH can be treated with 12 months of RIF and EMB.

If option 5 in Fig. 22–4 (initially INH, RIF, and EMB or SM) was chosen and included EMB, and INH resistance is demonstrated, a 12-month regimen of RIF and EMB should be completed. If EMB was not initially used, susceptibility tests should be repeated, INH should be discontinued, and two new drugs (eg, EMB and PZA) should be added. The regimen can then be adjusted when susceptibilities are available.

If initial susceptibility tests show that the TB strain is resistant to both INH and RIF (MDR-TB by definition), therapy needs to be individualized. The patient should receive three new drugs to which the strain is sensitive until cultures convert to negative. After culture conversion, the patient should receive at least 12 months of therapy with two drugs to which the TB strain is sensitive. Empirically, a total of 24 months of therapy is

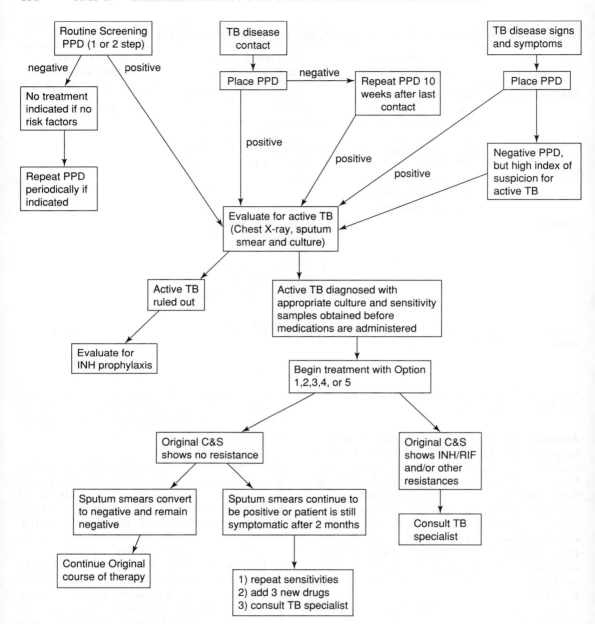

**Figure 22–3.** Algorithm for management of tuberculosis.

often given. Patients with MDR-TB may need to receive second-line agents for TB as well, which are often less effective and more toxic. *If MDR-TB is documented, experts on the treatment of TB should be consulted.*

***First-line agents.*** Isoniazid is the most widely used antituberculous agent. It is bactericidal against TB. INH penetrates well into all body fluids. The most serious adverse effects associated with INH are hepatitis and peripheral neuropathy. The risk of hepatitis increases with age, being rare at less than 20 years of age. Alcohol consumption, especially daily alcohol consumption, increases the risk of hepatitis. Peripheral neuropathy or neuritis is more likely to occur in

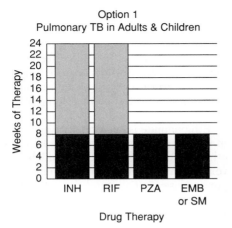

Option 1
Pulmonary TB in Adults & Children

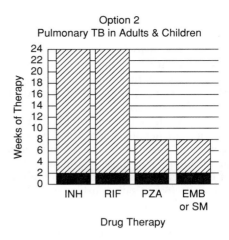

Option 2
Pulmonary TB in Adults & Children

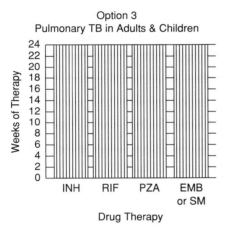

Option 3
Pulmonary TB in Adults & Children

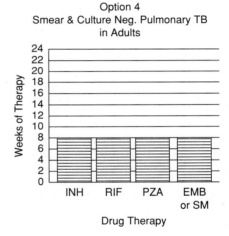

Option 4
Smear & Culture Neg. Pulmonary TB
in Adults

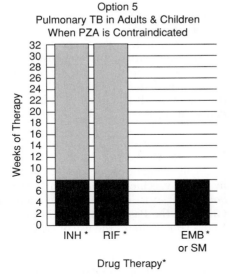

Option 5
Pulmonary TB in Adults & Children
When PZA is Contraindicated

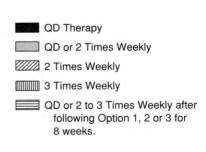

■ QD Therapy

▨ QD or 2 Times Weekly

▨ 2 Times Weekly

▥ 3 Times Weekly

▤ QD or 2 to 3 Times Weekly after
following Option 1, 2 or 3 for
8 weeks.

*Daily for 4 to 8 weeks; total treatment = 32 weeks.

**Figure 22–4.** Five treatment options for pulmonary tuberculosis.

patients predisposed to neuritis (eg, diabetics, alcoholics, malnourished individuals). To decrease the risk of peripheral neuropathy, patients should receive 10–50 mg of pyridoxine daily during INH therapy.

Rifampin is bactericidal against TB. RIF is a potent inducer of hepatic microsomal enzymes and accelerates the metabolism of numerous other medications. The most common adverse effect of RIF is GI upset. RIF turns all body secretions orange (tears, saliva, urine, sweat) and may permanently stain soft contact lenses and lens implants.

Pyrazinamide is bactericidal against TB in the acidic intracellular environment. The most serious adverse effect of PZA is hepatotoxicity, which is dose-related and can occur at any time during therapy. Hyperuricemia frequently occurs with PZA therapy, but acute gout is uncommon. Nongouty arthralgia may occur in up to 40% of patients. PZA-related arthralgia can be treated symptomatically with salicylates.

In doses of 15–25 mg/kg used for daily therapy, ethambutol is considered to be bacteriostatic. In higher doses used for intermittent therapy (30–50 mg/kg), EMB may be bactericidal. The most common and serious adverse effect of EMB is optic neuritis and is dose-related. The symptoms of neuritis include decreased visual acuity, loss of red-green color discrimination, and scotomas. With early detection and discontinuation, the visual effects are usually reversible over a period of weeks to months. EMB is not recommended for use in children, for whom it is difficult to assess visual acuity (ie, less than 6–8 years old).

Streptomycin is an aminoglycoside antibiotic that is bactericidal against TB in an alkaline environment. It must be given parenterally. The most common serious adverse effect of SM is ototoxicity manifested as vertigo and/or hearing loss. Ototoxicity is more likely if other ototoxic drugs are administered. Nephrotoxicity may also occur and is more likely in older patients and those who have underlying renal insufficiency.

**Second-line agents.**   Second-line agents are less effective against TB and sometimes more toxic. Second-line agents should only be used in consultation with experts on the treatment of TB.

Cycloserine is bacteriostatic against TB. The most frequent adverse effects involve the CNS (dizziness, drowsiness, headache, emotional disturbances, psychosis, seizures, neuropathy) and occur in approximately 30% of patients. Patients

with underlying psychiatric disorders are more likely to experience the CNS effects of cycloserine. Adverse CNS effects can be minimized by keeping serum levels <30 µg/mL and by concomitant administration of 150 mg of pyridoxine daily.

Ethionamide is bacteriostatic against TB. The most common adverse effects associated with ethionamide are GI distress, which can be severe. Many patients cannot tolerate full therapeutic doses initially and must be started at a lower dose and gradually increased to full doses. In some cases patients may need to have an antiemetic administered along with ethionamide.

Capreomycin is an aminoglycoside antibiotic. It has a higher incidence of ototoxicity and nephrotoxicity than streptomycin. The elderly are usually more susceptible to these toxicities. Patients should have an audiogram performed at baseline and every other month during therapy (AHFS, 1997; ATS, 1994).

Para-aminosalicylic acid (PAS) is bacteriostatic against TB. The minimum inhibitory concentration (MIC) for susceptible TB is 0.5–2.0 µg/mL.

Kanamycin and amikacin are aminoglycoside antibiotics. Auditory toxicity is greater with amikacin and kanamycin than with capreomycin. Both agents can cause nephrotoxicity, more often in elderly patients and in patients with underlying renal insufficiency (ATS, 1994).

Ciprofloxacin and ofloxacin are fluoroquinolone antibiotics and are not FDA-approved for TB treatment. Their use should be avoided in children and pregnant women because of the risk of arthropathy.

Clofazimine is a phenazine dye antiinfective that has an in vitro activity against many species of *Mycobacterium* (eg, *M. leprae, M. avium* complex, and *M. tuberculosis*). Its efficacy in the treatment of TB is unproven. It has a high incidence of adverse GI effects (up to 60%). Because it is a dye, reversible discoloration of skin occurs in the majority of patients (AHFS, 1997; USDHHS, 1994).

Bacille Calmette-Guérin (BCG) vaccines are live virus vaccines derived from a strain of *M. bovis* that was attenuated by Calmette and Guérin at the Pasteur Institute in Lille, France. In the United States the use of BCG vaccine has very few indications. It should be considered for infants and children who are living in households where the likelihood of becoming infected with TB is high and where other prevention strategies cannot be implemented. It may also be considered in a subset of health care workers who work in a setting where the risk of contracting MDR-TB is high. Practitioners considering the use of BCG vaccine should consult the TB control program in their area (Centers for Disease Control and Prevention [CDC], 1996b).

## Selecting Agents for Children

In general the selection of agents in pediatrics is the same as for adults.

*Prophylaxis.*  Infants exposed to TB disease should have a PPD and chest x-ray. If the initial PPD is negative and the chest x-ray is normal, then the PPD should be repeated at 3–4 months and then again at 6 months. Infants should receive INH prophylaxis even if the PPD and chest x-ray are negative because they may be anergic as late as 6 months of age. INH can be discontinued at 6 months if the PPD is negative *and* at least 10 weeks have passed since the infant was last exposed to infectious TB.

Prophylactic dosage regimens in children are the same as those for adults, but the minimum recommended duration of therapy is 9 months.

*Active disease.*  The treatment regimens for TB disease in children is the same as for adults. EMB is relatively contraindicated in children less than 8 years old because it is difficult to assess changes in visual acuity in this age group. Adequate sputum samples are difficult to obtain from children. It may therefore be necessary to base treatment regimens on the drug susceptibilities of the index adult case. Tuberculosis in children less than 4 years old is much more likely to be disseminated TB. Therefore, treatment needs to be initiated promptly when TB is suspected. Options 1, 2, 3, and 5 of Fig. 22–4 are also indicated for extrapulmonary TB in adults and children (ATS, 1994; USDHHS, 1994).

## Selecting Agents during Pregnancy and Lactation

The pregnant patient needs to be counseled on the teratogenic risk of the particular agent. Refer to Chapter 10 for a discussion of medication use in pregnancy.

*Prophylaxis.*  In general, pregnant women who are PPD-positive during routine screening do not need to start INH prophylaxis until after delivery. However, pregnant women who are likely to have been recently infected or have high-risk medical conditions, especially HIV, should be given INH prophylaxis as soon as TB infection is documented and TB disease has been ruled out. Pregnant patients receiving INH should also receive pyridoxine 10–50 mg PO daily to prevent peripheral neuropathy (USDHHS, 1994).

INH is excreted in breast milk, and the infant should be monitored for signs and symptoms of peripheral neuritis or hepatitis. INH is considered compatible with breast-feeding by the American Academy of Pediatrics. RIF is also considered compatible with breast-feeding by the AAP (Briggs et al, 1994). For more information on the risk of drugs to the developing fetus and to breast-fed infants, the patient should be referred to a specialist.

*Active disease.*  Treatment of TB disease in pregnancy should initially consist of a 9-month regimen of INH, RIF, and EMB. Pregnant women should receive daily pyridoxine. Further drug selection and regimens should be based on specific drug sensitivities obtained.

SM and the other aminoglycosides should be avoided because of fetal toxicity. PZA should also be avoided because of unknown effects on the fetus. Other drugs that should be avoided in pregnancy include fluoroquinolones, cycloserine, ethionamide, and clofazimine. If it is deemed necessary to treat a pregnant patient with one of these drugs, the patient should be counseled about potential teratogenic risks (ATS, 1994; USDHHS, 1994).

## Monitoring for Efficacy

All patients being treated for TB infection and TB disease should be assessed at least monthly. For patients at risk of not completing self-administered therapy, DOT should be strongly considered. DOT is initially more expensive, but from a public health standpoint it can be very cost-effective by preventing the spread of TB and by slowing the emergence of MDR-TB. DOT consists of twice-weekly or thrice-weekly regimens where the patients are actually observed taking their medications by a health care provider, public health worker, or responsible community or family member.

Patients with TB disease should be assessed for resolution of TB disease signs and symptoms including fever, night sweats, weight loss, cough, and hemoptysis. Patients with TB infection should also be assessed for symptoms of progression from TB infection to TB disease.

All patients should be instructed to bring all of their medications with them to every clinician visit to aid in assessment of medication compliance. Pill counts should be done at every visit. No more than a 1-month supply of medications should be given or prescribed at each visit.

Physical examinations should include a lung assessment to evaluate cough. Patients should be weighed periodically as an indicator of their nutritional status.

Patients with initially positive sputum smears should have sputum smears examined at least monthly. Preferentially, weekly sputum smears should be performed until conversion to negative smears is documented (ATS, 1994; US-DHHS, 1994).

Patients with positive sputum cultures prior to drug therapy should have monthly sputum cultures performed until the cultures are negative. Patients whose sputum cultures remain positive beyond 2 months need to be carefully reevaluated for continued drug susceptibility and/or drug resistance. Continued positive cultures may also suggest patient noncompliance with medication regimens. DOT regimens should be strongly considered for these patients if they are not already in such a program.

After initial drug sensitivities are determined, subsequent drug sensitivities should be determined if sputum cultures remain positive after 2 months (USDHHS, 1994).

Patients with pulmonary TB disease are considered infectious if they are coughing, if their sputum smears contain acid-fast bacilli, if they are not receiving therapy or have just started therapy, or if they have a poor clinical or bacterial response to drug therapy. Patients are not considered infectious if they have received adequate therapy for 2–3 weeks, *and* they have a favorable clinical response (eg, resolution of fever, night sweats, dyspnea, fatigue, and hemoptysis), *and* they have three consecutive negative sputum smears on samples from different days. Infectiousness may last several weeks to several months in patients with drug-resistant TB disease. Patients with drug-resistant TB disease need to be isolated until infectiousness is ruled out. Patients infected with MDR-TB should be considered for isolation throughout their hospitalization (USDHHS, 1994).

## Monitoring for Toxicity

Patients should be monitored monthly for signs and symptoms of drug toxicity. They should also be instructed to monitor themselves at home for toxicity and to report any symptoms immediately.

Gastrointestinal upset can be associated with any medication, but is more common with RIF and PZA. It is also reported with PAS, the fluoroquinolones, and clofazimine. GI upset can be minimized by taking the medication with a full glass of water. GI upset is not an indication for discontinuation of therapy unless the upset is so severe that the patient refuses to take the medication. Hepatotoxicity is the most common toxicity associated with drugs used to treat TB. Hepatotoxicity is usually associated with INH, RIF, and PZA. At each visit patients should be evaluated for symptoms of hepatitis including nausea, loss of appetite, vomiting, dark urine, jaundice, malaise, abdominal pain (especially RUQ pain), and unexplained fever for more than 3 days.

Patients should be questioned regarding symptoms of peripheral neuropathy at each visit. Ocular toxicity caused by EMB should also be assessed at each visit. Patients should be questioned regarding symptoms of decreased visual acuity, scotomas, and loss of red-green color discrimination.

Any patient on INH prophylaxis who develops symptoms of hepatotoxicity or peripheral neuropathy or whose LFTs are elevated 3–5 times above the upper limit of normal should discontinue therapy. Patients taking any aminoglycoside should be monitored for ototoxicity (vestibular dysfunction and/or hearing loss) and renal toxicity (increased BUN and serum creatinine). Patients receiving PZA may develop asymptomatic hyperuricemia and very rarely gout. Hyperuricemia and gout should only be treated if symptoms appear.

Signs of hepatitis (enlarged liver, RUQ tenderness, abdominal pain on palpation) should be followed up, as should signs of thrombocytopenia from RIF (easy bruising, bleeding tendency, blood in urine). A visual acuity examination for patients receiving EMB should be performed before initiating therapy and at any subsequent visit if the patient notes any symptoms or change in vision.

Patients who are suspected of developing liver toxicity should have liver function tests evaluated immediately. Monthly liver function tests (LFTs) are not indicated for all patients on INH prophylaxis. Baseline and monthly LFTs should be measured for those patients who are considered at high risk for hepatotoxicity (pregnant, history of alcohol abuse, chronic liver disease, IV drug user). For patients older than 35 years receiving INH prophylaxis monitor LFTs at baseline, at 1 month, and periodically thereafter if needed.

Patients being treated for TB disease should have pretreatment baseline measurements of LFTs (AST, ALT, bilirubin), renal function tests (serum creatinine and BUN), and CBC with platelets. If PZA is used, patients should have baseline serum uric acid levels measured. For patients being treated with EMB, a baseline visual acuity examination should be performed. For patients receiving streptomycin or any other aminoglycoside, baseline and periodic audiometry should be performed (USDHHS, 1994).

Patients at high risk for hepatotoxicity should have monthly LFTs assessed. Patients at higher risk of renal toxicity caused by aminoglycosides should have BUN and serum creatinine levels periodically assessed.

## Follow-up Recommendations

Patients who were infected with INH- and RIF-sensitive strains of TB and who satisfactorily completed a 6- or 9-month course of therapy that included INH and RIF do not need routine follow-up. They should, however, be educated to report the subsequent development of any symptoms of TB (eg, prolonged cough, fever, weight loss).

Patients who were infected with strains of TB resistant to INH and/or RIF need individualized follow-up (USDHHS, 1994).

## REFERENCES

Aboussouan, L. S. (1996). Acute exacerbations of chronic bronchitis. Focusing management for optimum results. *Postgraduate Medicine, 99,* 89–90, 95–98, 101–102, 104.

Agertoft, L., & Pedersen, S. (1993). Importance of the inhalation device on the effect of budesonide. *Archives of Diseases in Childhood, 69,* 130–133.

*AHFS Drug Information.* (1997). G. K. McEvoy (Ed.), Bethesda: American Society of Health-System Pharmacists, Inc.

Allen, D. B. (1996). Growth suppression by glucocorticoid therapy. *Endocrinology and Metabolism Clinics in North America,* 699–717.

Allen, D. B., Mullen, M., & Mullen, B. (1994). A meta-analysis of the effect of oral and inhaled corticosteroids in growth. *Journal of Allergy and Clinical Immunology, 93,* 967–976.

Allen, E. D. (1996). Opportunities for the use of aerosolized alpha-1 antitrypsin for the treatment of cystic fibrosis. *Chest, 110*(6)(Suppl), 256S–260S.

Alpha—New Therapeutic Bulletin. Background information about asthma and usage of serevent.

American Academy of Pediatrics Committee on Infectious Diseases. (1998). Red book: Report of the Committee on Infectious Diseases. Elk Grove Village, Ill: American Academy of Pediatrics.

American Thoracic Society. (1991). Lung function testing: Selection of reference values and interpretive strategies. *American Review of Respiratory Disease, 144,* 1202–1208.

American Thoracic Society. (1993). Guidelines for the initial management of adults with community-acquired pneumonia: Diagnosis, assessment of severity and initial antimicrobial therapy. *American Review of Respiratory Disease, 148,* 1418–1426.

American Thoracic Society. (1994). Treatment of tuberculosis and tuberculosis infection in adults and children. *American Journal of Respiratory and Critical Care Medicine, 149,* 1359–1374.

American Thoracic Society. (1995). Standards for the diagnosis and care of patients with chronic obstructive pulmonary disease. *American Journal of Respiratory and Critical Care Medicine, 152,* S77–S120.

Anderson, B. (1991). An overview of drug therapy for chronic adult asthma. *Nurse Practitioner, 16,* 39–46.

Areno, J., San Pedro, G., & Campbell, G. D. (1996). Diagnosis and prognosis in community-acquired pneumonia: When and where should the patient be treated. *Seminars in Respiratory and Critical Care Medicine, 17*(3), 231–236.

Arunabh, M. D., & Niederman, M. (1996). Prevention of community-acquired pneumonia. *Seminars in Respiratory and Critical Care Medicine, 17*(3), 273–280.

Austrian, R. (1992). Pneumococcal infections. *Harrison's Principles of Internal Medicine* (13th ed.). New York: McGraw-Hill.

Barnes, P. J., & Lee, T. H. (1992). Recent advances in asthma. *Postgraduate Medical Journal, 68*(806), 942–953.

Barnes, P. J., & Pawels, R. A. (1994). Theophylline in the management of asthma: Time for reappraisal. *European Respiratory Journal, 7,* 579–591.

Barnes, P. J., & Rederson, S. (1993). Efficacy and safety of inhaled corticosteroids in asthma. *American Review of Respiratory Disease, 148,* S1+.

Bartlett, J., & Mundy, L. (1995). Community-acquired pneumonia. *New England Journal of Medicine, 333*(24), 1618–1623.

Bender, B. G., Lerner, J. A., Ikle, E., Comer, C., & Szefler, S. (1991). Psychological changes associated with theophylline treatment of asthmatic children: A 6 month study. *Pediatric Pulmonology, 11*(3), 233–242.

Bender, B. G., Lerner, J. A., & Poland, J. E. (1991). Association between corticosteroids and psychologic change in hospitalized asthmatic children. *Annals of Allergy, 66,* 414–419.

Bender, B., & Milgrom, H. (1992). Theophylline-induced behavior change in children: An objective evaluation of parents' perceptions. *Journal of the American Medical Association, 267,* 2621–2624.

Bernstein, M. S. & Locksley, R. M. (1997). Infections due to gram-positive bacilli. Infectious Disease. *Scientific American,* 51.

Boucher, R. (1996). Cystic fibrosis. In *Nelson's Textbook of Pediatrics* (15th ed.). Philadelphia: WB Saunders.

Bousquet, J., Chanez, P., Vignola, A. M., & Michel, F. B. (1996). Asthma and chronic bronchitis: Similarities and differences. *Respiratory Medicine,* (90), 187–190.

Bozzoni, M., Radice, L., Frosi, A., Vezzoli, S., Cuboni, A., & Vezzoli, F. (1995). Prevalence of pneumonia due to Legionaella pneumophila and Mycoplasma pneumoniae in a population admitted to a Department of Internal Medicine. *Respiration,* (62):331–335.

Braman, S. S. (1993). Asthma in the elderly patient. *Pulmonary Disease in the Elderly Patient, 14*(3), 413–422.

Braman, S. S., & Davis, S. M. (1986). Wheezing in the elderly. Asthma and other causes. *Clinics in Geriatric Medicine, 2*(2), 269–283.

Briggs, G. G., Freeman, R. K., & Yaffe, S. J. (1994). *Drugs in pregnancy and lactation: A reference guide to fetal and neonatal risk* (4th ed.). Baltimore: Williams and Wilkins.

Briggs, R. G., Mahre, W. C., & Sibai, B. M. (1996). Community acquired pneumonia in pregnancy. *American Journal of Obstetrics and Gynecology, 174,* 389+.

Brown, R. B. (1993). Community-acquired pneumonia: Diagnosis and therapy of older adults. *Geriatrics,* (48), 43–50.

Broussard, R. C., Payne, D. K., & George, R. B. (1991). Treatment with acyclovir in varicella pneumonia in pregnancy. *Chest, 99*(4), 1045–1047.

Brunell, P. A. (1990). Varicella in the womb and beyond. *Pediatric Infectious Disease Journal, 9*(10), 770–772.

Burrows, B. (1987). The natural history of asthma. *Journal of Allergy and Clinical Immunology,* (3 Pt 2), 373–377.

Busse, W. W. (1993). Mechanisms of inflammation in the asthmatic patient. *Allergy Proceedings, 14*(1), 5–8.

Bye, M. R., Ewig, J. M., & Quittell, L. M. (1994). Cystic Fibrosis. *Lung, 172*(5), 251–270.

Carr, W., Zeitel, L., & Weiss, K. (1992). Variations in asthma hospitalizations and deaths in New York City. *American Journal of Public Health, 82*(1), 59–65.

Carter, R., Coast, J. R., & Idell, S. (1992). Exercise training in patients with chronic obstructive pulmonary disease. *Medicine and Science in Sports and Exercise, 24,* 281–291.

Cassell, G., Gray, G., & Maites, K. B. (1998). Mycoplasma infections. In Fauci, A., et al (Eds.), *Harrison's Principles of Internal Medicine.* New York: McGraw Hill.

Cassiere, H., Rodrigues, J. C., & Fein, A. M. (1996). Delayed resolution of pneumonia. *Postgraduate Medicine, 99*(1), 151–158.

Catanzaro, A. (1984). Pulmonary mycosis in pregnant women. *Chest, 86,* 145–195.

Centers for Disease Control and Prevention. (1996a). Control and prevention. Asthma mortality and hospitalizations among children and youth— United States. *MMWR, 45,* 350–353.

Centers for Disease Control and Prevention. (1996b). The role of BCG vaccine in the prevention and control of tuberculosis in the United States: A joint statement by the advisory council for the elimination of tuberculosis and the advisory committee on immunization practices. *MMWR, 45,* No. RR4.

Chanarin, N., & Johnston, S. L. (1994). Leukotrienes as a target in asthma therapy. *Drugs, 47*(1), 12–24.

Chan-Yeung, M., & Malo, J. L. (1994). Aetiological agents in occupational asthma. *European Respiratory Journal, 7*(2), 346–371.

Charlesworth, E. N. (1996). Late-phase inflammation: Influence on morbidity. *Journal of Allergy and Clinical Immunology,* (98), S291–S297.

Clark, B. (1993). General pharmacology, pharmacokinetics and toxicology of nedocromil sodium. *Journal of Allergy and Clinical Immunology, 92,* 200–202.

Clark, D. J., Grove, A., Cargill, R. I., & Lipworth, B. J. (1996). Comparative adrenal suppression with inhaled budesonide and fluticasone propionate in adult asthmatics. *Thorax, 51,* 262–266.

Connoly, M. J., Crowley, J. J., Charan, N. B., Nielson, C. P., & Vestal, R. E. (1992). Reduced subjective awareness of bronchoconstriction provoked by methacholine in elderly asthmatic and normal subjects as measured on a simple awareness scale. *Thorax, 47,* 410–413.

Conte, J. (1995). *Manual of antibiotics and infectious diseases* (8th ed.). Baltimore: Williams and Wilkins.

Costello, J., Meltzer, S., & Bleecker, E. R. (1994). Summary: The pharmacology of leukotrienes in asthma. *Advances in Prostaglandin Thrombaxone Leukotrones Research, 22,* 263–268.

Coultas, D. B., Gong, H., Jr., Grad R, Handler, A., McCurdy, S. A., Player, R., Rhoades, E. R., Samet, J. M., Thomas, A., & Westley, M. (1994). Respiratory diseases in minorities in the United States. *American Journal of Respiratory and Critical Care Medicine, 149*(3 Pt 2), S93–S131.

Cunha, B. A. (1996). Community-acquired pneumonia. Cost-effective antimicrobial therapy. *Postgraduate Medicine,* (99), 109–117.

Cunha, B. A., & Ortega, A. M. (1996). Atypical pneumonia. *Postgraduate Medicine,* (99), 123–132.

Davis, P. P., & Bayard, P. J. (1988). Relationships among airway reactivity, pupillary alpha-adrenergic and cholinergic responsiveness and age. *Journal of Applied Physiology, 65*(1), 200–204.

de Benedictis, F. M., Tuteri, G., Pazzeli, P., Bertotto, A., & R. Vaccaro. (1995). Cromolyn versus nedocromil: Duration of action in exercise-induced asthma in children. *Journal of Allergy and Clinical Immunology, 96,* 510–514.

deBenedictis, A. M., Martinati, L. C., Solinas L. F., Tuteri G., & Boner, A. L. (1996). Nebulized flunisolide in infants and young children with asthma: A pilot study. *Pediatric Pulmonology,* (21), 310–315.

Doull, I. J. M., Freezer, N. J., & Holgate, S. T. (1995). Growth of pre-pubertal children with mild asthma treated with inhaled beclomethasone dipropionate. *American Journal of Respiratory and Critical Care Medicine, 151,* 1715–1719.

Drug Facts and Comparisons. (1998). Ed. Erwin Kastrup. St. Louis, Mo.: Wolters Kluwer Co.

DuBuske, L. M. (1994). Asthma: Diagnosis and management of nocturnal symptoms. *Comprehensive Therapy, 20*(11).

Durie, P. R., & Pencharz, P. B. (1992). Cystic fibrosis: Nutrition. *British Medical Bulletin, 48*(4), 823–846.

Elkus, R., & Popovich, J., Jr. (1992). Respiratory physiology in pregnancy. *Clinical Chest Medicine, 13*(4), 555–565.

Fein, A. M. (1994). Pneumonia in the elderly: Special diagnostic and therapeutic considerations. *Medical Clinics of North America, 78*(5), 1015–1034.

Fein, A. M. (1996). Treatment of community-acquired pneumonia: Clinical guidelines or clinical judgment? *Seminars in Respiratory and Critical Care Medicine, 17*(3), 237–241.

Ferguson, G. T., & Cherniack, R. M. (1993). Management of chronic obstructive pulmonary disease. *New England Journal of Medicine, 328,* 1017–1022.

Fete, T. J., & Noyes, B. (1996). Common (but not always considered) viral infections of the lower respiratory tract. *Pediatric Annals, 25*(10), 577–584.

File, T. (1997). Management of community-acquired pneumonia. *Infectious Disease Practice, 21,* 9–12.

File, T. M., Tan, J. S., & Plouffe, J. F. (1996). Community-acquired pneumonia. What's needed for accurate diagnosis. *Postgraduate Medicine, 99*(1), 95–107.

Fineland, M., & Dublin, T. D. (1939). Pneumococcal pneumonias complicating pregnancy and the puerperium. *JAMA, 112,* 1027–1032.

Forstner, G. G., & Durie, P. R. (1996). Cystic fibrosis. In W. A. Walker, P. R. Durie, J. R. Hamilton, et al (Eds.), *Pediatric gastrointestinal disease* (2nd ed.) (pp. 1466–1487). St. Louis, Mo: Mosby.

Foucard, T. (1996). Aggressive treatment of childhood asthma with local steroids. Good or bad? *Allergy,* (51), 367–371.

Fragoso, C. A., & Miller, M. A. (1993). Review of the clinical efficacy of theophylline in the treatment of chronic obstructive pulmonary disease. *American Review of Respiratory Disease, 147,* S40–S47.

Fraser, D. (1993). Patient assessment: Infection in the elderly. *Journal of Gerontologic Nursing, 6,* 5–11.

Frederiksen, B., Lanng, S., Koch, C., & Hoiby, N. (1996). Improved survival in the Danish center-treated cystic fibrosis patients: Results of aggressive treatment. *Pediatric Pulmonology,* (21), 153–158.

Friedman, M. (1995). Changing practices in COPD. A new pharmacologic treatment algorithm. *Chest, 107,* S194–S197.

Gales, M., & McClain, P. (1997). Coccidioidomycosis. A mycotic infection on the rise. *Clinical Reviews, 7,* 71–84.

Gianaris, P. G., & Golish, J. A. (1994). Changing strategies in the management of asthma. *Postgraduate Medicine, 95*(5), 105–218.

Godden, D. J., Ross, S., Abdella, M., McMurray, D., Douglas, A., Oldman, D., Friend, J. A., Legge, J. S., & Douglas, J. G. (1994). Outcomes of wheeze in childhood: Symptoms and pulmonary function 25 years later. *American Journal of Respiratory Critical Care Medicine, 149*(1), 10–112.

Gold, D. R., Wypy, D., Wang, X., Speizer, F. E., Pugh, M., Ware, J. H., Ferris, B. G., & Dockery, D. W. (1994). Gender and race specific effects of asthma and wheeze on level and growth of lung function in children in 6 U.S. cities. *American Journal of Respiratory and Critical Care Medicine, 149*(5), 1198–1208.

Grant, C. C., Duggan, A. K., Santosham, M., & DeAngelis, C. (1996). Oral prednisone as a risk factor for infections in children with asthma. *Archives of Pediatric and Adolescent Medicine,* 58–63.

Granton, J., & Grossman, R. (1993). Community acquired pneumonia in the elderly patient. *Clinics in Chest Medicine, 14*(3), 537–553.

Green, M. (1997). Viral pneumonias. In Gillis & Kagan (Eds.), *Current pediatric therapy* (15th ed.) (pp. 637–638). Philadelphia: W. B. Saunders.

Green, M. A. R., Buchanan, E., & Weaver, L. T. (1995). Nutritional management of the infant with cystic fibrosis. *Archives of Disease in Childhood, 72,* 452–456.

Greenberger, P. A. (1992). Asthma in pregnancy. *Clinics in Chest Medicine, 13*(4), 597–605.

Groothius, J. R., Simoes, E. A., Hemming, V. G., & the Respiratory Syncytial Virus Immune Globulin Study Group. (1995). Respiratory syncytial virus (RSV) infection in preterm infants and the protective effects of RSV immune globulin (RSVIG). *Pediatrics 95,* 463–467.

Gross, N. J. (1995). Airway inflammation in COPD. Reality or myth. *Chest, 107,* S210–S213.

Haake, D. D., Zakowski, P. C., Haake, D. L., et al. (1990). Early treatment with acyclovir for varicella pneumonia in otherwise healthy adults: Retrospective controlled study and review. *Review of Infectious Diseases, 12,* 788–798.

Haas, D. W., & Des Prez, R. M. (1995). Mycobacterium tuberculosis. In G. L. Mandell, J. E. Bennett, & R. Dolin (Eds.), *Mandell, Douglas and Bennett's Principles and Practice of Infectious Diseases, 4th Ed.* (pp. 2213–2243). New York: Churchill Livingstone, Inc.

Hammerschlag, M. (1996). Chylamydia. In Behrman, et al (Eds.), *Textbook of pediatrics* (15th ed.) (pp. 827–830). Philadelphia: W. B. Saunders.

Hanson, M. A., & Midthun, D. E. (1992). Outpatient care of COPD patients. *Postgraduate Medicine, 91,* 89–95.

Hayes, F. J., O'Brien, A., O'Brien, C., Fitzgerald, M. X., & McKennon, M. J. (1995). Diabetes mellitus in an adult population with cystic fibrosis. *Irish Medical Journal, 88*(3), 102–104.

Hendeles, L., & Marshik, P. L. (1996). Zileuton: A new therapy for asthma or just the first of a new class of drugs? *Annals of Pharmacotherapy, 30,* 873–875.

Henderson, W. R., Jr. (1994). The role of leukotrienes in inflammation. *Annals of Internal Medicine, 121,* 684–697.

Hoiby, N. (1993). Antibiotic therapy for chronic infection of pseudomonas in the lung. *Annual Review of Medicine, 44,* 1–10.

Hopp, R. (1996). Evaluation of recurrent respiratory tract infections in children. *Current Problems in Pediatrics,* 148–151.

Horst, P. S. (1994). Bronchiolitis. *American Family Physician, 49*(6), 1449–1453.

Howarth, P. H., Redington, A. E., & Montefort, S. (1993). Pathophysiology of asthma. *Allergy, 48,* 50–56.

Ingram Jr., R. H. (1994). Chronic bronchitis, emphysema, and airways obstruction. In K. J. Isselbacher, E. Braunwald, G. D. Wilson, J. Martin, A. S. Fauchi, & D. L. Casper (Eds.), *Harrison's principles of internal medicine* (pp. 1197–1206). New York: McGraw Hill.

Irons, T. (1994). Respiratory infections in children. Highlights of the American Academy of Family Physicians' 46th Annual Scientific Assembly, *Audio Digest, 42*(48), 1–3.

Israel, E., Fischer, A. R., & Rosenberg, M. A., et al. (1993). The pivotal role of 5-lipoxygenase products in the reaction of aspirin-sensitive asthmatics to aspirin. *American Review of Respiratory Disease, 148,* 1447–1451.

James, J. (1995). Day care admissions. *Pediatric Nursing, 7*(1), 25–29, 37.

Janwetz, E. (1995). Principles of antimicrobial drug action. In Katzung, (Ed.), *Basic and Clinical Pharmacology* (6th ed.) (pp. 671–680). Norwalk, CT: Appleton & Lange.

Jarjour, N., Gelfand, E., McGill, K., & Busse, W. W. (1996). Alternative anti-inflammatory and immunomodulatory therapy. In Szefler J., Leung, D. Y. M., (Eds.), *Severe asthma. Pathogenesis and clinical management* (pp. 333–369). New York: Marcel Dekker.

Jenne, J. W. (1995). Two new roles for theophylline in the asthmatic? *Journal of Asthma, 32*(2), 89–95.

Johnson, C., Lawlor, M., & Weiner, M. (1994). The airway in the obstetrical patient. *American Association of Nurse Anesthetists Journal. 62*(2), 149–159.

Johnson, D. H., & Cunha, B. A. (1993). Atypical pneumonias. Clinical and extrapulmonary features of Chlamydia, Mycoplasma, and Legionella infections. *Postgraduate Medicine, 93*(7), 69–82.

Johnson, M. (1996). Pharmacodynamics and pharmacokinetics of inhaled glucocorticoids. *Journal of Allergy and Clinical Immunology, 97*(1 Pt 2), 169–176.

Kaliner, M. (1995). Asthma management during pregnancy. *The Female Patient, 20,* 54–70.

Kaliner, M., & Lemanske R. (1992). Rhinitis and asthma. *JAMA, 268*(20), 2807-2829.

Kamada, A. K., & Szefler, S. J. (1995). Glucocorticoids and growth in asthmatic children. *Pediatric Allergy and Immunology, 6,* 145–154.

Kamada, A., Szefler, S. J., Martin, R. J., et al. and the Asthma Clinical Research Network. (1996). Issues in the use of inhaled glucocorticoids. *American Journal of Respiratory Critical Care Medicine, 153,* 1739–1748.

Kendall, M. J., Dean, S., Bradley, D., Gibson, R., & Warthington, D. J. (1982). Cardiovascular and metabolic effects of terbutaline. *Journal of Clinical Hospital Pharmacy, 7*(1), 31–36.

Kerstjens, H. A. M., Brand, P. L. P., Hughes, M. D., et al. (1992). A comparison of bronchodilator therapy with or without inhaled corticosteroids therapy for obstructive airway disease. *New England Journal of Medicine, 327*, 1413–1419.

Klassen, T. P. (1997). Recent advances in the treatment of bronchiolitis and laryngitis. *Pediatric Clinics in North America, 44*(1), 249–259.

Klassen, T. P., Watters, L. K., Feldman, M. E., et al. (1996). The efficacy of budesonide in dexamethasone-treated outpatients with croup. *Pediatrics, 97*, 463.

Klein, J. (1997). Pneumonias. In Gellis & Kagan, *Current Pediatric Therapy* (15th ed.) (pp. 572–574). Philadelphia: W. B. Saunders.

Klein, N. C. (1991). Fluoroquinolones in respiratory infections. *Seminars in Respiratory Infections, 6*(3), 131–135.

Konstans, M., Byrard, P., Hoppel, C., & Davis, C. (1995). Effect of high dose ibuprofen in patients with cystic fibrosis. *New England Journal of Medicine, 332*–348.

Krieger, B. (1996). Respiratory tract infections in the elderly. *Pulmonary Perspectives, 8*, 1–4.

Krilov, L., Mandel, F. S., Barone, S. R., Fagin, J. C., & the Bronchiolitis Study Group. (1997). Followup of children with respiratory syncytial virus bronchiolitis in 1986 and 1987: Potential effect of ribavirin on long-term pulmonary function. *Pediatric Infectious Disease Journal, 16*, 237–276.

Laitinen, A., & Laitinem, L. A. (1994). Airway morphology: Endothelium/basement membrane. *American Journal of Respiratory and Critical Care Medicine, 150*, S14–17.

Laitinen, L. A., Laitinen, A., & Haahtela, T. (1992). A comparative study of the effects of an inhaled corticosteroid, budesonide and a beta-agonist, terbutaline, on airway inflammation in newly diagnosed asthma: A randomized, double-blind, parallel-group controlled trial. *Journal of Allergy and Clinical Immunology, 90*, 32–42.

Landau, L. I. (1996). Risks of developing asthma. *Pediatric Pulmonology, 22*, 314–318.

Lanng, S., Thorsteinsson, B., Nerupo J., & Koch, C. (1992). Influence of the development of diabetes mellitus on clinical status in patients with cystic fibrosis. *European Journal of Pediatrics, 151*(9), 684–687.

Lapin, C., & Cloutier, M. M. (1995). Outpatient management of acute exacerbations of asthma in children. *Journal of Asthma, 32*(1), 5–20.

Larsen, G. L. (1992). Asthma in children. *New England Journal of Medicine, 326*, 1540–1545.

LaVia, W. V., Marks, M. I., & Stutman, H. R. (1992). Respiratory syncytial virus puzzle: Clinical features, pathophysiology, treatment and prevention. *Journal of Pediatrics, 121*, 503–510.

Leeper, K. (1996). Severe community acquired pneumonia. *Seminars in Respiratory Infections, 11*(2), 96–108.

Levison, M. (1998). Pneumonia, including necrotizing pulmonary infections. In A. Fauci et al (Eds.) *Harrison's principles of internal medicine* (14th ed.) New York: McGraw-Hill.

Li, J. T., & O'Connell, J. O. (1996). Clinical evaluation of asthma. *Annals of Allergy, Asthma & Immunology, 76*, 1–15.

Long, S. (1997). Pertussis. In Gellis & Kagan (Eds.), *Current Pediatric Therapy* (15th ed.) (pp. 611–613). Philadelphia: W. B. Saunders.

Luskin, A. (1994). Asthma therapy: What really works. Highlights of the American Academy of Family Physicians 45th Annual Scientific Assembly. *Audio Digest, 42*, 1–2.

Luskin, A. T. (1990). Recalcitrant asthma: An allergist's approach. *Allergy Proceedings, 11*(6), 281–294.

Macato, M. L. (1991). Respiratory insufficiency due to pneumonia in pregnancy. *Obstetrics and Gynecology, 16*, 417–430.

MacDonald, A. (1996). Nutritional management of cystic fibrosis. *Archives of Disease in Childhood, 74*, 81–87.

Madinger, N. E., Greenspoon, J. S., & Ellrodt, A. G. (1989). Pneumonia during pregnancy: Has modern technology improved maternal and fetal outcome. *American Journal of Obstetrics and Gynecology, 161*, 657–662.

Mandell, L. A. (1996). Community-acquired pneumonia. *New England Journal of Medicine, 334*(13), 861–864.

Marcus, E. B., MacLean, C. J., Curb, J. D., Johnson, L. R., Vollmer, W. M., & Buist, A. S. (1988). Reference values for FEV1 in Japanese-American men from 45 to 68 years of age. *American Review of Respiratory Disease, 138*, 1393–1397.

Marrie, T. J. (1994). Community-acquired pneumonia. *Clinical Infectious Diseases, 8*(4), 501–503.

Marrie, T. J. (1996). Atypical pneumonia revisited. *Seminars in Respiratory and Critical Care Medicine, 17*(3), 221–229.

Martin, R. J. (1994). Nocturnal asthma. *Annals of Allergy, 72*, 5–13.

Martin, R. J. (1996). Managing the patient with intractable asthma. *Hospital Practice*, 61–80.

Martin, R. J., Cicutto, L. C., & Ballard, R. D. (1990). Factors related to the nocturnal worsening of asthma. *American Review of Respiratory Diseases, 141*, 33–38.

Martinez, F. D., Wright, A. L., Taussig, L. M., Holberg, C. J., Halonem, M., Morgan, W. J., Group Health Medical Associates. (1995). Asthma and wheezing in the first six years of life. *New England Journal of Medicine, 332*, 133–138.

Mascali, J. J., Cvietusa, P., Negri, J., & Borish, L. (1996). Antiinflammatory effects of theophylline: Modulation of cytokine production. *Annals of Allergy, Asthma & Immunology, 77*, 34–38.

Mason, C. M., & Nelson, S. (1996). Pathophysiology of community-acquired pneumonia and treatment strategies based on host-pathogen interactions: The inflammatory interface. *Seminars in Respiratory and Critical Care Medicine, 17*(3), 213–219.

Matthews, L. W., & Drotar, D. (1994). Cystic fibrosis—A challenging long-term chronic disease. *Pediatric Clinics of North America, 31*(1), 133–149.

Mays, M. & Leiner, S. (1995). Asthma—A comprehensive review. *Journal of Nurse-Midwifery, 40*(3), 256–268.

McColgin, S. W., Glee, L., & Brian, B. A. (1992). Pulmonary disorders complicating pregnancy. *Obstetrics & Gynecology Clinics of North America, 19*(4), 697–717.

McFadden, E. R., Jr., & Gilbert, I. A. (1994). Exercise-induced asthma. *New England Journal of Medicine, 330*, 1362–1367.

McKay, S. E., Howie, C. A., Thompson, A. H., Whiting, B., & Addis, G. J. (1993). Value of theophylline treatment in patients handicapped by chronic obstructive lung disease. *Thorax, 48*, 227–232.

Menon, K., Sutcliffe, T., & Klassen, T. P. (1995). A randomized trial comparing the efficacy of epinephrine to salbutamol in acute bronchiolitis. *Journal of Pediatrics, 126*, 1004+.

Milgrom, H., & Bender, B. (1995). Behavioral side effects of medications used to treat asthma and allergic rhinitis. *Pediatrics in Review, 16*(9), 333–335.

Mittl, R. L., Jr., Schwab, R. J., Duchin, J. S., et al. (1994). Radiographic resolution of community-acquired pneumonia. *American Journal of Respiratory and Critical Care Medicine, 149*, 630–635.

Morgan, W. J., & Martinez, F. D. (1992). Risk factors for developing wheezing and asthma in childhood. *Pediatric Clinics of North America, 39*(6), 1185–1203.

Moroney, C. (1996). Pharmacologic Update: Management of pneumonia in elderly people. *Journal of the American Academy of Nurse Practitioners, 6*(5), 237–241.

Mortenson, J., Falk, M., Groth, S., & Jensen, C. (1991). The effects of postural drainage and positive expiratory pressure physiotherapy on tracheobronchial clearance in cystic fibrosis. *Chest, 100*(5), 1350–1357.

Mouton, J. W., & Kerrebijn, K. F. (1990). Antibacterial therapy in cystic fibrosis. *Medical Clinics of North America, 74*(3), 837–850.

Murphy, S. J., & Kelly, H. W. (1996). Advances in the management of acute asthma in children. *Pediatrics in Review, 17*(7), 227–234.

Musher, D. (1998). Pneumococcal infections. In A. Fauci et al, (Eds.), *Harrison's Principles of Internal Medicine.* New York: McGraw-Hill.

Natasi, K. J., Heinly, T. L., & Blaiss, M. S. (1995). Exercise-induced asthma and the athlete. *Journal of Asthma, 32*(4), 249–257.

National Asthma Education and Prevention Program. (1991). Expert Panel Report. Bethesda, MD: National Institutes of Health, National Health Blood Institute.

National Asthma Education and Prevention Program. (1997). Expert Panel Report. Bethesda, MD: National Institutes of Health, National Health Blood Institute.

National Center for Health Statistics. (1997). *Monthly Vital Statistics Report, 45,* S1–S80.

National Institutes of Health/National Heart, Lung and Blood Institute. (1993). *Executive summary: Management of asthma during pregnancy.* National Institute of Health/National Heart, Lung, and Blood Institute, NIH publication #93-3279A.

Newman, S. R., & Clarke, S. W. (1993). Bronchodilator delivery from gentlehaler, a new low-velocity pressurized aerosol inhaler. *Chest, 103*(5), 1442–1446.

Newson, T., & McKenzie, S. (1996). Cough and asthma in children. *Pediatric Annals, 25*(3), 156–161.

Niederhauser, U. P. (1997). Prescribing for children: Issues in pediatric pharmacology. *Nurse Practitioner, 22*(3), 16–18.

Niederman, M. S., Bass, J. B., & Campbell, G. D., et al. (1993). Guidelines for the initial management of adults with community-acquired pneumonia: Diagnosis, assessment of severity and initial antimicrobial therapy. American Thoracic Society. Medical Section of the American Lung Association. *American Review of Respiratory Disease, 148*(5), 1418–1426.

Nixon, P. A. (1996). Role of exercise in the evaluation and management of pulmonary disease in children and youth. *Medicine & Science of Sports & Exercise, 28*(4), 414–420.

O'Byrne, P. M., & Kerstjens, H. A. M. (1996). Inhaled B2-agonists in the treatment of asthma. *New England Journal of Medicine, 12*, 886–888.

Odeh, M., Oliven, A., & Bassan, H. (1991). Timolol eyedrops-induced fatal bronchospasm in an asthmatic patient. *Journal of Family Practice, 32*(1), 97–98.

Okamoto, L. J., Noonan, M., DeBoisblanc, B. P., & Kellerman, D. J. (1996). Fluticasone propionate improves quality of life in patients with asthma requiring oral corticosteroids. *Annals of Allergy, Asthma, & Immunology, 76*, 455–461.

Orenstein, D. M. (1986). Exercise tolerance and exercise conditioning in children with chronic lung disease. *Journal of Pediatrics, 112*(6), 1043–1047.

Orenstein, S. R. (1994). GERD. *Seminars in Gastrointestinal Diseases, 5*(1), 2–14.

Oswald, H., Phelan, P. D., Lanigan, A., Hibbert, M., Carlin, J. B., Bowes, G., & Olinsky, A. (1997). Childhood asthma and lung function in mid-adult life. *Pediatric Pulmonology, 23*, 14–20.

Oxman, A. D., Muir, D. C. F., Shannon, H. S., Stock, S. R., Hnizdo, E., & Lange, H. J. (1993). Occupational dust exposure and chronic obstructive pulmonary disease. *American Review of Respiratory Disease, 148*, 38–48.

Pallares, R., Linares, J., Vadillo M., et al. (1995). Resistance to penicillin and cephalosporins and mortality from severe pneumococcal pneumonia in Barcelona, Spain. *New England Journal of Medicine, 333*, 474–480.

Panitch, H., Callahan, C., & Schidlow, D. (1993). Bronchiolitis in children. *Clinics in Chest Medicine, 14*(4), 715–727.

PDR Generics. (1996). 2nd ed. *Medical Economics.* Montvale, NJ.

Pearson, D. A., Pumariega, A. J., & Seilheimer, D. K. (1991). The development of psychiatric symptoms in patients with cystic fibrosis. *Journal of the American Academy of Child-Adolescent Psychiatry, 30*(2), 290–297.

Pedersen, S. (1996). Inhalers and nebulizers: Which to choose and why. *Respiratory Medicine, 90*, 69–77.

Peloquin, C. A., & Berning, S. E. (1994). Infection caused by *Mycobacterium tuberculosis. Annals of Pharmacotherapy, 28*, 72–84.

Perlman, P. E., & Ginn, D. R. (1990). Respiratory infections in ambulatory adults. Choosing the best treatment. *Postgraduate Medicine, 87*(1), 175–184.

Piedra, P. A. (1995). Influenza virus pneumonia: Pathogenesis, treatment and prevention. *Seminars in Respiratory Medicine, 10*(4), 216–223.

Pomilla, P. V., & Brown, R. B. (1994). Outpatient treatment of community-acquired pneumonia in adults. *Archives of Internal Medicine, 154*, 1793–1802.

Powell, D. (1996). Mycoplasmal infections. In Behrman et al (Eds.), *Textbook of pediatrics* (15th ed.) (pp. 824–827). Philadelphia: W. B. Saunders.

Prakash, U. (1996). Pulmonary diseases. In *Mayo International Medicine Board Review.* Rochester, MN: Mayo Foundation for Medicine.

Prober, C. (1996). Pneumonia. In Behrman et al (Eds.), *Textbook of pediatrics* (15th ed.) (pp. 716–721). Philadelphia: W. B. Saunders.

Puchelle, E., de Bentzmann, S., & Zahm, J. M. (1995). Physical and functional properties of airway secretions in cystic fibrosis—Therapeutic approaches. *Respiration, 62*(suppl. 1), 2–12.

Pulmonary Disorders. (1997). In E. Cunningham et al, *Williams obstretrics* (20th ed.) (pp. 1103–1121). Norwalk, CT: Appleton & Lange.

Rachelefsky, G. S. (1995a). Asthma update: New approaches and partnerships. *Journal of Pediatric Health Care, 12*–21.

Rachelefsky, G. S. (1995b). Helping patients live with asthma. *Hospital Practice, 15*, 51–63.

Rachelefsky, G., Fitzgerald, S., Page, D., & Santamaria, B. (1993). An update on diagnosis and management of pediatric asthma. *Nurse Practitioner, 18*, 51–61.

Ramsdell, J. (1995). Use of theophylline in the treatment of COPD. *Chest, 107*, S206–S209.

Ramsey, B. W., Farrell, P. M., P. Pancharz, & The Consensus Committee. (1992). Nutritional assessment and management in cystic fibrosis: A consensus report. *American Journal of Clinical Nutrition 55*(1), 108–116.

Reijonen, T., Kroppi, M., Kukka, L., & Remes, K. (1996). Antiinflammatory therapy reduces wheezing after bronchiolitis. *Archives of Pediatric and Adolescent Medicine, 150*, 512–517.

Reilly, K., & Clemenson, N. (1993). Infections complicating pregnancy. *Primary Care, 20*(3), 665–684.

Relman, D., & Schwartz, M. (1994). Diseases due to chlamydia. *Scientific American, 9*, 4–9.

Richey, S. D., Roberts, S., Ramin, K. D., Ramin, S. M., & Cunningham, F. G. (1994). Pneumonia complicating pregnancy. *Obstetrics and Gynecology, 84*(4), 525–691.

Rice, S. G., Bierman, C. W., Shapiro, G. G., Furukawce, C. T., & Pierson, W. E. (1985). Identification of exercise-induced asthma among intercollegiate athletes. *Annals of Allergy, 55*, 790–793.

Rigby, F., & Pastorek, J. G., II. (1996). Pneumonia during pregnancy. *Clinical Obstetrics and Gynecology, 39*(1), 107–119.

Robinson, D. S., & Geddes, D. M. (1996). Inhaled corticosteroids: Benefits and risks. *Journal of Asthma, 33*(1), 5–16.

Roche, W. R. (1991). Fibroblasts and asthma. *Clinical and Experimental Allergy, 21*(5), 545–548.

Rodrigues, J. & Niederman, M. S. (1992). Pneumonia complicating pregnancy. *Pulmonary Disease in Pregnancy, 13*(4), 679–685.

Rodriquez, W. J., Gruber, W. C., Welliver, R. C., Groothuis, J. R., Simoes, E. A. F., Meissner, H. C.,

Hemming, V. G., Hall, C. B., Lepow, M. L., Rosas, A. J., Robertsen, C., & Virus Immune Globulin Study Group. (1997). Respiratory syncytial virus (RSV) immune globulin intravenous therapy for RSV lower respiratory tract infection in infants and young children at high risk for severe RSV infections. *Pediatrics, 99*(3), 454–460.

Roncolli, M., & Dempster, J. S. (1996). Continuing education forum: Asthma medications for children: Guidelines for the primary care practitioner. *Journal of the American Academy of Nurse Practitioners, 8*(5), 243–255.

Roorda, R. J., Gerritsen, J., Van Aalderen, W. M., Schouten, J. P., Veltman, J. C., Weiss, S. T., & Knol, K. (1993). Risk factors for the persistence of respiratory symptoms in childhood asthma. *American Review of Respiratory Disease 148*(6 Pt 1), 1490–1495.

Roosevelt, G., Sheehan, K., Grupp-Phelan, J., et al. (1996). Dexamethasone in bronchiolitis: A randomized controlled trial. *Lancet, 348*, 292.

Rosen, M. J. (1992). Treatment of exacerbations of COPD. *American Family Physician, 45*, 693–697.

Rosenstein, B. J., & Eigen, H. (1991). Risks of alternate day prednisone in patients with cystic fibrosis. 1. *Pediatrics, 87*(2), 245–246.

Ruben, F. L. (1993). Viral pneumonias. The increasing importance of high index of suspicion. *Postgraduate Medicine, 93*(7), 57–64.

Rubin, R. H. (1996). Mycotic infections. *Scientific American,* 6–12.

Rubin, R. H., & O'Hanley, P. (1995). Infections due to gram-negative bacilli. *Scientific American,* 24–27.

Sanchez, I., & Guiraldes, E. (1995). Drug management of noninfective complications of cystic fibrosis. *Drugs, 50*(4), 626–635.

Schaffer, S. D. (1991). Current approaches in adult asthma: Assessment, education and emergency management. *Nurse Practitioner, 16*(12), 18–32.

Schatz, B. S., Karavokiros, K. T., Taeubel, M. A., & Ilokozu, G. S. (1996). Comparison of cefprozil, cefpodoxime proxetil, locarabef, cefixime and ceftibuten. *Annals of Pharmacotherapy, 30*(3), 258–268.

Schatz, M., Zeiger, R. S., Harden, K. M., Hoffman, C. P., Forsythe, A. B., Chilinger, L. M., et al. (1988). The safety of inhaled beta agonist bronchodilators during pregnancy. *Journal of Allergy and Clinical Immunology, 82*, 686–695.

Schatz, M., Zeiger, R. S., Hoffman, C. P. & the Kaiser-Permanente Asthma and Pregnancy Study Group. (1990). Intrauterine growth is related to gestational pulmonary function in pregnant asthmatic women. *Chest, 98*(2), 389–392.

Schidlow, D. V., & Callahan, C. W. (1996). Pneumonia. *Pediatrics in Review, 17*(9), 300–309.

Schreiber, J. R., & Jacobs, M. R. (1995). Antibiotic-resistant pneumococci. *Antimicrobial Resistance in Pediatrics, 42*(3), 519–532.

Seidel, J. (1996). Delivering nebulized medication to infants and toddlers. *Pediatrics in Review, 17*(9), 327.

Selroos, O., Pietinalho, A., Lofroos, A., & Riska, H. (1995). Effect of early versus late intervention with inhaled corticosteroids in asthma. *Chest, 108*, 1228–1234.

Shulman, V., Alderman, E., Ewig, J. M., & Bye, M. R. (1996). Asthma in the pregnant adolescent: A review. *Journal of Adolescent Medicine, 18*, 168–176.

Shuttari, M. F. (1995). Asthma: Diagnosis and management. *American Family Physician, 52*(8), 2225–2235.

Simon, H. B. (1995). Infections due to gram-positive cocci. *Scientific American, 7*, 2–4.

Simons, F. E., Persaud, M. P., Gillespie, C. A., Cheang, M., & Schuckett, E. P. (1993). Absence of posterior subcapsular cataracts in young patients treated with inhaled glucocorticoids. *Lancet, 342*, 776–778.

Singulair (1998). Drug Product Information Sheet, Merck and Company.

Skorodin, M. S. (1993). Pharmacotherapy for asthma and chronic obstructive pulmonary disease. *Archives of Internal Medicine, 153*, 814–828.

Smith, A. L., & Ramsey, B. (1995). Aerosol administration of antibiotics. *Respiration, 62*(suppl 1), 19–24.

Spahn, J. D., & Kamada, A. K. (1995). Special considerations in the use of glucocorticoids in children. *Pediatrics in Review, 16*(7), 266–272.

Sporik, R., Holgate, S. T., Platts-Mills, T. A., & Cogswell, J. J. (1990). Exposure to house-dust mite allergen (Der p1) and the development of asthma in childhood. A prospective study. *New England Journal of Medicine, 323*, 502–507.

St. John, R. C., Gadek, J. E., & Pacht, E. R. (1993). Chronic obstructive pulmonary disease: Less common causes. *Journal of General Internal Medicine, 8*, 564–572.

Stauffer, J. L. (1995). Lung. In L. M. Tierney, Jr., S. J. McPhee, & M. A. Papadakis (Eds.), *Current medical diagnosis and treatment* (pp. 203–280). Norwalk, CT: Appleton & Lange.

Thompson, A. (1997). Pneumonia. In R. Hoekelman, S. Friedman, et al. (Eds.), *Primary pediatric care* (pp. 133–145). St. Louis: Mosby-Year Book.

Toogood, J. H. (1993). Making better—and safer—use of inhaled steroids. *The Journal of Respiratory Diseases, 14*(2), 221–237.

U.S. Department of Health and Human Services, Public Health Service, Centers for Disease Control and Prevention, National Center for Prevention Services, Division of Tuberculosis Elimination. (1994). *Treating Tuberculosis: A Clinical Guide.* Atlanta, GA.

U.S. Department of Health and Human Services, Public Health Service, National Institutes of Health, National Heart, Lung, and Blood Institute. (1995). *Pocket guide for asthma management and prevention.*

Vathenen, A. S., Knox, A. J., Wisniewski, A., & Tattersfield, A. E. (1991a). Effect of inhaled budesonide on bronchial reactivity to histamine, exercise and eucapnic dry air hyperventilation in patients with asthma. *Thorax, 46*(11), 811–816.

Vathenen, A. S., Knox, A. J., Wisniewski, A., & Tattersfield, A. E. (1991b). Time course of change in bronchial reactivity on inhaled corticosteroids in asthma. *American Review of Respiratory Disease, 143*(6), 1317–1321.

Virant, F. S. (1991). Exercise-induced bronchospasms: Epidemiology, pathophysiology and therapy. *Medicine & Science of Sports & Exercise, 24,* 851–855.

Waalkens, H. J., Merkus, P. J., van Essen Zandvliet, E. E., Brand, P. L., Gerritsen, J., Duiverman, E. J., Kerrebyn, K. F., Knol, K. K., & Quangler, P. H. (1993). Assessment of bronchodilator response in children with asthma. Dutch CNSLD Study Group. *European Respiratory Journal, 6*(5), 645–651.

Waalkens, H. J., van Essen Zandvliet, E. E., Gerritsen, J., Duiverman, E. J., Kerrebyn, K. F., & Knol, K. (1993). The effect of an inhaled corticosteroid (budesonide) on exercise-induced asthma in children. Dutch CNSLD Study Group. *European Respiratory Journal, 6*(5), 614–616.

Walker, C., Bode, E., Boer, L., Hansel, T. T., Blaser, K., & Virchow, J. C., Jr. (1992). Allergic and nonallergic asthmatics have distinct patterns of T-cell activation and cytokine production in peripheral blood and bronchoaveolar lavage. *American Review of Respiratory Disease, 146*(1), 109–115.

Webb, A. K. (1995). The treatment of pulmonary infections in cystic fibrosis. *Scandinavian Journal of Infectious Disease, 96*(Suppl), 24–27.

Welliver, R. C. (1997). Therapy for bronchiolitis: Help wanted. *Journal of Pediatrics, 130,* 170–172.

Wenzel, S. E., & Kamada, A. K. (1996). Zileuton: The first 5-lipoxygenase inhibitor for the treatment of asthma. *The Annals of Pharmacotherapy, 30,* 858–864.

White, K. R., Munro, C. L., & Boyle, A. H. (1996). Nursing management of adults who have cystic fibrosis. *Medsurg Nursing, 5*(3), 163–167.

Williams, D. M. (1995). Chronic Obstructive Airway Disease. In L. L. Young & M. A. Koda-Kimble (Eds.), *Applied therapeutics: The clinical use of drugs* (pp. 20-1 to 20-12). Vancouver, WA: Applied Therapeutics, Inc.

Wilmott, R. W., & Fiedler, M. A. (1994). Recent advances in the treatment of cystic fibrosis. *Respiratory Medicine* II, *41*(3), 431–447.

Wolthers, O. D. (1996). Long-, intermediate-, and short-term growth studies in asthmatic children treated with inhaled glucocorticosteroids. *European Respiratory Journal, 9*(4), 821–827.

Woolcock, A., Lundbeck, B., Ringdal, N., & L. A. Jacques. (1996). Comparison of addition of salmneterol to inhaled steroids with doubling of the dose of inhaled steroid. *American Journal of Respiratory Critical Care Medicine, 153,* 1481–1488.

Yang, E., & Rubin, B. K. (1995). "Childhood" viruses as a cause of pneumonia in adults. *Seminars in Respiratory Infections, 10*(4), 232–243.

Yu, N. C., & Maurer, J. R. (1996). Community-acquired pneumonia in high-risk populations. *Seminars in Respiratory and Critical Care Medicine, 17*(3), 255–257.

# 23

## EYE DISORDERS

*Joanne K. Singleton and Robert V. DiGregorio*

The eye is a sophisticated and sensitive organ. Eye disorders occur across the lifespan, with the most common disorders resulting from inflammation, infection, trauma, or increased intraocular pressure. The following common eye disorders seen in primary care will be reviewed in this chapter: corneal abrasion, disorders of *the eyelid* (hordeolum, chalazion, and blepharitis), conjunctivitis, glaucoma, and uveitis. Primary care providers should be able to diagnose and treat many of these conditions; however, several, once suspected, require an immediate ophthalmology consultation. For those conditions in which treatment is initiated and managed by an ophthalmologist, primary care providers must be fully aware of current management plans and expected outcomes.

## CORNEAL ABRASION

The cornea is a transparent, avascular, biconvex structure of the eye, which receives rich sensory innervation from the trigeminal, or fifth, cranial nerve. Major functions of the cornea include refraction of light and protection of the eye from injury and infection. The epithelium is the outermost layer of the five layers that comprise the cornea. Corneal abrasion is the result of localized loss of the epithelium. Common causes of corneal abrasion include direct trauma, foreign bodies, and contact lenses. Differentiation of

traumatic corneal abrasion from that associated with contact lens wear is critical in the treatment and management of this condition.

The baseline history should include a thorough assessment of the injury: when it occurred, where it occurred, and especially what occurred. Common symptoms associated with corneal abrasion include pain, reduced visual acuity, lacrimation, photophobia, foreign body sensation, and blepharospasm (involuntary movement of the eyelids). Additionally, question patients about known drug allergies or sensitivities, past and current medical conditions, family history of glaucoma, head injury, hypermetropia (farsightedness), presbyopia (inability to focus on near objects), and current medications.

The following signs should be evaluated on physical examination: lid swelling, visual acuity measured by the Snellen chart, conjunctival injection, circumcorneal injection, anterior chamber depth, and fluorescein dye uptake by damaged corneal tissue. To evaluate the corneal defect, fluorescein dye 2% is topically applied to the affected eye, and the eye is examined using Wood's lamp or a cobalt blue slit lamp. Contact lenses must be removed before applying the fluorescein dye. Damaged corneal epithelium tissue will take up the fluorescein, and fluorescein will react with the light, thereby outlining the affected area. Short-acting topical anesthetic drops may be required to facilitate the examination (Bertolini & Pelucio, 1995; Jampel, 1995; Knox & McIntee, 1995).

## SPECIFIC CONSIDERATIONS FOR PHARMACOTHERAPY

### When Drug Therapy Is Needed

Treatment should relieve pain, reduce the risk of or prevent bacterial infection, and promote healing. Corneal abrasions usually heal within 48 h, whether left untreated or covered with an eye patch (Jampel, 1995). Pharmacotherapy, while not absolutely necessary, is often used for pain relief related to ciliary muscle spasm and the prevention of secondary infections (Jampel 1995; Knox & McIntee, 1995). Steroids should be avoided since their use is associated with enhanced bacterial replication and herpes simplex activation. The use of mydriatic eye drops is contraindicated in patients with a positive family history of narrow-angle glaucoma, head injury, hypermetropia, or presbyopia. Before using mydriatic eye drops, the anterior chamber depth must be evaluated to avoid precipitating an attack of acute angle-closure glaucoma.

### Short-Term and Long-Term Goals of Pharmacotherapy

The short-term goal of treating corneal abrasions is pain relief. The long-term goals of treating corneal abrasions are complete cure and prevention of infection. In the context of corneal abrasion therapy, these long-term goals should be attainable within 24–48 h.

### Nonpharmacologic Therapy

Controversy exists in the literature regarding the role of immobilizing the eyelids with a patch. Although commonly done, there is no definitive evidence that patching an eye results in faster healing. Patching the eye for 24–48 h may provide greater comfort for the patient because the immobilized eyelids will not rub against the abrasion. The patch is usually combined with adjunctive cycloplegic agents as well as ophthalmic antibiotics. *It must be noted that corneal abrasions associated with contact lens injuries should not be managed with an eye patch and must be treated with ophthalmic antibiotics* (Bertolini & Pelucio, 1995; Jampel, 1995; Knox & McIntee, 1995).

### Time Frame for Initiating Pharmacotherapy

Since corneal abrasions are associated with a significant amount of pain and infections can develop rapidly, treatment should be initiated as soon as possible. Corneal abrasions generally heal within 48 h because the epithelium regenerates rapidly; thus, cycloplegic therapy should not be needed beyond 48 h. Antibiotics are generally empirically utilized for approximately 1 week.

Pain relief due to cilliary spasm is generally achieved within 30–60 min after cycloplegic preparations are administered (*Ophthalmic Drug Facts*, 1996). However, patients may still have pain from exposed corneal nerve endings. General healing occurs within 48 h.

See Drug Table 401.1, 2.

### Patient/Caregiver Information

Patients should be advised how to prevent future corneal abrasions; for example, if corneal abrasions are due to work-related trauma or a foreign body, use of protective eye wear should be encouraged. Contact lens wearers should be reminded to clean their lenses more frequently.

## OUTCOMES MANAGEMENT

### Selecting Appropriate Agents

Topical steroids should be avoided. Homatropine hydrobromide 2–5% or cyclopentolate 0.5–2% are appropriate cycloplegic agents based on a 30-min onset of action and moderate duration of action (1–3 days). Homatropine is a more cost-effective agent than other cycloplegics. The usual dose of these agents is one or two drops of the solution prior to antibiotic instillation, and patching is used when indicated. Patients with a heavily pigmented iris may require higher doses. The lower-percentage solutions are reserved for pediatric use.

Choice of an antibiotic agent should be based on the type of abrasion, with antipseudomonal agents used exclusively for contact lens wearers and sulfacetamide for all others. Although gentamicin is the most inexpensive of the antipseudomonal agents, an increased resistance of *Pseudomonas aeruginosa* to gentamicin has made tobramycin and ciprofloxacin the preferred agents (*Ophthalmic Drug Facts*, 1996). Efficacy is established by the relief of pain, decreased inflammation, and absence of infection.

### Monitoring for Toxicity

Prolonged use of cycloplegic products may produce irritation and edema in the eyelid.

Systemic toxicity presents as anticholinergic poisoning with dryness of the mouth, blurred vision, tachycardia, fever, urinary retention, dysarthria, vasodilation, coma, and even death.

## Follow-up Recommendations

Follow-up examinations for patients with corneal abrasions should be scheduled for 24 h after the initial examination and treatment. Follow-up should include evaluation of common complications of corneal abrasion: recurrent erosion, corneal ulceration, and secondary iritis.

# DISORDERS OF THE EYELID: HORDEOLUM, CHALAZION, AND BLEPHARITIS

Eyelids, accessory organs of the eye, are lined with elongated sebaceous glands called *meibomian* glands, the smaller sebaceous glands of Zeis at the edge of the lid, and the modified sweat glands of Moll at the border of the lids. Projecting from the margin of the eyelids are eyelashes that are lubricated by fluid from these glands.

A hordeolum, or the common stye—an acute inflammation of a hair follicle of the eyelash or a gland of the eyelid—forms when there is infection and blockage of the gland(s). The cause of infection is usually *Staphylococcus aureus*. A hordeolum resembling a pimple appears on the lid margin, and may be internal with pointing onto the conjunctival surface of the lid. It is red, tender, and painful, and may be accompanied by moderate conjunctival injection (Crouch & Berger, 1995).

A chalazion results from a chronic inflammation of a meibomian gland. It is not usually preceded by acute inflammation, and appears approximately 2 mm or more from the margin of the eyelid, with pointing of the lesion inside the lid (Diegel, 1986). Secondary infection may develop in surrounding tissue.

Blepharitis is an inflammation of the eyelid margins and associated structures. It is a chronic condition, usually bilateral, and is seen in all age groups, but especially in the elderly population. Although there are elaborate classification schemes for blepharitis, the two basic classifications are *seborrhea* and *infectious*, which may be found together. Patients often identify a history

of hordeola or chalazia. Blepharitis may present with an associated conjunctivitis and tear deficiency, which is a risk factor for this condition. Factors that may contribute to acute phases of blepharitis and cause inflammation and irritation include: eye makeup, contact lens buildup, smoke, smog, and chemicals (Raskin, Speaker, & Laibson, 1992; Smith & Flowers, 1995; Wittpenn, 1995).

The usual organism found in blepharitis is staphylococcus, primarily *S. aureus* and secondarily *S. epidermidis*. Patients present with inflamed eyelids, moderate erythema, fibrinous scaling and crusts, and may have loss of lashes.

Eyelid inflammation in patients with seborrheic blepharitis is less prominent and is accompanied by greasy or oily scaling. There is a high incidence of other seborrheic dermatoses in these patients, ie, rosacea, psoriasis, seborrhea, and dandruff (Wittpenn, 1995).

Patients who present with blepharitis often complain of itching, burning, and a chronic foreign body sensation. There is no cure for blepharitis since those affected by staphyloccus are most likely susceptible to the organism and suffer from reinfection; those with seborrhea blepharitis have other underlying dermatologic pathologies.

The baseline history in patients with conditions of the eyelid should include identification of onset, symptoms, and previous occurrences, response to treatment; and known drug sensitivity. Common symptoms of hordeolum include pain, redness, and tenderness on palpation of the affected eyelid. In addition to the baseline history for hordeolum, the patient with chalazion should be asked about changes in visual acuity, a feeling of pressure on the affected eye, and tenderness or pain of the affected eyelid. In patients with blepharitis, the baseline history should also include presence of skin problems and exposure to eye makeup, contact lens buildup, smoke, chemicals, or smog.

On physical examination, evaluate the following signs for disorders of the eyelid: visual acuity, eyelid abnormalities, pointing of the lesion, abnormalities of the sclerae and conjunctivae, and adenopathy, particularly in the preauricular area. In patients with blepharitis, use a magnifier to inspect the eyelids and assess erythema, scaling, and ulcers.

Diagnostic tests are not indicated for either a hordeolum or chalazion; in refractory cases of blepharitis a culture should be obtained.

## SPECIFIC CONSIDERATIONS FOR PHARMACOTHERAPY

### When Drug Therapy Is Needed

The initial treatments of hordeolum, chalazion, and blepharitis are primarily nondrug regimens. The aim of treatment for a hordeolum is to stimulate drainage of the gland and to eliminate the infectious bacteria. Patients need to be aware that there is currently no cure for blepharitis and that the goals of treatment are to control symptoms and prevent secondary complications.

Chalazia that are large or persist for several months may require treatment. Local or systemic treatment is generally not successful, and incision and curettage are recommended.

Antibiotic ointment is valuable in the treatment of blepharitis because it adheres to the eyelid margin; however, if more than small amounts are used, it can cause blurring of vision and therefore should be used at night. Antibiotic drops can be used during the daytime but may not be as effective as the ointment.

The drugs of choice are bacitracin and erythromycin. Gentamicin and tobramycin may also be used, although they may not be well tolerated in chronic treatment. In patients with coexisting conditions, additional treatment directed at the concomitant condition is necessary.

Topical antibiotics may be useful for refractory cases, and systemic antibiotics may be substituted if topical therapy fails. Topical antibiotics are more commonly used in the treatment of blepharitis, with therapy focused on the eradication of *S. aureus*.

### Short-Term and Long-Term Goals of Pharmacotherapy

The short- and long-term goals of treating a hordeolum or chalazion are reversal of the blocked meibomian gland(s). Blepharitis is a disorder without a cure; the goals of therapy are geared towards a reduction in episode frequency. During the acute phase, direct the therapy at controlling the disease process. This first phase usually lasts 2–8 weeks. Over the long term, a reduction in episode frequency is achieved by determining the minimal amount of therapy necessary to maintain control.

### Nonpharmacologic Therapy

Nonpharmacologic therapy centers on warm compresses applied to the affected area, several times a day. The refractory chalazion can be removed surgically. Meticulous lid hygiene is essential for managing blepharitis. Lid hygiene should consist of warm eyelid scrubs with a cotton-tipped applicator, with either a 1:5 dilution of baby shampoo or a commercial eye scrub. Identification and removal of contributing factors, ie, cosmetics, are essential to reducing the frequency of episodes.

### Time Frame for Initiating Pharmacotherapy

Nonpharmacologic and pharmacologic therapy should begin as soon as possible. Therapy should be continued until the hordeolum or chalazion is relieved. Antibiotics are generally used for 5–7 days. Blepharitis treatment consists of two phases; the acute phase lasts from 2–8 weeks, and the maintenance phase lasts indefinitely.

Relief of these disorders varies. Chalazia resolve spontaneously after 3–4 months without therapy. If the hordeolum or chalazion persists, the patient should be referred to an ophthalmologist. Blepharitis may be controlled in as little as several days to 8 weeks; however, chronic therapy is needed to maintain the therapeutic goal (Dreyer, 1996; Raskin et al, 1992; Smith & Flowers, 1995).

See Drug Table 401.2.

### Patient/Caregiver Information

Patients or their caregivers should apply the antibiotic ointment evenly over the margins of the eyelid. Ointment can cause blurring and loss of binocular vision; patients should be advised not to drive.

Patients who present with hordeolum need to be instructed in eye hygiene. Makeup should not be worn until the stye has resolved, current eye makeup should be discarded, and the same eye makeup should not be used for long periods of time.

## OUTCOMES MANAGEMENT

### Selecting Appropriate Agents

Infection of the meibomian glands is usually caused by staphylococcus. The agent of choice for treating this infection is bacitracin. Alternative therapies have included aminoglycosides (gentamicin, tobramycin), vancomycin, and quinolones (ciprofloxacin, norfoxacin). The quinolones and the aminoglycosides have shown equal efficacy in several studies (Bloom et al, 1994; Gwon, 1992; Miller, Vogel, Cook, & Wittreich, 1992). The quinolones typically are the most expensive of the available therapies. Thus, these agents are reserved for refractory cases or for patients who cannot tolerate aminoglycoside preparations. Systemic therapy, if warranted, is generally initiated by an ophthalmologist and can be accomplished cost-effectively with oxacillin, amoxicillin, or occasionally tetracycline (contraindicated in pregnant women and young children).

## Monitoring for Efficacy and Toxicity

Efficacy is primarily judged by the eradication of the hordeolum or chalazion. Efficacy in blepharitis therapy is observed when the apparent lid dermatitis has disappeared and reported symptoms have resolved. There is no need to monitor for toxicity.

## Follow-up Recommendations

Since a hordeolum should resolve within 2 weeks of treatment, follow-up is usually not required. Chalazia that have not resolved after 3–4 months should be evaluated by an ophthalmologist for possible surgical excision. Sometimes a chronic chalazion may actually turn out to be a misdiagnosed carcinoma. Patients who present with chalazia and secondary infection should be treated and reevaluated in 2 weeks, whereas patients with small chalazia do not need follow-up care.

Chronic blepharitis should be followed closely until a maintenance phase is clearly established. Patients with mild cases of blepharitis can receive follow-up care at regularly scheduled appointments to evaluate effectiveness of maintenance treatment. In more severe cases, patients should be reevaluated in 10–14 days.

# GLAUCOMA

The term *glaucoma* actually refers to a group of optic disorders reflecting a variety of changes that alter the functional anatomy of the eye, leading to increased internal pressure of the eye, cupping of the optic nerve, optic nerve atrophy, and visual field loss. Blindness may occur if the pressure is not controlled. The two major types of glaucoma are *open-angle* and *closed-angle*.

Both types can be *primary*, or inherited, or *secondary*, related to injury or underlying disease or precipitated by medications. Glaucoma is the second most common cause of blindness in the United States, and the most common cause of blindness in the black population. Risk factors include; age, race, heredity, and myopia (Bensinger, 1994; Gelvin, 1994; Long & Long, 1994; Rosenberg, 1995; Tucker, 1993). This section only discusses primary open-angle glaucoma, the most prevalent form of glaucoma.

Primary open-angle glaucoma—often called the "silent blinder"—is an inherited, bilateral disorder, usually seen after the age of 40, with the greatest incidence in those over 75. In primary open-angle glaucoma, there is a slow, gradual increase in intraocular pressure due to a low-grade outflow obstruction of the aqueous fluid from the anterior chamber. This causes a gradual loss in peripheral vision; if untreated, it will lead to a reduction of the central field of vision. In the early stages of the disease, midperipheral field vision may be affected; however, irreversible damage has occurred before the patient experiences visual changes. Medical management using drug therapy is usually initiated by an ophthalmologist and comanaged by the primary care provider (Bensinger 1994; Gelvin, 1994; Long & Long, 1994; Rosenberg, 1995; Tucker, 1993).

The baseline history should include identification of risk factors as well as loss of peripheral vision, one or both eyes are involved, and onset. Medication history and known drug sensitivities must also be identified.

The physical examination should include measurement of intraocular pressure (the acceptable range is 10–21 mm Hg) a fundoscopic examination to assess the disk for cupping, and gross measurement of visual fields by direct confrontation. Patients in whom open-angle glaucoma is suspected should be referred to an ophthalmologist for a complete examination (Bensinger, 1994; Long & Long, 1994; Uphold & Graham, 1994).

Current diagnostic tests used to screen for open-angle glaucoma include tonometry, ophthalmoscopy, and perimetry (evaluation of visual fields). Sensitivity and specificity of tonometry and ophthalmoscopy are poor for predicting open-angle glaucoma. Such a diagnosis is best made by perimetry, which has good sensitivity and specificity in identification of visual field damage in open-angle glaucoma. It is not an effective screening tool since it detects irreversible field loss rather than early disease (Tucker, 1993).

## SPECIFIC CONSIDERATIONS FOR PHARMACOTHERAPY

### When Drug Therapy Is Needed

The goal of therapy is to reduce the intraocular pressure to prevent further damage to the optic nerve and vision loss. Glaucoma is primarily medically managed, although surgical interventions are possible. Medical management centers on reducing ocular hypertension and minimizing drug-induced adverse reactions. The choice of a medication regimen is usually made by an ophthalmologist (Gelvin, 1994). It also should be noted that glaucoma can be aggravated or induced by medications such as anticholinergics, benzodiazepines, phenothiazines, tricyclic antidepressants, and corticosteroids (Abel, 1995). Patients with a history suggestive of glaucoma should have a thorough medication history taken for possible drug association.

### Short-Term and Long-Term Goals of Pharmacotherapy

The short- and long-term goal in comanaging the glaucoma patient is to lower intraocular pressure and stave off resultant ocular atrophy and loss of vision.

### Nonpharmacologic Therapy

Modern surgical techniques such as laser surgery and filtration surgery serve as alternatives to medical therapy in unresponsive patients.

### Time Frame for Initiating Pharmacotherapy

Medical therapy should be initiated when the optic disk exhibits pathologic changes in addition to an increase in intraocular pressure. An increase in intraocular pressure of less than 30 mm Hg with a normal optic disk does not warrant therapy. Glaucoma management is chronic, despite a relative lack of symptoms in the patient. Significant reductions in intraocular pressure can be seen within 1–2 weeks of therapy initiation. However, pressures may increase slightly before stabilizing. It may take 4–6 weeks for intraocular pressure to stabilize.

See Drug Table 401.1.

### Patient/Caregiver Information

Ocular hypertension is similar to cardiovascular hypertension in that it is a silent disease, with successful management dependent upon the patient's participation in her or his medication regimen. Patients and caregivers should receive extensive counseling regarding the importance of regular use of their prescribed medical therapy regardless of a disappearance of symptoms. See Table 23–1 for basic information both patients and caregivers can use to help administer eyedrops.

## OUTCOMES MANAGEMENT

### Selecting Appropriate Agents

Medical management of glaucoma, usually prescribed by an ophthalmologist, is most often initiated with a beta-adrenergic antagonist, such as timolol 0.25%, one drop twice daily. Therapy

---

## TABLE 23–1. PATIENT AND CAREGIVER INFORMATION FOR ADMINISTERING OPHTHALMIC SOLUTIONS AND SUSPENSIONS

1. Wash hands thoroughly prior to administration.
2. Tilt the patient's head backward or have the patient lie down.
3. Gently grasp the lower eyelid and pull the eyelid away from the eye, forming a pocket.
4. Without coming in contact with fingers or the eye itself, position the dropper over the eye and instill a drop.
5. Have the patient look down.
6. Release the eyelid.
7. Using a fingertip, gently apply pressure to the inside corner of the eye for several minutes.
8. Do not rub the eye.
9. Do not rinse the dropper.
10. Do not use eyedrops if their color has changed.
11. Wait 3–5 min between medications when administering multiple eye preparations.

*Source: Adapted from* Ophthalmic Drug Facts *(1996).*

can be limited to one eye until an efficacy and side-effect profile is established. Alternatives to beta-adrenergic blockers include pilocarpine or epinephrine. Dorzolamide, the new topical carbonic anhydrase inhibitor, may also be used alone or in combination with a beta-adrenergic antagonist (Serle, 1994).

Beta-adrenergic antagonists have proven efficacy with 20–30% reductions in intraocular pressure. The products available differ slightly from one another. Timolol, the oldest of the ophthalmic products, is inexpensive relative to the other agents but may not be as well tolerated as carteolol. Metipranolol and levobunolol are newer agents that are as effective as timolol. Currently they are used less often, probably only because of practitioner comfort and experience with the traditional agent, timolol. Betaxolol is slightly less effective than timolol, but offers beta$_1$ selectivity for use in patients for whom beta-adrenergic antagonists are typically contraindicated (Brooks & Gillies, 1992; Frichman, Fuksbrumer, & Tannenbaum, 1994; Zimmerman, 1993).

Parasympathomimetics, such as pilocarpine, may be substituted for beta-adrenergic blockers in those patients unable to tolerate the latter. Therapy may be initiated with a 0.5–1% solution (one drop three to four times daily) and titrated up until efficacy is achieved. Epinephrine ophthalmic solution or the related compound, dipivefrin, also may be used as initial therapy.

If a patient is unresponsive to a medication, therapy can generally be switched to an alternative agent rather than combining therapies. Each medication should undergo dose titration first, and should then be switched to an alternative agent with a 1-day overlap of the old and new therapies (Lesar, 1997).

## Monitoring for Efficacy

Symptomatic relief usually occurs within 2–6 h after beta-adrenergic antagonist administration. However, it may take 3 weeks to 3 months for intraocular pressure to be lowered. Pilocarpine and the parasympatholytics may decrease intraocular pressure within 10–30 min.

## Monitoring for Toxicity

In cases of acute overdosage with these preparations, the eye should be flushed with warm tap water or saline solution. Many of these products contain benzalkonium chloride as a preservative agent and should be avoided in soft contact lens wearers (Chapman, Cheeks, & Green, 1990).

## Follow-up Recommendations

Follow-up care should be provided by a ophthalmologist. Follow-up should occur at 2-week intervals initially, followed by 3-month intervals once stabilization has occurred. Patients must continue therapy even after symptoms have resolved. Primary care providers comanage through their understanding of the antiglaucoma medications, of their potential for systemic effects, and of the high frequency with which patients either do not use their eye medications or do not administer them correctly.

## CONJUNCTIVITIS

Conjunctivitis is an inflammation of the conjunctiva. The classification of conjunctivitis is primarily based on cause: allergic, bacterial, chemical, fungal, parasitic, and viral.

Ocular allergy is often the cause of allergic conjunctivitis. It is usually differentiated from infectious conjunctivitis based on seasonality, intense itching, and recurrence.

Bacterial conjunctivitis is seen worldwide and occurs in all age groups. Common bacterial pathogens include: Staphylococcus aureus, Streptococcus species; Haemophilus influenzae, Neisseria gonorrhoeae, Proteus species, and Klebsiella. Contamination with the invading organism causes an acute inflammatory response that is most often self-limiting. However, in patients whose immune status is compromised, bacterial conjunctivitis can progress to a sight-threatening infection.

Gonococcal conjunctivitis may be seen in individuals who come in contact with infected genital secretions. Presenting as a copious purulent discharge that may result in corneal perforation, gonococcal conjuntivitis is considered an ophthalmologic emergency. Gonococcal ophthalmia neonatorum—gonococcal infection in the neonate—presents as a serosanguinous discharge, which rapidly changes to purulent exudate 24–48 hours after delivery. Instillation of silver nitrate drops or erythromycin ointment at birth has resulted in a significant decrease in this infection.

Viral conjunctivitis is usually caused by adenoviruses. The more benign condition, commonly seen in children, is pharyngoconjunctival fever, caused by adenovirus types 3 and 7. Adenovirus types 8 and 9 cause epidemic keratoconjunctivitis, which is highly contagious. Treatment for viral conjunctivitis caused by adenoviruses is aimed at relief of symptoms. Viral ocular infection can also occur with the herpes simplex virus; when suspected, an immediate ophthalmologic consultation is required (Bertolini & Pelucio, 1995).

Fungal conjunctivitis is rare. It is seen most often in patients who are immunosuppressed or who are receiving broad-spectrum antibiotic therapy or glucocorticoid therapy.

*Chlamydia trachomatis* causes ocular and genital disease in humans. *C. trachomatis* is most often transmitted venereally and through contaminated eye makeup, and may also be associated with unsanitary conditions and poorly chlorinated swimming pools. The coexistence in women of chlamydial conjunctivitis and genital disease is extremely high—over 90%; for men, over 60% will have genitourinary symptoms (Bertolini & Pelucio, 1995). Trachoma, a chronic contagious form of conjunctivitis, is the leading cause of blindness in humans and generally is seen in the southwest United States.

Chemical conjunctivitis can be caused by any offending agent that comes in contact with the eye. The most common offending agents are chemicals found in eyedrops. Additional offending agents may include: eye makeup, household cleaning agents, and insect bites in the periorbital area.

Characteristics of conjunctivitis include loss of pupillary vision or intraocular pressure changes; itching, tearing, and diffuse conjunctival hyperemia will be present. Distinguishing features in bacterial conjunctivitis include mucopurulent discharge, with morning matting of the eyes, usually unilateral at onset but after a few days becoming bilateral; in viral conjunctivitis foreign body sensation, excessive tearing, mucoid discharge, preauricular adenopathy, and corneal infiltrates or punctate staining may be present; and in allergic conjunctivitis excessive itching is present with a clear discharge. Treatment is directed at the specific organism. Gram staining is the gold standard for determining the cause in bacterial conjunctivitis; however, it is reserved for cases that do not respond after 48–72 h of treatment.

A baseline history should include onset of symptoms; contact with anyone with pinkeye; upper respiratory symptoms; type of discharge; matting of eyelids upon awaking; photophobia; history of allergies, *Chlamydia*, herpes simplex, or herpes zoster; and chemical irritants or insect bites in the area of the eye. Known drug sensitivities must also be identified.

On physical examination visual acuity should be measured, preauricular nodes should be evaluated, and a complete examination of the external structures of the eye should be performed. In addition, evaluate discharge and culture if purulent and perform a fundoscopic examination. Patients with conjunctivitis who have changes in visual acuity, photophobia, and pain should be referred for ophthalmologic consultation.

Bacterial conjunctivitis should improve with treatment within several days; the viral version may not resolve for several weeks and is contagious, so patients must be advised not to rub their eyes and cross-contaminate the other eye or another person. Allergic conjunctivitis is relieved with treatment, and chemical conjunctivitis is relieved after identification and removal of the offending agent.

## SPECIFIC CONSIDERATIONS FOR PHARMACOTHERAPY

### When Drug Therapy Is Needed

Conjunctivitis is usually a self-limiting inflammatory disorder associated with multiple causes, including bacteria, viruses, allergens, chemicals, and mechanical irritants. Although it is self-limiting, the use of medical therapies shortens the time to resolution by about 75% (Dreyer, 1996). Since it may be difficult to ascertain the etiology of the conjunctivitis, therapy is geared toward bacterial conjunctivitis with topical antibiotics (Bertolini & Pelucio, 1995). Allergic conjunctivitis is differentiated by the presence of itching in addition to seasonal recurrence. The treatment of allergic conjunctivitis includes antihistamines, decongestants, mast-cell stabilizers, and cold compresses. If bacterial and allergic conjunctivitis are ruled out, viral conjunctivitis may be considered and treated with antiviral agents.

### Short-Term and Long-Term Goals of Pharmacotherapy

The primary goal in managing conjunctivitis is achieving comfort for the patient, followed by cure.

### Nonpharmacologic Therapy

Warm compresses and eye scrubs are considered as adjunctive therapies to antibiotics for bacterial conjunctivitis. Cold compresses and identification and eradication of causative allergens are beneficial for allergic conjunctivitis. Conjunctivitis secondary to chemical or foreign body exposure should be treated with copious amounts of water, saline, or eyewash solution.

## Time Frame for Initiating Pharmacotherapy

Therapy should be initiated as soon as possible for patient comfort. Antibiotics are generally used for approximately 5–7 days. Antivirals are generally used for 14–21 days. Therapy for allergic conjunctivitis may be necessary for several months if the allergen cannot be eliminated. Bacterial conjunctivitis usually resolves in 48–72 h with treatment and in 2 weeks without treatment. Viral conjunctivitis responds to therapy in 2–3 weeks. Response to allergic conjunctivitis therapies should be seen within a few days.

See Drug Table 401.3, 4, 5.

## Patient/Caregiver Information

Patients and caregivers should be advised that overuse of over-the-counter (OTC) sympathomimetic decongestants can lead to rebound vasodilation, worsening the conjunctivitis. Additionally, patients with open-angle glaucoma should be instructed not to use sympathomimetics. Patients and caregivers should be warned that viral conjunctivitis is highly contagious; hand washing must be used as a means to prevent spread of the infection to others, as well as not sharing bed linens. When ophthalmic ointments are used, patients should be advised not to drive because of loss of binocular vision.

## OUTCOMES MANAGEMENT

### Selecting Appropriate Agent

Antibiotic therapy is generally aimed at eradicating *Staphylococcus* and *Streptococcus* bacteria. Therapy may be initiated in a cost-effective manner with erythromycin or bacitracin ophthalmic ointments; however, many practitioners also use fortified aminoglycoside and cephalosporin preparations. These fortified antibiotics are not commercially available and must be compounded by a pharmacist familiar with sterile product preparation. Topical quinolones, such as ciprofloxacin and norfloxacin, have been shown to have comparable efficacy to the aminoglycosides and present a more costly alternative.

Therapy should be guided by local resistance patterns and experience.

Neonatal conjunctivitis (ophthalmia neonatorum) occurs in the first month of life. Historically, this was an important cause of blindness prior to prophylactic regimens of silver nitrate and/or erythromycin ointment. The causative bacterium in this form of conjunctivitis is usually *N. gonorrhoea*, the consequence of maternal venereal disease. The U.S. Centers for Disease Control currently recommend topical erythromycin ointment at birth for prophylaxis.

The treatment of viral conjunctivitis is aimed at inactivating the sight-threatening herpes simplex virus. Infections of adenovirus types 3 and 8 are not sight-threatening and are usually self-limiting. The treatment of the herpes simplex virus consists of either vidarabine 5% or idoxuridine 0.5% ointment five times a day, or trifluridine 1% solution nine times per day. Each regimen should be followed by acyclovir 3% ophthalmic ointment five times daily until 3 days after healing is complete (Dreyer, 1996).

The most cost-effective therapy for allergic conjunctivitis is removal of the causative allergen. Unfortunately, this is not always possible. Symptoms may be managed by ophthalmic decongestants, oral antihistamines, and agents such as ophthalmic cromolyn, lodoxamide, or levocabastine. These agents should be chosen based on individual response. The newer agents, lodoxamide and levocabastine, have been noted to be at least as effective as cromolyn with less frequent administration necessary.

## Monitoring for Efficacy

Efficacy can be seen with a reduction and overall elimination of symptoms.

## Monitoring for Toxicity

There are many minor toxicities associated with the agents used for symptomatic treatment of conjunctivitis. These include rebound hyperemia with overuse (more than 48 h) of the decongestant. Use of decongestants may also lead to pigment floaters in the iris 30–45 min after administration of the product. These floaters usually resolve in 12–24 h and are not associated with inflammation. Prolonged use of topical decongestants may also cause corneal edema and maculopathy, which may resolve in 6 months or more. Antihistamines are associated with anticholinergic side effects, including dilated pupils, flushing, dry mouth, fever, ataxia, and hallucinations 30–120 min after administration. Ophthalmic cromolyn may be associated with a transient stinging or burning sensation.

## Follow-up Recommendations

Bacterial conjunctivitis should be followed closely for response in 48–72 h. If no response is seen, a Gram stain should be obtained to determine etiology. Patients should be reevaluated within 48 h if there is no improvement. Severe cases, after response to treatment, should be followed up in 10–14 days; in mild cases no follow-up is necessary if symptoms resolve.

## UVEITIS

Uveitis is inflammation in any part of the uveal tract, which includes the iris, ciliary body, and choroid. Adjacent ocular structures may also be involved. Uveitis is categorized as: *anterior uveitis*, which involves the iris (iritis) or both the iris and the ciliary body (iridocyclitis); *intermediate uveitis*, which affects the retinal vessels and the peripheral area of the retina and uveal tract; and *posterior uveitis*, which involves the posterior choroid (choroiditis), the retina (retinitis), or both (chorioretinitis). In *Panuveitis* inflammatory signs are both anteriorly and posteriorly distributed. Uveitis may be caused by infectious and noninfectious disorders, is associated with numerous systemic diseases, or may be idiopathic (McCannel, 1996).

The most common conditions associated with anterior uveitis include sarcoidosis, ankylosing spondylitis, Reiter's syndrome, juvenile rheumatoid arthritis, inflammatory bowel disease, herpes simplex, tuberculosis, and trauma. Posterior uveitis is most commonly caused by toxoplasmosis and is also associated with syphilis, HIV/AIDS, tuberculosis, and cytomegalovirus. Posterior uveitis may also be associated with sarcoidosis (Dunn & Nozik, 1994).

Uveitis may be acute or chronic. It may be asymptomatic or present with decreased visual acuity, pain, photophobia, tearing, small and irregular pupils, diffuse conjunctival hyperemia with ciliary flush, and complaint of vision with floaters. Early diagnosis of chronic anterior uveitis is more likely to be made in patients who have associated systemic conditions and have had ongoing ophthalmic evaluations. *If uveitis is suspected, the patient should be immediately referred for an ophthalmology consultation.*

A baseline history must include the following: symptoms and their onset, circumstances surrounding their onset, occupational and environmental exposure, social and sexual history, and current illnesses and their symptoms.

On physical examination the following should be evaluated: visual acuity; pupil size, shape, and response to light; conjunctiva for flush or perilimbal injection; fundoscopic examination; and consensual photophobia. A slit-lamp examination should be performed to confirm the presence of any inflammatory cells in the anterior chamber. If a systemic condition is present, additional physical assessment may be indicated.

## SPECIFIC CONSIDERATIONS FOR PHARMACOTHERAPY

### When Drug Therapy Is Needed

Therapy is aimed at symptom relief, reduction of inflammation, and restoring or preserving vision. Uveitis is a self-limiting disorder and typically resolves in approximately 2–4 weeks. Treatment is based on severity, as well as the general health of the patient. The need for therapy is usually determined upon referral to an ophthalmologist (Anglade & Whiteup, 1995; Bertolini & Pelucio, 1995).

### Short-Term and Long-Term Goals of Pharmacotherapy

The initial management of uveitis is geared toward the reduction of symptoms and pain related to inflammation. Long-term goals of therapy are directed toward treatment of the underlying causative systemic disease, and prevention of complications such as permanent synechiae—adhesion of parts, especially the iris to the lens and cornea—and the preservation of vision (Bertolini & Pelucio, 1995).

### Time Frame for Initiating Pharmacotherapy

Therapy, if needed, should be initiated upon diagnosis. The duration of therapy is determined by the patient's response and resolution of underlying disease states. The time it will take for a therapeutic response depends on the underlying cause.

See Drug Table 401.6, 7.

## Patient/Caregiver Information

Soft contact lens wearers should avoid using diclofenac and ketorolac. These products contain benzalkonium chloride as a preservative. Benzalkonium chloride is readily absorbed into soft contact lenses, which may allow for prolonged exposure to the preservative, resulting in physiological and morphological changes to the corneal epithelium (Chapman, Cheeks, & Green, 1990). Patients who are experiencing photophobia should wear sunglasses.

## OUTCOMES MANAGEMENT

### Selecting Appropriate Agents

Treatment, when necessary, is usually initiated with a long-acting cycloplegic agent followed by a topical steroid. Topical steriods are contraindicated if the causal agent is infection. The choice of cycloplegic agent is made based on the severity of disease, with homatropine 5% for mild to moderate disease and atropine 1–4% for moderate to severe disease. Cyclopegic agents are avoided if the client has or is at risk for glaucoma. Cyclopentolate should be avoided since it may further aggravate the uveitis (Dreyer, 1996). The corticosteroid of choice is prednisolone acetate 1% ophthalmic suspension used four times daily (Bertolini & Pelucio, 1995). Systemic corticosteroids and immunosuppressants are reserved for unresponsive cases or for those cases in which the disease manifests systemically and visual acuity is affected. Prednisone is the oral corticosteroid of choice. Immunosuppressants used include cyclosporine, azathioprine, and mercaptopurine. NSAIDs are also used.

### Monitoring for Efficacy

Relief of pain should be seen within 3 days of initiating corticosteroids along with resolution of photophobia and maintenance or improvement of visual acuity.

### Monitoring for Toxicity

Corticosteroid use is associated with a multitude of systemic adverse effects including cataract formation, glaucoma, retinopathy, activation of herpes, depression, psychosis, mania, euphoria, headache, diabetes and glucose intolerance, growth suppression in children, Cushing's syndrome, abnormal hair growth, nausea, peptic ulcers, sodium retention and edema, hypokalemia, myopathies, osteoporosis, acne, and poor wound healing.

## Follow-up Recommendations

Serious and sight-threatening uveitis should be followed by an ophthalmologist. Some sources advise that all uveitis should be seen first by an opthalmologist, with comanagement by other providers for underlying causes and treatment.

## REFERENCES

Abel, S. (1995). In L. Young & M. A. Koda-Kimble, *Applied therapeutics: The clinical use of drugs* (6th ed.) (pp. 49-1–49-23). Vancouver, WA: Applied Therapeutics.

Anglade, E., & Whitcup, S. (1995). The diagnosis and management of uveitis. *Drugs, 49*(2), 213–233.

Bensinger, R. (1994). Glaucoma: A general perspective. *Journal of the Florida Medical Association, 81*(4), 243–247.

Bertolini, J., & Pelucio, M. (1995). The red eye. *Emergency Medicine Clinics of North America, 13*(3), 561–578.

Bloom, P. A., Leeming, J. P., Power, W., Laidlaw, D. A., Collum, L. M., & Easty, D. L. (1994). Topical ciprofloxacin in the treatment of blepharitis and blepharoconjunctivitis. *European Journal of Ophthalmology, 4*(1), 6–12.

Brooks, A., & Gillies, W. (1992). Ocular beta-blockers in glaucoma management. *Drugs and Aging, 2*(3), 208–221.

Chapman, J., Cheeks, L., & Green, K. (1990). Interactions of benzalkonium chloride with soft and hard contact lenses. *Archives of Ophthalmology, 108*(2), 244–246.

Crouch, E., & Berger, A. (1995). Ophthalmology. In Rakel, R. E., *Textbook of family practice* (pp. 1345–1379). Philadelphia: W. B. Saunders.

Diegel, J. T. (1986). Eyelid problems: Blepharitis, hordeola, and chalazia. *Postgraduate Medicine, 80*(2), 271–272.

Dreyer, A. (1996). In E. Herfindal & D. Gourley, *Textbook of therapeutics: Drug and disease management* (6th ed.) (pp. 437–450). Baltimore: Williams & Wilkins.

Dunn, J. P., & Nozik, R. A. (1994). Uveitis: Role of the physician in treating systemic causes. *Geriatrics, 49*(8), 27–32.

Frichman, W., Fuksbrumer, M., & Tannenbaum, M. (1994). Topical ophthalmic beta-adrenergic blockade for the treatment of glaucoma and ocular hypertension. *Journal of Clinical Pharmacology,* 34(8), 795–803.

Gelvin, J. (1994). Co-management of patients with glaucoma. *Optometry Clinics,* 4(2), 81–100.

Gwon, A. (1992). Ofloxacin vs tobramycin for the treatment of external ocular infection. *Archives of Ophthalmology,* 110(9), 1234–1237.

Jampel, H. (1995). Patching for corneal abrasions. *JAMA,* 272(19), 1504.

Knox, K., & McIntee, J. (1995). Nurse management of corneal abrasion. *British Journal of Nursing,* 4(8), 440–442, 459–460.

Lesar, T. (1997). Glaucoma. In J. DiPiro et al (eds.), *Pharmacotherapy: A pathophysiologic approach* (3rd ed.). Norwalk, CT: Appleton & Lange.

Long, K., & Long, R. (1994). Treating open-angle glaucoma. *Nurse Practitioner Forum,* 5(4), 205–206.

McCannel, C. A., Holland, G. N., Helm, C. J., Cornell, P. J., Winston, J. V., & Rimmer, T. G. (1996). Causes of uveitis in the general practice of ophthalmology. *American Journal of Ophthalmology,* 121(1), 35–46.

Miller, I., Vogel, R., Cook, T., & Wittreich, J. (1992). Topically administered norfloxacin compared with topically administered gentamicin for the treatment of external ocular bacterial infections.

American *Journal of Ophthalmology,* 113(6), 638–644.

*Ophthalmic drug facts.* (1996). St. Louis, MO: Facts and Comparisons.

Raskin, E., Speaker, M., & Laibson, P. (1992). Blepharitis. *Infectious Disease Clinics of North America,* 6(4), 777–787.

Rosenberg, L. (1995). Glaucoma: Early detection and therapy for prevention of vision loss. *American Family Physician,* 52(8), 2289–2298.

Serle, J. (1994). Pharmacological advances in the treatment of glaucoma. *Drug Therapy,* 5(3), 156–170.

Smith, R., & Flowers, C., Jr. (1995). Chronic blepharitis: A review. *CLAO Journal,* 21(3), 200–206.

Tucker, J. (1993). Screening for open-angle glaucoma. *American Family Physician,* 48(1), 75–80.

Uphold, C., & Graham, M. (1994). *Clinical guidelines in family practice.* Gainsville, FL: Barmarrae Books.

Wittpenn, J. (1995). EyeScrub: Simplifying the management of blepharitis. *Journal of Ophthalmic Nursing and Technology,* 14(1), 25–28.

Zimmerman, T. (1993). Topical ophthalmic beta blockers: A comparative review. *Journal of Ocular Pharmacology,* 9(4), 373–384.

# 24

# EAR DISORDERS

*Jeanette F. Kissinger, Kathleen J. Sawin, and Debra S. Israel*

Ear conditions are some of the most frequently occurring problems treated in primary care, especially among infants and children. This chapter reviews the treatment of selected ear conditions across the age span: acute otitis media, otitis media with effusion (serous otitis media), otitis externa, labrynthitis, and perforated tympanic membrane.

The Agency for Health Care Policy and Research (AHCPR) guidelines on otitis media (Stool et al, 1994), after a comprehensive meta-analysis of the literature, generated the following definitions of these selected types of otitis:

- *Acute otitis media* (AOM) is inflammation of the middle ear with signs or symptoms of middle ear infection.

- *Otitis media with effusion* (OME) is fluid in the middle ear without signs or symptoms of infection.

- *Persistent acute otitis media* (PAOM) is middle ear inflammation with signs of infection that do not resolve after initial treatment.

- *Otitis externa* (OE) is inflammation of the external auditory canal.

- *Perforated tympanic membrane* (PTM) is alteration of the integrity of the tympanic membrane caused by internal pressure or external trauma.

## OTITIS MEDIA

Otitis media (inflammation of the middle ear) encompasses a number of clinical conditions with a variety of names. The National Center for Health Statistics and others (Schappert, 1992; Teele, Klein, Rosen & The Greater Boston Media Study Groups, 1983) indicate that otitis media (OM) is the most frequent primary care illness diagnosed in infants and children younger than 15 years of age, accounting for 24.5 million visits in 1990 alone. By the age of 3, approximately 80% of children have been diagnosed with otitis media, with 40% having had three or more infections (Richer & LeBel, 1997; Teele, Klein, & Rosen, 1989). For adults, otitis media accounted for 4 million yearly visits. Data on otitis media are not separated by type of condition and include otitis externa, acute otitis media, and otitis media with effusion. The most common causative organisms in children over 1 month, as well as adults are *Streptococcus pneumoniae*, 30–35%; *Haemophilus influenzae*, 20–25%; and *Moraxella catarrhalis*, 10–15% (Richer & LeBel, 1997), Resistance of these bacteria to commonly used antibiotics is a growing concern (see discussion under Selecting Appropriate Agents below). It is estimated that in 8–25% of cases of OM, viruses such as influenza A virus, respiratory syncytial virus, and coxsackievirus may be implicated (Eden, Fireman, & Stool, 1995).

Certain populations seem to be at greater risk for otitis media. HIV-infected children with decreased T4 lymphocytes, in the first 3 years of life, have a threefold increase in risk for recurrent OM infection. Barnett, Klein, Pelton, &

Luginbahl (1992) reported that 80% of the children in their study with low T4 counts experienced more than six recurrent OM infections before the age of 3. Adesman, Altshuler, Lipkin, & Walco (1990) reported that in a sample of 138 children with a mean age of 9.5, middle ear disease was associated with hyperactivity (attention deficit disorder with hyperactivity). It is suggested that day care for children poses a special risk for OM and its adverse complications. A multinational study reported by Froom and Culpepper (1991) included 1335 children ranging in age from 0 to 60 months that showed a higher frequency of recurrent OM, hearing problems, and tonsillectomies in the day care children than in the cohort cared for at home.

## SPECIFIC CONSIDERATIONS FOR PHARMACOTHERAPY

### When Drug Therapy Is Needed

Some data suggest that up to 30% of patients would clear the OM without the use of antibiotics, although we generally use antimicrobial therapy since we do not have a way to identify those patients who might not need treatment. According to the guidelines developed for otitis media with effusion, the use of antibiotics is optional. The meta-analysis found only a 14% increase in the resolution of fluid or hearing loss with antibiotic treatment, with 85% of the cases resolved without treatment in 3 months (Stool et al, 1994). In the algorithm for treatment of children 1–3 years of age with OME, antibiotic treatment is an option at initial diagnosis, at 6 weeks, and at a 3-month follow-up. Observation and hearing evaluation are also an option. Decongestants and antihistamines are not supported in the treatment of this condition in any age population (Richer & LeBel, 1997, p. 2023; Stool et al, 1994). If OME persists after 3 months, especially with hearing loss, aggressive treatment is indicated (Stool et al, 1994; Terris, Magit, & Davidson, 1995). The guidelines recommend that health care providers need to inform patients fully as to the side effects and costs of antibiotic therapy as well as the benefits and harms of other options for care.

Teele, Klein, Chase, Menyuk, and Rosner (1990) conducted a fairly large study of children, with controls for confounding variables, and found that the number of recurring or lasting otitis media with effusion during the first 3 years

of life predicted lower scores on tests of cognitive, speech, and language ability and school performance at 7 years of age. In contrast, there was no such outcome if the otitis media with effusion occurred after 3 years of life. Ruben, Wallace & Gravel (1997) found that children who had multiple episodes of OM in their first year of life suffered consequential hearing loss that negatively affected their development of communication skills through age 9. They suggest that this effect may extend throughout childhood.

## Short-Term and Long-Term Goals of Pharmacotherapy

The short-term goal of treatment for AOM is to resolve the infection in the middle ear and to restore normal, painless hearing. This is in contrast to OME treatment for which the short-term goal is to eliminate fluid in the middle ear and restore normal hearing. The short-term goal of treatment of OE is to resolve the local inflammation of the ear canal and prevent the extension of the inflammation to the pinna. AOM can be accompanied by OME, but OME can occur without AOM.

Long-term goals of treatment for AOM include prevention of recurrent episodes, intracranial complications (Munz, Farmer, Auger, O'Gorman, & Schloss, 1992), and hearing loss and the resulting speech, language, and cognitive developmental delays (Terris et al, 1995). The long-term goal of treating OME is principally the prevention of hearing loss and the resulting speech, language, and cognitive developmental delays (Terris et al, 1995). Although the casual relationship between sensorineural hearing loss and language is well established, a causal relationship between conductive hearing loss with OME and subsequent language and speech delays has not been established (Berman, 1995). The AHCPR panel did find a weak relationship between OME and abnormal speech and language development in children under 4 and a weak relationship between OME and expressive language, behavior, and development in children over 4. The lack of clarity regarding the role of OME in these delays contributes to the variability in treatment options. In each of the conditions of the middle ear, the goals of treatment are frequently achieved by antibiotic treatment. This discussion is aimed at the treatment of otherwise healthy patients with no craniofacial or neurologic abnormalities or sensory deficits. See Table 24–1 for nonpharmacologic therapy and prevention for OME and OM.

## Time Frame for Initiating Pharmacotherapy

AOM should be treated at the time of diagnosis to prevent the serious sequelae discussed. A full course of antibiotics will be needed to fully treat the infection; however, significant improvement should be seen in 48 h. AOM caused by a virus may spontaneously resolve. Follow-up of all cases of AOM needs to be scheduled in 2–3 weeks (Barnett & Klein, 1995). The timing of OME treatment is complicated particularly in children and involves the possibility of antimicrobial treatment at one of several decision points (Stool et al, 1994). There is evidence that spontaneous resolution occurs for many children under age 3 with asymptomatic OME (Zeisel et al, 1995).

See Drug Table 102.

## ASSESSMENT AND HISTORY

A history of pain, fever, prior episodes of AOM and/or OME, upper respiratory infection (UR), hearing difficulties, speech delays, exposure to passive smoking, placement in a child-care center, and packs per year smoked by teenagers and adults are important aspects of the history of AOM. OME can be asymptomatic and highly prevalent in children under 2 in group day-care settings (Zeisel et al, 1995). The hallmark of AOM is the inflamed tympanic membrane (TM). Changes in the landmarks and/or diminished landmarks secondary to a bulging TM may also be present. The clinician has to be alert to the possibility that a red TM when a child is actively crying may be a normal response and not an indicator of AOM. A pneumatic otoscope can be used to test the mobility of the TM, which is

---

## TABLE 24–1. NONPHARMACOLOGIC THERAPY AND PREVENTION FOR OME AND OM

Tympanostomy tubes
Adenoidectomy
Tonsillectomy
Equilibrating pressure techniques
Change of day-care setting

*Source: Linder et al. (1997)*

---

reduced when exudate or fluid collects behind it. However, pneumatic otoscope evaluation is not necessary when it is evident that the TM is inflamed and bulging. Forced movement of the TM would only cause unnecessary pain to the patient. A pneumatic evaluation requires that the examiner obtain a tight seal. In many adults and some children, using a ear speculum with a specifically designed cuff will aid in achieving an airtight seal.

Fluid behind the TM without signs of inflammation is the hallmark of OME. Bubbles or a fluid line may be seen, or the short process of the umbo can be prominent if the drum is retracted. Pneumatic otoscope evaluation is preferable to otoscope evaluation alone whenever OME is suspected (Belkengren & Sapala, 1995). A tympanogram, when available, can quantify the mobility of the TM and can be a valuable tool in accurately assessing response to treatment.

It is common for AOM to occur concomitantly with other infections such as viral URI, pharyngitis, sinusitis, and influenza. Ear pain may occur without AOM or OME from a source other than the ear. Failure to treat AOM may result in meningitis, lateral sinus thrombosis, and chronic suppurative otitis media (Poole, 1995) as well as hearing loss and possible speech delay (Canafax & Geibink, 1994). Labrynthitis can be a complication of acute or chronic otitis media, and is often overlooked in children (Sun, Parnes, & Freeman, 1996).

## Patient/Caregiver Information

Use of a pacifier by children in day-care centers under 2 years of age increases AOM risk 1.6 times, and for children 2–3 years old, the risk increases 2.9 times. One study by Niemela, Uhari, and Mottonen (1995) failed to show a strong association between AOM and breast-feeding, parental smoking, thumb sucking, use of a bottle, or social class. The panel of experts who developed the AHCPR guidelines found that while bottle-feeding and placement in child care are associated with increased incidence of OME, removal from child-care facilities does not decrease incidence (Stevenson & Brooke, 1995; Stool et al, 1994).

The absorption of some newer broad-spectrum antibiotics that are prodrug esters, such as cefpodoxime proxetil (Vantin) or cefuroxime axetil (Ceftin), requires metabolism to become an active agent. Thus, their absorption is enhanced when given with food (Gerchufsky, 1995).

There is some evidence that children in day care who have been given a flu shot have decreased incidence of AOM and OME during the flu season (Clements, Langdon, Bland, & Walter, 1995). If prednisone (a corticosteroid) is used for children, the tablets can be crushed and added to jelly to make the bitter taste more palatable (Berman, 1995). A common practice, meant to reduce ear pain, is to instill warm olive oil in the affected ear. In a comparative study, Hoberman, Paradise, Reynolds, & Urkin (1997) found that Auralgan provided greater pain relief within 30 minutes.

In a small but important study of nurse practitioner (NP) outcomes when treating OM, Matas, Brown, and Holman (1996) found the NP very effective. Parents reported 93% achieved completion of the medication regime. However, parents and providers can have different perceptions about information shared in a health care visit for AOM. Even when teaching is documented in the chart, parents may not hear or may not perceive getting important information about the care of their child. Health care providers need to develop multiple strategies to share critical information such as the rationale for completing the antibiotic course of treatment and the need for follow-up and behavioral changes helpful for prevention of future episodes of OM.

## OUTCOMES MANAGEMENT

### Selecting an Appropriate Agent

Antibiotics are the mainstay of therapy for the treatment of acute otitis media, although disagreement exists as to which agent(s) should be first-line. Selection of an agent to treat AOM requires consideration of factors such as the patient's age, OM history, drug hypersensitivity, prior antimicrobial response, and associated illness. Drug therapy should be active against the common middle ear pathogens (including *S. pneumoniae, H. influenzae*, and *M. catarrhalis*).

Amoxicillin and trimethoprim-sulfamethoxazole (TMP-SMX) are the most commonly prescribed first-line drugs. Concerns exist about the increasing incidence of beta-lactamase–producing strains of *H. influenzae*: regional variation exists in the percentage of resistance (10–30%), and studies have shown good clinical results for amoxicillin

despite the presence of beta-lactamase–producing organisms (Hughes, 1995). Practitioners should also be aware that *M. catarrhalis* exhibits a high rate of beta-lactamase production (70–90%). Many agents are effective against beta-lactamase–producing strains of *H. influenzae* and *M. catarrhalis*. See the in vitro spectrum of activity of antibiotics used in upper respiratory tract infections shown in Table 24–2. TMP-SMX is often first-line because of low cost and twice-daily dosing although in the non-penicillin-allergic patient, amoxicillin is also a reasonable first choice.

Amoxicillin is still regarded by many as the drug of choice (Barnett & Klein, 1995; Swanson & Hoecker, 1996). The other antimicrobials are considered second-line for patients with persistent or recurrent AOM, for patients in other high-risk groups, or for special situations (Canafax & Geibink, 1994; Hughes, 1995). There is no evidence for children free from AOM symptoms after the initial course of antibiotic treatment that further treatment results in faster resolution of effusion (Mandel, Casselbrant, Rockette, Bluestone, & Kurs-Lasky, 1995).

Of growing concern is the increase of resistant strains of *S. pneumoniae* in Europe and in areas of the United States. This has lead to treatment failures with such commonly used antimicrobials as TMP-SMX, beta-lactams, and macrolides. Clinicians should be aware of the resistance patterns in their communities and prescribe accordingly.

Some older antibiotics that have poor activity against *H. influenzae* (erythromycin, penicillin, and first-generation cephalosporins) should not be used to treat AOM. Sulfonamides alone are not effective because of poor activity against pneumococcus and group A streptococcus. In penicillin-allergic patients, TMP-SMX or erythromycin-sulfisoxazole (EES-SSX) are reasonable choices. These drugs should be avoided in patients with known sulfonamide allergies (Hughes, 1995).

Infants younger than 4–6 weeks of age are likely to be infected with *Staphylococcus aureus* and gram-negative enteric bacilli. These infants often need to be hospitalized for evaluation of systemic infection and generally require parenteral antibiotics for initial therapy (Canafax & Geibink, 1994; Hughes, 1995). Infants younger than 6 months may be infected with *Chlamydia trachomatis* since it is a common cause of acute respiratory infections in that age group (Klein, 1995). The treatment of meningogenic labryn-

## TABLE 24–2. IN VITRO SPECTRUM OF ACTIVITY OF ANTIBIOTICS USED IN UPPER RESPIRATORY TRACT INFECTIONS

| Antibiotic | Streptococcus pneumoniae | Haemophilus influenzae | | Moraxella catarrhalis | | Group A Beta-Hemolytic Streptococci |
| | | Beta-Lactamase Negative | Positive | Beta-Lactamase Negative | Positive | |
| --- | --- | --- | --- | --- | --- | --- |
| Ampicillin or amoxicillin | + | + | − | + | − | + |
| Azithromycin | + | + | + | + | + | + |
| Clarithromycin | + | + | + | + | + | + |
| Erythromycin | + | − | − | + | − | + |
| Erythromycin-sulfisoxazole | + | + | + | + | + | + |
| Trimethoprim-sulfamethoxazole | + | + | + | + | + | − |
| Amoxicillin-clavulanate | + | + | + | + | + | + |
| Cefaclor | + | + | ± | + | + | + |
| Cefixime | + | + | + | + | + | + |
| Cefpodoxime proxetil | + | + | + | + | + | + |
| Cefprozil | + | + | + | + | + | + |
| Cefuroxime axetil | + | + | + | + | + | + |
| Loracarbef | + | + | + | + | + | + |

+ = organism highly susceptible to antibiotic; ± = moderately susceptible to antibiotic; − = nonsusceptible to antibiotic.
*Source: DiPiro et al. (1997)*

thitis complicating acute or chronic otitis media is most effectively achieved by cephalosporins. Of the cephalosporins, there is evidence that ceftazidime may be the optimum choice (Sun, Parnes, & Freeman, 1995; Sun et al, 1996).

**Amoxicillin versus amoxicillin-clavulanate for first-line therapy.** Many practitioners are tempted to start a patient on amoxicillin-clavulanate for first-line therapy since it is "broader-spectrum" than amoxicillin. This raises concern for a number of reasons. First, the amoxicillin-clavulanate is more expensive and likely to cause more adverse gastrointestinal effects than amoxicillin. Second, overuse of drugs like amoxicillin-clavulanate contributes to the growing problems of bacterial resistance. It is estimated that approximately 30% and 10% of cases of otitis media are due to *H. influenzae* and *M. catarrhalis*, respectively. If 30% of *H. influenza* and 90% of *M. catarrhalis* are beta-lactamase–producing, then 16% of cases of AOM are due to beta-lactamase–producing strains. It is clear that the incidence of resistance is not high enough to warrant abandonment of amoxicillin as first-line therapy (Klein, 1995). The caveat is that if a patient does not improve within 48–72

h, switching therapy from amoxicillin is reasonable. *Please note*: Some antibiotics may not be approved for use in certain age groups. Refer to Drug Table 102 for specific information.

**Alternative initial therapies.** Amoxicillin-clavulanate failure has been related to nontypeable *H. influenzae*, history of previous episodes, gender (boys), and race (nonwhite) in a study of 99 children, mean age 21.4 months. This study found no relationship between compliance and drug failure (Patel et al, 1995). The use of broad-spectrum antibiotics as a first-line therapy should be deferred except for patients who have three or more previous episodes of AOM, who have polymicrobial infections (Patel et al, 1995), who are in conditions or situations that preclude sequential dosing for multiple days, who have not responded previously to amoxicillin, or who are considering air travel within the next 3 days. In addition, regional antimicrobial susceptibility may influence the clinician's decision (Canafax & Geibink, 1994). In these cases several options may be considered. Traditional dosing of a broader-spectrum antibiotic (ie, Ceclor t.i.d. 10–14 days), use of a broader-spectrum antibiotic with less frequent dosing (ie, Suprax given once daily for 10 days), or the use of nontraditional dosing of some agents has been shown to be safe and effective.

Recent studies of nontraditional dosing have supported the use of the following:

- A one-time intramuscular injection of ceftriaxone (50 mg/kg) in children 5 months to 5 years with uncomplicated AOM (Green & Rothrock, 1993)
- A 5-day treatment with cefpodoxime proxetil (8 mg/kg per day) for children 5 months to 12 years old (Cohen, 1995)
- A daily dose of azithromycin, 10 mg/kg per day for 3 days in children 6 months to 12 years (Daniel, 1993; Principi, 1995), faster resolution of symptoms was reported with azithromycin use in both studies

Cefpodoxime proxetil was found to be one of the most active compounds against *H. influenzae* and *S. pneumoniae*. Children who are very ill, who have recently been hospitalized, who have already had antibiotic treatment, who have had known exposure to resistant pneumococci, or who have an immunodeficiency are candidates for initial treatment with second-line agents (Barnett & Klein, 1995). There is also some evidence that ibuprofen alters the disease pathogenesis of AOM. When given with an antimicrobial agent, the incidence of effusion and the degree of mucosal thickness at day 10 is less (Diven, Evans, Swarts, Burckart, & Doyle, 1995).

In most cases OME resolves spontaneously within 3 months. The AHCPR guidelines discuss treatment of uncomplicated OME in children under 3 by the use of observation or antibiotic therapy, but recommend environmental risk factor control counseling for all. The use of antibiotics at the initial diagnosis only achieved 16% increased resolution of the OME. If the patient still has OME 3 months after diagnosis, by pneumatic otoscopy and tympanometry, the patient needs to be referred for hearing evaluation. The algorithm developed by AHCPR tracks each decision point and the considerations for antibiotics at several stages. Presence of speech and/or hearing problems in children may accelerate the treatment plan (Stool et al, 1994). An alternative interpretation of the meta-analysis of OME treatment suggests a third option for treatment: an antibiotic plus a corticosteroid. Limited data suggest this combination is significantly more effective than an antibiotic alone. However, if this option is used, it is critical to as-

sess the exposure of the child to varicella. Children who have been exposed within the last month should not be treated with steroids due to risk of disseminated disease (Berman, 1995).

When the clinician determines that OME needs to be treated with antibiotics, the same parameters used to identify the drug of choice for AOM can generally be used to determine the drug of choice for OME. There is no evidence that antihistamines or decongestants are effective in treatment of OME in children (Stevenson & Brooke, 1995). However, they are frequently used in adults to control symptoms of URI. Their effect on prevention or treatment of OME is unknown.

## Monitoring for Efficacy

A typical course of treatment for AOM is 10–14 days. Signs and symptoms should improve within 48–72 h. Common reasons for lack of improvement include noncompliance, adverse effects, short duration of therapy, or the presence of resistant organisms. These factors should be taken into account before switching to another agent. If there is no improvement in 48–72 h, some investigators suggest, if the initial therapy was amoxicillin, change to TMP-SMX is often successful, and conversely, if TMP-SMX was used first-line, a switch to amoxicillin may prove to be successful (Canafax & Geibink, 1994). Other practitioners feel that if no improvement is seen within 48 h, switching to an agent with a broader spectrum of activity is recommended (Hughes, 1995).

When there is still no improvement, some clinicians suggest a culture of the middle ear effusion by tympanocentesis to guide antimicrobial selection. Antimicrobial prophylaxis may be reasonable in patients who have a clearing of the middle ear effusion between episodes.

If there is recurrence within 1 month of the initial episode, the clinician can assume the same organisms caused the infection. However, resistance to initial therapy can also be assumed and a second-line antibiotic should be prescribed. If, however, the recurrence occurs more than 1 month following the initial episode in a child free of symptoms, the same treatment can be repeated. If children have more than four episodes of AOM in 6 months or six episodes in 12 months, prophylaxis treatment should be considered (Richer & LeBel, 1997).

There is some evidence that recurrent infections can be prevented by daily use of either amoxicillin 20 mg/kg daily or sulfisoxazole 75 mg/kg per day for 3–6 months (Berman, 1995). However, Goldstein and Sculerati (1994) found that only 46% of the patients they studied claimed compliance with this regimen. It would be important to monitor the status of children on this regimen for recurrent infections. Qualitative investigations may be helpful in understanding the experience of maintaining a preventive antimicrobial regimen in families and identifying the barriers to consistent achievement of prophylactic treatment.

Surgical treatment with placement of ear tubes is considered in patients who continue to have middle ear infections despite prophylactic treatment (Berman, 1995). Most healthy children will outgrow OM by the age of 6 or 7 years. There is some evidence that children 2 years old and older who have recurrent disease may benefit from pneumococcal vaccine (Barnett & Klein, 1995).

### Monitoring for Toxicity

Data support up to 30% incidence of diarrhea in children with antibiotic treatment of AOM. Skin care and fluid replacement strategies need to be reviewed (Mitchell, Van, Mason, Norris & Pickering, 1996). In addition, spacing of medication evenly throughout the day may decrease the incidence of diarrhea.

Some antimicrobials may aggravate gastrointestinal symptoms that may already be present in an ill patient. These drugs include amoxicillin-clavulanate, EES-SSX, cefuroxime axetil, and cefixime. Side effects such as skin rash, diarrhea, and nonspecific gastrointestinal complaints are reported in as many as 20% of patients. These effects are thought to be due to an associated viral infection. General guidelines suggest that if the symptoms are severe or the rash urticarial, further use of the drug should be avoided.

### Follow-up

A follow-up evaluation for AOM is recommend within 1–2 weeks of completing a course of therapy. In OM with effusion, follow-up will depend on the plan the provider has chosen.

## OTITIS EXTERNA

The incidence of otitis externa (swimmer's ear) is higher in the summer months but overall incidence is unknown. This infection is usually bacterial, commonly caused by *Pseudomonas aeruginosa* and *S. aureus*, although occasionally fungus may be involved. When otitis externa (OE) is very localized, it is usually due to an infected hair follicle in the external canal. OE is termed malignant or necrotizing when it extends into the soft and bony tissues surrounding the ear canal. This condition has been classically seen in diabetic patients. Only since 1990 has it been seen in immunosupressed patients (Weinroth, Schessel, & Tuazon, 1994).

## SPECIFIC CONSIDERATIONS FOR PHARMACOTHERAPY

### When Drug Therapy Is Needed

The identified organisms usually require topical antibiotic treatment or antifungal treatment. The short-term goal is resolution of pain, inflammation, and edema with the restoration of normal hearing. In recurrent OE, the goal is prevention of repeat episodes and prevention of extension to periauricular tissue.

### Nonpharmacologic Therapy

Use of preventive ear plugs and swimming caps is common but of unknown value. There is no known nonpharmacologic treatment of the disease. If the condition is secondary to a furuncle, an adjunct treatment can be the application of heat.

### Time Frame for Initiating Pharmacotherapy

Treatment should be initiated at the time of diagnosis. The medication should be continued for 1 week (Hoole, Pickard, Ouimette, Lohr, & Greenberg, 1995). If this is a recurrent infection, the medication should be continued for 10–14 days after cessation of symptoms.

See Drug Tables 102 and 402.

### Assessment Needed Prior to Therapy

Otitis externa is suggested by a history of pain on movement of the external ear and decreased unilateral hearing on the affected side; it is confirmed by visualization of the canal with an otoscope. Exudate, inflammation, or narrowing of the canal secondary to edema is usually present. Occasionally otorrhea is present. Pain can be reproduced by manipulation of the pinns and pressure on the tragus. If systemic symptoms such as fever, joint pain, paresis, or palsy are present, a complete neurologic exam is indicated.

Ask the patient if he or she was swimming. Even when swimming in waters that have passed environmental standards, OE still occurs. Persons with recurrent OE should take precautions (Van Asperen et al, 1995). No controlled studies were found, but current clinical practice is to use two to three drops of a 1:1 solution of white vinegar and 70% ethyl alcohol in the ear canal before and after swimming (Hay, Groothuis, Hayward, & Levin, 1995, p. 465). Swimming should be avoided during the acute phase. If on the otoscope examination the TM is clearly abnormal with no landmarks visualized and an apparent hole, or if a portion of the TM is missing, a diagnosis of perforated TM exists. If the TM looks somewhat abnormal and there is a question about a localized perforation in a child, a pneumatic otoscope can be used to clarify the diagnosis. A drum that moves, even slightly, cannot be perforated.

Assessment for malignant otitis externa includes a thorough history that may be characterized by persistent ear pain following treatment for OE in individuals with a compromised immune system. Increased drainage and/or odor or visible growth in the canal is frequently present. In addition, the clinician needs to assess the cranial nerves. Extensive cranial nerve paresis may be present (Boringa, Hoekstra, Roos, & Bertelsmann, 1995).

## Patient/Caregiver Information

When the ear canal is very edematous, the insertion of a wick, on which the treatment solution is dropped, is effective in distributing the medication in the canal. The wick will spontaneously drop out of the canal when the edema resolves. The patient then drops the medication directly into the ear canal for the remainder of the treatment regime.

## OUTCOMES MANAGEMENT

### Selecting an Appropriate Agent

OE treatment is usually local and consists of Cortisporin otic solution four drops four times a day for adults and three drops four times a day for children. If perforation is suspected, Cortisporin otic suspension needs to be used. In addition, the canal needs to be kept dry and pro-

tected from the wind. There is no evidence to support the addition of oral antibiotics to the topical treatment in mild to moderate OE (Cantor, 1995). If the TM perforation coexists with AOM, oral antibiotics need to be included in the plan.

Some alternative drugs have been found to be helpful: 2% acetic acid in propylene glycol (VoSol or VoSolH) has been found to be an effective alternative for uncomplicated OE (Mengel & Schwiebert, 1993). When OE is accompanied by a chronic suppurative OM, Sumitsawan, Tharavichitkul, Prawatmuang, Ingsuwan, and Sriburi (1995) and Supiyaphun, Tonsakulrungruang, Chochaipanichnon, Chongtateong, and Samart (1995) recommend the use of 0.3% ofloxacin otic solution for 2 weeks. Drugs recommended for malignant OE are the cephalosporins, penicillins, and aminoglycosides for a prolonged duration. In several studies, ciprofloxacin has demonstrated to be effective as an oral agent (Weinroth et al, 1994). Although initial assessment and treatment of malignant OE is appropriate for the primary care provider, referral to the appropriate specialist is recommended.

### Monitoring for Efficacy

If the OE does not respond to medication within 48 hours, a fungal organism needs to be considered. Nystatin otic solution is the choice if the clinician suspects a fungal causation. If symptoms are not resolved in 7 days, referral to your collaborating physician is recommended. If normal hearing is not restored, referral to an ENT specialist is indicated.

### Monitoring for Toxicity

Toxicity of topical treatment is unusual. If there is any increase in drainage/odor or urticaria, the drug should be discontinued. In cases of malignant OE, refer immediately to a specialist for consideration of a gallium scan and hospitalization for treatment (Boringa et al, 1995). Follow-up is generally not needed if symptoms resolve.

### REFERENCES

Adesman, A. R., Altshuler, L. A., Lipkin, P. H., & Walco, G. A. (1990). Otitis media in children with learning disabilities and in children with attention deficit disorder with hyperactivity. *Pediatrics, 85* (3, Pt. 2), 442–446.

Barnett, E. D., & Klein, J. O. (1995). The problem of resistant bacteria for the management of acute otitis media. *Pediatric Clinics of North America, 42* (3), 509–517.

Barnett, E. D., Klein, J. O., Pelton, S. I., & Luginbuhl, L. M. (1992). Otitis media in children born to human immunodeficiency virus-infected mothers. *Pediatric Infectious Disease Journal, 11* (5), 360–364.

Belkengren, R, & Sapala, S. (1995). Pediatric management problems. *Pediatric Nursing, 21* (3), 304–305.

Berman, S. (1995). Otitis media in children. *New England Journal of Medicine, 332* (23), 1560–1565.

Boringa, J. B., Hoekstra, O. S., Roos, J. W., & Bertelsmann, F. W. (1995). Multiple cranial nerve palsy after otitis externa: A case report. *Clinics of Neurology and Neurosurgery, 97* (4), 332–335.

Canafax, D. M., & Geibink, G. (1994). Antimicrobial treatment of otitis media. *Annals of Otology, Rhinology and Laryngology, 103,* 11–14.

Cantor, R. M. (1995). Otitis externa and otitis media. A new look at old problems. *Emergency Medicine Clinics of North America, 13* (2), 445–455.

Clements, D. A., Langdon, L., Bland, C., & Walter, E. (1995). Influenza A vaccine decreases the incidence of otitis media in 6 to 30 month old children in day care. *Archives of Pediatric Adolescent Medicine, 149,* 1113–1117.

Cohen, R. (1995). Clinical experience with cefpodoxime proxetil in acute otitis media. *Pediatric Infectious Disease Journal, 14* (4 Suppl.), S12–18.

Daniel, R. R. (1993). Comparison of azithromycin and co-amoxiclav in the treatment of otitis media in children. *Journal of Antimicrobial Chemotherapy, 31* (Suppl. E), 65–71.

DiPiro, J. T., Talbert, R. L., Yee, G. C., Matzke, G. R., Wells, B. G., & Posey, L. M. (1997). *Pharmacotherapy: A Pathophysiologic Approach.* Stamford, CT: Appleton & Lange.

Diven, W. F., Evans, R. W., Swarts, J. D., Burckart, G. J., & Doyle, W. J. (1995). Effect of ibuprofen treatment during experimental acute otitis media. *Auris Nasus, Larynx, 22* (2), 73–79.

Eden, A. N., Fireman, P., & Stool, S. E. (1995). The rise of acute otitis media. *Patient Care, 29* (16), 22–24, 29–30, 32, 35–36, 39–41, 46–52.

Froom, J., & Culpepper, L. (1991). Otitis media in day-care children. A report from the international primary care network. *Journal of Family Practice, 32* (3), 289–294.

Gerchufsky, M. (1995). Understanding upper respiratory tract infections. *Advance for Nurse Practitioners, 3* (3), 25–27.

Goldstein, N. A., & Sculerati, N. (1994). Compliance with prophylactic antibiotics for otitis media in a New York city clinic. *International Journal of Pediatric Otorhinolaryngology, 28* (2–3), 129–140.

Green, S. M., & Rothrock, S. G. (1993). Single-dose intramuscular ceftriaxone for acute otitis media in children. *Pediatrics, 91* (1), 23–30.

Hay, W. H., Groothuis, J. R., Hayward, A. R., & Levin, M. J. (1995). *Current pediatric diagnosis and treatment.* Norwalk, CT: Appleton & Lange.

Hoberman, A., Paradise, J. L., Reynolds, E. A., & Urkin, J. (1997). Efficacy of Auralgan for treating ear pain in children with acute otitis media. *Archives of Pediatric Adolescent Medicine, 151*(7), 675–678.

Hoole, A. J., Pickard, C. G., Jr., Ouimette, R. M., Lohr, J. A., & Greenberg, R. A. (1995). *Patient care guidelines for nurse practitioners* (4th ed.). Philadelphia: J. B. Lippincott.

Hughes, G. B. (1995). Otitis media. In R. E. Rakel (Ed.) *Conn's current therapy* (pp. 172–174). Philadelphia: W. B. Saunders.

Klein, J. O. (1995). Otitis externa, otitis media, mastoiditis. In G. L. Mandel, J. E. Bennett, and R. Dolin (Eds.), *Bennett's principles and practice of infectious diseases* (4th ed) (pp. 579–585). New York: Churchill Livingston.

Linder, T. E., Marder, H. P., & Munzinger, J. (1997). Role of adenoids in the pathogenesis of otitis media: A bacteriologic and immunohistochemical analysis. *Annals of Otology, Rhinology, and Laryngology, 106*(8), 619–623.

Mandel, E. M., Casselbrant, M. L., Rockette, H. E., Bluestone, C. D., & Kurs-Lasky, M. (1995). Efficacy of 20- versus 10-day antimicrobial treatment for acute otitis media. *Pediatrics, 96* (1 Pt. 1), 5–13.

Matas, K. E., Brown, N. C., & Holman, E. J. (1996). Measuring outcomes in nursing centers. *Nurse Practitioner, 21* (6), 116–125.

Mengel, M. B., & Schwiebert, L. P. (1993). *Ambulatory medicine: The primary care of families* (pp. 119–125). Norwalk, CT: Appleton & Lange.

Mitchell, D. K., Van, R., Mason, E. H., Norris, D. M., & Pickering, L. K. (1996). Prospective study of toxigenic clostridium difficile in children given amoxicillin/clavulanate for otitis media. *The Pediatric Infectious Disease Journal, 15* (6), 514–519.

Munz, M., Farmer, J. P., Auger, L., O'Gorman, A. M., & Schloss, M. D. (1992). Otitis media and CNS complications. *Journal of Otolaryngology, 21* (3), 224–226.

Niemela, M., Uhari, M., & Mottonen, M. (1995). A pacifier increases the risk of recurrent acute otitis media in children in day care centers. *Pediatrics, 96* (5 Pt. 1), 884–888.

Patel, J. A., Reisner, B., Vizirinia, N., Owen, M., Chonmaitree, T., & Howie, V. (1995). Bacteriologic failure of amoxicillin-clavulanate in treatment of acute otitis media caused by nontypeable *Haemophilus influenzae*. *Journal of Pediatrics, 126* (5 Pt. 1), 799–806.

Poole, M. D. (1995). Otitis media complications and treatment failures: Implications of pneumococcal resistance. *Pediatric Infectious Disease Journal, 14* (4 suppl), S23–26.

Principi, N. (1995). Multicentre comparative study of the efficacy and safety of azithromycin compared with amoxicillin/clavulanic acid in the treatment of paediatric patients with otitis media. *European Journal of Clinical Microbiology and Infectious Diseases, 14* (8), 669–676.

Richer, M., & LeBel, M. (1997). Upper respiratory tract infections. In J. T. DiPiro, R. L. Talbert, G. C. Yee, G. R. Matzke, B. G. Wells, & L. M. Posey (Eds), *Pharmacotherapy: A pathophysiologic approach* (3rd ed). Stamford, CT: Appleton & Lange.

Ruben, R. J., Wallace, I. F., & Gravel, J. (1997). Long-term communication deficiencies in children with otitis media during their first year of life. *Acta Otolaryngologica (Stockholm) 117*(2), 206–207.

Schappert, S. M. (1992). *Office visits for otitis media: United States, 1975–90. Advance data from vital and health statistics of the Centers for Disease Control/National Center for Health Statistics*, (p. 214). Washington, DC: U.S. Department of Health and Human Services.

Stevenson, L., & Brooke, D. S. (1995). Managing otitis media with effusion in young children. *Journal of Pediatric Health Care, 9* (1), 36–39.

Stool, S. E., Berg, A. O., Berman, S., Carney, C. J., Cooley, J. R., Culpepper, L., Eavy, R. D., Feagans, L. V., Finitzo, T., Friedman, E. M., et al. (1994). *Otitis media with effusion in young children: Clinical practice guideline* (12), AHCPR publication no. 94-0622. Rockville, MD: Agency for Health Care Policy and Research, Public Health Service, U.S. Department of Health and Human Services.

Sumitsawan, Y., Tharavichitkul, P., Prawatmuang, W., Ingsuwan, B., & Sriburi, P. (1995). Ofloxacin otic solution as treatment of chronic suppurative otitis media and diffuse bacterial otitis externa. *Journal of the Medical Association of Thailand, 78* (9), 455–459.

Sun, A. H., Parnes, L. S., & Freeman, D. J. (1995). Pharmacokinetic profiles of ceftazidime in cochlear perilymph, cerebrospinal fluid and plasma: A high-performance liquid chromatographic study. *ORL Journal of Oto-rhino-laryngology and Related Specialties, 57* (5), 256–259.

Sun, A. H., Parnes, L. S., & Freeman, D. J. (1996). Comparative perilymph permeability of cephalosporins and its significance in the treatment and prevention of suppurative labyrinthitis. *Annals of Otology, Rhinology and Laryngology, 105* (1), 54–57.

Supiyaphun, P., Tonsakulrungruang, K., Chochaipanichnon, L., Chongtateong, A., & Samart, Y. (1995). The treatment of chronic suppurative otitis media and otitis externa with 0.3 percent ofloxacin otic solution: A clinico-microbiological study. *Journal of the Medical Association of Thailand, 78* (1), 18–21.

Swanson, J. A., & Hoecker, J. L. (1996). Concise review for primary-care physicians. *Mayo Clinic Proceedings, 71* (2), 179–183.

Teele, D. W., Klein, J. O., Chase, C., Menyuk, P., & Rosner, B. A. (1990). Otitis media in infancy and intellectual ability, school achievement, speech, and language at age 7 years. *Journal of Infectious Diseases, 162* (3), 685–694.

Teele, D. W., Klein, J. O., & Rosen, B. (1989). Epidemiology of otitis media during the first seven years of life in children in greater Boston. *Journal of Infectious Diseases, 160*, 83–94.

Teele, D. W., Klein, J. O., Rosen, B., & The Greater Boston Otitis Media Study Group. (1983). Middle ear disease and the practice of pediatrics. Burden during the first five years of life. *JAMA, 249* (8), 1026–1029.

Terris, M. H., Magit, A. E., & Davidson, T. M. (1995). Otitis media with effusion in infants and children. Primary care concerns addressed from an otolaryngologist's perspective. *Postgraduate Medicine, 97* (1), 137–138, 143–144, 147.

Van Asperen, I. A., de Rover, C. M., Schijven, J. F., Oetomo, S. B., Schellekens, J. F., van Leeuwen, N. J., Colle, C., Havelaar, A. H., Kromhout, D., & Sprenger, M. W. (1995). Risk of otitis externa after swimming in recreational fresh water lakes containing *Pseudomonas aeruginosa*. *British Medical Journal, 311* (7017), 1407–1410.

Weinroth, S. E., Schessel, D., & Tuazon, C. U. (1994). Malignant otitis externa in AIDS patients: Case report and review of the literature. *Ear, Nose, and Throat Journal, 73* (10), 772–774, 777–778.

Zeisel, S. A., Robert, J. E., Gunn, E. B., Riggins, R., Evans, G. A., Roush, J., Burchinak, M. R., & Henderson, F. W. (1995). Prospective surveillance for otitis media with effusion among black infants in group child care. *Journal of Pediatrics, 127* (6), 875–880.

# 25

# GASTROINTESTINAL DISORDERS

*Patricia J. Kelly and Candice Smith-Scott*

This chapter covers the pharmacotherapy of selected common and uncommon gastrointestinal (GI) problems seen in primary care settings. Common symptoms such as nausea, vomiting, diarrhea, constipation, hemorrhoids, and flatus will be reviewed as well as the treatment and diagnosis of inflammatory bowel syndrome, peptic ulcer disease, gastroesophageal reflux, and hepatitis.

## NAUSEA AND VOMITING

Nausea and vomiting (N & V) are common but annoying problems experienced by virtually all patients and providers. Although seldom life-threatening conditions in the primary care setting, these symptoms can result in considerable concern, discomfort, and time lost from daily activities.

Nausea and vomiting may present as primary symptoms or they may be part of a complex clinical presentation. Symptoms may be self-induced, as in cases of bulimia or anorexia nervosa; caused by external stimuli such as acute infection, drug toxicity, food intake, and emotional stress; the result of metabolic conditions such as myocardial infarction, pregnancy, and diabetic ketoacidosis; or gastrointestinal disorders such as obstruction, peptic ulcer disease, or motility disorders.

## SPECIFIC CONSIDERATIONS FOR PHARMACOTHERAPY

### When Drug Therapy Is Needed

For many patients, N & V are self-limiting conditions that resolve without medical or drug therapy. When N & V are the predominant symptoms, the primary care provider's main concern is dehydration, especially with pediatric and geriatric patients. Intervention will be directed toward (1) maintenance or return of hydration status with oral replacement therapy or parenteral fluids that may be administered in the office and (2) cessation of symptoms with antiemetics. With these two intervention goals, severe dehydration and hospitalization can be avoided. For patients whose symptoms are caused by life-threatening illnesses such as bowel obstruction or myocardial infarction, immediate referral is indicated. If the symptoms of N & V are secondary symptoms of a systemic disease process, assessment and treatment of the underlying disease is usually indicated for relief of symptoms.

### Short- and Long-Term Goals of Pharmacotherapy

Pharmacotherapy for N & V has two goals: to provide symptomatic relief for the patient and to maintain his or her hydration status.

## Nonpharmacologic Therapy

Nonpharmacologic therapy consists of GI rest with gradual increases in bland foods. See also Table 25–1.

For morning sickness in the first trimester of pregnancy, avoidance of foods that provoke symptoms is the preferred treatment. Suggestions for relief include minimizing of odors, eating desired food (regardless of the time of day), and small morning feedings. Traditional recommendations are saltines and ginger ale; alternatively, potato chips and lemonade in the morning may allow women to eat regular meals for the remainder of the day (Erick, 1994). Vitamin $B_6$ (25 mg/day) PO is thought to be useful (Goroll, May, & Mulley, 1995).

In children with vomiting and/or diarrhea, volume depletion can occur rapidly. A solution of oral rehydration therapy (ORT) can be easily made in the home—see Table 25–2—or offer commercial ORT solutions, ie, Pedialyte.

## Time Frame for Initiating Pharmacotherapy

After ensuring that N & V are not indicative of an underlying condition needing immediate atten-

---

### TABLE 25–1.  WHAT THE PATIENT CAN DO TO TREAT NAUSEA AND VOMITING

- No solids for 8 h.
- Clear liquids only (no milk) until 8–12 h have passed without vomiting. Start with 1 tbsp (15 cc) every 10 min. If vomiting does not occur, double the amount each hour. If vomiting does occur, allow stomach to rest 1–2 h and then start again. The key is to gradually increase the amount of fluid until taking 8 oz every hour.
  Older children and adults: Gatorade, Pedialyte, or Ricelyte may be combined with flavored gelatin to make them more palatable.
  Pedialyte, Ricelyte, or Kao Lectrolyte should be given to infants and small children since they tend to become dehydrated quickly. Resume breast/bottle feeding as soon as possible.
- Bland food after 8 h without vomiting:
  Saltines, bland soups (chicken noodle), rice, mashed potatoes
  Also acceptable is BRAT (bananas, rice, applesauce, toast)
- Resume normal diet as soon as possible

Adapted from Uphold and Graham (1994) with permission.

---

### TABLE 25–2.  HOMEMADE ORAL REHYDRATION THERAPY (ORT) SOLUTION

1/2 or 1 tsp salt
1/2 tsp baking soda
4 tbsp sugar
1 L (or 4-1/3 cups) water

Mix or shake together all ingredients until the salt, baking soda, and sugar have dissolved in the water. Water should be kept at room temperature. Give frequent small sips to prevent dehydration and loss of electrolytes.

Adapted from Sears and Sack (1995).

---

tion, it is reasonable to wait 24 h to see if symptoms abate on their own. For motion sickness and travel-related prophylaxis, patients should be instructed to take medication 20–30 min before initiation of travel. Transdermal patches should be applied 2–3 h prior to travel.

Metoclopramide PO should be started 15–30 min before specific migraine therapy and repeated in 4–6 h (DiPiro & Bowden, 1997).

Chemotherapy–associated nausea and vomiting can be classified as acute, delayed, or anticipatory, depending upon the chemotherapeutic agent. Initiation of treatment should be based on the type of N & V as well as the agent used. Acute N & V usually occur within 1–4 h after the start of chemotherapy and resolve within 24 h. Delayed N & V may not begin for 24 h and may last for several days (Morrow, Hickok, & Rosenthal, 1995). Some chemotherapeutic agents may have both an acute and a delayed phase (Morrow et al, 1995). Anticipatory N & V are associated with provoking stimuli, such as sight, smell, sound, and remembrance of past experiences. Antiemetic agents should be started prior to chemotherapy for acute and anticipatory N & V and continued until the emetogenic potential of the chemotherapeutic agent has passed—usually 48 h for the vomiting and up to 72 h for the nausea (Rhodes, Watson, & Johnson, 1985).

See Drug Table 502.

## Assessment and History Taking

The determination of whether or not to initiate therapy should be based on a targeted medical history and physical examination. The history should include the following information:

- Timing of symptoms; relation to meals or other activities
- Self-treatments initiated and results
- Related signs/symptoms such as diarrhea and chest pain
- Current medications
- Presence of other medical problems, especially diabetes, renal disease, pregnancy, or peptic ulcer disease
- Recent history of travel (especially to areas with poor sanitation)
- Ingestion of foods commonly causing vomiting

The physical examination should include:

- Vital signs, including blood pressure and orthostatics
- Assessment of skin turgor and mucous membranes
- Abdominal examination to assess for distention, organ enlargement, visible peristalsis, abnormal bowel sounds, organ enlargement, and flank tenderness
- Screening neurological examination to assess for weakness

Consider the following diagnostic tests if symptoms are prolonged or especially severe:

- Serum chemistry (to check BUN/creatine; check glucose and anion gap, especially if the patient is diabetic)
- Liver function tests or AST and ALT (to rule out hepatitis)
- EKG (if myocardial infarction is suspected)
- Serum drug levels if an overdose is suspected (especially digitalis and theophylline)
- Pregnancy test if last menstrual period was more than 1 month ago
- X-ray to rule out obstruction (if symptoms present with acute abdominal pain)

Antiemetics have been implicated in contributing to or altering the course of Reye's syndrome and are not recommended for use in children. Their use should be limited to episodes of prolonged vomiting whose etiology is known.

Drug therapy should be minimized with pregnancy. No antiemetic is approved for used during pregnancy, although metoclopramide has been used without reports of fetal problems (Goroll et al, 1995).

Use of antiemetic drug therapy may make the diagnosis of acute abdomen more difficult.

Therefore, it is important to rule out emergency conditions such as myocardial infarction, paralytic ileus, or bowel obstruction before starting antiemetics.

## Patient/Caregiver Information

Primary emphasis should be on maintenance of hydration status, especially when diarrhea is also present. Giving very small sips of rehydration solution can assist. Instruct the patient and caregiver on Uphold and Graham's (1994) therapy regimen (Table 25–1). A reduction of personal and environmental activity and stimuli such as household smells and loud noises can serve as comfort measures. Teach patients to rinse their mouths after vomiting to minimize bad taste and corrosion of tooth enamel.

## OUTCOMES MANAGEMENT

### Selecting An Appropriate Agent

*Motion Sickness.* The differences in onset and duration of action of each drug should be kept in mind when selecting a drug for the prevention of motion sickness. Patients with mild to moderate motion sickness generally respond well to antihistamines such as dimenhydrinate (50–100 mg PO every 4–6 h, with a maximum dose of 400 mg a day), diphenhydramine (25–50 mg PO three to four times a day, up to 300 mg a day), and scopolamine. Scopolamine is more effective against motion sickness, with a faster onset of action but a relatively short duration compared to the antihistamines. By releasing drug constantly, at a rate of 0.5 mg every 72 h transdermal scopolamine (Transderm-Scop) provides an effective drug concentration over a prolonged period while minimizing the adverse effects. Scopolamine is also effective after nausea has started (Mitchelson, 1992).

*Migraine Headaches and Pain.* Migraines require treatment of the headache as well as therapy for the N & V. Metoclopramide increases the absorption or effectiveness of concurrent analgesic therapy and also acts as an antiemetic (Mitchelson, 1992). Phenothiazines such as prochlorperazine may be helpful in suppressing vomiting that is the result of migraines.

*Chemotherapy-Associated Nausea and Vomiting.* When choosing an agent for patients receiving chemotherapy, consider the mechanism of action of the drug and the pathological process causing the N & V. For example, chemotherapy-associated N & V may be the result of stimulation of the chemoreceptor trigger zone (CTZ) and also GI tract inflammation or irritation. Consequently, combination therapy with different mechanisms of antiemetic action is frequently required (Kris, 1992). A prokinetic drug like metoclopramide acts both centrally and peripherally by blocking dopamine receptors in the CTZ and gastrointestinal tract and, at high doses, serotonin receptors (Follet-Veryrat, Farinott, & Palmer, 1997). Therefore, this agent is helpful for migraines as well as chemotherapy-associated N & V. Metoclopramide, delivered via the oral, parenteral, or rectal route, has been effective in controlling highly emetogenic chemotherapeutic agents (Agostinucci, Gannon, Schauer, & Wallers, 1986; Anthony et al, 1986; Tami & Waite, 1988). High-dose metoclopramide (1–3 mg/kg) has been shown to be more effective in preventing emesis than prochlorperazine or cannabinoids in patients receiving cisplatin chemotherapy (Gralla et al, 1984, 1981). One major disadvantage of metoclopramide is the extrapyramidal side effects. However, intravenous diphenhydramine 50 mg usually prevents or eliminates these adverse effects (Morrow et al, 1995).

The antiemetic activity of corticosteroids (dexamethasone or methylprednisolone) has been beneficial when they are employed as single agents in mild or moderate emetogenic chemotherapy, but they are less effective against highly emetogenic agents (Cersosimo & Karp, 1986). Therefore, combination therapy with corticosteroids is a good choice when a single agent fails (Morrow et al, 1995). Large, single doses of corticosteroids are as effective as divided doses (Tortorice & O'Connell, 1990).

Phenothiazines are helpful in mild to moderate emetogenic chemotherapy, but have limited efficacy against highly emetogenic agents. Therefore, they are generally used in combination with other agents or as alternative agents. The piperazine compounds (thiethylperazine, prochloperazine, and perphenazine) as a class have the greatest antiemetic activity and produce less sedation and hypotension; however, they have the highest incidence of extrapyramidal effects (Seigel & Longo, 1981; Wampler, 1983).

The butyrophenones, haloperidol and droperidol, are potent inhibitors of the CTZ and more effective in controlling highly emetogenic chemotherapy (Krebs, 1988). At antiemetic doses, the frequency of extrapyramidal, cardiovascular, and respiratory effects may be less than that seen with phenothiazines. Butyrophenones are generally inferior to high-dose metoclopramide but may be useful as an alternative therapy for patients intolerant of the side effects or refractory to metoclopramide.

The cannabinoids, dronabinol and nabilone, have been effective in patients refractory to other antiemetic therapy. Because of their high frequency of side effects and abuse potential, cannabinoids are not first-line antiemetics and should be used as alternative antiemetics or in combination therapy. Younger patients are more tolerant of cannabinoid-induced psychologic effects (Sallen, Cronin, Zellen, & Zimberg, 1980).

Serotonin antagonists, such as ondansetron and granisetron, have been very effective in the treatment and prevention of chemotherapy-associated N & V. Comparative studies have shown that granisetron is as effective as high-dose metoclopramide plus dexamethasone, and superior to combinations of phenothiazines plus dexamethasone in the treatment of cisplatin-induced N & V (Chevallier, 1990; Marty, 1990).

Ondansetron, 8 mg orally, either as a divided dose given 1 h prior to chemotherapy and 12 h after the start of chemotherapy, or as a single dose 1 h prior to chemotherapy, has demonstrated effectiveness against high-dose metoclopramide in controlling emesis in patients receiving moderate and highly emetogenic chemotherapy (Ettinger et al, 1996; Marty et al, 1990). Studies comparing the two serotonin antagonists have found them to be comparable (Ruff et al, 1994). The combination with dexamethasone has been shown to increase the effectiveness of the serotonin antagonist in patients receiving highly emetogenic chemotherapy (Roila & The Italian Group, 1995). However, serotonin receptor antagonists do not appear to be superior to conventional therapy (metoclopramide plus dexamethasone) in the treatment of delayed chemotherapy-induced N & V (DeMulder et al, 1990). In addition, these agents are very expensive. Therefore, these agents are considered the drug of choice only for patients who are receiving highly emetogenic chemotherapy, those unable to tolerate the adverse effects, or those refractory to other antiemetic therapy.

Benzodiazepines (lorazepam and midazolam) are agents with anxiolytic and amnestic properties; therefore, they are helpful in the prevention of anticipatory N & V associated with chemotherapy (Kris, 1992).

**Mechanical Obstruction or Motility Disorders.** Prokinetic agents are very effective in the treatment of mechanical obstruction or motility disorders. Cisapride, as well as metoclopramide, can stimulate the GI tract in patients with diabetic gastroparesis. However metoclopramide has been shown to decrease N & V more than cisapride (Agostinucci et al, 1986; Gralla et al, 1981; Tami & Waite, 1988).

**Postoperative Vomiting.** The incidence of postoperative N & V depends upon the anesthesia used, the age of the patient, and the concurrent medications used. Benzquinamide, phenothiazines, and butyrophenones are very helpful. Metoclopramide has not been shown to be effective possibly because of its short duration of action compared to the duration of the anesthetic agent (Mitchelson, 1992).

## Monitoring for Efficacy

Symptoms should improve within a short period of time, usually with one or two courses of medication. If symptoms do not resolve after maximum, frequent doses of antiemetic medication, the patient should be switched to a different agent with a different mechanism of action. N & V associated with an underlying process may require correction of the underlying cause before complete resolution of symptoms can occur. If the N & V are the result of a drug toxicity, symptoms should abate after the serum concentration of the offending drug starts to fall within the therapeutic range. If the symptoms continue despite a normal serum concentration, the drug should not be restarted. Select an alternative agent. Signs and symptoms of dehydration, electrolyte disturbances, and volume depletion should be monitored with frequent evaluation of mucous membranes and skin turgor. Fluid replacement should be initiated if necessary. Follow-up is not usually indicated after resolution of symptoms.

Migraine headache associated emesis requires time for the underlying condition to abate. If the patient does not show improvement with metoclopramide or the patient cannot take the drug orally, prochlorperazine suppositories can be used.

Prolonged N & V can occur following chemotherapy; other antiemetic agents should be added to the regimen if chemotherapy-associated N & V fail to respond adequately to the initial treatment. A patient's prior history with chemotherapy-associated N & V greatly affects the emetic control of subsequent therapy. Use of benzodiazepines may be beneficial to prevent subsequent anticipatory N & V. If good control is obtained with a particular regimen, maintain the regimen for successive therapy. If pharmacotherapy is not effective, behavioral interventions may help prevent anticipatory N & V and reduce posttreatment symptoms (Morrow et al, 1995). Behavioral methods include relaxation techniques, hypnosis, distraction, and biofeedback (Burish & Jenkins, 1992; Morrow et al, 1995).

## DIARRHEA

Diarrhea, or the abnormal frequency and liquidity of bowel movements, is another familiar condition in primary care practices. Virtually all diarrhea seen in an outpatient setting is due to infection, has an antibiotic association, is food- or drug-induced, or is the result of inflammatory bowel disease. Diarrhea can be classified as acute or chronic, depending on whether or not it persists for more than 3 weeks (McQuaid, 1997). Most patients have simple diarrhea manifested by watery stools, low-grade fever, mild malaise, abdominal cramps, and nausea (Nathwani & Wood, 1993). Although most episodes are short-term and self-limiting, serious effects such as dehydration, perforation, perianal skin breakdown, weight loss, and nutritional compromise can result if symptoms do not resolve and the condition becomes chronic. Approximately 5–10% of patients who seek medical care for diarrheal illness present with dysentery (Nathwani & Wood, 1993). Travelers' diarrhea is the passage of at least three unformed stools in a 24-h period, together with nausea, vomiting, fecal urgency, and abdominal pain or cramps (DuPont & Ericsson, 1993).

## SPECIFIC CONSIDERATIONS FOR PHARMACOTHERAPY

### When Drug Therapy Is Needed

In general, diarrhea is self-limiting. If an infectious etiology is present, there is an associated morbidity and mortality, especially in populations of children and the elderly. The most disastrous consequences of infectious diarrhea (dysentery) are related to dehydration and toxic megacolon, and are seen with *Clostridium difficile*. All patients with dysentery should receive antibiotic therapy (McQuaid, 1997). In travelers' diarrhea, symptoms are usually mild and short-lived, lasting 1–5 days—just enough to spoil a vacation.

## Short- and Long-Term Goals of Pharmacotherapy

The short-term goal of treatment for diarrhea is prevention or reversal of fluid and electrolyte disturbances and any resultant metabolic complications. Long-term goals of treatment include prevention of recurrent episodes and prevention of antibiotic-resistant organisms.

## Nonpharmacologic Therapy

Oral rehydration therapy in either homemade (see Table 25–2) or commercial forms, such as Pedialyte, should precede or accompany all other therapies. This is especially important in children and the elderly to prevent loss of fluids and electrolytes.

Persons who develop travelers' diarrhea should practice good food hygiene. This includes avoiding tap water and ice cubes, unreliable restaurants, raw seafood, uncooked foods, and unpeeled fruits. Bottled or boiled water should be used even for tooth brushing.

Discontinue any antibiotics that are associated with the development of *Clostridium difficile* or change to another antibiotic with less incidence of causing this problem.

Regular dietary intake should be maintained. A BRAT diet (bananas, rice, applesauce, tea/toast) can assist in maintaining nutrition status and avoiding dehydration. In adults, dairy products should be avoided during the time of symptoms and for several days after resolution because lactose intolerance accompanies many cases of diarrhea (Richter, 1995). Children can continue to receive lactose-containing products (Brown, 1994).

Good perianal hygiene can avoid skin irritation and breakdown. After each loose stool, rinsing the perineum with warm water and patting the area dry with a cotton towel will minimize discomfort. Toilet paper should be avoided. Witch hazel pads (Tucks) are soothing. Apply hydrocortisone cream or an emollient such as petrolatum jelly to the perineum. Sitz baths for 10 min, two or three times a day, are a comfort measure.

## Time Frame for Initiating Pharmacotherapy

Assurance of adequate hydration is the initial step in treatment. Consideration of whether or not antibiotics would be useful can be based on the epidemiological setting and the medical history. Empiric antibiotic treatment for diarrhea in otherwise healthy adults in industrialized countries is not recommended (Scott & Edelman, 1993).

Prophylaxis for travelers' diarrhea should be initiated on the day of arrival at the risk location and continued for 1–2 days after leaving the country, to a maximum of 3 weeks (DuPont et al, 1987). The decision to initiate treatment for travelers' diarrhea will depend on the severity and duration of the diarrhea, and the past medical history of the traveler. Mild diarrhea is generally self-limiting and requires only symptomatic treatment. If the patient is dehydrated, rehydration should be initiated promptly and antidiarrheal agents initiated for relief of symptoms. If the diarrhea is severe or the patient high-risk (ie, is immunocompromised or has gastro-intestinal disease or low gastric acidity), antibacterial agents should be started.

The use of antidiarrheal drugs is not recommended for treatment of acute diarrhea in children.

See Drug Table 501.8.

## Assessment and History Taking

To determine the kind or even desirability of therapy a targeted medical history and physical examination are needed. The history and examination should include the following:

- Timing of symptoms; relation to meals; acute or chronic condition
- Related signs and symptoms
- Current medications, especially antibiotics
- Presence of other medical problems, especially diabetes, renal disease, pregnancy, peptic ulcer disease, HIV infection
- Recent history of travel (especially to areas with poor sanitation)
- Ingestion of foods commonly causing diarrhea
- Self-treatments initiated and results

The physical examination should include assessment of:

- Vital signs, including BP for postural hypotension, temperature, weight
- Skin turgor, mucous membranes
- Abdomen to check for tenderness, distention, guarding, rebound, abnormal bowel sounds, organ enlargement or masses, visible peristalsis
- Rectal exam and fecal occult blood check (if positive, do CBC with differential to determine if infectious process or occult bleed)
- Screening neurologic examination to assess for weakness

Consider the following diagnostic tests if symptoms do not resolve within 3 days:

- Stool bacterial culture
- Stool examination for ova and parasites
- *Clostridium difficile* toxin assay (if recent history of antibiotics)
- CBC with differential (to rule out infectious process or if fecal occult blood test is positive)

## Patient/Caregiver Information

The importance of thorough hand washing with soap and water after each episode of loose stool should be stressed. Hand lotions can minimize dryness and towels used for hand drying should be changed daily.

Education about the importance of maintaining nutritional input should be provided. Many patients have misconceptions about the use of ORT agents and should be instructed that their use is to prevent dehydration, not to reduce the actual symptoms of diarrhea. Also, since food products like Gatorade or Jello do not contain the proper ratios of essential elements, they should not be used as a treatment for diarrhea. (See Table 25–1 for recommendations.)

## OUTCOMES MANAGEMENT

### Selecting An Appropriate Agent

Antibiotics are the mainstay of therapy for the treatment of diarrhea of infectious etiology. Selection of an agent requires consideration of the patient's allergy history, previous drug history, age, whether the patient is pregnant, the severity of the diarrhea, antibiotic resistance pattern in the community, and suspected pathogen.

The management of travelers' diarrhea can be divided into prophylaxis and treatment. Many investigators feel that prophylaxis with antibiotics is not indicated in the majority of people because it may lead (1) to the development of antibiotic-associated diarrhea, (2) other adverse effects, and (3) antibiotic resistance (DuPont & Ericsson, 1993; Johnson et al, 1986). Antibiotic prophylaxis may be considered in people with (1) a previous history of travelers' diarrhea, (2) an underlying illness that would be worsened with the development of diarrhea, or (3) travel plans to an area with poor sanitation for less than 3 weeks. Fluoroquinolones (ciprofloxacin, ofloxacin, or norfloxacin) ("Advice for Travelers," 1996) or trimethoprim-sulfamethoxazole (DuPont et al, 1987) is recommended when prophylaxis is used. Other approaches to the prevention of travelers' diarrhea are the use of lactobacillus preparations or bismuth subsalicylate (DuPont et al, 1987; Oksanen et al, 1990). Bismuth subsalicylate should not be used in persons allergic to salicylates or with coagulopathies. Bismuth subsalicylate is not as effective when given twice daily as when given four times a day with meals (DuPont et al, 1987).

For treatment of mild diarrhea, travelers can use antimotility drugs (loperamide or diphenoxylate plus atropine) or bismuth subsalicylate (Pepto-Bismol) to shorten symptom time (Johnson et al, 1986). Bismuth subsalicylate may be preferred because of its antisecretory and antimicrobial activity (Gorbach, 1990). Bismuth subsalicylate should not be taken with doxycycline or fluoroquinolones, since it can prevent the absorption of the latter. Although the onset of action of the antimotility drugs is faster than bismuth subsalicylate, antimotility drugs may aggravate diarrhea that is caused by enteropathogens such as *Shigella* and *Campylobacter* (Danziger & Itakazu, 1995; DuPont & Hormick, 1973). In addition, caution should be exercised in using opiate-based antimotility drugs because they can cause sedation, nausea, and vomiting. Therefore, antimotility drugs should not be used in patients with high fever or bloody stools, and they should be discontinued if symptoms persist for greater than 48 h. They can serve as an alternative agent in nondysenteric travelers' diarrhea. Antimicrobial therapy is recommended if symptoms worsen or continue for more than 24 h, for diarrhea associated with fever, for severe diarrhea, and for symptoms that recur when symptomatic therapy is discontinued. Antibacterial drug therapy should be active against the principle pathogens responsible for travelers' diarrhea. *Escherichia coli* is the most frequently isolated pathogen (30–70%) in all parts of the world, with *Shigella* species occurring 5–20% of the time (Nathwani & Wood, 1993). Salmonella, *Vibrio parahaemolyticus* and campylobacter species are less common (Nathwani & Wood, 1993). *Campylobacter* species are subject to seasonal variation, predominating in the winter months.

Trimethoprim-sulfamethoxazole (Bactrim, Septra) and doxycycline are two effective agents for both prophylaxis and treatment for travelers' diarrhea for most areas. However, trimethoprim-sulfamethoxazole may not be effective in the treatment of *Campylobacter*-associated diarrhea and, therefore, should not be used if traveling in the winter or to known areas of resistance. Resistance is also found in many areas of the world to doxycycline (Dupont et al, 1987). Because photosensitivity is an adverse effect of doxycycline, this drug should be avoided in persons traveling to sunny areas or engaged in outdoor activity.

Fluoroquinolones are the drugs of choice for adults traveling to high-risk parts of the world, or areas with very poor sanitation (Ericsson et al, 1987). All fluoroquinolone drugs (ciprofloxacin, norfloxacin, ofloxacin, and fleroxacin) have similar efficacy; the choice should depend upon concurrent medications and cost. Doxycycline and the fluoroquinolones should not be given to pregnant women or children under the age of 12 years.

Up-to-date detailed information for travelers is available from the Centers for Disease Control's annual bulletin *Health Information for International Travel*, or the CDC phone line (401-332-4559).

The drug of choice for treatment of *Clostridium difficile* pseudomembranous colitis is metronidazole. It is as effective as vancomycin and much lower in cost. It addition, with the widespread use of vancomycin, resistance has developed to this antibiotic. Vancomycin can be considered as backup therapy if there is no response to metronidazole. Although antimotility drugs promote relief of diarrheal symptoms, they should be avoided in these patients.

Intestinal parasites such as *Giardia lamblia* Microsporidia, *Entamoeba histolytica*, *Isospora belli*, and *Cryptosporidium parvum* are all frequent causes of waterborne diarrheal outbreaks in humans. Infections with these organisms are generally self-limiting except in children, the el-

derly, and immunocompromised patients. Stool cultures should be done to determine appropriate, organism-specific treatment. Empiric therapy is not recommended (Liu & Weller, 1996).

Immunocompromised patients will require more aggressive therapy. Approximately 50% of patients with HIV infection will have a diarrhea infection, although the etiology may be elusive. Evaluations to identify the causative organisms may include sigmoidoscopy and/or upper and lower endoscopy.

Cholera, a serious diarrheal disease in both children and adults caused by *Vibrio* species, requires aggressive rehydration. Two days of tetracycline have been effective in clearing the stool of vibrios (Islam, 1987). For tetracycline-resistant cholera, erythromycin and norfloxacin have been used successfully (Scott & Edelman, 1993); furazolidone is an alternative antibiotic for children.

## Monitoring for Efficacy

For travelers' diarrhea, after the initiation of antimicrobial therapy, diarrhea should subside within 24–36 h. Temperature should return to normal within 24 h. For *Clostridium difficile* diarrhea, relapse is frequent despite the extreme sensitivity of the organism to antibiotic therapy. Relapses respond well to retreatment with vancomycin or metronidazole. Similarly, those who fail to respond to metronidazole may respond to vancomycin.

# CONSTIPATION

Constipation is defined as the infrequent or difficult evacuation of feces. It results from delayed colonic transit time, usually the consequence of a sedentary lifestyle, inadequate intake of fluids and high-fiber foods, or the habitual ignoring of the urge to defecate. This common problem, which is one of the most frequent reasons for self-medication, is usually without serious underlying cause.

## SPECIFIC CONSIDERATIONS FOR PHARMACOTHERAPY

### When Drug Therapy Is Needed

The normal frequency of bowel movements can vary greatly, and the usual pattern of the individual must be taken into account. For some, daily or even two to three times a day may be the norm, while others will have bowel movements only every 3–5 days. Individual differences may be the result of diet and/or exercise. A change in the patient's usual pattern may be reason for intervention. Although not common, metabolic and endocrine disturbances can be the reason for the constipation, and they must be ruled out.

## Short- and Long-Term Goals of Pharmacotherapy

The establishment of normal bowel patterns, that is, the comfortable passage of formed stool on a regular basis, should be the goal of pharmacotherapy.

## Nonpharmacologic Therapy

The primary prevention of constipation consists of adequate dietary intake of fluids and fibrous foods, moderate exercise, and recognition of the urge to defecate. Nonpharmacologic therapy consists of changing a sedentary lifestyle, increasing dietary fiber (bran cereal, whole grain breads, fruits, and vegetables), and maintaining an adequate fluid intake, usually a minimum of six to eight glasses of noncaffeinated beverages daily.

## Time Frame for Initiating Pharmacotherapy

Conservative therapy for constipation can be initiated when a patient complains of feeling bloated or having difficulty moving his or her bowels.

See Drug Tables 501.9, 501.10.

## Assessment and History Taking

A screening history and physical examination should determine that intestinal obstruction, drug-induced constipation, and metabolic and endocrine disorders are not the causes of the patient's constipation. The history should include the following:

- Patient's usual bowel habits (if alternating with diarrhea, consider irritable bowel syndrome)
- Recent dietary intake
- Activity level
- Other medications (including OTCs, such as iron)
- Previous use of laxatives, enemas

- Other medical problems
- Signs of hypothyroidism
- Somatic complaints that might indicate depression
- History of current pregnancy, postpartum status, or recent abdominal surgery

The physical examination should include:

- Abdominal examination checking for bowel sounds, distention, tenderness, rebound
- Anal check for fissures, irritation, and hemorrhoids; rectal examination for hemorrhoids, fecal impaction, and occult blood

Diagnostic tests to consider to rule out obstruction and metabolic and endocrine disorders as causes of constipation include:

- Abdominal x-ray (if the constipation is of acute onset, accompanied by abdominal pain)
- Thyroid stimulating hormone (TSH) (if there are other signs of hypothyroidism)
- Serum chemistry (if diabetes, hypokalemia, or hypercalcemia is suspected)

If the patient with constipation also has nausea, vomiting, or abdominal pain, do not give laxatives.

## Patient/Caregiver Information

For prevention and for initial therapy, a change in dietary habits to include foods high in fiber should be a priority for patients with constipation. The adequate intake of foods such as fruits, vegetables, and whole grain breads will result almost immediately in decreased GI transit time. Over the long term, such a diet is correlated with decreased colon cancer and diverticulosis.

Urge patients to avoid long-term or chronic use of laxatives and enemas. Although they are generally safe and well-tolerated drugs, the potential for dependence exists if laxatives are used regularly over long periods of time. Patients should work toward lifestyle changes including increased exercise, increased fluid intake, and increased dietary fiber.

## OUTCOMES MANAGEMENT

## Selecting An Appropriate Agent

Bulk-forming agents, such as wheat bran, absorb water and make soft, bulky stools without systemic side effects. They are taken by mixing with a full glass of water or juice and must not be chewed or swallowed dry. These agents are quite effective if taken on a regular basis. They can be purchased in bulk at health food stores or supermarkets and are inexpensive for daily use.

Psyllium preparations are more expensive but also effective with regular use. They may contain large amounts of dextrose and should be avoided by patients who have diabetes. These agents are excellent choices, as are stool softeners, for patients with hemorrhoids, for women who are pregnant, or for patients in whom Valsalva's maneuvers can be difficult or harmful, such as post-MI patients or patients who have had recent surgery.

Stool softeners or emollients work by allowing water in the intestine to enter the stool. They are used for prevention of constipation and are less useful in its treatment. Emollients are useful in patients who are pregnant and post-MI patients, in whom straining should be avoided.

Mineral oil or liquid petrolatum lubricates and softens the stool. Its long-term use should be avoided because of the potential for impairing the absorption of vitamins A and D. They should not be given to children under 6 years of age.

Enemas are used only in cases of fecal impaction and seldom indicated in the primary care setting. Stimulants increase GI peristalsis but can often also cause GI cramping.

Saline laxatives should be used with caution in patients with decreased ambulatory ability, because they may experience incontinence as the result of laxative use. These laxatives usually work within 2–6 h and are indicated when fast, complete bowel evacuation is needed. Saline laxatives can result in considerable fluid loss, so they should not be used in the elderly or in patients with hypertension or cardiac conditions.

Nonpregnant patients showing no result from conservative therapy might find symptom relief with the use of cisapride 10 mg three to four times a day (Gardner, Beckwith, & Heyneman, 1995).

## Monitoring for Efficacy

Moderate exercise, increasing noncaffeinated fluids to six to eight glasses daily, prune juice, bulk-forming agents, or stool softeners should show effects within 2 days. If there is no effect within 1 week, a more thorough workup is indicated.

# INFLAMMATORY BOWEL DISEASE

The two inflammatory bowel diseases (IBDs)—Crohn's disease (CD) and ulcerative colitis (UC)—have similar symptoms but also important differences. UC is a mucosal disease and confined to the colon. In contrast, Crohn's disease affects any part of the gastrointestinal tract. UC causes a cascade of abdominal cramping, diarrhea, rectal bleeding, and weight loss. CD is characterized by chronic intestinal inflammation and periodic exacerbations with a variety of local and systematic manifestations (Ruymann & Richter, 1995). The chronic nature of the symptoms of IBD makes management a challenge; however, the majority of patients can be managed in a primary care setting, with referral to gastroenterologists necessary only for the most severe cases.

## SPECIFIC CONSIDERATIONS FOR PHARMACOTHERAPY

### When Drug Therapy Is Needed

Drug therapy acts at multiple sites, locally—depending on the location of the intestinal lesions—and systemically—to minimize inflammation. Drug therapy for UC and CD is indicated to enable patients to maintain as normal a lifestyle as possible, prevent nutritional deficiencies, and minimize the physiologic and social impact of the disease. Such treatment offers most patients relief from the symptoms of diarrhea, bleeding, abdominal cramps, flatulence, and pain. Drug therapy is the first line of defense against both diseases for patients with uncomplicated disease. Surgical intervention is reserved for patients with drug- or disease-related complications or for whom medical treatment has failed.

### Short- and Long-Term Goals of Pharmacotherapy

The long-term goal of pharmacotherapy is to control mucosal inflammation and minimize the systemic impact of disease. Short-term goals are to induce and maintain remission of symptoms and to assist in the maintenance of an adequate nutritional status. However, clinical signs of remission are often difficult to interpret because they are so varied and subjective.

## Nonpharmacologic Therapy

A positive therapeutic alliance between patient and provider is essential in the care of patients with long-term, frequently relapsing conditions such as IBD. Patients can experience a sense of trust and caring by working together with a provider to monitor the ups and downs of symptom exacerbation and medication efficacy and side effects common in IBD.

For all patients with cramping and diarrhea, an empiric trial of a milk-free diet will eliminate symptoms that may be due to lactose intolerance (DiPiro & Bowden, 1997). The constipation symptoms that may be a part of IBD can be treated with bulk-type laxatives. However, fiber should be reduced when patients have active disease symptoms of cramping and diarrhea (Ruymann & Richter, 1995).

Nutritional support is important to prevent or minimize weight loss, or inadequate intake of vitamins and minerals. Multiple therapies are used to ensure an adequate nutritional status and minimize inflammation. In UC, therapy must make up for the increased nutritional loss as a result of diarrhea and the often decreased intake. Large doses of fish oil capsules (Max-EPA, Purepa) three times a day have been found to reduce the number of relapses or the need for steroids (Belluzzi et al, 1996; Stenson et al, 1992); however, some patients dislike the taste and resultant fishy breath.

In CD, bowel rest can be obtained with the preparations of an elemental diet such as Ensure, Sustacal, or Magnacal. In severe cases, total parenteral nutrition (TPN) for short periods of time may be indicated to improve symptoms, inflammation, and nutritional status (DiPiro & Bowden, 1997). Children and adolescents can alternate these nutritional therapies with steroids to allow them to obtain the nutrients needed for normal growth and development (DiPiro & Bowden, 1997). TPN should only be used for patients with severe malnutrition and/or intolerance to an elemental diet. Patients with steatorrhea should reduce their overall fat intake.

All patients with CD should take a multivitamin with minerals. Patients on long-term steroid therapy should supplement it with vitamin D and calcium supplements. Patients on sulfasalazine should supplement with folic acid (1 mg/day) (Ruymann & Richter, 1995). Patients who have had ileal resections should supplement with vitamins A, $B_{12}$, and D. Oral or parenteral iron supplements will be necessary if anemia is present.

Smoking, acetaminophen use, and increased sugar intake have been associated with increased symptoms of CD (Podolsky, 1991) so avoiding or minimizing use can be suggested to patients.

Nonsmoking has been positively correlated with the incidence of UC, and a role for nicotine has been suggested. Transdermal nicotine patches have been found to improve symptoms for some patients (Pullan et al, 1994), although nicotine gum was less helpful (Lashner, Hanauer, & Silverstein, 1990).

The National Ileitis and Colitis Foundation can provide patient education and support; check for the availability of local chapters. Exploration of sources of stress and their relationship to symptom manifestation may be productive for some patients, along with support for individualized stress relief and relaxation activities.

## Time Frame for Initiating Pharmacotherapy

Because of the relapsing nature of IBD, treatment depends on the patient's clinical picture. Pharmacotherapy should be instituted when symptoms occur. CD can present in an insidious manner; fever, weight loss, perianal disease, and fistulas indicate the need to start treatment. Sulfasalazine, aminosalicylic acid (5-ASA) preparations, or antibiotic therapy are used to treat mild CD. For disease of the colon, sulfasalazine is generally given for 4–8 weeks; if there is a positive response, therapy is continued for 4–6 months (Ruymann & Richter, 1995) and then stopped if the patient has no symptoms. Corticosteroid therapy is indicated for the short-term induction of remission in patients with moderate or severe symptoms. Immunosuppressive therapy can be used in CD patients who are dependent on corticosteroids or have persistent perianal disease or fistulas (Hanauer, 1996).

In patients with mild cases of UC, which are less associated with rectal bleeding, urgency, frequency, and rectal pain, treatment should be based on severity of symptoms and location of disease. Patients with mild to moderate disease can generally be treated with either oral or topical 5-ASA compounds or sulfasalazine. Patients with severe symptoms need close monitoring and may require hospitalization for treatment and observation of toxic megacolin. Costicosteroids are generally required to bring the acute disease under control. As in CD, immunosuppressive therapy is indicated for long-term treatment in patients with UC who are dependent on corticosteroids or do not respond to aminosalicylate corticosteroid therapy (Hanauer, 1996).

Patients with ulcerative proctitis should be differentiated from patients with more extensive disease. Ulcerative proctitis can generally be treated with topical compounds. Oral or topical therapy also can be used for disease of the distal colon or rectum.

With immunosuppressive drugs, therapy may take up to 6 months to show a positive effect. Aminosalicylates such as mesalamine can take several weeks to months to show effects (Shah & Peppercorn, 1995).

See Drug Tables 102.9, 102.10.

## Assessment and History Taking

Since the laboratory workup that will give a definitive diagnosis is based on the patient's symptoms, a thorough history about the onset, timing, and nature of symptoms is essential. Ask about extracolonic disease manifestations, which can be seen in both UC and CD, such as blurred vision, headaches, eye pain, photophobia, mouth sores, and joint pain. Ask also about the associated signs and symptoms of active hepatitis, cholelithiasis, or kidney stones that are often seen in patients with IBD (Ruymann & Richter, 1995). History about family disease, recent travel, and/or antibiotic use is also helpful in ruling out other causes of symptoms.

In the physical examination, focus on the following areas:

- Vital signs, weight, body mass index
- Skin surfaces, especially of extremities and tibial surfaces of arms and legs for lesions of erythema nodosum
- Mouth, checking for lesions
- Thorough eye examination
- Thorough abdominal examination
- Rectal and perianal examination

To diagnose UC, flexible sigmoidoscopy without cleansing preparation is useful; if this gives only nonspecific findings, a stool culture and sensitivity and/or rectal biopsy may be more helpful (Ruymann & Richter, 1995). A barium enema or colonoscopy can assist in an uncertain diagnosis, but should not be performed during acute attacks since the risk of bowel perforation is increased.

In CD, a barium enema or air contrast barium enema can show the characteristic skip patterns of CD and provide a definitive diagnosis. In difficult to diagnose cases, sigmoidoscopy or colonoscopy also can be helpful. Radiologic tests should be minimized during pregnancy. A CBC, sedimentation rate, serum chemistry, and stool exam for occult blood can provide useful baseline information.

## Patient/Caregiver Information

Sulfonamide drugs can result in hypersensitivity reactions of rash and fever or the dose-related side effects of nausea, vomiting, and headaches (Hirschfeld & Clearfield, 1995). Titrating the dose of the sulfasalazine can help to minimize headaches; taking these drugs with food will minimize other side effects (Hanauer & Baert, 1994). Sulfonamides also interfere with the bioavailability of digoxin so patients should be warned of signs and symptoms of inadequate digoxin dosing. Sulfa should not be taken at the same time as iron preparations (Ruymann & Richter, 1995).

Patients given metronidazole should be warned to avoid all alcohol and alcohol-containing products.

Patients should be told to contact their provider if they experience fever, increased diarrhea, rectal bleeding, or increased abdominal pain.

## OUTCOMES MANAGEMENT

The primary end points of therapy should be the induction and remission of disease. In UC, the severity of disease can be assessed on the basis of clinical features using endoscopy and the criteria of Truelove and Witts (Hanauer, 1996). The Gastrointestinal Advisory Panel of the Food and Drug Administration has defined remission of UC as "absence of inflammatory symptoms (ie, rectal bleeding) along with mucosal healing" (Hanauer, 1991). Assessing disease activity in patients with CD is more difficult because the clinical pattern and complications are more heterogeneous (Hanauer, 1996). The Crohn's Disease Activity Index has been used and consists of clinical variables and assessment of a patient's well-being. However, these end points are often difficult to define in IBD (Hodgson & Hazlan, 1991).

Maintenance therapy should be aimed at preventing recurrence of active disease.

## Selecting An Appropriate Agent

Treatment options are determined by the location, the extent, and the severity of disease, and by the patient's response to current or past therapy.

Corticosteroids have been the most widely used and efficacious agents for the induction of remission of both moderate to severe active ulcerative colitis and Crohn's disease (Griffin & Miner, 1995). These agents are not useful as maintenance therapy for disease in remission or prophylaxis (Peppercorn, 1990; Shah & Peppercorn, 1995). The addition of corticosteroids to sulfasalazine for the treatment of patients with active Crohn's disease results in more rapid initial improvement, but not better overall results (Linn & Peppercorn, 1992). Therefore, corticosteroids are used primarily in severely ill patients or in patients who have failed with sulfasalazine or mesalamine. Once symptomatic improvement has been induced, steroids should be tapered to avoid their associated ill effects. The corticosteroid of choice should be one that is low in mineralocorticoid activity and high in antiinflammatory activity, such as prednisone or methylprednisolone.

Rectal administration of steroids has proven effective in patients with localized distal colitis, whereas oral corticosteroids are active against mild to moderate disease (Peppercorn, 1990). The use of topical rectal corticosteroids can minimize the adverse-effect profile as well as tenesmus and the urgent call to stool in patients with mild UC that is limited to the distal colon and rectum (Geier, Miner, Danielsson, Hellers, & Lyrenas, 1987). Foam preparations and suppositories are easier to administer than hydrocortisone enemas. However, even local administration can lead to Cushing's syndrome and adrenal suppression (Hanauer, Meyers, & Sachar, 1995; Mulder & Tygat, 1993). Newer oral and topical steroids with minimal side effects are currently used in Europe and expected to become available soon in the United States. In children, steroid therapy, using an alternating dose schedule, has minimized the effect on growth hormone. Since there may be better absorption of gluccocorticoid from intact than from inflamed mucosa, a lower dose can be used as healing occurs (Petitijean et al, 1992). In patients with severe UC, the absorption of oral corticosteroids may be decreased, requiring parenteral therapy. Corticotropin has been shown to be superior to hydrocortisone in patients naive to corticosteroid therapy; hydrocortisone is superior in patients previously treated with corticosteroids (Meyers, Sachar, Goldberg, & Janowitz, 1983).

The initial and subsequent dose of corticosteroid therapy should be individualized based upon the severity of symptoms and disease, and the corticosteroid used. Corticosteroid therapy should not be abruptly stopped, but gradually tapered as symptoms are controlled.

Sulfasalazine, a combination of 5-ASA and sulfapyridine, is effective for the initial treatment of UC and CD; it also is useful in preventing relapses. In CD this drug is only effective in patients with disease involving the colon or the ileum; it is not effective in patients with only small bowel disease (Malchow, 1984). Sulfasalazine will induce remission in up to 75% of patients with UC. Remission will be maintained in 70% of patients compared to 24% of those receiving placebo (Linn & Peppercorn, 1992). Since sulfasalazine is generally considered less effective than steroids, it is reserved for mild cases. It can also be combined with oral steroids for early treatment. Relapse rates appear to be dose-related, with higher doses resulting in lower frequencies of relapse (Griffin & Miner, 1995). For both UC and CD, a sulfasalazine dose of 500 mg q.i.d. PO can be initiated and increased rapidly to 4 g daily. As symptoms are relieved, decrease to the lowest dose necessary to control symptoms, usually 2–4 g/day (Ruymann & Richter, 1995). Doses greater than 4 g/day tend to increase side effects.

Despite its widespread acceptance, the usefulness of sulfasalazine has been limited by its adverse-effect profile (Peppercorn, 1990), which is a dose-related function of the sulfapyridine moiety (Hanauer, 1996; Geier et al, 1987). To counter this, the active component of sulfasalazine, 5-aminosalicylate, was isolated. Mesalamine, the generic name for 5-aminosalicylate, is hydrolyzed quickly in the stomach and well absorbed in the proximal small intestine. It does not reach disease sites in the distal colon and rectum. However, mesalamine can be administered via retention enemas or suppositories. Studies with patients with distal colitis have shown this form of administration to be more effective than placebos and as effective as sulfasalazine (Biddel & Miner, 1990; Campieri et al, 1990; Sutherland et al, 1987). Because local contact is necessary for therapeutic efficacy, rectal administration of mesalamine should be used only in patients with disease confined to the distal colon (Hanauer, 1996). For long-term prophylaxis, oral forms of therapy are preferable to enemas or suppositories (Peppercorn, 1990).

In an attempt to increase the area of treatment, controlled-release (Pentasa) and delayed-release (Asacol) versions of mesalamine and a dimer of 5-aminosalicylic acid (olsalazine) have been developed for the treatment of disease in the small intestine and colon. In general, these oral aminosalicylates are therapeutically equivalent to sulfasalazine in the treatment of active disease or the maintenance of remission in mild or moderate UC. However, they may be better tolerated than sulfasalazine and can be used in patients unable to tolerate sulfasalazine (Linn & Peppercorn, 1992; "Olsalazine for Ulcerative Colitis," 1990). Pentasa has been shown to be useful as well in achieving and controlling remission in patients with active CD (Hanauer, 1993; Hanauer et al, 1990). Asacol also may prove useful in maintaining Crohn's disease in remission (Pallone et al, 1991). The recommended dose for Pentasa is 1.5–4 gs/day PO, in four divided doses; Asacol doses are 800–2400 mg/day PO, in three divided doses. For the maintenance of remission with olsalazine, the dose is 500 mg twice daily.

A switch to metronidazole 250–500 mg PO, three times a day may be helpful for patients with mild to moderate CD who are unresponsive to sulfasalazine or olsalazine (Ruymann & Richter, 1995). Metronidazole 750–2000 mg PO per day is also effective for perianal complications in CD; treatment needs to be long-term (Ruymann & Richter, 1995). Many clinicians are using other antibiotics, especially ciprofloxacin in patients with CD who are intolerant or unresponsive to metronidazole (Hanauer & Baert, 1994; Peppercorn, 1993). Antibiotics, including metronidazole, have not been shown to be reliably effective in UC unless the patient has a concurrent infection with *Clostridium difficile*. Research findings do not support their use (Hanauer & Baert, 1994).

For CD patients who are refractory to aminosalicylates and/or steroids or who are steroid-dependent, the use of immunosuppressive therapies such as azathioprine (2.0–2.5 mg/kg per day PO) and 6-mercaptopurine (1–1.5 mg/kg per day PO) are indicated (Hanauer & Baert, 1994) and may allow tapering of the steroids (Ewe, Press, & Singe, 1993). Azathioprine has been shown to prolong remission in corticosteroid-dependent

patients with UC (Hawthorne, Logan, & Gawkey, 1992). Caution is needed in the use of these agents because of their toxicity. The incidence of hematologic adverse effects is relatively low with initiating doses of 50 mg per day for both agents (Griffin & Miner, 1995). Parenteral methotrexate (25 mg intramuscularly or subcutaneously per week) has allowed significant reduction in steroid use in chronically active CD and UC (Geier & Miner, 1992; Hanauer & Baert, 1994).

Both steroids and sulfasalazine have been successfully used in pregnancy (Hanan, 1993). Steroids do not appear to have an effect on the fetus. There is some concern about the effect of sulfasalazine and congenital abnormalities (Willoughby & Truelove, 1980). Sulfasalazine can also lower sperm counts in men, a reversible effect (Toovey, Hudson, Herdry, & Levy, 1981).

## Monitoring for Efficacy

Patients requiring parenteral corticosteroid therapy should see symptomatic relief within 72 h. They should then be changed to oral therapy. Remission should be achieved within 2–4 weeks; steroids should then be slowly tapered (Hanauer, 1996). If the disease recurs during the taper, the steroid dose should be increased for several days and a slower taper then started.

Improvement shown by a decrease in pain and severity of diarrhea, with an increase in appetite and overall quality of life, should be seen with 4–6 weeks of maintenance therapy. Treatment should continue as the patient improves, even after resolution of symptoms (Hanauer & Baert, 1994).

Patients requiring immunosuppressive therapy (azathioprine, 6-mercaptopurine) may require 25-mg-per-day PO increases over the 50-mg initial doses to a maximum of 2 mg/kg per day (Hirschfeld & Clearfield, 1995). Therapeutic benefit from immunomodulators may require 3–6 months of therapy (Hanauer & Baert, 1994).

For patients placed on metronidazole, if there is no response within 4–8 weeks, the drug should be discontinued. If patients do respond to metronidazole, the drug can be continued for 3–4 months and then tapered (Peppercorn, 1990).

## Monitoring for Toxicity

Sulfa drugs often cause nausea and headaches. Their allergic manifestations include hemolytic anemia, bone marrow suppression, and generalized hypersensitivity reactions which can be fatal (Hanauer, 1996). Sulfasalazine's effects are dose-related and can be minimized by administering less than 4 g per day. To minimize gastrointestinal effects, administer the drug with meals, initiate therapy at low doses, and titrate up slowly. If adverse effects occur, discontinue the drug until the effects abate and reinstitute at a lower dose. Patients should also be monitored for rash, fever, hematologic reactions, lupus-like syndrome, and hepatotoxicity.

Watery diarrhea is the most common adverse effect of olsalazine and can be avoided by starting with low doses and titrating up.

Anal irritation and pruritus have been associated with rectally administered mesalamine.

For patients on steroid therapy, be alert for cataracts, metabolic bone disease, and osteonecrosis. Monitor blood pressure and serum glucose levels.

Bone marrow suppression is dose-related when using immunomodulators. Monitor with a complete CBC with differential weekly for the first month and then monthly thereafter (Hirschfeld & Clearfield, 1995). The drug should be discontinued or dose decreased if the white blood cell count or platelets decrease. Because azathioprine and mercaptopurine have been associated with pancreatitis in 3–15% of patients, monitor amylase and lipase and be alert to patients' complaints of abdominal pain (Hanauer, 1996; Hanauer & Baert, 1994). Symptoms usually occur after several weeks of therapy.

Be alert for perforation or severe bleeding in all patients. Some patients may be refractory to treatment and need referral to gastroenterologists. Patients with UC who have high-grade dysplasia or suspected cancer or who are unresponsive to maximum treatment should be referred for surgery, which is curative. In CD, surgery is not curative but necessary when patients have an obstruction.

### Follow-Up Recommendations

Initial therapy may require a follow-up evaluation every 2–8 weeks. Maintenance therapy for at least 6 months to 1 year may be necessary for patients with UC, based on the severity of attacks, the response to treatment, and the history of relapse (Hanauer & Baert, 1994; Ruymann & Richter, 1995). At least annual follow-up with a primary care provider is indicated for patients with currently asymptomatic IBD.

# PEPTIC ULCER DISEASE

Peptic ulcer disease (PUD) is a heterogeneous group of disorders involving the upper gastrointestinal tract. Duodenal and gastric ulcers are the most common types of peptic ulcer; however, ulcers of other areas of the gastrointestinal tract do occur. It is a disease that results from an imbalance between the body's aggressive forces and its defensive factors. PUD can be acute and short-lived or chronic and characterized by remission and recurrences. There are three etiologic groups into which PUD can be divided: (1) massive acid hypersecretion, for example, Zollinger-Ellison syndrome; (2) drug-induced, for example, from the intake of nonsteroidal antiinflammatory agents; or (3) infectious, from *Helicobacter pylori*.

A number of factors can predispose someone to PUD. The hypersecretion of gastric acid in individuals with increased parietal cell mass can lead to the development of ulcers. Through direct mucosal irritation and prostaglandin inhibition, drugs such as nonsteroidal antiinflammatory agents and aspirin can induce ulcer formation. The disruption of the architecture of the gastroduodenal mucosa from an inflammation associated with *H. pylori* can cause ulcers. Cigarette smoking, alcohol intake, and psychological stress have been implicated in ulcer formation. Age and family history may also play a role in the development of certain types of ulcers (Katz, 1991).

## SPECIFIC CONSIDERATIONS FOR PHARMACOTHERAPY

### When Drug Therapy Is Needed

The mortality of PUD has declined over the last decade. Less than 2% of patients with ulcers receiving therapy are expected to have a complication such as bleeding, perforation, or obstruction (Katz, 1991). However, PUD remains one of the most common GI diseases that results in loss of work and high medical costs. The natural history of PUD is associated with ulcer recurrence. The recurrence rate within the first year after healing is approximately 50–90%; however, eradication of the *H. pylori* organism significantly decreases the recurrence rate (Greenberger, 1997). Approximately 35% of duodenal ulcers are asymptomatic, and about 20% eventually result in complications such as bleeding and perforation (Sontag, 1988). Complications are reported to develop every year in 2.7% of patients without a history of bleeding or perforation and in 5% of those with previous complications.

## Short- and Long-Term Goals of Pharmacotherapy

The short-term goal of treatment for PUD is resolution of pain or symptoms, promotion of ulcer healing, and prevention of complications. In Zollinger-Ellison syndrome, the goal of therapy is symptomatic pain relief and control of gastric acid secretion. The long-term goal of PUD treatment is the prevention of ulcer recurrence.

## Nonpharmacologic Therapy

Patients should be counseled to avoid the following:

- Completely cease and avoid cigarette smoking
- Decrease caffeine-containing foods
- Avoid or limit corticosteroids and nonsteroidal antiinflammatory drugs
- Avoid foods that cause discomfort
- Abstain from foods late in the evening that will stimulate nocturnal acid secretion
- Develop a personal stress reduction program

## Time Frame for Initiating Pharmacotherapy

Patients should be treated at the time of diagnosis to prevent the complications of bleeding or perforation. H. pylori–infected patients without symptoms need not be treated. Patients infected with H. pylori and with a gastric or duodenal ulcer should be treated with a full course of antibiotics along with an antisecretory agent (Berardi, 1997). For drug-induced ulcers, the offending drug should be discontinued and treatment with an antisecretory agent should be initiated. For patients who require continued NSAID therapy, enteric-coated formulations taken with meals may minimize recurrence but concurrent omeprazole (40 mg per day PO) administration may be necessary (Berardi, 1997; Goroll et al, 1995). In patients with Zollinger-Ellison syndrome, control of the excess amount of gastric acid output is important. Successful medical management can be achieved by titrating the 60-mg-per-day PO initial dose of omeprazole according to patient response (Berardi, 1997).

See Drug Tables 501.5, 501.6.

## Assessment and History Taking

Assessment of the patient should include evaluation of pain—including the type, timing (ie, episodic or continuous), and duration of pain, its association with meals, and what relieves the pain. The history should also include:

- Presence of related symptoms such as intermittent nausea, vomiting, belching
- Past medical history, including previous PUD occurrence, hyperparathyroidism, cirrhosis, pancreatitis, arthritis
- Medication history
- Smoking history
- Family history of ulcers

The physical examination should include:

- Abdominal examination, checking for rebound, tenderness, bowel sounds
- Rectal examination, checking for occult blood

Diagnostic tests should include:

- Radiologic and endoscopic tests
- Cultures and stains of endoscopically obtained specimens if H. pylori is suspected
- Acid-secreting tests for those unresponsive to therapy and/or if gastrinoma or other hypersecretory states are suspected

Laboratory tests should include:

- Hemoglobin, hematocrit
- BUN and creatinine
- Stool occult blood test

## Patient/Caregiver Information

Patients should be counseled to:

- Avoid cigarette smoking
- Decrease caffeine-containing foods
- Minimize foods which cause symptoms
- Avoid corticorsteroids, aspirin, and nonsteroidal antiinflammatory drugs
- Develop a personal stress management plan

## OUTCOMES MANAGEMENT

### Selecting an Appropriate Agent

Presently, $H_2$-receptor antagonists, sucralfate, omeprazole, antacids, and antibiotics are all indicated for the treatment of PUD. The therapeutic regimen should be chosen based upon etiology of the ulcer, comparative efficacies, adverse-effect profiles, pharmacokinetic properties, potential drug interactions, and cost.

$H_2$-receptor antagonists are indicated for the treatment of both duodenal and gastric ulcers. $H_2$-receptor antagonists have comparable healing rates of 70–95% after 4–8 weeks of therapy, respectively. Famotidine and nizatidine are the most potent and possess the longest duration of action; however, all the $H_2$-receptor antagonists can be administered once daily for the treatment of acute duodenal ulcers (Gitlin et al, 1987). Although studies comparing single, large nighttime doses of $H_2$-receptor antagonists to morning doses found them equally effective, the FDA recommends nighttime administration for single-dose therapy (Bianchi Porro & Sangaletti, 1990; Marenco, Menardo, Pallini, Rossini, & Saggioro, 1989). All $H_2$-receptor antagonists are eliminated by a combination of hepatic metabolism, glomerular filtration, and renal tubular secretion. Renal excretion is the major route of elimination for famotidine and nizatidine; therefore, dosage adjustments are recommended for patients with moderate to severe renal insufficiency (creatinine clearance < 50 mL/min). In ulcers associated with Zollinger-Ellison syndrome, larger doses of $H_2$-receptor antagonists and more frequent dosing are required (Wolfe & Jensen, 1987).

Sucralfate is a nonsystemic agent that has been approved only for the treatment of duodenal ulcers. It is not approved for the treatment of gastric ulcers, despite studies showing its efficacy (Blum et al, 1990). This drug should not be used in a patient who may have a compliance problem because it must be administered four times a day. Sucralfate may be helpful for patients who have difficulty in swallowing because it is available as a suspension.

Antacids serve two roles in the treatment of PUD: pain relief and healing. Because one of the goals of PUD therapy is elimination of symptoms, antacids can be given on an "as needed" basis to provide pain relief. Antacids have a rapid onset of action (5–15 min); however, the duration of action is only 2 h. Therefore, these agents are *not* recommended for patients who might have difficulty taking medications on a frequent and regular basis. Because of the adverse-effect profile and the multiple daily dosing, antacids are primarily used for symptomatic relief of pain or for patients unable to tolerate other therapies.

Omeprazole and lansoprazole are potent and highly specific inhibitors of gastric acid secretion. These agents are effective in the treatment of duodenal ulcers, Zollinger-Ellison syndrome, and *H. pylori*–associated ulcers. Because hypersecretion and resistance develop with the use of $H_2$-receptor antagonists, these drugs are the drugs of choice for the treatment of Zollinger-Ellison syndrome. They relieve symptoms and heal ulcers faster in PUD than $H_2$-receptor antagonists (2–4 versus 4–8 weeks). Because of the prolonged achlorhydria caused by these agents, they should be reserved for patients who have severe disease, a greater likelihood of complications, refractory PUD disease, or *H. pylori*–associated ulcers (Bardham et al, 1991; Hixson et al, 1992).

In the treatment of *H. pylori* ulcers, the combination of a $H_2$-receptor antagonist with bismuth subsalicylate, 525 mg qid, plus two antibiotics (metronidazole, 250 mg q.i.d., plus tetracycline 500 mg q.i.d. (Helidac) or amoxicillin 500 mg q.i.d.) for 14 days has produced an eradication rate of approximately 90% (Labenz & Borsch, 1995). Alternative regimens that have similar results include clarithromycin 500 mg b.i.d., metronidazole 250 mg q.i.d., and a proton pump inhibitor (omeprazole 20 mg b.i.d. or lansoprazole 15 mg b.i.d.) for 7 days. (Taylor, Zagari, & Murphy, 1997). In patients unable to tolerate metronidazole's side effects, clarithromycin 500 mg b.i.d., amoxicillin 1 gram b.i.d. and a proton pump inhibitor for 14 days were equally efficacious and cost-effective.

Other regimens which include amoxicillin or clarithromycin, for two weeks, along with a proton pump inhibitor for four weeks, have shown a less than 70% cure rate. As well, Tritec (ranitidine bismuth citrate) for 4 weeks plus clarithromycin for two weeks has a 70% cure rate; therefore it is suggested to add amoxicillin or tetracycline to the regimen (Soll, 1996).

Currently the four FDA approved regimens for the treatment of *H. pylori* associated ulcers include standard triple therapy (Bismuth subsalicylate, metronidazole and tetracycline), Tritec™ (Ranitidine bismuth citrate, Prevpac™ (lansoprazole, amoxicillin, and clarithromycin), and Helidac™ (Bismuth subsalicylate, metronidazole and tetracycline).

## Monitoring for Efficacy

The treatment course is dependent upon the type of ulcer and its etiology. Duodenal ulcers should show improvement and healing within 4–8 weeks. Gastric ulcers generally require more time, up to 12 weeks of therapy. If the ulcer has not healed within the specified period of time, retreatment for an additional 4 weeks is indicated. Patients who do not heal with 3–4 months of therapy are considered refractory and should be evaluated for noncompliance or other causes for impaired healing (ie, smoking, nonsteroidal drug use, alcohol use). Therapeutic options available for refractory ulcers include higher doses and more frequent dosing of $H_2$-receptor antagonists, or proton pump inhibitors. Omeprazole has been shown to work better than continued $H_2$-receptor antagonists for the treatment of refractory PUD (Bardham et al, 1991; Guerreiro, 1990).

Eradication of the *H. pylori* organism has been shown to decrease the recurrence and accelerate the healing process of many ulcers (Fennerty, 1995). *H. pylori* therapy has been shown to be effective when administered as a 14-day course; however, a 7-day course of triple therapy (omeprazole plus clarithromycin, amoxicillin, metronidazole, or bismuth) may be sufficient (Labenz & Borsch, 1995; Markham & McTavish, 1996).

Patients with diagnosed drug-induced ulcers should see improvement rapidly when the causative agent is removed (Howden, Jones, Peace, Burget, & Hunt, 1988). $H_2$-receptor antagonists will heal small ulcers (< 0.5 cm) within 8 weeks; larger ulcers may require 12 weeks of therapy. Continued NSAID therapy may delay healing of small ulcers but does not appear to prevent healing. Misoprostol 200 µg q.i.d. PO can prevent NSAID-associated ulcers in patients who require continuous NSAIDs.

The medical goal of therapy for Zollinger-Ellison syndrome is pain relief and control of gastric secretion, which can be achieved by titrating the drug dosage to a postdrug gastric acid secretion of less than 10 mEq/h PO for the last hour before the next dose of medication (Raufman et al, 1983). If large once-daily dosing does not control acid secretion, administer the total daily dose in two divided doses for better gastric acid control (Frucht, Maton, & Jensen, 1991).

## Monitoring for Toxicity

All $H_2$-receptor antagonists have a similar adverse-effect profile: all cause rashes, central nervous system alterations (ie, confusion) and gastrointestinal disturbances. Famotidine has been associated with headaches and should be avoided in patients with a history of migraines. Because of its antiandrogenic effects, cimetidine has been associated with gynecomastia and impotence. Thrombocytopenia has been associated with the use of ranitidine and famotidine, and patients should be monitored for this periodically. With long-term use, proton pump inhibitors has been associated with hypergastrinemia, which may lead to carcinoid tumors of the stomach (Maton, 1991). With short-term therapy, omeprazole and lansoprazole are well tolerated despite gastrointestinal discomforts.

All antibiotics can cause gastrointestinal disturbances and rashes. Alcohol must be avoided in patients taking metronidazole.

Misoprostol is contraindicated in women of childbearing age unless contraceptive measures are utilized. The diarrhea associated with misoprostal is dose-related, but with reduced dosage the protection against drug-associated ulcers is impaired.

## Follow-Up Recommendations

Healing of the ulcer and/or eradication of *H. pylori* should be documented via endoscopy at least 4 weeks after completion of therapy for patients who are of high risk for complications or patients who are candidates for long-term maintenance therapy. For low-risk patients, documentation is optional because the recurrence of symptoms will identify those with reappearing ulcers or in whom infection has not been eradicated (Fennerty, 1995). The breath test (Meretek UBT) can be used to screen symptomatic patients suspected of having recurrent ulcers. However, a delay of one month is required following antibiotic therapy to avoid false negative results (Soll, 1996). If positive, these patients should undergo endoscopy for visualization of ulcers, and histological and culture testing.

Patients not responsive to antibiotic therapy can receive a second course of therapy. These patients should also have a fasting gastrin secretion test done to rule out Zollinger-Ellison syndrome. Consultation with a gastroenterologist should be considered to rule out gastric cancer, especially for patients over 50 (Berardi, 1997; Goroll et al, 1995; Katz, 1995).

# GASTROESOPHAGEAL REFLUX

Gastroesophageal reflux disease (GERD) is a disorder in which the gastric contents are regurgitated into the esophagus, leading to irritation and injury to the esophageal mucosa. Heartburn, or pyrosis, is the primary symptom. Gastroesophageal reflux events have been shown to occur by three mechanisms: (1) transient lower esophageal sphincter (LES) relaxation, (2) abdominal strain, and (3) a low resting LES pressure (Fennerty, Castell & Fendrick, 1996).

## SPECIFIC CONSIDERATIONS FOR PHARMACOTHERAPY

### When Drug Therapy Is Needed

Although lifestyle modification may alleviate the symptoms of mild disease, drug therapy is necessary for patients with more severe disease. The long-term exposure of the esophagus to refluxed material can result in serious complications, including hemorrhage, strictures, and ulceration (Katz, 1995).

### Short- and Long-Term Goals of Pharmacotherapy

The initial goal of therapy is to eliminate the symptoms of retrosternal pain and diminish the frequency and duration of esophageal reflux. The long-term goal is to prevent relapse, recurrence, and esophageal injury.

### Nonpharmacologic Therapy

Lifestyle modifications remain the cornerstone of initial therapy. These include the following:

- Dietary restrictions (ie, avoid fatty foods and large meals, peppermint, onions, garlic, chocolate)
- Not eating for a least 3 hours before lying down; no bedtime snacks
- Sleeping with the head of the bed elevated to decrease nocturnal esophageal acid contact time
- Weight reduction
- No cigarette smoking

### Time Frame for Initiating Pharmacotherapy

Lifestyle modifications alone remain limited, and pharmacotherapy for GERD is indicated when symptoms continue or are severe.
    See Drug Tables 501.1, 501.5, 501.6.

### Assessment and History Taking

The medical history should include specific questions about:

- Nature and frequency of pain and its relationship to sleep and meals
- Anorexia and recent weight loss
- Presence of symptoms of dysphagia, regurgitation, increased salivation, odynophagia, bleeding
- Dietary precipitants such as coffee, tomato or orange juice, spicy foods
- Use of antiinflammatory drugs
- Smoking history
- Alcohol use
- Conditions such as pregnancy, scleroderma, achalasia

During the physical examination look for:

- Presence of cough, hoarseness, hiccups
- Presence of occult or frank blood in the stool

    Laboratory tests that may be useful in the diagnosis of GERD include:

- 24-hour ambulatory esophageal pH study to quantitate and document reflux of gastric contents
- Barium swallow and/or an endoscopy may be the best initial test; the latter is the most sensitive test for detecting esophageal strictures
- Endoscopy is useful in assessing mucosal damage or documenting the presence of Barrett's epithelium, hiatal hernia, and/or strictures (Katz, 1995)

### Patient/Caregiver Information

Patients should be counseled to:

- Avoid or stop smoking; consider use of nicotine gum or patches
- Lose weight if necessary
- Wear loose-fitting clothes to prevent abdominal or sternal pressure
- Avoid lying flat while watching television or sleeping

- Avoid foods that irritate the gastric mucosa (ie, spicy food) or foods that stimulate acid production (ie, alcohol)
- Avoid foods that lower the esophageal sphincter (ie, fatty meals, chocolate, peppermint)
- Avoid eating prior to going to bed
- Avoid bending over after eating
- Elevate head of bed with blocks

## OUTCOMES MANAGEMENT

### Selecting an Appropriate Agent

For patients with mild symptoms and nonerosive disease, therapy can include antacids, prokinetics, or H$_2$-receptor antagonists. The use of antacids is effective in relieving symptoms (DeVault & Castell, 1995). Because antacids have a short duration of action and do not heal esophagitis, they are recommended for use only with other therapies to provide symptomatic relief.

For patients with moderately severe symptoms and nonerosive or mildly erosive disease, prokinetics and H$_2$-receptor antagonists are usually efficacious. Response to an H$_2$-receptor antagonist depends upon dose, duration of therapy, and severity of the disease. Overall, 50–70% of symptomatic patients will respond with complete or partial resolution of symptoms when treated with H$_2$-receptor antagonists (Fennerty et al, 1996). The healing rates of esophagitis will vary depending upon the severity of the disease as well as the duration and dosage of the drug therapy. Studies have shown variable results (0–82%) in endoscopic healing of esophagitis with these agents (DeVault & Castell, 1995). For those with moderate symptoms and nonerosive disease, H$_2$ receptors can be administered in standard doses but on a more frequent basis (twice daily) (DiPiro & Bowden, 1997). For those with more severe disease or those who fail standard therapeutic doses, 1.5 to 2 times the standard doses should be utilized. Only twice-daily administration and high doses of H$_2$-receptor antagonists will suppress acid approximately to the levels attained by proton pump inhibitors (Hatlebakk & Berstad, 1996). These results appear to depend upon the severity of the esophageal lesions and the dose given.

The role of prokinetic drugs (ie, metoclopramide, cisapride) in the treatment of GERD is limited. Metoclopramide has shown minimal symptomatic improvement in promoting endo-scopic healing, and because of the side-effect profile, its use is limited (Ramirez & Richter, 1993). The recommended regimen for metoclopramide orally is 10 mg taken 20–30 min prior to meals and at bedtime (Hatlebakk & Berstad, 1996). In contrast, cisapride has been shown to be as effective as H$_2$-receptor antagonists, with comparable improvement of both symptoms and endoscopic healing in patients with GERD (DeMicco et al, 1992; Geldof, Hazelhoff, & Otten, 1993). A randomized trial involving patients with reflux esophagitis demonstrated that cisapride 20 mg q.i.d. PO provided better endoscopic healing (69%) than 10 mg q.i.d. PO (57%) (Faruqui et al, 1992). However, because cisapride has no clinical advantage over H$_2$-receptor antagonists and is more expensive, it is not recommended as a sole agent for the treatment of GERD. A study comparing single-drug regimens (cisapride, ranitidine, and omeprazole) and two combined drug regimens (ranitidine plus cisapride and omeprazole plus cisapride) in patients with erosive reflux esophagitis found that omeprazole alone or in combination with cisapride was more effective than ranitidine alone or cisapride alone (Greenberger, 1997). Cisapride also may be beneficial in combination with an H$_2$-receptor antagonist in patients with delayed gastric emptying.

For patients with moderate to severe erosive esophagitis, a proton pump inhibitor is considered the drug of choice. These agents have a greater antisecretory effect and have been shown to be superior to the H$_2$-receptor antagonists. Omeprazole has been shown to heal approximately 60% of patients with esophagitis compared to 30% healing with H$_2$-receptor antagonist after 4 weeks (Bianchi Porro et al, 1992; Havelund, Laursen, & Lauritsen, 1994). After 8 weeks of therapy, healing rates further increased to 35% and 80% for ranitidine and omeprazole, respectively. The higher healing rate for omeprazole was also accompanied by faster and more substantial symptom relief.

Patients with GERD without esophagitis or who have frequent recurrent symptoms should be placed on a maintenance program with an antisecretory agent or prokinetic agent if delayed gastric emptying is present. Other patients may have symptomatic relapses and failure of healing of esophagitis.

Proton pump inhibitors have been shown to be more effective than other therapies in controlling acid and in preventing recurrence of erosive esophagitis (Dent et al, 1994; Hallerback et al, 1994). Unfortunately, after the pharmacotherapy is discontinued, rapid return of symptoms generally occurs and may be a problem for long-term maintenance therapy.

## Monitoring for Efficacy

Patients should see relief of symptoms such as heartburn within 4 weeks. If patients continue to have symptoms or there is incomplete healing of the esophagitis, consider increasing the dose and/or the frequency of the drug. For patients with resistant GERD who are already on a proton pump inhibitor and have gastroparesis, cisapride may be a helpful addition. Effective maintenance therapy depends on the severity of the disease and may require only lifestyle changes and antacids (Lieberman, 1987), or continuous maintenance therapy with acid-suppressing medications may be necessary (Howden et al, 1995). For many patients, esophagitis is a chronic relapsing disease, and the majority of patients will have a recurrence within 6–12 months after therapy is discontinued (Fennerty et al, 1996).

## Monitoring for Toxicity

Cisapride has been associated with gastrointestinal upset and rhinitis. Therefore, patients with chronic sinusitis should be monitored for an exacerbation of this condition. $H_2$-receptor antagonists have a similar adverse-effect profile, which includes rash and gastrointestinal disturbances. Cimetidine is associated with impotence and gynecomastia, and famotidine has been associated with headaches. Thrombocytopenia can occur with all $H_2$-receptor antagonists but is more common with famotidine and ranitidine.

With long-term use, omeprazole has been associated with hypergastrinemia, which has the potential to lead to carcinoid tumors of the stomach. Therefore, patients placed on long-term proton pump inhibitors should be monitored for this.

## Follow-Up

Patients should be followed up within 4 weeks after diagnosis and initial treatment. Because this condition is associated with a high relapse and recurrence rate, patients should be followed closely.

# EXCESSIVE FLATUS

Flatus, or the passage of intestinal gas through the anus, is a natural byproduct of digestion. Differing physiology and/or dietary intake, however, can result in excessive, noisy, or malodorous eruptions that can be embarrassing. Several over-the-counter preparations are available to minimize excessive flatus or bloating, none of which are considered highly effective.

## SPECIFIC CONSIDERATIONS FOR PHARMACOTHERAPY

### When Drug Therapy Is Needed

Based on personal criteria, patients generally decide when to initiate therapy. Generally, their immediate and longer-term goals of elimination of all flatus are not able to be met; minimizing the number and/or intensity of events is a more realistic goal.

The most important nonpharmacologic therapy for flatus is simple dietary modification, which is generally indicated for all patients. To minimize swallowed air in the stomach, patients should eliminate carbonated beverages and gum chewing, avoid rapid eating or drinking, and ensure that dentures fit well. Alternatives to anticholinergic drugs should be found; these drugs cause dry mouth which can also lead to aerophagia ("Simethicone for Gastrointestinal Gas," 1996).

See Drug Table 501.2.

### Assessment and History Taking

Before therapy, patients should be evaluated for history or signs and symptoms of other GI disorders, such as diverticulosis, irritable bowel syndrome, or inflammatory bowel disease. Symptoms such as abdominal pain, alternating diarrhea and constipation, and passage of mucus or bloody stools should be considered together and not treated individually. Provider discretion should determine if a physical examination is indicated. Consider an abdominal examination checking for tenderness, rebound, and masses; a rectal exam to rule out impaction, and a stool guaiac test to check for occult blood.

Patients and caregivers should be reassured that their symptoms are not unusual. A daily chart of flatus events, noting specifics and timing of food ingestion and time and quantification of eruptions, can be helpful in determining which foods might be eliminated. Provide patients with education about the most common causes of flatus and appropriate dietary modification. Carbonated beverages, lactose-containing foods, beans, and certain vegetables such as cabbage, cauliflower, and broccoli are common causes of flatus.

## SELECTING AN APPROPRIATE AGENT

Antibiotics are not recommended for the treatment of flatus. Although there was at one time hope that antibiotic manipulation of the intestinal flora could assist in the elimination of flatus, results have not proven successful (Danzl, 1992; Murphy & Calloway, 1972).

Simethicone, a combination of dimethylpolysiloxanes and silica gel, acts as an antifoaming agent. It causes gas bubbles to coalesce by lowering their surface tension. Although simethicone-containing products (Maalox Anti-Gas, Mylanta Gas Relief, Mylicon, etc.) are heavily advertised for treatment of flatus, well-controlled, double-blind studies in infants, postoperative patients, and healthy volunteers found no significant differences between subjects and controls ("Simethicone," 1996).

Alpha-galactosidase preparations (Beano) contain an enzyme intended to break down indigestible oligosaccharides found in high-fiber foods. Although minimal studies have been done with these products, they are considered generally safe and do provide relief for some patients (Ganiats, Norcross, Halverson, Burford, & Palinkas, 1994). The breakdown of the oligosaccharides produces galactose, so these products should be avoided in patients with galactosemia.

Anticholinergic agents decrease colonic contractions. These agents are not recommended because such contractions cannot be suppressed indefinitely; their resultant pressure must have an eventual outlet.

Activated charcoal works in the GI tract by absorption of surrounding substances. Studies demonstrating the effectiveness of activated charcoal products (Charcoal Plus) have not been able to be replicated (Potter, Ellis, & Leavitt, 1985).

## HEMORRHOIDS

Hemorrhoids are a common condition in the population over age 50 and in women of all ages

who have been pregnant. They result from the pressure of large, firm stool, from partial blockage of the anal canal, and/or from increased venous pressure from conditions such as congestive heart failure or pregnancy. Hemorrhoids generally present with painless rectal bleeding, rectal itching, or anal discomfort.

## SPECIFIC CONSIDERATIONS FOR PHARMACOTHERAPY

### When Drug Therapy Is Needed

Patients can experience considerable pain, pressure and discomfort from symptomatic hemorrhoids. Therapeutic interventions can provide prompt relief for many patients.

Alleviation of the patient's discomfort, promotion of healing, and prevention of future attacks are the goals of therapy.

### Nonpharmacologic Therapy

Local application of a cold pack can provide symptomatic relief. Finding a sitting position that avoids direct pressure on the symptomatic hemorrhoid is essential. This may be facilitated by the use of donut-shaped inflatable rings or soft foam pillows that distribute the pressure evenly. Warm sitz baths two or three times a day for 15–20 min are often soothing. A high-fiber diet and bulk-forming agents can result in soft, easily passed stools, minimizing local pressure on the anus. These should be continued after resolution of the acute problem as preventive measures against recurrence.

### Time for Initiating Pharmacotherapy

Preventive therapy in the form of a high-fiber diet and bulk-forming agents can be suggested to all patients as a preventive measure. Localized therapy for hemorrhoids can be initiated at onset of acute symptoms.

See Drug Table 304.

### Assessment and History Taking

The history of the patient with hemorrhoids should include questions about the nature, onset, and duration of symptoms; the usual nature of his or her bowel movements; and whether the patient has had a history of constipation or hemorrhoids in the past. Also determine if the patient is pregnant, has any systemic illnesses, has a history of anorectal surgery, or is taking any medications that might cause constipation or increased venous pressure. The physical examination should include a thorough inspection of the anal area and a digital rectal exam. Thrombosed or prolapsed hemorrhoids found on examination should be referred for surgical intervention. Anal fissures should receive antibiotic treatment and/or surgery.

## Patient/Caregiver Information

Reduction of rectal pressure, constipation, and straining with defecation is the best long-term method for prevention of future hemorrhoids.

## OUTCOMES MANAGEMENT

### Selecting an Appropriate Agent

External creams or ointments are preferable to medicated suppositories inserted into the rectum with less local effect.

Most over-the-counter preparations contain topical anesthetics that provide relief from pain or pruritus. Benzocaine, one of the commonly used anesthetics, can give relief in several minutes but also produces local allergic reactions that can be worse than the original symptoms. Pramoxine is a less sensitizing anesthetic (Goroll et al, 1995). Astringents such as witch hazel provide inexpensive relief for some patients.

During pregnancy products such as Preparation H and Anusol Hc are acceptable (Remick, 1994). Topical steroids should be minimized because of the possibility of systemic absorption through the rectal mucosa.

### Monitoring for Efficacy

If a patient complains of continued pain after all attempts at symptom relief, referral to a surgeon can be made for surgical treatment. Hemorrhoids that prolapse produce severe symptoms, reoccur repeatedly, or bleed heavily despite local treatments should also be referred to a surgeon for evaluation.

### Monitoring for Toxicity

Patients should be warned that any increased symptoms after using the OTC or prescribed medications may be the result of local irritation and medication reaction. The medication should be discontinued and an alternative used that does not contain the offending product's main ingredient.

### Follow-Up

Patients should be encouraged to return for alternative medication within 1 week if the initial recommendations offered no relief. Surgical consultation may be necessary.

## HEPATITIS

Hepatitis is an acute or chronic inflammation of the liver as a result of viral infection from one of five distinct viruses (A, B, C, D, and E) or chemical exposure, including alcohol.

## SPECIFIC CONSIDERATIONS FOR PHARMACOTHERAPY

### When Drug Therapy Is Needed

Pharmacotherapy in the primary care setting is limited to prophylactic immunizations for specific risk groups. Hepatitis A (HAV) viral-specific immunization is available for international travelers and children in day care; immune globulin (IG) is indicated for household contacts of known cases of hepatitis A. Hepatitis B (HBV) vaccine, given in a series of three doses, is indicated for sexually active adults, health care workers, and the children of chronic carriers. An HBV prophylaxis regimen is suggested after percutaneous or mucous membrane exposure to known carriers of hepatitis B surface antigen (HBsAg). For more complete guidelines on immunization and postexposure prophylaxis against hepatitis A and B, see the guidelines from the U.S. Preventive Services Task Force (1995).

### Short- and Long-Term Goals of Pharmacotherapy

The goals of pharmacotherapy are the prevention of infection in individuals who are exposed to any of the known hepatitis viruses.

### Nonpharmacologic Therapy

Since hepatitis A and E are transmitted primarily by the fecal-oral route, meticulous attention to hygiene and hand washing after use of the toilet and changing diapers is indicated.

Condoms, either male or female, should be used with all sexual encounters to prevent spread of HBV. To prevent parenteral HBV spread, counsel patients to avoid injection drug use and not to share needles or drug apparatus. Universal precautions should be practiced by health care workers when in contact with blood and fluids. Family members of known HBV carriers should be educated about universal precautions.

## Time Frame for Initiating Pharmacotherapy

Injections of HAV IG can be given immediately before travel exposures and last up to 3 months. For longer exposures, IG can be repeated every 4–6 months. IG should be given as soon as possible after exposure to household, sexual, and daycare center contacts; its use after 2 weeks is not effective. HAV vaccine is effective 14 to 21 days after IM administration (Benenson, 1995).

The hepatitis B vaccine series is recommended for all infants. Special attention should be given to vaccinating children from populations with high rates of hepatitis B infection, including Alaskan Natives, Pacific Islanders, and immigrants from countries with endemic HBV infection (Committee on Infectious Diseases, 1994). Immunization against HBV is also recommended for all adolescents. Emphasis should be on adolescents and adults who (Committee on Infectious Diseases, 1994):

1. Have sexually transmitted diseases
2. Have more than one sex partner
3. Are injecting drug users
4. Are homosexual men or bisexual men or women
5. Are sexual contacts of high-risk individuals
6. Work in contact with blood or body fluids

There are two timetables for administration of HBV vaccine: a three-dose schedule, which is initial, 1–2 months later, and 6–18 months later; or a four-dose schedule with the first dose at birth, followed at 1, 2, and 6 months of age (Benenson, 1995).

Hepatitis B immune globulin (HBIG) IM is indicated as soon as possible, but within 24 h, after percutaneous or mucous membrane contact with blood that may contain HBsAg. An HBV vaccine series should be started at the same time in unimmunized persons. If the vac-

cine series cannot be started at the time of HBIG administration, a second dose of HBIG should be given 1 month after the first (Benenson, 1995). Sexual contacts of patients with acute HBV infection should also receive HBIG and initiation of an HBV vaccine series within 2 weeks of exposure.

See Drug Table 106.

## Assessment and History Taking

The medical history should include specific questions about:

- Common presenting symptoms, including jaundice, fatigue, muscle pain, decreased appetite, nausea, vomiting, diarrhea, right upper quadrant abdominal pain, and low-grade fever
- Illnesses in household and sexual contacts
- Presence of darkened urine and white, chalky-colored stool
- History of recent travel
- Substance use, including alcohol and injection drugs
- Sexual partners and practices
- Work-related exposures
- Medication history, including OTCs

The physical examination should include:

- Skin examination to document the presence of jaundice on skin, sclerae, or mucous membranes
- Abdominal examination, checking for liver and spleen enlargement and/or tenderness

Laboratory tests should include (Uphold & Graham, 1994):

- CBC
- Liver function tests
- Prothrombin time
- Urinalysis
- Total and direct bilirubin
- Hepatitis screening panel, which will include HAV IgM antibody (IgM anti-HAV), HBV surface antigen (HBsAg), and HBV core antibody (anti-HBc)

## Patient/Caregiver Information

Education should be provided about hand washing, condoms, and nonsharing of parenteral drug apparatus, as discussed above.

# OUTCOMES MANAGEMENT

## Selecting an Appropriate Agent

Two formulations of HBV vaccine are available: a plasma-derived version (Heptavax-B), which has been extensively tested and found safe, and a recombinant vaccine (Recombivax HB); both result in high rates of conversion. To avoid unnecessary prophylaxis in those already immune, prevaccination testing for anti-HBs may be done. There is no adverse effect in giving HBV vaccine to individuals with previous HBV infection. One-milliliter (10 μg of the recombinant vaccine or 20 μg of the plasma-derived vaccine) (or 0.5 mL in children less than 10 years old) intramuscular injections should be given in the deltoid region. Hemodialysis patients should receive higher doses because of less effective antibody response (Jacobs, 1997).

For postexposure prophylaxis of HBV, 0.06 mL/kg IM of HBIG should be given, with a second dose 1 month later (Benenson, 1995). For infants of mothers who are HBsAg positive, HBIG 0.5 mg intramuscularly is indicated within 12 h of birth (U.S. Preventive Services Task Force, 1995).

Human leukocyte alpha-interferon and adenine arabinoside (ara-A) have been shown to inhibit serum viral markers in patients with chronic HBV infection. Patients that are HBsAg carriers for over 1 year and symptomatic should be referred to a gastroenterologist for liver biopsy and possible treatment.

## Monitoring for Efficacy

Testing for anti-HBs after vaccination should be done to ascertain that seroconversion has occurred. Revaccination with the same three-dose schedule is indicated for individuals who have no detectable antibody response. Protection against chronic HBV infection remains for at least 10 years even though anti-HBs becomes undetectable (Committee on Infectious Diseases, 1994).

## Monitoring for Toxicity

As for all immunizations, pain at the injection site and occasional mild constitutional symptoms (Jacobs, 1997) may be experienced.

## Follow-Up

After an HBV vaccine series, immunity is maintained for an indeterminant time. Future recommendations for booster doses may be required to ensure immunity through adolescence and adulthood.

# IRRITABLE BOWEL SYNDROME

Irritable bowel syndrome (IBS) presents as a combination of abdominal pain and altered bowel habits (either diarrhea or constipation) that is not explained by any detectable pathology. Symptoms are often aggravated by stress and begin in the second and third decades (McQuaid, 1997).

## SPECIFIC CONSIDERATIONS FOR PHARMACOTHERAPY

### When Drug Therapy Is Needed

Patients are frequently concerned about their condition and request drug therapy for relief of the distressing symptoms of IBS. However, drugs should be cautiously initiated since many patients are taking multiple medications prescribed from various attempts to alleviate symptoms. One suggestion is to initially stop all nonessential medications that may affect bowel habits and reintroduce them in a stepwise, selective manner (Goroll et al, 1995).

### Short- and Long-Term Goals of Pharmacotherapy

The goal of pharmacotherapy is to work as an adjunct to diet and emotional support of the patient to minimize the disruptive symptoms of IBS.

### Nonpharmacologic Therapy

A food/symptom diary can allow patients to see relationships among symptoms, food choices, and life events and assist in making dietary changes. However, a balance must be struck between avoidance of foods that provoke symptoms and becoming a slave to diets and food choices. Even if fruits and vegetables provoke symptoms, they should be eaten in small amounts. A trial of a lactose-free diet is indicated for all patients. The limiting of simple sugars, including sorbitol and fructose, has lessened symptoms in up to one third of patients (Greenberger, 1995). These sugars are found in large amounts in colas, "sugar-free" gum, apples, cherries, and several special diet foods. Flatulence-producing foods such as beans, cabbage, and cauliflower can be minimized. Many patients are unable to tolerate caffeine (McQuaid, 1997). A high-fiber diet (20–30 g per day) and bulking agents can be useful in breaking the diarrhea-constipation pattern and should be recommended for most patients (McQuaid, 1997). Regular exercise and an increase in the intake of fluids, especially water and dilute juices, can often help minimize symptoms of constipation.

The development of a personal stress management plan and, if necessary, psychological counseling can be useful to many patients.

## Time Frame for Initiating Pharmacotherapy

At the initial visit for IBS complaints, discontinue previous medications related to GI symptoms and initiate dietary changes as discussed above. Follow up with patient in 2 weeks. Drug therapy should be reserved for patients who do not respond to these conservative measures (McQuaid, 1997).

See Drug Tables 311.1, 501.3, 501.4, 501.8.

## Assessment and History Taking

The goal of assessment is to rule out organic causes of the patient's symptoms before the initiation of drug therapy. The baseline history should elicit specific information on:

- Full constellation of GI symptoms, including pain, flatus, bloating, distension, diarrhea, and constipation and their pattern of occurrence; disappearance of symptoms is common with IBS (Uphold & Graham, 1994)

- Recent history of weight loss (a positive answer to this usually rules out IBS) (Uphold & Graham, 1994)

- Diet, specifically for foods with diarrheogenic potential, including nonabsorbable sugars such as sorbitol (Greenberger, 1995)

- Relationship of life stress to symptom occurrence

The physical examination should document weight loss and the presence of any masses, organ enlargement, tenderness, rigidity, or guarding of the abdomen. A rectal examination and fecal occult blood test should also be performed.

Routine laboratory tests should include CBC, sedimentation rate, thyroid function tests, and stool occult blood test. With predominant diarrhea symptoms, consider stool for ova and parasites, 24-h stool collection, flexible sigmoidoscopy (in patients less than 40 years old), or barium enema/colonoscopy (in patients over age 40) (McQuaid, 1997).

## Patient/Caregiver Information

Primary care providers should reassure patients about the functional nature of their symptoms and stress the ongoing nature of both the symptoms and the provider relationship.

## OUTCOMES MANAGEMENT

### Selecting an Appropriate Agent

Antispasmodic drugs such as dicyclomine 10–20 mg PO, three to four times a day; propantheline 15 mg PO, three times a day; and hyoscyamine 0.125 mg PO or S have anticholinergic effects that may be useful in relieving intermittent cramping pain. They are useful on a short-term or as-needed basis, or can be given 30–60 min before meals to relieve postprandial pain. They should not be used on a long-term basis (Garoll et al, 1995; McQuaid, 1997).

Antidiarrheal agents such as loperamide 2 mg PO, three to four times a day, or diphenoxylate with atropine 2.5 mg PO, four times a day, can be used prophylactically when diarrhea would be socially inconvenient. For patients in whom constipation is the main symptom even after dietary changes and bulking agents, cisapride 5–10 mg a day PO may be useful (McQuaid, 1997).

Patients with chronic, unremitting abdominal pain may benefit from antidepressants. The tricyclic amitriptyline 50–100 mg PO, once a day, is worth a trial because of its anticholinergic activity (Goroll et al, 1995).

### Monitoring for Efficacy

The chronic nature of the disease should be stressed along with the waxing and waning of symptoms regardless of pharmacotherapy. Try dietary changes and a bulking agent for 2-week trial. Consultation with a gastroenterologist can be considered for patients in whom a reasonable trial of dietary changes, bulking agents, and dicyclomine are unsuccessful.

## Monitoring for Toxicity

Chronic use of antispasmodics can make constipation and pain worse.

## REFERENCES

Advice for travelers. (1996). *Medical Letter, 38,* 17–20.

Agostinucci, W., Gannon, R., Schauer P., & Walters, J. (1986). Continuous infusion of metoclopramide for prevention of chemotherapy-induced emesis. *Clinical Pharmacy* 5(2), 150–153.

Anthony L. B., Krozely, M. G., Woodward N. J., Hinsworth, J., Hande, K., & Brenner, D. (1986). Antiemetic effect of oral versus intravenous metoclopramide in patients receiving cisplatin: A randomized double-blind trial. *Journal of Clinical Oncology, 4* (1), 98–103.

Bardham, K., Naesdal, J., Bianchi, P., Petrillo, M., Lazzaroni, M., & Hinchliffe, R. (1991). Treatment of refractory peptic ulcer with omeprazole or continued $H_2$ receptor antagonists: A controlled clinical trial. *Gut, 32* (4), 435–438.

Belluzzi, A., Brignola, C., Campieri, M., Pera, A., Boschi, S., & Miglioli, M. (1996). Effect of an enteric-coated fish-oil preparation on relapses in Crohn's disease. *New England Journal of Medicine, 334* (24), 1557–1560.

Benenson, A. (Ed.). (1995). *Control of Communicable Diseases Manual* (16th ed.). Washington, D.C.: American Public Health Association.

Berardi, R. (1997). Peptic ulcer disease and Zollinger-Ellison syndrome. In J. Dipiro, R. Talbert, G. Yee, G. Matzke, B. Wells, & L. Posey (Eds.), *Pharmacotherapy: A pathophysiologic approach* (3rd ed.). Stamford, CT: Appleton & Lange.

Bianchi Porro, O., Pace, F., Peracchia, A., Bonavina, L., Vigneri, S., & Scialabba, A. (1992). Short-term treatment of refractory reflux oesophagitis with different doses of omeprazole or ranitidine. *Journal of Clinical Gastroenterology, 15* (3), 192–198.

Bianchi Porro, O., & Sangaletti O. (1990). Inhibition of nocturnal acidity is important but not essential for duodenal ulcer healing. *Gut, 31* (4), 397–400.

Biddle, W., & Miner, P. (1990). Long-term use of mesalamine enemas to induce remission in ulcerative colitis. *Gastroenterology, 99,* 113–118.

Blum, A. L., Bethge, H., Bode, J. C., Domschke, W., Feurle, G., & Hackenberg, K. (1990). Sucralfate in the treatment and prevention of gastric ulcer: A multicentre double-blind placebo controlled study. *Gut, 31*(7), 825–830.

Brown, K. (1994). Dietary management of acute diarrheal disease: Contemporary scientific issues. *Journal of Nutrition, 124* (8 Suppl.), 1455S–1460S.

Burish, T., & Jenkins, R. (1992). Effectiveness of biofeedback and relaxation training in reducing the side effects of cancer chemotherapy. *Health Psychology, 11*(1), 17–23.

Campieri, M., DeFranchis, R., Bianchi Porro, G., et al. (1990). Mesalamine (5-ASA) suppositories in the treatment of ulcerative proctitis or distal proctosigmoiditis: A randomized controlled trial. *Scandanavian Journal of Gastroenterology, 25,* 663–668.

Cersosimo, R., & Karp, D. (1986). Adrenal corticosteroids as antiemetics during cancer chemotherapy. *Pharmacotherapy, 6*(3), 118–127.

Chevallier, B., on behalf of the Granisetron Study Group (1990). Efficacy and safety of granisetron compared with high-dose metoclopramide plus dexamethasone in patients receiving high-dose cisplatin in a single-blind study. *European Journal of Cancer, 15*(Suppl.1), 33–36.

Committee on Infectious Diseases, American Academy of Pediatrics (1994). *1994 Red book.* Elk Grove Village, IL: AP.

Cutler A., Schubert, A., & Schubert, T. (1993). Role of *Helicobacter pylori* serology in evaluating treatment success. *Digestive Diseases and Sciences, 38*(12), 2262–2266.

Danziger, L., & Itakazu, G. (1995). Gastrointestinal infections. In L. L. Young & M. Koda-Kimble (Eds.), *Applied therapeutics: The clinical use of drugs* (6th ed.). Vancouver, WA: Applied Therapeutics.

Danzl, D. (1992). Flatology. *Journal of Emergency Medicine, 10,* 79–88.

DeMicco, M., Berenson, M., Wu, W., et al. (1992). Oral cisapride in GERD: A double-blind, placebo-controlled multicenter dose-response trial [abstract]. *Gastroenterology, 102,* A59.

DeMulder, P. H., Seynaeve, C., Vermorken, J. B., vanLiessum, P. A., Mols-Jevdevic, S., & Allman, E. L. (1990). Ondansetron compared with high-dose metoclopramide in prophylaxis of acute and delayed cisplatin-induced nausea and vomiting. *Annals of Internal Medicine, 113*(11), 834–840.

Dent, J., Yeomans, N., Mackinoon, M., Reed, W., Narielvala, F., & Hetzel, D. (1994). Omeprazole vs ranitidine for prevention of relapse in reflux oesophagitis: A controlled double-blind trial of their efficacy and safety. *Gut, 35*(5), 590–598.

DeVault, K., & Castell, D. (1995). Guidelines for the diagnosis and treatment of gastroesophageal reflux disease. *Archives of Internal Medicine, 155*(20), 2165–2173.

DiPiro, J., & Bowden, T. (1997). Inflammatory bowel disease. In J. Dipiro, R. Talbert, G. Yee, G. Matzke, B. Wells, & L. Posey (Eds.), *Pharmacotherapy: A pathophysiologic approach* (3rd ed.). Stamford, CT: Appleton & Lange.

DuPont, H. L., & Ericsson, C. D. (1993). Prevention and treatment of traveler's diarrhea. *New England Journal of Medicine, 328*(25), 1821–1827.

DuPont, H. L., Ericsson, C. D., Johnson, P. C., Biitsura, J. A., DuPont, M. W., & de la Cabada, F. J. (1987). Prevention of travelers' diarrhea by the tablet formulation of bismuth subsalicylate. *JAMA, 257*(40), 1347–1350.

DuPont, H. L., & Hormick, R. (1973). Adverse effects of Lomotil therapy in shigellosis. *JAMA, 226*(13), 15–25.

Erick, M. (1994). Battling morning (noon and night) sickness. *Journal of the American Dietetic Association, 94*(2), 147–148.

Ericsson, C., Johnson, P., DuPont, H., Morgan, D., Bitsura, J., & de la Cabada, F. J. (1987). Ciprofloxacin or trimethoprim-sulfamethoxazole as initial therapy for travelers' diarrhea: A placebo-controlled, randomized trial. *Annals of Internal Medicine, 106*(2), 216–220.

Ettinger, D., Eisenberg, Fitts, D., Friedman, C., Wilson-Lynch, K. & Yocom, K. (1996). A double-blind comparison of the efficacy of two dose regimens of oral granisetron in preventing acute emesis in patients receiving moderately emetogenic chemotherapy. *Cancer, 78*(1), 144–151.

Ewe, K., Press, A., & Singe, C. (1993). Azathioprine combined with prednisolone or monotherapy with prednisolone in active Crohn's disease. *Gastroenterology, 105*, 367–372.

Faruqui, S., Sigmund, C., Smith, R., et al.. (1992). Cisapride in the treatment of GERD: A double-blind placebo-controlled multicenter dose-response trial. *Gastroenterology, 102*(4), A66.

Fennerty, B. (1995). "Cure" of Helicobacter pylori. *Archives of Internal Medicine, 155*, 1929–1931.

Fennerty, M., Castell, D., & Fendrick, M. (1996). The diagnosis and treatment of gastroesophageal reflux disease in a managed care environment. *Archives of Internal Medicine, 156*, 477–484.

Follett-Veryrat, C., Farinott, R., Palmer, J. (1997). Physiology of chemotherapy-induced emesis and antiemetic therapy. *Drugs, 53*, 206–234.

Frucht, H., Maton, P., & Jensen, R. (1991). Use of omeprazole in patients with Zollinger-Ellison syndrome. *Digestive Diseases and Sciences, 36*(4), 394–404.

Ganiats, T., Norcross, W., Halverson, A., Burford, P., & Palinkas, L. (1994). Does Beano prevent gas? A double-blind crossover study of oral alpha-galactosidase to treat dietary oligosaccharide intolerance. *Journal of Family Practice, 39*(5), 441–445.

Gardner, V., Beckwith, J., & Heyneman, C. (1995). Cisapride for the treatment of chronic idiopathic constipation. *Annals of Pharmacotherapy, 29*(11), 1161–1163.

Geier, D., & Miner, P. (1992) New therapeutic agents in the treatment of irritable bowel syndrome. *American Journal of Medicine, 93*, 199–208.

Geier, D., Miner, P., Danielsson, A., Hellers, G. O., & Lyrenas, E. (1987). A controlled randomized trial of budesonide versus prednisolone retention enemas in active distal ulcerative colitis. *Scandanavian Journal of Gastroenterology, 22*, 987–992.

Geldof, H., Hazelhoff, B., & Otten, M. (1993). Two different dose regimens of cisapride in the treatment of reflux oesophagitis: A double-blind comparison with ranitidine. *Alimentary Pharmacology and Therapeutics, 7*(4), 409–415.

Gitlin, N., McCullough, A., Smith, J., et al. (1987). A multicenter, double blind, randomized, placebo-controlled comparison of nocturnal and twice-a-day famotidine in the treatment of active duodenal ulcer disease. *Gastroenterology, 92*, 48–53.

Gorbach, S., (1990). Bismuth therapy in gastrointestinal diseases. *Gastroenterology, 99*, 863.

Goroll, A., May, L., & Mulley, A. (1995). *Primary care medicine: Office evaluation and management of the adult patient.* Philadelphia: J. B. Lippincott.

Gralla, R., Itri, L., Pisko, S., Squillante, A., Kelsen, D., & Braun, D. (1981). Antiemetic efficacy of high-dose metoclopramide: Randomized trials with placebo and prochlorperazine in patients with chemotherapy-induced nausea and vomiting. *New England Journal of Medicine, 305*(16), 905–906.

Gralla, R., Tyson, L., Bordin, L., Clark, R., Kelsen, D., & Kris, M. (1984). Antiemetic therapy: A review of recent studies and a report of a randomized assignment trial comparing metoclopramide with delta-9-tetrahydrocannabinol. *Cancer Treatment Reports, 68*(1), 163–172.

Greenberger, N. (1995, Summer). Chronic diarrhea: When is it irritable bowel? *Contemporary Nurse Practitioner*, 32–39.

Greenberger, N. (1997). Update in gastroenterology. *Annals of Internal Medicine, 126*, 221–225.

Griffin, M., & Miner, P. (1995). Conventional drug therapy in inflammatory bowel disease. *Gastroenterology Clinics of North America, 24*(3), 509–521.

Guerreiro, A. (1990). Omeprazole in the treatment of peptic ulcers resistant to $H_2$ receptor antagonists. *Alimentary Pharmacology and Therapeutics, 4*(3), 309–313.

Hallerback, B., Unge, P., Carling, L., Edwin, B., Glise, H., & Havu, N. (1994). Omeprazole and ranitidine in long-term treatment of reflux oesophagitis. *Gastroenterology, 107*(5), 1305–1311.

Hanan, I. (1993). Inflammatory bowel disease in the pregnant woman. *Comparative Therapeutics, 19*, 91–95.

Hanauer, S. (1991). Guidelines for the clinical evaluation of drugs for patients with inflammatory bowel disease. *Federal Register, 56*, 27.

Hanauer, S. (1993). Long-term management of Crohn's disease with mesalamine capsules (Pentasa). *American Journal of Gastroenterology, 881*, 343–351.

Hanauer, S. (1996). Inflammatory bowel disease. *New England Journal of Medicine, 334*(13), 841–847.

Hanauer, S., & Baert, F. (1994). Medical therapy of inflammatory bowel disease. *Medical Clinics of North America, 78*(6), 1413–1426.

Hanauer, S., Belker, M., Giltrick, G., et al. (1990). Multi-center, placebo-controlled, dose-ranging study of oral Pentasa for active Crohn's disease: Preliminary results. *Gastroenterology, 98*, 173.

Hanauer, S., Meyers, S., & Sachar, D. (1995). The pharmacology of anti-inflammatory drugs in inflammatory bowel disease. In J. Kirsner, & R. Shorter (Eds.), *Inflammatory bowel disease*, (4th ed.). Baltimore: Williams & Wilkins.

Hatlebakk, & Berstad, A. (1996). Pharmacokinetic optimisation in the treatment of gastro-esophageal reflux disease. *Clinical Pharmacokinetics, 5*, 386–406.

Havelund, T., Laursen, L., & Lauritsen, K. (1994). Efficacy of omeprazole in lower grades of gastro-oesophageal reflux disease. *Scandanavian Journal of Gastroenterology, 201*(Suppl.), 69–73.

Hawthorne, A., Logan, R., & Gawkey, C. (1992). Randomized controlled trial of azathioprine withdrawal in ulcerative colitis. *British Medical Journal, 305*, 20–22.

Hirschfeld, S., & Clearfield, H. (1995). Pharmacologic therapy for inflammatory bowel disease. *American Family Physician, 51*(8), 1971–1975.

Hixson, L., Kelley, C., Jones, W., et al. (1992). Current trends in the pharmacotherapy for peptic ulcer disease. *Archives of Internal Medicine, 152*, 726–732.

Hodgson, H., & Hazlan M. (1991). Assessment of drug therapy in inflammatory bowel disease. *Alimentary Pharmacology and Therapeutics, 5*, 555–584.

Howden, C., Castell, D., Cohen, S., Freston, J., Orlando, R., & Robinson, M. (1995). The rationale for continuous maintenance treatment of reflux esophagitis. *Archives of Internal Medicine, 155*(14), 1465–1471.

Howden, C., Jones, D., Peace, K., Burget, D., & Hunt, R. (1988). The treatment of gastric ulcer with antisecretory drugs. *Digestive Diseases and Sciences, 33*(5), 619–624.

Islam, M. R. (1987). Single dose tetracycline in cholera. *Gut, 28*(8), 1029–1032.

Jacobs, R. (1997). General problems in infectious diseases. In L. Tierney, S. McPhee, & M. Papadakis (Eds.). *Current Medical Diagnosis & Treatment* (36th ed.). Stamford, CT: Appleton & Lange.

Johnson, P., Ericsson, C., DuPont, H., Morgan, D., Bitsura, J., & Wood, L. (1986). Comparison of loperamide with bismuth subsalicylate for the treatment of acute travelers' diarrhea. *JAMA, 255*(6), 757–772.

Katz, J. (1991). The course of peptic ulcer disease. *Medical Clinics of North America, 75*(4), 831–841.

Katz, P. (1995). Disorders of the esophagus: Dysphagia, noncardiac chest pain and gastroesophageal reflux. In L. Barker, J. Burton, & P. Zieve (Eds.), *Principles of ambulatory medicine* (4th ed.). Baltimore: Williams & Wilkins.

Kelly, W. (1994). Approach to the patient with diarrhea. In *Essentials of internal medicine*. Philadelphia: J. B. Lippincott.

Krebs, H. (1988). Control of chemotherapy-induced nausea and vomiting by combination antiemetic therapy. *Resident and Staff Physician, 34*(1), 75–82.

Kris, M. (1992). Rational for combination antiemetic therapy and strategies for the use of ondansetron in combinations. *Seminars in Oncology, 19*(4), 61–66.

Labenz, J., & Borsch, G. (1995). Toward an optimal treatment of *Helicobacter pylori*-positive peptic ulcers. *American Journal of Gastroenterology, 90*(5), 692–694.

Lashner, B., Hanauer, S., & Silverstein, M. (1990). Testing nicotine gum for ulcerative colitis patients: Experience with single-patient trials. *Digestive Diseases and Sciences, 35*, 827–832.

Lieberman, D. A. (1987). Medical therapy for chronic reflux esophagitis: Long-term follow-up. *Archives of Internal Medicine, 147*(10), 717–720.

Linn, F., & Peppercorn, M. (1992). Drug therapy for inflammatory bowel disease. *American Journal of Surgery, 164*, 85–89.

Liu, L., & Weller, P. (1996). Antiparasitic drugs. *New England Journal of Medicine, 334*(18), 1178–1184.

Malchow, H. (1984). European cooperative Crohn's disease study: Results of drug treatment. *Gastroenterology, 86*, 249–254.

Marenco, G., Menardo, G., Pallini, P., Rossini, F.P., & Saggioro, A. (1989). Comparison between single morning and bedtime doses of 40 mg famotidine for the treatment of duodenal ulcer. *Alimentary Pharmacology and Therapeutics, 3*(3), 285–291.

Markham, A., & McTavish, D. (1996). Clarithromycin and omeprazole. *Drugs, 1,* 161–178.

Marty, M., on behalf of the Granisetron Study Group. (1990). A comparative study of the use of granisetron, a selective 5-HT$_3$ antagonist, versus a standard anti-emetic regimen of chlorpromazine plus dexamethasone in the treatment of cytostatic-induced emesis. *European Journal of Cancer, 25*(Suppl. 1), 28–32.

Marty, M., Pouillart, P., Scholl, S., Droz, J., Azab, M. & Brion, N. (1990). Comparison of the 5-hydroxytryptamine$_3$ (serotonin) antagonist on-dansetron (GR 38032F) with high-dose metoclopramide in the control of cisplatin-induced emesis. *New England Journal of Medicine, 322*(12), 816–821.

Maton, P. N. (1991). Omeprazole. *New England Journal of Medicine, 324*(14), 965–975.

McQuaid, K. (1997). Alimentary tract. In L. Tierny, S. McPhee, & M. Papadakis (Eds.), *Current medical diagnosis and treatment, 1997.* Stamford, CT: Appleton & Lange.

Meyers, S., Sachar, D., Goldberg, J., & Janowitz, H. (1983). Corticotropin versus hydrocortisone in the intravenous treatment of ulcerative colitis: A prospective, randomized, double-blind clinical trial. *Gastroenterology, 85,* 351–357.

Mitchelson, F. (1992). Pharmacological agents affecting emesis. *Drugs, 43*(4), 443–463.

Morrow, G., Hickok, J., & Rosenthal, S. (1995). Progress in reducing nausea and emesis. *Cancer, 76,* 343–357.

Mulder, C., & Tygat, G. (1993). Topical corticosteroids in inflammatory bowel disease. *Alimentary Pharmacology and Therapeutics, 7*(2), 125–130.

Murphy, E., & Calloway, D. (1972). The effect of antibiotic drugs on the volume and composition of intestinal gas from beans. *American Journal of Digestive Disease, 17,* 639–642.

Nathwani, D., & Wood, M. (1993). The management of travellers' diarrhoea. *Journal of Antimicrobial Chemotherapy, 31*(5), 623–626.

Oksanen, P., Salminen, S., Saxelin, M., Hamalainen, P., Ihantola-Vormisto, A., & Muurasniemi-Isoviita, L. (1990). Prevention of travellers' diarrheoea by *Lactobacillus* GG. *Annals of Medicine, 22*(1), 53–56.

Olsalazine for ulcerative colitis. (1990). *Medical Letter, 32,* 105–106.

Pallone, F., Prantera, C., Cottone, M., et al. (1991). Maintenance treatment of Crohn's disease with oral 5-ASA. *Gastroenterology, 100,* A237.

Peppercorn, M. (1990). Advances in drug therapy for inflammatory bowel disease. *Annals of Internal Medicine, 112,* 50–60.

Peppercorn, M. (1993). Is there a role for antibiotics as primary therapy in Crohn's? *Clinical Gastroenterology, 17,* 14.

Petitijean, O., Wendling, J., Tod, M., et al. (1992). Pharmacokinetics and absolute rectal bioavailability of hydrocortisone acetate in distal colitis. *Alimentary Pharmacology and Therapeutics, 6,* 351–357.

Podolsky, D. (1991). Inflammatory bowel disease. *New England Journal of Medicine, 325*(13), 928–937.

Potter, T., Ellis, C., & Levitt, M. (1985). Activated charcoal. In vivo and in vitro studies of effect on gas formation. *Gastroenterology, 88*(3), 620–624.

Pullan, R., Rhodes, J., Ganesh, S., Mani, V., Morris, J., Williams, G., Newcombe, R., Russell, M., et al. (1994). Transdermal nicotine for active ulcerative colitis. *New England Journal of Medicine, 330*(12), 811–815.

Ramirez, B., & Richter, J. (1993). Review article: Promotility drugs and the treatment of gastroesophageal reflux disease. *Alimentary Pharmacology and Therapeutics, 7*(1), 5–20.

Raufman, J., Collins, S., Pandol, S., Korman, L., Collen, M., & Cornelius, M. (1983). Reliability of symptoms in assessing control of gastric acid secretion in patients with Zollinger-Ellison syndrome. *Gastroenterology, 84*(1), 108–113.

Remick, M. (1994). Promoting a healthy pregnancy. In E. Youngkin & M. Davis (Eds.), *Women's health: A primary care clinical guide.* Norwalk, CT: Appleton & Lange.

Rhodes, V., Watson, P., & Johnson, M. (1985). Patterns of nausea and vomiting in chemotherapy patterns: A preliminary study. *Oncology Nursing Forum, 12*(2), 42–48.

Richter, J. (1995). Evaluation and management of diarrhea. In A. Goroll, L. May, & A. Mulley (Eds.), *Primary care medicine: Office evaluation and management of the adult patient.* Philadelphia: J. B. Lippincott.

Roila, R., and The Italian Group for Antiemetic Research. (1995). Dexamethasone, granisetron or both for the prevention of nausea and vomiting during chemotherapy for cancer. *New England Journal of Medicine, 332,* 1–5.

Ruff, P., Paska, W., Goldhals, L., Pouillart, P., Riviere, A., & Vorobiof, D. (1994). Ondansetron compared with granisetron in the prophylaxis of cisplatin-induced acute emesis: A multicentre double-blind, randomized, parallel-group study. *Oncology, 51*(1), 113–118.

Ruymann, F., & Richter, J. (1995). Management of inflammatory bowel disease. In A. Goroll, L. May, & A. Mulley (Eds.), *Primary care medicine.* Philadelphia: J. B. Lippincott.

Sallan, S., Cronin, C., Zellen, M., & Zimberg, N. (1980). Antiemetics in patients receiving chemotherapy for cancer. *New England Journal of Medicine, 302*(3), 135–138.

Scott, D., & Edelman, R. (1993). Treatment of gastrointestinal infections. *Baillieres Clinical Gastroenterology, 7*(2), 477–499.

Sears, S., & Sack, D. (1995). Medical advice for the international traveler. In L. R. Barker, J. Burton, & P. Zieve (Eds.), *Principles of ambulatory medicine* (4th ed.). Baltimore: Williams & Wilkins.

Seigel, L., & Longo, D. (1981). The control of chemotherapy-induced emesis. *Annals of Internal Medicine, 95*, 352.

Shah, S., & Peppercorn, M. (1995). Inflammatory bowel disease therapy: An update. *Comprehensive Therapy, 21*(6), 296–302.

Simethicone for gastrointestinal gas. (1996). *Medical Letter, 38* (977), 57–58.

Slapak, C., & Kufe, D. (1998). Principles of cancer therapy. In A. Fauci, E. Braunwald, K. Isselbacher, et al. (Eds.). *Principles of internal medicine* (4th ed.). New York: McGraw-Hill.

Soll, A. (1996). Medical treatment of peptic ulcer disease: Practice guidelines. *JAMA, 275*, 622–629.

Sontag, S. (1988). Current status of maintenance therapy in peptic ulcer disease. *American Journal of Gastroenterology, 83*, 607–617.

Stenson, W., Cort, D., Rodgers, J., Rubakoff, R., DeSchryver-Keeskemeti, K., Gramlich, T., & Becken, W. (1992). Dietary supplementation with fish oil in ulcerative colitis. *Annals of Internal Medicine, 116*(8), 609–614.

Sutherland, L., Martin, F., Greer, S., et al. (1987). 5-aminosalicylic acid enemas in the treatment of distal ulcerative colitis, proctosigmoiditis, and proctitis. *Gastroenterology, 92*, 1894.

Tami, J. A., & Waite, W. W. (1988). Metoclopramide suppository considerations. *Drug Intelligence in Clinical Pharmacology, 22*(3), 268–269.

Taylor, J., Zagari, M., & Murphy, K. (1997). Pharmacoeconomic comparison of treatments for the eradication of *Helicobacter pylori*. *Annals of Internal Medicine, 157*, 87–94.

Toovey, S., Hudson, E., Herdry, W., & Levy, A. (1981). Sulphasalazine and male infertility: Reversibility and possible mechanism. *Gut, 22*(6), 445–451.

Tortorice, P., & O'Connell, M. (1990). Management of chemotherapy-induced nausea and vomiting. *Pharmacotherapy, 10*(2), 129–145.

Uphold, C., & Graham, M. (1994). *Clinical guidelines in family practice*. Gainesville, FL: Barmarrae Books.

U.S. Preventive Services Task Force. (1995). *Guide to clinical preventive services*. Baltimore: Williams & Wilkins.

Wampler, G. (1983). Pharmacology and clinical effectiveness of phenothiazines and related drugs for managing chemotherapy-induced emesis. *Drugs, 25*(Suppl. 1), 35–51.

Willoughby, M., & Truelove, S. (1980). Ulcerative colitis and pregnancy. *Gut, 21*(16), 469.

Wolfe, M., & Jensen, R. (1987). Zollinger syndrome. *New England Journal of Medicine, 317*(19), 1200–1209.

# 26

## MUSCULOSKELETAL DISORDERS

*Sharon L. Sheahan, Aimee Gelhot, and Angela B. Hoth*

Annually, the incidence of the major musculoskeletal conditions varies from 1% for gout (Star & Hochberg, 1994), 1–2% for rheumatoid arthritis (Symmons et al, 1995), 15–20% for persons seeking back pain treatment (U.S. Department of Health and Human Services [USDHHS], 1994), 80% for osteoarthritis for persons over age 75 (Brandt & Slemenda, 1993), and 30% for osteoporosis-related fractures for persons 65 and over (Ott, 1993). Numerous others seek treatment for muscle strains, sprains, bursitis, and tendinitis.

The prevalence of arthritic and musculoskeletal conditions is likely to increase as the U.S. census shifts toward an aging high-risk society. The baby boomer cohort, historically the largest middle-aged cohort, is expected to account for increased prevalence rates for all conditions. In an era of managed care systems and cost containment, health care providers are challenged to support and maintain optimum functioning for individuals afflicted with musculoskeletal conditions by utilizing preventive measures and the most cost-effective treatment regimens. This chapter discusses the pharmacological and nonpharmacological management of the major arthritic and musculoskeletal conditions encountered in primary care.

## RHEUMATOID ARTHRITIS

The incidence (number of new cases occurring annually) of rheumatoid arthritis (RA) increases with age, with a peak incidence seen in persons aged 50 and older. By 2020, it is projected that arthritis will affect 59.4 million (18.2%) persons in the United States (CDC, 1996). Females in all age groups are afflicted more than males (Symmons & Silman, 1994).

### ETIOLOGY

The exact etiology of RA, a systemic autoimmune disorder, is unknown, but both genetic and environmental factors are involved (Ollier & MacGregor, 1995). There is a growing consensus that the disorder may be induced in genetically predisposed adults (specifically, the HLA-DR4 and HLA-DR1 genotypes) by more than one arthritogenic agent (Nepom, 1994; Ollier & MacGregor, 1995). Viruses, human T-cell lymphotrophic virus type 1, retroviruses, Epstein-Barr virus, herpes viruses, rubella virus, and paraviruses are being investigated as etiologic agents along with the bacterial candidates mycoplasma, mycobacteria, and various enteric organisms (Wilder, 1993). There is consensus among researchers and rheumatologists that CD4+ T cells seem to play a major role in the pathogenesis of RA by accumulating in the synovium and by recruiting other inflammatory cells (Salmon & Gaston, 1995; Tak et al, 1995; Viner, 1995). It is suggested that the disease-triggering agent is transmitted to the synovium via the bloodstream. The result is an activation and/or injury to the synovial microvascular endothelial cells. With disease progression, the synovium becomes hypertrophic and edematous with projection of synovial tissue into the joint cavity (Wilder, 1993). This process results in joint immobilization, muscle spasm and shortening, bone and cartilage destruction, ligamentous laxity, and altered tendon function (Palmer, 1995). The disease course is characterized by remissions and exacerbations.

## SPECIFIC CONSIDERATIONS FOR PHARMACOTHERAPY

### When Drug Therapy Is Needed

Treatment of rheumatoid arthritis (RA) remains a challenge. Since no known cure or preventative measures exist, the focus of therapy lies in optimal disease management (American College of Rheumatology [ACR], 1996b).

### Short-Term and Long-Term Goals of Pharmacotherapy

Goals of pharmacotherapy are to (1) achieve complete remission of disease (rarely successful), (2) control disease activity, (3) alleviate pain, (4) maintain joint function, (5) maximize quality of life, and (6) slow disease progression (ACR, 1996b). Unfortunately, no single agent used in the treatment of RA achieves all six goals. The ultimate practice goal is to initiate disease-modifying therapy before joint damage occurs.

### Nonpharmacologic Therapy

In addition to the standard pharmacologic therapies, a variety of treatment options exist, ranging from self-medication and self-help groups, yoga, water exercise and hydrotherapy, heat and paraffin baths, and referral to surgical intervention with joint replacement. Surgery is an option for patients with intractable pain or loss of function that ultimately interferes with activities of daily living. Many mechanical assistance devices are available to improve physical functioning.

### Time Frame for Initiating Pharmacotherapy

Pharmacologic therapies available for the treatment of RA include the nonsteroidal anti-inflammatory drugs (NSAIDs), corticosteroids (CSs), and disease-modifying antirheumatic drugs (DMARDs) also known as slow-acting antirheumatic drugs (SAARDs). According to the American College of Rheumatology, optimum management requires an early diagnosis and timely institution of disease-modifying therapy prior to joint destruction (ACR, 1996b). Unfortunately, the optimal initiation strategy for these medicines is not known. The response to currently available therapies varies between patients.

See Drug Tables 306, 307, and 319.

### Assessment and History Taking

Baseline parameters recommended prior to initiation of pharmacotherapy for RA are given in Table 26–1. Contraindications to therapy and concomitant disease states warranting caution when using certain drugs will be addressed below.

The typical history of the RA-afflicted individual is an insidious onset of peripheral joint pain and stiffness over a period of several weeks. In addition to morning stiffness, joint pain, and swelling, many patients experience constitutional symptoms of fatigue, malaise, or weight loss (Semble, 1995). Acute disabling polyarticular arthritis can occur, but disabling nonarticular presentation is rare. "By definition RA cannot be diagnosed until the condition has been present for at least several weeks" (Anderson, 1993). During the first month or two the extraarticular features, symmetrical inflammation, and the serologic findings may be absent. The differential diagnosis of RA includes osteoarthritis, gout, septic arthritis, and systemic lupus erythematosus. Table 26–2 shows the revised 1987 American Arthritis Association (AAA) diagnostic criteria, which are widely used (Macgregor, 1995).

A complete physical examination with particular attention to the musculoskeletal system is essential since RA can afflict any joint, with the wrist and hand, specifically the metacarpal phalangeal (MCP) and proximal interphalangeal (PIP) joints, most involved. The distal interphalangeal (DIP) joints are usually spared, but not always. The swan-neck deformity with ulnar deviation of MCP joints along with radial deviation of the wrist is a classic RA deformity. Other classic deformities are the boutonnière, with flexion of the PIP and hyperextension of the DIP joints of the fingers, and hammertoes, which occur with metatarsophalangeal joint subluxation.

***Diagnostic tests.***    No specific laboratory test, histologic, or radiographic finding diagnoses RA.

The rheumatoid factor is found in 85% of patients, and its presence tends to correlate with increased disease severity and poorer prognosis. Additional, nonspecific laboratory markers are an elevated erythrocyte sedimentation rate (ESR) and a C-reactive protein, which are used to monitor acute inflammatory stages. Synovial fluid leukocytosis (WBC > 2000/mm), histologic findings of chronic synovitis, and radiologic erosions, which do not occur until after 2 years, may be seen. A routine urinalysis and chemistry profile to determine kidney function should be performed prior to therapy. A uric acid level should be obtained to differentiate RA from gout. C-reactive protein, which is present in all individuals, is elevated in RA.

Radiographic findings associated with RA include soft tissue swelling, osteoporosis, narrowed joint spaces, and marginal erosions. The finding of osteoporosis, marginal erosions, and reactive bone formation distinguishes RA from other arthritic conditions (Brown & Deluca, 1995). A baseline chest x-ray and electrocardiogram are needed to detect the development of extraarticular manifestations.

**Extraarticular Manifestations.** RA is a systemic disease, and individuals will need to be monitored for development of extraarticular signs and symptoms (Halverson, 1995). The rheumatoid nodule is the most common extraarticular sign, occurring in 40% of seropositive patients (Snowden & Kay, 1995). The nodules form subcutaneously, in crops, over the bursae and along a tendon sheath and are more prevalent during the active phase. Although they can be found anywhere including the viscera, they are commonly seen over the olecranon, the extensor surface of the forearm, and the Achilles tendon. Vasculitic lesions with splinter hemorrhages and necrotic areas on the fingertips and around the nails may be present. A disproportionate number of men are afflicted with severe extraarticular symptoms, eg, vasculitis and Felty's syndrome (Snowden & Kay, 1995).

Baseline and periodic eye examinations are needed. Ocular involvement, including keratoconjunctivitis sicca, episcleritis, scleritis, and necrotizing scleritis (NS); marginal furrows; peripheral ulcerative keratitis (PUK); choroidal lesions; and retinal vasculitis, will afflict 25% of RA clients. The development of NS or PUK and vasculitis elsewhere in the body is a grim prognostic sign (Messmer & Foster, 1995).

A baseline CBC is needed, since a common hematologic manifestation is a hypochromic-microcytic anemia with a low iron and low or normal iron-binding capacity. RA-associated anemic patients fail to respond vigorously to iron therapy with a brisk reticulocytosis. A significant confounder for gastrointestinal bleeding is that the ulcerogenic antiinflammatory medications for treatment can produce a positive occult stool blood. Ferritin levels are not helpful in the differential diagnosis, and the clinician must restrict a detailed workup (bone marrow, x-ray, and endoscopy) to selected cases. Another hematologic manifestation is Felty's syndrome, which is a combination of RA, splenomegaly, leukopenia, and leg ulcers.

A baseline electrocardiogram is warranted to assess cardiac-associated extraarticular manifestations including involvement of the valves, pericardium, myocardium, and aorta. Inflammatory pericarditis and effusion usually develop during an acute exacerbation. Inflammatory lesions similar to the RA nodules can promote conduction defects, valvular dysfunction, embolic processes, and possibly myocardiopathy. Fifty percent of autopsied RA patients exhibited some cardiac pathology, as did 50% of RA cardiac asymptomatic patents undergoing echocardiography (Anderson, 1993).

Common neurologic manifestations include cervical spine–related myopathies with neck pain and associated bilateral sensory paresthesias of the hands. Entrapment neuropathies occur when a peripheral nerve passes through a compartment also occupied by a scarred synovium or tendon sheath. The severity of symptoms depends upon the degree of inflammation and the posture and stress on the joint. Nerves most frequently involved are the posterior interosseous nerve in the antecubital fossa, the femoral nerve anterior to the hip joint, the peroneal nerve adjacent to the fibular head, and the interdigital nerve at the metatarsal phalangeal (MTP) joint (Anderson, 1993).

Common respiratory associated involvement is manifested by inflammation of the cricoarytenoid joint. The symptoms are episodic laryngeal pain, dysphonia and occasional pain with swallowing. Symptomatic pleuritis may occur when nodules develop on the lung parenchyma. Small effusions may be seen on chest x-ray. Along with the extraarticular manifestations, there is a general consensus that comorbid conditions (cardiovascular, pulmonary, and renal diseases) are increased in RA patients and RA it-

## TABLE 26-1. RECOMMENDED MONITORING STRATEGIES FOR TREATMENT OF RHEUMATOID ARTHRITIS

| Drugs | Toxicities Requiring Monitoring[a] | Baseline Evaluation | Monitoring System review/examination | Monitoring Laboratory |
|---|---|---|---|---|
| Salicylates, nonsteroidal antiinflammatory drugs | Gastrointestinal ulceration and bleeding | CBC, creatinine, AST, ALT | Dark/black stool, dyspepsia, nausea/vomiting, abdominal pain, edema, shortness of breath | CBC yearly, LFTs, creatinine testing may be required[b] |
| Hydroxychloroquine | Macular damage | None unless patient is over age 40 or has previous eye disease | Visual changes, funduscopic and visual fields every 6–12 months | |
| Sulfasalazine | Myelosuppression | CBC, and AST or ALT in patients at risk, G-6PD | Symptoms of myelosuppression,[c] photosensitivity, rash | CBC every 2–4 weeks for first 3 months, then every 3 months |
| Methotrexate | Myelosuppression, hepatic fibrosis, cirrhosis, pulmonary infiltrates or fibrosis | CBC, chest radiography within past year, hepatitis B and C serology in high-risk patients, AST or ALT, albumin, alkaline phosphatase, and creatinine | Symptoms of myelosuppression,[c] shortness of breath, cough, DOE, nausea/vomiting, lymph node swelling, jaundice, dark urine | CBC, platelet count, AST, albumin, creatinine every 4–8 weeks |
| Gold, intramuscular | Myelosuppression, proteinuria | CBC, platelet count, creatinine, urine dipstick for protein | Symptoms of myelosuppression,[c] edema, rash, oral ulcers, diarrhea | CBC, platelet count, urine dipstick every 1–2 weeks for first 20 weeks, then at the time of each (or every other) injection |
| Gold, oral | Myelosuppression, proteinuria | CBC, platelet count, urine dipstick for protein | Symptoms of myelosuppression,[c] edema, rash, diarrhea | CBC, platelet count, urine dipstick for protein every 4–12 weeks |
| D-penicillamine | Myelosuppression, proteinuria | CBC, platelet count, creatinine, urine dipstick for protein | Symptoms of myelosuppression,[c] edema, rash | CBC, urine dipstick for protein every 2 weeks until dosage stable, then every 1–3 months |
| Azathioprine | Myelosuppression, hepatotoxicity, lymphoproliferative disorders | CBC, platelet count, creatinine, AST or ALT | Symptoms of myelosuppression,[c] | CBC and platelet count every 1–2 weeks with changes in dosage, and every 1–3 months thereafter |

530

| Agent | Toxicities | Baseline evaluation | Symptoms to inquire about[a] | Monitoring |
|---|---|---|---|---|
| Corticosteroids (oral ≤ 10 mg of prednisone or equivalent) | Hypertension, hyperglycemia | BP, chemistry panel, bone densitometry in high-risk patients | BP at each visit, polyuria, polydipsia, edema, shortness of breath, visual changes, weight gain | Urinalysis for glucose yearly |
| Agents for refractory RA or severe extraarticular complications | | | | |
| Cyclophosphamide | Myelosuppression, myeloproliferative disorders, malignancy, hemorrhagic cystitis | CBC, platelet count, urinalysis, creatinine, AST or ALT | Symptoms of myelosuppression,[c] hematuria | CBC and platelet count every 1–2 weeks with changes in dosage, and every 1–3 months thereafter, urinalysis and urine cytology every 6–12 months after cessation |
| Chlorambucil | Myelosuppression, myeloproliferative disorders, malignancy | CBC, urinalysis, creatinine, AST or ALT | Symptoms of myelosuppression,[c] | CBC and platelet count every 1–2 weeks with changes in dosage, and every 1–3 months thereafter |
| Cyclosporin A | Renal insufficiency, anemia, hypertension | CBC, creatinine, uric acid, LFTs, BP | Edema, BP every 2 weeks until dosage stable, then monthly | Creatinine every 2 weeks until dose is stable, then monthly; periodic CBC, potassium, and LFTs |

[a] Potential serious toxicities that may be detected by monitoring before they have become clinically apparent or harmful to the patient. This list mentions toxicities that occur frequently enough to justify monitoring. Patients with comorbidity, concurrent medications, and other specific risk factors may need further studies to monitor for specific toxicity.

[b] Package insert for diclofenac (Voltaren) recommends that AST and ALT be monitored within the first 8 weeks of treatment and periodically thereafter. Monitoring of serum creatinine should be performed weekly for at least 3 weeks in patients receiving concomitant angiotensin converting enzyme inhibitors or diuretics.

[c] Symptoms of myelosuppression include fever, symptoms of infection, easy bruisability, and bleeding.

CBC = complete blood cell count (hematocrit, hemoglobin, white blood cell count) including differential cell and platelet counts; ALT = alanine aminotransferase; AST = aspartate aminotransferase; LFTs = liver function tests; BP = blood pressure.

*Source: Used with permission from American College of Rheumatology (1996a).*

**TABLE 26–2. THE AMERICAN RHEUMATISM ASSOCIATION 1987 REVISED CRITERIA FOR THE CLASSIFICATION OF RHEUMATOID ARTHRITIS**

| Criterion | Definition |
|---|---|
| 1. Morning stiffness | Morning stiffness in and around the joints, lasting at least 1 h before maximal improvement |
| 2. Arthritis of three or more joint areas | At least three joint areas simultaneously have had soft tissue swelling or fluid (not bony overgrowth alone) observed by a physician. The 14 possible areas are right or left PIP, MP, wrist, elbow, knee, ankle, and MTP joints |
| 3. Arthritis of hand joints | At least one area swollen (as defined above) in a wrist, MCP, or PIP joint |
| 4. Symmetric arthritis | Simultaneous involvement of the same joint areas (as defined in item 2) on both sides of the body (bilateral involvement of PIPs, MCPs, or MTPs is acceptable without absolute symmetry) |
| 5. Rheumatoid nodules | Subcutaneous nodules, over bony prominences, or extensor surfaces, or in juxtaarticular regions, observed by a physician |
| 6. Serum rheumatoid factor | Demonstration of abnormal amounts of serum rheumatoid factor by any method for which the result has been positive in <5% of normal control subjects |
| 7. Radiographic changes | Radiographic changes typical of rheumatoid arthritis on posteroanterior hand and wrist radiographs, which must include erosions or unequivocal bony decalcification localized in or most marked adjacent to the involved joints (osteoarthritis changes alone do not qualify) |

For classification purposes, a patient shall be said to have rheumatoid arthritis if he or she has satisfied at least four of these seven criteria. Criteria 1 through 4 must have been present for at least 6 weeks. Patients with two clinical diagnoses are not excluded. Designation as classic, definite, or probable rheumatoid arthritis is not to be made.
*Source: From Schumacher et al (1993, p. 328). Used with permission from the Arthritis Foundation.*

self may be a marker for increased risk for these problems (Pincus, Wolfe, & Callahan, 1994).

### Patient/Caregiver Information

Symptoms of drug toxicity necessary for self-monitoring are listed for each drug in Table 26–1.

Patients receiving long-term corticosteroids should be advised to wear a medical alert bracelet. Any changes in vision must be reported immediately by patients taking hydroxychloroquine (HCQ). Sulfasalazine therapy results in discoloration of body fluids, namely urine and sweat, and may lead to permanent discoloration of contact lenses. Avoidance of alcohol is recommended during any course of drug therapy, but is especially important in patients receiving methotrexate (MTX). Women of child-bearing potential must be counseled on effective methods of contraception while receiving DMARD therapy. All drugs have unique effects on fetal development, and the benefits and risks of use should be individually evaluated.

Patient education remains the cornerstone of RA management. Patients and families need in-formation about the disease course, therapeutic options, medication toxicity, and available community resources. Arthritis self-help and group support courses have been effective in increasing efficacy. The local chapter of the Arthritis Foundation can be an excellent resource.

## OUTCOMES MANAGEMENT

### Selecting an Appropriate Agent

The drug classes mentioned above are commonly used in the treatment of RA. Guidelines for monitoring each therapy are provided in Table 26–1. Adverse effects may be listed as rare (occurring in <1% of patients), uncommon (1–10%), and common (>10%) as described by the ACR in its Guidelines for Monitoring Drug Therapy in Rheumatoid Arthritis (ACR, 1996a).

*Nonsteroidal Antiinflammatory Drugs.* Nonsteroidal antiinflammatory drugs are used for treatment and symptomatic relief of many musculoskeletal conditions. An overview of NSAIDs as a class is provided here, and each is discussed individually as it is applicable to each disease state. This drug class includes aspirin, nonacetylated salicylates, and nonsalicylate NSAIDs.

The exact mechanism of NSAIDs' anti-inflammatory and analgesic properties that are beneficial in musculoskeletal disorders remains unknown but may be related to the ability of NSAIDs to inhibit cyclooxygenase, decrease prostaglandin synthesis in inflamed tissue, and potentially interfere with other proinflammatory substances (Furst, 1994; Greene & Winickoff, 1992). Cyclooxygenase inhibition by NSAIDs leads to decreased prostaglandin synthesis. Prostaglandins play an important part in inflammation, gastrointestinal (GI) protection, and maintenance of renal perfusion. In addition, NSAIDs affect the activity of other inflammatory mediators such as bradykinins and leukotrienes and the production of oxygen radicals, influence cellular processes, and inhibit leukocyte migration and lymphocyte activation (Furst, 1994).

In RA, NSAIDs alleviate pain, reduce joint swelling, and maintain joint function. This class of drugs has not been shown to alter the disease course or slow the progression of joint destruction.

Pharmacokinetic parameters of the various NSAIDs are given in the NSAID Drug Table 306. Absorption of NSAIDs is rapid and complete. Coadministration with food interferes with the rate, but not the extent of absorption. Theoretically, analgesia onset may be slightly delayed with food ingestion, but this may not be clinically significant. All NSAIDs exhibit high protein binding. This becomes clinically significant in hypoalbuminemic patients who cannot clear the excess free drug, ie, those with renal failure. The majority of NSAIDs are metabolized by the liver to either active or inactive metabolites, which are then eliminated via the kidney. Aspirin and the nonacetylated salicylates also undergo metabolism in the gastric mucosa (Furst, 1994).

Table 26–3 lists the currently available NSAIDs according to chemical class. With the numerous NSAIDs available, choosing an agent becomes a challenge. Parameters to be considered in selecting an NSAID for a patient are given in Table 26–4. Phenylbutazone and meclofenamate are rarely used in practice due to severe toxicities and should not be considered for initial therapy.

The majority of NSAIDs available are prescription products. NSAIDs currently available

in nonprescription strength include ibuprofen, naproxen, and ketoprofen. Although few direct comparative data exist; the NSAIDs appear to be equally effective in the treatment of the majority of muscoskeletal disorders (ACR, 1996a; Furst, 1994; Williams, 1993). On an individual

## TABLE 26–3. NSAID CHEMICAL CLASSES

**Acetylated Salicylates**
Aspirin

**Nonacetylated Salicylates**
Choline magnesium trisalicylate
Diflunisal
Magnesium salicylate
Salsalate
Sodium salicylate

**Nonsalicylate NSAIDs**

| Propionic Acids | Acetic Acids | Fenamates |
|---|---|---|
| Fenoprofen | Diclofenac | Meclofenamate |
| Flurbiprofen | Etodolac | Mefenamic Acid |
| Ibuprofen | Indomethacin | |
| Ketoprofen | Ketorolac | Oxicams |
| Naproxen | Nabumetone | Piroxicam |
| Naproxen sodium | Sulindac | |
| Oxaprozin | Tolmetin | |

## TABLE 26–4. USE OF NONSTEROIDAL ANTIINFLAMMATORY DRUGS FOR RA

**Goal**
Symptomatic relief of pain and swelling

**Limitation**
Unlikely to prevent damage

**Factors for Selecting Drugs**
Dosing regimen
Efficacy
Tolerance
Costs
Patient's age
Presence of comorbid disease(s)
Concurrent drugs
Patient preferences

**Monitoring Efficacy**
Symptoms and signs of active synovitis

**Monitoring Toxicity**

Source: Used with permission from American College of Rheumatology (1996b).

basis, however, great variability exists in both clinical response and tolerability among the various agents. Failure to respond to one NSAID does not indicate a failure of the entire class. Selection of an NSAID from a different or even the same chemical class and trials of many NSAIDs may be required to achieve an adequate clinical response.

Aspirin remains a reasonable and inexpensive RA treatment option, although higher doses may be necessary (3900–6500 mg/day). Blood levels can be monitored and a target level of 20–30 mg/dL correlates with an antiinflammatory response. Levels higher than 30 mg/dL may produce significant toxicity.

Nonacetylated salicylates, including choline salicylate, choline magnesium trisalicylate, salsalate, and diflunisal are also effective. These agents are weak inhibitors of cyclooxygenase, which allows for fewer gastrointestinal side effects, less renal toxicity, and little to no antiplatelet effect (Atkinson, Menard, & Kalish, 1995). A potential disadvantage of these agents, however, is their relatively high cost. The usual maintenance dose for the nonacetylated salicylates is 3–4.5 g/day.

Nonsalicylate NSAIDs are reasonable alternatives to aspirin, equally efficacious, generally better tolerated, and do not require blood level monitoring. Selection of a particular NSAID product, whether aspirin, nonacetylated salicylate, or nonsalicylate NSAID, is based on trial and error and patient-specific response.

Consider cost when selecting an NSAID. Using a stepped-care approach, prescribe the least expensive NSAIDs initially and then progress to more expensive agents if necessary for substantial cost savings to patients and institutions without compromising adequate patient care (Jones et al, 1996).

The analgesic effect of NSAIDs occurs immediately, whereas antiinflammatory actions may take 1–2 weeks. Two weeks at an appropriate dose is considered an adequate trial before changing the patient to another NSAID. Concomitant use of more than one NSAID is not advised since simultaneous use increases the risk for toxicity as well as consumer cost.

Adverse effects associated with the use of NSAIDs include dyspepsia, peptic ulcer disease (PUD), renal insufficiency, hepatotoxicity, and central nervous system (CNS) effects such as headache (HA), dizziness, confusion, or depression. Aspirin irreversibly affects platelet function, thus prolonging bleeding time. The nonsal-

icylate NSAIDs, on the other hand, exhibit reversible platelet effects once the drug has been removed. Patients with aspirin sensitivity should use NSAIDs with caution as cross-sensitivity has been reported (Williams, 1993).

Dyspepsia, the most common adverse effect reported with NSAID use, may be avoided by advising that the drug be taken with food. Buffered and enteric-coated aspirin preparations may decrease GI discomfort. Other less common, yet more severe GI complications include ulceration, bleeding, perforation, and gastric outlet obstruction. Greene and Winickoff (1992) report that the treatment of NSAID-related GI toxicity adds 45% to the cost of arthritis care. Risk factors for severe GI toxicity include advanced age, prior history of PUD or GI bleeding, cardiovascular (CV) disease, higher NSAID dosage, and concurrent corticosteroid use (ACR, 1996a; Cryer & Feldman, 1992; Furst, 1994; Silverstein et al, 1995). Excess alcohol intake and smoking may also increase the risk of GI toxicity. Misoprostol, a prostaglandin analog, decreases NSAID-induced GI ulceration (Graham et al, 1993; Raskin et al, 1995). GI complications are reduced in high-risk patients receiving misoprostol 200 µg four times daily (Silverstein et al, 1995). High-risk patients (the elderly and patients with a history of PUD, GI bleeding, or CV disease) should receive GI prophylaxis to prevent potentially life-threatening complications (Silverstein et al, 1995). Other RA patients receiving long-term NSAID treatment may benefit from misoprostol therapy. However, the overall benefit in decreasing GI complications in this population is less clear. Taha et al (1996) demonstrated the efficacy of high-dose famotidine (40 mg b.i.d.) in preventing gastric and duodenal ulcers in patients receiving long-term NSAID therapy. However, it is unknown whether this therapy also prevents further GI sequelae in high-risk patients (Taha et al, 1996). Other $H_2$ antagonists, sucralfate, and antacids have not been shown to provide adequate GI protection or prevent complications in patients receiving NSAID therapy (Cryer & Feldman, 1992).

Renal toxicity may also occur as a result of NSAID use. All NSAIDs have the potential to cause reversible renal insufficiency, interstitial nephritis, and nephrotic syndrome. Although these complications are relatively uncommon, the elderly and patients with preexisting renal disease, congestive heart failure (CHF), cirrhosis, atherosclerosis, or any underlying condition affecting renal blood flow are at higher risk for developing NSAID-induced renal insufficiency (ACR, 1996a; Furst, 1994; Schlondorff, 1993). Patients taking diuretics may also be at risk. Monitoring renal function weekly for several weeks is indicated in high-risk patients following initiation of NSAID therapy (ACR, 1996a).

NSAIDs may induce a transient elevation in liver enzymes. Routine laboratory monitoring is generally not indicated unless the patient has underlying liver disease or receives diclofenac therapy (ACR, 1996a).

**Corticosteroids.**    Corticosteroids (CSs) effectively relieve symptoms associated with RA. Because of the toxicities associated with high doses and long-term use, continuous use of CSs is indicated only for life-threatening complications or refractory RA. Corticosteroids in low doses (10 mg/day of prednisone or equivalent) are generally adequate to reduce joint swelling, relieve pain, and allow patients to resume activity (ACR, 1996b). They are also used as interim therapy while waiting for DMARDs to take effect. Tapering the CS or discontinuation should be initiated as early as possible, but this may be difficult in many RA patients.

Intraarticular CS injections are a safe and effective method to provide relief and improve function, especially in patients with a limited number of affected joints (ACR, 1996b). The same joint should not be injected more than once within a 3-month period (ACR, 1996b). If this schedule is not adequate to control joint symptoms, reevaluate the treatment regimen.

Potential adverse effects associated with low-dose CS use include skin thinning, bruising, increased appetite, weight gain, fluid retention, acne, hypertension (HTN), hyperglycemia, atherosclerosis, gastric ulcers and associated bleeding, glaucoma, cataract formation, osteoporosis, avascular necrosis, impaired wound healing, increased susceptibility to infection, and development of a cushingoid appearance (ACR, 1996a; "Drugs for Rheumatoid Arthritis," 1994). Hypothalamic-pituitary axis (HPA) suppression is also a concern with long-term use. Adequate patient counseling is important regarding adverse effects, duration of therapy, risks of long-term administration and difficulties with tapering, and the dangers of suddenly stopping CS therapy.

**Hydroxychloroquine.**    Hydroxychloroquine, an antimalarial compound, is effective in treating mild to moderate RA. It is one of the least toxic

and least costly DMARDs to monitor (ACR, 1996a, Prashker & Meenan, 1995). Initiated at a single daily dose of 400 mg, HCQ may then be decreased to 200 mg per day once efficacy has been established. Dosage adjustments are indicated in patients with decreased renal function. Retinal damage (rare) is the major toxicity associated with HCQ use and is preventable with appropriate monitoring (Table 26–1). Patients older than 70 years of age who have received a cumulative dose of more than 800 g are at the greatest risk of developing retinal toxicity (ACR, 1996a). Other rare and less serious toxicities associated with HCQ include GI symptoms, myopathy, blurred vision, accommodation difficulty, abnormal skin pigmentation, and peripheral neuropathy.

**Sulfasalazine.**    Sulfasalazine (SSZ), a drug consisting of sulfapyridine and 5-aminosalacylic acid (5-ASA), is a well-established treatment for inflammatory bowel disease. SSZ has various immunomodulatory and antiinflammatory effects that may contribute to slowing the progression of joint damage (Smedegard & Bjork, 1995). Initial dosing in RA patients consists of 500 mg daily, increased by 500 mg weekly to a target dose of 2–3 g per day. SSZ has shown an efficacy equal to gold and penicillamine (Van Riel, Van Gestel, & Van De Putte, 1995). It has been proven to be more efficacious and have a faster onset of action than HCQ and auranofin (Van Riel et al, 1995).

Common adverse effects include skin rash, photosensitivity, HA, and GI symptoms (ACR, 1996a; "Drugs for Rheumatoid Arthritis," 1994; Gittoes, 1994; Van Riel et al, 1995). Administration of enteric-coated SSZ increases tolerability. Patients with sulfa allergy should not receive sulfasalazine. Myelosuppression, unrelated to dose, generally manifests as leukopenia in 1–3% of patients during the first 3–6 months of therapy (ACR, 1996a; Amos, 1995). Early detection by routine monitoring (Table 26–1) and drug discontinuation reverses the bone marrow suppression. Oligospermia may also occur and normalizes upon discontinuation of the drug. Routine monitoring of liver function tests (LFTs) is unnecessary unless the patient has underlying liver disease.

**Azathioprine.**    Azathioprine (AZA), a purine analog, is initiated at 1.25–1.5 mg/kg per day and then increased to 2–2.5 mg/kg per day after 3 months if necessary. Dosage adjustments are necessary in patients with renal failure. Severe toxicity is uncommon with the low doses used in RA. The most common adverse effect of AZA is GI intolerance, which leads to discontinuation of the drug in ~10% of patients (ACR, 1996a). Other adverse effects include reversible bone marrow suppression; rarely hepatitis and pancreatitis, and an increased risk of lymphoma with long-term use. Concomitant administration of allopurinol increases AZA concentrations and the risk of toxicity. If concurrent administration is necessary, decrease the AZA dose by 75%. Simultaneous use of angiotensin-converting enzyme inhibitors (ACEIs) or allopurinol in the presence of renal insufficiency increases the risk of AZA-associated bone marrow suppression (ACR, 1996a).

**Gold.** The injectable gold products gold sodium thiomalate and aurothioglucose are administered intramuscularly starting with a test dose of 10 mg. If no adverse effects occur, a 25-mg dose is given the next week, followed by 50 mg administered weekly until a total cumulative dose of 1 g is reached, toxicity appears, or remission occurs. Once the patient improves, the dosing interval is increased to 2 weeks and then to 3–4 weeks as tolerated. Disease exacerbations may require reinstitution of weekly injections.

Stomatitis and rash occur commonly with gold therapy (ACR, 1996a). Pruritis without rash may also occur. A nitritoid reaction consisting of flushing, weakness, nausea, and dizziness has been reported within 30 min of injecting gold thiomalate ("Drugs for Rheumatoid Arthritis," 1994). Hematologic, renal, and pulmonary toxicities are serious enough to require frequent monitoring (Table 26–1), but occur rarely (ACR, 1996a; Williams, 1993).

Oral gold, auranofin, is more convenient than the injectable form and causes fewer side effects, but is also less efficacious (Wood, 1994). Diarrhea resulting from auranofin therapy is generally dose-related and may necessitate discontinuation of the drug.

**ᴅ-Penicillamine.** A metabolite of penicillin, ᴅ-penicillamine is initiated at 250 mg given daily on an empty stomach. Doses may be increased 125–250 mg per day every 1–2 months to a maintenance dose of 750 mg per day.

Common, less severe side effects include pruritic rash, stomatitis, nausea, anorexia and transient decreased or altered taste (ACR,

1996a; "Drugs for Rheumatoid Arthritis," 1994). Dysguesia is temporary and may resolve even if the drug is continued (Gittoes, 1994). More severe but rare toxicities include myelosuppression (especially leukopenia and thrombocytopenia), renal toxicities including proteinuria, renal failure, and nephrotic syndrome, and autoimmune syndromes such as myasthenia gravis, Goodpasture's syndrome, or a lupus-like illness. Titrating the dose decreases the incidence of thrombocytopenia (ACR, 1996a). Bronchiolitis, cholestatic hepatitis, dermatomyositis, and polymyositis rarely have been reported ("Drugs for Rheumatoid Arthritis," 1994). Two types of rash have been reported. A rash occurring early in therapy (<6 months) is generally mild and represents a reaction that will resolve when the drug is discontinued. ᴅ-Penicillamine may be restarted once the rash has resolved. A rash occurring late in therapy (>6 months) is usually more severe and requires permanent discontinuance of the drug (Gittoes, 1994).

**Methotrexate.** Methotrexate, a cytotoxic agent inhibiting dihydrofolate reductase, is the DMARD of choice for initial therapy by many rheumatologists. MTX is available both orally and parenterally for use as a single dose of 7.5–15 mg per week. Intramuscular (IM) injections of MTX are reserved for patients intolerant to oral MTX or in whom efficacy has decreased over time.

Toxicities associated with MTX include GI symptoms (common), pulmonary toxicity and hypersensitivity pneumonitis (uncommon), bone marrow suppression (uncommon), and hepatic fibrosis (rare) (ACR, 1996a; "Drugs for Rheumatoid Arthritis," 1994; Sandoval, Alarcon, & Morgan, 1995). Toxicity risks increase in patients with renal insufficiency, folate deficiency, concomitant use of antifolate drugs (eg, Co-Trimoxazole), alcohol abuse, diabetes, and obesity (ACR, 1996a; Williams, 1993). There is also the concern of increased risk of lymphomas with long-term use (Moder et al, 1995).

Lung toxicity may be increased in smokers and patients with underlying lung disease. Pulmonary hypersensitivity presenting as fever, cough, and dyspnea may lead to pulmonary fibrosis. This toxicity can occur at any time regardless of dose or duration of therapy (ACR, 1996a; Sandoval et al, 1995).

Hepatotoxicity may present as irreversible fibrosis or cirrhosis. Transient increases of LFTs commonly occur with MTX therapy, but correlate poorly with the development of hepatic fibrosis. An increase of LFTs to greater than three times the baseline level requires discontinuation of MTX. Risk factors for MTX-associated liver disease include age, duration of therapy, obesity, diabetes mellitus (DM), alcohol use, and a history of hepatitis B or C (Walker et al, 1993). Patients with known liver disease should avoid using MTX; however, if MTX must be used in this patient population, a pretreatment biopsy is recommended. Liver biopsy is also recommended in patients with persistent LFT abnormalities while receiving or following discontinuation of the drug (ACR, 1996a; Williams, 1993). Routine liver biopsies are not cost-effective for patients receiving MTX with normal LFTs (Sandoval et al, 1995).

Myelosuppression, generally presenting as leukopenia, may also occur. Folate deficiency, renal insufficiency, and use of antifolate drugs increase the risk of cytopenias (ACR, 1996a). Severe bone marrow suppression is uncommon with recommended doses.

Common toxicities include mucositis, mild alopecia, and GI symptoms such as anorexia, nausea, vomiting, dyspepsia, and diarrhea. These adverse effects may be precipitated by an underlying folate deficiency. Concurrent administration of folic acid 1 mg/day or as a single dose of 7 mg/week is recommended to prevent toxicity (Dijkmans, 1995; "Drugs for Rheumatoid Arthritis," 1994; Sandoval et al, 1995). Folinic acid, or leucovorin, may also be used but is more expensive than folate.

MTX is also teratogenic, as well as an abortifacient, and can lead to infertility in both men and women. Couples wishing to become pregnant should wait a minimum of 3 months or one ovulatory cycle following discontinuation of MTX therapy by men or women, respectively (ACR, 1996a).

Concurrent administration of drugs affecting immune function should be avoided due to additive risks of bone marrow suppression. MTX concentrations may increase in patients with renal insufficiency also receiving NSAIDs, thus increasing the risk of toxicity ("Drugs for Rheumatoid Arthritis," 1994).

***Chlorambucil.***    Chlorambucil is an alkylating agent reserved for refractory RA. Myelosuppression is the most common toxicity. Monitoring is similar to that of AZA (Table 26–1).

***Cyclophosphamide.***    Also an alkylating agent reserved for the treatment of refractory RA, cy-clophosphamide is administered as a single dose of 1–1.5 mg/kg per day. Hemorrhagic cystitis is a complication of cyclophosphamide therapy; therefore patients should maintain good urine flow by drinking six to eight glasses of water per day to decrease the risk of toxicity (Williams, 1993). Long-term use is also carcinogenic.

***Cyclosporin A.***    Cyclosporin A is currently being evaluated for use in RA. Early clinical trials have indicated benefit, although toxicity is a major concern, especially renal toxicity (Wells & Tugwell, 1993). Results from ongoing trials will provide further information on the place of cyclosporin A in the treatment of RA.

***Capsaicin.***    Capsaicin may be an effective topical analgesic for some patients with mild to moderate disease. Refer to the osteoarthritis section for a more detailed description of capsaicin.

***Future Therapy.***    Other therapies currently under investigation include monoclonal antibodies to tumor necrosis factor (TNF), dietary manipulation, collagen, and minocycline.

***Approach to Therapy.***    Historically, a pyramid approach was used in managing RA in which NSAIDs constituted first-line therapy, CSs were used for temporary relief of disease flares, and DMARD therapy was added later in the disease course, starting with the least toxic drug (Blackburn, 1996; Williams, 1993). This approach has undergone much criticism and has generally fallen out of favor (Bensen, Bensen, Adachi, & Tugwell, 1990; Blackburn, 1996; Wilske & Healey, 1989). Current practice guidelines recommend starting DMARDs early (within 3 months of diagnosis) in active disease to prevent joint erosion (ACR, 1996b; Emery, 1995). The ACR (1996b) defines active disease as ongoing joint pain, significant morning stiffness or fatigue, active synovitis, or persistent increases in ESR or C-reactive protein. NSAIDs and nonpharmacologic therapy are also initiated at this time in order to alleviate pain and inflammation and maintain joint function.

As previously mentioned, an optimal initiation strategy of DMARDs for the treatment of RA is not known. Considerations for selecting a DMARD are listed in Table 26–5. All DMARDs have a slow onset of action and are associated with significant toxicity requiring frequent monitoring. Risks and benefits of DMARD therapy must be evaluated and presented to each patient prior to drug initiation.

A less toxic drug, such as HCQ or SSZ, is generally started in patients diagnosed with mild disease. Methotrexate may provide benefit in patients with more severe disease and is used as first line-therapy by many rheumatologists. Continuance rates are highest with MTX therapy, with >50% of patients continuing therapy >5 years (Pincus, Marcum, & Callahan, 1992). Most courses of other DMARDs are continued <2 years as a result of toxicity or loss of efficacy (Pincus et al, 1992). An adequate drug trial, provided in Table 26–6, is required before the patient is considered a nonresponder or therapy is changed. Currently, no consensus exists as to the sequence of DMARD initiation in patients who fail primary therapy. Controversy also exists as to the benefits of monotherapy versus combination DMARD therapy. Once a patient fails initial therapy, the option exists to either change to another DMARD, add a DMARD, or institute a new DMARD combination (ACR, 1996b; Blackburn, 1996; Emery, 1995; Gittoes, 1994; Williams, 1995). Discontinuing the DMARD may lead to a flare in disease activity. Tapering the drug being discontinued may allay this problem.

## TABLE 26–5. USE OF DISEASE-MODIFYING ANTIRHEUMATIC DRUGS FOR RA

### Goal
Remission or optimal control of inflammatory joint disease

### Limitations
May not prevent damage inspite of apparent clinical control
May not have lasting efficacy
May not be tolerated due to toxicity

### Factors for Selecting Drugs
Convenience and cost of medication and monitoring for toxicity
Risk of adverse reactions, including frequency and seriousness
Physician estimate of efficacy and disease prognosis

### Monitoring Efficacy
Is disease in remission or optimally controlled?

Source: Used with permission from American College of Rheumatology (1996b).

## TABLE 26–6. DISEASE-MODIFYING ANTIRHEUMATIC DRUGS USED IN TREATMENT OF RA

| Drug | Time to Response | Adequate Trial |
|---|---|---|
| Hydroxychloroquine | 2–4 months | 6 months |
| Sulfasalazine | 3 months | 6 months |
| Auranofin | 4–6 months | 6 months |
| Methotrexate | 4–6 weeks | |
| IM gold salts | 2–6 months | 1 g-cumulative dose |
| Azathioprine | 2–3 months | 6 months |
| D-penicillamine | 2–3 months | 6 months |

Source: Adapted with permission from American College of Rheumatology (1996b).

## Monitoring for Efficacy

There has been a paradigm shift from the traditional value placed on laboratory tests and radiological findings to assess RA status and therapeutic response. Currently, more emphasis is placed on the patient's self-report of functional status (Boers, Van Riel, Felson, & Tugwell, 1995; Pincus, Wolfe, & Callahan, 1994). Table 26–7 shows the categories used to measure disease activity and therapeutic response.

The Health Assessment Questionnaire (HAQ), Arthritis Impact Measurement Scales (AIMES), Modified Health Assessment Questionnaire (MHAQ), and McMaster Toronto Arthritis Questionnaire (MACTAR) are the most frequently used self-assessment tools. Data from these instruments are similar and if used consistently during each visit, the disease course can be easily followed (Meenan, 1994).

*Psychosocial factors.* Arthritis patients frequently report disease activation with stressful events. Relationships among stress, the immune system, and other biologic variables are being researched. There is some evidence that neural structures in the hypothalamus, which are associated with stress responses, may be related to the RA inflammatory response (Bradley, 1993). The current RA management paradigm includes the assessment of the psychosocial constructs of learned helplessness, self-efficacy, and mood affect. The learned helplessness construct is measured by the five-item Rheumatology Attitudes Index (RIA). The scale measures the degree to

## TABLE 26–7. DISEASE ACTIVITY MEASUREMENT CATEGORIES FOR RA

1. Global assessments of status by both patient and provider with a visual analog rating (VAS) scale.
2. Grading of symptoms (pain, morning stiffness, and fatigue).
3. Physical function measured with a scale, grip strength, and walk time.
4. Physical signs including joint counts of tender, swollen joints or both along with joint circumference.
5. Laboratory measures including ESR, C-reactive protein, hemoglobin, platelet count, and rheumatoid factor.

*Source: Adapted from Boers et al (1995, p. 308)*

which the individual feels he or she can cope with a stressful event. Changes in functional status have been highly correlated with RIA scores. Additional widely used psychosocial status assessment tools include the Beck Depression Inventory (BDI) and the Center for Epidemiologic Studies Depression Index (CES-D). Optimal management includes a comprehensive, coordinated, and multidisciplined approach (Bradley, 1993).

### Monitoring for Toxicity

Potential toxicities, baseline evaluations, monitoring parameters, and frequency of monitoring as recommended by the A&R are given in Table 26–1 for each therapy discussed above (ACR, 1996a).

### Follow-up

Patients should be assessed for relief of symptoms and medication toxicity at 2-week intervals until stabilized with optimal results.

## OSTEOARTHRITIS

Osteoarthritis (OA) is the most common joint disease afflicting the majority of persons aged 65 and older; over 80% of those age 75 and older are affected. With the demographic shift to an aging society, the economic impact of OA will increase. Compared with RA, OA with its increased prevalence has a 30-fold greater economic impact when work days lost, health care

visits, diagnostic testing (arthroscopy), and joint replacement (arthroplasty) are considered (Brandt & Slemenda, 1993). Gabriel, Crowson, and O'Fallon (1995) analyzed the population-based Rochester Project data and found that persons with OA, adjusted for age and sex, incurred substantial incremental medical costs due to comorbid conditions and experienced significantly greater work disability than non-OA persons.

The knee is the major joint affected and is associated with most disability cases. The hip joint is less commonly affected, and gender differences are not appreciable. There is a definite gender link with knee OA. Felson et al (1995) concluded that new onset knee OA is more common in women than men, with a 1.7 higher incidence rate for women. Progressive disease was experienced slightly more often by women, but rates did not vary by age in this sample of Framingham cohorts. In the National Health and Nutrition Examination Survey (NHANES), women were twice as likely as men to be afflicted, and African-American women were twice as likely to have knee OA than caucasian women (Brandt & Slemenda, 1993).

Besides age and gender, other risk factors associated with OA include obesity, mechanical stress, genetic disposition, and previous inflammatory diseases. Longitudinal and cross-sectional data demonstrate an association with OA and obesity, particularly knee OA. The Framingham data showed that over a 36-year span, persons in the highest quartile for body mass index at the baseline examination had a relative risk of 1.5 for males and 2.1 for females of developing knee OA. It seems that obese individuals who have not yet developed knee OA can significantly reduce their risk by 50% with a 5-kg weight loss (Felson, Zhang, & Anthony, et al, 1992). According to Felson (1995), data from the Framingham osteoarthritis study showed that for women, weight is the predominate risk factor for OA; for men, obesity is second to major knee injury as a preventable risk factor.

Genetic factors with autosomal dominant transmission in women and recessive inheritance in men are present with OA. The mother of a woman with DIP joint OA is twice as likely to have Heberden's nodes, and the patient's sister has a threefold chance compared with the mother and sister of a nonaffected woman (Brandt & Slemenda, 1993; Jimenez & Dharmavaram, 1994). Major trauma and repetitive use are strongly associated with OA. Human and animal studies show that damage to the anterior cruciate ligament or meniscus can result in knee OA. Occupations at risk for OA include jackhammer operators, cotton mill workers, coal miners, shipyard workers, and others who are subjected to repetitive stressful movement throughout the day. Farmers have a propensity for hip OA (Cooper, 1995). According to Lane's (1995) review of the literature, low-impact exercise activity does not increase the risk for OA. However, persons who participate in high-impact sports or on a competitive level seem to be at greater risk. Longitudinal studies need to be conducted with a cohort of lifelong exercisers.

## PATHOGENESIS

OA occurs when there are excessive loads (stress and weight) on the joint and when the biomaterial of the cartilage or bone is damaged. Although joint cartilage is the primary target, OA involves the articular cartilage, synovium, subchondral bone, ligaments, and neuromuscular system. Growth factors counteract this process in younger persons.

## SPECIFIC CONSIDERATIONS FOR PHARMACOTHERAPY

### When Drug Therapy Is Needed

Because of the current inability to reverse the underlying structural abnormalities associated with osteoarthritis, the primary objective of pharmacotherapy is to control the pain associated with the condition, and thus improve the patients' overall quality of life (Hochberg et al, 1995a,b; Moskowitz & Goldberg, 1993; Oddis, 1996). Standard pharmacologic agents used in the treatment of osteoarthritis include NSAIDs, analgesics, and occasionally intraarticular corticosteroids. In addition to standard therapy, a number of experimental agents are currently being evaluated. These agents are aimed at interrupting the disease process by preventing or inhibiting further cartilage destruction (Blackburn, 1996; Brandt, 1995; Hochberg et al, 1995a; Oddis, 1996). Examples include growth peptides that stimulate cartilage metabolic activities, tamoxifen (which inhibits estrogen responses), and a polysulphated glycosaminoglycan that inhibits proteolytic enzymes (Moskowitz & Goldberg, 1993).

## Short- and Long-Term Goals of Pharmacotherapy

The primary goal of pharmacotherapy in the management of osteoarthritis is to minimize the painful symptoms associated with the underlying degenerative process. Controlling the pain allows the patient to maintain joint mobility, thereby maintaining or improving the patient's overall quality of life.

## Nonpharmacologic Therapy

Weight reduction is essential for obese individuals. There is most likely an interaction between weight and OA since persons with OA may be reluctant to engage in physical activity due to discomfort. With increased age and obesity, other comorbid conditions including cardiovascular problems are present. A modified exercise program to improve mobility and psychological well-being should be individualized (Hocherg et al, 1995a,b). Short-term studies show that persons with knee OA report less pain and increased physical capacity with exercise training (Ettinger & Afable, 1994). Quadricep and hamstring muscles can be strengthened with isometric exercises. This strengthening permits better knee control and even weight distribution on the knee. Straight leg raises do not stress the knee joint and are an effective way to strengthen quadriceps (Bradley, 1994). A stationary bicycle, swimming, or water aerobics may be substituted for running. Hydrotherapy with hot tubs or heat applications (paraffin wax) relieves pain. The role of physical therapy is to relieve pain and associated muscle spasm and regain range of motion. The use of canes on the contralateral extremity can alleviate some joint stress (Hooker, 1996).

In terms of surgery, replacement procedures are available for all extremity joints. However, the knee and hip joint replacements have demonstrated the best mobility and pain relief outcomes. Earlier surgical interventions are possible with advanced arthroscopic techniques. Other surgical procedures employed in the early stages include joint abrasion, wash out, and debridement (Edelson, Burks, & Bloebaum, 1995).

Yoga exercises have demonstrated benefits for pain relief and relaxation for all types of arthritis (Galas, 1996). The exercise is a gentle modality for decreasing joint stiffness and improving flexibility. The deep breathing and gentle stretching exercises are a mental, physical, and spiritual pathway to improved overall functioning.

## Time Frame for Initiating Pharmacotherapy

Once the diagnosis of osteoarthritis has been made, pharmacotherapy can be initiated and is typically used in conjunction with nonpharmacologic therapy.

See Drug Tables 301, 306, 307, and 601.1.

## Assessment and History Taking

Joint pain associated with increased use is the hallmark symptom of OA. The pain is relieved by rest in the initial stages. With later-stage disease, the pain occurs with rest and is frequently present at night. Localized joint stiffness is present for a short time during acute inflammatory flares. The ACR has devised criteria for the classification and reporting of osteoarthritis; (see Table 26–8) (Schumacher, Klippel, & Koopman, 1993).

Physical findings include pain on passive motion and crepitus. The patient with OA of the knee or hip usually presents with an antalgic gait favoring the affected joint (Hooker, 1996). Joint enlargement may be present because of increased synovial fluid or proliferative cartilage and bone changes. Joint tenderness may be elicited with acute synovitis. Joints commonly afflicted include the knee, hands, hip, foot, and spine. The elbow, shoulders, and toes are usually spared, and occupational or metabolic problems should be considered when these joints are involved (Moskowitz & Goldberg, 1993).

A common finding is *Heberden's nodes*: spurs formed on the dorsolateral and medial aspects of the distal interphalangeal joints. These nodes usually develop slowly over months or years. They can, however, develop suddenly with an acute inflammatory process. Other common findings are: flexor and lateral deviations of the distal phalanx; Bouchard's nodes at the PIP joint; and the squared hand appearance, which results from involvement and tenderness of the first carpometacarpal joints. The trapezoid-scaphoid joint is frequently involved.

Persons affected with hip OA experience localized groin, anterior, or lateral thigh pain, and morning stiffness. On physical examination they have pain and limited range of motion (Hochberg et al, 1995a). With knee involvement, there is pain in and around the knee, which increases with weight bearing and im-

### TABLE 26–8.  THE AMERICAN COLLEGE OF RHEUMATOLOGY CRITERIA FOR THE CLASSIFICATION AND REPORTING OF OSTEOARTHRITIS OF THE HAND

**Classification criteria for osteoarthritis of the hand, traditional format[a]**

Hand pain, aching, or stiffness
  and
3 or 4 of the following features:
  Hard tissue enlargement of 2 or more of 10 selected joints
  Hard tissue enlargement of 2 or more DIP joints
  Fewer than 3 swollen MCP joints
  Deformity of at least 1 of 10 selected joints

---

[a] The 10 selected joints are the second and third distal interphalangeal (DIP), the second and third proximal interphalangeal, and the first carpometacarpal joints of both hands. This classification method yields a sensitivity of 94% and a specificity of 87%.
MCP = metacarpophalangeal.
*Source: Partial table reproduction with permission of The Arthritis Foundation from Schumacher et al (1993, p. 331).*

proves with rest, along with the morning stiffness and the gel phenomenon. On physical examination, there is tenderness upon palpation, bony enlargement, crepitus, and diminished range of motion (Hochberg et al, 1995b). There may be signs of inflammation since inflammation is now generally accepted as a component in the disease course of most symptomatic OA patients (Schumacher, 1995).

*Diagnostic tests.*    An erythrocyte sedimentation rate that may be slightly elevated and CBC rules out acute infection. A rheumatoid factor may be considered when the primary affected site is the hands. Diagnostic radiographic findings of OA include joint space narrowing in mild cases and the presence of osteophytes with subchondral bony sclerosis (eburnation) in advanced cases (Hooker, 1996). Standing anterior-posterior knee x-rays are superior to plain knee views in detecting subtle joint space narrowing. Other x-ray findings in OA include cysts. Arthroscopy, CT, and MRI are helpful in the differential diagnosis of nonosteoarthritic lesions (Moskowitz & Goldberg, 1993). Joint aspiration may be performed when the signs of inflammation or joint effusion are present. Future tests may include immunoassay to detect molecular markers of cartilage matrix metabolism.

## Patient/Caregiver Information

In addition to taking medications for the relief of pain, patients afflicted with osteoarthritis need to maintain an exercise and weight-monitoring program. Many household and lifestyle modifications can improve mobility and well-being for the arthritis patient. "Arthritis Today," published by the Arthritis Foundation, lists helpful tips to help make daily tasks for these patients more manageable (Schwartz, 1996). Examples include using a large plastic bag or piece of lining fabric on upholstered car seats to make sliding into the car easier, asking for a table near the entrance of a restaurant to reduce walking, and asking the newspaper carrier to hang the paper in a plastic bag on the front doorknob.

## OUTCOMES MANAGEMENT

### Selecting an Appropriate Agent

*Analgesics.*    Acetaminophen is currently considered first-line therapy in the treatment of osteoarthritis (Hochberg et al, 1995a; Moskowitz & Goldberg, 1993; Oddis, 1996). Potential advantages of acetaminophen over NSAIDs include comparable efficacy with fewer adverse effects and lower overall cost. Clinical trials evaluating the efficacy of acetaminophen for the treatment of osteoarthritis of the knee have found that, at doses up to 4000 mg/day, acetaminophen is comparable to naproxen and to both analgesic and antiinflammatory doses of ibuprofen (Bradley et al, 1991; Williams et al, 1993). For adequate control of symptoms, acetaminophen is typically dosed between 3000–4000 mg/day (Hochberg et al, 1995a; Moskowitz & Goldberg, 1993; Oddis, 1996). At therapeutic doses, acetaminophen is generally well tolerated. Potential adverse effects include rash, renal failure, and hepatotoxicity. Renal failure is typically associated with long-term use, and hepatotoxicty to excessive consumption of acetaminophen or use of acetaminophen in conjunction with regular alcohol intake. To minimize the risk of toxicity, a total daily dose of 4000 mg should not be exceeded and the patient should be advised to avoid alcohol consumption. Infrequently, not more than two or three alcohol-containing drinks should be consumed per day while taking acetaminophen.

Topical analgesics also can be used in the management of osteoarthritis either as sole therapy or in conjunction with systemic therapy. Commonly used agents include methysalicylate creams or capsaicin cream (Altman et al, 1994; Deal et al, 1991). These agents are typically applied to the affected joint three or four times a day. Capsaicin cream reduces the pain associated with osteoarthritis by acting on substance P, a neurotransmitter which communicates painful stimuli from the peripheral to the central nervous system. Capsaicin depletes substance P at sensory nerve terminals and prevents its further synthesis and reaccumulation in the neuron. With the use of capsaicin cream, a local stinging or burning sensation is common; however, this sensation usually dissipates after several days of therapy (Altman et al, 1994; Deal et al, 1991). Symptomatic relief is usually experienced after approximately 1–2 weeks of therapy.

Opioid analgesics also are occasionally used in the management of osteoarthritis; however, they are only used short-term to control acute, severe exacerbations of pain (Hochberg et al, 1995a).

*Nonsteroidal antiinflammatory drugs.*    The inflammatory component of osteoarthritis, although minimal in comparison to other rheumatic diseases, often becomes more evident as the disease progresses. When painful symptoms are not adequately controlled with acetaminophen, the use of an NSAID or an antiinflammatory dose of a salicylate or a nonacetylated salicylate is indicated (Hochberg et al, 1995a,b). If aspirin is used, the average dose required to obtain an adequate antiinflammatory effect is between 3.6–4.8 g/day. Unfortunately, at these doses gastrointestinal intolerance and blood loss in stool are more common. Nonacetylated salicylates including choline salicylate, choline magnesium trisalicylate, salsalate, and diflunisal provide another treatment option.

In addition to aspirin and nonacetylated salicylates, there are a variety of NSAIDs available for the treatment of osteoarthritis. The choice of an NSAID is largely empiric and based on individual response, tolerability, dosage frequency, and cost. Refer to the rheumatoid arthritis section for a general discussion of NSAIDs, including mechanism of action, pharmacokinetics, precautions, and adverse effects, and for a review of the antiinflammatory options.

*Corticosteroids.*    In the treatment of osteoarthritis, there is no indication for oral or intravenous administration of corticosteroids. Intraarticular injections of corticosteroids may be used and are particularly useful in large joints with effusions (Hochberg et al, 1995b). An intraarticular injection of a corticosteroid preparation such as triamcinolone acetonide may be given at a dose of 10–40 mg depending on joint size (Hochberg et al, 1995b; Moskowitz & Goldberg, 1993). Injections more frequent than every 3–4 months are generally not recommended because of possible acceleration of joint deterioration in weight-bearing joints (Hochberg et al, 1995b; Moskowitz & Goldberg, 1993). Accelerated joint deterioration may occur either from overuse of the affected joint because of alleviation of pain or from a direct effect of the corticosteroid on the joint (Moskowitz & Goldberg, 1993).

***Experimental Agents.***   A number of experimental therapies are also being evaluated in the treatment of osteoarthritis (Blackburn, 1996; Brandt, 1995; Creamer & Dieppe, 1993; Hochberg, et al, 1995a; Oddis, 1996). These agents are targeted toward both the prevention of further cartilage degradation and the reversal of preexisting structural abnormalities. There are currently no disease-modifying antiosteoarthritic drugs approved for use in the United States.

## Monitoring Efficacy

Therapeutic drug efficacy is monitored by an improvement in the individual's range of motion and activity level. Along with the physical activity tolerance, the psychosocial dimension should improve.

## Monitoring Toxicity

The Drug Tables on NSAIDs and analgesics (301, 306, 307, and 601.1) provide the potential toxicities, baseline evaluations, and frequency of monitoring for the therapeutic agents prescribed for OA.

## Follow-up

Initially, the individual should be assessed at 2–3 week intervals until pain relief and activity levels have improved. Clients should be encouraged to increase activity levels and maintain a weight reduction program during follow-up visits. Exploration of the psychological dimension is important during the follow-up visit.

# OSTEOPOROSIS

Osteoporosis, the most common metabolic bone disease, primarily afflicts postmenopausal women. However, the condition is seen in men (Peris et al, 1995; Seeman, 1995), pregnant women (Dunne et al, 1993), and juveniles (Smith, 1994). One third of women between ages 60–70 have osteoporosis [2.5 standard deviations (SDs) below the young adult mean] with or without fracture, and the remaining two thirds have osteopenia (decreased mineral density). Half of all causcasian postmenopausal women in the United States have osteopenia, and another 30% have osteoporosis (Ross, 1996). Osteoporosis is a major U.S. health problem that is implicated in more than 1.5 million fractures, with an annual cost of at least $10 billion (Riggs & Melton, 1992). The risk for hip fractures increases for women at age 50 and for men at age 60, with 90% occurring after age 70 (Silver & Einhorn, 1995). It is projected that 30% of women aged 80 or older will sustain a hip fracture, and the lifetime risk for women is 15%. The prevalence of vertebral fracture in postmenopausal women is 20% (Ott, 1993).

## CLASSIFICATION AND PATHOGENESIS

Osteoporosis is defined by two categories: primary and secondary. Primary, the most common form, is subdivided into two categories, types I and II. Type I develops as a result of diminished circulating estrogen, and type II is a consequence of aging. With type I, most bone loss occurs in the trabecular bone compartment. The horizontal connecting trabeculae are thinned and diminished, resulting in weakness of the cancellous bone regions. This type predisposes the patient to vertebral compression fractures, distal radial fractures, and intertrochanteric femoral fractures. In type II osteoporosis, bone loss is more global, affecting cortical and cancellous bone. Type II commonly affects the femoral neck. Types I and II may coexist. With secondary osteoporosis, an external factor is responsible for the bone density loss, such as steroid medications and the endocrine conditions of thyroid disease and hyperparathyroidism (Silver & Einhorn, 1995).

The basic pathology of osteoporosis is that bone resorption exceeds bone formation. Bone remodeling is the process that constitutes a homeostatic balance between bone formation and resorption. Annually, adults replace 25% of their cancellous bone mass via activation of the bone remodeling units (Rungby, Hermann, & Mosekilde, 1995). This process involves osteoblasts (cells that secrete osteoid) and osteoclasts (cells that remove bone by degradation of mineral and organic matrix moieties) (Khosla & Riggs, 1995; Silver & Einhorn, 1995). Other factors that regulate this process include vitamin D, calcium, parathyroid hormone (the major regulator of calcium and phosphate homeostasis), calcitonin, growth hormone of the anterior pituitary, and estrogen. Researchers are discovering new insights in the cellular, biochemical, and molecular mechanisms involved in osteoporosis (Manolagas, Bellido, & Jilka, 1995). Among the factors contributing to osteopenia among normal individuals, age is the most important factor, with the onset of diminishing bone density starting at age 30. After age 30, bone loss occurs at a rate of 0.3–1% per year until the first menopausal years, when the rate increases to 2–3% (Holmes-Walker, Prelevic, & Jacobs, 1995). Being female is the second most important factor, since the rate of bone density loss doubles every decade for women. Eighty percent of an individual's peak bone mass can be attributed to hereditary factors, and it is thought that heredity also influences bone density loss rate (Sambrook, Kelly, Morrison, & Eisman, 1994). African-Americans have higher bone density and mass and experience less bone turnover as they age.

Hormonal factors, specifically estrogen or testosterone deficiencies, influence bone mass. Women with irregular menses for whatever reason—including excessive exercise and anorexia—and postmenopausal women are at increased risk for osteoporotic fractures (Fruth & Worrell, 1995; Putukian, 1994; Thein & Thein, 1996).

Many women are at increased risk because of the medication they take. Use of corticosteroids, heparin, thyroid medications and possibly furosemide medications is associated with bone loss. Although thiazide diuretics may decrease calcium loss, they also may cause orthostasis in elderly patients. Lifestyle habits including smoking, alcohol use, and lack of exercise are associated with osteoporosis. Nutritional factors such as decreased lifetime intake of calcium and vitamin D and increased caffeine use have been linked with osteoporosis. Increased weight seems to be a negative risk factor, whereas being thin and tall as a young woman is an increased risk (Cummings, McClung, & Cummings, 1994; Murray & O'Brien, 1995). This may be due to the higher estrogen production with increased body fat. Additional risk factors include associated renal, hepatic, and endocrine diseases.

## SPECIFIC CONSIDERATIONS FOR PHARMACOTHERAPY

### When Drug Therapy Is Needed

Prescription medications, in combination with mineral supplementation and nonpharmacologic therapy, play an important role in the overall management of osteoporosis. Pharmacotherapy available for prevention and treatment of osteoporosis includes calcium, vitamin D, estrogen, alendronate, calcitonin, and sodium fluoride preparations.

### Short-Term and Long-Term Goals of Pharmacotherapy

Goals of pharmacologic therapy are to optimize bone mass and preserve skeletal integrity, relieve symptoms resulting from fractures and skeletal deformity, and ultimately, reduce the incidence of fractures and maintain normal physical function (Hodgson & Johnston, 1996). Prevention of osteoporosis and subsequent fractures becomes the primary focus when assessing patients at risk for osteoporosis.

### Nonpharmacologic Therapy

Modification of lifestyle controllable risk factors such as smoking cessation, reducing alcohol consumption, increasing exercise, and maintaining adequate nutritional intake of calcium and vitamin D remains the hallmark of management (Putukian, 1994). Regular activity of weight-bearing exercise enhances bone formation and may decrease bone loss (Rungby et al, 1995). Nelson et al (1994) reported, in a study of 40 sedentary and estrogen-depleted women, that high-intensity strength training exercises are an effective and feasible means to preserve bone density, muscle mass, strength, and balance. The National Osteoporosis Foundation recommends an exercise program (45–60 min, four times a week) consisting of walking, stair climbing, jogging, dancing, or tennis (Gamble, 1995).

For patients with established osteoporosis, the preventive measures listed in Table 26–9 may be suggested to decrease the risk of falls and potential fractures (Galsworthy & Wilson, 1996). Eliminating the use of drugs that increase the risk for falls, such as sedatives, antihypertensives, and diureticss, is another important preventive measure.

## Time Frame for Initiating Pharmacotherapy

Prevention of osteoporosis begins early in life by maintaining adequate calcium balance to preserve skeletal integrity. Initiation of estrogen therapy at the time of natural or surgical menopause (MP) provides the greatest benefit as is discussed below. Other pharmacologic therapy is generally instituted once the diagnosis of osteoporosis has been made.

See Drug Tables 605, 606.

## Assessment and History Taking

A detailed family history for evidence of osteoporotic trends (multiple fractures after age 50) is essential. A personal lifestyle history including dietary, smoking, and alcohol habits and exercise participation is mandatory. A history of comorbid conditions must be elicited. Frequently, detection of osteoporosis occurs when the high-risk patient presents with a fracture sustained under low-stress conditions. Screening of the patient for osteoporosis should include a height and weight baseline. An evaluation for risk of falls should be performed by assessing gait, muscle strength, medication use, and visual acuity (Murray & O'Brien, 1995). Cummings and colleagues (1994) cite four risk factors that predisposed persons to hip fractures:

- Inability to rise from a chair
- Decreased depth perception
- Decreased contrast sensitivity
- Resting heart rate over 80 beats per minute

A household assessment should be performed to identify unsafe conditions such as small rugs, lack of grab bars, and slippery floors. A thorough medication and alcohol use history is essential. Black (1995) and Kanis (1995) advocate that the most cost-effective time to screen and treat elderly women should be moved to age 65 or 15 years after menopause, since recent studies suggest bone loss at menopause is less accelerated than previously thought and that a more

### TABLE 26–9. TIPS FOR PREVENTING FALLS BY ROOM

#### Bedroom

- Keep the thermostat set to 65°F or above at night. Prolonged exposure to cold room temperatures can cause body temperature to drop, leading to drowsiness and increased risk of falling when getting out of bed.
- Get up slowly after lying down or sitting. Changing positions can cause blood pressure to decrease, resulting in dizziness.
- Place a lamp at the bedside. Have a night light somewhere between the bedroom and the bathroom.
- Wear shoes with a low, broad heel, a soft sole, and good flexibility.
- Avoid wearing loose-fitting slippers, high heels, or socks without shoes. And be aware that sneakers can actually give you too much traction and cause you to trip.

#### Living Room

- To avoid tripping over stray objects, keep your home free of clutter. Electrical cords and telephone wires should be kept out of walkways.
- Position small pieces of furniture, such as low coffee tables or stools, out of usual traffic pathways.
- Avoid throw rugs and lightweight area rugs, or make sure that they are anchored firmly to the floor with nonskid rubber backing.

#### Kitchen

- Store frequently used items in accessible cupboards to avoid unnecessary reaching, bending, or stooping.
- Cover linoleum floors with a nonskid floor wax.

#### Bathroom

- Install grab bars on walls along the tub and shower and beside toilets.
- Use nonskid mats, adhesive strips, or carpet on all surfaces that may get wet.
- Install a padded shower seat and a hand-held shower head to allow you to sit while bathing.

*Source: Adapted with permission from Galsworthy and Wilson (1996, p. 29).*

precise estimate of hip fracture risk can be made.

***Diagnostic tests.*** Several laboratory tests may be used to identify bone disease including serum levels of calcium, phosphate, and magnesium, acid-base status, and renal and liver function tests. A 24-hr urine specimen is used to evaluate calcium balance. Vitamin D deficiency is measured with a serum 25-hydroxyvitamin D level. Bone density of the lumbar spine, hip, and forearm is most accurately determined by radiographic bone densitometry since patients who have lost 30% of their bone mineral may have normal x-rays. Bone densitometry is indicated for patients who sustain fractures with minimal trauma and those who have increased risk factors for osteoporosis. Dual-energy x-ray absorptiometry (DEXA) of the spine, a noninvasive low-radiation technique, is currently the most precise method of assessing trabecular bone status.

## Patient/Caregiver Information

Information should be given to the patient on how to prevent falls and decrease fractures (Table 26–9). Other preventive measures include wearing sturdy low-heeled shoes and maintaining adequate lighting throughout the house. An active exercise program is essential to maintain adequate bone mass. Calcium supplements should be taken on an empty stomach between meals. The exception is calcium carbonate, which is taken with food. Avoid foods, such as spinach, that decrease calcium absorption. Foods high in calcium include low-fat or skim milk (1 cup = 300 mg of calcium), swiss cheese (1 oz = 272 mg), canned sardines with bones (3 oz = 375 mg), low-fat fruit yogurt (1 cup = 300–400 mg), sesame seeds (3 tbsp, whole = 300 mg), and broccoli (1 stalk, cooked = 150 mg) (Galsworthy & Wilson, 1996). Take alendronate with a glass of plain water 30 min prior to any other food or drink and avoid lying down for 30 min following dose administration. Calcitonin nasal spray doses are administered in one nostril, alternating nostrils daily.

## OUTCOMES MANAGEMENT

### Selecting an Appropriate Agent

*Calcium and Vitamin D Supplementation.* The recommended daily intake of calcium is given in Table 26–10. Dietary sources of calcium include dairy products, green vegetables, nuts, and some fish. Supplementation is recommended for men and women not meeting daily requirements through diet alone and those receiving the pharmacotherapy mentioned above (Hodgson & Johnston, 1996). Increasing age and ingestion of

certain foods (eg, oxalate-containing foods such as spinach) are associated with decreased calcium absorption. Vitamin D added to calcium supplementation enhances calcium bioavailability. This therapy is especially important in populations at risk for vitamin D deficiency such as the elderly.

Numerous calcium and vitamin D products are available without a prescription. Table 26–11 lists the various salts and calcium content per product. Calcium carbonate is generally recommended because of high calcium content and low cost. Because over-the counter (OTC) calcium products are not regulated by the Food and Drug Administration (FDA), the use of brand name products is suggested to ensure adequate bioavailability. With the exception of calcium carbonate, which requires an acid environment for absorption, other calcium products should be taken between meals to increase bioavailability (Hodgson & Johnston, 1996; Bradley, 1993; National Institutes of Health [NIH], 1994). Absorption is greatest with single doses of 500 mg or less (NIH, 1994). Side effects occur infrequently, with constipation being the most common complaint. Hypercalciuria rarely occurs at recommended doses (Hodgson & Johnston, 1996; NIH, 1994).

Vitamin D in recommended doses of 400–800 IU daily may be obtained from supplements, sunlight, vitamin D–fortified liquid dairy products, cod liver oil, and fatty fish (NIH, 1994). Calcitriol, a vitamin D analog, is currently not recommended for the treatment of osteoporosis.

### TABLE 26–10. OPTIMAL CALCIUM REQUIREMENTS RECOMMENDED BY THE NATIONAL INSTITUTES OF HEALTH CONSENSUS PANEL

| Age Group | Optimal Daily Intake of Calcium, mg |
|---|---|
| **Women** | |
| 25–50 | 1000 |
| >50 (PMP) on estrogens | 1000 |
| >50 (PMP) not on estrogens | 1500 |
| >65 ± estrogens | 1500 |
| **Men** | |
| 25–65 | 1000 |
| >65 | 1500 |

*Source: From National Institutes of Health (1994).*

## TABLE 26–11.  CALCIUM SUPPLEMENTATION PRODUCTS

| Calcium Salt | Elemental Calcium, % |
| --- | --- |
| Calcium carbonate | 40 |
| Calcium phosphate, tribasic | 39 |
| Calcium acetate | 25 |
| Calcium citrate | 21 |
| Calcium lactate | 13 |
| Calcium gluconate | 9 |
| Calcium glubionate | 6.5 |

The greatest effects of calcium supplementation have been shown in elderly women 10–20 years following menopause. Increased bone mineral density and a decreased risk of vertebral and nonvertebral fractures have been demonstrated in this population (Hodgson & Johnston, 1996; NIH, 1994; Chapuy et al, 1992). Calcium supplementation alone cannot counter the loss of bone mass during the early post-menopausal years, but is recommended as an adjunct to estrogen replacement therapy (NIH, 1994). Lifetime administration of calcium and vitamin D is recommended for optimal effect.

***Estrogen.***    Estrogen therapy is the most effective preventive strategy for postmenopausal osteoporosis. Administration of unopposed estrogen [estrogen replacement therapy (ERT)] or estrogen in combination with a progestin [hormone replacement therapy (HRT)] increases bone mineral density and decreases fracture rates (Cauley et al, 1995; Folsom et al, 1995, Grady et al, 1992; Kanis, 1995). Estrogen, acting through estrogen receptors on osteoclasts, inhibits bone resorption, thus decreasing bone turnover (Kanis, 1995).

Early initiation of ERT or HRT provides the greatest effect on preventing bone loss and decreasing fracture rates (Cauley et al, 1995). A minimum of 5–7 years of therapy may be necessary to obtain substantial benefits to decrease fracture risk, and lifelong therapy is necessary for maximum protection (Lobo, 1995). Discontinuation of ERT or HRT results in bone loss occurring at rates similar to nonusers and fracture rates returning to baseline approximately 5–7 years later (Cauley et al, 1995; Kanis, 1995). Recent clinical trials have shown that estrogen is beneficial when started later in life (ie, 10–20 years after menopause) and in women

with established osteoporosis (Cauley et al, 1995). Although BMD increases with estrogen therapy, restoration of bone mass to premenopausal levels is virtually impossible.

Oral and transdermal estrogens administered in a continous or cyclic fashion are effective as preventive therapy (Grady et al, 1992; Lufkin et al, 1992; Rosenfeld, 1994). Other benefits of postmenopausal ERT/HRT include favorable effects on lipid profile, prevention of coronary heart disease, and decreases in menopause-related symptoms (Folsom et al, 1995; Grady et al, 1992; Lobo, 1995; Stampfer & Colditz, 1991; Writing Group for the PEPI Trial, 1995). Common side effects associated with HRT include premenstrual symptoms such as breast tenderness, bloating, irritability, spotting or bleeding, and possible potentiation of migraine headaches.

Hormone replacement, although administered at physiologic doses, is not benign. Endometrial hyperplasia occurs in 20–40% of nonhysterectomized women taking unopposed estrogen (Grady et al, 1992; Lobo, 1995; Writing Group, 1996). Addition of a progestin at least 10 days per month decreases this risk and the risk of endometrial cancer. Gallbladder disease incidence also increases with supplemental estrogen therapy (Lobo, 1995). The most significant concern of long-term ERT or HRT is the question of an increased incidence of breast cancer. The literature regarding breast cancer risk remains unclear. It is estimated that the risk of breast cancer increases 15–30% after 10 years of ERT, but overall mortality from breast cancer does not appear to increase (Grady et al, 1992; Lobo, 1995; Colditz et al, 1995).

Patient education and discussion of the risks and benefits of HRT is vital in the long-term continuance of HRT. Contraindications to the use of estrogen include known or suspected pregnancy, presence or history of an estrogen-dependent tumor, undiagnosed vaginal bleeding, active thrombophlebitis or thromboembolic disease or a history of either with previous estrogen use, and acute liver disease or chronic impaired liver function.

***Bisphosphonates.***    Alendronate (Fosamax), an aminobisphosphonate similar to etidronate and pamidronate, inhibits osteoclast activity, decreases bone turnover, and alters bone metabolism to favor bone formation rather than resorption ("New Drugs for Osteoporosis," 1996). Indicated for the treatment of osteoporosis, alendronate is considered an alternative therapy for postmenopausal women who have contraindications to or cannot tolerate estrogen therapy (Hodgson & Johnston, 1996). Etidronate and pamidronate are not indicated for treatment of osteoporosis in the United States.

The alendronate product package insert states that alendronate is to be administered as a 10-mg dose taken with plain water 30 min prior to food, beverages, or any other medications and that patients should be instructed not to lie down for at least 30 min following administration in order to reduce the potential for esophageal irritation. Other adverse effects associated with alendronate include mild GI symptoms and headache. Concurrent administration of calcium 1000–1500 mg/day and vitamin D 400 IU daily is recommended with alendronate therapy, but administration must be separated by at least 30 min (Hodgson & Johnston, 1996). The package insert also states that hypocalcemia and other mineral deficiencies must be corrected prior to therapy initiation. Alendronate should be avoided in severe renal impairment.

For patients with established osteoporosis, alendronate leads to significant increases in vertebral, femoral neck, and trochanter bone mass, and appears to decrease the incidence of vertebral fractures (Chesnut et al, 1995; Liberman et al, 1995). Unfortunately, safety and efficacy data do not exist beyond 3 years. Pending completion of ongoing clinical trials, alendronate may play a role in primary prevention of osteoporosis in healthy postmenopausal women unable to take estrogen and in the treatment of steroid-induced osteoporosis.

**Calcitonin.** Salmon calcitonin, a peptide hormone, interferes with osteoclast function, reverses rapid bone turnover, and increases bone mass ("New Drugs for Osteoporosis," 1996; Rungby et al, 1995). Calcitonin therapy is recommended for patients who cannot tolerate or fail estrogen and alendronate therapy. Efficacy is more pronounced in patients with high bone turnover and loss (eg, steroid-induced osteoporosis) (Avioli, 1992). Calcitonin also possesses analgesic effects and is often used following osteoporosis-related fractures (Lyritis et al, 1991). Recommended doses for the injectable and intranasal calcitonin formulations are 50–100 IU daily or every other day subcutaneously or as an intramuscular injection and 200 IU (1 spray) daily, respectively. Parenteral calcitonin is dispensed in a concentration of

200 IU/mL; therefore, it is important to instruct patients on proper dosing using an insulin syringe. The nasal spray should be administered as one dose in the same nostril, alternating nostrils daily. Common dose-dependent side effects include nausea, vomiting, local inflammation at the site of injection, facial flushing, and tingling in the hands (Hodgson & Johnston, 1996).

Increased bone mineral density and decreased vertebral fracture rates have been shown with both routes of administration (Overgaart, Hansen, Jensen, & Christiansen, 1992; Reginster et al, 1995; Rico, Hernandez, Revilla, & Gomez-Castrensana, 1992).

**Sodium Fluoride.** Sodium fluoride has also been studied for treatment of osteoporosis. Unlike the previously mentioned drugs, sodium fluoride stimulates osteoblast proliferation, leading to increased bone formation ("New Drugs for Osteoporosis," 1996). High doses of regular-release sodium fluoride significantly increase bone mass, but have also been associated with increased fracture rates as a result of inadequate bone formation (Riggs et al, 1990). It is also associated with significant adverse effects such as gastritis, GI bleeding, and arthralgias. An alternative fluoride preparation that may find a role in the treatment of osteoporosis is slow-release sodium fluoride (SRSF). SRSF, by maintaining fluoride serum concentrations within the therapeutic range of 95–190 ng/mL, increases the formation of normal rather than fragile bone ("New Drugs for Osteoporosis," 1996). Tolerability is also increased, with mild GI toxicity predominating. SRSF dosed as 25 mg b.i.d. up to 4 years has demonstrated efficacy in decreasing vertebral fractures (Pak et al, 1995). The use of fluoride greatly increases calcium demand; adequate calcium and vitamin D supplementation are essential to prevent bone resorption. The long-term efficacy and safety of SRSF have yet to be evaluated.

**RALOXIFENE.** Raloxifene, recently approved by the FDA for postmenopausal osteoporosis, is a selective estrogen receptor modulator. It has an estrogen agonist effect on bone and an antagonist effect on both the breast and the uterus. Current clinical studies report that it increases bone mineral density, decreases LDL cholesterol, and may be effective in prevention and treatment of breast cancer. Long-term safety and effectiveness of Raloxifene have not yet been established (The Medical Letter, 1998). For dose and adverse effects see Drug Table 606.

**Combination Therapy.**  Currently few data exist regarding the use of combination therapy for the prevention and treatment of osteoporosis. The American Association of Clinical Endocrinologists (AACE) guidelines discourage the use of combination therapy (Hodgson & Johnston, 1996). Unsubstantiated use of combination therapy results in increased treatment costs and potentially increased adverse effects without evidence of additional efficacy.

## Monitoring for Efficacy

Measuring osteoporosis drug efficacy is a long-term process. Optimal efficacy is achieved by increasing bone mass, preventing fractures, and maintaining activity levels.

## Monitoring for Toxicity

Drugs used in the prevention and treatment of osteoporosis are generally well tolerated. Routine monitoring for adverse effects is important in maintaining patient compliance with long-term therapy.

## Follow-up Recommendations

Appropriate follow-up is necessary following initiation of drug therapy. A return visit 4–6 weeks later is important for assessing compliance and adverse effects (Kleerekoper & Avioli, 1993). Once the patient is stable, annual follow-up is recommended. Women receiving hormone replacement therapy need to be instructed on monthly breast self-examination. Yearly gynecologic exams and mammography are also recommended. Bone mineral density studies are indicated for monitoring where appropriate, but should not be a routine monitoring parameter in asymptomatic prevention patients (Hodgson & Johnston, 1996). The elderly patient with co-morbid conditions is often seen more frequently. All patients should be queried about their alcohol intake and smoking and encouraged to cease these behaviors.

## GOUT

Gout is an arthritic disease characterized by tissue deposition of monosodium urate crystals. One or more of the following clinical manifestations may exist (Terkeltaub, 1993):

1. Gouty arthritis with recurrent severe or chronic attacks of articular and periarticular inflammation

2. Tophi with accumulation of articular, osseous, soft tissue, and cartilaginous crystalline deposits

3. Gouty nephropathy

4. Presence of uric acid calculi in the urinary tract

Calcium pyrophosphate dihydrate (CPPD), another crystal-producing arthropathy formerly defined as pseudogout, must be differentiated from gout (Beutler & Schumaker, 1994; Joseph & McGrath, 1995).

## EPIDEMIOLOGY

A higher standard of living over the last few decades may contribute to the increased prevalence of gout. Middle-aged men in their fifth decade are most often afflicted, with post-menopausal women comprising the second highest-risk population. Gout is the most common cause of inflammatory arthritis in men over age 30 and is rarely seen in women prior to menopause. The incidence of gout is about twice that of CPPD. For gout, the male-to-female ratio of persons aged 58 is about 7:1. The male-to-female ratio for CPPD is equally distributed. Approximately 20% of younger gout-afflicted persons demonstrate a familial pattern (Beutler & Schumaker, 1994).

Acute gout may be precipitated by medications (see Table 26–12), alcohol abuse, minor trauma, or acute illness. Persons with gout have a higher incidence of poorly controlled chronic diseases associated with renal insufficiency, such as hypertension and diabetes mellitus (Terkeltaub, 1993). CPPD is frequently seen after trauma or surgery or with ischemic heart disease (Joseph & McGrath, 1995).

Older persons are more at risk for developing gout due to the increased number of medications they consume. They must be managed carefully since they usually have some degree of diminished renal functioning (Gonzalez, Miller, & Agudelo, 1994). The increased number of elderly women presenting with gout has been attributed to the almost 25% of Americans over aged 65 taking thiazide diuretics (Star & Hochberg, 1994; Terkeltaub, 1993). Although the current use of thiazide diuretics has decreased among this population, the incidence of alcohol use has risen among older women (Gomberg, 1995).

## TABLE 26–12. DRUGS THAT MAY CAUSE GOUT AND HYPERURICEMIA

Alcohol (ethanol)
Cyclosporin (kidney and heart transplant recipients)
Cytotoxics
Didanosine [2′,3′-dideoxyinosine (ddl)]
Diuretics
Laxatives (when abused)
Levodopa
Methoxyflurane
Nicotinic acid
Pyrazinamide
Salicylates (low doses)
Theophylline (pharmacological doses)

*Source: Reproduced with permission from Gonzalez et al. (1994, p. 129).*

## PATHOGENESIS

Gout results from a complex system that fails to balance uric acid and clearance. Uric acid production in humans occurs from the ingestion of purine-containing foods and from the endogenous synthesis of nucleic acids. Uric acid is derived from nucleic acids and free purine nucleotides in a complex degradation through the purine nucleoside intermediates of hypoxanthine and xanthine. The kidney is the major route of uric acid excretion and under normal conditions accounts for 60% of the disposal. The gut, through bacterial oxidation, is the major extrarenal disposal of urate. Compared with the kidney, the gut has a limited capability to deal with an increased urate load. Insufficient renal excretion of uric acid is responsible for the majority (90%) of patients with primary hyperuricemia. Individuals whose kidneys underexcrete uric acid (the majority of gout patients) maintain inappropriately high serum urate concentrations (Joseph & McGrath, 1995; Terkeltaub, 1993).

The exact mechanism that promotes spontaneous limited gouty inflammation remains elusive. The presence of monosodium salt crystals in oversaturated joint tissues in the acute attack is responsible for tophi in the first metatarsophalangeal joint or the ear lobes. The fact that uric acid crystals are found in asymptomatic joints substantiates that gout exists in an asymptomatic state.

## SPECIFIC CONSIDERATIONS FOR PHARMACOTHERAPY

### When Drug Therapy Is Needed

Once gout has been diagnosed, treatment is relatively straightforward and in the majority of cases can be handled on an outpatient basis. The primary objective of the treatment of acute gouty arthritis is the resolution of severe pain commonly associated with the attack. Agents available for the treatment of an acute attack of gouty arthritis include colchicine, NSAIDs, corticosteroids, and adrenocorticotropic hormone (ACTH). Agents used to manage symptomatic hyperuricemia include allopurinol and the uricosuric agents. Selection of an appropriate therapeutic regimen should be based on an assessment of efficacy versus toxicity through evaluation of patient-specific parameters.

### Short- and Long-Term Goals of Pharmacotherapy

The major short- and long-term goals of therapy include alleviation of pain associated with the acute attack as well as prevention of recurrent attacks and extraarticular manifestations of the disease (Pratt & Ball, 1993). Educate the patient regarding correctable factors, such as obesity, diet, use of thiazide diuretics, and alcohol consumption, as well as compliance with medications (Star & Hochberg, 1993).

### Nonpharmacologic Therapy

Gout attacks can be prevented by decreasing alcohol intake and avoidance of dehydration. Dietary modifications with low-purine-containing foods have not demonstrated marked efficacy. The patient should, however, avoid specific foods and medications that may have precipitated previous attacks. The patient should maintain enough hydration to produce a urinary output of 2 L per day. This amount will aid urate excretion and decrease urate precipitation in the urinary tract.

### Time Frame for Initiating Pharmacotherapy

In treating an acute attack of gouty arthritis, pharmacotherapy should be initiated at the first sign of symptoms. Delay in initiating palliative therapy typically results in a reduction of the medications' effectiveness. Any therapy that alters serum urate concentrations, such as allopurinol or the uricosurics, should not be initiated during an acute episode. If the patient is already on antihyperuricemic therapy, the dose should not be adjusted. Use or adjustment of these agents during an acute attack may cause exacerbation of symptoms or precipitation of a relapse due to changes in plasma urate concentrations (Emmerson, 1996; Star & Hochberg, 1993). If necessary, antihyperuricemic therapy should be initiated 1–2 weeks following the resolution of an acute attack with a prophylactic agent on board.

See Drug Tables 306, 316, and 601.1.

## Assessment and History Taking

There are four basic stages of gout: asymptomatic hyperuricemia, acute gouty arthritis, intercritical gout, and chronic tophaceous gout. It may be a misnomer to label asymptomatic hyperuricemia as gout since not all individuals who have hyperuricemia will develop gout. Acute gouty arthritis is characterized by an acute onset of intense pain usually in the first metatarsophalangeal joint, but the midfoot, ankles, knees, and wrists can be affected. The attack commonly occurs during the night. The individual reports being awakened by the pain and unable to stand the weight of bed covers touching the affected joint. The joint is tender, swollen, warm, and erythematous. Chills and mild fever may accompany the pain. Early in the disease process, attacks tend to subside spontaneously in 3–10 days with or without treatment. Another attack may occur months or years later. Acute attacks may be precipitated by trauma, alcohol, drugs, surgical stress, and acute medical illness.

Gout can have an atypical subclinical presentation without the acute signs and symptoms. These presentations are often misdiagnosed as rheumatoid arthritis, septic arthritis, or other rheumatic conditions (Uy, Nuwayhid, & Saadeh, 1996). Gout is frequently misdiagnosed in females since they present 70% of the time with polyarticular symptoms (Joseph & McGrath, 1995).

Intercritical gout is the interval occurring between attacks. The patient is asymptomatic and exhibits no abnormal physical findings. Monosodium urate (MSU) crystals are present in 97% of synovial fluid aspirated from previously affected joints.

Chronic tophaceous gout develops gradually over a 10-year period. The synovium, subchondral bone, olecranon bursa, Achilles tendon, and subcutaneous tissue on the extensor forearm surfaces are the usual sites for tophi development (Beutler & Schumaker, 1994). Diagnostic aspiration may be necessary since tophi can be confused with rheumatoid or other nodules.

Individuals who overexcrete uric acid may present with an acute episode of flank pain as a consequence of urolithiasis. With long-standing untreated disease, patients may present initially with an acute urinary tract infection caused by stone formation and blockage.

Prior to the initiation of therapy, assessment of renal and hepatic function is recommended for the elderly patient.

***Diagnostic Tests.*** Radiographs are useful to show soft tissue swelling and exclude septic joint changes, calcifications, and spur formations from other processes. A finding of calcified tophi may be difficult to differentiate. With chronic disease states, intraarticular or periarticular asymmetric round or oval bony erosions with sclerotic margins are seen (Beutler & Schumaker, 1994).

The presence of MSU crystals in aspirated synovial fluid is considered the diagnostic marker for gout (Beutler & Schumaker, 1994; Star & Hochberg, 1994). The serum uric acid level may not be elevated in some patients with acute gout and is considered to be of limited value since 30% of patients have normal levels during an acute attack (Joseph & McGrath, 1995; McCarty, 1994). However, serial measurements to follow treatment response are helpful. Synovial fluid leukocyte cell counts are elevated from 20,000–100,000/mm and are predominately neutrophils (Tate, 1993). Additional tests may include a 24-hour urine uric acid measurement to assess renal stone risk, to detect underlying factors in the gout, and to determine the treatment. Urinary uric acid excretion greater than 750–1000 mg/day on a regular diet suggests uric acid overproduction. Aspirin, phenylbutazone, alcohol consumption, and contrast dye can affect uric acid excretion and should be withheld prior to testing (Tate, 1993).

## Patient/Caregiver Information

Patients must avoid dehydration and large amounts of alcohol. They should be encouraged to drink enough fluids to maintain an urinary output of at least 2 L per day. Their fluid intake will need to be increased during hot dry weather. In order to obtain maximum pain relief, it is important to start pharmacotherapy at the first sign of an attack. Patients should contact their health care provider as soon as symptoms begin.

## OUTCOMES MANAGEMENT

### Selecting an Appropriate Agent for Acute Gout

*Colchicine.* Colchicine is an antimitotic agent that has been used for years in the treatment of gout. Although the mechanism by which colchicine exerts its effect has not been fully elucidated, it appears to inhibit the migration and phagocytosis by leukocytes. With phagocytosis decreased in the tissues, there is less lactic acid, which limits the deposition of the crystals in joint tissue and diminishes the inflammatory response. Colchicine also appears to decrease the release of chemotactic factors (Emmerson, 1996; Moreland & Ball, 1991). It has no analgesic or antihyperuricemic activity.

At one time, colchicine was considered the drug of choice for the treatment of acute gouty arthritis. However, since less toxic alternatives are now available, colchicine has decreased in use as first-line therapy (Moreland & Ball, 1991; Roberts, Liang, & Stern, 1987). In treating an acute attack, colchicine can be given either orally or intravenously. Unfortunately, the oral dose necessary for symptomatic relief almost inevitably leads to the development of gastrointestinal side effects, such as nausea, vomiting, diarrhea, and abdominal cramping (Agarwal, 1993).

To effectively abort an acute attack, the medication should be initiated at the first sign of symptoms. Delay in initiating therapy reduces the medication's effectiveness. The usual oral dosage is 1.0–1.2 mg initially, followed by 0.5–0.6 mg every 1–2 h until pain is relieved or until abdominal discomfort, nausea, vomiting, or diarrhea develops. A total dose of 8 mg should not be exceeded, and at least 3 days should pass before initiating another course of therapy. In elderly patients and patients with renal or hepatic dysfunction, a decrease in dose is necessary (Emmerson, 1996; Pratt & Ball, 1993; Wallace et al, 1991). Due to impaired elimination, these patients are more likely to develop cumulative toxicity to colchicine. A general guideline is to decrease the dose by approximately 50% in this patient population (Emmerson, 1996; Pratt & Ball, 1993).

Intravenous administration of colchicine is typically reserved for patients who are unable to take oral medications or for situations where gastrointestinal side effects must be avoided (Roberts et al, 1987). The use of intravenous colchicine has been associated with a greater incidence of serious systemic toxicity than oral therapy and, therefore, is not routinely used in practice. Toxicity, which has been found to be attributable primarily to improper intravenous administration, includes bone marrow suppression, renal and hepatocellular damage, disseminated intravascular coagulation, and tissue necrosis from local extravasation (Pratt & Ball, 1993; Roberts et al, 1987; Wallace & Singer, 1988). If administered according to guidelines, intravenous colchicine may be a safe and effective alternative for specific patients in the treatment of gout (Moreland & Ball, 1991; Wallace & Singer, 1988). In patients with normal renal and hepatic function, an initial dose of 2 mg may be followed by two additional doses of 1 mg given at 6–12-h intervals until the desired response is obtained. A total dose of 4 mg in 24 h should not be exceeded (Wallace & Singer, 1988). After a full intravenous dose has been administered, additional colchicine should not be given by either the intravenous or oral route for at least 7 days in order to prevent cumulative toxicity (Wallace & Singer, 1988). A total intravenous dose of 2 mg should not be exceeded in geriatric patients who appear to have normal serum creatinine levels, patients with renal or hepatic impairment, and patients who have been receiving oral prophylactic therapy of colchicine (Pratt & Ball, 1993; Roberts et al, 1987; Wallace & Singer, 1988). Intravenous colchicine should not be used in patients with combined renal and hepatic dysfunction, a creatinine clearance of <10 mL/min, extrahepatic biliary obstruction, and immediate prior use of oral colchicine (Pratt & Ball, 1993; Roberts et al, 1987; Wallace & Singer, 1988). In order to prevent local tissue reaction or sclerosis, colchicine should be diluted with 20 mL of normal saline and delivered through an intravenous catheter over approximately 10 min. Colchicine is incompatible with dextrose and, therefore, should only be diluted with normal saline to prevent precipitation.

***Nonsteroidal Antiinflammatory Drugs.*** Nonsteroidal antiinflammatory drugs have been a mainstay in the treatment of acute gout and, unless contraindicated, are often the drugs of choice. NSAIDs should not be given to patients with active peptic ulcer disease or with a recent history of gastrointestinal bleeding (Star & Hochberg, 1993). Risk versus benefit must be carefully assessed before using NSAIDs in patients with other comorbid conditions, including renal dysfunction, congestive heart failure, uncontrolled hypertension, asthma, and inflammatory bowel disease (Pratt & Ball, 1993; Star & Hochberg, 1993). Use of NSAIDs in these patient populations can potentially lead to a worsening of their underlying disease state. Patients who appear to be at higher risk of developing gastrointestinal bleeding secondary to NSAID use include the elderly, patients receiving high-dose therapy, those with a prior history of gastrointestinal bleeding, and patients receiving concomitant anticoagulation therapy (Cryer & Feldman, 1992; Polisson, 1996; Pratt & Ball, 1993).

Although few direct comparative data are available, it appears that most NSAIDs are effective in the treatment of gout. Among individual patients, however, there may be variability in both clinical response and tolerability among the various agents (Brooks & Day, 1991; Furst, 1994). In the treatment of gout, NSAIDs are typically given at high doses for the first several days and then tapered down over the next 5–7 days as the symptoms of the acute attack resolve. Indomethacin is one NSAID that has been used extensively over the years in the treatment of acute gout. A typical regimen of indomethacin is 50 mg three to four times a day for 1–2 days, reduced to 25 mg two to three times a day for 5–7 days. Other NSAIDs may be used and are dosed in a similar fashion; start high, taper down gradually, and discontinue the agent when the symptoms resolve (Pratt & Ball, 1993). Common side effects associated with the use of NSAIDs include headache, dizziness, gastrointestinal complaints, and renal impairment (Brooks & Day, 1991; Furst, 1994; Simon, 1995). Administering the agents with food may decrease the incidence of gastrointestinal intolerance.

**Corticosteroids.**    Corticosteroids and ACTH have been shown to be beneficial in the treatment of acute gouty arthritis. In most cases, these agents are reserved for refractory cases or cases where the use of colchicine and NSAIDs is contraindicated (Pratt & Ball, 1993). At the relatively low doses and short duration of therapy used in the treatment of gout, the corticosteroids and ACTH are generally well tolerated. Potential

side effects include fluid retention, hyperglycemia, and CNS effects.

Corticosteroids may be administered either orally, parenterally, or intraarticularly. Presence of a septic joint should be ruled out prior to the use of corticosteroids. In the treatment of acute gout, often involving multiple joints, oral doses of prednisone from 20–40 mg/day are recommended. This dose is administered for the first 3–5 days and then gradually tapered off over a 1- to 2-week period (Pratt & Ball, 1993; Star & Hochberg, 1993). For patients unable to take oral medications, particularly those in the hospital setting, an equivalent intravenous dose of methylprednisolone may be given. Intraarticular administration of corticosteroids is useful in cases involving one or two large joints. Triamcinolone acetonide at a dose of 10–40 mg, depending on the size of the joint, may be used for intraarticular injections (Pratt & Ball, 1993).

Studies evaluating ACTH have found it to be useful in the treatment of gout, particularly in patients whose multiple medical conditions prevent the use of colchicine and NSAIDs (Ritter et al, 1994). ACTH appears to exert its effect, at least in part, through stimulation of the adrenal gland, thus increasing secretion of endogenous corticosteroids (Star & Hochberg, 1993). Intramuscular injection of ACTH at a dose of 40–80 IU may be given followed by 40 IU every 6–12 h as needed for 1–3 days (Pratt & Ball, 1993). The use of ACTH at 40 IU IM as a single dose also has been shown to be effective in providing rapid relief of symptoms when given within 24–48 h of symptom onset (Axelrod & Preston, 1988).

**Prophylactic Treatment of Acute Gout.**    Although no strict guidelines exist regarding the ideal time to initiate prophylactic therapy, it is typically reserved for patients with recurrent attacks and is not initiated following the first attack of gout (Pratt & Ball, 1993). Other variables to consider include potential toxicity, drug cost, patient compliance, and patient tolerance of acute attacks (Pratt & Ball, 1993). Nonpharmacologic intervention is often considered first-line therapy in preventing recurrent attacks. This consists of weight reduction, restriction of dietary purine and alcohol intake, and avoidance of drugs known to increase serum urate concentrations (low-dose salicylate, niacin, pyrazinamide, and thiazide and loop diuretics) (Fam, 1995). Compliance with these measures may circumvent the need for daily drug therapy.

Patients with recurrent attacks, despite compliance with nonpharmacologic intervention, are typically started on prophylactic drug therapy. Small daily doses of oral colchicine or NSAIDs are effective. One of these agents also should be started prior to initiating therapy with an antihyperuricemic agent to prevent precipitation of an attack. For prophylactic therapy, colchicine is usually dosed at 0.5–0.6 mg one to two times daily. To minimize the chance of toxicity, the smallest effective dose should be used (Pratt & Ball, 1993). In patients with no other comorbid conditions affecting the elimination of colchicine, prophylactic doses are generally well tolerated. In patients with impaired renal function (creatinine clearance < 50 mL/min), reversible myopathy and neuropathy have been observed with long-term use (Kuncl, Duncan, & Watson 1987; Wallace et al, 1991). NSAIDs can also be used as prophylactic therapy, but their long-term use may be associated with a higher incidence of gastrointestinal adverse effects (Kot, Day, & Brooks, 1993). No consensus exists regarding the duration of prophylactic therapy; however, recommendations range from 6 months to 1 year of an attack-free interval following the normalization of serum urate concentrations (Emmerson, 1996; Kot et al, 1993).

## Selecting an Appropriate Agent for Hyperuricemia

For patients with symptomatic hyperuricemia, the goal of treatment is to reduce and maintain the serum urate concentration below 6.0 mg/dL in order to prevent recurrent attacks and reverse the deposition of urate crystals in tissues (Pratt & Ball, 1993). Lower concentrations may be needed for resorption of tophi. There are currently two classes of drugs which can effectively lower serum urate concentrations: uricosuric agents and allopurinol. The uricosuric agents act to lower serum urate concentrations by inhibiting the reabsorption of uric acid from the proximal tubule, thus increasing its excretion. Allopurinol decreases the production of uric acid through inhibition of the enzyme xanthine oxidase, which is responsible for the breakdown of purines to uric acid. Selection of an agent is based on patient-specific parameters including the overproduction or underexcretion of uric acid, renal function, and the presence of tophaceous gout. Allopurinol is the preferred agent in cases of overproduction of uric acid, renal impairment, and chronic tophaceous gout (Pratt &

Ball, 1993; Star & Hochberg, 1993). Uricosuric agents are preferred in cases of normal or underexcretion of uric acid, normal renal function, and nontophaceous gout (Pratt & Ball, 1993; Star & Hochberg, 1993). The presence of both overproduction (high purine intake) and underexcretion (low clearance) of uric acid is fairly common. In this case, allopurinol may be the preferred agent because it is effective in handling both problems (Emmerson, 1996). To reduce the risk of precipitating an acute attack of gout, these agents should not be initiated until 1–2 weeks have passed following the resolution of an attack and a prophylactic agent (colchicine or NSAID) has been on board for several days.

***Probenecid and Sulfinpyrazone.***  Probenecid and sulfinpyrazone are two uricosuric agents that have long been used in the management of hyperuricemia. These agents should be avoided in patients with excessive uric acid excretion, impaired renal function (creatinine clearance <50–60 mL/min), inadequate urine flow (<1 mL/min), and a history of renal calculi (Emmerson, 1996; Pratt & Ball, 1993). Probenecid is initiated at a dose of 500 mg once daily and increased as needed to a maintenance dose of 1–2 g/day in divided doses to maintain serum urate concentrations <6 mg/dL. Common adverse effects include gastrointestinal intolerance, rash, and nephrolithiasis. Formation of renal calculi may be minimized by starting with low-dose therapy and titrating slowly, maintaining high urine output, and alkalinizing the urine during initial therapy (Emmerson, 1996; Pratt & Ball, 1993; Star & Hochberg, 1993). The risk of developing renal calculi occurs each time therapy is restarted; therefore, compliance with uricosuric therapy must be emphasized. Due to its site of action, probenecid inhibits the excretion of a number of medications, thus enhancing their efficacy and/or toxicity. Some of these agents include penicillins, indomethacin, dapsone, acyclovir, and methotrexate. Concomitant use of salicylates may interfere with the uricosuric effect of probenecid.

Sufinpyrazone, a more potent uricosuric agent, is initiated at a dose of 100 mg/day and titrated as needed up to 800 mg/day given in divided doses. Potential adverse effects include gastrointestinal intolerance, nephrolithiasis, platelet dysfunction, and rarely bone marrow suppression. When initiating therapy, the same precautions must be taken as with probenecid.

***Allopurinol.***   The xanthine oxidase inhibitor allopurinol effectively lowers serum and urinary uric acid concentrations and facilitates resorption of tophi (Day et al, 1994). In cases of renal insufficiency, allopurinol is preferred over the uricosurics. However, due to potential toxicity secondary to accumulation of the active metabolite, oxypurinol, the dose must be adjusted. Allopurinol is typically started at a dose of 100 mg/day and titrated up to a maintenance dose of 300 mg/day as needed to effectively lower serum urate concentrations (Kot et al, 1993). Smaller daily doses are recommended for patients with glomerular filtration rates <50 mL/min (Pratt & Ball, 1993). Depending on the degree of renal insufficiency, doses as low as 100 mg every other day or every third day may be necessary. As with the uricosurics, prophylactic therapy with colchicine or NSAIDs should be started prior to initiating allopurinol in order to minimize the risk of precipitating an acute attack of gout (Day et al, 1994; Emmerson, 1996; Pratt & Ball, 1993; Star & Hochberg, 1993).

Common adverse effects associated with allopurinol use include gastrointestinal intolerance, hypersensitivity reactions, and skin rash. Use of allopurinol with ampicillin is associated with an increased frequency of skin rash. Fairly rare, yet serious adverse effects include toxic epidermal necrolysis, fever, leukopenia, vasculitis, interstitial nephritis, and hepatotoxicity. These effects tend to occur more commonly in patients receiving concomitant thiazide diuretic therapy and in those with renal insufficiency. Important drug interactions associated with allopurinol include increased serum concentrations of methotrexate, azathioprine, and theophylline secondary to inhibition of their metabolism.

### Monitoring for Efficacy

Therapeutic drug efficacy is monitored by improvement in the patient's symptoms. Following prompt initiation of therapy for an acute attack, resolution of severe pain commonly occurs within several hours. Initially, the patient should be assessed in 1 week to verify that the acute attack has resolved. Residual pain is common; therefore, therapy is typically continued for 5–7 days. After the acute attack has resolved, the need for prophylactic therapy must be evaluated. Nonpharmacologic interventions should be emphasized.

### Monitoring for Toxicity

Toxicity may occur with any of the agents used in the treatment and prevention of gouty arthritis. See the discussions of individual drugs for potential toxicities.

### Follow-up Recommendations

Initially, the individual should be assessed at a 1- or 2-week interval to verify that the acute attack has resolved. If it is not the patient's first attack, the need for prophylactic therapy must be evaluated. Nonpharmacologic interventions also must be emphasized.

## LOW BACK PAIN

Low back pain is the most frequent musculoskeletal complaint for adults, with 80% of adults experiencing at least one lifetime episode (Borenstein, 1993). Annually, 50% of working adults will have an acute episode for which 15–20% will seek health care (USDHHS, 1994). Back pain disorders are responsible for 20% of work-related injuries and account for 40% of disability claims (Marras et al, 1995).

### ETIOLOGY

Ninety percent of back pain in adults is attributed to a mechanical disorder, and the remaining 10% stems from one of 60 nonmechanical etiologies: rheumatologic, infectious (urinary tract, prostatitis, pelvic inflammatory disease, herpes zoster, epidural abscess), neoplastic, endocrine (diabetes), hematologic, referred from the abdomen (abdominal aortic aneurysm, perforated ulcer, pancreatitis, and endometriosis), and miscellaneous causes (Deen, 1996). Mechanical back pain is caused by overuse or strain, trauma, or spinal anatomic deformity. Common mechanical disorders associated with low back pain include muscle strain, osteoarthritis of the apophyseal joints, spinal stenosis, herniated disk with or without radiculopathy, or spondylolisthesis. Most back pain results from the pain-sensitive areas, including anterior and posterior ligaments, vertebral bodies, facet synovial lining, paraspinal muscles, sacroiliac joint, and neural tissue within the neural canal and foramen. The intervertebral disk is not sensitive to pain; therefore pain from a damaged disk must result from irritation or entrapment of pain-sensitive structures and tissue (Hainline, 1995).

## SPECIFIC CONSIDERATIONS FOR PHARMACOTHERAPY

### When Drug Therapy Is Needed

Attempts to prove the efficacy of pharmacologic agents used in the treatment of back pain is difficult since as many as 80% of patients with acute low back pain symptomatically improve within 2 weeks without intervention (Brody, 1996). Pharmacologic agents commonly used in the management of low back pain include acetaminophen, NSAIDs, and muscle relaxants. Other agents used to provide symptom control include opioid analgesics, corticosteroids, and antidepressants; however, the efficacy of these agents in the treatment of low back pain is debated (Agency for Health Care Policy and Research [AHCPR], 1994).

### Short-Term and Long-Term Goals of Pharmacotherapy

The primary short-term goal of pharmacotherapy is to provide symptom control to allow for activity tolerance until recovery occurs. Achieving this goal permits the patient to continue functioning normally both at work and home. Long-term management of back pain focuses primarily on nonpharmacologic therapy rather than prolonged drug therapy. Among other things, goals of long-term therapy include adequately educating the patient regarding low back problems and recommending activity modification (AHCPR, 1994).

### Nonpharmacologic Therapy

Many therapeutic options with varying efficacy are utilized for relief of back pain. The management goal of back pain has shifted from a focus on the pain toward helping the patient improve activity tolerance (Bigos, Deyo, Romanowski, & Whitten, 1995; USDHHS, 1994). Limited physical activity for 2 days is recommended for patients without neurological deficits (USDHHS, 1994). Most patients will recover faster when they resume their normal activities (Peate, 1994). Malmivaara et al (1995) found in a controlled trial of back pain patients, in an occupational health setting in Finland, that continuing ordinary activities within the pain threshold limits led to more rapid recovery than either bed rest or back-mobilizing exercises.

A commonly utilized treatment modality is spinal manipulation. Short-term (1 month) spinal manipulation is recommended for patients with uncomplicated low back pain. Continuous long-term therapy has no proven benefit (Bigos et al, 1995).

Physical therapy also is widely used for mechanical back pain. Typically, a 1- to 2-week physical therapy program in conjunction with pharmacological agents is effective. Some patients benefit from exercise and being taught improved body mechanics by the physical therapist.

Relaxation and stress management modalities, including yoga, meditation, imagery, and counseling, are employed with the patient afflicted with chronic back pain. Frequently, the patient's psychological status is a major factor contributing to the condition. Relationship conditions in marriage, at home, or at work may be intolerable for the patient, and stress management is an important aspect of treatment. For these patients, all stress, tensions, and frustrations are psychologically channeled to the back muscles. Traction, which was once widely used, has demonstrated no significant results other than keeping the patient passive and nonfunctional. Transcutaneous electrical nerve stimulation (TENS) is another treatment modality that has demonstrated equivocal efficacy in a few controlled studies (Hadler, 1993). An ice pack (wrapped in a towel) placed on the back for 10–20 min every hour provides relief for some patients. For those who can not tolerate the ice therapy, moist heat is very effective. The heat should be applied for 20 min five to six times a day (Peate, 1994). A moist hot towel applied to the back covered with plastic and a heating pad is very effective.

Most low back pain resolves within 4 weeks with conservative management (Deen, 1996). Only 1–2% of patients will require surgery. According to outcome studies, surgery has demonstrated no appreciable efficacy (Bigos et al, 1995; USDHHS, 1994). Back pain prevention education programs by employers are a key element of management (Gustafson, 1995; Ross, 1994).

### Time Frame for Initiating Pharmacotherapy

Once the diagnosis of back strain or musculoskeletal pain has been made, pharmacotherapy can be initiated and typically is used in conjunction with nonpharmacologic therapy. See Drug Tables 301, 302, and 306.

## Assessment and History Taking

The management plan for most back pain patients is derived from a detailed history and physical. Three basic questions should guide the workup of the patient with back pain (Connelly, 1996):

1. Is there an underlying systemic problem such as cancer, abdominal aneurysm, or infection?

2. Is there a neuro-deficit present that warrants a consultation?

3. Is there a psychosocial component that may amplify or prolong the pain?

Plain x-rays are indicated for a few selected cases: pain sustained by a fall or forceful trauma, pain that does not improve with conservative therapy, possible metastatic cancer, older osteoporotic high-risk patients, patients over age 70, and patients using steroids (USDHHS, 1994). Patients with neurological signs and symptoms should receive an MRI and/or CT scan. The history begins with a description of the circumstances associated with the onset of pain. This includes the type of work and usual position. Does the patient primarily sit or stand throughout the day? For possible litigation purposes, the exact location, conditions, wet or slippery floor, exact height of the fall, or force of the injury must be documented. Most work-related low back pain is due to mechanical strain (Peate, 1994). A previous history of back pain and its sequelae should be elicited. A detailed description of the pain is mandatory. Is the pain worse with activity or rest? Pain worse at night is usually indicative of disk disease. Is the pain localized or does it radiate? Be specific as to the radiation of the pain. Is it above or below the knee and which aspect of the leg? Neurological deficits should be ascertained by asking about the presence of extremity weakness or numbness and bowel or bladder deficits. Infectious processes can be detected by asking about fever, chills, dysuria, frequency, or vaginal discharge for females. Males over age 50 should be asked about prostate problems such as difficulty with stream and frequent voiding.

A history of coexisting predisposing factors should be elicited. For example, hypertension is a risk factor for an aortic aneurysm, and postmenopausal status poses a risk for vertebral fractures. Both conditions produce back pain. The psychological status of all patients should be assessed by inquiring about their life stressors and ability to cope (Seimon, 1995).

The physical examination begins by observing the patient ambulate to detect list or leg lag. Next, to rule out neurological deficits, the patient is asked to walk on his or her toes (S1) and heels (L4,5). The spine, paravertebral muscles, and costovertebral angles are palpated for tenderness. The patient should perform range of motion as tolerated. The patient's ability to squat and rise tests strength of the quadriceps and L4 innervation. Against resistance, dorsiflexion of the great toe tests L5. Testing for straight leg raising is performed with the patient sitting and lying. Pain below the knee at 70 degrees or less is indicative of L5 and/or S1 nerve root irritation. Pain that is relieved by plantar flexion of the ankle or external limb rotation suggests a herniated disk. A possible herniated disk diagnosis is further confirmed with the cross-over strength leg raising (SLR) test. With this test, pain occurs when the elevated uninvolved leg produces similar pain distribution. Next, deep tendon reflexes and peripheral pulses are compared. Dorsiflexion and extension strength of the great toe is elicited to determine muscle weakness associated with neurological deficit. Hip range of motion and abdominal examination are performed with the patient supine. Pelvic and rectal examinations may be indicated by the history (Calliet, 1995).

## Patient/Caregiver Information

Patients need to be instructed to refrain from operating moving vehicles or operating machines while taking narcotic analgesics and muscle relaxants. The patient should sleep on a firm mattress or place a board under the mattress to provide additional back support. When the back pain subsides, back stretching and abdominal strengthening exercises are preventive measures for subsequent episodes. In appropriate cases weight reduction is advisable. When lifting heavy objects, the patient should bend the knees and use the large quadriceps and hamstring muscles. Back rehabilitation classes that teach back exercises are very beneficial. Yoga is another modality that enhances back muscle stretching and mind/body relaxation. It is important to emphasize tension and stress management and reduction and the role they play in reducing back pain. Patients should always be instructed to seek care immediately for increased extremity numbness or weakness or decreased ability to void or move their bowels.

## OUTCOMES MANAGEMENT

### Selecting an Appropriate Agent

*Analgesics.*  Acetaminophen, a primarily centrally acting analgesic with little to no antiinflammatory activity, is considered a safe, effective, and low-cost agent for initial treatment of acute low back pain. Patients who experience inadequate pain relief with acetaminophen are often given a trial of NSAIDs. Use of an NSAID provides both analgesic and antiinflammatory activity. As in the treatment of other musculoskeletal disorders, no one NSAID has been found to be superior to the others. There may, however, be great variability in efficacy among agents on an individual basis. Therefore, a patient may be given a trial of another NSAID, typically from a different class, if little to no pain relief is obtained after a 2-week period.

Short-term use of oral opioid analgesics provides another option for the treatment of severe, acute low back pain (AHCPR, 1994). The use of opioid analgesics should rarely extend beyond a 1- to 2-week period. Risk versus benefit must be assessed before initiating therapy with opioids because of potential CNS side effects and the potential for developing tolerance and physical dependence with this class of drugs. Commonly prescribed agents include codeine-containing products and synthetic opioids (eg, hydrocodone, oxycodone). See the Drug Table 303 for further information on dosing and side effects.

*Muscle Relaxants.*  Muscle relaxants are another class of agents commonly used in the treatment of various painful musculoskeletal conditions, including low back problems. These agents are targeted toward the relief of muscle spasm, which may or may not be associated with the pain. Based on findings in the literature, the efficacy of muscle relaxants remains somewhat inconclusive. Although they appear to be more effective than a placebo in controlling back pain symptoms, they have not been shown consistently to be more effective than NSAIDs or to provide an additive benefit when used in combination (AHCPR, 1994).

For treatment of low back problems, the centrally acting skeletal muscle relaxants are frequently prescribed. Rather than causing direct relaxation of skeletal muscle, these agents appear to act centrally through a sedative effect, which ultimately results in depression of neu-

ronal activity (Waldman, 1994). Commonly used skeletal muscle relaxants include carisoprodol, chlorzoxazone, cyclobenzaprine, metaxalone, methocarbamol, and orphenadrine citrate.

Although these agents may provide some symptomatic relief, their use is associated with a number of potential adverse effects. The side effect most commonly reported with these agents is drowsiness, which occurs in up to 30% of patients (AHCPR, 1994). Other reported CNS side effects include dizziness, headache, confusion, and agitation. Use of these agents in conjunction with alcohol or other CNS depressants may lead to cumulative toxicity.

Caution must be exercised with the use of chlorzoxazone. The FDA-approved labeling changes for chlorzoxazone warn of the rare idiosyncratic and unpredictable hepatotoxicity associated with its use (Nightingale, 1995). Early signs and symptoms of hepatotoxicity patients should be aware of include fever, rash, anorexia, nausea, vomiting, fatigue, right upper quadrant pain, dark urine, or jaundice (Nightingale, 1995). With long-term use, liver function tests should be monitored and if abnormality develops, the drug should be discontinued. Hepatotoxicity has also been associated with the use of metaxalone.

Both cyclobenzaprine, which is structurally similar to the tricyclic antidepressants, and orphenadrine, which is an analog of diphenhydramine, have anticholinergic properties. Use of these agents may be associated with the presence of dry mouth, blurred vision, urinary retention, and constipation. These agents should be avoided in patients with prostatic hypertrophy, angle-closure glaucoma, and underlying cardiac abnormalities. See Drug Table 314 for other commonly reported adverse effects and precautions.

In addition to adverse effects, concern exists over the potential for dependence and abuse of some of the centrally acting skeletal muscle relaxants secondary to their CNS effects (Waldman, 1994). Dependence and withdrawal have been observed with the use of carisoprodol and cyclobenzaprine. To minimize the risk of dependence and abuse, ideally, these agents should be prescribed only for brief periods to provide acute symptomatic relief and discontinued gradually to avoid possible withdrawal symptoms. They typically can be limited to a 1- to 2-week course of therapy.

Other agents used with relaxant properties include diazepam (benzodiazepine), baclofen (antispasmodic), and dantrolene sodium (peripherally acting skeletal muscle relaxant). Diazepam appears to exert its muscle relaxant properties through augmentation of the inhibitory effect of the neurotransmitter gamma-aminobutyric acid (GABA) at spinal and supraspinal sites. Although diazepam has not shown superiority over centrally acting skeletal muscle relaxants in the treatment of muscle spasm and pain, it may provide some advantage in treating anxiety associated with painful conditions (Waldman, 1994). The prolonged use of diazepam in the treatment of musculoskeletal disorders is limited because of its CNS depressant properties and its potential for dependence and abuse.

The antispasmodic agent baclofen which is chemically related to GABA, elicits its effect through inhibition of the transmission of both monosynaptic and polysynaptic reflexes at the level of the spinal cord. This agent is indicated primarily for the relief of muscle spasticity associated with multiple sclerosis and spinal cord lesions (Waldman, 1994). It is not indicated for the treatment of muscle spasms associated with rheumatic disorders. In patients with severe spasticity unresponsive to maximum oral therapy, baclofen may be administered by the intrathecal route. When initiating therapy with baclofen, it should be titrated up slowly to minimize the risk of side effects.

Dantrolene sodium appears to produce skeletal muscle relaxation through a direct peripheral effect rather than a central effect. This agent inhibits the release of calcium ions from the sarcoplasmic reticulum, ultimately leading to skeletal muscle relaxation. It is indicated for the treatment of muscle spasticity associated with upper motor disorders such as spinal cord injury, stroke, cerebral palsy, and multiple sclerosis. Like baclofen, it is not indicated for the relief of spasms associated with rheumatic disorders. Dantrolene use has been associated with hepatotoxicity caused by an idiosyncratic or hypersensitivity reaction to the medication. The risk for hepatotoxicity appears to be greatest for females over the age of 35 who are receiving other medications, in particular, estrogen therapy (Waldman, 1994).

***Corticosteroids.*** In the treatment of low back pain, there is no indication for the use of oral or intravenous corticosteroids (AHCPR, 1994). The use of corticosteroids for trigger point, facet joint, and epidural injections has been evaluated; however, their efficacy is still being de-

bated (AHCPR, 1994). Because of potential complications, use of these invasive measures is typically not recommended for the treatment of acute low back problems.

## Monitoring for Efficacy

The typical course of treatment for acute low back problems is 1–2 weeks with up to 80% of patients symptomatically improving within this time period.

## Monitoring for Toxicity

With many of the agents used in the management of low back pain, the most common and use-limiting side effects are CNS-related. These CNS effects include drowsiness, dizziness, headache, agitation, and confusion. Often, tolerance develops to these side effects; however, if they persist or are intolerable, the agent should be discontinued. The use of a number of centrally acting skeletal muscle relaxants has been associated with the development of hepatotoxicity. If one of these agents is used, the patient must be warned of early signs and symptoms of hepatotoxicity, and liver function tests should be monitored regularly. See Drug Tables 301, 302, 306 and 314 for specific agents associated with hepatotoxicity.

## Follow-up Recommendations

The patient should be instructed to return for a follow-up visit immediately if bladder or bowel problems occur or if there is increased extremity numbness or weakness. Patients with acute injuries covered by workman's compensation are usually reevaluated within 1 week to determine the ability to resume full or partial work activities.

# TENDINITIS, BURSITIS, SPRAINS, AND STRAINS

Persons experience muscle, tendon, or ligament strains or sprains as a result of trauma and overuse. During the past decade, reported workplace-associated overuse injuries have escalated, and the repetitive movement syndrome accounts for 30–50% of workplace injuries (Schwartz & Weinstein, 1996). In addition, the increased numbers of persons engaged in exercise activities (running and aerobic exercise) have produced a variety of musculoskeletal complaints. The most common problems are discussed below.

*Stiff neck syndrome*, which results when patients are subjected to strenuous positions (plumbers and others who must work in awkward positions). *Tension neck syndrome* is experienced by patients who sit at a desk and have poor posture (computer operators and accountants). These problems are not associated with an injury, but result from maintaining an incorrect posture for a prolonged time. The patient has neck pain and stiffness, often with a dull headache. The pain may spread to the upper thoracic regions, and the trapezius and levator muscles are tender with palpation. Radicular symptoms are usually absent, and if tingling sensations are present, consider other causes. *Occipital cephalalgia* results from restricted motion of the occipital-cervical joints. It commonly occurs from prolonged tucking of a telephone under the chin, from extended desk or computer work or from when a person lays on a couch watching television with a pillow propping the head. These patients have intense unilateral pain, sometimes associated with migraine-like headaches (nausea and photosensitivity) and dizziness. The occipital muscular triangle is tender.

*Tendinitis* is an inflammation of a tendon sheath as a result of overuse or injury. Common areas afflicted include the elbow (epicondylitis), the shoulder (rotator cuff and adhesive capsulitis with frozen shoulder), the extensor tendon of the wrist and thumb, or the lower extremity (hamstring or Achilles tendon). Diabetics and arthritic patients are prone to developing tendinitis of the hands, and wrists (carpal tunnel syndrome) and shoulder (adhesive capsulitis). Patients experience pain with motion and occasionally paresthesia of the affected area. The affected area is usually tender, occasionally minimally swollen, but usually with no erythema.

*Bursitis* resulting from trauma, overuse, crystal-induced diseases (eg, gout), connective tissue disease (eg, rheumatoid arthritis), and infections (eg, gonorrhea) commonly involves the elbow, shoulder, and the hip. Trochanteric bursitis of the hip, which is frequently underdiagnosed, is characterized by a chronic, intermittent aching pain in the lateral aspect of the hip. It results from inflammation of the four trochanter bursae and often secondarily from tendinous calcification (Shbeeb & Matteson, 1996). The pain

can be sharp and intense and increases with external rotation and abduction along with other hip movements. The pain can be reproduced by resisted abduction and external rotation. Patients will have localized tenderness over the greater trochanter and may have a positive Patrick's fabere test (Shbeeb & Matteson, 1996).

Patients with bursitis of the shoulder complain of nocturnal diffuse shoulder pain in addition to specific abduction pain ranging from 70–110 degrees (painful arc). The pain is poorly localized to the deltoid area and may radiate down the arm. There should be no neurovascular compromise.

Musculoskeletal injuries with sprains and strains are among the most common complaints in primary care (Onieal, 1996). When an injury is sustained, a specific inflammatory process initiates the symptoms of redness, swelling, heat, and pain. Ninety percent of ankle sprains involve the anterior or posterior talofibular ligament of the lateral malleolus. Injury to the medial malleolus is more likely to result in a fracture. There is usually a history of ankle inversion or eversion with or without a "pop." The presence of an audible sound indicates more serious injury, and the patient may be nauseated, lightheaded, and diaphoretic (Onieal, 1996). With more serious injuries, the patient is unable to ambulate after the injury and there is immediate swelling and redness. With less serious injuries, swelling and pain may not occur until 8–12 hours after the injury. Neurovascular intactness and point tenderness, which are more specific for fracture, must be assessed. Ankle sprains are graded from I to III (Onieal, 1996). A grade I sprain is mild with minimal swelling and ecchymosis, no instability or functional disability, and full range of motion. A grade II sprain has moderate to severe pain, decreased range of motion, and swelling and ecchymosis with an incomplete ligament tear. A grade III sprain is more severe with a complete ligamentous tear and must be referred to an orthopedic surgeon for management. An x-ray can rule out fracture and is warranted for all high-risk injuries and for patients with severe pain or who are unable to ambulate.

## NONPHARMACOLOGICAL TREATMENT

An effective simple treatment for tendinitis, bursitis, and ligamentous injuries is described by the acronym RICE (rest, ice, compression, and elevation). Put the affected area to rest to diminish swelling and inflammation. Compression can be attained with ace bangages, elastic bands, or an ankle air splint. Elevation of the extremity by sling or simply propping the foot higher than the heart will aid in recovery. Persons with grade II and III ankle injuries will need crutches for 2–5 days. Most patients with grade I injuries can ambulate with an ace bandage or air splint. Cold therapy application, 15–30 min three to five times a day during the initial 24–72 h after an injury or work-induced syndrome reduces cellular metabolism and allows marginally viable cells to survive. Cold therapy is also applied to prevent reactive swelling after rehabilitative exercises (Baumert, 1995). During the subacute and chronic stages of the pain, when the swelling has subsided, moist heat application, 15–30 min three to five times a day, increases blood flow, promotes tissue healing, and loosens stiff joints and muscles. Moist heat may be applied, as suggested for back pain. A whirlpool bath is also an effective way to apply moist heat. Ultrasound transmits high-frequency acoustic energy deep heat waves to the injury and is used in the rehabilitative stage after the acute inflammation has subsided (Baumert, 1995). The use of a supportive device such as an elastic wrist band or carpal splint during the acute inflammatory phase of tendinitis is often therapeutic.

See Drug Table 306 for pharmacological treatment of these conditions.

## REFERENCES

### Rheumatoid Arthritis

American College of Rheumatology Ad Hoc Committee On Clinical Guidelines. (1996a). Guidelines for monitoring drug therapy in rheumatoid arthritis. *Arthritis and Rheumatism, 39*(5), 723–731.

American College of Rheumatology Ad Hoc Committee on Clinical Guidelines. (1996b). Guidelines for the management of rheumatoid arthritis. *Arthritis and Rheumatism, 39*(5), 713–722.

Amos, R. S. (1995). The history of the use of sulphasalazine in rheumatology. *British Journal of Rheumatology, 34*(Suppl. 2), 2–6.

Anderson, R. J. (1993). Rheumatoid arthritis: Clinical features and laboratory. In H. R. Schumacher, Jr., J. H. Klippel & W. J. Koopman (Eds.), *Primer on the rheumatic diseases* (10th ed.). Atlanta: Arthritis Foundation.

Atkinson, M. H., Menard, H. A., & Kalish, G. H. (1995). Assessment of salsalate, a nonacetylated salicylate, in the treatment of patients with arthritis. *Clinical Therapeutics, 17*(5), 827–837.

Bensen, W. G., Bensen, W., Adachi, J. D., & Tugwell, P. X. (1990). Remodeling the pyramid: The therapeutic target of rheumatoid arthritis. *Journal of Rheumatology, 170,* 987–989.

Blackburn, W. D. (1996). Managment of osteoarthritis and rheumatoid arthritis: Prospects and possibilities. *American Journal of Medicine, 100*(Suppl. 2A), 2A-24S–2A-30S.

Boers, M., Van Riel, P. L., Felson, D. T., & Tugwell, P. (1995). Assessing the activity of rheumatoid arthritis. *Baillieres Clinical Rheumatology, 9*(2), 305–317.

Bradley, L. A. (1993). Psychosocial factors and arthritis. In H. R. Schumacher, Jr., J. H. Klippel & W. J. Koopman (Eds.), *Primer on the rheumatic diseases* (10th ed.). Atlanta: Arthritis Foundation.

Brown, J. H., & Deluca, S. A. (1995). The radiology of rheumatoid arthritis. *American Family Physician, 52*(5), 1372–1380.

CDC (1996). Factors associated with prevalent self-reported arthritis and other rheumatic conditions—United States, 1989–1991. *MMWR, 45*(23), 487–491.

Cryer, B., & Feldman, M. (1992). Effects of nonsteroidal anti-inflammatory drugs on endogenous gastrointestinal prostaglandins and therapeutic strategies for prevention and treatment of nonsteroidal anti-inflammatory drug-induced damage. *Archives of Internal Medicine, 152,* 1145–1155.

Dijkmans, B. A. C. (1995). Folate supplementation and methotrexate. *British Journal of Rheumatology, 34,* 1172–1174.

Drugs for rheumatoid arthritis. (1994). *Medical Letter on Drugs and Therapeutics, 36,* 101–106.

Emery, P. (1995). Therapeutic approaches for early rheumatoid arthritis. How early? How aggressive? *British Journal of Rheumatology, 34*(Suppl 2), 87–90.

Furst, D. E. (1994). Are there differences among nonsteroidal antiinflammatory drugs? Comparing acetylated salicylates, nonacetylated salicylates, and nonacetylated nonsteroidal antiinflammatory drugs. *Arthritis and Rheumatism, 37,* 1–9.

Gittoes, N. J. L. (1994). Therapeutic progress I: Current treatment of rheumatoid arthritis. *Journal of Clinical Pharmacy and Therapeutics, 19,* 147–162.

Graham, D. Y., White, R. H., Moreland, L. W., et al. (1993). Duodenal and gastric ulcer prevention with misoprostol in arthritis patients taking NSAIDs. *Annals of Internal Medicine, 119*(4), 257–262.

Greene, J. M., & Winickoff, R. N. (1992). Cost-consious prescribing of nonsteroidal anti-inflammatory drugs for adults with arthritis: A review and suggestions. *Archives of Internal Medicine, 152,* 1995–2002.

Halverson, P. B. (1995). Extraarticular manifestations of rheumatoid arthritis. *Orthopedic Nursing, 14*(4), 47–50.

Jones, D. L., Kroenke K., Landry, F. J., et al. (1996). Cost savings using a stepped-care prescribing protocol for nonsteroidal anti-inflammatory drugs. *JAMA, 275,* 926–930.

MacGregor, A. J. (1995). Classification criteria for rheumatoid arthritis. *Baillieres Clinical Rheumatology, 9*(2), 287–304.

Meenan, R. F. (1994). Health status assessment. In F. Wolfe & T. Pincus (Eds.), *Rheumatoid arthritis, pathogenesis, assessment, outcome and treatment.* New York: Marcel Dekker, 191–205.

Messmer, E. M., & Foster, C. S. (1995). Destructive corneal and scleral disease associated with rheumatoid arthritis. *Cornea, 14*(4), 408–417.

Moder, K. G., Tefferi, A., Cohen, M. D., et al. (1995). Hematologic malignancies and the use of methotrexate in rheumatoid arthritis: A retrospective study. *American Journal of Medicine, 99,* 276–281.

Nepom, G. T. (1994). HLA-DR4 and Rheumatoid arthritis. In F. Wolfe & T. Pincus (Eds.), *Rheumatoid arthritis, pathogenesis, assessment, outcome and treatment* (chap. 3). New York: Marcel Dekker.

Ollier, W. E. R., & MacGregor, A. (1995). Genetic epidemiology of rheumatoid disease. *British Medical Bulletin, 51*(2), 267–285.

Palmer, D. G. (1995). The anatomy of the rheumatoid lesion. *British Medical Bulletin, 51*(2), 286–295.

Pincus, T., Marcum, S. B., & Callahan, L. F. (1992). Longterm drug therapy for rheumatoid arthritis in seven rheumatology private practices: II. Second line drugs and prednisone. *Journal of Rheumatology, 19*(12), 1885–1894.

Pincus, T., Wolfe, F., & Callahan, L. F. (1994). Introduction: Updating a reassessment of traditional paradigms concerning rheumatoid arthritis. In F. Wolfe & T. Pincus (Eds.), *Rheumatoid arthritis, pathogenesis, assessment, outcome and treatment.* New York: Marcel Dekker.

Prashker, M. J., & Meenan, R. F. (1995). The total costs of drug therapy for rheumatoid arthritis. A model based on costs of drug, monitoring, and toxicity. *Arthritis and Rheumatism, 38,* 318—325.

Raskin, J. B., White, R. H., Jackson, J. E., et al. (1995). Misoprostol dosage in the prevention of nonsteroidal anti-inflammatory drug-induced gastric and duodenal ulcers: A comparison of three regimens. *Annals of Internal Medicine, 123*(5), 344–350.

Salmon, J., & Gaston, J. (1995). The role of T-lymphocytes in rheumatoid arthritis. *British Medical Bulletin, 51*(2), 332–345.

Sandoval, D. M., Alarcon, G. S., & Morgan, S. L. (1995). Adverse events in methotrexate-treated rheumatoid arthritis patients. *British Journal of Rheumatology, 34*(Suppl. 2), 49–56.

Schlondorff, D. (1993). Renal complications of nonsteroidal anti-inflammatory drugs. *Kidney International, 44,* 643–653.

Schumacher, H. R., Jr., Klippel, J. H., & Koopman, W. J. (Eds.). (1993). *Primer on the rheumatic diseases* (10th ed.). Atlanta: Arthritis Foundation.

Semble, E. L. (1995). Rheumatoid arthritis: New approaches for its evaluation and management. *Archives of Physical Medicine and Rehabilitation, 76,* 190–201.

Silverstein, F. E., Graham, D. Y., Davies, H. W., et al. (1995). Misoprostol reduces serious gastrointestinal complications in patients with rheumatoid arthritis receiving nonsteroidal anti-inflammatory drugs. *Annals of Internal Medicine, 123*(4), 241–249.

Smedegard, G. & Bjork, J. (1995). Sulphasalazine: Mechanism of action in rheumatoid arthritis. *British Journal of Rheumatology, 34*(suppl. 2), 7–15.

Snowden, N., & Kay, R. A. (1995). Immunology of systemic rheumatoid disease. *British Medical Bulletin, 51*(2), 437–448.

Symmons, D. P. M., Hassell, A. B., Gunatillaka, K., Jones, P. J., Schollum, J., & Dawes, P. T. (1995). Development and preliminary assessment of a simple measure of overall status in rheumatoid arthritis (OSRA for routine clinical use). *OJM, 88,* 429–437.

Symmons, D. P., & Silman, A. J. (1994). The epidemiology of rheumatoid arthritis. In F. Wolfe & T. Pincus (Eds.), *Rheumatoid arthritis, pathogenesis, assessment outcome and treatment* (chap. 4). New York: Marcel Dekker.

Taha, A. S., Hudson, N., Hawkey, C. J., et al. (1996). Famotidine for the prevention of gastric and duodenal ulcers caused by nonsteroidal antiinflammatory drugs. *New England Journal of Medicine, 334,* 1435–1439.

Tak, P. P., Van Der Lubbe, P. A., Cauli, A., et al. (1995). Reduction of synovial inflammation after anti-CD4 monoclonal antibody treatment in early rheumatoid arthritis. *Arthritis and Rheumatism, 38*(10), 1457–1465.

Van Riel, P. L. C. M., Van Gestel, A. M., & Van De Putte, L. B. A. (1995). Long-term usage and side-effect profile of sulphasalazine in rheumatoid arthritis. *British Journal of Rheumatology, 34*(Suppl. 2), 40–42.

Viner, N. J. (1995). Role of antigen presenting cells in rheumatoid arthritis. *British Medical Bulletin, 51*(2), 359–367.

Walker, A. M., Funch, D., Dreyer, N. A., et al. (1993). Determinants of serious liver disease among patients receiving low-dose methotrexate for rheumatoid arthritis. *Arthritis and Rheumatism, 36,* 329–335.

Wells, G., & Tugwell, P. (1993). Cyclosporin A in rheumatoid arthritis: Overview of efficacy. *British Journal of Rheumatology, 32*(Suppl. 1), 51–56.

Wilder, R. L. (1993). Rheumatoid arthritis: Clinical features and laboratory. In H. R. Schumacher, Jr., J. H. Klippel, & W. J. Koopman (Eds.), *Primer on the rheumatic diseases* (10th ed.). Atlanta: Arthritis Foundation.

Williams, H. J. (1993). Rheumatoid arthritis: Treatment. In: H. R. Schumacher, J. H. Klippel, & W. J. Koopman (Eds.), *Primer on the rheumatic diseases* (10th ed.). Atlanta: Arthritis Foundation.

Williams, H. J. (1995). Overview of combination second-line or disease-modifying antirheumatic drug therapy in rheumatoid arthritis. *British Journal of Rheumatology, 34*(Suppl. 2), 96–99.

Wilske, K. R., & Healey, L. A. (1989). Remodeling the pyramid—A concept whose time has come. *Journal of Rheumatology, 165,* 565–567.

Wood, A. J. J. (1994). Second-line drug therapy for rheumatoid arthritis. *New England Journal of Medicine, 330,* 1368–1375.

## Osteoarthritis

Altman, R. D., Aven, A., Holmburg, C. E., et al. (1994). Capsaicin cream 0.025% as monotherapy for osteoarthritis: A double-blind study. *Seminars in Arthritis and Rheumatism, 23*(6), 25–33.

Blackburn, W. D. (1996). Management of osteoarthritis and rheumatoid arthritis: Prospects and possibilities. *American Journal of Medicine, 100*(Suppl. 2A), 24S–30S.

Bradley, J. D. (1994). Nonsurgical options for managing osteoarthritis of the knee. *Journal of Musculoskeletal Medicine, 11*(8), 14–26.

Bradley, J. D., Brandt, K. D., Katz, B. P., et al. (1991). Comparison of an antiinflammatory dose of ibuprofen, an analgesic dose of ibuprofen, and acetaminophen in the treatment of patients with osteoarthritis of the knee. *New England Journal of Medicine, 325*(2), 87–91.

Brandt, K. D. (1995). Toward pharmacologic modification of joint damage in osteoarthritis. *Annals of Internal Medicine, 122,* 874–875.

Brandt, K. D., & Slemenda, E. W. (1993). Osteoarthritis, epidemiology, pathology, and pathogenesis. In H. R. Schumacher, Jr., J. H. Klippel, & W. J. Koopman (Eds.), *Primer on the rheumatic diseases* (10th ed.). Atlanta: Arthritis Foundation.

Cooper, C. (1995). Occupational activity and the risk of osteoarthritis. *Journal of Rheumatology, 22*(1)(Suppl. 43), 10–12.

Creamer, P., & Dieppe, P. A. (1993). Novel drug treatment strategies for osteoarthritis. *Journal of Rheumatology, 20*(9), 1461–1464.

Deal, C. L., Schnitzer, T. J., Lipstein, E., et al. (1991). Treatment of arthritis with topical capsaicin: A double-blind trial. *Clinical Therapeutics, 13*(3), 383–395.

Edelson, R., Burks, R. T., & Bloebaum, R. D. (1995). Short-term effects of knee washout for osteoarthritis. *American Journal of Sports Medicine, 23*(3), 345–349.

Ettinger, W. H., Jr., & Afable, R. F. (1994). Physical disability from knee osteoarthritis: The role of exercise as an intervention. *Medicine and Science in Sports and Exercise, 26*(12), 1435–1440.

Felson, D. T. (1995). Weight and osteoarthritis. *Journal of Rheumatology, 22*(1), 7–9.

Felson, D. T., Zhang, Y., Anthony, M., et al. (1992). Weight loss reduces the risk for symptomatic knee arthritis in women. *Annals of Internal Medicine, 117,* 535–539.

Felson, D. T., Zhang, Y., Hannan, M. T., et al. (1995). The incidence and natural history of knee osteoarthritis in the elderly: The Framingham Osteoarthritis Study. *Arthritis and Rheumatism, 38*(10), 1500–1505.

Gabriel, S. E., Crowson, C. S., & O'Fallon, W. M. (1995). Costs of osteoarthritis: Estimates from a geographically defined population. *Journal of Rheumatology, 22*(Suppl. 43), 23–25.

Galas, J. (May–June 1996). Yoga all gain no pain. *Arthritis Today,* 30–32.

Hochberg, M. C., Altman, R. D., Brandt, K. D., et al. (1995a). Guidelines for the medical management of osteoarthritis. Part I. Osteoarthritis of the hip. *Arthritis and Rheumatism, 38*(11), 1535–1540.

Hochberg, M. C., Altman, R. D., Brandt, K. D., et al. (1995b). Guidelines for the medical management of osteoarthritis. Part II. Osteoarthritis of the knee. *Arthritis and Rheumatism, 38*(11), 1541–1546.

Hooker, R. S. (1996). Osteoarthritis of the hip and knee: Managing a common joint disease. *Clinician Reviews, 6,* 54–68.

Jimenez, S. A., & Dharmavaram, R. M. (1994). Genetic aspects of familial osteoarthritis. *Annals of Rheumatic Diseases, 53,* 789–797.

Lane, N. E. (1995). Exercise: A cause of osteoarthritis. *Journal of Rheumatology, 22*(1)(Suppl. 43), 3–6.

Moskowitz, R. W., & Goldberg, V. M. (1993). Osteoarthritis: Clinical features and treatment. In H. R. Schumacher, Jr., J. H. Klippel, & W. J. Koopman (Eds.), *Primer on the rheumatic diseases* (10th ed.). Atlanta: Arthritis Foundation.

Oddis, C. V. (1996). New perspectives on osteoarthritis. *American Journal of Medicine, 100*(Suppl. 2A), 10S–15S.

Schumacher, H. R., Jr. (1995). Synovial inflammation, crystals, and osteoarthritis. *Journal of Rheumatology, 22*(1)(Suppl. 43), 101–103.

Schumacher, H. R., Jr., Klippel, J. H., & Koopman, W. J. (1993). *Primer on the rheumatic diseases* (10th ed.). Atlanta: Arthritis Foundation.

Schwartz, S. P. (1996, July–August). 25 more tips to simplify your life. *Arthritis Today*, 34–35.

Williams, H. J., Ward, J. R., Egger, M. J., et al. (1993). Comparison of naproxen and acetaminophen in a two-year study of treatment of osteoarthritis of the knee. *Arthritis and Rheumatism, 36*(9), 1196–1206.


## Osteoporosis

Avioli, L. V. (1992). Heterogeneity of osteoporotic syndromes and the response to calcitonin therapy. *Calcified Tissue International, 51*, 105–110.

Black, D. M. (1995). Why elderly women should be screened and treated to prevent osteoporosis. *American Journal of Medicine, 98* (Suppl. 2A), 2A-67S–2A-75S.

Cauley, J. A., Seeley, D. G., Ensrud, K., et al. (1995). Estrogen replacement therapy and fractures in older women. *Annals of Internal Medicine, 122*, 9–16.

Chapuy, M. C., Arlot, M. E., Duboeuf, F., et al. (1992). Vitamin $D_3$ and calcium to prevent hip fractures in elderly women. *New England Journal of Medicine 27*, 1637–1642.

Chesnut, C. H., III, McClung, M. R., Ensrud, K. E., et al. (1995). Alendronate treatment of the postmenopausal osteoporotic woman: Effect of multiple dosages on bone mass and bone remodeling. *American Journal of Medicine, 99*, 144–152.

Colditz, G. A., Hankinson, S. E., Hunter, D. J., et al. (1995). The use of estrogens and progestins and the risk of breast cancer in postmenopausal women. *New England Journal of Medicine, 332*, 1589–1593.

Cummings, K. G., McClung, M., & Cummings, S. R. (1994). Risk factors for hip fracture in white women. *New England Journal of Medicine, 332*, 767–773.

Dunne, F. P., Walters, B. A., Marshall, T., et al. (1993). Pregnancy associated osteoporosis. *Clinical Endocrinology, 39*, 487–490.

Folsom, A. R., Mink, P. J., Sellers, T. A., et al. (1995). Hormonal replacement therapy and morbidity and mortality in a prospective study of postmenopausal women. *American Journal of Public Health, 85*, 1128–1132.

Fruth, S. J., & Worrell, T. W. (1995). Factors associated with menstrual irregularities and decreased bone mineral density in female athletes. *Journal of Orthopaedic and Sports Physical Therapy, 22*(1), 26–38.

Galsworthy, T. D., & Wilson, P. L. (1996). Osteoporosis: It steals more than bone. *American Journal of Nursing, 96*(6), 27–33.

Gamble, C. L. (1995). Osteoporosis: Drug and nondrug therapies for the patient at risk. *Geriatrics, 50*(8), 39–43.

Grady, D., Rubin, S. M., Petitti, D. B., et al. (1992). Hormone therapy to prevent disease and prolong life in postmenopausal women. *Annals of Internal Medicine, 117*, 1016–1037.

Hodgson, S. F., & Johnston, C. C. (1996). AACE clinical practice guidelines for the prevention and treatment of postmenopausal osteoporosis. *Endocrine Practice, 2*(2), 155–169.

Holmes-Walker, J., Prelevic, G. M., & Jacobs, H. S. (1995). Effects of calcium and exercise on bone mineral density in premenopausal women with osteoporosis. *Current Opinion in Obstetrics and Gynecology, 7*, 323–326.

Kanis, J. A. (1995). Treatment of osteoporosis in elderly women. *American Journal of Medicine, 98* (Suppl. 2A), 2A-60S–2A-66S.

Khosla, S., & Riggs, B. L. (1995). Treatment options for osteoporosis. *Mayo Clinic Proceedings, 70*, 978–982.

Kleerekoper, M., & Avioli, L. V. (1993). Evaluation and treatment of postmenopausal osteoporosis. In M. J. Favus (Ed.), *Primer on metabolic bone diseases*, New York: Raven Press.

Liberman, U. A., Weiss, S. R., Broll, J., et al. (1995). Effect of oral alendronate on bone mineral density and the incidence of fractures in postmenopausal osteoporosis. *New England Journal of Medicine, 333*(22), 1437–1443.

Lobo, R. A. (1995). Benefits and risks of estrogen replacement therapy. *American Journal of Obstetrics and Gynecology, 173*, 982–990.

Lufkin, E. G., Wahner, H. W., O'Fallon, W. M., et al. (1992). Treatment of postmenopausal osteoporosis with transdermal estrogen. *Annals of Internal Medicines, 117*, 1–9.

Lyritis, G. P., Tsakalakos, N., Magiasis, B., et al. (1991). Analgesic effect of salmon calcitonin in osteoporotic vertebral fractures: A double-blind placebo-controlled clinical study. *Calcified Tissue International, 49*, 369–372.

Manolagas, S. C., Bellido, T., & Jilka, R. L. (1995). New insights into the cellular, biochemical, and molecular basis of postmenopausal and senile osteoporosis: Roles of IL-6 and gp130. *International Journal of Immunopharmacology, 17*(2), 109–116.

The Medical Letter. (1998). Raloxifene for post-menopausal osteoporosis. *The Medical Letter* 1022(40).

Murray, C., & O'Brien, K. (1995). Osteoporosis workup: Evaluating bone loss and risk of fractures. *Geriatrics, 50*(9), 1–53.

National Institutes of Health Consensus Development Panel on Optimal Calcium Intake. (1994). *JAMA, 272*(24), 1942–1948.

Nelson, M. E., Fiatarone, M. A., Morganti, C. M., et al. (1994). Effects of high-intensity strength training on multiple risk factors for osteoporotic fractures. *JAMA, 272*(24), 1909–1914.

New drugs for osteoporosis. (1996). *Medical Letter on Drugs and Therapeutics, 38*, 1–3.

Ott, S. M. (1993). Metabolic bone diseases. In H. R. Schumacher, Jr., J. H. Klippel, & W. J. Koopman (Eds.), *Primer on the rheumatic diseases* (10th ed.). Atlanta: Arthritis Foundation.

Overgaard, K., Hansen, M. A., Jensen, S. B., & Christiansen, C. (1992). Effect of salcatonin given intranasally on bone mass and fracture rates in established osteoporosis: A dose-response study. *British Medical Journal, 305*, 56–61.

Pak, C. Y. C., Sakhaee, K., Adams-Huet, B., et al. (1995). Treatment of postmenopausal osteoporosis with slow-release sodium fluoride. *Annals of Internal Medicine, 123*, 401–408.

Peris, P., Guanabens, N., Monegal, A., et al. (1995). Aetiology and preventing symptoms in male osteoporosis. *British Journal of Rheumatology, 34*, 936–941.

Putukian, M. (1994). The female triad: Eating disorders, amenorrhea, and osteoporosis. *Medical Clinics of North America, 78*(2), 345–356.

Reginster, J. Y., Deriosy, R., Lecart, M. P., et al. (1995). A double-blind, placebo-controlled, dose-finding trial of intermittent nasal salmon calcitonin for prevention of postmenopausal lumbar spine loss. *American Journal of Medicine, 98*, 452–468.

Rico, H., Hernandez, E. R., Revilla, M., & Gomez-Castrensana, F. (1992). Salmon calcitonin reduces vertebral fracture rate in postmenopausal fracture syndrome. *Bone and Mineral, 16*, 131–138.

Riggs, B. L., Hodgson, S. F., O'Fallon, W. M., et al. (1990). Effect of fluoride treatment on the fracture rate in postmenopausal women with osteoporosis. *New England Journal of Medicine, 322*, 802–809.

Riggs, B. L., & Melton, L. J., III. (1992). The prevention and treatment of osteoporosis. *New England Journal of Medicine, 327*, 620–627.

Rosenfeld, J. (1994). Update on continuous estrogen-progestin replacement therapy. *American Family Physician, 50*, 1519–1522.

Ross, P. D. (1996). Osteoporosis: Frequency, consequences, and risk factors. *Archives of Internal Medicine, 156*, 1399–1411.

Rungby, J., Hermann, A. P., & Mosekilde, L. (1995). Epidemiology of osteoporosis: Implications for drug therapy. *Drugs and Aging, 6*(6), 470–478.

Sambrook, P. N., Kelly, P. J., Morrison, N. A., & Eisman, J. A. (1994). Genetics of osteoporosis. *British Journal of Rheumatology, 33*, 1007–1011.

Seeman, E. (1995). The dilemma of osteoporosis in men. *American Journal of Medicine, 98*(Suppl. 2A), 2A-76S–2A-88S.

Silver, J. J., & Einhorn, T. A. (1995). Osteoporosis and aging. *Clinical Orthopedics and Related Research, 316*, 10–20.

Smith, R. (1994). Idiopathic juvenile osteoporosis: Experience of twenty-one patients. *British Journal of Rheumatology, 34*, 68–77.

Stampfer, M. J., & Colditz, G. A. (1991). Estrogen replacement therapy and coronary heart disease: A quantitative assessment of the epidemiologic evidence. *Preventive Medicine, 20*, 47–63.

Thein, L. A., & Thein, J. M. (1996). The female athlete. *Journal of Orthopaedic and Sports Physical Therapy, 23*(2), 134–148.

Writing Group for the PEPI Trial. (1995). Effects of estrogen or estrogen/progestin regimens on heart disease risk factors in postmenopausal women: The postmenopausal estrogen/progestin interventions (PEPI) trial. *JAMA, 273*, 199–208.

Writing Group for the PEPI Trial. (1996). Effects of hormone replacement therapy on endometrial histology in postmenopausal women. *JAMA, 275*, 370–375.

## Gout

Agarwal, A. K. (1993). Gout and pseudogout. *Primary Care, 20*, 839–855.

Axelrod, D., & Preston, S. (1988). Comparison of parenteral adrenocorticotropic hormone with oral indomethacin in the treatment of acute gout. *Arthritis and Rheumatism, 31*, 803–805.

Beutler, A., & Schumaker, R. (1994). Gout and pseudogout. *Postgraduate Medicine, 95*(2), 103–116.

Brooks, P. M., & Day, R. O. (1991). Nonsteroidal antiinflammatory drugs—Differences and similarities. *New England Journal of Medicine, 324*(24), 1716–1725.

Cryer B., & Feldman, M. (1992). Effects of nonsteroidal anti-inflammatory drugs on endogenous gastrointestinal prostaglandins and therapeutic strategies for prevention and treatment of nonsteroidal anti-inflammatory drug-induced damage. *Archives of Internal Medicine, 152*, 1145–1154.

Day, R. O., Birkett, D. J., Hicks, M., et al. (1994). New uses for allopurinol. *Drugs, 48*(3), 339–344.

Emmerson, B. T. (1996). The management of gout. *New England Journal of Medicine, 334*(7), 445–451.

Fam, A. G. (1995). Should patients with interval gout be treated with urate lowering drugs? *Journal of Rheumatology, 22*(9), 1621–1623.

Furst, D. E. (1994). Are there differences among nonsteroidal antiinflammatory drugs? Comparing acetylated salicylates, nonacetylated salicylates, and nonacetylated nonsteroidal antiinflammatory drugs. *Arthritis and Rheumatism, 37*, 1–9.

Gomberg, E. S. (1995). Older women and alcohol: Use and abuse. *Recent Developments in Alcoholism, 12*, 61–79.

Gonzalez, E., Miller, S. B., & Agudelo, C. A. (1994). Optimal management of gout in older patients. *Drugs and Aging, 4*(2), 128–134.

Joseph, J., & McGrath, H. (1995). Gout or pseudo-gout: How to differentiate crystal-induced arthropotis. *Geriatrics, 50*(4), 33–39.

Kot, T. V., Day, R. O., & Brooks, P. M. (1993). Preventing acute gout when starting allopurinol therapy: Colchicine or NSAIDs? *Medical Journal of Australia, 159*(2), 182–184.

Kuncl, R. W., Duncan, G., & Watson, D. (1987). Colchicine myopathy and neuropathy. *New England Journal of Medicine, 316*(25), 1562–1568.

McCarty, D. J. (1994). Gout without hyperuricemia. *JAMA, 271*(4), 302–303.

Moreland, L. W., & Ball, G. V. (1991). Colchicine and gout. *Arthritis and Rheumatism, 34*(6), 782–786.

Polisson, R. (1996). Nonsteroidal anti-inflammatory drugs: Practical and theoretical considerations in their selection. *American Journal of Medicine, 100* (Suppl. 2A), 31S–36S.

Pratt, P. W., & Ball, G. V. (1993). Gout—Treatment. In: H. R. Schumacher, Jr., J. H. Klippel, & W. J. Koopman (Eds.), *Primer on the rheumatic diseases* (10th ed.) (pp. 216–219). Atlanta: Arthritis Foundation.

Ritter, J., Kerr, L. D., Valeriano-Marcet, J., et al. (1994). ACTH revisited: Effective treatment for acute crystal induced synovitis in patients with multiple medical problems. *Journal of Rheumatology, 21*, 696–699.

Roberts, W. N., Liang, M. H., & Stern, S. H. (1987). Colchicine in acute gout: Reassessment of risks and benefits. *JAMA, 257*(14), 1920–1922.

Simon, L. S. (1995). Actions and toxicity of non-steroidal anti-inflammatory drugs. *Current Opinion in Rheumatology, 7*, 159–166.

Star, V. L., & Hochberg, M. C. (1993). Prevention and management of gout. *Drugs, 45*(2), 212–222.

Star, V. L., & Hochberg, M. C. (1994). Gout: Steps to relieve acute symptoms, prevent further attacks. *Consultant, 34*, 1697–1706.

Tate, G. A. (1993). Gout: Clinical and laboratory features. In H. R. Schumacher, Jr., J. H. Klippel, & W. J. Koopman (Eds.), *Primer on the rheumatic diseases* (10th ed.). Atlanta: Arthritis Foundation.

Terkeltaub, R. (1993) Gout: Epidemiology, pathology, and pathogenesis in rheumatic diseases. In H. R. Schumacher, Jr., J. H. Klippel, & W. J. Koopman (Eds.), *Primer on the Rheumatic Diseases* (10th ed.). Atlanta: Arthritis Foundation.

Uy, J. P., Nuwayhid, N., & Saadeh, C. (1996). Unusual presentations of gout: Tips for accurate diagnosis. *Postgraduate Medicine, 100*(1), 253–268.

Wallace, S. L., & Singer, J. Z. (1988). Review: Systemic toxicity associated with the intravenous administration of colchicine—Guidelines for use. *Journal of Rheumatology, 15*, 495–499.

Wallace, S. L., Singer, J. Z., Duncan, G. J., et al. (1991). Renal function predicts colchicine toxicity: Guidelines for the prophylactic use of colchicine for gout. *Journal of Rheumatology, 18*, 264–269.

## Low Back Pain

Agency for Health Care Policy and Research. (1994). Acute low back problems in adults. AHCPR Publication No. 95-0642 Rockville, MD: U.S. Department of Health and Human Services.

Bigos, S. J., Deyo, R. A., Romanowski, T. S., & Whitten, R. R. (1995). The new thinking on low-back pain. *Patient Care, 29*, 140–177.

Borenstein, D. (1993). Medical therapy of low back pain. *Orthopaedic Review, 22*(1), 20–25.

Brody, M. (1996). Low back pain. *Annals of Emergency Medicine, 27*, 454–456.

Cailliet, R. (1995). *Low back pain syndrome* (5th ed.). Philadelphia: F. A. Davis.

Connelly, C. (1996). Patients with low back pain. *Postgraduate Medicine, 100*, 143–156.

Deen, H. G., Jr. (1996). Diagnosis and management of lumbar disk disease. *Mayo Clinic Proceedings, 71*, 283–287.

Gustafson, M. C. (1995). To prevent back injury, change behavior. *Occupational Health and Safety, 64*, 67–80.

Hadler, N. M. (1993). Disorders of the back and neck. In R. H. Schumacher, Jr., J. H. Klippel, & W. J. Koopman (Eds.), *Primer on the rheumatic diseases* (10th ed.). Atlanta: Arthritis Foundation.

Hainline, B. (1995). Low back injury. *Clinics in Sports Medicine, 14*(1), 241–265.

Malmivaara, A., Hakkinen, U., Aro, T., et al. (1995). The treatment of acute low back pain—Bed rest, exercises, or ordinary activity? *New England Journal of Medicine, 332*(6), 351–355.

Marras, W. S., Lavender, S. A., Leurgans, S. E., et al. (1995). Biomechanical risk factors for occupationally related low back disorders. *Ergonomics, 38*(2), 377–410.

Nightingale, S. L. (1995). Chlorzoxazone warning on hepatotoxicity is strengthened. *JAMA, 274*(24), 1903.

Peate, W. F. (1994). Occupational musculoskeletal disorders. *Primary Care, 21*(2), 313–327.

Ross, P. (1994). Ergonomic hazards in the workplace: Assessment and prevention. *AAOHN Journal, 42*(4), 171–176.

Seimon, L. P. (1995). *Low back pain clinical diagnosis and management* (2nd ed.). New York: Denos Vermande.

U.S. Department of Health and Human Services. (1994). Acute low back problems in adults: Assessment and treatment (AHCPR Publication No. 95-0643). *Orthopaedic Nursing, 14*(5), 37–52.

Waldman, H. J. (1994). Centrally acting skeletal muscle relaxants and associated drugs. *Journal of Pain and Symptom Management, 9*(7), 434–431.

## Tendinitis, Bursitis, Sprains, and Strains

Baumert, P. W., Jr. (1995). Acute inflammation after injury: Quick control speeds rehabilitation. *Postgraduate Medicine, 97*(2), 35–49.

Onieal, M. (August, 1996). Common wrist and ankle injuries. *Advance for Nurse Practitioners*, 31–36.

Schwartz, R. G., & Weinstein, S. M. (1996). Getting a handle on cumulative trauma disorders. *Patient Care, 30*, 118–142.

Shbeeb, M. I., & Matteson, E. L. (1996). Trochanteric bursitis (greater trochanter pain syndrome). *Mayo Clinic Proceedings, 71*, 565–569.

# 27

# DERMATOLOGIC DISORDERS

*Candace M. Burns and Douglas F. Covey*

Approximately 7% of patients treated in primary care settings have dermatological problems. Conditions are seen across the life cycle and those addressed in this chapter include: bacterial, fungal, viral, and yeast infections of the hair, skin, and nails; infestations, bites, and stings; dermatitis; acne; sunburn, minor burns, and recognition of possibly cancerous skin lesions; and psoriasis and pityriasis rosea.

Treatment is dependent upon accurate diagnosis. Thorough examination of the skin requires inspection and palpation of the entire body, nails, scalp, and hair in good light. The sequence of the appearance, onset, and duration of lesions—both primary and secondary changes—is very important. It is beyond the scope of this chapter to detail assessment of the skin and appendages.

## BACTERIAL INFECTIONS

Bacterial infections usually develop in skin that has been damaged by chemical, mechanical, or thermal trauma, infection, or inflammation. The two most common organisms causing infection are *Staphylococcus aureus* and *Streptococcus pyogenes* (group A streptococcus) (Barker, Burton, & Zieve, 1995; Dockery, 1997; Goroll, May, & Mulley, 1995; Hirschmann, 1996; Sauer & Hall, 1996). Bacterial skin infections may be divided into *primary infections*—impetigo, ecthyma, folliculitis, furuncle, carbuncle, cellulitis,

sweat gland infections—and *secondary infections*—cutaneous diseases with secondary infection, infected ulcers, infected eczematoid dermatitis. Systemic bacterial infections such as chancroid and gonorrhea are dealt with elsewhere in the text. Refer to Chapter 36.

## PRIMARY INFECTIONS

*Impetigo* is a superficial but contagious skin infection usually caused by S. *pyogenes* and S. *aureus*. Although common in children, it may be seen at any age or among those living in close quarters. Lack of good hygiene is a predisposing factor, and it is common in hot, humid climates. There are two forms:

- *Nonbullous impetigo* lesions are small thin-walled vesicles or pustules on an erythematous base that rupture and discharge a honey-colored serous fluid that forms yellow-brown crusts when dried. Lesions are most commonly seen on the face and extremities. Impetigo develops in skin damaged by previous minor trauma such as cuts, abrasions, or insect bites. The involved areas may be pruritic, and regional lymph node enlargement may be present. A rare complication (<1% cases) of nonbullous impetigo is acute poststreptococcal glomerulonephritis. It occurs with selected strains of S. *pyogenes* (Dockery, 1997; Hirschmann, 1996).

- *Bullous impetigo* is less common. The characteristic lesions are thin-walled bullae usually less than 3 cm in diameter that rupture easily. The lesions may form on untraumatized skin, and the fluid may be amber, white, or yellow pus. Once the blister ruptures, the erythematous base dries to a shiny "varnish-like" crust (Dockery, 1997). The usual causative organism is *S. aureus*.

*Ecthyma,* another superficial bacterial infection, is deeper than impetigo and commonly seen in children, usually on the buttocks and thighs. It is commonly caused by beta-hemolytic streptococci. The primary lesion is characterized by a vesicle or vesicopustule arising on an erythematous base. The lesion enlarges to a diameter of 3 cm but proceeds to deep erosions in the epidermis covered by a thick, dry, hard crust (Dockery, 1997; Hirschman, 1996; Orkin & Maibach, 1991).

*Folliculitis* is a common bacterial infection of the hair follicle usually caused by coagulase-positive staphylococci. The infection may be superficial or deep. In the superficial form, the erythema and swelling are limited to the shallow portion of the hair follicle. The lesion is characterized by a red, elevated, slightly tender pustule. Deeper infections involving the entire hair follicle usually have a larger area of erythema and are quite painful. Pseudodomal folliculitis is a form of folliculitis that develops after exposure to a contaminated hot tub. The infection can occur several hours or days after the exposure and is most commonly seen on the legs, buttocks, and arms.

*Cellulitis* and *erysipelas* occur when the superficial streptococcal infection spreads to the deeper dermis and subcutaneous fat, cellulitis, and dermal lymphatics. Systemic symptoms of fever, tachycardia, confusion, regional lymphadenitis, and hypotension may also occur. Predisposing factors include edema, inflammation, tinea pedis, and skin permanently damaged by trauma, ie, burns, radiation, or surgery. Facial cellulitis in young children 6–36 months may develop from *Haemophilus influenzae.* Periorbital cellulitis—infection of the tissues around the eye—is commonly seen as edema and pain and often accompanied by mild fever. Orbital cellulitis is generally due to a contagious sinus infection characterized by proptosis, restricted eye movement, pain with eye movement, and high fever (Eisenbaum, 1997). Cellulitis may also occur in normal skin. It is characterized by erythema and brawny edema that is tender with poorly defined borders.

*Furunculosis* is an acute staphylococcal infection of the hair follicle in which the cellulitis has spread into adjacent dermis accompanied by a greater degree of pain and inflammation. The lesion is characterized by an inflamed nodule with a pustular center through which the hair emerges.

A *carbuncle* is an extensive infection of several adjoining hair follicles (furuncles) with several openings onto the surface of the skin. Carbuncles are more commonly seen in adults on the neck and back and are more common in patients with diabetes mellitus.

*Sweat gland* infection is quite rare; however, prickly heat, a sweat retention disease, frequently develops secondary infection (Sauer & Hall, 1996).

## SECONDARY INFECTIONS

Secondary bacterial infection of the skin is a complicating factor of another skin disease, including ulcers. Delay in treating the primary disease can predispose the patient to secondary infection. The presence of a secondary bacterial infection can also make correct diagnosis of the primary disease more challenging.

*S. aureus,* including methicillin-resistant *S. aureus* (MRSA); streptococci; enterococci; Enterobacteriaceae; and anaerobes are common organisms causing secondary infection of skin disorders, including diabetic foot ulcers. The increased prevalence of these infections may be due to antimicrobial overuse (Goldstein, Citron, & Nesbit, 1996).

## SPECIFIC CONSIDERATIONS FOR PHARMACOTHERAPY

### When Drug Therapy Is Needed

Bacterial skin infections should be treated as soon as possible to prevent spread and to contain the progression to a more serious condition. Cleanliness and correct treatment of superficial skin trauma may help prevent infections such as impetigo. The affected area should be cleansed regularly with antibacterial soaps and topical antiseptics, or antibiotics should be applied to cuts, bites, and abrasions.

### Short- and Long-Term Goals of Pharmacotherapy

The goal of treatment is to prevent acute and long-term complications. Eradication of the offending organism and supportive therapy are of immediate concern while avoiding superinfection, systemic infection or other complications, scarring, or disability as well. Open ulcers colonized by bacteria share the treatment goal of resolving the infection and addressing the cause of the ulcer as well.

## Nonpharmacologic Therapy

Primary prevention is an important part of overall treatment. Patients should be encouraged to improve their hygiene with more frequent bathing and use of a bactericidal soap. Pustules and crusts of lesions should be removed during bathing to facilitate penetration of topical medications. Warm compresses may be applied to furuncles to promote drainage of the pus; large furuncles and carbuncles may require incision for drainage.

Clothing and bedding should be changed frequently and washed with hot, soapy water. The health history should include use of drugs that can cause lesions that mimic or cause pyodermas, such as iodides, bromides, testosterone, corticosteroids, and lithium (Dockery, 1997; Sauer & Hall, 1996). Patients with chronic skin infections should be assessed to rule out diabetes mellitus or other predisposing systemic diseases and immunosuppression. Patients should also be instructed to avoid oily hair care products and tanning oils as appropriate. Furuncles, if fluctuant, require incision and drainage. Squeezing can cause bacteremia (Middleton, 1996).

## Time Frame for Initiating Pharmacotherapy

Treatment should be initiated as soon as the diagnosis is made. Instructing the patient/caregiver about interventions to prevent future infections is an important part of therapy. In cases in which the infection is contagious, the patient should use separate towels and wash cloths, bedding, etc.

## Overview of Drug Classes for Treatment

Since the normal skin flora is generally responsible for primary infections, antibiotics to treat coagulase-positive staphylococci or beta-hemolytic streptococci are the mainstays of therapy. They include the macrolide antibiotics (erythromycin, neomycin), penicillins, cephalosporins, and mupirocin. Secondary infection medications will need to be directed at those organisms found in primary infections, as well as organisms such as *Proteus*, *Pseudomonas*, and *Escherichia coli*.

See Drug Tables 102, 805.

## Assessment and History Taking

Bacterial skin infections are generally characterized by pain at the site of infection, with significant individual variability. However, impetigo is often painless. Pruritis is generally present with impetigo, cellulitis, folliculitis, and erythrasma. Scratching may cause further trauma to the skin and lead to secondary infection. Chills, fever, and malaise may develop acutely and signify spread of the infection to deeper tissues or the bloodstream.

Cultures of the skin and biopsies have marginal value. However, Gram's stain and culture of pus or deeply necrotic material may be of value. Magnetic resonance imaging (MRI) or computerized tomographic (CT) scans are useful with severe cellulitis in diabetics and can distinguish preseptal from postseptal cellulitis. Bone scans and bone biopsies with culture may be indicated in selected cases of cellulitis to reveal concomitant osteomyelitis. Wood's lamp is useful in erythasma since the infected skin fluoresces coral red (Middleton, 1996).

## Patient/Caregiver Information

Symptoms of common adverse drug reactions (ADRs) and drug toxicity, administration issues, and contraindications are listed in Drug Tables 102 and 805. Information should be taught to each patient and caregiver as appropriate and applicable. Information relative to significant food and drug interactions as discussed below should also be included in patient/caregiver education. Patients are generally placed on bed rest; getting up to use the bathroom is generally permitted. The importance of not scratching the affected areas must be stressed with the patient and caregiver. Also, it is important to teach the patient to take or use the medication(s) as indicated. The patient should be instructed to report progress or lack thereof to the primary care provider.

## OUTCOMES MANAGEMENT

### Selecting an Appropriate Agent

***Impetigo and ecthyma.*** Superficial impetigo, if mild, can be treated with topical erythromycin, neosporin, or mupirocin. Moderate to severe impetigo and ecthyma require a 10-day course of a beta-lactamase–resistant drug such as erythromycin or dicloxacillin, in addition to the topical therapy. Ecthyma lesions can produce scarring so should be treated more aggressively, even for mild cases.

**Folliculitis.**    Following warm soaks to aid the extraction of the pustule and reduce the inflammation, folliculitis may be treated with topical antiinfective agents such as bacitracin, neomycin, or mupirocin. In superficial folliculitis, this is all that may be necessary. For more widespread or deeper lesions, oral antibiotics directed at *S. aureus* organisms are required (cloxacillin, dicloxacillin, erythromycin).

**Cellulitis.**    In addition to the application of cool wet compresses, oral antibiotic therapy is required for cellulitis. Penicillinase-resistant penicillins or cephalosporins are generally used. Dicloxacillin seems to be particularly beneficial.

**Furunculosis and carbuncles.**    Treatment with warm wet compresses will relieve the pain and assist in both relieving the pustule and in penetration of topical agents. Topical and systemic therapy is necessary and mimics that used for more widespread folliculitis.

## Monitoring for Efficacy

Resolution of the infection is the primary endpoint. If improvement or eradication is not seen in 1 week, cultures may be necessary.

## Significant Food and Drug Interactions and Management

Food interactions relate to the oral antibiotics used for these conditions. Erythromycin absorption is quicker without food, but many patients do not tolerate the GI side effects of this drug. In that case, food may be taken without losing overall effectiveness. Dicloxacillin should be given on an empty stomach for maximal absorption.

## Monitoring for Toxicity

Neosporin ointment may have a potential for causing a contact dermatitis if used long-term. The macrolide antibiotics (erythromycin) may cause GI intolerance as mentioned above.

## Follow-up Recommendations

If after a week of treatment for impetigo, the lesions have not resolved, antibiotic resistance or poor compliance should be suspected. At this point, a new culture should be obtained from the base of the lesion below the crust. Antibiotic therapy should be adjusted accordingly. Ecthyma lesions are slower to heal, but can be evaluated at 1 week as well. If improvement is not seen at that point, cultures should be done.

# FUNGAL AND YEAST INFECTIONS

Superficial fungal infections are common, infecting and surviving on dead keratin, ie, the top layer of the skin (stratum corneum or keratin layer). Dermatophytes are responsible for the vast majority of skin, hair, and nail fungal infections. Lesions vary in appearance and should be verified for appropriate diagnosis and treatment.

## DERMATOPHYTES

Superficial fungal infections of the skin affect various sites of the body. Therefore, fungal diseases of the skin are classified according to the location of the infection into the following clinical types: tinea of the feet (tinea pedis), tinea of the hands (tinea manus), tinea of the nails (onychomycosis), tinea of the groin (tinea cruris or "jock itch"), tinea of smooth skin (tinea corporis), tinea of the scalp (tinea capitis), and tinea of the beard and moustache (tinea barbae) (Skinner & Baselski, 1996).

*Tinea pedis,* or "athlete's foot," is common. Blisters occur between the toes and on the soles and sides of the feet. In chronic infections, the entire sole is dry and covered with a fine silvery white scale. The skin is pink, tender, and pruritic. Secondary bacterial infection, maceration, and fissures are common. The diagnosis of tinea pedis in the prepubertal child is uncommon; atopic or contact dermatitis is a more likely diagnosis in this age group (Morelli & Weston, 1997).

Primary prevention should be taught to all patients: Wear shower shoes or thongs in public or communal showers and locker rooms and footwear made of natural fibers (eg, leather shoes, cotton or wool socks), avoid going barefoot, and change socks daily.

*Acute vesicular tinea pedis* is a highly inflammatory fungal infection of the foot. It is seen in individuals who wear occlusive shoes. This acute infection often develops after a chronic infection. Vesicles from a few to many form on the sole and dorsum of the foot. The vesicles may fuse into bullae or remain as collections of fluid under the thick scale on the sole of the foot. Secondary bacterial infection is common.

*Tinea of the hands* is quite rare. Careful differential diagnosis—ie, contact dermatitis, atopic eczema, psoriasis—is essential. The primary lesions appear as blisters on the palms and fingers at the edge of red areas with clear borders. It is frequently seen in association with tinea pedis.

*Onychomycosis* of the toenails is quite common and frequently accompanies tinea of the foot, whereas fungal infection of the finger nails is rather uncommon. The nail detaches distally and laterally with subsequent thickening and deformity. Secondary infection is common.

*Tinea cruris* is a common fungal infection of the groin area, mostly in men, and is seen on the crural fold, scrotum, penis, thighs, perianal area, and buttocks. The primary lesions appear bilaterally as fan-shaped, red, scaly patches with a sharp, slightly raised border. Small vesicles may be seen in the active border (Sauer & Hall, 1996). Secondary bacterial infection may occur. It is especially common in the summer months as it thrives in warm, moist areas.

*Tinea of the smooth skin*—ringworm of the skin—is most commonly seen in children, can occur at any age, and is highly contagious. The primary lesions are round, oval, or semicircular scaly patches with slightly raised borders that are usually vesicular. Secondary infection can occur.

*Tinea capitis* can occur in two forms, noninflammatory and inflammatory. The noninflammatory type occurs most frequently in children aged 3 to 8, usually in the posterior scalp, causing gray, scaly round patches with broken hairs appearing as bald areas. Secondary bacterial infection is rare (Sauer & Hall, 1996). The inflammatory type is characterized by pustular, scaly, round patches with broken hairs resulting in patchy baldness and frequently is seen in children and farmers. Secondary bacterial-like infection is common (Sauer & Hall, 1996). Fungal culture is recommended in cases of suspected tinea capitis (Morelli & Weston, 1997). Health care providers should consult the local health department regarding guidelines for school attendance.

*Tinea of the beard and moustache* appears as follicular, pustular, or sharp-bordered ring-worm-type lesions or deep, boggy inflammation masses (Sauer & Hall, 1996). Secondary infection is common.

## CANDIDIASIS

Candidiasis (moniliasis) is a fungal infection caused by *Candida albicans*, resulting in lesions in the mouth, vagina, skin, nails, lungs, and gastrointestinal tract. The organisms live in the normal flora of the mouth, vaginal tract, and gastrointestinal system. Pregnancy, oral contraceptives, antibiotic therapy, certain endocrinopathies (eg, diabetes mellitus), and factors related to immunosuppression allow the yeast to become pathogenic (Habif, 1996). The specific appearance of the lesion varies with the location of the infection.

*Oral candidiasis,* or "thrush," is common in neonates, young children, and immunocompromised adults. It is characterized by discrete or confluent white patches on the buccal mucosa, tongue, gingiva, palate, and or oropharynx. Thrush develops in 5–10% of neonates, who usually acquired it during delivery (Ray, 1996). Prolonged wearing of dentures (especially all night long), poor dental hygiene, and factors associated with aging increase the risk of developing thrush in the older adult. Broad-spectrum antibiotic, systemic corticosteroids, and cytotoxic and/or radiation therapy are common predisposing factors (Ray, 1996).

*Candida vulvovaginitis* and *balanitis* are covered in Chap. 35.

*Candida intertrigo* commonly occurs on the surfaces of the gluteal, perineal, and inguinal folds; scrotum; axillae; inframammary regions; and pannus folds of the abdomen. Moisture, heat, and friction lead to maceration and erythema. Lesions are characterized by vesicopustules, bright erythema, and superficial erosions, surrounded by peripheral scaling; satellite pustules are usually seen (Ray, 1996). Diaper dermatitis is a variation of intertrigo. The warm, moist, occluded environment and the ammoniacal urine contribute to the process (Ray, 1996).

*Candidal paronychia* and *onychia* develop in individuals who have their hands in water or do other wet work for prolonged periods of time, eg, dishwashers, bartenders, and food handlers. The infection develops in the nail plate and nail folds. The disease is characterized by swollen, erythematous, painful nail folds and mild serous or purulent discharge (Ray, 1996). Secondary infection may occur.

*Congenital* and *neonatal candidiases* are commonly seen in the newborn. Congenital candidiasis usually occurs within 12 h of birth and is characterized by a generalized erythema and vesiculopustules over the head, neck, hands, feet, and trunk. Oral thrush may develop with time. Neonatal candidiasis is acquired during birth, but lesions do not manifest until several days after delivery. Erythema, vesiculopustules, and erosive lesions resembling intertriginous candidiasis are diffuse and accentuated in the skin folds.

## SPECIFIC CONSIDERATIONS FOR PHARMACOTHERAPY

### When Drug Therapy Is Needed

Fungal and candidal infections can be disfiguring if left untreated and allowed to progress. Nail infections can be particularly difficult to resolve if the entire nail and bed are involved. Tinea versicolor will leave hypopigmented spots on the skin that will take sunlight or UV radiation to recolor. Additionally, these infections can be contagious, so quick resolution prevents spread of infection to others.

### Short- and Long-Term Goals of Pharmacotherapy

Stopping the spread of infection, both on the patient and to others, and eradication of infectious agent should be high on the priority list. In the more difficult cases, such as onychomycosis, maintaining remission and managing outbreaks when they occur may be all that can be done.

### Nonpharmacologic Therapy

Since fungal infections are contagious, patients should be taught to avoid sharing combs, headgear, and other personal items. Candidiasis thrives best in warm, moist environments, so the keys to prevention are to maintain good hygiene and ventilation and to keep the skin as dry as possible. Caregivers should remind patients to remove dentures at night and brush teeth daily; wear clean, cotton clothing or other fabrics that "breathe"; wear cotton underwear, socks, and cotton gloves inside rubber gloves when hands are wet for long periods of time; and change diapers frequently. Cornstarch powder should be avoided since it provides nutrients for *Candida* growth (Ray, 1996).

### Time Frame for Initiating Pharmacotherapy

Treatment should be initiated as soon as possible after proper diagnosis.

### Overview of Drug Classes for Treatment

Topical antifungal agents may be divided into (1) polyene antibiotics, such as nystatin, which is effective against *Candida* but not dermatophytes; (2) imidazoles, such as clotrimazole, sulconazole, and ketoconazole, which are fungistatic at low concentrations and fungicidal at high concentrations; and (3) allylamines, such as terbinafine, which is fungicidal. The latter two classes are effective against yeasts as well as dermatophytes. Selenium sulfide shampoos are also very effective in certain tinea infections.

Oral agents include nystatin for candidal infections, griseofulvin for tinea infections, and ketoconazole, fluconazole, and itraconazole for either of these or mixed infections.

See Drug Tables 102.10, 103.

### Assessment and History Taking

Correct diagnosis is essential to proper treatment. Refer to the specific description of each type of lesion. Direct visualization under the microscope showing the branching hyphae in keratinized material is the most important test for correct diagnosis (Habif, 1996). Hyphae may be difficult to find in a potassium hydroxide (KOH) wet mount. Chlorazol fungal stain, Swartz Lamkins fungal stain, or Parker's blue-black ink clearly stain hyphae, making them visible under the microscope (Habif, 1996). Fungal culture is necessary for fungal infections of the hair and nails (Habif, 1996). A sterile cotton swab moistened with sterile water or on an agar plate and rubbed vigorously over the lesion yields good results and is preferable for use with children (Jones, 1991; Cohn, 1992; Elewski & Weil, 1996; Habif, 1996).

### Patient/Caregiver Information

Information about correct application of medications as described in the relevant drug tables should be taught to the patient and caregiver as appropriate. Refer above by disorder for patient education relative to prevention. Ketoconazole and itraconazole should not be taken within 2 h of use of antacids. Both medications should be taken with a full meal. Patients and caregivers should also be instructed about common adverse drug reactions (ADRs) and toxic effects.

## OUTCOMES MANAGEMENT

### Selecting an Appropriate Agent

Selecting an agent is based on location, causative organism (or likely causative organism if a KOH prep or culture evaluation is not done), and severity. Topical therapy is relatively ineffective for *tinea capitis*. Therefore, treatment includes selenium sulfide for 1 to several days to reduce spore shedding *and* oral griseofulvin to eradicate the fungus. Griseofulvin is only effective against dermatophytes. It also has slight antiinflammatory activity. Since the infection will require a few months of therapy with an oral agent, it is a good idea to confirm the diagnosis with a scraping or culture. After 6 weeks, KOH preparation cultures should be repeated. Treatment should continue for 2 weeks after cultures are negative.

*Tinea corporis* treatment consists of topical imidazole antifungals twice daily (clotrimazole, miconazole) or once daily (ketoconazole, sulconazole) for 4–6 weeks. The preparation should be placed thinly over the lesion and the surrounding skin about 1 cm out from the area. For more widespread infection, the treatment of choice is griseofulvin. Patients whose infection is resistant to treatment or who cannot tolerate griseofulvin can use oral ketoconazole. Note that miconazole is not effective against *Microsporum* and sulconazole is only effective against *Trichophyton*.

*Tinea cruris* and mild *tinea pedis* usually subside with a few days of topical imidazoles. *Tinea manus* may also respond well to topical imidazoles, but will require 6–8 weeks of therapy. Refractory tinea pedis or manus requires oral griseofulvin or ketoconazole.

*Candidiasis* may be treated with topical nystatin cream or an imidazole cream. Do not use the ointments. Topicals are applied two times a day until complete clearing is seen, generally in 2–3 weeks. In resistant cases amphotericin B 3% lotion or cream four times daily, or oral ketoconazole (10–14 days) may be necessary. Topical drying powders (such as dry talc) may be helpful in preventing recurrences.

*Paronychial Candida* infections are best treated with liquid clotrimazole or cyclopirox since delivery to areas is difficult. Concurrent *Pseudomonas* infection is not uncommon and should be treated appropriately.

*Tinea versicolor* treatment should be initiated with topical selenium sulfide 2.5% lotion lathered and left on for 15–20 min every night for 2 weeks. Alternatively, some evidence exists that applying selenium sulfide to the body after an evening shower, sleeping overnight with the lotion on the body, and rinsing it off in the morning may resolve the infection. A reapplication 1 week later may be required in resistant cases. Alternative therapies include ketoconazole shampoo daily for 2 weeks, sodium thiosulfate applied daily for 2 weeks, zinc pyrithione 1% daily for 2 weeks, or imidazoles twice daily for 2 weeks. Sulfur soaps are effective prophylactically. Repigmentation of the hypopigmented spots is necessary to totally visualize the resolution. Ketoconazole orally, 200–400 mg depending on the extent, once and repeated in 1 week may be needed.

There are several other agents available for treatment of these conditions. Cyclopirox is as effective as imidazoles for all three types of fungi and is effective against all species of dermatophytes. It is applied twice daily. The allylamines (naftifine, terbinafine) may be alternative agents for candidiasis and tinea versicolor. Haloprogin, an older agent, is only effective for tineas. Tolnaftate, undecylenic acid, and Whitfield's ointment are over-the-counter alternatives.

### Monitoring for Efficacy

Monitoring will require visual inspection, and repeating a KOH preparation and culture.

### Significant Food and Drug Interactions and Management

Ketoconazole and itraconazole should not be taken within 2 h of antacids. Both should be taken with a full meal. Griseofulvin is better absorbed if given with milk or food. This may also reduce side effects. Griseofulvin may also decrease the effectiveness of oral contraceptives, anticoagulants, and barbiturates. A disulfiram-like reaction may also occur if this drug is taken with alcohol. Ketoconazole should not be given with antacids since it needs an acid medium to be absorbed; ketoconazole can increase blood levels of both digoxin and cyclosporine, so proper monitoring is important.

### Monitoring for Toxicity

Topical therapy is rarely a problem in terms of toxicity. In some instances irritation and stinging have been noted. If burning, erythema, or pruritis occur, switching to another agent may prove beneficial. Skin discoloration with amphotericin B can occur. Discontinuing the offending agent will resolve the problem.

The most common side effects of griseofulvin include diarrhea and headache. Both usually resolve after the initial week of therapy; however, persistence requires a dose reduction. Nausea, vomiting, urticaria, and photosensitivity occur occasionally. *Candidal* infections, and rarely leukopenia and proteinuria, may occur. Note that griseofulvin is teratogenic and impairs absorption of birth control pills. Young women who are sexually active need to be made fully aware of this and instructed to use two forms of birth control during treatment.

Ketoconazole may elevate liver function tests, so pretreatment and periodic analysis during treatment is necessary. All the oral antifungal agents may alter the pharmacokinetics of several other drugs, so care should be taken when concomitantly prescribing these agents.

## Follow-up Recommendations

Depending on the circumstances and location and extent of involvement, follow-up can be once, at 6–8 weeks, or every few months.

## ACNE

Acne vulgaris is a disease of the pilosebaceous unit of the skin. It is the most common skin disease in the United States, affecting 85% of the population between the ages of 12 and 25 years and frequently persisting or recurring in the third, fourth, and fifth decades (Whitmore, 1996). Eight percent of adults 25 to 34 years of age and 3% of 35- to 44-year-olds experience some form of acne (Bergfeld, 1995; Clark, 1993; Kaminer & Gilchrist, 1995; Thiboutot & Lookingbill, 1995). Men and women are affected nearly equally (Clark, 1993). Neonatal acne occurs in response to maternal androgen, first appears at 4–6 weeks of age, and lasts until 4–6 months (Morelli & Weston, 1997). The disease can contribute to psychosocial problems such as clinical depression, anxiety, self-imposed isolation, low-self-esteem, and negative body image (Whitmore, 1996).

Acne vulgaris is a chronic disorder of the sebaceous glands, particularly those on the face, chest, and back, where the glands are the largest and most dense. Sebum from the glands reaches the surface by emptying into the hair follicle and flowing along the hair shaft; the two skin appendages form the pilosebaceous unit (Whitmore, 1996).

There are two primary types of acne lesions: noninflammatory and inflammatory. Noninflammatory acne lesions are further subdivided into closed comedones and open comedones. Inflammatory acne lesions are comprised of papules or pustules and nodules.

The initial acne lesion is the comedo, a plug formed by the impaction of the opening of the pilosebaceous duct by keratin debris and dried sebum. The closed comedones are also known as "whiteheads." The open comedones—"blackheads"—are due to oxidation of melanin and sebum in the plugs (Whitmore, 1996). Erythematous tender papules form when comedones become inflamed as the normal skin bacteria, *Propionibacterium acnes,* proliferate in response to increased sebum. Pustules form as the inflammation progresses and in severe cases become cystic due to abscess formation deep in the dermis. Scarring may occur from acne and is usually of the pitted type.

Four conditions must be present for acne to occur: (1) androgen-stimulated sebum production; (2) *P. acnes,* the anaerobic diphtheroid that constitutes most of the normal follicular flora and proliferates in response to increased sebum; (3) altered keratinization and desquamation of the cells lining the follicles; and (4) a host inflammatory response (Whitmore, 1996).

Neonatal acne may occur in the newborn shortly after birth or in infancy. Acneiform lesions generally occur on the nose and cheeks. The large sebaceous glands are stimulated by maternal androgens. The lesions generally clear without treatment.

## When Drug Therapy Is Needed

Due to the external nature of this disorder, it can have profound psychological sequelae. Further, if the more severe cases are left untreated, scarring and chronic infection can occur.

## Short- and Long-Term Goals of Pharmacotherapy

The goals of treating acne are to reduce the acute inflammation and redness, minimize recurrences, and eliminate the potentially disfiguring consequences.

## Nonpharmacologic Therapy

Patients should be instructed to gently wash the face with the fingertips two times a day using a mild soap. Avoid oil-based skin care, makeup, and hair care products.

Certain medications—hormonal contraceptives, corticosteroids, lithium, iodides, phenytoin, anabolic steroids, and high doses of vitamin $B_2$ (riboflavin), $B_6$ (pyridoxine), and $B_{12}$ (cyanocobalamin)—have been associated with acne (Whitmore, 1996).

Natural sun exposure and ultraviolet light therapy have not been found to affect the course of the disease. There is no evidence that particular foods are acnegenic. Therefore, food restrictions are not indicated.

Surgery removes open comedones, closed comedones, and occasionally very small pustules. The instrument used (comedo extractor) has a flat surface with a central orifice. The contents of the lesion are expressed when firm even pressure is exerted around the lesion. The orifices of closed comedones may need to be enlarged by the use of vitamin A acid topically for 3–4 weeks to soften the closed comedones. Removal of closed comedones is important because they are the precursors of inflammatory lesions (Strauss, 1991).

## Time Frame for Initiating Pharmacotherapy

Treatment should be initiated as soon as acne develops.

## Overview of Drug Classes for Treatment

Effective treatments include topical antiinflammatory agents, antibiotic and peeling agents, oral antibiotics, topical and oral retinoids, and hormonal agonists and antagonists. Mild cases of comedonal acne may respond to a topical retinoid or benzoyl peroxide, whereas inflammatory lesions benefit from topical antibiotics. More severe inflammatory acne is treated with systemic antibiotics. Recalcitrant cases often require oral isotretinoin or hormonal therapies.

See Drug Tables 102, 605, 801.

## Assessment and History Taking

The type of acne, inflammatory or noninflammatory, and severity of the condition influence the treatment plan. The history should include duration, location of lesions, seasonal variation, aggravation by stress, current treatment of the condition (topical, systemic) and treatment of other coexisting conditions, over-the-counter medication use, past treatment and outcomes, family history of skin disorders, drug and other allergies, general health, impact of the disease including psychosocial, and for women premenstrual exacerbation, menstrual history, pregnancy status and history, use of oral contraceptives, and use of cosmetics, moisturizers, and hair care products. The physical examination should include type and number of lesions, location, gradation, complications, and other associated findings (Habif, 1996).

## Patient and Caregiver Information

The information regarding medication use, common ADRs, and toxic effects (refer to Drug Tables 102, 605, 801) should be taught to patients and caregivers as appropriate. Explain the mechanism of acne to the patient and caregiver. The treatment plan and a realistic time table also should be presented. Since acne often causes significant psychosocial effects, patients are often impatient and want immediate results. The treatment of acne and improvement of appearance generally takes several weeks. Patients and caregivers often require reassurance and emotional support.

## OUTCOME MANAGEMENT

### Selecting an Appropriate Agent

For the typical case of mild to moderate acne vulgaris, a clinician may begin by recommending exclusively topical therapy. Erythromycin or clindamycin may be applied either once or twice a day when the acne is predominately inflammatory. These antibiotics may be used alone or combined with tretinoin cream 0.025–0.05% applied sparingly at bedtime. Although more involved, the latter regimen treats both the comedonal and inflammatory phases of the disease. Alternatives include topical erythromycin or clindamycin in the morning and benzoyl peroxide 2.5–10% in a lotion base applied in the evening. The combination drug containing benzoyl peroxide and erythromycin (benzamycin) may be applied twice a day and gives very good clinical results.

Other agents may be substituted for erythromycin or clinidamycin when appropriate (ineffectiveness or adverse reactions). Tetracycline

0.25% is modestly effective. Meclocycline sulfosalicylate 1% cream is somewhat more effective than tetracycline and less staining.

More severe inflammatory acne is best treated using oral rather than topical antibiotics. Systemic agents useful in treating acne include estrogens, antiandrogens, tetracycline, erythromycin, minocycline, and clindamycin. Historically, the first choice of oral antibiotic has been one of the tetracyclines, such as tetracycline 250 mg four times a day, doxycycline 100 mg twice a day, or minocycline 50 mg or 100 mg once or twice a day depending upon the severity of the acne. Erythromycin is a good choice if the patient appears to be tetracycline-resistant. The dose is the same as for tetracycline. Tetracycline or erythromycin should be continued for 2–3 months until the lesions are suppressed (Morelli & Weston, 1997). Generally, the patient will respond to therapy within 6 weeks. Clindamycin 150 mg daily may also be used. Penicillins and cephalosporins are of little use in acne. The quinolones, such as ciprofloxacin, are effective in acne, but are quite costly and have not been demonstrated to be superior to less expensive antibiotics. Sulfanilamide drugs, such as Co-Trimoxazole, are often effective in acne that is resistant to tetracyclines or erythromycin. Tretinoin cream should be used concomitantly at bedtime.

Patients with severe nodular acne or those who do not respond to topical and oral therapy may be considered for oral isotretinoin therapy. This drug can actually cure acne after a 20-week course, but has considerable precautions associated with it. Most notable is the danger to a fetus. Women of childbearing age should be made aware of the well-documented teratogenic effects of the retinoids and use dual methods of birth control during therapy (Sykes & Webster, 1994).

Estrogens have been given to female patients with severe, recalcitrant, pustulocystic acne (Abel & Farber, 1993). Estrogens reduce sebum secretion and therefore may reduce the formation of acne. There may also be an indirect action on the sebaceous gland. Women for whom oral contraception is not contraindicated may be prescribed ethinyl estradiol at 80–100 μg. Smaller doses appear to be much less effective. A temporary flare of acne may occur during the initial cycles of therapy and upon discontinuation, and patients should be forewarned of this possibility (Strauss, 1991). The antiandrogen spironolactone has been used for short-term

control of acute acne at 100 mg daily with promising results.

Corticosteroids have been shown useful for men and women with androgen excess caused by a variety of endocrine disorders. Patients with resistant cystic acne should be tested for androgen excess. If apparent, therapies should be directed at lowering adrenal androgen production without totally suppressing the pituitary-adrenal axis. It is best to turn this form of treatment over to an endocrinologist for further workup and treatment.

In the interest of completeness, there are other therapies not as well studied but available. Acne surgery to remove the comedones may be cosmetically desirable, but will not affect the course of the acne. Injection of steroids into a cystic or nodular lesion has met with limited success. The use of x-ray or ultraviolet light therapies was once popular, but due to their carcinogenic effects, these therapies are now out of favor. Finally, the use of liquid nitrogen and solid carbon dioxide (cryotherapy) may accelerate the resolution of cystic and inflammatory acne lesions (Able & Farber, 1993).

## Significant Food and Drug Interactions and Management

Caution is necessary when prescribing oral antibiotics to patients with acne. Erythromycin and the sulfa drugs can upset the stomach and although their absorption is more rapid on an empty stomach, food may minimize the irritation. Tetracycline, doxycycline, and minocycline should not be taken with dairy products or products (such as antacids) containing magnesium, aluminum, or calcium, all of which bind to the drug and reduce the extent of absorption. Tetracycline is best taken on an empty stomach. Minocycline is not affected by food.

## Monitoring for Efficacy

Acne is a common self-limiting disease for which there are several effective therapeutic modalities. Concepts of therapy should be conveyed to the patient, and the importance of compliance should be emphasized. Achievement of clinical effectiveness by any given therapeutic regimen may require 6–8 weeks. Patients may also notice an exacerbation of acne after initiation of therapy. Inflammatory acne lesions may take approximately 4 weeks to surface; thereafter, new follicular plugging should be under control after 2 months of effective therapy. For topical agents, all acne-prone areas should be treated because the purpose of therapy is to prevent or minimize the formation of new lesions and to minimize the risk of scarring, a permanent endpoint for moderate to severe disease.

### Monitoring for Toxicity

Many of the topical agents used contain alcohol, which may dry and irritate the skin, causing redness and inflammation. A similar outcome can be expected with the use of topical corticosteroids. Since inflammation promotes new skin growth and may actually aid in the healing process, remind the patient that it will pass. In most cases, reducing the number of applications per day will help. If irritation continues, discontinuing use may be necessary. Switching to a gel or cream-based topical agent should be considered. Maintaining adequate fluid intake may also be of benefit.

Tetracycline antibiotics should not be prescribed to patients under 9 years old to avoid the risk of bone and tooth pigmentation. Long-term therapy with tetracyclines has been associated with the development of skin pigmentation and pigmented osteoma cutis (bluish or skin-colored, firm dermal lesions, typically on the face) (Walter & Macknet, 1991).

Sulfa drugs are known to cause hypersensitivity to the sun, and patients should be warned to use sunscreen. Rarely, blood dyscrasias have been noted, so a periodic CBC (every 6 months) would be appropriate.

Adverse effects with the use of oral isotretinoin and all other oral retinoids are particularly bothersome. The most common include generalized dryness of the skin and mucous membranes and hair loss. These all resolve after discontinuing the drug. Patients may experience myalgias and arthralgias. Abnormalities in laboratory parameters may also occur, such as elevation in triglycerides, cholesterol, and sometimes liver transaminases. But the greatest concern regarding oral retinoids is their extraordinary teratogenicity (Lammer, Chen, & Hoar, 1985; Stern, Rosa, & Baum, 1984).

## VIRAL INFECTIONS

Common viral diseases of the skin include herpes simplex, warts (verrucae), varicella and herpes zoster, and exanthematous diseases (measles, German measles, roseola, and erythema infectiosum). Since these disorders are distinct, treatment varies for each disease. There is no specific antiviral drug yet available.

Primary care providers have a major responsibility to ensure that all individuals receive primary prevention for the common viral diseases for which there is an FDA-approved vaccine. Refer to Chap. 11 for specific guidelines about immunization administration.

## HERPES SIMPLEX

The herpes simplex virus (HSV) is a member of the herpesvirus family that includes varicella (herpes zoster), cytomegalovirus, and Epstein-Barr virus (infectious mononucleosis). Herpes simplex viruses are divided into two major groups: type 1 (HSV-1) and type 2 (HSV-2). In general, HSV-1 causes diseases above the waist and HSV-2 causes diseases below the waist. However, either virus can infect any site on the skin or mucous membranes.

Herpes simplex viruses are transmitted through close personal contact via mucous membranes and broken epithelium. Primary infection in adults is usually through sexual contact. Primary infection in children is usually through close personal contact with infected adults or other children. In general, herpes simplex is characterized by recurring, localized painful vesicles that progress into erosions with crusts. The primary signs and symptoms vary with the location of the vesicles as follows (Jarratt & Dahl, 1991; Sams & Lynch, 1996; Sauer & Hall, 1996):

1. *Primary herpetic gingivostomatitis* is characterized by sore throat and fever. Painful vesicles and erosions occur on the tongue, palate, pharynx, gingivae, buccal mucosa, and lips. Incubation time from exposure ranges from 3–10 days, and it may persist for 2–6 weeks before resolving.

2. *Recurrent herpes labialis* occurs after the primary herpetic gingivostomatitis and is characterized by periodic localized vesicles on the vermilion border of the lip, commonly known as "fever blisters" or "cold sores." They usually resolve in 5–7 days. Recurrences may be triggered by trauma, sunburn, emotional stress, fatigue, menses, and upper respiratory infections.

3. *Herpetic whitlow* is herpes simplex infection of the fingers and hands. It is estimated that 2–5%

of the normal adult population shed the virus in saliva (Jarratt & Dahl, 1991); thus dental technicians, dentists, nurses, and physicians are at risk for acquiring the virus. Incubation time is 5–7 days. The primary infection is characterized by painful, deep, clustered vesicles; fever and regional lymphadenopathy may be present.

4. *Genital herpes* usually occurs within 5–10 days after sexual contact. Painful vesicles occur on the penis, vulva, or anus and rupture after a few days. Healing occurs usually within 2 weeks. Fever, headache, fatigue, and lymphadenopathy may accompany the vesicles. Patients may shed the virus prior to the eruption of lesions or development of symptoms.

5. *Neonatal herpes simplex* generally occurs in the presenting part of the newborn initially. Clusters of vesicles and bullae erode and crust. Mothers of the infants may be asymptomatic of the disease, making anticipation difficult even in high-risk pregnancies. The incubation period is 2–4 weeks. Neonatal herpes simplex may be fatal due to rapid progression to systemic infection. Early diagnosis is essential for the infant to receive appropriate intravenous therapy with acyclovir.

## WARTS

Warts (verrucae) are caused by the human papillomavirus (HPV). They can occur on any cutaneous or mucosal surface and have varying appearances depending upon the specific site and type of human papillomavirus. Human papillomavirus is transmitted by direct contact or indirectly by contact with infected surfaces, eg, shower floors or swimming pools (Jarratt & Dahl, 1991). Incubation averages 3 months.

The contagiousness of warts varies with the type of wart, the amount of virus it contains, and host susceptibility. Genital warts are particularly contagious, with contact infectivity rates higher than 60% (Stone & Lynch, 1996).

Most warts occurring in immunologically normal individuals remain benign. However, several types of HPV predispose infected individuals to the development of squamous cell carcinoma and cutaneous carcinomas of renal transplant patients (Stone & Lynch, 1996).

Children 6–12 years of age commonly develop warts. It is estimated that 65% of warts in children resolve spontaneously within 2 years (Jarratt & Dahl, 1991).

The characteristics of warts vary with location and specific type of HPV as follows:

1. *Common warts* (verrucae vulgaris) generally occur on the hands and distal forefingers. Initially, they appear as translucent vesicles and progress to hyperkeratotic papules 0.25–1+ cm in diameter. The warts may demonstrate punctate hemorrhages or "black dots" representing thrombosed dermal capillaries (Jarratt & Dahl, 1991; Stone & Lynch, 1996).

2. *Flat warts* (verrucae planae) are flat, skin-colored papules usually a few millimeters in diameter and occurring most commonly on the face, neck, forearms, knees, and backs of the hands. They may be quite numerous.

3. *Plantar warts* appear as circumscribed, thickened, slightly elevated papules with surface callus and thrombosed capillaries often visible. The entire heel or plantar surface of the foot may be covered with warts in severe infections. Confluent plaques called mosaic warts may also appear.

   Plantar warts may be confused with corns and calluses. A callus does not have tiny black dots representing hemorrhages, and a corn has a central nonbleeding core; warts demonstrate punctate bleeding points.

4. *Genital warts* (condylomata acuminata) most commonly occur as pale pink warts with numerous discrete narrow to wide projections on a broad base. The surface is smooth and moist and lacks hyperkeratosis. Warts may coalesce in the rectal or perianal area to form large, cauliflower-like masses. Another type of genital wart seen primarily in young, sexually active patients is multifocal, often with bilateral, red- or brown-pigmented, slightly raised, smooth papules (Habif, 1996). Lesions may occur in the external genitalia, perianal and pubic areas, intravaginally, and in the anal canal. Cervical lesions in women and anal lesions in men predispose to intraepithelial neoplasia. Genital warts in children should raise the question of sexual abuse although warts can be transmitted by the child or by a caregiver with warts on the hands.

## VARICELLA

Varicella—chicken pox—is a highly contagious viral infection transmitted through airborne droplets or vesicular fluid. Patients are contagious from 2 days prior to onset of the rash until all lesions have crusted. The incubation period averages 2 weeks with a range of 9–21 days. The prodromal symptoms may be absent or consist of low-grade fever, chills, malaise, and headache.

The rash begins on the trunk and spreads to the face and extremities. The severity of the disease varies greatly from mild to very severe. Lesions at different stages appear at the same time in any body area. Lesions begin as 2–4-mm red papules that gradually develop irregular borders (rose petal) as a thin-walled vesicle appears on the surface (dew drop). The lesions break within 8–12 h and crust. Pruritus accompanies the vesicular stage of the lesion.

Complications include secondary bacterial infection, encephalitis, Reye's syndrome, pneumonia, hepatitis (immunocompromised patients), and thrombocytopenia. Patients with defective, cell-mediated immunity or those on immunosuppressive drugs, especially systemic corticosteroids, generally experienced a prolonged course of the disease, more extensive eruption of lesions, and a greater incidence of complications (Habif, 1996). Pregnant women should be immediately referred to their obstetrical care provider for follow-up.

Varicella vaccine is available and approved for children and adults as primary prevention.

## HERPES ZOSTER

Herpes zoster—shingles—is a common viral disease believed to be caused by the same virus as chickenpox. It results from the reactivation of the virus and is seen in 10–20% of people in the United States (Elliott & Sams, 1996). It can occur at any age but is more common in older adults. When seen in children, it most often occurs in cases in which the mother had varicella during pregnancy, at which time the infant became infected and a latent infection was established (Elliott & Sams, 1996). Although not as contagious as the primary infection (varicella), it can cause varicella in unimmunized individuals.

The virus may spread to motor root ganglia and cause peripheral muscle weakness, leading to ophthalmoplegia or Bell's palsy. Involvement of sacral dermatomes can occasionally lead to urinary retention, frequency, and hematuria that generally resolve with time (Elliott & Sams, 1996).

The primary lesion is characterized by painful, multiple groups of vesicles or crusted lesions usually unilateral along one or two dermatomes. The prodrome consists of fever, malaise, headache, and localized pain and paresthesia lasting 1–4 days. Resolution occurs in approximately 2 weeks.

Pain is the most common problem in herpes zoster. Postherpetic neuralgia, defined as pain lasting longer than 1 month, is seen in 10–15% of patients. It resolves within 2 months in 50% of patients and within 1 year in 75%, but it may persist for many years in a small percentage (Elliott & Sams, 1996).

## VIRAL EXANTHEMS

Viral exanthems include rubeola (measles), roseola, rubella (German measles), and erythema infectiosum. They are common causes of generalized rashes, especially in children. Historically, exanthems were referred to by the order in which they were differentiated from other exanthems, ie, measles "first," scarlet fever "second," rubella "third," erythema infectiosum "fifth." More than 50 agents are known to cause viral exanthems (Frieden, 1996). The common exanthems are described as follows:

1. *Rubeola* (measles) is caused by infection with a paramyxovirus. A vaccine is available for primary prevention immunization. There are three forms of measles: typical, modified, and atypical. The incubation period averages 14 days. Typically, measles is characterized by a prodrome of 2–4 days of high fever, upper respiratory tract congestion, conjunctivitis, and cough. A pathognomonic lesion appears during the prodrome consisting of Koplik's spots, small white or blue-gray dots on an erythematous, granular base located on the buccal mucosa. The dots begin to fade within 2–3 days after the onset of the exanthem.

   The measles exanthem typically begins behind the ears at the hairline and spreads to involve the total body. Lesions begin as discrete erythematous papules and then become confluent, lasting about 4–7 days. Fever may persist for several days in addition to adenopathy, pharyngitis, and splenomegaly. Complications include pneumonia, otitis media, laryngotracheobronchitis, myocarditis, and encephalitis (rare).

   Modified measles generally occurs in partially immune hosts such as infants less than 9 months of age, persons with partial immunization failure, and those with secondary infection (Frieden, 1996). The course of the disease is generally shorter and milder than typical measles.

   Atypical measles is a characteristic syndrome that occurs in individuals previously immunized with killed virus vaccine (not used in the United

States since 1967) and is now quite rare. The disease is more abrupt; pneumonia is common and may be life-threatening.

2. *Rubella* (German measles) is a common viral infection that is usually benign in children. However, if a pregnant women contracts the disease during the first trimester, it can cause birth defects in the fetus. The incubation period averages 17 days. The prodrome consists of fever and malaise. The rash is similar to the measles rash but is usually less intense and of shorter duration, 2–3 days. Lymphadenopathy is common.

3. *Roseola* (exanthema subitum) is a common childhood rash. It is caused by the human herpesvirus 6 or herpesvirus 7 (Leach, Sumaya, & Brown, 1992). It most commonly occurs in children between the ages of 6 months to 3 years. The incubation period is 5–15 days. The prodrome is a high fever of 3–5 days' duration, followed by the appearance of the rash. The lesions are characterized by maculopapules 2–5 mm in size with irregular configurations most commonly on the neck and trunk with a duration of 1–2 days. Pruritus is uncommon.

4. *Erythema infectiosum* is caused by human parvovirus B19. It primarily affects children, but during epidemics may affect adults. The incubation period is 1–7 days. The prodrome may consist of headache, fever, malaise, nausea, and muscular aches. The rash begins on the cheeks as pink macules or papules that coalesce to form confluent erythematous patches resembling "slapped cheeks." The rash on the body is measles-like with a duration of 6–10 days. Itching is usually present. The presence of petechiae or purpura in an acral distribution may occur (Frieden, 1996). Infection of pregnant women during the first trimester can result in hydrops fetalis or fetal death in up to 19% of the cases (Frieden, 1996).

## SPECIFIC CONSIDERATIONS FOR PHARMACOTHERAPY

### When Drug Therapy Is Needed

The need for drug therapy varies with the specific viral infection. Herpes, varicella, and measles viruses are highly contagious and require prompt attention to limit the spread of infection. Some warts, such as condylomata acuminata, are also contagious. In some instances, failure to adequately treat a topical viral infection can result in scarring.

## Short- and Long-Term Goals of Pharmacotherapy

The goals of treatment of viral infections are to prevent secondary infection when applicable, minimize itching and discomfort, and address the social concerns, stigma, and altered body image that may occur with some of the diseases, eg, genital infections or warts.

## Nonpharmacologic Therapy

*Herpes simplex.* Primary gingivostomatitis is often accompanied by a painful mouth. Pain can be minimized with frequent mouthwashes of sodium bicarbonate in warm tap water or rinsing the mouth with a topical anesthetic such as viscous lidocaine. Systemic analgesics may be used if the infection is severe. If the infection is protracted and the individual is likely to become dehydrated, referral for hospitalization for rehydration and treatment with intravenous acyclovir may be indicated.

Herpetic lesions of the body and extremities can be treated with Burrow's compresses 20 min three times per day. Fever may be treated with acetaminophen unless contraindicated. Sunscreens (specifically formulated for the lips) can be applied to the lips to help prevent sun-induced herpes simplex.

*Warts.* There are several surgical procedures that may be used to remove common warts. However, care must be taken to avoid scarring that may be more painful and problematic than the wart itself. Surgical procedures include electrosurgery and liquid nitrogen applied to the wart with a cotton-tipped applicator. Freezing of plantar or palmar warts may cause painful hemorrhagic blisters. Both techniques require specific training and equipment of the primary care provider.

## Time Frame for Initiating Pharmacotherapy

Therapy should be initiated promptly with the earliest symptomatology after proper diagnosis has been made.

## Overview of Drug Classes for Treatment

Warts may be treated with simple noninvasive methods, such as topical application of keratolytics, and/or soaking and filing. More extensive or resistant warts may require cryosurgery with liquid nitrogen, or laser surgery. Podophyllin is generally reserved for condylomata acuminata, and acyclovir for herpes.

For pain resolution, primarily with herpes zoster, topical capsaicin or oral tricyclic antidepressant medications are used.

See Drug Tables 106, 301, 306, 311.1.

## Assessment and History Taking

Herpes simplex often follows a history of infection, trauma, stress, or sun exposure. Physical examination may reveal regional lymph nodes as swollen and tender. A Tzanck smear is positive for large multinucleated cells; immunofluorescence tests are positive (Berger, Goldstein, & Odom, 1997).

The pain of herpes zoster generally follows along a nerve, followed by painful grouped vesicular lesions. Upon physical examination, the lesions are usually unilateral although some lesions may occur outside the affected dermatome. Lesions are usually on the face and the trunk; regional lymph node swelling is inconsistent (Berger et al, 1997). Herpes zoster in children may not be painful and usually has a mild course (Morelli & Weston, 1997).

## Patient and Caregiver Information

Patients and caregivers should be instructed in nonpharmacologic interventions for care as previously described. The indication for use of the medications, ADRs, and toxic effects of the drug therapies (refer to Drug Tables 106, 301, 306, 311.1) should be taught as appropriate. Primary prevention through immunization should be encouraged when applicable.

Cloths or towels used for compresses by the patient may contain infectious viruses for several hours after use. Family members should be taught not to use these items before they are laundered in hot, soapy water.

## OUTCOMES MANAGEMENT

### Selecting an Appropriate Agent

Appropriate therapy for warts requires consideration of the patient's age and underlying health status as well as the number of warts and their location. According to a task force of the American Academy of Dermatology's Committee on Guidelines of Care (Drake et al, 1995), acceptable indications for treatment of warts include (1) the patient's desire for therapy; (2) presence of such symptoms as pain, bleeding, itching, or burning; (3) lesions that are disabling or disfiguring; (4) large numbers of lesions or large-sized lesions; (5) a desire to prevent spread to unblemished skin; and (6) an immunocompromised state.

Treatment of common, flat, and plantar warts is typically daily self-application of topical 17% salicylic acid. If possible, the wart should be soaked for several minutes in warm water and then gently scraped with a file or pumice stone before applying the salicylic acid. The salicylic acid should be applied and left on overnight under occlusion. The next day the site should be washed and pared with an emery board. If the wart has not resolved after 6 weeks, the patient should be referred to a dermatologist for cryotherapy. Also available are transdermal patches, generally provided with securing tape and an emery board.

Salicylic acid 40% plaster is the product of choice for plantar warts. The process used is to trim the wart down, apply the plaster for 5 days, trim again, and repeat until resolution.

Condylomata acuminata are successfully treated with a solution of podophyllin 25% in tincture of benzoin applied weekly. Care should be given to applying the mixture only to the affected surface since it can cause irritation of the surrounding tissue from its antimitotic action. The mixture is left on for 4 h and then washed off. Following a few applications, the mixture may be left on for up to 24 h. Resolution can occur after a few applications, or it may take as many as 25 applications. If podophyllin is ineffective, cryosurgery is the next line of therapy.

Herpes infection treatment consists of topical antiviral therapy, with or without oral therapy, and pain medication if necessary. With severe cases, intravenous infusions may be necessary, but this is beyond the scope of this book. For initial herpes simplex treatment, acyclovir 200 mg five times daily for 10 days is necessary. Recurrent bouts will need only 5 days of therapy. The dose is doubled in immunocompromised patients and duration is 14 days. Ongoing prophylactic acyclovir therapy can be given at 400 mg twice daily for up to 12 months for those patients having six or more episodes yearly.

Varicella (chickenpox) is treated symptomatically with calamine lotion, acetaminophen, and acyclovir. The dose of acyclovir is 20 mg/kg per day for 5 days. A vaccine is available now that is given between the ages of 12–18 months. Whether protection lasts until adulthood is yet to be determined. Herpes zoster is symptomatically treated with calamine lotion, hot soaks, and capsaicin cream. Prednisone 60 mg daily for 2 weeks may also be needed along with acyclovir 800 mg five times daily for 10 days. This should be started as soon as the diagnosis is made. Valacyclovir 1 g three times daily for 7 days is indicated for zoster in the immunocompetent patient. Famciclovir 500 mg three times daily for 7 days is also available. If more than 48 h have elapsed since the outbreak began, this therapy will only be marginally beneficial. The therapy reduces the development of new lesions, which may be beneficial in patients experiencing excruciating pain.

Rubeola and rubella are treated with rest and acetaminophen for relief of discomfort. Vaccine is available and indicated in rubeola.

Pain may be managed by nonpharmacologic means (wet to damp dressings to reduce the dry, cracking nature of the lesions) and by pharmacologic means. Analgesics such as NSAIDs and acetaminophen help. Narcotics may be necessary. Topical capsaicin cream applied four times daily to the affected dermatome has been proven useful in diminishing the pain. Relief comes slowly, however, with days to weeks before full pain relief. Oral amitriptyline in doses of 12.5–150 mg per day also may decrease the discomfort of postherpetic neuralgia (Max et al, 1988).

### Monitoring for Efficacy

Elimination of the virus is not always possible when treating these disorders. They are notorious for their recurrence, with remission and less frequent occurrences being the goals. Absolute resolution does happen and should be the aim of therapy.

### Significant Food and Drug Interactions and Management

Oral acyclovir may be taken without regard to meals.

### Monitoring for Toxicity

Nausea and vomiting have been reported with patients taking acyclovir oral capsules. It is generally considered safe and effective with minimal side effects.

Topical application of salicylic acid can be irritating to surrounding unaffected tissue, causing some burning and irritation. Podophyllin causes stinging and burning as local wart necrosis occurs. Capsaicin, derived from peppers, causes discomfort in the initial 1–3 days as substance P is depleted.

Nonsteroidal antiinflammatory drugs should not be used in patients with renal failure and have several notable drug interactions. GI upset may also occur, so they should be taken with food.

Amitriptyline should be used with caution in elderly patients and those with cardiac abnormalities.

### Follow-up Recommendations

Most warts may be followed at the patient's discretion. Because of the frequent application and potential toxicity of podophyllin, daily application and observation should be the norm for condylomata acuminata, unless the over-the-counter brand is used. It has a lower strength and is applied twice daily for a longer period of time. Patients may choose to follow this themselves.

Follow-up for herpes simplex and zoster infections is done with each outbreak. Herpes zoster may require closer supervision of disease progression, but herpes simplex requires more patient education to avert the spread of infection.

# INSECT INFESTATIONS, BITES, AND STINGS

This section addresses the treatment of common dermatologic disorders caused by infestations, namely scabies (mite infestation), pediculosis (lice infestation), and the bites and stings from commonly encountered arthropods.

## SCABIES

Scabies is caused by an infestation with the female *Sarcoptes scabiei* mite. It is transmitted through close personal contact and affects all socioeconomic levels, both sexes, and individuals of all ages. The disease accounts for 2–4% of all dermatologic visits in the United States (Orkin & Maibach, 1991). The adult mite is approximately ⅓ mm in length and has a flattened, oval body with wrinkled, transverse corrugations and eight legs (two are brush-like) (Habif, 1996). The female mite attaches to the skin, digs a burrow (primary lesion), and lays approximately two or three eggs per day for the duration of her 1-month life. The eggs hatch within 3–4 days and mature within 14 days. Fecal pellets (scybala) are deposited along with the eggs and appear as dark, oval masses. Secondary lesions of excoriations of the burrows may be the only visible lesion. In severe, chronic infestations, secondary bacterial infection may develop in the form of impetigo, cellulitis, or furunculosis.

In adults the most common areas affected are the waist, pelvis, elbows, hands (especially finger webs), feet and ankles, penis and scrotum, buttocks, and axillae. Infants, young children, and the elderly may have lesions on the head and neck. Atypical (crusted or Norwegian) scabies may occur in patients who are immunocompromised [eg, have human immunodeficiency virus (HIV)].

The initial phase of the disease is asymptomatic, with the pruritic rash developing in about 14–28 days. The primary symptom is intense itching, especially at night. The pathognomonic lesion is the burrow appearing as a pink-white linear or curved ridge with a tiny vesicle at one end. A skin scraping with an oil or potassium hydroxide mount reveals a mite, eggs, or fecal pellets.

Scabies may be overlooked in elderly patients in nursing homes. The inflammatory reaction may be muted although the patient itches intensely and may be misdiagnosed as "senile pruritus" (Orkin & Maibach, 1991).

## PEDICULOSIS

Infestations with lice have been documented for thousands of years. More deaths have occurred from diseases transmitted by lice than from any insect-borne disease other than the malaria mosquito (Orkin & Maibach, 1991).

The louse is a wingless, dorsoventrally flattened, bloodsucking insect. There are three types: *Pediculus humanus corporis,* which infests the body and clothing, *P. humanus capitis,* which infests the head, and *Phthirus pubis,* which infests the pubic area and is considered a sexually transmitted disease (Orkin & Maibach, 1991; Sauer & Hall, 1996). Pediculosis is most commonly seen in individuals with poor hygiene, and head lice are commonly seen in school children.

The louse is 3–4 mm in length and transmitted by contact with infested clothing, bedding, and combs. Since lice bite the skin and live on the blood, they cannot live without human contact and die within 2–3 weeks. The oval eggs, or "nits," are deposited on hairs or fibers of clothing by the female louse. Eggs hatch within 30 days. The female louse lives for about 30 days and deposits a few eggs daily. Body lice are most commonly seen as linear excoriations on the trunk. Secondary infection often masks the primary lesions. Nits and lice can often be found in the seams of the infested clothing.

In head and pubic pediculosis, the nits are generally found attached to hairs; lice are rarely found. Erythema and scaling of the scalp may be present. Cervical lymphadenopathy (eg, posterior) and febrile episodes are also common. *Pthirus pubis* on the eyelashes or hair of children should alert the primary care provider to the possibility of sexual abuse, but other modes of transmission do occur.

The bites of lice are relatively painless and often go unnoticed. The clinical signs and symptoms are caused by the patient's reaction to the saliva or anticoagulant injected into the dermis by the louse during feeding (bloodsucking). Individual sensitivity varies greatly. The sites of feeding may exhibit 2–3-mm erythematous macules or papules within hours to days of the bite. Others may develop an almost immediate reaction with flare and wheal formation (Orkin & Maibach, 1991).

## ARTHROPOD BITES AND STINGS

Bites and stings from common arthropods such as mosquitos, fleas, ticks, hymenoptera (ants, bees, wasps), and spiders are common. Prior to treatment in the nonallergic individual, assessment will usually find local swelling, papule or wheal formation, pruritis, erythema, and mild discomfort. An allergic individual may experience a more severe local reaction or a systemic reaction of urticaria, hypotension, respiratory distress, angioedema, anaphylaxis, and death.

Two species of spiders have a venom strong enough to produce toxic reactions: the brown recluse spider (*Loxosceles reclusa*) and the black widow spider (*Latrodectus mactans*). The brown recluse spider commonly inhabits old buildings, storage sheds, wood piles, garages or basement storage areas, and occasionally closets. Therefore, the victim commonly reports being bitten while working around one of these areas or after donning boots, jackets, etc., that have been stored for a period of time. The venom of the brown recluse spider contains sphingomyelinase, which acts on the cell membranes resulting in dermonecrotic activity and a lipase that induces disseminated intravascular hemolysis (Dockery, 1997). The brown recluse spider bite generally has two types of responses, a localized cutaneous reaction and a systemic reaction marked by intravascular hemolysis, acute vasculitis, platelet thrombi, and leukocyte infiltrates (Dockery, 1997). The more severe reaction most frequently occurs in children and debilitated patients. A blue-gray halo develops around the site of the bite, and a cyanotic vesicle or bulla may appear. Pain may be severe. The necrotic tissue may extend deep into muscle. Within 12–24 h after the bite, the patient commonly reports fever, chills, nausea, vomiting, and urticaria. The patient may not have seen the spider; therefore, the history of activities when the bite occurred facilitates diagnosis.

In mild reactions, treatment is symptomatic with rest, ice compresses, pain control, and antibiotics to prevent secondary infection; warm compresses and exercise worsen the lesion. Tetanus toxoid may be indicated. Dapsone may be required in more severe cases, and referral of the patient to a hospital emergency room may be indicated. Surgical excision of the wound and skin grafting also may be required for severe reactions.

The black widow spider bite, although commonly believed to be a fatal bite, has a mortality of less than 1% (Dockery, 1997). The bite itself may not have been felt, and there may be minimal local reaction. The venom is a neurotoxin that produces symptoms of general toxemia 10–15 min after the bite, including muscle spasms and cramps, especially of the legs and abdomen; numbness that gradually spreads from the site of the bite to the entire torso; headache; sweating; increased salivation; nausea and vomiting; and a diffuse macular rash (Dockery, 1997). The acute phase generally subsides within 48 h and gradually resolves in 2–4 days. The patient should be referred to an emergency room for treatment. An antivenom is available for bites in the very young, the debilitated, or for those with severe reactions. Mild reactions can be treated with cool compresses, analgesics for pain, and muscle relaxants.

Hymenoptera, ants, bees, wasps, and hornets commonly sting adults and children. The bite of the fire ant usually causes immediate pain that quickly subsides. The small red wheal becomes a vesicle over several hours. After 24 h, the vesicles become pustules that usually resolve in about 10 days. Multiple ant stings can cause severe allergic reactions requiring emergency treatment. Individuals with mild local reactions can be treated with cool compresses, antipruritic lotions, oral antihistamines, and thorough cleansing of the bites to prevent secondary infection.

The honeybee is the only stinging insect that leaves its barbed stinger and venom sac in the victim (Dockery, 1997). The venom of stinging insects contains histamines and vasoactive agents that are hemolytic and neurotoxic. The nonallergic patient generally reports moderate to severe pain at the time of the bite and a localized wheal, erythema, pruritis, and edema. Systemic reactions vary from mild to severe as previously described. Localized stings in nonallergic individuals are treated with cool compresses and mild analgesics for the pain. Antihistamines may be indicated in more severe localized reactions.

Prepackaged bee-sting kits including epinephrine 1:1000 in prefilled syringes and antihistamine tablets are available for allergic individuals. Patients should be instructed to carry them when participating in activities during which a sting might occur and in the use of the kit. Parents and caregivers should be taught how to care for allergic children and the elderly. The allergic individual also should be instructed to wear a medical alert tag or bracelet.

Tick bites are usually self-limiting; however, ticks can carry organisms that cause serious disease, eg, Lyme disease or Rocky Mountain spotted fever. Prevention of tick bites is important. Patients who camp in woods or hike in tall grasses are at risk. Therefore, remind them to wear long pants with the cuffs tucked into boots, long-sleeved shirts, turned-up collars, and hats with brims and to treat clothing with repellents.

## SPECIFIC CONSIDERATIONS FOR PHARMACOTHERAPY

### When Drug Therapy Is Needed

Treatment is required to eradicate the infestation of both scabies mites and lice. Patients should be questioned about itching in family members and close personal contacts, including classmates of school children. Selective treatment of asymptomatic family members at high risk for acquiring the infestations from a confirmed case may be appropriate, eg, if the infested patient shares a bed with another individual. Sexual contacts should also be treated.

Most common bites and stings should be thoroughly washed with soap and water to cleanse the wound to prevent secondary infection. The area should be kept clean and itching avoided until the wound has healed.

## Short- and Long-Term Goals of Pharmacotherapy

The goals of therapy are to eradicate the infestation, relieve the itching, treat secondary infection as needed, and educate the patient about the transmission of the disease to minimize the possibility of future infestations. Instruction in good personal hygiene should be conducted as appropriate. Individuals, especially school children, should be taught to avoid sharing combs, clothing, caps, etc., with others.

Patients should be instructed that the treatment destroys the insects and eggs, but the response to the sensitizing substances may last for several weeks; ie, itching may persist for several weeks. If the rash persists and itching is intense, requiring treatment, topical corticosteroids and oral antihistamines may be necessary.

Patients must be cautioned not to overtreat themselves or family members, since these drugs can be toxic. Patients should be instructed NOT to repeat the treatment unless it is specifically prescribed by their health care provider.

## Nonpharmacologic Therapy

*Scabies.*   At the conclusion of therapy, all articles of clothing, bedding, and towels should be laundered with hot, soapy water and rinsed in hot water. Alternatives to this would be to dry-clean the clothes or place them in a sealed plastic bag for 30 days. Outerwear and furniture do not need to be cleaned because mites survive only a short time when deprived of the human host. Spraying upholstery with pyrethrin may help.

*Pediculosis.*   Good hygiene, frequent bathing, use of clean clothing (including underclothing), and proper nutrition are important nonpharmacologic aspects of therapy. All clothing and bedding should be thoroughly washed in hot, soapy water and rinsed in hot water. Dry cleaning destroys lice in wool garments. Pressing woolens at home is also effective, but pay special attention to the seams of clothing. If items cannot be laundered or dry-cleaned, placing the items in plastic bags tightly sealed for at least 2 weeks will also kill the lice. Brushes and combs should be soaked in hot soapy water for 15–20 min.

Floors, furniture, play areas, etc., should be thoroughly vacuumed to remove hairs that contain nits with viable eggs.

*Arthropod Bites and Stings.*   Cleansing of the wound with a mild soap and water should be done as soon as possible. The wound should be checked for the presence of a stinger, foreign body, or the insect itself (a tick), and it should be removed if needed. Local reactions are generally treated with ice compresses, topical antipruritics, oral antihistamines, and mild analgesics as needed. Scratching should be avoided to prevent secondary infection. For secondary infection, topical or oral antibiotics may be required. Systemic allergic reactions necessitate the use of epinephrine, antihistamines, and supportive care. Primary prevention should include use of appropriate repellents, barrier clothing, and avoidance of areas containing the arthropods.

## Time Frame for Initiating Pharmacotherapy

Treatment should be instituted as soon as a diagnosis is made. Treatment for scabies should be preceded by a tepid bath or shower and drying with a towel.

Cutaneous manifestations of bites and stings often will be the only clinical expressions of an acute systemic allergic reaction. Therefore, individuals allergic to bites and stings should be instructed to carry a kit containing self-injecting epinephrine and oral antihistamines at all times when exposure might occur and taught how to use it. Allergic individuals should also be instructed to wear a medical alert tag or bracelet.

## Overview of Drug Classes for Treatment

There are three major forms of medications for the treatment of scabies: lindane, crotamiton, and sulfur (see Drug Table 806). Sulfur is generally not used in adults because it is messy and odoriferous, and it stains clothing easily. It is good for infants and is used by applying a 10% ointment to the site for 24 h on three consecutive nights. Alternative medications for the treatment of scabies include permethrin, thiabendazole, and coal tar. Lindane and pyrethrins are commonly used for pediculosis infestations. The applications of the drugs when treating scabies and pediculosis are different, as noted below. Urticaria and redness may require topical corticosteroids, antihistamines, or antibiotics.

Insect bites and stings are generally benign, but in some patients can lead to serious consequences. Antihistamines are effective for mild cases. Corticosteroids may be necessary for more severe or prolonged cases.

See Drug Tables 102, 601, 705, 807.

## Assessment and History Taking

Infestations, stings, and bites are characterized by a history of localized rash with pruritis. Specific signs and symptoms were described previously for each vector.

## Patient and Caregiver Information

Specific patient and caregiver information is discussed in the section on nonpharmacologic treatment for each vector. The patient and caregiver should be taught the correct use of medications and encouraged to complete the course of drug therapy as prescribed. Patients and caregivers also should be taught about ADRs and the toxic effects of the drugs.

## OUTCOMES MANAGEMENT

### Selecting an Appropriate Agent

*Scabies.* Patients and family members should be treated with an overnight application of lindane or permethrin cream. The application should be from the neck down, left on for 8–12 h (generally overnight), and then washed off. Emphasize that all areas must be treated, especially between the fingers and toes, the groin, and the axilla. One fluid ounce (lindane) or 30 g (permethrin) should suffice. If there are scabetic lesions on the head and neck (usually seen only in children), they are also treated, but great care is needed to avoid the eyes, nose, and mouth. Permethrin and lindane are safe for children over 2 years of age. Alternatively, crotamiton is used and applied in the same fashion as lindane, but reapplied in 24 h. It is then left on for an additional 24 h. Permethrin 5% cream (Elimite) may be substituted for lindane in infants (Morelli & Weston, 1997).

*Pediculosis.* Treatment consists of the application of pyrethrins or permethrin (over-the-counter), or lindane or malathion (prescription). The shampoo formulation should be used for hairy areas; the cream or lotion can be used elsewhere. The formulation should be left on for 5 min and then rinsed off. A repeat application 1 week later is necessary for lindane since it does not kill the nits. Since nits attach to the hair shaft, a fine-tooth comb should be used to remove them once they have been treated.

Secondary infection may be treated with topical mupirocin 2% ointment applied three times daily or with appropriate oral antibiotics.

Eyelash involvement is treated with petrolatum applied twice daily for 9 days followed by removal of any nits.

*Arthropod bites and stings.* Simple acute urticaria may be treated with an antihistamine such as diphenhydramine. In some cases, a short course of a glucocorticoid in a moderate dose may be necessary (eg, prednisone 40 mg PO once daily for 4 days). In low doses for short periods of time, glucocorticoids seldom cause difficulties in an otherwise healthy subject or in an individual with other diseases that are properly treated (Sullivan, 1986). A similar treatment can be used for angioedema unless it is associated with upper airway obstruction.

Venom immunotherapy may be recommended as the treatment of choice for the prevention of recurrent systemic sting reactions. Treatment of this nature should be referred to the appropriate specialty practitioner.

### Monitoring for Efficacy

Resolution of the infestation or diminishing of the erythema and urticaria is the primary endpoint to treating these conditions.

### Significant Food and Drug Interactions and Management

Agents used for pediculosis and scabies are topical and have no food interactions. Corticosteroids should be taken with food.

### Monitoring for Toxicity

Lindane is a neurotoxin and therefore should be avoided in infants, pregnant or lactating women, and persons with seizure disorders or numerous excoriations, which potentiate absorption.

## Follow-up Recommendations

Patients may choose to monitor themselves without follow-up, but should be warned to return at the first sign of infection or continued symptoms.

# DERMATITIS

Common dermatitis includes asteatotic dermatitis, atopic and contact dermatitis ("eczema"), and seborrheic dermatitis. Eczematous dermatitis is an inflammatory response of the skin to a wide variety of external and internal agents. The cause of the dermatitis often is unknown.

*Eczematous dermatitis* is classified according to general appearance, location, and presenting symptoms and acute, subacute, and chronic stages. The acute stage is characterized by vesicles, blisters, or bullae; erythema; and moderate to severe pruritis. The subacute stage is characterized by erythema, scaling and fissuring with a scalded appearance, mild to moderate pruritis, and discomfort commonly described as "burning" in character. The chronic stage is characterized by lichenification (thickening and dryness giving a "washboard" appearance to the skin) with fissures and excoriations.

*Asteatotic dermatitis* is a common condition also known as chronic "winter itch" because it is frequently seen during the winter and in geographical areas of low humidity. It is characterized with dehydration, erythema, dry scaling, and fine superficial cracking of the skin. It results from a decrease in skin surface lipids (Dockery, 1997; Sauer & Hall, 1996). Frequent bathing in hot water and use of deodorant soaps can aggravate the condition. Elderly individuals are most commonly affected.

*Atopic dermatitis* is a chronic inflammation of the skin. Patients often have associated allergic rhinitis and approximately 70% report a family history of atopy (Barker et al, 1995; Dockery, 1997; Sauer & Hall, 1996; Anderson, 1991). Atopic dermatitis can be divided into subtypes based on the age of onset: infantile (2 months to 2 years), childhood (2 years through adolescence), and adult. Areas of involvement are typically those that the patient can scratch: infantile (cheeks, extensor arms, and legs), childhood (flexural arms, legs, neck, wrists, and ankles), and adult (flexural surfaces, face, wrists, knees, hands, and feet) (Barker et al, 1995). Acute lesions are characterized by erythema, edema, papules, vesicles, erosions, crusts, and scale. Chronic lesions are characterized by lichenified plaques. Secondary bacterial infections may also occur.

*Contact dermatitis* may present as primary irritant contact dermatitis, allergic contact dermatitis, and photoallergic contact dermatitis. Lesions are seen in any of the stages from mild erythema or vesicles to large bullae with a significant amount of oozing. In primary irritant dermatitis, the patient is usually exposed to the irritant for a relatively short period of time and is not immunologically mediated. About 80% of all cases of contact dermatitis are of the irritant variety (Barker et al, 1995). Irritant contact dermatitis is characterized by a scalded, erythematous appearance of the skin with peeling of the most superficial epidermis. Common agents causing irritant dermatitis include agents with extremes of pH such as harsh soaps and cleansers.

Allergic contact dermatitis is caused by a delayed hypersensitive reaction. The most common cause of allergic contact dermatitis is plant dermatitis caused by the *Rhus* genus, which includes poison ivy, oak, and sumac. It is the oleoresin oil within the plants that is the allergen. Sensitive individuals may continue to develop lesions for up to 3 weeks after exposure. Other common allergens include nickel compounds (costume jewelry), neomycin, benzocaine, fragrances and preservatives in cosmetics and personal hygiene products, paraphenylenediamines (shoe dyes), rubber products, ethylenediamines, and the chromates (Dockery, 1997).

Occupational allergic contact dermatitis frequently occurs. It is estimated that 65% of all industrial diseases are dermatoses (Sauer & Hall, 1996). Common allergens include potassium dichromate in cement, dyes, or textiles; epoxy resins in adhesives, finishing products, and casings for electrical devices; rosin in adhesive materials; thiuram, mercaptobenzothiazole, and carbamates in rubber products; glycerol monothioglycolate and paraphenylenediamine in hair wave and dye formulations; and acrylates in methylmethacrylate used in orthopedic surgery, dentistry, and nail sculpturing (Barker et al, 1995). A very detailed history is important for correct diagnosis, including questions regarding improvement when away from work or while on vacation.

Allergic contact dermatitis is unusual in children under the age of 3 years since this type of dermatitis occurs after a variable number of exposures with a sensitizer (Dockery, 1997). However, in children, the foot may be a site for allergic contact dermatitis to occur. Children frequently wear shoes for extended periods of time and the increased heat and perspiration can exacerbate an allergic contact dermatitis from shoe materials (Dockery, 1997). Differential diagnosis from tinea pedis is essential for initiation of correct therapy.

Photoallergic dermatitis may be seen with drugs such as chlorpromazine, promethazine, p-aminobenzoic acid, phenothiazines, tincture of benzoin, and povidone-iodine solutions.

*Contact urticaria,* although not strictly a dermatitis, is a contact reaction to latex that is very prevalent, especially in health care workers. Reactions vary from itching after wearing latex gloves to anaphylaxis.

*Nummular eczema* (discoid eczema) is characterized by coin-shaped papulovesicular lesions on the arms and legs and is of unknown etiology. It is most frequently seen in middle-aged and older adult men. Itching usually is quite severe (Vickers, 1991).

*Seborrheic dermatitis* is a common idiopathic dermatitis occurring in about 3–5% of the population (Barker et al, 1995). It is characterized by inflammatory hyperproliferation of the skin affecting areas of the body where sebaceous glands are plentiful (ie, scalp, facial hair areas, presternal chest, axilla, umbilicus, inguinal folds, gluteal cleft, and perianal skin). The lesions appear as scaly, reddish, and brown patches. (Note: Dandruff is a similar but noninflammatory erythematous scaling of the skin in the seborrheic areas.) The etiology of seborrheic dermatitis is not known; however, it has been associated with the presence of *Pityrosporum ovale,* a yeast commonly present on the skin (Barker et al, 1995; Faergemann, Jones, Hettler, & Loria, 1996). Treatment with antifungal agents (eg, terbinafine) has proven very successful. Infants frequently present with seborrheic dermatitis commonly called "cradle cap," which is characterized by greasy adherent scale on the vertex of the scalp. Secondary infection can occur.

## SPECIFIC CONSIDERATIONS FOR PHARMACOTHERAPY

### When Drug Therapy Is Needed

Treatment should be initiated as soon as the condition is diagnosed. However, drug therapy may not be indicated in asteatotic dermatitis. Rather, educate the patient about skin care and decreasing the number of baths or showers and encourage the use of topical emollients containing lanolin, glycerine, urea, and lactic acid or other alpha-hydroxy acids.

### Short- and Long-Term Goals of Pharmacotherapy

Try to determine the causative nature of the dermatitis so the patient can avoid the antigen source. Education is important in preventing future occurrences. Caution the patient to remove the antigen as soon as possible after exposure and rinse with warm, soapy water. Ultimately, it is hoped that more severe reactions, more widespread coverage, and scarring can be avoided. Prevention of secondary infections, caused by excoriating the skin, is also important.

### Nonpharmacologic Therapy

The source(s) of the irritant(s) should be determined in contact dermatitis and photodermatitis, and the patient should be instructed about interventions to avoid future exposure. When a medication is determined to be the causative factor, the medication should be discontinued under the supervision of a health care provider and alternative drug therapy initiated as appropriate. Patients should be instructed about their drug allergy and to wear a medical alert tag or bracelet.

### Time Frame for Initiating Pharmacotherapy

Removing the causative agent and rinsing with warm soapy water in appropriate circumstances should be done immediately. Prevention of long-term complications should then be addressed.

### Overview of Drug Classes for Treatment

Treatment of dermatitis reflects the inflammatory nature of the disorder. Management with low- to midstrength corticosteroids may be all that is necessary. For more severe dermatitis, higher-strength topical or oral corticosteroids are available. Treating pruritus with diphenhydramine or hydroxyzine and treating secondary infections with antibiotics also may be necessary.

See Drug Tables 601, 803, 807, 808.

## Assessment and History Taking

A thorough health history, including a detailed occupational history, is essential to the effective treatment of dermatitis. Exposure(s) to the irritant(s) must be identified so that the patient and caregiver can be taught to avoid future exposure as much as possible. Elimination of the offending irritant is essential to optimal treatment. Assessment should include mechanism of response, number of exposures, nature of the substance, mode of onset, and distribution (Habif, 1996).

## Patient and Caregiver Information

Once the offending irritants have been identified, patients and caregivers should be taught to avoid future exposure. If the offending agent is a medication, the health care provider who prescribed the medication should be notified immediately, the offending medication discontinued, and an alternative medication prescribed. Patients with drug allergies or other life-threatening allergies should wear a medical alert tag or bracelet to identify themselves as allergic.

The patient should be instructed to take oral corticosteroid medications with food to minimize stomach irritation.

## OUTCOMES MANAGEMENT

### Selecting an Appropriate Agent

Mild cases of contact dermatitis are usually treated with topical corticosteroids. Newer, more potent corticosteroids control both the symptoms and the spread of dermatitis. It is rarely necessary to use antipruritics. Adjunctive use of menthol and camphor lotions, cool soaks, and wet-to-dry soaks may be helpful in controlling pruritus (Millikan & Shrum, 1992). When the face is involved, only low-potency corticosteroids (like hydrocortisone 1% cream) should be used.

For more lichenified lesions that are not on the face, midpotency (eg, triamcinolone, betamethasone valerate) to high-potency (eg, fluocinonide, betamethasone) fluorinated steroids must be used. Use of systemic corticosteroids is generally reserved for patients who have a history of severe, widespread reactions or those in whom more than 30% of the body is involved. Patients with involvement of the hands, face, or genitals also are candidates for aggressive sys-

temic corticosteorid therapy (Millikan & Shrum, 1992).

Some patients also require oral antibiotics for recurrent infection. Coverage should include S. aureus.

For patients unresponsive to therapy, other therapies, including phototherapy or photochemotherapy with UVB radiation or psoralen and UVA radiation, may be prescribed by a dermatologist.

Nummular dermatitis and asteatotic eczema are treated in a similar fashion to that described for contact dermatitis. Seborrheic dermatitis requires the addition of tar and antiyeast shampoos (eg, selenium or ketoconazole) to the regimen. Since selenium sulfide shampoo is readily available in over-the-counter products, at a lower cost, recommend this first.

## Monitoring for Efficacy

Relief of symptoms and resolution of the dermatitis are realistic goals for managing most of these patients. Temporary remission may be all that can be expected with seborrheic dermatitis.

## Significant Food and Drug Interactions and Management

Most of the products used to treat dermatitis are topical, thus eliminating the food and drug interaction potential. Corticosteroids should be taken with food to minimize GI irritation.

## Monitoring for Toxicity

All the topical corticosteroids can cause burning, itching, irritation, and erythema of the skin. The higher the potency, the higher is the likelihood of this occurring. The highest-potency corticosteroids can also cause skin atrophy and hypothalamic-pituitary-adrenocortical (HPA) axis suppression with long-term use.

Oral corticosteroids will cause HPA axis suppression with continued use at modest dosages. Patients who are at risk for complications of fluid retention caused by the mineralocorticoid effects of prednisone may benefit from the substitution of dexamethasone. This may be useful in older patients with cardiac problems and patients taking diuretics.

Diphenhydramine and hydroxyzine can cause drowsiness, but this side effect decreases with continued use. Patients driving or operating heavy equipment should be treated cautiously.

## Follow-up Recommendations

Depending on severity, follow-up may be determined by the patient. In those patients requiring systemic therapy (corticosteroid or antibiotic), follow-up is in 1 week.

# SUNBURN, SUNSCREENS, AND MINOR BURNS

Primary prevention of sunburn, the use of sunscreens, and the clinical management of minor burns will be described in this section. Sunburn—excessive exposure to ultraviolet radiation (UVR)—causes multiple health problems in addition to skin cancers. Skin cancer is the most common and also the most preventable cancer (American Cancer Society [ACS], 1998).* It is estimated that 50% of all people who live to age 65 will have at least one form of skin cancer.

There are approximately 1 million cases a year of highly curable basal cell or squamous cell cancers. It is projected that there will be 41,600 cases of the most serious skin cancer, melanoma, in 1998. It is estimated that 9200 deaths will be due to skin cancer, 7300 from malignant melanoma and the remainder from other skin cancers. About 90% of skin cancers can be prevented by protection from the sun's rays (ACS, 1998).

A relationship between ultraviolet B (UVB) exposure and the development of basal cell and squamous cell carcinoma has been documented. High-dose exposure to UVR generally increases the risk for development of malignant melanoma. Chronic exposure to ultraviolet A (UVA) and UVB increases the rate of skin aging and wrinkling. The cumulative effect of repeated sunburns in childhood is also a major risk factor for melanoma (Whiteman & Green, 1994).

Patients should be taught the long-term consequences of sun exposure (ie, photoaging) and the benefits of regular sunscreen use and avoidance of sunburns. Appropriate use of sunscreens and reduction of the risk for skin cancer can be

accomplished through aggressive patient teaching and counseling by the primary care provider.

Of the total solar radiation that reaches the earth, ultraviolet (UV) light accounts for about 3% and visible and infrared comprise the remainder. UV light is further divided into three subgroups: UVC, UVB, and UVA. UV radiation is measured as wavelengths of light in units of nanometers (nm).

UVC (200–290 nm) is considered potentially the most carcinogenic, but is almost completely absorbed by the ozone layer of the atmosphere. The UVB spectrum (290–320 nm) causes most sunburns. UVA (320–400 nm) can be up to 1000 times more intense than UVB, penetrates much deeper into the skin than any other UV wavelength, and can potentiate the carcinogenic effects of UVB (ACS, 1998; Farmer & Naylor, 1996). In addition, significant UV damage occurs prior to the development of perceptible UV-induced erythema (Farmer & Naylor, 1996). UVA contributes substantially to photoaging (wrinkling, drying) and may cause immunologic effects (ACS, 1998; Griffiths, 1992).

DNA damage is required before the tanning mechanisms are activated, specifically, pyrimidine dimer formation. DNA damage thus appears to be the trigger for the tanning response, meaning one cannot begin to tan until there is at least some damage. This suggests that there is no safe form or degree of tanning and that all UV radiation causes some skin damage (ACS, 1998; Eller, Yaar, & Gilchrist, 1994). Repeated miniexposures should not be overlooked since this type of incidental exposure accounts for 80% of the total exposure over a lifetime (Engle, 1995). In addition, the use of artificial tanning lamps and booths that use exposure to UVR should be avoided.

The ability to tan is largely determined genetically. Individuals with darker constitutive (ie, non-sun-induced) pigmentation require different levels of UV protection. There are six skin types based on the relative amount of constitutive pigmentation. See Table 27–1 for a general guide to skin type.

The incidence of melanomas in light-complected individuals (skin types I–III) is several times greater than those with darker skin types (types IV–VI) even in similar geographic regions (Farmer & Naylor, 1996; Wentzell, 1996; Miller & Weinstock, 1994).

Regular sunscreen use has been shown to reduce the formation of precancerous actinic ker-

---

* The American Cancer Society has a national toll-free number (1-800-ACS-2345) for obtaining general information as well as patient education materials about sun exposure, skin cancers, and skin examination guidelines for both the primary care provider and the patient.

## TABLE 27–1. A GENERAL GUIDE TO SKIN TYPE

Type I
- Low levels of constitutive pigmentation; very fair
- Never tan; always burn
- Redheads, light-complected blonds
- Freckled; Celtic descent

Type II
- Slightly higher levels of constitutive pigmentation; fair
- Always burn; able to tan small amounts after multiple sun exposures
- Light-skinned individuals; blue-eyed
- Slavic and Germanic descent

Type III
- Moderate levels of constitutive pigmentation
- Infrequently burn; tan readily
- Caucasians with brown/black hair (NOTE: most white individuals fall into pigmentation types II and III.)

Type IV
- Moderate levels of constitutive pigmentation
- Rarely burn; tan heavily with moderate sun exposure
- Individuals of Asian, Native American, Mediterranean, and Latin American descent

Type V
- Dark constitutive pigmentation
- Individuals become measurably darker with sun exposure
- Light-complected African-Americans, East Indian descent

Type VI
- Heaviest constitutive pigmentation
- Dark-skinned African-Americans

atoses (AKs) by 36%. A dose-response–specific relationship has been found between the amount of sunscreen used and AK formation (Farmer & Naylor, 1996).

The development of benign nevi, one of the known risk factors for melanoma, is associated with personal sun exposure, especially multiple sunburns (Garbe, Buttner, & Weiss, 1994; Richard, Grob, & Gouvernet, 1993).

## SPECIFIC CONSIDERATIONS FOR PHARMACOTHERAPY

### When Drug Therapy Is Needed

The problem is summarized by this statement: "The skin never forgets an injury. . . . The even-

tual condition of the skin results from a summation of all the injuries it has received" (Farmer & Naylor, 1996). Prevention is the key to maintaining healthy skin throughout one's life.

Sunscreens act either physically or chemically. Physical sunscreens provide a mechanical barrier to sunlight; for example, zinc oxide paste and titanium dioxide scatter ultraviolet light. Clothing and beach umbrellas are also effective as physical sunscreens, but ultraviolet light may be reflected from sand and water to reach under a beach umbrella and cause burning.

Chemical sunscreens absorb a specific portion of the ultraviolet light spectrum. When the light is absorbed by the sunscreen, several changes may occur in the absorbing compound:

- Light energy is converted to heat.
- The sunscreen molecule may dissociate into atoms or radicals.
- The molecule may be excited to higher energy levels and its energy transferred through collision with another molecule, followed by a chemical reaction.
- The compound may become excited and lose its energy immediately by fluorescence or later by phosphorescence.

The literature shows disagreement on the value of sunscreen agent protection. However, there is evidence that these products provide some protection, depending on the degree of photosensitization. A photoallergic response is characterized by a delayed onset, occurs in sensitized skin, and recurs with subsequent exposures to ultraviolet light. Ultraviolet light above 320 nm can elicit a photoallergic response, so compounds that absorb energy throughout the ultraviolet region may be the most desirable for this purpose if they are used in adequate amounts. The following are sunscreen compounds known to have the propensity to cause a photoallergic response: barbiturates, chlorothiazide, chlorpromazine, demeclocycline, erythromycin, phenylsulfonylurea, promethazine, psoralens, quinidine, quinine, sulfas, and tetracycline.

### Short- and Long-Term Goals of Pharmacotherapy

Sunscreen agents should be considered for protection against sunburn and premature aging of the skin. They also may reduce actinic or solar keratosis and some types of skin cancer.

Treatment of first-degree burns is aimed at healing with minimal scarring, preventing infection, and minimizing pain and discomfort.

## Nonpharmacologic Therapy

Requirements for protection from UVR are generally based on pigmentation skin type, presence of precancerous skin lesions, usual extent of UVR exposure, and history of skin cancer. It is important for the health care provider to obtain a thorough health history, including occupational and avocational/recreational history, as well as to conduct a thorough assessment of the skin in accordance with ACS guidelines (ACS, 1998).

For example, outdoor workers (eg, construction workers, farmers, military personnel) and individuals whose recreation takes them out of doors (eg, golfers, cyclists) require specific teaching and counseling relative to their extensive sun exposure. However, it is generally believed that most individuals should develop the positive health behavior of routinely using a sunscreen whenever they spend any time outside. Patients should be taught the following:

- Avoid sun exposure during the period when the UVR is most intense, ie, from 10 A.M. to 3 P.M.
- UVA remains constant throughout the day (ACS, 1996).
- UVA is not blocked by glass; UVB is.

- UVR intensity increases by 4% for every 1000 ft of increase in elevation.
- Approximately 60–80% of UV radiation can penetrate a thin cloud.
- Snow reflects as much as 85% of the sun's rays.
- Shade and clouds do not provide adequate protection from UVR. Rays bounce from all directions off sand, water, patio floors, and snow. Approximately 70–80% of the UVR burning power penetrates clouds, and rays can even penetrate the surface of the water (ACS, 1998).

There are several ways to protect the skin from UVR, including clothing, physical sunscreens, and chemical sunscreens such as the ones with SPF values. Patients should be instructed to wear protective clothing that provides good physical coverage to high-exposure areas (eg, hats with 2–3-in brims to shade the face, neck, and ears and long sleeves to cover the arms). A general guide is that if one can see light through the fabric, then UVR can penetrate it (ACS, 1998).

Physical sunscreens (eg, zinc oxide and titanium dioxide) and chemical sunscreens (eg, ones with SPF values) will be discussed in the drug therapy section. Table 27–2 summarizes recommendations for protection from sun exposure for adults.

A common misconception among many people is that after applying a SPF 15 sunscreen and staying out in the sun for 4 h, they can reapply

## TABLE 27-2. UVR PROTECTION RECOMMENDATIONS FOR ADULTS

| Risk | Nonpharmacologic Therapy | Pharmacologic Therapy |
|------|--------------------------|------------------------|
| **High**<br>Skin types I–III; outdoors more than ⅓ day; history of precancerous lesions, skin cancer, recreational and occupational exposure; individuals wanting to decrease photoaging, photosensitivity disorders/drugs | Maximum protection; long-sleeve heavy cotton shirt, long pants, hat with wide brim; avoid sun from 10 A.M. to 3 P.M. when possible | SPF 30 sunscreen |
| **Moderate**<br>Skin types III–IV; minimum occupational and recreational exposure | Hat and shirt to cover face, ears, and arms; avoid sun from 10 A.M. to 3 P.M. when possible | SPF 15 sunscreen |
| **Minimum**<br>Skin types V and VI | Hat and shirt to cover face, ears, and arms; avoid sun from 10 A.M. to 3 P.M. when possible | SPF 8–15 sunscreen |

the sunscreen and stay out in the sun another 4 h. At the end of 4 h, they have received their dose of sun for the day! They should go indoors or cover up so as not to receive *any* additional sun exposure. To increase exposure time, apply a sunscreen with a higher SPF initially.

Infants and children require special consideration. It is believed that people may receive up to 80% of their total life's exposure to UV light by the age of 18, and that by using sunscreens during that time, the number of skin pathologies can be reduced by up to 80% (American Academy of Pediatrics [AAP], 1995; ACS, 1998). The American Academy of Pediatrics (AAP) and the American Academy of Dermatology (AAD) (1995) cite the dangers of sunburn in infants and children. A baby's sensitive skin is thinner than adult skin, so a baby will burn more easily than an adult. In addition, sunburn can cause fever and dehydration in children. Sunburn in a child can be very dangerous, and severe sunburn in a child under 1 year of age is an emergency; parents should be instructed to notify their health care provider immediately (AAP, 1995). Infants under 6 months of age should be kept out of direct sunlight and placed in shade. In addition, the child's clothing should cover the total body; use long, lightweight pants, long-sleeved shirts, and hats with brims that shade the face and cover the ears. Clothing should be made of tightly woven fabrics that do not allow light to penetrate. Hold clothing up to a lamp or window and see how much light shines through: the less light, the better. Clothing made of cotton is both cool and protective. The bill of a hat should be facing forward to cover the child's face. Child-sized sunglasses with UV protection should be used to protect the child's eyes (AAP, 1995; Pion, 1996; Battan, Dart, & Rumack, 1997).

**Burn Classification.**    Sunburn is usually a *first-degree* burn characterized by a delayed response to the UVR developing approximately 3–6 h after exposure and peaking within 12–24 h. The response is characterized by erythema, pruritus, tenderness, and pain, and may progress to edema, vesiculation, and even blistering. It involves the superficial layers of the epidermis. It blanches with pressure and shows little edema. A *second-degree* burn involves the epidermis and dermis. Generally, a distinction is made between superficial and deep second-degree burns based on the amount of dermis involved. Deep second-degree burns involve the entire papillary dermis with penetration to some or all of the

reticular dermis. Second-degree burns are characterized by painful red blisters or broken epidermis with a weeping edematous surface. *Third-degree* burns involve all the layers of the epidermis and dermis with penetration into underlying fat and muscle. Third-degree burns are generally painless because the nerve tissue in the area has been destroyed.

All second-degree burns greater than 5–10% of the body, all third-degree burns, all burns associated with electrical current, and all burns of the ears, eyes, face, hands, feet, and perineum should be referred to a hospital prepared to handle burn patients. The remaining first-degree and second-degree burns less than 5% of the body should receive wound care and close follow-up. The goals of therapy are to decrease inflammation, prevent infection, relieve pain, and promote healing.

Nonpharmacologic treatment for first-degree burns includes application of cool, wet compresses of water, milk, or oatmeal to reduce discomfort and edema and mild analgesics for discomfort. Dressings or prophylactic antibiotics are not required. Infants and children should be referred to a physician or emergency room for initial treatment as previously described.

Second-degree burns require protection of the wound from potential infection. If the skin is intact, the burn should be washed with water and a mild antiseptic soap. Chemical burns should be flushed with running water for 15–30 min. A syringe or dental water device can be used to remove embedded debris. Management of blisters is somewhat controversial. Some believe blisters provide a protective barrier and should remain intact. Others suggest that the fluid beneath blisters is a medium for bacterial growth.

Silver sulfadiazine is the topical antibiotic of choice. (Refer to Drug Table 805.) Dressings are prepared by applying nonadherent gauze saturated in sterile saline to the burn and covering with a thick dressing to facilitate drainage. Follow-up is in 2 days to evaluate for infection. The patient should be instructed about the signs of infection and when to call the health care provider. Pain relief is accomplished with a nonsteroidal agent. Tetanus prophylaxis is indicated, and previously immunized patients should receive a booster as needed (Monafo, 1996; Peate, 1992).

## Time Frame for Initiating Pharmacotherapy

The vast majority of individuals should be taught to use a sunscreen any time their skin is exposed to UVR because of the effects of miniexposures over time and long-term consequences of UV exposure. In addition, those individuals taking drugs with photosensitivity side effects and individuals with photosensitive disorders should be taught to use maximum UVR protection strategies.

Typically, burns managed in the outpatient setting are small, superficial thermal burns that do not effect areas of critical function (eg, hands, joints) or of cosmetic concern (eg, face). These wounds usually meet the criteria for first-degree or minor second-degree burns. Persons with larger or deeper burns, circumferential burns of an extremity, burns complicated by an underlying medical condition, or burns of the hands, joints, or face and infants and children with burns are best treated as inpatients (Clayton & Solem, 1995).

## Overview of Drug Classes for Treatment

Initial outpatient management of burns includes pain control, cleansing of the wound, debridement of blisters or bullae, and application of a suitable dressing. An up-to-date tetanus immunization should be confirmed.

See Drug Table 805.

## Assessment and History Taking

Assessment of the skin is an essential component of all patient visits. A thorough history of the patient's habits of sun exposure is important, including hobbies, occupations, and other activities that take the patient outdoors. This is essential to the accurate determination of overall sun exposure of the patient and prescription of appropriate sunscreens, including protective clothing. Sensitivity to sunscreen preparations should also be assessed.

The primary health care provider should perform a thorough physical examination of the patient's skin to detect any suspicious lesions that may be cancerous or precancerous. The patient may require referral to a dermatologist or oncologist as appropriate.

Accurate assessment of burns is essential to appropriate treatment. Referral to a hospital prepared to care for burn patients may be indicated as previously described.

## Patient and Caregiver Information

Patients and caregivers should be taught the optimal methods of protecting their skin from harmful exposure to the sun during periods of outdoor activities. This includes correct selection and use of sunscreen preparations as well as the use of protective clothing and actual avoidance of sun exposure during the times of the day when the rays are most harmful. Special precautions for infants and children should also be taught to caregivers.

Patients with burns should be taught the correct way to care for the burn at home. Signs and symptoms of infection should also be taught to the patient and caregiver.

Patients and caregivers should be taught to examine their skin once a month in accordance with ACS guidelines. Literature is available from the ACS for use with patients.

## OUTCOMES MANAGEMENT

### Selecting an Appropriate Agent

Before recommending a sunscreen or suntan product, one should know the active ingredient and its maximum absorption, molar absorptivity, and concentration. Actual effectiveness in patients is difficult to determine precisely because individuals react in varying degrees to sunlight. The minimal erythemal dose (MED), the amount of sunlight needed for a minimum perceptible erythema (redness), is used to gauge the degree of sensitivity of both protected and unprotected skin to sunlight. The protection factor (PF), the ratio of the MED for protected skin to that for unprotected skin, is used to measure the relative effectiveness of sunscreens (the larger the PF value, the greater is the protection).

Individuals should be taught to select a sunscreen that provides the appropriate amount of protection for their skin type and the extent of UVR exposure. The goal of therapy is to prevent sunburn and minimize UVR exposure to reduce the extent of photoaging. Table 7–2 summarizes UVR photoprotection in adults.

Self-tanning products consist primarily of dihydroxyacetone (DHA). They are nontoxic and have a protein-staining effect in the stratum corneum of the skin. They may accentuate freckles and seborrheic keratoses, which may not be cosmetically desirable. Tanning accelerators are generally nontoxic and are a natural component of the skin in the normal melanogenic process. Tanning promoters (eg, 5-methoxypsoralen) are not available over-the-counter in the United States and have been documented as highly phototoxic and carcinogenic. Tanning pills contain canthaxanthin and are toxic to both skin and eyes. They are not available over-the-counter in the United States.

## Management of Minor Burns

*Pain control.*   Most burn patients will experience intense pain because of the exposure of nerve endings that generally lie beneath the epidermal layer. Any manipulation of the wound, for instance during debridement, will further stimulate the pain response. Immediate cooling of the wound may lessen the severity, but rarely will diminish the pain to such a level that drugs are not necessary. Narcotics are almost always necessary and may be needed until the wound has healed over. Generally, the combinations of acetaminophen with codeine (eg, Tylenol with Codeine No. 3) or acetaminophen with oxycodone (eg, Percocet, Tylox) are the preferred choices, the latter being more potent. Aspirin products should be avoided since they have antiplatelet activity, which may impair the healing process.

*Cleansing and wound protection.*   Most wounds are cleansed and dressed once daily. More frequent changes increase patient discomfort without improving the clinical rate of healing. Many protective and antibacterial products have been marketed for wound healing, but all have similar outcomes. Silver sulfadiazine is most commonly used. After cleaning the wound with mild soap and water, silver sulfadiazine is spread over it in a thin layer and a dressing is applied. A less expensive and equally effective alternative is bacitracin ointment. It is important to use a protective agent with antibacterial properties early in management. Microorganisms proliferate rapidly in burn wounds, especially in those severe enough to impair immune function. Topical antimicrobial agents increase the interval between injury and colonization and maintain low levels of wound flora.

*Adjuvant therapies.*   As a wound heals, the skin dries and is prone to itching. Initially, it is best to use moisturizers without added ingredients since the skin is sensitive. Simple petroleum jelly (Vasoline) or lotions suffice. Other agents containing urea and fragrances may be used as the skin matures. If the itching is particularly bothersome and unrelieved by topical therapy, diphenhydramine (Benadryl) or hydroxyzine (Atarax, Vistaril) orally may be used. These do

have a tendency to cause drowsiness, so the patient should be duly warned of the side effects.

## Monitoring for Efficacy

Patients should be monitored for risk of excessive UVR exposure; correct use, sensitivity, and toxicity of sunscreens, and assessed for precancerous and cancerous lesions as previously described. Patients should be referred to a dermatologist for diagnosis and treatment for precancerous and cancerous lesions immediately. Patients also should be taught how to examine their skin monthly for changes in existing moles and appearance of new ones. The ACS has numerous patient education materials that can be used to assist in teaching patients about skin care and assessment.

Patients should be taught to apply sunscreens correctly. Sunscreens should be applied at least 30–60 min prior to sun exposure. This allows for penetration of the skin for maximum efficacy. They should be reapplied after sweating, swimming, or exercising. However, remind them that *reapplication does not extend the amount of time the individual can spend out in the sun.* Nine teaspoons of sunscreen are considered adequate to cover the average adult; ½ teaspoon each to the face, neck, arms, both shoulders, back, and torso, and 1 teaspoon to each of the legs and feet (ACS, 1998). The patient should be instructed to read the label of the sunscreen product carefully and follow the instructions and precautions.

Sunscreens for children should be selected by the caregiver rigorously. The sunscreen should screen out both UVA and UVB radiation. The SPF should be at least 15, and the sunscreen should be applied at least 30 min before going outside (AAP, 1995). The sunscreen should be water-resistant or waterproof. Waterproof sunscreens should be reapplied at least every 2 h. An adequate amount (refer to package directions) should be used and rubbed in well. Be sure to cover the baby's face, nose, ears, feet, and hands, and the backs of the knees. Zinc oxide, an effective sunblock, can be used as extra protection on the nose, cheeks, tops of the ears, and shoulders (AAP, 1995).

The sunscreen should be tested on the baby's wrist for any type of reaction before applying it all over; however avoid the eyes. If the child cries or complains that the sunscreen burns his or her eyes, a different brand of sunscreen may be tried or try a sunscreen stick or sunblock with titanium dioxide or zinc oxide. If a rash develops, the caregiver should be instructed to contact the health care provider (AAP, 1995).

Patients with first- or second-degree burns should be followed up within 2 days to evaluate for healing, pain control and infection. Thereafter, weekly office examinations help in the monitoring of healing rate and for early signs of infection. Wounds should heal within 2–3 weeks. If healing takes longer, concern over infection and the potential for scarring should guide the therapy.

## Significant Food and Drug Interactions and Management

Since all of the agents used to treat burns and minimize the effect of UVR are topical, food and drug interactions are not a problem.

## Monitoring for Toxicity

As previously described, sunscreens should be tested prior to application by using a small amount in the inner aspect of the arm and waiting 24 h to determine whether there is a reaction to the agent. Sunscreens should be removed with bathing or showering after UVR exposure, especially in children, to reduce the chance of absorption.

## Follow-up Recommendations

Patients should be followed up at least yearly when the annual skin examination is conducted. Use of sunscreens, protective clothing, and monthly skin self-assessment can be evaluated at that time.

# PSORIASIS AND PITYRIASIS ROSEA

## PSORIASIS

Psoriasis is a common, chronically recurring papulosquamous skin disease of multifactorial etiology and about 5 million Americans (1.5–2% of the population) have the disease (Stern, 1996; Zanolli, 1996). The annual cost of treating psoriasis exceeds $1.6 billion. There is an equal sex incidence although females may be affected earlier in life than males (Camisa, 1995). Psoriasis occurs more often in whites than in Asians or African-Americans and only rarely in Native American Indians (Abel & Morhenn, 1996). Most patients with psoriasis are treated in primary care settings; psoriasis is the third most common reason for patients to visit a dermatologist (Stern & Nelson, 1993).

Psoriasis is characterized by whitish, scaly patches of varying size most commonly seen on the elbows, knees, and scalp. However, there is wide variation in severity and distribution of the skin lesions and the disease is marked by exacerbations and remissions.

Adults account for 84% of the office visits for psoriasis (Stern, 1996). Although lesions may occur just after birth, onset is most common in the second to fourth decades of life, with a mean age of onset of 27.8 years (Abel & Morhenn, 1996).

The disease is influenced by environmental, immunological, and genetic factors. The exact modes of inheritance are unknown. Certain HLA antigens are more common among populations of psoriasis patients, so a gene linked to or related to HLA genes may be one predisposing factor (Roenigk, 1991). Kinetic cell studies have shown that in psoriasis the epidermal cells proliferate rapidly, completing a germinative cell cycle more rapidly than do the cells of normal skin. The normal epidermal turnover time is 28–56 days. In psoriasis, the epidermis renews itself in just 3–4 days. Psoriasis is not contagious, and is often worse in the winter due to low indoor humidity and relative absence of sunlight.

There are four major subtypes of psoriasis based on the appearance of the lesions:

1. *Chronic plaque psoriasis* is the most common type. Patients exhibit one to many erythematous, clearly demarcated, oval plaques several centimeters in diameter. The plaques are covered by silvery-white scales.

2. *Guttate psoriasis* is the second most common type. It is characterized by an acute exanthum-like eruption with flat-topped scaly papules usually 1 mm to 1 cm in diameter over the entire body. It frequently follows an infection such as streptococcal pharyngitis or a viral upper respiratory infection, especially in children and young adults.

3. *Erythrodermic psoriasis* is infrequently seen. It is characterized by a generalized exfoliative erythroderma.

4. *Pustular psoriasis* is also uncommon. It is characterized by a generalized scaly plaque. In addition, small, superficial nonfollicular pustules develop. The pustules generally resolve in a few days, but usually recur.

The two major clinical characteristics of psoriasis are:

1. The primary lesions are papules or maculopapules.
2. The majority of the lesions are covered with imbricated scale.

The scale is usually silver-white, silver-gray, or mother-of-pearl in color and occurs in thin mica-like layers. If the scale is removed, minute bleeding points are exposed (Auspitz's sign). Once the initial lesion forms, it continues to enlarge by peripheral extension and gradually becomes more indurated and slightly more elevated, becoming a plaque. A plaque may cover several centimeters and gradually join other plaques to cover large areas. Other common sites of involvement are the sacral and perianal areas, genitalia, and nails. The patient may experience a burning sensation and pruritus in acute exacerbations of the disease.

Physical trauma in the active phase results in development of linear patterns of psoriasis in the injured areas (Koebner's phenomenon). Such isomorphic lesions also may be seen on the hands of factory workers in jobs requiring extensive use of the hands; they also occur in golf and tennis players (Roenigk, 1991).

Approximately 30% of psoriasis patients have nail involvement characterized by pitting of the nail plate, onycholysis (separation of the nail from the nail bed with resulting white color caused by air between the plate and the bed), and subungual hyperkeratosis (scale between the plate and the bed). Secondary bacterial or fungal infections may result in black or green discoloration of the nail plate.

## PITYRIASIS ROSEA

Pityriasis rosea is a common skin disease that occurs primarily on chest and trunk of young adults and is characterized by papulosquamous, oval, erythematous discrete lesions. It is mildly to moderately pruritic and occurs most often in the spring and fall. Face lesions are rare in white adults but are rather common in children and patients of African-American descent (Sauer & Hall, 1996). A "herald patch" lesion 2–10 cm round to oval resembling a patch of "ringworm" may precede the general rash by 2–10 days. The lesions are salmon-colored in Caucasians and hyperpigmented in African-Americans. The etiology is unknown, contagiousness is unknown,

and recurrence is not usual (2%). However, there is some belief that the rash is viral in origin (Habif, 1996). The disease is benign and self-limited.

## SPECIFIC CONSIDERATIONS FOR PHARMACOTHERAPY

### When Drug Therapy Is Needed

Although the exact causes of psoriasis and pityriasis rosea are unknown, treatment approaches are reliable and offer good control of the disorder. Since the disorders are visually apparent, emotional and psychological considerations warrant intervention in even the mildest of cases.

### Short- and Long-Term Goals of Pharmacotherapy

Psoriasis is often a lifelong relapsing and remitting disease, so modes of therapy should be selected with long-term consequences in mind. The goal of therapy is to achieve complete clearing of lesions (partial clearing is acceptable at times), using regimens with minimal toxicity and maximum patient acceptability. Consideration should be given to the patient's ability to maintain an active home and work environment with little interference from this disorder.

Pityriasis rosea is generally self-limiting. Treatment of pruritis with oral antihistamines and topical corticosteroids may be appropriate.

### Nonpharmacologic Therapy

Factors that tend to exacerbate psoriasis include alcohol use, obesity, emotional upsets or stress, infection, trauma to the skin, and certain drugs (ie, lithium, beta blockers, antimalarials, indomethacin). Patients should be instructed to eat a balanced diet to attain and maintain optimal weight and to avoid stress and fatigue. They should also be told that it can be controlled, it is completely epidermal, and they should continue therapy until it is clear.

Natural sunlight is effective adjunctive therapy for psoriasis in many patients. Psoriasis often improves in the summer months. Some patients move to warm, sunny climates to maximize sun exposure year round.

Phototherapy in the form of artificial ultraviolet light exposure is a specialized treatment. Ultraviolet therapy (UVB) in increasing suberythema doses, once or twice a week, can be used after a daily thin application of a 2% tar salve, similar to the Goeckerman regimen (Able & Morhenn, 1996; Roenigk, 1991; Sauer & Hall, 1996).

Psoralen plus ultraviolet A (PUVA) therapy uses a combination of oral psoralen and UVA for persistent or extensive psoriasis. It requires a special UVA light source, equipment, and specially trained personnel. PUVA therapy increases an individual's risk for nonmelanoma (but not melanoma) skin cancer. Therefore, patients should be followed indefinitely for the later development of skin cancer. There are numerous precautions when administering PUVA therapy. A detailed discussion of this therapy is beyond the scope of this chapter.

Erythrodermic and pustular psoriasis may be very difficult to treat, and such patients should be referred to a dermatologist as soon as possible for initial treatment (Whitmore, 1996).

Pityriasis rosea lesions have been found to resolve more quickly when exposed to direct sunlight or UVB administered in five consecutive treatments when used during the first week of the rash (Habif, 1996).

## Time Frame for Initiating Pharmacotherapy

Psoriasis is a lifelong disease and therefore will never be cured. To minimize the extent of skin involvement and to decrease the likelihood of progression beyond the epidermal layer, pharmacotherapy should be started at the earliest evidence of disease.

See Drug Table 802.

## Assessment and History Taking

Patients should be assessed for return of the lesions, overall disability, and discomfort. The Psoriasis Area and Severity Index quantifies disability and discomfort. This disease is characterized by remissions and exacerbations and cannot be cured. However, there have been reported cases of spontaneous remission with no recurrence that have not been explained.

Arthritis has been reported to affect nearly one third of psoriasis patients. Many view psoriasis and psoriatic arthritis as one disease affecting two organ systems. However, others believe the two are separate disorders. Regardless of etiology, the patient should be treated aggressively to minimize progression of the disease (Whitmore, 1996). Referral to a rheumatologist should be considered.

## Patient/Caregiver Information

Although there is no cure for psoriasis, the disease can be managed. The overall goal of therapy is to achieve remission in which most or all of the lesions resolve. However, exacerbations and remissions are the typical course of the disease. There is also significant variability in the extent of the disease and the psychological and social response to the disease.

## OUTCOMES MANAGEMENT

### Selecting an Appropriate Agent

Selection of specific therapies depends upon the degree of body surface involvement and the clinical subtype of the disease. In many cases, combination therapy may be used to enhance the efficacy and to enable the use of lower doses, thereby decreasing the toxicity of each individual agent.

For chronic plaque psoriasis, mild emollients and keratolytics with low-potency topical corticosteroids are usually all that is necessary. Over-the-counter products available are plain white petrolatum or mineral oil, hydrocortisone 1%, coal tar ointments or shampoos (5%), zinc pyrithione shampoo, and salt water. If the plaque becomes more generalized, topical agents become less useful and can become quite expensive. Therefore, consideration must be given to oral psoralen therapy in combination with ultraviolet A radiation. This therapy is generally given three times weekly until the outbreak clears, and is repeated as necessary.

Topical corticosteroids may be necessary. Products with triamcinolone 0.1% (ointment) or fluocinonide with 10% salicylic acid are particularly useful. However, tachyphylaxis can develop to these products.

Trigel, anthralin, and ketoconazole shampoo have been successful for scalp psoriasis, or ketoconazole 400 mg daily for 1 month may be tried.

Guttate psoriasis may be treated in the same fashion as described above and usually responds very well. Conversely, erythrodermic and pustular psoriasis may be very difficult to treat. Initial therapy includes bed rest, warm baths, and bland emollients, generally in combination with systemic therapy with etretinate, methotrexate, or cyclosporine. Systemic agents may be continued or the patient switched to PUVA therapy as tolerated once the disease is controlled. Many patients exhibit signs and symptoms of sepsis (vasodilation, increased cardiac output, fever, elevated white blood cell count with neutrophilia).

Methotrexate should be reserved for severe recalcitrant psoriasis. It has been used since the late 1950s with some success. There are currently 30,000 patients using it for psoriasis. It is contraindicated in liver disease. Oral administration is more convenient for the patient, but produces more nausea and compliance may be an issue. Intramuscular administration is less convenient for the patient, but minimizes these problems. The oral dose is 2.5 mg every 12 h for three doses; the intramuscular injection is given once as a 7.5-mg dose. The dose is increased as needed with the effective range being 7.5–25 mg. The average dose is 15 mg. After 1.5–2.0 g, a biopsy of the liver should be considered. Duration of therapy is dependent on cumulative dose and biopsy; a 3-year maximum is recommended.

Etretinate (ethyl ester of retinoic acid) and acitretin (metabolite of etretinate) are particularly effective in pustular psoriasis.

Calcipotriene (synthetic analog of vitamin D) is approved for plaque psoriasis. It should not be used on the face and is applied twice daily for up to 8 weeks. A maximum of 300 g a week is suggested. Improvement is usually seen in 2 weeks. Only 10% of patients show complete clearing. It has shown superiority to anthralin and topical steroids. It is better tolerated than anthralin but not as well tolerated as topical steroids.

Each patient should be assessed as an individual relative to disease severity, symptom, and level of physical, psychological, and social disability.

## Monitoring for Efficacy

Psoriasis is a common hyperproliferative epidermal disorder for which several effective therapeutic modalities control rather than cure the condition. Recognition of the pathogenic factors associated with psoriasis, selection of an appropriate treatment regimen, and monitoring for adverse effects as well as disease progression often lead to a satisfactory outcome.

Achievement of clinical efficacy by any given therapeutic regimen requires days to weeks. Initial dramatic response may be achieved with some agents such as corticosteroids; however, sustained benefit with pharmacologically specific antipsoriatic therapy usually requires about 2–4 weeks for noticeable response.

## Significant Food and Drug Interactions and Management

Oral corticosteroids and methotrexate may be taken with food if GI upset is noted. It is suggested that etretinate always be taken with food.

Drugs which may cause toxic levels of methotrexate include barbiturates, phenylbutazone, phenytoin, probenecid, salicylates, and sulfonamides. Severe bone marrow suppression can occur when methotrexate is combined with trimethoprim. It is ineffective with concomitant folic acid.

## Monitoring for Toxicity

For most of the agents used to treat psoriasis, hypersensitivity and photosensitivity are the major concerns. If acute inflammation, rash, burning, and/or blistering lesions occur at the area of application, discontinue use. Calcipotriene is 6% systemically absorbed, so when used regularly over a large area patients may demonstrate signs of hypercalcemia or vitamin D toxicity.

The most important side effects of methotrexate are acute cytopenias and chronic hepatitis and cirrhosis. The most important side effect of etretinate is the induction of mutations in a developing fetus. Because it has been detected in tissue many years after dosing, it should never be used in women of childbearing potential. It can also lead to hepatotoxicity. Cyclosporine's side effects include hypertension, nephrotoxicity, paresthesias, hypertrichosis, hyperuricemia, and anergy.

Over a long period of time, PUVA therapy increases an individual's risk of nonmelanoma skin cancer. Therefore, patients should be followed indefinitely to evaluate for these occurrences.

## Follow-up Recommendations

Follow-up is determined by the type of therapy and the recurrence of lesions. Patients should be monitored closely for efficacy of treatment and side effects and toxicity specific to the drug therapy prescribed (Abel & Morhenn, 1996; Barker et al, 1995). Vitamin and mineral deficiencies may occur because of the increased epidermal cell turnover rate of all the skin (Barker et al, 1995).

## REFERENCES

Abel, E., & Farber, E. (1993). Acne vulgaris and acneiform eruptions. In *Dermatology*. Scientific American.

Abel, E., & Morhenn, V. (1996). Psoriasis. In D. Demis (Ed.), *Clinical dermatology*. Philadelphia, PA: Lippincott-Raven.

American Academy of Pediatrics and the American Academy of Dermatology. (1995). *Fun in the sun: Keep your baby safe. Guidelines for parents*. Elk Grove, IL: AAP.

American Cancer Society. (1998). *Facts & Figures: Skin cancer*. Atlanta: American Cancer Society.

Anderson, K., & Maibach, H. (1991). Contact dermatitis. In M. Orkin, H. Maibach, & M. Dahl (Eds.), *Dermatology*. Norwalk, CT: Appleton & Lange.

Barker, L., Burton, J., & Zieve, P. (1995). *Principles of ambulatory medicine*. Baltimore: Williams & Wilkins.

Battan, F., Dart, R., & Rumack, B. (1997). Emergencies, injuries, and poisoning. In W. Hay, J. Groothius, A. Hayward, & M. Levin (Eds.), *Current pediatric diagnosis and treatment*. Stamford, CT: Appleton & Lange.

Berger, T., Goldstein, S., & Odom, R. (1997). Skin and appendages. In L. Tierney, S. McPhee, & M. Papadakis (Eds.), *Current medical diagnosis and treatment*. Stamford, CT: Appleton & Lange.

Bergfeld, W. (1995). The evaluation and management of acne: Economic considerations. *Journal of the American Academy of Dermatology, 32* (Suppl.), S52–S56.

Camisa, C. (1995). Treatment of severe psoriasis with systemic drugs. *Dermatology Nursing, 8*(2), 107–118.

Clark, C. (1993). Acne: General practice management. *The Practitioner, 237*(2), 160–164.

Clayton, M., & Solem, L. (1995). No ice, no butter. *Postgraduate Medicine, 97*(5), 151–165.

Cohn, M. (1992). Superficial fungal infections. *Postgraduate Medicine, 91*(2), 239–252.

Dockery, G. (1997). *Cutaneous disorders of the lower extremities*. Philadelphia: W. B. Saunders.

Drake, L., Ceilley, R., Cornelison, R., et al. (1995). Guidelines of care for warts: Human papillomavirus. *Journal of the American Academy of Dermatology, 32*(1), 98–103.

Eisenbaum, A. (1997). Eye. In W. Hay, J. Groothuis, A. Hayward, & M. Levin (Eds.), *Current pediatric diagnosis and treatment*. Stamford, CT: Appleton & Lange.

Elewski, B., & Weil, M. (1996). Dermatophytes and superficial fungi. In W. Sams & P. Lynch (Eds.), *Principles and practice of dermatology*. New York: Churchill Livingstone.

Eller, M., Yaar, M., & Gilchrist, B. (1994). DNA damage and melanogenesis. *Nature, 372*, 413–414.

Elliott, G., & Sams, W. (1996). Viral vesicular diseases. In W. Sams & P. Lynch (Eds.), *Principles and practice of dermatology*. New York: Churchill Livingstone.

Engle, J. (1995). Choosing sunscreen products. *American Druggist, 212*(2), 36.

Faergemann, J., Jones, T., Hettler, O., & Loria, Y. (1996). Pityrosporum ovale (*Malassezia furfur*) as the causative agent of seborrhoeic dermatitis: New treatment options. *British Journal of Dermatology, 134* (Suppl. 46), 12–15.

Farmer, K., & Naylor, M. (1996). Sunexposure, sunscreens, and skin cancer prevention: A year-round concern. *Annals of Pharmacotherapy, 30*, 662–673.

Frieden, I. (1996). Viral exanthems. In W. Sams & P. Lynch (Eds.), *Principles and practice of dermatology*. New York: Churchill Livingstone.

Garbe, C., Buttner, P., & Weiss, J. (1994). Associated factors in the prevalence of more than 50 common melanocytic nevi, atypical melanocytic nevi, and actini lentigines: Multicenter case-control study of the Central Malignant Registry of the German Dermatological Society. *Journal of Investigative Dermatology, 102*, 700–705.

Goldstein, E., Citron, D., & Nesbit, C. (1996). Diabetic foot infections: Bacteriology and activity of 10 oral antimicrobial agents against bacteria isolated from consecutive cases. *Diabetic Care, 19*(6), 638–641.

Goroll, J., May, L., & Mulley, A. (1995). *Primary care medicine*. Philadelphia: J. B. Lippincott.

Griffiths, C. (1992). The clinical identification and quantification of photodamage. *British Journal of Dermatology, 127* (Suppl. 41), 37–42.

Habif, T. (1996). *Clinical dermatology*. St. Louis: Mosby–Year Book.

Hirschmann, J. (1996). Bacterial infections of the skin. In W. Sams & P. Lynch (Eds.), *Principles and practice of dermatology*. New York: Churchill Livingstone.

Jarratt, M., & Dahl, M. (1991). Viral infections. In M. Orkin, H. Maibach, & M. Dahl (Eds.), *Dermatology*. Norwalk, CT: Appleton & Lange.

Jones, H. (1991). Fungal infections. In M. Orkin, H. Mailbach, & M. Dahl (Eds.), *Dermatology*. Norwalk, CT: Appleton & Lange.

Kaminer, M., & Gilchrist, B. (1995). The many faces of acne. *Journal of the American Academy of Dermatology, 32* (Suppl.), S6–S14.

Lammer, E., Chen, D., & Hoar, R. (1985). Retinoic acid embryopathy. *New England Journal of Medicine, 313*, 837–841.

Leach, C., Sumaya, C., & Brown, N. (1992). Human herpesvirus-6: Clinical implications of a recently discovered ubiquitous agent. *Journal of Pediatrics, 121*, 173–181.

Max, M., Schafer, S., Culnane, M., et al. (1988). Amitriptyline, but not lorazepam, relieves postherpetic neuralgia. *Neurology, 38,* 1427.

Middleton, D. (1996). Cellulitis and other bacterial infections. In M. Mengel & L. Schwiebert (Eds.), *Ambulatory medicine in the primary care of families.* Stamford, CT: Appleton & Lange.

Miller, D., & Weinstock, M. (1994). Nonmelanoma skin cancer in the United States: Incidence. *Journal of the American Academy of Dermatology, 30*(5), 774–778.

Millikan, L., & Shrum, J. (1992). An update on common skin diseases. *Postgraduate Medicine, 91*(6), 103–104, 107–108.

Monafo, W. (1996). Initial management of burns. *New England Journal of Medicine, 335*(21), 1581–1585.

Morelli, J., & Weston, W. (1997). Skin: General principles and diagnosis. In W. Hay, J. Groothius, A. Hayward, & M. Levin, (Eds.), *Current pediatric diagnosis and treatment.* Stamford, CT: Appleton & Lange.

Orkin, M., & Maibach, H. (1991). Ectoparasitic diseases. In M. Orkin, H. Maibach, & M. Dahl (Eds.), *Dermatology.* Norwalk, CT: Appleton & Lange.

Peate, W. (1992). Outpatient management of burns. *American Family Physician, 45*(3), 1321–1330.

Pion, I. (1996). Educating children and parents about sun protection. *Dermatology Nursing, 8*(1), 29–36.

Ray, T. (1996). Candidiasis and other yeast infections. In W. Sams & P. Lynch (Eds.), *Principles and practice of dermatology.* New York: Churchill Livingstone.

Richard, M., Grob, J., & Gouvernet, J. (1993). Role of sun exposure on nevus. First study in age-sex phenotype-controlled population. *Archives of Dermatology, 129,* 1280–1285.

Roenigk, H. (1991). Papulosquamous diseases. In M. Orkin, H. Maibach, & M. Dahl (Eds.), *Dermatology.* Norwalk, CT: Appleton & Lange.

Sams, W., & Lynch, P. (1996). *Principles and practice of dermatology.* New York: Churchill Livingstone.

Sauer, G., & Hall, J. (1996). *Manual of skin diseases.* Philadelphia: J. B. Lippincott.

Skinner, R., & Baselski, V. (1996). Dermatophytes and superficial fungi. In W. Sams & P. Lynch

(Eds.), *Principles and practice of dermatology.* New York: Churchill Livingstone.

Stern, R. (1996). Utilization of outpatient care for psoriasis. *Journal of the American Academy of Dermatology, 35,* 543–545.

Stern, R., & Nelson, C. (1993). The diminishing role of the dermatologist in the office-based care of cutaneous diseases. *Journal of the American Academy of Dermatology, 29,* 773–777.

Stern, R., Rosa, F., & Baum, C. (1984). Isotretinoin and pregnancy (Review). *Journal of the American Academy of Dermatology, 10,* 851–854.

Stone, M., & Lynch, P. (1996). Viral warts. In W. Sams & P. Lynch (Eds.), *Principles and practice of dermatology.* New York: Churchill Livingstone.

Strauss, J. (1991). Acne and rosacea. In M. Orkin, H. Maibach, & M. Dahl (Eds.), *Dermatology.* Norwalk, CT: Appleton & Lange.

Sullivan, T. (1986). Treatment of reactions to insect stings and bites. In L. Levin & J. Lockey (Eds.), *Monograph on insect allergy* (2nd ed.). Pittsburgh: American Academy of Allergy and Immunology.

Sykes, N., & Webster, G. (1994). Acne: A review of optimum treatment. *Drugs, 48*(1), 59–70.

Thiboutout, D., & Lookingbill, D. (1995). Acne: Acute or chronic disease? *Journal of the American Academy of Dermatology, 32* (Suppl.), S2–S5.

Vickers, C. (1991). Eczematous disease. In M. Orkin, H. Maibach, & M. Dahl (Eds.), *Dermatology.* Norwalk, CT: Appleton & Lange.

Walter, J., & Macknet, K. (1991). Pigmentation of osteoma cutis caused by tetracycline. *Archives of Dermatology, 110,* 113–114.

Wentzell, J. (1996). Sunscreens: The ounce of prevention. *American Family Physician, 53*(5), 1713–1715.

Whiteman, D., & Green, A. (1994). Melanoma and sunburn. *Cancer Causes and Control, 5,* 564–572.

Whitmore, E. (1996). Common problems of the skin. In L. Barker, J. Burton, & P. Zieve (Eds.), *Principles of ambulatory medicine.* Baltimore: Williams & Wilkins.

Zanolli, M. (1996). Psoriasis and Reiter's disease. In W. Sams & P. Lynch (Eds.), *Principles and practice of dermatology.* New York: Churchill Livingstone.

# 28

## HEMATOLOGIC DISORDERS

*Margaret A. Fitzgerald*

This chapter focuses on the assessment and management of anemias—iron, folate, and vitamin $B_{12}$ deficiencies—along with information on thrombus formation and the treatment of selected disorders of coagulation, encountered in primary care practice.

## ERYTHROPOIESIS

Red blood cell (RBC) production (erythropoiesis) occurs in marrow located in the vertebrae, ribs, sternum, skull, sacrum, pelvis, and proximal epiphyses of long bones such as the femur and humerus. In the child, nearly all marrow is active in RBC production (Spruill & Wade, 1993).

RBCs arise from undifferentiated stem cells containing DNA needed for mitosis and RNA needed for protein synthesis. Stem cells can be committed to developing into certain cell lines by the influence of growth factors, a group of glycoproteins that influence the differentiation of stem cells to their mature forms and regulate the number of these cells produced. Erythropoietin, a glycoprotein growth factor produced primarily by the kidney, influences the undifferentiated stem cell to form the RBC precursor (Hoffbrand & Pettit, 1993).

For erythrocytes to form, a number of conditions must be present. The marrow must be intact and capable of cell production with adequate supplies of micronutrients critical to RBC production. These micronutrients include vitamins $B_{12}$, C, E, $B_6$, thiamin, riboflavin, pantothenic acid, and folic acid. Also, certain metals such as iron, manganese, and cobalt as well as amino acids must be present in the marrow (Hoffbrand & Pettit, 1993; Spruill & Wade, 1993).

In addition, factors influencing bone marrow stimulation, such as the erythropoietin mechanism, should be intact. The continued production of RBCs is in great part regulated by erythropoietin, a hormone primarily produced by the kidney (90%) and the liver (10%). Erythropoietin production is stimulated by the presence of low blood oxygen tension in the renal tissue. The kidney then interprets this as a situation consistent with anemia or other clinical conditions indicating the oxygen-carrying capability of the blood is diminished, such as hypoxia, poor cardiac output, or acute blood loss. As a result, erythropoietin excretion is increased and the number of stem cells committed to RBC formation increases. When adequate blood oxygen tension is detected, erythropoietin excretion is limited, thus promoting homeostasis (Hoffbrand & Pettit, 1993). Critical to erythropoietin production is the function of the kidney. In end-stage renal failure, kidney tissue damage severely limits erythropoietin production. As a result, anemia is a significant problem. This can be treated with recombinant erythropoietin (Grossman & Brody, 1994). Also, adequate amounts of androgens and thyroxin—other hormones contributing to erythropoiesis—must be present (Hoffbrand & Pettit, 1993). Normal hematologic values are shown in Table 28–1.

## THE LIFE CYCLE OF THE RED BLOOD CELL

The length of time from development of the committed stem cell to circulating young RBC is about 1 week (Spruill & Wade, 1993). These young forms, known as reticulocytes, mature in about 24 h in circulation. The normal RBC life span is 120 days. During that time, 85% will be engulfed by the macrocyte-macrophage system. In this system, the hemoglobin is broken down into its components. The iron is largely extracted for reuse and placed back in plasma circulation. The amino acids in the globin chains are conserved. The remaining 15% of RBCs undergo hemolysis in circulation (Hardy, 1996). The presence of chronic infection can shorten the life span of the RBC. In addition, conditions causing chronic inflammation, such as in rheumatoid arthritis, cancer, and liver disease, can truncate the RBC life span (Linker, 1996).

## ANEMIA: DEFINITION AND CAUSES

Anemia is defined as a decrease in the number of circulating RBCs (Grossman & Brody, 1994). This results in decreased oxygen-carrying capability of the blood (Spruill & Wade, 1993). Equally important, with an anemia, there is a reduction in the reverse transport function of the RBC in carrying carbon dioxide waste away from the cell.

An important concept to bear in mind is that anemia is simply a sign of an underlying disease and only occurs when the hematologic reserves are exceeded. For example, in the healthy adult, the marrow reserve allows for new RBC production at two to three times normal in the face of acute blood loss. This can rise to six to eight times normal in the face of hemolysis (Hardy, 1996). Thus, anemias occur in the presence of a clinical insult severe enough to disturb the normal homeostatic mechanisms and exceed reserves.

An anemia is usually classified by its underlying etiology. For example, the problem may be decreased RBC production related to a lack of a vital micronutrient, such as in iron, folate, or vitamin $B_{12}$ deficiency. Reduced RBC production also can be seen in clinical situations when the RBC synthesis is reduced in the presence of chronic infection and/ or inflammation. Bone marrow can be suppressed due to the use of certain drugs, such as large doses of alcohol. As normal RBC cell death occurs without the production of new RBC forms, anemia can occur (Linker, 1996)

The classification of anemia also includes those caused by premature RBC destruction, or hemolysis. Intrinsic factors precipitating hemolysis include certain inherited hemoglobinopathies such as sickle cell anemia and G6PD deficiency. Less common is hemolysis caused by extrinsic factors such as immune responses and thrombotic thrombocytopenia (Linker, 1996).

Anemia can also be caused by blood loss. Generally, blood loss in an adult needs to be greater than 1 L before there is an appreciable drop in hemoglobin (Treseler, 1995). Severe trauma can, of course, cause sudden, acute blood loss. More common in primary care is an anemia caused by chronic lower-volume blood loss, as from heavy menstrual flow or a small volume gastrointestinal bleed. This scenario may also lead to a combined anemia: the patient not only loses RBCs at a level exceeding replace-

### TABLE 28–1. NORMAL HEMATOLOGIC VALUES

|  | Female Adult | Male Adult | Neonatal | Infant | Childhood |
|---|---|---|---|---|---|
| Hemoglobin | 12–15 g/dL | 13–17 g/dL | 14–24 g/dL | 10–15 g/dL | 11–16 g/dL |
| Hematocrit | 36–45% | 39–51% | 48–70% | 30–45% | 32–42% |
| RBC count | 4–5.3[a] | 4.4–5.7[a] | 4.8–7[a] | 4.1–6.4[a] | 4–5.3[a] |
| MCV | 81–100 fL | 81–100 fL | 96–108 fL | 82–91 fL | 82–91 fL |
| MCHC | 32–37% | 32–37% | 32–33% | 32–36% | 32–36% |
| RDW | 11.5–14.5% | 11.5–14.5% |  | 11.5–14.5% | 11.5–14.5% |

[a] measured in millions/mm³.
MCV = mean cell volume; MCHC = mean corpuscle hemoglobin concentration; RDW = red cell distribution width.
*Source: Adapted from Treseler (1995).*

ment but also develops iron deficiency. Since the iron from the RBC wasted via blood loss cannot be recycled, a vital source of iron is forfeited (Duffy, 1996).

As a result of the mechanisms causing anemia, remember that pharmacologic intervention to correct the presenting hematologic disorder is only part of the treatment plan. Correcting or modifying the underlying disease process is critical. When the diagnosis of anemia is established, the underlying cause can usually be identified by determining the following:

- *What is the cell size?* Is the RBC unusually small (microcytic)? Since hemoglobin is a major contributor to cell size, microcytosis is usually seen in anemia in which hemoglobin synthesis is impaired, such as iron deficiency anemia and the thalassemias (Linker, 1996). Is the RBC unusually large (macrocytic)? Macrocytosis is most commonly caused by impaired RNA and DNA synthesis in the young erythrocyte. Folic acid and vitamin $B_{12}$ contribute significantly to this process. Thus, a lack of either or both of these micronutrients can cause a macrocytic anemia (Spruill & Wade, 1993). Is the RBC of normal size (normocytic)? Generally, in these anemias there is no problem with RNA, DNA, or hemoglobin synthesis. Acute blood loss is one of a variety of reasons for a normocytic anemia (Linker, 1996).

- *What is the RDW?* RDW is the degree of variation in RBC width. This also may be noted as anisocytosis on RBC morphology (Treseler, 1995). RDW measurement is elevated when red blood cells are of varying sizes, implying that cells were synthesized under varying conditions. For example, in an iron deficiency anemia, normal-sized cells produced prior to the iron depletion will continue to circulate until their 120-day life span ends. At the same time, the new, smaller, iron deficient cells containing less hemoglobin are produced. Therefore, there will be wide variation in cell size and an increase in RDW. Since minor variation in cell size is normal, RDW is only considered increased when it is above 15% (Treseler, 1995).

- *What is the hemoglobin content (color) of the cell?* The hemoglobin content of the cell is reflected in the mean (average) corpuscle hemoglobin concentration (MCHC). It is reported as a percentage of the cell's volume. Since hemoglobin gives the RBC its characteristic red color, the suffix *-chromic* is used to describe the MCHC. Thus, when a cell has a normal MCHC, it is a normal color, or normochromic. When there is an impairment of hemoglobin synthesis, such as in iron deficiency anemia or thalassemia, the cells are pale, or hypochromic, and the MCHC is low. RBCs are seldom hyperchromic, or containing excessive amounts of hemoglobin (Treseler, 1995).

## CLINICAL PRESENTATION OF ANEMIA

The clinical presentation of anemia is highly variable as compensation is common because most anemias are gradual in onset. In addition, the oxyhemoglobin dissociation curve is moved to the right as the hemoglobin drops. As a result, the oxygen molecule is given up more freely by the RBC. Thus, symptoms of anemia seldom present unless the hemoglobin is below 10 g/dL. (Hoffbrand & Pettit, 1993).

Complaints of deep, sighing respiration with activity, often associated with a sensation of rapid, forceful heart rate, may be reported. This reflects the decreased oxygen-carrying capability of the blood and a corresponding compensatory mechanism. Fatigue and headache may also present. In the patient at risk or with coronary artery disease, angina may be reported. In the infant and younger child, the caregiver may report irritability and delay of large motor skills, primarily due to poor muscle tone (Lane, Armstrong, Ingrim, & Lance, 1995).

The physical examination usually contributes little to a diagnosis of anemia unless the anemia is severe. Pallor of the skin and mucous membranes is not reliable and usually only seen when anemia is severe (hemoglobin below 8 g/dL) (Hoffbrand & Pettit, 1993). In the elderly or patients with coronary artery disease, congestive heart failure signs (distended neck veins, rales, tachycardia, right upper quadrant abdominal tenderness, hepatomegaly) may be seen in severe anemia (Lindenbaum, 1996). An early systolic murmur may be heard, owing to the increase of blood flow over the heart valves (Grimes & Burns, 1992). Neurologic findings such as paresthesia or difficulty with balance and, in extreme cases, confusion may be found in vitamin $B_{12}$ deficiency anemia (Linker, 1996). Findings for specific anemias are found in their corresponding section, in this chapter.

## IRON DEFICIENCY ANEMIA

Iron deficiency is the most common reason for anemia worldwide (Hoffbrand & Pettit, 1993). A number of factors contribute to the development of iron deficiency anemia (IDA). In the adult, diet is rarely a cause of iron deficiency. An estimated 8 years of poor iron intake in an adult would be needed to elicit IDA (Hoffbrand & Pettit, 1993). Rather, chronic blood loss, causing a wasting of the RBCs' recyclable iron, is the most common cause. In premenopausal women, blood loss from the reproductive tract is a significant contributor to IDA (Ries & Santi, 1995). The average woman loses 50 mL of blood monthly, increasing five- to sevenfold in the presence of heavy menstrual flow. In these women with menorrhagia, replacing wasted iron with diet alone would be unlikely, as 3–4 mg/day is needed (Linker, 1996). Pharmacologic iron supplementation to avoid anemia probably is necessary.

Normal daily iron losses equal absorption, so iron balance is a tightly regulated system. Adult males and postmenopausal women require 1 mg iron per day. The woman during reproductive years requires 1.5–3mg/day, in part because of the monthly loss of RBCs with the menses. Children have higher iron demands due to growth and increase in blood volume. In all these circumstances, iron requirements are achievable with a well-balanced diet.

Blood loss from the gastrointestinal tract is also a common cause of IDA in adults (Ries & Santi, 1995). This blood loss is usually low-volume and chronic, such as from aspirin or other NSAID use or peptic ulcer disease (Duffy, 1996). One milliliter of packed red blood cells contains 1 mg of iron (Linker, 1996), so even losses of 2–3 ml of blood via the gastrointestinal tract can lead to iron deficiency.

The term infant is born with iron stores that will be exhausted by age 4 months if no dietary iron supplementation is given. Preterm infants will deplete their stores more rapidly since fetal iron storage is primarily an activity of the third trimester. Iron-enriched formula and/or breast milk used as the major caloric source in the first year of life assists in meeting the rapidly growing infant's iron needs and largely prevents the development of IDA in early childhood. However, early childhood is a period of high iron use. As a result, dietary iron deficiency is a significant cause of IDA in the child aged 6–24 months. In the child over 2, the most common cause of IDA is chronic blood loss (Lane, Armstrong, Ingrim, & Lance, 1995).

## SPECIAL CONSIDERATIONS FOR PHARMACOTHERAPY

### When Drug Therapy Is Needed

The diagnosis of iron deficiency anemia must be established before initiating iron therapy. A number of other conditions, such as thalassemia trait and plumbism (lead poisoning), can mimic IDA. Misinterpretation of laboratory data can lead to the inappropriate treatment of a benign condition (thalassemia trait) or a potentially life-threatening disease (plumbism). The laboratory diagnosis of IDA is supported by the following findings:

- *Early disease:* Low normal hemoglobin, hematocrit, and total RBC count and normocytic, possibly hypochromic, RDW >15%.
- *Later disease:* Microcytic, hypochromic anemia with low RBC count and elevated RDW >15%.
- *Low serum iron:* Reflects iron concentration in circulation. This level may be falsely elevated due to recent high iron intake.
- *Elevated total iron-binding capacity (TIBC):* A measure of transferrin, a plasma protein that easily combines with iron. When more transferrin is available for binding, the TIBC rises, reflecting iron deficiency.
- *Iron saturation less than 15%:* Calculate by dividing the serum iron by the TIBC.
- *Low serum ferritin:* The body's major iron storage protein.
- *Absence of iron from bone marrow,* if aspiration is done (Treseler, 1995).

In IDA, the order of the fall of the laboratory markers is as follows: Ferritin, marrow, serum iron, TIBC (rise), RDW (rise), hemoglobin, RBC indices. As a result, a drop in hemoglobin or RBC indices is a late rather than early marker of disease.

***Prevention of IDA in Pregnancy.***    Fifteen to 25% of all pregnancies are complicated by anemia, with IDA accounting for 95% (Biswas & Perloff, 1994). During the first half of pregnancy, iron requirements are only slightly increased and likely can be met by diet. However, during the later half of pregnancy and the postpartum period, iron requirements for RBC replacement increase dramatically because of increased red cell mass, and rapid fetal growth, and anticipated blood loss at the time of the birth (Biswas & Perloff, 1994).

Iron absorption by the duodenum doubles during pregnancy (Spruill & Wade, 1993). In spite of this, iron needed by the woman in the second half of pregnancy is equivalent to 3.5 mg/day, likely exceeding what can be supplied by even the most prudent diet. Total pregnancy iron needs are about 1000 mg (500 mg for fetal use, 300mg for maternal RBC use, and 200 mg to compensate for loss). As a result, prescription prenatal vitamins usually contain 60 mg of elemental iron as ferrous sulfate 300 mg.

## Short- and Long-Term Goals of Pharmacotherapy

The short-term goal of pharmacotherapy is resolution of the iron deficiency–induced anemia and treatment of the underlying cause of the IDA. The long-term goal is restoration and maintenance of iron stores.

## Nonpharmacologic Therapies

The rate of iron absorption from the duodenum and proximal jejunum increases significantly during times of great iron needs (pregnancy, childhood growth spurts) as well as disease states such as IDA (Hoffbrand & Pettit, 1993). Those with the greatest iron needs should receive nutritional counseling so as to minimize the risk of IDA development and make use of this natural adaptive process.

Iron is found in abundance in meat protein, the most available dietary iron source. Animal source iron is easily extracted for use. Plant sources of iron are much more tightly bound and thus less available (Ries & Santi, 1995).

## Time Frame for Initiating Pharmacotherapy

Iron therapy should be initiated as soon as the IDA diagnosis is made. Usually iron therapy is continued for 2–3 months after hemoglobin correction to ensure that iron stores have been replenished.

See Table 28–2.

## Assessment and History Taking

The primary assessment needed is the definitive diagnosis of IDA: the presence of a microcytic, hypochromic anemia with abnormal iron studies consistent with the diagnosis. There are no specific contraindications to treating IDA. However, the issue of iron's ability to interact with many medications (see Table 28–3) needs to be considered before its initiation. The condition causing IDA, such as chronic blood loss and poor diet, must also be treated.

## OUTCOMES MANAGEMENT

### Selecting an Appropriate Agent

Supplemental or pharmacologic iron is available in a number of forms. Ferrous sulfate ($FeSO_4$) is the most commonly used and represents an inexpensive, effective treatment option. Each 325-mg tablet contains 65 mg of elemental iron, with an absorption rate of approximately 25%. Since the person with IDA can absorb a maximum of 50–100 mg of iron daily, a dose range of 200–400 mg of elemental iron is recommended (Ries & Santi, 1995). However, the duodenum remains relatively refractory to iron absorption for 6 h after a large dose is ingested. Therefore, for the multiple doses that fit within this recommendation (three to six tablets), dosing would need to be on a rigid, round-the-clock schedule. The most commonly recommended regime for adults is ferrous sulfate 325 mg three times a day (Linker, 1996).

In children, 4–6 mg/kg per day of elemental iron in three divided doses daily is needed to correct IDA. Less severe IDA can be treated with 3mg/kg per day (Lane, Armstrong, Ingrim, & Lance, 1995). For the preterm infant receiving iron therapy as prophylaxis to compensate for low iron stores, the recommended dose is 0.5–2 mg/kg per day as a single dose (Dupuis, Smith, & Kowalczyk, 1995). The most commonly used pediatric iron forms are ferrous sulfate elixir 220 mg/5 mL for toddlers and preschoolers and ferrous sulfate liquid 75 mg/0.6 mL for use in infants.

Alternative oral iron forms include ferrous gluconate and ferrous fumarate, each containing a different amount of elemental iron per tablet. The prescriber must adjust the recommended number of tablets per day to ensure that the appropriate dose of elemental iron is being taken; see Table 28–2. Sustained-release and enteric-coated iron products should be avoided. These products are less likely to release iron in the proximal jejunum and duodenum, the area of best iron absorption (Ries & Santi, 1995). Iron

### TABLE 28-2. IRON PREPARATIONS

| Form | % Elemental Iron | Recommended Dose Range |
| --- | --- | --- |
| Ferrous fumarate | 33 | Adult: 200 mg b.i.d.–q.i.d. |
| Ferrous gluconate | 11.6 | Adult: 325–650 mg q.i.d.<br>Child: 16mg/kg/day |
| Ferrous sulfate | 20 | Adult: 300 mg b.i.d.–q.i.d.<br>Child: 10 mg/kg t.i.d. |

Source: Ries and Santi (1995).

deposited in the alkaline environment of the small intestine, common when sustained-release products are used, forms an insoluble complex and is not utilized (Spruill & Wade, 1993). In addition, the cost of sustained-release products usually is considerably higher.

Iron also is available in an injectable form as iron dextran. Indications for its use include intestinal diseases, such as sprue, that limit ability to absorb oral preparations, and for those receiving parenteral nutrition only. Resolution of IDA is not more rapid when using injectable iron, although stores may be replenished more rapidly.

Using injectable iron can cause an allergic reaction ranging from local inflammation to anaphylaxis. For that reason, a test dose of 0.5 mL IM (using the Z track technique to minimize the risk of tissue staining and/ or irritation) should be administered over 5 m IV. If no reaction is noted, the needed therapeutic dose is calculated by body weight or through the use of a formula to calculate the iron dose needed to correct the anemia. Caution must continue to be used with injectable iron therapy since allergic reactions have been noted in those who have previously received the product without difficulty (Hillman, 1996).

### Patent/Caregiver Information

Drug interactions with iron are numerous and potentially serious; see Table 28–3. In general, the iron dose should be separated by at least 2 h from any other medication.

Optimally, ferrous sulfate should be taken on an empty stomach to enhance iron absorption (Hoffbrand & Pettit, 1993). In addition, taking vitamin C 200 mg or more with the iron dose increases its absorption by at least 30% (Hillman, 1996). However, both these strategies significantly increase the risk of gastrointestinal upset.

Iron staining of the teeth may be seen when liquid preparations are used (Lane, Armstrong, Ingrim, & Lance, 1995). In addition, children may find the taste objectionable. Mixing the medication with orange juice to mask its taste and having the child sip the mixture through a straw placed toward the back of the mouth may help with both problems. Since the staining is superficial, it will resolve after iron therapy is complete. Brushing the teeth after an iron dose may also minimize this problem.

### Iron Therapy Side Effects

Gastrointestinal irritation, epigastric pain, nausea, and vomiting are reported by more than 10% of those who take iron (Lane, Armstrong, Ingrim, & Lance, 1995). Although this can be largely eliminated by taking the drug with a meal, recognize that this will reduce iron absorption. Length of treatment may need to be extended as a result. Another strategy to reduce iron-induced GI upset is to initiate the therapy with a single dose once a day (Duffy, 1996), and then add additional doses on a weekly basis until the desired dose is reached. Changing from one iron source to another, particularly to a form with a lower amount of elemental iron per tablet, can be helpful (Ries & Santi, 1995). Prescribing the needed dose in elixir form may help with gastrointestinal irritation because of its rapid dispersion.

Constipation is also reported in more than 10% of those on iron therapy (Lane, Armstrong, Ingrim, & Lance, 1995). Adding extra fiber and liquid to the diet can often help. If constipation persists, lower the dose and extend the length of treatment so the patient can complete the needed therapeutic course.

## TABLE 28–3.  DRUG INTERACTIONS WITH IRON THERAPY

| Drug | Effect | Comment |
|---|---|---|
| Calcium carbonate antacids | Decreased iron absorption | Al, Mg antacids do not interact |
| Cimetidine | Decreased iron absorption | Avoid concurrent use |
| Caffeine | Decreased iron absorption | Separate by at least 2 h |
| Fluoroquinolones (ciprofloxacin, norfloxacin, ofloxacin, lomefloxacin) | Decreased fluoroquinolone effect | Avoid concurrent use |
| Levodopa | Decreased levodopa effect | May not be noted with carbodopa |
| Methyldopa (Aldomet) | Decreased antihypertensive effect | Monitor BP |
| Penicillamine | Decreased penicillamine absorption | Increase penicillamine dose when iron added |
| Tetracycline | Decreased tetracycline effect; decreased iron absorption | Do not use concurrently if possible, interaction not noted with doxycycline |
| Thyroid hormones | Decreased thyroxine effect | Take thyroid hormones at least 2 h before or 4 h after iron dose |
| Zinc | Decreased zinc absorption | Avoid concurrent use |

*Source: Rizack (1996).*

## Monitoring for Efficacy

Reticulocytosis begins quickly after initiation of iron therapy, with the reticulocyte count peaking 7–10 days into therapy. Hemoglobin rises at a rate of 2 g/dL every 3 weeks in response to iron therapy (Hoffbrand & Pettit, 1993) and will likely take 2 months to correct (Duffy, 1996). As a result, the following laboratory tests may be used to evaluate the resolution of IDA: reticulocytes at 1–2 weeks to ensure marrow response to iron therapy, hemoglobin at 6 weeks to 2 months to ensure anemia recovery, and ferritin at 2 months after measure of normal hemoglobin (or 4 months after initiation of iron therapy) to ensure documentation of replenished iron stores.

## Monitoring for Toxicity

In children, iron overdose is common and potentially life-threatening. The most common source of this poisoning is maternal prenatal vitamins. In addition, ferrous sulfate tablets may resemble candy (Nolan, 1997). Although the lethal level of poisoning has not been established, ingestion of elemental iron of 25 mg/kg will likely cause symptoms, of 50mg/kg potentially serious reactions, and of 75mg/kg severe signs and symptoms. In large doses, iron is corrosive to the gastric mucosa, allowing a large amount of systematic absorption. Virtually every body system is negatively affected by this toxic level of iron exposure.

When a child presents with a history consistent with iron overdose, a plain x-ray of the abdomen will reveal iron tablet fragments ingested within the past 2 hours. The film will not, however, reveal the multivitamins with low iron doses, nor, due to its rapid dispersion, iron elixir. Iron does not bind with activated charcoal nor can it be lavaged from the upper gastrointestinal system. Bowel decontamination with a polyethylene glycol solution given via nasogastric means may help remove undissolved tablets.

Deferoxamine is a specific agent for the management of iron overdose, acting as a chelating agent. Its use is continued until iron levels are reduced. Supportive care for airway and circulatory maintenance is critical.

## Follow-up Recommendations

Iron deficiency anemia occurs secondary to another condition, such as pregnancy, bleeding, or poor nutrition. Follow-up care for the person recovering from IDA should include care for the underlying condition.

# MEGALOBLASTIC ANEMIAS CAUSED BY FOLATE OR VITAMIN B$_{12}$ DEFICIENCIES

Folate (the reduced form of folic acid) and vitamin B$_{12}$ are essential for DNA synthesis. When deficiencies of either of these micronutrients exist, DNA synthesis in the RBC is impaired, leading to distinctive changes in the RBC and bone marrow (Allen, 1996; Ries & Santi, 1995). The most clinically distinct change is the development of macrocytosis caused in part by the cell's high RNA:DNA ratio. This change is reflected in an increase in RBC mean cell volume (MCV). Since hemoglobin production is unaffected (Ries & Santi, 1995), cell color is maintained, yielding a normochromic cell, reflected in the measure of mean corpuscular hemoglobin concentration (MCHC).

## FOLATE DEFICIENCY ANEMIA

Through a complex reaction, folic acid is reduced to folate. Folate donates one carbon unit to oxidation at various levels, reactions vital to the proper DNA synthesis (Hillman, 1996). Folic acid (pteroylglutamic acid) is a water-soluble B-complex vitamin found in abundance in peanuts, fruits, and vegetables (Linker, 1996). The standard diet contains approximately 50–500 µg/day as absorbable folate. During times of accelerated growth, such as childhood growth spurts and pregnancy and hemolytic anemia, the folic acid requirements increase from the baseline of 50 µg/day to 100–200 µg/day (Hillman, 1996). Folate is absorbed throughout the gastrointestinal tract (Linker, 1996).

The usual nonspecific findings in anemia may be present in folate deficiency. Diarrhea, sore tongue, and anorexia are common, with forgetfulness and irritability seen less often. Scleral icterus and splenomegaly may be seen. These findings also are seen in pernicious anemia (Grossman & Brody, 1994).

### Special Consideration for the Woman Who Is Pregnant or Planning a Pregnancy

About 1% of all pregnancies are affected by folate deficiency, accounting for 10% of pregnancy-related anemias. Given that normal stores of folic acid last 3–4 months, the condition is usually diagnosed in the later part of pregnancy (50%) or in the postpartum period (50%) (Cruickshank, 1994). Folic acid transfers readily through the placenta to the fetus, with fetal levels usually higher than maternal levels. Thus, there is evidence that pregnancy is a maternal folate-depleting event. Repeated or multiple pregnancies, in particular, cause depletion of

the maternal RBC folate levels (Briggs, Freeman, & Yaffee, 1994).

Folic acid has been assigned pregnancy risk category A (Briggs, Freeman, & Yaffee, 1994). Folate deficiency during pregnancy can be largely avoided through the consistent use of prescriptive prenatal vitamins, each tablet usually containing 0.8–1 mg of folic acid. Over-the-counter prenatal vitamins contain significantly less of this micronutrient, usually about 0.4 mg per tablet.

Supplementation should continue through lactation since approximately 0.5 mg of folic acid per day is transferred to breast milk (Hillman, 1996). Accumulation of the vitamin in human milk takes preference over maintaining maternal folate levels. The folic acid level is low in colostrum, with levels rising as true milk production is established. Refrigerating breast milk for short periods of time does not appear to alter its folic acid content, whereas protracted frozen storage (up to 3 months) causes a progressive drop in levels to below the recommended daily folate requirement for an infant (Briggs, Freeman, & Yaffee, 1994).

Maternal folic acid deficiency is likely a teratogenic state, particularly during neural tube formation. To reduce the rate of neural tube defects in their offspring, women planning a pregnancy should be advised take additional folic acid, 0.4 mg daily for 3 months, prior to conception. This recommendation should be extended to all women capable of conception. Over-the-counter multivitamin or diet supplementation with vitamin-fortified foods can easily supply the recommended folate dose. If the woman has a history of giving birth to a child with a neural tube defect, the folic acid dose should be increased to 4 mg daily 3 months preconception (Olson, 1995) and continued at least through the first 12 weeks of pregnancy (Briggs, Freeman, & Yaffee, 1994).

If the pregnancy is unplanned or preconception counseling was not sought, initiating folic acid supplementation during the first 7 weeks of pregnancy appears to offer some neural tube protection (Briggs, Freeman, & Yaffee, 1994). This can be supplied by a prescription prenatal vitamin supplement. However, if the pregnant woman cannot tolerate the prenatal vitamin supplement because of nausea, a common condition, she likely will be able to take folic acid alone without difficulty.

Phenytoin (Dilantin) use in pregnancy presents a particularly difficult situation. As a result of pregnancy-related changes in drug metabolism and excretion, phenytoin doses usually need to be increased 30–50% above the prepregnancy dose in order to maintain seizure control. In addition, the pregnant woman requires folic acid supplementation to avoid developing anemia and to assist in neural tube formation in the fetus, thus potentially reducing phenytoin levels and negatively affecting seizure control. In this situation, monitoring free phenytoin levels is critical to the health of the mother and unborn child. In addition, the woman taking phenytoin should have serum and RBC folate levels measured preconception and during the period of organogenesis to ensure the best pregnancy outcome (Briggs, Freeman, and Yaffee, 1994).

## Short- and Long-Term Goals of Pharmacotherapy

The short-term goal of pharmacotherapy is resolution of the folate deficiency–induced anemia and treatment of the underlying cause of the folate deficiency. The long-term goal is restoration and maintenance of folate stores.

## Nonpharmacologic Therapies

Folic acid deficiency often can be avoided or, if present, treatment enhanced by a high folic acid diet. The most common causes of folic acid deficiency anemia are inadequate dietary intake, seen in the elderly, alcoholics, and the impoverished as well as those with a decreased ability to absorb folic acid, patients with malabsorption syndromes such as sprue and celiac disease. Also, children given folic acid–poor goat's milk in place of cow's milk may become folate-deficient. As it is heat-labile, up to 90% of folic acid can be destroyed through excessive cooking or food reheating (Hillman, 1996), leaving those who eat little fresh food at higher risk. In addition, unusually high folic acid utilization can be seen when cell division is high—during pregnancy, childhood growth spurts, hemolytic anemia, inflammation, and rheumatoid arthritis—leading to folic acid deficiency (Hoffbrand & Pettit, 1993; Spruill & Wade, 1993). Thus diet counseling for these high risk groups is critical.

## Time Frame for Initiating Pharmacotherapy

Intervention is initiated when the diagnosis is established. Folic acid supplementation should be continued until the anemia is resolved (1–2 months) and continued as long as the risk for its development exists.

## Assessment and History Taking

Folic acid deficiency anemia takes some months to develop. In the absolute absence of dietary folic acid, the body stores are exhausted within a few months, with liver stores depleted in 4–6 weeks. At that time, the serum folate drops. In an additional 5 weeks, hypersegmented neutrophils develop, again reflecting the contribution of folic acid to cellular DNA synthesis. The RDW rises. In 17 weeks, reduced RBC folate levels and macrocytosis are noted, with megaloblastic bone marrow changes at week 19 and the appearance of anemia at week 20 (Samuels, 1991). These changes may take longer to occur when folic acid intake is decreased but not absent, or when it is available but demands are increased.

When a megaloblastic anemia is found, screening needs to be performed for both folic acid and vitamin $B_{12}$ deficiency by obtaining serum levels of both micronutrients. Since vitamin $B_{12}$ deficiency can cause irreversible neurologic damage if not promptly treated, ruling out its presence is critical to safe practice.

Phenytoin can cause a macrocytic anemia reversible with folic acid supplementation. At the same time, folic acid supplementation in large doses causes increased metabolism of phenytoin, possibly reducing its therapeutic efficacy. As a result, phenytoin levels should be carefully monitored when folic acid supplementation is required (Rizack, 1996).

## Patient and Caregiver Information

Informing the patient and/or caregiver about folic acid dietary supplementation is important in obtaining the anemia's resolution. Pharmacologic folic acid supplements require no specific advice on timing of dose.

## Outcomes Management

***Selecting an Appropriate Agent.***   Folic acid is supplied primarily in an inexpensive generic form. Recommended doses for folic acid replacement in the adult range from 0.5–1 mg/day (Olson, 1995) to 5 mg/day (Hoffbrand & Pettit, 1993), with the usual dose being 1 mg/day (Linker, 1996). Folic acid is generally well tolerated, with doses of 50–100 recommended daily amounts (RDA) needed before toxic effects are noted (Olson, 1995). The underlying cause of the folate deficiency also must be treated.

***Monitoring for Efficacy.*** Reticulocytosis occurs rapidly, with a peak at 7–10 days into folic acid therapy. The hematocrit rises by 4–5% per week and generally returns to normal in 1 month. Leukopenia and thrombocytopenia resolve within 2–3 days of therapy (Waterbury, 1995). A repeat hemogram in 1–2 months assists in the monitoring of therapeutic effect. Resolution of the related signs and symptoms generally follows the time frame needed for the resolution of the anemia.

***Monitoring for Toxicity.*** Folic acid is a water-soluble vitamin that is easily excreted. As a result, even in overdose, toxicity is seldom seen.

***Follow-up Recommendations.*** Folate deficiency anemia occurs secondary to another condition. Follow-up care for the person recovering from folate deficiency anemia should include care for the underlying condition.

## VITAMIN B₁₂ DEFICIENCY

Vitamin $B_{12}$, a member of the cobalamin family, is found in abundance in foods of animal origin and is essential to the development of the red blood cell. When vitamin $B_{12}$ is ingested orally, it binds with intrinsic factor, a glycoprotein produced by the gastric parietal cells and transported systematically. Within the portal blood flow, the vitamin is attached to transcobalamin II, a polypeptide synthesized in the liver and ileum. Intrinsic factor is not absorbed, and the new compound is transported to the bone marrow and other sites where it is available for use in red blood cell formation. Two additional glycoproteins, transcobalamin I and III, combine with $B_{12}$ and are used in the formation of granulocytes (Linker, 1996). In synergy with folic acid, vitamin $B_{12}$ plays a role essential to RBC DNA synthesis. When deficiencies of either of these micronutrients exist, DNA synthesis in the RBC is impaired, leading to the distinct changes in the RBC and bone marrow (Allen, 1996; Ries & Santi, 1995). The most clinically distinctive change is the development of macrocytosis caused in part by the cell's high RNA:DNA ratio. This change is reflected in an increase in RBC

MCV. Since hemoglobin production is unaffected (Ries & Santi, 1995), cell color is maintained, yielding a normochromic cell, reflected in the measure of MCHC.

The most common form of vitamin $B_{12}$ deficiency is *pernicious anemia*, a disorder that causes atrophy of the stomach and is probably autoimmune in nature. With this atrophy, secretion of the intrinsic factor ceases and achlorhydria is present (Hoffbrand & Pettit, 1993). Without intrinsic factor, a vital link of $B_{12}$ delivery is lost. Rarely, vitamin $B_{12}$ deficiency can be caused by a highly restricted vegan-type diet in which all animal products are omitted and no supplementation is taken (Linker, 1996).

Physical manifestations of vitamin $B_{12}$ deficiency include those noted with other anemias. However, this anemia can be particularly severe, with presenting hematocrits as low as 10–15%, since the disease is slow in developing and compensation is common. Vitamin $B_{12}$ deficiency can cause a characteristic group of neurologic problems, including peripheral neuropathy, difficulty with balance, and memory changes (Linker, 1996), as well as oral irritation and icterus (Hoffbrand & Pettit, 1993). Without treatment, these neurologic changes may become permanent. Since the disease is most common in elderly women, an older woman presenting with a sore tongue, fatigue, new-onset forgetfulness, and a gait disturbance should be tested for this disorder.

### When Drug Therapy Is Needed

As the neurologic complications can be irreversible if left untreated, prompt treatment of pernicious anemia is essential. In addition, the degree of anemia is often severe, necessitating swift intervention to prevent cardiac decompensation.

### Short- and Long-Terms Goals of Pharmacotherapy

The short-term goals of treatment include the reversal of neurologic signs and the reversal of anemia. Long-term goals include maintenance of a normal blood count and an intact neurologic status.

### Nonpharmacologic Therapies

As mentioned, most individuals have ample dietary $B_{12}$ and need no supplementation. However, those who do not eat animal products should be advised either to supplement the diet with vitamin $B_{12}$ orally or to use $B_{12}$-rich foods, such as brewer's yeast.

## Time Frame for Initiating Pharmacotherapy

Vitamin $B_{12}$ therapy should be initiated when the diagnosis is made. Usually there is a brisk hematologic response, and the anemia is resolved within 2 months. Reversal of neurologic abnormalities is generally slower, but improvement is seen quickly.

See Table 28–4.

## Assessment and History Taking

As with folate deficiency anemia, vitamin $B_{12}$ deficiency anemia is a macrocytic (elevated MCV) normochromic (normal MCHC) anemia. However, the degree of macrocytosis is generally marked (MCV 110–160), exceeding that seen in folate deficiency. Additional hematologic changes include the presence of hypersegmented neutrophils, often with leukopenia. The platelet count is often reduced as well (Linker, 1996).

Any person presenting with a macrocytic anemia should be assessed by history and physical examination for the neurologic changes seen in vitamin $B_{12}$ deficiency. In addition, serum folate and $B_{12}$ should be measured as part of the initial evaluation of macrocytic anemia to ensure that $B_{12}$ and not folate deficiency is the problem. In vitamin $B_{12}$ deficiency, the serum $B_{12}$ will be low, whereas serum folate is elevated or normal. However, RBC folate is often low, reflecting the interaction of these micronutrients during RBC formation (Hoffbrand & Pettit, 1993).

If the serum $B_{12}$ level is abnormally low, a Schilling's test is usually done. This is an indirect test of intrinsic factor deficiency, used to confirm the etiology of the vitamin $B_{12}$ deficiency (Treseler, 1995).

## Patient/Caregiver Information

The importance of treatment and appropriate follow-up must be stressed. With pernicious anemia, lifelong intervention is needed to avoid recurrence and relapse.

## Outcomes Management

**Selecting an Appropriate Agent.**  Vitamin $B_{12}$, usually supplied as cyanocobalamin or hydroxocobalamin, is available in generic form both orally and parenterally. Vitamin $B_{12}$ injections may be given by the patient, family member, or health care provider's office or with the assistance of the visiting nurse. If the oral form is used, absolute adherence to a daily dosing schedule is critical in order to avoid relapse and development of neurologic sequelae. There are no other therapeutic equivalents available. Oral $B_{12}$ drug interactions are shown in Table 28–4.

The usual initial $B_{12}$ dose is 100 μg/day IM for the first week, weekly for the first month, and then monthly for the rest of the life span. Orally, a higher dose, 1000 μg/day, is needed (Linker, 1996). When the etiology of the macrocytic anemia has not yet been established, a prudent course of action is to initially give parenteral vitamin $B_{12}$ while giving folic acid 1–2 mg/daily. With this plan, no intervention time is lost. Once the appropriate diagnosis is established, the correct vitamin supplement is continued (Hoffbrand & Pettit, 1993).

**Monitoring for Efficacy.**  The hematologic response is generally rapid once therapy is given. Reticulocytosis is brisk and peaks at 5–7 days. Hypokalemia, caused by serum to intracellular potassium shifts, is common if the anemia was particularly severe (Linker, 1996) and will be most likely seen with the peak of reticulocytosis. Full hematologic recovery usually takes about 2 months.

## TABLE 28–4. ORAL VITAMIN $B_{12}$ DRUG INTERACTIONS

| Drug | Effect |
| --- | --- |
| Aminoglycosides | With concomitant use, decreased $B_{12}$ absorption |
| Colchicine | With concomitant use, decreased $B_{12}$ absorption |
| Potassium supplements | With concomitant use, decreased $B_{12}$ absorption |
| Ascorbic acid | May destroy $B_{12}$ if taken within 1 h |

*Source: Rizack (1996).*

Reversal of vitamin $B_{12}$ deficiency signs and symptoms is generally rapid. A sense of improved well-being is usually reported within 24 h of the onset of treatment. Neurologic changes, if present under 6 months, reverse quickly. However, if these changes have been present for a protracted period, neurologic reversal is likely not possible (Linker, 1996).

***Monitoring for Toxicity.*** Vitamin $B_{12}$ is a water-soluble compound, with excess drug being easily eliminated by the kidney. As with most therapeutic vitamin replacements, it is well tolerated and has virtually no side effects other than localized irritation at the site of injection. On rare occasions, reaction may be seen in the person who has a cobalt allergy. An intradermal test dose may be given before initiating therapy (*Nurse practitioner drug handbook*, 1996).

***Follow-Up Recommendations.*** Recovery from pernicious anemia is usually rapid and without complications. However, if hematologic recovery is not achieved or is unusually slow, the presence of a second anemia should be investigated. Increasing the vitamin $B_{12}$ dose is seldom needed. Patient follow-up is usually dictated by the presence of other health problems.

## ANEMIA ASSOCIATED WITH RENAL FAILURE

Anemia occurs commonly in the person with select chronic health problems, such as acute and chronic inflammatory conditions (infection, arthritis), renal insufficiency, and hypothyroidism. In part, the anemia is caused by reduced erythropoietin response in the marrow, resulting in hypoproliferation of RBCs. These anemias are second only to iron deficiency in oc-

currence (Hillman & Ault, 1995). Treatment of the underlying cause is usually sufficient in all but anemia associated with renal failure.

With end-stage renal disease (ESRD), there is reduced erythropoietin response because of limited supply; that is, as the kidney fails, erythropoietin production declines. In addition, as is common in chronic illness, RBC life span is shortened. These factors result in a normocytic, normochromic anemia in the presence of a low reticulocyte count (Hillman & Ault, 1995)

## ERYTHROPOIETIN THERAPY

Recombinant human erythropoietin, known as epoetin alfa, can be used for treatment of anemia in ESRD, with its use recommended for those with hematocrits below 30%. It also has been used for the treatment of HIV-related anemias (Grossman & Brody, 1994). The drug is administered parenterally (SC or IV) three times a week. The expected rise in hematocrit is about 4% per week, a level that should not be exceeded since a rapid expansion of circulating volume may induce hypertension. If this level is exceeded, the dose is lowered. Coexisting hematologic problems, such as micronutrient deficiencies, also must be treated (Hillman & Ault, 1995). The annual cost of treatment exceeds thousands of dollars (*Physician GenRx*, 1996). See Table 28–5 for specific information about epoetin alfa.

## THROMBUS FORMATION AND ANTITHROMBOTIC THERAPY

Pathologic thrombus formation, leading to blood vessel occlusion, causes a variety of clinically significant conditions. With arterial thrombi, the tissue supplied by the vessel may

| TABLE 28–5. THERAPEUTIC FORM OF ERYTHROPOIETIN | | | | |
|---|---|---|---|---|
| Drug | Dose Range | Pharmacology | Drug Interaction | Common ADR |
| Epoetin alfa | 50–100 U/kg TIW IV/SC until hct≥36% or increased by 4% in a 2-week period; titrate therapeutic dose to maintain hct 30–36% | Same action as endogenous erythropoietin | None noted | HTN, HA, arthralgia, edema, fatigue, GI Sx |

become necrotic, such as in myocardial infarction. With venous thrombosis, the tissue drained by the affected vein usually becomes edematous and/or inflamed, such as in deep vein thrombophlebitis in the leg (Majerus, Broze, Miletich & Tollefsen, 1996). Intervention aimed at preventing and treating thrombosis is a critically important part of primary care practice.

## NORMAL CLOTTING MECHANISM

Thrombus formation is an important component of the normal hemostatic mechanism. When a vessel is injured, its normally smooth surface becomes uneven. Platelets adhere to this, aggregating and forming a hemostatic plug. Plasma coagulation factors are stimulated by the platelets, leading to further activation of the clotting process. Platelet factors combine with the protein prothrombin as well as with calcium and other substances, resulting in the formation of thrombin. Thrombin then combines with fibrinogen, another naturally occurring protein. Fibrinogen combines with thrombin to form a fibrous gel-like material, fibrin. The presence of fibrin increases platelet aggregation. As the site of the injury heals, the fibrin and platelet clots are broken down, allowing resumption of the normal hemostatic mechanisms (Majerus et al, 1996).

In arterial disease, thrombosis formation usually occurs in response to atherosclerotic changes and decrease in arterial lumen size. In addition, thrombi formed at a distant location can be carried by the arteries, causing such clinical conditions as transient ischemic attacks and cerebral infarct (Hoffbrand & Pettit, 1993).

With venous thrombosis, a systemic increase in coagulability is usually seen, commonly as a sequela of immobility, as local production of thrombin is increased in immobile limbs. An additional mechanism is stasis of blood flow, in which fibrin production is enhanced. Localized venous thrombus formation may also occur as a result of venous damage (Hoffbrand & Pettit, 1993).

## SPECIFIC CONSIDERATIONS FOR PHARMACOTHERAPY

### When Drug Therapy Is Needed

Drug therapy includes preventive measures as well as treatment for acute thrombotic conditions. With drug therapy, these are largely accomplished by the use of heparin and warfarin.

### Short- and Long-Term Goals of Pharmacotherapy

The short- and long-term goals of anticoagulant therapy are to prevent or minimize the negative effects of thrombus formation, thus minimizing negative outcome. Since this is often associated with a potentially life-threatening condition, accurate assessment and swift, appropriate intervention are critical.

### Time Frame for Initiating Therapy

Anticoagulant therapy should be initiated immediately upon the recognition of its need. Inappropriate delay may lead to unnecessary morbidity and mortality.

### Assessment and History Taking

Accurate diagnosis of thrombosis or assessment of thromboembolic risk is crucial prior to initiating anticoagulant therapy. The type of diagnostic testing will vary according to the site of the thrombus.

### Patient/Caregiver Information

In order to avoid problems with warfarin therapy, the patient and caregiver must be well aware of the drug–drug and drug–food interactions. Reading labels on over-the-counter medications is critical to avoid unintentional drug interactions. In addition, the patient must inform all health care providers about warfarin therapy. Additional advice concerning activities of daily living must also be addressed. These include using a soft tooth brush to avoid gum trauma, shaving with an electric razor to avoid nicking, providing household and workplace safety, and wearing a medical alert bracelet. As cigarette smoking will likely increase thrombotic risk while reducing warfarin's efficacy, developing a smoking cessation plan is important (Kee & Hayes, 1997).

Warfarin therapy is contraindicated during pregnancy. Freely crossing the placenta, warfarin is a potent teratogen. A recognizable pattern of facial, skin, bone, and central nervous system deformity is found in up to 30% exposed fetuses. If anticoagulant therapy is needed during pregnancy, heparin, with a large molecule

**TABLE 28–6. INDICATIONS FOR LOW-DOSE VERSUS HIGH-DOSE HEPARIN THERAPY**

Low-dose UFH therapy—usually 500 U SC every 8–12 h as prophylaxis for deep venous thrombus formation:
- Higher-risk surgical patients, such as orthopedic
- Acute myocardial infarction
- Ischemic stroke with lower extremity paralysis
- Patients with congestive heart failure or pneumonia
- Pregnant women with previous thrombotic disease or with antiphospholipid antibody

High-dose UFH therapy—IV or SC administration to maintain a therapeutic APTT:
- Deep vein thrombophlebitis
- Pulmonary embolus
- Unstable angina
- Those receiving thrombolytic therapy
- Perioperative management of those on warfarin therapy

APTT = Activated partial thromboplastin time.

incapable of placental transfer, is the preferred agent (Hillman & Ault, 1995).

Warfarin has a narrow therapeutic range and requires careful monitoring. The importance of regular monitoring of laboratory parameters and provider visits should be stressed.

## OUTCOMES MANAGEMENT

### Selecting an Appropriate Agent

Although other oral anticoagulants are available, warfarin is the preferred form. Dicumarol was the first available oral anticoagulant, but it carries a high gastrointestinal side-effect profile as well as slow and unpredictable absorption. Other forms present no advantage over warfarin (Majerus et al, 1996).

*Heparin.* Heparin is an acidic carbohydrate that occurs naturally. Heparin combines with anti-thromboplastin III, a naturally occurring antithrombotic agent, and inhibits the activity of a number of coagulating factors. Its effect on thrombus formation is immediate (Silverstein, 1995). Table 28–6 gives indicators for low-dose versus high-dose heparin therapy.

Available as standard unfractionated heparin (UFH), molecular weight ranges from 3000–30,000 d, with an average of 15,000 d. UFH has been the heparin form most commonly used in North America. However, low-molecular-weight heparin (LMWH, molecular weight 4000–6500 d) is now also available and may prove to offer certain advantages. See Table 28–7 for comparisons.

*Warfarin.* As a result of vitamin K antagonism, warfarin acts against coagulation factors II, VII, IX, and X. Given orally, it is widely used for the long-term prevention of thromboembolic disease. Warfarin is highly (99%) protein-bound, primarily to albumin, and has a narrow therapeutic range (Majerus et al., 1996).

Drug interactions with warfarin are numerous; see Table 28–8. The mechanism of action varies from displacement of warfarin from the protein-binding site to induction of hepatic enzymes, decreased drug metabolism, and others (Majerus et al., 1996).

**TABLE 28–7. LOW MOLECULAR WEIGHT (LMWH) VERSUS STANDARD UNFRACTIONATED HEPARIN (UFH)**

| Property | UFH | LMWH |
|---|---|---|
| Bioavailability | Variable | Good to excellent |
| Half-life | Dose-dependent, 1–2 h | Long, allows for BID dosing |
| Able to be used in pregnancy? | Yes | No |
| Dosing | Variable, usually titrated in response to APTT | Usually a fixed, weight-based dose |
| Antiplatelet effect | Significant | Limited |

APTT = Activated partial thromboplastin time.

## TABLE 28–8.  WARFARIN DRUG AND FOOD INTERACTIONS

### Increased Anticoagulant Effect

| | |
|---|---|
| Acetaminophen (inconsistent effect) | H$_2$ blockers |
| | Fluconazole, ketoconazole, miconazole (oral or parenteral) |
| Acute alcohol use | Metronidazole |
| Allopurinol | Narcotics |
| Amiodarone | NSAIDs |
| Cisapride | Penicillins |
| Cephalosporins | Propanolol |
| Chloral hydrate | Quinidine |
| Disopyramide | SSRIs |
| Disulfiram | Sulfonylureas |
| Erythromycin | Tetracycline |
| Ethacrynic acid | Trimethoprim-sulfamethoxasole |
| Fluoroquinolones | Valproate |
| Gemfibrozil | Vitamins A, C, E |

### Decreased Anticoagulant Effect

| | |
|---|---|
| Barbiturates | Griseofulvin |
| Carbamazepine | Oral contraceptives |
| Chronic alcohol abuse | Rifampin |
| | Spironolactone |
| Cholestyramine | Sucralfate |

### Variable Effects

Phenytoin (Both increased and decreased effects noted, as well as increase in phenytoin level)

*Source: Rizack (1996).*

## Monitoring for Efficacy

To achieve the anticoagulant effect with warfarin, 3–4 days of therapy is needed. The dose may be initiated in the nonurgent situation as 5 mg (a common maintenance dose) or with a higher dose of 10 mg daily for 2 days, followed by a lower maintenance dose. The latter regimen affords greater anticoagulation effect in the first 48 h of intervention. Daily doses range from 2–15 mg (Hillman & Ault, 1995). If rapid anticoagulation is needed, heparin should be given initially and then discontinued after 5 days of warfarin therapy (Stauffer, 1996).

The prothrombin time (PT) is used as the measure of warfarin's efficacy. It is commonly measured in an International Normalized Ratio (INR). After the first warfarin dose, PT prolongation is seen in about 48–72 h. Daily PT measurement is generally done until the desired INR is reached, and then weekly to monthly testing continues throughout therapy (Treseler, 1995). Table 28–9 shows recommendations for different conditions and lengths of treatment with warfarin.

## Monitoring for Toxicity

Approximately 2 to 10% of those taking warfarin will develop hemorrhage. This complication, however, is rarely seen in those with an INR of 2.0–3.0 (Stauffer, 1996). In the presence of significant bleeding in the person taking warfarin, the drug should be discontinued and vitamin K given promptly. However, vitamin K will have little effect on hemostasis for 24 h. If more prompt action is needed, such as in the case of hemorrhage or bleeding into an enclosed space, fresh frozen plasma must be given. After the bleeding crisis, if anticoagulation therapy is continued, response to warfarin may fluctuate, necessitating close monitoring (Majerus et al, 1996).

## TABLE 28–9.  INDICATIONS AND LENGTH OF WARFARIN TREATMENT

| Condition | Recommended Length of Treatment | INR range |
|---|---|---|
| • Acute venous thrombosis | 3–6 months | 2.0–3.0 |
| • Prevention of venous thrombus in high-risk patient | Chronic | 1.5–2.5 |
| • Prevention of emboli in atrial fibrillation | Chronic | 1.5–2.5 |
| • Stoke prevention in the high-risk patient | Chronic | 2.0–4.0 |
| • Prosthetic heart valves | Chronic | 2.0/2.5 (tissue valves); 3.0–4.0 (mechanical valve) |
| • Prevention of emboli after myocardial infarction | 2–3 months | 2.0–3.0 |

*Source: Hillman and Ault (1995).*

## Follow-up Recommendations

Follow-up is recommended as needed to monitor INR and the underlying clinical condition.

## REFERENCES

Allen, R. (1996). Megaloblastic anemias. In J. Bennett & F. Plum, *Cecil's textbook of medicine* (20th ed.) (pp. 843–851). Philadelphia: W. B. Saunders.

Biswas, M., & Perloff, D. (1994). Cardiac, hematologic, pulmonary, renal, and urinary tract disorders. In A. DeCherney & M. Pernoll, *Current obstetric and gynecologic diagnosis and treatment* (pp. 428–467). Norwalk, CT: Appleton & Lange.

Briggs, G., Freeman, R., & Yaffee, S. (1994). *Drugs in pregnancy and lactation* (4th ed.). Baltimore: Williams & Wilkins.

Cruikshank, D. (1994). Cardiovascular, pulmonary, renal, and hematologic diseases in pregnancy. In J. Scott, P. DiSaia, C. Hammond, & W. Spellacy, *Danforth's obstetrics and gynecology* (7th ed.) (pp. 367–392). Philadelphia: J. B. Lippincott.

Duffy, T. (1996) Microcytic and hypochromic anemias. In J. Bennett, & F. Plum, *Cecil's textbook of medicine* (20th ed.) (pp. 838–843). Philadelphia: W. B. Saunders.

Dupuis, L., Smith, J., & Kowalczyk, A. (1995). Drug dosing in infants, children and adolescents. In L. Pagliaro & A. M. Pagliaro, *Problems in pediatric drug therapy* (3rd ed.) (pp. 815–920). Hamilton, IL: Drug Intelligence.

Grimes J., & Burns, E. (1992). Health assessment in nursing practice (3rd ed.). Boston: Jones & Bartlett.

Grossman, B., & Brody, T. (1994) Drugs to treat anemia. In T. Brody, J. Larner, K. Minneman, & H. Neu, *Human pharmacology* (2nd ed.) (pp. 861–870). St. Louis: C. V. Mosby.

Hardy, W. (1996). Common hematologic-oncologic problems. In R. Rubin, C. Vos, D. Derksen, A. Gately, & R. Quenzer, *Medicine: A primary care approach* (pp. 311–316). Philadelphia: W. B. Saunders.

Hillman, R. (1996). Hematopoietic agents. In J. Hardman, L. Limbird, P. Molinoff, & R. Ruddon, *Goodman & Gillman's The pharmacologic basis for disease* (9th ed.) (pp. 1311–1340). New York: McGraw-Hill.

Hillman, R., & Ault, K. (1995). *Hematology in clinical practice: A guide to diagnosis and management.* New York: McGraw-Hill.

Hoffbrand, A., & Pettit, J. (1993). *Essential hematology.* London: Blackwell Scientific.

Kee, J., & Hayes, E. (1997). Drugs for circulatory disorders. In J. Kee & E. Hayes, *Pharmacology: A nursing process approach* (pp. 518–536). Philadelphia: W. B. Saunders.

Lane, C., Armstrong, L., Ingrim, N., & Lance, L. (1995). *Drug information handbook.* Hudson, OH: Lexi-Comp.

Lindenbaum, J. (1996). An approach to anemias. In J. Bennett, & F. Plum, *Cecil's textbook of medicine* (20th ed.) (pp. 823–830). Philadelphia: W. B. Saunders.

Linker, C. (1996). Blood. In L. Tierney, S. McPhee, & M. Papadakis, *Current medical diagnosis and treatment* (35th ed.) (434–488). Norwalk, CT: Appleton and Lange.

Majerus, P., Broze, B., Miletich, J., & Tollefsen, D. (1996). Anticoagulant, thrombolytic and antiplatelet drugs. In J. Hardman, L. Limbird, P. Molinoff, R. Ruddon, *Goodman & Gillman's The pharmacologic basis for disease* (9th ed.) (pp. 1341–1359). New York: McGraw-Hill.

Nolan, R. (1997). Poisoning. In R. Hoekelman, S. Friedman, N. Nelson, H. Siedel, & M. Weiztman, *Primary pediatric care* (pp. 1738–1750). St. Louis: C. V. Mosby.

*Nurse practitioner drug handbook.* (1996). Springhouse, PA: Springhouse.

Olson, R. (1995). Water soluble vitamins. In P. Munson, R. Mueller, & G. Breeze, *Principles of pharmacology* (pp. 949–979). New York: Chapman and Hall.

*Physician GenRx.* (1996). St. Louis: C. V. Mosby.

Ries, C., & Santi, D. (1995). Agents used in anemias: Hematopoietic growth factors. In B. Katzung, *Basic and clinical pharmacology* (pp. 493–506). Norwalk, CT: Appleton & Lange.

Rizack, M. (1996). *Handbook of adverse drug interactions.* New Rochelle, NY: The Medical Letter.

Samuels, P. (1991). Hematologic disorders. In S. Gabbe, J. Niebyl, & J. Simpson, *Obstetrics: Normal and problem pregnancies* (2nd ed.) (pp. 1137–1150). New York: Churchill and Livingstone.

Silverstein, R. (1995). Drugs affecting hemostasis. In P. Munson, R. Mueller, & G. Breeze, *Principles of pharmacology* (pp. 1123–1143). New York: Chapman and Hall.

Spruill, W., & Wade, W. (1993). Hematologic disorders. In J. DiPiro, R. Talbert, P. Hayes, G. Yee, G. Matzke, & L. Posey. *Pharmacotherapy: A pathophysiologic approach* (2nd ed.) (pp. 1423–1442). Norwalk, CT: Appleton & Lange.

Stauffer, J. (1996). Lung. In L. Tierney, S. McPhee, & M. Papadakis, *Current medical diagnosis and treatment* (35th ed.) (pp. 215–294). Norwalk, CT: Appleton & Lange.

Treseler, K. (1995). *Clinical laboratory and diagnostic tests: Significance and nursing implications* (3rd ed.). Norwalk, CT: Appleton & Lange.

Waterbury, L. (1995). Anemias. In R. Barker, J. Burton, & P. Zieve, *Principles of ambulatory medicine* (4th ed.) (593–607). Baltimore: Williams & Wilkins.

# 29

# NEUROLOGIC DISORDERS

*Jessie Drew-Cates and Robert A. Gross*

Conditions affecting the nervous system remain one of the great frontiers in health care, with gains in basic neuroscience beginning to create new pharmacologic interventions to improve the quality of life in what were once considered nontreatable conditions. The focus of this chapter is on the more common neurologic problems encountered in primary care, usually managed by the primary care provider in conjunction with a consulting neurologist.

The chapter focuses on the current common drugs utilized in specific conditions so the primary care provider is knowledgeable regarding their use, concurrent drug interactions, toxicities, and systemic changes that they bring about.

## TRAUMATIC HEAD INJURY

Traumatic brain injury (TBI) is defined as observed or reported loss of consciousness, amnesia to the traumatic event, skull fracture, and objective neurologic or neuropsychologic abnormalities. The reported incidence of head trauma is approximately 152 to 367 per 100,000 with two to three times more males than females (Elovic & Antoinette, 1996). Another name given to this condition, in individuals with mild to moderate traumatic brain injury, is postconcussion syndrome.

## PATHOPHYSIOLOGY

The specific pathophysiology of any head injury (HI) can be complex. There are three specific causes of head injury. The first, diffuse axonal injury (DAI), occurs when rapid deceleration of the head causes inertial forces that dissipate through widespread microscopic shearing of long-axis structures, affecting axons, synapses, and blood vessels. The rupture of capillaries and small veins may or may not show up on a computed tomography (CT) scan. DAI always causes at least a transient alteration of consciousness in which there is no lucid interval; this altered state varies in duration from a few moments to weeks (Alexander, 1994).

The second type of injury is called focal cortical contusion (FCC). FCC is related to the effect of inertial forces on the rough bony surfaces and dural attachments inside the skull. Sudden force causes surface abrasions on the outside cortex and surface vessels, particularly in the inferior frontal and anterior temporal regions, which can result in localized intracerebral hemorrhage, infarction, and edema and acute subdural hematomas (Alexander, 1994).

The third type of injury is called hypoxic-ischemic injury (HII) and occurs when whole-body system injury occurs and cerebral perfusion is compromised. Focal HII can also occur in local regions as a result of a local pressure change from subdural hematomas, or it can occur more diffusely as a result of brain edema and temporal herniation from pressure on the posterior cerebral arteries (Alexander, 1994).

## PROGNOSIS

The recovery from even mild head injury can take longer than most professionals anticipate. Patients with only minutes of time lost to unconsciousness report difficulty with divided attention to tasks and problems with sustained attention lasting weeks to months (Cope, 1994). Individuals with post concussive syndrome with neck and spine injury report clearing of overt balance and vestibular symptoms in days to weeks but persistent movement-induced symptoms that persist for months, as well as difficulty with neck whiplash. Often the patient is bothered by persistent headaches that may be migrainous and require treatment as such (Alexander, 1995). In addition, the fatigue and difficulty of carrying out multiple tasks can create great anxiety, short temper, and even depression. Referral to a psychologist trained in head injury is often helpful in treating these symptoms (Stein, Glasur, & Hoffman, 1994).

Individuals with moderate to severe head injury can continue to recover for years following the event. By 12–18 months, patients with moderate head injury may plateau on standard neuropsychologic tests yet show improvement in daily executive and memory function over longer periods of time (Alexander, 1995).

DAI can produce motor deficits, particularly vestibular problems, as well as a combination of bradykinesia, rigidity, postural change, and ataxia, all of which are responsive to aggressive therapy. Both DAI and FCC can present with blunted awareness, poor executive function, and forgetfulness, but the outcome of the two conditions can be very different. Over time, focal lesions often heal because patchy cortical deafferentation is very different from the complete cortical loss occurring in DAI. HII initially looks very much like DAI or FCC. In HII, a coma of more than 2 days' duration is associated with poor recovery, as is the presence of visual impairment, amnesia, and extrapyramidal movements.

Persons in a coma or persistent vegetative state who do not respond to their environment may be treated at home or in an extended care facility by primary care providers. These patients require excellent nursing care to carry out adequate nutrition, bowel and bladder management, skin care, positioning, range of motion exercises,

and transfers. Interval assessment is necessary to consider responsiveness and cognitive abilities and to determine the benefit of increased therapeutic interaction. As patients come out of a vegetative state, they enter an acute confusional state with agitation and amnesia. Generalized learning can take place at this time with motor patterns and repeating activities.

Once patients reach a degree of independence in activities of daily living, they are candidates for outpatient therapy. If the deficits are primarily motor, a general rehabilitation setting may be helpful. But individuals with cognitive "executive deficits" in planning and organization benefit from programs emphasizing repetition with schedules, shopping, finances, and specific problems related to the workplace. Behavioral problems may require a specific program addressing uninhibited behaviors that are inappropriate in specific settings, often with a strong psychiatric flavor (Alexander, 1994).

For individuals with psychotic and anxious behaviors, a structured environment with structured interventions carried out consistently is helpful in supplying the external structure many head-injured individuals need to guide them through their days. Routine becomes a blessing, giving consistency and meaning to a time frame not yet totally meaningful for someone recovering from posttraumatic amnesia. Many individuals need the assistance of a log book to act as a calendar for the events of the day as well as a short-term memory for the names of familiar individuals they wish to recall (Long and Novack, 1986).

## SPECIFIC CONSIDERATIONS FOR PHARMACOTHERAPY

### When Drug Therapy Is Needed

The aim of treatment is currently focused on symptom management. In mild to moderate head injury, there can be a complete "cure" for all the symptoms of the injury over time. However, focal deficits continue to exist for the duration of life, and in severe head injury permanent changes are the norm. The more common deficits seen in head injury are listed in Table 29–1.

### Short- and Long-Term Goals of Pharmacotherapy

The aim of pharmacotherapy is to manage the physical, cognitive, and emotional changes oc-

## TABLE 29–1. COMMON DEFICITS SEEN IN HEAD INJURY

| | |
|---|---|
| Anxiety | Field cuts |
| Ataxia | Headaches |
| Cognitive dysfunction | (vascular or migraines) |
| Depression | Hearing loss/tinnitus |
| Diplopia | Hemiparesis |
| Dysphagia | Sleep problems |
| Emotional lability and/or irritability | Spasticity |
| | Tremor |
| Fatigue | |

*Adapted from Horn and Zasler (1996).*

curring as a result of the injury. With rehabilitation, patients can regain function in their activities of daily living, family relationships, and working lives.

### Nonpharmacologic Therapy

Nonpharmacologic treatment in head injury is aimed at restoring all levels of function the individual possessed prior to the event. This is best carried out by a rehabilitation team specifically trained in head injury care encompassing cognitive therapy, memory retraining, community reintegration, and vocational counseling. This care is in addition to traditional rehabilitation services concerned with restoration of limb function, activities of daily living, and communication skills through physical therapists, occupational therapists, and speech pathologists. In the absence of a full rehabilitation team, specific professionals who are most helpful are neurologists, neuropsychologists, and speech therapists trained in head injury.

Even in mild head injury, fatigue may persist for weeks to months, necessitating a curtailment of usual activities. Patients are often overwhelmed by multiple tasking, as well as prioritizing of tasks, and are unable to retain new memories, which interferes with learning. In terms of general guidelines for care, head-injured persons require regular sleep, exercise, no alcohol, and avoidance of stress in order to function at their previous capacity. Applying daily structured organization is often very helpful.

### Time Frame for Initiating Pharmacotherapy

In mild to moderate head injury it is better to delay drug therapy for a number of weeks after

injury. There is some evidence that the brain recovers better without using medications that may interfere with its own neurotransmitters (Honing and Albers, 1994). Consequently, the usual first line of treatment is the elimination of drugs that have sedating effects, particularly benzodiazepines and antipsychotics (Cope, 1994). Because of the sedating effect of many seizure medications, carbamazepine "may be the anticonvulsant of choice for TBI . . ." (Cope, 1994, p. 579) if the individual requires seizure medication.

At 6–8 weeks postinjury, it is safe to consider drug therapy for specific symptom management. In severe head injury, especially in the acute hospital setting, sedatives are often prescribed for agitation. This may interfere with alertness and potentially harm neurotransmitters, but does allow ongoing use of ventilatory support and other life-enhancing equipment. Short-acting sedatives are preferred over long-acting drugs.

### Overview of Drug Classes for Treatment of Head Injury

As in many neurologic problems, medications used in head injury are prescribed in conjunction with a physician, usually a neurologist or physiatrist trained in head injury (Cope, 1994). In addition, many of the medications currently used were not specifically developed for use in head injury, and references may actually state that their use is contraindicated in head injury or seizure. However, for some individuals the gains far outweigh the risks of treatment (Cope, 1994). Table 29–2 lists medications that may impede brain injury recovery.

Specific medications may influence recovery in head injury. For example, specific drugs may facilitate the learning process dependent on specific neurotransmitter systems. In focal brain injury pharmacologic enhancement of recovery is possible.

## TABLE 29–2. DRUGS THAT MAY IMPEDE RECOVERY FROM BRAIN INJURY

| | |
|---|---|
| Benzodiazepines | Phenothiazines |
| Clonidine | Phenoxybenzamine |
| GABA | Phenytoin |
| Haloperidol | Prazosin |
| Phenobarbital | |

*Adapted from Dombovy (1997).*

Symptom management in head injury is complex because of the new knowledge regarding neurotransmitters and behaviors. It is estimated that only 10–15% of the neurotransmitters are known. Different receptors in different parts of the brain transmit different kinds of information. Through interaction with brain receptors neuropeptides may influence brain plasticity and enhance recovery. However, there are as yet no good guidelines regarding specific agents, their dosages, and the timing of their use. Factors influencing the effects of these pharmacologic agents include anatomic localization of the lesions, lesion size, and age of the patient.

In addition, two individuals who may exhibit very similar behavior may respond very differently to the same drug because the lesion foci are different (Cope, 1994). Silver and Yudofsky (1994) argue for combinations of therapeutic interventions administered simultaneously, which may make tailoring a useful regimen even more challenging. It is useful to have a resource clinician (usually a neurologist or physiatrist) who is knowledgeable about head injury pharmacotherapeutics when prescribing these medications (Cope, 1994).

The drugs utilized in head injury are primarily from seven major groups: stimulants, dopaminergics, antipsychotics, antidepressants, anticonvulsants, and antianxiety agents including beta blockers. Many of the drugs are used for several different groups of symptoms. Drug utilization in this section is addressed by symptom: attention and arousal, psychosis, agitation and aggression, cognition, affective disorders (particularly depression), and seizures.

## Assessment

The primary care provider will see individuals who present for follow-up if the injury was severe enough to warrant hospitalization. The primary care provider may also be consulted by individuals following a traumatic event for complaints of headaches, irritability, depression, difficulty thinking clearly, and inability to work. In many cases, these are individuals who were not hospitalized after the trauma; the provider may also be unaware that the new symptoms may be related to a head injury. Often on the initial head CT scan, damage is absent, although magnetic resonance imaging (MRI) performed months after the event may show focal punctate densities. The changes in cognition, personality, and memory are often subtle, requiring a careful history.

Use of a neurobehavioral rating scale such as the one shown in Table 29–3 is often helpful in determining the behaviors and cognitive skills that are impaired. Frequently head injured persons lack insight into their own deficits, necessitating careful consideration of family members description and reaction to the change in behavior and thinking.

At this point in their use, the prescription of medications is on a case-by-case basis. In about half the cases, medications are effective in alleviating symptoms from head injury. It is important to assess previous drug and alcohol abuse as well as previous use of psychotropic medications for underlying medical conditions such as schizophrenia and bipolar disease. In most cases, medications used previously are reintroduced at lower levels to ascertain their influence on behavior prior to introducing new medications. A dose schedule of one third to one half the previous dose is not unusual.

### Patient/Caregiver Information

Initially, the person who suffered the injury may have little insight into his or her own changed behaviors. Often it is weeks to months before the effect of the injury becomes known to the person. Family members may choose not to see differences as well, but generally the changes in behavior, subtle or dramatic, become clear (Kreutzer, Gervasio, and Camplair, 1994). Basic information about head injury is essential and available through the Head Injury Foundation. However, information about specific medications for symptom management is best done by contrast on a case-by-case basis.

## OUTCOMES MANAGEMENT

The aim of drug utilization is symptom management. The common drugs used in head injury are listed in Table 29–3A, with dosages, side effects, and other information given in the drug tables. The symptoms and drug use and monitoring are individually addressed below.

### Attention and Arousal

***Selecting an appropriate agent.***    General arousal is mediated by the reticular activating system, which projects to the entire cerebrum, midbrain, and lower brain, as well as the spinal cord. Damage to one or both cerebral hemispheres

## TABLE 29–3. NEUROBEHAVIORAL RATING SCALE

| | Not Present | Very Mild | Mild | Mod Severe | Severe | Extremely Severe |
|---|---|---|---|---|---|---|
| 1. *Inattention/reduced alertness:* Fails to sustain attention, easily distracted, fails to notice aspects of environment, difficulty directing attention, decreased alertness. | ___ | ___ | ___ | ___ | ___ | ___ |
| 2. *Somatic concern:* Volunteers complaints or elaborates about somatic symptoms (eg, headache, dizziness, blurred vision) and about physical health in general. | ___ | ___ | ___ | ___ | ___ | ___ |
| 3. *Disorientation:* Confusion or lack of proper association for person, place, or time. | ___ | ___ | ___ | ___ | ___ | ___ |
| 4. *Anxiety:* Worry, fear, overconcern for present or future. | ___ | ___ | ___ | ___ | ___ | ___ |
| 5. *Expressive deficit:* Word-finding disturbance, anomia, pauses in speech, effortful speech, circumlocution. | ___ | ___ | ___ | ___ | ___ | ___ |
| 6. *Emotional withdrawal:* Lack of spontaneous interaction, isolation, deficiency in relating to others. | ___ | ___ | ___ | ___ | ___ | ___ |
| 7. *Conceptual disorganization:* Thought processes confused, disconnected, disorganized, disrupted, tangential social communication, perseverative. | ___ | ___ | ___ | ___ | ___ | ___ |
| 8. *Disinhibition:* Socially inappropriate comments and/or actions, including aggressive/sexual content, or inappropriate to the situation, outbursts of temper. | ___ | ___ | ___ | ___ | ___ | ___ |
| 9. *Guilt feelings:* Self-blame, shame, remorse for past behavior. | ___ | ___ | ___ | ___ | ___ | ___ |
| 10. *Memory deficit:* Difficulty learning new information, rapidly forgets recent events, although immediate recall (forward digit span) may be intact. | ___ | ___ | ___ | ___ | ___ | ___ |
| 11. *Agitation:* Motor manifestations of overactivation (eg, kicking, arm flailing, picking, roaming, restlessness, talkativeness). | ___ | ___ | ___ | ___ | ___ | ___ |
| 12. *Inaccurate insight and self-appraisal:* Poor insight, exaggerated self-opinion, overrates level of ability and underrates personality change in comparison with evaluation by clinicians and family. | ___ | ___ | ___ | ___ | ___ | ___ |
| 13. *Depressive mood:* Sorrow, sadness, despondency, pessimism. | ___ | ___ | ___ | ___ | ___ | ___ |
| 14. *Hostility/uncooperativeness:* Animosity, irritability, belligerence, disdain for others, defiance of authority. | ___ | ___ | ___ | ___ | ___ | ___ |
| 15. *Decreased initiative/motivation:* Lacks normal initiative in work or leisure, fails to persist in tasks, is reluctant to accept new challenges. | ___ | ___ | ___ | ___ | ___ | ___ |
| 16. *Suspiciousness:* Mistrust, belief that others harbor malicious or discriminatory intent. | ___ | ___ | ___ | ___ | ___ | ___ |

*(continues on next page)*

**TABLE 29–3. NEUROBEHAVIORAL RATING SCALE** (continued from previous page)

| | Not Present | Very Mild | Mild | Mod Severe | Severe | Extremely Severe |
|---|---|---|---|---|---|---|
| 17. *Fatigability:* Rapidly fatigues on challenging cognitive tasks or complex activities, lethargic. | — | — | — | — | — | — |
| 18. *Hallucinatory behavior:* Perceptions without normal external stimulus correspondence. | — | — | — | — | — | — |
| 19. *Motor retardation:* Slowed movements or speech (excluding primary weakness). | — | — | — | — | — | — |
| 20. *Unusual thought content:* Unusual, odd, strange, bizarre thought content. | — | — | — | — | — | — |
| 21. *Blunted affect:* Reduced emotional tone, reduction in normal intensity of feelings; flatness. | — | — | — | — | — | — |
| 22. *Excitement:* Heightened emotional tone, increased reactivity. | — | — | — | — | — | — |
| 23. *Poor planning:* Unrealistic goals, poorly formulated plans for the future, disregard prerequisites (eg, training), fails to take disability into account. | — | — | — | — | — | — |
| 24. *Lability of mood:* Sudden change in mood which is disproportionate to the situation. | — | — | — | — | — | — |
| 25. *Tension:* Postural and facial expression of heightened tension, without the necessity of excessive activity involving the limbs or trunk. | — | — | — | — | — | — |
| 26. *Comprehension deficit:* Difficulty in understanding oral instructions on single or multistage commands. | — | — | — | — | — | — |
| 27. *Speech articulation defect:* Misarticulation, slurring, or substitution of sounds which affects intelligibility (rating is independent of linguistic content). | — | — | — | — | — | — |

and/or the reticular activating system results in disorders of attention and arousal.

The arousal medications used in head injury primarily act on the catecholaminergic system. The traditional stimulant, dextroamphetamine, blocks the reuptake of norepinephrine, and higher doses can block the reuptake of dopamine. In the presence of psychomotor retardation, antiparkinsonian drugs are utilized. Amantadine acts on the dopamine receptor both before and after the synapse and probably increases cholinergic and GABAergic activity. Bromocriptine is both a dopamine receptor antagonist and agonist. In its midrange dose it primarily acts as an agonist.

The amphetamines, methylphenidate, and levodopa all improve arousal level. Antidepressants may also have a stimulating effect. Levodopa and bromocriptine have had successful use in patients with long-term loss of arousal.

Cholinergic agonists have a detrimental effect in the acute stage of HI, but are therapeutic in some persistent vegetative states.

Two drugs commonly used are methylphenidate (0.3 mg/kg b.i.d.) or dextroamphetamine (0.2 mg/kg b.i.d.). They tend to increase alertness and improve mood as well as task performance. These medications may require titration upward to 60 mg/day b.i.d. or t.i.d. with dosage increases every 5–7 days (Silver & Yudofsky, 1994).

The dopamine agonist Sinemet (L-dopa/carbidopa) is used to improve alertness and concentration; decrease fatigue, sialorrhea, and hypomania; and improve memory. The dosage used is 10/100–25/250 q.i.d. Another dopamine agonist, bromocriptine, is used to treat cognitive initiation problems with a starting dose of 2.5 mg/day and treatment for at least 2 months. The drug is thought to help with increasing goal-directed behaviors.

## TABLE 29–3A. COMMON DRUGS USED IN BRAIN INJURY

| Generic (Trade) Name | Uses for Specific Behaviors in Head Injury |
|---|---|
| **Drugs Used in Cognitive Function and Arousal[a]** | |
| Dextroamphetamine (Dexadrin) | Cognitive function and arousal (stimulant) |
| Methylphenidate (Ritalin) | Cognitive function and arousal (stimulant) |
| Amantadine (Symmetrel) | Cognitive function and arousal (dopamine agonist), Parkinsonian symptoms |
| Bromocriptine (Parlodel) | Cognitive function and arousal (dopamine agonist) |
| L. Dopa/Carbidopa (Sinemet) | Cognitive function and arousal (dopamine agonist) |
| Trazadone (Desyrel) | Sleep and antidepressant |
| **Drugs Used in Psychosis, Anxiety and Aggression[b]** | |
| Haloperidol (Haldol) | Anti-psychotic |
| Fluphenazine (Prolixin) | Anti-psychotic |
| Clozapine (Clozaril) | Anti-psychotic, anxiolytic |
| Buspirone (Buspar | Anxiety, especially post-aggressive syndrome |
| Propanolol (Inderal) | Anxiety, especially post-aggressive syndrome |
| **Mania Therapeutic Drugs** | |
| Lithium carbonate (Lithobid) | Mania/manic depression, aggressive behavior and agitation |
| Clonidine (Catapres) | Mania |
| **Mania & Anti-Seizure Drugs** | |
| Carbamazepine (Tegretol) | Mania, anti-seizure, aggression/agitation, lancinating neurogenic pain |
| Valproic acid (Depakene, Depakote) | Mania, mood lability, seizures, aggression/agitation, myoclonus |
| **Other Anti-Seizure Medications[c]** | |
| Clonazepam (Klonopin) | Anti-seizure (myoclonic) |
| Phenytoin (Dilantin) | Anti-seizure |
| Phenobarbital (Phenobarb) | Anti-seizure |
| **Antidepressants[d]** | |
| Fluoxetine (Prozac) | Antidepressant, mood lability, "emotional incontinence" |
| Sertraline (Zoloft) | Antidepressant |
| Paroxetine (Paxil) | Antidepressant, mood lability |
| Nortriptyline (Aventyl or Pamelor) | Antidepressant, mood lability |
| Desipramine (Norpramin) | Antidepressant |

*Please refer to Drug Tables for further information on mechanism of action, dosages, toxicity, side effects, and interactions.

[a]As a group, can increase dopamine activity, paranoia, euphoria, agitation, irritability.

[b]Anti-psychotic drugs as a group can cause hypertension, sedation and confusion, Parkinsonian syndrome, acute dystomia. May impede neuronal brain recovery in subacute stage.

[c]As a group, can decrease cognition and cause depression.

[d]All antidepressants can increase seizure frequency. Continue this drug group six months after remission of symptoms. Some anti-convulsants increase therapeutic blood levels of the antidepressants.

Another medication used in head injury to improve impulsivity, emotional lability, and general arousal is amantadine at initial dosages of 50 mg b.i.d. to 400 mg/day, increasing the dose at 3-day to weekly intervals by 100 mg/day.

***Monitoring for efficacy and toxicity.*** The major risk of the stimulant drugs is the increase in dopamine activity, leading to symptoms of overstimulation. The symptoms of overstimulation with dextroamphetamine and methylphenidate include paranoia, dysphoria, agitation, and irritability; bromocriptine can cause sedation, nausea, psychosis, headaches, and delirium; and amantadine can cause confusion, hallucinations, edema, and hypotension (Silver & Yudofsky,

1994). Because depression can arise with sudden withdrawal, slow titration off dextroamphetamine and methylphenidate is as important as slow titration at their initiation. Several recent studies cite little increased risk of seizures with methylphenidate, dextroamphetamine, and bromocriptine, but amantadine appears to lower the seizure threshold in some subjects.

## Psychosis

*Selecting an appropriate agent.* Acute posttraumatic psychosis and anxiety following traumatic brain injury is common. Antipsychotic drugs are used only when other measures of environmental management are not appropriate or fail. These drugs as a group produce significant side effects at very small doses. Consequently, the recommended doses are often one third to one half of what might normally be prescribed in traditional psychosis. In addition, manufacturers may warn prescribers not to give these drugs to individuals with head injury.

Antipsychotics are indicated when the behaviors resemble classic schizophrenia, such as hallucinations, paranoid or bizarre ideations, and loose associations. The drugs to avoid are those with a high anticholinergic effect, which can impair memory and new learning, as well as cause constipation, urinary retention, and blurred vision.

The drugs most commonly used are Haldol, Clozaril, lorazepam, BuSpar, and Inderal. Their mechanisms of action, specific use, dosage, and interactions are listed in Drug Tables 205.5, 308.6, 309.2, 312.2, 312.3.

*Monitoring for efficacy and toxicity.* Although the risk is small, the use of neuroleptics may promote seizure activity. Other more common risk factors include the development of tardive dyskinesia and neuroleptic malignant syndrome.

As a group, the drugs can cause hypertension, hypotension, sedation, confusion, parkinsonian syndrome, and acute dystonia. In the acute phase, the drugs may impede brain recovery.

## Agitation and Aggression

*Selecting an appropriate agent.* In early head injury, agitation is expected, and in the majority of patients this symptom subsides as recovery proceeds. In a minority of long-term patients agitation and aggression remain. Another source of aggression and agitation is improper use of medications that aggravate this behavior. The most common offenders are Haldol, Ativan, and Valium, which can lead directly to aggressive behaviors or indirectly as a rebound effect once the medication begins to wear off. Nonpharmacologic interventions include removing the source of frustration by controlling the environment, by reducing the amount of stimulation, and by setting a lower level of expected behavior. An aggressive approach to both structure and medication use is helpful in the small number of patients in whom the behavior becomes chronic.

The traditional approach to this behavior in other diseases is the use of neuroleptics, but in head injury these drugs appear to have little efficacy. Tricyclic antidepressants (TCAs) are used in agitation in TBI. The rationale for their use is similar to the rationale for their use in attention deficit hyperactivity disorders in that they curb distractibility, impulsivity, and irritability.

Benzodiazepines are used, but their efficacy in the long term is in doubt. In the short term they are very effective, particularly Ativan. The beta blockers are more widely known for their use as antihypertensives. The drug propranolol is useful with unprovoked rage and aggression in chronic TBI. The suggested dose is quite high, so use of other drugs first is suggested because of the hypotensive effect.

## Cognition

Cognition is the process of learning, including memory and information processing. Cognitive impairment affects multiple areas of the brain but particularly the hippocampus, cerebral cortex, and cerebellum. The neurotransmitters involved include the ACh (acetylcholine) amino acid neurotransmitters such as gamma-aminobutyric acid (GABA), neuropeptides, and ACTH fragments, as well as opioids. The cholinergic agents show promise in treating cognitive deficits, but no studies currently exist to support their use in memory and learning disorders. Clonidine is also used to improve attention and cognition.

The effective utilization of any of these drugs can change with time, as the brain changes in relationship to the injury. The drugs should all receive a weaning trial.

## Affective Disorders

*Selecting an appropriate agent.* The two common affective disorders in head injury are mania and depression. The mania is often viewed in terms of agitation and aggression and treated as such. There is some thought that the depression seen in brain injury may be a straightforward chemical defect from the brain injury itself or a superimposed depression from the event of the head injury. In any case, the depressive behaviors are similar, with psychomotor slowing, sparse speech, and changes in sleep and appetite. In head injury the depression can be acute or delayed and is often dependent on the amount of insight an individual may have at different times regarding the brain injury.

The drugs of choice in treating depression in head injury are the serotonin selective reuptake inhibitors (SSRIs), particularly sertraline and fluoxetine. These drugs have fewer anticholinergic side effects with a lower incidence of dyskinesias. In addition, lability of mood (excessive crying or laughing) is often treatable with SSRIs and other antidepressant medications such as amitriptyline (Elavil) and sertaline (Zoloft) (Cope, 1994). Other drugs used to treat depression in head injury include the neuroleptics.

## Seizures

***Selecting an appropriate agent.***   The incidence of seizures in moderate closed head injury (CHI) is 4–7%. Penetrating injuries, depressed skull fractures, intracranial hemorrhage, prolonged duration of posttraumatic amnesia, and loss of consciousness all increase the risk of seizures (Yablon, 1996). Consequently, seizures are more frequent in individuals treated in a rehabilitation setting, and the incidence of seizures is higher the first 5 years postinjury. Focal seizures are more common than generalized seizures. Those with mild head injuries have no greater seizure incidence than the general population. Additional predisposing factors to seizure development are alcoholism, epilepsy, and age. Children may have seizures immediately after injury but are not as predisposed to develop epilepsy as adults.

If an individual has a seizure, early use of antiseizure medications is warranted to prevent increasing cerebral pressure or hypertension, but prolonged use of anti-seizure medications after the first 6 months may only increase the risk of further seizures. The use of antidepressant medications may also increase the risk of seizures.

To determine if a patient can discontinue seizure medications, an EEG is helpful only if epileptiform activity is seen; a normal EEG does not guarantee seizures will not occur once the medication is withdrawn. If necessary, long-term monitoring of EEG can be done on an inpatient or outpatient basis (Yablon, 1996).

Although phenytoin (Dilantin) is often prescribed during the early acute phase of injury to the brain, it may not be the drug of choice in long-term use. If a patient never had a seizure during the acute event and has a normal EEG, it is safe to consider discontinuing the drug. This decision is usually left to the prescribing physician. The antiseizure medications, particularly phenytoin, phenobarbital, and carbamazepine, can impair cognition and behavior at subtherapeutic and therapeutic levels. Conversely, in some patients, carbamazepine may improve mood, attention, information processing, and general functioning because this drug, as well as valproic acid, has mood-stabilizing properties. These two drugs are the two drugs of choice with seizure activity in CHI (Cope, 1994, p. 586). In some cases aggressive or agitated behavior may be related to seizures or a postictal state and may thus respond to antiseizure medication.

***Monitoring for efficacy and toxicity.***   See the seizure section of this chapter for a fuller discussion of efficacy and toxicity in antiseizure medications.

## ATTENTION DEFICIT/ HYPERACTIVITY DISORDER

### BACKGROUND

Attention deficit disorder was originally thought to be the inability to pay attention. Although still controversial, the condition is currently more commonly believed to be a biologically based condition. More recently, attention deficit hyperactivity disorders (AD/HD) are thought to be disorders of self-regulation. The major manifestation of these conditions is the inability to use a sense of time in the present and in the future to guide behavior (Barkley, 1995).

This inability to use time results in the inability to be organized, to plan, to be goal-directed, and to control impulses. The classic behaviors are poor attention, impulsive action, and hyperactivity. Adults exhibit similar behaviors, with an inability to inhibit or modulate behaviors, emotion, or attention (Fargason & Ford, 1994). Table 29–4 lists the DSM IV criteria for the five AD/HD diagnoses. The first three are the most commonly used.

## TABLE 29–4. DSM IV DIAGNOSIS AND CRITERIA FOR AD/HD

### Approved Diagnosis

1. AD/HD, predominately inattention (Criteria A1, B, C, D, E met)
2. AD/HD, predominately hyperactive/impulsive (Criteria A2, B, C, D, E met)
3. AD/HD, mixed (Criteria A1 and A2, B, C, D, E met)
4. AD/HD, not otherwise specified (prominent symptoms that do not meet criteria)
5. (In partial remission) a suffix used for individuals, especially adults and some adolescents whose present symptoms do not fully meet criteria

### Criteria

For any ADHD related diagnosis all of the following need to be present:

A. Six or more symptoms of inattention (A1) or hyperactivity/impulsivity (A2) (see below) present for 6 months to a degree that is maladaptive and inconsistent with developmental level
B. Symptoms that caused impairment present before age 7
C. Impairment from symptoms present in two or more settings (home, school, work)
D. Evidence of clinically significant impairment in social, academic or occupational functioning
E. Symptoms do not occur only during course of pervasive developmental disorder or other psychotic disorder and are not better accounted for by another mental disease diagnosis

### A1. Criteria for Inattention

a. Often fails to give close attention to details or makes careless mistakes in school work or other activities.
b. Often has difficulty sustaining attention in tasks or play activities.
c. Often does not seem to listen when spoken to directly.
d. Often does not follow through with instructions and fails to finish schoolwork, chores, or duties in the workplace (not due to oppositional behavior or failure to understand instructions).
e. Often has difficulty organizing tasks and activities.
f. Often avoids, dislikes, or is reluctant to engage in tasks that require sustained mental effort (such as schoolwork or homework).
g. Often loses things necessary for tasks or activities (toys, school assignments, pencils, books or tools).
h. Is often easily distracted by extraneous stimuli.
i. Is often forgetful in daily activities.

### A2. Criteria for Hyperactivity/Impulsivity

*Hyperactivity*

a. Often fidgets with hands or feet or squirms in seat.
b. Often leaves seat in classroom or in other situations in which remaining seated is expected.
c. Often runs about or climbs excessively in situations in which it is inappropriate (in adolescents or adults may be limited to subjective feelings of restlessness).
d. Often has difficulty playing or engaging in leisure activities quietly.
e. If often "on the go" or often acts as if "driven by motor."
f. Often talks excessively.

*Impulsivity*

g. Often blurts out answers before questions have been completed.
h. Often has difficulty awaiting turn.
i. Often interrupts or intrudes on others (butts into conversations or games).

*APA (1994), pp. 83–85.*

## CURRENT ISSUES IN ADHD

The DSM IV incorporates the current research on the five AD/HD conditions and concludes that common criteria are needed (see Criteria, A–E, Table 29-4). However, some clinicians find select criteria problematic. The most problematic is "B," as some symptoms may not emerge until the complexity of school increases, especially for children with AD/HD, primarily inattention.

Adolescents are likely to have academic underachievement due to these behaviors, exhibiting immaturity, excessive "fooling around," inappropriate silliness, or overreaction to teasing or normal peer interaction. Their talking back, frequent fighting, disobedience, and low frustration tolerance can be mistaken for delinquency behavior (Wender, 1995).

AD/HD is the most common childhood school related behavior problem (Wolraich &

Baumgaertel, 1997). Epidemiologic studies reveal a prevalence of AD/HD of 5% of children, with one Canadian study showing a 9% prevalence in boys and 3.3% prevalence in girls (Rappley, Gardiner, Jetton, & Houang, 1995). AD/HD does decline with aging, showing a 50% decline in age groupings every 5 years. The prevalence in childhood is 4%, and the estimated prevalence in adulthood ranges from 0.8% at 20 years to 0.05% at 40 (Hill & Schoener, 1996).

Both children and adults with AD/HD may manifest opposition, defiance, and hostile behavior towards others, particularly parents and teachers, a behavioral syndrome called oppositional-defiant disorder. This in turn can increase the risk for antisocial and drug-abusive disorders, as well as lost educational and vocational opportunities as the child grows to adulthood (Mannuzza, Klein, Bessler, Malloy, & LaPadula, 1993).

Symptoms of AD/HD can overlap with depression, anxiety, personality disorders, thought disorders, seizures, traumatic brain injury, and sensory deficits (particularly hearing losses). In AD/HD the symptoms can vary, being particularly dependent on the level of interest in the subject at hand; the syndrome is also marked by rapid mood shifts, no vegetative symptoms, clear thinking, and capacity for caring.

## CURRENT ISSUES IN TREATMENT

It is probable that biology rather than environment is at the heart of this disorder. A recent study notes a difference in central serotonergic function (Halperin et al, 1994). As some individuals mature, the chemical/behavioral deficit becomes less apparent; in others the changes are lifelong. Children with acquired sensorineural disorders have a higher rate of AD/HD. Children born with mental retardation also show a higher incidence of AD/HD (Mercugliano, 1993). The increased incidence of thyroid deficits in children with AD/HD also lends credence to a biologic etiology (Weiss, Stein, Trommer, & Refetoff, 1993). The possible change in uptake of neurotransmitters may lend credence to the apparent effect of certain foods on the behavior of individuals with AD/HD, because objective assessment has shown a change in behaviors in relation to the ingestion of specific foods (Carter et al, 1993).

The clinician needs to consider the following differential in establishing the AD/HD diagnosis (Baren, 1994; Wolraich & Baumgaertel, 1997).

- Fetal alcohol syndrome
- Fragile X syndrome
- Chronic lead poisoning/anemia
- Pervasive developmental disorders
- Seizure disorder
- Postinfectious or posttraumatic encephalopathy
- Hearing/vision problems
- Thyroid dysfunction
- Allergy and effects of medicines to treat allergy
- Psychiatric conditions
- Learning disorders

If treatment is ineffective, the diagnosis needs to be reconsidered.

The following co-morbid conditions need to be considered (Baren, 1994; Blondis, 1996; Wolraich & Baumgaertel, 1997).

- Learning disabilities
- Anxiety or mood disorders
- Language and communication disorders
- Other developmental disorders
- Tourette's syndrome or chronic tic disorder
- Generalized unresponsiveness to thyroid hormone
- Oppositional defiant or chronic disorder
- Chronic conditions (cerebral palsy, spina bifida, autism)

A subset of children will have co-morbid conditions. Treatment that does not address both conditions will be ineffective. Collaboration with a specialist is critical for management of these children.

There is a documented association of children with AD/HD having anxiety and behavioral and mood disorders, particularly depression and learning disabilities. Consequently, the workup for AD/HD should consider comorbid psychiatric diagnoses (Biederman et al, 1996) and include specific measures of anxiety and depression. Families of children with AD/HD are significantly more likely to have a parent affected by alcoholism, other drug abuse, learning disabilities, delinquency, and other cases of AD/HD (Roizen et al, 1996). One of the strongest associations is between adults with AD/HD and their children having a higher incidence of AD/HD than in the general population (Biederman et al, 1995).

There is also a link between hyperactive disorders and tics or dyskinesias, particularly Tourette's syndrome. Individuals under treatment for AD/HD may manifest tics and Tourette's behaviors such as sudden loud vocalizations. The incidence of tics and dyskinesias in children under treatment for AD/HD was 9% in one study, with

1 child in 122 developing Tourette's syndrome (Lipkin, Goldstein, & Adesman, 1994).

There is currently no research showing that using stimulant medication will produce a lasting tic disorder in children who were not predisposed to the condition. In low doses the tics and other symptoms of Tourette's syndrome may be alleviated (Mercugliano, 1993).

Adults with AD/HD present with similar behaviors as children with AD/HD and with more propensity for mood disorders. Adults and adolescents with AD/HD may also show an increased incidence of driving accidents and poor driving habits (Barkley, Guevremont, Anastopoulos, DuPaul, & Shelton, 1993). Children and adults with AD/HD can have other disorders of higher-level cortical functioning, including disturbances in social competence, communication, and cognition and movement disorders.

The parent of a child with AD/HD may come to the primary care office complaining about the child's behavior at home and in school. The child is described as unable to listen, unable to retain information in school, frequently daydreaming, and quickly going from one activity to another without finishing the first. The child is impulsive as well as hyperactive, constantly on the move, and forgetting in a few minutes what the adult has just told him or her in regard to a specific behavior.

The parent may describe other additional behaviors. In a general way these children are hyperresponsive to their environments. In an environment where multiple persons are completing multiple tasks, the child may seem even more hyperactive. When promised a future activity, the child may constantly badger the adult during the waiting period, demonstrating little regard for the normal passage of time.

In social and educational settings this behavior is seen as rude and inconsiderate. AD/HD children show an inability to maintain a consistent pattern of work productivity. The child's school work is often inconsistent, with one paper showing a failing grade and the next showing good work. The hallmark of the school work is its inconsistency.

## SPECIFIC CONSIDERATIONS FOR PHARMACOTHERAPY

### When Drug Therapy Is Needed

Medications in AD/HD should not be used prior to a complete diagnostic evaluation completed by a team of health care professionals, psychologists, speech pathologists, and educators. Prior to prescription, evidence must be present that social, learning, and behavioral difficulties are present that interfere with a child's or adult's ability to relate to others and learn or perform required tasks.

If the resources are limited and the clinician elects to place the child on medication before testing is completed, close monitoring is essential. If the child's behavior is not changed on the first medication selected, a referral to a specialist in the management of AD/HD is imperative. The management of this condition, especially in the presence of co-morbid conditions, can be complex and needs the close collaboration of primary care and specialist providers.

### Short- and Long-term Goals of Pharmacotherapy

The aim of pharmacotherapy is to improve attention and control impulsivity and excessive motor behaviors that interfere with daily life and to treat concomitant anxiety and depression. Assessing problem behaviors prior to treatment and outlining targeted tasks is necessary to establish outcome measures specific to the individual. Examples of outcome measures include the amount of time a child can attend to specific school-related tasks, the ability to complete homework in a reasonable amount of time, the ability to play with schoolmates in appropriate ways, and sleeping with fewer interruptions. For the adult it may mean the ability to complete work assignments in shorter periods, and better sleep patterns.

### Nonpharmacologic Therapy

The key treatments in AD/HD are control of the environment and education. Establishing a partnership with the adults who work with the person with AD/HD is a primary goal. The team around the child with AD/HD works together to provide consistent structure, counsel about specific detrimental and alternative behaviors, and control environmental stimulation to maximize success. This may require special placement within the educational system.

Education and counseling, individually or in groups and before and during pharmacological therapy, can be useful for children, teens, and adults with AD/HD. Local support groups are helpful. Educational information should include a discussion of the biologic aspect (rather than character disorder) of the disease. Coping behaviors may help with organizational skills; avoiding fatigue may improve social skills. Open communication by family members to the AD/HD person is helpful since the individual often lacks self-awareness (Fargason & Ford, 1994).

## Time Frame for Initiating Pharmacotherapy

Once one of the five diagnoses of AD/HD has been established, it is appropriate to start treatment. In very young, preschool-age children medications are rarely needed and should be instituted only with consultation of a specialist. Medication may begin during elementary education when the behaviors may interfere with learning. Periodic reappraisals for the need of medication are important, given the potential changes in AD/HD symptoms with maturity.

## Overview of Drug Classes

The primary medications used in AD/HD are the stimulants methylphenidate hydrochloride (Ritalin), amphetamines (methamphetamine and dextroamphetamine), and pemoline (Cylert). When stimulants are not efficacious, the tricyclic antidepressants desipramine (Norpramin) and imipramine (Tofranil) and the antihypertensive agent clonidine (Catapres) are often used, but with less success than the stimulants. The monoamine oxidase inhibitors and neuroleptics are also used in AD/HD.

## Assessment Prior to Therapy

A comprehensive developmental history and physical exam precede treatment. Diagnosis may be aided by use of family/teacher/child questionnaires. The most frequently used questionnaire is the Conner, a 28-item teacher version and a 48-item parent version (Wender, 1995). The examiner needs to assess for dysmorphic features, especially single palmer crease, epicanthal folds, low set ears, third toe longer than second, high arched palate, hypertelorism, or adherent ear lobes (Blondis, 1996).

Methylphenidate (MPD) use may require a preliminary complete blood and platelet count, and large doses of the medication may require yearly review of laboratory studies (AHFS, 1996, p. 1672). The amphetamines and pemoline are not recommended in children younger than 6 years old in the treatment of AD/HD (AHFS, 1996, pp. 1664, 1674). Because of common side effects such as decreased appetite and nausea, baseline weight is necessary before using any of the stimulants. Pemoline has also shown an adverse effect on hepatic function, so baseline studies of AST (SGOT) and ALT (SGPT) are necessary.

Adults with AD/HD may require utilization of rating scales, collateral reports, and neuropsychological testing before medication use. The tricyclic antidepressants are not given to individuals with a history of respiratory (asthma) or cardiac disorders (new acute myocardial infarction), hypertension, urinary retention, and known seizure disorders. These drugs should not be given in conjunction with antihypertensives or MAO inhibitors. Using desipramine necessitates a cardiac history, EKG, and lab studies prior to starting medication. Like other tricyclic antidepressants, imipramine (Tofranil) has cardiogenic side effects that may necessitate EKG monitoring.

## Patient/Caregiver Information

Children treated with stimulants and antidepressants need educated parents and teachers knowledgeable about the primary and secondary effects of these medications. The two most common side effects of methylphenidate are lethargy and appetite suppression, so weight monitoring is necessary. In general, these drugs require tapering dosages prior to discontinuation in order to maintain treatment gains.

## OUTCOMES MANAGEMENT

### Selecting an Appropriate Agent

AD/HD diagnoses are generally treated with the same medications. However, lower doses may be effective in the treatment of AD/HD, especially inattention. The drug of choice used in over 80% of AD/HD children is methylphenidate. All of the stimulants have about a 70% response rate. The use of methylphenidate is highest in children 8–11 years old, representing 45% of the use of the drug (Rappley et al, 1995). There has been a 2.5-fold increase in the drug's use from 1990 to 1995. In the United States it is estimated that the drug was used in 1.5 million youths in 1995, with an increased duration of drug use into the teenage years and more girls receiving the drug (Safer, Zito, & Fine, 1996). Methylphenidate has rapid onset, high efficacy, and few side effects. Sustained-release forms of dextroamphetamine and methylphenidate are available, with one study suggesting better drug usage with no increase in side effects (Kessler, 1996).

If methylphenidate is not effective, amphetamines or pemoline may be tried. In many cases the depression or anxiety that may occur concurrently with AD/HD necessitates the use of tricyclic antidepressants of clonidine. Pemoline should be used with caution due to reported deaths (see Follow-up Recommendations).

Baltimore school nurses reported an increase in the proportion of public school students on medication for hyperactive/inattentive disorders from 11% in 1985 to 30% in 1993. Many more students remained under treatment as teenagers, with more girls now under treatment (Safer & Krager, 1994). One study did point out that a small group of physicians may be abusing the prescribing of methylphenidate. Michigan has one of the highest per capita utilizations of methylphenidate, with relatively few pediatricians accounting for the largest number of prescriptions (Rappley et al, 1995).

The effects of both methylphenidate and dextroamphetamine are seen fairly quickly but require titration monitoring. In children the recommended starting dose of methylphenidate is 0.3–0.8 mg/kg; with schoolage children dosages start at 5 mg in the morning and 5 mg at noon with gradual increases in dosage as needed.

Teens start on 10 mg b.i.d. with 5 mg increases as needed (Wender, 1995). Sustained release dextroamphetamine has been helpful in select children (Blondis & Roizen, 1996). Most children benefit from a two-to-three-times-a-day dosing daily and on weekends. Children on twice-a-day dosing have been reported to have a "rebound hyperactivity," and if this occurs dosing three times a day is indicated (Blondis & Roizen, 1996). Preliminary studies suggest children often sleep better on two doses of medication, but some children do better on three (Blondis & Roizen, 1996). The need for drug holidays is unclear. If the child is being treated for AD/HD predominantly inattentive type, medication may not be needed in home over weekends or summer break. The clinician needs to assess each case individually.

Children who are mentally retarded have a less beneficial response to methylphenidate and may require a higher drug dose (0.6 mg/kg) (Mercugliano, 1993). The standard dose range for dextroamphetamine is 0.4–1.3 mg/kg. If a child does not respond well to one stimulant or

experiences unacceptable side effects, it is appropriate to try another stimulant.

The dosing range for desipramine is 1 mg/kg per day to more than 4.5 mg/kg per day with greater effect on attention and behaviors at the higher doses (Mercugliano, 1993).

Clonidine is used in children who do not respond well to the stimulants and who show repetitive, compulsive behaviors and anxiety. Clonidine, an alpha-adrenergic agonist, binds to the autoreceptors on norepinephrine-releasing neurons, resulting in a reduction of norepinephrine released throughout the brain. The starting dose of clonidine is 0.05 mg given initially at night with increases at weekly intervals because of its sedating effects. Dosing may need to be increased to t.i.d. or q.i.d. The dosing range is 3–6 µg/kg per day.

Robust doses of methylphenidate have shown efficacy in the treatment of AD/HD in adults (Spencer et al, 1995). Methylphenidate dosing in adults starts at 5 mg at 8 A.M. and noon with increasing dosing by 5-mg increments every 2–3 days. Therapeutic benefits last from 1½–4 h. Some adults may require dosing 4–6 times a day, up to 40–90 mg daily, to control symptoms.

Desipramine, a tricyclic antidepressant, was also found to significantly reduce symptoms of AD/HD in adults using a randomized, placebo controlled study (Wilens et al, 1996).

See Drug Tables 311.1 and 313.

## Monitoring for Efficacy and Toxicity

Efficacy is monitored by behavioral control, social and academic performance as well as nutritional status (including weight, height, and blood pressure). The patient, family and sometimes school personnel need to be included in monitoring efficacy. Rating questionnaires are often helpful. Some centers will do a blind trial of medications (one–two weeks on medicine and one–two weeks off medicine, with the child/family/school and sometimes even the clinician blinded to the treatment order). Co-morbid conditions may develop after initial diagnosis and continued assessment for emerging symptoms is critical.

Although often not prescribed in the late afternoon for fear of sleep abnormalities, methylphenidate was found to create marked symptom reduction in the evenings with no untoward effects on sleeping in an inpatient study with children. Prior to attempting this dosage alteration, however, it is helpful to chart the sleep behavior of the child before the evening dose and again after the evening dose is initiated. No relation between dosing size and sleep disorder was found (Kent, Blader, Koplewicz, Abikoff, & Foley, 1995). Liver function tests should be done periodically for all persons on pemoline.

## Follow-up Recommendations

Adults with AD/HD require utilization of rating scales, collateral reports, and neuropsychological testing before medication use.

The Barkley Side Effects Questionnaire (BSEQ) was developed to monitor the effects of stimulant therapy in AD/HD. Each symptom is rated from 0 (absent) to 9 (severe). The behaviors associated with stimulant therapy noted to positively decrease are daydreaming, irritability, anxiety, and nailbiting. Common side effects that increase with stimulant therapy are insomnia, decreased appetite, stomachache, headache, and dizziness. Other side effects noted by the Barkley Questionnaire to occur with stimulant therapy are euphoria, sadness, crying, talking less, disinterest, drowsiness, nightmares, and vocal tics. In the Ahmann et al (1993) study the reason for discontinuing the drug desipramine was the occurrence of rapid heartbeat, difficulty breathing, significantly decreased appetite, and insomnia.

Common side effects of desipramine and imipramine are dry mouth, constipation, and lethargy. The cardiovascular side effects include increased heart rate and increased blood pressure, as well as changes in baseline EKG with prolonged PR or QT intervals and nonspecific T-wave changes. If EKG changes occur, the medication should be discontinued because of the potential for fatal arrhythmias. Prior to using antidepressants, it is necessary to obtain a family history involving sudden death, arrhythmias, cardiomyopathy, and mitral valve disease, and to obtain an electrocardiogram (EKG).

Pemoline has been associated with fatal liver failure in two cases. In a third case study reporting a fatal liver failure, the authors argue for causality and urge further studies to quantify the risk in AD/HD children receiving this drug (Berkovitch, Pope, Phillips, & Koren, 1995). Careful monitoring of liver function is recommended.

Methylphenidate is a Schedule 2 controlled medication, requiring a collaborative signature in some states prior to prescription. Methylphenidate dosing should be increased slowly (at weekly intervals) in children after assessing side effects. Increasing adult doses can be done at 3-day intervals. Children are followed initially at 1-month intervals, then at 6 months, and then yearly.

## STROKE

Cerebrovascular accident (CVA), or stroke, is a general term referring to neurovascular events causing loss of neuronal circulation in one of three ways. Infarction of a cerebral vessel accounts for 75–80% of strokes; intracerebral or subarachnoid hemorrhage accounts for 15%; and 10% of strokes are from other or unknown causes including cerebral ischemia, artery dissection, coagulopathy, infection, and amyloid angiopathy. Approximately 550,000 Americans suffer a stroke every year, with more than 3 million at any given time living with stroke and its concomitant disabilities (Gresham, 1995).

The incidence of stroke doubles with every decade after age 55. Stroke occurrence is highest in men and African-Americans. Mortality ranges from 17–30% in the first 30 days to 25–40% in the first year. Declines in stroke mortality are due to reduction in stroke severity, better acute care, and modifying the risk factors known to cause stroke. The size of the stroke lesion and its location are key factors in the specific neurologic losses.

In acute stroke, permanent cerebral damage can affect a certain number of neuronal cells directly. The resulting swelling can cause further damage to surrounding neuronal tissue, some of which can recover spontaneously within hours to weeks following the acute event. The most common site of stroke is the middle cerebral artery (MCA) or one of its smaller tributaries. The MCA is the primary vascular source for the cerebral cortex, and damage to the MCA can result in loss of motor function to the opposite side of the body, as well as loss of sensory function and a loss of language (aphasia) if the stroke affects the predominant left hemisphere.

The unmodifiable risk factors for stroke are age, gender, prior stroke, race, and family history. Almost three quarters of strokes occur in individuals over 65 years of age. Males have a higher risk in all but the oldest age groups, and African-Americans have a twofold risk over whites, attributed to higher cardiovascular risk factors, lower family income, and other undetermined factors (Gresham, 1995).

The modifiable risk factors are hypertension, diabetes, high cholesterol levels, coronary heart disease, cocaine use, obesity, and heavy alcohol use (Gresham, 1995).

Particular cardiovascular conditions that increase the risk for stroke include hypertension, endocarditis, valve replacement, atrial fibrillation, left ventricular hypertrophy, known cardiac thrombi, ventricular aneurysm, mitral regurgitation, mitral valve prolapse, coronary artery disease, and congestive heart failure.

Blood pressure readings above 160/95 mm Hg have a 10- to 12-fold risk of stroke compared to blood pressure in the 140/90 range (Margolis & Wityk, 1997).

Diabetes carries a two- to threefold risk of stroke which can be reduced by good hypertension control, good daily glucose control, and monitoring of glycohemoglobin levels (Margolis & Wityk, 1997). The relationship between cholesterol level and stroke is not as direct, although increased lipid levels are seen in stroke and in some studies low lipid levels are seen in cerebral hemorrhage.

Drug use is a significant cause of stroke. Smoking increases the risk of stroke and hemorrhage by 50% in all gender and age groups, and the risk is directly related to the number of cigarettes smoked. Alcohol consumption at more than two drinks per day carries a 50% increased risk of cardiac arrhythmias, increased blood pressure, abnormal blood clotting mechanisms, and a higher risk of cerebral hemorrhage (Margolis & Wityk, 1997). Cocaine use and obesity, particularly abdominal obesity with a waist-hip ratio over 1, increase stroke risk (Margolis & Wityk, 1997).

The result of acute vascular changes can be a transient ischemic attack (TIA) with complete resolution of all neurologic losses within 24 h. A TIA is a short-lived (5- to 20-min) neurological deficit with no permanent neurologic loss that can act as a warning sign to other neurologic changes.

Full recovery from a stroke can occur for up to a year and beyond, although most recovery occurs in the first 1–3 months. Recovery is due to spontaneous neurologic recovery as well as the individual learning new skills in daily functioning through rehabilitation. Recent studies have shown that physical rehabilitation undertaken 3 years following stroke can improve functional skill in dressing, bathing, and transfers, freeing the individual of the need for physical assistance (Margolis & Wityk, 1997).

The most common deficits following stroke are hemiparesis, sensory deficits, dysarthria, visual-perceptual deficits, cognitive deficits (particularly memory impairment), bladder control, and hemianopsia (Gresham, 1995).

Comorbid conditions of hypertension, heart disease, diabetes mellitus, obesity, and arthritis all predispose the individual with a stroke to a recurrent stroke and can compromise the ability to participate in rehabilitation as well as life in general. Good medical management of the comorbidities often improves the quality of life.

## SPECIFIC CONSIDERATIONS FOR PHARMACOTHERAPY

The aim of this section is threefold: First, a general overview of medications used to treat modifiable risk factors; second, a discussion of medications used in the treatment of acute TIA and stroke including the new antithrombolytic agents; and third, a general review of medications commonly used for the relief of symptoms following stroke.

### When Drug Therapy Is Needed

Modifying risk factors to prevent further stroke is the first goal. The second goal is to understand the newer pharmacologic treatments available at the time of acute stroke. The specific sequelae of the stroke, including but not limited to spasticity, mood disorders (particularly depression), alterations in bowel and bladder function, and attention deficits, amenable to drug therapy are covered below.

### Short- and Long-Term Goals of Pharmacotherapy

Recently, new therapies have radically changed the acute care of strokes. In embolic stroke, about 33% of patients may regain some or all of their previous function if treated within 3 h of stroke onset with a thrombolytic agent.

The long-term goals of pharmacotherapy are the prevention of stroke and of recurrent stroke through modification of known risk factors. There is a 5% incidence per year of stroke following TIA and a 10% incidence of further stroke following mild stroke (Gasecki & Hachinski, 1993). The second long-term goal is appropriate use of pharmaceuticals for disability symptom relief.

### Nonpharmacologic Therapy

Nonpharmacologic prevention of stroke therapy is similar to that directed toward coronary artery disease. In addition to obesity prevention by maintaining a low-fat, high-fiber diet, appropriate stress management and aerobic exercise of a minimum of 20 min three times weekly are recommended. One study found a 22% reduction in stroke risk for every increase in three servings of fruits and vegetables per day (Margolis & Wityk, 1997).

Individuals with a high degree of carotid stenosis (70–99% stenosis of any carotid vessel) show a better outcome with surgery because the risk of stroke without surgery is higher than the 5% risk with surgery (Gasecki & Hachinski, 1993). The key to a better outcome with carotid endarterectomy is a technically competent surgeon who performs the procedure frequently and has a low rate of complication.

Stroke occurs in 5–10% of individuals following coronary artery bypass surgery. The skill of the surgeon and his complication rate are factors in the outcome as well as close monitoring of oxygen levels.

In the event of a new acute stroke, pharmacologic treatment within 3 h of the event may decrease the neurologic losses or eliminate any stroke symptoms. This necessitates a real reeducation process within the American public to treat stroke as a "brain attack," with immediate transport to an emergency unit capable of administering the new agents.

Once an individual is outside the 3-h window for acute antithrombolytic therapy or is not a candidate for such therapy, the acute care should be given in a setting allowing coordinated, multidisciplinary services emphasizing early rehabilitation and early mobility. Acute care stroke teams have made a significant change in the length and cost of hospitalization as well as the prevention of stroke complications. Acute stroke teams have expertise in stroke etiology, brain areas involved, specific neurologic deficits, and complications that occur with stroke (Gresham, 1995, p. 4). The stroke team decreases mortality and shows better maintenance of blood pressure, better treatment of hyperthermia, and better control of hyperglycemia than traditional care. Hyperthermia with an increase in temperature of 2.7°F doubles the risk of poor outcome after stroke (Margolis and Wityk, 1997).

Following stroke, the services of a full rehabilitation team are useful, including speech pathologists, certified rehabilitation or neurologic nurses, physical therapists, occupational therapists, neuropsychologists, and recreational therapists, as well as consulting neurologists and physiatrists.

## Time Frame for Initiating Pharmacotherapy

With the exception of a new acute stroke, the time frame for initiation of pharmacotherapy for stroke prevention and for symptom relief is within a day or week depending on the particular symptoms being addressed.

However, with a new acute stroke time to pharmacologic intervention is crucial. Within 3 h of the acute stroke event, the person must undergo a head CT scan to determine if hemorrhaging is occurring with the stroke, as well as emergency blood work to determine normal blood clotting capabilities prior to treatment with thrombolytic agents. Those individuals who wake up in the morning with a stroke and are unable to determine the specific time in the night the stroke occurred are usually not eligible for acute therapy. The presenting symptom in stroke is often hemiparesis, as well as slurred speech and in some cases total inability to speak or understand what is said. If the specific event is witnessed and the individual can get treatment early, thrombolytic agents may be effective in ameliorating or lessening stroke sequelae.

## Overview of Drug Classes for Treatment

Many drug groups are utilized in treating the modifiable risk factors in stroke. In treating the modifiable risk factors, antihypertensive agents, lipid-reducing agents, agents to treat obesity, and smoking cessation agents are all utilized.

In acute stroke, treatment is dependent on the diagnosis of ischemic stroke, the presence of ischemia, and the use of thrombolytic agents, as well as the necessity of treating concurrent hypertension accompanying the stroke and other forms of coronary artery disease.

In treating the sequelae of acute stroke the drug classes include antispasmolytics, drugs to control incontinency, drugs for anxiety and depression, and pain relievers.

## Assessment Needed Prior to Therapy

Assessment of stroke risk is recognizing the unmodifiable risk factors of age and sex and assessing those risk factors that can be modified. This assessment includes elevation of systolic blood pressure, general hypertension, diabetes mellitus, obesity, use of oral contraceptives, cigarette smoking, cardiovascular disease (particularly atrial fibrillation, left ventricular hypertrophy, and carotid artery stenosis), and alcohol or drug abuse.

In acute stroke or possible TIA, assessment starts with a full history, general physical examination, and full neurologic examination including overall mental status, cranial nerve status, motor strength, sensory changes, coordination, and communication. The next step is a brain CAT scan to rule out cerebral hemorrhage, neoplasms, and other causes of TIA or stroke not of ischemic origin. CAT scans within hours to days of an ischemic stroke may not show new lesions. To rule out other metabolic etiologies and the possible presence of infection as a cause of the stroke requires an electrocardiogram, full chemical lab analysis (SMA-18), complete blood count, urinalysis, and urine culture and sensitivity (Margolis and Preziosi, 1996).

In assessing treatment after stroke, the pharmacologic agents utilized are for symptomatic relief. For the long-term treatment of these stroke sequelae, see the sections covering spasticity, incontinency, pain relief, depression, and anxiety.

## Patient/Caregiver Information

The patient needs to understand the role he or she can play in stroke prevention through good control of modifiable risk factors and compliance with prescribed drug routines. At the same time patients and families need to realize that age, gender, race, and concurrent disease out of their control can lead to the development of stroke.

At the time of an acute stroke families need education in treating stroke as a "brain attack." This entails understanding the symptoms of TIA or stroke and appropriate transport to a medical facility for further treatment. The symptoms of TIA or stroke include limb weakness, speech slurring, loss of sensation in a limb, acute confusion, incoordination, incontinency, inability to speak, facial weakness, loss of vision to loss of consciousness, and impaired breathing.

If the onset of symptoms is within 3 h and a protocol for the use of thrombolytic agents is available at a local facility, then the patient and family need to be directed to that facility. Regardless of time frame, transfer to a facility with a stroke team in place may improve acute treatment, prevent complications, lessen the length of an acute hospital stay, and lessen stroke care costs.

Patient and caregiver information following a stroke includes specific guidelines for general and rehabilitation care, as well as measures needed to try and prevent further strokes. This includes information and treatment plans to modify further risk factors; the goals and pharmacologic treatment of spasticity, incontinency, cognitive impairments, speech, and dysphagia, and basic rehabilitation measures in daily as well as extended activities of daily living. In some cases caregivers need information regarding skilled care facilities, assisted living programs, home health services, financial issues, and health care proxies.

## OUTCOMES MANAGEMENT

This section considers pharmacologic agents in three groups: the drugs used in the prevention of stroke, the drugs used in acute stroke, and the drugs used after a completed stroke.

### Drugs Used in Stroke Prevention

The objectives for stroke prevention are similar to those for cardiovascular disease and many of the same drugs are utilized. In treating hypertension, the systolic and diastolic blood pressure from the initial contact in a physician's office is the most reliable indicator of cerebral infarction risk. In the Framingham Study, repeated blood pressure, pulse pressure, and mean arterial pressure measurement provided little overall further prognostic value (Arnold, 1993).

*Acetylsalicylic acid (Aspirin).*   ASA use reduces stroke incidence by 22%. ASA acts by inhibiting platelet buildup at the site of vascular plaque abnormalities primarily in the arterial system by preventing platelet aggregation. Chemically, it has irreversible acetylation of cyclo-oxygenase and inhibits the formation of endothelial prostacyclin (Unwin & Greenlee, 1993). ASA is more effective in men than women, and the dose varies from 36–1300 mg per day. In the United States the most common dosing recommendation is 360 mg twice a day. The chief side effect of ASA therapy is gastric irritation and consequent GI bleeding. ASA is not as effective in atrial fibrillation as warfarin.

*Ticlopidine.*   Ticlopidine (Ticlid) is another antiplatelet medication that acts by inhibiting adenosine diphosphate pathways for platelet activation, showing a 2% absolute reduction and 12% relative risk reduction using Ticlid over

ASA. The drug is utilized more in women, those failing ASA therapy, and with vertebrobasilar symptoms and does not cause the gastric irritation seen with ASA. There is a reduction in nonfatal or fatal stroke of 21% at 3 years as reported in the Ticlopidine Aspirin Stroke Study (TASS) and a 30% reduction in the Canadian-American Ticlid study (Teasell & Gillen, 1993). However, Ticlid carries its own side effects of diarrhea and rash in 2% of patients as well as the serious side effect of neutropenia in 10%, 1% of which can be fatal. Ticlid use requires monitoring with CBCs every 2 weeks for the first 3 months and monthly thereafter.

**Warfarin.**   Warfarin (Coumadin) is used to prevent cardioembolic stroke in individuals with atrial fibrillation. It acts by inhibiting the clotting cascade, as in the left atrium in a fibrillating heart. In the Chimowitz et al (1995) study, warfarin was significantly better than ASA for stroke prevention in patients with symptomatic stenosis of a major intracerebral artery. In terms of stroke prevention, warfarin is more effective and less costly overall than ASA in patients with nonvalvular atrial fibrillation (Gage et al, 1995). Warfarin use requires careful management by following INR levels daily at first and then weekly and monthly once an individual is stabilized. The INR therapeutic range is generally 2.0–4.0. Thus, a cooperative patient and adequate laboratory facilities are required. Contraindications to its use may include heavy use of alcohol, history of GI bleeding, risk of falls, underlying hepatic or renal disease, use of antiplatelet agents, and thyrotoxicosis (Silva-Smith, 1994).

**Nimodipine.**   In cerebral hemorrhage, and more specifically in subarachnoid hemorrhage (SAH), the drug nimodipine shows a trend toward prevention of infarction. It is started in the acute care setting and may be continued for a period of time in the outpatient setting. This calcium channel blocker prefers the central nervous system and probably inhibits the uptake of calcium into damaged neurons and consequent neurocellular damage and cerebral vasoconstriction. The drug is given orally at 60 mg every 4 h for 21 days following a cerebral hemorrhage. The chief side effect is hypotension, and in some cases this may necessitate discontinuing the drug. Other less common side effects include thrombocytopenia, rash, abdominal cramping, and elevated liver enzymes (AHFS, 1996).

## Drugs Used in Acute Stroke Care

**Thrombolytic agents.**   In June 1996 the FDA approved the use of tissue plasminogen activator (t-PA) to reduce the acute deficit in ischemic stroke. National studies (National Institute of Neurological Disorders and Stroke [NINDS], 1995) found t-PA reduced neurologic deficit and improved functional outcome by 30% in the treatment group. Streptokinase has not shown the same results (Donnan et al, 1996). The efficacy is time-based to within 3 h of the acute stroke. It requires a CT scan with no hemorrhage, normal blood coagulation studies, normal platelet count, normal blood glucose levels, easily controlled hypertension, and informed consent. Use of ASA or Ticlid does not preclude the use of t-PA. The inpatient hospital setting must have the ability to care for cerebral hemorrhage, which can occur following its use. The usual dose is 0.9 mg/kg with a maximum dose of 90 mg; it is infused by a 10% bolus with the rest over 60 min.

**Hypertension management.**   In ischemic stroke, acute hypertension will usually resolve and begin to fall within hours of the event. The initial rise in systemic blood pressure is protective to ensure adequate blood flow to cerebral vessels. Stroke due to hemorrhage and initial hypertension in ischemia may, however, require aggressive treatment to prevent end-organ damage (heart, liver, and kidneys). The aim of reducing systemic hypertension is the maintenance of cerebral perfusion to prevent further brain ischemia. If brain cerebral pressure autoregulation is impaired, an elevated blood pressure will increase cerebral blood volume, increase cerebral blood flow, and increase intracerebral pressure. If blood pressure is reduced too quickly or by drugs inducing cerebral vessel dilatation, the increase in cerebral edema causes cerebral blood vessel damage with vascular leakage and more cerebral edema.

Hypertension should be treated if the calculated mean blood pressure (sum of systolic blood pressure plus diastolic blood pressure times 2 and divided by 3) is over 130 mm Hg or systolic pressure is over 220 mm Hg. The recommended drugs are labetalol and enalapril. Labetalol acts by decreasing systolic vascular resistance without reflex tachycardia by beta-adrenergic receptor blockage and improves cerebral perfusion pressure by a decrease in intracerebral pressure. The dose of labetalol is 0.05 mg/kg IV with response in 5–10 min. The dose can be repeated every 10 min or continuously infused at 0.5–2 mg/min. Enalapril is an angiotensin-converting enzyme inhibitor that does not produce a reflex sympathetic stimulation and so retains favorable end-organ perfusion (Kay et al, 1996).

In the office setting, if the patient's blood pressure is over 180/100 with a new stroke, hospital treatment is required. If blood pressure is mildly elevated, the oral agents used most frequently are captopril and nicardipine. The calcium sublingual agents can precipitously lower blood pressure, inhibiting cerebral pressure.

***Management of acute myocardial infarction.*** In acute stroke, there is a 12% incidence of acute MI that accompanies the stroke, as well as a higher rate of EKG changes, some of which are thought to be neuronal in origin. If EKG changes occur with stroke, patient survival is decreased by 50% in the first 3 years. Consequently, following stroke, appropriate ASA treatment at 325 mg per day in asymptomatic stroke survivors is recommended. If the individual has symptoms of cardiac disease, other treatment is recommended depending on their cardiac status (Arnold, 1993).

***Congestive heart failure.*** Congestive heart failure can occur with stroke and requires appropriate acute treatment (see Chapter 20).

***Seizure management.*** Utilization of antiseizure medications will not prevent the onset of seizures. Seizures can occur with stroke in 7–42% of patients depending on the study reviewed. About 10% of patients present with a new acute seizure at the time of stroke. However, a much smaller number go on to develop recurrent seizures or epilepsy requiring antiseizure medications. Consequently, single seizures at stroke onset may not require antiseizure medications.

Most epilepsy development occurs in the first year following stroke. Injury to the cortex carries a higher risk of seizure than injury to deeper cortical areas, both in infarction and hemorrhage, as does metabolic imbalance and multiple cerebral infarction. If recurrent seizures do occur, they are often well controlled with monotherapy in a low therapeutic range. Metabolic clearance for antiepileptic drugs does decline in the elderly, so frequently this group of patients needs less drug than a younger popula-

tion. Initially, frequent screening of blood levels, every 2 weeks to monthly, is necessary. Weaning off seizure medications can be done at 1 year given a normal EEG and no recurrent seizure (Wiebe-Velazquez & Blume, 1993).

## Drug Use Following Stroke

***Incontinency.*** Incontinency and bladder retention can occur after stroke. Medication use is delayed until specific diagnosis is made and behavioral therapies are initiated. The most common cause of initial incontinency in a previously hospitalized patient is a urinary tract infection. It is important to eliminate the cause before other therapy is initiated. If the patient remains persistently incontinent, assessing any previous history of incontinence and prostate disease is imperative, followed by a cystometrography study. If detrusor instability and hyperreflexia are found, specific medications are helpful as well as the utilization of incontinence devices.

***Urinary retention.*** Males with existing prostate disease can develop retention, which is most clearly indicated by a high postvoid residual (over 100 cc) if catheterized immediately. It is not uncommon for individuals with a mild stroke to present in the office setting with a large retentive bladder. Specifics for medication treatment are in Chapter 34.

***Spasticity.*** Spasticity is a motor neuron disorder indicated by an increase in stretch reflexes and objectively noted by an increase in muscle tone. It occurs within hours to up to 38 days after a stroke, first in the proximal muscles of the hip and shoulder, and then more distally. The presenting pattern is usually flexor then extensor synergy. The extensor synergy in the leg can help with gait. Spasticity can resolve with the return of voluntary muscle control. The specifics of treatment and pharmacotherapeutics are in Chapter 14. Pharmacologic treatment can be difficult with this population because of the sedating properties of many of the drugs (Harburn & Potter, 1993).

***Upper extremity pain.*** Reflex sympathetic dystrophy (RSD), or shoulder-hand syndrome, is a clinical syndrome occurring in acute paralysis with distal limb pain, edema, vasomotor instability (swelling and redness), and hyperalgia. It is commonly seen 1–5 months after stroke and is primarily diagnosed by a positive bone scan that shows an elevated nuclear uptake. The cause of the condition is not clear; however, it may be related to reduced sympathetic outflow to the affected extremity. Secondary signs of RSD include osteoporosis, muscle atrophy, temperature changes, and vasomotor instability. In addition to aggressive physical therapy, optimal limb positioning, and decreased stimulus to the limb, pharmacologic interventions include oral steroids, acupuncture, and NSAIDs (Teasell & Gillen, 1993).

**Deep vein thrombus.** Immobility or a stroke that limits ambulation to less than 30 ft per day requires prophylactic treatment with heparin; 5000 units every 12 h is recommended. A newer form of heparin, low molecular weight, is also being tested for use in acute ischemic stroke (Chan et al, 1995). Twenty percent of individuals on low-dose heparin still develop DVT, and 10% of these individuals will develop pulmonary emboli, which carry a 10% fatality rate (Potter, 1993).

**Depression.** Depression in completed stroke is very common; upwards of 30% of the stroke population suffer from acute or long-term depression. It is often underdiagnosed and undertreated. The two primary causes are changes in neurotransmitters caused by local damage and diaschisis (the interruption of normal neural networks via axons and dendrites, as well as changes in neurochemical transmission), which can affect neurons distant from the original stroke site, as well as depression from the physical and psychological trauma accompanying the stroke (Swartzman & Teasell, 1993).

Regardless of the etiology, depression should be treated. Standard depression scales and the DSM-IV criteria are helpful in diagnosis. In stroke the serotonin reuptake inhibitors are a first-line drug choice, because they produce less lethargy. In addition, Zoloft may have cognitive benefits as well. A second choice is tricyclic antidepressants. They require monitoring of cardiac conduction, heart rate, and blood pressure, particularly if left ventricle dysfunction is present. Tricyclics can also be more sedating.

**Anxiety.** A recent stroke review (Margolis, 1997) showed an increase in general anxiety disorders of 25% following stroke. The symptoms were insomnia, excessive fatigue, and irritability.

This group benefited by treatment with antidepressant rather than anxiolytic medications, which tended to be too sedating. The serotonin reuptake medications were the recommended medications because of fewer side effects.

**Dementia.** Stroke can cause, contribute to, or coexist with dementia. In some elderly patients with mild dementias, the compensatory capacity of the brain may be overcome with the stroke. The prevalence of dementia in stroke is 26–52% if the individual is over 80 (Erkinjuntti & Hachinski, 1993). See the dementia section of this chapter regarding specifics of pharmacologic treatment.

**Sexuality.** Many changes can occur in sexual relationships and functioning after a stroke. The alterations can be related to physiologic and cognitive changes, use of medications, alterations in autonomic nervous system function, fear of another stroke, and diminished self-image.

**Drugs not to use in stroke.** In a retrospective analysis of the Sygen in Acute Stroke Study (Goldstein, 1995), a small but significant relationship between certain drug classes and a poor functional and motor outcome was noted. The drugs showing poorer outcome at 84 days after stroke were all given in the first month after stroke. The classes included benzodiazepines (phenytoin and phenobarbital) and dopamine. It is postulated that these drugs may inhibit stroke recovery by impairing the use of associated neurons at the site of the stroke, as well as inhibiting resolution of diaschisis.

### Follow-up Recommendations

Follow-up in the office setting is based on the medication regimes of patients and their medical stability. Prior to stroke, follow-up is dependent on general medical status. After stroke follow-up may be at 6-week intervals depending on other medical conditions and symptoms of stroke that remain.

## MULTIPLE SCLEROSIS

Multiple sclerosis (MS) is the most common neurologic diagnosis of young adults. Evidence suggests that this is an autoimmune condition, affecting 250,000–350,000 young adults less than 40, with one peak in the mid-20s and another peak in the mid-40s. More women than men are affected with prevalence ranging from 1.1–2.8, and it is more common in Caucasians. The disease is more prevalent in North America and Northern Europe and migration after age 15 shows a prevalence to the country of origin (Donohoe, 1995).

The exact etiology is unknown. A proposed etiology is an autoimmune regulation abnormality. Two genetic markers, HLA-DR2 on chromosome 6 and immunoglobulin GM on chromosome 14, are found more frequently in MS. There is a familial tendency with identical twins showing a 26% chance of both twins having the disease if one develops it, and 2.5% in fraternal twins and first-degree relatives, a 5–15 times greater ratio than the general population. Although a viral infection is suspected, no active or latent virus has been located in brain or spinal cord tissue. There is a decreased risk of exacerbation in pregnancy, but there is an increased risk of exacerbation postpartum. The family's ability to carry out child care should play a role in the decision of women to bear children (Donohoe, 1995).

The pathophysiology of MS is one of CNS demyelination of nerve fibers, sparing of axons, gliosis, and development of inflammatory cells. Plaques ranging from 1 mm to 4 cm, are scattered throughout white matter and to some degree in grey matter. The areas usually showing early pathology are the optic nerves and chiasm, the areas surrounding the blood vessels in the cerebellum, cerebrum, and cervical spinal cord. Plaques that are actively forming create increased edema with a number of lymphs, macrophages, and plasma cells. The chronic lesions show astrocyte hyperplasia and a reduced number of oligodendrocytes that appear as scars. The disease is thought to be initiated by an immune response against a virus that cross-reacts with myelin or oligodendrocyte cells; the antigen that is produced is still unknown.

One current hypothesis is that a defect in suppressor T-cell function lowers the threshold of T-cell activity. Cytokines (tumor necrosis factor and interleukin-2), interferon, and prostaglandins are present in MS and implicated in the regulation of the immune system and in autoimmune reactions. The use of MRI in judging the development of new plaques that may be clinically silent allows an objective measure of drug utilization and drug suppression of new plaque formation as a marker of drug efficacy (Donohoe, 1995).

The clinical manifestations of MS are in Table 29–5 and the diagnostic test studies are in Table 29–6. Patients may appear in the office with an acute "attack" or exacerbation. They may present with complaints of visual changes, fatigue, heat intolerance, sensory disturbance, weakness and spasticity in the legs, bowel and bladder dysfunction, ataxic gait, paresthesias in the extremities, and sexual dysfunction. On clinical neurologic examination these patients show

## TABLE 29–5. CLINICAL SIGNS AND SYMPTOMS OF MULTIPLE SCLEROSIS

| Area of Dysfunction | Signs and Symptoms |
| --- | --- |
| Cranial nerves | Blurred central vision, faded color, blind spots (optic neuritis), diplopia, dysphagia, facial weakness, numbness, pain |
| Fatigue | Overwhelming weakness, not overcome by increased physical effort |
| Motor dysfunction | Weakness, paralysis, spasticity, abnormal gait |
| Cerebellar dysfunction | Dysarthria, tremor, incoordination, ataxia, vertigo |
| Cognitive dysfunction | Impaired short-term memory, difficulty learning new information, word-finding trouble, short attention span, decreased concentration, mood alterations (depression) |
| Sensory dysfunction | Paresthesia, decreased proprioception and temperature perception, Lhermitte's sign (electric shock sensation down spine into legs) |
| Bowel and bladder dysfunction | Fecal urgency, constipation, bladder urgency, incontinence |
| Sexual dysfunction | Women: decreased libido and orgasmic ability, decreased genital sensation<br>Men: erectile, orgasmic, and ejaculation dysfunction |

*Adapted from Donohoe (1995).*

**TABLE 29–6.  DIAGNOSTIC TESTS AND RESULTS FOR MULTIPLE SCLEROSIS**

| Test | Result |
| --- | --- |
| Magnetic resonance imaging | White matter lesions (plaques) of brain, brainstem, and spinal cord |
| CSF analysis (lumbar puncture) | Presence of oligoclonal bands and an increase in protein, lymphocytes, and IgG |
| Evoked potentials (visual, brainstem, somatosensory) | Prolonged impulse conduction |
| Urodynamic studies | Neurogenic bladder |
| Myelogram, skull and spine x-rays, CT scan | Rule out other neurologic disease |

*Adapted from Donohoe (1995).*

changes in ocular movement, changes in visual acuity, trigeminal neuralgia and optic neuritis, increased tone in the legs, a decrease in motor strength, bilateral clonus of knees and ankles, upgoing toes bilaterally, decreased appreciation of position, and decreased appreciation of vibration. A significant number of patients have cognitive impairment and emotional changes. Cognitively, in 50–60% there is difficulty processing new information, difficulty recalling new information, and deficits in nonverbal problem solving. There may be deficits in sequencing and organizational skills, along with poor judgment, impulsivity, and inability to appreciate the consequences of an action. The Mini Mental Status Examination is helpful in assessing mental status. Emotional changes range from depression to a pseudobulbar affect that is often seen as euphoria, as well as significant amounts of fatigue, anxiety, and mental confusion.

The clinical course is marked by great variability and is unpredictable. The number and frequency of the acute "attacks" do not predict future disability. There are two major phases of disease: exacerbating-remitting and chronic-progressive. Patients in the first group average one attack per year, but after several years the disease usually becomes more chronic-progressive in 50% of MS patients. The attacks or exacerbations consist of new signs or worsening of old clinical signs or symptoms that last more than 24 h in the absence of fever or infection. Some individuals who present with chronic-progressive disease then change to an exacerbating-remitting disease pattern. Twenty percent present with chronic-progressive disease and are usually over 40 years of age.

## SPECIFIC CONSIDERATIONS FOR PHARMACOTHERAPY

### When Drug Therapy Is Needed

As with other neurologic conditions, MS is managed with the assistance of a consulting neurologist who has in-depth training in the disease and its manifestations. Although not necessarily prescribing, the primary care provider needs an understanding of the drugs and their usual efficacy as well as side effects.

### Short- and Long-Term Goals of Pharmacotherapy

The aim of drug therapy is to delay progression of the disease, manage the chronic symptoms associated with the disease, and treat exacerbations.

### Nonpharmacologic Therapy

The timing of therapy and specific goals are less clear in MS because of the unpredictability of the condition. Third-party payers are less familiar with the disease and somewhat reluctant to pay for therapy unless specific goals of treatment are established and met in an appropriate time frame. The goal of rehabilitation is to minimize functional loss despite the possibility of progressive neurologic impairments. This means the prevention of further hospitalization and preventing or delaying long-term care by adapting energy, skills, home modification, continuing employment, and cognitive rehabilitation (see the section on head injury) as needed (Dombovy, 1997).

Symptomatic treatment areas include fatigue, spasticity, ataxia, pain, dysarthria, respiratory dysfunction, and bowel and bladder dysfunction. Learning energy conservation techniques from a physical and occupational therapist is helpful. Spasticity, muscle weakness, and ataxia often benefit from gait analysis and the use of assistive devices to ensure safety in ambulation, the necessity of wheelchair use, and proper transfer techniques. The key to reimbursement for these therapies is specificity in prescription with clear-cut goals. Pain in MS is often helped by relaxation techniques and electric stimulation. Dysarthria and respiratory dysfunction are often improved through the use of short-term speech therapy, as well as respiratory therapy to teach appropriate breathing techniques.

Bowel dysfunction is often related to constipation. It is the result of decreased exercise and consequent low motility as well as lesions or plaques on nerves that control normal bowel motility. The goal of therapy is regular bowel movements. Nonpharmacologic techniques include drinking 8–10 glasses of water per day (this can be problematic in bladder dysfunction). Other diet considerations include a high-bulk diet with fruits, vegetables, and whole grain cereals. Establishing a regular evacuation time is helpful, allowing 15 min of relaxation is necessary, and this may require 2–3 weeks to establish. Avoiding the use of a bedpan is helpful because the bowel is more active in an upright position. Exercising without causing extreme fatigue is helpful. Not having a bowel movement for 3–4 days and having very hard bowel movements or liquid bowel movements can result in further problems. Early intervention is helpful, so patients need to feel free to call the primary care provider with these kinds of problems. It is important to assess bowel function and use the nonpharmaceutical treatments as well as pharmaceutical treatments to maintain good bowel function.

Bladder dysfunction due to poor positioning and plaque formation on nerves and brain also is common. The bladder problems need follow-up with a urologist to obtain cystometric studies of bladder function. High residual urine is often a cause of urinary tract infections. If possible individuals with MS can be taught intermittent catheterization to maintain low residual urine. This may require catheterization up to 4–6 times a day, depending on the ability of the bladder to void and empty. Techniques to prevent urinary tract infection include the minimum intake of 2–3 qt of fluid per day, limiting caffeine to 2 cups per day, drinking cranberry juice, which inhibits bacteria from implantation on the bladder wall, and washing the genital area with warm water and soap twice a day. Bladder emptying may require more relaxation and time than usual in the face of dysfunction and more frequent emptying. Depending on the results of urine cystometric studies, some patients are taught to perform Credé's maneuver on their bladders. Patients need to know the symptoms of bladder infection to act appropriately and seek guidance. These symptoms include increased frequency, urgency to urinate, pain, burning with urination, and foul-smelling or cloudy urine. Because of the increased bacterial resistance to antibiotic treatment, urine cultures are necessary prior to starting treatment; prolonged prophylactic antibiotic use is not necessarily an appropriate alternative in this group of patients because of this increased resistance to antibiotics.

## Time Frame for Initiating Therapy

The time frame for therapy is dependent on the specifics of treatment. In an acute exacerbation, it usually begins within a day of symptom relief or long-term prevention of new attacks. Symptomatic relief does not require such a strict time frame.

## Overview of Drug Classes for Treatment

To prevent new plaque formation or acute exacerbations, patients are now placed on immunomodulators; the ones currently approved by the FDA are both derivatives of interferon. The two commonly used are interferon beta-1a (Avonex) and interferon beta-1b (Betaseron). During an acute exacerbation, steroids are used to decrease inflammation and may be given orally (prednisone) or IV (methylprednisolone). The nitrogen mustard derivative cyclophosphamide (Cytoxan) and methotrexate are now also used (off label) to prevent acute inflammation. These oncology chemotherapy drugs have been shown to slow the rate of progression of MS in some people and are used when individuals do not respond to steroid use.

Symptomatically, treatment class is dependent on the symptom. The antispasm medications include baclofen, diazepam, and dantrolene. Options in the treatment of tremors include isoniazid, propranolol, and clonazepam. Bladder dysfunction may require oxybutynin and propantheline bromide. Bowel dysfunction may require bulk additives, stool softeners, and stimulants. Fatigue is treated with amantadine and pemoline, whereas mood alterations may require antidepressants, both SSRIs, and tricyclics.

## Assessment Needed Prior to Drug Therapy

Once the diagnosis of MS is confirmed by a neurologist, appropriate follow-up by the primary provider is helpful in understanding the patient's baseline of disease so that the new acute exacerbation can be adequately treated. A thorough neurologic examination is helpful to rate both baseline and function at exacerbation. Symptomatic treatment also will require regular visits to ascertain the effectiveness of drug treatment.

## Patient and Caregiver Information

The unpredictability of the disease and its cycle of remission and exacerbation (and in some individuals, progressive nature) make information necessary and helpful. Patients need both physical and emotional support with the disease and assessment of family systems is helpful to ascertain the need for outside support (Rudick, 1993). In addition, health care proxies and at some point placing financial affairs in order is necessary. A recommended support source is the local Multiple Sclerosis Society as well as the regional neurologic clinic treating individuals with multiple sclerosis. Symptomatic intervention will require specific teaching as the medications are utilized.

## OUTCOMES MANAGEMENT

This section focuses on the treatments to prevent the continued development of MS and those used in acute exacerbations, and briefly reviews the drugs used in symptomatic therapy.

## Drugs Used to Prevent Exacerbations

*Interferon beta-1b (Betaseron).*  The interferons are from a large protein family, the cytokines, which "interfere" with viral infection on tissue culture. The drugs have antiviral, antiproliferative, and immunomodulatory activities. Inter-

ferons are naturally occurring agents in humans, primarily manufactured by white blood cells. The drugs appear to inhibit exacerbations in the first 2 years of therapy but have less benefit in years 3–5, although the rate of change over placebo is significant. The drugs' efficacy is judged by the number of new plaques seen on MRI. However, plaque formation does not always correlate with clinical signs and symptoms (Kelly, 1996).

Betaseron was released by the FDA in July of 1993 for the treatment of relapsing MS. This immunomodulator is thought to act by augmenting suppressor cell function, increasing cytotoxicity of natural killer cells, and increasing macrophage activity. Interferon beta reduces the activity of interferon gamma, which decreases the inflammation produced in MS by its autoimmune response (Gidal et al, 1996).

The current dosage is 8 million units given subcutaneously every other day. Therapy is often begun at 4 million units and increased to 8 million after 1–2 weeks to diminish the initial side effects. The side effects are flu-like symptoms with fever, chills, and myalgias as well as injection site redness and swelling in almost all users. The drug can increase temperature, causing a loss of motor function in some MS patients, so it is better given at night. At times walking may be difficult, and patients may need temporary assistance in transfers and toileting due to adverse drug effects (Kelly, 1996). Nonsteroidal antiinflammatory agents taken before and 24 h after administration are helpful, as is applying ice to the local injection site. Other adverse effects include shortness of breath, tachycardia, and depression, which requires close monitoring for suicide risk. Blood work before therapy includes baseline hemoglobin, complete blood counts, platelets, and liver function tests (RMSC, 1995).

*Interferon beta-1a (Avonex).*  This drug was released for general use in 1994. It is given by IM injection once weekly at 4 million units (30 µg) and can be given by the patient or a family member. It has similar side effects with flu-like symptoms, muscle aches, fever, chill, and weakness, and use of nonsteroidal antiinflammatory agents before and for 24 h after the injection is suggested, as well as ice application to the injection site. The drug may cause abortion and is not recommended for women trying to become pregnant; birth control must be practiced. It requires the same baseline hemoglobin, complete blood counts, platelet, and liver function tests; these are repeated after 1, 2, and 3 months on drug and then every 3 months. Its adverse effects can include exacerbation of seizures and heart disease, so some individuals may not be candidates for this treatment. Depression may also increase, requiring frequent monitoring and examination for suicide risk. The drug needs refrigeration, but not freezing, at home once reconstituted (RMSC, 1993).

**Copolymer 1.** This drug is not yet FDA-approved. Copolymer 1 is a mixture of polypeptides from four amino acids, L-alanine, L-glutamic acid, L-lysine and L-tyrosine. It is thought to act by decreasing cell-mediated immune response against myelin basic protein. In relapsing-remitting MS, the drug showed a reduction in relapse rate over placebo in patients who are in early stages of the disease. The side effects include site reaction and systemic reactions of brief chest tightness and flushing (Gidal et al, 1996). It has few long-term side effects on initial testing. The drug is given daily at 20 mg subcutaneously (Johnson, 1996).

**Methotrexate.** This chemotherapeutic agent slows the rate of progression in MS in some patients. It is thought to work by suppressing the immune system so it does not attack myelin. Patients with worsening disease who are not responsive to steroids can be given this drug. The oral dose is 7.5 mg per week usually taken as three tablets of 2.5 mg each in the morning with food. In the first 6 months side effects can include nausea, loss of appetite, mouth sores, mood alteration, dizziness, fatigue, hair loss, easy bruising, diarrhea, headaches, rash, and photosensitivity. It also requires blood monitoring before treatment; at 1 month, 2 months, and 3 months; and thereafter for decreases in red and white cell production, as well as altered liver and kidney function. The drug also can produce immunosuppressant diseases such as pneumonias, fungal infections, and herpes zoster (shingles). It can produce birth defects during and 6 months following treatment so birth control should be practiced. Folic acid 1 mg per day may reduce some of the side effects. Using aspirin or its derivatives and drinking alcoholic beverages is contraindicated. Use of nonsteroidal antiinflammatories should be under the direction of a primary care provider. Patients are advised to report dry cough over 2 days, mouth sores, signs of infection, and unusual bleeding (RMSC, 1995).

**Cyclophosphamide (Cytoxan).** Cytoxan is another chemotherapeutic medication used in MS when the condition worsens and is unresponsive to steroid therapy. It is given IV in a clinic setting and dosing is based on height and weight. Usually the drug is given monthly for 6 months. The drug kills rapidly dividing cells (blood cells, hair cells, and mucous membrane cells). The side effects include nausea, vomiting, and loss of appetite at 6–8 h after the dose, diminishing over 1–2 days. Other side effects are hair loss, changes in taste, lowered blood cell counts with slow healing and increased bleeding times, bladder irritation, mouth sores, and facial tingling or burning during the injection. It also affects reproduction both during and for 4 months posttreatment, requiring the use of birth control. Patients and family need to call the provider if fever is greater than 100°F and the patient has burning on urination, frequent or foul-smelling urine, sore throat, cough, swelling or redness at the injection site, and worsening of MS symptoms (RMSC, 1996).

**Estrogen.** Although no double-blind studies have tested the effect of estrogen therapy in women with MS, it is postulated that estrogen may stabilize clinical manifestations of MS, particularly cognitive impairments. Serotonin function is felt to be a part of memory function, and estrogen modulates the effects of serotonins. Women who are menopausal and postmenopausal with MS are advised to seek estrogen replacement for the prevention of cognitive deterioration (Sandyk, 1996; Neurocommunications, 1996).

**Corticosteroids.** Steroid use appears to reduce the intensity and duration of an exacerbation but does not change the overall loss of function. There is no consensus on dose, administration route, or duration of steroid therapy in MS. One protocol calls for methylprednisolone 1 g IV given each day for 3–5 days followed by oral prednisone at 60 mg and tapered over the next 11–18 days in patients with a substantial increase in their disability due to an exacerbation (Anderson & Goodkin, 1996).

**Bee stinging.** There are centers using bee stinging and its antibody response to limit disease exacerbation as an alternative therapy. It appears to be therapeutic in some individuals for a period of months.

### Drugs Used in Symptomatic Treatment of MS

The primary care provider will spend the most time with MS patients in order to treat their symptoms and for counseling. Symptom management primarily centers around urinary tract infections, urinary incontinence, constipation, and spasticity. In a Dutch study family counseling focused on disease explanation, emotional support, and coping strategies (Donker, Foets, & Spreeuwenberg, 1996). MS is costly, with patients over 65 on alpha blockers, anticholinergics, cholinergics, tricyclic antidepressants, anticonvulsants, antifatigue agents, antispasticity agents, and antibiotics for UTI in one Nova Scotia study. The average drug costs were 65% greater for MS patients than in comparable age groups (Sketris, Brown, Murray, Fisk, & McLean, 1996).

The symptoms reviewed here include spasticity, fatigue, bowel and bladder dysfunction, tremors, and mood dysfunctions.

**Spasticity.**   Spasticity is an increase in resistance to movement. Range of motion exercises two to three times daily remain a mainstay of treatment. Spasticity can also be effective in allowing ambulation of a weakened extremity, and removal of the spasticity can impair gait. Excess spasm is debilitating and needs treatment. Treatment of spasticity is usually done on an ambulatory patient. The primary drug is oral baclofen given two to three times daily, increased by 5 mg every 3 days as tolerated. Many patients easily tolerate 60–80 mg per day. Telephone contact is helpful in establishing dosage parameters. The adverse effects increase with higher doses and include weakness, drowsiness, leg swelling, confusion, and sedation. Monitoring for liver function is necessary. The drug requires weaning since abrupt termination can lead to agitated behavior, paranoid ideation, and seizures. Supplemental doses of diazepam (Valium) 1–2 mg or clonidine 0.1–2 mg are often helpful and well tolerated.

Dantrolene sodium often is not effective in MS because it causes weakness and sedation, but it is used in nonambulatory patients (Marshall & Ragland, 1996). The dosage is 25 mg daily and is gradually increased to 100 mg four times daily. The adverse effects are diarrhea and toxic hepatitis.

Intrathecal baclofen administered through a subcutaneous pump has had good results in selected patients with intractable spasticity, allowing a fraction of the oral dose. This requires implantation of an abdominal pump, with tubing placed into the spinal canal. The cost, locating the proper surgeon to carry out the procedure, and ongoing maintenance limit its usefulness. Even after pump removal lasting reduction of severe spasticity has been documented, and

lower dosing is often achieved after months of therapy (Dressnandt & Conrad, 1996).

**Fatigue.**   Over three quarters of individuals with MS complain of excessive fatigue, which worsens during afternoon hours and with an increase in ambient temperature. It requires the patient to sit, lie down, and sleep. Training in energy conservation techniques is helpful. The drug of choice in excessive fatigue is amantadine hydrochloride in doses of 100 mg once or twice daily, and it is effective in about half the MS patient population. Pemoline 37.5 mg and fluoxetine hydrochloride 10–20 mg once or twice a day are also used. The adverse effects are anxiety and insomnia. Patients who respond do so within several days, and 1-week drug holidays every month are effective in diminishing drug tolerances.

**Tremor or ataxia.**   This is a most disabling symptom and one of the least responsive to treatment. The drug that seems to be effective is clonazepam 0.5 mg at bedtime and increasing slowly to 2 mg four times per day, given to an end-point of sedation or effective control of cerebellar tremor. Another recommended drug is primidone 125–250 mg daily in two to three doses. Oblative cerebellar surgery is done in some individuals with poor results (Rudick, 1993).

**Bowel dysfunction and bladder dysfunction.**   Over half of MS patients experience constipation, evacuation urgency, and incontinence. High fluid intake, bulk laxatives, and stool softeners with a regular evacuation time are helpful. In addition to the nonpharmacologic objectives outlined earlier, there are medications that can improve bladder function once a diagnosis is established. Detrusor spasticity will respond to anticholinergic agents, such as oxybutynin chloride at 2.5–5 mg two to three times daily or propantheline bromide at 15 mg orally three to four times each day. Dry mouth and constipation are common side effects. Bladder retention usually is best treated by intermittent catheterization but may also respond to terazosin hydrochloride 5 mg orally three to four times a day.

**Mood alterations.**   The most common disorder is depression, but bipolar affective disease and anxiety disorders also can occur more commonly in MS than the general population. The risk of suicide is higher in this population, requiring a routine review of suicide risk. One third of the MS population will experience a major depression requiring treatment, usually in younger patients with less overall disability. The patients respond better to a combined regime of pharmacotherapy and psychotherapy. Medical treatment for depression in this group is often prolonged, requiring treatment for 18 months before successful medication withdrawal.

The current first-line drug of choice for depression in MS is the SSRI agent fluoxetine, at 10–20 mg per day each morning, because the side effects are less. The traditional tricyclic agent used is amitriptyline 25 mg at bedtime and increased by 25 mg each week to 75–100 mg daily. Adverse effects of tricyclics include dry mouth, urinary retention, and drowsiness (Scott, Allen, Price, McConnell, Lang, 1996). The anticholinergic properties of amitriptyline is helpful in individuals with bladder spasm.

MS patients can present with manic-depression as the first sign of the disease. These individual do respond well to lithium (Scott, Allen, Price, McConnell, & Lang, 1996).

**Other symptoms in MS.** Chronic pain and acute pain in extremities is reported and tricyclic antidepressants are used. Lumbar pain is often related to mechanical stress on the spine, spasticity, and weakness and may benefit from NSAIDs. Degenerative disc disease can also occur mechanically from the weakened back structure. Trigeminal neuralgias also occur in MS and may respond to carbamazepine 100–200 mg two to three times each day (Anderson & Goodkin, 1996).

Labile behavior with a persistent euphoria is not unknown in MS. The euphoria is thought to be the result of structural brain damage and dementia as well. The display of emotion without subjective content can be disabling. Some patients respond well to antidepressants to treat this condition.

Psychosis can also occur, probably due to temporal lobe and frontal lobe plaque formation. Lack of insight and persecutory delusions may ensue, as well as visual hallucinations. Follow-up with a psychiatrist familiar with MS may be helpful in treatment (Rodgers & Bland, 1996).

### Follow-up Recommendations

In the office setting for individuals with stable disease, medical follow-up may be dependent on other disease states in the MS patient. For in-

dividuals with chronic remitting disease, 3-month follow-up visits may be necessary to keep abreast of symptom relief. Alternating visits with the consulting neurologist also may be helpful.

## VERTIGO

Vertigo and dizziness are symptoms that require diagnosis before treatment. Vertigo is defined as a "sensation of turning or spinning," either of the person or environment, and dizziness is a "sensation of light-headedness, giddiness, or uneasiness in the head." The two are often difficult to separate and are often treated as one entity. The associated signs and symptoms also help in determining the diagnosis. These include cranial nerve symptoms and signs, fluctuating hearing loss, ringing in the ears, facial paralysis, headache, recent head trauma, circulatory system impairment, and medication use (Baloh, 1994).

Less than half of the patients who complain of dizziness actually have diseases of the vestibular system (Baloh, 1994). Generally there are five etiologies of dizziness (see Table 29–7). The

### TABLE 29–7.  ETIOLOGIES OF VERTIGO

- Cardiovascular and respiratory
    Cardiac arrhythmias
    Hypotension
    Hypertension
    Congestive heart failure
    Pneumonia
    Asthma
- Eighth cranial nerve deficits
    Viral infections
    Ototoxicity from medications (eg, aminoglycosides)
- Central nervous system disease with CNS changes
    Cerebellar ataxia
    Vertebrobasilar artery insufficiency
    Medications affecting the CNS (tranquilizers, anticonvulsants, antihypertensives
- Psychological
    Anxiety
    Phobias
    Panic
- Dizziness without other focal or general signs
    Otitis
    Benign paroxysmal positional vertigo
    Meniere's disease

first is a systemic cardiovascular or respiratory etiology. Cardiac arrhythmias, hypotension, hypertension, congestive heart failure, anemia, pneumonia, and asthma can all present as dizziness, with or without other accompanying symptoms. The dizziness can be constant and is not necessarily related to movement. It is most frequently seen in older adults.

The second etiology is peripheral nervous system disease associated with eighth cranial nerve deficits, which can present with associated nausea, tinnitus, and deafness, but no central nervous system signs. One cause is viral infection, with symptoms clearing as the virus runs its course. Another cause is ototoxicity brought on by medication use, particularly with aminoglycoside antibiotics.

A third etiology is central nervous system disease accompanied by cerebellar ataxia and other cranial nerve abnormalities such as diplopia, dysarthria, and nystagmus. If other nervous system deficits accompany the vertigo, the clinician is not just dealing with simple vertigo but a more complex problem. The presence of marked nystagmus with little vertigo is often a symptom of central disease. The CNS disturbance also can be of vascular origin with vertebrobasilar artery insufficiency. This type of dizziness can last minutes to hours and be positional and directly related to vasodilator use and arterial occlusive disease. It can also be a symptom of migraine headache.

Medications that act on the central nervous system can be the general cause of dizziness due to depression of the CNS and cerebellar dysfunction from tranquilizers, anticonvulsants, and alcohol use. Antihypertensives can elicit postural hypotension and subsequent dizziness if the blood pressure is too low to maintain adequate blood supply to the posterior cerebellar and cerebral blood vessels.

A fourth etiology is of psychological origin. Vertigo presents as a symptom of anxiety, phobias, or panic syndrome. In this condition, the dizziness is not episodic, but a constant condition with no remission during waking hours. Body movement can improve the dizziness, which is usually the opposite of vestibular dizziness, and the vertigo may appear only in certain situations such as a crowded room.

The fifth etiology is the presentation of vertigo with no other neurologic signs and symptoms caused by the circulatory system, neurologic system, or drugs. There are commonly three causes. The first is otitis, resulting in swelling that disturbs normal endolymph flow. Even impacted wax can cause dizziness if the surrounding tissue begins to swell. Removal of the wax and treating the otitis, if present, may be all that is necessary to treat the vertigo.

The second is benign paroxysmal positional vertigo (BPPV), which is diagnosed by the presence of peripheral nystagmus after taking a new head position, accompanied by severe vertigo and nausea with symptoms quickly fading, usually in seconds to minutes once the head is in a new position. BPPV is not accompanied by hearing loss, and caloric testing is normal. In many cases, BPPV is thought to be the result of clogging in the labyrinth processes, resulting in the inability of endolymph tissue to move freely. BPPV can also accompany head trauma.

Thirdly, if the vertigo is accompanied by tinnitus (ringing in the ears), fluctuating hearing loss, and aural fullness, the condition is Meniere's disease. In Meniere's disease, the dizziness is episodic and described as a whirling or spinning sensation. Physiologically there is swelling of the endolymph of the middle ear. It commonly occurs in 30- to 60-year-olds, and over many years can cause residual tinnitus, initially low-frequency sensorineural hearing loss, and eventual deafness. It too can accompany head trauma (Knox & McPherson, 1997).

The duration of the vertigo is a clue to its etiology with BPPV lasting only seconds, vertebrobasilar insufficiency and migraine vertigo lasting minutes to hours, Meniere's disease vertigo lasting hours, and dizziness of days duration due to viral neurolabyrinthitis, vascular occlusion, and trauma.

The pharmacotherapy and other treatments discussed below are only specific to BPPV and Meniere's disease. Like other diseases in this section, referral to a neurologist or otolaryngologist may be necessary, with concurrent treatment.

## SPECIFIC CONSIDERATIONS FOR PHARMACOTHERAPY

### When Drug Therapy Is Needed

The treatment of vertigo is aimed at symptom alleviation, and cure in some cases. There are as yet no drugs known to absolutely cure vertigo without the possibility of serious side effects, the most common being permanent hearing loss.

## Short- and Long-Term Goals of Pharmacotherapy

The aim is symptom relief in short-term treatment of vertigo. Direct injection of medications into the inner ear is aimed at cure in the case of Meniere's disease.

## Nonpharmacologic Therapy

Vestibular training with symptomatic medication use is more effective than drug use alone in BPPV (Fujino et al, 1996). Nonpharmacologic therapy is directed to two goals. The first is aimed at removing any clogs within the endolymph, and the second is to carry out vestibular retraining, desensitizing the individual to movement that causes the dizziness. In some cases of BPPV, otolithic debris is thought to be attached to the posterior canal, plugging the canal. Dislodging the plug through a repositioning maneuver can cure BPPV often in just one to three treatments, so that the clot falls into the utricular vestibule (Gans, 1996).

The treatments can be given by a neurologist, an ENT specialist, or a physical therapist trained in the maneuvers, variously called the Semont maneuver or the Epley maneuver. In these maneuvers, the patient is initially sitting. The head is turned to one side and then the patient assumes a lying position, the head remaining to the side and upward. The patient then resumes the upright position and the maneuver is repeated with the head and body to the opposite side. The maneuver is repeated until the vertigo subsides, which may require treatment over several days (Grizzi, 1995).

In habitual training, the etiology of the vertigo may not be a clog in the endolymph canal. The goal is habituation treatment through excessive stimulation of the labyrinth canal and the use of balance retraining. Several studies show that physical therapy is more efficacious than the use of medications (Grizzi, 1995), showing a 63–70% improvement rating with therapy and only a 37% improvement with medications. Nonmedicinal treatment works even in vertigo of many years duration. Vestibular training shows better results in individuals with unilateral vestibular disease.

Avoidance of some drug classes is also effective for a minority of persons with vertigo. Caffeine, alcohol, and nicotine should be avoided, as well as a diet high in sodium. The initial treatment for Meniere's disease is a low-salt diet of 1–2g of sodium per day, with or without the addition of a diuretic (Knox & MacPherson, 1997). In cases of severe Meniere's disease, surgical obliteration of the endolymph canals is a traditional treatment that results in permanent deafness. This corresponds to direct injection of aminoglycosides via the tympanic membrane into the ear, a newer ablative treatment for Meniere's disease.

## Time Frame for Initiating Pharmacotherapy

In terms of immediate symptomatic relief, the treatment should begin immediately. As a last resort, in unremitting vertigo, it may be necessary to destroy the endolymph canals through injection of neurotoxins.

## Overview of Drug Classes for Treatment

The drug classes used in vertigo include steroids as antiinflammatories, diuretics to reduce the amount of fluid within the inner ear, antiemetics for nausea, antidepressants for symptomatic relief, vestibular suppressants (including the calcium channel blockers nimodipine and Antivert), and aminoglycosides to destroy the endolymph in severe cases of vertigo.

## Assessment Needed Prior to Therapy

The initial workup begins with a brief general examination, including careful attention to the cardiovascular, lung, and abdominal systems, noting tachycardia, arrhythmias, shortness of breath, and abdominal swelling and bruits. The examination includes the head, with attention to the ear canal and hearing, as well as eliciting specifics on subjective ringing of the ear. In addition to the cranial nerves, the examination needs to include cerebellar function and the presence of nystagmus. Checking for vertical and horizontal nystagmus, assessing the fatigue and latency of response in eye movements, and checking for positional nystagmus by having the patient go quickly from sitting to supine and turning the head, noting the presence of nystagmus, fatigue, and accompanying vertigo, should be done routinely. A modified caloric test may be helpful in establishing the differentiation of central and peripheral nystagmus, but it is not necessary to establish the diagnosis.

In some instances, sudden or fluctuating hearing loss, vertigo, and ringing in the ears can be a presentation of otosyphilis and/or AIDS; testing for both diseases and a screening CBC may be warranted (Linstrom & Gleich, 1993). Another cause of vertigo can be vertebral artery insufficiency, which may warrant further ultrasound testing if the condition is suspected.

## Patient/Caregiver Information

Once a diagnosis is established, thorough education about the various treatments is helpful, including vestibular and balance retraining through a physician specialist or physical therapist. Information on the action and side effects of medications for symptomatic relief is necessary. The patients and caregivers should understand that some cases of vertigo can improve over time, but in Meniere's disease the condition is chronic and may require ongoing treatment.

## OUTCOMES MANAGEMENT

### Selecting an Appropriate Agent

Pharmaceutical use in BPPV and Meniere's disease does not have high efficacy, with less than half of the patient population obtaining relief from medication. For both Meniere's disease and BPPV, using nonpharmaceutical therapeutics along with attempting symptom relief with medications can improve outcome. Traditionally, the first-line drug group is the vertigo suppressants with newer treatments including direct injection of steroids into the middle ear to reduce the inflammation. Steroid use does not cause the hearing loss that accompanies the use of the aminoglycosides.

The traditional first-line drug is meclizine hydrochloride (Antivert), classified as an antiemetic and used to treat the nausea accompanying vertigo. It is an antihistamine, suppressing labyrinth excitability and acting centrally to depress vestibulo-cerebellar pathways. It is long-acting, having a half-life of 6 h and single-dose effect of 8–24 h. It will depress the CNS, with resulting drowsiness among other side effects. For the control of vertigo, the usual dose is 25–100 mg per day in divided doses (ASHSP, 1996).

The calcium channel blocker nimodipine was successful in 50% of patients within a small sample in relieving vertigo in Meniere's disease. Calcium channel blockers are a common form of treatment in Europe and may act as vestibular suppressants because vestibular hair cells are rich in calcium channels. The drug may also act because of its general sedating properties (Rascol et al, 1995).

The neuroleptics (Haldol, Thorazine) act by blocking dopaminergic receptors in the brainstem, reducing the neurovegetative symptoms paralleling vertigo. They act in 4–12 h given as oral agents or suppositories (Rascol et al, 1995).

Another drug group commonly used (with little proven efficacy) is the benzodiazepines, which produce sedation, hypnosis, decreased anxiety, muscle relaxation, and amnesia but are not known to actually reduce vertigo. Their use is not recommended for true vertigo, but they may have a place in psychological etiologies of vertigo.

Other oral medications used in Meniere's disease include diuretics (Lasix, Diuril) to reduce the inner ear endolymph swelling and antidepressants to inhibit CNS response to the sensation of dizziness.

Otolaryngologists also use direct injection of medications through the tympanic membrane into the inner ear to control unremitting vertigo. Some physicians, viewing Meniere's disease as an immune-mediated disease, advocate initial treatment with steroids to decrease endolymph swelling; this does not cause any hearing loss. Dexamethasone is injected directly into the inner ear through the round window and accompanied by IV injection of dexamethasone. The drug decreases and restores normal fluid balance (Shea & Gee, 1996).

Initially, direct injection of streptomycin was used, which did cure the vertigo but also left the patient with complete hearing loss to the treated ear. More recently, intratympanic gentamicin instillation in small doses is used and modifications to the amount of drug strength and injection techniques have allowed better control for hearing loss and stabilization of the vertigo, with one third of the patients experiencing hearing loss as a result of the injections (Driscoll, Kasperbauer, Facer, Harner, & Beatty, 1997; Hirsch and Kamerer, 1997). There are other reported cases of gentamicin treatment in peripheral vestibular disorder other than Meniere's disease (Brantberg, Bergenius, & Tribukait, 1996). For many individuals hearing loss is a small price to pay for return of function and relief from the disability of severe vertigo.

### Monitoring for Efficacy

Although effective in some cases, the long-term use of meclizine with concurrent CNS depression must be kept in mind when attempting use of heavy machinery or driving, so the drug itself can cause a significant change in daily function. Meclizine use in children has not been studied.

## Monitoring for Toxicity

Additive CNS depression can occur with meclizine when used with alcohol, barbiturates, or tranquilizers. The anticholinergic effects of the drug can cause increased symptoms of angle-closure glaucoma and prostatic hypertrophy. Like other antihistamines it can cause systemic dermatitis, CNS depression, changes in cardiac function, and interaction with other depressants.

Although now off the market, scopolamine was used in the treatment of vertigo. There are cases of reported addiction to scopolamine in the literature, and the drug manufacturers warn of easy addiction (Luetje & Wooten, 1996). Extended use over weeks to months may lead to withdrawal symptoms of nausea, vomiting, headache, and dizziness, requiring treatment to allow for drug withdrawal. Primary addictive signs are the nausea, vomiting, and headache rather than the occurrence of dizziness. Some patients require hospitalization for symptom control for 72 h while the drug is cleared from their systems. The other adverse effects of scopolamine include dry mouth, drowsiness, blurred vision, dry eyes, dizziness, disorientation, restlessness, giddiness, hallucinations, and confusion. Skin rashes and contact dermatitis can also occur.

## Follow-up Recommendations

The important treatment breakthrough for vertigo is the positional maneuvers that can cure benign positional vertigo. Finding a clinician who understands the condition and is skilled in the maneuvers can lead to cure. The association of BPPV and Meniere's disease requires follow-up on all patients with vertigo. In both conditions, vestibular rehabilitation can help the brain reorganize its visual, vestibular, and proprioceptive signals to allow full function once again. Newer dosing of intratympanic steroids or gentamicin at lower doses can give relief without further hearing loss in many patients with intractable vertigo and Meniere's disease.

## DEMENTIA

Although commonly associated with a loss of memory, the term *dementia* refers to a loss in cognitive functioning and in thinking abilities that include memory, planning, perception of relationships, problem solving, abstraction, and recognition of consequences and safety. In the late stages of the disease, it can interfere with attention and consciousness. This disorder of memory, cognition, and personality gradually interferes with ability to perform in social or occupational situations. At any given time, well over 4 million Americans have some form of dementia that limits their capacity to live independently, creating an immense financial, social, and emotional burden on families and society in general (Kawas & Morrison, 1997). In most early to middle stages of dementia, the individual is alert and has the physical capacity to be independent but may be unable to process information and plan and carry out safe actions (Costa et al, 1996).

Most forms of dementia are progressive, creating a subtle, slow decline in function that does not become apparent until a specific event draws attention to the cognitive dysfunction. The diagnosis of dementia is made by history, patterns of cognitive losses, neurologic and physical examination, and laboratory and radiologic testing. It is important to exclude treatable secondary causes.

Changes characteristic of dementia in general are changes in cognition, function, and behavior. The hallmark of many dementias is memory disorder, particularly immediate recall and declarative memory (ie, who is the president of the United States?). Word-finding difficulties are also a common cognitive complaint, as is sentence syntax in later stages. Losses in recognizing visual spatial relationships can also accompany dementias. These losses result in functional impairment in dealing with the basic activities of daily living and instrumental activities of daily living (banking, using the telephone, taking medications, meal planning, and shopping). Although personality symptoms are a late sign in Alzheimer's disease, other dementias can cause early personality changes, mood disturbances, delusions, hallucinations, and psychosis. The earliest symptom can be depression. The most difficult behavioral change is the occurrence of verbal and physical aggression, which can be progressive and pose serious stress on caregivers (Costa et al, 1996).

Dementia can be of primary or secondary origin. Examples of primary degenerative dementias are the dementias of Alzheimer's disease (AD), Parkinson's disease, Pick's disease, and

Huntington's disease. Other irreversible causes of dementia include the vascular dementias, traumatic dementias, and cerebral infections. Until recently, there was little but symptomatic treatment available for the primary dementias. Reversible or secondary dementias can be of iatrogenic, vascular, infectious, metabolic, neurophysiologic, or psychological origin. They include such conditions as neurosyphilis, vitamin $B_{12}$ deficiency, hypothyroidism, chronic drug ingestion, chronic subdural hematomas, brain tumors, and depression. The most common iatrogenic causes are medications, and the drug classes known to cause dementia are listed in Table 29–8. The secondary dementias are often improved or completely resolved by treating the underlying cause(s) (APA, 1997).

As with other neurologic conditions, determining the cause of the loss in cognitive functioning is the key to therapeutic interventions. In addition, it is not uncommon for an individual to have more than one cause of dementia; for example, multi-infarct dementia can occur along with Alzheimer's disease (Hollister & Gruber, 1996).

The diagnosis of Alzheimer's disease requires a progressive loss in memory (either new recall or recalling previously learned functions), loss in one or more cognitive areas (aphasia, apraxia, agnosia, and decline in executive thinking), no disturbance in consciousness, onset between ages 40–90 (most often after age 65), and absence of any systemic disorder or brain disease accounting for other causes of the dementia (Costa et al, 1996; Woo & Lantz, 1995). The pathology in Alzheimer's disease is the formation of neurofibrillary tangles and dendritic plaques in the cerebral cortex and hippocampal formation with a resultant loss in choline acetyltransferase in those areas (Woo & Lantz, 1995). AD affects more women than men at a rate greater than the longer life span of women.

## SPECIFIC CONSIDERATIONS FOR PHARMACOTHERAPY

### When Drug Therapy Is Needed

In all dementias, both primary and secondary, there is a need for appropriate symptomatic relief. In the reversible or secondary dementias, the drug therapy is often directed at alleviating the primary problem and consequently the changes in cognitive functioning. In the primary, irreversible dementias there are now drugs that can slow down the disease progression in select individuals and may stabilize functional losses, allowing the individual to maintain a higher level of cognitive functioning for a longer duration of time.

### Short- and Long-Term Goals of Pharmacotherapy

The drug therapy in primary dementias, particularly in Alzheimer's disease, is aimed at slowing the cognitive impairments present in individuals with mild to moderate AD. The second treatment aim in all the dementias is relief of symptoms.

### Nonpharmacologic Therapy

Frequent office follow-up at 3- to 4-month intervals is helpful in reviewing the functional and behavioral limitations seen with progressive dementias for the patient as well as the primary caregivers. Because many individuals with dementia have a progressive form and their problems change over time, frequent follow-up is helpful to treat symptoms and behaviors. This alone may encourage enough problem solving so individuals with progressive dementias can be maintained in a home setting for appropriate lengths of time.

Nonpharmacologic symptom relief can incorporate a multitude of interventions. There is evidence that continuous reassessment of patient problems in dementia renders better quality of life and improved patient survival (Applegate & Burns, 1996). Specific interventions include

## TABLE 29–8. DRUG CLASSES KNOWN TO CAUSE DEMENTIA

| | |
|---|---|
| Antiarrhythmic agents | Antipsychotic (neuroleptic) agents |
| Antibiotics | |
| Anticholinergic agents | Corticosteroids |
| Anticonvulsants | Decongestants |
| Antidepressants | $H_2$ receptor agonists |
| Antiemetics | Hypnotics |
| Antifungal agents | Nonsteroidal anti-inflammatory drugs |
| Antihistamines | |
| Antihypertensive agents | Narcotic analgesics |
| Antimanic agents | Radiocontrast media |
| Antineoplastic agents | Sedative/hypnotic agents |
| Antiparkinsonian agents | Skeletal muscle relaxants |

elder day care for socialization, exercise, stimulation, medical follow-up and physical therapy and to meet nutritional needs. Having a stable routine and environment with limited distractions and consistent behaviors is often a key to consistent behavior in the early to middle stages of dementia.

Specific problem behaviors can be eliminated through good planning. For example, limiting fluids after 7 P.M. may eliminate evening incontinence, and daily walking and limiting daytime napping may be helpful in eliminating nocturnal behaviors. Ensuring respite care via specific health care workers and other family members may eliminate stress for the primary caregiver. Reexploring all local options in terms of day care, assisted care, and nursing home care should be attempted at periodic intervals. Lastly, health care proxies and living wills need addressing while individuals can still participate in these decisions.

## Time Frame for Initiating Pharmacotherapy

The time frame for initiating symptom relief in dementias is symptom-dependent. However, individuals with severe vegetative signs of primary dementia do not respond well to drug therapy nor do individuals who show minimal impairments, such as in higher-order abstract reasoning, calculation deficits, and immediate recall.

Outcome measures for any therapy directed at cognitive stability, functional impairment, or behavioral instability should include retesting cognitive function by using the Mini-Mental Status Scale, a functional impairment measure such as the Functional Independence Measure, and behavioral assessments, as well as caregiver burden. Caregiver burden is often the factor leading to nursing home placement, not only the losses in cognition, function, and behavior.

Specific cholinesterase inhibitor therapy usually is initiated when an individual is diagnosed with mild to moderate Alzheimer's disease, usually defined as a score of 10–24 on the Mini-Mental Status Examination or a similar scale. This drug group is not effective in individuals with very mild or very severe Alzheimer's disease.

## Overview of Drug Classes for Treatment

The drug classes used to treat the primary dementias include neurotransmitter inhibitors and estrogen to women as primary therapy in AD as well as antidepressants, anxiolytics, nonsteroidal antiinflammatory drugs, antipsychotics, and sedatives for symptom relief in all the dementias.

## Assessment Needed Prior to Therapy

Individuals who present with memory changes, difficulty with abstract thinking, disorientation, and confusion require a full and careful history as well as laboratory and physical assessment before determining a diagnosis. The classic symptoms of dementia are new difficulties with learning and retaining new information, handling complex tasks, reasoning ability, spatial ability and orientation, and language and behavior (Costa et al, 1996). In the preliminary assessment, ascertaining the temporality of behavioral and cognitive changes from both the patient and significant others is very helpful. Specific questions regarding falls and recent trauma, changes in the home environment, and information related to new and/or changes in medication need asking to rule out head trauma, medication toxicity, or psychological stressors as the cause of behavioral change. Alzheimer's disease presents with an insidious onset, gradual progression, and absence of focal findings, and it remains primarily a diagnosis of exclusion.

For a thorough and complete assessment of dementias and Alzheimer's disease see the AHCPR Guideline Number 19 on *Recognition and Initial Assessment of Alzheimer's Disease and Related Dementias* (Costa et al, 1996) or the *Alzheimer's Disease Assessment Scale* (Mohs, 1996). A physical examination of all systems is necessary as well as a valid mental status examination, such as the Mini-Mental Status Examination or other valid and reliable dementia screens, such as the Alzheimer's Disease Assessment Scale (Hollister & Gruber, 1996). Repeating the screening test over time is helpful in quantifying the effects of both pharmacologic and nonpharmacologic treatment. A full neuropsychologic evaluation can help characterize the type of dementia and help rule out depression as part of the etiology. A short group of four neuropsychologic tests have proven reliable in determining the diagnosis of Alzheimer's disease. In addition to the Mini-Mental Status Examination, they are the Blessed Information-Memory Concentration Test, the Blessed Orientation-Memory-Concentration Test, and the Short Test of Mental Status. All are available in AHCPR Guideline 19 (Costa et al, 1996).

The two common differential diagnoses to consider in assessing for dementia are delirium and depression. Acute delirium can indicate the development of an acute medical condition. It is marked by disturbances in consciousness, behavioral changes over hours to days (but not months), evidence of physical signs on focused examination, and alteration in cognition, which it shares with dementia. Although depression can coexist with dementia, it can also lead in itself to significant cognitive changes. In depression the individual gives a feeling of being down or irritated at all times with a decreased interest in most activities. There is significant weight gain or loss, with daily insomnia or hypersomnia. There is not a good external reason for the depression (ie, loss of spouse).

If radiology examination is necessary for the diagnosis, it is usually a brain CT or MRI. The brain MRI or CT can determine white matter changes, presence of infarction or neoplasm, or hydrocephalus and determine demyelinating diseases. The location of brain atrophy can also give clues to etiology. The blood tests for persons presenting with possible dementia include CBC, serum $B_{12}$ level, TSH, HIV, and VDRL serologies. If indicated, it may be necessary to obtain CSF testing to rule out meningitis or encephalitis. Even if a secondary cause of dementia is found, further assessment following treatment may be necessary to rule out a concomitant dementia.

The second most common cause of dementia after Alzheimer's disease is multiinfarct dementia. In this group the cognitive losses may be more focal. In order to prevent further disease, especially if large cerebral arterial vessels are involved, anticoagulation treatment may be started or carotid endarectomy addressed. Another possible reversible cause of dementia is normal pressure hydrocephalus with the cognitive changes accompanied by incontinence and balance and gait changes. If the patient responds well to withdrawal of 50 cc of CSF, with improvement in gait 1 and 24 h after the lumbar puncture, the patient may respond well to ventricular shunting to allow normal flow of CSF within the brain (Chan & Hachinski, 1997). An electroencephalogram may be indicated if seizures are considered.

Another helpful guideline to consider in cases of dementia with an uncertain diagnosis is the use of neuropsychologic testing. It can serve several purposes: to give information to patients and their families on the specifics of cognitive deficits, assist in diagnosis, contribute to treatment recommendations, and provide a baseline measure for treatment and disease progression (Costa et al, 1996).

## Patient/Caregiver Information

Once a diagnosis is established, there are several resources available for families, including the local Council on Aging, the local Alzheimer's Disease Foundation, and the local Parkinson's Disease Foundation. A classic reference for families is *The 35-Hour Day* (Mace, 1981). The Alzheimer's Association also publishes pamphlets on newer drugs (Alzheimer's Association, 1996).

## OUTCOMES MANAGEMENT

The pharmacologic treatments listed in this section are limited to the newer medications used to treat Alzheimer's disease and those for symptom treatment in all dementias.

### Selecting an Appropriate Agent

Recently, drug agents have been developed to compensate for cerebral damage through the use of cholinesterase inhibitors to preserve the decreasing amount of acetylcholine found in the brains of individuals with Alzheimer's disease (Gidal et al, 1996). Higher concentrations of acetylcholine may increase communication between nerve cells and temporarily improve the symptoms of the disease (Alzheimer's Association, 1996). More recently, it is postulated that cholinesterase inhibitors may be neuroprotective, slowing down or preventing formation of amyloid fragments (Schneider, 1996).

The first cholinesterase inhibitor approved in Alzheimer's disease treatment is tacrine (Cognex), which showed a dramatic improvement in 5–10% of the patients who took it and a 30–40% modest improvement in cognitive function for the remainder of the test groups (Knopman et al, 1996). The improvements are in memory, social interaction, and attention. Tacrine is titrated up to a maximum of 160 mg per day, or until toxicity. The drug is started at 40 mg per day (10 mg q.i.d.) and titrated upward after 6 weeks, adding 40 mg per day in q.i.d. doses every 6 weeks. Most patients can only tolerate 80–120 mg per day because of side effects (Woo & Lantz, 1995).

The major side effect is liver transaminase elevation, requiring blood testing every 1–2 weeks for 4–6 months after starting the drug. Up to 28% of the experimental subjects developed liver transaminase elevations at three times normal. The manufacturer recommends stopping the drug if the liver transaminase levels rise to

10 times normal. Other side effects leading to drug withdrawal are nausea, vomiting, and diarrhea, occurring in over 50% of patients at the drug's higher dosing. Side effects of the medication can abate after 10 weeks of use, and are most common in the third to sixth week of treatment. If the patient has no discernible benefit from treatment, the medication is usually stopped (Woo & Lantz, 1995).

A second cholinesterase inhibitor, Aricept (donepezil hydrochloride), was FDA-approved in January 1997. This group is thought to be more stable, longer-acting, and provide higher concentrations of cholinergic transmitters in the central nervous system. This drug does not at present raise liver enzyme levels according to the manufacturer's description. It is given to individuals with mild to moderate Alzheimer's disease initially at 5 mg per day, advancing to 10 mg per day in A.M. doses when it is determined the individual will have few side effects from the 5-mg dose. The side effects of diarrhea, nausea, vomiting, insomnia, fatigue, and anorexia are usually mild, lasting 1–3 weeks and declining with continuing drug use. No stated interactions with other drugs are currently listed. Other drugs under consideration in this class include ENA 713 and metrifonate.

Estrogen therapy is postulated to act as a neurotransmitter modifier by enhancing the action of cholinesterase transmission and through improved blood flow to the brain, which inhibits arteriosclerotic plaque buildup (Birge, 1996). One recently published trial showed greater improvement in women with Alzheimer's disease who received tacrine and estrogen together over groups receiving just tacrine or placebo (Schneider, Farlow, Henderson, & Pogoda, 1996). The effect of receiving estrogen before, during, or just after menopause in the prevention or delay of Alzheimer's disease is not yet established.

The other area of drug treatment in the dementias is symptomatic treatment for agitation, psychosis, and depression. In all symptomatic treatment, the smallest dose that alleviates the symptom should be used with frequent monitoring and periodic drug withdrawal to ascertain that the drug is actually effective in symptomatic relief.

Individuals with advanced dementias, particularly with AD, may show signs of frank psychosis. The symptoms may include delusional episodes, agitation, hallucinations, hostility, and hyperactivity along with diminished independence in ADLs and loss of language skills. Using neuroleptics for symptom control is often attempted. However, if the patient is in a nursing home setting and subject to OBRA guidelines, a diagnosis of psychosis must be made prior to treatment. At this time there are no controlled studies on the efficacy of neuroleptics in the treatment of dementias. Many of the drugs may alleviate the symptoms but can lead to further cognitive decline, increased sedation, tardive dyskinesias, and parkinsonian symptoms. In a review of several studies, Trazodone at 150 mg per day carried the least side effects (Sunderland, 1996). One drug frequently used is haloperidol at 1–2 mg per day, and it can cause imbalance with rigidity with falls. For some, substituting clozapine is effective in reducing psychotic symptoms, but the mental status of the patient was not as sharp. The reduction in psychotic symptoms may allow a patient to stay longer in the home setting (Clipp & Moore, 1995).

Another common symptom in dementias is depression, occurring in 20% of AD patients. Traditionally, the tricyclic antidepressants are used, such as nortriptyline (Pamelor) at 10–30 mg or more per day, as well as desipramine (25–75 mg per day) and trazodone at 75–200 mg per day. More recently, better relief has been found with the selective serotonin reuptake inhibitors, such as sertraline (Zoloft) at 50 mg (up to 200) per day, paroxetine (Paxil) at 20 mg (up to 50) per day, and fluoxetine (Prozac) at 20 mg per day, which tend to produce fewer side effects, particularly sedation (Chan & Hachinski, 1997).

The agitation in dementia can actually be depression and more responsive to antidepressants than traditional medications prescribed for agitation. The medications used in agitation, particularly in Alzheimer's disease, are thioridazine (Mellaril) at 10–20 mg per day (up to 80 mg) and haloperidol (Haldol) at 0.25–0.50 mg once or twice daily up to 3–5 mg per day. Haldol in particular can cause associated movement disorders and further cognitive losses; it requires careful use and frequent trials off the medication. Active delusions also may respond to Haldol and Mellaril (Chan & Hachinski, 1997).

Another common symptom in dementia is anxiety. The medication treatment includes lorazepam (Ativan) 0.5–1.0 mg per day, alprazolam (Xanax) at 0.25–0.5 mg up to b.i.d. and oxazepam (Serax) 10 mg up to b.i.d. (Chan & Hachinski, 1997).

Insomnia can become the caregiver's burden. Preventing reversal of the sleep-wake cycle is important, and daily exercise is often helpful. Treatment can include warm milk at bedtime, trazodone 50–20 mg, diphenhydramine 25–50 mg, temazepam (Restoril) 7.5–15 mg, and chloral hydrate 500 mg all given at bedtime or 1–2 h before bedtime (Chan & Hachinski, 1997). Temazepam may induce daytime sedation due to its long half-life.

Another treatment under review is the use of agents to prevent or inhibit neuronal degeneration (Thal et al, 1996). Experimental treatments include giving neuronal growth factors (cholinergic neurotropin). There are several other experimental agents under study, including antioxidants, monoamine oxidase-B inhibitors, antiinflammatory agents, and estrogen. The support for the use of nonsteroidal antiinflammatory agents and estrogen is primarily through survey research. Many of the newer drugs used in dementias are without large-scale double-blind placebo trials, making their use more empirical than scientific at present (Wilcock & Harrold, 1996). Lastly, it is postulated that genetic gene transfer may eliminate some forms of Alzheimer's disease.

## Monitoring for Efficacy

Given the lack of reliable testing and the use of symptomatic treatment, a brief cognitive test like the Mini-Mental Status Examination (Smucker, 1996), levels of independence in ADLs, specific symptom relief, and caregiver burden are good vehicles for assessing drug efficacy.

## Monitoring for Toxicity

Tacrine and concurrent use of cimetidine is not recommended because cimetidine raises the level of tacrine and increases the side effects. If the patient has asthma and uses theophylline, this drug will also increase tacrine blood levels and side effects. Tacrine is contraindicated in individuals with a history of sensitivity to cholinesterase drugs, history of elevated liver function tests and liver disease, history of strokes, hydrocephalus, subdural hematomas, and central nervous system tumors. Using tacrine in patients with Parkinson's disease may increase movement disorders, but it is used in some patients already on a levodopa-carbidopa regime, which may relieve the movement disorder (Woo & Lantz, 1995).

## Follow-up Recommendations

In very stable patients with dementia, follow-up is recommended twice per year. In patients under symptomatic treatment, follow-up every 4–8 weeks may be necessary. Patients receiving tacrine or Aricept may need follow-up biweekly with blood monitoring weekly or biweekly. Dementia is a dynamic, progressive disease and keeping abreast of new problems, eliminating drug therapy when symptoms subside, and providing support for the caregivers enhances the quality of life of the patient and the caregivers.

# HEADACHE

Head pain is a symptom and in some persons also a chronic condition. Headaches are common, with over 90% of men and 95% of women reporting at least one headache annually. Headaches are episodic and can be classified by the type of pain (ie, tension-type or migraine) or by pattern of occurrence (ie, chronic daily headache or cluster headaches) with overlap noted between all groups (Goadsby, 1997). Additionally, some individuals may suffer from more than one type of headache. The amount of physical dysfunction in activities of daily living produced by a headache is also a classification parameter. In this country serious headaches have a huge economic and social impact due to lost work, lost income, difficulty with daily living activities, and social dysfunction. Although most individuals do not seek health care for their headaches, it is one of the most common presenting symptoms in primary care (de Lissovoy & Lazarus, 1994).

Diagnosis of headache is difficult due to its episodic nature, with occurrence and remission and the need to rely on the patient's description. Careful history and assessment are necessary in order to rule out serious underlying disease. A classification of headaches is contained in Table 27–9. Migraine headaches with or without aura once were thought to be at one end of a continuum with tension-type headaches being at the other end. More recently, rather than the description of the headache leading to a diagnosis of migraine, the severity and frequency of headache may determine its classification as migraine. Cluster headaches are sometimes classified as a migraine variant. Chronic daily headaches can be of migraine or tension-type origin and are particularly common in analgesia over-

## TABLE 29–9. DIAGNOSTIC CRITERIA OF HEADACHES

- Chronic daily headache
  1. Lasts 4–15 h per day, occurs daily or near daily (over 15 days per month), occurs over 180 days per year
  2. Transformed migraine (with or without analgesic overuse)
  3. Transformed tension-type headache (with or without analgesic overuse)
  4. New persistent daily headache
  5. Cervicogenic headache
     Idiopathic
     After neck trauma
  6. Post-head-trauma headache
     With migrainous features
     Without migrainous features
- Migraine headache
  1. Migraine without aura (history of five previous attacks)
     Lasts 4–72 h untreated or unsuccessfully treated
     Has at least two of the following:
       Unilateral location
       Pulsating quality
       Moderate to severe intensity (inhibits/prohibits daily activities)
       Aggravated by walking, stair climbing, or other physical activity
     Has one of the following:
       Nausea and/or vomiting
       Photophobia or phonophobia
  2. Migraine with aura (history of two attacks)
     Has three or more of the following:
       One or more reversible aura symptoms of focal, cerebral, cortical, or brainstem dysfunction

One aura over 4 min or two or more auras in succession
Each aura limited to 60 min
Headache after aura or simultaneously with aura
- Tension-type headache
  1. Has two of the following:
     Pressing or tightening quality
     Mild to moderate intensity that does not prohibit activities
     Not aggravated by physical exercise
  2. Has both of the following:
     No nausea or vomiting, but anorexia can occur
     Photophobia and/or phonophobia generally absent and do not occur together
- Cluster headache (history of five previous attacks)
  1. Severe unilateral, orbital, supraorbital, and/or temporal pain lasting over 15 min to 180 min
  2. Headache associated with one of the following:
     Conjunctival injection
     Lacrimation
     Nasal congestion
     Rhinorrhea
     Forehead and facial sweating
     Eyelid edema
     Miosis
     Ptosis
  3. Frequency is one every other day to eight a day
- Other headaches
  1. Knife-blade
  2. TMJ headache
  3. Occipital neuralgia
  4. Exertional headache
  5. Paroxysmal hemicrania

For all of the types, the history and physical examination show no other organic causes of headache and if another disorder is present it does not coincide with the headache.
*Adapted from Solomon (1997), Mathew (1997), and Silberstein, Young, & Lipton (1997).*

use, resulting in a rebound headache response (Lipton & Stewart, 1997).

In primary care practice, it is appropriate to refer patients to a headache clinic or at least for neurologic assessment when they have worsening headaches or headaches that evolve to daily events and are unresponsive to pharmacotherapy or when they present with focal neurologic signs.

Migraine headaches are a chronic disease with episodic exacerbations marked by nausea, possible vomiting, photophobia, and phonophobia. An aura, a focal neurologic symptom, can precede migraine. Migraine may also have prodromes, changes in mood or behavior. Migraines as an episodic disorder produce changes in gastrointestinal and autonomic functions as well as cause head pain.

A popular myth is that migraine is a disorder of higher socioeconomic status. The truth is that individuals with higher incomes are more likely to seek medical care for migraines. In large population studies, migraines are more prevalent among the poor, but remain more common in Caucasians than African-Americans or Asian-Americans (Lipton & Stewart, 1997).

The significant dysfunction of migraine headaches may lead the patient to the health care provider. One third of individuals experiencing migraines require bedrest, and 50% account for 90% of the lost work time caused by migraines, leading to an economic cost in the billions of dollars per year. Migraines can occur in children, being described by children as young as 8 years old. In males the prevalence is steady at 6%, with a much higher percentage (17%) in females, peaking at 25% for women in their 40s and then declining. The female decline does coincide with declining estrogen levels and approaching menopause, but women still experience more migraine than men even into their 80s.

A small percentage of women (6%) have migraine associated with the onset of menses (plus or minus 2 days) (MacGregor, 1997). Falling estrogen levels are postulated to be related to changes in neurotransmitters through one or more of four ways: a decrease in serum dopamine beta-hydroxylase, a dysfunction in opioid control of the hypothalamic-pituitary-adrenal axis, a decrease in magnesium levels, and a platelet dysfunction. In patients with known migraine headaches, using oral contraceptives can be contraindicated, although some studies show the association is weak. However, if an individual has migraines and smokes, the use of oral contraceptives is definitely contraindicated. In some women with migraines pregnancy abates the migraines, but 10% of pregnant women experience their first migraine with pregnancy (MacGregor, 1997).

There is a familial component to migraine headaches, particularly to the occurrence of familial hemiplegia accompanying the headache. There is some indication of an ion channel gene abnormality in some families. In addition, some individuals have emotional trigger features to their migraine headaches. The pathophysiology of migraine headaches does indicate a reduced cortical blood flow in migraines with or without aura. About 3% of the population with migraines may also experience seizures associated with their migraines. These seizures may be due to spreading changes in electrical or chemical potential brought on by the migraine headache (Welsh & Lewis, 1997). Migraine headaches have a documented association with psychiatric disorders, particularly depression and anxiety. It is not clear which is the antecedent to the other (Merikangas & Stevens, 1997).

Tension headaches are also commonly called stress headaches. These headaches are not severe, are usually bilateral, and are not exacerbated by increased physical activity. They are not marked by nausea and vomiting, photophobia, or phonophobia. The pericranial muscles are usually tense, and the headache is not brought on by systemic or organic disease.

Cluster headaches are marked by sharp, severe, unilateral pain lasting 15–180 min in the orbital, supraorbital, or temporal area. The attacks can be one to eight a day and have a higher occurrence in heavy smokers. Accompanying autonomic signs include tearing, conjunctival redness, nasal congestion, facial sweating, and ptosis.

The majority of individuals who seek help from headache clinics do so because they are experiencing headaches daily. Although chronic tension headaches initially were described as the only form of daily headache, recent work tends to point to more than one type of headache becoming daily and chronic, either from a migrainous or tension type and often related to analgesic overuse. Headaches can evolve into daily events, often starting as occasional headaches while individuals are in their teens. About 20% of daily headache sufferers have a sudden onset possibly due to trauma, viral illness, septic meningitis, surgery, or other illness.

Individuals with chronic excessive analgesia use experience related rebound headaches characterized by daily headaches. The headache can vary in severity, location, and type with a low threshold of intellectual or physical activity bringing on the headache. Patients complain of many related symptoms: asthenia, nausea, restlessness, anxiety, irritability, decreased memory, decreased concentration, decreased attention, and depression. If using daily ergotamine medications, they can complain of cold extremities, tachycardia, paresthesias, decreased pulse, hypertension, light-headedness, extremity muscle pain, or leg weakness. Daily headaches often occur from 2–5 A.M. and with decreased REM sleep, and individuals awaken with a severe headache.

## SPECIFIC CONSIDERATIONS FOR PHARMACOTHERAPY

### When Drug Therapy Is Needed

Drug therapy in headaches is aimed at treating the headache at the time it occurs and aimed at prophylactic treatment to prevent headaches.

The aim of drug use is to start with milder and then more potent analgesics as needed. The use of prophylactic medication is usually reserved for moderate to severe headaches and those occurring more than twice a week. Unfortunately with analgesic and some prophylactic medications, there can be a rebound dependency effect with headache recurrence; thus frequent medication use can lead to more frequent headaches.

## Short- and Long-Term Goals of Pharmacotherapy

The goals of medication use are the relief of headache and, in more severe, frequent headaches, the prevention of headache. A secondary goal in frequent headaches is prevention of drug dependency and more rebound headaches.

## Nonpharmacologic Therapy

Regular patterns of sleep, exercise, and eating are helpful in preventing headaches. Headache sufferers, particularly those with migraine, often can identify trigger factors that should be avoided in preventing headaches. Some foods can trigger migraines, such as tyramine-containing food (red wine, aged cheese), monosodium glutamate, alcoholic beverages, and caffeine. Some individuals also find it helpful to avoid milk products, citrus products, and chocolate. Some medications can also cause headache, and stress management might be helpful in curbing frequent headaches. Stress management techniques include biofeedback, acupuncture, and behavioral counseling.

One known cause of headaches is sleep deprivation, which is curable with enough sleep. This may mean changing behaviors to establish a regular sleep schedule, using the bed primarily for sleeping (not reading or watching TV) and developing a set presleep routine. Other behaviors that help sleep are regular exercise, investing in a good bed and mattress, and avoiding large meals before bedtime. If unable to sleep, getting up and carrying out other activities in another room and trying to deal with stressful concerns before going to bed are also helpful (Bristol-Myers, 1995).

## Time Frame for Initiating Pharmacotherapy

With all headaches, the earlier the pharmacotherapy is initiated, the easier it is to treat the headache. In headache treatment it is impera-

tive to take enough drug when the headache begins to abort it; the longer it takes to obtain relief (requiring more than one drug dose), the longer is the headache and its disability. In prophylactic headache relief, it is important to be consistent with medication and not forget to take the medication. Prophylactic treatment is considered when two or more headaches per month produce disability lasting 3 or more days per month and when symptomatic medications are ineffective.

## Overview of Drug Classes for Treatment

There are many drug classes used in the treatment of headache. In treating headache the analgesic groups for mild to moderate headache include aspirin, acetaminophen, and NSAIDs (Naprosyn, Anaprox, ibuprofen, Voltaren); analgesic combinations including caffeine (Excedrin, Anacin) and butalbital (Fiorinal, Midrin); combination analgesics with narcotics (Fiorinal with Codeine, Tylenol with Codeine); and narcotics (Darvon, Darvocet, Dilaudid, Demerol, morphine). Acute migraine and cluster headaches are treated with serotonin agonists (ergotamine and dihydroergotamine, D.H.E., sumatriptan). Headache prophylaxis includes beta-adrenergic blocking agents (propranolol, timolol), ergot alkaloids (methysergide), NSAIDs, antidepressants, and valproic acid.

## Assessment Needed Prior to Therapy

A sudden onset of severe headache in a person with or without a history of severe headaches can be a medical emergency. Frequently, the person will call and say, "This is the worst headache of my life," and with or without focal symptoms this person should be seen by a health care provider within a short period of time to evaluate the possible etiology with appropriate diagnostic aids. Headaches that worsen over a period of weeks or months or headaches that occur three or more times a week may also justify emergent laboratory and radiology diagnostics to rule out other diseases.

A careful history is necessary in routine workups on headaches. This includes careful description of the headache and if more than one type of headache occurs. For each type it is helpful to know its location, duration, temporality, warning symptoms, associated symptoms, alleviation or palliation of pain, medication use, and familial headache history. Asking the patient what she or he thinks causes the headaches is also helpful. Two types of headache may mean one is a rebound headache from prolonged, daily use of medication (which may or may not be for the headache itself), particularly if used prophylactically. Common medications known to cause headache include estrogens, vasodilators, and oral contraceptives.

If it is difficult for the patient to give this kind of specific information regarding the headache episodes, keeping a headache diary for 1 month may be helpful. For each headache ask the person to write out the warning signs, time the headache began and ended, type of pain, location, and intensity of pain on a 1–10 scale. Logging events prior to the headache (exercise, conflicts), foods eaten, hours of sleep, and treatment attempted is also helpful. Because headaches can be a symptom of other disease, a careful general examination and specific neurologic examination looking for focal symptom is also necessary.

## Patient/Caregiver Information

Individuals seeking headache relief need assistance in treatment for pain relief. They also need advice on headache etiology and headache prevention. These patients can be anxious and need reassurance that their chronic recurring headaches are usually benign. Making patients partners in headache relief enhances their success in treatment.

## OUTCOMES MANAGEMENT

### Selecting an Appropriate Agent

The order of medication use in mild to moderate headaches is analgesics; combination analgesic drugs with caffeine (potentiates the analgesic), butalbital, and/or narcotics; and NSAIDs, which work by blocking the synthesis of prostaglandins through inhibition of cyclooxygenase (Silberstein, 1993). For moderate to severe headaches, ergot derivatives and sumatriptan are used, but not at the same time. D.H.E. is more effective in headache relief and associated autonomic symptoms and rebound headaches are less likely; there also is less nausea. To prevent migraine, beta blockers, ergot alkaloids, NSAIDs, antidepressants, and valproic acid are used.

Combination drugs are often used to enhance the analgesic action, reduce the total amount of medication, relieve anxiety, and for product convenience. Opiates can be used to prevent needless suffering, and most individuals are careful with their use. Some individuals find other combinations and higher doses of medications other than opiates taken early in the headache as effective with less side effects (Sheftell, 1997).

### Monitoring for Efficacy

In acute migrainous headache the use of oral medications can be delayed due to decreased gastric motility. The side effects of many of these medications may also limit their effectiveness. Aspirin can potentiate nausea, and opioids can induce sedation. Ergot derivatives can lead to nausea, vomiting, and dependency (rebound headache). Rebound headache can occur with ergotamine with as little as 3 mg three times per week. Both ergot and sumatriptan are effective in relieving acute migraine (Mathew, 1997). However, sumatriptan, which causes less nausea, has a higher incidence of rebound headache (Drugs for migraines, 1995).

### Monitoring for Toxicity

Children younger than 15 should not use aspirin for headache because of the risk of Reyes's syndrome, making acetaminophen preferable. Patients with a history of gastritis and ulcers or other bleeding disorders should also use acetaminophen. NSAIDs, used symptomatically and prophylactically, need careful monitoring because of occult gastric disease. Ergotamine can cause vascular occlusion and gangrene with overdosage (over 6 mg in 24 h or 10 mg per week), and the action is potentiated by beta-adrenergic blockers, dopamine, erythromycins or troleandomycin, liver disease, and fever (Drugs for migraines, 1995). D.H.E. is less toxic. Ergotamine and D.H.E. are contraindicated in renal failure, liver failure, pregnancy, coronary artery disease, peripheral vascular disease, hypertension, and sepsis. Sumatriptan use is associated with chest pain and one report of myocardial infarction. Both sumatriptan and ergot derivatives are vasoconstrictive and can be additive. Their use needs to be sequentially separated by 24 h.

### Follow-up Recommendations

Chronic headache sufferers need routine follow-up at 3- to 6-month intervals, primarily because of the frequent development of rebound headache. Warning signs of rebound headaches include increased medication tolerance and increased headaches. Limiting dosages to lower than the dosage producing the daily headache is useful, as is using different classes of medications to limit headaches. Educated, informed patients will often work with the provider to help themselves counter the effects of this disabling symptom and chronic disease. Referral to a headache clinic is appropriate if the individual does not respond to headache relief measures and the number of headaches is increasing.

## PARKINSON'S DISEASE

The neuronal degenerative syndrome termed Parkinson's disease (PD) typically occurs when a loss of 80–90% of the dopaminergic cells occurs in substantia nigra. This results in an imbalance between dopamine and acetylcholine with resulting difficulty in controlling skeletal muscle and autonomic nervous system activity. There is also a genetic component to the disease. The early treatment of PD involved the inhibition of acetylcholine. In the 1960s levodopa (L-dopa) was introduced as replacement therapy.

The majority of causes of PD are unknown but some causes are known, such as repeated trauma (pugilistic syndrome), carbon monoxide poisoning, heavy metal poisoning, illicit drug use, encephalitis, and medications which interfere with the dopamine brain function in the brain such as tranquilizers and antipsychotic medications (see Table 29–10). Theoretically, the release of oxygen radicals generated by oxidation reactions from dopamine metabolism may also play a role in the development of PD (Stern, 1997).

Patients with PD with good health management can now live 10 or more years with a relatively normal life and much longer with physical limitations (Silberstein, 1996).

### TABLE 29–10. DRUG THAT CAN CAUSE PARKINSONISM

| | |
|---|---|
| Calcium channel blockers | Phenothiazines/ |
| Captopril | butyrophenones |
| Chlorpromazine | Phenytoin |
| Diltiazem | Prochlorperanine |
| Haloperidol | Valproate |
| Lithium | Verapamil |
| Metaclopramide | Vincristine |
| Methyldopa | |

The idiopathic, often insidious onset of PD is between ages 40–70 with a progressive course. The classic presentation is of a tremor at rest, first seen in the hands, face, and tongue and a stiffness (rigidity) marked by slowness or paucity of movement (bradykinesia). The early tremor is usually unilateral, unintentional, and slow with a pill-rolling motion seen in the hands. There is a loss of facial expression, decreased blinking, and gait changes marked by shuffling steps, little arm swing, and stooped posture.

Other signs include frequent falls, micrographia, hypophonia, excess salivation, and altered tendon reflexes (but downward toes). Concurrent symptoms can include depression, dysarthria, and fatigue. Numerous changes in the autonomic nervous system (impotence, increased salivation, orthostatic hypotension, paroxysmal sweating, seborrheic dermatitis, and urinary frequency) also occur.

Cognitive impairment is present in 15–30% of individuals who present with PD and is more prominent in individuals without tremor. Dementia is present in 15–30% of individuals who present with PD, often in those with little tremor. Consequently, cognitive testing is necessary for any individual who presents with PD symptoms. The dopaminergic medications used in treatment may also produce hallucinations or psychosis more readily in this population as well as toxic delirium (agitation, confusion, and worsening of the PD symptoms), necessitating lower doses of medications.

## SPECIFIC CONSIDERATIONS FOR PHARMACOTHERAPY*

### When Drug Therapy Is Needed

Because the cause is unknown and there is no cure, the primary treatment is symptomatic relief. Because of the probable role the release of oxygen free radicals plays in the development of the disease, medications to prevent their release are now advocated early in treatment. As the stiffness, tremor, slow movement, and gait difficulties worsen, dopaminergic drug treatment becomes necessary. In the late stages of the disease, the autonomic nervous system changes and possible occurrence of psychosis and dementia require symptomatic treatment (Stacy & Brownlee, 1996).

---

*See additional note, page 682.

## Short- and Long-Term Goals of Pharmacotherapy

The short-term goal of therapy is symptomatic control. The long-term goal is careful use of medications to prevent side effects and to some extent the necessity of adding further medications to control the side effects of the dopaminergic agents. Side effects of levodopa usually develop within 3 years of starting therapy.

## Nonpharmacologic Therapy

Although the mainstay of treatment is drug use, other treatments are available. If patients have severe depression with their PD, electroconvulsive therapy (ECT) may be indicated. A beneficial side effect of ECT is improvement in PD, which may last 6 months or more.

Direct neurologic surgical interventions may also be indicated. Stereotactic surgery is done to create a lesion in the anterior lateral thalamus, which reduces the severe tremor that can occur. Another surgical option is ventrolateral thalamotomy or medial pallidotomy to treat contralateral rigidity, dystonia, or levodopa- or other drug-induced dyskinesias. All these procedures continue to require antiparkinsonism medication. On an experimental basis, neural fetal tissue and adrenal medullary tissue are implanted in the striatum to alleviate the disease (Alexander, 1997).

Patient education allowing patient choice in medication treatment can produce better outcomes. Long-term decisions include employment, financial concerns, caregiving decisions, health care proxies, and the use of self-help strategies.

## Time Frame for Initiating Pharmacotherapy

Patients usually complain of the impairment related to movement slowness and imbalance more than the tremor, although the tremors can be socially embarrassing. A mild tremor not interfering with daily activities does not usually require treatment. Pharmacologic treatment of PD is usually initiated when daily functioning becomes impaired.

## Overview of Drug Classes for Treatment

The drug classes used in PD include using the dopamine precursor levodopa to replace the lost dopamine. Levodopa and carbidopa (Sinemet) are given together to prevent peripheral uptake and enhance brain absorption of levodopa. Dopamine agonists act directly on the receptor, bypassing the need for replenishment or release from dying terminals. Monoamine oxidase B (MAO-B) inhibitors are used to inhibit the catabolic breakdown of dopamine, and the MAO-B inhibitor selegiline is often used prior to major symptomatic control because of its probable effects as an antioxidant agent. One class of anticholinergics, the antimuscarinics, block the effects of the unopposed acetylcholine activity and are used as second-line drugs to counteract tremor. Amantidine, classified as an antiviral medication, is used to increase the effects of dopamine levels at the nerve ending. If psychotic symptoms induced through levodopa and MAO-B use cannot be controlled by limiting or withdrawing drugs, then antipsychotic agents may be utilized.

## Assessment Needed Prior to Therapy

The nature of this disease leads to easy misdiagnosis, and the treatment of the disease has become a neurologic subspecialty. The most common misdiagnosis by the primary care provider is essential familial tremor. For the neurologist, misdiagnosis can also occur with patients actually having other conditions such as progressive supranuclear palsy, multiple system atrophy, corticobasal ganglionic degeneration, and vascular parkinsonism.

Dementia is a common finding (approximately 20% on initial assessment) with the diagnosis of PD, and a screening mental status examination (Mini-Mental Status Examination) at initial assessment is often helpful. If the disease is accompanied by dementia, the differential diagnosis then includes Alzheimer's disease and Pick's disease. The current changes in drug therapy in PD are very dynamic, and individuals with rapidly progressing disease may be best managed by a neurologist or special PD clinic aware of current treatment modalities.

## Patient/Caregiver Information

Current treatment of PD is changing rapidly, and there are local chapters of the national Parkinson's disease organization in almost all areas of the country. In addition to group support, current information on family and patient educational materials, nutritional guidance, and exercise can be offered. Patients who are educated about their disease and medications usually fare better and are able to manipulate their medications to allow maximum possible functioning. Functionally, great gains can be made to help with gait, balance, ADLs, and speech problems (dysphagia, hypophonia) through referral to physical, occupational, and speech therapists. Because PD is a chronic disease, counseling regarding occupation, caregiving decisions, and financial concerns needs addressing by appropriate therapists.

The four major organizations involved are the American Parkinson's Disease Association, Inc., the National Parkinson's Foundation, the Parkinson's Disease Foundation, and the United Parkinson's Foundation and International Tremor Foundation. They are helpful in addressing medical treatment, self-help strategies, and research advances.

## OUTCOMES MANAGEMENT

Each of the major groups of drugs used in PD are presented below with its specific action, side effects, monitoring issues, toxicities, and follow-up recommendations. Please see Fig. 29–1 for an overview of medications used in Parkinson's disease. As patients become functionally dis-

abled, symptomatic treatment is started. The drug choice is also based on the presence of cognitive disease, age, extent of disability, symptoms, and response to initial drug therapy (Silberstein, 1996). Drugs known to release dopamine may be indicated either before or in conjunction with levodopa to allow the use of less levodopa. Over time and with disease progression, L-dopa almost universally develops side effects limiting its efficacy because of "on-off" phenomena. Depression, dementias, and psychosis are common problems in Parkinson's disease. A section outlining common drugs used for these problems in PD follows the discussion on antiparkinsonian medications.

### Neuroprotective Agents

After initial diagnosis and before there is any functional deficit interfering with daily life, early use of selegiline (Eldepryl, L-deprenyl), an MAO-B inhibitor dopamine agonist, is recommended. Selegiline is neuroprotective by reducing free oxygen radical production through diminished oxidative metabolism of dopamine. It also has mild dopaminergic effects. Both effects allow delayed use of levodopa, necessary because of its long-term side effects of motor fluctuation and "on-off" phenomena (Ahlskig, 1996).

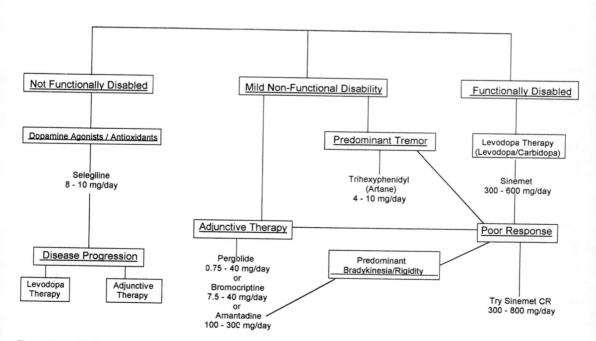

**Figure 29–1.** Medications used in Parkinson's disease.

Selegiline is also used as an adjunct medication, primarily to cut down on the amount of dopa therapy and resulting motor fluctuations, usually allowing a 10–30% decrease in L-dopa therapy. Some patients do not tolerate both drugs well because of the combined dopaminergic effects with hallucinations and nausea, but a 5-year study showed good results with combined therapy (Myllyla, Sontaniemi, Hakulinen, Maki-Ikola, & Heinonen, 1997) in contrast to the earlier 2-year DATATOP study (Hely & Morris, 1996).

The usual dose is 5–10 mg per day. The drug should be taken early in the day since it has a mild amphetamine metabolite that may cause sleep disturbance and anxiety. The drug can also cause increased sedation when given with narcotics. Overdosing may be dangerous because of the MAO inhibition with a "cheese response" (or red wine or chocolate) producing hypertension, increased heart rate, headaches, and vomiting from too much gut absorption of tyramine. A new form of selegiline given transdermally, Desmethyl-selegiline (DMS), is under development and showing fewer side effects than oral dosing.

Although the manufacturer of Selegiline now warns against its use with SSRIs, commonly given in PD for depression, a new review of 2000 patients on combined selegiline and SSRI, found that the incidence of SSRI reaction with selegiline was 0.24% with no deaths (Richard et al, 1997). The reported reaction is one of seizures, anxiety, LOC, or remotely, pseudo-pheochromocytoma.

Another side effect of the drug is its effect on the cardiovascular system. Patients with Parkinson's disease have changes in their cardiovascular systems over other groups with hypotension, slowing of heart rate, and decreased autonomic vascular regulation with position change. Selegiline tends to exacerbate this condition in some individuals, especially under stressed conditions such as the tilt table, Valsalva's maneuver, and sudden standing with a delay in autonomic response of over 2 min from the stressor onset, suggesting an increased risk for orthostatic hypotension in selegiline users and a need to test BP lying, sitting, and standing during routine office visit follow-up. Selegiline at present is often a very expensive drug, currently costing $1,200 per year. That factor should be discussed at the time of prescription.

## Dopamine Agonists

The dopamine agonists directly stimulate specific subclasses of dopamine receptors. By re-

ducing the turnover of dopamine, these drugs may reduce the toxic byproducts of dopamine metabolism, hydrogen peroxide and free radical accumulation. If a patient has only mild functional disability and it is appropriate to delay the use of levodopa therapy, then adjunctive therapy can be tried. These drugs are also used in combination with levodopa when the response to levodopa begins to fade. Drug Table 318 also lists other adjunctive medications not as commonly used as the ones described below. All of the dopamine agonists can cause nausea, vomiting, and orthostatic hypotension so slow titration is a key in treatment, and the drugs must be weaned slowly to prevent a rebound worsening of symptoms. Drugs specifically contraindicated when using dopaminergic agents in PD are neuroleptics, centrally active dopamine antagonist antiemetics (prochlorperazine, promethazine), and catecholamine-depleting agents such as reserpine. The dopamine agonists are also more expensive than Sinemet, but their use may delay the onset of motor fluctuations, reducing levodopa requirements and decreasing the disability from motor fluctuations.

Bromocriptine (Parlodel) is an ergot alkaloid, with D2 receptor agonist activity. The drug is also used in conjunction with levodopa and by itself in the early stage of Parkinson's disease. In conjunction therapy the dose is 1.25 mg per day with a slow increase to 7.5–10 mg per day in three to four divided doses until adequate control is achieved. The dose may go as high as 30 mg per day. Its side effects include nausea, somnolence, orthostatic hypotension, back pain, confusion, and hallucinations.

Pergolide (Permax) also is an ergot preparation that is 10 times more potent than bromocriptine, stimulating the D2 receptors and having a partial effect on the D1 receptors. It is used early on as initial therapy and as adjunctive therapy in later Parkinson's disease with L-dopa. The early titrating dose is 0.125 mg per day, increased by 0.125 mg every 5 days to a total dose of 0.75–1.0 mg per day in three or four divided dosages. The usual dose in conjunction therapy is 0.05 mg daily, increased slowly to 0.2–0.6 mg per day until adequate control is achieved, or reachieved as the disease progresses. The drug's side effects are somnolence, nausea, orthostatic hypotension, confusion, back pain, and hallucinations.

Many more specific dopamine agonists are under development as researchers try to specifically match dopamine receptor subtypes (characterized by anatomic location, link to enzyme systems, and pharmacologic response) and prolong their action, such as cabergoline, a D2 dopamine agonist given at 2–6 mg each morning. Transcutaneous preparations are also being developed, and subcutaneous dopamine agonists (apomorphine) are useful in specific cases for advanced PD and severe unpredictable "off" periods (Stern, 1994).

## Anticholinergics

Anticholinergics were the first drugs used to treat PD and primarily provide relief of severe tremor with less effect on bradykinesia, rigidity, and postural instability. These compounds block muscarinic receptors, thus restoring the balance between dopaminergic and cholinergic influence in the basal ganglia. Artane (trihexyphenidyl) is primarily used in disabling tremor in younger patients without many other disease symptoms. Its side effects include dry eyes, dry mouth, urinary retention, loss of concentration, and hallucinations. It is poorly tolerated in the elderly. The starting dose is 1 mg/day, increased by 1-mg increments to 5–12 mg per day in three or four divided doses, raising the dose every 3–5 days. The drug is usually effective for only 3–6 months. A less potent anticholinergic agent, procyclidine, can be tried if the Artane has too many adverse effects.

Benztropine (Cogentin) is also used in the treatment of tremor, either alone or with other agents. The dosage is 0.5–6 mg per day, and it can also produce confusion, sleepiness, blurred vision, and dry mouth.

## Amantadine

Amantadine (Symmetrel) is a known antiviral agent that enhances dopamine release, has antimuscarinic effects, and may increase dopamine synthesis and inhibit dopamine reuptake. The drug has a modest effect on bradykinesia and rigidity with less effect on tremor. The drug is also a mild psychostimulant. The drug's effect is time-limited, usually 3–6 months. Amantadine is usually well tolerated in doses of 100–300 mg per day given in two or three divided doses. The common adverse effects are dose-dependent ankle edema and livedo reticularis (a purple mottling of the skin), as well as anticholinergic side effects of confusion, sleepiness, blurred vision, and dry mouth. The medication is available in an elixir (50mg/5 mL) for smaller dosing and

use in severe dysphagia. The drug is cleared by the kidney and needs reduction in impaired renal function.

## Levodopa Therapy

Levodopa, combined with carbidopa (Sinemet) to block peripheral breakdown of the drug outside the brain, is the cornerstone of PD therapy. Levodopa is an intermediate byproduct of tyrosine. Carbidopa, a peripheral amino acid decarboxylase inhibitor, eliminates many of the severe GI effects of levodopa metabolized outside the brain. Levodopa is absorbed in the gut and transported by neutral amino acids into the brain to the substantia nigra by dopaminergic neurons, peaking in 1 h and lasting 3–8 h. The progression of PD, with fewer dopaminergic neurons available to take up the levodopa, contributes to the erratic clinical response of levodopa in long-term treatment. The effect is simple and complex motor fluctuations marked by dyskinesias, end-of-dose deterioration (wearing-off effect), and random fluctuations (on-off effect).

Treatment with levodopa begins when the disability affects social or occupational function with as low a dose as needed. The drug may be started alone or in conjunction with dopamine agonists to enable low-dose levodopa for as long as possible. Over time and with disease progression, individuals may require more medication in order to continue their daily functioning. Two controlled-release levodopa preparations are also in use, Sinemet-CR and Madopar HBS (hydrodynamically balanced system). The bioavailability of the drugs is less than in Sinemet so the drug dosages are actually higher, despite fewer daily doses. In advanced disease, patients like better control of their dyskinesias and on-off and wearing-off phenomena and will use a combination of controlled-release and regular Sinemet.

The treatment goal is not abolishing of all symptoms, but relieving functional disability. Initial treatment may begin with Sinemet 25/100 (25 mg carbidopa and 100 mg levodopa), one-half tablet once daily, increasing by one-half tablet every 3 to 5 days to one tablet three times daily. Sinemet usually starts working in 30 min. The last dose should be given in mid- to late afternoon as it is not needed during sleep and may cause vivid dreams or nightmares. If nausea occurs, the drug may be given with meals.

The steady state of levodopa in the controlled-release format may in itself prevent response fluctuations so that Sinemet-CR is prescribed as the first-line drug in levodopa therapy using 50/200, one-half tablet twice daily, titrating up to two full tablets daily. As the disease progresses, the dosing may go to t.i.d. Treatment response to Sinemet-CR usually takes 1 h. Because the actual bioavailability of Sinemet-CR is less than plain Sinemet, the controlled-release forms require higher doses. As the disease progresses, the dosage may then be titrated to two to four tablets daily. Keeping a diary of dose response is helpful in establishing a better response to dosing. A dosage of 1000 mg per day with no response implies the diagnosis is other than Parkinson's disease.

Adding standard Sinemet, dopamine agonists, or other secondary drugs when symptom control is inadequate (Stern, 1997) may be necessary with disease progression. The early morning bradykinesia and later dyskinesia complications of levodopa therapy have many approaches. One approach is the use of a combination of regular and controlled-release Sinemet early in the morning and perhaps again at midafternoon to shorten the time of drug efficacy. Patients over time may find only minutes of time that are free from the bradykinesia of too little Sinemet and the dyskinesias of higher levels of Sinemet if on the Sinemet for a number of years. Another treatment option is to add dopamine agonists and reduce the amount of Sinemet used. Still another approach is to dilute the Sinemet to a liquid form and take it every 2–3 h to ensure a drug steady state.

Keeping a very time-specific log of drug dosing and side effects is helpful in altering drug therapy to produce better function and "smooth" the transitions. If predominant tremor is an issue, anticholinergics are used in addition to Artane. The anticholinergics can cause hallucinations, and patients must be monitored carefully for behavioral changes. The fluctuations in drug effect may also be related to food intake. The levodopa/carbidopa competes with large amino acids for transportation across the blood-brain barrier. Thus, it is helpful to coordinate protein intake with medication use.

## Drugs Used for Depression, Dementia, and Psychosis in Parkinson's Disease

*Depression.* The classic symptoms of depression—psychomotor retardation, insomnia, poor concentration, and anorexia—are often overlooked in PD because the symptoms resemble the signs of PD. Approximately 40% of patients with PD will suffer from depression. The depression should be treated aggressively using tricyclics, serotoninergic uptake blockers (SSRIs), psychotherapy, and possible electroshock therapy.

A drug commonly used is amitriptyline (Elavil, Endep) with starting doses of 12.5–75 mg per day given at hour of sleep, which may be increased up to 100–300 mg per day. Its effects include improving mood, helping with sleep fragmentation, and possibly aiding in the control of tremor. Some patients have an early morning dystonia, or leg cramping, that is also helped by this drug. The side effects include early morning lethargy, dry mouth, hallucinations, and confusion so starting with low doses and slow titration is often necessary.

The SSRIs are another choice in treating the depression because they cause fewer extrapyramidal side effects than tricyclic agents. Both Prozac and BuSpar are in common use.

*Dementia.* Loss in cognitive function is common. The usual dementia medications to improve memory have traditionally shown a poor clinical response in this patient population.

*Psychosis.* Hallucinations both visual and auditory, are common in PD. Some patients may also become paranoid. Infrequent hallucinations not altering the patient's functioning are usually not treated. Recording hallucinations before drug treatment is necessary to ascertain if hallucinations are related to just the disease or the drug treatment as well. The drugs used in the treatment of PD, particularly anticholinergic and dopaminergic compounds, can also cause confusion, sleep disturbance, frightening nightmares, and hallucinations. If the hallucinations are drug-related, titrating down dosages and eliminating their use late in the day may be effective. If the reaction is severe enough, it may require hospitalization.

The antipsychotic medication clozapine (Clozaril) is the cited drug of choice in psychosis. It can be used with a starting dose of 12.5–50 mg h.s. to treat the insomnia, hallucinations, and psychosis from dopaminergic medications and occasionally helps with tremor. Patients who present with hallucinations that are not drug-induced alone may require doses of up to 200 mg per day. This drug does not have the severe extrapyramidal side effects associated with traditional neuroleptics. However, it can cause agranulocytosis in 1% of patients so weekly monitoring of neutrophil count is necessary if a patient is on this drug.

Other medications used to treat psychosis include molindone starting at 2.5 and up to 20 mg per day. However, this drug may worsen the symptoms of PD.

## Follow-up Recommendations

Careful monitoring of Parkinson's disease symptoms and drug therapy every 3–6 months and even sooner if the disease is rapidly progressive is necessary. A daily log of symptoms and drug use is helpful for the clinician and patient to establish optimum drug utilization. If the disease is refractory to medication and presents in an atypical manner, referral to a neurologist specializing in Parkinson's disease is helpful.

# SEIZURE DISORDERS

The brain has characteristic electrical activity that can be recorded on an EEG. A seizure is a paroxysmal discharge of synchronously firing cortical neurons, which is the symptom of an epilepsy syndrome. The seizure source can be any one of numerous causes, which presumably result in altered synaptic anatomy, physiology, or pharmacology. The discharge originating within the seizure focus can then spread to other cortical neurons, accounting for seizure generalization. In some cases, seizures can be generalized at the outset.

Epilepsy is the condition in which seizures recur and may be self-perpetuating. More than 4 million Americans take medication to prevent recurrent seizures. In the majority of patients these medications are effective, although a small percentage are intractable. The drugs as a group can be called anticonvulsant, antiseizure, or antiepileptic medications. Patients with epilepsy can have more than one type of seizure. In order to use antiseizure medications, it is necessary to have an understanding of seizures, mechanisms of seizure generation, the mechanism of drug action, and how the drugs are metabolized by the body and their interaction with other drugs.

Up to 5% of the population may suffer a seizure at one time or another, but only 10% go on to develop recurrent seizures, or epilepsy, requiring drug therapy. All the available medications to treat seizures do not influence the development of epilepsy. Thus, they would be more properly thought of as antiseizure drugs (ASDs). However, the current commonly used abbreviation for medications used to treat seizures and epilepsy is AEDs (anti-epileptic drugs).

In children, epilepsy is not necessarily a chronic progressive disorder, with 70–80% of children who may have required treatment as young children going into remission and discontinuing medication after 2–3 years of remaining seizure-free. Neonatal seizures are considered too complex for this text and referral to a specialist is expected. Children can experience seizures from fever, but only a few go on to need ASD treatment. Two to four percent of all children may experience febrile seizures, but only 1% of these children go on to develop epilepsy. Even a second febrile seizure does not substantially raise the risk of a seizure disorder if no other neurologic abnormalities are present (Berg & Shinnar, 1994).

Idiopathic seizures that occur in adulthood may require medical treatment. Seizure incidence rises steadily in persons over 60, concurrently with the rise of other neuronal disorders and changes in the cerebrovascular system. Adults can also have seizures from metabolic disorders, particularly alcoholic withdrawal and metabolic abnormalities such as diabetes, renal failure, drug overdose, and drug interactions in addition to alcoholism. The latter seizures do not usually require ongoing antiseizure medications, with treatment being aimed at the underlying condition.

Epilepsy syndromes can be classified as partial or generalized with variants of each type. These syndromes are either primary or acquired (secondary). Usually the history is used to determine the syndrome (see Table 29–11). Seizures

---

### TABLE 29–11.  SEIZURE SYNDROMES

**Partial (Focal) Seizures**
Simple partial with motor, sensory, autonomic, and psychic symptoms (without impaired consciousness at onset)
Complex partial with impaired consciousness at onset
Simple partial evolving to secondarily generalized
Complex partial evolving to secondarily generalized

**Generalized Seizures**
**(Convulsive or Nonconvulsive)**
Absence with brief lapses in consciousness
Myoclonic
Clonic-tonic
Atonic

**Unclassified**

can be convulsive or nonconvulsive. Convulsive seizures are those with tonic-clonic motor activity, and nonconvulsive seizures can present with sensory, autonomic, or psychic symptoms. Partial seizures can originate in temporal or nontemporal areas, such as the frontal or occipital lobe. Simple partial seizures present with a single symptom or sign and preserved awareness. The most common type of seizures, affecting 55% of adults, are complex partial seizures; more than one symptom or sign is present, and an alteration in consciousness occurs.

Complex partial seizures can become secondary generalized tonic-clonic (convulsive) seizures if the neuronal discharge spreads to both sides of the brain usually with disruption of awareness caused by bilateral cortical involvement.

Primary generalized nonconvulsive seizures are called absence seizures (formally petit mal seizures) with diffusely abnormal cortical electrical activity and no focal onset. These seizures typically last seconds and are most common in children, occurring less commonly in adults. There is a lapse in consciousness often associated with eye fluttering and automatisms.

Status epilepticus, a true neurologic emergency, is a condition in which epileptic seizures are so frequently repeated or prolonged that they create a fixed and lasting condition (Pellock, 1993). This condition commonly lasts up to 30 minutes, or even longer. It is a medical emergency usually treated in an emergency setting. It will only be discussed here in relationship to one new pharmaceutic agent now available for use in the home to treat status epilepticus.

Classification of epilepsy syndromes is not comprehensively discussed in this text, and the reader is referred to neurology texts for a full discussion of epilepsy syndromes.

## SPECIFIC CONSIDERATIONS FOR PHARMACOTHERAPY

### When Drug Therapy Is Needed

Seizures can markedly interfere with activities of daily living, particularly driving, and some types can be life-threatening. Persons with intractable seizures of any kind can show a worsening of their seizures as well as memory and cognitive function decline over time. Drug treatment of seizures involves targeting ion channels to suppress the abnormal electrical discharges. Persons with any recurrent seizures not caused

by a readily treated primary condition (such as hypoglycemia) should be administered antiseizure drugs.

### Short- and Long-Term Goals of Pharmacotherapy

The goal of treatment is to prevent the greatest number of seizures with minimal toxicity and side effects. Table 29–12 outlines the plan for an anticonvulsant regimen.

### Nonpharmacologic Therapy

Intractable seizures in childhood may be treated with a ketogenic diet, usually in combination with AEDs, if medical therapy fails and surgery is not possible.

Another nonpharmacologic treatment is epilepsy surgery for well-localized seizure foci found in partial epilepsy, usually temporal in origin. This is not necessarily a procedure of last resort but should be considered as an early treatment option in medically intractable partial seizure disorders. Patients undergo a comprehensive outpatient evaluation including neuropsychometry, speech-language testing, MRI, and visual perimetry testing. The surgical procedures include an anterior temporal lobectomy, or in bilateral temporal epilepsy, a partial resection of epileptic brain tissue, a corpus callostomy, or even a hemispherectomy. Potential surgical candidates can be identified and surgery performed usually within 1 year after diagnosis in a comprehensive epilepsy treatment center (Cascino, 1994).

A vagal nerve stimulator has just been approved for adjunctive treatment of partial epi-

### TABLE 29–12.  PLANNING AN ANTICONVULSANT REGIMEN

1. Select the proper drug for the seizure type.
2. Determine the initial dosage based on weight and potential toxicity or interactions.
3. Increase the dosage until the therapeutic effect is achieved or until limited by side effects or toxicity.
4. Monitor levels as indicated (total/free; metabolites).
5. Use the highest tolerated dosage and add a second drug if the therapeutic level is inadequate.
6. If possible, taper the first drug off.
7. NEVER stop an antiepileptic drug abruptly.

lepsy with or without generalization. Its mechanism of action is not known.

## Time Frame for Initiating Pharmacotherapy

A first seizure is usually not treated with antiseizure drugs unless there is clear evidence of pathology. No drugs currently in use can prevent the development of epilepsy, and a diagnosis of epilepsy is not proven until the presentation of another seizure. The course of action following the first seizure is a diagnostic workup. If a focus for the seizure is found on MRI or EEG, then treatment may be initiated since the likelihood of a seizure recurrence is high.

In febrile children, a generalized seizure of less than 15 min with normal neurologic status and a normal lumbar puncture is usually not treated with medication. A focal onset and seizure lasting over 15 min is treated acutely and further evaluated with EEG, brain imaging, and cerebral spinal fluid examination and, if warranted, treatment is begun. An afebrile child with normal neurologic status and a normal EEG is usually followed with no medical treatment. If the afebrile child has abnormal neurologic signs, with abnormalities on EEG and brain imaging, the child is usually treated. Persons with abnormal EEGs showing generalized discharges or focal spikes are usually treated with medications. An exception is rolandic epilepsy in childhood.

## Overview of Drug Classes for Treatment

Antiseizure medications may work in one of two ways: by preventing "bursting" of individual neurons (a nonsynaptic action) or by altering neuronal communication (a synaptic action), both effects mediated through actions on ion channels. Nonsynaptic action is carried out by inhibition of voltage-dependent sodium or calcium channels, thereby preventing action potentials. Drug action on calcium channels (T-type) is a special case relevant to absence epilepsy. The spread of seizures can be prevented by enhancing inhibition or by decreasing excitation by acting on GABA or glutamate channels, respectively.

## Assessment Needed Prior to Therapy

The initial workup and treatment for recurrent seizures is usually done in consultation with a neurologist. Stabilization at times of seizure breakthroughs and treatment of the patient with intractable epilepsy are best done by a neurologist with an interest in epilepsy and neurophysiology (Derrigan & Fisher, 1997). When a seizure occurs, the workup includes a history, eliciting information pertinent to the development of seizures, a general screening physical examination, a complete screening neurological examination, and diagnostic tests. Patients with a partial seizure disorder may relate a history of meningitis, head trauma, or complex febrile seizures as children.

It is helpful to interview the caretakers of children to determine the possibility of a seizure disorder. The behaviors that may indicate a seizure disorder include the following: does not remember what happened; moves mouth funny; jerks, or twitches; becomes stiff; has a change in breathing pattern; stares off and bites or chews tongue; eyes look glassy; does not respond; mumbles or slurs words; and eyes or head turn to one side. Other behaviors, such as fidgeting in the seat, are not associated with having a seizure (Williams et al, 1996). In most cases a neurologist should be involved if behaviors are of uncertain etiology.

Eliciting information regarding alcohol use is imperative in adults and adolescents since alcohol withdrawal seizures are one of the most common causes of seizure disorders (McMicken & Freedland, 1994). Alcohol can produce seizures by its partial or absolute withdrawal following chronic inebriation, by direct neurotoxic effects, and by inducing metabolic abnormalities such as hypoglycemia. This group is also predisposed to cerebrovascular insults and infections. Seizure risk is linearly related to the daily intake of absolute alcohol, with the consumption of 1.5 pt of whiskey or its equivalent raising the risk of seizures to 20-fold that of nondrinkers (McMicken & Freedland, 1994).

The diagnostic tests for all patients are a CBC, electrolytes, and liver function tests, as well as an EEG and MRI inclusive of coronal sections through the temporal lobes. In partial seizures, it is important to obtain an EEG during sleep because the abnormalities may not appear in a wakeful state. Some patients may require a video EEG or an ambulatory EEG to classify types of seizures before therapy is initiated. The MRI can suggest the location of an epileptogenic zone as well as rule out foreign tissue lesions (vascular and tumor). A lumbar puncture is usually done routinely in infants to rule out meningitis and in others if focal neurologic symptoms and the general condition warrant the procedure.

The differential diagnosis for a seizure disorder includes paroxysmal disorders such as TIAs, syncope, migraine, transient global amnesia, psychiatric disorders, and sleep disorders.

## Patient/Caregiver Information

Patients and caregivers need to know the correct drug for the epilepsy syndrome and have a basic understanding of the type of seizure and its treatment in order to increase compliance with drug therapy. In most cases, the brand name of an antiepilepsy or antiseizure drug is necessary to ensure consistency and bioavailability of the drug. The patient and family need to understand if the drug they use is generic or brand name and ought not to substitute one for the other, as they may lose control of the seizures or develop toxicity because the bioavailability of the drug may differ from preparation to preparation.

Misinformation about epilepsy, eg, that it is a mental illness or a form of mental retardation, needs to be discussed. Critical issues regarding lifestyle also need discussion, including the need to avoid sleep deprivation, and limiting if not eliminating alcohol and caffeine intake. The other large social issue affecting persons with seizure disorders is driving. Although dependent on state law, most physicians recommend that persons initially suffering seizures be seizure-free 6–12 months before beginning driving again. Primary care providers need to know and understand their responsibility in relation to driving and seizure disorders in their practicing state(s).

Women of childbearing age need to understand that seizure medications that enhance metabolism (e.g. Tegretol) can interfere with the effectiveness of oral contraceptives and that some antiseizure medications are teratogenic, particularly in the first month of conception. Folic acid is prescribed before attempting conception at a daily dose of 1–5 mg to reduce the possibility of neural tube defects.

As with all medications, the patient and family need to know the risks and benefits of treatment, the side effects and toxicity of the particular therapy, and the common drug interactions. The person taking the drug should carry information or an ID bracelet regarding the condition and inform others (eg, a child's teacher) of the condition if necessary for safety. Showering is preferred over bathtub use, and the use of ladders or being in high places should be avoided.

An invaluable resource for patients and families is the Epilepsy Foundation of America (EFA); the toll free number is 1-800-EFA-1000 and the Internet address is http://www.efa.org. Educational materials are available there and at local epilepsy support groups in many areas throughout the United States.

## OUTCOMES MANAGEMENT

General information about antiseizure medications is followed by specific information on the most commonly used seizure medications.

### Selecting an Appropriate Agent

Treatment of seizures is dependent on the patient's symptoms and seizure type. If possible, patients are started on monotherapy and maintained on monotherapy. Single medications reduce the potential for side effects toxicity, drug interactions, and cost. Because 5–20% of the population require two-drug therapy to remain seizure-free, it is best to consider using drugs with complementary mechanisms of action. About 60% of individuals can become seizure-free with drug therapy, but up to 30% may continue to have breakthrough seizures. The longer the seizures remain uncontrolled, the more difficult it may be to control seizures over the long term.

Some patients can enter remission, allowing the gradual discontinuation of seizure medications after 2–3 years of being seizure-free. However, for some individuals the risk of seizure recurrence for socioeconomic reasons is greater than the risk of ongoing medication use, so they remain on seizure medications. One of the primary issues in this regard is the potential loss of driving privilege or job dismissal (although this is illegal under the ADA Act of 1990). Risk of seizure recurrence is higher in individuals with identifiable neurologic abnormalities by EEG or MRI, longer duration of the seizure disorder, multiple seizure types, and onset of seizure after age 12 (Zacharowicz & Moshe, 1995).

Seizures refractory to a particular antiseizure drug are only considered refractory when the first medication is either ineffective, causes side effects, or induces symptomatic toxicity. If a second medication is utilized, the first is then tapered and discontinued if possible. If seizures recur during the changeover, the first medication can be reinstituted, or a third medication may be started and a wean of the second begun. Normally, switching medications is a 1- to 2-month process, achieving a therapeutic level of the second drug before withdrawing the first, unless there are serious side effects or toxicity necessitating an abrupt withdrawal. A general rule for tapering is reducing the medication by one tablet for every three half-lives of the medication (Swartz, 1997). Patients who are on two medications can switch to a new one by simultaneously withdrawing one and increasing the dose of the new medication. Patients requiring more than one antiseizure medication are better managed, at least initially, by a neurologist.

Drug levels are used to help as a monitor to therapy, but the goal of treatment is the prevention of seizures. The therapeutic level of a drug is the level that provides adequate control without undue side effects or toxicity. This may mean giving "subtherapeutic" drug levels if an individual is seizure-free and above-therapeutic levels in an individual who remains seizure-free, without reported symptomatic side effects or toxicity. In the case of drugs which bind strongly to plasma protein (Dilantin, Depakote), monitoring unbound levels, preferably at plasma troughs gives a more accurate assessment. Some drugs produce active or toxic metabolites that may also be monitored (Tegretol).

Any change in medication (increasing, tapering, adding a medication, or switching medications) needs to be discussed with the patient and family. Although no rule exists, tapering a medication and discontinuing it is usually contemplated when the person has been seizure-free for at least 2 years.

## Monitoring for Efficacy

Seizure history, primarily through the use of a seizure diary, is one way to ascertain medication efficacy. Dosages of medications are then adjusted according to seizure occurrence, side effects, and blood levels. The factors affecting the efficacy of ASDs are outlined in Table 29–13. The first and second choices of drugs for specific seizure disorders are outlined in Table 29–14.

Serum levels are obtained when clinically indicated. The levels are effective in establishing compliance with anticonvulsant regimes, in establishing current levels when contemplating a change to a higher medication dose because of a seizure breakthrough, and in correlation of blood level with clinical toxicity when a decrease

---

### TABLE 29–13. FACTORS AFFECTING ANTIEPILEPTIC DRUG EFFICACY

- Compliance
- Indication for drug
- Bioavailability
  - Formulation/absorption
    - Food
    - Enteral feeding
    - Antacids
  - Distribution: protein binding
    - Salicylates
    - Other AEDs
- Metabolism and excretion
  - Age
  - Genetic factors
  - Volume of distribution
  - Drug half-life dosing
  - Renal and liver disease
- Drug interactions
  - Metabolism induction
    - Carbamazepine
    - Phenobarbital
    - Phenytoin
    - Rifampin
  - Metabolism inhibition
    - Cimetidine
    - Erythromycin
    - Felbamate
    - Fluoxetine
    - Nimodipine
    - Fantidine
    - Verapamil
- Mechanism of action

---

in dose is contemplated. Serum levels do not mandate a change in dose; that decision is primarily dependent on seizure control, toxicity, and side effects.

Some of these medications require monitoring of the CBC, differentials, liver function, and electrolytes initially monthly, and then every 3 months, 6 months, and yearly. This is probably just as important for the newer drug as the older ones only because long-term experience has not determined all known side effects.

Substituting generic name antiseizure medications for brand name drugs remains controversial. The long-term effect of less bioavailability in generic drugs may cause the redevelopment of seizures in a previously controlled person. In the case of generic carbamazepine, reinstating the

## TABLE 29–14. SEIZURE TYPE AND DRUG CHOICE

| | First Options | Second Options |
|---|---|---|
| Partial seizures | Carbamazepine (Tegretol)<br>Phenytoin (Dilantin)<br>Valproate | Gabapentin<br>Lamotrigine |
| Generalized seizures | | |
| Tonic-clonic seizures | Valproate<br>Phenytoin | Carbamazepine<br>Phenobarbital<br>Primidone<br>Felbamate |
| Absence seizures | Ethosuximide<br>Valproate | Acetazolamide<br>Lamotrigine<br>Felbamate |
| Myoclonic seizures | Valproate<br>Clonazepam | Lamotrigine<br>Phenobarbital<br>Felbamate |
| Tonic, clonic, and atonic seizures | Valproate | Carbamazepine |
| Multiple seizure types | Valproate | Carbamazepine |

brand name drug was unsuccessful in reestablishing seizure control in two cases (Welty, Pickering, Hale, and Aruzi, 1992).

### Monitoring for Toxicity

A review of mental status is needed on each visit as well as questioning the patient about the side effects and toxicities of each specific drug. The drug level is not as important as the patient's symptoms. There is a triad of similar side effects with almost all the seizure medications, which includes sedation, nausea, and ataxia. These side effects can be transient or occur only at high doses (Swartz, 1997). Allergic reactions include skin rash (common in 10% of patients), hepatitis, pancreatitis, and toxic epidermal necrolysis (Stevens-Johnson syndrome).

### Overview of Commonly Used Antiepileptic Drugs

Seizures can be controlled through two primary methods: by blocking or inhibiting neurotransmitters or by blocking voltage-dependent channels. The drugs' action either blocks the action of the excitatory neurotransmitter glutamate or enhances the inhibitory neurotransmitter GABA. Blocking the voltage-dependent sodium or calcium channels that participate in action potentials is the second method. The drug choice,

however, is primarily by seizure type. If more than one drug is required for seizure management, the prescriber may wish to choose drugs with different actions.

*Drugs that act on sodium channels.* Phenytoin, carbamazepine, lamotrigine, and topiramate all are sodium channel blockers that act by stabilizing the inactivated state of the channel and thus limiting sustained repetitive firing. Topiramate has additional actions than may enhance its efficacy.

*PHENYTOIN.* This drug was introduced in 1938 and remains one of the best-tolerated anticonvulsants for partial and generalized seizures. Phenytoin (Dilantin) acts by limiting sustained repetitive firing by enhancing sodium channel inactivation. It is taken orally, in capsule form, or IV but not given IM because of poor absorption. A new drug, an ester of phenytoin called fosphenytoin, is now used in acute therapy for seizure management and can be given IM. It is converted to phenytoin by platelet action (phosphatases) in the blood.

The usual maintenance dosage is 4–7 mg/kg. It has a long half-life (24 h) and although traditionally given t.i.d., it can be given b.i.d. and some neurologists even give it once a day. The drug readily binds with protein so it should not be given with gastric feedings, which inhibit its uptake. Binding with plasma proteins can be the cause of significant interactions particularly with drugs that compete for binding sites (eg, Depakote and Lamictal).

Alcohol or any inducer of metabolism such as the drug Tegretol can increase phenytoin clearance. Individuals who consume alcohol and use other metabolism inducers must have careful monitoring of blood levels to ensure therapeutic doses of the medication. The drug also alters metabolism of vitamin D, resulting in the bone disorders osteomalacia and hypocalcemia. The risk factors are increased with sun exposure, therapy with other anticonvulsants, and use of exogenous male hormones. Blood dyscrasias (leukopenia) and bone marrow suppression are rare but can occur, necessitating CBC monitoring on a routine basis. Some neurologists recommend giving folic acid 1–5 mg daily with this drug to counteract some of its known side effects.

The common side effects include diplopia, rash (especially on sun-exposed surfaces), and adenopathy. A more serious side effect is Stevens-Johnson syndrome. Other chronic effects of the drug include gingival hyperplasia, hirsutism, cerebellar atrophy, and coarsening of facial features.

**CARBAMAZEPINE.** This drug (Tegretol) is used for generalized tonic-clonic seizures as well as simple and complex partial seizures. It acts by limiting sustained repetitive neuronal firing. This drug is pharmacologically related to tricyclic antidepressants and is used in the affective disorders. The usual daily dosage is 4–20 mg/kg with a half-life of 12 h and it requires t.i.d. to q.i.d. dosing. At toxic levels it can produce ataxia, nystagmus, and lethargy.

The side effects of the drug include bone marrow suppression with resulting blood dyscrasias and aplastic anemia, bleeding, and liver function abnormalities giving rise to jaundice. The drug can also cause exfoliative dermatitis.

Carbamazepine is a metabolism inducer increasing the clearance of many drugs (itself included) resulting in higher dosage requirements. Propoxyphene and erythromycin significantly increase the blood levels of carbamazepine, so careful monitoring is required with these combinations. Aspirin, acetaminophen, and ibuprofen can be given with this drug.

**LAMOTRIGINE.** Lamotrigine (Lamictal) is used as an adjunct or second drug in the treatment of generalized tonic-clonic seizures, and in com-

plex partial seizures. It is also beneficial in primary generalized seizures. It acts to block sodium channels and reduces sustained repetitive firing, consequently reducing glutamate release. The usual dosage is 300–700 mg/day, maintaining a plasma level of 0.5–3.0. It has a half-life of 24 h and is less than 50% protein-bound. The drug is titrated up very slowly, usually over several weeks, because its use can result in a rash (a tender rash is a poor clinical sign). If the rash is in conjunction with a fever, hospitalization may be necessary. The primary interaction is with valproate, which roughly triples the half-life of lamotrigine, necessitating a reduction in dosage. Concurrent valproate use also increases the risk of rash.

**TOPIRAMATE.** This drug (Topamax) is a sodium channel blocker, but it also increases GABA-mediated chloride flux, and is a weak blocker of AMPA receptors (a subtype of glutamate receptors). It is an adjunct in the treatment of partial seizures and a second-choice drug in the treatment of generalized tonic-clonic seizures. It is rapidly absorbed. The dose is 400–600 mg per day. It shows minimal protein binding and has a long half-life of 21 h. Independent of dose its toxic effects include lethargy, ataxia, headache, paresthesias, and dysarthria. The dose-dependent effects include cognitive impairment, confusion, visual dysfunction, and nervousness. It can also cause lability, weight loss, and renal stones.

**Drugs that act on GABAa receptors.** Barbiturates, benzodiazepines, gabapentin, vigabatrin, tiagabine, and topiramate enhance the GABAa-mediated inhibition by either increasing receptor activation (barbiturates and benzodiazepines), decreasing the breakdown of GABAa (vigabatrin), decreasing its synaptic uptake (gabapentin and tiagabine), or by enhancing synaptic release (gabapentin).

**PHENOBARBITAL.** This barbiturate enhances GABA action. The drug is used for generalized tonic-clonic seizures as well as complex partial seizures. The usual dose is 2–3 mg per day. The half-life can be up to 96 h; daily dosing is sufficient. The side effects include rash and osteomalacia as well as the toxic effects of fatigue, lethargy, and ataxia. Giving the drug once a day at the hour of sleep may alleviate some of the drowsiness. In terms of its interactions, it induces drug metabolism. Drugs that increase hepatic enzyme activity may lower phenobarbital levels, such as Coumadin, hydrocortisone and digoxin. When these drugs are given together, monitoring for lowered blood phenobarbital levels is necessary.

**PRIMIDONE.** Primidone (Mysoline) is a desoxy-barbiturate, and is also used for generalized tonic-clonic seizures and complex partial seizures. This drug is usually given as an adjunct or a second-line drug when an individual is refractory to other drugs. It acts to reduce sustained firing. The dosage is usually 10–15 mg/kg and the half-life is 12 h give or take 6 h. It has two active metabolites, phenobarbital and PEMA, which share the same toxicity, side effects, and drug interactions as phenobarbitol.

**BENZODIAZEPINES.** This class includes diazepam (Valium), lorazepam (Ativan), clonazepam (Klonopin), and clorazepate (Tranxene). They are used for status epilepticus and myoclonic seizures or as an adjunctive for generalized tonic-clonic seizures, complex partial seizures, and absence seizures. The drug group enhances GABA action. The drug class has few side effects. Toxic reactions are marked by sedation and fatigue. This class of drug has high fat solubility and protein binding. In primary care practice, clonazepam is used for myoclonic seizures.

Diazepam can be used orally and in IV dosing for status epilepticus. A new dosing method is diazepam administered rectally for prophylactic treatment of febrile seizures in children (Diastat). It can also be used as an adjunctive with severe convulsive seizure clusters. The usual dose is 0.5 mg/kg every 8 h when the fever is above 38.5° C. It is effective in reducing febrile seizures by approximately 30% (Morton, Rizkallah, & Pellock, 1997).

**GABAPENTIN.** This drug (Neurontin) is used as an adjunctive therapy in generalized tonic-clonic seizures and in complex partial seizures. Its mechanism of action is unknown, but it may act by blocking amino acid transport as well as inhibiting the breakdown of GABA and enhancing its release. A typical dosage is 2400 mg per day given in three divided doses. Its half-life is 5–7 h, and it is excreted unchanged in the urine; hence it has virtually no drug interactions. Toxic effects are fatigue, somnolence, ataxia, and dizziness. There are reports of irritability and dysphoric mood swings, requiring stoppage of this drug (Swartz, 1997). This is a relatively new drug with as yet no known side effects and no major reported drug interactions. It is also used to treat chronic pain.

**TIAGABINE.** Tiagabine (Gabitril) is useful as an adjunctive therapy for partial seizures with or without secondary generalization. It acts by blocking GABA uptake into neurons and glia, thus increasing the synaptic concentration of GABA and increasing inhibition. It is rapidly absorbed, reaching peak plasma concentrations within 2 hours, but its plasma concentration is affected as well by its reabsorption through the enterohepatic route. It is highly protein bound, and thus may interact with other drugs that are strongly protein bound, such as Dilantin and Depakote. It is extensively metabolized, and has a half-life of 5–8 hours. The usual dosing is from 32 to 56 mg/day in three divided doses. The major interactions are with metabolism inducers, such as Tegretol.

Toxicity is similar to other anti-seizure drugs, with dizziness, altered thinking, sedation, and tremulousness being the most common. Headache has also been reported. Recently released, few serious adverse events have been reported.

**VALPROATE SODIUM.** The mechanism of action of valproate sodium (Depakote) is unknown, although it does reduce repetitive firing and may also block T-type calcium currents. This drug is considered a drug of choice in primary generalized seizures; however, it also is useful in partial seizures. The dosage is 20–60 mg/kg. The half-life is 12 h. The drug binds with protein and has inactive metabolites.

The toxic effects are tremor, lethargy, and weight gain, and the side effects are nausea, vomiting, chemical hepatitis, and alopecia. Using sprinkles on food as an alternative dosing form is one way to prevent the nausea. L-carnitine 300 mg t.i.d. may help alleviate the low blood count. The hair loss and hair color and hair consistency change may be helped by using zinc and magnesium supplements. The weight gain can be alleviated by exercise and diet control. If polyuria occurs at high doses, avoiding dehydration is necessary. Valproate can decrease platelet count and function, resulting in increased bleeding. Aspirin and ibuprofen are consequently contraindicated. Because it binds protein strongly, it interacts with phenytoin, resulting in higher fractions of unbound drug, which may produce toxicity.

**VIGABATRIN.** This drug (Sabril), not yet released by the FDA, acts as a GABA analog that irreversibly inhibits GABA-T, the catabolic enzyme, reversibly inhibits GABA uptake, and enhances release of GABA. The net effect is to increase GABA-mediated inhibition. It is effective in a wide range of seizure models except absence and myoclonic seizures. It is rapidly and completely absorbed and is not significantly affected by other medications with little protein binding. The toxicity and side effects are high with one third of patients reporting adverse symptoms and over 5% having fatigue, dizziness, tremor, blurred vision, agitation, rash, anxiety, and possible psychosis. Drug levels and guidelines are not yet established.

***Drugs that act on glutamate receptors.*** Felbamate (Felbatol) and tapiramate (Topomax) are the only approved drugs available in the United States in this group. Felbatol acts by blocking NMDA receptors by inhibiting glycine modulation. Topiramate is a blocker at another glutamate receptor subtype, the AMPA receptor. Felbamate is used for generalized tonic-clonic seizures, either alone or as an adjunct drug. It is the drug of choice in children with Lennox-Gastaut syndrome. The dosage is 15–45 mg/kg. Toxic effects include weight loss, headaches, and insomnia. The side effects are nausea and aplastic anemia. Because the anemia can be fatal, informed consent and rigorous neurologic monitoring are required when this drug is prescribed. The drug increases levels of phenytoin, valproate, and carbamazepine by inhibiting their metabolism. The dose of any hepatically-metabolized drug may thus need to be reduced.

***Drugs that act on calcium channels.*** Ethosuximide (Zarontin) blocks T-type channels, interrupting oscillatory thalamocortical activations, the basis of primary generalized nonconvulsive (absence) seizures. Valproate may share this action.

Ethosuximide is used for absence seizures but has a "narrow spectrum" of activity, reducing its effectiveness in many patients (Derrigan & Fisher, 1997). The dosage is 20–60 mg/kg. Ethosuximide has a very long half-life of 30 h in children, and 50 h in adults. It does not easily bind to protein and has inactive metabolites. The toxic effects are headache, fatigue, dizziness, and hiccoughs. The side effects are rash and blood dyscrasias. The drug does interact with valproate and can precipitate absence status epilepticus.

Barbiturates, at very high dosages (status epilepticus) block peripheral high-voltage-activated calcium channels, which may result in cardiovascular suppression.

## Follow-up Recommendations

For 20% of epilepsy patients who have intractable seizures, referral from a neurologist to a comprehensive epilepsy center is warranted. Epilepsy centers can deal with difficult diagnoses and treat complicated seizure disorders of more than one type, try newer and experimental medications, and determine if surgical intervention (resection, implantation of vagal nerve stimulators) may be helpful in controlling the seizures.

## AUTHORS' NOTE

The authors would like to thank Mary Dombovy, MD, Stephanie Metzger, MS, Pediatric Nurse Practitioner, and Paddy Coates, MS, Family Nurse Practitioner, for their comments on sections of this chapter in an earlier draft.

## REFERENCES

### Traumatic head injury

Alexander, M. P. (1994). Survivors of traumatic brain injury. In *Current therapy in neurologic disease.*

Alexander, M. P. (1995). Mild traumatic brain injury: Pathophysiology, natural history, clinical management. *Neurology 45*, 1253–1260.

Cope, N. D. (1994). Head trauma destiny. In A. Christenson & B. P. Uzzell (Eds.), *Interactions of neuropharmacology and personality in brain injury and neuropsychological rehabilitation international perspectives.* Hillsdale, NJ: Laurence Erlbaum Associates.

Dombovy, M. L. (1997). Mechanisms of recovery following neurological injury and the role of rehabilitation. *Continuum: Lifelong Learning in Neurology, 3*(2).

Elovic, E., & Antoinette, T. (1996). Epidemiology and primary prevention of traumatic brain injury. In L. J. Horn and N. D. Zasler (Eds.), *Medical Rehabilitation of Traumatic Brain Injury.* Philadelphia: Hanley & Belfus.

Honing, L. S., & Albers, G. W. (1994). In J. M. Silver, S. C. Yudofsky, & R. E. Hales (Eds.), *Neuropharmacological treatment for acute brain injury.* Washington, DC: American Psychiatric Press.

Horn, L. J., & Zasler, N. D. (1996). *Medical rehabilitation of traumatic brain injury.* Philadelphia: Hanley and Belfus.

Kreutzer, J. S., Gervasio, A. H., & Camplair, P. S. (1994). Primary caregivers' psychological status and family functioning after traumatic brain injury. *Brain Injury, 8,* 197–210.

Levin, H. S., High, W. M., Goethe, K., Sisson, R. A., Overall, J. E., Rhoades, H. M., Eisenberg, H. M., Kalisky, Z., & Gary, H. E. (1987). The neurobehavioral rating scale: Assessment of the behavioral sequelae of head injury by the clinician. *Journal of Neurology, Neurosurgery and Psychiatry, 50,* 183–193.

Long, C. J., & Novack, T. A. (1986). Postconcussion symptoms after head trauma: Interpretation and treatment. *Southern Medical Journal, 79,* 728–732.

Serio, C. D., Kreutzer, J. S., & Gervasio, A. H. (1995). Predicting family needs after brain injury: Implications for intervention. *Journal of Head Trauma and Rehabilitation, 10*(2):32–45.

Silver, J. M., & Yudofsky, S. C. (1994). Pharmacology. In J. M. Silver, S. C. Yudofsky, & R. E. Hales (Eds.), *Psychopharmacology in neuropsychiatry of traumatic brain injury.* Washington, DC: American Psychiatric Press.

Stein, D. G., Glasier, M. M., & Hoffman, S. W. (1994). Pharmacological treatments for brain-injury repair. In A. Christenson & B. P. Uzzell (Eds.), *Progress and prognosis in brain injury and neuropsychological rehabilitation international perspectives.* Hillsdale, NJ: Laurence Erlbaum Associates.

Yablon, S. A. (1996). Posttraumatic Seizures. In L. J. Horn and N. D. Zasler (Eds.), *Medical Rehabilitation of Traumatic Brain Injury.* Philadelphia: Hanley & Belfus.

## Attention Deficit Disorder/Attention Deficit Hyperactivity Disorder

AHFS (1996). Drug Information. Gerald K. McEvoy, Ed. American Society of Health System Pharmacists.

Ahmann, P. A., Waltonen, S. J., Olson, K. A., Theye, F. W., Van Erem, A. J., LaPlant, R. J. (1993). Placebo-controlled evaluation of Ritalin side effects. *Pediatrics, 91*(6), 1101–1106.

American Psychiatric Association. (1994). *Diagnostic and Statistical Manual of Mental Disorders (DSM-IV).* Washington, DC: American Psychiatric Association.

Baren, M. (1994). ADHD: Do we finally have it right. *Contemporary Pediatrics, 11*(11), 96–124.

Barkley, R. A. (1995). *Taking charge of ADHD: The complete, authoritative guide for parents.* New York: The Guilford Press.

Barkley, R. A., Guevremont, D. C., Anastapoulos, A. D., DuPaul, G. J., & Shelton, T. L. (1993). Driving-related risks and outcomes of attention deficit hyperactivity disorder in adolescents and young adults: A 3- to 5-year follow-up survey. *Pediatrics, 92*(2), 212–219.

Berkovitch, M., Pope, E., Phillips, J., & Koren, G. (1995). Pemoline-associated fulminant liver failure: Testing the evidence for causation. *Clinical Pharmacology and Therapeutics, 57*(6), 696–698.

Biederman, J., Faraone, S., Milberger, S., Guite, J., Mick, E., Chen, L., Mennin, D., Marrs, A., Ouellette, C., Moore, P., Spencer, T., Norman, D., Wilens, T., Kraus, I., & Perrin, J. (1996). A prospective 4-year follow-up study of attention-deficit hyperactivity and related disorders. *Archives of General Psychiatry, 53,* 437–446.

Biederman, J., Faraone, S. V., Spencer, T., Wilens, T., Norman, D., Lapey, K. A., Mick, E., Lehman, B. K., Doyle, A. (1995). Patterns of psychiatric comorbidity, cognition, and psychosocial functioning in adults with attentional deficit hyperactivity disorder. *American Journal of Psychiatry, 1993; 150,* 1792–1798.

Blondis, T. A. (1996). Attention-deficit disorders and hyperactivity. In A. J. Capute & J. A. Pasquale, *Developmental Disabilities in Infancy and Childhood* (2nd ed.). Baltimore: Paul H. Brookes, pp. 417–436.

Blondis, T. A., & Roizen, N. J. (1996). Management of attention-deficit disorders and hyperactivity. In A. J. Capute & J. A. Pasquale, *Developmental Disabilities in Infancy and Childhood* (2nd ed.). Baltimore: Paul H. Brookes, pp. 437–449.

Carter, C. M., Urbanowicz, M., Hemsley, R., Mantilla, L., Strobel, S., Graham, P. J., & Taylor, E. (1993). Effects of a few food diets in attention deficit disorder. *Archives of Diseases of Childhood, 69,* 564–568.

DuPaul, G. J., & Castillo, A. (1995). The stimulants. In R. A. Barkley (Ed.), *Taking Charge of ADHD.* New York: Guilford Press.

Fargason, R. E., & Ford, C. V. (1994). Attention deficit hyperactivity disorder in adults: Diagnosis, treatment and prognosis. *Southern Medical Journal, 87*(3), 302–309.

Feifel, D. (1996). Attention-deficit hyperactivity disorder in adults. *Postgraduate Medicine, 100*(3), 207–218.

Halperin, J. M., Sharma, V., Siever, L. J., Schwartz, S. T., Matier, K., Wornell, G., & Newcorn, J. H. (1994). Serotonergic function in aggressive and nonaggressive boys with attention deficit hyperactivity disorder. *American Journal of Psychiatry, 151*(2), 243–248.

Hill, J. C., & Schoener, E. P. (1996). Age-dependent decline of attention deficit hyperactivity disorder. *American Journal of Psychiatry, 153,* 1143–1146.

Kent, J. D., Blader, J. C., Koplewicz, H. S., Abikoff, H., & Foley, C. A. (1995). Effects of late-afternoon methylphenidate administration on behavior and sleep in attention-deficit hyperactivity disorder. *Pediatrics* 96(2), 320–325.

Kessler, S. (1996). Drug therapy in attention-deficit hyperactivity disorder. *Southern Medical Journal*, 89(1), 33–38.

Lipkin, P. H., Goldstein, I. J., & Adesman, A. R. (1994). Tics and dyskinesias associated with stimulant treatment in attention-deficit hyperactivity disorder. *Archives of Pediatric Adolescent Medicine*, 148(8), 859–861.

Mannuzza, S., Klein, R. G., Bessler, A., Malloy, P., & LaPadula, M. (1993). Adult outcome of hyperactive boys. *Archives of General Psychiatry, 50*, 565–576.

Mercugliano, M. (1993). Psychopharmacology in children with developmental disabilities. *Pediatric Clinics of North America, 40*, 593–616.

Rappley, M. D., Gardiner, J. C., Jetton, J. R., & Houang, R. T. (1995). The use of methylphenidate in Michigan. *Archives of Pediatrics and Adolescent Medicine, 149*, 675–679.

Roizen, N. J., Blondis, T. A., Irwin, M., Rubinoff, A., Kieffer, J., & Stein, M. A. (1996). Psychiatric and developmental disorders in families of children with attention-deficit hyperactivity disorder. *Archives of Pediatrics and Adolescent Medicine, 150*, 203–208.

Safer, D. J., & Krager, J. M. (1994). The increased rate of stimulant treatment for hyperactive/inattentive students in secondary schools. *Pediatrics, 94*(8), 462–464.

Safer, D. J., Zito, J. M., & Fine, E. M. (1996). Increased methylphenidate usage for attention deficit disorder in the 1990s. *Pediatrics, 98*(6), 1084–1088.

Spencer, T., Wilens, T., Biederman, J., Faraone, S. V., Abion, S., & Lapey, K. (1995). A double-blind, crossover comparison of methylphenidate and placebo in adults with childhood-onset attention-deficit hyperactivity disorder. *Archives of General Psychiatry, 52*, 434–443.

Tirosh, E., Sadeh, A., Munvez, R., & Lavie, P. (1993). Effects of methylphenidate on sleep in children with attention-deficit hyperactivity disorder. *AJDC, 147*, 1313–1315.

Weiss, R., Stein, M. A., Trommer, B., & Refetoff, S. (1993). Attention-deficit hyperactivity disorder and thyroid dysfunction. *Journal of Pediatrics, 123*, 539–545.

Wender, E. H. (1995). Attention-deficit hyperactivity disorders in adolescence. *Journal of Developmental and Behavioral Pediatrics, 16*(3), 192–195.

Wilens, T. E., Biederman, J., Prince, J., Spencer, T. J., Faraone, S. V., Warburton, R., Schleifer, D., Harding, M., Linehan, C., & Geller, D. (1996). Six-week, double-blind, placebo-controlled study of disipramine for adult attention deficit hyperactivity disorder. *American Journal of Psychiatry, 153*, 1147–1152.

Wolraich, M. L., & Baumgaertel, A. (1997). The practical aspects of diagnosing and managing children with attention deficit hyperactivity disorder. *Clinical Pediatrics, 36*(9), 497–504.

## Stroke

American Hospital Formulary Service. (1996). Drug Information. Gerald K. McEvoy, Ed. American Society of Health System Pharmacists.

Arnold, M. O. (1993). Cardiovascular associations of stroke. In R. W. Teasell (Ed.), Long-term consequences of stroke. Physical medicine and rehabilitation. *State of the Art Reviews, 7*, 55–72.

Chan, F. L., Fong, K. Y., Law, C. B., Wong, A., & Woo, J. (1995). Low-molecular-weight heparin for the treatment of acute ischemic stroke. *New England Journal of Medicine, 333*(24), 1588–1593.

Chimowitz, M. I., Kokkinos, J., Strong, J., Brown, M. B., Levine, S. R., Silliman, S., et al. (1995). The warfarin-aspirin symptomatic intracranial disease study. *Neurology, 45*, 1488–1493.

Donnan, G. A., Davis, S. M., Chambers, B. R., Gates, P. C., Hankey, G. J., McNeil, J. J., Rosen, D., Stewart-Wayne, E. G., & Tuck, R. R. (1996). The Australian streptokinase (AKS) trial study group. *JAMA, 276*, 961–966.

Erkinjuntti, T., & Hachinski, V. C. (1993). Dementia post stroke. In R. W. Teasell (Ed.), Long-term consequences of stroke. Physical medicine and rehabilitation. *State of the Art Reviews, 7*, 195–212.

Gage, B. F., Cardinalli, A. B., Albers, G. W., & Owens, D. K. (1995). Cost-effectiveness of warfarin and aspirin for prophylaxis of stroke in patients with nonvalvular atrial fibrillation. *JAMA, 274*, 1839–1845.

Gasecki, A. P., & Hachinski, V. C. (1993). Stroke recurrence and prevention. In R. W. Teasell (Ed.), Long-term consequences of stroke. Physical medicine and rehabilitation. *State of the Art Reviews, 7*, 43–54.

Goldstein, L. B., & Sygen in Acute Stroke Study Investigators. (1995). Common drugs may influence motor recovery after stroke. *Neurology, 45*, 865–871.

Gresham, G. E. (Editor) and the Post-Stroke Rehabilitation Guideline Panel. (1995). *Post-stroke rehabilitation*. Clinical Practice Guideline No. 16, AHCPR Publication No. 95-0662. Rockville, MD: U.S. Department of Health and Human Services.

Grotta, J. C., Norris, J. W., Kamm, B., & the TASS Baseline and Angiographic Data Subgroup (1992). Prevention of stroke with ticlopidine: Who benefits most? *Neurology, 42*, 111–115.

Hacke, W., Kaste, M., Fieschi, C., Toni, D., Lesaffre, E., Kummer, R. V., Boyson, G., Bluhmki, E.,

Hoxter, G., Mahagne, M. H., & Hennerici, M. (ECASS Study Group). (1995). Intravenous thrombolysis with recombinant tissue plasminogen activator for acute hemispheric stroke. *JAMA, 274*(13), 1017–1025.

Harburn, K. L., & Potter, P. J. (1993). Spasticity and contractures. In R. W. Teasell (Ed.), Long-term consequences of stroke. Physical medicine and rehabilitation. *State of the Art Reviews, 7*, 113–132.

Kay, R., Wong, K. S., Ling, Y., Chan, Y. W., Tsoi, T. H., Ahuja, A. T., & Kenton, E. J. (1996). Diagnosis and treatment of concomitant hypertension and stroke. *JAMA, 88*, 364–368.

Margolis, S., & Preziosi, T. J. (1996). *Stroke.* Baltimore: The Johns Hopkins Medical Institutions.

Margolis, S., & Wityk, R. J. (1997). *Stroke.* Baltimore: The Johns Hopkins Medical Institutions.

National Institute of Neurological Disorders and Stroke rt-PA Stroke Study Group. (1995). Tissue plasminogen activator for acute ischemic stroke. *New England Journal of Medicine, 333*(24), 1581–1587.

O'Connell, J. E., & Gray, C. S. (1996). Atrial fibrillation and stroke prevention in the community. *Age and Aging, 25*, 307–308.

Potter, P. J. (1993). Lower extremity disorders. In R. W. Teasell (Ed.), Long-term consequences of stroke. Physical medicine and rehabilitation. *State of the Art Reviews, 7*, 147–160.

Silva-Smith, A. (1994). Reducing the risk of stroke in patients with chronic, nonvalvular atrial fibrillation. *Nurse Practitioner, 19*(2), 38–44.

Swartzman, L., & Teasell, R. W. (1993). Psychological consequences of stroke. In R. W. Teasell (Ed.), Long-term consequences of stroke. Physical medicine and rehabilitation. *State of the Art Reviews, 7*, 179–194.

Teasell, R. W., & Gillen, M. (1993). Upper extremity disorders and pain following stroke. In R. W. Teasell (Ed.), Long-term consequences of stroke. Physical medicine and rehabilitation. *State of the Art Reviews, 7*, 133–146.

Unwin, D. H., & Greenlee, R. G. (1993). Prophylactic drug therapy in cerebrovascular disease. *American Family Physician, 48*, 85–90.

Wiebe-Velazquez, S. & Blume, W. T. (1993). Seizures. In R. W. Teasell (Ed.), Long-term consequences of stroke. Physical medicine and rehabilitation. *State of the Art Reviews, 7*, 73–88.

## Multiple Sclerosis

Anderson, P., & Goodkin, D. E. (1996). Current pharmacologic treatment of multiple sclerosis symptoms. *Western Journal of Medicine, 165*, 313–317.

Dombovy, M. L. (1997). Neuro-rehabilitation. *Continuum: Lifelong Learning in Neurology, 3*(2), 130–132.

Donker, G. A., Foets, M., & Spreeuwenberg, P. (1996). Multiple sclerosis: Management in Dutch general practice. *Family Practice, 13*(5), 439–444.

Donohoe, K. M. (1995). Autoimmune disorders. In E. Barker (Ed.), *Neuroscience nursing* (pp. 559–585). St. Louis: C. V. Mosby.

Dressnandt, J., & Conrad, B. (1996). Lasting reduction of severe spasticity after ending chronic treatment with intrathecal baclofen. *Journal of Neurology, Neurosurgery and Psychiatry, 60*, 168–173.

Gidal, B. E., Wagner, M. L., Privetera, M. D., Dalmady-Isreal, C., Crismon, M. L., Fagan, S. C., & Graves, N. M. (1996). Current developments in neurology, part I: Advances in the pharmacotherapy of headache, epilepsy, and multiple sclerosis. *Annals of Pharmacotherapy, 30*, 1272–1276.

Jacobs, L. D., Cookfair, D. L., Rudick, R. A., Herndon, R. M., Richert, J. R., Salazar, A. M., et al. (1996). Intramuscular interferon beta-1a for disease progression in relapsing multiple sclerosis. *Annals of Neurology, 39*, 285–294.

Johnson, K. P. (1996). A review of the clinical efficacy profile of copolymer 1: New U.S. phase III trial data. *Journal of Neurology, 243* (Suppl. 1), S3–S7.

Kelly, C. L. (1996). The role of interferons in the treatment of multiple sclerosis. *Journal of Neuroscience Nursing, 24*, 114–120.

Marshall, L. L., & Ragland, D. (1996). Therapeutic management of multiple sclerosis. *Pharmacist*, 41–55.

NeuroCommunications Research Laboratories and Department of Neuroscience at the Institute for Biomedical Engineering and Rehabilitations Services of Touro College. (1996). Estrogen's impact on cognitive functions in multiple sclerosis. *International Journal of Neuroscience, 86*, 23–31.

Rochester Multiple Sclerosis Clinic Patient Information Sheet. (1993). Beta interferon (Betaseron) Strong Memorial Hospital, Rochester, NY.

Rochester Multiple Sclerosis Clinic Patient Information Sheet (1995). Methatrexate as a treatment for multiple sclerosis. Strong Memorial Hospital, Rochester, NY.

Rochester Multiple Sclerosis Clinic Patient Information Sheet. (1996). Cytaxan. Strong Memorial Hospital, Rochester, NY.

Rodgers, J., & Bland, R. (1996). Psychiatric manifestations of multiple sclerosis: A review. *Canadian Journal of Psychiatry, 41*, 441–445.

Rudick, R. A. (1993). Multiple sclerosis. In R. T. Johnson & J. W. Griffin, (Eds.). *Current therapy in neurologic disease*, (pp. 158–163). St. Louis: C. V. Mosby.

Sandyk, R. (1996). Estrogen's impact on cognitive functions in multiple sclerosis. *International Journal of Neuroscience, 86*, 23–31.

Scott, T. F., Allen, D., Price, T. R. P., McConnell, H., & Lang, D. (1996). Characterization of major depression in symptoms in multiple sclerosis patients. *Journal of Neuropsychiatry and Clinical Neurosciences, 8*, 318–323.

Sketris, I. S., Brown, M., Murray, T. J., Fisk, J. D., & McLean, K. (1996). Drug therapy in multiple sclerosis: A study of Nova Scotia senior citizens. *Clinical Therapeutics, 18*(2), 303–318.

Swain, S. E. (1996). Multiple sclerosis primary health care implications. *Nurse Practitioner, 21*, 40–54.

## Vertigo

*American Hospital Formulatory Service* (1996). Drug Information. Bethesda, Maryland. American Society of Health Systems Pharmacists.

Baloh, R. W. (1994). Approach to the dizzy patient. *Baillieres Clinical Neurology, 3*(3), 453–465.

Brantberg, K., Bergenius, J., & Tribukait, A. (1996). Gentamicin treatment in peripheral vestibular disorders other than Meniere's disease. *ORL, 58,* 277–279.

Driscoll, C., Kasperbauer, J. L., Facer, G. W., Harner, S. G., & Beatty, C. W. (1997). Low-dose intratympanic gentamicin and the treatment of Meniere's disease: Preliminary results. *Laryngoscope, 107,* 83–89.

Fujino, A., Tokumasu, K., Okamoto, M., Naganuma, H., Hoshino, I., Arai, M., & Yoneda, S. (1996). Vestibular training for acute unilateral vestibular disturbances: Its efficacy in comparison with antivertigo drug. *Acta Oto-laryngologica,* (Suppl. 524), 21–26.

Gans, R. E. (1996). *Vestibular rehabilitation: Protocols and programs.* San Diego: Singular Publishing Group.

Grizzi, M. (1995). The efficacy of vestibular rehabilitation for patients with head trauma. *Journal of Head Injury Trauma, 10*(6), 60–77.

Hain, T. C. (1997). Vertigo and dysequilibrium. In R. T. Johnson, & J. W. Griffin (Eds.), *Current therapy in neurologic disease* (pp. 8–13). St. Louis: C. V. Mosby.

Hirsch, B. E., & Kamerer, D. B. (1997). Intratympanic gentamicin therapy for Meniere's disease. *American Journal of Otology, 18,* 44–51.

Knox & McPherson (1997)

Linstrom, C. J., & Gleich, L. L. (1993). Otosyphilis: Diagnostic and therapeutic update. *Journal of Otolaryngology, 22*(6), 401–408.

Luetje, C. M., & Wooten, J. (1996, April). Clinical manifestations of transdermal scopolamine addiction. *Ear, Nose and Throat Journal,* 210–214.

Rascol, O., Hain, T. C., Brefel, C., Benazet, M., Clanet, M., & Mostastruc, J-L. (1995). Antivertigo medications and drug-induced vertigo: A pharmacological review. *Drugs, 50*(5), 777–791.

Shea, J. J., Jr., & Gee, X. (1996). Dexamethasone perfusion of the labyrinth plus intravenous dexamethasone for Meniere's disease. *Otolaryngolic Clinics of North America, 29*(2), 358–368, April.

## Dementia

Alzheimer's Association (1996). Facts about donepezil hydrochloride and Alzheimer's disease.

American Psychiatric Association. (1997). Practice guideline for the treatment of patients with Alzheimer's disease and other dementias of late life. *American Journal of Psychiatry, 154*(5 Suppl.), 1–33.

Applegate, W. B., & Burns, R. (1996). Geriatric medicine. *JAMA, 275*(23), 1892–1893.

Birge, S. J. (1996). Is there a role for estrogen replacement therapy in the prevention and treatment of dementia? *Journal of the American Geriatric Society, 44,* 865–870.

Chan, R. K. T., & Hachinski, V. C. (1997). The other dementias. In *Current therapy in neurologic disease* (pp. 311–314). St. Louis: C. V. Mosby.

Clipp, E. C., & Moore, M. J. (1995). Caregiver time use: An outcome measure in clinical trial research on Alzheimer's disease. *Clinical Pharmacology and Therapeutics, 58,* 228–236.

Costa, P. T., Williams, T. F., Albert, M. S., Butters, N. M., Folstein, M. F., Gilman, S., et al. (1996). *Recognition and initial assessment of Alzheimer's disease and related dementias.* Clinical Practice Guideline No. 19. AHCPR No. 97-0702. Rockville, MD: U.S. Department of Health Care Policy Research.

Gidal, B. E., Crismon, M. L., Wagner, M. L., Fagan, S. C., Privitera, M. D., Dalmady-Isreal, C., & Graves, N. M. (1996). Current developments in neurology, Part II: Alzheimer's disease, Parkinson's disease and stroke. *Annals of Pharmacotherapy, 30,* 1446–1451.

Hollister, L., & Gruber, N. (1996). Drug treatment of Alzheimer's disease. Effects on caregiver burden and patient quality of life. *Drugs and Aging, 8*(1), 47–56.

Kawas, C., & Morrison, A. (1997). Alzheimer's disease and other dementias. In *Current therapy in neurologic disease* (pp. 303–311). St. Louis: C. V. Mosby.

Knopman, M. D., Schneider, L., Davis, K., Talwalker, S., Smith, F., Hoover, T., Gracon, S., & the

Tacrine Study Group (1996). Long-term tacrine (Cognex) treatment: Effects on nursing home placement and mortality. *Neurology, 47,* 166–177.

Mace, N. L. (1981). *The 35-hour day.* Baltimore: Johns Hopkins University Press.

Mohs, R. C. (1996). The Alzheimer's Disease Assessment Scale. *International Psychogeriatrics, 8*(2), 195–203.

Schneider, L. S. (1996). New therapeutic approaches to Alzheimer's disease. *Journal of Clinical Psychiatry, 57* (Suppl. 14), 30–36.

Schneider, L. S., Farlow, M. R., Henderson, V. W., & Pogoda, J. M. (1996). Effects of estrogen replacement therapy on response to tacrine in patients with Alzheimer's disease. *Neurology, 46,* 1580–1584.

Smucker, W. D. (1996). Maximizing function in Alzheimer's disease: What role for tacrine? *American Family Physician, 54*(2), 645–652.

Sunderland, T. (1996). Treatment of the elderly suffering from psychosis and dementia. *Journal of Clinical Psychiatry, 57* (Suppl. 9), 53–56.

Thal, L. J., Schwartz, G., Sano, M., Weiner, M., Knopman, D., Harrell, L., Bodenheimer, S., Rossor, M., Philpot, M., Schor, J., & Goldberg, A. for the Psysostigmine Study Group. (1996). A multicenter double-blind study of controlled-release physostigmine for the treatment of symptoms secondary to Alzheimer's disease. *Neurology, 47,* 1389–1395.

Wilcock, G. K., & Harrold, P. L. (1996). Treatment of Alzheimer's disease: Future directions. *Acta Neurologica Scandinavica,* (Suppl. 165), 128–136.

Woo, J. K., & Lantz, M. S. (1995). Alzheimer's disease: How to give and monitor tacrine therapy. *Geriatrics, 50*(5), 50–53.

## Headache

Bristol-Myers Products. (1995). *The Excedrin headache relief update.* West Caldwell, NJ: Bristol-Meyers.

de Lissovoy, G., & Lazarus, S. S. (1994). The economic cost of migraine. *Neurology, 44* (Suppl. 4), S56–S62.

Drugs for Migraines. (1995). *The Medical Letter, 37*(943), 17–20.

Goadsby, P. J. (1997). Concepts of the pathophysiology of migraine. In N. T. Mathew (Ed.), *Neurologic Clinics, 15*(1), 27–42.

Lipton, R. B., & Stewart, W. F. (1997). Prevalence and impact of migraine. In N. T. Mathew (Ed.), *Neurologic Clinics, 15*(1), 2–14.

MacGregor, E. A. (1997). Menstruation, sex hormones, and migraine. In N. T. Mathew (Ed.), *Neurologic Clinics, 15*(1), 126–141.

Mathew, N. T. (1997). Serotonin 1d (5-HT1d) agonists and other agents in acute migraine. In N. T. Mathew (Ed.), *Neurologic Clinics, 15*(1), 61–84.

Mathew, N. T. (1997). Transformed migraine, analgesic rebound, and other chronic daily headaches. In N. T. Mathew (Ed.), *Neurologic Clinics, 15*(1), 167–185.

Merikangas, K. R., & Stevens, D. E. (1997). Comorbidity of migraine and psychiatric disorders. In N. T. Mathew (Ed.), *Neurologic Clinics, 15*(1), 115–124.

Raskin, N. H. (1994). Headache. *Western Journal of Medicine, 161,* 299–302.

Rothner, A. D. (1997). Headache in children and adolescents. In R. T. Johnson & J. W. Griffin (Eds.), *Current therapy in neurologic disease* (pp. 95–99). St. Louis: C. V. Mosby.

Sheftell, F. D. (1997). Role and impact of over-the-counter medications in the management of headache. In N. T. Mathew (Ed.), *Neurologic Clinics, 15*(1), 187–198.

Silberstein, S. D. (1993). Office management of benign headache. *Postgraduate Medicine, 93*(1), 223–240.

Silberstein, S. D., Young, W. B., & Lipton, R. B. (1997). Migraine and cluster headaches. In R. T. Johnson & J. W. Griffin (Eds.), *Current therapy in neurologic disease* (pp. 85–92). St. Louis: C. V. Mosby.

Solomon, S. (1997). Diagnosis of primary headache disorders: Validity of the International Headache Society criteria in clinical practice. In N. T. Mathew (Ed.), *Neurologic Clinics, 15*(1), 15–26.

Welsh, L. M. A., & Lewis, D. (1997). Migraine and epilepsy. In N. T. Mathew (Ed.), *Neurologic Clinics, 15*(1), 107–114.

## Parkinson's Disease

Ahlskig, J. E. (1996). Treatment of early Parkinson's disease: Are complicated strategies justified? *Mayo Clinic Proceedings, 71,* 659–670.

Alexander, G. E. (1997). Parkinson's disease. In R. T. Johnson & J. W. Griffin (Eds.), *Current therapy in neurologic disease* (pp. 268–274). St. Louis: C. V. Mosby.

Hely, M. A., & Morris, J. G. L. (1996). Controversies in the treatment of Parkinson's disease. *Current Opinion in Neurology, 9,* 308–313.

Myllyla, V. V., Sotaniemi, D. A., Hakulinen, P., Maki-Ikola, O., & Heinonen, E. H. (1997). Selegiline as the primary treatment of Parkinson's disease—A long-term double-blind study. *Acta Neurologica Scandinovica, 95,* 211–218.

Olanow, C. W., & Koller, W. C. (1998). An algorithm for the management of Parkinson's disease: treatment guidelines. *Neurology, 50* (suppl 3), s1–s57.

Richard, I. H., Kurlan, M. D., Tanner, C., Factor, S., Hubble, J., Suchowerski, M. D., Waters, C., the Parkinson Study Group (1997). Serotonin syndrome and the combined use of deprenyl and an antidepressant in Parkinson's disease. *Neurology, 48,* 1070–1077.

Silberstein, P. M. (1996). Moderate Parkinson's disease. Strategies for maximizing treatment. *Postgraduate Medicine, 96*(1), 52–68.

Stacy, M., & Brownlee, H. J. (1996). Treatment options for early Parkinson's disease. *American Family Physician,* 1281–1287.

Stern, M. B. (1994). Movement disorders. In R. T. Johnson & J. W. Griffin (Eds.), *Current therapy in neurological disease* (pp. 242–246). St. Louis: C. V. Mosby.

Stern, M. B. (1997). Contemporary approaches to the pharmacotherapeutic management of Parkinson's disease: An overview. *Neurology, 49* (Suppl. 1), 82–89.

## Seizure Disorders

Berg, A., & Shinnar, S. (1994). The contributions of epidemiology to the understanding of childhood seizures and epilepsy. *Journal of Child Neurology,* 9 (Suppl.), 2S19–2S26.

## ADDITIONAL NOTE: PARKINSON'S DISEASE

The most recent complete guidelines for the comprehensive treatment of Parkinson's disease, usually conducted in collaboration with a neurologist, can be found as a supplement in the journal *Neurology*, published in March 1998. These guidelines include algorithms for pharmacologic and nonpharmacologic treatment, in-

Cascino, G. D. (1994). Epilepsy: Contemporary perspectives on evaluation and treatment. *Mayo Clinic Proceedings, 69,* 1199–1211.

Derrigan, J. F., & Fisher, R. S. (1997). Recurrent generalized and partial seizures. In R. T. Johnson & J. W. Griffin (Eds.), *Current therapy in neurologic disease* (pp. 47–60). St. Louis: C. V. Mosby.

McMicken, D. B., & Freedland, E. S. (1994). Alcohol-related seizures. *Emergency Medicine Clinics of North America, 12*(4), 1057–1073.

Morton, L. D., Rizkallah, E., & Pellock, J. M. New drug therapy for acute seizure management. *Seminars in Pediatric Neurology, 4*(1), 51–63.

Pellock, J. M. (1993). Status epilepticus. In W. E. Dodson & J. M. Pellock. *Pediatric Epilepsy: Diagnosis and Therapy.* New York: Demos Publications.

Swartz, B. E. (1997). Complex partial seizures. In R. T. Johnson & J. W. Griffin (Eds.), *Current therapy in neurologic disease* (pp. 55–60). St. Louis: C. V. Mosby.

Welty, T. E., Pickering, P. R., Hale, B. C., & Aruzi, R. (1992). Loss of seizure control associated with generic substitution of carbamazepine. *Annals of Pharmacotherapy, 26,* 775–777.

Williams, J., Grant, M., Jackson, M., Sherma, S. J., Sharp, G., Griebel, M., et al. (1996). Behavioral descriptors that differentiate between seizure and nonseizure events in a pediatric population. *Clinical Pediatrics,* 243–249.

Zacharowicz, I., & Moshe, S. L. (1995). Antiepileptic drug therapy in younger patients: When to start, when to stop. *Cleveland Clinic Journal of Medicine, 62,* 176–183.

cluding algorithms for exercise, support, nutrition, and problems associated with Parkinson's disease, such as dysautonomias, falls, motor complications, neuropsychiatric problems, and sleep disorders. In the pharmacologic treatment plan, algorithms are presented for no response, suboptimal peak response, "wearing off" response, unpredictable "on" and "off" response, and freezing (motor blocks) (Olanow & Koller, 1998).

# 30

# ENDOCRINE DISORDERS: THYROID AND ADRENAL CONDITIONS

*Jeanne Archer and Michael S. Monaghan*

The endocrine system helps the body respond to changes from stressors like temperature, injury, electrolyte imbalances, changes in osmolality, or shock (Toto, 1994). Its purpose is to maintain a steady internal state in response to stimuli. Two components of the endocrine system, the thyroid gland and the adrenal gland are discussed in this chapter as well as the conditions that may arise from disorders associated with these glands.

## THYROID CONDITIONS

Metabolically, the thyroid gland and thyroid hormones influence virtually all cellular function. Normal growth and development depend on appropriate production of thyroid hormones. Conditions affecting the thyroid are common, occurring in approximately 10% of the general population (Sawin, Castelli, Hershman, McNamara, & Bacharach, 1985). Women are more frequently affected, at a three to four times greater rate. Further, the prevalence of thyroid conditions increases significantly with age (Shetty & Duthie, 1995). The first part of this chapter addresses the two major divisions of thyroid conditions: hypothyroidism and hyperthyroidism. Thyroid conditions as they pertain to children, the pregnant, and the elderly are then discussed, followed by drug-induced changes in thyroid function.

## NORMAL THYROID FUNCTION

Thyroid hormones, thyroxine ($T_4$) and triodothyronine ($T_3$), are iodinated complexes synthesized and stored in the thyroid. $T_3$ is more physiologically active, having a biological half-life of approximately 1.5 days. $T_4$ is the major hormone circulating in blood, but is less physiologically active. $T_4$ has a longer biological half-life, up to 1 week (Reasner & Talbert, 1997; Wartofsky, 1994). $T_4$, though active, serves mainly as a reserve for $T_3$. $T_4$ can be converted to $T_3$ peripherally when increased thyroid hormone activity is required. Only about 20% of circulating $T_3$ is secreted by the thyroid; the majority is peripherally converted from $T_4$ (Reasner and Talbert, 1997; Wartofsky, 1994).

Production and release of thyroid hormones are minutely regulated by the hypothalamic-pituitary-thyroid axis; see Figure 30–1. Changes in concentration of circulating $T_3$ and $T_4$ produce positive or negative stimuli to the hormonal regulation of the thyroid gland. Thyrotropin-releasing hormone (TRH) is released by the hypothalamus when concentrations of $T_3$ and $T_4$ drop below normal. TRH then stimulates the release of thyrotropin, also known as thyroid-stimulating hormone (TSH), which stimulates thyroid synthesis and release of $T_3$ and $T_4$. When adequate concentrations of circulating $T_3$ and $T_4$ are achieved, negative feedback stops further TSH release (Fig. 30–1) (Larsen, 1982). Again, the majority of circulating $T_3$ is generated through peripheral conversion. Peripheral conversion of

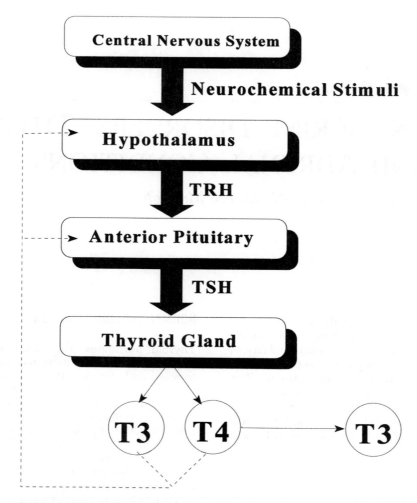

**Figure 30–1.** Hypothalamic-pituitary-thyroid axis illustrating the positive (heavy black arrows) and negative feedback (dashed arrows) stimuli that affect the hormonal regulators thyrotropin-releasing hormone (TRH) and thyrotropin (ie, thyroid-stimulating hormone, TSH).

$T_4$ to $T_3$ is stimulated by cold temperatures. Peripheral conversion is inhibited by acute illness, chronic illness, starvation, and some medications, see Table 30–1 (Vanderpump & Tunbridge, 1993). Together, the negative feedback process and peripheral conversion allow acute regulation of thyroid hormone synthesis and activity.

## THYROID FUNCTION TESTS

Thyroid function tests (TFTs) are used to evaluate thyroid function and as a screening mechanism for the detection of thyroid conditions. Table 30–2 lists the common TFTs, their normal ranges, and findings in hypo- and hyperthyroidism (Hershman, Ladenson, & Paulshock, 1992). The initial laboratory test for evaluating thyroid conditions is the sensitive TSH assay (Brody & Reichard, 1995). The result from this measurement may then be used to determine which, if any, additional tests should be performed. One possible algorithm for use of TFTs in evaluating thyroid conditions is given in Figure 30–2 (Hershman et al, 1992). Once an abnormality in TSH is detected, a review of the patient's medications may provide the explanation (Smith, 1995). A number of medications can affect thyroid function, both clinically and subclinically. A drug-induced cause for the ab-

## TABLE 30–1. ADVERSE EFFECTS OF DRUGS ON THYROID FUNCTION

| Thyroid Function Affected | Drug | Comments |
|---|---|---|
| TSH response to TRH | Phenytoin | Decreases TSH response to TRH by up to 50%. Mechanism: enhancing cellular uptake and metabolism of $T_4$. |
| | High-dose salicylates | Doses of about 4.0 g suppress TSH response. Mechanism: displacement of thyroid hormones from thyroid-binding globulin (TBG). |
| | Levodopa | Chronic therapy suppresses TSH response. Mechanism: displacement of thyroid hormones from TBG. |
| | Glucocorticoids | Impair basal and TRH-stimulated TSH concentrations. |
| | Dopamine blockers (ie, neuroleptics) | Increase basal TSH and enhance TSH response to TRH. |
| | Theophylline | Increase TSH response through beta-adrenergic stimulation of the hypothalamus. |
| Euthyroid hypothyroxinemia (clinically insignificant) | Phenytoin | Therapeutic doses decrease total $T_4$ ($TT_4$) by increasing metabolism of $T_4$. High doses can also impair binding of $T_4$ and $T_3$ to TBG. |
| | Carbamazepine | Decreases $TT_4$ by increasing metabolism of $T_4$. |
| | High-dose salicylates | Inhibit binding of $T_4$ and $T_3$ by TBG and prealbumin. |
| Euthyroid hyperthyroxinemia (clinically insignificant) | Cholecystographic agents (ie, gallbladder dyes) | Inhibit peripheral conversion of $T_4$ to $T_3$. |
| | Propranolol, nadolol | Inhibit peripheral conversion of $T_4$ to $T_3$. |
| | Amiodarone | Inhibit peripheral conversion of $T_4$ to $T_3$. |
| | Estrogen preparations | Cause an increase in TBG values. |
| Hypothyroidism | Amiodarone | Release of iodine as drug is metabolized. Clinically significant in up to 10% of patients. |
| | Lithium | Blocks iodine uptake by the thyroid and release of thyroid hormones. Clinically significant in about 2% of patients. |
| Hyperthyroidism | Amiodarone | Released iodine can induce thyrotoxicosis. Clinically significant in about 3% of patients on long-term therapy. |

*Adapted from Vanderpump & Tunbridge (1993) with permission.*

normal TSH measurement must be ruled out before further diagnostic investigation is pursued. [Refer back to Table 30–1 for common medications known to adversely affect thyroid function (Vanderpump & Tunbridge, 1993).]

Thyroid conditions may be classified as clinical or subclinical, based on presenting signs and symptoms in conjunction with TFT results (Smith, 1995). A patient with clinical or overt disease presents with signs and symptoms typically associated with hypo- or hyperthyroidism.

Generally, *subclinical* implies an asymptomatic or presymptomatic status based on the measurements of TFTs. For example, a symptomatic patient with a high TSH and a low $T_4$ is classified as having clinical or overt hypothyroidism. A symptomatic patient with a low TSH and a high $T_4$ is classified as having overt hyperthyroidism. An asymptomatic patient with a high TSH and a normal $T_4$ has subclinical hypothyroidism. An asymptomatic patient with a low TSH and a normal $T_4$ has subclinical hyperthyroidism. Again,

## TABLE 30–2. COMMON THYROID FUNCTION TESTS (TFTs) USED FOR EVALUATION

| Test | Normal Range[a] | Comments |
|---|---|---|
| Thyrotropin (thyroid stimulating hormone, ie, TSH) | 0.5–5.5 mU/L | Elevated in primary hypothyroidism (may be >10); low or normal in pituitary/hypothalamic-related disease; low or undetectable in hyperthyroidism. |
| Total (free and bound) thyroxine ($TT_4$) | 5.0–11.0 µg/dL | Elevated in hyperthyroidism; low in hypothyroidism. |
| Free thyroxine ($FT_4$) | 0.6–2.1 ng/dL | Elevated in hyperthyroidism; low in hypothyroidism. |
| Total (free and bound) triiodothyronine ($TT_3$) | 88–160 ng/dL | Useful in detecting mild hyperthyroidism; less so for mild hypothyroidism. |
| Triiodothyronine resin uptake ($RT_3U$) | 26–35% | Estimates the number of unoccupied binding sites (inverse relationship, ie, a high $RT_3U$ indicates few unoccupied binding sites). Elevated in hyperthyroidism; low in hypothyroidism and thyroxine-binding globulin (TBG) excess. |
| Free thyroxine index ($FT_4I$) | 1.3–3.9 µg/dL | Calculated as the product of $RT_3U \times T_4$. Aids in interpreting abnormal $T_4$ levels due to elevation or depression of thyroid binding globulin levels (eg, if total $T_4$ levels are elevated due to increase TBG, $RT_3U$ will be depressed, indicating a high amount of binding sites and the $FT_4I$ will be normal). |

[a] Normal values may vary based on the laboratory.

*Adapted from Hershman et al (1992) with permission.*

medications may produce TFT abnormalities in asymptomatic patients (Table 30–1). TFTs in patients on phenytoin or high-dose salicylates show a normal TSH and a low $T_4$. In patients on amiodarone or estrogen preparations, LFTs show a normal TSH and a high $T_4$ (Smith, 1995).

## HYPOTHYROIDISM

Hypothyroidism refers to the clinical syndrome caused by undersecretion of thyroid hormone from the gland ("AACE Clinical Practice Guidelines," 1995). Hypothyroidism may be classified as primary or secondary, based on the etiology. Primary hypothyroidism, by far the more common of the two, is caused by thyroid gland dysfunction. Secondary hypothyroidism, a relatively rare occurrence, is caused by failure of the hypothalamic-pituitary-thyroid axis due to pituitary or hypothalamic disease. Patients with secondary hypothyroidism generally present with other endocrine abnormalities such as adrenal insufficiency or hypogonadism. Table 30–3 lists major causes of hypothyroidism.

Symptoms of hypothyroidism may be nonspecific and vary among patients depending on gender, age, duration and severity of disease, and rapidity of onset of the deficiency ("AACE Clinical Practice Guidelines," 1995). Table 30–4 lists common signs and symptoms of hypothyroidism (Dong, 1995).

## HYPERTHYROIDISM

Hyperthyroidism refers to the clinical syndrome produced by the body's exposure to the excessive action of thyroid hormone ("AACE Clinical Practice Guidelines," 1995). Common causes of hyperthyroidism are listed in Table 30–5 (Franklyn, 1994). Graves' disease is the most common cause of hyperthyroidism. Like Hashimoto's thyroiditis, it is an autoimmune disorder thought to be inherited secondary to familial clustering (Johnson & Felicetta, 1992).

Symptoms of hyperthyroidism are caused by the action of supraphysiologic thyroid hormone and vary among patients depending on age, duration of disease, and the magnitude of circulat-

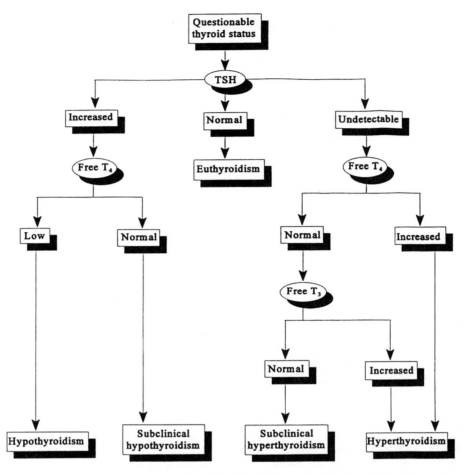

**Figure 30–2.** An algorithm for the evaluation of thyroid conditions using laboratory data, including measurements of serum thyrotropin (ie, thyroid stimulating hormone, TSH), free $T_4$, and free $T_3$.

**Source:** Adapted from Caldwell et al (1985) with permission.

ing hormonal excess ("AACE Clinical Practice Guidelines," 1995). Elderly patients often present without classic signs and symptoms of hyperthyroidism, but almost always present with some cardiac manifestation (eg, congestive heart failure, atrial fibrillation, and angina) (Gambert, 1995). Table 30–6 lists common signs and symptoms of hyperthyroidism (Dong, 1995).

## SPECIFIC CONSIDERATIONS FOR PHARMACOTHERAPY

### When Drug Therapy Is Needed

The benefits of drug therapy must always outweigh risks before therapy is instituted. The need for drug therapy is based on the answers to two questions: (1) Is the patient experiencing signs and symptoms of disease? (2) What is the magnitude of abnormalities in TFTs? Once a diagnosis of clinical disease or subclinical disease is reached (refer to Fig. 30–2), the decision to institute drug therapy must be individualized.

*Hypothyroidism.* In children with hypothyroidism, growth and mental development depend on adequate hormonal therapy (Rogers, 1994). Since the function of virtually all organ systems depends on the euthyroid state, prompt treatment of clinical hypothyroidism is necessary. Treatment of subclinical hypothyroidism, common in the elderly, is more controversial

**TABLE 30–3. MAJOR CAUSES OF PRIMARY AND SECONDARY HYPOTHYROIDISM**

| Classification | Mechanism | Etiology |
|---|---|---|
| **Primary** | | |
| | Thyroid destruction | Chronic inflammation (ie, Hashimoto's thyroiditis) |
| | | Surgical thyroid gland removal |
| | | Radioiodine thyroid gland ablation |
| | | External irradiation |
| | Thyroid deficiency | Iodine deficiency—lack of hormonal substrate |
| | | Iodine excess—interference with hormone release |
| | | Drug-induced (ie, amiodarone, lithium) |
| **Secondary** | | |
| | Deficiency of TSH | Pituitary disease |
| | Deficiency of TRH | Hypothalamic disease |

(Sawin, 1991). Poor left ventricular function and an increase in serum cholesterol are associated with thyroid dysfunction. Subclinical hypothyroidism may be associated with thyroid dysfunction. Subclinical hypothyroidism may be associated with coronary heart disease in both men and women (Bansal, Sahi, Basu, and Old, 1986; Tieche et al, 1981). Although irrefutable benefit has yet to be demonstrated, most endocrinologists treat subclinical hypothyroidism ("AACE Clinical Practice Guidelines," 1995). An individualized approach to the introduction of drug therapy must be taken. For example, thyroid replacement may aggravate preexisting myocardial ischemia in the elderly, and some cardiac intervention (eg, coronary artery bypass graft) may be necessary prior to initiating replacement therapy to ensure benefit from drug therapy (Stockigt, 1993). Hypothyroidism in pregnancy is associated with gestational hypertension, premature labor, and low-birth-weight infants (Bishnoi & Sachmechi, 1996). Therapy can decrease neonatal morbidity.

*Hyperthyroidism.*    Again, to maximize organ function, treatment of clinical hyperthyroidism is necessary. Hyperthyroidism can produce cardiomegaly and heart failure in newborns, as well as interfering with normal growth during adolescence (Rogers, 1994). In the elderly, untreated

**TABLE 30–4. COMMON SIGNS AND SYMPTOMS OF HYPOTHYROIDISM**

| Signs | Symptoms |
|---|---|
| Thin brittle nails | Weakness, tiredness, lethargy, fatigue |
| Thinning of skin | Cold intolerance |
| Pallor | Headache |
| Puffiness of face | Loss of taste and/or smell |
| Yellowing of skin | Deafness |
| Thinning of outer eyebrows | Hoarseness |
| Thickening of tongue | Absence of sweating |
| Peripheral edema | Modest weight gain |
| Decreased deep tendon reflexes | Muscle cramps |
| Pleural/peritoneal/pericardial effusions | Slow speech |
| Bradycardia | Angina |
| Hypertension | Constipation |
| Goiter | Menorrhagia and/or galactorrhea |

*Adapted from Young and Koda-Kimble (1995) with permission.*

## TABLE 30–5. MAJOR CAUSES OF HYPERTHYROIDISM

- Graves' disease (diffuse toxic goiter)
- Toxic adenoma (Plummer's nodule)
- Toxic multinodular goiter
- Painful subacute thyroiditis (viral etiology, de Quervain's thyroiditis)
- Silent thyroiditis (lymphocytic and postpartum variations)
- Iodine-induced hyperthyroidism
- Excessive pituitary TSH or trophoblastic disease
- Excessive therapy with thyroid hormone

*Adapted from Franklyn (1994) with permission.*

hyperthyroidism is associated with heart failure and atrial fibrillation (Hefland & Crapo, 1990). Hyperthyroidism, too, complicates pregnancy. Inadequately treated hyperthyroidism increases the risk of first-trimester spontaneous abortion, still births, and neonatal mortality (Bishnoi & Sachmechi, 1996).

Again, drug therapy for hyperthyroidism must be individualized. The selection of adjuvant therapy (eg, beta-adrenergic blocking drugs) in an elderly person with heart failure secondary to hyperthyroidism must be done with great care so as to not worsen cardiac output (Stockigt, 1993). During pregnancy, some treatment modalities are absolutely contraindicated (eg, radioiodine) secondary to fetal risks (Bishnoi & Sachmechi, 1996).

## Short- and Long-Term Goals for Pharmacotherapy

***Hypothyroidism.*** The short-term goal for the treatment of hypothyroidism is to relieve signs and symptoms experienced by the patient. Long-term goals are to restore TSH concentration to within the normal range and reverse biochemical abnormalities (ie, lipid abnormalities) of hypothyroidism (Hefland & Crapo, 1990).

***Hyperthyroidism.*** Goals of therapy for hyperthyroidism are to minimize symptoms, eliminate excess circulating thyroid hormone, and prevent long-term sequelae caused by hyperthyroidism (Reasner & Talbert, 1997).

## Time Frame for Initiating Pharmacotherapy

***Hypothyroidism.*** For clinical hypothyroidism, pharmacotherapy is initiated at the time of diagnosis. Whether replacement therapy should be initiated at the time of detecting subclinical hypothyroidism is less certain. In a patient with an elevated TSH and a normal $T_4$, progression from subclinical to overt hypothyroidism occurs at a rate of less than 5% per year (Stockigt, 1993). Therefore, some clinicians recommend repeat-

## TABLE 30–6. COMMON SIGNS AND SYMPTOMS OF HYPERTHYROIDISM

| Signs | Symptoms |
|---|---|
| Thinning of hair | Heat intolerance |
| Proptosis, lid lag, lid retraction, periorbital edema | Weight loss common (or weight gain due to increased appetite) |
| Diffusely enlarged goiter | Increased sweating |
| Thyroid bruits, thrills | Palpitations |
| Flushed, moist skin | Pedal edema |
| Palmar erythema | Diarrhea |
| Increased deep tendon reflexes | Light menses or amenorrhea |
| Pretibial myxedema | Weakness, fatigue |
| Wide pulse pressure | Tremor, nervousness, irritability, insomnia |

*Adapted from Young and Koda-Kimble (1995) with permission.*

ing TFTs in 6 months and annually thereafter. Replacement therapy is begun only if there is a clear trend in the TFTs toward clinical hypothyroidism.

**Hyperthyroidism.** For clinical hyperthyroidism, pharmacotherapy is initiated at the time of diagnosis. For subclinical hyperthyroidism caused by toxic goiter, toxic adenoma, or toxic multinodular goiter, therapy is generally initiated at diagnosis. Subclinical hyperthyroidism caused by glucocorticoid use, severe illness, and pituitary dysfunction does not require standard therapeutic intervention ("AACE Clinical Practice Guidelines," 1995). See Drug Table 607.

### Assessment and History Taking

A complete history and physical examination should be aimed at uncovering the signs and symptoms relevant to thyroid disease, listed in Tables 30–3 through 30–6. Baseline TFTs are

necessary prior to drug therapy since these measurements will be used to determine the adequacy of treatment. Both pregnancy and certain medications can affect normal, expected TFT values. During pregnancy, circulating estrogen increases. Estrogen stimulates a 2.5-fold increase in thyroxine-binding globulin (TBG). This increased TBG results in increased total serum $T_4$ and $T_3$ concentrations, but no change in serum free $T_4$. Also, because of the increased binding, $T_3$ resin uptake will be decreased. Generally, no change in TSH concentration is seen (Bishnoi & Sachmechi, 1996). These changes must be taken into consideration when deciding when and if drug therapy is introduced and during the assessment of treatment.

### Patient/Caregiver Information

Examples of patient information for drug treatment of hypo- and hyperthyroidism are given in Tables 30–7 and 30–8, respectively.

---

**TABLE 30–7. EXAMPLE OF PATIENT INFORMATION FOR THE TREATMENT OF HYPOTHYROIDISM CAUSED BY HASHIMOTO'S THYROIDITIS**

**Levothyroxine**

- Levothyroxine is a thyroid medicine belonging to the group of medications called hormones. It is used when the thyroid gland does not produce enough hormone.

- When you get this medicine refilled, make sure your pharmacist uses the same manufacturer's brand each time. This will help the medicine work best for you.

- Use this medicine only as directed. Do not use more or less of it, and do not take it more often than ordered. If you take a different amount than prescribed for you, you may experience symptoms of overactive or underactive thyroid. Take the medicine at the same time each day to make sure it always has the same effect.

- You may have to take this medicine for the rest of your life. It is very important that you do not stop taking this medicine without first checking with your health care professional.

- If you miss a dose of this medicine, take it as soon as possible. However, if it is almost time for your next dose, skip the missed dose and go back to your regular dosing schedule. Do not double doses.

- Make sure all health care professionals you see know you are taking this medicine. Also, make sure they are aware of other medicines you now take. If you start taking a new medicine, make sure you state that you take levothyroxine.

- It is very important that your health care professional check your progress at regular visits, to make sure this medicine is working properly. Any dose changes you may need are based on these visits.

- Report any problems such as chest pain, fast or irregular heartbeats, or shortness of breath.

- This medicine usually takes several weeks to have a noticeable effect on your condition. If you do not improve in about 3 weeks, check with your health care professional.

---

*Abstracted from United States Pharmacopeial Convention (1996) with permission.*

**TABLE 30-8. EXAMPLE OF PATIENT INFORMATION FOR THE TREATMENT OF HYPERTHYROIDISM CAUSED BY GRAVES' DISEASE**

**Methimazole**

- Methimazole is used when the thyroid gland makes too much thyroid hormone. It works by slowing down your body's production of thyroid hormone.

- Use this medicine only as directed. Do not use more or less of it and do not use it for a longer time than prescribed. If you do, you increase the chances of side effects.

- This medicine works best when there is a constant amount in the blood. To help keep the amount constant, do not miss any doses. Also, if you are taking more than one dose a day, it is best to take the doses at evenly spaced times day and night.

- Usually you have to take this medicine for 6 months to a year. It is very important that you do not stop taking this medicine without first checking with your health care professional.

- If you miss a dose of this medicine, take it as soon as possible. If it is almost time for your next dose, take both doses together. Then go back to your regular dosing schedule.

- If you wish to become pregnant or become pregnant while taking this medicine, notify your health care professional.

- Make sure all health care professionals you see know you are taking this medicine. Also, make sure they are aware of other medicines you now take. If you start taking a new medicine, make sure you state that you take methimazole.

- It is very important that your health care professional check your progress at regular visits, to make sure this medicine is working properly and to check for unwanted effects.

- Check with your health care professional immediately if you develop a rash, cough, fever, or chills that do not go away within a week.

- This medicine usually takes several weeks to have a noticeable effect on your condition. If you do not improve in a month, check with your health care professional.

*Abstracted from United States Pharmacopeial Convention (1996) with permission.*

## OUTCOMES MANAGEMENT

### Selecting an Appropriate Agent

*Hypothyroidism.* Although several thyroid replacement agents are available, the American Association of Clinical Endocrinologists advocates the use of a high-quality brand preparation of levothyroxine ("AACE Clinical Practice Guidelines," 1995). Levothyroxine possesses consistent activity while having a long half-life. Desiccated products are available, but their potency is based on iodine content rather than hormone activity, and therefore they provide less predictable activity (Reasner & Talbert, 1997). Other products listed in Drug Table 607.3, liothyronine, liotrix, and thyroglobulin, offer no advantage over levothyroxine and should not be used to initiate therapy ("AACE Clinical Practice Guidelines," 1995). Generic levothyroxine brands may be used, but therapy should be initiated with one brand and that brand used to control and maintain thyroid replacement therapy. Available brands are not bioequivalent; the use of a single brand will prevent under- or overtreatment.

The initial dose (range 12.5–100 μg) for adults is based on the age, weight, and cardiac status of the patient, as well as the duration and severity of hypothyroidism ("AACE Clinical Practice Guidelines," 1995). Also, the duration and speed with which replacement therapy is attempted will be patient-specific. An appropriate initial dose of levothyroxine for most patients is 50 μg/day for 1 month, which is then increased to 100 μg/day (Toft, 1994). The appropriate maintenance dose also will vary, but the mean replacement dose of levothyroxine is 1.6 μg/kg per day ("AACE Clinical Practice Guidelines," 1995). The following examples illustrate initial and maintenance dosing. In young adults with no risk factors limiting rapid replacement (eg, advanced age, cardiac disease, long-standing hypothyroidism), a conservative maintenance dose of 100 µg/day may be initiated. For elderly patients or those with a history of heart disease, the starting dose is 25 µg/day, which is then increased by 12.5 µg to 25 µg/day each month until the appropriate maintenance dose is achieved. This slower increase prevents aggravation of preexisting ischemic heart disease (Farwell & Ebner, 1996). Also, maintenance dosing in the elderly is generally less than 1.6 µg/kg per day (Rosenbaum & Barzel, 1982; Sawin, Herman, Molitch, London, and Kramer, 1983), with adequate maintenance doses of 50 µg/day not uncommon in those over 60 years of age.

Levothyroxine tablets are also the agent of choice for the treatment of pediatric hypothyroidism. Tablets may be crushed and added to bottle contents for treatment of infants. The suggested replacement dose for pediatric patients, like adults, varies according to age and presence of risk factors (LaFranchi, 1987; Fisher & Foley, 1989). These risk factors are preexisting cardiac disease or extreme sensitivity to the effects of levothyroxine. In these patients, one quarter to one third the recommended dose should be initiated and slowly increased until a therapeutic dose is achieved. The recommended dosing for pediatric patients, based on age, is shown in Table 30–9. Normal TFT values vary in early life and may be difficult to interpret without experience (American Academy of Pediatrics [AAP] & American Thyroid Association [ATA], 1993). Therefore, diagnosis and treatment of congenital hypothyroidism may require referral to a specialist.

During pregnancy, women will require an approximate 45% increase in levothyroxine dosing over their usual maintenance dose (Mandel, Larsen, Seely, & Brent, 1990). Maintenance dosing returns to prepregnancy requirements after delivery.

Minimal amounts of levothyroxine are excreted into breast milk. No dosage adjustments are necessary secondary to breast-feeding (Briggs, Freeman, & Yaffe, 1994). Further, any amounts reaching the breast milk are insufficient to treat neonatal hypothyroidism.

***Hyperthyroidism.*** Three treatment modalities exist for the management of hyperthyroidism caused by Graves' disease: radioiodine, surgery, and antithyroid drugs (Klein, Becker, and Levey, 1994). Radioiodine is currently the therapy of choice. Surgery is used when radioiodine or antithyroid agents are not optimal for patient-specific reasons. The antithyroid agents methimazole and propylthiouracil (PTU) are utilized to induce a remission. These agents are easy to use, have somewhat predictable therapeutic effects, and are inexpensive (Klein et al, 1994). They inhibit binding of iodine and inhibit coupling of reactions during thyroid hormone formation. PTU, unlike methimazole, also inhibits peripheral conversion of $T_4$ to $T_3$. This additional mechanism makes PTU useful in the treatment of severe hyperthyroidism (ie, thyroid storm), when lowering serum $T_3$ aids in treatment.

**TABLE 30–9. RECOMMENDED LEVOTHYROXIINE REPLACEMENT DOSING IN PEDIATRIC PATIENTS BASED ON AGE**

| Patient Age | Recommended Dose | Comments |
|---|---|---|
| 0–3 months | 10–15 µg/kg/day | Maintain total serum $T_4$ concentrations between 10–14 µg/dL to ensure adequate replacement therapy. At this age, serum $T_4$ is more accurate than serum thyrotropin (ie, thyroid-stimulating hormone, TSH). |
| 3–6 months | 6–8 µg/kg/day | |
| 6–12 months | 5–7 µg/kg/day | |
| 1–10 years | 3–6 µg/kg/day | TSH should be used to determine adequacy of therapy in children. May take 3–4 months to see a complete resolution to normal range. |
| < 10 years | 2–4 µg/kg/day | |

*Adapted from LaFranchi (1987) and Fisher and Foley (1989).*

Other differences between the two agents exist (Klein et al, 1994). Methimazole possesses a longer half-life, permitting once-daily dosing and potentially increasing compliance. PTU has a shorter half-life and must be dosed three times daily. PTU does not cross the placenta well and is the drug of choice for hyperthyroidism in pregnancy and breast-feeding. These agents are given until TFTs are within the normal range (ie, euthyroid) or a remission occurs. The ideal duration of therapy is not well defined; the length of therapy is usually 6 months to 2 years. A reasonable treatment course should be up to 18 months to maximize the chance of inducing a remission (Klein et al, 1994). Once the patient is euthyroid, the dose is decreased to the lowest possible dose that will maintain normal TFT values (Klein et al, 1994). For those experiencing severe hyperthyroidism, for children, and for patients who are pregnant or breast-feeding, PTU is the agent of choice (Burrow, 1985). The effectiveness of both agents depends on patient compliance ("AACE Clinical Practice Guidelines," 1995). If the patient has a history of noncompliance, methimazole may be the preferred agent since the longer half-life permits once-daily dosing, particularly during maintenance therapy.

Iodine products (see Drug Table 607.2) are used as short-term adjuvant therapy in the treatment of hyperthyroidism (Farwell & Ebner, 1996). These products acutely block thyroid hormone release, inhibit thyroid hormone biosynthesis (ie, Wolff-Chaikoff paradoxical effect), and decrease the vascularity of the gland (Dong, 1995). Therefore, they are most useful as adjuvants to surgery or emergent radiation administration since they are capable of producing a short-term (7–14 day) euthyroid state and decrease gland vascularity.

Both radioiodine and antithyroid agents take several weeks to produce symptomatic relief. Because many of the symptoms caused by hyperthyroidism mimic excess beta-adrenergic activity (eg, palpitations, tremor, sweating, heat intolerance), beta-adrenergic blocking drugs (beta blockers) may be used to control these symptoms until the gland-modifying agent takes action (Geffner & Hershman, 1992). Propranolol and nadolol are the agents of choice since they can block peripheral conversion of $T_4$ to $T_3$ as well as beta-receptor-mediated effects of catecholamines (see Table 30–1). Doses are titrated to a pulse less than 100 beats/min. Propranolol, the drug of choice for thyroid-induced atrial fib-

rillation, is initiated at dosages of 20 mg four times daily and titrated to pulse; very large doses may be required.

## Monitoring for Efficacy

**Hypothyroidism.**   Two to three weeks after the initiation of therapy, subjective benefit is experienced (Toft, 1994). But other signs and symptoms (eg, weight gain, increased pulse, hoarseness, skin changes) may take months to correct.

Approximately 3 months after the initiation of therapy, TFTs [ie, TSH and free $T_4$ ($FT_4$)] should be obtained (Toft, 1994). These measurements will then be used to make adjustments in replacement therapy. Also, after any dosage adjustment, TFT measurements should not be obtained for at least 6 weeks. This is because of the long half-life of levothyroxine and the length of time necessary to reach a steady state.

The appropriateness of replacement therapy for pediatric patients is discussed in Table 30–9.

In pregnancy, as previously stated, elevated estrogen stimulates an increase in TBG, altering total $T_4$ ($TT_4$) values but not $FT_4$. Therefore, the adequacy of replacement therapy in pregnancy also should be based on TSH and $FT_4$ laboratory values (Kaplan, 1992). Laboratory measurements should be made at 8 weeks' and 6 months' gestation. The goal of therapy is to normalize TSH values while maintaining $FT_4$ at the upper limits of normal.

**Hyperthyroidism.**   Several weeks after the initiation of therapy, most patients experience subjective benefit (Klein et al, 1994). Beta blockers may be added to provide immediate symptomatic relief. If symptomatic improvement does not occur within this time frame, consider increasing the dose of the antithyroid agent.

Dosage adjustments are based on TFTs (ie, TSH and $TT_4$) (Farwell & Ebner, 1996). With appropriate dosing, TSH will increase to within the normal range and $TT_4$ will decrease to within the normal range. Laboratory assessment should occur monthly until a euthyroid state is achieved.

## Monitoring for Toxicity

**Hypothyroidism.**   With excessive thyroid replacement, symptoms of hyperthyroidism will occur (Toft, 1994). These symptoms—weight loss, increased sweating and palpitations—are similar to those listed in Table 30–6. Explain this to patients so they will contact a health care professional if these symptoms occur. Generally, laboratory assessment is not performed at less than 6-week intervals, again because of the long half-life of levothyroxine.

**Hyperthyroidism.**    Adverse effects associated with the antithyroid agents are skin reactions, leukopenia, and rarely, agranulocytosis (Werner, Romaldini, Bromberg, Werner, & Farah, 1989). Agranulocytosis is the most serious adverse effect and generally occurs within the first 3 months of therapy. Patients should be instructed to report the development of a rash, cough, fever, or chill that does not resolve within a week (see Table 30–8).

To determine if antithyroid agents are affecting leukocytes, a baseline white blood cell count (WBC) should be performed prior to the initiation of therapy. Frequent monitoring of the WBC does not predict who will develop agranulocytosis (Tajiri, Noguchi, Murakami, & Murakami, 1990). Therefore, WBC should only be performed if the patient complains of flu-like symptoms and during TFT assessment.

### Follow-up Recommendations

**Hypothyroidism.**    Once a patient is euthyroid (as determined by TSH concentrations), a 6-month laboratory assessment should be performed. Patients should then be assessed, using TFTs, annually. At the time of laboratory assessments, an appropriate interim history (assessing symptoms of under- or overtreatment) and physical examination also should be performed ("AACE Clinical Practice Guidelines," 1995).

**Hypothyroidism.**    Once a patient is euthyroid (as determined by TSH and $TT_4$), a 6-month laboratory assessment should be performed. Patients should then be assessed, using TFTs, annually. The risk of relapse is high, as well as the risk of developing hypothyroidism. At the time of laboratory assessments, an appropriate interim history (assessing symptoms of under- or overtreatment) and physical examination also should be performed.

## ADRENAL CONDITIONS

Adrenal conditions are rarely encountered by general clinicians, particularly compared to thyroid conditions. The adrenal glands rest above the kidneys and are composed of the adrenal medulla and the adrenal cortex. The adrenal medulla comprises 10% of the gland and secretes catecholamines. The hormones produced by the adrenal medulla are not essential for life. The adrenal cortex makes up the majority of the gland and secretes three classes of steroid hormones: the glucocorticoids, the mineralocorticoids, and the androgens. The glucocorticoids and mineralocorticoids are necessary for subsistence; in fact, life is not possible without adrenocortical function (Ganong, 1997). Glucocorticoids regulate carbohydrate and protein metabolism. Mineralocorticoids regulate sodium, potassium, and fluid balance. A lack or overabundance of either steroid class produces disease. Androgens contribute to the pubertal growth of body hair, particularly the pubic and axillary hair of women (Porth, 1994). Excess androgen production can result in hirsutism and virilization. This section of the chapter addresses the two major divisions of adrenocortical disorders: hypofunction (eg, adrenal insufficiency, or Addison's disease, and hypoaldosteronism) and hyperfunction (eg, Cushing's syndrome, aldosteronism, and hirsutism). Where appropriate, adrenal conditions as they pertain to children and pregnancy are discussed.

## NORMAL ADRENAL CORTEX FUNCTION

The major role of the adrenal cortex is the production of glucocorticoid and mineralocorticoid hormones (Tyrrell & Baxter, 1992). The major physiologic glucocorticoid synthesized and secreted is cortisol. Cortisol influences numerous processes in the body including: the regulation of intermediary metabolism (ie, glucose and lipid metabolism), inflammatory and immunologic responses, cardiac and hemodynamic function, calcium homeostasis, and normal growth and development. Normal cortisol secretion follows a diurnal pattern, with burst production occurring in response to stress, such as illness or trauma (Ganong, 1997). Therefore, normal cortisol production is necessary for the appropriate reaction to stress. The major physiologic mineralocorticoid is aldosterone. Aldosterone mainly affects the kidney's ability to regulate fluid and electrolyte balance (Tyrrell & Baxter, 1992). Aldosterone increases sodium reabsorption and potassium secretion. Water passively follows sodium movement; therefore, aldosterone affects extracellular fluid volume. Aldosterone also causes hydrogen ion secretion, thus affecting acid-base status.

Cortisol production and secretion are regulated by the hypothalamic-pituitary-adrenal axis (Fig. 30–3) (Tyrrell & Baxter, 1992). Changes in concentration of cortisol produce positive or negative stimuli to the hormonal regulation of the adrenal cortex. Corticotropin-releasing hormone (CRH) is released by the hypothalamus when increased concentrations of cortisol are required. CRH then stimulates the release of corticotropin [ie, adrenocorticotropic hormone (ACTH)], which stimulates the adrenal cortex to release cortisol. When adequate concentrations of circulating cortisol are achieved, negative feedback stops further production and release of cortisol by the adrenal cortex (Fig. 30–3).

Aldosterone production and secretion are governed mainly by the renin-angiotensin system (Tyrrell & Baxter, 1992). Four predominant factors influence aldosterone release: changes in renal tubular sodium chloride concentration, renal perfusion pressure, angiotensin II, and

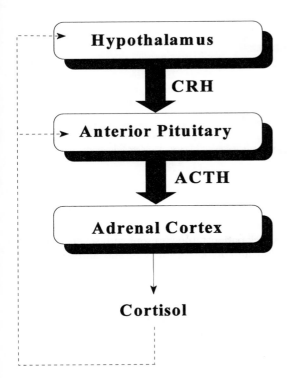

**Figure 30–3.** Hypothalamic-pituitary-adrenal axis illustrating the positive (heavy black arrows) and negative feedback (dashed arrows) stimuli that affect the hormonal regulators corticotropin-releasing hormone (CRH) and corticotropin (ie, adrenocorticotropic hormone, ACTH).

serum potassium concentration. When sodium chloride concentration falls, when intravascular volume is low, or when blood pressure falls, renin is released from the juxtaglomerular cells of the afferent renal arteriole. Renin stimulates angiotensin II production and release. Angiotensin II is a potent stimulator of aldosterone release. The presence of angiotensin II also blocks further renin release, thus providing feedback to inhibit the system. High serum potassium concentrations can also stimulate aldosterone release, whereas decreases in serum potassium inhibit aldosterone release.

Androgens include testosterone, androstenedione, and dehydroepiandrosterone sulfate (DHEAS). Testosterone, the most potent androgen in women, is derived from direct ovarian secretion (60%) and from peripheral conversion of androstenedione (40%).

The majority of testosterone (98%) circulates in a bound state and only 2% of the total is biologically active (Fitzgerald, 1994; Schneyer, 1996). The active testosterone is able to enter target cells to exert androgenic effects. It is in the skin that testosterone is converted by $5\alpha$-reductase to dihydrotestosterone to regulate androgen-dependent hair growth (Schneyer, 1996). Androgens exert little influence on the daily control of body functions, but do impact the development of body hair in women. Androstenedione is secreted equally by the adrenals and ovaries. DHEAS is secreted totally by the adrenals (Fitzgerald, 1994).

## ADRENOCORTICAL HYPOFUNCTION: ADRENAL INSUFFICIENCY

Adrenal insufficiency, by definition, is characterized by inadequate production of cortisol, aldosterone, or both. Adrenal insufficiency may be classified as primary or secondary, based on the etiology. Primary adrenal insufficiency, or Addison's disease, is caused by the destruction of the adrenal cortex (Muir, Schatz, & Maclaren, 1993). Primary adrenal insufficiency is associated with deficiencies in both cortisol and aldosterone. Secondary adrenal insufficiency stems from a hypothalamic-pituitary defect resulting in insufficient ACTH. Aldosterone production is usually adequate in secondary adrenal insufficiency. The differentiation between a primary and secondary etiology can be made through laboratory evaluation; see Figure 30–4. Table 30–10 lists major causes of primary and secondary adrenal insufficiency (Werbel & Ober, 1993).

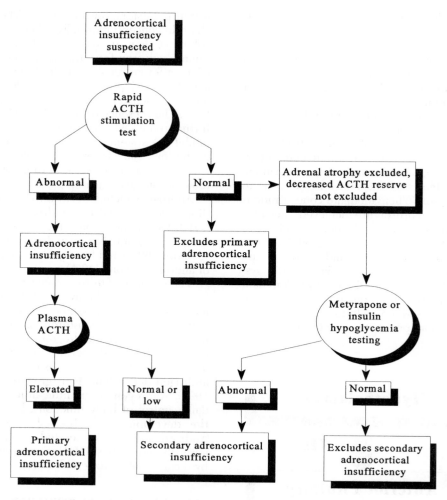

**Figure 30–4.** An algorithm for the evaluation of suspected adrenal insufficiency utilizing serum corticotropin (ie, adrenocorticotropic hormone, ACTH).

**Source:** Adapted from Baxter and Tyrrell (1987, p. 609) with permission.

Symptoms common to both primary and secondary adrenal insufficiency are weakness, easy fatiguability, and weight loss. Table 30–11 lists common signs and symptoms of primary adrenal insufficiency (Werbel & Ober, 1993). In comparison, patients with secondary adrenal insufficiency tend to have less hyperpigmentation and retain aldosterone activity, and therefore do not present with severe dehydration and electrolyte abnormalities. The clinical presentation of adrenal insufficiency depends on the rate and degree of loss of adrenocortical function. With acute stress, patients may present with addisonian crisis, a life-threatening emergency. Resembling

shock patients, they present with severe dehydration and hypotension. Chronic adrenal insufficiency is associated with an insidious onset, and the symptoms at presentation are nonspecific.

## ADRENOCORTICAL HYPOFUNCTION: HYPOALDOSTERONISM

Hypoaldosteronism is rare. This disorder can occur with Addison's disease or as the sole adrenocortical defect (Tyrrell & Baxter, 1992). When it is the sole defect, hypoaldosteronism is usually caused by hyporeninemic hypoaldoste-

**TABLE 30–10.  MAJOR CAUSES OF PRIMARY AND SECONDARY ADRENAL INSUFFICIENCY**

| Classification | Etiology | Comments |
|---|---|---|
| **Primary** | | |
| | Autoimmune | Accounts for approximately 80% of all cases |
| | Infections | Examples: tuberculosis—accounts for approximately 15–20% of all cases; fungal infections (ie, histoplasmosis); HIV |
| | Adrenal hemorrhage | |
| | Metastatic disease | Examples: lung, gastric, breast, malignant melanoma |
| | Drugs | Two mechanisms: decreased steroid synthesis (ie, ketoconazole) and increased clearance (ie, rifampin) |
| **Secondary** | | |
| | Glucocorticoid use | Major cause: synthetic steroids suppress adrenocorticotropic hormone (ACTH) release |
| | Pituitary disease | |
| | Hypothalamic disease | |

*Adapted from Werbel & Ober (1993) with permission.*

ronism, a defect in the secretion of renin. Hyporeninemic hypoaldosteronism generally occurs concurrently with renal disease, but also may occur in patients with normal renal function who have malignancies (Chung, Tanaka, & Fujita, 1996). Patients present with low serum sodium and high serum potassium concentrations.

## ADRENOCORTICAL HYPERFUNCTION: CUSHING'S SYNDROME

Cushing's syndrome is caused by chronic exposure to supraphysiologic glucocorticoids

**TABLE 30–11.  COMMON SIGNS AND SYMPTOMS OF PRIMARY ADRENAL INSUFFICIENCY (ADDISON'S DISEASE) AND PERCENT OCCURRENCE OF EACH**

| Sign or Symptom | Percentage |
|---|---|
| Weakness and fatigue | 74–100 |
| Weight loss | 56–100 |
| Hyperpigmentation | 92–96 |
| Hyponatremia | 88–96 |
| Hypotension | 59–88 |
| Hyperkalemia | 52–64 |
| Gastrointestinal symptoms | 56 |
| Postural dizziness | 12 |

*Adapted from Werbel and Ober (1993) with permission.*

(Ganong, 1997). The syndrome is most commonly due to excessive administration of exogenous glucocorticoids or may occur endogenously (Gabrilove, 1992). Major endogenous causes of Cushing's syndrome, classified as either ACTH-dependent or ACTH-independent, and their prevalence are listed in Table 30–12 (Orth, 1995). The etiology generally can be determined through laboratory evaluation (see Fig. 30–5). Most endogenous cases, up to 68%, are caused by excessive pituitary secretion of ACTH and are termed Cushing's disease. In Cushing's disease, pituitary adenomas are the etiology for hypersecretion in more than 90% of cases. The cause of these adenomas is unknown, but CRH may play a role in their development (Kovacs, 1993).

Signs and symptoms of Cushing's disease, listed in Table 30–13, develop over years (Tyrell & Baxter, 1992). Their development is thought to be caused by catabolic or antianabolic effects of cortisol (Gabrilove, 1992). Two of the more common ones, facial rounding and fat accumulation around the supraclavicular areas, are generally referred to as *moon face* and *buffalo hump*. Striae are most commonly on the lower trunk and are red to purple in color. The hypertension seen in approximately 70% of patients is thought to be due to a combination of glucocorticoid and mineralocorticoid effects (Danese & Aron, 1994).

Presentation in children may differ, with growth failure as the most common presenting

**TABLE 30–12. CAUSES OF CUSHING'S SYNDROME AND THEIR PREVALENCE, CLASSIFIED AS CORTICOTROPIN (ie, ANDRENOCORTICOTROPIC HORMONE, ACTH)-DEPENDENT AND ACTH-INDEPENDENT**

| Classification | Etiology | Percentage of Patients |
| --- | --- | --- |
| **ACTH-dependent** | | |
| | Cushing's disease | 68 |
| | Ectopic ACTH syndrome | 12 |
| | Ectopic CRH syndrome | <1 |
| **ACTH-independent** | | |
| | Adrenal adenoma | 10 |
| | Adrenal carcinoma | 8 |
| | Micronodular hyperplasia | 1 |
| | Macronodular hyperplasia | <1 |

*Adapted from Orth (1995) with permission.*

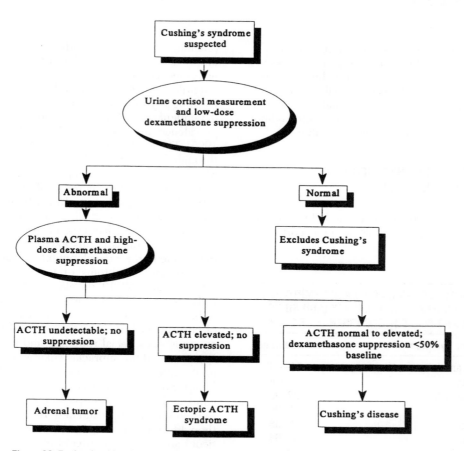

**Figure 30–5.** An algorithm for the evaluation of suspected Cushing's syndrome utilizing laboratory measurements, including serum corticotropin (ie, adrenocorticotropic hormone, ACTH).

**Source:** Adapted from Baxter and Tyrrell (1987, p. 609) with permission.

**TABLE 30–13. COMMON SIGNS AND SYMPTOMS OF CUSHING'S DISEASE AND PERCENTAGE OCCURRENCE OF EACH**

| Sign or Symptom | Percentage |
|---|---|
| Obesity | 94 |
| Facial rounding | 84 |
| Hirsutism | 82 |
| Menstrual complications | 76 |
| Hypertension | 72 |
| Muscular weakness | 58 |
| Back pain | 58 |
| Striae | 52 |
| Acne | 40 |
| Psychiatric changes | 40 |

*Adapted from Baxter and Tyrell (1987, p. 606) with permission.*

abnormality (Leinung & Zimmerman, 1994). Other signs and symptoms common in adults (see Table 30–13) are also present. Although Cushing's disease in adults is more common in women (at a ratio of 8:1), in children there is no female predominance.

Because of the adverse effects of cortisol on the reproductive state, pregnancy is rare in women with Cushing's disease (Sheeler, 1994). To date, approximately 70 cases are reported. Presentation is essentially the same in pregnancy as in nonpregnancy.

## ADRENOCORTICAL HYPERFUNCTION: ALDOSTERONISM

Primary aldosteronism, caused by an increased production of aldosterone, is a rare disorder characterized by sodium retention, suppression of renin activity, hypokalemia, and hypertension (Tyrrell & Baxter, 1992). The usual pathogenesis is an aldosterone-producing adrenocortical adenoma or bilateral adrenocortical hyperplasia (White, 1994). Patients are commonly identified by detection of hypertension on a routine physical examination.

## ADRENOCORTICAL HYPERFUNCTION: HIRSUTISM AND VIRILIZATION

Hirsutism, the presence of excess body hair in women, is primarily an androgen-dependent process. The definition of excess hair growth varies among ethnic groups and is more common in women of Mediterranean ancestry and least common in women of Japanese or North American Indian ancestry (Gilchrest, 1996). Hirsutism can be caused by drugs or pathologic conditions involving the ovaries, adrenals, or skin; see Table 30–14.

Virilization, the masculinization of women, is associated with androgen-secreting tumors (Gilchrest, 1996). The condition includes hirsutism, temporal balding, deepening of the voice, pectoral muscle development, and clitoral enlargement (Schneyer, 1996).

## SPECIFIC CONSIDERATIONS FOR PHARMACOTHERAPY

### When Drug Therapy Is Needed

*Adrenocortical Hypofunction.* Appropriate production of adrenocortical hormones is essential. Before replacement therapy was available, most patients died within 2 years of diagnosis (Tyrrell & Baxter, 1992). Drug therapy to replace insufficient cortisol and aldosterone production (ie, Addison's disease) is essential to restore quality of life. Patients are suspected of having adrenal insufficiency based on signs and symptoms at presentation, and diagnosis is confirmed through laboratory evaluation (see Fig. 30–4). The rapid ACTH stimulation test also distinguishes primary from secondary adrenal insufficiency (Dluhy, Himathongkam, & Greenfield, 1974). This differentiation is important to define drug therapy. Patients with secondary adrenal insufficiency generally do not require mineralocorticoid replacement.

In hypoaldosteronism not associated with Addison's disease, drug therapy can correct abnormalities in blood pressure, electrolytes, and acid-base status.

*Adrenocortical Hyperfunction.* Excessive production of cortisol (ie, Cushing's disease) is associated with significant morbidity and mortality. Patients without medical therapy will develop comorbid conditions such as cardiovascular disease and diabetes mellitus, further adding to a poor prognosis. Medical therapies decrease morbidity. Like adrenal insufficiency, Cushing's syndrome may be suspected based on the clinical presentation. Laboratory evaluation is then used to confirm the diagnosis (see Fig. 30–5).

## TABLE 30–14.  COMMON CAUSES OF HIRSUTISM

| Causes | Clinical Clues |
|---|---|
| **Ovarian** | |
| Idiopathic hirsutism | Pubertal onset, regular menses |
| Polycystic ovary syndrome | Pubertal onset, irregular menses, family history |
| Androgen-producing ovarian neoplasms | Explosive course, virilization, abdominal or pelvic pain |
| Insulin resistance syndromes | Diabetes, acanthosis nigricans, skin tags |
| **Adrenal** | |
| Nonclassic 21-hydroxylase deficiency | Family history, Ashkenazic Jews |
| Androgen-producing adrenal neoplasms | Explosive course, virilization, abdominal or flank pain |
| Cushing's syndrome | Hypertension, muscle weakness, easy bruisability |
| Hyperprolactinemia | Headaches, seizures, weight gain, visual field cut, extraocular muscle disturbances, gynecomastia, fatigue, cold intolerance, constipation, muscle cramps, spinal cord lesions, herpes zoster, chest wall trauma, breast disease |
| **Medications** | |
| Anabolic steroids | Virilization |
| Phenytoin, minoxidil, cyclosporine, glucocorticoids | Growth of fine, nonpigmented hair in androgen-independent areas |

*Adapted from Schneyer (1996, p. 306), with permission.*

Delineating the etiology defines the medical therapy of choice.

In primary aldosteronism, medical therapy depends on the etiology (Siragy & Carey, 1986). Drug therapy is used only in primary aldosteronism caused by bilateral adrenal hyperplasia. Differentiating the etiologies can be done through the use of computed tomography (CT).

Therapy for women with hirsutism or virilization depends on the extent of the condition and etiology. Short-term measures may include waxing, bleaching, electrolysis, or shaving, whereas longer-term solutions like weight loss may help to decrease hair growth. In more severe cases, drug treatments can include oral contraceptives and antiandrogen drugs such as spironolactone, flutamide, or finasteride. Second- or third-line treatment includes GnRH analogs given in combination with estrogen-progestin therapy (Schneyer, 1996).

## Short- and Long-Term Goals for Pharmacotherapy

***Adrenocortical Hypofunction.***   The short-term goal for the treatment of adrenal insufficiency and hypoaldosteronism is to relieve patient signs and symptoms (including laboratory abnormalities) using the lowest effective dosing regimen that mimics normal physiologic adrenocortical function. The long-term goal is to improve quality of life (Stoffer, 1993).

***Adrenocortical Hyperfunction.***   Goals for the treatment of Cushing's disease and aldosteronism are to alleviate symptoms, cure the hypercortisolism or aldosteronism, eliminate any tumor which threatens the patient's health, and minimize the risk of secondary endocrine deficiency and long-term dependence on medications (Orth, 1995).

Goals for the treatment of hirsutism/virilization may include cosmetic or medical treatment.

The decision to utilize medical treatment may depend on the severity and degree of distress to the patient.

## Time Frame for Initiating Pharmacotherapy

For all adrenocortical disorders, medical intervention is begun at the time of diagnosis. In acutely ill patients with suspected adrenal insufficiency (ie, addisonian crisis), drug therapy is begun before laboratory confirmation of the suspected diagnosis is received because of patient acuity. Drug treatment may be lifelong, particularly in adrenal insufficiency.

See Drug Table 601.

## Assessment and History Taking

*Adrenocortical Hypofunction.* Laboratory data are less useful in monitoring the adequacy of adrenocortical replacement therapy than in monitoring thyroid condition (Stoffer, 1993). Regardless, a number of laboratory tests are recommended for the diagnosis and treatment of adrenocortical hypofunction. The tests are serum concentrations of ACTH, cortisol, aldosterone, and electrolytes. Blood pressure is used to assess treatment of aldosterone disorders and therefore should be measured prior to the initiation of drug therapy. A baseline patient weight is also helpful.

*Adrenocortical Hyperfunction.* Prior to initiating therapy for adrenocortical hyperfunction, serum concentrations of ACTH, cortisol, aldosterone, and electrolytes should be obtained. Also, a urinary cortisol concentration should be measured. Baseline measurements of blood pressure and patient weight are necessary. Urine electrolytes levels are useful if primary aldosteronism is suspected.

## Patient/Caregiver Information

Examples of patient information for drug treatment of Addison's disease and Cushing's syndrome are given in Tables 30–15 and 30–16, respectively. See also the discussion of patient education for adrenocortical hypofunction in the next section for additional information.

## OUTCOMES MANAGEMENT

### Selecting an Appropriate Agent

*Adrenocortical Hypofunction.* Treatment of adrenal insufficiency differs depending on the onset of symptoms. In acute adrenal insufficiency, a patient is exposed to a major stressor (ie, surgery, trauma) that requires an increased cortisol response. Because of adrenal insufficiency, the

---

**TABLE 30–15. EXAMPLE OF PATIENT INFORMATION FOR THE TREATMENT OF ADDISON'S DISEASE**

**Hydrocortisone**

• Your body naturally produces cortisone-like hormones that are necessary to maintain good health. Hydrocortisone is like those hormones. Because your body is not producing enough, you must take this medicine to make up the difference.

• Use this medicine only as directed. Do not use more or less of it and do not use it for a longer time than prescribed. If you do, you increase the chances of side effects. Take the medicine at the same time each day to make sure it always has the same effect.

• Take this medicine with food to help prevent stomach upset.

• You may have to take this medicine for the rest of your life. It is very important that you do not stop taking this medicine without first checking with your health care professional.

• If you take several doses of this medicine a day and you miss a dose, take it as soon as possible. If it is almost time for your next dose, take both doses together. Then go back to your regular dosing schedule.

• It is very important that your health care professional check your progress at regular visits to make sure this medicine is working properly. Any dose changes you may need are based on these visits.

• You should carry a medical identification card stating you have Addison's disease and you are taking this medicine.

*Abstracted from United States Pharmacopeial Convention (1996) with permission.*

## TABLE 30–16. EXAMPLE OF PATIENT INFORMATION FOR THE TREATMENT OF CUSHING'S SYNDROME

**Ketoconazole**

- Even though this medicine is usually for the treatment of serious fungus infections, that is not why you are taking it. Your body naturally produces cortisone-like hormones that are necessary to maintain good health. Because you have Cushing's disease, your body makes too much cortisone. This medicine reduces the body's production of cortisone and helps treat Cushing's disease.

- Use this medicine only as directed. Do not use more or less of it, and do not take it more often than ordered. If you take a different amount than prescribed for you or you take it longer than prescribed, you increase the chances of side effects. Take the medicine at the same time each day to make sure it always has the same effect.

- If you miss a dose of this medicine, take it as soon as possible. However, if it is almost time for your next dose, skip the missed dose and go back to your regular dosing schedule. Do not double doses.

- Make sure all health care professionals you see know you are taking this medicine. Also, make sure they are aware of other medicines you now take. If you start taking a new medicine, make sure you state that you take ketoconazole.

- Liver problems are more likely to occur if you drink alcoholic beverages while you take this medicine. Therefore, you should not drink alcoholic beverages or use alcohol-containing products while you are taking this medicine.

- Talk with your health care professional before you take any over-the-counter stomach medicines such as antacids.

- This medicine may cause your eyes to become more sensitive to light than they are normally. Wearing sunglasses and avoiding too much exposure to bright light should help.

- Check with your health care professional immediately if you develop a rash, cough, fever, or chills that do not go away within a week. Also, check with your doctor if your urine becomes dark or your stools become lighter than normal.

- This medicine usually takes several weeks to have a noticeable effect on your condition. If you do not improve in a month, check with your health care professional.

*Abstracted from United States Pharmacopeial Convention (1996) with permission.*

patient cannot adequately respond and a life-threatening condition ensues. Again, treatment is begun before laboratory confirmation is received. One potential protocol for the treatment of acute adrenal insufficiency is listed in Table 30–17 (Stoffer, 1993). Because of the severity of illness, hospitalization is required with intravenous glucocorticoids. The underlying stressor must be identified and corrected to prevent future complications.

Treatment of chronic adrenal insufficiency differs slightly based on classification of the condition as primary or secondary. Primary therapy requires both glucocorticoid and mineralocorticoid replacement, whereas secondary usually requires only glucocorticoid replacement. Table 30–17 includes one potential treatment regimen. A goal of drug therapy is to mimic normal physiologic adrenal secretion. Without disease, endogenous cortisol secretion follows a diurnal rhythm, with 75% of the daily production occurring between 4 and 10 A.M. and another peak occurring in late afternoon or early evening

(Ganong, 1997). Dosing regimens should be designed taking this diurnal rhythm into account. Therefore, the total daily dose must be given in two to three divided doses. A suggested daily glucocorticoid replacement is the equivalent of hydrocortisone 12–15 mg/m$^2$, given two thirds in the morning and one third in the afternoon or evening (Wand & Cooper, 1996). All regimens must be individualized based on the lowest effective dose possible. Some patients may subjectively improve using a three-times-a-day dosing regimen, hence improving their quality of life (Groves, Toms, Houghton, & Monson, 1988).

Patient education is extremely important. Patients must understand drug therapy is lifelong. Patients should understand the normal action of cortisol and how production increases in response to stress caused by illness, trauma, etc. They must then be able to adjust their glucocorticoid replacement therapy in response to personal need, similar to the way a person with diabetes increases insulin dosing in response to illness (ie, sick-day management). A rule of

**TABLE 30–17. SUGGESTED PROTOCOLS FOR THE TREATMENT OF ACUTE AND CHRONIC ADRENAL INSUFFICIENCY**

**Acute Crisis**
- Correct dehydration, sodium depletion, hypotension, and hypoglycemia with intravenous 5% dextrose and normal saline solution at a rate of 500 mL/h or faster as needed for the first 4 h. Adjust subsequent solution composition and rate as indicated.
- Give parenteral hydrocortisone 100 mg intravenous bolus followed by 100 mg every 8 h for 24–48 h.
- When the patient improves, convert hydrocortisone to 50 mg orally every 8 h for another 24–48 h.
- Taper oral hydrocortisone to a maintenance dose, usually 30–50 mg/day in divided doses.
- Identify and correct underlying factor (ie, infection) that triggered the crisis.

**Chronic Therapy**
- Hydrocortisone 15–20 mg orally every morning (by 8 A.M., approximately) and 5–10 mg orally between 4 and 6 P.M.
- Fludrocortisone 0.05–0.2 mg orally every morning.
- Patient education: Increase hydrocortisone dose during stress (ie, sick-day management).

*Adapted from Tables 12–17 and 12–18 in Baxter and Tyrrell (1987) with permission.*

thumb is to double their usual dose for illness associated with vomiting and/or diarrhea (Brunt & Melby, 1996) not requiring medical attention. Patients must be aware of the adverse effects associated with therapy and how to recognize them (eg, weight gain, edema). Also, patients must know what to do about missed doses (refer back to Table 30–15).

In the treatment of hypoaldosteronism, fludrocortisone alone is used in the same manner as listed in Table 30–17. Dosing is individualized based on response.

***Adrenocortical Hyperfunction.*** Medical treatment of Cushing's syndrome is based on the etiology of hypercortisolism (Gabrilove, 1992; Orth, 1995; Trainer & Besser, 1994). Although the causes of Cushing's syndrome, as shown in Table 30–12, are many, surgery is the therapy of choice. Drug therapy plays only a palliative or adjunctive role. A number of medications have been used for these purposes (Engelhardt & Weber, 1994; Miller & Crapo, 1993). When drug therapy is used, the goal of therapy is to lower the mean serum cortisol concentration throughout the day into the range of 150–300 nmol/L (Trainer et al, 1993). Four classes of agents are available: steroidogenic blocking drugs, adrenolytic drugs, neuromodulators, and steroid receptor antagonists.

The steroidogenic agents are metyrapone, aminoglutethimide, and ketoconazole. These agents inhibit the adrenal enzymes necessary for the production of cortisol. Currently, ketoconazole appears to be the most effective. Further, it has been recommended as the initial agent of choice for most patients (Klibanski & Zervas, 1991). Effective dosages range from 800–1200 mg/day divided in two doses. Overall, few patients experience adverse effects. The major adverse effect seen is hepatotoxicity, which occurs in about 12% of patients.

The adrenolytic agent, mitotane, selectively inhibits adrenocortical function without being cytotoxic. Adverse effects are common, occurring in approximately 75% of patients. The recommended dose is 6–12 g/day in divided doses.

Neuromodulators used in Cushing's syndrome are bromocriptine, cyproheptadine, and valproate sodium. These agents are thought to decrease ACTH release through their effect on neurotransmitters. Limited success is seen with these agents. A new investigational agent, mifepristone (RU-486), is a glucocorticoid receptor antagonist. Theoretically, patients treated with mifepristone may develop glucocorticoid insufficiency. Because signs and symptoms of adrenal insufficiency are the only means of assessing excessive therapy, this agent may see limited use in the future. How mifepristone impacts the treatment of Cushing's syndrome remains to be demonstrated.

One of the major causes of Cushing's syndrome is Cushing's disease. Again, Cushing's disease is typically caused by a pituitary adenoma. The therapy of choice for Cushing's disease is transsphenoidal adenomectomy (TSA). It is curative in approximately 80–85% of cases. Postsurgically, patients require daily glucocorticoid replacement therapy (same as in Table

30–17) for 6–12 months, until the hypothalamic-pituitary-adrenal axis recovers. In children, the therapy of choice has been pituitary irradiation with success rates up to 80% (Cappa et al, 1987). However, newer reports suggest TSA is as effective as irradiation with fewer side effects. Therefore, TSA may be the preferred mode of therapy in children (Leinung & Zimmerman, 1994).

If TSA fails, pituitary irradiation is suggested. A lag time of 3–12 months occurs before hypercortisolism is controlled. Therefore, adjunctive drug therapy is used to control hypercortisolism during this time. In the authors' opinion, ketoconazole will probably become the agent of choice.

Ectopic ACTH syndrome is caused by nonpituitary tumors that secrete ACTH. The therapy of choice is surgical resection, but localization of the tumor with a cure is successful in only about 10% of cases. Therefore, 90% of cases require drug therapy. Again, ketoconazole will probably become the drug of choice. Serum and urinary cortisol concentrations can be measured and used to adjust drug therapy.

In patients with ACTH-independent disease caused by an adrenal adenoma, adrenal carcinoma, or adrenal hyperplasia, surgical resection or removal of the gland is the therapy of choice. If both adrenals are removed, lifelong replacement therapy is indicated (see Table 30–17). With unilateral adrenalectomy, contralateral gland atrophy is common and glucocorticoid replacement therapy is required up to 12 months. Adrenal carcinomas may not be completely resected and require palliative therapy. The drug of choice, at present, is mitotane.

Because so few pregnancies have occurred in women with Cushing's syndrome, no definitive recommendations regarding treatment can be made (Buescher, McClamrock, & Adashi, 1992; Sheeler, 1994).

As in the case of Cushing's syndrome, medical management of primary aldosteronism depends on the etiology. When the cause is an adrenocortical adenoma, surgical resection is the therapy of choice. When bilateral adrenocortical hyperplasia is the cause, drug therapy is indicated. The therapy of choice is spironolactone (Siragy & Carey, 1986). In this particular indication, spironolactone appears to inhibit adrenal gland synthesis of aldosterone (Weinberger et al, 1979). The effective dosage range is 200–400 mg/day. It may take 4–8 weeks to see the full effect of therapy. Therefore,

dosage adjustments usually are not performed until this time. Blood pressure is the primary monitoring parameter used to assess the appropriateness of therapy. In most patients, the drug is well tolerated.

## Monitoring for Efficacy

Unlike hypothyroidism, no one test is available to appropriately assess adrenal insufficiency replacement therapy (Stoffer, 1993). Most clinicians assess the adequacy of therapy clinically. Patients without sufficient replacement retain or develop signs and symptoms of adrenal insufficiency. Patients with excessive replacement develop signs and symptoms of Cushing's syndrome. Thus, subjective improvement and questions regarding symptoms of disease are important markers in assessing drug therapy. Objectively, patient weight, blood pressure, signs of disease, and serum electrolytes are monitored and used to adjust replacement therapy. Most clinicians do not include measurements of serum cortisol and ACTH.

Symptoms usually subside within days from the initiation of therapy. Strength and hyperpigmentation generally take longer to improve (weeks vs. days) (Tyrrell & Baxter, 1992). Hyperpigmentation will ameliorate with appropriate replacement, and a lack of improvement may be used to assess the adequacy of therapy.

Adverse drug effects are monitored as well. Symptoms such as dyspepsia, edema, hypertension, hypokalemia, insomnia, and glucose intolerance all indicate an excess of glucocorticoid and/or mineralocorticoid therapy.

In hypoaldosteronism, dosage adjustments are based on serum electrolytes, particularly potassium, and blood pressure response.

## REFERENCES

AACE clinical practice guidelines for the evaluation and treatment of hyperthyroidism and hypothyroidism. (1995). *Endocrine Practice, 1,* 54–62.

American Academy of Pediatrics & American Thyroid Association. (1993). Newborn screening for congenital hypothyroidism: Recommended guidelines. *Pediatrics, 91,* 1203–1209.

Bansal, S. K., Sahi, S. P., Basu, S. K., & Old, J. M. (1986). Hypothyroidism in elderly males–An under diagnosis. *British Journal of Clinical Practice, 40,* 17–18.

Baxter, J. D., & Tyrrell, J. B. (1987). The adrenal cortex. In P. Felig, J. D. Baxter, A. G. Broadus, L. A.

Frohman (Eds.), *Endocrinology and metabolism*, (2nd ed.). New York: McGraw-Hill.

Bishnoi, A., & Sachmechi, I. (1996). Thyroid disease during pregnancy. *American Family Physician, 53*, 215–220.

Briggs, G. G., Freeman, R. K., & Yaffe, S. J. (Eds.). (1994). *Drugs in pregnancy and lactation* (4th ed.) (pp. 483–486). Baltimore: Williams & Wilkins.

Brody, M. B., & Reichard, R. A. (1995). Thyroid screening: How to interpret and apply the results. *Postgraduate Medicine, 98*, 54–68.

Brunt, M. J., & Melby, J. C. (1996). Adrenal gland disorders. In J. Noble (Ed.), *Primary care medicine*. St. Louis: C. V. Mosby.

Buescher, M. A., McClamrock, H. D., & Adashi, E. Y. (1992). Cushing syndrome in pregnancy. *Obstetrics and Gynecology, 79*, 130–137.

Burrow, G. N. (1985). The management of thyrotoxicosis in pregnancy. *New England Journal of Medicine, 313*, 562–565.

Caldwell, G., Kellett, H. A., Gow, S. M., Sweeting, V. M., Kellett, H. A., Becket, G. J., Seth, J., & Toft, A. D. (1985). A new strategy for thyroid function testing. *Lancet, 1*, 1117–1119.

Cappa, M., Stoner, E., DiMartino-Nardi, J., Pang, S., Temeck, J., & New, M. I. (1987). Recurrence of Cushing's disease in childhood after radiotherapy-induced remission. *American Journal of Child Diseases, 141*, 736–740.

Chung, U., Tanaka, Y., & Fujita, T. (1996). Association of interleukin-6 and hypoaldosteronism in patients with cancer. *New England Journal of Medicine, 334*, 473.

Danese, R. D., & Aron, D. C. (1994). Cushing's syndrome and hypertension. *Endocrinology and Metabolism Clinics of North America, 23*, 299–324.

Dluhy, R. G., Himathongkam, T., & Greenfield, M. (1974). Rapid ACTH test with plasma aldosterone levels: Improved diagnostic discrimination. *Annals of Internal Medicine, 80*, 693–696.

Dong, B. J. (1995). Thyroid disorders. In Young, L. Y., & Koda-Kimble, M. A., *Applied therapeutics: The clinical use of drugs*, (6th ed.). Vancouver, WA: Applied Therapeutics.

Engelhardt, D., & Weber, M. M. (1994). Therapy of Cushing's syndrome with steroid biosynthesis inhibitors. *Journal of Steroid Biochemistry and Molecular Biology, 49*, 261–267.

Farwell, A. P., & Ebner, S. A. (1996). Thyroid gland disorders. In J. Noble (Ed.), *Primary care textbook*. St. Louis: C. V. Mosby.

Fisher, D. A., & Foley, B. L. (1989). Early treatment of congenital hypothyroidism. *Pediatrics, 83*, 785–789.

Fitzgerald, P. A. (1994). Endocrine disorders. In L. M. Tierney, S. J. McPhee, & M. A. Papadakis,

*Current medical diagnosis and treatment*. Norwalk, CT: Appleton & Lange.

Franklyn, J. A. (1994). The management of hyperthyroidism. *New England Journal of Medicine, 330*, 1731–1738.

Gabrilove, J. L. (1992). Cushing's syndrome. *Comprehensive Therapy, 18*, 13–16.

Gambert, S. R. (1995). Hyperthyroidism in the elderly. *Clinics in Geriatric Medicine, 11*, 181–188.

Ganong, W. F. (1997). The adrenal medulla and adrenal cortex. In W. F. Ganong, *Review of medical physiology*. Stamford, CT: Appleton & Lange.

Geffner, D. L., & Hershman, J. M. (1992). Beta adrenergic blockade for the treatment of hyperthyroidism. *American Journal of Medicine, 93*, 61–68.

Gilchrest, V. (1996). Hirsutism. In C. A. Johnson, B. E. Johnson, J. L. Murray, & B. S. Apgar (Eds.), *Women's health care handbook*. St. Louis: C. V. Mosby.

Groves, R. W., Toms, G. C., Houghton, B. J. & Monson, J. P. (1988). Corticosteroid replacement therapy: Twice or thrice daily? *Journal of Royal Society of Medicine, 81*, 514–516.

Hefland, M., & Crapo, L. M. (1990). Monitoring therapy in patients taking levothyroxine. *Annals of Internal Medicine, 113*, 450–454.

Hershman, J. M., Ladenson, P. W., & Paulshock, B. Z. (1992). A savvy approach to thyroid testing. *Patient Care, 26*(3), 134–151.

Johnson, J. L., & Felicetta, J. V. (1992). Hyperthyroidism: A comprehensive review. *Journal of the American Academy of Nurse Practitioners, 4*(1), 8–14.

Kaplan, M. M. (1992). Monitoring thyroxine treatment during pregnancy. *Thyroid, 2*, 147–152.

Klein, I., Becker, D. V., & Levey, G. S. (1994). Treatment of hyperthyroid disease. *Annals of Internal Medicine, 121*, 281–288.

Klibanski, A., & Zervas, N. T. (1991). Diagnosis and management of hormone-secreting pituitary adenomas. *New England Journal of Medicine, 324*, 822–831.

Kovacs, K. (1993). The pathology of Cushing's disease. *Journal of Steroid Biochemistry and Molecular Biology, 45*, 179–182.

LaFranchi, S. (1987). Diagnosis and treatment of hypothyroidism in children. *Comprehensive Therapy, 13*(10), 20–30.

Larsen, P. R. (1982). Thyroid-pituitary interaction: Feedback regulation of thyrotropin secretion by thyroid hormones. *New England Journal of Medicine, 306*, 23–32.

Leinung, M. C., & Zimmerman, D. (1994). Cushing's disease in children. *Endocrinology and Metabolism Clinics of North America, 23*, 629–639.

Mandel, S. J., Larsen, P. R., Seely, E. W., & Brent, G. A. (1990). Increased need for thyroxine during pregnancy in women with primary hypothyroidism. *New England Journal Medicine, 323,* 91–96.

Miller, J. W., & Crapo, L. (1993). The medical treatment of Cushing's syndrome. *Endocrinology Reviews, 14,* 443–458.

Muir, A., Schatz, D. A., & Maclaren, N. K. (1993). Autoimmune Addison's disease. *Springer Seminars in Immunopathology, 14,* 275–284.

Orth, D. N. (1995). Cushing's syndrome. *New England Journal of Medicine, 332,* 791–803.

Porth, C. M. (1994). *Pathophysiology.* Philadelphia: J. B. Lippincott.

Reasner, C. A., & Talbert, R. L. (1997). Thyroid disorders. In J. T. DiPiro, R. L. Talbert, G. C. Yee, G. R. Matzke, B. G. Wells, & L. M. Posey (Eds.), *Pharmacotherapy: A pathophysiologic approach* (3rd ed.) (pp. 1521–1546). Stamford, CT: Appleton & Lange.

Rogers, D. G. (1994). Thyroid disease in children. *American Family Physician, 50,* 344–350.

Rosenbaum, R. L., & Barzel, U. S. (1982). Levothyroxine replacement dose for primary hypothyroidism decreases with age. *Annals of Internal Medicine, 96,* 53–55.

Sawin, C. T. (1991). Thyroid dysfunction in older persons. *Advances in Internal Medicine, 37,* 223–248.

Sawin, C. T., Castelli, W. P., Hershman, J. M., McNamara, P., & Bacharach, P. (1985). The aging thyroid: Thyroid deficiency in the Framingham study. *Archives of Internal Medicine, 145,* 1386–1388.

Sawin, C. T., Herman, T., Molitch, M. E., London, M. H., & Kramer, S. M. (1983). Aging and the thyroid. Decreased requirement for thyroid hormone in older hypothyroid patients. *American Journal of Medicine, 75,* 206–209.

Schneyer, C. R. (1996). Gonadal disorders. In J. D. Stobo, D. B. Hellmann, P. W. Ladenson, B. G. Petty, & T. A. Thraill (Eds.), *Principles and practice of medicine.* Stamford, CT: Appleton & Lange.

Sheeler, L. R. (1994). Cushing's syndrome and pregnancy. *Endocrinology and Metabolism Clinics of North America, 23,* 619–627.

Shetty, K. R., & Duthie, E. H. (1995). Thyroid disease and associated illness in the elderly. *Clinics in Geriatric Medicine, 11,* 311–325.

Siragy, H., & Carey, R. M. (1986). Management of primary aldosteronism. *Drug Therapy, 16,* 89–103.

Smith, S. A. (1995). Concise review for primary-care physicians: Commonly asked questions about thyroid function. *Mayo Clinic Proceedings, 70,* 573–577.

Stockigt, J. R. (1993). Prescribing for the elderly: Thyroid disease. *Medical Journal of Australia, 158,* 770–774.

Stoffer, S. S. (1993). Addison's disease. How to improve patients' quality of life. *Postgraduate Medicine, 93,* 265–278.

Tajiri, J., Noguchi, S., Murakami, T., & Murakami, N. (1990). Antithyroid drug-induced agranulocytosis. The usefulness of routine white blood cell count monitoring. *Archives of Internal Medicine, 150,* 621–624.

Tieche, M., Lupi, G. A., Gutzwiller, F., Grob, P. J., Studer, H., & Burgi, H. (1981). Borderline low thyroid function and thyroid autoimmunity: Risk factors for coronary heart disease? *British Heart Journal, 46,* 202–206.

Toft, A. D. (1994). Thyroxine therapy. *New England Journal of Medicine, 331,* 174–180.

Toto, K. H. (1994). Endocrine physiology: A comprehensive review. *Critical Care Nursing Clinics of North America, 6,* 637–653.

Trainer, P. J., & Besser, M. (1994). Cushing's syndrome. Therapy directed at the adrenal glands. *Endocrinology and Metabolism Clinics of North America, 23,* 571–584.

Trainer, P. J., Eastment, C., Grossman, A. B., Wheeler, M. J., Perry, L., & Besser, G. M. (1993). The relationship between cortisol production rate and serial serum cortisol estimation in patients on medical therapy for Cushing's syndrome. *Clinical Endocrinology, 39,* 441–443.

Tyrrell, J. B., & Baxter, J. D. (1992). Disorders of the adrenal cortex. In J. B. Wyngaarden, L. H. Smith, J. C. Bennett (Eds.), *Cecil's textbook of medicine* (19th ed.) (pp. 1271–1291). Philadelphia: W. B. Saunders.

United States Pharmacopeial Convention. (1996). Advice for the Patient USP DI Vol. II (17th ed.). The United States Pharmacopeial Convention, Inc.

Vanderpump, M. P. J., & Tunbridge, M. G. (1993). The effects of drugs on endocrine function. *Clinical Endocrinology, 39,* 389–397.

Wand, G. S., & Cooper, D. S. (1996). Adrenal disorders. In J. D. Stobo, D. B. Hellman, P. W. Ladenson, B. G. Petty, & T. A. Traill (Eds.), *Principles and practice of medicine.* Norwalk, CT: Appleton & Lange.

Wartofsky, L. (1994). Diseases of the thyroid. In K. J. Isselbacher, E. Braunwald, L. D. Wilson, J. B. Martin, A. S. Fauci, & D. L. Kasper (Eds.), *Harrison's principles of internal medicine* (13th ed.) (pp. 1930–1953). New York: McGraw-Hill.

Weinberger, M. H., Grim, C. E., Hollifield, J. W., Kem, D. C., Ganguly, A., Kramer, N. J., Yune, H. Y., Wellman, H., & Donohue, J. P. (1979). Primary aldosteronism: Diagnosis, localization, and treatment. *Annals of Internal Medicine, 90,* 386–395.

Werbel, S. S., & Ober, K. P. (1993). Acute adrenal insufficiency. *Endocrinology and Metabolism Clinics of North America, 22,* 303–328.

Werner, M. C., Romaldini, J. H., Bromberg, N., Werner, R. S., & Farah, C. S. (1989). Adverse effects related to thionamide drugs and their dose regimen. *American Journal of the Medical Sciences, 297,* 216–219.

White, P. C. (1994). Disorders of aldosterone biosynthesis and action. *New England Journal of Medicine, 331,* 250–258.

Young, L. Y. & Koda-Kimble, M. A. (Eds.). (1995). *Applied therapeutics: The clinical use of drugs* (6th ed.). Vancouver, WA: Applied Therapeutics.

# 31

# ENDOCRINE DISORDERS: DIABETES MELLITUS

*Martha J. Price and Daniel Kent*

The treatment of diabetes mellitus has been dramatically influenced in the past 25 years by improved diagnosis and classification of the disease, first by the National Diabetes Data Group in 1979, and most recently by an expert committee's review of the current state of the diabetes diagnostic and classification evidence (American Diabetes Association, 1997). Both classification efforts have helped to track and synthesize the most relevant information to better understand diabetes' etiology, pathophysiology and progression. The pharmaceutical market, too, has kept pace with these changes, and the projected treatment for the 21st Century suggests that therapies, as we now know them, will give way to new and combined agents, including preventative therapies.

## CHARACTERISTICS OF DIABETES MELLITUS

Diabetes mellitus is a metabolic syndrome characterized by glucose intolerance from an absolute or relative lack of the pancreatic hormone, insulin. Insulin is an essential hormone that allows glucose, the body's principal energy source, to enter insulin-dependent tissue—skeletal muscle, liver, fat cells. Elevated blood glucose and associated symptoms, such as polydipsia (increased thirst) and polyuria (increased urinary frequency) are diagnostic markers. More specifically, using the aforementioned American Diabetes Asso-

ciation (1997) criteria, a casual plasma glucose *>200 mg/dl or a fasting plasma glucose of >126 mg/dl supports the diagnosis of diabetes mellitus.* Normal fasting glycemia range is 70–110 mg/dl. Weight loss and fluid and electrolyte imbalance may also accompany the onset, particularly in type 1 diabetes which is caused by pancreatic beta cell destruction. Type 2, the most common type of diabetes, may present more subtly over a period of years with symptoms of fatigue, blurred vision, and persistent infections, such as vaginal candidiasis. Classification of diabetes types, as accepted by the World Health Organization (1985) include: type 1 diabetes, type 2 diabetes, secondary diabetes, gestational diabetes, and impaired glucose tolerance (IGT). In the short term, very elevated hyperglycemia may pose a threat to stable fluid and electrolyte balance. Long term complications of diabetes result in chronic macrovascular, microvascular and neurologic changes, increasing the risk of disability and death from myocardial infarction, stroke, and end organ damage to eyes, kidneys, extremities and autonomic functioning, such as gastrointestinal and sexual disorders.

## THE TWO MOST COMMON TYPES OF DIABETES

### Type 1 Diabetes

In type 1 diabetes the pathophysiology lies in the autoimmune destruction of the pancreatic beta cells, thus insulin replacement is the critical component of treatment. Hyperglycemia associated with this type of diabetes is often accompanied by elevated triglycerides, insulin resistance during very elevated hyperglycemia (over 250 mg/dl), production of ketones, alteration of counterregulatory hormone production, and weight loss. Failure to treat adequately with insulin results in catabolism, ketoacidosis and death. If treatment is sufficient to prevent ketoacidosis, but not adequate to control continuous hyperglycemia, the risk of microvascular disease resulting in nephropathy, retinopathy, and neuropathy is increased. The Diabetes Control and Complications Trial (DCCT) (Diabetes Control and Complications Trial Research Group, 1993) conclusively demonstrated that those with type 1 diabetes who achieve and maintain near-normal glycemia can prevent or markedly slow such microvascular complications. These results pertained to both of the study's experimental cohorts—those with type 1 diabetes and no evidence of complications, as well those with type 1 diabetes in very early stages of microvascular changes.

The current pharmacological goal of treating type 1 diabetes is to 1) replace insulin; 2) achieve a balance of insulin, food, and activity compatible with the individual's growth and development; and 3) achieve an average range of fasting blood glucose between 70–110 mg/dl. In addition to available insulin treatment, newer therapies are emerging that include insulin analogs, potential alteration and/or reduction in the rate or onset of pancreatic beta cell destruction, and altering metabolism via carbohydrate absorption.

## Type 2 Diabetes

Hyperglycemia is also the hallmark of *type 2 diabetes mellitus*, however, the etiology of this form of diabetes differs markedly from type 1. Its etiology includes a progression of events that includes alteration in beta cell production of insulin, resistance to insulin uptake at the target cells (skeletal muscle, liver, fat), and increased hepatic secretion of glycogen (DeFronzo, 1988). When insulin cannot link up with the insulin receptors along the target cell rim, glucose is prevented from entering the cell. It is not uncommon for relatively high doses of exogenous insulin to be required to overcome this insulin resistance. In contrast, smaller amounts of exogenous insulin are needed to suppress hepatic release of glycogen stores.

Type 2 diabetes is more likely to have associated obesity and hypertension, and the major mortality risks are from cardiovascular events—myocardial infarction and stroke. The common blood lipid pattern in this type of diabetes is very similar to those at risk for CVD—elevated total cholesterol and LDL-cholesterol, and lower HDL-cholesterol.

Not all people with type 2 are overweight (about 20%), and this may actually be another variation in the genetic expression of diabetes as a disease. These individuals are more likely to exhaust their endogenous insulin supply, fail sulfonylurea therapy and need insulin therapy to prevent severe hyperglycemia.

## DIABETES AND PHARMACOLOGICAL AIMS

To understand the rationale of pharmacologic approaches for diabetes treatment, it is important to first understand what occurs when diabetes is *not* present. In the non-diabetes state, insulin and accompanying counter-regulatory hormones—glucagon, growth hormone, glucocorticoids, and norepinephrine—exist in a continuous rising and falling balance to keep blood glucose contained within a narrow range (fasting of 70–100 mg/dl (4–6 mmol/l); casual plasma glucose < 200 mg/dl (11.1 mmol/l). When this balance is upset because of lack of insulin (type 1 diabetes) or inability to use endogenous insulin (type 2 diabetes), the treatment must be targeted to the areas of deficiency and/or defect.

Any attempt to artificially reproduce what the body would normally do if diabetes were not present brings with it the potential for untoward side effects of treatment. Diabetes therapies that directly reduce hyperglycemia also pose the risk of hypoglycemia. Hypoglycemic danger exists because insulin and oral hypoglycemic agents must be offered as *open-loop therapy, meaning that there is no automatic feedback loop for controlled release of counterregulatory hormones to keep blood glucose within a physiologic normal and safe range.* The body will be unable to respond with an automatic reduction in the agent's action if blood glucose begins to fall below normal (i.e., 70 mg/dl). Keeping the balance between a sufficient metabolically stable blood glucose level and avoiding hyperglycemia or hypoglycemia requires near constant vigilance and self-management. For this reason, food is an essential factor in the treatment of diabetes management. Sufficient calories and nutrients to sustain normal weight and activity will be required, and appropriate timing of both has to be coordinated with hypoglycemic drugs. Activity and exercise are also critical cornerstones of treatment, because diabetes mellitus, as a disease of metabolism, will effect how the body is able to access quick energy and store/release energy for activity needs. For these reasons, pharmacotherapeutics for diabetes will necessarily require concurrent attention to food and activity patterns as essential components of any treatment equation.

As more information becomes available about the pathophysiology of diabetes, the question for clinicians will be necessarily expanded from *"how can blood glucose control be achieved"* to how will this particular therapy affect *"the processes and outcomes of the disease known as diabetes?"* This perspective is so important that it is suggested that the clinician view ALL pharmacological therapies with the questions posed in Table 31-1 in mind.

## SETTING GLYCEMIC GOALS

In addition to targeting therapies to reduce the damage of diabetes, whether microvascular or macrovascular, it is important to set safe, therapeutic targets for blood glucose. Setting glycemic goals needs to be considered within what is safest, in the short term, and most beneficial, in the long term, for the individual patient. Current science should guide this decision. The Diabetes Control and Complications Trial (DCCT) results indicate that the glycemic level is positively correlated to degree of rate of microvascular damage. That is, when glycemia levels are persistently above normal (HbA1c > 7%), the rate of damage to eyes, kidneys, and nerves rises exponentially (Diabetes Control and Complications Trial Research Group, 1993). Those DCCT data also show that even modest reductions in HbA1c can reduce the rate of eye, kidney, and nerve damage. With glycated hemoglobins (HbA1c assay) of 7.0% or less, the rate of damage is reduced substantially; *however*, the *risk of hypoglycemia* increases. For that reason, and because those data show that the additional effort to move HbA1c much below 8% may yield only minimal reduction in the rate of diabetes damage to small blood vessels, the glycemic goal should be evaluated carefully for each individual. HbA1c below 8% may be contraindicated for some patients whose quality of life and safety (i.e. risk of hypoglycemia) would be adversely affected.

Although the DCCT evidence verifies the protective effect that good glycemic control has on microvascular damage from diabetes, the science is less clear about glycemic control's effect on macrovascular disease, i.e. risk of heart attack and stroke. Therefore, an essential focus of treatment for diabetes must continue to give concentrated attention to reducing cardiovascular risks—diet and exercise; no smoking or tobacco use; controlling hypertension; and use of aspirin when possible to prevent CVD events. Overall treatment is targeted to support maintenance of desired body weight, control of blood lipids and reduction of hyperglycemia. These recommended risk reductions are often difficult to treat because they require, for the most part, lifestyle or major behavioral change.

Type 1 therapy should be aimed at insulin replacement via regimens that afford the best glycemic control given the patient's capacity and willingness to attend to multiple self-management behaviors and problem-solving techniques.

The treatment for Type 2 is targeted to supporting endogenous insulin production and utilization, a reduction in insulin resistance, and suppression of hepatic glucose release during nocturnal fasting (sleep), rather than replace-

---

### TABLE 31-1.   QUESTIONS TO ASK WHEN SELECTING ANTIDIABETES THERAPY

1. How will this agent affect blood glucose? (Does it exert a direct effect on lowering glucose and is severe hypoglycemia a possible side effect?)
2. How will this agent affect blood lipids?
3. How will this agent affect end-organs most frequently affected by diabetes?
4. How will this agent affect body weight?
5. How will this agent affect hepatic glucose production?
6. How will this agent affect counterregulatory hormones?
7. Will this agent likely be altered by over-the-counter, self-prescribed therapies?
8. What is the science base to support use of this agent within specific age ranges?
9. What food, activity, and monitoring conditions must be met for this agent to be safely administered? Can the patient or family meet these conditions?
10. Even if the agent is the drug of choice, is it the drug of choice for THIS patient given the pharmacodynamics and associated self-management requirements and costs?

ment. Thus, type 2 diabetes may actually require a combination of several therapies to achieve the desired physiologic balance and lifestyle change outcomes. A stepped approach to type 2 treatment is aimed towards reducing cardiovascular risks, and safe blood glucose control through first diet and exercise, then monotherapy of either a sulfonylurea or metformin (ADA Consensus Statement, 1996). Monotherapy can be advanced to a combination therapy of oral agents and, then, if necessary, single bedtime dose of intermediate insulin can be added to augment daytime oral agent therapy. If these approaches fail to control blood glucose to the safe target goal, then twice a day intermediate insulin or twice a day, split-mixed insulin may be required. The reader is encouraged to be informed about the many newer oral diabetes agents rapidly becoming available and to discern whether or not the agents are intended as monotherapy or for combination therapy. For example, a newer agent, troglitazone, has been approved by the Federal Food and Drug Administration for use with type 2 diabetics currently using insulin. It is likely that this agent will have approval as a monotherapeutic agent in the near future. Throughout all attempts at pharmacological control, the type 2 patient must be encouraged to continue with meticulous diet and exercise involvement.

Consistent, ideal blood glucose levels (70–110 mg/dl for fasting blood glucose; a random blood glucose of 70–140 mg/dl) corresponds to a glycated hemoglobin (HbA1c) of approximately 6% or less. However, factors such as age, cognitive skills, accompanying co-morbidities, and psycho-social characteristics all need to be taken into consideration. For example, the glycemic targets for a 72 year old man with pre-existing cardiovascular disease and who lives alone, will not be the same as for a 27 year old, healthy mother of two active pre-schoolers. Near-normal glycemic control predisposes to as much as a three-fold risk of severe hypoglycemia, and for the elderly this would increase their risk of confusion, falls and broken bones, hospitalization, and pneumonia.

## THE IMPORTANT ROLE OF SELF-MANAGEMENT IN EFFECTIVE DIABETES THERAPY

Whether the treatment plan is limited to diet and exercise or includes one or more pharmacotherapeutic agents, self-management is an essential

on-going activity for successful outcomes. Self-management will depend upon diabetes acuity, end organ damage, and perceived treatment goals. The actual activities prescribed for self-management will depend upon the age, cognitive and psycho-motor skills, psycho-social resources and the value that the patient and/or his or her family place on treatment and self-management.

Obviously, there is no 'easy' age at which to be diagnosed with diabetes. Each developmental level in life presents its own demands and challenges. The child, adolescent or young adult in whom type 1 diabetes is most common, requires a treatment schedule that most mimics the insulin production and glucose utilization in the non-diabetic person. Without proper treatment, growth and development can be adversely affected. Yet near euglycemia targets place the type 1 patient at risk for hypoglycemia.

In the child under age 13, the treatment goals should target promotion of healthy growth and development while avoiding severe hyperglycemia and diabetic ketoacidosis and severe hypoglycemia. For the older child, she or he will need to learn diabetes management skills that avoid acute complications and sustain the best possible glycemic control.

A tighter glycemic control regimen requires multiple decisions to be made during the course of the day regarding types and amounts of food, as well as types and amounts of insulin. These decisions must be made on a variety of data: blood glucose test results, physical signs and symptoms, and knowledge of which factors can or have affected blood glucose levels. Couple these treatment demands with the child's need to develop his/her own self-identity and social self, and the challenges for patients and their families come into sharper focus.

Questions abound of when to give the child responsibility and how much. Most of the family literature regarding diabetes has been focused on type 1 diabetes and the special challenges of the diabetic child and diabetic family. The available evidence clearly shows that children who are provided with loving parental guidance, as well as caring and patient teaching per their own readiness, can succeed in learning to take on self-management (Giordano, Petrila, Banion, and Neuenkirchen, 1992; Hentinen & Kyngäs, 1996; Grey, Cameron & Thurber, 1991). Child and parents will need accurate and supportive information from their health care provider. It will not be sufficient for the provider to know and prescribe the various diabetes pharmacotherapeutics; he or she will also be required to skillfully guide and support the patient and family in the application of therapy and determine the readiness of the child to assume responsibility for tasks and decision-making. This includes being aware of the support resources available to patients and families in the care setting, community, or region.

## OTHER IMPORTANT PHARMACOTHERAPEUTICS FOR DIABETES MANAGEMENT

Although the remainder of this chapter is dedicated to discussion of those agents that specifically lower blood glucose, the reader is referred to Chapter 20 for information on the agents used to control cardiovascular disease and lipoprotein management as well as discussion of ACE-inhibitors as the drug of choice to reduce the progression and/or onset of diabetes renal disease. Diabetes pharmacotherapeutics are changing rapidly. Development and availability of new glucose lowering agents will likely increase the complexity of designing effective diabetes treatment regimens. At the same time, the 'tried and true' elements of diet and exercise remain powerful tools in the treatment of type 2 diabetes and should not be minimized or replaced entirely with drug therapy.

## SPECIFIC CONSIDERATIONS FOR PHARMACOTHERAPY

### NONPHARMACOLOGIC THERAPY

Because diabetes mellitus is a metabolic disease, nutrition and exercise remain the most essential part of diabetes management. In Type 2 diabetes, weight management and exercise are the initial focus because insulin resistance can be initially dramatically improved with minimal weight loss (10 to 20 pounds), and drug therapy is reserved for those requiring additional glycemic management (Franz, 1994). Even though type 1 diabetes will require insulin replacement, that replacement regimen will require coordination with meal planning, meal patterns, and adjusting insulin to match activity level and food intake. Establishing individual caloric needs necessary to maintain desired body weight is best achieved by balancing carbohydrate, fat, and protein in-

take. The American Diabetes Association recommends dietary intake of these nutrients to be individualized to the particular patient. However, the following can be used as a guide to plan nutrition therapy: carbohydrate intake of 50–60% with a fiber content of 10–30 gm daily, fat comprising less than 30% of calories, and protein 10–20% of the total daily calorie content. Goals of therapy remain the same—euglycemia, optimal lipid management, weight management, and maintenance of self-management behaviors. Even before or along with a dietary referral, the primary care provider can easily reinforce good nutrition principles of quality or balance in healthy, low-fat food choices (the Food Guide Pyramid is an easy place to start), in appropriate quantities or serving sizes, and, if on glucose-lowering drugs, being consistent in the timing of meals and amounts of carbohydrates (Powers, 1996). The general benefits of exercise apply to all humans, including those with diabetes, and the primary care provider can promote participation in consistent, planned physical exercise (American Diabetes Association, 1994a).

### WHEN DRUG THERAPY IS NEEDED

Type 1 diabetes must be treated by replacing insulin.The ideal insulin replacement regimen would be to try to approximate the normal, physiological pattern of insulin release and glucose utilization. For the older adult with type 1 diabetes, this regimen may necessarily be modified to prioritize safety and quality of life. In type 1 diabetes, nutrition and exercise are important adjuncts to successful insulin therapy.

In type 2, dietary management and exercise are the cornerstones of treatment. About 80% of those with type 2 diabetes are likely to require weight reduction and effort at maintaining a desirable body weight. Depending on presenting symptom severity, it is appropriate to begin type 2 diabetes treatment with sole attention to diet and exercise for six weeks to three months (Franz, 1994). This effort cannot be underemphasized! For most patients, carbohydrate balance and control are the most difficult and unsuccessful part of diabetes management.

Diet and exercise alone may not be sufficient therapy for someone with type 2 diabetes, and if target glycemic goals are not attained by these requisite steps, then adding (not displacing diet and exercise) drug therapy must be considered. Each therapy is tried as monotherapy first, and given sufficient trial and careful follow-up to see if glycemic targets (HbA1c and FPG goals) can be attained. This means careful attention to diet, exercise, and blood glucose monitoring and glycated hemoglobin data. The choice of therapy is matched to the specific pathophysiology defect, and, in the case of type 2 is usually targeted at decreasing insulin resistance and improving endogenous insulin production. Thus, begin with monotherapy of either a sulfonylurea or metformin (White, 1996). Then, if goals are not achieved after a full 3 to 6 month trial, or fail after a time, combination therapy is the next step. More specifics are given below by drug agent. Monitor each step as carefully as any scientific experiment. Keep as many glucose influencing factors as constant and controlled for as long as possible. The art of this treatment approach cannot be underestimated. To find a therapeutic regimen for each patient requires a full partnership between the patient and health care provider.

## SHORT-TERM AND LONG-TERM GOALS OF PHARMACOTHERAPY

Setting specific glycemic goals using intermediate and longer-term markers of success are critical for patient motivation and accomplishment of desired health outcomes. Short-term markers include monitoring for improvement in blood lipids: cholesterol, low density lipoproteins (LDLs), high density lipoproteins (HDLs), and triglycerides; body weight reduction; and a trend toward the targeted hemoglobin A1c. The patient should be encouraged to participate in daily self-blood glucose monitoring frequently enough to discern whether or not treatment is effective. For type 2 patients on either monotherapy or two oral agents, a fasting and pre-evening meal testing schedule may be sufficient. The patient who wants to achieve and maintain normal glycemic control will require blood tests and decision-making throughout the day. Longer-term goals will focus on overall weight management, evidence of lipid control, and reduction of microvascular and macrovascular complications.

## TIME FRAME FOR INITIATING AND MODIFYING PHARMACOTHERAPY

For those with type 1 diabetes, insulin therapy is initiated at the time of diagnosis. Primary care team support should target not only finding the most effective insulin dose, but also helping the patient incorporate this therapy into daily living. The challenge with this therapy is most often learning how to achieve pattern management. Pattern management is both collecting and using information from blood glucose test results along with the type of and timing of meals and the influence of varying levels of activity or exercise. When glycemic management is modified, it is useful to apply and monitor the changes for at least 1 to 2 weeks. Overall glycemic changes can be evaluated by laboratory data of a glycated hemoglobin as often as every 2 to 3 months. The major guide is whether or not the treatment approach is bringing about glycemic shifts towards the preferred targeted range.

In type 2 diabetes, initiating drug therapy depends first on an individual's ability to successfully use nutrition and exercise. A reasonable trial period, during which concerted effort is applied, is 2–3 months. If the target glycemic goal has not been reached by then, it is reasonable to consider adding oral drug therapy to the continued diet and exercise program. As with type 1, the glycemic targets will guide the therapeutic approach and determine over time if changes are needed.

## ASSESSMENT AND HISTORY TAKING

The same principles of general health screening apply to persons with diabetes. However, special monitoring of changes to the end organs commonly affected by diabetes is necessary. The American Diabetes Association publishes information on clinical practice recommendations for those providers who may encounter patients with diabetes (American Diabetes Association, 1997). General assessment for type 1 and type 2 diabetes should include review of current cardiovascular risks (smoking status, blood pressure, weight, exercise, and nutrition habits), routine retinal screening, evaluation of the presence of microalbuminuria, foot ulcer risk, as well as establishing a glycemic management plan appropriate to the individual patient's targeted treatment goals.

Laboratory evaluation should include glycated hemoglobin, fasting lipid profile, serum creatinine, urinalysis, albumin/creatinine ratio for microalbuminuria, thyroid function tests if indicated, and electrocardiogram in adults.

The frequency of visits thereafter need to be determined by treatment goals and the requisite monitoring to assess treatment effectiveness. At the very least an annual examination would be wise to repeat evaluation of cardiovascular risk factors and assessment of eyes, kidneys, feet, and glycemic control. In addition, an evaluation of the patient's self-management skills and behaviors as pertain to the treatment plan and patient's goals needs to occur. This can be done by careful review of hyper and hypoglycemia symptoms and frequency, the blood glucose test results record, current medication regimen and how administered, and review of typical day's meals, work, and exercise times.

Encourage the patient to self-manage and self-monitor to help determine the effectiveness of a specific treatment approach. The questions in Table 31-2 can help both the patient and the healthcare provider determine treatment self-management requirements and effectiveness. For example, if insulin is prescribed, the patient has to know how to prepare and administer an injection, how to store insulin, how and when to test blood glucose, what and when to eat, and how to detect and treat mild or severe hypoglycemia. It may also be helpful for the patient to understand what insulin is intended to accomplish in terms of successful treatment. For example, the intention of therapy with insulin for a type 1 diabetic who makes no endogenous insulin is quite different from the prescription for a type 2 diabetic of a single bedtime dose of intermediate acting insulin to suppress nocturnal hepatic glucose release.

Although there are many literature resources for patients with diabetes mellitus, none of these is likely to be effective unless the healthcare provider or team can integrate the information into the specific patient's overall management plan. The American Diabetes Association (1660 Duke Street, Alexandria, VA 22314) has many kinds of educational materials—pamphlets, tapes, video, and so on—to assist patients and professionals in learning about and managing diabetes. Because much of the information is generalized, the health care team can assist with interpretation to make it most meaningful for the individual. The pharmaceutical industry also can help with developing disease management programs, setting up specific delivery approaches, and providing specific diabetes product aids. These products range from specific drug agents to durable goods, such as insulin delivery devices, including pens, air-jet injectors, glucose measuring monitors, test monitoring strips, and visual (large-type, Braille) devices.

---

**TABLE 31–2. QUESTIONS TO HELP THE PATIENT EVALUATE THE EFFECTIVENESS OF ANTI-DIABETES THERAPIES**

1. How will this agent affect my blood glucose? (Does it exert a *direct effect* on lowering glucose and is severe hypoglycemia a possible side effect?)
2. How often do I need to test my blood glucose? What can/should I do with the information?
3. What are the short-term effects (including side effects) of the agent?
4. What are the long-term side effects of the agent?
5. How will this agent affect me in preventing or slowing diabetes complications?
6. How will this agent affect my weight?
7. How will this agent affect my cholesterol and lipid levels?
8. How will this agent affect hepatic glucose production?
9. How will this agent affect counterregulatory hormones?
10. Will this agent likely be changed by over-the-counter, self-prescribed therapies?
11. Is this the best agent for someone of my age, physical condition, and living situation?
12. Do I have to be careful about when and what I eat because of this agent?
13. Do I have to watch how exercise affects this agent? How can I prevent my blood glucose from going too high or too low because of exercise effects?
14. Does my family or live-in partner need to be taught how to treat a reaction to this agent? What if there is no one to do this for me?
15. How will I know if this treatment is not working? When or how often should I be in touch with the provider?

---

## OUTCOMES MANAGEMENT

### SELECTING AN APPROPRIATE AGENT

Because hyperglycemia depends on the specific pathology, it is important to try to match the pharmacological agent with the targeted defect. In type 1 diabetes this choice is always insulin replacement. In type 2 diabetes, the disease can express in varying degrees of insulin resistance, compensated insulin production by the pancreatic beta cell, and hepatic glucose secretion. Individuals with type 2 diabetes and obesity generally have greater insulin resistance and require agents to improve this problem. Also, these individuals may benefit from small bed-time doses of an intermediate acting insulin to suppress the release of hepatic glucose and con-comitant use of daytime sulfonylureas or biguanide, or both, to handle glucose loads from food intake. Those type 2 diabetics who are non-obese are more likely to progress from oral agent therapy alone to daytime insulin supple-ments. The important caveat is that all diabetes changes over time and requires monitoring to assess its progress and effect on overall systemic health. Thus, therapies need to be evaluated over time.

At present, the best way to determine glycemic control is to obtain glycated hemoglo-bin measures (HbA1c values) to determine the average blood glucose level during the past 2 to 3 months. Equally important is the patient's daily blood glucose monitoring record. Because the HbA1c is an average, which incorporates but does not reveal specific instances of glucose ex-cursions, it is important to evaluate both pieces of information together to see the patterns. For example, if someone has a HbA1c of 7.0 but is experiencing frequent hypoglycemic episodes or wide fluctuation (highs and lows), reassess the approach to glycemic control by reviewing when and how much medication is being used and how consistent other factors—food and activ-ity—are in the patient's daily schedule. Pattern review always considers how these three vari-ables—food, activity/exercise, and medica-tions—interact.

One additional caveat to consider is that giv-ing the maximum dose of an agent is not always warranted. The decision to increase dosage should be accompanied by careful evaluation of whether or not the increase improves overall glycemic control and diabetes health. If not, then the therapy is both ineffective and expen-sive, and another treatment approach should to be considered.

## Alpha-Glucosidase Inhibitors

Alpha-glucosidase inhibitors are one of sev-eral classes of drugs that work to slow or delay the absorption of carbohydrates prior to their di-gestion to glucose and other monosaccharides. They exert their action on the brush border in-testinal cells by binding to pancreatic amylase and alpha glucosidase to prevent hydrolysis of complex carbohydrates. An alpha-glucosidase inhibitor competes with carbohydrates for bind-ing these enzymes in the small intestine, and the

result is the slowing of the absorption of the monosaccharides from the gut. This delayed ab-sorption lowers the characteristically high post-prandial peak of blood glucose that is seen in pa-tients with diabetes (Gavin III, et al., 1998).

*Acarbose.*     The first of its class to become avail-able in the U.S. is acarbose (Precose). Systemic absorption of this drug is less than 1%. The sec-ond agent is miglitol (Glyset), and it is absorbed from the gut and is excreted via the kidneys (Sels, et al., 1994). The FDA has approved use of these drugs in type 2 diabetes. Their action decreases the peak postprandial rise in serum glucose by delaying and more evenly distribut-ing the absorption of glucose. This gradual delay in absorption then allows a sluggish endogenous insulin response to a meal (as in type 2 diabetes) to "catch up" to and better manage the glucose load of the meal. Of course, this assumes that the dietary carbohydrate burden is controlled by appropriate type and amounts of carbohydrates, i.e., that the meal contains complex carbohy-drates of prescribed proportions. Absorption of monosaccharides, or sucrose will be delayed by acarbose, so oral treatment of hypoglycemia must be accomplished with dextrose (com-mercially prepared glucose tablets) (Bayer Corporation, 1995).

Acarbose and miglitol induce action in the in-testinal tract in the brush border cells starting proximal and continuing distally to the ascend-ing colon. This action has been responsible for the most significant side effects and has led to dose-dependent flatulence, abdominal cramp-ing, distention, belching and diarrhea. These ef-fects are due in part to the fermentation of the unabsorbed carbohydrates as they travel through the colon (Baliga and Fonseca, 1997; Conniff, 1995c). As more of the border cells are induced, the side effects tend to diminish with time; however, approximately 11% of patients will seek relief from this major side effect.

Before treating the uncomfortable side ef-fects of abdominal bloating and flatulence, the practitioner needs to be aware that some prod-ucts for flatulence relief also contain alpha glu-cosidase (an example is "Beano") and prevent the therapeutic action of acarbose or miglitol and therefore are contraindicated in combina-tion. Antacids and bismuth are appropriate al-ternatives for treating abdominal side effects. Patients with chronic abdominal and intestinal diseases should avoid the use of acarbose due to its action on intestinal border cells.

Side effects may be minimized by dosing to acclimatize acarbose within the colon. The starting dose for both acarbose and miglitol should begin at 25mg three times daily and taken at the beginning of the meal for maximal effect. At 4–6 week intervals the dose can be increased, depending on postprandial blood glucose levels and patient tolerance (May, 1995). The maximal dose for acarbose is 50 mg three times daily for patients less than 60 kg, and 100 mg three times daily if the person is over 60 kg. The usual maintenance dose for miglitol is 50 mg three times a day. Some patients may require 100 mg three times daily for maximal benefit (Bischoff, 1995). Clinical response to acarbose is defined as consistent 1 hour postprandial glucose lowering. This effect is experienced by 35–50% of type 2 patients with diabetes. Acarbose is indicated in treatment for:

- Type 2: Primary treatment for mild to moderate hyperglycemia
- Type 2: Adjunct therapy for those on sulfonylureas, biguanides, and/ or insulin
- Type 1: *Not yet FDA approved for this group*: Potential adjunct therapy with insulin for postprandial glucose excursions with insulin

The effectiveness of acarbose to reduce postprandial glucose serum concentrations and glycosylated hemoglobin has been demonstrated in patients managed by diet alone, diet plus metformin, diet plus sulfonylurea, and diet plus insulin therapy (Chaisson, 1994). Insulin treated type 2 patients taking acarbose have been able to reduce insulin intake by 20%. Study subjects have experienced at least an additional 0.4% reduction in glycosylated hemoglobin levels while continuing to focus on diet and exercise (Coniff, 1995a). Combination tolbutamide plus acarbose has shown greater reduction in serum glucose concentrations than either will alone (Baliga and Fonseca, 1997; Coniff, 1995a), and so suggests that acarbose has better overall glycemic effect when combined with another hypoglycemic agent.

Lipid management may actually be improved slightly with acarbose, with enhancements seen in total cholesterol levels and the HDL-to-cholesterol ratio. It is likely that lipid reduction is a consequence of a reduction in hyperinsulinemia while on acarbose (Leonhardt, 1994).

Potentially significant elevations in hepatic transaminase levels may occur while on acarbose and should be monitored regularly. Transaminase levels usually return to normal once acarbose has been discontinued (Conniff, 1995, Baliga and Fonseca, 1997).

Caution is necessary when selecting an alpha-glucosidase inhibitor because of potential systemic absorption. If the agent is absorbed from the small intestine, it is prudent to exclude patients whose serum creatinine is > 2.0 mg/dL. And, although the agents do not directly cause hypoglycemia when used as a monotherapy, there is a risk of hypoglycemia when they are used in combination with sulfonylureas or insulins (Johnson and Taylor, 1996). Treatment of hypoglycemia must be modified to use dextrose, NOT sucrose (table sugar) products, because the alpha-glucosidase inhibitor will inhibit conversion of sucrose to glucose (Bayer Corporation, 1995). Mild hypoglycemia would be best treated with dextrose tablets which are commercially available as glucose tablets. More severe hypoglycemia will require either glucagon administration or intravenous dextrose solution.

## Biguanides

Compounds synthesized from the amino acid *guanidine* have been available in European markets for over 40 years. Of these, two have been removed (phenformin and butformin) because of the incidence of lactic acidosis. Metformin, however, is one biguanide with minimal propensity towards lactic acidosis, except in persons whose renal and cardiac function have been compromised. Metformin became available in the United States market in 1995.

Metformin acts in at least two ways to lower plasma glucose. Without altering insulin secretion or releasing or depleting insulin stores, at the cellular level, metformin has been shown to increase muscle and adipose cell receptor sensitivity to glucose, thereby making glucose uptake more efficient. It also acts to suppress hepatic output of glycogen, a phenomenon common to type 2 pathology. In a study reported by Riddle, et al., (1996), low dose metformin (500mg) at bedtime was sufficient to suppress hepatic glucose release, while higher doses (1 to 2 grams) during the day were required to handle prandial glucose. Because metformin can affect (reduce) glucose absorption from the gastrointestinal tract, some individuals may experience transient anorexia and weight loss. This weight loss is usually a modest 3–5 kilograms (Calle-Pascual, 1995; Dunn, 1995).

An advantage of metformin seems to be that it provides little risk of hypoglycemia in either patients with or without diabetes. The incidence of hypoglycemia is greater when metformin is combined with a sulfonylurea or insulin than when it is used separately (DeFronzo, 1995; Baliga and Fonseca, 1997). Metformin has also been shown to improve the lipid profiles by decreasing LDL-cholesterol, triglycerides, and increasing HDL-cholesterol.

Metformin is appropriate for patients who have Type 2 diabetes, whose serum creatinine is less than 1.4, and in whom diet and exercise alone have not achieved desired blood glucose levels. There is an advantage to using metformin with those eligible patients who are obese or would benefit from modest weight reduction (Chong, 1995).

The addition of metformin to diet alone, or with a sulfonylurea or with insulin have been successful in controlling blood glucose in those with Type 2 diabetes (UKPDS, 1995; Hermann, 1994).

The limiting side effects of metformin are predominantly those associated with gastrointestinal disturbances. These disturbances are prevalent in 10–35% of the patients and consist of bloating, nausea, abdominal cramping, diarrhea, and flatulence. These effects are controlled by slowly initiating therapy, starting with the lowest dose tolerated, usually 250 or 500 mg daily, then increasing the dosage every 1–3 weeks until the maximum effective dose is reached. Maximum dose is 1–2.5 grams divided into 2–3 doses per day (Dunn, 1995). This slow-dosing approach often circumvents gastrointestinal side effects and enables patients to achieve full dose ranges with the benefit of optimal glycemic control.

Glycemic targets and benefits of metformin therapy are realized within 3–6 months once the patient is cycled to an optimal dose. During this time it is prudent to have the patient self-monitoring and recording blood glucose levels. This is especially important for those who are combining metformin therapy with that of a sulfonylurea or insulin regimen. When used in combination, metformin is more likely to improve the body's sensitivity to insulin and thereby lower blood glucose. Hypoglycemia may occur, and the dose of sulfonylurea and/or insulin may need to be reduced, or sometimes even stopped.

Metformin is the least likely of the biguanides to precipitate lactic acidosis. Even though lactic acidosis is rare, it has a high mortality rate and the use of concomitant drugs that can alter systems function (i.e. kidney, liver, cardiac) have the potential for complicating therapy (Lalau, 1995). Patients who are at risk for kidney, liver, cardiovascular, and electrolyte imbalances are at risk for lactic acidosis, and metformin is not appropriate therapy for these individuals.

Because metformin excretion is through tubular secretion in the kidneys, lactic acidosis is more likely in those patients whose renal function has been diminished. **Metformin should not be prescribed for individuals with a serum creatinine of 1.4 or higher.** The possibility of lactic acidosis may also be increased when contrast dyes for radiological procedures are required for those diabetic patients on metformin. In that circumstance, the practitioner needs to be alert to the potential for short-term kidney failure and lactic acidosis. Therefore, in addition to keeping the patient well hydrated, metformin should be discontinued for 48 hours following the procedure until full renal functioning is apparent. Similar situations apply also to hospitalizations or procedures where changes in renal function are likely to occur. This problem can be avoided by frequent monitoring of renal function and appropriate selection of patients for metformin therapy who are not expected to have major shifts in fluids, electrolytes, and kidney, cardiac, or respiratory function (Lalau, 1995).

Metformin is effective in reducing blood glucose for patients with type 2 diabetes who have failed diet and exercise alone. Comparison studies have shown that metformin is more likely to be effective in patients who are 120% or higher in their recommended body weight. It is more likely to provide the best glycemic control when used in combination with sulfonylurea (DeFronzo, 1995; UKPDS, 1995; Baliga and Fonseca, 1997). At least 80–90% of patients experience a decrease in fasting plasma glucose and overall HbA1c level—58 mg/dL and 1.8%, respectively (DeFronzo, 1995).

## Insulin

Insulin is a hormone that is made and secreted by the pancreas. It is essential for metabolism of nutrients—particularly carbohydrates. At present, insulin can only be replaced by injecting commercially prepared insulins. Available insulin preparations are biogenetically engineered using yeast or E. coli bacteria. This recombinant DNA technology has replaced insulins prepared from animals sources (beef and pork). Not only are these sources purified to less than 10 ppm of extraneous materials, but they are also molecularly the same as human insulin. All insulin preparations contain protein components and none are antigenic, although biogenetically engineered human source insulin may be somewhat less immunogenic than animal source insulin.

Originally insulin was derived from the extraction of animal pancreas—either pork, beef, or beef-pork combinations. In the early 1980's, so-called human insulin became available through semi-synthetic recombinant DNA technology. Most animal source insulins have been replaced with the human insulin product. Further DNA sequencing has lead to new insulin products (analogs) with altered pharmacokinetic properties to improve potential for the duration of action and shortening the time to onset of action.

Insulin preparations are also available by varying unit-dose concentrations, the most common of which is U-100, which means that 1 cc will equal 100 units of insulin. For special use situations, Regular insulin is also available in a concentration of U-500. (Note: Regular insulin will be denoted as a proper noun to avoid confusion of the term 'regular.') For convenience, insulin is available in fixed ratios of either 70/30 or 50/50, meaning that the solution contains 70% of an intermediate acting insulin and 30% of a shorter action insulin, or, as in the 50/50, equal parts of each.

*Insulin actions.* Insulin preparations can be further categorized by duration of action: very fast acting insulin analogs, short acting insulins, intermediate acting insulins, and long acting insulins. By adding either protamine or zinc to pure insulin (Regular, clear insulin), the action of insulin can be prolonged, and administration regimens can be prescribed that more nearly mimic the body's physiological secretion of inuslin. Basically, there are two physiologic insulin secretion patterns that insulin regimens try to duplicate: 1) a continuous basal level which provides continuous 24 hour insulin availability to match metabolic glucose requirements, and 2) bolus-released insulin in direct response to meal or glucose intake (see Figure 31-1). The second action also serves the purpose of stimulating glucose utilization and storage of glucose, fat and protein.

In type 1 diabetes, when insulin is no longer produced by the pancreas, the goal of insulin regimens is to provide both components of action-basal and meal-stimulated glucose utilization. For this reason, patients usually require a combination of insulins that can provide varied length of action.

In type 2 diabetes, in which there is some residual insulin production, the goal is often to suppress hepatic glucose release, particularly that which occurs at night during fasting, and to improve utilization of insulin at the cell receptor. For these reasons, longer acting insulins at bedtime can support the hepatic suppression, while mealtime glucose utilization may be achieved through administration of a sulfonyl-

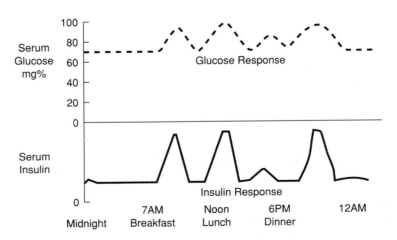

**Figure 31–1.** Physiologic insulin secretion in response to a meal or glucose intake.

urea, metformin, or an alpha glucosidase in-hibitor. However, because type 2 diabetes does not present in an homogenous pattern, some type 2 patients may require a combination of in-sulins and a regimen more similar to those advo-cated for type 1 patients in order to control blood glucose throughout the day and night.

*Short acting insulins* include Regular and lispro (trade name, Humalog). These are the most rapid acting insulins, with lispro having the fastest time to onset of action (see Figure 31-2). Both of these insulins are clear and colorless and can be administered by intravenous, intramus-cular, or subcutaneous route.

For daily use, all injections of insulin are most commonly self-administered into the subcuta-neous tissue, and for this reason there is a 'lag-time' between absorption and action. Regular insulin should be given 30 to 60 minutes prior to meals to maximize onset to peak of action. Because its molecular structure allows for very quick subcutaneous absorption, lispro can be given just 15 minutes prior to meals (Howey, 1995; Anderson, 1995), providing patients with the flexibility to more accurately match insulin requirements to the quantity and types of carbo-hydrate in the meal. Lispro's quick onset and action can also reduce the post-prandial blood glucose rise.

*Intermediate acting insulins* are used to pro-vide the basal level insulin release and are admin-istered as a single or twice-a-day injection. Twice-a-day injections of intermediate acting insulin are given about 10 to 12 hours apart, in the morning and either with the evening meal or at bedtime, depending on existing or targeted glucose pat-terns. Administering the intermediate evening dose at the evening meal may predispose the pa-tient to nocturnal hypoglycemia about 2 or 3 a.m. If that occurs, the first step is to move the admin-istration of the intermediate insulin to later in the evening, for example at 10 p.m.

When patients require total dosages of in-sulin greater than 30 units/day it is recom-mended by the American Diabetes Association that the dose be split and administered twice daily (American Diabetes Association, 1994b). This split administration regimen may not only provide more consistent insulin coverage throughout a 24 hour period, but may reduce the total volume of the insulin depot placed within a subcutaneous site. A larger insulin vol-ume is likely to be more slowly and unpre-dictably absorbed.

Theoretically, the onset of action of interme-diate insulin is 1–2 hours with peak action oc-curring in 6–8 hours and lasting 10–14 hours (as seen in Fig. 31-2). When NPH and/or Lente in-sulins are mixed with Regular insulin, the rapid action of the Regular may be blunted, and in-stead of two action peaks, the action is sustained as one intermediate action peak. Patients expe-riencing otherwise inexplicable glucose variation may want to try separating these two insulins as separate injections to see if glycemic excursions become more manageable.

Intermediate insulins, when combined with a short acting insulin, offer patients more flexibil-ity in meal planning and closer physiological in-sulin patterns with potentially better glucose control. Certain insulins mix well and are stable for extended periods of time. For example, NPH

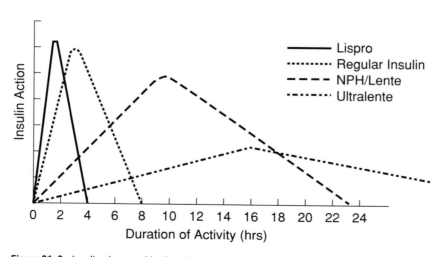

**Figure 31–2.** Insulin pharmacokinetic action.

and Regular can be mixed and used up to 7–14 days (Peters, 1986), while Lente and Regular are stable for just 5 minutes before the Regular insulin bonds to the Lente and loses its rapid action (Heine, 1984). Lispro has similar mixing compatabilities and actions as Regular insulin.

*Long acting insulins* include Ultralente insulin, which has an extended action that can last as long as 36 hours. Unlike the other insulins, Ultralente essentially has no peak effect but rather provides continued low levels of insulin activity (see Fig 31-2). Unfortunately, experience has shown that Ultralente, especially human Ultralente, produces a variation effect in basal control and may require at least two injections per day along with boluses of shorter acting insulin, such as lispro or Regular. Ultralente given as a single daily injection offers better basal control when given later in the evening (Riccio, 1994). To meet basal level insulin requirements about 40–50% of the total daily insulin dose will need to be provided by Ultralente for adequate insulin coverage.

***Insulin dosing.***   For adults with type 1 diabetes who present with normal body weight, without infection, concurrent disease, or illness, the recommended beginning dose is 0.6–0.75 units per kg per day (American Diabetes Association, 1994b). To meet growth and hormonal changes, higher dosages for children (0.6–0.9 units/kg per day) and adolescents (up to 1.5 units/kg per day) may be needed. Patients who also have hyperglycemia and some degree of ketoacidosis may require higher doses of insulin (1.0–1.5 units/kg per day) until the hyperglycemia and accompanying insulin resistance improves. During times of illness or stress, insulin dosages as high as 2.5 units/kg/day may be required to compensate for inadequate blood glucose control, and must be changed as the patient's condition changes.

When taken along with Regular insulin or lispro insulin, the dosage of intermediate insulin is approximately 60% of the total daily insulin requirement. This is often given as two thirds in the morning and one third of the total in the evening. Intermediate acting insulin doses should be adjusted no more frequently than every 5 to 7 days, and preferably with adequate supportive and guiding blood glucose data to provide sufficient pattern discernment of insulin requirements at various points throughout the day.

In type 1 diabetes, the person who is newly diagnosed may find that s/he enters a remission of sorts, referred to as the "honeymoon" period.

Insulin dosage may be dramatically reduced, with requirements being as little as 0.1 to 0.3 units per kg per day (American Diabetes Association, 1994b). During this phase, it is recommended that the patient be continued on a low dose of insulin.

Women who have diabetes and become pregnant will require careful and, usually increased, insulin dose adjustment. Those who plan to become pregnant should try to achieve excellent pre-conception glucose control to secure the best possible outcome of the pregnancy. This level of control prior to conception is best achieved via multiple insulin injections per day, as well as four to six blood glucose tests per day. Consultation with a diabetologist and diabetes educator can help design an effective, individualized approach.

Patients with type 2 diabetes, on oral agents, usually begin insulin therapy with a small bedtime dose of intermediate insulin. A common starting dose for adults is 6–10 units of intermediate insulin, depending on the suspected degree of insulin resistance. The aim is to suppress hepatic glucose release during the night, and this suppression requires less insulin than that required to control prandial glucose loads. To assess the effectiveness of this regimen and the dose, the patient can be asked to test and average a week's worth of fasting blood glucose values. The bedtime insulin dose can be adjusted according to whether or not the average fasting test value is within the targeted fasting blood glucose range. Doses of 40 units or more will require re-evaluation of therapy, as larger boluses of insulin may be unpredictably absorbed. If the fasting blood glucose is at target, but daytime targets cannot be achieved with sulfonylureas and/or metformin and/or acarbose, then the practitioner may need to consider adding daytime administration of insulin as well.

Type 2 patients using insulin as the principal therapy for blood glucose control may need high doses, even at or greater than 100 units per day. This will be determined by degree of obesity and associated insulin resistance (American Diabetes Association, 1994c).

The need for self-management of insulin therapy with continual blood glucose monitoring cannot be overemphasized, and recommendations for target blood glucose testing should be individualized to meet the patient's need for insulin, meals, exercise, and glycemic homeostasis. For target blood glucose levels see Table 31-3. These targets may require adjustment for safety and feasibility for the patient.

## TABLE 31–3. OPTIMAL BLOOD GLUCOSE LEVELS

| Time | Level, mg/dL |
|---|---|
| Preprandial (30–60 min before meal) | 70–120 |
| 1 h postprandial | 100–180 |
| 2 h postprandial | 80–120 |
| 3 A.M. | 70–120 |

**Insulin regimens.**   There are many dosage regimens for designing optimal insulin therapy. Depending on the type of diabetes and severity of insulin impairment, regimens may range from a single injection per day to 4–5 injections per day.

The simplest regimen is one injection per day. This may be given as a single pre-breakfast injection, or, as in the case of type 2 diabetes with elevated fasting blood glucose values, a single bedtime dose of intermediate acting insulin. Seldom is a single injection of insulin per day sufficient for glycemic management of type 1 diabetes.

If two injections of insulin are required per day, they may consist of only intermediate or longest acting insulin. However, a common insulin regimen of two injections per day is that of a 'split-mixed' regimen. The morning injection contains intermediate- or long-acting insulin, with a bolus of regular insulin or lispro. If inter-

mediate and regular insulins are used, they should be injected 30–60 minutes prior to meal time for maximal results. The evidence supports mixing these two insulins together, however, if a patient is experiencing fluctuating blood glucose levels while keeping food (amounts of carbohydrate and timing) consistent, the patient can try using two separate injections: the intermediate- or long-acting in the thigh or buttock, and the regular or insulin lispro administered in the abdomen. Also, if the ratio of regular to intermediate or longer-acting insulin is greater than 1:2, and/or glucose variation is inexplicable, separate injections may be beneficial in achieving predictable absorption and desired duration.

The use of multiple insulin administrations per day (three or more) is often referred to as 'intensive insulin therapy.' Table 31-4 outlines three regimens that may be used.

Intensive regimens of multiple administrations of insulin require that the patient be testing his/her blood glucose at least four times a day and be able to make decisions about adjusting the dose of the shorter-acting insulins based on individual activity and eating patterns. These intensive regimens can help achieve near euglycemia, but they are not for everyone. Because of the concurrent blood glucose testing and insulin adjustments necessary, the patient also requires ongoing support and guidance from a knowledgeable, confident provider. An individualized "sliding scale," or algorithm, for adjusting the

## TABLE 31–4. THREE MODELS FOR INTENSIVE INSULIN THERAPY

| Method | Insulin Ratio | Types of Insulins Used | Number of Injections |
|---|---|---|---|
| Model 1 | Insulin dosage dependent on blood glucose | Regular insulin (or) lispro | Three injections daily before meals |
| Model 2 | Two thirds of daily dose of intermediate insulin in the morning along with a bolus of fast-acting insulin<br>Fast-acting insulin before dinner<br>One third of daily dose of intermediate insulin at consistent bedtime hour | NPH or Lente, and Regular insulin (or) lispro | Three injections daily<br>• Intermediate + Regular before breakfast<br>• Regular before dinner<br>• Intermediate at bedtime |
| Model 3 | Ultralente along with fast-acting insulin before breakfast<br>Fast-acting insulin dose before lunch<br>Ultralente along with fast-acting insulin dose with evening meal | Ultralente, Regular insulin, (or) lispro | Three injections daily |

dose of the shorter-acting insulins is needed, and patients must learn to use it. See the example of an adjustment guide for regulating Regular or lispro in Table 31-5.

If the multiple injections do not achieve the targeted blood glucose goals, consider other methods of insulin delivery, such as an insulin pump. This equipment is expensive to obtain and maintain, requiring access to health personnel well versed in its use. For select patients, it may help to achieve near normal glycemic control.

***Storing insulin.*** All unopened insulin should be stored in the refrigerator and kept from freezing. Patients should keep the bottle currently being used at room temperature away from exposure to heat and sunlight. Injectable medicine kept at room temperature causes less pain. Vials of insulin, once opened, can be used up to 6 months, if refrigerated. The exception is lispro insulin. This insulin analog should be used within 28 days, even if refrigerated. Check the expiration date stamped on the vial. If traveling, patients should always keep insulin with them at a constant temperature. Because it is a protein, insulin is similar to egg whites (also protein) and can be easily affected by very hot or very cold temperatures. The insulated thermal packs or thermos bottles can be used to transport insulin while traveling. Remind the insulin-using patients to carry a letter from their health care provider when traveling abroad, in case care is needed at the arrival destination and to avoid problems with transporting syringes and insulin through customs.

***Insulin injection preparation.*** Visual inspection of each vial should be performed prior to withdrawing an insulin dose. Short-acting insulin should always be clear and all intermediate-acting, long-acting or combination insulins should be homogenous without clumping or flocculation. After inspection and prior to withdrawing a dose of suspension (intermediate, long-acting) insulin from a vial, the vial should be gently rolled between the palms, not shaken.

***Administration of insulin.*** Commercially available insulin needles are of such a fine gauge and short length that the injection can be made by inserting the insulin needle at a 90 degree angle into the adipose tissue of the abdomen, arms, thigh, or buttocks. A very lean person may find it necessary to pinch the skin and insert the needle into the adipose at a 30 degree angle. It is not necessary to prepare clean skin with alcohol or any other cleansing lotion or fluid. Insert entire length of needle, then deliver the contents of syringe quickly. Aspiration is not necessary. Do not apply pressure or rub the site after injecting. To avoid stinging and discomfort use insulin that is at room temperature.

Acceptable injection areas include the abdomen, upper back of the arms, and thigh and buttocks. Since there is as much as 25% variation of insulin absorption intraindividually, injections should be consistently rotated *within* these areas and *not from area to area*. Absorption is fastest from the abdomen, then the arms, then the thighs and slowest from the buttocks (American Diabetes Association, 1994b). Of course, absorption rates will be affected by increased or decreased blood flow to the injection site. For example, insulin is absorbed faster if, after injection, the patient has a hot shower or sits in a hot tub. Or, if after injecting into the thigh, the patient goes jogging, the absorption will likely be much quicker.

---

**TABLE 31–5. SAMPLE OF AN ALGORITHM/SLIDING SCALE FOR ADJUSTING REGULAR OR LISPRO INSULIN ONLY**

**Basic Insulin Dose**[a]

| 7 A.M. breakfast: | 12 noon lunch: | 6 P.M. dinner: |
|---|---|---|
| 12 Ultralente | | 12 Ultralente |
| 6 Regular insulin | 3 Regular insulin | 6 Regular insulin |

Test blood glucose (BG) before each meal and adjust Regular or lispro (only) insulin as follows:

- If BG is less than 70 mg/dL, eat right away and take 2 units less of basic Regular or lispro insulin dose.
- If BG is between 71 and 140, take the basic dose of Regular or lispro insulin.
- If BG is between 141 and 180, take 1 extra unit of Regular or lispro insulin.
- If BG is between 181 and 220, take 2 extra units of Regular or lispro insulin.
- If BG is between 221 and 300, take 3 extra units of Regular or lispro insulin.
- If BG is over 300, take 4 extra units of Regular or lispro insulin, drink plenty of calorie-free fluids, check for ketones in urine and symptoms of illness.

[a] Refers to the prescribed usual dose. Adjustments to regular or lispro are made by adding or subtracting units to or from the basic dose. Without establishing a basic dose, it is very difficult to determine how to reliably and predictably adjust Regular or lispro insulin for diet and/or exercise changes.

Other factors that will influence onset, peak, and duration of action include whether administration is into dermis/adipose/muscle; current blood glucose level; insulin sensitivity; metabolic state; insulin antibodies. These multiple factors can best be controlled by consistent administration in both selected sites and by keeping food and exercise consistent.

To accommodate delivery convenience, most patients administer through devices known as *insulin pen*. These products consist of insulin cartridges (as opposed to the usual vials), the pen device, and disposable needles. In most instances, the cartridges cost more than the ordinary vial insulin, but busy, on-the-go people may prefer this option. Other convenient—and more costly—products include air-jet injectors instead of the standard insulin syringe, which individuals who are needle phobic may prefer. Insulin pumps are expensive in terms of cost for the technology (approximately $4,000+) and require further education and follow-up. However, they allow some individuals to achieve a more near-normal insulin delivery when the other intensive, multiple injection regimens have been unsuccessful.

**Side effects of insulin.** Adverse reactions from insulins are essentially those associated with hypoglycemia, especially in patients with type 1 diabetes who are active and intent on achieving near-euglycemia (The DCCT Research Group, 1993). A severe hypoglycemic reaction can result in coma, seizure and the need for intravenous glucose or glucagon. Hypoglycemia can be strictly defined as blood glucose <50 mg/dl, and patients with clinical symptoms of hypoglycemia—tachycardia, palpitations, shakiness, sweating, dizziness, hunger—can reverse the symptoms with 10–15 gm of quick acting carbohydrate (see Table 31-6).

Hypoglycemia can be caused by three main factors, or a combination of all three: 1) too much insulin; 2) delay of food intake; 3) increase in activity or exercise. Alcohol consumption without concurrent carbohydrate intake may also predispose to hypoglycemia. Query patients to determine if they have recently started a new bottle of insulin, changed injection technique or major sites, experienced hormonal changes or symptoms of gastroparesis (delay in stomach emptying and reduction in intestinal peristalsis).

Patients intent on maintaining euglycemia will experience a near three-fold increase in episodes of hypoglycemia. Unrealistic glycemic goals can endanger patients, so negotiate healthy

---

### TABLE 31–6. SUGGESTED FAST-ACTING CARBOHYDRATES TO TREAT HYPOGLYCEMIA

**Symptomatic Mild Hypoglycemia**
Goal: Administer 10–15 gm glucose:
   2–3 glucose tablets
   1/2 tube of glucose gel
   4 oz of orange juice
   1 small tube of cake icing
   4 oz of regular (sweetened) soda
   4–6 Lifesavers

**Unresponsive Severe Hypoglycemia**
Glucagon (kit)—1 dose injected subcutaneously
50% dextrose and water administered intravenously

---

patterns of control with them. Family, friends, school and work associates should be instructed on appropriate treatment for hypoglycemia and shown how to administer glucagon injection in the event the patient becomes unconscious.

Hypoglycemia-unawareness can occur in patients who have had type 1 for many years, and in those patients who have employed a regimen of very tight glucose regulation (Edleman, 1997). For those with long duration of the disease, it can become increasingly difficult to recognize and self treat hypoglycemic symptoms. Monitoring and a readily available glucose source is essential for these individuals, as is renegotiating blood glucose targets to a safer range. Those experiencing hypoglycemia due to tight glycemic control regimens, may be able to improve symptom detection by meticulously avoiding hypoglycemia and allowing the blood glucose to run in the mid to high 100's mg/dL for several days (Edleman, 1997).

Nocturnal hypoglycemia that occurs in the early morning hours (around 3 or 4 a.m.) is more common in those patients who are trying to achieve near-euglycemia and/or in those who take intermediate-acting insulin with the evening meal. Patients may not awaken during these episodes, but may recall nightmares or awaken with a headache. Have the patient monitor the 3 a.m. blood glucose and adjust the regimen. For example, moving the intermediate-acting insulin to a bedtime hour (and being consistent in this administration), may avoid the middle of the night peak that occurs from evening meal intermediate-acting insulin.

Other side effects of insulin may occur through immunological effects. Lipoatrophy and lipohypertrophy can occur with repeated injections to the same puncture site. Injection rotation within the site area will help to prevent these changes to the adipose tissue, and subsequent variation in absorption.

***Situations requiring immediate insulin therapy.***
Two metabolic situations increase insulin requirements, and both are often precipitated by illness or infection. *Diabetic Ketoacidosis (DKA)* is most common in type 1 diabetes. Illness, trauma, or infection can create a need for more energy and more insulin. Because of the absolute absence of insulin, type 1 patients are more likely to begin experiencing a breakdown of fat into fatty acids when their insulin and energy requirements are in higher demand. These acid by-products, along with the release of counter-regulatory hormones (further elevating hyperglycemia) create a metabolic state of ketoacidosis. The result is major fluid and electrolyte shift, and the treatment is immediate replacement of insulin.

In type 2 diabetes, since some insulin production capability remains, fat breakdown does not occur. This condition is called *non-ketosis, hyperglycemic, hyperosmosis (NKHH)*. Hyperglycemia is severe in NKHH, and, so too, are the fluid and electrolyte shifts. The comparative difference is that ketosis is not present, the hyperglycemia may be significantly high (over 500 mg/dl), and osmolality is greater than 320 mOsm. Treatment calls for insulin replacement, along with fluid and electrolyte administration. Both conditions are life-threatening.

Illness is the common precipitator of both of these metabolic conditions, so it is essential that the patient with diabetes be aware of this potential when ill and take steps to prevent symptoms from progressing.

## Meglitinides

The newest class of drugs for type 2 are the "meglitinides." This category of drug has just received FDA approval, but is not yet available for use as an oral agent. It is one of several new classes of drugs making their way through phase III clinical trials. With the generic name of repaglinide, it is the first of the meglitinide class that is soon to be available.

It works in a fashion similar to the sulfonylurea agents in that it stimulates insulin secretion from pancreatic beta cells (Wolffenbuttel & Graal, 1996). A possible therapeutic advantage,

which is yet unsubstantiated, is that repaglinide action is diminished when glucose levels drop to near hypoglycemia. Also, unlike sulfonylureas that tend to have time-limited effectiveness of two to five years, repaglinide's ability to 'switch-off' during conditions of hypoglycemia may also promote resensitization and preservation of the beta cells. This action would, theoretically, offer more years of effective oral therapy for glycemic control. Long-term clinical studies have not been completed to support this theory.

Repaglinide has pharmacokinetic properties that require the drug be given just prior to meals 2–4 times daily (Wolffenbuttel, 1996). If a meal is missed or added then so is the drug. This requires a rather intensive adherence schedule and may be difficult for some patients who have had problems structuring meals or remembering to take their medications. The most common adverse effects from repaglinide include influenza symptoms, respiratory infections, and rhinitis.

Weight gain on average was 3.3% in those treated with the agent. One potential advantage is that this drug has a kidney sparing effect and may be used by patients with altered renal function. Because the drug is metabolized in the liver, frequent monitoring of liver function may be necessary.

In very short and limited clinical trials, the reported clinical benefits from this new oral hypoglycemic agent are improvements in glycemic control, ranging from 1–2% drop in glycosolated hemoglobin. In patients on oral combination therapy the glycemic response appears to be slightly less. The dosing range is 0.5–4 mg given as 0.5 mg, 1 mg, or 2 mg tablets with each meal, and the maximum total daily dose is 16 mg. The starting dose is 1 mg with each meal. Repaglinide is due to be released by the manufacturer in late spring 1998.

## Sulfonylurea Drugs

The class of sulfonylurea drugs has expanded to 2 generations, with each generation showing unique differences in their kinetic and dynamic actions. Sulfonylureas are commonly referred to as 'oral hypoglycemic agents' (OHAs). The first generation of these agents included tolbutamide (Orinase), chlorpropamide (Diabinese), tolazamide (Tolinase), and acetohexamide, and these are still in use today. The second generation agents are glyburide (DiaBeta, Glynase PresTab, Micronase), glipizide (Glucotrol, Glucotrol XL) and glimepiride (Amaryl).

The mechanism of action of sulfonylureas is complex and still not completely understood. Study evidence shows that pharmacological actions can be seen both within the pancreas, where there is an increase in insulin release, and at the cellular receptor level, where an increase in the sensitivity and binding of insulin can be measured. A combination of these mechanisms probably produces the intended hypoglycemic effect (American Diabetes Association, 1996)

The major utility of the sulfonylurea class has been their ability to more efficiently and effectively increase circulating insulin levels to bring about reduced blood glucose levels. About 20% of patients will experience no therapeutic response to these agents, a condition called 'primary failure.' Another portion of users will initially respond with increased beta cell stimulation and resultant increased insulin secretion; however, over time (5–7 years) this effect may diminish, insulin levels fall and secondary failure will occur. The former is known as 'primary failure,' in which the sulfonylureas immediately fail to produce any change in glycemic control. The latter, 'secondary failure,' is the term applied to that category of patients for whom sulfonylureas worked for a time.

The therapeutic decision for what agent would be the best choice for a particular patient will necessarily stem from the kinetic profile of the drug, the patient's metabolic condition, and the therapeutic goal. This means it is best to consider the drug's metabolism and excretion, along with the duration of activity (see chart) and the patient's blood glucose control targets. For example, tolbutamide, with its short half life, may be most appropriate for patients in whom hypoglycemia is to be avoided if possible. This group includes those who frequently experience hypoglycemia, are renally compromised or elderly (Lebovitz, 1991). Acetohexamide and tolazamide have intermediate duration of activity but contain active metabolites that can accumulate in those patients with renal failure and who are elderly (The DCCT Research Group, 1993; American Diabetes Association, 1996). Chlorpropamide has the longest duration of action with active metabolites. Chlorpropamide is the least expensive OHA product available, yet its long action combined with the potential for hyponatremia, can complicate therapy in the elderly and renal-compromised patient.

Of the second generation sulfonylurea agents, glimepiride, is similar in kinetics and therapeutic action to glyburide. Generally the onset of action for the second generation agents is 1–4 hours and is best given 30 minutes to an hour prior to the breakfast and/or dinner meal. The duration of action for glyburide is 24 hours while glipizide's approaches 10–24 hours. When the patient reaches greater than 50% of the maximum daily dose, it may become necessary to split the daily dose. Once the total daily dose reaches 15 mg of glyburide or 30 mg of glipizide, the efficacy of blood glucose reduction decreases with increased dosing (Cefalu, 1996; Stenman, 1993). When the patient has reached maximum benefit from the sulfonylureas, additional blood glucose reduction can be achieved by adding agents from other glucose lowering classes, such as metformin and/or acarbose. Glyburide has shown to be more effective over the 24 hour period in reducing blood glucose and longer term glucose control, while glipizide has been more effective in reducing postprandial glucose levels, but circulating insulin levels tend to be elevated. High circulating levels of insulin have been suggested to be associated with advancing atherosclerosis (Lebovitz, 1991).

Approximately 25–60% of patients who fail a sulfonylurea agent will respond to the addition of another sulfonylurea and/or another oral antidiabetic. Patients who fail on oral hypoglycemic agents have been shown to do better on combination oral and insulin therapy in reducing long-term glucose levels. Specifically, the BIDS regimen (bedtime intermediate insulin and daytime sulfonylurea) has been demonstrated to be effective in those type 2 patients who have persistently elevated fasting blood glucose levels (Riddle, 1990; Pugh et al., 1992; Groop et al., 1992).

The side effects of sulfonylurea drugs are not extensive. The most common side effect (and therapeutic effect) that all sulfonylurea agents share is *hypoglycemia*. Depending on the duration of activity of the specific agent and the age and morbidity status of the patient, hypoglycemia can usually be easily treated with ingestion of simple carbohydrates, such as juice, hard candy, honey, or syrup. However, in the longer acting agents or those with active metabolites, the hypoglycemia may be significantly and seriously prolonged. The elderly tend to be more susceptible to it because of declining renal and liver function. This is true for even those agents with weak metabolites, such as glyburide. Elderly patients (>70 yrs) most likely to be at risk are those with poor nutritional status, fragile states of health, chronic diseases where fluid shifts occur and any compromised renal and hepatic function. Any of those conditions will warrant OHA's that are shorter acting and less likely to evoke a prolonged hypoglycemic reaction. In fact, a single dose of long acting insulin such as Ultralente may be the preferred agent for glucose control in those susceptible individuals.

Hypoglycemia can be a very serious complication with significantly poor outcomes, and treatment should include aggressive glucose replacement for as long as 24–48 hours with intravenous therapy. To avoid hypoglycemia for patients receiving OHA's, consider using the agent with the shortest duration of action, appropriate to existing renal and hepatic function, avoiding drug interactions, and thoroughly reviewing the patients potential for changes in fluid and nutrition status or shifts.

Renal function can be an important consideration when starting a patient on an oral hypoglycemic agent. Most sulfonylurea's have some diuresis action. However, acetohexamide and tolazamide have more than most, and all can cause fluid retention. Electrolyte imbalance can occur more frequently with the first generation agents, with hyponatremia being especially a risk with chlorpropamide use. Cholestatic jaundice is particularly a problem with chlorpropamide as well; however the agents have this potential, too, and it is recommended that patients be switched to insulin or an alternative non-sulfonylurea agent if this should occur.

Less common, but equally significant are hematological reactions such as thrombocytopenia, leukopenia, hemolytic anemia; maculopapular rashes; pulmonary reactions; and decrease in thyroid function (Hermann, 1994). Drug interactions can be an important cause of poor glycemic control and can change metabolism, elimination and actions of the sulfonylurea agents. In general, the second generation sulfonylurea agents will have less potential for interactions that produce significant glycemic changes.

The sulfonylurea drugs have been effective in reducing blood glucose in patients who have some inherent circulating and stored insulin. Of patients who use OHA's, 60–70% will have an initial response to therapy. Glycemic control will generally continue for 2 or more years; failures after this period of time occur 5–20% of the time. Excluding patient compliance problems, failure usually requires increasing the dose, fre-

quency, or administration; switching to alternative agents; or adding an agent from a different class of OHA's. The success rate of oral combination therapy is time- and disease progression-dependent and may necessitate insulin therapy (Hermann, 1994; Lebovitz, 1991). Insulin therapy may be used during periods of stress, illness, or major life changes until stabilization of blood glucose is established and oral therapy can be reinstated. Changes in drug management should not preclude appropriate emphasis on dietary and exercise management and should complement lifestyle changes.

## Thiazolidinediones

Troglitazone, the first agent in a new class of glucose lowering drugs, acts to lower blood glucose by reducing insulin resistance and improving insulin sensitivity in muscle and adipose tissue (Whitcomb, Saltiel, & Lockwood, 1996). Hepatic glucose output is also suppressed, much like the biguanides, but to a much lesser extent. Endogenous or exogenous insulin is required for troglitazone to be effective and is currently approved for use in type 2 patients as monotherapy or in combination therapy (Spencer, 1997).

Since there is still little clinical experience with troglitazone, its precise role in diabetes management is yet to be determined. Currently it is approved for use as monotherapy, or in combination with a sulfonylurea when glycemic response has not been adequate (Iwamoto, 1996). Combination therapy with troglitazone has been shown to be more effective when combined with sulfonylurea drugs than when given as monotherapy (Iwamoto, 1996). On average, glycosolated hemoglobin can be expected to drop by 1.8% when used together with a sulfonylurea compared to 0.7% when used alone (Spencer, 1997). Results of glycemic improvement when insulin and troglitazone are used are slightly less than that seen with combination oral agents including troglitazone.

The thiazolidinedione class of antidiabetic agents by themselves do not contribute to hypoglycemia, such as may occur with either insulin or sulfonylurea therapy. Nor does this agent contribute to the development of hyperinsulinemia. By itself, troglitazone, like the biguanides, generally does not cause significant weight gain like insulin and sulfonylurea drugs. Troglitazone has a positive affect on triglycerides and high density lipoproteins (HDL) levels, decreasing triglyceride levels by an average of 13%–20%

and increasing HDL by 5%–11% (Spencer, 1997; Wolffenbuttel, 1996). However, it also increases low density lipoproteins (7%–10%), but has a neutral effect on lipid ratios (Spencer, 1997).

Early reports showed that this agent was generally well tolerated and that primary side effects from troglitazone are fluid retention and minor abdominal cramping, nausea, and back pain. However, there are increasing concerns about this agent because 1.9% (n = 48) of those treated in clinical trials of troglitazone experienced transaminase elevation, compared to 0.6% of the subjects in the placebo group. Of the 48, 20 subjects were discontinued on troglitazone and their liver function tests (LFTs) returned to normal; 20 continued on troglitazone and LFTs returned to normal. The remaining 8 were discontinued for other reasons, and in all cases the LFTs returned to normal. Once the agent was released for market use, 35 reports of elevated LFTs were made, and 2 of the 35 sustained severe clinical outcomes when LFTs were elevated but the drug was not discontinued. One died of liver failure and one received a liver transplant (Olefsky, 1997).

Adverse effects may be minimized by careful selection of patients for troglitazone. Those who have predisposing congestive heart failure or hepatic impairment are not appropriate candidates for troglitazone use. LFTs should be done prior to starting therapy, then monthly for the first six months, then bimonthly for a year. The drug should be discontinued if LFTs show abnormal elevations.

## TABLE 31–7. DRUGS CAUSING HYPERGLYCEMIA

| | |
|---|---|
| Acetazolamide | Indapamide |
| Alpha blockers | L-Asparaginase |
| Beta blockers | Niacin-nicotinic acid |
| Butmetanide | Nicotine |
| Caffeine | Nonsteroidal |
| Calcium channel blockers | antiinflammatory |
| Cyclophosphamide | drugs |
| Diazoxide | Oral contraceptives |
| Epinephrine | Pentamidine |
| (sympathomimetics) | Phenobarbital |
| Fish oils | Phenytoin |
| Furosemide | Sugar-containing drug |
| Hormones (glucagon, | products |
| estrogens, thyroid, | Thiazide diuretics |
| steroids) | |

## TABLE 31–8. DRUGS CAUSING HYPOGLYCEMIA

| | |
|---|---|
| Alcohol | Insulin |
| Alpha glucosidase inhibitors | MAO inhibitors |
| Anabolic steroids | Phenylbutazone |
| Beta blockers | Salicylates |
| Biguanides | Sulfinpyrazone |
| Clofibrate | Sulfonylureas |
| Fenfluramine | Tetracycline |
| Guanethidine | Thiazolidinediones |

To initiate monotherapy or combination therapy, the following guidelines are provided: Combination therapy of troglitazone with insulin or sulfonylurea drugs generally requires that a reduced dose of 200mg be initiated and be administered once daily with careful monitoring for hypoglycemia over 2 to 4 weeks. A reduction in total daily insulin dosage (10–25%) can be made several days to weeks after troglitazone is started. In 15% of patients, insulin therapy can be discontinued. The usual maintenance dose of troglitazone when using insulin is 400 mg daily taken with meals.

## Drug Combinations

Drugs that can cause hyperglycemia or complicate treatment for hyperglycemia are not necessarily contraindicated in patients with diabetes, but they may require more attention for monitoring glucose levels and appropriate adjustment of the patient's drug regimen. The drugs that contribute to hyperglycemia and hypoglycemia are shown in Tables 31-7 and 31-8, respectively.

## REFERENCES

Ahern, J.A., & Grey, M. (1996). New developments in treating children with IDDM. *Journal of Pediatric Health Care, 10*(4), 161–166.

American Diabetes Association. (1994a). *Maximizing the role of nutrition in diabetes management.* Alexandria, VA: American Diabetes Association.

American Diabetes Association (1994b). *Medical management of insulin-dependent (Type 1) diabetes (2nd Ed.).* Alexandria, VA: American Diabetes Association Clinical Education Series.

American Diabetes Association (1994c). *Medical management of non-insulin-dependent (Type II) diabetes* (3rd Ed.). Alexandria, VA: American Diabetes Association Clinical Education Series.

American Diabetes Association. (1996). Consensus Statement: The pharmacologic treatment of hyperglycemia in NIDDM. *Diabetes Care, 19*(Suppl. 1), S 54–61.

American Diabetes Association. (1997). Clinical Practice Recommendations 1997. *Diabetes Care, 20*(1) (Suppl. 1).

American Diabetes Association Position Statement. (1995). Standards of medical care for patients with diabetes mellitus. *Diabetes Care, 12*(12), 365–368.

Anderson, J. H., et al. (1995). Insulin lispro compared to regular insulin in a crossover study involving 1,037 patients with type I diabetes. *Diabetes, 44*(Suppl 1), Abstract No. 228A.

Bailey, C. J., Path, M.R.C., & Turner, R.C. (1996). Drug therapy: Metformin. *New England Journal of Medicine, 334*(9) 574–579.

Baliga, B. S. & Fonseca, V. A. (1997). Recent advances in the treatment of type II diabetes mellitus. *American Family Physician*, pp. 817–824

Bayer Corporation, Pharmaceutical Division (1995). Precose package insert.

Bischoff, H. (1995). The mechanism of alpha-glucosidase inhibition in the management of diabetes. *Clin. Invest. Med, 18*, 303–311.

Calle-Pascual, A. L. (1995). Comparison between acarbose, metformin, and insulin treatment in type II diabetic patients with secondary failure to sulfonylurea treatment. *Diabetes Et Metabolism, 21*(4), 256–260

Cefalu, W.T. (1996). Treatment of type II diabetes. *Postgraduate Medicine, 99*(3), 109–119.

Chaisson, J. L. (1994). The efficacy of acarbose in the treatment of patients with non-insulin-dependent diabetes mellitus. *Annals of Internal Medicine. 121*, 928–935.

Chong, P. K. (1995). Energy expenditure in type II diabetic patients on metformin and sulfonylurea therapy. *Diabetic Medicine, 2*(5), 401–408.

Conniff, R. F. (1995a). A double-blind placebo-controlled trial evaluating the safety and efficacy of acarbose for the treatment of patients with insulin-requiring type II diabetes. *Diabetes Care, 18*(7), 928–932.

Conniff, R. F. (1995b). Multicenter, placebo-controlled trial comparing acarbose with placebo, tolbutamide, and tolbutamide plus-acarbose in non-insulin-dependent diabetes mellitus. *American Journal of Medicine, 98*, 443–451.

Conniff, R. F. (1995c). Reduction of glycosylated hemoglobin and postprandial hyperglycemia by acarbose in patients with NIDDM. *Diabetes Care, 18*(6), 817–824.

DeFronzo, R.A. (1988). The triumvirate: B-cell, muscle, liver. A collusion responsible for NIDDM. *Diabetes. 37*, 867–887.

DeFronzo, R. A. (1995). Efficacy of metformin in patients with non-insulin-dependent diabetes mellitus: The multicenter metformin study group. *New England Journal of Medicine, 333*(9), 541–549.

The Diabetes Control and Complications Trial Research Group. (1993). The effect of intensive treatment of diabetes on the development and progression of long-term complications in insulin-dependent diabetes mellitus. *New England Journal of Medicine, 329*, 977–986.

Dunn, C. J. (1995). Metformin: A review of its pharmacological properties and therapeutic use in non-insulin-dependent diabetes mellitus. *Drugs, 49*(5), 721–749.

Edleman, S. (1997). *Diabetes Interview*: Beware of hypoglycemia unawareness. Issue #61. (Available from *Diabetes Interview, 3715 Balboa Street, San Francisco, CA 98121*.)

Franz, M. (Ed). (1994). *Maximizing the role of nutrition in diabetes management*. Alexandria, VA: American Diabetes Association.

Ganda, O. P. (1996). Rational therapy: Non-insulin-dependent diabetes mellitus. *ICPR*.

Gavin III, J.R., Reasner, C.A., Weart, C.W., & Labso, L. (1998). Oral antidiabetic drugs: One size does not fit all. *Patient Care, 32*(3), 40–68.

Ghazzi, M.N., Perez, J.E., & Antonucci, T. (1997). Cardiac and glycemic benefits of troglitazone treatment in NIDDM. *Diabetes, 46*, 433–439.

Giordano, B.P., Petrila, A., Banion, C.R., & Neuenkirchen, G. (1992). The challenge of transferring responsibility for diabetes management from parent to child. *The Journal of Pediatric Health Care. 6*(5), 235–239.

Goo, A.K.Y., Carson, D.S., & Bjelajac, A. (1996). Metformin: A new treatment option for NIDDM. *The Journal of Family Practice. 42*(6), 612–618.

Grey, M., Cameron, M.E., & Thurber (1991). Coping and adaptation in children with diabetes. *Nursing Research, 1*(40), 144–149.

Groop, L.C., et al. (1992). Morning or bedtime NPH insulin combined with sulfonylurea in treatment of NIDDM. *Diabetes Care, 15*(7), 831–834.

Heine, R. J. (1984). Absorption kinetics and action of mixtures of short and intermediate-acting insulins. *Diabetologia, 27*, 558–562.

Hentinen, M., & Kyngäs, H. (1966). Diabetic adolescents' compliance with health regimens and associated factors. *International Journal of Nursing Studies, 33*(3), 325–337.

Hermann, L. S. (1994). Therapeutic comparison of metformin and sulfonylurea, alone and in various combinations: A double-blinded controlled study. *Diabetes Care, 17*(10), 1100–1109.

Howey, D. C., et al. (1994). A rapidly absorbed analogue of human insulin. *Diabetes, 43*(3), 396–402.

Howey, D. C., et al. (1995). Effect of injection time on postprandial glycemia. *Clinical Pharmacology Therapy, 58,* 459–469.

Iwamoto, Y., et al. (1996). Effect of combination therapy of troglitazone and sulphonylureas in patients with type 2 diabetes who were poorly controlled by sulphonylurea therapy alone. *Diabetes Med, 13:* 365–370.

Johnson, A. B., & Taylor, R. (1996). Does suppression of postprandial blood glucose excursions by the alpha-glucosidase inhibitor miglitol improve insulin sensitivity in diet-treated type II diabetic patients? *Diabetes Care, 19*(6), 559–563.

Krolewski, A.J., et al. (1995). Glycosylated hemoglobin and the risk of microalbuminuria in patients with insulin-dependent diabetes mellitus. *New England Journal of Medicine, 332,* 1251–1255.

Lalau, J. D. (1995). Role of metformin accumulation in metformin-associated lactic acidosis. *Diabetes Care, 18*(6), 779–784.

Lebovitz, H. (1991). *Therapy for diabetes mellitus and related disorders.* Alexandria, VA: American Diabetes Association.

Lee, T., et al. (1994). Incidence of renal failure in NIDDM. *Diabetes. 43,* 572.

Leonhardt, W. (1994). Efficacy of alpha-glucosidase inhibitors in lipids in NIDDM subjects with moderate hyperlipidaemia. *European Journal of Clinical Investigation, 24*( Suppl. 3), 45–49.

May, C. (1995). Efficacy and tolerability of stepwise increasing the dosage of acarbose in patients with non-insulin-dependent diabetes, treated with sulfonylureas. *Diabetes Und Stoffwechsel, 4,* 3–8.

National Diabetes Data Group. (1979). Classification and diagnosis of diabetes mellitus and other categories of glucose intolerance. *Diabetes, 28,* 1039–1057.

NCEP. (1993). Expert Panel on Detection, Evaluations, and Treatment of High Blood Cholesterol in Adults: Summary of the second report of the national cholesterol education program (NCEP) expert panel on detection, evaluation, and treatment of high blood cholesterol in adults. *Journal of the American Medical Association, 269,* 3015–3023.

Olefsky, J. (Personal communication to diabetes professional community of National Diabetes Education Initiative Faculty, November 12, 1997.)

Peters, A. L. (1986). Effect of storage on action of NPH and regular insulin mixtures. *Diabetes Care, 14,* 180–183.

Powers, M. (1996). *Handbook of diabetes medical nutrition therapy.* Gaithersburg, Maryland: Aspen Publishers.

Pugh, J.A., et al. (1992). Is combination sulfonylurea and insulin therapy useful in NIDDM patients? *Diabetes Care, 15*(8), 953–959.

Riccio, A. V. (1994). Improvement of basal hepatic glucose production and fasting hyperglycemia of type I diabetic patients treated with human recombinant ultralente insulin. *Diabetes Care, 17*(6), 535–540.

Riddle, M.C. (1990) Evening insulin strategy. *Diabetes Care, 13,* 676–686.

Riddle, M.C., McDaniel, P.A., Mitchell, M.C., Ahmann, A.J., & Karl, D.M. (1996). Lowdose metformin added to sulfonylurea: Comparison of two regimens. Scientific presentation at 56th Annual Meeting & Scientific Sessions of ADA, June 1996, San Francisco, CA.

Sambol, N. C. (1995). Kidney function and age are both predictors of pharmacokinetics of metformin. *Journal of Clinical Pharmacology, 35*(11), 1094–1102.

Sels, J. P., et al. (1994). Effect of miglitol (BAY m-1099) on fasting blood glucose in type 2 diabetes mellitus. *Netherlands Journal of Medicine. 44*(6): 198–201.

Spencer, C.M., & Markham, A. (1997). Troglitazone. *Drugs, 54*(1); 89–101.

Stenman, S., et al. (1993). What is the benefit of increasing the sulfonylurea dose? *Annals of Internal Medicine, 118*(3), 169–172.

United Kingdom Prospective Diabetes Study (UKPDS). (1995). Relative efficacy of randomly allocated diet, sufonylurea, insulin, or metformin in patients with newly diagnosed non-insulin-dependent diabetes followed for 3 years. *British Medical Journal, 310*(69–72), 83–88.

Vignati, L., et al. (1995). Treatment of 722 patients with type II diabetes with insulin lispro in a 6 month crossover study. *Diabetes, 44*(Suppl 1), Abstract No. 229A.

Whitcomb, R.W., Saltiel, A.R., & Lockwood, D.H. (1996). New therapies for NIDDM: Thiazolidinediones. In LeRoith, D., Taylor, S.I., Olefsky, J.M. (eds). *Diabetes mellitus: A fundamental & clinical text.* Philadelphia, PA: Lippincott-Raven, pp. 661–668.

White, J. R. (1996). The pharmacologic management of patients with type II diabetes mellitus in the era of new oral agents and insulin analogs. *Diabetes Spectrum, 9,* 227–234.

Wolffenbuttel, B.H.R., & Graal, M.B. (1996). New treatments for patients with type 2 diabetes mellitus. *Postgraduate Medical Journal, 72,* (853).

World Health Organization (1985). *Diabetes mellitus: Report of a WHO study group.* Geneva, Switzerland: World Health Organization (Tech. Rep. Service., No. 727).

# 32

# OBESITY

*Ellis Quinn Youngkin and Jeanette F. Kissinger*

With 25–34% of all adults and 18–30% of adolescents and prepubertal children in the United States significantly overweight, obesity is one of the most concerning as well as one of the most common problems plaguing this country today (Atkinson & Hubbard, 1994; Carek, Sherer, & Carson, 1997; Keller & Stevens, 1996; National Center for Health Statistics [NCHS], 1987). C. Everett Koop, former surgeon general of the United States, refers to the problem as an epidemic (Fraser, 1997). It is reported as the second leading cause of preventable death behind cigarette smoking with 58 million afflicted and contributing to 300,000 deaths annually (Davis & Feller, 1997). McMillan (1994) estimates the total number of obese Americans at more than 10% of the population. Thirty-one percent of adults in Canada are said to be obese (Stevens & Craig, 1988).

## DEFINITIONS AND PREVALENCE OF OBESITY

Obesity is defined by the National Institutes of Health as "an excess of body fat frequently resulting in a significant impairment of health" (McMillan, 1994, p. 17). *Healthy People 2000*, (USDHHS, 1992), however, admits that there is no real definition based on degree of excess body fat at this time. Thus, the more accepted definition for adult obesity is being 20% over ideal weight ("The Triumph of Obesity," 1997,

"Weight Management," 1996). The breakdown for men and women in the United States for obesity is reported as 27% of women and 24% of men. Forty-four percent of African-American women are obese compared to 25% of Caucasian women (NCHS, 1987). Rates for men are similar by race.

In children, obesity is defined with more difficulty because reference data on morbidity and mortality used for defining the problem in adults are less clear in children (Keller & Stevens, 1996). Sherman and Alexander (1990) support the use of triceps skin-fold thickness and weight for height, age, and sex in defining obesity for children, saying that if the triceps skin-fold thickness is greater than or equal to the 85th percentile, and the weight for height, age, and sex is greater than or equal to the 85th percentile, the child is obese. Corresponding approximately to 120% of ideal weight, which is the adult definition of obesity, the 85th percentile is a useful guideline with children (Whitaker, Wright, Pepe, et al, 1997). It is estimated that 5–25% of children and adolescents in America are obese, and about 80% of adolescents who are obese become obese adults.

The number of overweight and obese individuals in this country has climbed steadily in the last 20 years ("Update," MMWR, 1997; "Weight Management," 1996). According to surveys, 33–40% of adult women and 20–24% of adult men are seeking to lose weight at any one time. Many more are trying to maintain their current weight. African-American and Hispanic women have a greater prevalence of being overweight than Caucasian women ("Weight Management," 1996). More Hispanic men are trying to lose weight than any other group of men.

A Tufts University report mapped obesity levels in the 33 largest U.S. metropolitan areas ("Mapping U.S. Obesity," 1997). New York had the largest percentage of obese residents (38%); Denver had the lowest (22%). The report blamed overconsumption secondary to the many restaurants and corner food vendors in New York; however, this would not explain the second highest ranking city's rate—34% for Norfolk, Virginia. Cities with higher percentages of obese individuals were found to have the following in common: higher unemployment rates, a higher number of food stores per person, larger African-American populations, lower per capita income, and higher annual precipitation.

## RISKS OF OBESITY

Multiple studies have verified that obesity puts the individual at risk for a number of serious physical conditions, as well as for psychosocial disadvantages. The March 7, 1997, *MMWR Weekly Report* ("Update," 1997) and Carek, Sherer, and Carson (1997) state that being overweight or obese puts individuals at increased risk for morbidity and mortality associated with hypertension, hyperlipidemia, coronary heart disease, diabetes mellitus, gallbladder disease, respiratory disease, some types of cancer, gout, and arthritis. Additionally, children and adolescents who are overweight will more likely be overweight in adulthood. Men who are at 150–300% of ideal body weight die at 12 times the rate of nonobese men (Isselbacher, Braunwald, Wilson, et al, 1995). Van Itallie (1985) found that the relative risk (RR) for several diseases was significantly elevated in overweight people. The RR for hypertension is 2.9 overall, with an RR of 5.6 in the 20–44-year-old age group, and 1.9 in the 45–74-year-old age group. The RR for hyperlipidemia was 1.5 overall, 2.1 in the 20–44-year-old age group, and 1.1 for the 45–74-year-old age group. Individuals with diabetes mellitus in the 20–44-year-old age group had an RR of 3.8; 45–74-year-olds had an RR of 2.1; and the overall RR was 2.9.

People who are obese are 50% more likely to have serum cholesterol levels of at least 250 mg/dL, as well as other lipid abnormalities

(Pi-Sunyer, 1993; Van Itallie, 1985). Hypertension is much more common in obese individuals, as is coronary heart disease (CHD) (Bray, 1992; Pi-Sunyer, 1993). There is a five times greater incidence of non-insulin-dependent diabetes mellitus (type II) in individuals who are moderately obese, and this rises to ten times greater with severe obesity (Carek, Sherer, & Carson, 1997). A 15-year follow-up study of middle-aged men and women in Finland found that mortality from CHD and body mass index (BMI) were positively associated, and smoking further increased the risk ratio (Jousilahti, Tuomilehto, Vartianinen, et al, 1996). Obesity was said to be an independent risk factor for CHD mortality among men and a contributing factor among women.

The risk of morbidity such as stroke, ischemia, heart disease, and diabetes mellitus, is 3 to 4 times greater in people with a BMI greater than 28 than it is in the population generally (Rosenbaum, Leibel, & Hirsch, 1997). According to one study, BMI increased until age 50 in men, then plateaued (Lamon-Fava, Wilson, & Schaefer, 1996). BMI increased in women up to the 70s. Based on BMI, 72% of men and 42% of women had BMIs higher than 25, the traditional cutoff point for overweight (see Fig. 32–1). Reduced HDL cholesterol levels and hypertension were found to be the more strongly associated risk factors associated with higher BMI for both sexes. For women, elevated triglyceride levels, small LDL particles, and diabetes mellitus also were strongly associated with higher BMI. The "apple" figure (a central distribution of body fat) is a significant risk factor as opposed to a waist:hip ratio (WHR) that shows a more peripheral fat distribution ("pear shape") (Rosenbaum, Leibel, & Hirsch, 1997). Both men and women increase their WHRs as they age. An increased health risk is associated with a WHR of 0.95 or more for men and 0.80 or more for women (Cerulli, Lomaestro, & Malone, 1998).

Troiano, Frongillo, Sobal, and Levitsky (1996) estimated the relationship between BMI and all-cause mortality in a meta-analysis. They concluded that a comparable increased mortality existed at both moderately low BMI levels and at extreme overweight levels for white men, which was related to smoking or existing disease. According to Dr. Koop, a study out of Harvard by Mason found that even mild to moderate overweight was associated with an increased risk of premature death (Fraser, 1997). One British study found that fatter or overweight children had higher blood pressure levels and higher cholesterol concentrations than normal-weight children, and advised reducing obesity in children as one appropriate action to prevent CHD in adulthood (Rona, Qureshi, & Chinn, 1996).

Death rates from colorectal cancer and prostatic cancer were reported to be higher in overweight men; death rates from endometrial, cervical, ovarian, breast, and gallbladder cancers were higher in obese women (Garfinkel, 1985). Rates of renal disease and pregnancy complications, as well as those conditions mentioned previously, also are reported to be higher in overweight people (Brownell, 1982; McMillan, 1994; Pi-Sunyer, 1993).

Studies confirm that maternal obesity is associated with congenital malformation risks, especially neural tube defects (Prentice & Goldberg, 1996). This factor is an independent risk factor of other possible covariant confounders such as folate intake, smoking, socioeconomic status, maternal age, or maternal education. Some suggest that overweight or obese status influences folate to lose its protective influence in pregnancy.

Besides the physical risks, obesity causes serious social stigmata, with the obese person often being blamed for his or her own illness, labeled as lacking willpower, gluttonous, and lazy (McMillan, 1994). Often, people who are normal weight are repulsed by obese individuals, leading to anger and withdrawal by the obese person. Consequently, depression and social isolation are common. Obese people have a lesser chance for employment and advancement; acceptance into colleges may be affected (McMillan, 1994).

Children who are obese have particularly serious sequelae psychologically and socially (Keller & Stevens, 1996). In one study of adolescent overweight girls, after 7 years they were less likely to be married, had lower household incomes, and higher poverty rates regardless of aptitude scores or socioeconomic status at the beginning of the study (Gortmaker et al, 1993). An increased risk of later morbidity is associated with childhood obesity even if the person is not obese as an adult (Rosenbaum, Leibel, & Hirsch, 1997).

The emphasis in developed countries on being attractive and thin is so great that huge amounts of money are spent by Americans annually to try to become or stay thinner, or for products associated with conditions caused by being overweight. For example, just the sale of products to help decrease cellulite or fat ripples earned $50 million for cosmetic companies in 1992 (McMillan, 1994).

The estimated cost of diseases related to obesity in the United States is $70 billion annually. Gorsky, Pamuk, Williamson, Shaffer, and Koplan (1996) found that over the next 25 years the cost of treating health conditions associated with overweight in middle-aged women in the United States will be an estimated $16 billion and recommended prevention of excess weight gain as a main strategy for reducing health costs.

## CAUSES OF OBESITY

As a chronic condition, obesity is rooted in many areas: inherited traits, lifestyle, and environment (McMillan, 1994). Behavior is unlikely to be the only cause of obesity based on responses of lean and obese people to experimental perturbation of body weight (Rosenbaum, Leibel, & Hirsch, 1997). Recidivism occurs almost inevitably in lean and obese people who lose weight. The body acts to maintain its usual weight. There is a great diversity of opinion over the relative importance of factors related to obesity. A simple causal statement about obesity might be that "obesity results from excess energy intake and inadequate energy expenditure over an extended period of time," but this simplifies it too much (McMillan, 1994, p. 31). Because of differences in age, race, gender, activity level, metabolic rate, and habits like smoking and/or drinking, overeating in some people leads to obesity but in others to no weight change. Hunger and the hypothalamic satiety centers, regulated by the cerebral cortex, ultimately control eating (Isselbacher, Braunwald, Wilson, et al, 1995). Some studies support that obese people eat no more calories than thinner people (Braitman, Adlin, & Stanton, 1985; Romiue, Willet, Stampfer, et al, 1988). McMillan notes that the problem of obesity may more likely be the overconsumption of foods high in fat than simply overeating in general. However, as more data are obtained about overeating, it is evident that even low fat intake with high caloric intake of carbohydrates contributes to weight gain. In addition, sedentary lifestyle is a major contributor to obesity, and Americans lead very inactive lives (McMillan, 1994). Obesity that is mild to moderate is usually seen beginning in later life,

Height (ft, in)

| Weight (lb) | 4'10" | 4'11" | 5'0" | 5'1" | 5'2" | 5'3" | 5'4" | 5'5" | 5'6" | 5'7" | 5'8" | 5'9" | 5'10" | 5'11" | 6'0" | 6'1" |
|---|---|---|---|---|---|---|---|---|---|---|---|---|---|---|---|---|
| 130 | 27 | 26 | 25 | 25 | 24 | 23 | 22 | 22 | 21 | 20 | 20 | 20 | 19 | 18 | 18 | 17 |
| 135 | 28 | 27 | 26 | 25 | 25 | 24 | 23 | 22 | 22 | 21 | 21 | 20 | 19 | 19 | 18 | 18 |
| 140 | 29 | 28 | 27 | 27 | 26 | 25 | 24 | 23 | 23 | 22 | 21 | 21 | 20 | 19 | 19 | 19 |
| 145 | 30 | 29 | 28 | 27 | 27 | 26 | 25 | 24 | 23 | 23 | 22 | 21 | 21 | 20 | 20 | 19 |
| 150 | 31 | 30 | 29 | 28 | 27 | 27 | 26 | 25 | 24 | 24 | 23 | 22 | 22 | 21 | 20 | 20 |
| 155 | 32 | 31 | 30 | 29 | 28 | 28 | 27 | 26 | 25 | 24 | 24 | 23 | 22 | 22 | 21 | 20 |
| 160 | 34 | 32 | 31 | 30 | 29 | 28 | 28 | 27 | 26 | 25 | 24 | 24 | 23 | 22 | 22 | 21 |
| 165 | 35 | 33 | 32 | 31 | 30 | 29 | 28 | 28 | 27 | 26 | 25 | 24 | 24 | 23 | 22 | 22 |
| 170 | 36 | 34 | 33 | 32 | 31 | 30 | 29 | 28 | 28 | 27 | 26 | 25 | 25 | 24 | 23 | 22 |
| 175 | 37 | 35 | 34 | 33 | 32 | 31 | 30 | 29 | 28 | 27 | 27 | 26 | 25 | 24 | 24 | 23 |
| 180 | 38 | 36 | 35 | 34 | 33 | 32 | 31 | 30 | 29 | 28 | 27 | 27 | 26 | 25 | 24 | 24 |
| 185 | 39 | 37 | 36 | 35 | 34 | 33 | 32 | 31 | 30 | 29 | 28 | 27 | 27 | 26 | 25 | 25 |
| 190 | 40 | 38 | 37 | 36 | 35 | 34 | 33 | 32 | 31 | 30 | 29 | 28 | 27 | 26 | 26 | 25 |
| 195 | 41 | 39 | 38 | 37 | 36 | 35 | 34 | 32 | 32 | 31 | 30 | 29 | 28 | 27 | 26 | 26 |
| 200 | 42 | 40 | 39 | 38 | 37 | 36 | 34 | 33 | 32 | 31 | 30 | 30 | 29 | 28 | 27 | 26 |
| 205 | 43 | 41 | 40 | 39 | 38 | 36 | 35 | 34 | 33 | 32 | 31 | 30 | 29 | 28 | 28 | 27 |
| 210 | 44 | 43 | 41 | 40 | 38 | 37 | 36 | 35 | 34 | 33 | 32 | 31 | 30 | 29 | 28 | 28 |
| 215 | 45 | 44 | 42 | 41 | 39 | 38 | 37 | 36 | 35 | 34 | 33 | 32 | 31 | 30 | 29 | 28 |
| 220 | 46 | 45 | 43 | 42 | 40 | 39 | 38 | 37 | 36 | 35 | 34 | 33 | 32 | 31 | 30 | 29 |
| 225 | 47 | 46 | 44 | 43 | 41 | 40 | 39 | 38 | 36 | 35 | 34 | 33 | 32 | 31 | 31 | 30 |
| 230 | 48 | 47 | 45 | 44 | 42 | 41 | 40 | 38 | 37 | 36 | 35 | 34 | 33 | 32 | 31 | 30 |
| 235 | 49 | 48 | 46 | 44 | 43 | 42 | 40 | 39 | 38 | 37 | 36 | 35 | 34 | 33 | 32 | 31 |
| 240 | 50 | 49 | 47 | 45 | 44 | 43 | 41 | 40 | 39 | 38 | 37 | 36 | 35 | 34 | 33 | 32 |
| 245 | 51 | 50 | 48 | 46 | 45 | 43 | 42 | 41 | 40 | 38 | 37 | 36 | 35 | 34 | 33 | 32 |
| 250 | 52 | 51 | 49 | 47 | 46 | 44 | 43 | 42 | 40 | 39 | 38 | 37 | 36 | 35 | 34 | 33 |
| 255 | 53 | 52 | 50 | 48 | 47 | 45 | 44 | 43 | 41 | 40 | 39 | 38 | 37 | 36 | 35 | 34 |
| 260 | 54 | 53 | 51 | 49 | 48 | 46 | 45 | 43 | 42 | 41 | 40 | 38 | 37 | 36 | 35 | 34 |
| 265 | 55 | 54 | 52 | 50 | 49 | 47 | 46 | 44 | 43 | 42 | 40 | 39 | 38 | 37 | 36 | 35 |
| 270 | 56 | 55 | 53 | 51 | 49 | 48 | 46 | 45 | 44 | 42 | 41 | 40 | 39 | 38 | 37 | 36 |
| 275 | 57 | 56 | 54 | 52 | 50 | 49 | 47 | 46 | 44 | 43 | 42 | 41 | 40 | 39 | 37 | 36 |
| 280 | 58 | 57 | 55 | 53 | 51 | 50 | 48 | 47 | 45 | 44 | 43 | 41 | 40 | 39 | 38 | 37 |
| 285 | 59 | 58 | 56 | 54 | 52 | 51 | 49 | 48 | 46 | 45 | 43 | 42 | 41 | 40 | 39 | 38 |
| 290 | 60 | 59 | 57 | 55 | 53 | 51 | 50 | 48 | 47 | 46 | 44 | 43 | 42 | 41 | 39 | 38 |
| 295 | 61 | 60 | 58 | 56 | 54 | 52 | 51 | 49 | 48 | 46 | 45 | 44 | 42 | 41 | 40 | 39 |
| 300 | 62 | 61 | 59 | 57 | 55 | 53 | 52 | 50 | 49 | 47 | 46 | 44 | 43 | 42 | 41 | 40 |

Figure 32–1. Body mass index (BMI) self-assessment chart. An adult with a BMI over 25 is considered obese.

and can be attributed to a combination of genetic predisposition, diet high in fat and calories, infrequent exercise, and inadequate stress management (Andersen, 1996; Cerulli, Lomaestro, & Malone, 1998).

These behavioral problems also are seen with children, as more data link the patterns of physical activity, hours watching television and videos, intake of saturated fats, and body fatness (Obarzanek, Schrieber, Crawford, et al, 1994). The patterns for later life, including risk factors, are begun in childhood as the result of family behavioral patterns (Cunnane, 1993; Gutin & Manos, 1993; Serdula, Ivery, Coates, et al, 1993; Wolf, Gortmaker, Cheung, et al, 1993). Approximately one quarter of people suffering from severe obesity are said to have a binge-eating disorder (Andersen, 1996). These individuals graze or binge without purging.

The genetic influence is debatable in that studies demonstrate a total genetic transmission effect ranging from 5–35% across generations (Bouchard & Perusse, 1993). There is not a single gene that has been identified as causing obesity. There is a significant genetic influence, however, and obese parents are more likely to have obese children, although many more factors influence the outcome (Keller & Stevens, 1996). When both parents are obese, the child's chance of being obese is 80–90%; it is 40% with one obese parent, and 7–10% with no obese parents (Andersen, 1996; Eck, Klesges, Hanson, et al, 1992; Paige, 1986; Story & Alton, 1991). Women in the Nurses' Health Study who were overweight were more likely to have mothers who were in the heaviest of nine weight groups ("Birth Weight," 1996).

In utero, overnutrition or undernutrition may influence the development and capabilities of the hypothalamic centers' control of food (Dietz, 1994). There is some speculation that overnutrition in the third trimester and postnatal periods may influence adipose tissue cellularity, promoting obesity (Bray, 1992). Research from the Nurse's Health Study "Birth Weight," found that women who weighed more than 10 lb at birth were 62% more likely to become obese in midlife than those who weighed under 8.5 lb ("Birth Weight," 1996).

Some conditions occasionally cause a secondary obesity. These include endocrine disease (hypothyroidism, Cushing's syndrome, hypogonadism, insulinoma), hypothalamic hyperphagia (Prader-Willi syndrome seen in children), genetic alterations (beta$_3$-adrenergic receptor coding gene mutation), neurologic disorders, and some drugs, such as prednisone (Carek, Sherer, & Carson, 1997; Andersen, 1996).

The reader is referred to the review of the regulation of energy storage, intake, and expenditure, neurophysiology of feeding, metabolic effects of weight perturbation as well as futile cycles, chemical mediators of energy homeostasis, and genetic factors in Rosenbaum, Leibel, and Hirsch (1997). The discussion of these areas is beyond the scope of this chapter.

## SPECIFIC CONSIDERATIONS FOR PHARMACOTHERAPY

### WHEN DRUG THERAPY IS NEEDED

Pharmacotherapy may be needed as an adjunct to behavioral modification therapy. The literature, however, overwhelmingly supports behavioral, dietary, and activity modification therapies as the primary means toward long-lasting weight loss. Since these behavioral modifications are difficult for many people to begin or to maintain, and despite the fact that behavior therapy has proven to be a better way to maintain weight loss than pharmacotherapy, drug therapy may be indicated (Carek et al, 1997). Drug therapy has been shown to lead to a faster beginning weight loss; thus, this method as an adjunct to behavioral therapies is commonly accepted for initial cotherapy by many practitioners. However, providers must remember that "the history of weight-reduction efforts as aided by drug treatments is not a bright or happy one," as will be discussed later in this chapter (Davis & Feller, 1997, p.114). Children and adolescents are most successfully treated with realistic goals, a diet balanced in low-fat and high-fiber foods, moderate caloric reduction of 20–25%, increased physical activity, strong parental support, and behavioral therapy (Williams, Campanaro, Squillace, et al, 1997). Drug therapy in these age groups is not advised.

### SHORT- AND LONG-TERM GOALS OF PHARMACOTHERAPY

Of great importance is helping the obese person set realistic short-term goals, not impossible goals based on societal thinness standards (Rosenbaum, Leibel, & Hirsch, 1997). Pharmacotherapy, as a short-term therapy, is aimed at helping the individual get off to a faster start with weight loss, as well as promoting a more positive initial emotional response to therapy. The slower response to behavioral therapies that is the rule with behavioral, diet, and activity modifications may lead people to lose interest and motivation. When reducing morbidity and mortality risks are the long-term aims of weight loss, the use of drug therapy may be necessary.

If the weight level is mildly to moderately elevated and the patient has no serious complications, or worsening of complications, some providers feel any cycling of weight gain and loss is worse in promoting cardiovascular disease than remaining at a stable though somewhat increased weight (Andersen, 1996). Also, although anoretic drugs have some limited benefits, regaining of lost weight occurs rapidly once they are discontinued without continued maintenance of primary behavioral modification therapies concerning diet and exercise (Carek, Sherer, & Carson, 1997).

## NONPHARMACOLOGIC THERAPY

Behavioral, diet, and exercise therapies are the mainstays of weight-loss and maintenance programs today. When drug therapy is used, it should be used in conjunction with these where possible, and monitoring should occur around the combination of therapy.

### Behavioral Modifications

The initiation of any weight-loss program must begin with a mental and emotional dedication by the patient to change his or her behavior. Such alterations include lifestyle, dietary habits, and activity levels but most of all, they include a mental framework that encourages and enhances continuing with the modifications. Behavioral changes are said to progress through stages, whatever the health adaptation or cessation behavior (Pender, 1997). The transtheoretical model, developed by Prochaska and DiClemente, is applicable to modifying one's life and behavior. The reader is referred to Pender (1997) for more information on this topic. A continued close relationship with the group and therapist is advised after the weight is lost to help the person maintain (Rosenbaum, Leibel, & Hirsch, 1997).

### Dietary Modification

This is the most preferred therapy (Bray, 1993; "NIH Consensus," 1991). Numbers of diet plans are touted to produce weight loss, with everything from decreased caloric intake to low fat intake as the primary factors for loss. A huge, multibillion dollar market exists for such diet plans and for food products to enhance weight loss. This chapter does not review dietary behavioral therapy or diet plans. The reader is referred to appropriate references for this information. However, suffice it to say that a diet that is lower in calories than daily activity requires, low in fat (especially saturated fat), high in vegetables and fruits; adequate in complex carbohydrates, and adequate in vitamins and mineral requirements and provides protein from low-fat dairy products, vegetable sources, or fish and chicken (no more than 5–6 oz a day) is considered a healthy nutritional plan. Low-fat diets are associated with short-term weight loss, which can be maintained if the diet is continued (Rosenbaum, Leibel, & Hirsch, 1997). The heart-healthy step 1 diet recommended by the National Cholesterol Education Program (1993) lists 30% of caloric intake from fat (with only 8–10% from saturated fat), 55% from carbohydrates, and 15% from protein. Diet therapy involves not only modification of intake of foods, but changes in all the contextual elements surrounding eating, such as environment and emotional states that are more conducive to controlling intake. It also must take into account the sociocultural influences that will have to change after years of habituation and familial influence. No other activity of daily living in the lives of individuals is so ensconced with who one is as an individual. Changing the habits related to eating is no small or easy task for anyone.

### Physical Activity

Energy expenditure must be increased along with dietary modifications to attain the most success in weight loss. Without the congruence of these two methods, the needed calorie deficit cannot be achieved (Carek, Sherer, Carson, 1997). Again, this chapter does not cover the myriad of exercise and fitness therapies suggested as successful, but the reader is urged to seek readings in appropriate references in planning and counseling individuals about weight loss and fitness. Needless to say, a thorough history and physical examination are indicated prior to the initiation of any concerted fitness regimen to make sure the person is not at risk for illness or injury related to such activities. Any exercise program must be geared to the individual's abilities and interests to be maintained, and should be monitored by the provider for safety. Walking, cycling slowly, cleaning the house, dancing, raking leaves, and gardening are among the lower energy-expending activities that are generally safer for older individuals. For those who are safely able, running, fast cycling, skating, skiing, and rowing offer higher energy expenditure, but require better physical fitness to begin with. Exercise that is of high intensity followed by low intensity (intermittent) leads to more weight and fat loss than exercise that is the same low to moderate intensity even though both continuous and intermittent expend the same number of calories (Rosenbaum, Leibel, & Hirsch, 1997). Again, developing a safe exercise plan requires assessment and incorporation of all facets of the person's life.

## Surgical Therapy

The reader is referred to appropriate references for surgical therapy information. A BMI of more than 40 (defined as severe obesity) or a BMI of 35 to 40 (defined as less severe obesity) with co-existing conditions are indications for considering surgical therapy (Rosenbaum, Leibel, & Hirsch, 1997).

## TIME FRAME FOR INITIATING PHARMACOTHERAPY

When to initiate drug therapy for obesity depends on the individual patient. The provider can offer such therapy after an initial evaluation to rule out contraindications, but the patient must be ready emotionally to try it. If the patient has tried and relapsed using nonpharmacologic therapies, she or he may be more ready to try a drug regimen to assist with weight loss. Also, if the patient has complications of obesity, such as hypertension, CHD, or arthritis pain, these diseases become strong motivators to begin a plan comprised of behavioral change, as well as dietary, exercise, and drug therapy. The sooner an obese person can begin a safe weight-loss plan, the better the chances are of decreasing risks of serious consequences.

Drug therapy is contraindicated in children and pregnant or lactating women. Nonpharmacologic combination therapy plans are advised for children and adolescents. Nonprescribed and unsupervised dieting in pregnancy and lactation may be dangerous to the fetus.

How long it takes to achieve the goals with drug therapy depends on the individual. Some people will need a "boost" for a few months or more, whereas others will need longer support. There is evidence that some drug therapies do promote and maintain long-term weight loss, but they have to be taken long-term (Carek et al, 1997).

See Drug Table 1002.

## ASSESSMENT PRIOR TO THERAPY

### Baseline History, Physical Examination, and Diagnostic Test Data

Anyone who is being evaluated for obesity needs a complete history and physical examination. Pulmonary and cardiac status need to be determined as well as a lipid profile. Causes of secondary obesity, such as thyroid disease, as well as complications of obesity itself need to be ruled out; thus, an extensive history and physical examination are indicated. Treatments will hinge on the these findings.

A diagnosis of obesity is based on comparison of the patient's weight to standard tables for height and frame (see Table 32–1), ideal body weight (see Table 32–2), or by calculation of body mass index (BMI). An adult with a BMI over 25 is considered obese. A BMI self-assessment chart is provided in Fig. 32–1. A gross calculation of obesity can be made by calculating percentage of ideal body weight. The actual body weight is divided by ideal body weight, and the product is multiplied by 100. The ideal result is 100; over 120 is considered obese.

For children, see the previously discussed measurements of triceps skin folds and growth above the 85th percentile. For adults, skin-fold measurements of the triceps and subscapular sites with skin calipers (anthropometry) can provide more precise measures, when these are coupled with BMI, an accurate diagnosis can be made (see Table 32–3 for skinfold measures). Three skin-fold measurements are taken at each site (triceps and subscapular), and the median values are summed. Marked deviations above or below the 50th percentile for young adults indicates abnormality. The normal for young men is 21 or 9.45% of body fat; normal for young women is 30 or 22.8% of body fat. Pender (1997) states that the "gold standard" for indirect body fat estimates is hydrostatic weighing,

## TABLE 32–1. WEIGHT TABLE ACCORDING TO HEIGHT AND FRAME

| Height | | Weight in Pounds (Frame) | | |
|---|---|---|---|---|
| Feet | Inches | Small | Medium | Large |
| **Adult Man** | | | | |
| 5 | 2 | 128–134 | 131–141 | 138–150 |
| 5 | 3 | 130–136 | 133–143 | 140–153 |
| 5 | 4 | 132–138 | 135–145 | 142–156 |
| 5 | 5 | 134–140 | 137–148 | 144–160 |
| 5 | 6 | 136–142 | 139–151 | 146–164 |
| 5 | 7 | 138–145 | 142–154 | 149–168 |
| 5 | 8 | 140–148 | 145–157 | 152–172 |
| 5 | 9 | 142–151 | 148–160 | 155–176 |
| 5 | 10 | 144–154 | 151–163 | 158–180 |
| 5 | 11 | 146–157 | 154–166 | 161–184 |
| 6 | 0 | 149–160 | 157–170 | 164–188 |
| 6 | 1 | 152–164 | 160–174 | 168–192 |
| 6 | 2 | 155–168 | 164–178 | 172–197 |
| 6 | 3 | 158–172 | 167–182 | 176–202 |
| 6 | 4 | 162–175 | 171–187 | 181–207 |
| **Adult Woman** | | | | |
| 4 | 10 | 102–111 | 109–121 | 118–131 |
| 4 | 11 | 103–113 | 111–123 | 120–134 |
| 5 | 0 | 104–115 | 113–126 | 122–137 |
| 5 | 1 | 106–118 | 115–129 | 125–140 |
| 5 | 2 | 108–121 | 118–132 | 128–143 |
| 5 | 3 | 111–124 | 121–135 | 131–147 |
| 5 | 4 | 114–127 | 124–138 | 134–151 |
| 5 | 5 | 117–130 | 127–141 | 137–155 |
| 5 | 6 | 120–133 | 130–144 | 140–159 |
| 5 | 7 | 123–136 | 133–147 | 143–163 |
| 5 | 8 | 126–139 | 136–150 | 146–167 |
| 5 | 9 | 129–142 | 139–153 | 149–170 |
| 5 | 10 | 132–145 | 142–156 | 152–173 |
| 5 | 11 | 135–148 | 145–159 | 155–176 |
| 6 | 0 | 138–151 | 148–162 | 158–179 |

From Pender (1997, p. 122).

but this requires complex equipment and time and often causes anxiety to the patient.

## Concomitant Disease States and Contraindications

As mentioned previously, secondary obesity may be caused by a number of diseases. The management of these diseases is not covered in this chapter. Readers are referred to appropriate chapters in this book or other references for this information. Conditions contraindicating the use

of the drugs for treating obesity are provided in Drug Table 1002 or in the subsequent sections dealing specifically with drug therapy for obesity.

## PATIENT/CAREGIVER INFORMATION

All the literature agrees that pharmacotherapy for weight loss must be accompanied by an exercise regimen and a reduction in caloric intake. This requires, for most, a change in lifestyle. If the patient is committed to change, then the health care provider can work out a plan for the individual based on BMI, usual daily activity, and what the patient is willing to do for physical activity (energy expenditure). This will determine the amount of energy intake in calories that is needed to meet nutritional requirements but with sufficient deficit to provide for weight loss.

The patient should know that the medication will give him or her a "fast start" on losing weight, but will not continuously maintain weight loss. That will depend on the lifestyle changes made by the patient. If a patient is not losing weight while on medication, reassess readiness for change. They may benefit from learning strategies to *prevent weight gain*.

## TABLE 32–2. METROPOLITAN 1983 WEIGHTS FOR AGES 25–59

| Height (ft-in) | Men | Women |
|---|---|---|
| 4-10 | — | 100–131 |
| 4-11 | — | 101–134 |
| 5-0 | — | 103–137 |
| 5-1 | 123–145 | 105–140 |
| 5-2 | 125–148 | 108–144 |
| 5-3 | 127–151 | 111–148 |
| 5-4 | 129–155 | 114–152 |
| 5-5 | 131–159 | 117–156 |
| 5-6 | 133–163 | 120–160 |
| 5-7 | 135–167 | 123–164 |
| 5-8 | 137–171 | 126–167 |
| 5-9 | 139–175 | 129–170 |
| 5-10 | 141–179 | 132–173 |
| 5-11 | 144–183 | 135–176 |
| 6-0 | 147–187 | — |
| 6-1 | 150–192 | — |
| 6-2 | 153–197 | — |
| 6-3 | 157–202 | — |

Note: The weight range is the lower weight for small frame and the upper weight for large frame.
Adapted from Melkus (1994).

## TABLE 32–3.  TRICEPS SKIN-FOLD THICKNESS INDICATING OBESITY (mm)

| Age (yr) | Males | Females |
|----------|-------|---------|
| 5 | ≥12 | ≥15 |
| 10 | ≥13 | ≥17 |
| 15 | ≥15 | ≥20 |
| 20 | ≥16 | ≥28 |
| 25 | ≥20 | ≥29 |
| 30 and above | ≥23 | ≥30 |

*From Pender (1997, p. 122).*

Patients should know when and how to take their medications (see Drug Table 1002). They should be told the possible side effects and how to counteract them when possible. A common irritating side effect is dry mouth and/or thirst. Tell them to chew sugarless gum or suck on sugarless lemon drops and increase fluid intake.

Patients taking serotonergic agents should be warned not to abruptly stop the medication, as this could cause depression.

Patients taking dexfenfluramine or fenfluramine should be aware of the risk they are taking in increasing their odds ratio to 23 for primary pulmonary hypertension if they remain on the drug over 3 months. These drugs are now off the market. Those patients on fen-phen (fenfluramine-phentermine) also should be advised of the possible damage to heart valves if on the medication over a long period of time. A risk-benefit ratio needs to be considered for the individual patient.

## OUTCOMES MANAGEMENT

### SELECTING AN APPROPRIATE AGENT

The two major classes of anorectic drugs are noradrenergic and serotonergic agents (Carek et al, 1997). Noradrenergic drugs act on the appetite center, and serotonergic agents affect the satiety center.

### Noradrenergic Agents

These agents act by activating central beta and/or dopaminergic receptors in the hypothalamus (Carek et al, 1997). All except mazindol are related chemically to the prototype agent, amphetamine. Because amphetamine has such a high potential for abuse, its chemical structure has been modified to reduce stimulant effects, and the resulting newer agents are safer. Amphetamine, dexamphetamine, and phendimetrazine are now illegal for obesity treatment, and are controlled substances Schedule II. Abuse of the newer agents is rare if used according to the manufacturer's recommendations (Jung & Chong, 1991; Silverstone, 1992).

Leaders in the field of obesity treatment believe that true tolerance to a noradrenergic agent does not develop; however, patients reach a point in weight loss where they plateau at about 6 months after beginning therapy (Carek et al, 1997). They then must continue taking the drug even to maintain that weight, and no more weight is lost. This occurs, most likely, in response to the body's compensatory action of decreasing the metabolic rate as it senses the weight loss.

Specific noradrenergic agents (see the Monitoring for Toxicity section that follows for the typical noradrenergic side effects seen with these drugs; all are taken by mouth) are the following:

- *Phenylpropanolamine* is sold over-the-counter as Acutrim or Dexatrim. The typical daily dose is 25 mg t.i.d.; the extended-release dose is 75 mg q.d. There have been no trials lasting more than 3 months. Benzocaine in combination with this drug does not enhance weight loss (Carek et al, 1997).

- *Diethylpropion* (Tenuate) is a Schedule IV prescription medication. The typical daily dose is 25 mg t.i.d.; the extended-release dose is 75 mg q.d. It causes side effects more rarely than other drugs in this class (Carek et al, 1997).

- *Mazindol* (Mazanor, Sanorex) is a Schedule IV prescription medication. The typical daily dose is 1 mg t.i.d. or 2 mg q.d. This drug enhances insulin secretion and may have hypolipidemic action that is independent of weight loss. This is the most expensive of the noradrenergic agents (Carek et al, 1997).

- *Phentermine* (Fastin or Ionamin) is a Schedule IV prescription medication. The typical daily dose is 15–37.5 mg once q.d. Works equally well if given alternate months or continuously (Carek et al, 1997).

- *Phendimetrazine tartrate* (Bontril, Plegine, PreM-2) is a Schedule III prescription medication. The typical dose is 35 mg b.i.d. or t.i.d.; the extended-release dose is 105 mg once q.d. This drug increases free fatty acids and/or glycerol (Carek et al, 1997).

- *Benzphetamine* (Didrex) is a Schedule III prescription medication. The typical dose is 50 mg q.d. to t.i.d. (Carek et al, 1997).

## Serotonergic Agents

Since August 1997, serious adverse effects resulting from the treatment of some obese individuals with two popular serotonergic agents have been verified, leading to banning of dexfenfluramine (Redux) and fenfluramine (Pondimin) by states, and voluntary withdrawal from the market of both drugs by Wyeth-Ayerst, the manufacturer. Patients taking either drug were advised by the FDA to discontinue the drug immediately (Redux and Pondimin, 1997). A Mayo Clinic cardiologist, Dr. Heidi M. Connolly, and colleagues found that 24 women who had taken the popular combination of drugs, known as fen-phen (fenfluramine and phentermine), for an average of 12 months had developed fibrous thickening of one or more cardiac valves, preventing complete closure of the valve and resulting in regurgitation (Connolly, Crary, McGoon, et al, 1997). Valves on both sides of the heart were involved, and eight women had developed new pulmonary hypertension. Upon histopathological examination, the leaflets and chordal structures had plaque-like encasement. So serious were the findings that *The New England Journal of Medicine* allowed an early release of this study. The women in the study had no previous histories of heart disease and were young; the average age was 44 years. An advisory issued by the FDA warned the public and professionals of the results of this study and of 9 similar cases (Off-label drug use, 1997). By September 1997, Florida had banned use of the drugs for 90 days, and other states followed suit. As of October 1997, more than 45 additional cases had been reported to the FDA, leading the manufacturer to withdraw the drugs from the market. Phentermine was not implicated in the complications (Napier, 1997).

Interestingly, both fenfluramine (a serotonergic agent) and phentermine (an adrenergic agent) were approved by the FDA years before problems arose with fenfluramine, simply because the two were not prescribed together; when used alone, neither was particularly hailed, thus both were prescribed at low rates (Davis & Feller, 1997). Phentermine, when used alone, is limited as an effective weight loss agent because of intolerance to its stimulatory activity (Cerulli, Lomaestro, & Malone, 1998).

The introduction of dexfenfluramine in 1996 with an accompanying flurry of publicity not only increased its use but fenfluramine's as well. As research showed that fen-phen actually helped obese persons lose weight more effectively than nutritional alterations alone, the prescribing of the two drugs "became a veritable medical craze" (Davis & Feller, 1997, p. 177). Not soon enough did the realization come that significant complications resulted in some people from use.

Serotonergic agents are structurally very similar to noradrenergic agents, but they work by a different mechanism (Carek, Sherer, & Carson, 1997). A racemic mixture of dexfenfluramine and levofenfluramine, fenfluramine was a highly selective serotonin agonist. It enhanced serotonin release into nerve synapses and inhibited its reuptake. Dexfenfluramine was the active form and was found to be effective in half the dose of fenfluramine (Voelkel et al, 1997).

With the loss of these drugs for treating obesity, weight-loss clinics, providers, and consumers looked to fluoxetine (Prozac) to replace the "fen," and "phen-pro" was born (Davis & Feller, 1997). Although fluoxetine is believed to be an anorectic agent, it is not approved by the FDA for this purpose. In fact, Eli Lilly & Co., the manufacturer, does not endorse its use with phentermine for weight loss, a combination many have turned to as a replacement for fen-phen. Much research is needed before such a combination can be endorsed as safe or effective.

What is known about fluoxetine is that weight loss occurs in nonobese individuals as well as those who are obese or overweight (Carek, Sherer, & Carson, 1997). Weight loss is promoted for at least 5 to 6 months in people being treated for depression (Rosenbaum, Leibel, & Hirsch, 1997). After 16 to 20 weeks of using 10 to 20 mg q.d. of fluoxetine, some patients regain weight (Carek, Sherer, & Carson, 1997). Fluoxetine is approved for depression, bulimia, and obsessive-compulsive disorder. It raises basal body temperature and may increase energy expenditure as well as inhibit serotonin reuptake. Mean weight loss between control and treatment groups in a 1-year double-blind, randomized study of white women was not significantly different with fluoxetine 60 mg daily and placebo, although a clinically significant amount of weight was lost by the fluoxetine group (Goldstein, Rampey, Enas, et al, 1994). The treatment group reported adverse effects significantly more often; controls reported "allergic reactions" significantly more often. Side effects of the drug therapy were asthenia, diarrhea, sweating, insomnia, somnolence, bronchitis, nervousness, nausea and vomiting, tremor, and thirst. Less than half of the patients in both groups completed the study. Of those who did, the treatment group had significantly greater mean weight loss after 7 consecutive months than the placebo group, but maintenance of weight control beyond this point was not successful. Fluoxetine was used in a study with obese patients who had Type II diabetes (Gray, Fujioka, Devine, & Bray, 1992). These patients were receiving insulin. Those receiving fluoxetine lost significantly more weight than the placebo group, and their daily insulin dosage significantly decreased on active treatment. Both groups had similar adverse effects, but the sample was small. Goldstein, Hamilton, and associates (1997) found that fluoxetine used to treat older patients with major depression was not associated with statistically significant weight loss. Fluoxetine has been found effective and safe for up to 16 weeks when used to treat patients diagnosed with bulimia nervosa (Goldstein, Wilson, Thompson, Potvin, & Rampey, 1995).

Sertaline has a similar effect on appetite as fluoxetine, but paroxetine does not (Davis & Feller, 1997). Once again, the lack of data on the use of fluoxetine (and other similar drugs) with phentermine must lead providers to consider that a similar synergistic effect as with fen-phen may occur with phen-pro, and caution is urged.

## Herbal Weight Loss Products and Concerns

By October 1997, in the wake of the fen-phen demise, Nutri/System was suggesting that two herbal products, St. John's wort (active ingredient is Hypericum) and ephedra, were the answer to an obese person's dilemma to lose weight (see Chapter 9 for more on these herbs) (Hendren, 1997). The herbal combination was touted to be a safe replacement; however, no studies on the effectiveness or safety of these two herbs in combination are reported as of the writing of this book (Update '97, 1997). The largest U.S. manufacturer of St. John's wort, Twin Laboratories of Ronkonkoma, N.Y., sells St. John's wort as a nutritional supplement, and is barred from making health related claims by federal law. However, ads, stepping close to the line of allowable, trumpet the "garden" as a safe way to lose weight in selling the herb.

In the herbal plan, 250 mg of Hypericum in a capsule and 334 mg of ephedra extract in another capsule are given (Davis & Feller, 1997). The second capsule also may have additional herbs and substances in it supposed to increase fat metabolism, such as chromium, potassium and magnesium phosphates. The combination is supposed to have an anorexic effect (ephedra) and suppress compulsive eating urges by raising dopamine levels in the brain (Hypericum) (Davis & Feller, 1997).

In fact, ephedra, also called ma huang, epitonin, Sida cordifolia, or ephedrine, is associated with several deaths and many adverse health reports. Of additional importance for the consumer to know is the Federal Trade Commission's requirement that product labels for Herbal Ecstacy, an ephedra-containing herbal product, contain health warnings (FTC requires warning, 1997). The FDA cited 800 injuries and at least 17 deaths associated with ephedra. By November 1997, the FDA warned consumers that the combination of ephedra and St. John's wort could cause hypertension, insomnia, seizures, heart attacks, and stroke. Regulations that would limit the amount of ephedrine per dose and ban advertising recommending use of ephedra products for more than 7 days have been proposed by the FDA (Update '97, 1997). The FDA has warned companies that by advertising dietary supplements as weight loss products, they are violating federal law (Neergaard, 1997). Tyler (1998) attributes 22 deaths to ephedra. He states that the June 1997 FDA proposed limitation on ephedra use of no more than 8 mg of ephedra alkaloids in a 6 hour period, or 24 mg per day, for no longer than 7 days makes ephedra useless as a diet aid. His advice is that an emphatic "no" be given to the question, "Should I take ephedra." Besides the adverse reactions given earlier, Tyler lists nervousness, heart palpitations, headaches, dizziness, skin flushing, sleeplessness, and vomiting as side effects that may occur.

Davis and Feller (1997) issue special cautions to diabetics and hypertensives against taking the herbal combination. Some diabetics may be taking chromium already to enhance insulin action, and adding more may be excessive, and they also cite the dangers of ephedra. For the hypertensive, the ephedra may interfere with the action of prescribed medications putting the patient at risk.

Because so many people are turning to herbal alternatives to help with weight problems, Dr.

Tyler, dean emeritus of the Purdue University School of Pharmacy and Pharmacal Sciences, and distinguished professor emeritus of pharmacognosy, devoted an entire article in *Prevention* magazine to help the public have a better understanding of safety issues related to this topic (Tyler, 1998). In addition to discussing ephedra and St. John's wort, he discussed the following herbs being used for weight loss and the pros and cons of each:

- *Hydroxycitric acid (HCA)*: Obtained from the brindall berry (Garcinia cambogia), HCA seems to decrease appetite in animals and subsequent food intake. However, no rigorous human studies have been done. Tyler states that this product may work but recommends that many questions need to be answered by research before use, including substance activity and level after HCA is converted into a supplement; absorption efficiency; weight recidivism after stopping the herb; side effects; and length of time one can take the herb safely.

- *Diuretic and laxative herbs:* Listed are parsley, juniper, and dandelion leaves as diuretic herbs, and aloe, rhubarb root, buckthorn, cascara, and senna as laxative herbs. Many products have these herbs in them, so reading labels is important. Tyler warns that only water is lost with these herbs, thus weight is regained immediately upon stopping them. Using the laxative herbs indefinitely leads to dependence. They may cause diarrhea and severe abdominal cramping. Of greatest concern is potassium loss with low levels causing cardiac irregularities and possible heart failure (Tyler, 1998). Tyler reports the deaths of 4 women from these herbs in teas touted as teas for dieting. The use of these products to lose weight is discouraged.

One group of supplements that Tyler says may be helpful are dietary fiber products, although these are not approved or advertised as weight loss products (Tyler, 1998). He lists oat or barley bran, psyllium, or glucomanna capsules as ways to increase fiber which may decrease hunger and is known to decrease cholesterol, colon cancer risk, and reduce constipation. He cites a study where dieters either took a fiber supplement or not. The weight loss was nearly twice as great in the supplement group, who reported being less hungry. Tyler advises using small amounts to start (to decrease flatulence and diarrhea). Also, with psyllium and glucomannan capsules, patients need to be urged to drink additional fluids to be sure the product does not remain in the throat/esophagus, swell and obstruct.

## Investigational Agents

- *Monoamine reuptake inhibitor:* a drug with antiobesity activity, sibutramine (Meridia), was approved by the FDA for use in late 1997 (Davis & Feller, 1997). It has little or no monoamine oxidase effect but has a broad monoamine reuptake inhibitor action, interfering with reuptake of 5-HT, dopamine, and norepinephrine. It enhances the ability to regulate hunger. Because of its effect on elevating heart rate and blood pressure, it is not recommended for anyone who has poorly controlled or uncontrolled hypertension, a history of coronary artery disease, congestive heart failure, stroke, arrhythmia or is over the age of 60. It is recommended only for those whose BMI is 30, or 27 with other risk factors. The drug was approved by the FDA over the objection of its scientific advisors. The FDA, therefore, recommends that all persons taking the drug have their blood pressure and heart rate checked before initiating therapy and have reevaluations of same at regular intervals (Weighing in, 1998; NP Therapeutics, 1998; Diet drug, 1998). It is thought that it may be particularly helpful with obese Type 2 diabetics. Side effects, said to be mild, include dry mouth, headache, constipation, and insomnia (Davis & Feller, 1997). This drug is expected on the market in the spring of 1998, and will be available in 5, 10, and 15 mg capsules.

- *Lipase inhibitors:* A drug called tetrahydrolipstatin, formerly called orlistat, and also known as Xenical, under development, acts by reducing the amount of fat from the diet that is absorbed by the GI tract (Jung & Chong, 1991). As much as one third of dietary fat is not absorbed. Xenical, taken with each meal, binds to certain pancreatic enzymes to block the absorption of fat. It also causes a decreased absorption of fat-soluble vitamins. This results in soft stools and oily leakages ("Panel Recommends," 1997). Concerns focus on whether the decreased fat absorption will cause patients to take in more fat, offsetting any benefit (Carek, Sherer, & Carson, 1997). Side effects of orlistat create a defecation urgency and frequency that may be very bothersome (Davis & Feller, 1997). Abdominal pain may be present. The problems were reported to decrease in the second year of use. Of concern is that fat-soluble vitamins A, D, E, K, and beta-carotene, are not absorbed well when this drug is used, so multivitamin supplements should be taken at least 3 hours prior to taking the drug (Davis & Feller, 1997). Additionally, some concern about subjects developing neoplasms while on this drug have led to FDA approval being delayed.

- *Thermogenic agents:* Such agents act to strengthen trabecular bone (slowing bone loss), increase fatty acid oxidation potential by muscle, enhance cardiovascular fitness, and provide feedback signaling for food intake and body fat storage modulation (Bray, 1993). In these ways, they are similar to exercise (Carek et al, 1997). Ephedrine, the only thermogenic drug available, is not approved for weight loss because it is associated with tremor, adverse effects on glycemic control, elevated blood pressure, and minimal weight loss.

- *Selective beta₃-adrenergic agonists:* These agents are not approved for weight loss but have the potential for use in treating obesity (Howe, 1993). In animal studies, they increase thermogenesis, decrease body weight and improve metabolic profile (Carek, Sherer, & Carson, 1997). Trials in humans have found that weight loss is significant but the side effects are of concern: hand tremor, nervousness, and tachycardia (Davis & Feller, 1997).

- *Selective beta₂-adrenergic agonists:* In animal studies, these agents were useful for obesity treatment, but side effects interfered with their use in humans (Yang & McElligott, 1989). Tremor was the primary side effect. In humans, this agonist, either alone or in combination, is expected to have value by increasing lipolysis (Davis & Feller, 1997).

- *Thyroid hormone supplementation:* Although thyroid hormone supplementation is known to cause weight loss by reducing lean body mass, it should not be used unless the patient has hypothyroidism since it causes hyperthyroid side effects (Carek et al, 1997; Jung & Chong, 1991).

- *Gastric-emptying and carbohydrate digestion inhibitors:* Cholecystokinin (CCK) is a gastric-emptying inhibitor being studied (Jung & Chong, 1991). It is a peptide that signals the hypothalamus to decrease food intake (Cerulli, Lomaestro, & Malone, 1998). Acarbose is a carbohydrate digestion inhibitor that causes weight loss that is not sustained.

- *Recombinant leptin and leptin agonist:* Leptin, a 146-amino acid protein, is produced in obese mice by the obesity gene (Davis & Feller, 1997). In mice, the gene for diabetes expresses a mutated leptin receptor. Research is looking at agents that may be leptin agonists, crossing the blood-brain barrier to signal the satiety center in the hypothalamus.

- *Neuropeptide Y antagonist:* The neuropeptide Y (NPY) stimulates food intake and decreases thermogenesis. Antagonists are being studied as potential antiobesity treatments (Davis & Feller, 1997).

- *Melanocortin:* Research is examining melanocortin-like drugs that act to suppress the appetite. At this point, only animal studies are being done (Davis & Feller, 1997).

## MONITORING FOR EFFICACY

The patient should be weighed every week at first, then monthly as appropriate. If the patient is averaging a weight loss of 1–2 lb per week, reinforce the positive behaviors including accurate medication taking. Reassess medication-taking behavior, diet, physical activity, and readiness to change (Prochaska, DiClemente, & Norcross, 1992).

Evaluate the effect of weight loss on energy level, waist circumference and risk factors (blood pressure, hyperlipidemia, hyperglycemia, etc.). Even when patients are not able to attain ideal body weight, a reduction of 5–10% of weight often produces clinically relevant benefits (Davis & Faulds, 1996).

## MONITORING FOR TOXICITY AND FOLLOW-UP

### Noradrenergic Agents

Side effects of these agents include insomnia, headache, irritability, nervousness, dry mouth, sweating, nausea, elevations in heart rate and blood pressure, palpitations, and constipation (Carek, Sherer, & Carson, 1997; Silverstone, 1992). Diethylpropion, Phentermine, and mazindol can interfere with sleep (Carek, Sherer, & Carson, 1997). None of these agents should be given with a monoamine oxidase inhibitor due to the potential for interaction (Wellman, 1992). Physical and/or psychologic dependence is rare if noradrenergic agents are administered according to the manufacturer's advice.

### Serotonergic Agents

Side effects are similar to but usually more mild than the corresponding noradrenergic effects. They include sweating, nausea, vomiting, insomnia, diarrhea, somnolence, bronchitis, polyuria, asthenia, nervousness, tremor, and thirst. None of the serotonergic agents should be abruptly discontinued. Such cessation may result in depression. Fluoxentine's abrupt cessation may result additionally in muscle aches and paresthesias.

# REFERENCES

Andersen, A. E. (1996). Eating and weight disorders. In J. D. Stobo, D. B. Hellmann, P. W. Ladenson, B. G. Petty, & T. A. Traill, *The principles and practices of medicine*. Stamford, CT: Appleton & Lange.

Atkinson, R. L., & Hubbard, V. S. (1994). Report on the NIH workshop on pharmacologic treatment of obesity. *American Journal of Clinical Nutrition, 60*, 153–156.

Birth weight, hypertension, and obesity. (1996). *Harvard Women's Health Watch, IV*(4), 7.

Bouchard, C., & Perusse, L. (1993). Genetic aspects of obesity. *Annals of the New York Academy of Science, 699*, 26–35.

Braitman, L. E., Adlin, V., & Stanton, J. L. (1985). Obesity and caloric intake. *Journal of Chronic Diseases, 38*, 727.

Bray, G. A. (1992). Pathophysiology of obesity. *American Journal of Clinical Nutrition, 55*(Suppl. 2), 488–494.

Bray, G. A. (1993). Use and abuse of appetite-suppressant drugs in the treatment of obesity. *Annals of Internal Medicine, 119*(7 Pt. 2), 707–713.

Brownell D. D. (1982). Obesity: Understanding and treating a serious, prevalent, and refractory disorder. *Journal of Consulting and Clinical Psychology, 50*, 820–840.

Carek, P. J., Sherer, J. T., & Carson, D. S. (1997). Management of obesity: Medical treatment options. *American Family Physician, 55*(2), 551–558.

Cerulli, J., Lomaestro, B. M., & Malone, M. (January, 1998). Update on the pharmacotherapy of obesity. *The Annals of Pharmacotherapy, 32*, 88–102.

Connolly, H. M., Crary, J. L., McGoon, M. D., Hensrud, D. D., Edwards, B. S., Edwards, W. D., & Schaff, H. V. (1997). Valvular heart disease associated with fenfluramine-phentermine. *New England Journal of Medicine, 337*(9), 581–588.

Cunnane, S. C. (1993). Childhood origins of lifestyles-related risk factors for coronary heart disease in adulthood. *Nutrition and Health, 9*(2), 107–115.

Davis, R., & Faulds, D. (1996). Dexfenfluramine: An updated review of its therapeutic use in the management of obesity. *Drugs, 52*(5), 696–724.

Davis, W. M. & Feller, D. R. (December 8, 1997). Advances and retreats in the pharmacotherapy of obesity. *Drug Topics*, 114–121.

Diet drug to hit the shelves. (February 13, 1998). *Sun-Sentinel*. 11A.

Dietz, W. H. (1994). Critical periods in childhood for the development of obesity. *American Journal of Clinical Nutrition, 59*, 955–959.

Eck, L. H., Klesges, R. C., Hanson, C. L., et al. (1992). Children at familial risk for obesity: An examination of dietary intake, physical activity and weight status. *International Journal of Obesity and Related Metabolic Disorders, 16*(2), 71–78.

Fraser, L. (1997, March). C. Everett Koop, 1994 "Report Shape up America." *Reader's Digest*, 177–184.

FTC requires warning labels for Herbal Ecstacy. (October 18, 1997). *Sun-Sentinel*, 12A.

Garfinkel, L. (1985). Overweight and cancer. *Annals of Internal Medicine, 103*(6 Pt. 2), 1034–1036.

Goldstein, D. J., Hamilton, S. H., Masica, D. N., Beasley, C. M. Jr. (1997). Fluoxetine in medially stable, depressed geriatric patients: Effects on weight. *Journal of Clinical Psychopharmacology, 17*(5), 365–369.

Goldstein, D. J., Rampey, A. H., Jr., Enas, G. G., Potvin, J. H., & Fludzinski (1994). Fluoxetine: A randomized clinical trial in the treatment of obesity. *International Journal of Obesity and Related Metabolic Disorders, 18*, 129–135.

Goldstein, D. J., Wilson, M. G., Thompson, V. L., Potvin, J. H., & Rampey, A. H. (1995). Long-term fluoxetine treatment of bulimia nervosa. *British Journal of Psychiatry, 166*(5), 660–666.

Gorsky, R. D., Pamuk, E., Williamson, D. F., Shaffer, P. A., & Koplan, J. P. (1996). The 25-year health care costs of women who remain overweight after 40 years of age. *American Journal of Preventive Medicine, 12*(5), 388–394.

Gortmaker, S. L., Must, A., Perrin, J. M., et al. (1993). Social and economic consequences of overweight in adolescence and young adulthood. *New England Journal of Medicine, 329*(14), 1008–1012.

Gray, D. S., Fujioka, K., Devine, W., & Bray, G. A. (1992). A randomized double-blind clinical trial of fluoxetine in obese diabetics. *International Journal of Obesity and Related Metabolic Disorders, 16* Suppl 4, 567–572.

Gutin, B. & Manos, T. M. (1993). Physical activity in the prevention of childhood obesity. *Annals of the New York Academy of Science, 699*, 115–126.

Hendren, J. (October 18, 1997). Herb's popularity soars after ban on two diet drugs. *Sun-Sentinel*, 10A.

Howe, R. (1993). Beta$_3$-adrenergic agonists. *Drugs Future, 18*, 529–549.

Isselbacher, K. J., Braunwald, E., Wilson, J. D., Martin, J. B., et al. (1995). *Harrison's principles of internal medicine*, New York: McGraw-Hill.

Jousilahti, P., Tuomilehto, J., Vartianinen, E., Pekkanene, J., & Puska, P. (1996). Body weight, cardiovascular risk factors, and coronary mortality: 15-year follow-up of middle-aged men and women in eastern Finland. *Circulation, 93*(7), 1372–1379.

Jung, R. T. & Chong, P. (1991). The management of obesity. *Clinical Endocrinology, 35*, 11–20.

Keller, C., & Stevens, K. R. (1996). Assessment, etiology, and intervention in obesity in children. *NP, 21*(9), 31–42.

Lamon-Fava, S., Wilson, P. W., & Schaefer, E. J. (1996). Impact of body mass index on coronary heart disease risk factors in men and women. The Framingham Offspring Study. *Arteriosclerosis, Thrombosis, and Vascular Biology, 16*(12), 1509–1515.

Mapping U.S. obesity. (1997). Tufts University, *Health & Nutrition Letter, 15*(3), p 1.

McMillan, D. (1994). *Obesity*. New York: Venture Books.

Melkus, G. D. (1994). Obesity: Assessment and intervention for primary care practice. *Nurse Practitioner Forum, 5*(1), 28–33.

Napier, K. (December 1997). Special report: No more diet pills—What now? *Prevention,* 39–40.

National Center for Health Statistics (NCHS). (1987). *Anthropometric reference data: Prevalence of overweight, United States, 1976–1980* (DHHS Publication No. [PHS]87-1688). Washington, DC: U.S. Government Printing Office.

National Cholesterol Education Program. (1993). *Detection, evaluation, and treatment of high blood cholesterol in adults* (NIH Publication No. 93-3095). Rockville, MD: U.S. Department of Health and Human Services.

Neergaard, L. (November 7, 1997). FDA targets herbal fen-phen. *Sun-Sentinel,* 8A.

NIH consensus statement covers treatment of obesity. (1991). *American Family Physician, 44,* 305–306.

NP Therapeutics. (1998). *The Nurse Practitioner, 23,* 1, 94–95.

Obarzanek, E., Schrieber, G. B., Crawford, P. B., et al. (1994). Energy intake and physical activity in relation to indexes of body fat: The National Heart, Lung, and Blood Institute Growth and Health Study. *American Journal of Clinical Nutrition, 60*(1), 15–22.

Off-label drug use. (October 1997). *Harvard Women's Health Watch, V*(2), 2–3.

Paige, D. M. (1986). Obesity in childhood and adolescence. *Postgraduate Medicine, 62,* 233–238, 243–245.

Panel recommends anti-obesity drug. (1997, July 15). *Richmond Times Dispatch,* p. A3.

Pender, N. J. (1997). *Health promotion in nursing practice* (3rd ed.). Stamford, CT: Appleton & Lange.

Pi-Sunyer, F. X. (1993). Medical hazards of obesity. *Annals of Internal Medicine, 119*(7 Pt. 2), 655–660.

Prentice, A., & Goldberg, G. (1996). Maternal obesity increases congenital malformations. *Nutrition Reviews, 54*(5), 146–150.

Prochaska, J. O., DiClemente, C. C., & Norcross, J. C. (1992). In search of the structure of change. In Y. Klar, J. D. Fisher, J. M. Chinsky, et al (Eds), *Self-change: Social, psychological and clinical perspectives.* (pp. 87–114). New York: Springer-Verlag.

Redux and Pondimin withdrawn from market. (October 1997). *Nurses Drug News, 1*(11), 1.

Romieu, I., Willet, W. C., Stampfer, M. J., et al. (1988). Energy intake and other determinants of relative weight. *American Journal of Clinical Nutrition, 47,* 406.

Rona, R. J., Qureshi, S., & Chinn, S. (1996). Factors related to total cholesterol and blood pressure in British 9 year olds. *Journal of Epidemiology and Community Health, 50*(5), 512–518.

Rosenbaum, M., Leibel, R. L., & Hirsch, J. (1997). Obesity. *The New England Journal of Medicine, 337*(6), 396–407.

Serdula, M. K., Ivery, D., Coates, R. J., et al. (1993). Do obese children become obese adults? A review of the literature. *Preventive Medicine, 22*(2), 167–177.

Sherman, J. B., & Alexander, M. A. (1990). Obesity in childhood: A research update. *Journal of Pediatric Nursing, 5*(3), 161–167.

Silverstone, T. (1992). Appetite suppressants: A review. *Drugs, 43,* 820–836.

Stevens, T., & Craig, C. L. (1988). The well-being of Canadians: Highlights of the 1988 Campbell's survey. Ottawa, Ontario: Canada Fitness and Lifestyles Research Institute.

Story, M., & Alton, I. (1991). Current perspectives on adolescent obesity. *Journal of Clinical Nutrition, 6*(4), 51–60.

The triumph of obesity. (1997). In women and obesity: A preventable disease. *Women's Health Digest, 1*(4), 263.

Troiano, R. P., Frongillo, E. A., Jr., Sobal, J., & Levitsky, D. A. (1996). The relationship between body weight and mortality: A quantitative analysis of combined information from existing studies. *International Journal of Obesity and Related Metabolic Disorders, 20*(1), 63–75.

Tyler, V. E. (January 1998). Question: Since prescription diet pills are not on the market anymore, I'd like to try some of the herbal weight loss products. Do they work? *Prevention*, 81–85.

Update: Prevalence of overweight among children, adolescents, and adults—United States, 1988–1994. (1997). *MMWR, Morbidity and Mortality Weekly Report, 46*(9), 198–202.

Update '97: Weight-loss products: 'herbal' doesn't necessarily mean 'safe.' (December 1997). *Mayo Clinic Health Letter, 15*(12), 4.

U.S. Department of Health and Human Services. (1992). *Healthy people 2000: National health promotion and disease objectives*. Boston: Jones & Bartlett.

Van Itallie, T. B. (1985). Health implications of overweight and obesity in the United States. *Annals of Internal Medicine, 103*(6 Pt. 2), 983–988.

Voelkel, N. F., Clarke, W. R., & Higenbottam, T. (1997). Obesity, dexfenfluramine, and pulmonary hypertension. *American Journal of Respiratory and Critical Care Medicine, 155*, 786–788.

Weighing in on Meridia. (February 1998). *Harvard Women's Health Watch, 5*(6), 7.

Weight management: Making the leap to a healthy life. (1996). The Fitness Partner Connection. Reprinted from International Food Information Council & Food Insight (July/August 1992), 1–3.

Wellman, P. J. (1992). Overview of adrenergic anorectic agents. *American Journal of Clinical Nutrition, 55*(1 Suppl.), 193–198.

Whitaker, R. C., Wright, J. A., Pepe, M. S., Seidel, K. D., and Dietz, W. H. (1997). Predicting obesity in young adulthood from childhood and parental obesity. *The New England Journal of Medicine, 337*(13), 869–873.

Williams, C. L., Campanaro, L. A., Squillace, M., & Bollella, M. (1997). Management of childhood obesity in pediatric practice. *The Annals of the New York Academy of Science, 817*, 225–240.

Wolf, A. M., Gortmaker, S. L., Cheung, L., Gray, H. M., et al. (1993). Activity, inactivity, and obesity: Racial, ethnic, and age differences among school girls. *American Journal of Public Health, 83*(11), 1625–1627.

Yang, Y. T., & McElligott, M. A. (1989). Multiple actions of beta-adrenergic agonists on skeletal muscle and adipose tissue. *Biochemistry Journal, 261*(1), 1–10.

# 33

## MENTAL HEALTH DISORDERS

*B. J. Landis and Stephen G. Bryant*

Most individuals experiencing psychological distress go to their primary care providers rather than to mental health specialists, and over half of mentally ill patients in the United States receive their psychiatric care exclusively in primary care settings (Arean & Miranda, 1996; Engel, Kroenke, & Katon, 1994). This trend is likely to continue since the growing managed care systems limit patient access to specialists such as psychiatrists. However, treatment of mental illness has changed dramatically over the past 20 years. Many mental disorders have been linked to specific neurochemical imbalances that are amenable to pharmacologic intervention. Currently, pharmaceutical efforts are focused on developing more effective psychoactive drugs using new knowledge about neurotransmitters and receptors in the central nervous system. Mental health conditions covered in this chapter are the most common ones managed in primary care settings.

## DISORDERS OF MOOD

These disorders have a disturbance in mood as the predominant feature (American Psychiatric Association [APA], 1994a). Depression, a very prevalent condition seen in primary care, is associated with significant morbidity and mortality, lost productivity, diminished quality of life, and increased health care costs (Greensberg, Stiglin, Finkelstein, & Berndt, 1993; Hales,

Rakel, & Rothschild, 1994). Depressive illnesses cost the U.S. economy almost $12 billion in 1990; over $12 billion was spent on direct costs of diagnosis and treatment (Jessen, 1996). About 30% of the general population will suffer from a major depressive episode at some time. Although 85% of depressed patients can be successfully treated, surveys indicate that 70% of these do not get the treatment they need. Despite its high prevalence, depression is underdiagnosed and consequently undertreated in primary care settings, the place that patients most likely first seek help (Depression Guideline Panel [DGP], 1993a). The disorder is a common psychiatric problem in the elderly population, and the incidence of childhood depression is receiving increased attention (Jessen, 1996).

## MAJOR DEPRESSIVE DISORDER AND DYSTHYMIA

Clinical depression is a syndrome (a constellation of signs and symptoms) that is not a normal reaction to life's difficulties. Depression should not be confused with a sad mood that normally accompanies specific life experiences such as losses or disappointments. Also, a sad mood is only one of the many manifestations of depression, which may include apathy, anxiety, and irritability. These conditions tend to occur in families. Depressive disorders involve disturbances in emotional, cognitive, behavioral, and somatic regulation (DGP, 1993a). Suicide is the most serious consequence of depressive disorders, occurring at 30 times the rate of nondepressed individuals (Keller & Hanks, 1994; Wells, Mandos, & Hayes, 1997).

*Major depressive disorder* (MDD) consists of a discrete major depressive episode that can be distinguished from the patient's usual level of functioning and is classified into several subgroups (psychotic, melancholic, atypical, seasonal, and postpartum). The subtypes are not all-inclusive but may be useful in selecting treatment regimens.

MDD is a primary disease not associated with nonmood psychiatric conditions (such as eating disorders, panic attacks, or obsessive-compulsive disorder), substance abuse, or medical conditions. Major depression is an acute and sometimes severe episode of depression with unrelenting symptoms persisting for at least 2 weeks; it is not secondary to a medical illness, substance abuse, or other psychological disorders even though it may coexist with these conditions. It may be a chronic disorder that needs long-term follow-up attention and treatment (APA, 1994a; DGP, 1993a).

*Melancholic depression* is more common among older persons and is manifested by psychomotor retardation or agitation, anhedonia (inability to experience pleasure), worse depression in the morning, and early morning awakening.

*Atypical depression* is usually associated with younger age of onset and includes two broad categories of symptoms: (1) *vegetative*—marked overeating, oversleeping, and hypersensitivity to personal rejection; and (2) *anxious*—difficulty falling asleep, phobias, and sympathetic arousal along with marked anxiety.

*Seasonal depression* (seasonal affective disorder) is a well-documented mild to moderate chronic depressive disorder that recurs seasonally, most often during winter. It is more common in females and often presents with significant hypersomnia, lethargy, and weight gain. In addition to antidepressants, limited light therapy may be useful. The therapeutic response may be quick (4–7 days) or delayed up to 2 weeks (Bolen & Robbins, 1995; Millard, 1994b).

*Postpartum depression* occurs within 6 weeks to 6 months after childbirth and is more symptomatic than the "postpartum blues" that occur briefly within 1–5 days after delivery. It is characterized by irritability, anxiety, despondency, inability to cope, and tearfulness; suicide ideation is infrequent. Ten to twenty percent of postpartum women develop this disorder (Bolen & Robbins, 1995; Jermain, 1996).

*Psychotic depression* is characterized by hallucinations and delusions that are congruent with the patient's depressed mood. This psychotic variant is best managed in psychiatric settings.

*Dysthymic disorder* is characterized by a mild, insidious depressed mood and loss of interest or pleasure in customary activities with some additional signs and symptoms of depression. It is present most of the time for many years. This disorder rarely exists alone but often exists with a comorbid psychiatric or medical condition. Most often, major depressive disorder, personality disorders, social phobias, and prolonged stress are the most common comorbid psychiatric conditions. Cerebrovascular accident, multiple sclerosis, AIDS, hypothyroidism, and cardiac transplantation are common medical conditions coexisting with dysthymia (Sansone & Sansone, 1996). Many patients with dysthymia go on to develop a major depression (termed "double depression") that is difficult to treat. Dysthymia is usually manifested by sadness in adults and by either sadness or irritability in children and adolescents (DGP, 1993a; First, Donovan, & Frances, 1996; Freidman & Kocsis, 1996).

Depression commonly presents with symptoms of sleep and appetite disturbances, anhedonia, fatigue, decreased libido, diminished ability to concentrate, indecisiveness, feelings of worthlessness or hopelessness, suicidal ideation, and psychomotor agitation or retardation. Almost 90% of depressed patients also experience anxiety symptoms (Hales et al, 1994; Wells et al, 1997).

Children and adolescents may also suffer from depression. Depressed adolescents are at high risk for suicide or substance abuse, particularly if the depression is untreated. Although the diagnostic criteria for depression are the same for any age group, young patients may present differently. Unexplained pain and changes in school performance, mood, social aggressiveness, or athletic activities are often presenting symptoms. Also, youngsters who are withdrawn, angry, impulsive, or self-destructive should be evaluated for depression. Nursing home residents and elders with concomitant physical illnesses are also at risk for depressive disorders. Depression can mimic dementia, but usually psychological distress is present only in the depressed patient (DGP, 1993a; Rausch & Hyman, 1995).

# SPECIFIC CONSIDERATIONS FOR PHARMACOTHERAPY

## When Drug Therapy Is Needed

The foundation of treatment for MDD is an antidepressant agent to bring relief from the core symptoms. Most sources advocate using both pharmacotherapy and psychotherapy with frequent follow-up care by the primary clinician (DGP, 1993b; Kuzel, 1996; Miller & Keitner, 1996).

Basic principles for understanding and treating depression include the following:

1. Accurate diagnosis should rule out underlying physiologic causes.
2. Pharmacotherapy is only part of the treatment plan, which should include collaborative decision making with the patient and family and short-term psychotherapy.
3. No "magic bullet" exists.
4. Every drug has its side effects, and antidepressant choice depends on the drug's side-effect profile.
5. *Do not undertreat.*

Once the decision has been made to use an antidepressant drug, it is vital to use the proper dosage and duration of treatment. Factors to consider in drug selection include: age, family history, pattern of depression, suicidal potential, appetite, sleep habits, and coexistent diseases or other drugs being taken (Akiskal, Jensvold, Kramer, Paist, & Potter, 1994).

The treatment of depression occurs in three phases and gives direction for monitoring therapeutic outcomes: *acute, continuation,* and *maintenance* (DGP, 1993b). Acute phase goals are to eliminate symptoms of depression and restore psychosocial and occupational function. If treatment results in little or no symptom relief by 6 weeks or only partial relief by 12 weeks, the diagnosis and treatment plan should be reassessed. Substance abuse or underlying medical or psychiatric conditions may become apparent. The continuation phase is the middle stage in which the initially effective drug dosage is sustained. The treatment goal during the maintenance phase is to prevent recurrence of the depression. Some patients will require maintenance medication indefinitely. If depression responds to treatment, some sources recommend continuing the drug for at least 6 months and slowly tapering off over a 4-week period.

Should symptoms recur, the effective dose should be returned to its prior level and maintained for another 3–6 months. Reports indicate that patients do well when psychotherapy is continued during the maintenance phase. A therapeutic alliance with the patient and family and primary provider is important over the long term to lessen the likelihood of recurrence. Three or more depressive episodes greatly increase the chance of another, and these patients are good candidates for long-term maintenance phase therapy (Rausch & Hyman, 1995).

Depression is commonly associated with nonmood psychiatric disorders such as substance abuse and eating disorders. If present, these nonmood disorders should be treated first; if depression continues, then the depression is treated. Depression often coexists with anxiety; adequate treatment of the primary depression will alleviate secondary anxiety symptoms (Millard, 1994a). An algorithm for drug treatment of depression is shown in Fig. 33–1.

A number of current theories offer explanations for the complex etiology of depression. Some of these theories are shown in Table 33–1. The biogenic amine theory of depression explains its cause as a deficiency of brain neurotransmitters—primarily norepinephrine, serotonin, and dopamine. Antidepressants intensify neurotransmitter action by blocking reuptake inactivation into presynaptic nerve endings (eg, tricyclic antidepressants, selective serotonin reuptake inhibitors) or by preventing transmitter degradation (eg, monoamine oxidase inhibitors). Downregulation of norepinephrine and serotonin receptors occurs with persistent use of antidepressants, which would explain the delayed onset of the drug. Pharmacotherapy is the cornerstone of treatment for depression whether or not there is an identifiable psychological cause or stressor (Jessen, 1996; Wells et al, 1997).

## Short- and Long-Term Goals of Pharmacotherapy

Treatment goals include relieving signs and symptoms of depression, restoring psychosocial and occupational function, and avoiding relapse or recurrence of depression (DGP, 1993b). Current recommendations are to maintain effective drug therapy for up to 1 year at the same dosage level needed to achieve resolution of symptoms. Continuation therapy for at least 4 months after the acute episode is necessary to consolidate drug response and prevent relapse.

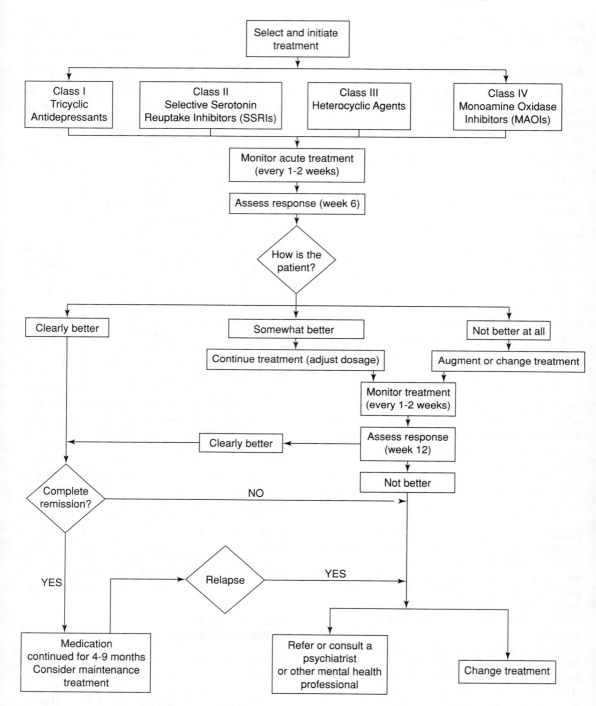

**Figure 33–1.** Algorithm for drug treatment of depression.

From Depression Guideline Panel (1993b).

## TABLE 33–1. THEORETICAL BASIS OF DEPRESSION

| Theory | Pathophysiology |
| --- | --- |
| Biogenic amine | Inadequate monoamine neuro-transmission produces depression, primarily from norepinephrine. |
| Receptor sensitivity | Downregulation of norepinephrine and serotonin receptors follows chronic administration of antidepressants. |
| Dysregulation | Failure of homeostatic regulation of the neurotransmitter system produces depression. |

*Adapted from Fankhauser and Benefield (1997).*

Some experts consider depression a chronic condition and recommend lifetime maintenance of drug therapy in selected patients. Most experts recommend psychotherapy with pharmacotherapy whenever practical. Any treatment program should include support, advice, reassurance, and hope as well as monitoring drug side effects and adjusting dosage for patients receiving medication (Bierer, 1995; Hales et al, 1994; Kuzel, 1996; Montgomery, 1994).

### Nonpharmacologic Treatment

All phases of treatment (acute, continuation, and maintenance) are carried out in the context of *clinical management,* which includes education and discussion with patients and their families about the nature of depression, its course, and relative costs and benefits of treatment options. The focus is on resolution of obstacles to treatment adherence, monitoring and management of treatment side effects, and outcome assessment. The primary provider is in a unique position to coordinate the care of a multidisciplinary treatment team and facilitate a therapeutic alliance among health professionals, patients, and their families (DGP, 1993b).

Psychotherapy is combined with medication for patients with partial responses to either treatment alone and for those with a chronic history of depressive disorder. Referral to a psychologist or mental health specialist is necessary for these interventions. Supportive therapy focuses on management and resolution of current difficulties and life decisions using the patient's

strengths and available resources. It includes supervision of more severe, complex, or chronic cases as well as active listening, education, reassurance, encouragement, and guidance. Short-term cognitive behavioral and interpersonal therapy, as well as social skills training (12–24 weeks), have demonstrated effectiveness in treating major depression. Postpartum depression responds to interpersonal therapy. Light therapy is a first-line treatment for well-documented seasonal affective disorder.

Hospitalization may be needed if psychosis is present, suicidal risk is significant, social support is inadequate, or a serious general medical condition exists. Electroconvulsive therapy (ECT) has proven effective in severely symptomatic patients who have failed to respond to medication trials or who are rapidly deteriorating. Patients are usually hospitalized, and referral to a psychiatrist is required (DGP, 1993b; Jermain, 1996; Miller & Keitner, 1996).

### Time Frame for Initiating Pharmacotherapy

Patients should be treated promptly after diagnosis to relieve symptoms and decrease suicide risk. The sooner antidepressant medication is started, the sooner patients will be afforded relief. Because all antidepressants may take up to 4–6 weeks to exert their effect and since short-term side effects may be common, patient support and encouragement to adhere to initial drug treatment recommendations are critical.

### Overview of Drug Classes for Treatment

- *Selective serotonin reuptake inhibitors* (SSRIs) exert selective effects on serotonin and are the first-line antidepressant agents in the primary care setting because of their proven efficacy, favorable adverse-effect profile, long-term tolerance, once-daily dosing, and wide therapeutic index. These agents also may be used as secondary choices for patients who do not respond well to a trial with tricyclic antidepressants (Friedman & Kocsis, 1996; Jessen, 1996; Kuzel, 1996).

- *Tricyclic antidepressants* (TCAs) have been used to treat depression in the United States for over 30 years and their efficacy has been well documented. TCAs inhibit reuptake of norepinephrine and/or serotonin; secondary amines primarily increase norepinephrine availability in the CNS. Tertiary amines have a greater effect on serotonin levels. All TCAs are equally effective antidepressant agents with major differences in degree of anticholinergic, sedative, and orthostatic side effects. Importantly, their narrow therapeutic index and potential for overdose may be life-threatening (Kuzel, 1996; Rausch & Hyman, 1995; Schlafer, 1993).

- *Monoamine oxidase inhibitors* (MAOIs) block monoamine oxidase from inactivating amine neurotransmitters, norepinephrine, dopamine, and serotonin in presynaptic neurons. MAOIs are potent antianxiety and antidepressant agents and may be very useful when anxiety is present with depression. However, the clinical utility of these drugs in primary care is limited by their adverse effects and drug-drug and drug-food interactions. Generally, a MAOI drug regimen is managed by a psychiatrist (Jessen, 1996; Kuzel, 1996).
- *Other antidepressants: Bupropion* is an antidepressant similar to SSRIs in its energizing effects. It is free of the cardiovascular and anticholinergic side effects of TCAs at both therapeutic doses and in the setting of overdose. Its mode of action is unclear, although it may be due to its reuptake blockade of dopamine. Bupropion has little or no effect on monoamine oxidase or the neurotransmitters serotonin and norepinephrine and, thus, is considered to be an antidepressant that affects different neural systems. For this reason, bupropion may be particularly useful in depressed patients who do not respond to or cannot tolerate SSRIs. Moreover, bupropion has no effect on sexual function and has gained utility in depressed patients treated with SSRIs who develop sexual dysfunction (impotence and delayed ejaculation in males and anorgasmia in females). Initial evidence indicates that bupropion may be especially useful in bipolar depressed patients because it may have less of a proclivity to induce hypomania in such patients.

    *Trazodone* and *nefazodone* are antidepressants that have in common triazolopyridine chemical structures. These drugs may be listed in some tables as tetracyclic antidepressants. Both of these agents tend to be sedative and orthostatic in their chemical effects. Trazodone is much more likely to cause these adverse effects than its more recently approved "cousin," nefazodone. However, nefazodone has the neurochemical properties of SSRIs, as well as some postsynaptic serotonergic effects. Given this profile, nefazodone can be used in patients who do not respond to SSRIs. *Venlafaxine* is another newer antidepressant that has a distinct neurochemical action among atypical agents (Guelfi et al, 1995). Termed a serotonergic noradrenergic reuptake inhibitor (SNRI), venlafaxine offers pa-

tients yet another alternative treatment to TCAs and may be used for the primary treatment of depression. Unlike some of the newer agents, venlafaxine has been shown to be effective even in severe depression compared to placebo and the SSRI fluoxetine. *Mirtazapine* is a more recently approved antidepressant available in the United States. Mirtazapine has multiple effects on serotonin and antagonizes alpha$_2$ presynaptic receptors, with a net effect of increasing both norepinephrine and serotonin. Its onset of action and efficacy are similar to the TCAs (Kehoe & Schorr, 1996).

## Assessment and History Taking

A detailed personal and family history is essential to selecting an appropriate treatment regimen. A depressed patient may present with a variety of somatic complaints such as insomnia, headache, musculoskeletal pain, GI disturbance, and vague abdominal pain.

Anxiety, insomnia, and substance abuse are often superimposed on the depression. Men are more likely to present with physical complaints, whereas women are more apt to report feelings of sadness. Cultural differences should be considered in assessing presenting symptomatology of depression. Depression is a potentially fatal disease given the propensity for suicide, and this risk needs to be carefully assessed (Rausch & Hyman, 1995). Approximately 60% of suicides can be attributed to major depression. Many experts maintain that the risk of attempted suicide is greatest as the patient begins to respond to treatment and has the psychic energy to act upon suicidal thoughts. Thus, a history of prior suicide attempts, suicidal ideation, sense of hopelessness, physical illness, or substance abuse places the patient at high risk, requiring psychiatric referral for treatment (Millard, 1994b). It is a myth that talking to a depressed patient about suicide may prompt the individual to act upon such self-destructive ideation. Rather, clinicians should routinely inquire about thoughts of suicide. If such thoughts are present, differentiate between fleeting thoughts of wishing life were over and recurrent suicidal ideation with a well-thought-out plan for self-injury. Seriously suicidal patients should always be referred immediately to a psychiatrist, and hospitalization is frequently required.

Determine if the depression is associated with a medical disease or an adverse drug response. Endocrine disorders (eg, diabetes mellitus, Cushing's disease), CNS disorders (eg,

Alzheimer's disease), CV disorders (eg, CHF, CVA), and other diseases (eg, cancer, malnutrition, lupus, AIDS) may be the underlying cause of depression. Antihypertensives and cardiovascular drugs (eg, clonidine, digitalis, guanethidine, hydralazine, prazosin, propanolol), sedative-hypnotic drugs (eg, alcohol, barbiturates, benzodiazepines), antiinflammatory and analgesic drugs (eg, indomethacin, opiates, phenylbutazone), steroids (eg, corticosteroids, estrogen withdrawal, oral contraceptives), and miscellaneous other drugs (eg, antineoplastics, antiparkinsonian agents, neuroleptics) may be associated with depression and should be reevaluated (DGP, 1993a).

A physical examination, CBC, chemistry panel, and thyroid function studies ($T_3$, $T_4$, TSH) are useful to rule out organic etiologies and guide selection of an antidepressant. A baseline EKG can detect cardiac conduction abnormalities prior to prescribing TCAs. Depression in the elderly may be difficult to distinguish from Alzheimer's disease and other dementia because their cognitive symptoms overlap. However, when depression is present without dementia, patients experience psychological distress and are aware of their cognitive deficits. Depression superimposed on chronic dementia may be responsible for agitation, insomnia, and apathy that frequently results in hospitalization. Controlling these behaviors may be the key to keeping patients home and out of the hospital (Hales et al, 1994; Schlafer, 1993).

See Drug Table 311.

## Patient/Caregiver Information

A caring family able to provide social and environmental support during treatment can be a real asset during recovery from any illness, including depression. Patients and families need to learn at the outset of treatment about the nature of depression and that treatment can be effective for most patients. Education and counseling needs to deal with issues of side effects and noncompliance. The primary clinician can instill a sense of hope. Inform patients and their families about target signs and symptoms that they can use to assess the therapeutic drug response (Citrome, 1994; Friedman & Kocsis, 1996).

The patient and family need to understand that medications should be taken regularly, that they may take several weeks to work, and that there may be side effects that usually resolve with time. Avoid using OTC medications or herbal remedies that may interact with the antidepressant. Reassure them that antidepressants are not addictive but they need to be taken as prescribed. Patient and caregiver need information about special dietary restrictions when MAOIs are prescribed; see, for example, Table 33–2. Caffeine intake should be limited because it tends to increase nervousness in patients taking TCAs and MAOIs and can precipitate cardiac arrhythmias or hypertension in patients taking MAOIs (Simmons, 1996). Table 33–3 contains patient, family, and health professional resources for managing depressive disorders.

## OUTCOMES MANAGEMENT

In assessing treatment outcomes remember that the major reasons for a poor response to antidepressant drug treatment are inadequate therapy, insufficient dosage, or inadequate duration of treatment.

### Selecting an Appropriate Agent

Selecting an antidepressant agent is based on the patient's age, general health status, clinical presentation, and past response to medication. Additional considerations include the drug's side-effect profile, potential drug interactions, and cost. If a patient has previously responded to a particular antidepressant, the same agent should be used again, unless it is contraindicated because of a newly diagnosed medical condition.

Some experts consider the key issues in selecting an antidepressant to be the side-effect profile of the drug and any comorbidities of the patient. The patient's target symptoms should be matched with the drug's side-effect profile to maximize potentially beneficial side effects and minimize the unwanted ones. For example, if symptoms include agitation and insomnia, choose a sedating antidepressant (amitriptyline, nortriptyline, doxepin, nefazodone, or mirtazapine). If symptoms include anhedonia, anergia, and psychomotor retardation, choose an activating antidepressant (desipramine, sertraline, or bupropion). No studies substantiate that such a selection leads to a better drug response; however, it should enhance compliance by decreasing unwanted side effects and making the patient more comfortable (Bierer, 1995; DGP, 1993b; Kuzel, 1996). The main differences among these antidepressant agents are their dif-

**TABLE 33–2.   DIETARY INFORMATION FOR PATIENTS TAKING MAO INHIBITORS**

**Prohibited Foods**

| | |
|---|---|
| Aged cheeses[a] | Meats: canned, aged or processed |
| Anchovies | Monosodium glutamate |
| Avocado, ripe | Pods or board beans (fava beans)[a] |
| Beer | Raisins |
| Fermented foods | Sardines |
| Figs, canned | Sauerkraut |
| Herring[a] | Snails |
| Licorice | Soy sauce |
| Liver (chicken or beef >2 days old) | Yeast products[a] |
| Marmite (meat extract) | |

**Limited Intake Permitted**

| | |
|---|---|
| American cheese: up to 2 oz daily | Sour cream: up to 2 oz daily |
| Chocolate: up to 2 oz daily | Wine (especially Chianti and sherry) and |
| Coffee: up to 2 oz daily; decaffeinated is unrestricted | spirits: 3 oz of white wine or a single cocktail |
| Cottage cheese: up to 2 oz daily | Yogurt: up to 2 oz daily |

[a] High tyramine content.
*Adapted from Wells, Mandos, and Hayes (1997).*

fering side-effect profiles—muscarinic, histaminergic, and alpha-adrenergic responses. Remember too that starting dosages for elderly patients should be approximately half the usual adult dose. Maximum tolerated doses within the therapeutic blood level guidelines should be used for 4–6 weeks at therapeutic serum levels before concluding that they are not effective for an individual patient (Miller & Keitner, 1996).

***Selective serotonin reuptake inhibitors.*** Fluoxetine, sertraline, and paroxetine are effective antidepressants and are first-line agents in primary care treatment of major depression. Fluoxetine is more likely to cause agitation and anxiety, whereas paroxetine causes dry mouth and sedation. Start fluoxetine at 10–20 mg and sertraline at 50 mg once daily in the morning. Sertraline is equally effective as imipramine for treating dysthymia; however, 51% of imipramine-treated patients dropped out of a recent study because of adverse side effects compared with only 25% of the sertraline-treated patients (Friedman & Kocsis, 1996; Jessen, 1996; Kocsis et al, 1994; Kuzel, 1996). In double-blind trials, paroxetine was about as effective as imipramine in treating major depression. However, like all SSRIs, paroxetine inhibits activity of cytochrome P-450

isoenzymes and thus interacts with other drugs such as phenytoin, digoxin, and warfarin. Begin paroxetine at 20 mg in the morning.

Venlafaxine (Effexor) and fluvoxamine (Luvox) are two additional SSRIs on the market. An extended-release form of venlafaxine is available (Effexor XR) for once-daily dosing. Dosing starts at 75 mg/d; it may be increased up to 225 mg/d by 75 mg/4 d increments. QT interval effects may occur in patients with heart problems.

Fluoxetine, paroxetine, and sertraline are first-line agents for treating postpartum depression. However, for the nursing mother, short- and long-term effects of SSRIs on the infant are not known and these drugs should be prescribed cautiously (Jermain, 1996). A reassuring preliminary study of fluvoxamine, paroxetine, and sertraline in pregnancy from nine medical centers indicates they do not cause birth defects. However, the 267 expectant mother sample was too small to establish safety in pregnancy definitively (Kulin, Pastuszak, & Sage, 1998).

Basically, the SSRIs have comparable efficacy, but subtle patterns of difference have been noted among the various agents. In general, SSRIs tend to be "energizing"; thus, they may be a good choice for patients presenting with lethargy and loss of energy. However, they can cause agitation, restlessness, and insomnia,

## TABLE 33–3. RESOURCES FOR MANAGING MOOD DISORDERS

The National Foundation for Depressive Illness, Inc.
  (NFDI)
P.O. Box 2257
New York, NY 10116-2257
1-800-245-4306

National Alliance for the Mentally Ill (NAMI)
200 N. Glebe Road; Suite 1015
Arlington, VA 22203-3754
Office: 703-524-7600
NAMI Helpline: 1-800-950-6264

National Mental Health Association (NMHA)
NMHA Information Center
1021 Prince Street
Alexandria, VA 23314-2071

AHCPR Clearinghouse
P.O. Box 8547
Silver Spring, MD 20907
1-800-358-9295

"Depression is a Treatable Illness: A Patient's Guide"
  (1993) from AHCPR is an excellent patient/family
  resource that uses the clinical practice guideline for
  treating depression in primary care.

National Depressive and Manic Depressive Association
  (NDMDA)
730 N. Franklin
Chicago, IL 60610
1-800-826-2632      1-800-82NDMDA

The Depressive and Related Affective Disorders
  Association
Johns Hopkins Hospital
600 North Wolfe Street
Baltimore, MD 21205
Internet: WWW site—http://infonet.welch.jhu.edu/
  departments/drada/default

*Adapted from Depression Guideline Panel (1993b).*

particularly if the patient presents with anxiety. Their advantage over TCAs are absence of weight gain, anticholinergic effects, and CV safety. Because SSRIs lack the CV toxicity of the TCAs, they present less danger from drug overdose. Some clinicians have found that SSRIs have better response rates with women, patients who are overweight, and those whose symptoms include overeating, oversleeping, or profound lethargy (Millard, 1994b).

Coadministration with an MAOI is hazardous, and the interaction can produce excitement, rigidity, diaphoresis, and hyperthermia (Jessen, 1996). There should be a 2-week "washout" before starting an MAOI after using an SSRI. A washout period of at least 5 weeks is recommended for fluoxetine because of its very long half-life. SSRIs inhibit cytochrome P-450 and may increase serum levels of benzodiazepines, anticonvulsants, antiarrhythmics, sulfonylureas, and warfarin (Preskorn, 1996).

The use of SSRIs in a pediatric population is not well studied, but clinical trials of these agents in childhood and adolescent depression and obsessive-compulsive disorder are under way at this time. Their relative CV safety and better tolerability augers well for possible future utility in younger populations (Janicak, Davis, Preskorn, & Ayd, 1993).

SSRIs are especially effective in treating elderly patients because they do not contribute to constipation, orthostatic hypotension, and potential cardiotoxicity as do the TCAs. Fluoxetine has a long half-life and would not be first choice for elderly patients because of increased risk of adverse effects. As noted above, the potential for causing drug interactions in the elderly, who take more medications in general, should be assessed.

The most frequently reported SSRI side effects are insomnia, nausea, headache, dizziness, agitation, and assorted sexual dysfunctions. Side effects are usually worse at the beginning of treatment, so if doses are kept low for the first 2–3 weeks, these can be minimized. Titrating dosages gradually can often keep these effects tolerable for the patient. Start with half the normal dose for the first week, especially with elderly patients. Benzodiazepines (eg, clonazepam) may be prescribed along with an SSRI to decrease anxiety and insomnia and can be tapered off as side effects are better tolerated (Friedman & Kocsis, 1996).

***Tricyclic antidepressants.***   Amitriptyline and doxepin have the greatest anticholinergic effects, are very sedating, and may be a good choice when the patient has psychomotor agitation and insomnia with the depression. Begin the medication at 50 mg taken at bedtime to minimize problems with side effects. Protriptyline is the least sedating TCA and is started at 10 mg at bedtime. Desipramine has an "energizing" effect and is a good choice for depression with psychomotor retardation and pronounced fatigue, but it may cause insomnia if taken too late in the day (Rausch & Hyman, 1995). Imipramine is the least costly with moderate sedative and anticholinergic activity.

Antidepressants should be avoided during pregnancy and lactation. If medication is necessary, nortriptyline and desipramine are preferred; however, these patients should be referred for pharmacologic management. Generally, only imipramine and clomipramine are recommended for children over 6 years of age. In children, adolescents, and young adults TCAs may produce tachycardia and mild hypertension ("Drugs for Psychiatric Disorders," 1994). Therefore, a pretreatment EKG in young depressed patients should be performed. Elderly patients and men with prostatic hypertrophy do best with a nonsedating TCA that has relatively mild anticholinergic effects such as nortriptyline or desipramine; these agents cause the least amount of postural hypotension. Overall, TCA use in elderly patients is limited because of anticholinergic, antihistaminic, antiandrenergic, and cardiac conduction side effects (Zisook, 1996).

TCAs may produce lethal cardiovascular toxicity if overdosed because of the quinidine-like effect of these agents that causes prolonged interventricular cardiac conduction complicated by severe anticholinergic and alpha-adrenergic blocking effects. *Because a TCA overdose may be lethal, no more than 1 week's supply (1 g) should be prescribed at a time to a depressed patient who could potentially use the drug to carry out a suicide plan.*

The most common side effects of TCAs are anticholinergic effects, orthostatic hypotension, sedation, sexual dysfunction, and weight gain. TCAs are contraindicated in patients with prostatic hypertrophy, narrow-angle glaucoma, and certain cardiac arrhythmias.

***Other antidepressants.*** Bupropion has a relatively short half-life and should be dosed three times a day. The minimally effective dose is from 225–300 mg/day. Begin with 100 mg b.i.d. and increase to 100 mg t.i.d. after 3 days. Early experience with bupropion revealed a somewhat greater potential for causing drug-induced seizures, especially in patients who have an existing seizure disorder or who are prone to experience seizures (eg, patients ingesting alcohol or benzodiazepines on a chronic basis, patients with recent head injury, and patients with other

neurological disorders). Bupropion should not be prescribed for patients with eating disorders because of a high seizure incidence at higher doses in that patient population. Drug-induced seizures from bupropion are dose-related as well as correlated with high peak plasma level concentrations achieved soon after a dose is administered. Therefore, no more than 150 mg should be taken at one time. Warn patients not to "double-up" for missed doses of bupropion but continue taking individual doses as prescribed. A sustained-release preparation has recently obtained FDA approval and now circumvents many of the dosing peculiarities of the agent. Bupropion probably should be avoided in depressed patients with psychotic features or in individuals with schizophrenia-like disorders because the dopaminergic effects of the agent may give rise to an increase in psychotic symptomatology (Akiskal et al, 1994).

Trazodone's sedative effects are prominent, and many patients cannot tolerate the doses of 200–400 mg/day needed for its antidepressant effect. For this reason, it now is primarily used as a hypnotic agent for insomnia in doses of 50–75 mg at bedtime. This sedative feature of trazodone has led to its concurrent use with other, more activating antidepressants, such as SSRIs, desipramine, and bupropion. Priapism (sustained, painful erection in males sometimes requiring surgical detumescence and resulting in permanent impotency) is a rare adverse effect of trazodone that occurs in approximately 1 in 6000 males treated with the drug (Wells et al, 1997). Men receiving trazodone should be counseled to stop the drug immediately if changes in erectile function are noticed and notify their clinician. Given its rarity, priaprism is not a reason to avoid its use in males. However, patient education is necessary.

Nefazodone's sedative effects, although not as prominent as those seen with trazodone, are useful in depressed patients who also have symptoms of anxiety. Begin with 100 mg b.i.d. and increase in increments of 100 mg/day each week up to the recommended dose. In older individuals, nefazodone's starting dose is 50 mg b.i.d. Progressive increases in dosage up to an average of approximately 300–400 mg/day are recommended for younger patients. Some patients will have difficulty tolerating its sedative and orthostatic effects and will complain of sleepiness, lightheadedness, and/or dizziness. The side effects of the agent can often be made more tolerable by gradual dose increases.

Priapism seems not to be a problem in men taking nefazodone, and sleep studies of nocturnal penile tumescence in normal volunteers serving as their control taking trazodone, nefazodone, or placebo at spaced time periods showed significant differences for trazodone compared to placebo, but no difference from placebo compared to nefazodone (Ware, Rose, & McBrayer, 1994).

Nefazodone is metabolized by the cytochrome P-450 isoenzyme system and inhibits the metabolism of other drugs. Therefore, nefazodone is contraindicated in patients taking the nonsedating antihistamines terfenadine and estimazole. Additionally, patients taking alprazolam or triazolam should have the dose of these benzodiazepines (BZDs) reduced by 50% if nefazodone is coadministered.

Venlafaxine has a short half-life and should be dosed twice daily. A starting dose of 25 mg b.i.d. or t.i.d. is recommended although some patients may experience early-onset side effects. Initial nausea and vomiting occasionally can be problematic, and slower introduction of the drug is necessary. It is better tolerated when the dose is gradually increased. Venlafaxine also can cause increased diastolic blood pressure, and blood pressure should be monitored, especially in hypertensive patients. It does not cause significant hypotension or sedation. Although venlafaxine is metabolized by the cytochrome P-450 enzyme system, it has a low potential for drug interactions and may be preferred in depressed patients taking multiple medications for other medical conditions that are metabolized by the liver (Holdcroft, 1994; Wells et al, 1997).

Mirtazapine's most common side effects are dry mouth, somnolence, asthenia, and constipation. Because of its relatively sedative pharmacology, it may be preferentially used in depressed patients with significant anxiety and/or insomnia. The recommended starting dose for mirtazapine is 15 mg at bedtime. After a few days, patients can be moved up to 30 mg/day. Some patients may require the maximal approved dose of 45 mg/day. Hepatic impairment of mild to moderate severity may cause up to a 33% decrease in hepatic clearance of mirtazapine and downward dosage adjustment is probably necessary if the patient has liver disease (Kehoe & Schorr, 1996).

MAOIs are usually prescribed by a psychiatrist; however, the primary care provider may monitor the treatment regimen. Common adverse effects include tachycardia, sedation,

insomnia, agitation, and sexual dysfunction (Jessen, 1996). MAOIs should not be administered with a TCA because of the potential for sudden, intense CNS and atropine-like effects.

If switching between SSRIs and MAOIs, allow a "washout" period because of the potential for serious interaction. When changing from a TCA to an MAOI, allow a drug-free interval of 1 week. When moving from fluoxetine to an MAOI, a drug-free interval of 5 weeks is recommended; when changing from sertraline or paroxetine, a 2-week interval is sufficient. When switching from an MAOI to an SSRI, a 2-week interval is recommended.

MAOIs are not recommended for patients under 16 years of age and contraindicated for patients over 60 years of age (Schlafer, 1993). The prevalence of CV disease in the elderly significantly increases the risk associated with MAOI therapy in this group of patients. Excessive hypotension from MAOI overdose and severe hypertension from drug or food interactions increase the risk with the elderly.

## Monitoring for Efficacy

Measuring treatment outcomes includes evaluation of target symptom relief and restoration of function. Symptom evaluation may be done through the clinical interview alone or in combination with a symptom-rating scale completed by the patient, such as the General Health Questionnaire (GHQ), Beck Depression Inventory (BDI), or Zung Self-Rating Depression Scale (ZSRDS). A rating scale allows both practitioner and patient to assess treatment response, determine if medication dosage should be adjusted, and clarify if and when alternative treatments are needed (DGP, 1993b).

Monitor drug response and provide clinical management every 1–2 weeks. Patients with more severe symptoms should be seen weekly for the first 6–8 weeks of the acute phase of treatment. Weekly psychotherapy sessions are useful. The clinician should be available by phone particularly during this phase of treatment. During the continuation phase of treatment, monitor for symptom resolution at least every 4 weeks. The goal here is to prevent relapse; this phase lasts about 9–12 months. During the maintenance phase, the goal of treatment is to prevent recurrence. If depression responds to treatment, some sources recommend continuing the drug for at least 6 months and always tapering off over a 4-week period. Should symptoms recur, return the dose to its prior level and maintain for another 3–6 months (DGP, 1993b).

If treatment results in little or no symptom relief by 6 weeks or only partial relief by 12 weeks, reassess the diagnosis and treatment plan. Substance abuse or underlying medical or psychiatric conditions may become apparent. Monitor adherence, check blood levels, raise the dose, or change the medication. Medication underdosing is a common cause of poor treatment response. Refractory depression that is not responsive to first-line treatment probably requires referral. Monitor for symptom resolution at least every 4 weeks during this phase.

A specific length of time for a monotherapy drug trial has not been established, but some response should be noted after 3–4 weeks and the patient should have substantial symptom relief after 6–8 weeks of treatment. If there is little or no response to antidepressant therapy after 4 weeks at the full recommended dose, the drug trial should be considered a failure. If the patient has not responded at all or has only minimal symptomatic response to the medication, two steps are recommended: (1) reassess the adequacy of the diagnosis and (2) reassess the adequacy of treatment (DGP, 1993b). The main reasons for failed drug therapy are inadequate dosing and insufficient length of treatment (Hales et al, 1994). Consider checking drug blood levels (generally available only for TCAs) and assess for adherence.

In general, monotherapy is preferred over a combination of drugs. Thus, switching medications is usually preferred over augmentation as an initial strategy. If the decision is to discontinue a medication, TCAs need to be tapered off over 2–4 weeks because patients may undergo gastrointestinal side effects caused by cholinergic rebound; MAOIs, bupropion, trazodone, nefazodone, venlafaxine, and mirtazapine do not require tapering. The shorter-acting SSRIs paroxetine and sertraline should be tapered off, whereas the longer-acting fluoxetine warrants no gradual reduction. After weaning off the medication, monitor the patient for 6–12 months for recurrence of symptoms. Inadequate treatment responses make chronic depression more likely and subsequent treatment more difficult (Millard, 1994b).

## Monitoring for Toxicity

Obtain a chemistry panel for liver and renal function when clinically indicated. Drug treatment regimens for patients with hepatic or renal impairment should be initiated by a psychiatrist or mental health specialist and managed collaboratively with the primary care provider.

SSRI toxicity may produce seizures, nausea, vomiting, excessive agitation, and restlessness. All SSRIs currently in use have been implicated in adverse drug interactions involving cytochrome P-450 enzymes. Most of these relate to elevated plasma levels of TCAs; fluoxetine is the most frequent offender. For this reason, SSRIs and TCAs should probably not be given concurrently unless the clinician is prepared to carefully monitor TCA plasma levels. Collaborative management with a psychiatrist or mental health specialist would be prudent. Fluoxetine has a longer half-life than other SSRIs and after withdrawing the drug, any TCA should be introduced at low dose (10–25 mg) and increased very slowly according to patient tolerance. Cimetidine and ketoconazole are strong cytochrome P-450 enzyme inhibitors and may interact with psychotropic drugs. Ranitidine could be substituted for cimetidine and fluconazole for ketoconazole because they are less likely to interact with psychotropic agents. Likewise, the antihistamines astemizole and terfenadine should not be taken with SSRIs (El-Mallakh, Wright, Breen, & Lippann, 1996; Taylor & Lader, 1996).

Serotonin syndrome (SS) is an occasionally fatal disorder characterized by symptoms such as mental status changes, seizures, myoclonus, and blood dyscrasias. Using OTC sympathomimetics, such as cold remedies or diet pills, can precipitate SS in patients taking SSRIs. For mild cases of SS, an oral benzodiazepine may be sufficient; however, a plan for emergency treatment should be in place if symptoms continue. Referral to a psychiatrist or mental health specialist for management is recommended (Brown, Skop, & Mareth, 1996).

TCAs can cause cardiac arrhythmias in toxic doses, and in patients with conduction disorders (bundle-branch disease), pose a serious risk for heart block even in normal therapeutic concentrations. Side effects include anticholinergic phenomena (dry mouth, constipation, blurred vision) and alpha blocking effects (sedation, orthostatic hypotension). They may lower the seizure threshold and can induce arrhythmias by increasing the heart rate and slowing cardiac conduction. High doses may produce severe postural hypotension, dizziness, tachycardia, palpitations, arrhythmias, and seizures. Amoxapine has caused extrapyramidal side effects.

Plasma TCA levels >1000 ng/mL indicate a major overdose and will generally cause EKG abnormalities; a prolonged corrected Q-T interval (Q-T$_c$) over 0.44 ms should cause concern. However, any elevated plasma level in conjunction with signs of toxicity should be regarded as potentially lethal. Nortriptyline has the most clearly defined therapeutic window for clinical response (50–150 ng/mL). Life-threatening CV symptoms include tachycardia and impaired conduction leading to AV block. At toxic levels, the EKG shows a prolonged QRS interval (Miller & Keitner, 1996).

Among the newer antidepressants, bupropion increases the risk of seizures in patients with bulimia or anorexia and in all patients at doses exceeding 450 mg/day or 150 mg/dose. Venlafaxine may increase diastolic blood pressure when used in high doses.

Mixed and indirect-acting sympathomimetics interact with MAOIs to produce a serious and potentially life-threatening hypertensive crisis. These sympathomimetics cause epinephrine to be abruptly released, which results in increased blood pressure. Patients need to be warned that many OTC preparations, particularly those for colds and weight loss (eg, pseudoephedrine and phenylpropanolamine), can interact with the MAOI, producing a serious hypertensive crisis. Taking meperidine or dextromethorphan with an MAOI may lead to delirium, hyperpyrexia, convulsions, coma, and even death. A low-tyramine diet also is required to avoid potential interactions. Refer again to Table 33–2. A hypertensive crisis presents with occipital headache, nausea, palpitations, tachycardia/bradycardia, and chest pain. Patients experiencing these symptoms should understand that this is an emergency situation and seek treatment promptly (Golwyn & Sevlie, 1993; Wells et al, 1997).

## Follow-up Recommendations

Support, reassurance, and hope are essential to effective management and follow-up care for depression in primary care settings. Collaborative decision making with the patient, family, and clinician generally improves adherence to treatment and provides better outcomes.

Establishing a working relationship with a psychiatrist and other mental health specialists can be helpful for patient consultation or referral. Prompt consultation or referral is needed in the following situations: uncertain diagnosis; severe, recurrent episodes; coexisting complex medical problems; poor adherence; partial response to initial treatment; suicidal ideation; need for hospitalization; or at the patient's request (DGP, 1993b; Millard, 1994b).

## BIPOLAR DISORDER

Bipolar disorder is formally known as manic-depressive illness. DSM-IV (APA, 1994a) classifies bipolar disorders into three types:

1. *Bipolar I* (manic-depressive) is characterized by the occurrence of at least one manic episode and at least one major depressive episode.
2. *Bipolar II* is characterized by the occurrence of at least one major depressive episode accompanied by at least one hypomanic episode.
3. *Cyclothymia* is characterized by chronic, fluctuating mood disturbances of both hypomania and depression that do not meet criteria for a manic or major depressive episode.

Bipolar disorder, affecting approximately 1% of the adult population or about 3 million persons in the United States, is chronic, with recurrent symptoms and relapses over the course of a lifetime and causes substantial psychosocial morbidity. Onset of the disorder usually begins in early adulthood (20–29 years of age) when the patient exhibits periods of abnormal mood swings that can be euphoric, depressed, or a combination of both. Although rare in preadolescent children, the second most common age range of onset is 15–19 years. It presents as silly, excited, hyperactive, irritable, withdrawn, angry, paranoid, or explosive behavior with mood lability among adolescent patient populations. Bipolar disorder differs from unipolar disorders in several ways: it occurs more commonly in families, presents with a more acute onset, and patients have more episodes over a lifetime than patients with unipolar depressive disorders (APA, 1994b).

Patients with bipolar disorder present with target symptoms that include: (1) mood disturbances (irritable, expansive, euphoric, manipulative, labile with depression), (2) hyperactivity (sleep disturbances, rapid speech, flight of ideas, distractibility), (3) delusional symptoms (sexual, persecutory, religious, grandiose, threatening), and (4) schizophreniform reactions (tangential associations, ideas of reference, catatonia, hallucinations). These symptoms are present almost daily for more than 1 week. The target symptoms are important for monitoring effects of drug therapy during the course of treatment (Weber, Saklad, & Kastenholz, 1992).

DSM-IV (APA, 1994a) describes a *manic episode* as a distinct period of abnormally and persistently elevated, expansive, or irritable mood that lasts at least a week. Mania is characterized in three stages: the initial stage is characterized by increased psychomotor activity and overconfidence; the intermediate stage is evidenced by greater psychomotor activity and delusional thoughts; and the final stage is evidenced by frenzied psychomotor activity, hallucinations, and disorientation. Not all patients progress from one stage to another, and often, the time between stages is short and difficult to recognize.

Patients may present with a mixed episode of bipolar disorder in which symptoms of both mania and depression occur almost daily for at least a week. Other patients may switch from a manic to a depressive mood quickly. This "rapid cycling" occurs four or more times a year and is difficult to distinguish from a mixed episode (Weber et al, 1992).

## SPECIFIC CONSIDERATIONS FOR PHARMACOTHERAPY

### When Drug Therapy Is Needed

Although major depression is frequently treated by primary care providers, bipolar disorder generally requires psychiatric referral for initial management of a manic episode. However, the treatment regimen may be monitored over time by the primary care provider. It is clinically important to distinguish between bipolar and unipolar mood disorders when selecting pharmacotherapeutic agents because antidepressants may precipitate mania in patients with bipolar disorder. Also, mania can be drug-induced from stimulants or adrenergic drugs, such as amphetamines, cocaine, levodopa, ephedrine, tricyclic antidepressants, and monoamine oxidase inhibitors, as well as by high doses of corticosteroids (Rausch & Hyman, 1995; Winokur, Coryell, Endicott, & Akiskal, 1994).

Treatment for bipolar disorder has three phases: (1) the acute phase involves treatment of the manic episode to afford the patient behavioral control; (2) the continuation phase further stabilizes the patient over time; and (3) the

maintenance phase has the goal of preventing recurrence. Primary care clinicians will generally be concerned with management of the continuation and maintenance phases of treatment (APA, 1994b). An algorithm for drug treatment of mania is presented in Fig. 33–2.

Bipolar disorder is a complex mood disorder because it appears to have multiple determinants and the clinical presentation differs significantly among individual patients. Several theories have been proposed to explain the underlying pathophysiology of the disorder and suggest the mechanism of various therapies. Some of these current theories are shown in Table 33–4.

### Short- and Long-Term Goals of Pharmacotherapy

Treatment goals are to decrease the frequency, severity, and psychosocial consequences of recurring episodes and to improve functioning between episodes. Initial treatment of a manic episode focuses on prompt symptom relief and behavioral control. Long-term goals focus on preventing recurrence of either manic or depressive episodes. Most patients remain on a mood stabilizer indefinitely (APA, 1994b).

### Nonpharmacologic Treatment

Psychotherapy can help patients learn how to manage their depression, fatigue, or obsessive ruminations and structure their daily activities to reduce mood lability during maintenance treatment. Psychotherapeutic modalities are most useful after mood episodes are stabilized. To reduce the incidence of relapse, patients can diminish psychosocial stress by carefully monitoring their sleep/wake/activity patterns. Family therapy is particularly useful for women, and all patients benefit from supportive therapy, which focuses on management and resolution of life difficulties using the patient's strengths and resources. It can significantly reduce nonadherence to medication regimens so prevalent among bipolar patients. Support groups are a beneficial and cost-effective strategy to decrease denial, increase adherence to pharmacologic treatment, and reduce the need for hospitalizations. Some self-help and advocacy groups are organized under the National Depressive and Manic-Depressive Association. Referral to a psychologist or mental health professional is necessary for specialized interventions.

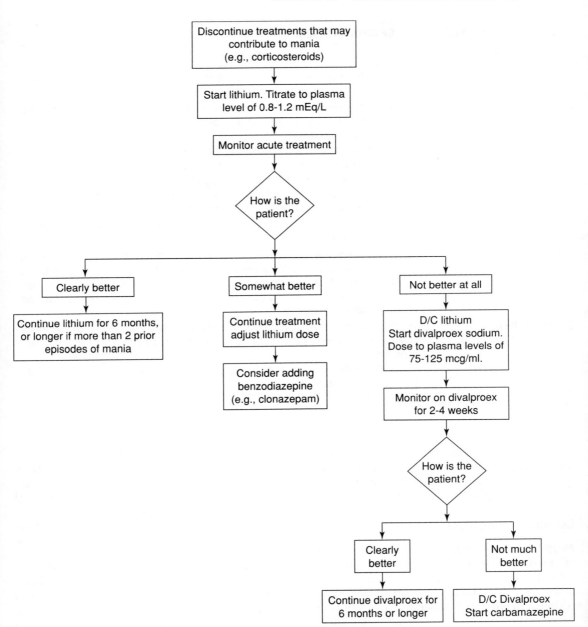

**Figure 33–2.** Algorithm for the treatment of mania.

Hospitalization may be necessary during the acute phase of a manic episode to control symptoms. Electroconvulsive therapy may be useful in severe mania or depression that does not respond to drug therapy. Patients are usually hospitalized and referral to a psychiatrist is required (APA, 1994b; Kahn, 1995).

## Time Frame for Initiating Pharmacotherapy

The key to managing bipolar illness is not aborting an acute episode but preventing recurrent manic and depressive episodes over time and diminishing the severity of those that do occur. However, treatment needs to be instituted

## TABLE 33–4. THEORETICAL BASIS OF BIPOLAR DISORDER

| Theory | Pathophysiology |
|---|---|
| Genetic | There is a high genetic risk for first-degree biological relatives of individuals with bipolar I disorder. Current research is focusing on chromosomal abnormalities. |
| Neurotransmitter | 1. There is a functional deficit of monoamine neurotransmitters (norepinephrine, serotonin) in the CNS, producing mood disorders. An excess results in mania, and a deficit results in depression. |
| | 2. Dysregulation between neurotransmitter systems (norepinephrine, serotonin) produces a cyclical disturbance in mood rhythms. Excessive catecholamine activity may contribute to manic episodes; deficits in dopamine may contribute to the disorder. |
| | 3. Deficiency of gamma-aminobutyric acid, a major inhibitory CNS neurotransmitter, causes excessive stimulation that produces mania. |
| Sensitization | Initial psychosocial or physical stressors trigger a bipolar episode, but later episodes occur spontaneously due to increased sensitization and kindling of the CNS. |
| Electrolyte | Alterations in electrolyte balance may cause the mood fluctuations of bipolar disorder. Calcium affects the excitability of neuronal firing and may account for bipolar mood vacillations. High levels of calcium have been found in the blood and cerebrospinal fluid of depressed patients; low calcium levels were found in the cerebrospinal fluid of manic patients. |
| Environmental or Circadian Rhythm | Environmental, psychosocial, and physical stressors may be factors that trigger mood changes in susceptible persons. Circadian or seasonal rhythms may cause diurnal variations in mood, sleep disturbances, and seasonal recurrences of bipolar episodes. Depression appears to be most prevalent during spring and mania most prevalent during summer. |

*Adapted from Fankhauser and Benefield (1997).*

promptly after diagnosis to relieve symptoms and manage manic behavior. A more rapid response can be obtained when drug treatment is begun in the early stage of mania (APA, 1994b).

## Overview of Drug Classes for Treatment

***Mood-stabilizing agents.*** These drugs are used in all phases of treatment of bipolar disorder. Lithium is the drug of choice for mania, but other agents (valproate, carbamazepine) have proven effective in managing manic episodes. Lithium, first reported to have antimanic effects in 1949, has been used for acute and preventive treatment of bipolar disorder in the United States since the mid-1960s. Lithium salts are chemically similar to sodium and alter reuptake of norepinephrine, serotonin, and dopamine. Lithium controls depressive as well as manic symptoms and is the initial drug of choice for treating bipolar disorder. It is an agent with a narrow therapeutic range, and patients frequently become toxic on the drug. Although lithium therapy is very useful, 40% of patients may fail to respond (Janicak et al, 1993).

***Anticonvulsants.*** Carbamazepine and valproate are anticonvulsant medications that have been used successfully as mood stabilizers for treatment of bipolar disorder. These agents are used primarily for treating acute mania in patients who respond poorly or are unable to tolerate lithium. Carbamazepine appears to increase norepinephrine and dopamine and enhance action of gamma-aminobutyric acid (GABA). It initially held much promise in controlling bipolar disorders; however, further study has shown it not to be as useful as lithium for many patients. Carbamazepine is a potent enzyme inducer of other drugs and also induces its own metabolism, making it difficult to regulate a therapeutic dosage. The agent does have some utility in rapid-cycling patients.

Although carbamazepine has a longer history of research as an antimanic drug, most experts prefer to use valproate (available as valproic acid or divalproex sodium), either in conjunction with or as a substitute for lithium (Bowden, Brugger, & Swain, 1994). The symptoms of mania and hypomania best treated by valproate are those of the "primary manic syndrome": increased activity, expansive mood, and decreased sleep. The agent appears to increase the action of GABA, which inhibits neurotransmitter stimulation. Valproate may be useful as a fourth-line antimanic agent (APA, 1994b; Bowden et al, 1994).

**Other agents.** Calcium channel blockers (CCBs) such as verapamil have been used to treat acute mania as an adjunct to neuroleptics and lithium or as a single agent. However, preliminary studies have not shown clearly positive results. Verapamil has a more acceptable side-effect profile than other agents, and it is useful for patients who are unable to tolerate other mood stabilizers (Dubovsky, 1995).

Antipsychotics and benzodiazepines (BZDs) are often required to augment treatment of an acute manic episode. These agents have a more rapid onset than lithium and allow faster symptom control. Clozapine and risperidone have been used with mood stabilizers because they cause less extrapyramidal side effects. When mania is controlled, these agents are gradually discontinued. Patients treated with antipsychotics require hospitalization. The BZDs (eg, clonazepam, lorazepam) are an alternative to antipsychotics and have minimal adverse effects with rapid sedation. BZDs are gradually tapered and discontinued when the manic episode is under control with the mood stabilizer (Fankhauser & Benefield, 1997).

Antidepressants (eg, MAOIs, bupropion) are often combined with a mood stabilizer during an acute depressive episode. MAOIs and bupropion are preferred agents; TCAs seem to initiate mania that is difficult to control. All antidepressants can precipitate a manic episode in patients with underlying bipolar disorder if they are not receiving a mood stabilizer (APA, 1994b; Kahn, 1995). Please see Chap. 29 for information on anticonvulsants (valproic acid and carbamazepine) in the treatment of epilepsy.

## Assessment and History Taking

A careful history and physical examination are essential to identify bipolar disorder. A positive family history of mood disorder is an important risk factor. The best predictor of mania is having a first-degree relative with bipolar I disorder. Talk with the family if possible because bipolar patients are usually unreliable reporters. Assess current medications and discontinue any precipitating drug such as a TCA, an MAOI, amphetamine, anticholinergic, antihypertensive, cocaine,

ephedrine, glucocorticosteroid, hallucinogen, or levodopa. Consider exposure to illegal drugs such as cocaine, amphetamines, or hallucinogens particularly in younger patients. More than 60% of patients with a history of mania also have a history of substance abuse. Keep in mind that obsessive-compulsive, panic, and eating disorders frequently accompany bipolarity (Gelenberg, Hirschfeld, Jefferson, Potter, & Thase, 1995b).

The baseline laboratory workup prior to starting lithium should include a CBC with differential, serum creatinine and electrolytes, thyroid function studies ($T_3$, $T_4$, TSH), urine specific gravity, and a pregnancy test for women of childbearing age. An EKG is recommended for patients with preexisting cardiac disease and those over age 40. In addition to the baseline workup, liver function studies are needed prior to prescribing carbamazepine or valproate (APA, 1994b).

See Drug Tables 205.6, 308, 309, 311, 312, 313.

## Patient/Caregiver Information

Psychoeducational programs for patients and their families are very important. Group sessions to discuss concerns about bipolar illness and drug treatment can help patients and their families adjust to this chronic condition. Denial and nonadherence are common among bipolar patients, so they need instructions repeated many times and written information is essential. Patients need to know how to recognize signs and symptoms of emerging mania or depression and when to seek prompt treatment. Keeping a diary of target symptoms is a useful way to identify mood changes.

Special instructions for lithium treatment include: (1) take lithium with meals to reduce nausea; (2) take the medication at about the same time each day to maintain serum levels; and (3) drink at least 8 glasses of fluid per day and avoid dehydration. Patients and their families need to know signs of lithium toxicity and to stop the drug at the first hint of sickness: diarrhea, vomiting, or a fever that could lead to dehydration. Have them stop the lithium for at least 24 h after the illness. Remind patients that the frequent use of NSAIDs may increase lithium levels and suggest aspirin or acetaminophen because these agents have minimal effect on serum levels and can be used with lithium. Sulindac is another good choice for an antiinflammatory agent because it does not decrease renal clearance of lithium. Regular use of thiazide diuretics can also increase lithium levels, while xanthines (coffee, theophylline, aminophylline) can decrease lithium levels (Price & Heninger, 1994). Refer to Table 33–3 for patient, family, and health professional resources.

## OUTCOMES MANAGEMENT

### Selecting an Appropriate Agent

The initial treatment plan for an acute manic episode should be determined by a psychiatrist or mental health specialist and usually requires referral and hospitalization. Neuroleptic drugs or BZDs are often required with a mood stabilizer to control the manic behavior until the antimanic agent (lithium, valproic acid, carbamazepine) begins to take effect in 1–2 weeks. Antipsychotics such as haloperidol and fluphenazine combined with lithium may produce neurotoxic syndromes and require careful monitoring. Clozapine and risperidone are less likely to cause extrapyramidal side effects than other antipsychotic agents when combined with lithium. However, use of antipsychotics is usually limited to psychotic patients who are under the care of a psychiatrist.

When bipolar depression occurs during maintenance treatment, add an antidepressant such as bupropion, desipramine, nortriptyline, fluoxetine, sertraline, or phenelzine cautiously and after consultation. Clinical trials regarding their use are limited. Initial reports suggested that bupropion was less likely to induce mania, but further study is needed. Generally, use the lowest effective dose for the shortest length of time (APA, 1994b, Price & Heninger, 1994).

*Mood-stabilizing agents.*    Lithium carbonate is the drug of choice for treatment and prophylaxis of bipolar disorder, but many patients in the manic phase do not respond to lithium or are intolerant of it. The drug is available in the United States as lithium carbonate in regular and extended-release tablets or capsules and lithium citrate in a syrup. The drug is contraindicated in patients with significant renal or CV disease and severe debilitation or dehydration. It should be used cautiously in patients with cardiac disease, decreased sodium intake (eg, low-sodium diets for hypertension) or increased sodium loss, and those on NSAIDs. For an acute manic episode, start lithium at 600 mg three times a day or 900 mg twice a day for the extended-release form.

Side effects of lithium include gastrointestinal distress, weight gain, tremors, polyuria, and fatigue. These symptoms usually can be managed by adjusting the dosages, and they gradually subside in the first few months of treatment; however, up to half of patients discontinue taking maintenance lithium therapy because of persistent unacceptable side effects (APA, 1994b; Fankhauser & Benefield, 1997).

Lithium is teratogenic and contraindicated in pregnancy and breast-feeding. There is no information about its safety for children under 12 years of age. Lithium should be used cautiously with elderly patients; the dosage needs to be reduced to account for decreased renal function, and fluid intake must be carefully monitored to avoid dehydration. Individual drug dosage should be determined by a mental health specialist and monitored collaboratively with the primary care provider.

Valproic acid is a good alternative for patients who do not respond to lithium or cannot tolerate its side effects. It has potent antimanic properties and minimal to moderate antidepressant properties. In controlled trials, valproic acid was found to be as effective as lithium (Bowden et al, 1994; "Drugs for Psychiatric Disorders," 1994). The drug is available in the United States as valproate, divalproex, and valproic acid. Valproate is rapidly converted to valproic acid in the stomach, whereas divalproex is converted more slowly in the small intestine. Valproate has few serious side effects other than a dose-related thrombocytopenia and rise in liver function tests that may require discontinuing the drug. Patients at risk for serious hepatitis are those with preexisting liver disease and those currently receiving enzyme-inducing anticonvulsants. Valproic acid is metabolized by the P-450 system but is not an enzyme inducer.

Nausea, vomiting, and diarrhea are common side effects during early therapy, but usually resolve and rarely require discontinuation of the drug. It has a short half-life and requires multiple daily dosing. For an acute manic episode start valproic acid at 250 mg three times a day. It is contraindicated in patients with hepatic disease or abnormal liver studies. Divalproex is a form of valproate that is better tolerated and causes fewer gastrointestinal side effects (Potter & Ketter, 1993).

Carbamazepine, a TCA compound similar to imipramine, is the most well-documented alternative to lithium and is used for patients who do not respond adequately to lithium and neuroleptics. It can be added to antidepressants, neuroleptics, or lithium in partial responders, but has been effective as a single agent. Unlike the TCAs, carbamazepine produces a better antidepressant response in patients with bipolar disorder than in those with unipolar depression. Carbamazepine appears to be effective in controlling both manic and depressive episodes.

For an acute manic episode, start at 100 mg twice a day and increase by 200 mg every 3 to 5 days up to 1200 mg/day four times a day. Give medication with meals to minimize gastrointestinal upset. Side effects include drowsiness, dizziness, unsteadiness, nausea, and diplopia. It is contraindicated in patients with a history of bone marrow depression or abnormal blood studies (Fankhauser & Benefield, 1997).

***Other agents.*** The calcium channel blocker verapamil, has been used to treat acute mania as an adjunct to neuroleptics and lithium or as a single agent. In some reported cases, the neuroleptic was discontinued and the patient successfully maintained on verapamil, which has a more acceptable side-effect profile (Dubovsky, 1995).

If the patient presents with a depressive episode, remember that all antidepressants have the potential to precipitate a manic episode in susceptible patients and may increase the risk of rapid cycling in bipolar patients. This risk is reduced if the patient is already taking a mood stabilizer such as lithium. Bupropion or an SSRI (paroxetine or sertraline) may be a better choice than a TCA if an antidepressant is added to the lithium. If the patient is already taking lithium prophylaxis and becomes manic, raise the dosage to prior therapeutic treatment levels in collaboration with the mental health specialist.

## Monitoring for Efficacy

For manic episodes, a BZD or antipsychotic agent may be required initially for prompt symptom relief and behavior control. Mania symptoms begin to resolve in 1–2 weeks after beginning lithium. Changes in the target symptoms (abnormal mood, hyperactivity, delusions, and schizophreniform reactions) are used to monitor response to drug therapy. Generally, the acute phase of mania is managed by a psychiatrist or mental health specialist; once control is achieved, the primary clinician can monitor mental status every 2 weeks, then once a month, then 2–4 times per year. Lithium levels take 4–5 days to stabilize after adjusting the dosage, so there is no need to monitor levels more fre-

quently. Serum levels should be drawn 12 h following the last dose of lithium.

Patients who respond only partially to lithium may benefit from adding either divalproex or carbamazepine to the treatment regimen. Unlike unipolar depression, antidepressants for bipolar depressive episodes are usually discontinued 1–2 months after symptoms are relieved (Gelenberg et al, 1995b).

## Monitoring for Toxicity

Lithium has a narrow therapeutic window, making it difficult to use; serum levels are necessary. Severe lithium toxicity can result in permanent neurologic damage or even death. Draw blood for drug levels as close as possible to 12 h after the last lithium dose. It is important to standardize timing to correctly interpret lab values. Monitoring serum lithium level assesses for toxicity and adherence to drug therapy. Lithium toxicity is manifested as follows: mild toxicity (serum level 1.0–1.5 mEq/L)—impaired concentration, lethargy, irritability, weakness, tremor, and nausea; moderate toxicity (serum level 1.6–2.5 mEq/L)—disorientation, confusion, drowsiness, restlessness, coarse tremor, muscle fasciculations, and vomiting; and severe toxicity (serum level >2.5 mEq/L)—impaired consciousness, delirium, extrapyramidal symptoms, convulsions, and coma.

During maintenance therapy with lithium, schedule weekly appointments until the patient is stable and then monthly for at least a year. Measure drug levels at each visit (draw blood sample 12 h after last dose). Check serum creatinine once or twice a year to assess renal function. If creatinine levels rise, consider a switch from lithium to divalproex or carbamazepine. This medication change should be done in collaboration with the mental health specialist. Monitor the patient more frequently to determine the response to any medication change. Some clinicians recommend assessing thyroid function periodically either by clinical findings or TSH assay because lithium can induce hypothyroidism and a nontoxic goiter. If hypothyroidism occurs and lithium is necessary, a thyroid supplement can be used (APA, 1994b; Gerchufsky, 1996).

Polyuria is a commonly reported side effect in maintenance therapy, and the patient should be encouraged to drink 8–12 glasses of fluids, preferably fruit juices containing electrolytes to avoid dehydration and possible lithium toxicity.

If lithium carbonate causes persistent GI distress, consider switching to lithium citrate syrup. Assess for possible dehydration because this can cause the body to conserve water, sodium, and lithium and increase the risk of toxicity.

Evidence suggests that most patients on maintenance therapy do not exhibit withdrawal or rebound symptoms if the drug is discontinued abruptly. Nevertheless, some clinicians prefer to gradually taper off lithium if it is to be stopped. Although there are conflicting reports about irreversible renal damage due to long-term lithium therapy, there is clear benefit from the medication for patients who have a significant number of manic episodes. Although nephrosis has been rarely reported, the most significant renal effect induced by lithium is a disability of urine concentration. Urine specific gravity should be monitored annually.

Valproic acid may produce profound CNS depression and possible coma. Hepatic dysfunction is most likely to occur during the first 6 months of therapy. Liver function studies are essential before beginning treatment with valproic acid, followed by once-monthly liver panels for 3 months and less frequent panels thereafter. Early signs of carbamazepine toxicity are neuromuscular disturbances, such as double vision, muscular restlessness, twitching, and involuntary movements. Large overdoses may cause coma or convulsions. Monitor liver enzymes for potential toxicity every 3 months after stabilization during the continuation phase of treatment. Another frequent toxicity of carbamazepine is neutropenia. Although usually transient, occasionally patients may experience a severe neutropenia. A CBC with differentials should be monitored routinely (once every 2 weeks initially, then once a month, and then 3–4 times per year). If decreases in granulocyte counts are seen, patients should be followed more carefully. In general, the discontinuation of carbamazepine is not necessary unless the absolute granulocyte count approaches 1000 or below (Joffie, 1993).

The concentration of calcium channel blockers can be increased if taken with grapefruit juice. The patient should be urged to take this medication with another fluid (Graedon & Graedon, 1995).

## Follow-up Recommendations

Encourage patients to establish a regular schedule for sleeping, eating, exercising, and socializing, which promotes maintenance of stable moods. During follow-up visits, nurture the therapeutic alliance with the patient and family, monitor the patient's mood and behavior, continue patient and family education, and promote adherence to the maintenance regimen.

Compliance is a major issue for patients with bipolar disorder. It is not unusual to hear patients complain that they feel less creative and productive when taking a mood stabilizer. To some extent, bipolar patients may enjoy their "high" episodes when they can perform at a more creative level. Whenever possible, the family should be involved in the patient's monitoring of the disorder. Often, patients themselves will not notice the onset of manic symptoms—such as increased talkativeness, "telephonitis," poor judgment in spending money, or increases in sexual activity—until these behaviors have taken their toll. Family members, once educated about the signs and symptoms of the disorder, can help control evolving decompensation, aid in early medical intervention, and prevent the need for hospitalization.

## ANXIETY DISORDERS

Although everyone experiences feelings of apprehension and uneasiness when facing a stressful situation, the fears of individuals with an anxiety disorder are abnormally intense and irrational and significantly interfere with their lives (APA, 1994a). Anxiety disorders are frequently encountered in primary care settings with an estimated lifetime prevalence rate of 24.9% of the U.S. population (Kessler et al, 1994). Characteristically a disorder of young adults, they affect women twice as often as men. As a complicating factor, 30–50% of patients with anxiety disorders are also clinically depressed. Substance abuse is frequently a complication of anxiety disorders because of patients' attempts at self-medication. Patients with untreated anxiety disorders are high utilizers of health care facilities for nonpsychiatric reasons and often have extensive workups for possible medical conditions (Kirkwood & Hayes, 1997).

Anxiety is a distressing experience manifested in one's affective, cognitive, behavioral, and somatic domains. The affective component is characterized by fear and feelings of dread and terror that are cognitively countered with attempts to make sense of the distress. Various behaviors reflect the anxiety state or evolve into avoidance behavior in response to the stress. Somatic complaints resulting primarily from autonomic nervous system hyperactivity include systemic, cardiopulmonary, gastrointestinal, urinary, and neurologic symptoms (Rausch & Rosenbaum, 1995). Generalized anxiety disorder, panic disorder, social phobia, obsessive-compulsive disorder, and post-traumatic stress disorder are the most common forms of anxiety seen in primary care settings.

*Generalized anxiety disorder* (GAD) is characterized by uncontrollable, chronic worry accompanied by insomnia, irritability, trembling, muscle tension, clammy hands, dry mouth, and palpitations. Unrealistic and excessive worry over physical conditions or circumstances persist for at least 6 months. The disorder is manifested in children by concern about their performance at school or in sporting events. GAD exhibits a chronic, prolonged course with a lifetime prevalence of 5% (APA, 1994a). It is often associated with drug and alcohol abuse, either as the underlying cause or as the patient's attempt to self-medicate the uncomfortable feelings. GAD includes both psychological (worry, tension), and somatic (tachycardia, palpitations, tremor, gastrointestinal upset) symptoms (Amsterdam, Carter, Holloway, & Schwenk, 1994).

*Panic disorder* is a series of discrete periods of intense fear or terror that are accompanied by somatic or cognitive symptoms lasting less than 30 min. The attacks have a sudden onset, build to a peak rapidly, and are often accompanied by a sense of imminent danger or impending doom accompanied by an urge to escape. The lifetime prevalence of the disorder is 3.5% (APA, 1994a). Onset usually occurs during adolescence or young adulthood. The patient experiences extreme apprehension, fear, terror, fear of death, and a desire to flee. Anticipatory anxiety and phobias usually follow one or more panic attacks. Agoraphobia (fear of being in places or situations from which escape might be difficult or embarrassing) often develops secondarily to the panic attacks. Patients begin to avoid situations that may precipitate panic attacks, which leads to restricted social interaction and occupational impairment (Turner, 1995).

*Social phobia* is characterized by extreme, persistent fear of social or performance situations. *Performance anxiety* is a discrete social phobia that can impair one's occupational or academic accomplishments. These individuals fear scrutiny, doing something embarrassing, or receiving a negative evaluation. Social phobia in children presents with crying, tantrums, clinging to familiar persons, and inhibited social interaction to the point of mutism. Young children may appear excessively timid in unfamiliar social situations, refuse to participate in group plans, and typically remain on the periphery of social activities. These children fail to achieve an expected level of functioning. When the onset is in adolescence, there may be a decline in social and academic achievement. Social phobia is a chronic and disabling condition with significant psychosocial, occupational, or academic morbidity. The lifetime prevalence rate of the disorder is 13% (APA, 1994a; Roy-Byrne, Wingerson, Cowley, & Dager, 1993).

*Obsessive-compulsive disorder* (OCD) is characterized by recurrent obsessions that cause marked anxiety and/or compulsions to neutralize the anxiety. Thoughts and images occur repeatedly, causing increased anxiety, which, in turn, fosters compulsive ritualistic behavior. The obsessions and compulsions are time-consuming and significantly interfere with the patient's normal daily activities. OCD has a lifetime prevalence of 2.5% for adults and 1% for children (APA, 1994a). Obsessional themes usually focus on contamination by germs, toxic materials, or dirt; orderliness; sexual thoughts and impulses; religion; doubts; and aggressive thoughts of harming self or others. Patients with OCD are aware that their thoughts and behaviors are aberrant, but are powerless to respond rationally. The mean age of onset is 17–20 years of age. In children, OCD presents with symptoms similar to those in adults. These children experience a gradual decline in their school work because they are unable to concentrate. Almost 20% of patients have a positive family history of the disorder. Most patients have a chronic waxing and waning course with exacerbations that may be related to stress. About 15% of OCD patients show progressive occupational and social dysfunction (APA, 1994a; Long & Long, 1995).

*Post-traumatic stress disorder* (PTSD) can occur when the patient has suffered or witnessed an event or events that involved actual or threatened death or serious injury to the self or others that is persistently reexperienced. Combat experiences, natural disasters, assault, and rape as well as emotional or physical abuse are typical traumatic events leading to the disorder. The patient has symptoms of avoidance, numbing, and increased arousal that endures for more than 4 weeks. PTSD often presents with depression, anxiety, or substance abuse symptoms. Children have nightmares about monsters or threats to self, or relieve the trauma through repetitive play. PTSD was previously recognized as "combat fatigue" or "shell shock." PTSD is considered acute if symptoms last less than 3 months and chronic if they last 3 months or longer. It is a serious disorder with significant associated psychiatric morbidity, functional impairment, and disability. The prevalence rates of PTSD from community-based studies range from 1–14%, whereas prevalence rates among at-risk populations (eg, combat veterans) range from 3–58% (APA, 1994a; Bursztajn, Joshi, Sutherland, & Tomb, 1995).

## SPECIFIC CONSIDERATIONS FOR PHARMACOTHERAPY

### When Drug Therapy Is Needed

Treatment of anxiety disorders occurs in two phases: stabilization and management. Pharmacotherapeutic agents are most needed during the stabilization phase to help the patient become more comfortable and to resume normal daily activities. Anxiolytics facilitate psychotherapy, which is the foundation of treatment in the management phase. During this phase, the patient learns to control fears and deal with residual phobias, cognitions, and psychosocial problems. The need for drug therapy may decrease during the management phase of treatment (Carter, Holloway, & Schwenk, 1994).

*Generalized anxiety disorder.* BZDs are the most frequently prescribed anxiolytic agents and are the drugs of choice for short-term or intermittent treatment of GAD. When long-term treatment is required, a non-BZD anxiolytic such as buspirone can be used. Drugs with secondary anxiolytic properties such as antihistamines, beta blockers, and antipsychotics are also prescribed for GAD (Kirkwood & Hayes, 1997; Valente, 1996).

*Panic disorder.* For years the BZD, alprazolam, was the only drug approved for treatment of panic disorder. Now, several other effective therapeutic options include SSRIs, TCAs, MAOIs, and other BZDs (Janicak et al, 1993).

An algorithm for drug treatment of panic disorder is shown in Fig. 33–3.

*Social phobia.* There is no approved drug for the treatment of social phobia; however, several agents are useful in alleviating the symptoms. Clonazepam and alprazolam are effective BZDs in treating the disorder; the MAOI phenelzine also has documented efficacy for generalized social phobia. Alprazolam may be used for occasional performance anxiety on an "as needed" basis. Although beta blockers are ineffective for treating generalized social phobia, they are quite effective for performance anxiety. A beta blocker given prior to the feared performance can eliminate the troublesome physical manifestations of anxiety, such as palpitations and tremor (Kirkwood & Hayes, 1997; Roy-Byrne et al, 1993).

*Obsessive-compulsive disorder.* Clomipramine, fluoxetine, and fluvoxamine are FDA approved for treatment of OCD. Although not approved for OCD, sertraline has demonstrated efficacy in managing the disorder (Wells et al, 1997).

*Post-traumatic stress disorder.* Prompt treatment following the precipitating traumatic event is necessary to prevent PTSD anxiety from becoming chronic and disabling. Personality changes may occur if the disorder becomes chronic. Selection of a pharmacotherapeutic agent focuses on the target symptoms to be treated, such as depression, anxiety, or panic. Antidepressants (TCAs, MAOIs, SSRIs), BZDs (clonazepam), and buspirone are most often used for PTSD. Clonidine is used to minimize the physiologic hyperreactivity associated with PTSD. Long-term treatment is best managed by a mental health specialist using individual, group, and family psychotherapy (Bursztajn et al, 1995; Sutherland & Davidson, 1994).

The underlying pathophysiology of anxiety disorders is unknown, but current evidence suggests it is a biologic illness with genetic factors. Anxiety is likely the result of multiple interactions among the central nervous system (CNS) neurotransmitters—norepinephrine, serotonin, and GABA—on which the anxiolytic drugs act. Both excitatory and inhibitory neurotransmitters function together to regulate CNS activity. Norepinephrine is an excitatory neurotransmitter; serotonin and GABA are inhibitory. The majority of norepinephrine in the brain is lo-

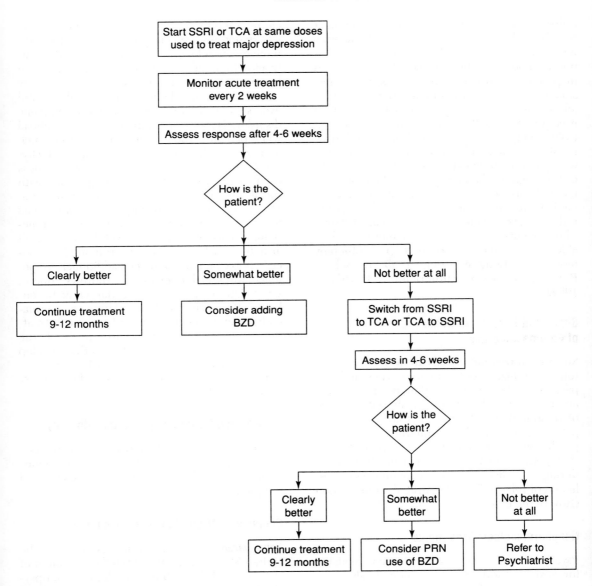

**Figure 33–3.** Algorithm for the treatment of panic disorder.

cated in the locus coeruleus (LC). When this area is stimulated, it activates the sympathetic nervous system, causing the characteristic somatic complaints accompanying the anxiety. When the GABA receptor is activated, it reduces the influx of chloride into the neuron, causing hyperpolarization that makes the neuron more difficult to fire when stimulated. BZDs enhance the actions of GABA, resulting in an anxiolytic effect. There are multiple subtypes of serotonin, which is located in the pons and

midbrain. BZDs, antidepressants, and alpha₂ antagonists inhibit LC firing, decrease noradrenergic activity, and reduce symptoms of anxiety (Olson, 1995).

Anxiolytics increase the action of the inhibitory neurotransmitter GABA and are most needed initially during the stabilization phase of treatment. GAD tends to be chronic and may require continued drug therapy during the management phase of treatment. Although psychotherapy is the mainstay for treating panic disorder and social phobias, anxiety is a prominent feature and amenable to pharmacotherapeutic intervention. The underlying cause for OCD is poorly understood, but it is thought to be caused in part by abnormal serotonin neurotransmission, particularly in the orbital gyri of the frontal lobes. Various types of psychotropics have been used to treat OCD although none have controlled symptoms completely. A combined treatment approach—pharmacotherapy combined with psychotherapy—for PTSD is most beneficial throughout the management phase of treatment. Pharmacotherapeutic agents provide relief from recurring nightmares or flashbacks and reduce psychological and physical distress. These agents make the patient more comfortable and enhance response to psychotherapy modalities (Long & Long, 1995; Rausch & Rosenbaum, 1995; Sutherland & Davidson, 1994).

## Short- and Long-Term Goals of Pharmacotherapy

Short-term treatment goals are to relieve symptoms, minimize anxiety with anxiolytics, and prepare the patient for psychotherapy. These goals are accomplished during the stabilization phase of treatment. Long-term goals are to have the patient gain control of symptoms and restore psychosocial and occupational function. Psychotherapeutic and nonpharmacologic treatments during the management stage minimize the likelihood of relapse following drug discontinuation (Roy-Byrne et al, 1993).

## Nonpharmacologic Treatments

Psychotherapy is the major treatment modality for anxiety disorders, either individually or in group settings. However, response to psychotherapy may be significantly enhanced if the anxiety is minimized with appropriate medication.

Supportive therapy should be offered by the primary care provider and includes empathic listening, education, reassurance, encouragement, and guidance, forming the basis for a therapeutic alliance between patient and clinician. Insight-oriented therapy helps the patient to understand the association between circumstances, emotions, and symptoms, which helps reduce the response to anxiety. Behavioral therapies are effective psychotherapeutics in reconditioning or modifying behaviors. These include: Relaxation techniques, such as progressive mus-

cle relaxation to help increase tolerance of anxiety symptoms, especially in GAD, and reconditioning, whereby gradual exposure and desensitization to the feared situation is made, useful in treating social phobia. Cognitive therapy stresses reframing the interpretation of stressful events and is used for OCD, phobias, and panic disorder. Hyperventilation control is beneficial when patients produce physical symptoms such as dizziness, shortness of breath, tingling, tachycardia, and feelings of suffocation. Assertiveness training is particularly useful for patients with social phobia who fear negative evaluation. Structured problem solving empowers patients to become more effective in their social functioning. This intervention is useful in treating all anxiety disorders. Social skills training helps social phobic patients who need additional competence for social interaction (Andrews, Rocco, Hunt, Lampe, & Page, 1994; Rausch & Rosenbaum, 1995; Turner, 1995). Although pharmacotherapeutic agents are useful in robustly treating panic disorder, they do not treat the agoraphobia or phobic avoidances that develop as a result of panic attacks nearly as well as nonpharmacologic interventions (Federici & Tommasini, 1992).

## Time Frame for Initiating Pharmacotherapy

Pharmacotherapy is initiated at the time of diagnosis during the stabilization phase to reduce anxiety and help the patient gain control of symptoms.

## Overview of Drug Classes for Treatment

**Benzodiazepines.** BZDs were first used in the United States during the 1960s for treatment of anxiety (Schlafer, 1993). They have no antipsychotic or analgesic action; however, they are powerful anxiolytics. Although serotonin, norepinephrine, and dopamine may be to some extent involved with BZDs, they primarily exert their antianxiety effects by potentiating the inhibitory action of GABA. Unlike other BZDs, lorazepam and oxazepam are metabolized solely by conjugation and thus are not affected by hepatic microsomal oxidation or liver disease. Other BZDs (eg, diazepam) are metabolized in the liver to an active metabolite with a very long half-life.

Chronic use of BZDs can cause a withdrawal syndrome upon abrupt discontinuation. If high doses of short-acting BZDs are suddenly stopped, the withdrawal symptoms include increased anxiety, restlessness, and irritability. Therefore, these shorter-acting BZDs (lorazepam, oxazepam, alprazolam) should be discontinued gradually. BZDs with longer half-lives (diazepam, chlorazepate, chlordiazepoxide) are more slowly eliminated from the body and less likely to cause severe withdrawal symptoms (Kirkwood & Hayes, 1997).

***Azapirones.***  Buspirone is the only azapirone currently available in the United States. Its anxiolytic action is not known, but it does not interact with the GABA complex. Buspirone acts as a partial agonist on serotonin ($5HT_{1a}$) receptors and as both an agonist and antagonist on dopamine receptors. This mode of action results in decreasing anxiety without the sedative effects of other antianxiety agents. Unlike BZDs, buspirone has no muscle-relaxant, anticonvulsant, or sedative effects. Moreover, it has no abuse potential and may be taken for an extended period of time without bringing about dependency or withdrawal upon discontinuation (Kaplan, Sadock, & Grebb, 1994). These characteristics make buspirone an attractive anxiolytic, particularly since substance abuse is frequently seen as a comorbid condition in anxiety disorders.

***Antidepressants.***  TCAs that are generally sedative in their pharmacology (eg, doxepin, amitriptyline) may be used as anxiolytics. Because of the sedative, orthostatic, and anticholinergic effects of these agents, tolerability may be a problem, especially in the elderly. Moreover, since GAD and clinical depression can coexist, special attention should be paid to the potential danger of a TCA overdose in depressed patients with suicidal ideation. Imipramine has been extensively studied in treating panic attacks. SSRIs were first introduced into the United States in 1988 for treatment of depression. Fluoxetine and fluvoxamine have been FDA-approved for treating OCD; paroxetine was approved in 1996 for treatment of panic disorder. MAOIs are potent antianxiety agents as well as antidepressants but are generally reserved for patients unresponsive to first-line drugs or who have medical problems that preclude using them. Because MAOIs have significant side effects and drug and food interactions, they may be difficult to monitor in a primary care setting.

***Other agents.***  Meprobamate was a widely used anxiolytic drug during the period prior to the advent of BZDs. For the most part it has fallen into disuse because other agents have become available. Still, occasional patients are seen who have taken meprobamate for years, and caution should be exercised if chronic high doses are suddenly stopped. Gradual discontinuation should be the rule. Antihistamines such as hydroxyzine and diphenhydramine can be useful in treating anxiety largely because of their sedative effects. Such agents are not substances of abuse and may be preferentially used for patients in whom anxiety is intermittent and the clinician is concerned about prescribing a BZD because of their abuse potential and "street value." Beta blockers (propanolol, atenolol) that blunt the physiologic response to anxiety are used for occasional performance anxiety and in some cases of panic disorder. Antihypertensives (clonidine) are used as an adjunctive medication to reduce hyperarousal symptoms of PTSD (Akiskal et al, 1994; Kaplan et al, 1994; Sutherland & Davidson, 1994).

See Drug Tables 309.1, 309.2, 311.1, 311.4.

## Assessment and History Taking

Most physiologic body systems are affected by anxiety (GI, GU, respiratory, CV), producing complaints of headache, fatigue, tremor, and general malaise. Consequently, patients present with a variety of unexplained physical symptoms such as dizziness, choking, chest pain, palpitations, trembling, paresthesias. An underlying medical problem may coexist with an anxiety disorder and must be appropriately recognized and treated (Federici & Tommasini, 1992). With numerous possible medical causes of anxiety, assessment should be focused on any medical conditions currently being treated.

The health history should center on the onset, quality, intensity, and duration of anxiety symptoms and what has been done to control them. A detailed history of present illness and family history are useful in predicting the patient's drug response. Anxiety may mask another psychiatric syndrome such as depression or psychosis. Any underlying medical or psychiatric disorder should be treated first. Obtain a history of current or past drug use (amphetamines, theophyllin, beta agonists, marijuana, OTC decongestants). CNS stimulants and depressants such as nicotine, caffeine, and OTC drugs containing phenylpropanolamine can induce anxiety. Up to 20% of panic disorder patients self-medicate with alcohol and have a coexisting drinking problem. All drinking should stop prior to using BZDs (Akiskal et al, 1994).

Laboratory studies may include an EKG, chemistry panel for hypoglycemia and electrolytes, CBC, and a thyroid profile if clinically indicated. A routine urine drug screen may be needed if substance abuse is suspected. A thorough physical examination is required.

### Patient/Caregiver Information

Patients need to understand that treatment of anxiety disorders is similar to that of any other complex, chronic health problem. Panic disorder and social phobia are fairly common conditions amenable to treatment. Reassure patients that they are not going to die during a panic attack, they are not losing their minds, and they can gain control of the disorder (Katon, Sheehan, & Uhde, 1992). Overcoming OCD is difficult and requires close collaboration with clinicians. Treatment success is directly related to patient motivation. Progress does not proceed in a straight line, but tends to fluctuate over time (Andrews et al, 1994; Hollander, Jenike, & Shahady, 1996). PTSD treatment response is relatively slow and may take up to 8 weeks or more to see beneficial effects. Good social and community support minimizes the likelihood of substance abuse during treatment. Remind patients that medication adherence is very important and troublesome side effects that occur with initial treatment usually decrease over time (Sutherland & Davidson, 1994). The primary provider should be available by phone particularly during the stabilization phase of treatment.

Often, simply educating patients about the nature of the disorder with reassurance that it can be treated is therapeutic. Also, advise patients to stop drinking caffeinated beverages and avoid excessive alcohol intake, and encourage patients who smoke to quit. Inform patients about relaxing techniques, such as deep breathing and progressive relaxation; imagery that focuses on a safe, pleasant mental picture; and positive self-talk to replace automatic negative thoughts. A regular exercise program (eg, walking) can relieve tension and enable patients to get sufficient sleep. Provide printed information and instructions on relaxation strategies and advise patients about appropriate community resources (Valente, 1996). Table 33–5 contains patient, family, and health professional information for managing anxiety disorders.

Again, treatment with MAOIs requires rather strict dietary and other drug restrictions. Refer

### TABLE 33–5. RESOURCES FOR MANAGING ANXIETY DISORDERS

Anxiety Disorders Association of America, Inc.
Dept. A, 6000 Executive Blvd.
Rockville, MD 20832-3801
301-231-9350

National Center for Post-Traumatic Distress Disorder
VAM & ROC 116D
Rural Route 5
White River Junction, VT 05009
802-296-5132

National Anxiety Foundation
3135 Custer Drive
Lexington, KY 40517-4001
606-272-7166

National Mental Health Consumers' Self-Help
Clearinghouse
1211 Chestnut Street
Philadelphia, PA 19107
1-800-553-4539

Phobics Anonymous
P.O. Box 1180
Palm Springs, CA 92263
619-322-2673

*From http://www.nimn.nih.gov/publicat/anxiety.html#anx7.*

to Table 33–2. Additional specific information is included in sections that follow.

### OUTCOMES MANAGEMENT

#### Selecting an Appropriate Agent

Benzodiazepines, azapirones, and sedating antidepressants are used for treating anxiety. Generally BZDs and TCAs are available in generic form and less expensive than newer agents. Cost should be a consideration in selecting an appropriate drug.

***Benzodiazepines.*** Diazepam is the oldest, most widely used of the BZDs and is a good choice for situational anxiety. Begin diazepam at 2 mg b.i.d. It has a rapid onset but has a high abuse potential in some patients, particularly those with a history of alcohol abuse. Alprazolam, the only BZD that is FDA-approved for treatment of panic disorder, has a rapid onset (20 min), peaks in 1–3 h without sedation, and wears off in about 6 h. It is useful for treating infrequent, predictable panic attacks. Begin alprazolam at 0.5 mg t.i.d. and increase by 1 mg/day every 3–4 days up to 10 mg if needed. Because depression usually accompanies panic disorder, therapy often begins with alprazolam in conjunction with an antidepressant (SSRI or TCA). The BZD is tapered off after 10–14 days as the antidepressant begins to take effect. During an acute exacerbation of panic attack or GAD, consider a short course of lorazepam 1 mg t.i.d. for 5 days either as a monotherapy or as adjuvant therapy to a TCA or SSRI being used as maintenance treatment.

Patients with performance anxiety who have an occasional public speaking engagement can benefit from pharmacotherapy an hour or two prior to the stressful event. A short-acting BZD, such as oxazepam (10–15 mg) or alprazolam (0.25–0.5 mg), about 1 h before the speech may be all that is needed. Because of the potential for CNS depression and memory impairment, the patient should be familiar with the effects of the drug before using it for a planned presentation. Chronic medication use may be necessary for patients whose phobias have had a significant psychosocial impact or if feared situations are frequently encountered and unscheduled. Low-dose clonazepam (0.5 mg t.i.d.) is a good choice to manage frequent or unpredictable attacks. Its onset occurs in about 60 min and lasts 8–12 h. When used for phobias, lorazepam (1 mg t.i.d.) provides a response within 2 weeks. Often patients are able to reduce their dose gradually over time, and some are able to stop the medication altogether after 6 months (Akiskal et al, 1994; Carter et al, 1994; Marshall et al, 1994).

If a BZD is selected, give an adequate dose to relieve symptoms; with careful patient selection and monitoring of compliance, dosage, and core symptoms, BZDs can be prescribed without fear of addiction. Dependency becomes a problem when BZDs are used more than three times per week or with daily use for more than 3 weeks. Moreover, patients with a history of substance abuse or unstable personalities are not good candidates for BZDs. The most common side effects are drowsiness, sedation, and psychomotor impairment (Shader & Greenblatt, 1993). Anecdotal reports suggest BZDs are effective in both generalized and discrete phobias such as performance anxiety; however, cognitive and psychomotor performance may be negatively affected. The tendency for abuse must be considered because of the high comorbidity of alcoholism with anxiety disorders.

Diazepam, alprazolam, and lorazepam are contraindicated in patients with narrow-angle glaucoma because of their anticholinergic side effects. BZDs must be used cautiously in patients with hepatic dysfunction and those who are elderly or debilitated. The elderly are much more sensitive to the side effects of BZDs and require lower doses. Elders are at risk for falls if BZDs with a long half-life such as diazepam are prescribed. Alprazolam (0.25 mg b.i.d. or t.i.d.), lorazepam (1–2 mg b.i.d.) or oxazepam (10 mg t.i.d.) are better choices for elderly patients and those with liver dysfunction. Hip fracture resulting from BZD-induced falls is an important concern. Safety and efficacy of BZD use in children under 18 years have not been established (Kirkwood & Hayes, 1997).

**Azapirones.** Buspirone is the drug of choice for GAD treatment because it has no abuse potential, can be used long-term, and is particularly beneficial when irritability and hostility are present (Wecker, 1994). Unlike other anxiolytic agents, buspirone should be taken on a regular, daily basis to exert its therapeutic effects, not periodically on an "as needed" basis. Like many other psychotropic drugs (eg, lithium, antidepressants), response to buspirone may not be seen until after 4–6 weeks of treatment. Adequate doses are necessary for efficacy to be seen: start it at approximately 7.5 mg b.i.d. and increase the dose up to 30 mg or more. Buspirone will not prevent withdrawal symptoms from BZDs; if a BZD is given initially, it should be tapered while buspirone is being increased. The subjective effects of buspirone are very different from BZDs, and it is not uncommon for patients who have taken BZDs to be disappointed in its effects and complain that it is not effective. Nevertheless, buspirone is effective when taken for an adequate length of time (4–6 weeks). The most commonly encountered side effects are nausea, headache, and dizziness, experienced early in the course of buspirone therapy and usually resolved with continued treatment. Patients should be encouraged to continue taking the medication if at all possible so that its anxiolytic effects can be evaluated. Safety and efficacy of buspirone use in children under 18 years have not been established (Kaplan et al, 1994).

*Antidepressants.*    TCAs, SSRIs, and MAOIs are effective drugs for treating core symptoms of anxiety disorders. Generally, the TCAs, imipramine or doxepin, are used for managing panic disorder especially if the patient has not responded to a trial of SSRIs. Begin imipramine or doxepin 100 mg daily and increase up to 300 mg/day, in divided doses, if necessary. Clomipramine was first marketed in 1990 for treating OCD. However, its success has been limited by adverse side effects and increased incidences of seizures and male sexual dysfunction. Start clomipramine at 25 mg daily and increase gradually as tolerated to 100 mg daily in divided doses within 2 weeks to a maximum total daily dose of 250 mg. Give clomipramine with meals to minimize gastrointestinal upset.

For elderly patients, start clomipramine at 25 mg daily, and increase as tolerated. Because it is very sedating, a bedtime dose with a snack may be safer for elders. For children over age 10, start at 25 mg daily, and increase to maximum total daily dose of either 200 mg or 3 mg/kg of body weight, whichever is less (Valente, 1996).

TCAs help decrease depressive and panic symptoms, nightmares, intrusive daytime thoughts, and flashbacks but have little effect on avoidance symptoms in patients with PTSD. Imipramine and amitriptyline have established efficacy for PTSD treatment. Response to TCAs is delayed for 4–6 weeks, so a BZD can be used during stabilization to bring prompt relief from anxiety. Later, taper off the BZD as the TCA becomes effective. Doses higher than recommended increase seizure risk. The most common side effects of TCAs include anticholinergic effects, orthostatic hypotension, sedation, sexual dysfunction, and weight gain (Jann, Jenike, & Lieberman, 1994; Long & Long, 1995; Rausch & Rosenbaum, 1995). TCAs are useful for patients unable to take BZDs or who have only partial response to buspirone. The more sedating TCAs (eg, doxepin, amitriptyline) may be used for their anxiolytic effects to treat GAD. Additionally, imipramine and trazodone are effective after 8 weeks of treatment (Rickles, Downing, Scheizer, & Hassman, 1993). Because of their sedative, orthostatic, and anticholinergic effects, tolerability may be a problem, especially in the elderly. Moreover, since GAD and clinical depression can coexist, special attention should be paid to the danger of TCA overdose in depressed patients with suicidal ideation.

SSRIs have a favorable side-effect profile making fluoxetine, sertraline, and paroxetine preferred agents in the treatment of panic disorder. Doses used should be similar to those used to treat depression. Occasional use of a BZD may be helpful early on in treatment to decrease anticipatory anxiety while the antipanic effects of the SSRI begin to be experienced (usually after 4–6 weeks of daily use). If an SSRI is not effective, imipramine may be used. Fluoxetine and fluvoxamine have been approved for treating OCD, although all SSRIs are probably effective; sertraline and paroxetine are currently being used investigationally for the disorder. Higher doses than used for antidepressants are frequently needed (eg, fluoxetine 40–50 mg/day rather than 20 mg for depression). They relieve symptoms without the histaminic, cholinergic, and alpha-adrenergic effects seen with the TCAs. Sertraline and paroxetine are being used investigationally for OCD treatment. Fluoxetine is slightly energizing, and the usual dose is 60–80 mg/day. Fluvoxamine is slightly calming; it has a short half-life, no proconvulsive effects, and is not associated with abuse. The initial dose of fluvoxamine is 50 mg h.s., increased 50 mg/day every 4–7 days up to 300 mg daily. Doses greater than 300 mg should be given in divided doses b.i.d. Safe use of fluvoxetine for children and adolescents has not been established. Although not approved for PTSD treatment, fluoxetine helps decrease the patient's withdrawal behavior and numbing symptoms. Several studies have shown fluoxetine particularly effective in social phobia (Roy-Byrne et al, 1993). Nausea, insomnia, anxiety, and sexual dysfunction are common SSRI side effects (Hollander et al, 1996; Kupsecz, 1995; Long & Long, 1995).

The MAOI agents phenelzine and tranylcypromine have been effective in treating social phobias in the short term, but improvement is not maintained when the medication is withdrawn. Phenelzine is effective in alleviating PTSD symptoms. However, its side effects and dietary and alcohol restrictions often preclude its use with this population of patients (Bursztajn et al, 1995; Federici & Tommasini, 1992; Roy-Byrne et al, 1993).

*Other agents.*    Beta blockers are effective in suppressing somatic and autonomic symptoms of anxiety, but do not alter the psychic symptoms. They blunt the peripheral catecholamine-mediated response of anxiety and thus are useful on an as-needed basis for "stage fright" or performance anxiety. Atenolol is effective for treating performance anxiety when given about 1 h prior to the feared performance (Rausch & Rosenbaum, 1995). Although not approved for treatment of panic disorder, propranolol 10–40 mg is helpful on an as-needed basis to alleviate autonomic symptoms of anxiety. Antihypertensives such as clonidine (an alpha agonist) have been used as adjunct agents for treating hyperarousal symptoms of PTSD (Sutherland & Davidson, 1994).

As a general rule, avoid prescribing any drug to a pregnant woman, particularly during the first trimester. The most teratogenic psychotropics are lithium and the anticonvulsants. If medication is required during a pregnancy, the patient should be referred to a specialist for management. Virtually all psychoactive drugs are excreted in breast milk, and mothers taking these medications should not breast-feed their infants (Kaplan et al, 1994).

## Monitoring for Efficacy

Patients and their families need an objective method of rating the severity of their symptoms so that improvement can be measured. Identify the core symptoms that are expected to improve and set treatment goals. Monitor anxiety symptoms and note the degree of dysfunction in social, occupational, and interpersonal activities (Roy-Byrne et al, 1993).

The stabilization phase of treatment may require up to 12 weeks to see maximum benefits from medications, and frequent contact with the patient is necessary to offer support during this time. It is important to monitor target symptoms and sufficiently alleviate anxiety to facilitate progress in psychotherapeutic interventions (Sutherland & Davidson, 1994). BZDs relieve symptoms of anxiety promptly, whereas the antidepressants (TCAs, SSRIs, and MAOIs) may take up to 12 weeks of treatment before maximum benefit is achieved; buspirone takes 4–6 weeks to become effective (Sussman, 1994).

## Monitoring for Toxicity

**Benzodiazepines.**  BZDs interact with all CNS depressants to produce additive effects. Although they have an extremely high margin of safety, even low doses of other CNS depressants such as alcohol dramatically increase the risk of toxicity. Coadministration with other sedative drugs (eg, antihistamines, TCAs, alcohol) should be avoided. Caution patients to be careful driving or operating dangerous machinery, especially when a BZD and another sedative agent are just beginning to be taken concurrently.

***Azapirones.***  Buspirone causes relatively few drug interactions and is generally well tolerated. Adverse effects include dizziness, drowsiness, dry mouth, headaches, fatigue, insomnia, and muscle spasms (Wecker, 1994).

***Antidepressants.***  TCAs can cause cardiac arrhythmias in toxic doses, and in patients with conduction disorders (bundle-branch disease) they pose a serious risk for heart block even in normal therapeutic concentrations. Side effects include anticholinergic phenomena (dry mouth, constipation, blurred vision) and alpha-blocking effects (sedation, orthostatic hypotension). They may lower the seizure threshold and can induce arrhythmias by increasing heart rate and slowing cardiac conduction. High doses may produce severe postural hypotension, dizziness, tachycardia, palpitations, arrhythmias, and seizures. Plasma TCA levels >1000 ng/mL indicate a major overdose; however, any elevated plasma level in conjunction with signs of toxicity should be regarded as potentially lethal. Life-threatening CV symptoms include tachycardia and impaired conduction leading to AV block. An EKG shows a prolonged QRS interval in the presence of a toxic serum level.

SSRI toxicity may produce seizures, nausea, vomiting, excessive agitation, and restlessness. All SSRIs currently in use have been implicated in adverse drug interactions involving cytochrome P-450 isoenzymes. Serotonin syndrome is an occasionally fatal disorder characterized by symptoms such as mental status changes, seizures, myoclonus, and blood dyscrasias. Ingesting OTC sympathomimetics such as cold remedies or diet pills can precipitate the serotonin syndrome in patients taking SSRIs. For mild cases of serotonin syndrome, an oral benzodiazepine may be sufficient; however, a plan for emergency treatment should be in place if symptoms continue. Refer the patient to a psychiatrist or mental health specialist for management (Brown et al, 1996).

## Follow-up Recommendations

If a BZD is used, the patient should be followed closely so as to avoid daily use of these potentially addictive agents. Try setting up a "contract" with the patient when the BZD is first prescribed, wherein the patient agrees not to use the drug more than 3 days a week.

Once an acute episode of GAD is controlled, patients should be encouraged to rely on non-pharmacologic aids to control anxiety on a long-term basis. Encourage continued exercise and relaxation techniques. Once patients with panic disorder are successfully treated, it is wise to follow up over time to ensure that medication adherence is maintained. Monitoring for concomitant alcohol use should be routine. Most importantly, patients should be encouraged to venture into previously feared situations. Panic disorder patients and their families should be advised to seek help early if panic attacks begin to reemerge to avoid a convoluted pattern of phobic avoidance. Most patients with OCD require prolonged follow-up to ensure continued benefit from drug therapy. Patients should be encouraged to seek psychotherapy from an individual familiar with the disorder.

## EATING DISORDERS

Disturbed eating behaviors are prevalent in Western societies because of a perceived link between beauty and thinness. Teenage and young adult women are most often affected (about 1.2 million in the United States); athletes, dancers, and models are at particular risk. The prevalence of anorexia nervosa among female adolescents and young adults is about 1.0%, whereas the prevalence for bulimia nervosa in the same population is about 3% (APA, 1994a). Eating disorders carry significant morbidity and a mortality rate that may be as high as 20% (Zerbe, 1996). Recognizing early signs of an eating disorder is essential if primary care providers are to intervene with preventive measures before a full-blown episode develops. Opportunities for recognition come during annual physical examinations for school, college, sports, or camp as well as family planning services (Rigotti, 1995a).

*Anorexia nervosa* is characterized by refusal to maintain a minimally normal body weight. These patients are obsessed with food and fearful of becoming obese even when thin and losing weight. A distorted body image, coupled with a rigorous need to control some part of their life, drives their constant desire to lose weight. Obsessive-compulsive features both related and unrelated to food are prominent in anorexia.

Weight loss is accomplished through fasting, dieting, excessive exercise (restrictive type), or purging with self-induced vomiting and misuse of laxatives, enemas, or diuretics after an eating binge (binge-purge type). Induced vomiting and laxative use are common purging methods. These patients commonly have an emaciated appearance and tend to withdraw from social activities. Females are usually amenorrheic. Over 90% of the patients are female with a mean age at onset of 17 years. This disorder is rarely seen in women over 40 years of age (APA, 1994a).

*Bulimia nervosa* is characterized by uncontrolled, repeated episodes of binge eating followed by inappropriate compensatory behaviors such as self-induced vomiting, laxative abuse, diuretics, fasting, or excessive exercise to prevent weight gain. There are two subtypes of bulimia: *purging type* (self-induced vomiting, laxatives, enemas) and *nonpurging type* (fasting, excessive exercise following a binge). Bingeing is triggered by dysphoric mood, stress, or hunger following a period of fasting. Individuals with bulimia usually are within a normal weight range, but may have frequent weight swings. They tend to be very sociable and outgoing. These patients often have depressive symptoms and are at increased risk for bulimia if they have a positive family history of an eating disorder. Bulimia usually begins in late adolescence or early adulthood (APA, 1994a).

Although not a diagnostic category, *compulsive overeating* covers a wide variety of overconsumption of food driven by emotions. Some authorities consider it a nonpurging form of bulimia. In many instances of compulsive overeating, the pattern is not to binge but to "graze" or overconsume food throughout the day. Compulsive overeating is likely a major cause of obesity in the United States. Patients may benefit from psychotherapy to resolve underlying psychosocial problems. A sensible eating plan, appropriate exercise program, and self-help group participation (eg, Overeaters Anonymous) offer the best strategies to control this behavior (APA, 1993; Lipscomb & Agostini, 1995).

## SPECIFIC CONSIDERATIONS FOR PHARMACOTHERAPY

### When Drug Therapy Is Needed

No pharmacologic agent has been found to remedy eating disorders, and psychotherapy remains the major therapeutic approach to treatment. Nutritional, cognitive, behavioral, and pharmacologic therapies should be integrated and coordinated with a mental health specialist, dietitian, gastroenterologist, and dentist as required.

Anorexia nervosa is a complex and often chronic disorder demanding a comprehensive treatment plan that coordinates medical management with individual and family psychotherapy. Medications should not be used routinely or as primary treatment for anorexia (APA, 1993). Because of the potentially grave complications of anorexia, these patients should be initially referred to a specialist for a treatment regimen and then monitored collaboratively by the primary care provider. Cyproheptadine, metoclopramide, and selected antidepressants may be used to treat target symptoms (Lipscomb & Agostini, 1995). Bulimia nervosa treatment strategies include nutritional and rehabilitation counseling, psychotherapy, family interventions, and pharmacotherapy. Anticonvulsants (eg, carbamazepine), antidepressants (TCAs, SSRIs, MAOIs), and other agents (eg, cyproheptadine, BZDs) may be necessary (APA, 1993; Rigotti, 1995a; Yager, 1994; Zerbe, 1996). If depression coexists, as it often does with compulsive overeating, consider an SSRI, which tends to decrease depression and suppresses appetite.

The pathogenesis of eating disorders is unknown, but it likely involves an array of physiologic, emotional, sociologic, genetic, and family factors. Central nervous system neurotransmitter abnormalities have been suggested as the physiologic pathogenesis of eating disorders and are amenable to drug intervention. Alterations in serotonin metabolism appear to affect central neurotransmitter activity related to eating behaviors. Serotonin-mediated eating activity is located primarily in the medial hypothalamus. Stimulation of serotonin receptors in the paraventricular and ventromedial nuclei decreases carbohydrate intake, enhances satiety, and terminates eating. However, stimulation of presynaptic serotonin receptors initiates eating, probably by inhibiting the release of serotonin. When there is decreased food intake, norepinephrine is released in the paraventricular nucleus, which inhibits satiety. Simultaneously, norepinephrine is inhibited in the lateral hypothalamus. Dopamine has been associated with self-stimulation behavior in other disorders and may be related to the eating binges observed in bulimia (Marken & Sommi, 1997).

## Short- and Long-Term Goals of Pharmacotherapy

The primary treatment goal for anorexia is to restore normal body weight (correct serious nutritional, fluid, and electrolyte imbalances, stop weight loss, and improve overall nutritional status) followed by establishment of healthy eating behaviors (Lipscomb & Agostini, 1995). Bulimia often presents with symptoms of major depression or bipolar disorder, and these patients should be started on appropriate medication. Long-term goals are directed at preventing relapse. Pharmacotherapeutic and psychotherapeutic interventions are directed at treating underlying psychological problems and changing disturbed eating behaviors (APA, 1993; Rock & Zerbe, 1995).

## Nonpharmacologic Treatment

Psychological and developmental issues, particularly regarding the role of family, are significant etiologic issues in eating disorders and are important considerations when selecting nonpharmacologic treatment strategies (APA, 1993). Although bulimic patients rarely require hospitalization, it may be necessary for the anorexic patient to restore weight and correct fluid and electrolyte imbalances. Criteria for hospitalization include (Rigotti, 1995a):

1. Weight loss greater than 40% of ideal weight or greater than 30% in 3 months
2. Rapid progression of weight loss
3. Cardiac arrhythmias
4. Persistent hypokalemia
5. Inadequate cerebral perfusion manifested by syncope, dizziness, and listlessness
6. Severe depression with suicide risk

All anorexic and bulimic patients require psychotherapy to reverse their abnormal eating patterns and distorted body image.

When the patient is not at medical risk, nonpharmacologic interventions are begun that include a refeeding regimen that begins with small increases in food intake. Add 200 calories to the diet every 2–3 days over several weeks. Anorectic patients need 3400 calories daily to begin gaining weight, but achieving this level of food intake will occur slowly. Supportive therapy, provided by the primary care clinician includes guidance on nutrition and exercise. Develop a therapeutic alliance with the patient, family, and treatment team. Cognitive therapy teaches the patient to identify irrational thoughts related to food, eating, and self-image. Behavior therapy helps the patient alter overt actions. Interpersonal psychotherapy helps the patient resolve role issues, social isolation, and prolonged grief reactions. Initially, treatment focuses on patient education about the disorder and, subsequently, on resolving interpersonal difficulties. Family therapy may be necessary, particularly if the patient is young, to change unhealthy family dynamics that could perpetuate the disorder. Psychotherapy may be individual or group-based and often includes the patient's family. Day treatment hospital programs, offered as an outpatient service, are less expensive than inpatient hospitalization yet give structured therapeutic care. The patient spends a half-day in a treatment program that includes one or two meals along with professionally supervised group therapy meetings (DGP, 1993b; Lipscomb & Agostini, 1995; Rock & Zerbe, 1995; Zerbe, 1996).

### Time Frame for Initiating Pharmacotherapy

Early intervention with counseling and medication is essential to achieving good treatment outcomes. The first treatment priority for patients with eating disorders is to correct any medical complication from severe malnutrition or harsh purging. Initiate appropriate pharmacotherapy promptly for underlying mood disorders or anxiety coexisting with the eating disorder.

### Overview of Drug Classes for Treatment

*Antidepressants.*    These drugs are used to improve depression and promote weight gain and have had some success in treating eating disorders. Studies show that the TCA clomipramine increases hunger and energy levels and maintains stable weight in anorexic patients. Imipramine and desipramine decrease the bingeing, vomiting, and depressive symptoms in bulimia. In one study anorexic patients taking the SSRI fluoxetine maintained their target body weight, regained normal eating behaviors, and reduced their obsessive and depressive symptoms. It also reduced the number of binges and purges in bulimic patients (Kay, Weltzin, Hsu, & Bulik, 1991). The fluoxetine dose used for treating eating disorders is higher than for

depression, and the cost of the drug may be prohibitive in some instances. Antidepressants should only be prescribed for anorexic patients who remain depressed after a target weight gain has been achieved. Phenelzine, an MAOI, reduces binge eating in bulimics; however, its severe dietary restrictions and potential for a hypertensive crisis limit its use in patients with eating disorders (APA, 1993).

*Anticonvulsants.*    These were the first drugs used specifically to treat bulimia nervosa after a relationship between binge eating and abnormal electroencephalography was noted. Carbamazepine and valproic acid have benefited patients who have symptoms of both bulimia and bipolar disorder (Herridge & Pope, 1985).

*Other agents.*    Cyproheptadine, an antihistamine and serotonin antagonist, has had variable success in improving appetite and decreasing depression in some anorexic patients. It has fewer side effects than antidepressants and, although not always effective, is a useful adjunctive treatment. Metoclopramide given before meals increases the rate of gastric emptying and relieves the gastrointestinal distress that often accompanies anorexia. Low-dose BZDs such as alprazolam given before meals reduces anxiety related to eating in both anorexics and bulimics. Lithium has been used for bipolar bulimics, but adverse side effects and toxicity risks from purging and laxative abuse limit its use (Marken & Sommi, 1997; Zerbe, 1996).

See Drug Tables 308, 311, 313, 502.2, 705.

### Assessment and History Taking

Anorexic patients often appear wasted and cachectic, making them easy to identify; bulimics are less immediately identifiable. Screening instruments may be helpful for detecting patients with eating disorders in a population at risk. However, two specific questions can be a quick predictor for detecting bulimia:

- Do you ever eat in secret?
- Are you generally satisfied with your eating patterns?

If the patient answers "yes" to the first and "no" to the second, explore further (Rock & Zerbe, 1995).

Initially, determine the degree of malnutrition, dehydration, and electrolyte disturbance, and determine if hospitalization and consultation or referral is needed. Explore the patient's attitude toward desired weight, weight loss, and eating habits; a 24-h diet recall is a useful tool for obtaining some of this information. Ask about bingeing, vomiting, laxatives, diuretics, diet pills, and daily exercise. Note symptoms of malnutrition and dehydration such as fatigue, skin changes, thirst, syncope, muscle cramps, and palpitations. Patients often present with complaints of amenorrhea, constipation, cold intolerance, lethargy, and heartburn.

Attention to family and psychosocial history may reveal a genetic link and/or a dysfunctional family that contributes to the eating disorder. Major life changes such as beginning college or a new job may trigger a bingeing episode. Low self-esteem or mood and anxiety disorders also affect eating behaviors. Look for indications of physical or sexual abuse because recent studies suggest a link with eating disorders (Zerbe, 1996).

The physical examination should assess for emaciation, severe hypotension, brittle hair, bradycardia, hypothermia, and very dry skin. There may be painless hypertrophy of the salivary glands, particularly the parotids. If the patient is inducing vomiting, dental enamel erosion may be noted as well as calluses on the dorsum of the hand from contact with teeth to induce vomiting. Broken blood vessels may be seen in the conjunctiva. Bulimics can induce vomiting with "tools" such as toothbrushes or spoons. Lanugo, fine downy hair, may be on the face and arms of the anorexic patient. A careful examination is required to rule out medical causes for weight loss and malnutrition such as malignancy, chronic infection, intestinal disorders, and endocrinopathies.

Laboratory studies should include a CBC, serum electrolytes, BUN, serum creatinine, urinalysis, and EKG. A thyroid profile is indicated because many symptoms mimic thyroid disorders. If the patient abuses laxatives, serum calcium and magnesium should be measured. Patients who have been underweight and amenorrheic for longer than 12 months may need a bone densitometry to assess for osteoporosis (Rigotti, 1995a).

## Patient/Caregiver Information

Educate the patient and family about eating disorders and particularly the dangers of insufficient protein and caloric intake, mental function impairment, lowered resistance to infection, heart arrhythmias, organ damage, and gastric or esophageal rupture. Inform the patient and family about community resources that can offer psychosocial support. Table 33–6 contains patient, family, and health professional resources for eating disorders.

## OUTCOMES MANAGEMENT

### Selecting an Appropriate Agent

***Anorexia nervosa.*** Individual, target symptoms of the anorexic patient guide selection of the ap-

---

**TABLE 33–6. EATING DISORDER RESOURCES**

American Anorexia/Bulimia Association
293 Central Park W., Suite #1R
New York, NY 10024
(212) 501-8351
http://members.aol.com/AMANBU

Anorexia Nervosa and Related Eating Disorders
Box 5102
Eugene, OR 97405
(503) 344-1144

National Association of Anorexia Nervosa and
   Associated Disorders
Box 7
Highland Park, IL 60035
(708) 831-3438

National Eating Disorders Organization
Laureate Psychiatric Clinic and Hospital
Box 470207
Tulsa, OK 74147-2027

Overeaters Anonymous
Box 44020
Rio Rancho, NM 87174-4020
(505) 891-2664

Eating Disorder Awareness & Prevention Inc.
603 Stewart Street, Suite 803
Seattle, WA 98101
(206) 382-3587

American Anorexia/Bulimia Association, Inc. (AABA)
425 East 61st Street, 6th Floor
New York, NY 10021
(212) 891-8686

---

*From http://www.nimh.nih.gov/publicat/eatdis/htm.*

propriate pharmacologic agent. However, many anorexic patients do not respond to any medication.

Cyproheptadine, an antihistamine/serotonin antagonist, is used to stimulate appetite and decrease depression in patients that do not exhibit bulimic symptoms (purging). It has few adverse effects and has been found effective in severe anorexia. Give cyproheptadine 8 mg q.i.d. Metoclopramide increases the rate of gastric emptying, which reduces the abdominal discomfort frequently seen in anorexic patients. Give 10 mg q.i.d. 30 min before meals. A short course of alprazolam 0.25 mg may be given before meals to reduce severe anxiety when it limits eating. Long-term use should be avoided because of abuse potential.

Antidepressants are used with varying success to decrease depression and promote weight gain. Generally, these agents are used only if depression continues after the target weight has been reached. Cardiac abnormalities may result from starvation or chronic purging behaviors, and a baseline EKG is essential to rule out potential impairment. Desipramine is a good first choice TCA because it has a preferred low anticholinergic profile and is better tolerated in this group of patients. It is "energizing" and may be useful in countering fatigue symptoms. Start desipramine at 25 mg in the morning and slowly titrate up to 150 mg/day given in divided doses. An alternative choice is clomipramine 100 mg at bedtime; it increases hunger and energy levels and aids in maintaining a stable weight. The SSRI fluoxetine reduces obsessions and depression, maintains target body weight, and restores normal eating behavior. The effective dosage for anorexia is higher than for treating depression and ranges from 20–60 mg/day. Begin fluoxetine at low doses (10 mg in the morning) and slowly titrate up to a therapeutic level. Give medication in divided doses in the morning and at noon. The cost for fluoxetine may limit its use for some patients. Bupropion has been linked with increased seizure risk in patients with eating disorders and should be avoided in these patients (APA, 1993; Janicak et al, 1993; Marken & Sommi, 1997).

**Bulimia nervosa.** Antidepressants reduce binge eating, vomiting, and depression as well as improve eating habits of bulimics. However, the adverse side effects of antidepressants limit their usefulness because bulimic patients have an increased sensitivity to them. The TCAs imipramine and desipramine and the MAOI phenelzine have been effective in treating bulimia (APA, 1993). The SSRI fluoxetine reduces vomiting, bingeing, depression, carbohydrate craving, and pathologic eating habits. It is well tolerated in bulimic patients (Fluoxetine Bulimia Nervosa Collaborative Study Group, 1992). Trazodone has fewer anticholinergic side effects than the TCAs but has limited controlled data reported. Desipramine and fluoxetine have a lower incidence of adverse side effects than the other agents and are good first-line drug choices. Dosages are the same for treating depression. Begin with a low dose and titrate up slowly to minimize initial side effects. Phenelzine should be used cautiously in bulimic patients because of its strict dietary requirements and potential for hypertensive crisis. A baseline EKG to rule out cardiac abnormalities is necessary prior to beginning an antidepressant. A personal or family history of seizures, cerebrovascular disease, and alcohol withdrawal puts a patient at risk for seizures when taking antidepressants.

Anticonvulsants are reserved for a subgroup of bulimic patients who also have symptoms of bipolar affective disorder and would benefit from mood stabilization. Dosages for carbamazepine and valproic acid are similar to those to treat seizure disorders, and prescribing information can be found in those sections (Marken & Sommi, 1997).

A short course of alprazolam 0.25 mg t.i.d. before meals can be used to reduce severe anxiety associated with eating. Avoid long-term use because of the potential for abuse (Marken & Sommi, 1997).

## Monitoring for Efficacy

**Anorexia nervosa.** Measure treatment outcomes by evaluating resolution of target symptoms. The aims of treatment are to restore healthy weight and healthy eating patterns, correct dysfunctional thoughts and behavior, improve family support, and prevent relapse (APA, 1993). Patients should be monitored every week until weight is stabilized, and there should be a 1–2 lb gain per week until the target weight is achieved. Check electrolyte balance and cardiac rhythm. Provide supportive therapy and help the patient and family assess treatment progress (Lipscomb & Agostini, 1995). During clinic visits, inquire about eating patterns, and review the patient's diet diary, feelings about eating, and any purging behavior. Regular menses should resume when the target weight is achieved.

Antidepressants should be tried for up to 8 weeks. If there is no improvement in mood, another antidepressant should be tried. If the medication is effective, it may be continued at the same dosage for up to 6 months. When TCAs are discontinued, they should be tapered off over a 2-week period to reduce anticholinergic rebound. No tapering is need for fluoxetine.

***Bulimia nervosa.***   Evaluate antidepressant effectiveness about 1 month after reaching therapeutic levels. Continue use for up to 12 months after the initial episode. Relapse following discontinuation of medication is prevalent, and long-term maintenance therapy should be considered (Marken & Sommi, 1997).

## Monitoring for Toxicity

Careful monitoring of TCA and SSRI antidepressant side effects is essential because anorexic and bulimic patients are particularly sensitive to their anticholinergic and cardiovascular side effects. Antidepressant medication toxicity is discussed in the section on depression and dysthymia above. Information on carbamazepine and valproic acid toxicity can be found in the section on bipolar disorder.

Cyproheptadine may cause anticholinergic side effects as well as drowsiness and should not be administered concurrently with MAOIs. Metoclopramide may produce dizziness and drowsiness and a hypertensive crisis may occur if it is given together with an MAOI.

## Follow-up Recommendations

Treatment of eating disorders is usually a long-term and complex undertaking that is best managed with the primary care provider working with a multidisciplinary team.

## INSOMNIA

Approximately 70 million Americans suffer from sleep disorders and for almost 60% of them it is chronic. Americans spend an estimated $15.9 billion on treating insomnia and related sleep disorders (Hahn, 1996). In 1993, the National Center on Sleep Disorders Research (NCSDR) was created to address this growing public health problem. In addition to supporting research, the NCSDR launched a major effort to educate both the public and primary care providers about sleep disorders.

*Insomnia* is defined as a persistent difficulty initiating or maintaining sleep or experiencing sleep that is nonrestorative (APA, 1994a). It implies fatigue, mood disturbance, or impaired performance. Basically, insomnia results from underlying physiologic or psychological processes. The disorder affects patients of all ages, especially the elderly because sleep patterns normally change with age. Problems are associated with sleep initiation (difficulty falling asleep), sleep maintenance (difficulty remaining asleep), or terminal sleep (difficulty with early morning awakening). The disorder may be considered as *primary* (idiopathic) or *secondary* (related to an underlying cause). About 10% of insomnia cases are due to a primary sleep disorder in which patients have objectively verified difficulty falling asleep or maintaining sleep in the absence of any identifiable underlying pathology. Transient insomnias related to acute situational factors such as stress are very common and affect about 85% of Americans at sometime in their lives (Hartman, 1995). Primary insomnia results from endogenous abnormalities in the normal 24-h wake-sleep cycle that may occur with rotating shift work or as "jet lag" from travel. Some patients have a conditional insomnia in which they associate bedtime with frustration, anxiety, and a variety of sleep-preventing behaviors. These patients typically sleep well away from their own bedroom, such as when on vacation or lying on the living room sofa. Primary insomnia is rare in childhood or adolescence and typically begins in young adulthood or middle age (APA, 1994a).

Secondary insomnia may be caused by multiple factors, such as drugs, alcohol, and caffeine use; psychiatric factors; or medical and neurologic illnesses. Stimulant drugs—amphetamines, cocaine, sympathomimetics, caffeine, and nicotine—may induce insomnia. Alcohol is a frequent cause for insomnia seen in primary care settings. Although alcohol induces sedation, the sleep is shallow, short, and not restorative. Activating antidepressants (SSRIs, phenelzine, bupropion) and phenylpropanolamine found in many OTC products can interrupt sleep. Caffeine intake may be an unsuspecting contributing factor. Common medications such as anticonvulsants, methylxanthines, antiarrhythmics, lipid-soluble beta blockers, and decongestants may interfere with sleep.

Up to half of all patients with chronic insomnia have underlying psychiatric disorders. Patients with depression have difficulty with falling asleep or early morning waking. Patients with agitated depression have diminished total sleep time and complain of overall exhaustion. During manic phases of bipolar disorder, patients have diminished total sleep time but do not feel tired. Patients with dysthymia may complain of feeling tired and irritable, of being unable to get enough sleep, and of never feeling rested. Patients with anxiety, particularly obsessive-compulsive disorder, often have great difficulty falling asleep because they lie in bed and ruminate. Those with post-traumatic stress syndrome fear going to sleep because of recurring, frightening nightmares, and sleep disturbances always accompany the psychoses. Medical problems such as chronic pain and cardiopulmonary dysfunction may cause orthopnea or paroxysmal nocturnal dyspnea, resulting in secondary insomnia. Urinary frequency associated with urinary tract infection or prostatism will prevent the patient from sleeping through the night. Patients with sleep apnea, a potentially serious breathing-related disorder, often present with a complaint of daytime sleepiness. *Sleep apnea* is caused by repeated periods of airway collapse followed by disruption of sleep. Most of these patients are unaware of how disrupted their sleep really is, but spouses report very loud snoring that interrupts their own sleep. Sleep apnea most often occurs in men over age 30, with a heavy upper body and a short, thick neck (APA, 1994a; Buysse & Reynolds, 1990).

## SPECIFIC CONSIDERATIONS FOR PHARMACOTHERAPY

### When Drug Therapy Is Needed

Management is determined by the underlying cause and duration of the insomnia. Treatment combines general measures to improve sleep, psychotherapeutic strategies, and pharmacotherapeutic agents. The treatment plan should be individualized based on underlying physiologic, psychological, or situational processes. General measures include treatment of any identified causes, patient education, and stress management techniques. Consider discontinuing all unnecessary medication and adjusting any unusually high drug dosages. Hypnotics are prescribed adjunctively for short-

term or intermittent insomnia; however, medication should be used carefully to avoid precipitating excessive drug use and habituation. Anxiolytics and hypnotics should be avoided in the patient with sleep apnea (Kirkwood & Sood, 1997; Weilburg, 1995).

The normal sleep-wake cycle is regulated by neuronal complexes located in the brainstem, basal forebrain, and hypothalamus with projections entering the cortex and thalamus. The reticular activating system maintains wakefulness; norepinephrine and acetylcholine in the cortex, and histamine and neuropeptides in the hypothalamus regulate neuronal activity during wakefulness. Sleep is promoted when the reticular activating system decelerates and serotonin neurotransmission in the raphe nuclei reduces sensory input, which inhibits motor activity. Norepinephrine is involved with dreaming, whereas serotonin is active during nondreaming periods. During sleep, the brain is extremely active and produces a pattern of stages that cycle throughout the night. The sleep pattern is altered with age, resulting in decreased overall sleep time (Kirkwood & Sood, 1997).

Hypnotics, drugs that facilitate or produce sleep, are used to treat short-term or intermittent insomnia. Anxiolytics such as BZDs can be used as hypnotics because they act on the GABA and BZD receptors that decrease neuronal firing. The non-BZD agent zolpidem selectively binds to BZD receptor sites to induce sleep. Other agents such as antihistamines produce drowsiness that facilitates sleep.

### Short- and Long-Term Goals of Pharmacotherapy

Basically, insomnia is a symptom and should be treated following these management principles: (1) any underlying medical or psychiatric disorder must be treated; (2) use nonpharmacologic treatment modalities; and (3) restrict use of hypnotics to transient or short-term insomnia only. Short-term insomnia is best managed by good sleep hygiene and other non-pharmacologic therapies. Patients with long-term or chronic insomnia will benefit from referral to a specialty sleep disorder clinic for evaluation and management (Pagel, 1994; Weilburg, 1995).

### Nonpharmacologic Treatment

Insomnia is a multidimensional problem requiring individualized treatment and nonpharmacologic behavioral interventions. The first-line insomnia treatment in the primary care setting is supportive therapy. Sleep hygiene measures center on environmental factors and behaviors that promote sleep. Stimulus control measures reinforce use of the bedroom only for sleeping or sexual activity, not for sleep-incompatible behaviors such as reading, eating, or watching television. Sleep restriction stresses no daytime napping. Relaxation techniques, such as progressive relaxation, guided imagery, and biofeedback, can help. Chronic insomnia responds well to psychotherapy and behavioral techniques. A sleep diary, found to correlate closely with polysomnography, is particularly useful in treating insomnia. Simply keeping the diary can improve one's sleep habits. Reviewing the patient's sleep diary and suggesting alterations may be all that is necessary to correct the problem. Sleep hygiene is an important treatment strategy and suggested measures are shown in Table 33–7. Stimulus control measures and sleep restriction are reported to be the most effective treatment modalities for chronic insomnia (Morin, Culbert, & Schwartz, 1994).

Referral to a psychologist or mental health specialist may be necessary for specialized psychological techniques, including cognitive restructuring, which encourages the patient to consider alternative, more rational beliefs about sleep and insomnia. In addition, psychotherapeutic interventions focus on assisting the patient to resolve conflicts and develop effective coping strategies.

## TABLE 33–7.  SLEEP HYGIENE MEASURES

1. Have regular hours for going to bed and waking up each day.
2. Don't take naps during the day.
3. Get regular exercise early in the day.
4. Avoid heavy evening meals. However, if hungry at bedtime, have a *light* snack.
5. Plan quiet evening activities.
6. Use bedroom only for sleeping or sexual activity.
7. Environment should be quiet, dark, and have a moderate temperature.
8. Avoid caffeine—coffee, tea, and colas—during evening.
9. Avoid alcohol, particularly in the evening.
10. Avoid chronic tobacco use.
11. Avoid excessive liquids in the evening.

*Adapted from Hartman (1995).*

Obstructive sleep apnea may respond to using plastic nasal strips placed across the bridge of the nose to keep the nasal passages open during sleep. Since obesity promotes the development of sleep apnea, weight management may be an important preventive intervention (Crismon, 1992; Hahn, 1996).

## Time Frame for Initiating Pharmacotherapy

Lack of sleep can impair work performance, reflex response, cognitive abilities, and one's sense of well-being. Patients with insomnia have undoubtedly tried various sleep-producing techniques, home remedies, and OTC sleep preparations before presenting to a clinic. However, pharmacologic agents generally are used only after nonpharmacologic interventions have failed. Sleep disturbances seem to be an important early indicator of psychiatric illness, allowing primary care providers the opportunity to diminish morbidity associated with new or recurrent mood disorders by prompt intervention or referral to mental health specialists (Gillin, 1992).

## Overview of Drug Classes for Treatment

Benzodiazepine hypnotics have sleep-producing effects similar to barbiturate hypnotics, but they are much safer to use and have become the drugs of choice for treatment of insomnia. They promote the onset of sleep, reduce awakenings, and increase total sleep time. Nevertheless, BZDs tend to alter the sleep stages and shorten restorative sleep. These agents are associated with development of tolerance and rebound insomnia after long-term continuous use.

The nonbarbiturate, nonbenzodiazepine hypnotic, zolpidem, has been approved for short-term use in treating insomnia and exerts minimal effects on the sleep stages. It is chemically unrelated to BZDs but is as effective in inducing sleep and increasing sleep quality. However, zolpidem is much more expensive to use than the BZDs.

Antidepressants such as amitriptyline, trazodone, and doxepin are prescribed for their hypnotic effects for patients who complain of nonrestorative sleep and should not receive BZDs.

Other agents may be used to avoid prescribing BZDs for insomnia. Some clinicians begin treatment with an OTC sleep preparation containing an antihistamine such as diphenhydramine or doxylamine. Melatonin is a hormone synthesized in the pineal gland that regulates sleep, mood, and ovarian cycles. Several small studies have linked melatonin supplements with improved sleep in elderly patients, but long-term studies have not been completed. Some reports suggest it is beneficial for "jet lag" and mild insomnia (Hahn, 1996; Kirkwood & Sood, 1997).

## Assessment and History Taking

A careful history is the most important part of assessment to differentiate between primary and secondary insomnia. Get a full description of the problem and have the patient keep a sleep diary for 2 weeks. Interview the patient's bed partner, especially if sleep apnea is suspected. During the interview, ask about specific symptoms, onset, duration, and exacerbating/alleviating factors; daytime symptoms; past treatment; past medical and psychiatric history; and sleep hygiene patterns. Rule out underlying medical or psychiatric conditions, drug/alcohol abuse, medication use, occupational situations, and travel patterns that may contribute to the insomnia. A complete physical examination is needed to rule out an underlying physiologic cause. Laboratory studies are rarely necessary and included only if clinically indicated. Continuous daytime sleepiness and fatigue suggests sleep apnea. It is important to recognize the possibility of sleep apnea because prescribing sedatives may increase the danger of respiratory difficulties in these patients. The bed partner or family members usually report that the patient snores loudly. Sleep apnea is ordinarily diagnosed with polysomnography in a specialized sleep laboratory (Hahn, 1996; Weilburg, 1995).

See Drug Table 310.

## Patient/Caregiver Information

Education related to sleep in general and to insomnia in particular is an important part of overall management. Explain how to keep a sleep diary: recording time in bed, estimated sleep time, any awakening, time of morning arousal, estimated sleep quality, any unusual events, and associated symptoms. Record information in the diary first thing each morning. The sleep diary is usually kept for 2 weeks prior to evaluation by the clinician and patient.

Correct any misconception that alcohol can improve sleep. Although alcohol may cause one to fall asleep more rapidly, sleep becomes rest-less in 2–4 h with frequent awakening and is not restorative. If patients are taking BZDs, remind them not to use these drugs for insomnia because of the high abuse potential, greater tolerance, and rebound insomnia when discontinued (Crismon, 1992).

## OUTCOMES MANAGEMENT

### Selecting an Appropriate Agent

*Benzodiazepine hypnotics.* Triazolam, temazepam, estazolam, quazepam, and flurazepam are used for managing short-term insomnia. Triazolam has the shortest duration of action (2-h half-life) and patients report less daytime sedation following its use. It is lipophilic, rapidly absorbed, and produces intense sedation in about 1 hour after administration. Begin with 0.125 mg h.s. Temazepam (15 mg h.s.) and estazolam (1 mg h.s.) are intermediate-acting BZD hypnotics used for patients who have difficulty remaining asleep. Temazepam and triazolam are most often used to induce sleep. Flurazepam (15 mg h.s.) and quazepam (7.5 mg h.s.) are long-acting agents because they form active metabolites with long half-lives. Flurazepam reduces both sleep-induction time and number of awakenings. All the BZD hypnotics, except temazepam, are metabolized in the liver and are affected by drugs that inhibit the cytochrome P-450 enzyme system (eg, erythromycin, nefazodone). Thus, temazepam may be a better choice for elderly patients and those with impaired liver function. BZDs are not prescribed to patients with a positive current or past history of drug abuse, and they generally are prescribed only for a short-term course of treatment.

Always use the lowest effective dose for the shortest length of time. Tolerance can develop when BZDs are used daily for over 4 weeks, so these drugs are best taken short-term or intermittently. Withdrawal may result in rebound insomnia, particularly with the short-acting agent triazolam. To avoid rebound insomnia following long-term use (greater than 6 months), gradually taper the dose to discontinuation. Elderly patients have an increased sensitivity to all the BZDs. Because there is an association between falls and hip fractures and the use of long-acting BZDs, flurazepam and quazepam should be avoided in this group of patients. BZDs should not be prescribed for patients with suspected sleep apnea or during pregnancy (Kirkwood & Sood, 1997; Sloan, 1995).

*Nonbenzodiazepine hypnotics.* Zolpidem, a newer hypnotic, selectively acts on the BZD receptor with minimal effect on sleep stages, consequently promoting a more natural sleep. It has little anxiolytic, muscle relaxant, or anticonvulsant effect. Although the potential for abusing zolpidem is minimized by the high incidence of nausea and vomiting at higher doses, its abuse and tolerance potential are unclear. It has a rapid onset and is useful for initiating and maintaining sleep. Begin with 10 mg h.s. for healthy adults, and this can be increased up to 20 mg per night as necessary. For the elderly and those with liver impairment, use 5 mg h.s. Zolpidem has not shown withdrawal effects, rebound insomnia, or development of tolerance with up to a year of use; however, studies are continuing (Holdcroft, 1993; Sloan, 1995).

*Antidepressants.* These drugs are effective alternatives for patients who complain of nonrestorative sleep but should not take BZDs. Some clinicians prescribe a sedating antidepressant such as trazodone 50 mg h.s. to avoid using a BZD hypnotic. Trazodone is particularly effective for treating insomnia secondary to fluoxetine or bupropion therapy (Nierenberg, Adler, Peselow, Zornberg, & Rosenthal, 1994). Anticholinergic side effects may limit use of the tricyclic antidepressants such as amitriptyline, particularly in elderly patients (Akiskal et al, 1994; Hartman, 1995; Kirkwood & Sood, 1997).

*Other agents.* OTC sleep preparations that contain diphenhydramine are readily available to patients. However, diphenhydramine alters sleep architecture and may cause confusion in the elderly. Melatonin, also available OTC, may be most beneficial for treating "jet lag" or mild insomnia in adults. Melatonin replacement therapy appears to be effective in treating insomnia in melatonin-deficient elderly patients (Haimov et al, 1995). The usual dose is 1–3 mg taken about 2 h before desired bedtime for at least 7 days. Lack of research on its long-term effects may limit recommending its use (Hahn, 1996). Table 33–8 contains a list of antianxiety agents often used in treating insomnia.

## Monitoring for Efficacy

Because insomnia is basically a subjective complaint, the patient's self-report is the most important determinant of improvement. If symptoms recur after a short-term drug course (2 weeks) for primary insomnia or if the patient is unresponsive to nonpharmacologic interventions, refer him or her to a specialist for management. Patients with chronic, long-term insomnia are best evaluated and treated by specialists at a sleep disorder clinic.

## Monitoring for Toxicity

For benzodiazepine hypnotics, refer to the section on anxiety disorders above. Among the nonbenzodiazepine hypnotics, zolpidem can produce headache, agitation, daytime drowsiness, and gastrointestinal upset. Further comparative studies are needed to assess effects of this drug. For antidepressants, refer to the section on major depression and dysthymia above. For antihistamines, refer to Drug Table 705. To date, little is known about the side effects of melatonin and its potential toxicity.

## Follow-up Recommendations

Patients should be evaluated after a week of treatment to assess drug effectiveness, any adverse effects, and adherence to nonpharmacologic interventions. The sleep diary should be evaluated after 2 weeks. Should a BZD be used for short-term treatment, follow-up is essential to monitor for appropriate use. Remind patients not to drink alcohol when taking BZDs. Provide printed information and counseling on precautions when using medications for sleep.

# SUBSTANCE ABUSE

Substance abuse is the harmful use of alcohol, tobacco, or other drugs knowing they cause psychosocial problems or are physically damaging. It is a leading cause of premature but preventable illness, disability, and death in the United States (Department of Health and Human Services [DHHS], 1994). The abuse of alcohol and nicotine, the most widely used legal psychoactive drugs in the United States today, is discussed in this section. Alcohol abuse alone costs society almost twice as much as all other drugs combined, for a total of about $86 billion annually. Adults as well as older children and adolescents are at risk. The potential for fetal alcohol syndrome makes alcohol abuse of particular concern among women of childbearing age (Bjornson, Fiore, & Logan-Morrison, 1996); DHHS, 1994).

**TABLE 33–8. ANTIANXIETY AGENTS USED IN TREATMENT OF INSOMNIA**

| Generic Name | Brand Name | Approved Indications | Usual Dose Range (mg/day)[a] |
|---|---|---|---|
| **Non-BZD Agents** | | | |
| Buspirone | BuSpar | Anxiety | 15–60[b] |
| Hydroxyzine | Vistaril Atarax Generics | Anxiety | 50–400 |
| Diphenhydramine | Benadryl | Not approved for anxiety | 25–200 |
| Propanolol | Inderal Generics | Not approved for anxiety | 80–160 |
| | | | |
| **BZD Agents** | | | |
| Alprazolam | Xanax Generics | Anxiety-depression Panic disorder | 0.75–4 1.5–10 |
| Chlordiazepoxide | Librium Generics | Anxiety Alcohol withdrawal | 25–200 |
| Chlorazepate | Tranxene Generics | Anxiety Seizure disorders | 7.5–90 |
| Diazepam | Valium Generics | Anxiety Alcohol withdrawal | 2–40 |
| Halazepam | Paxipam | Anxiety | 20–160 |
| Lorazepam | Ativan Generics | Anxiety | 0.5–10 |
| Oxazepam | Serax Generics | Anxiety-depression Alcohol withdrawal | 30–120 |
| Prazepam | Centrax | Anxiety | 20–60 |

[a] Dose for adults. Elderly patients are usually treated with half adult dose listed.
[b] Dose for elderly patients appears to be same, but is not established.
*Adapted from Kirkwood and Hayes (1997).*

Although tobacco use is the delivery system for the drug, nicotine, it is not thought of as substance abuse in the same way as other substances. However, any use of tobacco causes significant harm even when used in moderation. Tobacco dependence is a doubly serious problem not only because of health risks involved in its use but also because nicotine is an addictive psychoactive drug. *Smoking is the leading cause of preventable death in the United States today, with 430,000 tobacco-related deaths annually.* Exposure of nonsmokers to environmental tobacco smoke also poses a substantial health risk to these individuals. Infants and children exposed to environmental smoke have increased rates of chronic middle ear effusions, pneumonia, and other respiratory illnesses. Smoking cessation involves more than changing a habit because of the powerful addictive nature of nicotine. Counseling regarding alcohol and tobacco abuse should be included as a routine part of well-child care, and all complete health examinations for adults should include an in-depth history of alcohol and tobacco use (DHHS, 1994). Given the significant morbidity and mortality associated with alcohol and nicotine abuse, prevention should be the first-line intervention strategy in all primary care settings.

## ALCOHOL ABUSE

Alcohol abuse is a frequently encountered problem in primary care. Many individuals have suffered some adverse event in their lives from alcohol use and are able to modify their drinking behavior so that dependence and abuse do not become a problem (APA, 1994a). However, the psychiatric complications that may result from alcohol abuse and dependence are many, ranging from delirium to drug-induced mood and anxiety disorders. Additionally, individuals with mood or anxiety disorders may use alcohol as an attempt at self-treatment, only to complicate further the course of their underlying disorder. Prevention of alcohol abuse is the most important intervention strategy for primary care settings (DHHS, 1994). Ideally, primary care providers should try to screen for and treat an alcohol problem in its early phases routinely, before it becomes an addiction and more difficult to manage. As needed, treatment programs should be recommended. Generally, outpatient alcohol treatment programs combine pharmacotherapeutic and psychotherapeutic treatment modalities. Inpatient care is costly and reserved for patients with severe, acute withdrawal syndrome; those who have failed previous treatment programs; or those who have a poor social environment (Hanna, 1995).

## SPECIFIC CONSIDERATIONS FOR PHARMACOTHERAPY

### When Drug Therapy Is Needed

Because all the repercussions of alcohol use and abuse are well beyond the scope of this section, the management of outpatient alcohol withdrawal will be the focus. This disorder may require acute treatment and, left unattended, could result in serious medical (mostly neurologic) consequences such as seizures. Early detection and prompt intervention are essential for successful treatment outcomes.

Individuals who chronically abuse alcohol in large quantities expose themselves to the possibility of acute withdrawal upon abrupt cessation of drinking. The withdrawal syndrome is characterized by autonomic hyperactivity such as sweating, tachycardia, hand tremor, agitation, anxiety, and grand mal seizures (APA, 1994a). Such symptoms are the result of unmasking a hyperactive autonomic state that develops because of the chronic consumption of alcohol and its sedating effects. Thus, treatment of alcohol withdrawal consists of replacing alcohol with another sedative agent (such as a benzodiazepine) with a longer half-life, from which the patient can then be gradually withdrawn without such severe neurological sequelae. Further, because alcoholics may ignore the need for adequate nutrition, the body usually becomes deficient in the B vitamins.

Treatment of alcohol withdrawal syndrome requires patient monitoring, keeping an environment with minimal stimulation, and providing food, noncaffeinated fluids, rest, and reassurance.

### Short- and Long-Term Goals of Pharmacotherapy

The short-term goal of alcohol withdrawal is to prevent or minimize occurrence of withdrawal symptoms and related psychiatric and nutritional problems. Long-term goals include maximizing the patient's motivation for abstinence from alcohol and preventing relapse by assisting the individual to rebuild a substance-free lifestyle. It is increasingly recognized that achieving motivation for abstinence is a critical first step in achieving long-term treatment goals. The latter goal of maximizing multiple life-style changes so as to prevent relapse is the most formidable challenge (Schuckit, 1994).

### Nonpharmacologic Treatment

Over the years many nonpharmacologic treatment programs for alcoholism have evolved. Any successful program stresses both the importance of continued sobriety and basic life-style changes. Dealing with marital and other family issues, enhancing self-esteem, enriching job functioning and financial management, addressing relevant spiritual issues, and dealing with the possibility of homelessness are special issues for those in alcohol treatment programs (Schuckit, 1994). The primary care provider can offer supportive therapy, encouraging the patient to seek psychotherapeutic modalities such as cognitive-behavioral techniques, coping skills training, and relapse prevention. Psychotherapy is usually delivered in a group therapy setting. Self-help groups such as Alcoholics Anonymous (AA) are very successful because its members know all the tricks of the disease and the value of surrender and serenity. There are over 750,000 local chapters of AA in the United States. A treatment program that is negotiated with the individual patient and family, together with a multidisciplinary team approach, has the best chance of success. Table 33–9 contains patient, family, and health professional resources for managing alcohol abuse.

### Time Frame for Initiating Pharmacotherapy

Outpatient drug treatment for alcohol withdrawal can be achieved successfully and is less

## TABLE 33–9. RESOURCES FOR MANAGING ALCOHOL ABUSE

Alcoholics Anonymous
Check local telephone books for information on meetings

American Academy of Pediatrics
P.O. Box 927
Elk Grove Village, IL 60009-0927
1-800-433-9016
Ask for "Alcohol: Your Child and Drugs."

American Council on Drug Education
136 East 64th Street
New York, NY 10021
1-800-488-DRUG

National Clearing House for Alcohol and Drug
   Information
P.O. Box 2345
Rockville, MD 20847-2345
301-468-2600
1-800-729-6686

National Council on Alcoholism and Drug Dependence
12 West 21st Street
New York, NY 10000
212-206-6770

*Adapted from DHHS (1994).*

emergent if the patient's degree of withdrawal is relatively mild to moderate. The time frame for initiating drug treatment for alcohol withdrawal may vary, depending upon the severity of symptoms. Immediate treatment is necessary and should be carried out on an inpatient basis if there is a history of severe alcohol withdrawal symptoms or recent head trauma. Fever of over 101°F, delirium or hallucinations, significant malnutrition, or serious medical complications of alcohol use also would warrant hospitalization for withdrawal management (Janicak et al, 1993). Alcohol withdrawal symptoms occur after a period of abstinence or during a reduction in the amount of alcohol intake. The primary care provider should be cognizant of the fact that a withdrawal syndrome may occur inadvertently from a sometimes brief concurrent illness or during the course of a medical illness or trauma. Therefore, it is important to be aware of the possibility of alcohol withdrawal even though abuse may not have been previously recognized.

## Overview of Drug Classes for Treatment

Benzodiazepines have a central role in alcohol withdrawal treatment. These agents suppress signs and symptoms of uncomplicated alcohol withdrawal, seizures, and delirium. Chlordiazepoxide, diazepam, lorazepam, and oxazepam are most often prescribed (Bohn, 1993).

Adrenergic agents treat the autonomic hyperactivity seen during alcohol withdrawal. Clonidine and propanolol, although not considered first-line drugs, are sometimes used to control these symptoms.

Anticonvulsants, such as phenytoin and carbamazepine, may be given to prevent withdrawal seizures, particularly in patients with an underlying seizure disorder. Patients with a history of seizures are not good candidates for outpatient alcohol withdrawal and should be referred for management.

Nutritional supplements help restore nutritional deficiencies and facilitate the withdrawal process. These generally include multivitamins and thiamine supplements. Recently, the opiate antagonist naltrexone has been approved as an adjunctive treatment to lessen the craving for alcohol (Crabtree & Polles, 1997).

## Assessment and History Taking

Obtain a thorough history of previous alcohol use and have this information confirmed by family members, if possible. A complete health assessment can determine if the patient is an appropriate candidate for outpatient withdrawal. Vital signs should be measured to monitor for autonomic hyperactivity. Observe for symptoms of mild withdrawal, including insomnia, irritability, anxiety, headache, GI distress, mild hypertension, and tremulousness.

Laboratory studies should include a chemistry panel, liver panel, and CBC. Plasma albumin, serum folate, and vitamin $B_{12}$ level will aid in evaluating nutritional status. Consultation and collaboration with a specialist is recommended for outpatient withdrawal management.

The CAGE questionnaire, a brief screening instrument for alcohol abuse, is easily administered in a primary care setting (Mayfield, McLeod, & Hall, 1974). CAGE questions ask the patient about attempts to *c*ut down on drinking, being *a*nnoyed by criticism of drinking, feeling *g*uilty about drinking, and having an *e*ye-opener drink in the mornings for a hangover. Positive responses to two of the questions suggests possible alcohol abuse and further evaluation is indicated (Caulker-Burnett, 1994).

See Drug Tables 205.5, 308.2, 308.3, 309.1, 312, 313.

## Patient/Caregiver Information

Whenever significant alcohol abuse or dependency is suspected, address the issue directly with the patient. Explaining the difference between appropriate alcohol use and abuse is an important step. Refer the patient to various community resources, such as an alcohol treatment program or Alcoholics Anonymous.

A supportive family who can provide close supervision is essential for outpatient management of alcohol withdrawal (Hanna, 1995). Refer to Table 33–9 for resources. In addition, family members dealing with a problem alcoholic can get excellent support from their local Alanon, Alateen, and Adult Children of Alcoholics (ACOA) meetings.

## OUTCOMES MANAGEMENT

### Selecting an Appropriate Agent

***Benzodiazepines.*** BZDs have been the most frequently used agents to treat alcohol withdrawal symptoms of autonomic hyperactivity such as tremors, anxiety, sweating, tachycardia, and hypertension. Tremulousness is the earliest appearing symptom and can be seen 6–12 h after the patient's last drink. Chlordiazepoxide, a long-acting BZD, is a good choice; diazepam is a reasonable substitute. Begin withdrawal by tapering chlordiazepoxide starting with 50 mg t.i.d. for 1 day, 50 mg b.i.d. for 1 day, 25 mg t.i.d. for 1 day, 25 mg b.i.d. for 1 day, 25 mg daily for 1 day, and then discontinue. Tapering of the BZD can be accomplished over a 5–7-day period of time depending on symptom manifestations. Tapering an acute dose over a 2-week period may be indicated (Janicak et al, 1993). The longer-acting BZDs may be erratically absorbed from the gastrointestinal tract if the patient is experiencing nausea and vomiting, and an intramuscular BZD may be required. In such cases, lorazepam intramuscularly is the preferred agent for injection because chlordiazepoxide and diazepam are poorly absorbed from the muscle. However, patients requiring parenteral medications for withdrawal treatment should be referred for inpatient care.

If liver function tests suggest possible hepatic complications, intermediate-acting BZDs, which do not depend on the liver for their metabolism, would be prudent. Examples of such agents are oxazepam and lorazepam, which are good choices for treating elderly patients in alcohol withdrawal. Begin BZD withdrawal by tapering over a 5–7-day period. Start with lorazepam 2 mg t.i.d. for 2 days, 2 mg b.i.d. for 2 days, 2 mg daily for 1 day, and then discontinue (Bohn, 1993; Crabtree & Polles, 1997).

Antipsychotic agents may be needed for severe delirium and hallucinosis; low doses of haloperidol (1–10 mg/day) aid in the control of these symptoms (Gallant, 1994). However, should the patient exhibit such symptoms of a severe withdrawal syndrome, he or she should be immediately referred to a specialist for inpatient care.

***Adrenergic agents.*** Beta-adrenergic blockers such as propanolol or atenolol may be administered to treat the autonomic hyperactivity seen in alcohol withdrawal. Some clinicians prefer to use alpha-adrenergic agonists to treat alcohol withdrawal. Clonidine in doses as high as 0.2 mg t.i.d. may be prescribed. This agent is useful in lowering the hypertension seen in alcohol withdrawal. Careful monitoring should ensue (Gallant, 1994).

***Anticonvulsants.*** Phenytoin can be started at 300 mg orally each morning to manage seizures. Plasma blood levels should be monitored.

***Nutritional supplements.*** Thiamine 100 mg/day for 3 days should be taken. A multivitamin preparation is given to restore possible deficiencies due to poor nutrition. Often, a prenatal multivitamin preparation is recommended because of its folic acid content.

***Other agents.*** If naltrexone is used, give 50 mg orally b.i.d. However, naltrexone should only be one part of a more global alcohol treatment program (Blondell, Frierson, & Lippman, 1996; Bohn, 1993).

### Monitoring for Efficacy

***Benzodiazepines.*** The goal of BZD therapy is not to sedate patients but to treat for withdrawal. They should still be able to participate in other, nondrug therapeutic interventions.

*Adrenergic agents.*    When beta-adrenergic block-ers are used to treat withdrawal symptoms, blood glucose should be monitored, especially in the first 36 h after drinking since the patient's poor nutritional status may result in hypo-glycemia, which in turn could lower the seizure threshold.

*Anticonvulsants.*    Although BZDs have anticon-vulsant properties, alpha- and beta-adrenergic blockers do not prevent convulsions. Particularly in patients who have had withdrawal seizures in the past, anticonvulsant therapy is needed to prevent seizures. Phenytoin may be used, but long-term anticonvulsant therapy is rarely needed unless the patient has had a head injury. These patients should be referred for with-drawal treatment.

*Nutritional supplements.*    Supplements such as a prenatal multivitamin may be continued indefi-nitely to augment adequate dietary intake. A 24-h diet recall or 3-day diet diary may be useful to monitor nutritional status.

*Other agents.*    If naltrexone is prescribed, a daily dose of 50 mg orally is usually given. A weekly dose of 350 mg may be given in three divided doses, eg, 100 mg on Monday and Wednesday and 150 mg on Friday. Naltrexone is started after detoxification to avoid uninten-tional precipitation of withdrawal. Do not ad-minister naltrexone to polysubstance abusers since it can induce opiate withdrawal in heroin or other chronic opiate users. It is only adjunc-tive therapy for alcoholism (O'Malley et al, 1992).

On occasion, disulfiram (250–500 mg/day for 3 days as a loading dose and maintained on 125–200 mg/day) may be useful to prevent re-lapse following withdrawal. It should be used only by well-motivated patients who are physi-cally healthy. Patients must be warned of the re-actions that will occur if alcohol is ingested while taking disulfiram: headaches, nausea, vomiting, and facial flushing. For these reasons, many pri-mary care providers obtain written consent be-fore starting a disulfiram regimen.

## Monitoring for Toxicity

Benzodiazepine toxicity may be monitored by looking for oversedation. Patients undergoing

alcohol withdrawal, who are asleep most of the day, provide evidence that more than adequate doses are being administered.

Beta-adrenergic blockers may be monitored by a family member watching for bradycardia, level of alertness, mobility, and difficulty breath-ing (if emphysema or asthma is present). A blood glucose level may be obtained after the first 2 days of use, or earlier if indicated. Beta blockers can have adverse effects on comorbid conditions such as diabetes, chronic obstructive pulmonary disease (COPD), and cardiomyop-athies. Alpha-adrenergic agonists may be moni-tored by following the patient's blood pressure during clinic visits.

If phenytoin or another anticonvulsant is used, plasma levels should be monitored. If a loading dose is administered, a therapeutic level of 10–20 µg/mL is advisable. Signs and symp-toms of toxicity, including nystagmus and ataxia, should be checked daily.

The most commonly reported side effect of naltrexone is gastrointestinal disturbances. It is potentially hepatotoxic, so serum transaminases should be measured before initiating therapy and periodically throughout. The hepatotoxicity seems to be readily reversible on discontinuing the drug (Triolo, 1997). Serious disulfiram reac-tions can include chest pain, shock, and respira-tory depression.

## Follow-up Recommendations

Once alcohol withdrawal is controlled, patients and families both need to be counseled about obtaining help from a rehabilitation program for the patient and from support groups for family members, of which there are usually many in the community.

## NICOTINE ABUSE

Tobacco use is the single largest cause of preventable illness and death in the United States. Smoking is a known cause of heart and lung disease, cancer, and stroke in this country. It is a dangerous activity because of significant health risks associated with smoking, the addic-tive nature of nicotine, and the hazard to others in a smoking environment. Exposure to second-hand smoke is a potential health hazard to in-fants and young children. Since passive smoking can aggravate symptoms of asthma and allergies and decrease pulmonary function, exposed children have higher rates of lower respiratory tract infections, middle ear infections, and lung cancer. Primary health care providers can play a key role in helping smokers stop smoking and preventing others from starting (DHHS, 1994; Long, 1993).

## SPECIFIC CONSIDERATIONS FOR PHARMACOTHERAPY

The three stages of smoking cessation are: (1) preparing to quit, (2) initial cessation, and (3) maintenance of cessation. Pharmacotherapy is used when the patient stops smoking. Nicotine replacement therapy (NRT) along with cognitive-behavioral interventions has proven to be the most successful program in maintaining smoking cessation (Ockene & Kristeller, 1994). An algorithm for NRT is shown in Fig. 33–4.

### When Drug Therapy Is Needed

The nicotine found in tobacco causes the release of epinephrine and norepinephrine, producing a pleasurable feeling to smokers. Tolerance develops quickly, and users must increase their intake to obtain the desired effect. A typical one-pack-per-day smoker absorbs 20–60 mg of nicotine a day. Tobacco (nicotine) withdrawal syndrome begins within 24 h after smoking cessation. Common symptoms of withdrawal include craving for tobacco, anxiety, headaches, gastrointestinal upset, mood changes, irritability, difficulty concentrating, changes in appetite, and craving for sweets. Pharmacotherapy is used to relieve these symptoms so the patient can focus on changing the behavioral dependency during the smoking cessation program (APA, 1994a; Rigotti, 1995b).

### Short- and Long-Term Goals of Pharmacotherapy

The short-term goal of pharmacotherapy is to relieve symptoms of nicotine withdrawal so that patients can concentrate on behavioral change. The major long-term goal is to prevent risks of relapse by continued encouragement and discussion of strategies to maintain abstinence from smoking.

### Nonpharmacologic Treatment

Prevention is the first-line intervention strategy for all primary health care providers. It is particularly important for children and teenage patient populations because about 95% of adult smokers began smoking before age 20. Providers can use the National Cancer Institute's smoking prevention/cessation counseling principles:

- Anticipate a smoking risk
- Ask about smoke exposure
- Advise all smoking patients to quit
- Assist smokers in quitting
- Arrange for follow-up care

Antismoking strategies should begin in early preteen years with constant reinforcement and efforts to promote nonsmoking as the norm. Establish a smoke-free clinic environment and make educational materials related to the dangers of smoking and benefits of quitting available. Successful smoking cessation programs must include nonpharmacologic treatment along with pharmacotherapy. When smokers are preparing to quit, increase their motivation by discussing the risks and benefits of smoking cessation related to their physical, psychological, and social status. The health care professional's advice to stop smoking is a powerful motivator for some patients. During *every* clinic visit, providers should advise smokers to quit, offer brief smoking cessation counseling, give educational materials, prescribe NRT when appropriate, and refer to a stop-smoking program when the patient is ready to quit (DHHS, 1994; Schwartz, 1996).

Supportive therapy from the primary provider is important to the patient during a smoking cessation program. Personalizing reasons to quit improves the patient's motivation to begin a treatment program and maintain cessation. Supporting the patient's belief that he or she *can* stop smoking is key to beginning the change process of a smoking cessation program.

### Time Frame for Initiating Pharmacotherapy

Pharmacotherapy is begun on the day the patient stops smoking. NRT should be coupled with cognitive-behavioral interventions with self-help manuals, audiotapes, referral to a structured program, group therapy, and follow-up counseling. NRT alone will not change smok-

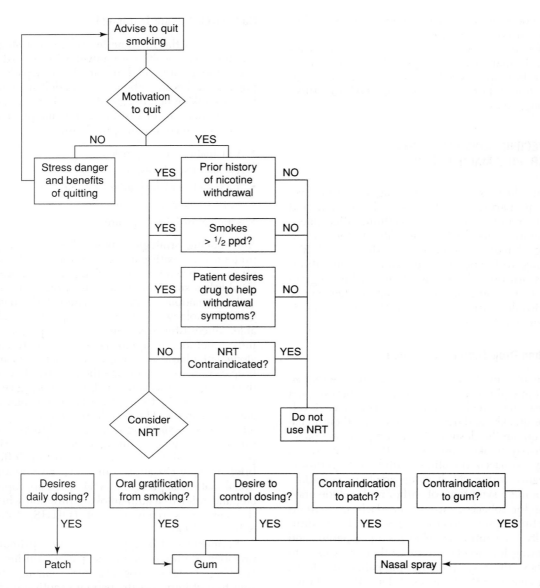

**Figure 33–4.** Algorithm for nicotine replacement therapy.

From Cox (1993).

ing behaviors; it only mitigates nicotine withdrawal symptoms.

## Overview of Drug Classes for Treatment

Nicotine withdrawal symptoms can be relieved by maintaining some exposure to nicotine other than by inhalation. Chewing gum, transdermal patches, and nasal sprays are available delivery methods for NRT. Other agents used for withdrawal symptoms include clonidine, a centrally acting adrenergic blocking agent; lobeline, a nicotine imposter; and antidepressants (Goroll, May, & Mulley, 1995).

## Assessment and History Taking

Ask every child and adult about tobacco use. Obtain a history of smoking in the patient's home and work environments. Determine if the patient has tried to quit previously and how successful the effort was. Assess for any coexisting psychiatric disorders that may contribute to continuation of smoking.

Assess cardiovascular and circulatory status to rule out any contraindications to NRT, such as recent MI, worsening angina, arrhythmias, active peptic ulcer, or pregnancy. Women who are pregnant or nursing infants should not use NRT. Discuss any physical findings that may be associated with tobacco use, which tends to "personalize" the need for smoking cessation and reinforce a commitment to quit.

See Drug Table 1003.

## Patient/Caregiver Information

Provide educational materials on the dangers of smoking, benefits of quitting, and community resources to help people stop smoking. Talk about nicotine addiction and smoking cessation program availability. Although nicotine gum and the patch became OTC products in 1996, patients still need a behavioral treatment program for the best smoking cessation outcomes. The nicotine nasal spray requires a prescription. Instruct patients not to smoke during NRT (gum, patch, or nasal spray) or use other nicotine products. Remind patients to wash their hands after applying nicotine patches or handling the nasal spray. Table 33–10 contains patient, family, and health professional resources for smoking cessation.

## OUTCOMES MANAGEMENT

### Selecting an Appropriate Agent

Patients who smoke more than one pack per day or smoke their first cigarette of the day within 30 min of waking are most likely to be addicted to nicotine and will benefit most from NRT. With nicotine chewing gum, the nicotine is absorbed through the oral mucosa while avoiding harmful effects of smoking. The gum comes in 2- and 4-mg strengths. Instruct the patient to pick a target date to quit smoking. After that date, chew the gum whenever there is an urge to smoke. Advise the patient to chew the gum slowly, just enough for a slight tingling taste, "park it" between the cheek and teeth for proper absorption, and chew for about 30 min. Up to 12 pieces of gum may be chewed at the beginning of withdrawal, but not more than 30 pieces of 2-mg gum should be used in 24 h. Common side effects of nicotine gum include mouth irritation, dizziness, nausea, headache, and excess salivation. Some patients have problems with the gum adhering to dental work. Remind patients to avoid coffee, tea, or colas immediately before or after using the gum to enhance nicotine absorption (Ockene & Kristeller, 1994).

The transdermal patch, available OTC, provides a means of maintaining a steadier level of nicotine replacement during the smoking cessation program. The patch is used with patients who are willing to set a stop date, have significant nicotine addiction (smoke more than one pack per day or have had withdrawal symptoms), are willing to refrain from smoking while using the patch, and will participate in a structured behavioral program. Patches may be used for 24 h a day or for 16 h a day and removed at bedtime. Instruct patients to apply the patch to a nonhairy area of the skin on the trunk or the upper, outer area of the arm. Rotate the sites to avoid skin irritation. The patch can be worn in the shower or while swimming; however, perspiration can loosen the patch.

Begin with a 21-mg/day patch (strongest) for 4–6 weeks, gradually taper down to a 14-mg/day patch for 2–4 weeks, and finally go to a 7-mg/day patch (lowest) for 2–4 weeks. If the patient weighs less than 100 lb, begin with a 14-mg/day patch. The most common side effect of the nicotine patch is skin irritation, so patients with psoriasis or atopic dermatitis should consider another NRT delivery system. Use cautiously in patients with severe renal impairment or insulin-dependent diabetes mellitus because nicotine increases release of catecholamines. Patients who complain of insomnia may do better with a 16-mg/day patch that is removed at bedtime. Headache, nausea, vertigo, and dyspepsia have been reported with using the patch ("Nicotrol," 1997).

Nicotine nasal spray delivers nicotine to the nasal mucosa and provides a rapid response to nicotine craving. Patients should not smoke while using the nasal spray or use other nicotine-containing products. One dose of the spray delivers 1 mg of nicotine in two sprays (one spray in each nostril). Patients start on one or two doses per hour, increasing up to 40 mg (80

## TABLE 33–10.  RESOURCES FOR MANAGING SMOKING CESSATION

American Academy of Family Physicians
8880 Ward Parkway
Kansas City, MO 64114-2797
1-800-944-0000
"Smoking: Steps To Help You Break the Habit" or
    "Stop Smoking Kit"

American Academy of Pediatrics
P.O. Box 927
Elk Grove Village, IL 60009-0927
1-800-433-9016
"Smoking Guidelines for Teens"; "Tobacco Abuse—A
    Message to Parents and Teens"

American Cancer Society
1559 Clifton Rd. NE
Atlanta, GA 30329-4251
1-800-ACS-2345
"How to Quit Cigarettes"; "The Fifty Most Often Asked
    Questions about Smoking and Health and the
    Answers"; and other materials

American College of Obstetricians and Gynecologists
409 12th St. SW
Washington, DC 20024
1-800-762-2264
Technical Bulletin AT180, "Smoking and Reproductive
    Health?"; "Smoking in Women"

*For professionals:*
Office of Cancer Communications
National Cancer Institute
Bldg. 31, Rm. 10A24
Bethesda, MD 20892
1-800-4-CANCER
"Clinical Interventions to Prevent Tobacco Use by
    Children and Adolescents"; "How to Help Your
    Patients Stop Using Tobacco: A National Cancer
    Institute Manual for the Oral Health Team"; "How to
    Help Your Patients Stop Smoking: A National Cancer
    Institute Manual for Physicians"; and other materials

*For consumers:*
National Cancer Institute
Superintendent of Documents
Consumer Information Center—3C
P.O. Box 100
Pueblo, CO 81002
"Chew or Snuff Is Real Bad Stuff"; "Why Do You Smoke?"

National Heart, Lung, and Blood Institute
Smoking Education Program
P.O. Box 30105
Bethesda, MD 20824-0105
(301) 251-1222
"Clinical Opportunities for Smoking Intervention—A Guide
    for the Busy Physician"; "How You Can Help Your
    Patients Stop Smoking: Opportunity for Respiratory
    Care Practitioners"; "Nurses: Help Your Patients Stop
    Smoking"; "Check Your Smoking IQ: An Important
    Quiz for Older Smokers"; and other materials

Nicotine Anonymous World Services
P.O. Box 591777
San Francisco, CA 94159-1777
(415) 750-0329

Check your phone directory for smoking cessation re-
    sources sponsored by local chapters of the American
    Cancer Society, American Lung Association, American
    Heart Association, or state health departments.

Internet
These are some of the web sites available for persons in-
    terested in smoking cessation.
AHCPR Home Page
    http://www.ahcpr.gov/guide
    "Smoking Cessation: Clinical Practice Guideline" (The
        "Clinical Guidelines" is an excellent document for
        implementing a smoking cessation program into
        your practice.)
"For Smokers Only"
    http://www.dental.uab.edu/pubs/factlin/tobac.html
"Nicotine Anonymous"
    http://www.slip.net/n~billh/nic2home.htm

*Adapted from DHHS (1996).*

sprays) as needed to control withdrawal symptoms. Common side effects include nasal and
throat irritation, watering eyes, sneezing, and
cough. Usually patients adjust to these symp-

toms during the first week of treatment.
Nicotine nasal spray is contraindicated in pregnant or nursing smokers and is not recommended for patients with asthma or allergic

rhinitis. Benefits of using NRT for patients with cardiovascular and peripheral vascular diseases must be weighed against the risks of continued smoking. Nicotine nasal spray should not be used for longer than 6 months.

Generally, NRT is contraindicated for patients with a history of recent MI, increasing angina, severe arrhythmias, pregnancy, or lactation. Safe use in children under 18 has not been determined ("Nicotrol NS," 1997). For heavy smokers who are pregnant, less uterine contractions may occur with the lower nicotine levels in replacement therapy than if the woman continues to smoke (Brideau, 1997).

Bupropion hydrochloride (Zyban) is now approved for aiding smoking cessation and has minimal side effects (Hurt, Sacks, Glover, et al, 1997). It is not recommended in pregnancy or lactation.

## Monitoring for Efficacy

Phone or write patients within 7 days of the initial visit to remind them of their quit date. Schedule a clinic visit within 1–2 weeks after the patient's stop date. Assess smoking cessation progress to provide support and help prevent relapse. Remind the patient that relapse is common, and if it should happen, to try again immediately. The nicotine gum dose should be tapered after about 3 months and used for not more than 6 months. Although the patch may be used for up to 16 weeks, a 3-step–10-week program is recommended and detailed instructions accompany the product. The nasal spray may be continued for up to 6 months (DHHS, 1994).

## Monitoring for Toxicity

Signs and symptoms of nicotine toxicity include pallor, nausea, salivation, vomiting, abdominal pain, diarrhea, vision disturbances, dizziness, and mental confusion. Nausea, heartburn, and palpitations are the most often reported side effects of NRT. Assess for adverse reactions at each clinic visit or phone contact.

## Follow-up Recommendations

Regular follow-up with patients is critical to their smoking cessation success. Providers should use every clinic encounter to encourage the smoker to quit, to support smoking cessation efforts, and to refer to appropriate community resources.

## REFERENCES

Akiskal, H. S., Jensvold, M. F., Kramer, P. D., Paist, S. S., & Potter, W. Z. (1994). The wise use of psychiatric drugs. *Patient Care, 28*(26), 83–117.

American Psychiatric Association. (1993). Practice guidelines for eating disorders. *American Journal of Psychiatry, 150*(2), 207–234.

American Psychiatric Association. (1994a). Diagnostic and statistical manual of mental disorders (4th ed.). Washington, DC: APA.

American Psychiatric Association. (1994b). Practice guideline for the treatment of patients with bipolar disorder. *American Journal of Psychiatry, 151*(12) (Suppl.), 1–29.

Amsterdam, E. A., Carter, C., Holloway, R., & Schwenk, T. L. (1994). Is it normal worry or pathologic anxiety? *Patient Care, 28*(26), 26–36.

Andrews, R. C., Rocco, C., Hunt, C., Lampe, L., & Page, A. (1994). *The treatment of anxieties disorders: Clinicians guide and patient manuals.* New York: Cambridge University Press.

Arean, P. A., & Miranda, J. (1996). Do primary care patients accept psychological treatments? *General Hospital Psychiatry, 18*(1), 22–27.

Bierer, M. T. (1995). Case studies. In *American Society of Consultant Pharmacists symposia highlights.* San Francisco: ASCP.

Bjornson, W. M., Fiore, M. C., & Logan-Morrison, B. A. (1996). The growing problem of smoking in women. *Patient Care, 30*(13), 143–165.

Blondell, R. D., Frierson, R. L., & Lippmann, S. B. (1996). Alcoholism: Taking a preventive, public health approach. *Postgraduate Medicine, 100*(1), 69–80.

Bohn, M. J. (1993). Alcoholism. *Psychiatric Clinics of North America, 16*(4), 679–692.

Bolen, J. D., & Robbins, M. (1995). Mood disorders. In D. P. Lemcke, J. Pattison, L. A. Marshall, D. Cowley. *Primary care of women.* Norwalk, CT: Appleton & Lange.

Bowden, C. L., Brugger, A. M., & Swain, A. C. (1994). Efficacy of divalproex vs lithium and placebo in the treatment of mania. *JAMA, 271,* 918–924.

Brideau, D. J., Jr. (1997). Using nicotine replacement therapies. *Patient Care, 31,* 31–44.

Brown, T. M., Skop, B. P., & Mareth, T. R. (1996). Pathophysiology and management of the serotonin syndrome. *Annals of Pharmacotherapy, 30,* 527–533.

Bursztajn, H. J., Joshi, P. T., Sutherland, S. M., & Tomb, D. A. (1995, March 30). Recognizing posttraumatic stress. *Patient Care,* 40–61.

Buysse, D. J., & Reynolds, C. F., III. (1990). Insomnia. In M. J. Thorpy (Ed.), *Handbook of sleep disorders.* New York: Dekker.

Carter, C., Holloway, R., & Schwenk, T. L. (1994, November 15). Treating anxiety: A collaborative approach. *Patient Care*, 36–52.

Caulker-Burnett, I. (1994). Primary care screening for substance abuse. *Nurse Practitioner*, 19(6), 42–48.

Citrome, L. (1994). Management of depression. *Postgraduate Medicine*, 95(1), 137–143.

Cox, J. L. (1993). Algorithms for nicotine withdrawal therapy. *American Journal of Health Behavior*, 17(2), 41–50.

Crabtree, B. L., & Polles, A. (1997). Substance-related disorders. In J. R. DiPalma, G. J. DiGregorio, E. J. Barbieri, & A. P. Ferko (Eds.), *Basic pharmacology in medicine* (4th ed.). West Chester, PA: Medical Surveillance.

Crismon, M. L. (1992). Insomnia. In M. A. Koda-Kimble, L. Y. Young, W. A. Kradjan, & B. J. Guglielmo (Eds.), *Applied therapeutics: The clinical use of drugs* (5th ed.). Vancouver, WA: Applied Therapeutics.

Department of Health and Human Services. (1994). *Clinician's handbook of preventive services*. Waldorf, MD: American Nurses Association.

Department of Health and Human Services. (1996). Quick reference guide for clinicians. Smoking cessation: Information for specialists. *Journal of American Academy of Nurse Practitioners*, 8(7), 317–322.

Depression Guideline Panel. (1993a). *Clinical practice guideline number 5. Depression in primary care: Volume 1. Detection and diagnosis* (AHCPR Publication No. 93-0550). Washington, DC: U.S. Government Printing Office.

Depression Guideline Panel. (1993b). *Clinical practice guideline number 5. Depression in primary care: Volume 2. Treatment of major depression* (AHCPR Publication No. 93-0551). Washington, DC: U.S. Government Printing Office.

Drugs for psychiatric disorders. (1994). *Medical Letter*, 36(933), 89–96.

Dubovsky, S. L. (1995). Calcium channel antagonists as novel agents for manic-depressive disorder. In *The American Psychiatric Press textbook of psychopharmacology*. Washington, DC: Author.

El-Mallakh, R. S., Wright, J. C., Breen, K. J., & Lippann, S. B. (1996). Clues to depression in primary care practice. *Postgraduate Medicine*, 100(1), 85–96.

Engel, C. C., Kroenke, K., & Katon, W. J. (1994). Mental health services in army primary care: The need for a collaborative health care agenda. *Military Medicine*, 159(3), 203–209.

Fankhauser, M. P., & Benefield, W. H. (1997). Bipolar disorders. In J. T. DiPiro, R. L. Talbert, G. C. Yee, G. R. Matzke, B. G. Wells, & L. M. Posey (Eds.), *Pharmacotherapy: A pathophysiologic approach* (3rd ed.) (pp. 1419–1441). Stamford, CT: Appleton & Lange.

Federici, C. M., & Tommasini, N. R. (1992). The assessment and management of panic disorder. *Nurse Practitioner*, 17(3), 20–34.

First, M. B., Donovan, S., & Frances, A. (1996). Nosology of chronic mood disorders. *Psychiatric Clinics of North America*, 19(1), 29–39.

Fluoxetine Bulimia Nervosa Collaborative Study Group (1992). Fluoxetine in the treatment of bulimia nervosa. A multicenter placebo-controlled double-blind trial. *Archives of General Psychiatry*, 49, 139–147.

Friedman, R. A., & Kocsis, J. H. (1996). Pharmacotherapy for chronic depression. *Psychiatric Clinics of North America*, 19(1), 121–132.

Gallant, D. (1994). Alcohol. In M. Galanter, & H. D. Kleber (Eds.), *The American Psychiatric Press textbook of substance abuse treatment* (pp. 69–90). Washington, DC: American Psychiatric Press.

Gelenberg, A. J., Hirschfeld, R. M., Jefferson, J. W., Potter, W. Z., & Thase, M. E. (1995a). Bipolar disorder: Easy to miss, essential to treat. *Patient Care*, 29(19), 50–68, 71–94.

Gelenberg, A. J., Hirschfeld, R. M., Jefferson, J. W., Potter, W. Z., & Thase, M. E. (1995b). Bipolar disorder: Managing lithium therapy. *Patient Care*, 29(19), 71–94.

Gerchufsky, M. (1996, March). The art and science of prescribing psychiatric medications. *ADVANCE for Nurse Practitioners*, 33–36.

Gillin, J. C. (1992). Relief from situational insomnia. *Postgraduate Medicine*, 92(2), 157–160, 163–165.

Golwyn, D. H., & Sevlie, C. P. (1993). Monoamine oxidase inhibitor hypertensive crisis headache and orthostatic hypotension. *Journal of Clinical Psychopharmacology*, 13(1), 77–78.

Goroll, A., May, L., & Mulley, A. (1995). *Primary Care Medicine*. Philadelphia: J. B. Lippincott.

Graedon, J. & Graedon, T. (1995). *The people's guide to deadly drug interactions*. New York: St. Martin's Press.

Greensberg, P. E., Stiglin, L. E., Finkelstein, S. N., & Berndt, E. R. (1993). The economic burden of depression in 1990. *Journal of Clinical Psychiatry*, 54(11), 405–418.

Guelfi, J. D., White, C., Hackett, D., Guichoux, J. D., & Magoni, G. (1995). Effectiveness of venlafaxine in patients hospitalized for major depression and melancholia. *Journal of Clinical Psychiatry*, 56, 450–458.

Hahn, M. S. (1996, May). In search of mr. sandman. *ADVANCE for Nurse Practitioners*, 36–42.

Haimov, I., Lavie, P., Laudon, M., Herer, P., Vigder, C., & Zisapel, N. (1995). Melatonin replacement therapy of elderly insomniacs. *Sleep, 18*(7), 598–603.

Hales, R., Rakel, R., & Rothschild, S. (1994). Depression: Practical tips for detection and treatment. *Patient Care, 28*(26), 60–80.

Hanna, E. Z. (1995). Approach to the patient with alcohol abuse. In A. H. Goroll, L. A. May, & A. G. Mulley (Eds.), *Primary care medicine: Office evaluation and management of the adult patient* (3rd ed.). Philadelphia: J. B. Lippincott.

Hartman, P. M. (1995). Drug treatment of insomnia: Indications and newer agents. *American Family Physician, 51,* 191–194.

Holdcroft, C. (1993). Zolpidem: A nonbenzodiazepine hypnotic. *Nurse Practitioner, 18*(9), 21–22.

Holdcroft, C. (1994). Vanlafaxine: A new antidepressant drug. *Nurse Practitioner, 19*(9), 21.

Hollander, E., Jenike, M. A., & Shahady, E. J. (1996). Help for hands that can't stop washing. *Patient Care, 30*(11), 66–85.

Hurt, R. D., Sacks, D. P., Glover, B. D., et al. (1997). A comparison of sustained release buproprion and placebo for smoking cessation. *The New England Journal of Medicine, 337,* 1195–1202.

Janicak, P. G., Davis, J. M., Preskorn, S. H., & Ayd, F. (1993). *Principles and practice of psychopharmacotherapy.* Baltimore: Williams & Wilkins.

Jann, M. W., Jenike, M. A., & Lieberman, J. A. (1994, January 30). The new psychopharmaceuticals. *Patient Care,* 47–50, 53–61.

Jermain, D. (1996). Treatment of postpartum depression. *American Pharmacy, NS35*(1), 33–38.

Jessen, L. M. (1996, May). Depression. *Pharmacist,* 57–70.

Joffie, R. T. (1993). Valproate in bipolar disorder: The canadian perspective. *Canadian Journal of Psychiatry, 38* Supplement 2, 546–550.

Kahn, D. A. (1995). New strategies in bi-polar disorder part II: Treatment. *Journal of Practical Psychiatry and Behavioral Health, 1,* 148–157.

Kaplan, H. I., Sadock, B. J., & Grebb, J. A. (1994). *Synopsis of psychiatry* (7th ed.). Baltimore: Williams & Wilkins.

Katon, W., Sheehan, D. V., & Uhde, T. W. (1992). Panic disorder: A treatable problem. *Patient Care, 26*(8), 81–107.

Kay, W. H., Weltzin, T. E., Hsu, G., & Bulik, C. M. (1991). An open trial of fluoxetine in patients with anorexia nervosa. *Journal of Clinical Psychiatry, 52,* 464–471.

Kehoe, W. A., & Schorr, R. B. (1996). Focus of mirtazopine. *Hospital Formulary, 31,* 455–469.

Keller, M. B., & Hanks, D. L. (1994). The natural history and heterogeneity of depressive disorders: Implication for rational antidepressant therapy. *Journal of Clinical Psychiatry, 55*(9) (Suppl. A), 25–31.

Kessler, R. C., McGonagle, K. A., Zhao, S., et al. (1994). Lifetime and 12-month prevalence of DSM-III-R psychiatric disorders in the United States. Results from the national comorbidity survey. *Archives of General Psychiatry, 51,* 8–19.

Kirkwood, C. K. & Hayes, P. E. (1997). Anxiety disorders. In J. T. DiPiro, R. L. Talbert, G. C. Yee, G. R. Matzke, B. G. Wells, & L. M. Posey (Eds.), *Pharmacotherapy: A pathophysiologic approach* (3rd ed.). Stamford, CT: Appleton & Lange.

Kirkwood, C. K., & Sood, R. K. (1997). Sleep disorders. In J. T. DiPiro, R. L. Talbert, G. C. Yee, G. R. Matzke, B. G. Wells, & L. M. Posey (Eds.), *Pharmacotherapy: A pathophysiologic approach* (3rd ed.). Stamford, CT: Appleton & Lange.

Kocsis, J. H., Thase, M. E., Koran, L., et al (1994). Pharmacotherapy for pure dysthymia: Sertraline vs imipramine and placebo. *European Journal of Neuropsychopharmacology, 4,* 204.

Kulin, N. A., Pastuszak, M. Sc., Sage, S. R., et al. (1998). Pregnancy outcome following maternal use of the new selective serotonin reuptake inhibitors. *Journal of the American Medical Association, 279*(8), 609–610.

Kupsecz, D. (1995). New antidepressants. *Nurse Practitioner, 20*(9), 64–67.

Kuzel, R. (1996). Management of depression. *Postgraduate Medicine, 99*(5), 179–195.

Lipscomb, P. A., & Agostini, R. (1995). Disordered eating. In D. P. Lemche & J. Pattison (Eds.), *Primary care of women.* Norwalk, CT: Appleton & Lange.

Long, K., & Long, R. (1995). Treating obsessive-compulsive disorder. *Nurse Practitioner Forum, 6*(3), 136–137.

Long, M. C. (1993). Overview of substance abuse: Implications for the primary care nurse practitioner. *Nurse Practitioner Forum, 4*(4), 191–198.

Marken, P. & Sommi, R. (1997). Eating disorders. In J. T. DiPiro, R. L. Talbert, G. C. Yee, G. R. Matzke, B. G. Wells, & L. M. Posey (Eds.), *Pharmacotherapy: A pathophysiologic approach* (3rd ed.). Stamford, CT: Appleton & Lange.

Marshall, R. D., Schneier, F. R., Fallow, B. A., et al. (1994). Medication therapy for the treatment of panic disorder. *Neuropsychobiology, 27,* 150–153.

Mayfield, D., McLeod, G., & Hall, P. (1974). The CAGE questionnaire: Validation of a new alcoholism screening instrument. *American Journal of Psychiatry, 131*(10), 1121–1123.

Millard, W. B. (Ed.). (1994a). Depression: Serious, prevalent, detectable. *Patient Care, 28*(3), 30–63.

Millard, W. B. (Ed.). (1994b). Depression: A treatable medical condition. *Patient Care, 28*(3), 65–87.

Miller, I. & Keitner, G. (1996). Combined medication and psychotherapy. *Psychiatric Clinics of North America, 19*(1), 151–171.

Montgomery, S. A. (1994). Antidepressants in long-term treatment. *Annual Review of Medicine, 45,* 447–457.

Morin, C. M., Culbert, J. P., & Schwartz, S. M. (1994). Nonpharmacological interventions for insomnia: A meta-analysis of treatment efficacy. *American Journal of Psychiatry, 151,* 1172–1180.

Nicotrol: Nicotine transdermal system. (1997). In *Physicians' desk reference* (51st ed.). Montvale, NJ: Medical Economics.

Nicotrol NS. (1997). In *Physicians' desk reference* (51st ed.). Montvale, NJ: Medical Economics.

Nierenberg, A. A., Adler, L. A., Peselow, E., Zornberg, G., & Rosenthal, M. (1994). Trazodone for antidepressant-associated insomnia. *American Journal of Psychiatry, 151,* 1069–1072.

Ockene, J. K., & Kristeller, J. L. (1994). Tobacco. In M. G. Galenter, & H. D. Kugin (Eds.), *The American Psychiatric Press textbook of substance abuse treatment.* Washington, DC: American Psychiatric Press.

Olson, J. (1995). *Clinical pharmacology made ridiculously simple.* Miami: MedMaster.

O'Malley, S. S., Jaffe, A. J., Chang, G., Schottenfeld, R. S., Meyer, R. E., & Rounsaville, B. (1992). Naltrexone and coping skills therapy for alcohol dependence: A controlled study. *Archives of General Psychiatry, 49*(11), 881–887.

Pagel, J. F. (1994). Treatment of insomnia. *American Family Physician, 49*(6), 1417–1421, 1423–1424.

Potter, W. Z., & Ketter, T. A. (1993). Pharmacological issues in the treatment of bipolar disorder. Focus on mood stabilizing compounds. *Canadian Journal of Psychiatry, 38*(3) (Suppl. 2), 551–556.

Preskorn, S. H. (1996). Reducing the risk of drug-drug interactions: A goal of rational drug development. *Journal of Clinical Psychiatry, 57* (Suppl. 1), 3–6.

Price, L. H. & Heninger, G. R. (1994). Lithium in the treatment of mood disorders. *Drug Therapy, 331*(9), 591–595.

Rausch, S. L., & Hyman, S. E. (1995). Approach to the patient with depression. In A. H. Goroll, L. A. May, & A. G. Mulley (Eds.), *Primary care medicine: Office evaluation and management of the adult patient* (3rd ed.). Philadelphia: J. B. Lippincott.

Rausch, S. L., & Rosenbaum, J. F. (1995). Approach to the patient with anxiety. In A. H. Goroll, L. A. May, & A. G. Mulley (Eds.), *Primary care medicine: Office evaluation and management of the adult patient* (3rd ed.). Philadelphia: J. B. Lippincott.

Rickles, K., Downing, R., Scheizer, E., & Hassman, H. (1993). Antidepressants for the treatment of generalized anxiety disorder. *Archives of General Psychiatry, 50,* 884–895.

Rigotti, N. A. (1995a). Eating disorders. In A. H. Goroll, L. A. May, & A. G. Mulley, (eds.). *Primary care medicine: Office evaluation and management of the adult patient* (3rd ed.). Philadelphia, J. B. Lippincott.

Rigotti, N. A. (1995b). Smoking cessation. In A. H. Goroll, L. A. May, & A. G. Mulley (Eds.), *Primary care medicine: Office evaluation and management of the adult patient* (3rd ed.). Philadelphia: J. B. Lippincott.

Rock, C. L., & Zerbe, K. J. (1995). Keeping eating disorders at bay. *Patient Care, 29*(18), 78–104.

Roy-Byrne, P., Wingerson, D., Cowley, D., & Dager, S. (1993). Psychopharmacologic treatment of panic, generalized anxiety disorder, and social phobia. *Psychiatric Clinics of North America, 16*(4), 719–735.

Sansone, R. & Sansone, L. (1996). Dysthymic disorder. *Postgraduate medicine, 99*(6), 233–249.

Schlafer, M. (1993). *The nurse, pharmacology, and drug therapy: A prototype approach* (2nd ed.). Redwood City, CA: Addison-Wesley.

Schuckit, M. A. (1994). Goals of treatment. In M. Galanter & H. D. Kleber (Eds.), *The American Psychiatric Press textbook of substance abuse treatment* (pp. 3–10). Washington, DC: American Psychiatric Press.

Schwartz, R. H. (1996). Let's help young smokers quit. *Patient Care, 30*(3), 45–51.

Shader, R. I., & Greenblatt, D. J. (1993). Use of benzodiazepines in anxiety disorders. *New England Journal of Medicine, 328,* 1398–1405.

Simmons, D. H. (1996). Caffeine and its effect on persons with mental disorders. *Archives of Psychiatric Nursing, 2,* 116–122.

Sloan, R. W. (1995). Drug treatment of insomnia: Indications and newer agents. *American Family Physician, 51*(1), 191–194.

Sussman, N. (1994). The uses of buspirone in psychiatry [Monograph]. *Journal of Clinical Psychiatry, 12,* 3–19.

Sutherland, S. M., & Davidson, R. T. (1994). Pharmacotherapy for post-traumatic stress disorder. *Psychiatric Clinics of North America, 17*(2), 409–423.

Taylor, D., & Lader, M. (1996). Cytochromes and psychotropic drug interactions. *British Journal of Psychiatry, 168,* 529–532.

Triolo, A. J. (1997). Opoid analgesics. In J. R. DiPalma, G. J. DiGregorio, E. J. Barbieri, & A. P. Ferko (Eds.), *Basic pharmacology in medicine* (4th ed.). West Chester, PA: Medical Surveillance.

Turner, D. M. (1995). Panic disorder. A personal and nursing perspective. *Journal of Psychosocial Nursing, 33*(4), 5–8.

Valente, S. (1996). Diagnosis and treatment of panic disorder and generalized anxiety in primary care. *Nurse Practitioner, 21*(8), 26–45.

Ware, J. C., Rose, F. V., & McBrayer, R. H. (1994). The acute effects of nefazodone, trazodone, and buspirone on sleep and sleep-related penile tumescence in normal subjects. *Sleep, 17,* 544–550.

Weber, S. S., Saklad, S. R., & Kastenholz, K. V. (1992). Bipolar affective disorders. In M. A. Koda-Kimble, L. Y. Young, W. A. Kradjan, & B. J. Guglielmo (Eds.), *Applied therapeutics: The clinical use of drugs* (5th ed.). Vancouver, WA: Applied Therapeutics.

Wecker, L. (1994). Antianxiety drugs. In J. R. DiPalma, G. J. DiGregorio, E. J. Barbieri, & A. P. Ferko (Eds.), *Basic pharmacology in medicine* (4th ed.). West Chester, PA: Medical Surveillance.

Weilburg, J. B. (1995). Approach to the patient with insomnia. In A. H. Goroll, L. A. May, & A. G. Mulley (Eds.), *Primary care medicine: Office evaluation and management of the adult patient* (3rd ed.). Philadelphia: J. B. Lippincott.

Wells, B. G., Mandos, L. A., & Hayes, D. E. (1997). Depressive disorders. In J. T. DiPiro, R. L. Talbert, G. C. Yee, G. R. Matzke, B. G. Wells, & L. M. Posey (Eds.), *Pharmacotherapy: A pathophysiologic approach* (3rd ed.). Stamford, CT: Appleton & Lange.

Winokur, G., Coryell, W., Endicott, J., & Akiskal, H. (1994). Further distinctions between manic-depressive illness (bipolar disorder) and primary depressive disorder (unipolar depression). *American Journal of Psychiatry, 151*(9), 1397–1398.

Yager, J. (1994). Psychosocial treatments for eating disorders. *Psychiatry, 57,* 153–164.

Zerbe, K. J. (1996). Anorexia nervosa and bulimia nervosa. *Postgraduate Medicine, 99*(1), 161–170.

Zisook, S. (1996). Depression in late life. *Postgraduate Medicine, 100*(4), 161–172.

# 34

## URINARY TRACT DISORDERS AND MALE SEXUAL DYSFUNCTION

*Linda D. Scott and David H. Nelson*

Urinary tract infections (UTIs) are some of the most frequently treated health problems in primary care. Infections of the upper and lower urinary account for 7 million visits to health care providers, contribute to more than 1 million hospital admissions, and cost approximately $1 billion annually. Statistical data in the literature rarely differentiate between lower and upper UTIs. UTI syndromes range from uncomplicated to complex, relate to an inflammatory response, and describe an anatomical site of infection (Barger & Woolner, 1995; Hassay, 1995; Hooton, 1995; Mullenix & Prince, 1997). Definitions of UTIs are listed in Table 34–1. This chapter addresses the treatment of selected urinary tract infections across the life span and covers lower UTIs; upper UTIs; stress urinary incontinence; and male urinary tract disorders, such as epididymitis, urethritis, prostatitis, benign prostatic hyperplasia (BPH), and male sexual dysfunction. It also presupposes that the treatment is for healthy patients who do not have renal complications or neurologic or urologic abnormalities.

## LOWER URINARY TRACT INFECTIONS

*Cystitis* and *urethritis* (inflammation of the bladder and urethra) are characterized by dysuria, frequency, urgency, hesitancy, back pain, nocturia, and suprapubic heaviness or pain (Barger & Woolner, 1995; Hassay, 1995; Hooton, 1995; Mullenix & Prince, 1997). The most common pathogen of community-acquired UTIs is the gram-negative bacillus *Escherichia coli* (80%), followed by gram-positive coccus *Staphylococcus saprophyticus* (5–15%), and less frequently, *Klebsiella pneumoniae*, *Proteus mirabilis*, *Pseudomonas aeruginosa*, and *Enterococcus faecalis* (Hassay, 1995; Mullenix & Prince, 1997; Stamm & Hooton, 1993).

The prevalence of UTIs relates to age and gender. In newborns and infants up to age 1, the prevalence of bacteriuria is 1%, more common in males, and relates to structural or functional abnormalities. UTIs in males after age 1 is rare, with incidence increasing after age 50 and relating to prostatic obstruction (Hooton, 1995; Howes, 1992; Mullenix & Prince, 1997; Stamm & Hooton, 1993).

The incidence of UTIs after age 1 year is most common in females (1–5%) and dramatically increases by 1–4% after puberty. Risk factors for UTIs include frequency of sexual intercourse, use of diaphragm and spermicide, delayed coital micturition, pregnancy, and history of recent UTIs. Symptomatic cystitis in females is commonly associated with chlamydia, *Neisseria gonorrhoeae*, herpes simplex infections, fungal infections, or mycobacterial (tuberculosis is the most common) infections. It is estimated that 20% of all females experience discomforts of UTIs in their lifetimes, accounting for 5–15% of annual visits to health care providers, with 20% of these experiencing recurrent UTIs. Morbidity, time lost at work, cost of medical care, and psychological and emotional stress are experienced with urinary dis-

---

**TABLE 34–1. DEFINITIONS OF UPPER AND LOWER URINARY TRACT INFECTIONS**

| Term | Definition |
| --- | --- |
| **Lower Urinary Tract** | |
| Uncomplicated cystitis | Infection in a healthy individual by a common pathogen. Presents with symptoms of fever, chills, nausea, vomiting, diarrhea, constipation, hematuria, abdominal and back pain, and vaginal or urethral secretions. |
| Asymptomatic cystitis | Infection with significant bacteria (>10$^5$ CFU/mL of urine) and the absence of symptoms. |
| Symptomatic cystitis | Complaints of frequency, urgency, and dysuria in the presence of significant bacteria. |
| Reinfection | Infection with no association to a previous infection and causation of a different organism. |
| Relapse | Infection within 2–3 weeks after a previous infection by the same organism. May be associated with pyelonephritis, stone, or anatomical abnormality. |
| Complicated cystitis | Infection associated with structural, neurologic, or congenital abnormalities or distortion of urinary tract. Associated conditions include diabetes, pregnancy, age >65 years, UTI in prior 6 weeks, urinary symptoms >7 days, use of a diaphragm, and symptoms of upper UTI. |
| **Upper Urinary Tract** | |
| Uncomplicated pyelonephritis | Infection in a healthy individual by a common pathogen. Varies from mild to severe state and characterized by systemic symptoms of acute onset of fever (101°F or 38.5°C), headache, frank shaking chills, CVA tenderness, and nausea or vomiting or both. |
| Complicated pyelonephritis | Infection by common pathogen and associated with structural, neurologic, or congenital abnormalities that interfere with normal urinary flow. Associated with diabetes, pregnancy, age >65 years, UTIs in prior 6 weeks, stones, prostatic hypertrophy, and indwelling catheter. Acute onset of systemic symptoms of fever (>101°F or 38.5°C), frank shaking chills, moderate to severe CVA tenderness, abdominal pains, nausea, vomiting, malaise, headache, dehydration, and possible hematuria. Varies from mild to severe state. |

---

comfort (Barger & Woolner, 1995; Hooton, 1995; Howes, 1992; Mullenix & Prince, 1997; Stamm & Hooton, 1993).

UTI, specifically asymptomatic bacteriuria, is the most common complication of pregnancy. It occurs in 4–7% of normal pregnancies and is comparable to the prevalence in sexually active nonpregnant females of reproductive age. UTI places the pregnant female at risk for adverse outcomes, such as preterm labor, low birth weight, preeclampsia, and chronic renal disease. Socioeconomic status, sickle cell trait, diabetes mellitus, and multiparity are factors that relate to increased prevalence, with a twofold increase during pregnancy (Kiningham, 1993; Mullenix & Prince, 1997).

The overall incidence of asymptomatic cystitis increases substantially after the age of 65 years and is approximately equal for both genders. The rate of incidence further increases for institutionalized and hospitalized elders. This relates to prostatic hypertrophy, poor bladder emptying with prolapse in females, absence of estrogen effects, fecal incontinence, neuromuscular diseases, and increased urinary instrumentation or catheterization (Howes, 1992; Mullenix & Prince, 1997; Stamm & Hooton, 1993).

## SPECIFIC CONSIDERATIONS FOR PHARMACOTHERAPY

### When Drug Therapy Is Needed

Cystitis needs to be treated with antibiotics when the patient presents with symptoms and/or the disease is confirmed with diagnostic testing. Prompt diagnosis is essential because the incidence of disease varies according to age and gender; may be symptomatic or asymptomatic; and has the potential for renal scarring or serious damage to the urinary system (Barger & Woolner, 1995; Hooton, 1995; Howes, 1992; Stamm & Hooton, 1993). The key to diagnosis is confirmation of significant numbers of pathogens in an appropriate urine specimen. The type and extent of laboratory examination depends on the clinical situation (Hooton, 1995; Howes, 1992; Mullenix & Prince, 1997; Stamm & Hooton, 1993). Health care providers need to educate patients fully to side effects and costs of antibiotic therapy as well as the benefits and harms of other options of care.

### Short- and Long-Term Goals of Pharmacotherapy

The short-term goals of treatment for uncomplicated and complicated cystitis are to resolve the infection, restore normal physiological function of the urinary tract, and prevent future recurrence of infection. The long-term goals of treatment for uncomplicated cystitis are to prevent recurrent episodes of infection and renal complications. The long-term goals of treatment for complicated cystitis are to correct any physiological abnormality when possible and prevent reinfection or renal complications.

In each condition of the lower urinary tract, treatment goals are achieved primarily by antibiotic therapy and patient education.

### Time Frame for Initiating Pharmacotherapy

Treatment for cystitis should be initiated when the patient presents with complaints or by laboratory confirmation of diagnosis to prevent the serious sequelae discussed. A course of antibiotics is the required therapy to eliminate causative bacteria. Significant improvement of symptoms is expected in 24–48 h (Barger & Woolner, 1995; Hooton, 1995; Howes, 1992; Kiningham, 1993; Mullenix & Prince, 1997; Stamm & Hooton, 1993).

See Drug Tables 102.1–102.7, 102.10, 903.

### Assessment and History Taking

Refer to Tables 34–2 and 34–3.

---

### TABLE 34–2. BASELINE DATA: HISTORY AND PHYSICAL EXAMINATION FOR URINARY TRACT INFECTIONS

**History**
Onset and duration of symptoms and voiding patterns
Sequence of dysuria in voiding pattern
Past medical history (drugs, allergies, chronic diseases, previous genitourinary problems and treatment)
Sexual (LMP, length of menopausal state, sexual behaviors, frequency of coitus, risk for STDs)
Contraception

**Physical Examination**
Vital signs: note elevation of temperature and hydration status
Complete abdominal examination: note suprapubic tenderness
Costovertebral tenderness (CVA)
Females: inspect perineum; complete pelvic, speculum, and rectal examinations
Males: inspect and palpate external genitalia; prostate, and rectal examination
Children: observe general appearance for pallor, diaphoresis, listlessness, signs of sepsis, and dehydration
Elders: usually asymptomatic and present with altered mental status, change in eating habits, or gastrointestinal
  symptoms

## TABLE 34–3. DIAGNOSTIC TESTS FOR URINARY TRACT INFECTIONS

**Urine Collection**
- Midstream clean-catch voided specimens (preferably first morning specimen or wait 2 hours after last voiding)
- Single-time catherization if unable to obtain clean midstream specimen

**Urinalysis**
- Dipstick
  Positive leukocyte esterase test indicates pyuria
  Positive nitrite denotes presence of gram-negative bacteria only
  Positive blood indicates infection
- Microscopic analysis
  Significant pyuria is >2–5 WBCs per high-power field in centrifuged specimen
  Complete Gram's stain to identify if positive or negative plus shape and pattern
  Presence of hematuria or RBCs
  Sterile pyuria suggests presence of STDs
- Urine culture and sensitivity
  Determine organism for type of cystitis
  Obtain with all children, all men, initial prenatal visits, and females with renal abnormalities, immunocompromise,
    diabetes mellitus, prolonged symptoms, three or more UTIs in past year, or pyelonephritis
  Significant hematuria is $\leq 10^2$ CFU/mL of urine
  Determine bacteria and antibiotic sensitivity

**Tests for STDs**
Wet mount for vaginal or urethral secretions
*Neisseria gonorrhoeae* culture
Chlamydia test

**CBC with Differential for Systemic Symptoms**

**Consider Erythrocyte Sedimentation Rate**

**Rule out Pregnancy When Indicated**

**For Complicated Cystitis or Complicated Pyelonephritis**
Refer for renal ultrasound, intravenous pyelogram (IVP), renal scan, renal biopsy, cystoscopy, voiding
    cystourethrogram

## Patient/Caregiver Information

Educating the patient concerning signs and symptoms of the disease, drug therapy, and prevention measures is critical for positive outcomes. Refer to Table 34–4.

## OUTCOMES MANAGEMENT

### Selecting an Appropriate Agent

Patient factors of age, gender, presence or absence of symptoms, pregnancy, drug or environmental hypersensitivities, adherence to therapy regimen, and recent antibiotic therapy must be considered in selecting an appropriate drug and regimen to treat UTIs. Drug features of cost, safety, urinary excretion, effects on bowel and vaginal flora, local sensitivity, and resistance patterns are important considerations (Hassay, 1995; Mullenix & Prince, 1997; Stamm & Hooton, 1993). Refer to Table 34–5 for antibiotic recommendations for the following lower and upper UTIs.

***Symptomatic Uncomplicated Cystitis.*** The diagnosis is based on symptoms, and a pretreatment urine culture is not required. Single-dose ther-

## TABLE 34–4. PATIENT/CAREGIVER INFORMATION FOR URINARY TRACT INFECTIONS

Drink adequate amounts of fluid, 2–4 L daily
Avoid excessive intake of carbonated beverages, coffee, tea, or alcohol
Ensure nutrition is adequate
Establish frequent, regular urinary elimination patterns
Avoid retention of urine or delay of elimination
Practice good perineal hygiene by wiping perineal area front to back
Wash hands before and after urination
Shower or bathe daily, taking particular attention to cleansing perineal area
Know the signs and symptoms of infection and how important it is to seek health care
   immediately

apy of trimethoprin-sulfamethoxazole (TMP-SMX) or fluoroquinolones (FQLNs) is not as effective and is associated with a higher failure rate than the 3-day course. Three-day courses are as effective as the traditional 7 to 10-day therapies and have fewer side effects (Barger & Woolner, 1995; Hassay, 1995; Hooton, 1995; Howes, 1992; Mullenix & Prince, 1997; Stamm & Hooton, 1993).

**Asymptomatic Uncomplicated Cystitis.** Therapy recommendations depend on the patient's age, presence of pregnancy, and urine culture ($\geq 10^2$ CFU/mL) (Barger & Woolner, 1995; Hassay, 1995; Mullenix & Prince, 1997, Stamm & Hooton, 1993). For therapy recommendations for children, pregnant females, and elders, refer to "Special Situations" in Table 34–5.

**Reinfection.** Differentiation between reinfection and relapse is critical for appropriate drug selection. Reinfection is viewed as a new UTI; however, serial reinfections require a review of the patient's health habits and risk factors. Changes in risk factors such as changing from a diaphragm to birth control pills or daily application of estrogen vaginal cream in postmenopausal females to decrease colonization of E. coli, and education about preventive measures may reduce the frequency of reinfection (Mullenix & Prince, 1997; Stamm & Hooton, 1993).

**Relapse.** Relapse or treatment failure requires resolution of the source of infection and potentially a change of drugs. Further diagnostic evaluation is needed to rule out prostatitis, stones, occult upper UTI, or a resistant organism. Urine cultures guide antibiotic selection (Mullenix & Prince, 1997; Stamm & Hooton, 1993).

**Complicated Cystitis.** The choice of antibiotics is guided by the pretreatment urine culture (Barger & Woolner, 1995; Hassay, 1995; Howes, 1992; Mullenix & Prince, 1997; Stamm & Hooton, 1993).

**Symptomatic Relief.** The patient needs to be aware that phenazopyridine changes the color of urine and other body fluids. Do not use antispasmodics, such as hyoscyamine, unless the patient's symptoms are severe because they exert strong systemic anticholinergic effects (Howes, 1992; Mullenix & Prince, 1997).

**Special Situations.** *Pregnant patients* with bacteriuria or pyuria must be treated aggressively, including close monitoring. Pretreatment urine cultures guide therapy. TMP/SMX is a good economic choice during the first two trimesters, but is contraindicated during the third trimester because of the risk of inducing kernicterus in the fetus. Nitrofurantoin appears safe for pregnancy and a reasonable choice in cases of penicillin allergies. FLQNs and tetracyclines are contraindicated in pregnancy because of potential adverse effects on fetal bone development (Kiningham, 1993; Mullenix & Prince, 1997).

Drug selection for *children* and *elders* is guided by pretreatment urine cultures as necessary (Howes, 1992; Sherbotie & Cornfield, 1991).

### Monitoring for Efficacy

**Symptomatic Uncomplicated Cystitis.** Symptom resolution within 24–48 hours is considered sufficient monitoring of outcomes. Persistence of symptoms or continued bacteriuria requires a urine culture before resuming therapy for 7–10 days. All patients with positive pretreatment cultures must have a posttreatment urine

**TABLE 34–5. EMPIRIC ANTIBIOTIC RECOMMENDATIONS FOR UPPER AND LOWER URINARY TRACT INFECTIONS**

| Diagnosis | Antibiotic | Regimen | Preference |
|---|---|---|---|
| **Lower Urinary Tract: Cystitis** | | | |
| **Uncomplicated** | | | |
| Symptomatic or | TMP-SMX | Give for 3 days[a] | 1st |
| asymptomatic | FLQN | Give for 3 days[a] | 2nd |
| Reinfection (single event) | Same as symptomatic or asymptomatic | | |
| Reinfection (serial— | TMP-SMX | Single dose postcoital[a] | 1st |
| associated with coitus) | FLQN | Single dose postcoital[a] | 2nd |
| Reinfection (serial— | TMP-SMX | For 3 days with onset of symptoms[a] | 1st |
| genetic risk) | FLQN | For 3 days with onset of symptoms[a] | 2nd |
| Relapse | Follow culture and sensitivity results | Treat for 14+ days | |
| **Complicated** | TMP-SMX | Give for 7–14 days[a] | 1st |
| | FLQN | Give for 7–14 days[a] | 2nd |
| **Symptomatic relief** | Phenazopyridine | 100–200 mg PO t.i.d. for maximum 3 days | |
| **Special Situations** | | | |
| Pregnancy | Amoxicillin | 500 mg PO t.i.d. for 14 days | 1st |
| | Cephalexin | 500 mg PO q.i.d. for 14 days | Alt |
| | Amoxicillin-clavulanate | 500 mg PO t.i.d. for 14 days | 2nd |
| | Third-generation cephalosporin | Give for 14 days[a] | Alt |
| Children | | | |
| <6 weeks | Amoxicillin | Give for 7–10 days[a] | 1st |
| | Cephalexin | Give for 7–10 days[a] | 2nd |
| >6 weeks | TMP-SMX | Give for 7–10 days[a] | 1st |
| All ages | Amoxicillin-clavulanate | Give for 7–10 days[a] | Alt |
| | Third-generation cephalosporin | Give for 7–10 days[a] | Alt |
| Elders | | | |
| Symptomatic | Same as for any adult | | |
| Asymptomatic | No treatment indicated | | |
| **Upper Urinary Tract: Pyelonephritis** | | | |
| **Uncomplicated** (Mild to moderate symptoms) | | | |
| Gram-negative bacilli | TMP-SMX | Give for 10–14 days[a] | 1st |
| | FLQN | Give for 10–14 days[a] | Alt |
| Gram-positive cocci | Amoxicillin | 500 mg po t.i.d. for 10–14 days | 1st |
| | Amoxicillin-clavulanate | 500 mg po t.i.d. for 10–14 days | Alt |
| (Moderate to severe symptoms) | Hospitalization | | |
| **Complicated** | | | |
| (Mild to moderate symptoms) | Same as uncomplicated | | |
| (Moderate to severe symptoms) | Hospitalization | | |

(continues on next page)

**TABLE 34–5.** *(continued)*

**Special Situations**

| | |
|---|---|
| Pregnancy | Hospitalization |
| Children | Hospitalization |
| Elders | Hospitalization |

[a]See drug table for specific doses for various agents or ages.
Alt = alternative; FLQN = fluoroquinolone; TMP-SMX = trimethoprim-sulfamethoxazole.

culture in 1–2 weeks on completion of therapy to verify sterilization of the urine (Hooton, 1995; Mullenix & Prince, 1997).

***Asymptomatic Uncomplicated Cystitis.*** A posttreatment urine analysis (UA) or dipstick assessment of asymptomatic UTIs is recommended. Continued bacteriuria requires a urine culture before resuming therapy for 7–10 days. All patients with positive pretreatment urine cultures must have a posttreatment urine culture 1–2 weeks after completion of therapy to verify sterilization of the urine (Hooton, 1995; Mullenix & Prince, 1997).

***Reinfection.*** Patients with infrequent reinfections need to be monitored as if they have separately occurring symptomatic or asymptomatic infections. Patients on chronic prophylaxis or self-directed therapy require periodic urine cultures during and on completion of 6–12 months of therapy. If symptoms redevelop after discontinuation of prophylaxis, initiate a full course of therapy and follow with continuous prophylaxis (Mullenix & Prince, 1997; Stamm & Hooton, 1993).

***Relapse.*** Monitor patients with relapse infections periodically with urine cultures. Efficacy of therapy is achieved with symptom resolution. If relapse infections continue, refer the patient for comprehensive urological evaluation (Mullenix & Prince, 1997; Stamm & Hooton, 1993).

***Complicated Cystitis.*** A urine culture in 1–2 weeks posttherapy is essential to demonstrate cure. A positive urine culture requires resolution of treatable risk factors and is followed by 2 weeks or more of antibiotic therapy. Urine culture results guide drug selection (Hooton, 1995; Mullenix & Prince, 1997).

***Special Situations.*** *Pregnant patients* with a positive urine culture must be screened for reinfec-

tion or relapse through the remainder of the pregnancy and at the 6-week postpartum examination. Serial reinfections or relapses require chronic prophylaxis with ampicillin 250 mg twice daily, nitrofurantoin 100 mg once daily, or cephalexin 250 mg twice daily. A comprehensive postpartum urological evaluation is essential (Kiningham, 1993).

*Children* with any treatment failure require a comprehensive urological diagnostic evaluation. Ureteral reflux in combination with infection may lead to permanent renal damage (Howes, 1992; Sherbotie & Cornfield, 1991).

## Monitoring for Toxicity

Refer to the Drug Tables 102.1–102.7, 102.10, 903.

## Follow-up Recommendations

Patient follow-up should be scheduled in 10–14 days if symptoms persist. Resolution of symptomatic and asymptomatic cystitis requires no follow-up. Reinfected cystitis and all patients with complicated cystitis require posttreatment urine cultures and correction of identified abnormalities on completion of antibiotic therapy or within 14 days. All pregnant patients require repeat urine cultures every 2 weeks until delivery and at postpartum examination (Barger & Woolner, 1995; Hassay, 1995; Hooton, 1995; Howes, 1992; Kiningham, 1993; Mullenix & Prince, 1997; Stamm & Hooton, 1993).

# UPPER URINARY TRACT INFECTIONS

## PYELONEPHRITIS

Pyelonephritis (inflammation of the renal parenchyma and collecting system) varies from mild to severe states and is characterized by systemic symptoms and lower urinary tract symptoms. Differentiation of pyelonephritis from cystitis is not always possible (Barger & Woolner, 1995; Hassay, 1995; Hooton, 1995; Howes, 1992; Johnson, 1992; Mullenix & Prince, 1997; Plattner, 1994; Stamm & Hooton, 1993). Clinical presentation, laboratory findings, and pathologic findings assist the clinician in determining a definitive diagnosis of pyelonephritis (Talner, Davidson, Lebowitz, Palma, & Goldman, 1994).

Pyelonephritis occurs when organisms ascend from the lower to upper urinary tract or arrive via the blood or lymphatic systems. The most common pathogen of pyelonephritis is the gram-negative bacillus E. coli (80–90%), with unique subgroups of specific virulence. Gram-positive S. saprophyticus accounts for 5–10% of cases and K. pneumoniae, P. mirabilis, P. aeruginosa, or E. faecalis present less frequently (Hooton, 1995; Mullenix & Prince, 1997; Stamm & Hooton, 1993).

The prevalence of pyelonephritis relates to age and gender. In newborns and infants up to age 1, the prevalence of bacteriuria is 1–5%, and it is more prevalent in febrile infants (5%), more common in males, and connected with structural or functional abnormalities. Pyelonephritis after age 1 is more common in females and dramatically increases by 1–4% after puberty. Risk factors for pyelonephritis include frequency of sexual intercourse, use of diaphragms and spermicide, delayed coital micturition, pregnancy, history of recent UTIs, and history of structural abnormalities (Hooton, 1995; Howes, 1992; Johnson, 1992; Mullenix & Prince, 1997; Plattner, 1994; Reynolds & Hoberman, 1995; Stamm & Hooton, 1993).

Pyelonephritis occurs in 1–2% of all pregnancies and is the most common nonobstetric cause of hospitalization. Untreated or unidentified asymptomatic cystitis progresses to pyelonephritis in 20–40% of all pregnant females. Pyelonephritis places the pregnant female at risk for adverse outcomes, such as preterm labor, septicemia, intrauterine growth retardation, anemia, altered renal function, and chronic renal disease. The prevalence of pyelonephritis directly relates to normal physiological changes of pregnancy and needs to be monitored through routine prenatal screenings (Plattner, 1994).

The overall incidence of pyelonephritis increases after the age of 65 years and is approximately equal for both genders. The rate of incidence further increases for institutionalized and hospitalized elders. This relates to prostatic hypertrophy, poor bladder emptying with prolapse in females, absence of estrogen effects, fecal incontinence, neuromuscular diseases, and increased urinary instrumentation or catheterization (Hooton, 1995; Howes, 1992; Johnson, 1992; Mullenix & Prince, 1997; Stamm & Hooton, 1993).

## SPECIFIC CONSIDERATIONS FOR PHARMACOTHERAPY

### When Drug Therapy Is Needed

Pyelonephritis is treated with antibiotics when the patient presents with symptoms or the disease is confirmed by diagnostic findings. Prompt diagnosis and treatment are essential because the incidence varies according to age and gender; the degree of systemic illness may advance rapidly; and the potential for renal scarring leads to chronic problems, such as hypertension or end-stage renal disease (Barger & Woolner, 1995; Hooton, 1995; Howes, 1992; Mullenix & Prince, 1997; Plattner, 1994; Reynolds & Hoberman, 1995; Stamm & Hooton, 1993).

The key to diagnosis is confirmation of significant numbers of pathogens in an appropriate urine specimen (Hooton, 1995; Howes, 1992; Johnson, 1992; Mullenix & Prince, 1997; Plattner, 1994; Reynolds & Hoberman, 1995; Stamm & Hooton, 1993). The type and extent of laboratory and radiological examinations depend on the clinical situation. Health care providers need to educate patients to side effects and costs of antibiotic therapy as well as benefits and harms of other options of care.

### Short- and Long-Term Goals of Pharmacotherapy

The short-term goals of treatment for uncomplicated and complicated pyelonephritis are to resolve the infection, restore normal physiological function of the urinary tract, and prevent further recurrence of infection. The long-term goals for uncomplicated pyelonephritis are to prevent recurrence of infection and renal complications. The long-term goals for complicated pyelonephritis are to correct the physiological abnormality when possible and prevent reinfection or renal complications. In each of the conditions of the upper urinary tract, the treatment goals are achieved primarily by antibiotic therapy and patient education.

### Nonpharmacologic Therapy

Patient education of prevention measures is located in Table 34–4.

## Time Frame for Initiating Pharmacotherapy

Pyelonephritis requires immediate treatment when patients present with complaints or laboratory confirmation of diagnosis to prevent the serious sequelae discussed. The clinician needs to determine the patient's degree of systemic illness (bacteremia) because that guides the treatment regimen of outpatient or inpatient care and the choice of oral or parenteral antibiotic therapy. The clinician should consider hospitalization of those patients who are pregnant, vomiting, dehydrating, and have a history of chronic disease or of nonadherence to therapies (Hooton, 1995; Howes, 1992; Johnson, 1992; Mullenix & Prince, 1997; Plattner, 1994; Reynolds & Hoberman, 1995; Stamm & Hooton, 1993; Talner et al, 1994).

See Drug Table 102.

## Assessment and History Taking

Refer to Tables 34–2 and 34–3.

## Patient/Caregiver Information

Education of the patient concerning signs and symptoms of the disease, drug therapy, and prevention measures is critical for positive outcomes. Refer to Table 34–4.

## OUTCOMES MANAGEMENT

### Selecting an Appropriate Agent

Consider age, gender, pregnancy, drug or environmental hypersensitivities, concurrent diseases, recent antibiotic therapy, recent institutionalization, adherence to therapy regimen, and presence, absence, or severity of symptoms when selecting appropriate drugs and regimen to treat pyelonephritis. Cost, safety, urinary excretion, effects on bowel and vaginal flora, local sensitivity, resistance patterns, and efficacy are drug features of importance. Laboratory findings guide antibiotic selection (Bergeron, 1995; Mullenix & Prince, 1997).

Empiric therapy is based on the Gram's stain results and directed toward specific bacteria groups. The degree of systemic disease determines whether oral or parenteral therapy is required. Patients with nausea and vomiting, who are acutely ill, under 5 years old, over 65 years, immunosuppressed, diabetic, or pregnant must be hospitalized for parenteral therapy (Bergeron,

1995; Mullenix & Prince, 1997; Stamm & Hooton, 1993).

Costs of failure to treat pyelonephritis promptly and aggressively often outweigh any potential drug costs. Pretreatment urine cultures allow for effective and economical antibiotic selection. With decreases in the patient's symptoms, a change from parenteral to oral therapy contributes to cost savings, such as an oral FLQN following parenteral aminoglycoside therapy (Bergeron, 1995; Mullenix & Prince, 1997; Stamm & Hooton, 1993).

***Uncomplicated and Complicated Pyelonephritis.*** Refer to Table 34–5. Patents with complicated pyelonephritis are generally hospitalized for parenteral therapy and resolution of the obstruction, stone, or complicating factor (Bergeron, 1995; Mullenix & Prince, 1997).

***Special Situations.*** Pregnant patients with pyelonephritis require hospitalization for parenteral therapy (Bergeron, 1995; Plattner, 1994). In *males*, pyelonephritis is considered a complicated infection unless the urologic diagnostic evaluation proves otherwise (Bergeron, 1995; Mullenix & Prince, 1997). *Elders* tend to have more bacteremia than other age groups; therefore, a blood culture is prudent before initiating therapy (Baldassarre & Kaye, 1991). For *children* and for all groups, refer to Table 34–5.

### Monitoring for Efficacy

***Uncomplicated Pyelonephritis.*** Assess all patients' clinical responses to drug therapy within 12–72 hours. Utilize follow-up urine culture results to modify antibiotic therapy as needed. Resolution of clinical symptoms and a sterile urine culture within 2 weeks indicate that further therapy is not needed. A final urine culture is performed 2 months after therapy completion. If the patient's symptoms persist, assess for antibiotic resistance and perform diagnostic evaluation to rule out complicated pyelonephritis or abscess (Bergeron, 1995; Mullenix & Prince, 1997).

***Complicated Pyelonephritis.*** Continue medical management and utilize urine culture results for modification of antibiotic therapy. Resolution of clinical symptoms and a sterile urine culture 2 weeks after completion of drug therapy indicate that further drug therapy is not needed. The clinician needs to monitor for complications or obstruction until a final urine culture is obtained 2 months after therapy completion. If symptoms persist, expand the diagnostic evaluation, assess for a drug-resistant organism strain, and consider surgical intervention. If urine cultures indicate S. aureus, determine if it is a real pathogen or urine sample contaminant. This organism presents in renal tissue by blood rather than ascending the urinary tract and requires that an abscess be ruled out (Bergeron, 1995; Stamm & Hooton, 1993).

*Special Situations.* For *pregnant patients*, a urine culture is essential on completion of drug therapy and every 2 weeks until delivery. Those with serial relapse or reinfection cystitis and recurrent episodes of pyelonephritis need extensive diagnostic evaluation during pregnancy and up to 3 months postpartum (Kiningham, 1993; Plattner, 1994).

*Children* under the age of 1 year are at risk for recurrence of pyelonephritis (30%) within 1 year. Close follow-up for this age group is critical. Obtain urine cultures every 3 months after the infection is resolved, monitor febrile episodes, and educate parents on prevention measures, potential complications, and the need to seek health care when signs and symptoms of pyelonephritis present (Reynolds & Hoberman, 1995).

Assess *elders'* response to drug therapy within 12 h and then as recommended for all adults. Treatment response may be affected by multiply resistant or nosocomial organisms, such as *P. aerguinosa* or *E. faecalis*. Increased rates of hospitalization, institutional care, or catheter use by elders enhances the opportunity for treatment failure from these organisms (Baldassarre & Kaye, 1991).

## Monitoring for Toxicity

Elders, diabetics, and patients with chronic disease or severe renal infections require blood urea nitrogen and serum creatinine tests to monitor renal function. Aminoglycoside doses are adjusted according to renal function as they are ototoxic and nephrotoxic. Low-dose, 3-day therapy of aminoglycosides does not routinely require serum level monitoring. Moderate aminoglycoside serum levels in pyelonephritis without systemic involvement are appropriate and avoid toxicity. Systemic infections require higher levels of therapy and mandate the monitoring of blood levels. Depending on renal clearance, aminoglycoside dosing intervals range from 8–48 h (Bergeron, 1995; Mullenix & Prince, 1997).

## Follow-Up Recommendations

*Uncomplicated Pyelonephritis.* An initial assessment of patients' symptoms is essential within 12–24 h by phone or office visit. Significant improvement of symptoms should occur in 12–48 h. A second assessment of the patient's symptoms needs to be scheduled in the office within 2–3 days. If symptoms persist or worsen in 24–48 h, the patient needs to be hospitalized for parenteral antibiotic therapy and diagnostic evaluation to determine etiology of complicated pyelonephritis. All patients with pyelonephritis require posttreatment urine cultures within 2 weeks of therapy completion and 2 months later (Bergeron, 1995; Hooton, 1995; Howes, 1992; Johnson, 1992; Mullenix & Prince, 1997; Plattner, 1994; Reynolds & Hoberman, 1995; Stamm & Hooton, 1993; Talner et al, 1994).

*Complicated Pyelonephritis.* After hospitalization, posttreatment urine cultures are required within 2 weeks of therapy completion and 2 months later. The urine culture guides further drug therapy to alleviate the infection. Further diagnostic evaluation to determine etiology and referral for correction of the problem is essential if this was not achieved during the hospital stay. Sufficient monitoring of complicated pyelonephritis may require 6–12 months to prevent reinfection or renal complications (Bergeron, 1995; Hooton, 1995; Howes, 1992; Johnson, 1992; Mullenix & Prince, 1997; Plattner, 1994; Reynolds & Hoberman, 1995; Stamm & Hooton, 1993; Talner et al, 1994). Refer to "Special Situations" for specific follow-up of pregnant patients, children, and elders.

# STRESS URINARY INCONTINENCE

Stress urinary incontinence (SUI) is defined as the involuntary loss of urine during activities that increase abdominal pressure, such as coughing, sneezing, laughing, or other physical activities. Pathophysiologic changes of SUI in females relate to increased intraabdominal pressure from neuromuscular changes and hypermobility of the bladder base and urethra associated with poor pelvic support or intrinsic urethral sphincter failure or weakness. In males, pathophysiologic changes relate to overflow from an underactive or acontractile detrusor and are associated with prostate gland problems, urethral stricture, neurologic problems, or idiopathic detrusor failure. SUI from intrinsic sphincter deficiency (ISD) is characterized by continuous leakage at rest or with minimal exertion, such as postural changes (Beckman, 1995; U. S. Department of Health and Human Services [USDHHS], 1996; Webb, 1994).

Risk factors for SUI include medications, smoking, fecal impaction, habitual straining during defecation, low fluid intake, high-impact physical activities, obesity, estrogen depletion, pelvic muscle weakness, pelvic floor trauma, vaginal infections, parity, pregnancy, vaginal delivery, episiotomy, and history of childhood sexual abuse. Urinary incontinence affects approximately 13 million Americans or 10–35% of adults and 50% of the 1.5 million nursing home residents. Females have twice the prevalence of incontinence (Beckman, 1995; Brooks, 1993; Pearce, 1994; USDHHS, 1996). Approximately 26% of females between the ages of 30 and 59 years experience SUI or a combination of SUI and urge incontinence (Webb, 1994). Approximately 5–10% of all community-dwelling individuals older than 60 years have urinary incontinence (UI). It is estimated that 53% of all homebound elders are incontinent. UI is the second leading cause of institutionalization of elders. Direct costs of caring for persons of all ages with UI are more than $15 billion annually (Beckman, 1995; Brooks, 1993; Pearce, 1994; USDHHS, 1996).

Patients underreport UI because of embarrassment, stress related to odor and appearance, and the belief that UI is normal, especially in females. Most affected individuals do not seek help for incontinence and may be reluctant to admit to their UI. Patients need to be asked if they are accidentally leaking urine, since 70% of UI is curable, but correct diagnosis is essential (Beckman, 1995; Brooks, 1993; Pearce, 1994; USDHHS, 1996).

## SPECIFIC CONSIDERATIONS FOR PHARMACOTHERAPY

### When Drug Therapy Is Needed

The first line of therapy for SUI is behavioral techniques, as they are the least invasive and have fewer potential side effects (USDHHS, 1996;

Webb, 1994; Wyman, 1994). Approximately 12–16% of patients are cured of stress and urge incontinence, and 54–75% of patients report improvement of symptoms with the use of behavioral techniques (Pearce, 1994).

The second line of therapy is pharmacotherapeutics. The purpose of drug therapy is to increase or decrease bladder contractility or urethral resistance. Alpha-adrenergic agents increase striated or smooth muscle tone to increase urethral resistance. Tricyclic agents decrease bladder contractility and increase urethral resistance. Estrogen in postmenopausal females stimulates squamous epithelium to decrease bladder contractility and improve periurethral vascularity, tone, and coaptation. Most commonly, drug therapy is combined with behavioral techniques for maximum patient outcomes (USDHHS, 1996; Webb, 1994; Wyman, 1994).

The elimination, dosage adjustment, or schedule change of drugs that precipitate or contribute to SUI is considered a therapeutic action. All patients need a comprehensive assessment of their over-the-counter or prescribed medications. Drugs that affect UI include anticholinergic agents, diuretics, caffeine, alcohol, antidepressants, psychotropics, sedatives, hypnotics, narcotics, antipsychotics, antispasmodics, antiparkinsonian agents, and phenothiazines (Beckman, 1995; Pearce, 1994; USDHHS, 1996; Wyman, 1994).

### Short- and Long-Term Goals of Pharmacotherapy

The short-term goals of treatment for SUI are to decrease incontinent symptoms or episodes, improve management of SUI, and prevent complications. The long-term goals of treatment of SUI are to eliminate incontinent symptoms or episodes and prevent complications. The goals of treatment are best accomplished by combining behavioral techniques and drug therapy.

### Nonpharmacologic Therapy

Refer to "Patient/Caregiver Information" for additional information. Behavioral techniques and/or mechanical to surgical interventions require education and positive reinforcement. They consist of the following

- Pelvic muscle exercise (PME) or Kegel exercises
- Voiding records

- Dietary modifications
- Fluid intake modification
- Eliminating constipation
- Smoking cessation
- Weight reduction
- Using absorbent pads or garments
- Biofeedback
- Physical, social, and environmental devices to facilitate toileting
- Penile clamps or external catheters or condoms
- Pessaries or vaginal cones for pelvic support
- Electrical stimulation
- Use of catheters (intermittent, indwelling, or suprapubic)
- Surgery on bladder neck or urethra obstruction, detrusor overactivity, intrinsic and sphincter deficiency, and urethral hypermotility (Beckman, 1995; Brooks, 1993; Pearce, 1994; USDHHS, 1996; Webb, 1994; Wyman, 1994).

### Time Frame for Initiating Pharmacotherapy

SUI should be treated at time of diagnosis to prevent increased symptomatology, patient embarrassment and discomfort, and complications. The degree of symptomatology, patient preference, and the clinician's judgment determine when drug therapy is initiated.

See Drug Tables 311.1, 501.10, 605, 703.

### Assessment and History Taking

Refer to Tables 34–6 and 34–7.

### Patient/Caregiver Information

Refer to Table 34–8.

## OUTCOMES MANAGEMENT

### Selecting an Appropriate Agent

Pharmacotherapy is secondary to behavioral therapy in SUI since it supplements behavioral therapy. Treatment success or failure with behavioral therapy, history of hypertension, history of cardiovascular disease, gender, and menstrual age are factors to consider in drug selection (USDHHS, 1996; Webb, 1994; Wyman, 1994).

Refer to Table 34–9. Alpha-adrenergic agonists are the drugs of choice because they increase bladder sphincter tone. Approximately 9–14% of

females report more dryness with use of phenylpropanolamine (PPA) while 31–60% report leakage reduction. Use these drugs cautiously in patients with hypertension, hyperthyroidism, diabetes, cardiac arrhythmias, and cardiac ischemia because of possible adverse effects (USDHHS, 1996; Webb, 1994; Wyman, 1994).

Oral or topical estrogen in postmenopausal females restores mucosal vascularity and tone and increases the alpha-adrenergic response of urethral tissue. Combination therapy of estrogen and an alpha-adrenergic agonist needs to be considered when treatment failure exists with an alpha-adrenergic agonist alone (USDHHS, 1996; Wyman, 1994).

Imipramine, a tricyclic antidepressant, possesses indirect alpha-adrenergic agonist activity and anticholinergic properties. Approximately 70% of females on imipramine 75 mg daily report continence (USDHHS, 1996; Webb, 1994; Wyman, 1994).

### Monitoring for Efficacy

Monitoring guidelines for drug efficacy in SUI therapy lack clarity because efficacy relates to subjective expectations and multiple effects of combined therapies. A paucity of empirical longitudinal studies provides few monitoring guidelines. Monitoring of drug efficacy is based on the pharmacological properties of selected drugs, sufficient time frames, such as weeks to months for optimum drug effects, and the reduction of incontinent episodes (USDHHS, 1996; Wyman, 1994).

### Monitoring for Toxicity

In using alpha-adrenergic agonists, monitor for adverse effects of hypertension, tachycardia, anorexia, insomnia, agitation, headache, sweating, and respiratory difficulty. Avoid the use of estrogen in females with thromboembolic disease, abnormal bleeding, pregnancy, or known or suspected breast or uterine cancer. Monitor anticholinergic effects of imipramine, such as increased constipation, blurred vision, dry mouth, and tachycardia, particularly in elderly patients (USDHHS, 1996; Wyman, 1994).

### Follow-Up Recommendations

All patients require periodic monitoring of behavioral therapy and drug efficacy. The degree of symptomatology, patient characteristics and compliance, and potential drug adverse reac-

## TABLE 34–6. BASELINE DATA: HISTORY AND PHYSICAL EXAMINATION FOR STRESS URINARY INCONTINENCE

### History

Onset of SUI, duration, and characteristics, such as stress, dribble, or urge

Patient's most bothersome symptom(s)

Urinary habits, such as frequency, timing, and volume of voiding; continent and incontinent episodes

Precipitating factors, such as cough, sneeze, laugh, "on way to bathroom," high-impact exercise, surgery, trauma, recent pregnancy, onset of illness, or new medications

Current management of SUI, including protective devices and use of pads or briefs

Previous treatment for SUI and its effect; patient expectations of treatment

Presence of UTI symptoms, such as dysuria, nocturia, hesitancy, sensation of incomplete bladder emptying, hematuria, or vaginitis

Bowel habits, frequency, consistency of stool, and changes in bowel habits

Alterations of sexual function related to SUI

Amount of daily fluid intake and use of any diuretic fluids or irritants, such as caffeine

Complete past medical and surgical history

Review all patient medications

History of genitourinary and neurological systems

   In females, comprehensive obstetrical history, such as episiotomy, length of labor, baby's birth weight, and complications

   In males, postvoid dribbling, urgency, and problems with prostate

Assess patient for SUI risk factors

Determine any physical, social, and environmental barriers, such as disability, access to bathroom, work restrictions, or living arrangements

Assess a voiding record or diary for frequency of voiding, time of day, and precipitating events; may be initial assessment measure and evaluation measure to determine effectiveness of treatment

### Physical Examination

Abdominal examination to detect masses, suprapubic tenderness or fullness, diastasis rectus, and estimation of postvoiding residual (PVR) urine

   In males, perform genital examination to detect abnormalities of the foreskin, glans, penis, and perineal skin; assess the consistency and contour of the prostate

   In females, perform a pelvic examination to assess perineal skin, urethra, pelvic prolapse (cystocele, vaginal vault prolapse, uterine prolapse), pelvic mass, perivaginal muscle tone, atrophic vaginitis, and to estimate PVR urine by abdominal palpation and percussion

Rectal examination to assess perineal sensation, resting and active sphincter tone, rectal mass, fecal impaction, and estimation of PVR

Neurologic examination and observe mobility

---

tions determine monitoring frequency. Positive reinforcement of the patient's efforts is critical to continuation and success of therapy (US-DHHS, 1996; Webb, 1994; Wyman, 1994).

# MALE URINARY AND RELATED PROBLEMS

## EPIDIDYMITIS

Epididymitis (inflammation of the epididymis) is the most common acute scrotal pain in post-pubertal males and accounts for more than 600,000 annual visits to health care providers in the United States. Pathogens reach the epididymis through the lumen of the vas deferens from infected urine, the posterior urethra, or seminal vesicles; underlying structural disorders are rare. Epididymitis is most commonly sexually transmitted and accompanied by asymptomatic urethritis, prostatitis, or cystitis in postpubertal boys and males under 35 years. *Neisseria gonorrhoeae* and more commonly *Chlamydia trachomatis* are the causative pathogens in 75% of all cases. In homosexual males, specifically the insertive partner, E. coli is the causative

## TABLE 34-7.  DIAGNOSTIC TESTS FOR STRESS URINARY INCONTINENCE

*Postvoiding residual (PVR) urine:* Catheterized specimen after patient voids; PVR <50 mL is adequate bladder emptying; PVR >200 mL is inadequate emptying.

*Provocative stress testing:* Client relax, then cough vigorously, observe for urine loss from urethra.

*Perineal pad test:* Objective measurement of volume of urine loss.

*Urinalysis:* Detect contributing conditions, such as hematuria, pyuria, bacteriuria, gylcosuria, and proteinuria (dipstick acceptable for screening; microscopic analysis helpful).

*Urine culture:* If bacteria present in urinalysis.

*Bedside cystometrogram* (bladder capacity): Volume of first sensation of bladder fullness and presence or absence of uninhibited detrusor contractions. Have patient void in privacy to empty a comfortably full bladder. Catheterize for postvoiding residual volume (14 French straight catheter). Fill bladder using a 50-mL syringe (without piston or bulb) with 25–50 mL of room temperature sterile water; hold syringe 15 cm above pubic symphysis. Have patient void with first sensation; maximum capacity assumed when patient cannot hold anymore. Upward movement of column fluid indicates presence of involuntary bladder contractions. Involuntary contractions or severe urgency at low bladder volumes, <250–300 mL, suggests detrusor instability, especially if consistent with patient symptoms.

*Suspected urinary obstruction, retention, or noncompliant bladder:* Blood urea nitrogen, creatinine, calcium levels.

*Uroflowmetry and other urine cytology:* If patient has recent onset of irritative voiding or hematuria.

## TABLE 34-8.  PATIENT/CAREGIVER INFORMATION FOR STRESS URINARY INCONTINENCE

Behavioral techniques
  Habit training or scheduled voiding
  Timed voiding
  Bladder training
  Prompted voiding
  Relaxation techniques
  Voiding or bladder record
Importance of daily pelvic muscle exercise (PME) or Kegel exercises to reduce SUI
Dietary modifications to include a decrease or elimination of alcohol, sweetener substitutes, and caffeine
Fluid intake modification by decreasing or increasing volume (individual needs and related health problems); recommend 48–64 oz per day to stimulate bladder's stretch receptors and dilute urine
Eliminate constipation with high-fiber foods and daily exercise, such as walking
Importance of smoking cessation
Develop a weight reduction plan
Proper use of absorbent pads or garments and meticulous skin care
Strategies to overcome physical, social, and environmental barriers to facilitate toileting, such as accessible toileting facilities, adequate lighting in bathroom, grab bars in the bathroom, elevated toilet seats, and walkers or mobility aids
In males, purpose and appropriate use of penile clamps or external catheters
In females, purpose and proper use of vaginal cones, pessaries, electrical stimulation, and vaginal creams
Signs and symptoms of UTI and to seek health care if these occur
Purpose, dosage, and side effects of drugs
Teach health promotion and prevention measures
  PME for all females in schools and clinics
  Weight reduction
  Birth control methods
  Consistent bladder and bowel habits
  Proper lifting techniques to avoid abdominal strain
  Postcoital voiding to prevent UTI

## TABLE 34-9. PHARMACOTHERAPY FOR STRESS URINARY INCONTINENCE

| Drug | Regimen |
|------|---------|
| **Alpha-adrenergic agonists** | |
| Phenylpropanolamine SR | 25–100 mg PO b.i.d. |
| Pseudoephedrine | 15–30 mg PO t.i.d. |
| | |
| **Hormones (in postmenopausal women)** | |
| Conjugated estrogen | 1–2 g vaginally, paraurethrally q.d. |
| Conjugated estrogen | 0.3–1.25 mg PO q.d., continuous or cyclic (days 1–25) |
| Medroxyprogesterone | 2.5–10 mg PO q.d., continuous or cyclic (days 16–25) (uterus present) |
| | |
| **Miscellaneous** | |
| Imipramine SR | 75 mg PO g.h.s; use stool softener for constipation |
| Docusate sodium | 100–200 mg once or twice daily, to avoid straining |

SR = sustained release.

pathogen (Centers for Disease Control and Prevention, 1994; Krieger 1995; Zahn & Craven, 1994).

Nonsexually transmitted epididymitis is generally seen in males older than 35 years or those who have recently experienced urinary tract surgery or instrumentation. It is commonly associated with UTI caused by gram-negative enteric organisms (CDCP, 1994; Krieger, 1995; Zahn & Craven, 1994). An underlying urinary abnormality or anomaly is often present in infants and children, such as a pathological connection between the urinary tract, genital duct system, or bowel that results in contamination of the epididymis with coliform bacteria (Kaler, 1990).

Epididymitis is characterized by gradual onset of pain, unilateral testicular pain and tenderness, fever, dysuria, urinary frequency, urgency, urethral discharge, and scrotum edema as the disease progresses. Nausea and vomiting are usually absent. Uncommon complications include testicular necrosis, testicular atrophy, and infertility. Common complications among immunocompromised patients include testicular cancer, tuberculosis epididymitis, and fungal epididymitis. Differentiation between epididymitis and testicular torsion must be made since the latter presents with sudden onset of severe pain and requires emergency treatment (CDCP, 1994; Krieger, 1995; Zahn & Craven, 1994).

A comprehensive analysis of the literature generates the following definitions (CDCP, 1994; Krieger, 1995; Zahn & Craven, 1994):

- *Sexually transmitted epididymitis* is an infection of the epididymis in a healthy individual by a sexually transmitted organism and associated with urethritis.

- *Nonsexually transmitted epididymitis* is an infection of the epididymis in a healthy individual by a common pathogen and associated with gram-negative enteric organisms

## SPECIFIC CONSIDERATIONS FOR PHARMACOTHERAPY

### When Drug Therapy Is Needed

Epididymitis is treated with antibiotics when the patient presents with symptoms. Prompt diagnosis and treatment are essential because of varying degree of illness, potential spread of sexually transmitted diseases, and potential urinary and renal complications. Bed rest and comfort measures are essential to provide relief of symptoms. Patients with severe symptomatology or who appear septic need to be hospitalized immediately for parenteral therapy (CDCP, 1994; Krieger, 1995; Zahn & Craven, 1994).

### Short- and Long-Term Goals of Pharmacotherapy

The short-term goals of treatment for sexually transmitted epididymitis are to resolve the infection, restore normal physiological function, and prevent the spread and recurrence of infection. For nonsexually transmitted epididymitis, they are to resolve the infection, restore normal physiological function, and prevent further recurrence of infection. The long-term goals of treatment for both types of epididymitis are to prevent recurrence of infection and potential renal complications. In each of the conditions of epididymitis, the goals of treatment are achieved primarily by antibiotic therapy and patient education.

## Time Frame for Initiating Pharmacotherapy

Epididymitis requires prompt diagnosis and treatment when patients present with clinical symptoms to prevent the serious sequelae discussed. Empiric treatment is indicated before culture results are available. Treatment failures require further evaluation, and culture results guide drug selection (Krieger, 1995). Differential diagnosis to rule out testicular torsion and abscesses is critical for positive patient outcomes (CDCP, 1994; Krieger, 1995; Zahn & Craven, 1994).

See Drug Tables 102.3–102.6, 102.10, 102.11, 306.

## Assessment and History Taking

Refer to Tables 34–10 and 34–11.

## Patient/Caregiver Information

Refer to Table 34–12.

## OUTCOMES MANAGEMENT

### Selecting an Appropriate Agent

Patient factors of age, sexual activity, sexual preference, drug or environmental allergies, concurrent diseases, degree of symptomatology, and adherence to therapy regimen guide antibiotic therapy selection. Empiric therapy is based on a patient's symptomatology and diagnostic findings. Treatment of males with HIV infection and epididymitis is the same as those without HIV (CDCP, 1994; Krieger, 1995; Zahn & Craven, 1994).

***Sexually Transmitted Epididymitis.*** Empiric therapy for patients with sexually transmitted epididymitis is directed at *C. trachomatis* and *N. gonorrhoeae*. See Table 34–13. The patient's sex partner(s), for the 30 days prior to diagnosis, needs diagnostic evaluation and treatment (CDCP, 1994; Krieger, 1995; Sanford, Gilbert, & Sande, 1996; Zahn & Craven, 1994). See Chapter 36 for treatment of STDs.

***Nonsexually Transmitted Epididymitis.*** Empiric therapy for nonsexually transmitted epididymitis is directed at enterobacteriaceae common in UTIs. Selection of oral or parenteral therapy is based on the severity of patient symptomatology (CDCP, 1994; Krieger, 1995; Sanford, Gilbert, & Sande, 1996; Zahn & Craven, 1994). Refer to Table 34–13 also.

---

**TABLE 34–10. BASELINE DATA: HISTORY AND PHYSICAL EXAMINATION FOR EPIDIDYMITIS**

**History**
Onset, duration, and course of symptoms of scrotal pain, dysuria, urinary frequency, urgency, and urethral discharge (color, amount, and consistency)
Associated diseases, such as fever, nausea, vomiting, and diagnosed urinary tract infections and structural or neurologic abnormalities
History of new sexual partners and complaints, if any, of dysuria, urinary frequency, or genitourinary discharges

**Physical Examination**
Vital signs; note any temperature elevation
Inspect scrotum for erythema, edema, and torsion; usually indurated, enlarged, and tender if epididymitis present
Testicular tenderness, position, size, and consistency; testes are generally normal
Elicit Prehn's sign (passive elevation of testicles) as it relieves pain
Suprapubic tenderness and CVA tenderness
Rectal examination to elicit prostatic tenderness and urethral discharge

## TABLE 34–11.  DIAGNOSTIC TESTS FOR EPIDIDYMITIS

Urinalysis
  Pyuria in 20–95% cases
Urine culture and sensitivity and Gram's stain smear of uncentrifuged urine for gram-negative bacteria
Postpubertal males with STD
  Gram's stain of urethral discharge or intraurethral swab for *N. gonorrhoeae* and nongonococcal urethritis
    ($\geq$5 polymorphonuclear leukocytes per oil immersion field)
  Urethral discharge or intraurethral swab for chlamydia
  Gonococcal culture of urethral discharge
CBC for elevation in leukocytes
Older males
  Culture of expressed prostatic secretions (EPS) unless acute prostatitis suspected
  Assess for an obstruction of the bladder outlet, such as an intravenous pyelography, doppler ultrasound, scrotal
    ultrasound, or radionuclide scrotal imaging

Drugs for comfort measures in epididymitis include nonsteroidal antiinflammatory drugs (NSAIDs), such as ibuprofen and naproxen. Opiates, such as hydrocodone and oxycodone in combination with acetaminophen or aspirin are for patients with severe symptomatology (Kaler, 1990; Zahn & Craven, 1994).

### Monitoring for Efficacy

Drug efficacy is determined by resolution of patient symptoms. Failure of symptoms to improve within 72 h requires reassessment of the patient (CDCP, 1994; Krieger, 1995; Zahn & Craven, 1994).

### Monitoring for Toxicity

Tetracyclines and FLQNs in males <17 years may cause abnormalities in cartilage and bone development (Mullenix & Prince, 1997).

### Follow-up Recommendations

Prepubertal boys and older males with bacteriuria require posttreatment cultures on completion of therapy. Delayed or further diagnostic evaluation for urological abnormalities needs to be completed. In postpubertal and <35-year-old males, no follow-up or test of cure is needed if symptoms resolve. Failure of symptoms to improve within 72 h requires reassessment of the patient's symptoms, diagnosis, and therapy. Males with tenderness and swelling that persist after completion of therapy need evaluation for testicular cancer and tuberculosis or fungal epididymitis. These diseases are common among patients who are immunocompromised (CDCP, 1994; Krieger, 1995; Zahn & Craven, 1994).

## URETHRITIS IN MALES

Urethritis (inflammation of the urethra) in males is known as nongonococcal or gonococcal

## TABLE 34–12.  PATIENT/CAREGIVER INFORMATION FOR EPIDIDYMITIS

Condom use during sexual intercourse to prevent risk of exposure to STDs
Bed rest with scrotal elevation and ice packs for pain
Scrotal support as needed
Warm sitz baths three times daily for relief of symptoms
Patients with STD epididymitis need to refer sex partners for evaluation and treatment
Avoid sexual intercourse until both patient and partner(s) have completed therapy and are without symptoms
Educate about signs and symptoms of septicemia or potential complications and the importance of seeking health
  care immediately

## TABLE 34–13. EMPIRIC DRUG THERAPY FOR EPIDIDYMITIS

| Drug | Regimen | Preference |
|------|---------|------------|
| **Sexually Transmitted** | | |
| | Age: 17–35 years | |
| Ceftriaxone | 250 mg IM once | 1st |
| and | | |
| Doxycycline | 100 mg PO b.i.d. for 10 days | |
| Ofloxacin | 300 mg PO b.i.d. for 10 days | Alt |
| **Nonsexually Transmitted** | | |
| | Age: >35 years | |
| TMP-SMX | 1 DS PO b.i.d. for 10–14 days | 1st |
| Ofloxacin | 400 mg PO b.i.d. for 10–14 days | Alt |
| Ciprofloxin | 500 mg PO/400 mg IV b.i.d. for 10–14 days | Alt |
| Third-generation cephalosporin | | Alt |
| Ampicillin with sulbactam | | Alt |

Alt = alternative; DS = double strength; TMP-SMX = trimethoprim-sulfamethoxazole.

urethritis (GU). Nongonococcal urethritis (NGU) is the most common STD syndrome and accounts for 4–6 million health care visits in the United States per year. The two major causative agents of NGU are *C. trachomatis* (35–45%) and *Ureaplasma urealyticum* (15–25%). Trichomonas vaginalis, herpes simplex, and the newly recognized genital *M. genitalium* account for the remaining cases. *N. gonorrhoeae* is the causative agent of GU; however, the patient may be co-infected with *C. trachomatis* (CDCP, 1994; Krieger, 1994, 1995; Schmid & Fontanarosa, 1995; Stamm et al, 1995).

Urethritis may be symptomatic or asymptomatic, with the latter being common. Urethritis is characterized by a mucoid or purulent discharge (yellow, white, or cloudy), dysuria, and urethral itching or tingling. Diagnosis of NGU is based on the presence of a urethral discharge and laboratory confirmation of leukocytes on a Gram's stain smear. GU is diagnosed by the presence of a urethral discharge and confirmation of gram-negative diplococci in a urethral secretion or an intraurethral swab (CDCP, 1994; Krieger, 1994, 1995; Schmid & Fontanarosa, 1995; Stamm et al, 1995).

Approximately 600,000 males develop recurrent or persistent urethritis annually because of lack of compliance with a therapeutic regimen or reinfection by untreated sex partner(s). Males with persistent or recurrent urethritis need to be retreated along with sex partners. Untreated urethritis may lead to severe complications, such as epididymitis, Reiter's syndrome, or infertility. The female sex partners of males with urethritis are at risk for mucopurulent cervicitis, chlamydial infections, pelvic inflammatory disease, ectopic pregnancy, and tubal infertility. The presence of STDs may facilitate transmission of the HIV virus. Early recognition and prompt, effective treatment may contribute significantly to decreasing potential complications and reducing heterosexual transmission of HIV (CDCP, 1994; Krieger, 1994, 1995; Schmid & Fontanarosa, 1995; Stamm et al, 1995).

A comprehensive analysis of the literature generates the following definitions:

- *Nongonococcal Urethritis* is an inflammation of the urethra not caused by gonococcal infection and diagnosed by ≥ 5 polymorphonuclear leukocytes per oil immersion field on a smear of an intraurethral swab specimen.

- *Gonococcal Urethritis* is an inflammation of the urethra caused by gonococci and diagnosed by the presence of intracellular gram-negative diplococci from an intraurethral swab.

## SPECIFIC CONSIDERATIONS FOR PHARMACOTHERAPY

### When Drug Therapy Is Needed

NGU and GU are treated with antibiotics when the patient presents with symptoms and diagnostic tests confirm identification of etiological organisms. Prompt diagnosis and treatment are essential to prevent serious renal, reproductive, and systemic complications. Therapy for a specific disease or infections is reportable to state health departments. Treatment compliance and partner notification are generally better with a specific diagnosis. If diagnostic tools are not available, the clinician should treat the patient for both types of infections; however, clinicians need to avoid the cost of treating two diseases (CDCP, 1994; Krieger, 1994, 1995; Schmid & Fontanarosa, 1995; Stamm et al, 1995).

## Short- and Long-Term Goals of Pharmacotherapy

The short-term goals for treatment of NGU and GU are to identify the causative agent, resolve the infection, restore normal physiological function, and prevent the spread and recurrence of the infection. The long-term goals are to prevent recurrence of infection and prevent potential complications. Both conditions respond to antibiotic therapy and patient education.

## Time Frame for Initiating Pharmacotherapy

Treatment of urethritis should be initiated when the patient presents with complaints and by laboratory confirmation of causative organisms to prevent the serious sequelae discussed.

See Drug Table 102.

## Assessment and History Taking

Refer to Tables 34–14 and 34–15.

## Patient/Caregiver Information

Education of the patient about the signs and symptoms of the disease, drug therapy, and prevention measures is critical for positive outcomes. Refer to Table 34–16.

## OUTCOMES MANAGEMENT

### Selecting an Appropriate Agent

Empiric therapy is based on laboratory results. In the absence of a definitive diagnosis, therapy for NGU and GU must be initiated. Lack of patient compliance with the prescribed therapeutic regimen is a barrier in the effective treatment of STDs. Monitored single doses enhance compliance as in the case of doxycycline and azithromycin; however, dosages of azithromycin cost five to six times more than the cost of a week's supply of doxycycline. Evaluation and treatment of the patient's sex partner(s) are critical to prevent the spread of the disease or reinfection (CDCP, 1994; Krieger, 1995; Sanford et al, 1996; Schmid & Fontanarosa, 1995). See Table 34–17.

Sex partners are treated with the same therapies except in the presence of pregnancy. Erythromycin is the therapy for pregnancy. Approximately 50% of patients with GU present with coinfections of *C. trachomatis* (CDCP, 1994; Krieger, 1995; Sanford et al, 1996; Schmid & Fontanarosa, 1995).

### Monitoring for Efficacy

Symptom resolution within 48–72 h is considered sufficient for monitoring of outcomes.

---

## TABLE 34–14. BASELINE DATA: HISTORY AND PHYSICAL EXAMINATION FOR URETHRITIS

### History

History of onset and duration of symptoms, such as presence and color of urethral discharge, presence of dysuria, and urethral itching along with associated symptoms of fever, chills, nausea, vomiting, diarrhea, constipation, abdominal and back pain, and hematuria

Sexual history, such as age of first intercourse, number of sexual partners, specifically within the last 30–60 days, frequency of sexual coitus, sexual behaviors (anal and vaginal coitus), and use of barrier methods

Past history of STDs, including characteristics, frequency, duration, and effectiveness of treatments

Past medical history including drug and environmental allergies; chronic diseases such as diabetes mellitus, multiple sclerosis, and cancer; and previous genitourinary problems and treatment

### Physical Examination

Vital signs, particularly noting temperature elevation

Inspect and palpate external genitalia

Examine urethra for mucopurulent discharge

## TABLE 34–15. DIAGNOSTIC TESTS FOR URETHRITIS

Gram's stain of an intraurethral swab specimen
    NGU confirmed with ≥5 polymorphonuclear leukocytes per oil immersion field
    GU confirmed by the presence of intracellular gram-negative diplococci
Asymptomatic males
    First 10–20 mL of urine to screen for GU or NGU with leukocyte estrase test (LET); positive LET indicates *T. vaginalis* and must be confirmed with an urethral swab specimen Gram's stain
*Neisseria gonorrhoea* cultures (GC) and chlamydia test
Blood tests for syphilis and HIV
Presence of systemic symptoms, order CBC with differential and consider erythrocyte sedimentation rate

Persistence or recurrence of symptoms requires further diagnostic evaluation (CDCP, 1994; Krieger, 1995; Schmid & Fontanarosa, 1995).

### Monitoring for Toxicity

Tetracyclines and FLQNs in pregnant patients or patients in the puberty stage may cause abnormalities in cartilage and bone development. Metronidazole is contraindicated in the first trimester of pregnancy (CDCP, 1994; Sanford et al, 1996).

### Follow-up Recommendations

Persistence or recurrence of symptoms requires diagnostic evaluation. Assess the patient's compliance with the selected therapeutic regimen and for possible reinfection by untreated sex partner(s). Treatment failure or reinfection of NGU or GU requires the same therapeutic regimen after laboratory confirmation of the specific organism. Evaluate the patient for *T. vaginalis* with a microscopic wet mount from an intraurethral swab. If the wet mount is positive for *T. vaginalis*, treat the patient and sex partner(s) with a single, oral dose of metronidazole 2 gm or 500 mg b.i.d. for 5 days. A negative wet mount indicates that a change to an alternative drug is needed, such as from doxycycline to

azithromycin (CDCP, 1994; Krieger, 1995; Schmid & Fontanarosa, 1995).

## PROSTATITIS

Prostatitis (inflammation of the prostate gland) is one of the most common urologic diseases in adult males, accounts for 25% of office visits for genitourinary complaints, and occurs in 25–50% of all males at some time (Table 34–18). It may result from (1) an ascending uretheral infection, (2) reflux of infected urine, (3) direct extension or lymphatic spread of a rectal infection, or (4) hematogenous spread (Criste, Gray, & Gallo, 1994; Moul, 1993; Mullenix & Prince, 1997).

In clinical practice, prostatitis is a general term to describe any unexplained symptoms that may occur with a disorder of the prostate gland (Criste et al, 1994; Moul, 1993).

In bacterial prostatitis, gram-negative enteric organisms are the causative pathogens, similar in type and prevalence to those in UTI. *Escherichia coli* occurs in 75% of diagnosed cases and is followed by *P. mirabilis*, *K. pneumoniae*, and species of *Enterobacter*, *Pseudomonas*, and *Serratia*. There is some evidence, though controversial, that gram-positive organisms may play a role in chronic bacterial prosta-

## TABLE 34–16. PATIENT/CAREGIVER INFORMATION FOR URETHRITIS

Condom usage during sexual intercourse to prevent the risk of exposure of STDs to self and partner(s)
Refer sex partner(s) for evaluation and treatment
Avoid sexual intercourse until the patient and partner(s) have completed therapy and are without symptoms
Know about signs and symptoms of reinfection, septicemia, or potential complications and the importance of
    seeking health care immediately

## TABLE 34–17. EMPIRIC DRUG THERAPY FOR URETHRITIS

| Drug | Regimen | Preference |
|------|---------|------------|
| **Nongonococcal Urethritis** | | |
| Azithromycin | 1 g PO once | 1st |
| Doxycycline | 100 mg PO b.i.d. for 7 days | Alt |
| Erythromycin base | 500 mg PO q.i.d. for 7 days | Alt |
| Erythromycin ethylsuccinate | 800 mg PO q.i.d. for 7 days | Alt |
| Ofloxacin | 400 mg PO b.i.d. for 7 days | Alt |
| | | |
| **Gonococcal Urethritis** | | |
| Add one of the following drugs to NGU therapy: | | |
| Ceftriaxone | 125 mg IM once | 1st |
| Cefixime | 400 mg PO once | Alt |
| Ciprofloxacin | 500 mg PO once | Alt |
| Ofloxacin | 400 mg PO once | Alt |

Alt = alternative.

## TABLE 34–18. DEFINITIONS OF PROSTATITIS

| Term | Definition |
|------|------------|
| Acute bacterial prostatitis (ABP) | Least common type of prostatitis, most easily diagnosed, and generally occurs in young males during times of greater sexual activity. Asystemic disease characterized by an acute onset of fever, chills, dysuria, frequency, retention, urgency, nocturia, low back and perineal pain, generalized malaise, arthralgia, myalgia, and suprapubic discomfort. Diagnosis confirmed by the presence of >10 WBCs per high-power field in a urine specimen. |
| Chronic bacterial prostatitis (CBP) | More common in older males and difficult to diagnose since the clinical presentation is less clear and often resembles other disorders. The hallmark feature of CBP is a history of recurrent UTIs by the same pathogen. CBP is characterized by dysuria, urgency, frequency, nocturia, dribbling, hesitancy, loss of stream volume and force, pain in various sites (low back, perineal, suprapubic, scrotal, or penile), hematuria, and hematospermia or painful ejaculation. CBP has periods of exacerbation and remission. Diagnosis is confirmed by the presence of >10–15 WBCs per high-power field in a urine specimen, serial segmented cultures of urine and EPS, and IgA and IgG antibody levels. |
| Nonbacterial prostatitis (NBP) | Most common type of prostatitis and occurs eight times more frequently than BP. Presents with symptoms similar to CBP, but in the absence of a UTI or history of UTI. Penile discharge is common and complaints are vague. Diagnosis is confirmed by excessive WBCs (>10) and macrophages containing fat in EPS, but urine cultures contain no bacterial growth. |
| Prostatodynia (PD) | A symptom complex of unknown etiology and difficult to diagnose. Patients present with subjective symptoms that mimic prostatitis, including a painful prostate and irritative or obstructive voiding symptoms. There is an absence of objective findings or inflammatory cells in urine and EPS cultures. Patients' ages range from 22 to 56 years. Stress, emotional problems, internal sphincter dyssynergia, and tension myalgia need to be considered in the differential diagnosis. |

titis (CBP). These gram-positive organisms include *S. epidermidis*, *S. aureus*, and diphtheroids. Over the last decade, sexually transmitted diseases have been associated with nonbacterial prostatitis (NBP) and UTI in males. These pathogens include *N. gonorrhoeae*, *T. vaginalis*, *C. trachomatis*, *Gardnerella vaginalis*, and *U. urealyticum* with *Chlamydia* being the most common. The clinician needs to consider the possibility of mixed infections that involve two or more pathogens (Criste et al, 1994; Moul, 1993; Mullenix & Prince, 1997).

## SPECIFIC CONSIDERATIONS FOR PHARMACOTHERAPY

### When Drug Therapy Is Needed

Bacterial prostatitis is treated with antibiotics when the patient presents with symptoms and diagnostic tests confirm identification of etiologic organisms. Prompt diagnosis and treatment are essential because of varying degrees of systemic illness and potential sequelae that may lead to prostatic edema with urinary retention, renal parenchymal infection, or bacteremia; chronic infections may produce prostatic stones. Diagnosis of acute bacterial prostatitis (ABP) requires immediate treatment with antibiotics, whereas CBP is less life-threatening and requires long-term antibiotic therapy of weeks to months. Many antibiotics fail to achieve the high concentrations that are needed to penetrate the prostatic fluid for an adequate cure rate. CBP is often frustrating to the patient with continuation of symptoms and frequently leads to nonadherence to the prescribed therapy regimen (Criste et al, 1994; Moul, 1993; Mullenix & Prince, 1997).

NBP requires an individualized approach since the etiologic organism cannot be identified and cures are rarely obtained. Current therapy consists of antibiotics to eradicate potential STD organisms and measures to control symptoms. Patients need reassurance that NBP is self-limiting and not a life-threatening situation. The persistence of symptoms requires referral to a urologist for diagnostic studies to rule out carcinoma of the bladder or interstitial cystitis. Prostatodynia (PD) treatment modalities vary with the individual and referral to a urologist is essential for a complete evaluation, such as urodynamic tests or cystoscopic examination, and diagnosis of etiology to determine the therapeu-

tic regimen (Criste et al, 1994; Moul, 1993; Mullenix & Prince, 1997).

Health care providers need to educate patients fully to side effects and costs of antibiotic therapy as well as to the benefits and risks of other options of care.

### Short- and Long-Term Goals of Pharmacotherapy

The short-term goals of treatment for bacterial prostatitis are to resolve the infection, restore normal physiological functioning, and prevent the spread and recurrence of the infection. The long-term goals are to prevent recurrence of infection and potential complications. The short-term goals for NBP and prostatodynia are to control individual symptoms and refer patients for a comprehensive diagnostic evaluation to determine the etiology of illness. The long-term goals are to implement the prescribed therapeutic regimen, provide individualized comfort measures, and prevent potential renal complications.

### Time Frame for Initiating Pharmacotherapy

Bacterial prostatitis requires prompt diagnosis and treatment. Treatment of ABP is based on clinical presentation, and therapy is adjusted according to urine culture results. Expressed prostatic secretion (EPS) is not always obtainable because massage of the prostate can cause bacteremia. The patient's degree of systemic illness guides the treatment regimen of outpatient or inpatient care and the choice of oral or parenteral antibiotic therapy. In CBP and NBP, treatment is based on serial segmented urine and EPS results. Treatment of prostatodynia requires differentiation of diagnosis and the elimination of life-threatening conditions (Criste et al, 1994; Moul, 1993; Mullenix & Prince, 1997).

See Drug Tables 102.4, 102.7, 102.10, 102.11, 306, 502.1.

### Assessment and History Taking

Refer to Tables 34–19 and 34–20.

### Patient/Caregiver Information

Education of the patient about the signs and symptoms of the disease, drug therapy, and prevention measures is critical for positive outcomes (Criste et al, 1994; Moul, 1993; Mullenix & Prince, 1997). See Table 34–21.

## TABLE 34-19. BASELINE DATA: HISTORY AND PHYSICAL EXAMINATION FOR PROSTATITIS

**History**

Onset and course of illness and associated symptoms, such as urethral discharge, urethral meatal itching, fever, perineal pain, hematuria, hesitancy, decreased stream, painful ejaculation, incontinence, back pain, and weight loss

History of previous urinary tract infections and STDs with successes and failures of treatment

Sexual partner has symptoms of dysuria or STDs

Any new sexual partners

**Physical Examination**

General appearance for signs of systemic illness

Vital signs; note for elevation of temperature and hydration status

Complete abdominal examination; note bladder distention and suprapubic pain

External genitalia and scrotum for edema

Prostatic evaluation:

   ABP: *Do NOT palpate the prostate.* Prostate is extremely tender, warm, swollen, irregular, and partially or totally firm, soggy, or boggy

   CBP and NBP: Carefully palpate prostate for size and shape; it usually feels normal, but may be irregular and mildly tender

## OUTCOMES MANAGEMENT

### Selecting an Appropriate Agent

Empiric therapy is based on the patient's symptomatology, laboratory findings, and presumptive diagnosis of ABP, CBP, NBP, or PD. Table 34–22 lists specific drug therapies. Effective antibiotic therapy in bacterial prostatitis is often difficult to attain because of poor prostatic tissue penetration by some agents commonly used in the treatment of UTI. Other

## TABLE 34-20. DIAGNOSTIC TESTS FOR PROSTATITIS

Serial segmented cultures of urine and expressed prostatic secretion (EPS)

   Urine collection

      In uncircumcised male, instruct patient to tape foreskin back, cleanse meatus with soap and water, and then dry.

      In circumcised male, instruct patient to cleanse meatus with soap and water, then dry.

   Patient collects first 5–10 mL of urine voided; label first bladder voiding as VB$^1$.

   Patient voids about 200 mL of urine, stops midstream and collects 50–100 mL of urine; label as VB$^2$.

   Clinician massages prostate from each lateral lobe to midline, about six to seven times on each side; milks urethra to produce secretion; collects secretions on swab, slide, or in cup; and labels as EPS.

   Patient voids first 5–10 mL of urine; label as VB$^3$ (voided urine post prostatic massage).

   If unable to obtain all specimens on command, interpretation of results may be confusing.

   Microscopic examination of all specimens

      Presence of >10 WBCs per high-power field in EPS indicates some type of prostatitis; Macrophages with oval fat bodies confirm this diagnosis

Culture all specimens

Bacteria growth in VB$^1$ and VB$^2$, but no growth in EPS and VB$^3$ indicates cystitis.

A 10-fold increase of bacteria in EPS and VB$^3$ indicates APB or CBP.

>10 WBCs in EPS and VB$^3$, but no growth of bacteria indicates NBP.

Testing for antibody levels of IgA and IgG in common pathogenic bacteria in EPS and VB$^3$ may diagnose CBP without serial segmented urine specimens. Elevation of antibody levels indicates bacterial prostatitis, especially CBP.

CBC

In CBP, consider transrectal ultrasound for prostate calculi.

Older males, consider urine cytologies to rule out bladder malignancy.

## TABLE 34-21.  PATIENT/CAREGIVER INFORMATION FOR PROSTATITIS

Bed rest as needed for symptom relief
Warm sitz baths three to four times daily
Adequate hydration (2–4 L daily)
Avoid irritants, such as alcohol, coffee, or tea
High-fiber diet for adequate bowel elimination to decrease abdominal pressure
Avoid spicy foods (decreases spasms)
Avoid urethral instrumentation
Use relaxation techniques daily
Educate about signs and symptoms of infection and importance of seeking health care
    immediately

agents penetrate the prostatic tissue, but are inactive against gram-negative rods. TMP-SMX and FLQN achieve reasonable tissue penetration. Treatment success in ABP is common because inflamed prostate tissue has increased permeability to drugs (Criste et al, 1994; Meares, 1992; Moul, 1993; Mullenix & Prince, 1997).

Treatment failure in CBP is common and indicates the need for long-term, low-dose suppressive therapy. Cure rates are 50–90% for FLQNs and 32–71% for TMP-SMX. Carbenicillin indanyl sodium is effective, with cure rates of 60–74%; however, it is expensive and usually reserved for treatment failure with FLQNs (Criste et al, 1994; Meares, 1992; Mullenix & Prince,

## TABLE 34-22.  EMPIRIC THERAPY FOR PROSTATITIS

| Drug | Regimen | Preference |
|---|---|---|
| **Acute Bacterial Prostatitis (ABP)** | | |
| FLQN | Oral 4–6 weeks | 1st |
| TMP-SMX | Oral 4–6 weeks | 1st |
| **Chronic Bacterial Prostatitis (CBP)** | | |
| FLQN | Oral 4–6 weeks; 3–4 months in treatment failure | 1st |
| TMP-SMX | Oral 4–6 weeks; 3–4 months in treatment failure | 1st |
| **Nonbacterial Prostatitis (NBP)** | | |
| | Client age <35 or suspect STDs | |
| Doxycycline | Oral 2–4 weeks | 1st |
| Erythromycin | Oral 2–4 weeks | Alt |
| | Not STD | |
| NSAIDs | Oral for symptomatic relief | |
| **Prostadynia (PD)** | | |
| Terazosin | Oral daily for sphincter dyssynergia; 1 mg titrated up for symptomatic relief; 8–10 mg maximum dose | 1st |
| Doxazosin | 1 mg titrated up for symptomatic relief; 8–10 mg maximum dose | 1st |
| Diazepam | Oral prn | 1st |
| NSAIDs | Oral prn for other symptoms | Alt |

Alt = alternative; FLQN = fluoroquinolone; NSAID = nonsteroidal antiinflammatory drug; TMP-SMX = trimethoprim-sulfamethoxazole.

1997). Prostatic calculi preclude a cure, and evaluation for surgical removal of prostatic stones is recommended (Moul, 1993).

Treatment of NBP is controversial. If a lack of therapeutic response occurs, antibiotics are discontinued and therapy focuses on symptomatic control with NSAIDs and anticholinergics. If the patient has a therapeutic response, the patient's sexual partner is referred for diagnostic evaluation and treatment for STD (Meares, 1992; Moul, 1993). Treatment of PD depends on the results of a comprehensive urodynamic evaluation. Tension myalgia of the pelvic floor requires antispasmodics, such as diazepam. NSAIDs are usually effective in controlling other symptomatology (Criste et al, 1994; Meares, 1992; Moul, 1993).

### Monitoring for Efficacy

*Acute and Chronic Bacterial Prostatitis.* Failure of symptoms to improve within 48–72 h requires reassessment of the patient. Posttreatment urine and EPS cultures are essential within 2–3 weeks of therapy completion (Meares, 1992; Moul, 1993; Mullenix & Prince, 1997).

*Nonbacterial Prostatitis and Prostadynia.* The patient's subjective report of symptom relief determines the effectiveness of drug therapy since all cultures are negative (Criste et al, 1994; Meares, 1992; Moul, 1993; Mullenix & Prince, 1997).

### Monitoring for Toxicity

Refer to Drug Tables.

### Follow-up Recommendations

*Acute Bacterial Prostatitis.* Posttreatment urine and EPS cultures are required within 2 weeks of therapy completion.

*Chronic Bacterial Prostatitis.* Posttreatment urine and EPS cultures are essential within 1–2 weeks of therapy completion. Patients unresponsive to antibiotic therapy require a referral to a urologist for comprehensive evaluation for the presence of prostatic stones or other complicating factors (Meares, 1992; Moul, 1993).

*Nonbacterial Bacterial Prostatitis.* Follow-up depends on the severity of symptoms and selected therapeutic agent. Patients using NSAIDs long-term need periodic evaluations for gastrointestinal bleeding, renal function, and adverse effects of NSAID therapy. Persistence or relapse of symptoms requires a referral to a urologist for a comprehensive evaluation (Meares, 1992; Moul, 1993).

*Prostadynia.* Patients with PD require close monitoring of symptoms. Refer for psychological evaluation if significant stress or emotional problems are present (Meares, 1992; Moul, 1993).

## BENIGN PROSTATIC HYPERPLASIA

Benign prostatic hyperplasia (BPH) or "prostatism" is a symptom complex defined as benign adenomatous hyperplasia of the periurethral prostate gland's stromal and glandular elements. The etiology of BPH is unclear; however, contributing factors include: (1) increased age, (2) increased 5-alpha-dihydrotestosterone (DHT), (3) increased estrogen, and (4) stimulation of alpha-adrenergic nerve endings that interfere with the opening of the bladder neck internal sphincter (Hicks & Cook, 1995; Long & Long, 1994; Madsen & Bruskewitz, 1995; McConnell, 1995; Oesterling, 1995; Shapiro & Lepor, 1995).

BPH is rare in males <40 years old and common in males >50 years (50%). Approximately 90% of males older than 85 years have microscopic evidence of BPH. It is estimated that approximately 25% of all males in the United States will require treatment for relief of symptoms of BPH during their lifetime (Hicks & Cook, 1995; Long & Long, 1994; Madsen & Bruskewitz, 1995; Oesterling, 1995; Roehrborn, 1995; Shapiro & Lepor, 1995; U.S. Department of Health and Human Services [USDHHS], 1994). Approximately 400,000 transurethral resections are performed annually, and this procedure is rated the second most common procedure after cataract extraction in males over 65 years. The associated expense is estimated at $5 billion per year (Madsen & Bruskewitz, 1995; Oesterling, 1995; Roehrborn, 1995). Significant health care costs, variance of therapeutic regimens, lack of guidelines for timing and treatment choices, uncertainty regarding etiology and natural history of the disease process, and ambiguous treatment outcomes are factors that influenced the development of clinical guidelines for BPH by the Agency for Health Care

Policy and Research (AHCPR) (Roehrborn, 1995).

BPH is characterized by obstructive or irritative symptoms or a combination of both in varying degrees with gradual worsening of symptoms. The enlarged prostate compresses the urethra to reduce or obstruct urinary flow, which results in obstructive symptoms of weak or decreased force of urinary stream, urinary hesitancy, postvoid or terminal dribbling, intermittency, abdominal straining to urinate, and incomplete bladder emptying. Irritative symptoms result from uninhibited smooth muscle contractions and detrusor instability and include nocturia, urinary frequency, urinary urgency, dysuria, and incontinence. BPH is the most common cause of hematuria. These symptoms frequently increase during periods of stress, exposure to cold, or use of sympathomimetic agents (Hicks & Cook, 1995; Long & Long, 1994; Madsen & Bruskewitz, 1995; Oesterling, 1995; Shapiro & Lepor, 1995).

Males seek health care for BPH because of worry, embarrassment, and progressive symptoms that affect their quality of life. Complications of BPH may vary from recurrent UTIs, UTIs with possible sepsis, acute urinary retention, and uremia. Postoperative complications from transurethral prostate resection include morbidity, retrograde ejaculation, impotence, urinary incontinence, repeat surgeries, and lack of satisfactory long-term outcomes. Differential diagnosis is critical to rule out prostatic cancer, vesical neck obstruction, hyperreflexia from inflammatory or infectious conditions, and impaired detrusor contractility related to neurogenic, myogenic, or psychogenic factors (Hicks & Cook, 1995; Long & Long, 1994; Madsen & Bruskewitz, 1995; Oesterling, 1995; Roehrborn, 1995; Shapiro & Lepor, 1995).

## SPECIFIC CONSIDERATIONS FOR PHARMACOTHERAPY

### When Drug Therapy Is Needed

Therapeutic regimens of BPH are in transition. The clinician needs to consider the degree of symptomatology, patient preference, pharmacologic agents, and surgical therapies in determining the best therapeutic regimen for each patient. The purpose of therapy in BPH is to decrease urological symptoms and to improve the rate of urinary flow. Urologists' primary

therapy preference remains transurethral prostate resection (Hicks & Cook, 1995; Long & Long, 1994; Madsen & Bruskewitz, 1995; Oesterling, 1995; Roehrborn, 1995; Shapiro & Lepor, 1995).

The degree of symptomatology is measurable by the American Urological Association (AUA) Symptom Index (USDHHS, 1994). It is a reliable, subjective tool for initial assessment of the patient's symptoms and periodic determination of disease progression or treatment effectiveness. The AUA Symptom Index is a self-administered seven-item questionnaire that rates the severity of symptoms on a scale from 0 (not at all) to 5 (almost always); items are summed to obtain a total score (Hicks & Cook, 1995; Madsen & Bruskewitz, 1995; Lepor, 1995a; Oesterling, 1995; Roehrborn, 1995; Shapiro & Lepor, 1995).

Males with minimal to moderate symptoms or an AUA Symptom Index score of ≤7 may safely be followed by the strategy of watchful waiting and stand to gain little from any treatment, including surgery. Males with moderate to severe symptoms or an AUA Symptom Index score ≥8 may be offered the various treatment alternatives (including watchful waiting) or be scheduled for additional tests. Tests include flow rate recording, residual urine measurement, and pressure flow urodynamic studies to confirm the presence of BPH, rule out other causes of the patient's symptoms, and assist in determining the proper time for therapeutic interventions. Patients with refractory urinary retention, recurrent UTIs, recurrent gross hematuria, and bladder or renal insufficiency clearly related to BPH are candidates for surgery and should be referred to a urologist for a comprehensive evaluation (Hicks & Cook, 1995; Long & Long, 1994; Madsen & Bruskewitz, 1995; Oesterling, 1995; Roehrborn, 1995; Shapiro & Lepor, 1995).

Patient preference is influenced by the degree of symptomatology, personal living circumstances, cost concerns, knowledge of therapeutic options, and probability of expected symptom improvement. Patient education includes the benefits and risks of watchful waiting and alternate therapies, such as behavioral techniques, drug therapy, balloon dilation, or surgery (Hicks & Cook, 1995; Long & Long, 1994; Oesterling, 1995; Roehrborn, 1995).

Ideal candidates for pharmacologic therapy are males with moderate symptoms, those unfit for surgery, or those who desire to avoid surgery.

Pharmacologic agents target two avenues of action: (1) reduction of prostate size by hormonal manipulation and (2) reduction of smooth muscle tone by adrenergic blockage. Hormonal therapies, such as the 5-alpha-reductase inhibitor, finasteride, block the enzyme that converts testosterone into DHT and result in atrophy of prostatic epithelium with shrinkage of the gland. Finasteride has few side effects, lowers the serum concentration of prostate-specific antigen (PSA), and has a low toxicity profile. It is moderately effective in the reduction of clinical symptoms. Because finasteride spares testosterone levels while lowering DHT, sexual potency and functioning are spared in 96–97% of patients (Hicks & Cook, 1995; Long & Long, 1994; McConnell, 1995; Oesterling, 1995; Roehrborn, 1995).

Alpha$_1$-selective adrenergic receptor blockers, such as terazosin and doxazosin, relax smooth muscle tone in prostatic tissue to produce immediate, significant improvement in urinary flow and irritative symptoms of BPH. There is greater patient compliance with one daily dosage and fewer side effects than with nonselective alpha blockers. Adverse reactions include dizziness, postural hypertension, and asthenia. There is no evidence that these drugs reduce complication rates or postpone future surgery (Hicks & Cook, 1995; Long & Long, 1994; Lepor, 1995a; Oesterling, 1995).

### Short- and Long-Term Goals of Pharmacotherapy

The short-term goals of therapy for BPH are to decrease the patient's symptoms and increase urinary flow. The long-term goals are to decrease the patient's symptoms, halt progress of the disease, increase urinary flow, and prevent complications of the disease to improve the patient's quality of life. The goals of treatment are achieved by watchful waiting, drug therapy, or surgery.

### Time Frame for Initiating Pharmacotherapy

BPH should be treated at the time of diagnosis to prevent worsening of urinary symptoms and potential complications. The clinician's treatment decision should be based on the degree of symptomatology, patient preference, etiology of the disease process, and pharmacological agents (Hicks & Cook, 1995; Long & Long, 1994; Lepor, 1995a; Madsen & Bruskewitz, 1995;

McConnell, 1995; Oesterling, 1995; Roehrborn, 1995).

See Drug Tables 205.3, 602.2, 1001.

### Assessment and History Taking

Refer to Table 34–23 and 34–24.

### Patient/Caregiver Information

Education of the patient about signs and symptoms of the disease, drug therapy, and palliative measures is critical for positive outcomes (Hicks & Cook, 1995; Madsen & Bruskewitz, 1995; Oesterling, 1995; Roehrborn, 1995). Refer to Table 34–25.

## OUTCOMES MANAGEMENT

### Selecting an Appropriate Agent

There is a lack of clarity in the literature regarding selection of definitive hormonal or alpha blockade therapy. Refer to Table 34–26. Patient preference, degree of symptomatology, and cost concerns are important factors in therapy selection. Clinical assessment of the static and dynamic prostate hyperplastic components provides guidance in drug selection. Hormonal therapy provides symptomatic relief by reducing testosterone and DHT to shrink the prostate gland. Alpha$_1$-selective blockade therapy reduces the dynamic component by decreasing smooth muscle tone (Hicks & Cook, 1995; Lepor, 1995a; Long & Long, 1994; McConnell, 1995; Oesterling, 1995).

The advantages of finasteride over most hormonal therapies include fewer adverse effects and a wide margin of safety. Disadvantages of finasteride therapy are high cost, moderate efficacy (35–50%), and PSA suppression (McConnell, 1995; Oesterling, 1995).

The short-acting alpha$_1$-selective blocker prazosin relaxes smooth muscle tone and increases uroflow. Multiple daily dosages decrease patient compliance and increase adverse effects despite its lower cost. The long-acting alpha$_1$-selective blockers doxazosin and terazosin are effective with single daily dosages. Advantages of alpha$_1$-selective blockers are more rapid onset, moderate cost, and potential for therapy in hypertensive patients. Disadvantages are frequent postural hypotension, drowsiness, dizziness, and lightheadedness (Lepor, 1995a; Long & Long, 1994; Oesterling, 1995).

## TABLE 34-23. BASELINE DATA: HISTORY AND PHYSICAL EXAMINATION FOR BENIGN PROSTATIC HYPERPLASIA

**History**

Onset and duration of symptoms

Initial assessment with the American Urological Association (AUA) Symptom Index: patient rates symptoms experienced over the past month, such as sensation of not emptying bladder after urination, occurrence of the need to urinate within 2 hours of last urination, episodes of having to start and stop during urination, difficulty postponing urination, weak urinary stream, occurrence of needing to push and strain to urinate, and the number of times got up from bed to urinate during the night

History of pain or discomfort, hematuria, recent onset of back or bone pain, anorexia, and weight loss

Patient records symptoms in a daily diary for a period of 1 week

Medical history, specifically about genitourinary problems and surgeries, such as urethral trauma, gonococcal urethritis, or urethral instrumentation; diabetes mellitus; and neurologic diseases that may cause a neurologic bladder dysfunction

Medication history: ask if cold or sinus medications aggravate their symptoms; use of drugs, such as anticholinergics that impair bladder contractility and sympathomimetics that increase outflow resistance

**Physical Examination**

Abdominal examination to detect a distended bladder from retention, renal tenderness, or a mass

Digital rectal examination (DRE) to estimate the size of the prostate, detect nodules or induration indicative of prostate cancer, and evaluate anal sphincter tone

Observe patient voiding or ask him to time urination to determine size and force of urinary stream (a male normally empties bladder of 300 mL of urine in 12–15 s)

Neurologic examination to detect neurogenic disease, such as multiple sclerosis

## Monitoring for Efficacy

Reassessment of the patient's symptoms using the AUA Symptom Index is essential after 6 months of *hormonal therapy*, along with peak uroflow diagnostic evaluation. The expectation is a decrease in the AUA Symptom Index Score from the initial assessment or scores from periodic monitoring. Reports show a mean score improvement of 2.7 points and peak flow improvement of 1.6 mL/s (Oesterling, 1995). For treatment failures consider alpha blockade therapy, watchful waiting, or surgical intervention (Hicks & Cook, 1995; Oesterling, 1995).

Reassessment of the patient's symptoms using the AUA Symptom Index is essential after obtaining optimal tolerated dosages of *alpha₁-selective blockers*. The expectation is a decrease in the AUA Symptom Index Score from the initial assessment or scores from periodic monitoring. Reports show a mean index score improvement of 4.5 points (Oesterling, 1995). For treatment failures consider hormonal therapy, watchful waiting, or surgical intervention (Hicks & Cook, 1995; Oesterling, 1995).

## Monitoring for Toxicity

Finasteride has significant adverse effects on a developing fetus. Patients need to avoid fathering children while on the medication and avoid exposing pregnant patients to semen fluid as it

## TABLE 34-24. DIAGNOSTIC TESTS FOR BENIGN PROSTATIC HYPERPLASIA

Urinalysis to rule out UTI and hematuria

Creatinine to assess renal function (renal insufficiency increases risk for postoperative complications)

Prostate serum antigen (PSA) is optional; serum values of PSA increase in direct proportion to the volume of BPH; thus PSA levels may be as high as 10 µg/L without being indicative of prostate cancer; digital rectal examination (DRE) and PSA are the best strategy for detecting prostate cancer

Moderate to severe symptoms, consider urinary flow rate, postvoid residual urine, pressure flow urodynamic studies, and urethrocystoscopy

## TABLE 34–25. PATIENT/CAREGIVER INFORMATION FOR BENIGN PROSTATIC HYPERPLASIA

- Limit fluid intake after dinner
- Avoid decongestants
- Void frequently
- Avoid sudden diuresis, which often occurs after drinking caffeine or alcohol
- Perform prostatic massage after intercourse
- Avoid certain medications, such as anticholinergics, tranquilizers, and antidepressants
- Educate how to assess for signs and symptoms of retention and obstruction and to seek health care if problems exist

can produce fetal abnormalities (McConnell, 1995). Alpha$_1$-selective agent therapy may be problematic in normotensive patients. Gradual tapering of dosage allows for adaptation to the loss of alpha tone. Future development of alpha$_{1a}$-selective blocking agents may reduce the incidence of adverse effects (Lepor, 1995b; Oesterling, 1995).

### Follow-up Recommendations

All BPH patients need periodic assessments to monitor for progression of disease. Time frames for assessment depend on mode of therapy, such as watchful waiting or drug therapy. Assessments include the determination of changes in symptomatology and diagnostic evaluation, such as urinalysis, uroflow, and renal function. Comparison of AUA Symptom Index scores clearly delineates symptom relief and delay of disease progression. Elderly males need an annual monitoring of PSA and a digital rectal examination (DRE) to check

for the development of prostate cancer. Patients undergoing surgery or balloon dilation are followed by a urologist (Hicks & Cook, 1995; Madsen & Bruskewitz, 1995; McConnell, 1995; Oesterling, 1995; Roehrborn, 1995; Shapiro & Lepor, 1995).

## ERECTILE DYSFUNCTION

Erectile dysfunction (ED) is a non-life-threatening disorder that is influenced by cultural, religious, and legal factors. The continual change of societal attitudes, lifting of taboos, and expansion of the media regarding human sexuality since the 1960s are factors that enhance open communication between patients and health care providers plus stimulate research. Early research findings lack clarity because of inconsistent definitions and poorly defined variables or parameters. Greater knowledge and under-

## TABLE 34–26. EMPIRIC THERAPY FOR BENIGN PROSTATIC HYPERPLASIA

| Drug | Regimen | Duration |
|---|---|---|
| **Alpha Blocker Categories** | | |
| Terazosin | 1 mg PO daily | 1–2 weeks then advance |
| | 2 mg PO daily | 1–2 weeks then advance |
| | 5 mg PO daily | 1–2 weeks then advance |
| | 10 mg PO daily | Continuously |
| Doxazosin | 1 mg PO daily | 1–2 weeks then advance |
| | 2 mg PO daily | 1–2 weeks then advance |
| | 4 mg PO daily | 1–2 weeks then advance |
| | 8 mg PO daily | Continuously |
| **Hormones** | | |
| Finasteride | 5 mg PO daily | Continuously |

Note: Advance dosage as tolerated. The goal of therapy is the largest tolerated dose listed for each drug.

standing of sexual pathophysiology encourage research, evaluation, and management of sexual problems (Baum & Rhodes, 1995; Benet & Melman, 1995).

Erectile dysfunction, also termed *impotence*, includes libidinal, orgasmic, and ejaculatory dysfunction. ED is defined as the inability of the male to attain and maintain an erection sufficient to allow sexual intercourse. An erection is a hemodynamic process mediated by neurogenic, endothelial, endocrine, and cortical (psychological) influences. Impairment of any element of the erectile apparatus or changes of its control leads to ED. It is estimated that 50% of ED is organic in nature (Baum & Rhodes, 1995; Benet & Melman, 1995; Linet & Ogrinc, 1996).

Approximately 10–20 million males are affected by ED in the United States. If males with minimal ED are included, the estimate increases to 30 million. Approximately 1% of males are affected by the age of 30, 6.7% by the age of 45–55, 25% by the age of 65, and 75% by the age of 80. Factors affecting the etiology of ED are diverse and may be hormonal, psychological, vasculogenic, or neurogenic (Table 34–27). The most common causes of ED are age, medications, diabetes (25–75% prevalence), and chronic health conditions. It is the main complaint of male partners that are evaluated in sex therapy clinics (Baum & Rhodes, 1995; Benet & Melman, 1995; Fallon, 1995; Georgitis &

Merenich, 1995; Linet & Ogrinc, 1996; Lipshultz, 1996; Nunez & Anderson, 1993).

Males are reluctant to seek health care for ED because of embarrassment, low self-esteem, myths regarding the aging process, and uncertainty in how to discuss concerns. The denial of problems with ED or omission of assessment for ED by health care providers leads to decreasing quality of life and lack of compliance with prescribed medication regimens. Patients at risk for ED need to be firmly and professionally asked if a problem with intimacy exists (Baum & Rhodes, 1995; Benet & Melman, 1995; Georgitis & Merenich, 1995).

## SPECIFIC CONSIDERATIONS FOR PHARMACOTHERAPY

### When Drug Therapy Is Needed

Therapeutic regimens of ED are in transition. Consider the degree of symptomatology, patient preferences, pharmacologic agents, and surgical therapies in determining the best therapeutic regimen for each patient. The aim is to decrease the symptoms of ED and improve the quality of life without interfering with prescribed health regimens for other health conditions. Effective therapy may be the simple adjustment of current medications, such as diuretics, hypertensives, or psychotropic agents by reducing dosage or switching to an angiotensin-converting enzyme inhibitor, calcium channel blocker, or cardiac-selective beta blocking agent. Urologists' primary therapy preference is intracavernosal injection therapy or penile implants (Baum & Rhodes, 1995; Benet & Melman, 1995; "Drug Induced," 1996; Fallon, 1995; Linet & Ogrinc, 1996; Lipshultz, 1996; Morales, Heaton, Johnston, & Adams, 1995).

The degree of symptomatology relies on the patient's and the sexual partner's perceptions and is subjectively defined. Patient preference is influenced by the degree of symptomatology, personal relationships, cost concerns, knowledge of therapeutic options, and probability of expected symptom improvement. Patient education includes the benefits and risks of all therapies (Baum & Rhodes, 1995; "Drug Induced," 1996; Fallon, 1995; Morales et al, 1995).

Ideal candidates for pharmacologic therapy are males with moderate symptoms, those unfit for surgery, or those who desire to avoid surgery.

## TABLE 34–27. ETIOLOGICAL FACTORS OF ERECTILE DYSFUNCTION

| | |
|---|---|
| Age | Fear of failure |
| Alcohol abuse | Hypertension |
| Atherosclerosis | Neurologic disease |
| Associated medications |   Multiple sclerosis |
|   Antihypertensives |   Spinal cord injury |
|   Antidepressants |   Stroke |
|   Analgesics | Peripheral vascular disease |
|   $H_2$ Blockers | Priapism |
|   Thiazide diuretics | Prostatic disease |
|   Tranquilizers |   Benign prostatic |
| Conflict with partner |     hypertrophy |
| Depression |   Cancer |
| Diabetes mellitus |   Prostatitis |
| Endocrine disease |   Vesiculoprostatitis |
|   Adrenal disorders | Penile and urethral lesions |
|   Hyperthyroidism | Radical pelvic surgery |
|   Hypothyroidism | Smoking |
|   Pituitary tumor | |

Pharmacologic agents act by inhibiting sympathetic tone and directly stimulating relaxation of the corporal smooth muscle to increase blood flow into the sinusoidal spaces of the cavernous bodies. An initial intracavernous injection needs to be performed in the office to determine the patient's response. If successful, the patient needs to be educated for self-injections at home (Baum & Rhodes, 1995; Fallon, 1995; Lipshultz, 1996; Morales et al, 1995).

## Short- and Long-Term Goals of Pharmacotherapy

The short-term goals of therapy for ED are to decrease the patient's symptoms and maintain compliance with any prescribed drug regimen for other health conditions. The long-term goals are to decrease the patent's symptoms, halt progress of disease, maintain compliance with any prescribed drug regimen for other health conditions, and prevent complications of diseases to improve the patient's quality of life.

## Time Frame for Initiating Pharmacotherapy

ED is treated at the time of diagnosis to prevent further symptoms and potential complications. The clinician's treatment decision is based on degree of symptomatology, patient preference, the etiology of the disease process, and pharmacologic agents (Baum & Rhodes, 1995; Benet & Melman, 1995; "Drug Induced," 1996; Fallon, 1995; Georgitis & Merenich, 1995; Linet & Ogrinc, 1996; Lipshultz, 1996; Morales et al, 1995).

## Assessment and History Taking

Refer to Tables 34–28 and 34–29.

## Patient/Caregiver Information

Education of the patient about signs and symptoms of the disease, drug therapy, and prevention measures is critical for positive outcomes and includes the following (Baum & Rhodes, 1995; Benet & Melman, 1995; Fallon, 1995;

---

## TABLE 34–28. BASELINE DATA: HISTORY AND PHYSICAL EXAMINATION FOR ERECTILE DYSFUNCTION

### History
Onset and duration of symptoms
Sexual history, such as age of first intercourse, number of sexual partners, frequency of sexual coitus, sexual behaviors (anal and vaginal coitus), sexual libido, and use of barrier methods
History of pain or discomfort, hematuria, recent onset of back or bone pain, anorexia, and weight loss
Frequency of early morning erections (sudden onset and preservation of erections on awakening or masturbation are characteristic of psychogenic disease whereas gradual onset and progressive loss of duration and strength of morning erections suggest organic disease)
Complete medical history, specifically about genitourinary problems and surgeries, such as urethral trauma, urethral instrumentation, or pelvic fracture, diabetes mellitus, neurologic diseases, and cardiovascular diseases
Complete medication history; any changes in ED while on medications

### Physical Examination
Vital signs; note if any postural fall in blood pressure
General appearance for loss of secondary sexual characteristics
Skin examination for spider angiomata, palmar erythema, excessive dryness, hyperpigmentation, and other dermatological signs of endocrinopathy
Flaccid penis examination for tumor, inflammation, discharge, and phimosis of the foreskin
Erect penis examination for degree of chordee to erectile weakness
Testicular examination for size, masses, nodules, and tenderness
Digital rectal examination (DRE) to estimate the size of the prostate and detect nodules, masses, or tenderness, and evaluate anal sphincter tone
Aorta and femoral arteries for rate, bruits, and other signs of occlusive disease, especially with history of claudication
Neurologic examination to detect neurogenic disease, such as multiple sclerosis that relates to etiology of ED
Pain sensation in genitalia and perianal areas

### TABLE 34-29. DIAGNOSTIC TESTS FOR ERECTILE DYSFUNCTION

Two-hour postprandial serum glucose to rule out diabetes mellitus
Serum total testosterone and luteinizing hormones with complaints of reduced libido
Lipid profile if evidence of peripheral vascular disease
TSH level if hypothyroidism a possibility
Nocturnal penile tumescence or "postage stamp" test to assess the intactness of erectile apparatus (most sensitive test available); Instruct client to wrap a ring of postage stamps snugly around a flaccid penis at bedtime and moisten overlapping stamps to seal the ring; positive test is confirmed with breakage along the perforations in the morning
Home monitoring of erections with Rigiscan for strength and number of erections
Other tests by urologist, such as doppler ultrasonography, intracavernosal injection, color flow tests, or sacral nerve reflex latency time

Linet & Ogrinc, 1996; Lipshultz, 1996; Morales et al, 1995; Nunez & Anderson, 1993):

- Etiology and progression of disease
- Use of coping mechanisms to reduce stress
- The purpose, dosage, and side effects of drugs
- Appropriate technique for self-administered injection prior to coitus
- Signs and symptoms of complications and importance of seeking health care

## OUTCOMES MANAGEMENT

### Selecting an Appropriate Agent

The key to therapy is having a complete history to be able to determine the etiology of ED. Discontinuing drugs or substituting alternative drugs is appropriate if ED is the result of a drug side effect (Abramowicz, 1992; "Drug Induced," 1996).

Antihypertensive drugs, such as thiazide diuretics, methyldopa, clonidine, and beta blockers, cause ED and loss of libido. Angiotensin-converting enzyme (ACE) inhibitors, calcium channel blockers, selective cardiac beta blockers, and peripheral alpha$_1$ blockers, such as prazocin and terazocin, are less likely to affect ED (Abramowicz, 1992; Benet & Melman, 1995; "Drug Induced," 1996).

Social or recreational drugs contribute significantly to ED. Chronic ethanol abuse results in feminization, gynecomastia, low libido, persistent impotence, testicular atrophy, and sterility. Opiates suppress LH secretion and stimulate prolactin secretion. Marijuana and amphetamines are possible offenders (Abramowicz, 1992; Benet & Melman, 1995; "Drug Induced," 1996).

Antipsychotics and antidepressants effect ED through the neurotransmitters. Dopaminergic and cholinergic stimulation of the central nervous system promote erectile function, whereas serotonergic stimulation inhibits sexual function. Reduction of dopamine blocker dosage or a trial use of another drug improves ED. Tricyclic antidepressants and selective serotonin reuptake inhibitors, such as fluoxetine, inhibit libido and orgasm by proserotonergic activity. Using fewer antimuscarinic antidepressants can offer some relief. Monamine oxidase inhibitors (MAOIs) have little association with ED (Abramowicz, 1992; Benet & Melman, 1995; "Drug Induced," 1996).

Urologists frequently prescribe intracavernous injections with a combination of drugs, such as alprostadil (PGE$_1$), papaverine, and phentolamine mesylate, whereas others prescribe PGE$_1$ alone (Baum & Rhodes, 1995; Fallon, 1995; Georgitis & Merenich, 1995; Linet & Ogrinc, 1996; Lipschultz, 1996; Morales et al, 1995; Nunez & Anderson, 1993). A trial of oral Yohimbine seeks to avoid the use of injections; however, it is often ineffective (Abramowicz, 1992; Benet & Melman, 1995). The new dosage form of alprostadil in a urethral suppository may replace the use of intracaverous injections because of better acceptance and comparable efficacy (Padma-Nathan et al, 1997). **See Drug Table 1001 for sildenafil citrate (Viagra).**

### Monitoring for Efficacy

Effects of drug therapy changes for ED range from a few days to several weeks. Frequent monitoring of blood pressure is essential when antihypertensive drugs are modified. The reduction of dosages for antipsychotics or the use of different antidepressants requires monitoring of therapeutic effects. Intracavernous injections for ED are initiated in the physician's office for observation of efficacy, duration of erection, and need of dosage adjustment to prevent priapism (Fallon, 1995; Linet & Ogrinc, 1996; Lipshultz, 1996; Morales et al, 1995).

## Monitoring for Toxicity

A prolonged erection or priapism is the most important toxic effect to monitor in intracavernous injections. Erections lasting longer than 4 h require immediate physician intervention (Fallon, 1995; Linet & Ogrinc, 1996; Lipshultz, 1996; Morales et al, 1995).

## Follow-up Recommendations

Dose adjustments of hypertensive, antidepressant, antipsychotic, or other drug therapies require follow-up recommendations for the respective treatment regimen. Patients using intracavernous injection therapy are evaluated every month for dosage adjustment, correct injection technique, and side effects (Baum & Rhodes, 1995; Fallon, 1995; Linet & Ogrinc, 1996; Lipshultz, 1996; Morales et al, 1995).

## REFERENCES

Abramowicz, M. (1992). Drugs that cause sexual dysfunction: An update. *Medical Letter, 34*(876), 73–78.

Baldassarre, J. S., & Kaye, D. (1991). Special problems of urinary tract infection in the elderly. *Medical Clinics of North America, 75*(2), 375–389.

Barger, M., & Woolner, B. (1995). Assessment and management of genitourinary tract disorders. *Journal of Nurse-Midwifery, 40*(2), 231–245.

Baum, N., & Rhodes, D. (1995). A practical approach to the evaluation and treatment of erectile dysfunction: A private practitioner's viewpoint. *Urology Clinics of North America, 22*(4), 865–877.

Beckman, N. J. (1995). An overview of urinary incontinence in adults: Assessments of behavioral interventions. *Clinical Nurse Specialist, 9*(5), 241–247.

Benet, A. E., & Melman, A. (1995). The epidemiology of erectile dysfunction. *Urology Clinics of North America, 22*(4), 699–709.

Bergeron, M. G. (1995). Treatment of pyelonephritis in adults. *Medical Clinics of North America, 79*(3), 619–649.

Brooks, M. J. (1993). Urinary incontinence: Assessment, treatment and reimbursement. *Home Healthcare Nurse, 11*(4), 41–46.

Centers for Disease Control and Prevention. (1994). *1993 sexually transmitted diseases treatment guidelines* (Publication No. 1994-533-001/80555). Washington, DC: U.S. Government Printing Office.

Criste, G., Gray, D., & Gallo, B. (1994). Prostatitis: A review of diagnosis and management. *Nurse Practitioner, 19*(7), 32–33, 37–38.

Drug induced sexual dysfunction (1996). *Micromedex, 89*, 1–19.

Fallon, B. (1995). Intracavernous injection therapy for male erectile dysfunction. *Urology Clinics of North America, 22*(4), 833–845.

Georgitis, W. J., & Merenich, J. A. (1995). Trial of pentoxifylline for diabetic impotence. *Diabetes Care, 18*(3), 345–352.

Hassay, K. A. (1995). Effective management of urinary discomfort. *Nurse Practitioner, 20*(2), 36, 39–40, 42–44, 46.

Hicks, R. J., & Cook, J. B. (1995). Managing patients with benign prostatic hyperplasia. *American Family Physician, 2*(1), 135–142.

Hooton, T. M. (1995). A simplified approach to urinary tact infection. *Hospital Practice*, 23–30.

Howes, D. S. (1992). UTI: Advances and controversies. *Emergency Medicine, 24*(11), 218–220, 223–224, 226–227.

Johnson, J. R. (1992). Recognizing and treating acute pyelonephritis. *Emergency Medicine, 24*(3), 24–26, 29–30, 33.

Kaler, S. R. (1990). Epididymitis in young adult males. *Nurse Practitioner, 15*(5), 10, 12, 14, 16.

Kiningham, R. B. (1993). Asymptomatic bacteriuria in pregnancy. *American Family Physician, 47*(5), 1232–1238.

Krieger, J. N. (1994). A burning issue. *Patient Care, 28*(11), 154, 156, 158.

Krieger, J. N. (1995). New sexually transmitted diseases treatment guidelines. *Journal of Urology, 154*(1), 209–213.

Lepor, H. (1995a). Alpha blockade for the treatment of benign prostatic hyperplasia. *Urology Clinics of North America, 22*(2), 375–386.

Lepor, H. (1995b). Combination medical therapy for benign prostatic hyperplasia. *Urology Clinics of North America, 22*(2), 401–405.

Linet, O. I., & Ogrinc, F. G. (1996). Efficacy and safety of intracavernosal alprostadil in men with erectile dysfunction. *New England Journal of Medicine, 334*(14), 873–877.

Lipshultz, L. I. (1996). Injection therapy for erectile dysfunction. *New England Journal of Medicine, 334*(14), 913–914.

Long, K., & Long, R. (1994). Treating benign prostatic hyperplasia with medication. *Nurse Practitioner Forum, 5*(3), 126–127.

Madsen, F. A., & Bruskewitz, R. C. (1995). Clinical manifestations of benign prostatic hyperplasia. *Urology Clinics of North America, 22*(2), 291–298.

McConnell, J. D. (1995). Benign prostatic hyperplasia. *Urology Clinics of North America, 22*(2), 387–400.

Meares, E. M. (1992). Prostatitis and related disorders. In *Campbell's Urology* (6th ed.). Philadelphia: W. B. Saunders.

Morales, A., Heaton, J. P., Johnston, B., & Adams, M. (1995). Oral and topical treatment of erectile dysfunction: Present and future. *Urology Clinics of North America, 22*(4), 879–886.

Moul, J. W. (1993). Prostatitis: Sorting out the different causes. *Postgraduate Medicine, 94*(5), 191–194.

Mullenix, T. A., & Prince, R. A. (1997). Urinary tract infections and prostatitis. In J. T. DiPiro, R. L. Talbert, G. C. Yee, G. R. Matzke, & L. M. Posey (Eds.), *Pharmacology: A pathophysiologic approach* (3rd ed.) (pp. 2173–2193). Stamford, CT: Appleton & Lange.

Nunez, B. D., & Anderson, D. C. (1993). Nitroglycerin ointment in the treatment of impotence. *Journal of Urology, 150*, 1241–1243.

Oesterling, J. E. (1995). Benign prostatic hyperplasia: Medical and minimally invasive treatment options. *New England Journal of Medicine, 332*(2), 99–109.

Padma-Nathan, H., Hellstrom, W. J. G., Kaiser, F. E., Labasky, R. F., Lue, T. F., Nolten, W. E., Norwood, P. C., Peterson, C. A., Shabsigh, R., Tam, P. Y., Place, V. A., & Gesundheit, N. (1997). Treatment of men with erectile dysfunction with transurethral alprostadil. *New England Journal of Medicine, 336*(1), 1–7.

Pearce, K. L. (1994). Levels I and II: Care in the outpatient setting. *Nurse Practitioner Forum, 5*(3), 146–151.

Plattner, M. S. (1994). Pyelonephritis in pregnancy. *Journal of Perinatal and Neonatal Nursing, 8*(1), 20–27.

Reynolds, E., & Hoberman, A. (1995). Diagnosis and management of pyelonephritis in infants. *Maternal Child Health Nursing, 20*, 78–84.

Roehrborn, C. G. (1995). The Agency for Health Care Policy and Research. *Urology Clinics of North America, 22*(2), 445–453.

Sanford, J. P., Gilbert, D. N., & Sande, M. A. (1996). *The Sanford guide to antimicrobial therapy, 1996* (26th ed.). Dallas, TX: Antimicrobial Therapy.

Schmid, G. P., & Fontanarosa, P. B. (1995). Evolving strategies for management of the nongonococcal urethritis syndrome. *JAMA, 274*(7), 577–579.

Shapiro, E., & Lepor, H. (1995). Pathophysiology of clinical benign prostatic hyperplasia. *Urology Clinics of North America, 22*(2), 285–290.

Sherbotie, J. R., & Cornfield, D. (1991). Management of urinary tract infections in children. *Medical Clinics of North America, 75*(2), 327–337.

Stamm, W. E., Hicks, C. B., Martin, D. H., Leone, P., Hook, E. W., Cooper, R. H., Cohen, M. S., Batteiger, B. E., Workowski, K., McCormack, W. M., Bolan, G., Douglas, J. M., Wong, E. S., Pappas, P. G., & Johnson, R. B. (1995). Azithromycin for empirical treatment of the nongonococcal urethritis syndrome in men. *JAMA, 274*(7), 545–549.

Stamm, W. E., & Hooton, T. M. (1993). Management of urinary tract infections in adults. *New England Journal of Medicine 329*(18), 1328–1334.

Talner, L. B., Davidson, A. J., Lebowitz, R. L., Palma, L. D., & Goldman, S. M. (1994). Acute pyelonephritis: Can we agree on terminology? *Radiology, 192*(2), 297–305.

U.S. Department of Health and Human Services. (1994). *Benign prostatic hyperplasia: Diagnosis and treatment* (AHCPR Publication No. 95-0583). Rockville, MD: Author.

U.S. Department of Health and Human Services. (1996). *Managing acute and chronic urinary incontinence* (AHCPR Publication No. 96-0686). Rockville, MD: Author.

Webb, M. L. (1994). Urinary incontinence in younger women. *Nurse Practitioner Forum, 5*(3), 164–169.

Wyman, J. F. (1994). Level 3: Comprehensive assessment and management of urinary incontinence by continence nurse specialists. *Nurse Practitioner Forum, 5*(3), 177–185.

Zahn, A. L., & Craven, R. A. (1994). The acute scrotum: Consider eight possibilities. *Emergency Medicine, 26*(1), 47–51.

# 35

# GYNECOLOGIC DISORDERS AND FEMALE SEXUAL DYSFUNCTION

*Linda O. Morphis and M. Sharm Steadman*

This chapter focuses on gynecological problems often seen in primary care. Vulvar conditions, including folliculitis, vulvar dermatitis, vulvodynia, vulvar vestibulitis, and lichen sclerosus are discussed. Amenorrhea, dysfunctional uterine bleeding, premenstrual syndrome, dysmenorrhea, endometriosis, adenomyosis, and sexual dysfunction are also covered.

## VULVAR CONDITIONS

In addition to vulvar tissue being under hormonal influence, the warm, moist environment makes it susceptible to many irritative and infectious conditions. To compound this susceptibility, the tissue is exposed to vaginal secretions, urine, and feces as well as nonabsorbent synthetic fibers and irritating products such as soaps, sprays, powders, daily use of peripads (scented ones are particularly irritating), and colored, scented toilet paper. It is little wonder that vulvar conditions are a common reason for visits to the practitioner.

Although some vulvar conditions may be difficult to diagnose and treat, careful assessment and management can relieve much discomfort and distress. Of paramount importance is the need to rule out serious conditions, realizing that premalignant and malignant vulvar lesions can, and do, occur. Consultation and referral are always warranted for any suspicious lesions.

## FOLLICULITIS

Folliculitis is an infection of the hair follicles, usually caused by *Staphylococcus* (Curry & Barclay, 1994). *Pseudomonas aeruginosa* has been identified as the offending organism in the development of folliculitis following hot-tub sessions, with pustules appearing within 1–4 days (Bartlett, 1996). Superficial trauma from chemical and mechanical factors also plays a role in the etiology, as with sycosis, a chronic form of folliculitis, which often results from shaving pubic hair (Goldstein & Odom, 1994). A nonbacterial type of folliculitis can be caused by the use of oils, cosmetics, cocoa butter, or coconut oil. Tight jeans or other restrictive clothing causes decreased air circulation, friction, and increased perspiration in the pubic or genital area, leading to folliculitis. *Candida albicans* can cause a yeast folliculitis (Bartlett, 1996).

### Specific Considerations for Pharmacotherapy

***When Drug Therapy is Needed.*** Drug therapy will be needed to treat the infection if self-care, non-pharmacotherapy-measures fail to clear the folliculitis.

***Short- and Long-Term Goals of Pharmacotherapy.*** The short-term goal is to treat infection and to relieve symptoms; the long-term goal is to prevent recurrence and complications.

***Nonpharmacologic Therapy.*** Warm, moist compresses to the vulvar area, using water or saline, or warm sitz baths, followed by patting dry with a clean towel and then thoroughly drying the area with a warm hair dryer setting can minimize discomfort. The prevention of predisposing causes is essential. Water in hot tubs and whirlpools must be properly treated (Goldstein & Odom, 1994). Other nonpharmacologic therapies include the elimination of irritating products; the use of an antibacterial soap only while infection is present and then changing to a nonalkaline, unscented, uncolored, pH-balanced soap; the use of a new or clean razor blade if shaving is continued; careful drying after bath or shower with a hair dryer on the warm setting; wearing all-cotton underwear; and leaving underwear off as frequently as possible, particularly at night.

***Time Frame for Initiating Pharmacotherapy.*** Depending on severity, nonpharmacologic treatment guidelines alone may be initiated when the patient presents for care, with the understanding that if symptom relief does not occur within 3 days, pharmacotherapy should be begun. If presenting symptoms warrant, pharmacological treatment should begin with initial patient contact, with expected symptom relief within several days to 1 week.

See Drug Tables 103, 805.

***Assessment and History Taking.*** On history, the patient will present with complaints of "bumps" in the area, mildly pruritic to nonpruritic. Questions related to shaving and use of irritating products, as well as presence of vaginal discharge should be included in history taking. Pelvic examination will show small superficial pustules at the base of the hair follicle, and mild erythema may be noted. Folliculitis lesions from *Pseudomonas* may be vesicular or pustular. Diagnostic tests for folliculitis are not indicated, as diagnosis is made by examining the area. Tests to rule out sexually transmitted infections, however, should be performed as indicated.

***Patient/Caregiver Information.*** Patients should be instructed in the nonpharmacologic and pharmacologic application of treatment. Inform the patient if any diagnostic test is pending, and when she should return for follow-up.

## Outcomes Management

***Selecting an Appropriate Agent.*** Bactroban (mupirocin 2%) topical antibiotic ointment applied sparingly b.i.d or t.i.d is the treatment agent of choice for folliculitis (Goldstein & Odom, 1994). Although this agent may be more costly than others, its effectiveness in the majority of cases justifies use. Creams and ointments containing neomycin also can be used (Sober, 1995). Unless pruritis is pronounced, oral antihistamines generally are not given. Yeast folliculitis requires treatment with an antifungal cream. Since underlying tissues are not affected in folliculitis, systemic antibiotics generally are not given. However, if the woman has chronic sycosis that is not responsive to local treatment, systemic antibiotics will be needed. Antistaphylococcal antibiotics for as long as 4 weeks may be indicated for recalcitrant infection (Goldstein & Odom, 1994).

***Monitoring for Efficacy.*** See "Time frame for initiating pharmacotherapy" above.

***Monitoring for Toxicity.*** Toxicity to mupirocin is rare. Neomycin is a known contact sensitizer, with sensitization developing with long-term use in denuded areas (Sober, 1995). See Drug Tables for antibiotic information.

***Follow-up Recommendations.*** Follow-up should be in 1 week to assess clearing of infection and adherence to guidelines for prevention. This could be by phone or office visit.

## VULVAR DERMATITIS

This vulvar condition is generally irritative but noninfectious in nature. It is a contact dermatitis, can be acute or chronic, and results from contact with allergens or chemicals, use of the previously noted irritants, as well as tight, restrictive clothing (Goldstein & Odom, 1994). Pruritis is very common and often severe, with risk of secondary infection from scratching.

### Specific Considerations for Pharmacotherapy

***When Drug Therapy is Needed.*** Discomfort and pruritis from vulvar dermatitis produces both physiological and psychological distress, warranting drug therapy.

***Short- and Long-term Goals of Pharmacotherapy.*** The short-term goal of pharmacotherapy is the relief of pruritis and irritation as quickly as possible, while the long-term goal is to prevent recurrence.

***Nonpharmacologic Therapy.*** Nonpharmacologic therapy includes cool to tepid sitz baths or compresses to the vulvar area, patting rather than rubbing dry, and careful drying using the warm hair dryer setting. This drying regimen, plus use of a mild, nonirritating soap, wearing all-cotton underwear, leaving underwear off as frequently as possible, and avoiding tight, restrictive clothing and irritating substances, will greatly reduce the risk of recurrence.

***Time Frame for Initiating Pharmacotherapy.*** Because of patient discomfort, treatment should be initiated with patient contact, and improvement in symptoms should be expected within 24 h after application of the topical agent.

See Drug Table 800.

***Assessment and History Taking.*** History taking should include specific questions related to use of irritants, as well as the presence of any chronic conditions, including liver disease. The woman will complain of itching, burning, and stinging of the affected area.

The vulva will be erythematous on exam. Mild edema, increased temperature scaling, and linear excoriations from scratching may also be present. A wet mount should be done to rule out infections such as *Candida*, and a culture for herpes simplex virus (HSV) also should be done if questionable lesions are present.

***Patient/Caregiver Information.*** Information should include instructions on how to use warm compresses and sitz baths. Avoidance of irritants is very important, and written information listing those products to avoid would be helpful. Patients should be told how to apply topical corticosteroids with emphasis placed on importance of short-term use. If oral corticosteroid therapy is indicated, appropriate information regarding side effects, interactions, and expected tapering regimen should be stressed (see Drug Table 601).

## Outcomes Management

***Selecting an Appropriate Agent.*** Appropriate topical corticosteroids include low-potency prescriptive preparations such as Aristocort or 0.5–1% OTC topical hydrocortisone, applied sparingly b.i.d. for 3–5 days (Lichtman & Duran, 1995). Oral antihistamines such as Atarax or Benadryl may also be used, particularly at bedtime if sleep is being disrupted. All these agents are fairly economical. For more severe acute problems, prednisone PO for 12–14 days can be used. One commonly used regimen is 60 mg for 4 days, 40 mg for 5 days, and 20 mg for 5 days (Goldstein & Odom, 1994). It is important to use a therapeutic dose early in therapy.

***Monitoring for Efficacy.*** Efficacy of treatment should be assessed in approximately 3 days. All symptoms, in mild cases, should be cleared in that time and physical examination should be negative. More severe cases may require a longer period to evidence healing.

***Monitoring for Toxicity.*** Local adverse reactions are reported infrequently with topical steroids when used short-term, but may include burning, irritation, dryness, and contact dermatitis. Skin atrophy, striae, and hypopigmentation especially are associated with long-term use, and therefore should be avoided. Short-term use of oral corticosteroids should not cause toxicity (see Drug Table 601, for possible negative effects from long-term use).

***Follow-up Recommendations.*** Stress the importance of continuing to avoid chemical or allergen irritants, nylon underwear, and tight-fitting garments. Lack of response to therapy requires referral to a specialist.

## VULVODYNIA

Vulvodynia is defined as "chronic vulvar discomfort characterized by the patient's complaint of constant burning, stinging, irritation, or feeling of rawness" (International Society, 1991). Although women have presented to health care providers with these symptoms and complaints for decades, in 1982 the International Society for the Study of Vulvar Disease at long last defined vulvodynia as a distinct clinical entity.

What seems to have confounded the defining of this condition, as well as the diagnosis and treatment, is the fact that it is virtually without visible evidence of vulvar pathology or abnormality, other than an occasional subtle redness. Sensitivity to touch will be noted on examination, but no proportional causative etiology will be detected initially.

Numerous disorders that result in chronic vulvar discomfort may be associated with vulvodynia. Discussion of two of these—vulvar vestibulitis and lichen sclerosus—follows.

## VULVAR VESTIBULITIS

Only recently recognized, vulvar vestibulitis is an inflammation of the minor vestibular glands at the introitus (Kaufman, 1995). The exact etiology is unknown, although many factors, including recurrent candidiasis (Mann, 1992), are probably causative. Other suggested causes include human papillomovirus (HPV) infection, elevated urinary levels of calcium oxalate, allergic reactions and chronic dermatitis, hormonal changes, and psychological responses.

### Specific Considerations for Pharmacotherapy

***When Drug Therapy is Needed.*** The psychic and physical pain of vulvar vestibulitis over months and even years can be tremendous. Activities of day-to-day life, work, and relationships are disrupted.

***Short- and Long-Term Goals of Pharmacotherapy.*** Short-term and long-term pharmacologic goals are to relieve pain and discomfort and to restore a semblance of normalcy to daily life, work, and relationships.

***Nonpharmacologic Therapy.*** Previously discussed nonpharmacologic therapies are included here. Needless to say, avoidance of irritants should be strictly observed, as they may not only aggravate the condition but also will add to discomfort. Additional nonpharmacologic therapies may include vaginal lubricants and a low oxalate diet along with the ingestion of calcium citrate tablets (Solomons, Melmed, & Heitler, 1991). Biofeedback could be investigated as a treatment modality. In addition, psychosocial support is extremely important, and consideration should be given to the formation of a support group for these women. Sexual counseling with emphasis on sexual gratification by means other than intercourse may be needed, as well as possible referral to a certified sex therapist for more intensive care.

***Time Frame for Initiating Pharmacotherapy.*** Pharmacologic intervention should be initiated with patient contact. Achievement of goals is extremely variable, and may not occur at all.

See Drug Tables 311, 809.

***Assessment and History Taking.*** Women often present with a history of postcoital vulvar burning lo-calized to the posterior fourchette. The painful burning may eventually become so constant and severe that intercourse, as well as insertion of tampons, is impossible. The history will also include discomfort with sitting, biking, snug-fitting clothing, or anything that touches or rubs the vulva. As with other vulvar problems, questions concerning past infections, especially *Candida*, HPV, and HSV should be asked. Ruling out the use of irritative products, douching, overbathing, and scrubbing also is very important.

With physical examination, redness may be seen around the vestibule, especially where the Skene's and Bartholin's ducts open (Kaufman, 1995). Staining with acetic acid will promote strong acetowhitening, and although some sources feel HPV is not currently considered a causative factor (Curry & Barclay, 1994), others differ. In 1988, Turner and Marinoff reported an association between HPV and vulvar vestibulitis. Umpierre et al (1991) further identified HPV in tissue specimens of a sample of women with the condition. Diagnostic tests to rule out other infectious processes should be done as needed. Colposcopy can be very helpful in identifying areas of inflammation, and the use of a moist cotton-tipped applicator in finding a pattern of localized point tenderness with touch is most diagnostic of vulvar vestibulitis. Any suspicious area should, of course, be biopsied.

***Patient/Caregiver Information.*** Women should be educated as much as possible concerning the known etiology of vulvar vestibulitis, emphasizing that it is a recognized physical entity. Encourage them to follow the recommended interventions, both pharmacologic and nonpharmacologic, and to avoid self-treatment until evaluation has been completed. If an antidepressant is prescribed, care should be taken to assure the patient that the prescription is not being given because the condition is "just in her head," but because of the antidepressant's effect on nerve endings and usefulness in treating chronic pain (Jones & Lehr, 1994). Ask her to keep a diary with notes about specific foods, activities, or events that seem to trigger discomfort, as well as any interventions that offer relief. Women should be informed of the possible long-term duration of this condition, as well as the possibility of spontaneous regression in 6 months to 1 year (Curry, 1995). Any available information concerning support groups should be given and the woman encouraged to attend.

## Outcomes Management

**Selecting an Appropriate Agent.** Since the psychological impact of vulvar vestibulitis cannot be overlooked, use of antidepressants is often a treatment choice (McKay, 1993). Amitriptyline (Elavil) is often given with an initial dosage of 10 mg/day. This is increased by 10 mg/week until the desired effect of pain reduction is achieved, or a maximum of 60 mg/day has been reached.

For management of pain, 2–5% lidocaine in an emollient base may be carefully applied in the specific area daily and before intercourse (Jones & Lehr, 1994).

The therapeutic success of intralesional injection of interferon is reported as 50% or higher. One million units of recombinant interferon alfa-2 is injected submucosally at a different location of the vestibule. The injections are three times per week for 4 weeks (a total of 12 injections) in a clockwise pattern, until the entire vestibule has been injected (Kaufman, 1995; Secor & Fertitta, 1992). This treatment is quite expensive. Although some studies have shown patient improvement, more research needs to be done to prove its efficacy. It is recommended that interferon be used only with consultation.

**Monitoring for Efficacy.** Women should be seen weekly if an antidepressant is ordered and if interferon injections are being given. Efficacy is determined by patient response, with the antidepressants being adjusted as previously noted, and interferon injections being given weekly. Since intercourse is not thought to have an effect on the prognosis of vulvar vestibulitis (Jones & Lehr, 1994), it need not be avoided during these treatments, and patient response can thus be monitored via degree of dyspareunia. Topical anesthetics may also be monitored in this way.

**Monitoring for Toxicity.** With amitriptyline, monitor for drowsiness, anticholinergic effects, and CNS overstimulation. Some women may experience galactorrhea with higher dosages (Weil, 1996); however, this response does not necessarily indicate toxicity.

Adverse reactions to interferon include flu-like symptoms. CBCs and liver function tests should be obtained to monitor for blood dyscrasias and hepatic problems (Weil, 1996), and although no set schedule seems to be available for these tests, it is prudent to obtain these tests at least every 4 weeks, and perhaps more frequently.

Topical lidocaine should be used with extreme caution since it may be a sensitizing agent in some patients if used over the entire vulva (Jones & Lehr, 1994).

**Follow-up Recommendations.** Follow-up appointments should be made weekly after initial contact, and treatment evaluated. Treatment outcomes are variable, and partial vulvectomy or vestibulectomy may be suggested to women with severe, long-term symptoms that fail to respond. This surgical intervention should be considered as a last resort, after all nonsurgical therapies have been ineffective.

## LICHEN SCLEROSUS

This condition is considered one of the vulvar dystrophies; it may also be characterized as a vulvar dermatosis. Vulvar dystrophies are generally characterized by hyperkeratotic or "white" lesions caused by a decrease in vascularity, chronic irritation with a resulting thicker than normal keratin layer, and changes in thickness of the epithelium (Curry & Barclay, 1994). All are pruritic and are seen primarily in the perimenopausal and menopausal years. The lesions may include areas of atypia and dysplastic cells, and malignancy may develop.

### Specific Considerations for Pharmacotherapy

**When Drug Therapy is Needed.** Intervention with drug therapy is indicated, since the discomfort resulting from severe, chronic pruritis can be debilitating.

**Short- and Long-Term Goals of Pharmacotherapy.** The primary short-term goal is to relieve pruritis and its concomitant rubbing, scratching, and inflammation. The long-term goal is to build up the atrophic epithelium, and to prevent recurrence.

**Nonpharmacologic Therapy.** Nonpharmacologic treatments are those noted previously, with strict attention paid to avoidance of irritants and hot baths. Leaving underwear off entirely is the best option; however, this may cause undue discomfort in some women. Encourage the patient to at least leave underwear off at night, and to wear loose-fitting, all-cotton, boxer-type underwear during the day.

***Time Frame for Initiating Pharmacotherapy.*** Treatment is initiated upon patient contact for care, after diagnosis has been confirmed.

See Drug Tables 705, 807, 810.

***Assessment and History Taking.*** Intense pruritis is the presenting complaint of women with lichen sclerosus, usually of long-term duration (Lichtman & Duran, 1995). Questions focused on previously prescribed treatments and self-treatment should be asked, as well as questions about the use of common irritants and chronic rubbing of clothes. Physical examination findings include a pattern of whitish, wrinkled, atrophic, parchment-like skin. Affected areas may include the vulva, clitoral hood, perineal area, skin-fold areas next to the thighs, buttocks, and a keyhole area around the anus (Kaufman, 1995). Excoriations and fissures may be present, and the introitus may be constricted. Topography is lost as the vulvar structures atrophy and contract and the labia minora blends with the labia majora. Intense pruritis leading to chronic scratching and rubbing results in lichenification, epithelial atrophy, and hyperkeratosis. Tentative diagnosis may be made from history and physical examination, but colposcopy with biopsy is necessary to confirm the diagnosis and to rule out dysplasia. Biopsy must always be done with any suspicious lesion of the vulva.

***Patient/Caregiver Information.*** The patient should be educated about the strict avoidance of irritants, medication use, and the etiology and chronic nature of this condition. She should be given support and encouragement, since beneficial effects depend largely on compliance with recommendations.

## Outcomes Management

***Selecting an Appropriate Agent.*** With the stated goals in mind, a combination of low-potency topical steroidal cream, oral antihistamines, and testosterone cream is used. The topical corticosteroid cream is used in the morning and the oral antihistamine at night in an effort to diminish itching. These medications include those discussed in the treatment of vulvar dermatitis, as well as fluocinolone acetonide 0.025% or 0.01%, triamcinolone acetonide 0.01%, or hydrocortisone cream 1% or 2.5%, applied two to three times daily. Clobetasol 0.05%, is applied b.i.d. for 1 month, daily for 2 months, then two times per week for 3 months (Kaufman, 1995). Beneficial

effects should be noticed by the patient within 24 h. Two percent testosterone propionate cream, which must be pharmacist-prepared, is prescribed to thicken the epithelium. It is applied at night. Benefits of this are much longer in occurring, possibly as long as 8 weeks. In time, however, a response rate of 90% is expected with this regimen (Curry, 1995). An alternative regime is to apply this cream two to three times daily for 3–6 months or until pruritis subsides, gradually decreasing the frequency of use over 1–2 years to a maintenance level of one to two times weekly (Kaufman, 1995).

***Monitoring for Efficacy.*** Subjective findings of decreased pruritis hopefully will be noted by the patient at the first follow-up visit, and as the weeks progress with adherence to pharmacologic and nonpharmacologic regimens, objective observations of decreased lichenification and atrophy should become evident. Testosterone propionate cream may be gradually decreased after epithelium is restored; however, it can be continued indefinitely (Kaufman, 1995).

***Monitoring for Toxicity.*** As previously noted, long-term use of topical corticosteroids in the vulvar area is not recommended; therefore, care must be taken to ensure proper use of this medication. The development of hirsutism, acne, and excessively oily skin may occur as androgenic side effects from testosterone. A serum testosterone level may be obtained if these problems are noted. They are annoying rather than posing an actual toxic effect, however, and should diminish if the treatment is discontinued.

***Follow-up Recommendations.*** Follow-up should be scheduled 1–2 weeks after the initial visit, and then monthly. With improvement of the condition, thought should be given to placing the patient on oral hormone replacement therapy if no contraindications exist. Estratest, with its combination of estrogen and testosterone, might be considered, thereby providing the benefits of estrogen (including alleviation of atrophic vaginitis) and continuing effects of testosterone to maintain epithelial thickness.

## MENSTRUAL DISORDERS

Much time, energy, thought, and money are given by women to the concerns of menstruation. Menses that are too frequent, too infrequent or absent, too scant, too heavy, too painful, or too bloating send women to pharmacies and health care providers every day. This section discusses four common menstrual problems: amenorrhea, dysfunctional uterine bleeding, premenstrual syndrome, and dysmenorrhea.

## AMENORRHEA

Amenorrhea is the absence of menses. It may be primary or secondary and either a physiologic function or caused by a pathologic condition. *Primary amenorrhea* is the absence of menarche by age 14 with the lack of secondary sex characteristics, or by age 16 regardless of the development of secondary sex characteristics (Skrypzak, 1995). Women with these presenting characteristics warrant thorough evaluation by a specialist, and this condition is beyond the scope of this chapter.

*Secondary amenorrhea* is the cessation of menses for at least 3 (some sources say 6) months in a woman who has previously had regular monthly menstrual cycles. Secondary amenorrhea is a frequent cause of concern for many women. Although secondary amenorrhea can be a sign of a serious problem such as a pituitary tumor, pregnancy and menopause are frequent causes of missed menses. The condition also may occur because of suppression of the hypothalamus, which can result from physical and emotional stress, strenuous exercise, use of hormonal therapy, and sudden weight loss or gain. Other causes include polycystic ovary disease, intrauterine scarring (Asherman's syndrome), and hypothyroidism (Hatcher et al, 1994).

## Specific Considerations for Pharmacotherapy

*When Drug Therapy is Needed.* Amenorrhea is generally associated with reduced estrogen levels, and estrogen is closely associated with bone density. Prolonged amenorrhea with reduced estrogen can result in bone loss and subsequent higher risk of fractures (Conviser & Fitzgibbon, 1997). Fertility is associated with regular ovulation and menses, and the lack of these two normal functions may indicate decreased fertility in women hoping to conceive. In addition, women with amenorrhea caused by anovulation are at risk for endometrial hyperplasia from unopposed estrogen. For these, as well as other psychological and physiological reasons, drug therapy is needed.

*Short- and Long-Term Goals of Pharmacotherapy.* Pharmacotherapy goals are to restore cyclic ovulation and menses in premenopausal women, to prevent problems associated with estrogen and progesterone deficit, and to eliminate the risk of endometrial hyperplasia.

*Nonpharmacologic Therapy.* If the absence of menses is determined to be due to nonpathologic hypothalamic suppression, lifestyle changes may correct the problem. Learning to manage stress, reducing intensity of exercise, and gaining weight are therapy options. If a serious eating disorder is diagnosed, referral to a specialist is essential as this can be a life-threatening condition.

*Time Frame for Initiating Pharmacotherapy.* Treatment should begin as soon as the cause of amenorrhea is established.
See Drug Tables 603, 605, 607.

*Assessment and History Taking.* Assessment through a complete history and physical examination is essential to rule out pathology prior to therapy. Careful history taking alone can often reveal the cause of missed menses; oral contraceptives, hormonal injections, and implants for contraception can all affect regularity of menstrual flow. It also is very important to ask questions concerning frequency and intensity of exercise, eating habits, significant changes in body weight, and stressful lifestyle events. The questions all relate to hypothalamic suppression. A history of headaches, nipple discharge (galactorrhea), and changes in vision could suggest a pituitary adenoma. Presence of hot flashes, night sweats, and vaginal dryness in a younger woman could indicate premature ovarian failure, and in an older woman, the common symptoms of approaching menopause.

Height, weight, and vital signs should be taken. A complete physical examination with pelvic and Pap smears is needed. If, by general appearance and history, an eating disorder is suspected, the percentage of body fat should be measured. Note any hirsutism. If present, androgen-producing tumors must be ruled out with testosterone and dehydroepiandrosterone sulfate levels. Additionally, polycystic ovarian syndrome (PCOS) may be the cause of amenorrhea evidenced by chronic anovulation and hyperandrogenemia (Skrypzak, 1995). A luteinizing hormone/follicle-stimulating hormone (LH/FSH) ratio greater than 3:1 (high LH and low to normal FSH) accompanied by low elevations of androgens indicates PCOS. The ovaries are usually enlarged (Gilchrist, 1996). The thyroid gland should be palpated for enlargement and/or nodules. Hypothyroidism can stimulate an increased prolactin level. A sensitive urine pregnancy test should be done on all women to rule out pregnancy, as this is a very frequent cause of amenorrhea. After pregnancy is ruled out, diagnostic tests, at a minimum, should include thyroid-stimulating hormone (TSH) and serum prolactin levels. FSH levels may also be obtained to rule out premature ovarian failure or menopause. A second FSH level should be drawn 2 weeks after the initial level as a mid-cycle FSH level may be elevated normally and mimic menopause (Skrypzak, 1995).

***Patient/Caregiver Information.*** Information should be given concerning physical examination findings and laboratory results. The etiology of amenorrhea should be reviewed, as well as the health risks associated with amenorrhea. If contraception is not currently being used and the pregnancy test is negative, the woman should be counseled on contraceptive techniques if pregnancy is unwanted. All pharmacologic and non-pharmacologic treatments should be discussed in detail, as well as the need for any follow-up testing, evaluation, and referral. Women placed on oral contraceptives should be told that amenorrhea will likely return if the medication is stopped (Hatcher et al, 1994).

## Outcomes Management

### Selecting an Appropriate Agent

- Pregnancy must first be excluded.
- If TSH is elevated, treat for hypothyroidism.
- If the serum prolactin level is elevated (greater than 100 ng/mL), a CT scan or MRI should be ordered to evaluate the sella turcica for pituitary adenoma. If the scan is abnormal, refer the patient for further evaluation and possible treatment with bromocriptine (Parlodel), a dopamine agonist (Mattox, 1995). If the scan is normal, hypothalamic suppression is responsible for the amenorrhea, and it should be treated with estrogen and progestin. Combined oral contraceptives are an appropriate choice, particularly if the woman desires birth control. Conjugated estrogen and medroxyprogesterone acetate (MPA) prescribed as for postmenopausal hormone treatment are also appropriate (Hatcher et al, 1994).

- If FSH is high, menopause (ovarian failure) is the cause of amenorrhea. Further evaluation of the younger woman less than 45 by an endocrinologist may be warranted. In any event, treatment to replace the loss of hormones, whether premature or expected, should be strongly encouraged (Hatcher et al, 1994).
- If TSH and serum prolactin levels are normal, administer a progestin challenge test. This consists of giving inexpensive MPA 10 mg PO daily for 5 days, or progesterone in oil 200 mg IM (Hatcher et al, 1994). If withdrawal bleeding occurs in 2–7 days after completion of medication, the diagnosis of anovulation is established. Assuming no contraindications, low-dose oral contraceptives are a good option for anovulatory patients. MPA 10 mg daily for 10 days each month is also an acceptable treatment (Baker, 1997).
- If withdrawal bleeding does not occur with the progestin challenge, the patient may be hypo-estrogenic and the endometrium should be "primed" for 21 days with conjugated estrogens 1.25 mg PO daily, followed by MPA 10 mg daily for 5 days (Goroll, May, & Mulley, 1995), or conjugated estrogens 2.5 mg daily for 21 days, with the addition of MPA 10 mg daily on days 12–21, the last 10 days (Skrypzak, 1995). If withdrawal bleeding occurs, then hypothalamic-pituitary dysfunction is indicated. Further assessment should be directed toward understanding why there was insufficient endogenous estrogen available (Skrypzak, 1995). An FSH level should be drawn if one has not previously been obtained. If this level is low or normal, order a CT scan or MRI evaluation of the sella turcica and proceed as previously discussed. High FSH levels again indicate ovarian failure with menopause and should be thus managed. If withdrawal bleeding still does not occur, referral should be made to evaluate for end-organ (uterine) problems, such as Asherman's syndrome.
- If physical findings, the LH/FSH ratio, and increased androgen levels indicate PCOS, low-dose oral contraceptives are used if the woman does not desire fertility (Gilchrist, 1996). Androgenic effects are opposed by the estrogen; testosterone clearance is increased by the progestogen; and testosterone levels should decrease in about 3 months, with an actual decrease in the ovaries' size in 6 months by ultrasound. Women who desire fertility will need ovarian stimulation. Consultation with or referral to a specialist is advised.

***Monitoring for Efficacy.*** Patient monitoring depends on the cause of amenorrhea and the treatment chosen. If hormonal therapy is used, patients should be seen in approximately 3 months to assess regulation of menses. It is recommended that the therapy be stopped after 6 months to assess spontaneous resumption of menses (Dambro, 1995).

***Monitoring for Toxicity.*** If oral contraceptives have been prescribed, patients should be seen in 3 months for a blood pressure check and to assess for any side effects. See Chap. 18 on contraceptives for further discussion. Likewise, in Chap. 19 on hormone replacement therapy monitoring is discussed for those women who have been given exogenous estrogen and progestin.

***Follow-up Recommendations.*** Follow-up should be as noted in monitoring for efficacy. Further workup for anovulatory women usually is not indicated unless the woman desires pregnancy. Women with chronic anovulation are at increased risk for endometrial carcinoma due to unopposed estrogen. Women with PCOS are at increased risk for cardiovascular disease, diabetes, and hypertension. Careful monitoring is indicated (Skrypzak, 1995).

## DYSFUNCTIONAL UTERINE BLEEDING

Dysfunctional uterine bleeding (DUB) is the abnormal, unpredictable bleeding of endometrial origin with no demonstrable organic pathology. Ninety percent of all DUB is caused by anovulation (Dambro, 1995). It occurs with conditions associated with anovulatory cycles, such as hypothyroidism, polycystic ovarian syndrome, and some of the other conditions previously discussed with amenorrhea. Since ovulation has not occurred, progesterone is not available to stabilize the endometrium. The endometrium, therefore, attains an abnormal height and is fragile, leading to spontaneous bleeding. As the endometrium from one site is shed, new sites break down in an asynchronous manner. There is no rhythmic vasoconstriction or orderly collapse to induce stasis and clotting. DUB is most commonly see in menarche, as regular ovulation is being established, and during perimenopause, as ovarian function is declining. However, it can occur at any time during a woman's reproductive years.

## Specific Considerations for Pharmacotherapy

***When Drug Therapy is Needed.*** Unpredictable menstrual bleeding is, at the very least, physi-

cally and emotionally disconcerting. Risks of unopposed estrogen have previously been discussed, notably endometrial hyperplasia. Anemia can result if bleeding is heavy and prolonged. Drug therapy is also needed for those women who are anovulatory and desire pregnancy.

***Short- and Long-Term Goals of Pharmacotherapy.*** Goals of therapy are to control bleeding and promote cyclic flow, prevent recurrences of irregular bleeding, prevent endometrial hyperplasia, and preserve fertility.

***Nonpharmacologic Therapy.*** For women whose bleeding cannot be controlled with hormonal therapy, surgical measures may be necessary. Options include dilatation and curettage (D&C), endometrial ablation by laser destruction, and, as a last resort, hysterectomy (Baker, 1997).

***Time Frame for Initiating Pharmacotherapy.*** Therapy should be instituted after pregnancy and pathology have been ruled out and a diagnosis made.
   See Drug Tables 306, 603, 605.

***Assessment and History Taking.*** A complete history and physical examination are needed. Menstrual history, contraceptive history, problems with infertility, fibroid tumors, obesity, hirsutism, and lifestyle changes are all important areas to explore, as are any possible systemic diseases that could cause bleeding. A sensitive urine test to rule out pregnancy should be done on every woman with irregular bleeding. If bleeding has been prolonged, a hemoglobin and hematocrit should be obtained. Other laboratory tests should be considered to rule out a thyroid disorder or coagulopathy. If the woman has symptoms of menopause, an FSH would be in order. Bleeding in a postmenopausal woman must always be investigated. An endometrial biopsy will rule out pathology. Other causes of bleeding, such as cervical cancer or infection, should also be ruled out. If history and examination suggest polycystic ovarian syndrome, a serum testosterone is indicated (Goroll et al, 1995).

***Patient/Caregiver Information.*** A thorough, easy-to-understand explanation of the etiology, diagnostic procedures, and treatment plan should be given. Techniques to manage stress may be discussed as well as good nutrition, including ways to increase iron in the diet.

## Outcomes Management

***Selecting an Appropriate Agent.*** To stop abnormal bleeding that is nonpathologic, MPA 10 mg daily for 10 days can be given orally, or 100 mg of progesterone can be given in a single intramuscular injection. This is frequently referred to as a medical D&C (Goroll et al, 1995). To prevent bleeding from again occurring because of withdrawal after the MPA, low-dose combination oral contraceptives may be started once treatment is completed and bleeding has stopped. Oral contraceptives may be continued for several months, after which time menses may regulate. If prevention of pregnancy is desired, oral contraceptives should be continued. An advantage of this approach is the improvement of the hyperandrogenism that accompanies some cases of anovulatory bleeding, primarily polycystic ovarian syndrome.

If contraception is not needed, oral MPA 10 mg may be taken every month on the first or last 10–12 days to ensure cyclic endometrial shedding (Fogel, 1995; Skrypzak, 1995), thereby protecting against cellular changes and the risk of endometrial cancer associated with long-term unopposed estrogen stimulation.

Prostaglandin synthetase inhibitors (PGSIs) and nonsteroidal antiinflammatory drugs (NSAIDs) are nonhormonal agents that may be helpful in decreasing flow. These include mefenamic acid (Ponstel) 500 mg PO t.i.d. for 3 days, or naproxen (Naprosyn) 500 mg PO stat, then 250 mg PO t.i.d. for 5 days (Baker, 1998). Ibuprofen is also included and is quite inexpensive. NSAIDs have been shown to decrease the endometrial blood flow by their antiprostaglandin effect. Alone, they may reduce blood loss by 30% (Baker, 1998).

***Monitoring for Efficacy.*** With progestin therapy, bleeding should stop within 24–48 hours, and a heavy withdrawal bleed can be expected several days to 1 week after completing the MPA. A telephone call should be made in that time to assess efficacy. If this therapy does not stop acute bleeding, referral for a surgical D&C is indicated (Goroll et al, 1995).

Ovulation can spontaneously resume when cyclic MPA is given; therefore, the treatment should be stopped for a month or two to evaluate for the return of regular cycles. Barrier con-

traception is indicated during this time if pregnancy is not desired. If this therapy is used, periodic visits, possibly every 6 months, should be scheduled.

***Monitoring for Toxicity.*** The side effects most often associated with progestin therapy include weight gain, fatigue, depression, and acne (Hatcher, et al, 1994). Also see Chapters 18 and 26 on oral contraceptives and NSAIDs use with musculoskeletal problems for side effects, as well as Drug Tables 306 and 603.

***Follow-up Recommendations.*** Patients should be seen in 3 months if started on oral contraceptives. The importance of annual Pap smears should be emphasized. Patients should be encouraged to keep a menstrual calendar and to return should irregular bleeding, as well as no bleeding, occur. If conception is desired, referral should be made to a reproductive specialist.

## PREMENSTRUAL SYNDROME

Premenstrual syndrome (PMS) is the cyclical recurrence of distressing physical, affective, and behavioral changes that can result in the deterioration of interpersonal relationships and personal health (Barnhart, Freeman, & Sondheimer, 1995). These symptoms tend to peak premenstrually and disappear after the beginning of menses. In addition, perimenopausal symptoms have been found to reduce work efficiency, increase absenteeism, and have an impact on family and personal relationships (Taylor, 1995).

Approximately 75% of women in the general population complain of some minor premenstrual symptoms (Freeman, 1993). However, depending on the criteria and population studied, only 20–50% of women experience moderate symptoms that prompt them to seek medical treatment. Only 3–5% of women have such severe symptoms that their level of functioning is significantly affected (American Psychiatric Association [APA], 1994; New approaches, 1998). Although cultural variations exist according to cross-cultural studies, African-American and Caucasian women in the United States report equal frequencies of various premenstrual symptoms, with frequency of symptom reported peaking in the 25–34-year-old group. Epidemiologic studies of PMS have not confirmed an unequivocal correlation between PMS symptoms and age, socioeconomic status, parity, diet or physical activity, menstrual characteristics, or personality (Rubinow, 1992).

## Symptoms

Although the most commonly reported perimenstrual symptoms may be complaints of physical discomfort (bloating, cramping), the reports of mood changes or negative affect symptoms are often the most distressing. Although symptoms are multiple and diverse, they are often grouped into categories such as somatic (mastalgia, bloating, headache, pelvic pain, fatigue), mood (irritability, depression, mood swings), cognitive (poor concentration, confusion), and behavioral (social withdrawal, impulsiveness, appetite changes); see Table 35–1. With more than 100 reported symptoms attributed to the menstrual cycle, delineation of symptoms into subtypes is an important step in understanding women's perimenstrual complaints (Taylor, 1995).

Although most clinicians and researchers generally agree that PMS is not a psychiatric disorder, a subtype with more severe behavioral symptoms, "Premenstrual Dysphoric Disorder" (PMDD), is included in the appendix of the *Diagnostic and Statistical Manual for Psychiatric Disorders (DSM-IV)*. Characteristics of PMDD include depression, anxiety, lability of mood, and irritability that are comparable to a major depressive episode (APA, 1994). Diagnostic criteria are seen in Table 35–2.

## Etiology

Although many theories have been proposed for the cause of premenstrual symptoms, none of the proposed etiological theories have been substantiated. Biologic theories have included hypotheses on neurotransmitter dysfunction, prostaglandin excess, estrogen/progesterone imbalance, vitamin deficiencies, and psychogenic factors (Servino & Moline, 1995). However, no significant differences in serum concentrations of estradiol, progesterone, FSH, or LH have been found in women with PMS compared to controls (Latassy & Sagraves, 1995).

Changes in prolactin concentrations have also not been found to be significantly different in women with or without PMS (Fankhauser, 1997). Alterations in gonadotropin-releasing hormone (GnRH) activity may play a key role in explaining some of the hormonal theories of PMS. Changes in GnRH and ovarian hormone production have been implicated in both the development or elimination of symptoms associated with PMS. GnRH must be released in the appropriate amounts and at the right pulse rate to stimulate gonadotropin secretion and to cause ovulation. Release of GnRH is regulated by positive and negative feedback from norepinephrine, dopamine, serotonin, ovarian hormones, and endogenous opiates. GnRH release is mediated by norepinephrine and serotonin, and its pulsating pattern is modified by endorphins, estrogen, and progesterone. Changes in any of these neurotransmitters may alter GnRH release, which eventually will downregulate LH and FSH release and prevent ovulation. Suppression of ovulation results in the reduction of the cyclical changes in moods and physical symptoms associated with PMS (Fankhauser, 1997).

## TABLE 35–1.  SYMPTOM CLUSTERS OF PERIMENSTRUAL COMPLAINTS

| Perimenstrual Negative Affect (PNA) | Perimenstrual Pain/ Discomfort (PPD) | Perimenstrual Dysphoric Symptoms (PDS) |
|---|---|---|
| Anger | Abdominal/pelvic pain | Depression |
| Irritability | Headache | Decreased sexual desire |
| Anxiety | Joint aches/pain | Fatigue |
| Guilt | | Decreased energy |
| Depression | | Decreased appetite |
| Feeling out of control | | Fluid retention |
| Tension | | |
| Hostility | | |
| Mood swings | | |
| Impatience | | |
| Tearfulness | | |

## TABLE 35–2. DIAGNOSTIC CRITERIA FOR PREMENSTRUAL DYSPHORIC DISORDER (PMDD)

1. Must have five or more of the following symptoms, including at least one of the first four:

   - Depressed mood, feelings of hopelessness, or self-deprecating thoughts
   - Marked anxiety or tension; feeling "keyed up" or "on edge"
   - Significant mood lability
   - Persistent anger or irritability; increased interpersonal conflicts
   - Decreased interest in usual activities
   - Lethargy, easy fatigability, or marked lack of energy
   - Changes in appetite; overeating or food cravings
   - Hypersomnia or insomnia
   - Subjective sense of difficulty in concentration
   - Physical symptoms such as breast tenderness, headache, joint or muscle pain, bloating, or weight gain

2. Symptoms occur during the last week of the luteal phase and remit within a few days after onset of menses.
3. Symptoms must seriously interfere with work or with usual social activities or relationships with others.
4. Symptoms not merely an exacerbation of another disorder (e.g., depressive, panic, dysthymic, or personality disorders).
5. Symptoms must be confirmed by prospective daily self-ratings during at least two symptomatic menstrual cycles.

*Adapted from APA (1994)*

Serotonin deficiency has also been proposed as a theory for the development of PMS. Depressed serotonergic activity has been associated with depressed mood, irritability, anxiety, impulsivity, aggressiveness, and increased appetite (Rapkin, 1992). Lower serotonin levels during the luteal phase of the menstrual cycle have been found in women with PMS compared to normal controls (Rapkin, 1992). These findings may explain the similarities in mood and behaviors associated with PMDD and depression. Lower blood levels of allopregnanolone, a by-product of progesterone thought to influence neurotransmitters and mood, may be implicated (New approaches, 1998).

Alternative theories have suggested stress as well as endorphin mediation as causal factors (Barnhart et al, 1995). The exact pathophysiologic abnormality of PMS has yet to be defined, but research efforts continue to focus on the influence of hormones on neurotransmitters, identification of biologic triggers, and behavioral modification (Latassy & Sagraves, 1995).

## Specific Considerations for Pharmacologic Therapy

***When Drug Therapy is Needed.*** Since a specific etiology for PMS has not been identified, a variety of pharmacological therapies have been tried without success. To date, many of the treatments in the pharmacologic trials have been no more effective than placebo. The FDA has approved no drug to date for the treatment of PMS (New approaches, 1998).

Pharmacologic interventions have been initiated in an effort to correct the theoretical endocrine or neurochemical imbalances that have been proposed as the causative factors for PMS. Various forms of progesterone have been prescribed based on the progesterone deficiency theory; oral contraceptives have been prescribed based on the need for ovarian suppression; aldosterone inhibitors have been used for excess aldosterone secretion and its role in premenstrual fluid retention; and prostaglandin inhibitors have been tried for imbalances in circulating prostaglandins. The latest research is focusing on selective serotonin reuptake inhibitors (SSRIs) because of the presumed role that an imbalance in the levels of the neurotransmitter serotonin may play in PMS (Rapkin, 1992).

Current pharmacologic therapy should be directed at the relief or prevention of symptoms to enable women to continue functioning with minimal interference with their activities of daily living. Symptomatic relief can be achieved with analgesics such as aspirin, acetaminophen or the NSAIDs, diuretics, anxiolytics, and antidepressants. GnRH agonists is a treatment used in extreme cases (New approaches, 1998).

A combination of treatments may be more effective than monotherapy if a woman is experiencing both incapacitating physical and behavioral symptoms. Drug therapy in combination with nonpharmacological interventions such as exercise, relaxation techniques, and dietary changes appears to hold the most promise in alleviating perimenstrual symptoms. Combination therapy may allow for lower doses of drugs, shorter duration of therapy, and less potential for adverse effects.

### Short- and Long-Term Goals of Pharmacotherapy.

The initial goal of therapy should be to understand the patient's perimenstrual experience and help her define and manage her symptoms and their related problems. Self-awareness of symptom severity and symptom patterns are the first steps of treatment. For some women, self-monitoring alone may be enough to assist them in making necessary changes in their relationships, stress load, and dietary and exercise routines. Only women with the most extreme manifestations of PMS are likely to require pharmacologic therapy. Initial symptom management should include multiple nonpharmacologic treatments. The woman should be included in the selection process as this promotes empowerment and a sense of self-control. An individualized treatment plan should be established initially and updated regularly until PMS severity is reduced and stabilized. The long-term goal of therapy is development of a treatment plan involving nonpharmacologic and pharmacologic agents and behavioral changes that lead to control of perimenstrual symptom severity and occurrence. This plan would allow the woman to continue her usual lifestyle without disruption.

### Nonpharmacologic Therapy.

Clinical experience indicates that patient education and support, stress reduction, a healthy diet, regular aerobic exercise, and vitamin supplements assist in relieving some of the symptoms associated with PMS and help a woman to feel more in control of her symptoms (Baker, 1998). Clinical data that demonstrate the clinical efficacy of these nonpharmacologic strategies are limited. For these strategies to be successful, results should be seen within a couple of months. Many women will see a marked reduction in perimenopausal symptoms with these interventions, and only women with more severe symptoms may require additional drug therapy (Taylor, 1995).

Acknowledging that the symptoms experienced by patients are real can be therapeutic. Information regarding PMS and the functioning of a normal menstrual cycle needs to be provided. A prospective calendar of menstrual symptoms should be kept for 2–3 months to enhance patient awareness and assist in planning and implementing an individualized treatment plan. The patients should be encouraged to identify personal and professional stresses that contribute to PMS and develop coping strategies or adjust their lifestyle to modify or remove these stresses from their lives. Patients may benefit from referral to a psychologist, counselor, or support group to assist them in stress management techniques (Baker, 1998).

Although there is no evidence that nutritional deficiencies cause PMS, poor dietary habits may exacerbate symptoms. Dietary changes that have been shown to reduce perimenstrual symptoms include reduction of sodium intake, limitation of foods high in simple sugars, and reduction or elimination of caffeine consumption in the 2 weeks prior to menses (Chuong & Dawson, 1992; Rossignol & Bonnlander, 1990). Recent studies contradict the long-held belief that women should resist carbohydrate cravings and suggest that carbohydrate-rich, low-protein foods, especially during the luteal phase, may improve mood symptoms (Sayeh et al, 1995). Increasing carbohydrates boosts levels of a precursor for serotonin, called tryptophan, thus affecting mood positively (New approaches, 1998). Women should be encouraged to eat smaller and more frequent meals high in complex carbohydrates and protein and low in simple sugars to reduce food cravings and "hypoglycemic episodes."

Vitamins, minerals, amino acids, and PMS-formula supplements have been suggested to relieve PMS symptoms, but actual clinical data to support their claims are limited. Pyridoxine (vitamin $B_6$) has been studied more thoroughly than other supplements. Pyridoxine is involved in the synthesis of the neurotransmitters serotonin and dopamine, which affect mood, affect, sleep patterns, and appetite. There is no evidence of pyridoxine deficiency in women with PMS, but supplementation is frequently recommended. Open-label trials have suggested that pyridoxine supplementation may help relieve PMS symptoms, but double-blind, placebo-controlled trials have produced inconsistent results (Chuong & Dawson, 1992; Kleignen, Ter Riet, & Knipschild, 1990). Doses should begin at 25–50 mg daily and not exceed 200 mg per day to avoid pyridoxine-induced peripheral neuropathy (Parry & Bredensen, 1985; Schaumberg et al, 1983).

Calcium and magnesium also have been reported to lessen perimenopausal symptoms. Calcium in doses of 1000 mg per day has been reported to reduce mood changes, fluid retention, and pain (Thys-Jacobs et al, 1989; Alvir & Thys-Jacobs, 1991). Supplementation with 360 mg of magnesium daily also has been shown to improve some of the mood symptoms associated with PMS (Facchinetti et al, 1991). Optivite, a high-dose multivitamin and mineral product, is being promoted as a nutritional supplement for PMS. The recommended dose is 6 to 12 tablets per day, which provides 300 mg of pyridoxine, 250 mg of magnesium, but only 125 mg of calcium. Limited data are available to support its beneficial effects in PMS (Fankhauser, 1997). The product is expensive and supplementation with the individual components is inexpensive and provides more appropriate doses.

Interest in vitamin E (alpha tocopherol) in treating PMS symptoms evolved from its use in the treatment of fibrocystic breast disease. High-dose vitamin E (400 IU) has been shown to reduce mood symptoms and food cravings but had no effect on physical symptoms, including breast tenderness (London, Bradley, & Chiamor, 1991). Low-dose vitamin E provided no symptom relief.

A deficiency of prostaglandin $E_1$ ($PGE_1$) has been proposed as a cause of some PMS symptoms, specifically mastodynia. Use of evening primrose oil has been advocated for relief of breast symptoms because it contains cis-linolenic acid, which is precursor to $PGE_1$. Limited data from clinical trials indicate inconsistent benefit in reduction of breast symptoms and no effect on mood or other physical symptoms (Collins, Cerin, Coleman, & Landgren, 1993).

Numerous commercial products including herbal supplements and teas, tryptophan supplements, amino acids, and PMS formula multivitamins have made claims that they relieve PMS symptoms. Phototherapy has also been reported to relieve some of the symptoms of PMS (Cerda & Parry, 1994). Studies have not substantiated these claims, however, and they probably provide a placebo effect at best. A new nonprescription dietary supplement, PMS Escape, has been marketed since 1997 for the changes in mood, appetite, and concentration associated with PMS (New approaches, 1998). PMS Escape is a powdered drink mix that contains a blend of carbohydrates, vitamins, and minerals that is claimed to restore the normal level of serotonin ("Nonprescription PMS Treatment," 1996). Decreased depression, anger, carbohydrate cravings, and confusion were reported in one trial with women with PMS, and results of a second trial are anticipated in 1998 (New approaches, 1998).

**Time Frame for Initiating Therapy.** Self-awareness of symptom severity and symptom patterns is the first step to treatment. For some women,

self-monitoring alone may be enough to assist them in making appropriate lifestyle changes. Monitoring stress in relationships and work and the individual's reaction to these stressors is also an important first step. A trial of nonpharmacologic interventions is recommended prior to changing to or adding drug therapy. Pharmacologic interventions should be targeted either at symptom relief or at correcting a presumed endocrine or neurotransmitter imbalance. Drug therapy can be initiated at any time based on the clinical assessment and patient preferences.

See Drug Tables 208, 301, 304, 306, 307, 309, 310, 311, 603, 605, 608, 705.

**Assessment and History Taking.** Before initiating either nonpharmacologic or pharmacologic treatment for PMS, it is necessary to obtain a thorough description of the patient's symptoms and their severity, as well as the effect that these symptoms have had on her ability to function. The initial evaluation should include an assessment of the patient's menstrual, obstetric, and gynecologic history, family history of PMS or other affective disorders, and a complete drug history. It is important to explore the impact that her symptoms have had on her relationships, professional activities, and family life.

Information gathered from the PMS history provides general information about the woman's symptom experience, but retrospective symptom severity reports are likely to overestimate severity and do not provide data about symptom patterns. A prospective menstrual or PMS calendar kept for a minimum of two menstrual cycles is useful for women to describe their unique symptoms and symptom clusters and help to visualize symptom severity patterns. Several validated PMS self-rating scales are available to help identify symptoms and quantify their severity (Fankhauser, 1997).

The diagnosis of PMS requires that symptoms appear or increase in severity during the luteal phase and disappear or return to baseline shortly after the onset of menses. The National Institute of Mental Health (NIMH) has recommended that the diagnosis of PMS be made only if the symptom severity scores change by at least 30% during the luteal phase.

A general physical examination is recommended to help rule out other causes for the symptoms that the woman is experiencing. Other gynecologic disorders, endocrine abnormalities, and psychiatric illnesses need to be ruled out as either the cause or as concomitant conditions exacerbating the woman's symptoms.

There are no specific laboratory tests that can confirm the diagnosis of PMS, but there are several tests that should be considered to rule out other causes. TSH, CBC, prolactin levels and FSH, urinalysis, and cultures for STDs may help establish the presence of another diagnosis. Routine measurements of serum estrogen and progesterone levels are not recommended.

***Patient/Caregiver Information.*** Women with PMS are usually relieved to learn that they have a recognized medical condition, that they are not crazy, and that there are effective treatments available to treat their symptoms. Education and support, along with self-monitoring of daily health and perimenstrual symptoms, are all the treatment some patients will need. Family members and coworkers also need to receive information on the condition to increase their awareness of the role that relationships play in symptom management. Many women find they can control their symptoms without pharmacologic intervention just by making changes in diet, exercise habits, and lifestyle. If pharmacologic therapy is indicated, the woman should receive complete information on how the drug works, potential adverse effects, and when to anticipate a therapeutic response. In addition, some women may benefit from participating in a self-help group where they can share problems and learn more effective strategies for self-management of PMS symptoms.

## Outcomes Management

***Selecting an Appropriate Agent.*** Pharmacologic interventions for PMS have been based on a number of theories that suggest that the symptoms of PMS are caused by imbalances or deficiencies of certain endogenously produced substances, including progesterone, estrogen, aldosterone, prostaglandins, and serotonin (Fankhauser, 1997). The current medical literature indicates a growing support for the role of serotonin imbalance in PMS and a lack of evidence confirming the role of progesterone deficiency as a causal mechanism (Rapkin, 1992; Rubinow & Schmidt, 1995).

Selection of an appropriate agent for treatment of PMS may be accomplished by taking a symptom-focused approach, especially for the physical symptoms. Many of the mild physical symptoms associated with PMS (cramps, head-

ache, and fluid retention) can be managed with nonprescription products, such as aspirin, acetaminophen, and nonprescription strength ibuprofen and naproxen.

NSAIDs may be effective in relieving breast and joint pain, abdominal cramps, and menstrual headaches but provide no relief from emotional or behavioral symptoms. Ibuprofen (Motrin) 200–400 mg every 4–6 h, or naproxen sodium (Anaprox) 550 mg followed by 275 mg every 6–8 h, should be begun at least 7 days prior to menses for maximum effectiveness (see Drug Table 306).

If menstrual headaches are not relieved by NSAIDs, other drugs such as beta blockers (see Drug Table 205) or tricyclic antidepressants (see Drug Table 311) may be given prophylactically to abort the occurrence of the headaches. Low-dose estradiol (see Drug Table 605), administered orally or by transdermal patch, may be helpful in decreasing the symptoms of a menstrual migraine if started within 3 days before menses and continued for 7 days through menstruation (Baker, 1998).

Increased breast tenderness and swelling may be relieved by bromocriptine, which suppresses prolactin secretion. Doses of 1.25–2.5 mg twice daily taken from ovulation until the start of menses have been shown to reduce breast engorgement and mastalgia. Severe symptoms not relieved by NSAIDs or bromocriptine may require treatment with danazol. Because of its significant antiestrogen effects, danazol 50–100 mg b.i.d. should be reserved for short-term use in refractory patients (Fankhauser, 1997).

Insomnia and complaints of restless sleep can be treated with nonprescription antihistamines such as diphenhydramine 25–50 mg at bedtime. Melatonin, a dietary supplement, may also help decrease sleep latency. Alternative treatments include low doses of sedative antidepressants such as trazodone, amitriptyline, or doxepin taken 1–2 h before bedtime. Chronic use of benzodiazepines as sedative hypnotics is not recommended because of the potential for physical dependence and rebound insomnia after discontinuation.

Diuretics (see Drug Table 208), such as the aldosterone inhibitor spironolactone (Aldactone) 25–50 mg b.i.d., q.i.d., have been used to treat the premenstrual fluid retention that may occur. Fluid retention or bloating generally responds well to nonpharmacologic measures such as decreased intake of high-sodium–containing foods and increased water intake.

Diuretics, if used, should be taken only during the week prior to menses (Taylor, 1995).

If an etiology-based approach is taken to the treatment of PMS, data seem to suggest that drugs that effect serotonin and/or hormone activity are important to consider when selecting an agent. If serotonin dysregulation is considered an etiology for PMS, selective serotonin reuptake inhibitors (SSRIs) should be strongly considered for first-line therapy.

Clinical trials indicate that women with PMS that receive SSRIs (see Drug Table 311) obtain significant relief from both behavioral and physical symptoms. Data from placebo-controlled trials indicate that fluoxetine (Prozac), sertraline (Zoloft), and paroxetine (Paxil) are all effective in the management of PMS (Frank et al, 1995; Freeman, Rickels, & Sondheimer, 1996; Steiner et al, 1995). In addition, nortriptyline, nefazodone, clomipramine (Anafranil), and fluvoxamine also have been shown to be effective based on limited clinical studies (Fankhauser, 1997).

Since the SSRIs are similar in efficacy, the choice of agent should be based on patient symptoms, side-effect profile, and cost. An activating drug, such as fluoxetine, may be a good initial choice for the woman who is depressed with low energy; if the woman is experiencing significant problems with insomnia, irritability, or anxiety, sertraline or paroxetine may be a better initial choice. If one agent does not work or is not tolerated, try another SSRI before declaring treatment a failure and switching to another class of drugs. Allow sufficient time for a trial of a drug.

If cost is an issue, prescribe a higher-dose pill and have the patient cut it in half. For example, the 100-mg sertraline (Zoloft) tablet costs the same as the 50-mg tablet. Another option could be to use a tricylic antidepressant, which is very inexpensive compared to the SSRIs. Limited efficacy data are available on the tricyclics, and they are less well tolerated because of their anticholinergic side effects (Fankhauser, 1997).

Therapy should be initiated at half the recommended dose for depression. If tolerated, increase the dose after 1–2 weeks. Clinical trials have studied both full menstrual cycle dosing starting on day 1, and others have limited treatment to the luteal phase only (Menkes et al, 1992; Wood et al, 1992). Another option is to use half the dosage for the first 2–3 weeks of the menstrual cycle and increase the dosage during the time when the woman becomes more symptomatic.

If an SSRI is ineffective, alprazolam (Xanax) is another option (see Drug Table 309). It is well tolerated and shown to be effective for PMS when taken only during the luteal phase (Freeman, Rickels, Sondheimer, & Polansky, 1995). Initiate therapy with 0.25 mg t.i.d., and increase to a total of 1–1.25 mg/day. Use should be limited to only the luteal phase (some women may require only 4–5 days of therapy), and the dose should be tapered at the start of menses to avoid withdrawal symptoms. If alprazolam is contraindicated or ineffective, buspirone (BuSpar) 10 mg t.i.d. taken during the entire menstrual cycle is an effective alternative (Rickels, Freeman, & Sondheimer, 1992).

Regardless of the lack of evidence confirming progesterone deficiency as a causal mechanism for PMS, progesterone is still prescribed by many practitioners and anecdotal reports suggest dramatic responses in some women. However, numerous randomized placebo-controlled clinical trials have shown that neither natural progesterone (in suppositories or micronized oral preparations) nor synthetic progestins are more effective than placebo for PMS (Freeman et al, 1995, 1990). Progesterone therapy for treatment of PMS is not FDA-approved, and the patient should be so informed (see Drug Table 605).

For women who experience symptoms that begin at ovulation or who have significant perimenstrual pain, suppression of ovarian function with low-dose oral contraceptives (see Drug Table 603) may decrease the severity of physical symptoms (Fankhauser, 1997). Affective symptoms may actually worsen in about one third of patients who take oral contraceptives (Moline, 1993).

GnRH agonists may be indicated in women who continue to be symptomatic and do not respond to other hormonal regimens (see Drug Table 608). GnRH agonists relieve symptoms of PMS by producing a chemical oophorectomy. Available products include goserelin acetate (Zoladex), leuprolide acetate (Lupron Depot), and intranasal nafarelin acetate (Synarel). Because these agents induce a "pseudomenopause" and increase the risk of osteoporosis, treatment is usually limited to 6 consecutive months (Barnhart et al, 1995). GnRH agonists may be given for longer periods of time if the patient is given oral contraceptives concurrently. These agents should only be prescribed in consultation with a specialist.

Many other pharmacological therapies have been tried for PMS (eg, clonidine, lithium, valproic acid, carbamazepine, verapamil), but few controlled studies are available to confirm either their efficacy or safety. Additional controlled clinical studies are needed before these alternative therapies become a part of standard practice (Fankhauser, 1997).

*Monitoring for Efficacy.* Determining efficacy or therapeutic failure with any of the pharmacologic treatments prescribed for the symptoms of PMS requires use for at least two menstrual cycles. Doses of SSRIs may be increased after 1 week of treatment if therapy was initiated with half the dose used for depression. After establishing a therapeutic response, doses may be reduced for the first 2–3 weeks of each menstrual cycle. An alternative would be to take just the SSRI during the luteal phase of the cycle. Assessment of the efficacy of NSAIDs and diuretics should be based on the patient's perception of the relief of physical symptoms.

Follow-up should be scheduled for 3 months for assessment of drug efficacy and lifestyle modifications. The patient should continue to keep her menstrual symptom calendar to provide objective documentation of treatment efficacy or failure.

*Monitoring for Toxicity.* Each of the therapies has its own unique side effects. Activating SSRIs, such as fluoxetine, may cause insomnia, irritability, and agitation, which may require a change to a less activating agent, such as sertraline or paroxetine. Loss of libido and anorgasmia have been reported with long-term use of some of the SSRIs (Steiner et al, 1995). A change to another agent or a drug holiday may restore sexual function. Benzodiazepines should be avoided in women with a history of alcohol or drug abuse. Abrupt discontinuation may produce withdrawal symptoms.

Oral contraceptives are generally well tolerated. However, depressive symptoms may be exacerbated in about one third of women. GnRH agonists may cause menopausal symptoms such as hot flushes, genitourinary changes, and mood changes and increase the risk of osteoporosis. These agents should be avoided in women who have a past or current history of depression. Treatment should be limited to 6 consecutive months to avoid adverse effects.

Overuse of NSAIDs may result in gastrointestinal irritation and bleeding, fluid retention, elevations in blood pressure, and renal insufficiency.

Chapters 19 on menopausal therapies and 18 on oral contraceptives contain more extensive discussions of the adverse effects associated with progesterone and estradiol. The Drug Tables also contain a more in-depth coverage of dosages, adverse effects, and drug interactions for all drugs discussed in this chapter.

# DYSMENORRHEA

Dysmenorrhea is one of the most frequently encountered gynecological disorders. In the United States over half of women of childbearing age experience some degree of painful menstruation. Approximately 10% of these women have dysmenorrhea severe enough to incapacitate them for 1–3 days each month, resulting in increased absenteeism and economic loss (Murphy, 1995). Dysmenorrhea is the leading cause of absenteeism for adolescent females and is reported to be one of the most frequent reasons for young females to seek medical advice.

Dysmenorrhea is classified as either primary or secondary. *Primary dysmenorrhea* occurs in the absence of pelvic pathology, whereas *secondary dysmenorrhea* occurs as the result of some other underlying gynecological condition, such as endometriosis, cervical stenosis, pelvic inflammatory disease (PID), or congenital malformations. Secondary dysmenorrhea should be considered when there is a history of recurrent PID, irregular menstrual cycles, menorrhagia, IUD use, or infertility (Klotz, 1995).

Primary dysmenorrhea usually presents within the first 6–12 months after menarche, when ovulatory cycles are established. The pain typically begins 1–2 h before the onset of menstrual flow and lasts several hours up to 1–2 days, usually diminishing with onset of menstrual bleeding. The pain is characteristically a dull, crampy ache located in the suprapubic area with radiation to the lower back and anterior thighs. The pain often is accompanied by nausea, vomiting, diarrhea, headache, dizziness, and fatigue. The severity of primary dysmenorrhea is associated with the duration of menstrual flow, cigarette smoking, and early menarche (Murphy, 1995).

The pathophysiology of primary dysmenorrhea is related to an increased production and release of prostaglandins ($PGF_{2\alpha}$) in the endometrial lining, resulting in increased uterine contractions, vasospasm, and cramping.

Secondary dysmenorrhea usually occurs either with the first menses or after age 25. The pain often begins earlier and lasts longer than with primary dysmenorrhea. The characteristics of the pain vary depending on the etiology of the secondary dysmenorrhea.

## Specific Considerations for Pharmacotherapy

**When Drug Therapy is Needed.** The pain and systemic symptoms associated with primary dysmenorrhea are thought to be prostaglandin-mediated so that the logical first-line treatment should involve prostaglandin inhibition with one of the NSAIDs. Another therapeutic option would be one of the low-dose combination oral contraceptives. This option could be considered as primary therapy if the woman also needs a method of birth control (Latassy & Sagraves, 1995).

By suppressing prostaglandin synthesis, NSAIDs decrease the concentration of $PGF_{2\alpha}$ in the endometrium, resulting in a decrease in uterine contractility, an increase in platelet aggregation, and a decrease in menstrual blood loss. Oral contraceptives suppress ovulation, which results in lower levels of prostaglandins in the endometrium and menstrual blood loss (Latassy & Sagraves, 1995).

Treatment of secondary dysmenorrhea should be based on the etiology of the dysmenorrhea.

**Short- and Long-Term Goals of Pharmacotherapy.** The short-term goal of therapy should be to relieve the pain of dysmenorrhea and other associated symptoms. An NSAID with a quick onset of effect, such as ibuprofen (Motrin, others), diclofenac potassium (Cataflam), or naproxen sodium (Anaprox, Aleve), provides the most rapid alleviation of symptoms. Diuretics may help relieve some of the symptoms of bloating and water retention.

The long-term goals should be to prescribe either an NSAID or oral contraceptives to prevent or diminish future episodes of dysmenorrhea. NSAIDs are more effective when they are started prior to or at the onset of menses.

**Time Frame for Initiating Therapy.** If the woman is symptomatic at the time of the office visit, drug therapy with an NSAID should be started immediately to relieve symptoms. If the woman is not currently experiencing dysmenorrhea, she should be given a prescription to be used with the onset of her next menstrual period. Oral contraceptives may be initiated either on the first day of menses or on the first Sunday after

the onset of menstrual bleeding. They will not provide acute relief of symptoms.

See Drug Tables 208, 306, 307, 603.

**Assessment and History Taking.** A complete menstrual history, sexual history, and description of symptoms should be taken prior to diagnosis or treatment. Physical findings are usually normal with primary dysmenorrhea and a pelvic examination may not be necessary in a non-sexually active adolescent with a typical presentation. Causes of secondary dysmenorrhea should be initially evaluated with a pelvic examination, Pap smear, pregnancy test, and cultures for STDs. Tests to identify specific pelvic pathology may include a pelvic ultrasound and exploratory laparoscopy.

**Patient/Caregiver Information.** Patients should be given information on the menstrual cycle and the causes of dysmenorrhea. Women with primary dysmenorrhea should be reassured that their symptoms are not caused by some other gynecological condition. Women with secondary dysmenorrhea may benefit from stress reduction and relaxation techniques or referral to a support group. Patient education should be provided on the medications prescribed including when they should be taken, when to expect pain relief, and potential side effects. This is particularly important if NSAIDs are prescribed since they are contraindicated in the first trimester of pregnancy. They are often started prior to the start of menses and a woman may not know if she is pregnant. Counseling on effective methods of contraception may be indicated. See Table 35–3.

## Outcomes Management

**Selecting an Appropriate Agent.** The initial choice of therapy for primary dysmenorrhea should be

---

### TABLE 35–3. WHAT PATIENTS NEED TO KNOW TO PREVENT OR TREAT DYSMENORRHEA

Education regarding normal menstrual cycle and causes of dysmenorrhea
Aerobic exercise should be continued, as possible
Advise cessation of cigarette smoking
Use heating pads or hot water bottles
Limit sodium and caffeine intake
TENS (transcutaneous nerve stimulation)
Use relaxation techniques and stress therapy
Contact support groups

one of the NSAIDs, which decrease both endometrial and menstrual fluid prostaglandin concentrations. NSAID selection should be based on overall effectiveness, onset of symptom relief, and side effects, as well having an FDA-approved indication for primary dysmenorrhea.

Certain classes of NSAIDs appear to be more effective than others in relieving the symptoms of dysmenorrhea. These include the indole acetic acids, propionic acids, salicylic acids, and fenamates (refer to Drug Tables 306, 307 for specific products). Mefenamic acid (Ponstel) may have a theoretical advantage over other NSAIDs because it appears to antagonize the action of formed prostaglandins at the receptor sites, in addition to inhibiting their production (Latassy & Sagraves, 1995). However, its clinical use is limited by a high incidence of GI side effects and cost.

NSAIDs with the FDA-approved indication for primary dysmenorrhea include ibuprofen, diclofenac potassium (Cataflam), ketoprofen (Orudis), naproxen and naproxen sodium (Aleve, Anaprox), meclofenamate sodium (Meclofen), and mefenamic acid (Ponstel). All of these have a rapid onset of effect within 30 min to an hour after administration.

All of the approved agents are effective if used as soon as the pain begins or at the onset of menses. The medication should be continued for the first 2–3 days of menstrual flow. Ibuprofen is usually the drug of choice because it is inexpensive, available in several strengths, and can be purchased without a prescription. If a clinical response is not seen with a particular agent, the subsequent doses should be increased or a change made to an alternative agent (Latassy & Sagraves, 1995).

If a woman also desires a method of contraception, a combination oral contraceptive may be the initial drug of choice. They are effective in controlling symptoms of dysmenorrhea in more than 90% of women (Murphy, 1995). If symptoms are relieved but still present after a trial of 3–4 months, an NSAID may be added to the regimen.

Narcotic analgesic combination products should be avoided unless all other options have been explored. If a woman requires a narcotic-containing product for more than 1–3 days of her cycle or if she requires increasing doses, the diagnosis of primary dysmenorrhea may be in question (Klotz, 1995).

There are numerous nonprescription products that are marketed for the relief or prevention of dysmenorrhea symptoms. Most of these products contain various combinations of aspirin, acetaminophen, ibuprofen, caffeine, and "natural" diuretics. The effectiveness of any of these expensive products is limited to, at most, a mild analgesic effect unless they contain ibuprofen.

***Monitoring for Efficacy.*** An appropriate NSAID should provide some symptomatic relief within 30 min to 1 h after ingestion. If pain relief does not occur, repeat and double the next dose. With the next menstrual cycle, start with the increased dose. If relief of symptoms does not occur, switch to another NSAID. A trial of 3–6 months should be adequate to determine the effectiveness of therapy. Therapy should be taken on a continuous basis through the first 48–72 h of menstrual flow rather than on an as-needed basis (Klotz, 1995).

Oral contraceptives should be taken for three to four menstrual cycles to determine their clinical effectiveness. An NSAID may be added at that time if symptoms are improved but still occurring.

***Monitoring for Toxicity.*** Adverse effects associated with NSAID use for primary dysmenorrhea should be uncommon except for gastrointestinal irritation, because of their limited, intermittent use. GI side effects can be reduced if NSAIDs are taken with food or an antacid. Other side effects that might occur include dizziness, visual disturbances, rash, tinnitus, fluid retention, and increased risk of bleeding. (Refer to Drug Table 306 for a more inclusive list of side effects and contraindications) Potential side effects and contraindications with oral contraceptives would be the same as those experienced when prescribed as a method of birth control (see Drug Table 603).

## ENDOMETRIOSIS AND ADENOMYOSIS

Endometriosis and adenomyosis are discussed together in this section as they have several similar characteristics. They both involve the growth of endometrial glands and stroma outside the uterine cavity; the etiology is essentially unknown; they both cause painful, heavy menses; and the treatment is generally the same for both conditions.

The most common sites of endometrial implants outside the uterine cavity are the ovaries, broad ligament, posterior cul-de-sac, bladder serosa, fallopian tubes, and large bowel. The degree of disease does not always correlate with the severity of symptoms (Adamson, 1990). With adenomyosis, endometrial tissue grows into the myometrium, or uterine wall (Forrest, 1994).

## SPECIFIC CONSIDERATIONS FOR PHARMACOTHERAPY

### When Drug Therapy Is Needed

Severe, or even moderate, dysmenorrhea can be life-disrupting. For this reason alone, drug therapy is needed since dysmenorrhea is a very common symptom of endometriosis and adenomyosis. Infertility, with all its emotional trauma, is associated frequently with endometriosis and occasionally with adenomyosis (Lichtman & Smith, 1995). Pharmacotherapy may be needed in the management and resolution of this stressful problem.

### Short- and Long-Term Goals of Pharmacotherapy

Pharmacotherapy goals are to halt stimulation of the endometrial implants, decrease severity of symptoms, and preserve fertility if the woman so desires.

### Nonpharmacologic Therapy

Herbal teas (such as that made from vitex berries, wild yam rhizome, and cramp bark), hot water bottles, and massage may help alleviate pelvic discomfort. Yoga, exercises to relieve pelvic congestion, warm tub baths, and biofeedback also may be useful.

In severe cases, surgical intervention may be necessary. Laparoscopic cautery or laser surgery is used for endometrial implants. Total hysterectomy and bilateral salpingo-oophorectomy may be done if all other medical and conservative surgical therapies have failed.

### Time Frame for Initiating Pharmacotherapy

Therapy should be initiated after a diagnosis has been made; however, medications are frequently given to alleviate dysmenorrhea before a definitive diagnosis by laparoscopy is made.

See Drug Tables 306, 603, 605, 608.

### Assessment and History Taking

A complete history and physical examination, with careful pelvic and rectovaginal assessment, is needed. A menstrual history, reproductive history, and sexual history should be obtained. Questions should be asked concerning dyspareunia, dysmenorrhea, STDs, and PID.

On pelvic examination, tender uterosacral ligaments or tender nodules in the posterior cul-de-sac may be palpated with endometriosis. The uterus may become fixed and retroverted as the disease advances (Richards, 1995). In adenomyosis, the uterus is globular and diffusely enlarged as much as two to three times normal size. It may have a fine granular or nodular surface. In both endometriosis and adenomyosis, the uterus may be tender with compression (Star, 1995).

Although no specific laboratory tests are available for the assessment of endometriosis and adenomyosis, cultures should be taken to rule out gonorrhea and chlamydia, and a pregnancy test and Pap smear should be done. The CA-125 level may be elevated with endometriosis, but this is neither specific nor sensitive enough to help with diagnosis (Adamson, 1990). Definitive diagnosis of endometriosis is made by laparoscopy. The diagnosis of adenomyosis is frequently made incidentally by the pathologist after hysterectomy or on autopsy (Star, 1995).

### Patient/Caregiver Information

Theories of etiology, diagnostic procedures, treatment options, and side effects should be discussed with the patient. Although various medical therapies may be effective, the definitive treatment of chronic pelvic pain associated with endometriosis and adenomyosis is total abdominal hysterectomy with bilateral salpingo-oophorectomy (Lu & Ory, 1995), and patients should be made aware of this. If pregnancy is desired, referral should be made to a competent fertility specialist.

## OUTCOMES MANAGEMENT

### Selecting an Appropriate Agent

If endometriosis or adenomyosis is suspected, the patient may be treated symptomatically as described in the section on dysmenorrhea. NSAIDs can offer symptomatic relief. Since endometriosis cannot be definitively diagnosed without a laparoscopy, referral to a gynecologist is needed not only for diagnosis but also for initial management and treatment (Klotz, 1995). Continued management should be in consultation with the gynecologist.

Oral contraceptives may be given continuously for 6–12 months to prevent ovulation and a state of "pseudopregnancy." Almost any combination oral contraceptive has been used with comparable success in promoting symptom relief (Lu & Ory, 1995).

Danazol, an androgen derivative that inhibits endometrial growth is one treatment modality. Although in the past danazol was given orally in two dosages of 400 mg/day, evidence shows that lower dosages of 400 mg/day can be used for less severe disease (Lu & Ory, 1995). Danazol is an appropriate treatment of endometriosis, but its side effects have decreased patient acceptance of this therapy (Klotz, 1995).

Progestin therapy has been shown to be as effective as danazol in the promoting the regression of endometriosis (Lu & Ory, 1995). The progestin most commonly used is medroxyprogesterone acetate (MPA) with the oral dosage being 10–30 mg/day for 6 months. It may also be given as an IM preparation (Depo-Provera) 100 mg every 2 weeks for four doses, followed by 200 mg/month for 4 months (Lu & Ory, 1995). With the lower cost of progestin therapy compared to danazol, the comparable effectiveness, and the potential for less serious side effects, it is frequently recommended over danazol.

The most recent class of drugs used to cause a regression in endometrial implants is the GnRH agonists. Although more costly, they are associated with better patient compliance (Klotz, 1995). These agents decrease the secretion of FSH and LH. Within 6 weeks the circulating levels of ovarian hormones subsequently become so low, the treatment is sometimes called a *medical oophorectomy*. The following medications may be used:

- Nafarelin (Synarel) intranasal spray, one spray (200 µg/spray) twice daily, administering the spray in a different nostril in the morning and in the evening. This should be continued for 6 months (Forrest, 1994).
- Leuprolide acetate (Lupron or Lupron Depot) 0.5–1.0 mg/day SC or 3.75–7.5 mg/month IM, respectively (Dambro, 1995).
- Goserelin acetate implant (Zoladex) 3.6 mg SC every 4 weeks for 6 months (Dambro, 1995).

## Monitoring for Efficacy

For oral contraceptives, monitoring for efficacy and side effects is the same as for women placed on cyclic oral contraceptive therapy. However, if breakthrough bleeding occurs, the tablet dosage may be increased to two per day, or additional conjugated estrogens, 1.25 mg/day for 2 weeks (Lu & Ory, 1995) or 2.5 mg/day for 1 week (Forrest, 1998).

If danazol therapy is being used, the patient should be seen in 6 weeks and if no improvement has occurred within that time, the dosage may be increased to 600–800 mg/day. Therapy usually is continued for 6 months, and up to 90% of patients will have alleviation of pelvic pain. A shorter treatment time also may be effective (Lu & Ory, 1995). Women should be seen every 1–2 months while receiving this therapy.

Efficacy for progestin therapy has been previously noted. As with danazol, women should be seen monthly or bimonthly and efficacy assessed.

Serum estradiol levels may be monitored when using GnRH. With nafarelin nasal spray, if the patient continues to have menses after 2 months of treatment, the dosage may be increased to 800 µg (Dambro, 1995).

## Monitoring for Toxicity

Side effects of danazol include those typically associated with androgenic agents, as well as those associated with low estrogenic states, oily skin, acne, weight gain, emotional lability, vaginal dryness, and hot flashes are the most common. Less frequent may be hirsutism, decreased breast size, and deepening of the voice. The drug also may cause a mild elevation of liver function tests, a decrease in high-density lipoprotein levels, and an increase in low-density lipoprotein levels. Although these side effects usually are reversible when danazol is discontinued, there have been reported cases of permanent voice changes (Klotz, 1995). It would be prudent to obtain LFTs and fractionated cholesterol levels prior to beginning therapy and every 6 months, and to avoid using this treatment in patients who have a history of hyperlipidemia.

Side effects of MPA have previously been discussed. Breakthrough bleeding with MPA is managed the same as with breakthrough bleeding with oral contraceptives, using conjugated estrogens. Untoward effects of estrogen should be monitored (see Chap. 18).

The primary concern with the GnRH ago-nists is osteoporosis secondary to low estrogen. Their use, therefore, is limited to 6 months. Although the loss of trabecular bone is measur-able, it also is reversible (Whitehouse, Adams, Bancroft, Vaughan-Williams, & Elstein, 1990). Hypoestrogenic effects such as atrophic vagini-tis, hot flashes, and others previously noted are certainly present with GnRH therapy.

## Follow-up Recommendations

Since medical therapy is seen as suppressive rather than curative and recurrence of symp-toms is common once the therapy has been dis-continued, close follow-up is recommended and is dependent on the chosen therapy. Referral to, or consultation with, appropriate specialists should occur as indicated.

## SEXUAL DYSFUNCTION

Sexual dysfunctions are currently classified into four major categories, according to the *Diagnostic and Statistical Manual of Mental Disorders* (DSM-IV). These categories are: (1) sexual desire disorders, including hypoactive sexual desire and sexual aversion disorder; (2) sexual arousal disorders, including female sexual arousal disorder and erectile disorder; (3) orgasmic disorders, including female and male orgasmic disorder, and premature ejacula-tion; and (4) sexual pain disorders, including dyspareunia and vaginismus (APA, 1994). Sexual dysfunction should be categorized as lifelong or acquired, general or situational, and affecting one or both partners (Rosen & Lieblum, 1995).

*Hypoactive sexual desire* (HSD) is a "defi-ciency or absence of sexual fantasies and desire for sexual activity and the disturbance must cause marked distress and interpersonal diffi-culty" (APA, 1994). The term is used when the etiology for low libido has not been determined. Other organic causes or other psychiatric dis-orders that may affect sexual desire such as de-pression need to be ruled out. HSD may be broken down into: (1) primary HSD: total lack of sexual desire throughout a woman's life; (2) secondary HSD: loss of previous desire, such as after childbirth; or (3) situational HSD: lack of desire in particular situations but not in others. Common etiologies for HSD include sexual trauma (sexual abuse, incest, or assault) and high amounts of hostility and/or resentment

in relationships. Physical causes include depres-sion, high stress levels, medications, and low testosterone levels (Ayres, 1995).

*Female orgasmic disorder* is diagnosed by a "persistent or recurrent delay in, or absence of, orgasm following a normal sexual excitement phase. The diagnosis should be based on the clinician's judgment that the woman's orgasmic capacity is less than would be reasonable for her age, sexual experience and the adequacy of sexual stimulation she receives" (APA, 1994). Female orgasmic disorder (or anorgasmia) can be categorized as: (1) primary anorgasmia: never experienced orgasm by any means including masturbation; (2) secondary anorgasmia: no longer experiences orgasms as a result of physi-cal illness, relationship problems, medications, or stress; (3) situational anorgasmia: achieves or-gasm only in certain situations; and (4) coital anorgasmia: can achieve orgasm by manual or oral stimulation but not from intercourse alone (Ayres, 1995).

*Dyspareunia* is a "recurrent or persistent genital pain in either a male or a female, which causes marked distress or interpersonal diffi-culty" (APA, 1994). Although one of the most common causes, it is not caused exclusively by lack of lubrication due to insufficient arousal. Lack of lubrication may also be caused by estro-gen deficiency, infection, or medications.

*Vaginismus* is a "recurrent or persistent in-voluntary spasm of the musculature of the outer third of the vagina that interferes with sexual in-tercourse" (APA, 1994). Involuntary contraction of the vaginal muscles is often a physical mani-festation of psychological or interpersonal fac-tors. Contributing factors may include sexual trauma or abuse, negative family and religious psychosexual messages, and sexual fears and phobia (Rosen & Leiblum, 1995). Pain associ-ated with PID or endometriosis, or fear of can-cer, pregnancy, HIV infection, or other STDs also may be associated with vaginismus (Ayres, 1995).

## SPECIFIC CONSIDERATIONS FOR PHARMACOTHERAPY

### When Drug Therapy Is Needed

Unless the sexual dysfunction is secondary to a medical condition that requires a specific drug for management, such as depression, diabetes, or menopause, pharmacologic interventions should not be considered first-line therapy. They can be adjunctive therapy to nonpharmacologic interventions such as stress management, individual counseling, or couples therapy.

Anxiolytics and/or antidepressants can help in certain cases of sexual dysfunction related to fear, previous sexual abuse, relationship problems, or preoccupation with other life stressors. Depending on the age of the woman, dyspareunia may be related to hormone deficiency and can be relieved with the use of vaginal lubricants and either oral or vaginal estrogen replacement. Anorgasmia may be related to medications that the woman may be taking for another medical indication, such as contraception or depression, which may require a change to an alternative agent with less effect on sexual functioning (Walker et al, 1993). Antibiotics may be necessary to treat genitourinary infections that may be causing pain or changes in lubrication that may interfere with sexual pleasure (Ayres, 1995).

## Short- and Long-Term Goals of Pharmacotherapy

The short-term goal of pharmacotherapy is to treat any medical condition that is causing pain or discomfort and interfering with normal sexual functioning. This could involve the use of antibiotics to treat genitourinary infections, use of vaginal lubricants, or use of vaginal estrogen creams. If the sexual dysfunction is related to stress or anxiety, short-term benzodiazepines could be prescribed along with behavior modification techniques.

Long-term goals involve appropriate treatment of medical conditions that have an association with sexual dysfunction, such as diabetes and depression. Efforts should be made to optimize management with appropriate drugs for those disease processes. Perimenopausal women should also be evaluated for signs and symptoms of estrogen deficiency that could be relieved with hormone replacement therapy.

Patients who present with a new onset of complaints of problems with sexual function or desire should always be questioned about their use of prescribed medications or substances of abuse. Common medications that can affect the various phases of sexual functioning include antihypertensives, antidepressants, antihistamines, neuroleptics, and histamine $H_2$ receptor antagonists. Excessive use of alcohol, cocaine, and narcotics may also interfere with the normal phases of sexual arousal (APA, 1994).

## Nonpharmacologic Therapy

Counseling is the primary nonpharmacologic therapy for sexual problems. This may take the form of instruction on stress management techniques, counseling for the woman and her partner, or intensive individual psychotherapy.

Of the various approaches, the classic PLISSIT model (Annon, 1976), with its varying levels of intervention, is one of the most widely used. Increased knowledge and skill are required of the practitioner as the levels of intervention are progressively more complex. The four levels are permission, limited information, specific suggestions, and intensive therapy. The following is a brief description of each level:

1. *Permission:* This level is the least complex and provides the patient with the reassurance that she is normal and has professional permission to continue with whatever she is doing, provided the activity is not harmful or detrimental to herself or her partner.

2. *Limited information:* Factual information that addresses the patient's problem or concern is given at this level, with the hope of changing attitude and/or behavior. An example of this could be providing to someone information on how stress affects libido if she is concerned about diminished sex drive during a time of upheaval and change.

3. *Specific suggestions:* Recommendations for behavior change are given here. Suggestions may range from recommending a vaginal lubricant to specific positional changes to increase clitoral contact during intercourse. The nature of the sexual difficulty treated here is limited in scope. For instance, sexual dysfunction that arises from long-term sexual abuse cannot be appropriately addressed at this level.

4. *Intensive therapy:* This is the most complex level. It is used when sexual problems have not been resolved with the first three levels of intervention. Practitioners must have advanced training and skills to intervene at this level; therefore, referral to a sex therapist generally is made at this point.

## Time Frame for Initiating Pharmacotherapy

Antidepressants and anxiolytics should only be initiated after nonpharmacologic interventions, such as stress management, counseling, and education about the normal sexual response cycle, have either been ineffective or refused by the patient. Treatment for genitourinary infections or hormone deficiency should be initiated as soon as the diagnosis is made.

Antibiotics should be given for the recommended number of days based on the causative organism and site of infection. Hormone replacement therapy must be taken continuously for symptomatic relief as well as for the long-term benefits on cardiovascular disease and osteoporosis prevention. Anxiolytics and antidepressants are intended for short-term use. An adequate trial to determine the benefit of antidepressants would be 4–6 weeks. If effective, the antidepressant should be continued for 6 months.

See Drug Tables 102, 309, 311, 605.

## Assessment and History Taking

Women who complain of any sexual dysfunction, no matter what the subsequent diagnosis, should be asked to complete a thorough history, including current health history, past medical and surgical history, and family history. This gains valuable information as to psychological contributors and rules out any organic cause for the dysfunction. The presence of physical symptoms should be explored; acute and chronic illnesses and current medications should be identified. Sexual habits and techniques should be discussed as well as any history of sexual assault and abuse. Lifestyle stressors, job/career stressors, financial stressors, and family and social support systems need to be identified as well as recent changes in the relationship that may contribute to the current problem. Since specific and intimate details are required, this interview must be handled in a respectful, professional manner, and the woman must feel comfortable and be assured that the information she supplies is totally confidential. She should be given a complete and thorough physical examination with careful attention to the thyroid gland. Pelvic examination should note any hooding (or covering) of the clitoris, which can result in decreased sensation, evidence of atrophy, and presence of discomfort at any time during the examination. Laboratory tests may include CBC, thyroid function tests, and any hormone studies deemed necessary.

## Patient/Caregiver Information

The patient should receive education about the different phases of the normal sexual response cycle and what physiological or psychological factors can affect them. In some instances, reassure patients that what they are experiencing is con-

sidered normal (Anderson & Cyranowski, 1995). The woman needs to become aware of specific situations, individuals, and/or relationships that may be contributing to her dysfunction. Recommend stress management techniques and improving coping skills. Participation in support groups should also be encouraged depending on the patient's comfort level. If the dysfunction is the result of a medical condition that is not well controlled, the importance of compliance with a prescribed therapeutic regimen should be strongly reinforced. If drug therapy is prescribed as part of the management of the sexual dysfunction, the patient needs to understand how the drug needs to taken and any special instructions, potential adverse effects, and drug interactions.

## OUTCOMES MANAGEMENT

### Selecting an Appropriate Agent

Selecting an appropriate pharmacologic agent and its duration depends on the etiology of the sexual dysfunction. The patient's medication list should be reviewed for optimal therapy of concomitant medical conditions and drugs that possibly may exacerbate sexual dysfunction. See Table 35–4.

Decreased or inhibited sexual desire can often be treated with a short-acting benzodiazepine, such as alprazolam, or one of the SSRIs, if the symptoms are stress- or depression-related. Select an antidepressant that has a low incidence of inhibition of libido and orgasm, such as bupropion (Wellbutrin) or nefazodone (Serzone), to ensure patient compliance.

### TABLE 35–4. SELECTED DRUGS THAT MAY DECREASE LIBIDO OR PREVENT ORGASM

Antihypertensives
   Thiazides
   Methyldopa(Aldomet)
   Clonidine (Catapres)
   Beta blockers
Tricyclic antidepressants
Selective serotonin reuptake inhibitors
   Fluoxetine (Prozac)
   Sertraline (Zoloft)
Phenothiazines
Narcotic analgesics

Additional agents may also cause erectile dysfunction.

If the woman is taking oral contraceptives, switching to an alternative product that contains a more androgenic progestin, such as Lovirg-Ovral, Ovral, or Loestrin 1.5/30, may have a positive effect on libido. With perimenopausal women, the addition of either oral or vaginal estrogen supplements may be helpful. If the woman is already receiving estrogen replacement, supplementation with testosterone may be beneficial. Testosterone can be given as methyltestosterone 1.25–5 mg PO daily, Depo-Testosterone 50 mg IM every 4 weeks, or in the conjugated estrogen 0.625 mg/methyltestosterone 1.25 mg combination product (Estratest).

If the woman is experiencing anorgasmia, the first-line therapy would involve discontinuing any medication that may decrease libido or interfere with the ability to achieve orgasm. Vaginal atrophy may require the use of vaginal lubricants or hormone replacement therapy.

Dyspareunia may be caused by inadequate lubrication, vaginal atrophy, or vaginal infections. Vaginal lubricants such as Lubrin or Astroglide may need to be used prior to intercourse. Vaginal estrogen creams, such as Premarin or Ogen, provide symptomatic relief of vaginal atrophy secondary to estrogen deficiency. The creams need to be used on a daily basis until symptoms begin to subside. They then may be continued on an intermittent basis, usually twice a week. Vaginal infections, urinary tract infections, and pelvic inflammatory disease need to be treated with appropriate antibiotics.

Symptoms of vaginismus can sometimes be relieved with vaginal lubricants and hormone replacement therapy, but the intense constriction of the vaginal muscles may require analgesics for the pain and discomfort. In addition to counseling, benzodiazepines may assist in relieving some of the underlying anxiety that may exist.

Clinical efficacy is based on the relief of signs and symptoms since there are no laboratory tests to follow and the physical examination is usually normal. The exceptions would be if there was an infection or evidence of vaginal atrophy present. Length of treatment will vary based on the underlying problem and the patient's response. The schedule for follow-up will depend on the etiology of the sexual dysfunction.

## Monitoring for Toxicity

The majority of the agents that are prescribed are well tolerated. However, it is important to assess whether the woman is pregnant before initiating therapy since all of the drugs that may be prescribed have a potential effect on pregnancy outcome. The exception is the vaginal lubricants, which have virtually no adverse effects. Chapters 18 and 19 on contraception and menopause contain a more extensive discussion of the adverse effects associated with the hormonal interventions. The benzodiazepines, antidepressants, and antibiotics are covered in depth in other chapters. The Drug Tables contain detailed coverage of drug dosages, adverse effects, and drug interactions for all the drugs discussed in this chapter.

## REFERENCES

Adamson, G. D. (1990). Diagnosis and clinical presentation of endometriosis. *American Journal of Obstetrics and Gynecology, 162,* 568.

Alvir, J., & Thys-Jacobs, S. (1991). Premenstrual and menstrual symptoms clusters and response to calcium treatment. *Psychopharmacology Bulletin, 27,* 145–148.

American Psychiatric Association. (1994). *Diagnostic and statistical manual of mental disorders* (4th ed.). Washington, DC: APA.

Anderson, B. L., & Cyranowski, S. (1995). Women's sexuality: Behaviors, response and individual differences. *Journal of Consulting and Clinical Psychology, 63*(6), 891–906.

Annon, J. S. (1976). The PLISSIT Model: A proposed conceptual scheme for the behavioral treatment of sexual problems. *Journal of Sex Education and Therapy, 2,* 1.

Ayres, T. (1995). Sexual dysfunction. In W. L. Star, L. L. Lommel, & M. T. Shannon (Eds.), *Women's primary health care: Protocols for practice.* Washington, DC: American Nurses Association.

Baker, S. (1998). Menstruation and related problems and concerns. In E. Youngkin & M. Davis (Eds.), *Women's health: A primary care clinical guide* (2nd ed.). Stamford, CT: Appleton & Lange.

Barnhart, K. T., Freeman, E. W., & Sondheimer, S. J. (1995). A clinician's guide to the premenstrual syndrome. *Medical Clinics of North America, 79*(6), 1457–1472.

Bartlett, J. G., III. (1996). Infections of skin, soft tissue, and bone. In J. Stoko, D. Hellman, P. Ladeuson, B. Petty, & T. Traill (Eds.), *The principles and practice of medicine.* Stamford, CT: Appleton & Lange.

Cerda, G. M., & Parry, B. L. (1994). The effects of bright light therapy on symptoms of depression, anxiety, and hibernation in patients with premenstrual syndrome. *Journal of Women's Health*, 3(1), 5.

Chuong, C. J., & Dawson, E. B. (1992). Critical evaluation of nutritional factors in the pathophysiology and treatment of premenstrual syndrome. *Clinics in Obstetrics and Gynecology, 35*, 679–692.

Collins, A., Cerin, A., Coleman G., & Landgren, B. M. (1993). Essential fatty acids in the treatment of premenstrual syndrome. *Obstetrics and Gynecology, 81*, 93–98.

Conviser, J. H., & Fitzgibbon, M. L. (1997). Eating disorders. In K. Allen & J. Phillips (Eds.), *Women's health across the lifespan*. Philadelphia: Lippincott.

Curry, S. L. (1995). Other disorders of the vulva, vagina, and uterus. In V. Seltzer & W. Pearse (Eds.), *Women's primary health care office practice and procedures*. New York: McGraw-Hill.

Curry, S. L., & Barclay, D. L. (1994). Benign disorders of the vulva and vagina. In A. DeCherney & M. Pernall (Eds.), *Current obstetric and gynecologic diagnosis and treatment*. Norwalk, CT: Appleton & Lange.

Dambro, M. (1995). *The 5 minute clinical consult*. Baltimore: Williams & Wilkins.

Facchinetti, F., Borela, P., Sances, G., et al. (1991). Oral magnesium successfully relieves premenstrual mood changes. *Obstetrics and Gynecology, 78*, 177–181.

Fankhauser, M. P. (1997). Premenstrual syndrome. In T. J. DiPiro, R. L. Talbert, G. C. Yee, G. R. Matzke, B. G. Wells, & L. M. Posey (Eds.), *Pharmacotherapy: A pathophysiologic approach* (3rd ed.). Stamford, CT: Appleton & Lange.

Fogel, C. I. (1995). Common symptoms. In C. I. Fogel & N. Woods (Eds.), *Women's health care*. Thousand Oaks, CA: Sage.

Forrest, D. E. (1998). Common gynecologic pelvic disorders. In E. Youngkin & M. Davis (Eds.), *Women's health: A primary care clinical guide* (2nd ed.). Stamford, CT: Appleton & Lange.

Frank, E., Hasket, R. F., Yonkers, K. A., Halbreich, U., Freeman, E. W., & Grady, T. A. (1995). *Efficacy of sertraline in premenstrual dysphoria*. Poster session presented at the 34th annual meeting of the American College of Neuropsychopharmacology, San Juan, Puerto Rico.

Freeman, E. (1993). Prevalence and risk factors of premenstrual syndrome. *Clinical Advances in Psychiatric Disorders, 7*, 13–16.

Freeman, E. W., Rickels, K., & Sondheimer, S. J. (1996). Sertraline versus dispramine in the treatment of premenstrual syndrome: An open-label trial. *Journal of Clinical Psychiatry, 57*, 7–11.

Freeman, E. W., Rickels, K., Sondheimer, S., & Polansky, M. (1995). A double-blind trial of oral progesterone, alprazolam, and placebo in treatment of severe premenstrual syndrome. *JAMA, 274*, 51–57.

Freeman, E. W., Rickels, K., Sondheimer, S., et al. (1990). Ineffectiveness of progesterone treatment for premenstrual syndrome. *JAMA, 264*, 349.

Gilchrist, V. (1996). Hirsuitism. In C. Johnson, B. Johnson, J. Murray, & B. Apgar. *Women's health care handbook*. Philadelphia: Hanley & Belfus.

Goldstein, S. M., & Odom, R. B. (1994). Skin and appendages. In L. Tierney, S. McPhee, & M. Papadakis (Eds.), *Current medical diagnosis and treatment*. Norwalk, CT: Appleton & Lange.

Goroll, A. H., May, L. A., & Mulley, A. G. (1995). *Primary care medicine*. Philadelphia: Lippincott.

Hatcher, R. A., Trussell, J., Stewart, F., Stewart, G. K., Kowal, D., Guest, F., Cates, W., Jr., & Policar, M. S. (1994). *Contraceptive technology* (16th ed.). New York: Irvington.

International Society for the Study of Vulva Disease. (1991). Issue Committee report on vulvodynia, vulva vestibulitus, and vestibular papillomatosis. *Journal of Reproductive Medicine, 36*, 413.

Jones, K. D., & Lehr, S. T. (1994). Vulvodynia diagnostic techniques and treatment modalities. *Nurse Practitioner, 19*(4), 34.

Kaufman, R. H. (1995). Disease of the vulva and vagina. In D. Lemcke, J. Pattison, L. Marshall, & D. Cowley (Eds.), *Primary care of women*. Norwalk, CT: Appleton & Lange.

Keville, K. (1996). *Herbs for health and healing*. Emmaus, PA: Rodale Press, Inc.

Kleignen, J., Ter Riet, G., & Knipschild, P. (1990). Vitamin $B_6$ in the treatment of the premenstrual syndrome: A review. *British Journal of Obstetrics and Gynecology, 97*, 847–852.

Klotz, M. M. (1995). Dysmenorrhea, endometriosis, and pelvic pain. In D. Lemcke, J. Pattison, L. Marshall, & D. Cawley (Eds.), *Primary care of women*. Norwalk, CT: Appleton & Lange.

Latassy, N. A., & Sagraves, R. (1995). Gynecological disorders. In M. A. Koda-Kimble & L. Y. Young (Eds.), *Applied therapeutics: The clinical use of drugs* (6th ed.). Vancouver, WA: Applied Therapeutics.

Lichtman, R., & Duran, P. (1995). The vulva and vagina. In R. Lichtman & S. Papera (Eds.), *Gynecology: Well-woman care*. Norwalk, CT: Appleton & Lange.

Lichtman, R., & Smith, S. M. (1995). Multiorgan disorders. In R. Lichtman & S. Papera (Eds.), *Gynecology: Well-woman care*. Norwalk, CT: Appleton & Lange.

London, R. S., Bradley, L., & Chiamor, N. (1991). Effect of nutritional supplement on premenstrual symptomatology in women with premenstrual syndrome: A longitudinal study. *Journal of the American College of Nutrition, 10,* 494–499.

Lu, P. Y., & Ory, S. J. (1995). Endometriosis current management. *Mayo Clinic Proceedings, 70,* 453.

Mann, M. (1992). Vulva vestibulitis: Significant clinical variables and treatment outcomes. *Obstetrics and Gynecology, 79,* 122.

Mattox, J. H. (1995). Disorders of menstruation. In V. Seltzer & W. Pearse (Eds.), *Women's primary health care office practice and procedures.* New York: McGraw-Hill.

McKay, M. (1993). Dysesthetic (essential) vulvodynia: Treatment with amitriptyline. *Journal of Reproductive Medicine, 38*(1), 9.

Menkes, D., Taghavi, E., Mason, D., et al. (1992). Fluoxetine treatment of severe premenstrual syndrome. *BMJ, 305,* 346–347.

Moline, M. (1993). Pharmacologic strategies for managing premenstrual syndrome. *Clinical Pharmacology, 12,* 181–196.

Murphy, J. R. (1995). Dysmenorrhea. In W. L. Star, L. L. Lommel, & M. T. Shannon (Eds.), *Women's primary health care: Protocols for practice.* Washington, DC: American Nurses Association.

New approaches to PMS. (February 1998). *Harvard Women's Health Watch, 5*(6), 6–7.

Nonprescription PMS treatment launched. (1996). *The Female Patient, 21,* 71.

Parry, G. J., & Bredensen, D. E. (1985). Sensory neuropathy with low-dose pyridoxine. *Neurology, 35,* 1466–1468.

Rapkin, A. J. (1992). The role of serotonin in premenstrual syndrome. *Clinics in Obstetrics and Gynecology, 35,* 629–636.

Richards, J. (1995). Endometriosis. In W. Star, L. Lommel, & M. Shannon (Eds.), *Women's primary health care: Protocols for practice.* Washington, DC: American Nurses Association.

Rickels, K., Freeman, E. W., & Sondheimer, S. (1992). Buspirone in treatment of premenstrual syndrome. *Lancet, 1,* 777.

Rosen, R. C., & Leiblum, S. R. (1995). Treatment of sexual disorders in the 1990s: An integrated approach. *Journal of Consulting and Clinical Psychology, 63*(6), 877–890.

Rossignol, A. M., & Bonnlander, H. (1990). Caffeine-containing beverages, total fluid consumption and premenstrual syndrome. *American Journal of Public Health, 80,* 1106–1110.

Rubinow, D. (1992). The premenstrual syndrome: New views. *JAMA, 268,* 1908.

Rubinow, D. R., & Schmidt, P. J. (1995). The treatment of premenstrual syndrome—forward into the past [editorial]. *New England Journal of Medicine, 332,* 1574–1575.

Sayeh, R., Schiff, I., Wurtman, J., et al. (1995). The effect of a carbohydrate-rich beverage on mood, appetite, and cognitive function in women with premenstrual syndrome. *Obstetrics and Gynecology, 86,* 520–528.

Schaumberg, H., Kaplan, J., Windebank, A., Vick, N., Rasmus, S., Pleasure, D., & Brown, M. (1983). Sensory neuropathy from pyridoxine abuse: A new megavitamin syndrome. *New England Journal of Medicine, 309,* 445.

Secor, R. M., & Fertitta, L. (1992). Vulva vesiculitis syndrome. *Nurse Practitioner Forum, 3*(3), 161.

Servino, S. K., & Moline, M. L. (1995). Premenstrual syndrome: Identification and management. *Drugs, 49*(1), 71–82.

Skrypzak, B. (1995). Approach to abnormal vaginal bleeding. In D. Lemcke, J. Pattison, L. Marshall, & D. Coley (Eds.), *Primary care of women.* Norwalk, CT: Appleton & Lange.

Sober, A. J. (1995). Dermatologic problems. In A. Goroll, L. May, & A. Mulley (Eds.), *Primary care medicine.* Philadelphia: Lippincott.

Solomons, C. C., Melmed, M. H., & Heitler, S. M. (1991). Calcium citrate for vulva vestibulitis. *Journal of Reproductive Medicine, 36,* 879.

Star, W. (1995). Pelvic masses. In W. Star, L. Lommel, & M. Shannon (Eds.), *Women's primary health care: Protocols for practice.* Washington, DC: American Nurses Association.

Steiner, M., Steinberg, S., Stewart, D., Carter, D., Berger, C., Reid, R., Grover, D., & Streiner, D. (1995). Fluoxetine in the treatment of premenstrual dysphoria. *New England Journal of Medicine, 332,* 1529–1534.

Taylor, D. (1995). Perimenstrual symptoms and premenstrual syndrome. In W. L. Star, L. L. Lommel, & M. T. Shannon (Eds.), *Women's primary health care: Protocols for practice.* Washington, DC: American Nurses Association.

Thys-Jacobs, S., Ceccarelli, S., Bierman, A., et al. (1989). Calcium supplementation in premenstrual syndrome: A randomized crossover trial. *Journal of General Internal Medicine, 4,* 183–189.

Turner, M. L. C., & Marinoff, S. C. (1988). Association of human papilloma virus with vulvodynia and the vulva vestibulitis syndrome. *Journal of Reproductive Medicine, 33,* 533.

Umpierre, S. A., et al. (1991). Human papilloma virus DNA in tissue biopsy specimens of vulva vestibulitis patients treated with interferon. *Obstetrics and Gynecology, 78,* 693.

Walker, P. W., Cole, J. O., Gardner, E. A., Hughes, A. R., Johnston, J. A., Batey, S. R., & Lineberry, C. G. (1993). Improvement in fluoxetine-associated sexual dysfunction in patients switched to bupropion. *Journal of Clinical Psychiatry, 54*(12), 459–465.

Weil, E. K. (Ed.). (1996). *Nurse practitioner's prescribing reference*. New York: Prescribing Reference.

Whitehouse, R. W., Adams, J. E., Bancroft, K., Vaughan-Williams, C. A., & Elstein, M. (1990). The effects of nafarelin and danazol on vertebral trabecular bone mass in patients with endometriosis. *Clinical Endocrinology, 33,* 365.

Wood, S. H., Mortola, J. F., Chan, Y., et al. (1992). Treatment of premenstrual syndrome with fluoxetine: A double-blind, placebo-controlled, crossover study. *Obstetrics and Gynecology, 80,* 344–347.

# 36

# SEXUALLY TRANSMITTED DISEASES, VAGINITIS, AND PELVIC INFLAMMATORY DISEASE

*Susan Rawlins, Robert L. Martin, and Mai Duong*

This chapter is an overview of the common sexually transmitted diseases (STDs) and pelvic inflammatory disease (PID), infestations, and vaginitis. An important viral pathogen, the human immunodeficiency virus (HIV) is covered in Chap. 37 of this book. From the clinician's perspective, comprehensive management of patients with sexually transmitted diseases is challenging. The clinician must be engaged in continuous reeducation to stay abreast of new developments such as emerging antibiotic resistance patterns, improved diagnostic tests, and new drugs and treatment regimens. In addition to being proficient at diagnosis and treatment, the clinician needs to be effective at prevention of the spread of these diseases, by educating and hopefully influencing change in the sexual behaviors that place patients at risk for acquiring or transmitting STDs.

The treatment regimens provided in this chapter closely follow the 1998 recommendations of the Centers for Disease Control and Prevention 1998 Guidelines for Treatment of Sexually Transmitted Diseases (CDC, 1998). However, additional current resources are used to supplement the CDC guidelines.

## SYPHILIS

Syphilis is a sexually transmitted disease caused by the anaerobic spirochete *Treponema pallidum.* An estimated yearly incidence as high as 200,000 cases per year is reported, with the greatest increase seen in the heterosexual population and users of crack cocaine (Johnson, 1996c). Women appear to be at a higher risk of contracting syphilis compared to men with similar high-risk behaviors (Johnson, 1996c). Once exposed to the mucous membrane, the spirochete penetrates the epithelial lining, resulting in spirochetemia. This fairly aggressive infectivity accounts for the 30% risk of infection after one exposure to a person with syphilis (Johnson, 1996c). If untreated, the individual remains contagious for about 1 year and may progress to a chronic systemic disease that can involve any organ in the body (Hook & Mara, 1992; Hutchinson & Hook, 1990; Johnson, 1996c).

## SPECIFIC CONSIDERATIONS FOR PHARMACOTHERAPY

### When Drug Therapy Is Needed

With all STDs, early therapy will prevent the spread of disease to others as well as prevent morbidity and mortality associated with disease progression. Untreated syphilis can potentially progress to involve the central nervous system (neurosyphilis) or other organ systems (aortitis, gumma syphilis) (Johnson, 1996c; Knodel & Kraynak, 1997). Congenital syphilis may lead to skeletal malformation, hepatitis, interstitial keratitis, or neurosyphilis (Johnson, 1996c; Knodel & Kraynak, 1997).

## Short- and Long-Term Goals of Pharmacotherapy

For all STD therapy, short-term goals are to relieve the acute symptoms and to halt the progression of any potential complications related to the disease. Preventing the spread of STDs to other individuals is also an immediate goal with long-term benefits.

The long-term goal is to prevent recurrence of sexually transmitted disease after treatment is complete. This may be accomplished through education on the prevention of STDs. See the section on nonpharmacologic therapy for a more thorough discussion of STD prevention.

## Nonpharmacologic Therapy

Education about transmission and prevention of STDs is fundamental and a crucial tool to break the cycle of transmission. However, the materials prepared should be specific for the targeted audience in order to be effective (Youngkin, 1995). Abstinence is a highly effective way to prevent STDs. However, in most situations, this method is impractical. A more reasonable and effective method to decrease the risk of STD transmission is the use of a condom during sexual intercourse. Using more than one barrier method (ie, condom, spermacide, and diaphragm) may be more effective than just one alone (American College of Obstetricians and Gynecologists [ACOG], 1995; Youngkin, 1995). More importantly, whichever method is employed, using it correctly and consistently is essential for effectiveness (Youngkin, 1995).

In addition to the male condom, a female condom (Reality™) was recently approved by the FDA as an effective alternative barrier contraceptive device. It is a lubricated polyurethane sheath with a diaphragm-like ring at each end and is an effective barrier against viral transmission (CDC, 1998). Therefore, it can be a useful barrier device for individuals who would not otherwise use a male condom.

Finally, notifying partners and the local health department of individuals diagnosed with STDs is important in preventing further transmission (CDC, 1998). In light of the asymptomatic nature of many STD infections, proper communication to any individual involved is crucial. Although viewed as a sensitive and private matter by some individuals, it is mandatory reporting that often enables sexual partners of STD-diagnosed individuals to receive appropriate evaluation and possible medical treatment.

## Time Frame for Initiating Pharmacotherapy

For all STDs, therapy should be initiated as soon as the diagnosis is confirmed. There is no need to delay treatment. Treatment delays provide a greater opportunity for transmission of the disease to sexual contacts and development of complications from disease progression.

Pharmacologic management should not be limited to the index patient, but extended to the sex partner(s) as soon as possible. For symptomatic patients with gonorrhea or chlamydia infection, current guidelines suggest evaluation and treatment of the sex partner if the last sexual contact is within 60 days of symptom onset. Individuals exposed within 90 days preceding the diagnosis of primary, secondary, or early latent syphilis should receive treatment even if seronegative. Individuals exposed greater than 90 days preceding the diagnosis of primary, secondary, or early latent syphilis should also receive treatment, even though test results are not available or follow-up is uncertain. Long-term sex partners of individuals with late syphilis should be completely evaluated and receive the appropriate treatment (CDC, 1998). Despite the specificity of the time frame of exposure, it is rather relative. Therefore, current CDC guidelines suggest treatment of sex partners even though there may be no clinical signs of infection or completion of diagnostic tests (CDC, 1998).

See Drug Tables 102.6, 102.11.

## Assessment and History Taking

The physical signs and symptoms of syphilis have been described for hundreds of years and appear to have changed little over time (Tartaglione & Celum, 1995). Basically, the clinical presentation of this disease can be described in three stages: primary syphilis, secondary syphilis, and latent syphilis.

***Primary syphilis.*** After an incubation period of about 10–90 days a painless chancre appears at the site of inoculation. Depending on the number of penetrating spirochetes, there may be more than one chancre. Common sites of penetrance are the fourchette, cervix, anus, labia, and nipples. The ulcer is usually round, painless, and red and has well-defined raised edges surrounding a granular base. The chancre is extremely infectious, but after about 3–8 weeks it heals spontaneously (Hook & Mara, 1992; Hutchinson & Hook, 1990; Johnson, 1996c).

**Secondary syphilis.** If untreated, the disease disseminates and symptoms of secondary syphilis appear 2–6 weeks after manifestation of primary syphilis. Unique to secondary syphilis is the occurrence of a maculopapular rash on the palms of hands and soles of feet. This mucocutaneous eruption may also occur throughout the body or remain localized to a particular area. Along with the dermatological manifestations, a low-grade fever, headache, malaise, pharyngitis, anorexia, and arthralgia are also commonly observed. Whether therapy is initiated or not, the rash resolves after about 4–10 weeks. Unless treatment is received, the rash could spontaneously reappear anytime within 4 years; therefore, these individuals are still considered infectious (Hutchinson & Hook, 1990; Johnson, 1996c).

**Latent syphilis.** Latent syphilis is divided into two stages: *early* latent and *late* latent. Early latent is defined by the U.S. Public Health Service as syphilis appearing within 1 year of the onset of infection (CDC, 1998; Knodel & Kraynak, 1997). However, some experts argue that this should be extended to 2–4 years because of the possible spontaneous mucocutaneous eruptions (Knodel & Kraynak, 1997). Late latent syphilis is defined as syphilis appearing more than 1 year after the onset of disease. With the exception of transplacental transmission, individuals in this stage remain as hosts to the organism, but are not infectious to others (Johnson, 1996c; Knodel & Kraynak, 1997). Interestingly, most patients with late latent syphilis will not progress to develop further sequelae. However, 25–30% will progress to tertiary syphilis, a slowly progressive inflammatory disease that can involve any organ system (Johnson, 1996c; Knodel & Kraynak, 1997). Tertiary syphilis may occur anywhere from 2–30 years after the initial infection and manifest as neurosyphilis (20%), benign gumma syphilis (50%), or cardiovascular syphilis (Johnson, 1996c; Knodel & Kraynak, 1997).

T. pallidum cannot be cultured in vitro; therefore, direct examination of the organism under darkfield microscopy or the use of serologic tests is necessary for laboratory diagnosis. Darkfield microscopy can be used to diagnose primary and secondary syphilis (Johnson, 1996c; Knodel & Kraynak, 1997; Youngkin, 1995). This method is fairly sensitive and specific for T. pallidum because it involves the organisms from chancres, cutaneous external lesions, or mucous patches, which are examined under a darkfield microscope for motile treponemes. However, it requires the specimens to be examined immediately. The direct fluorescent antibody test–T. pallidum (DFA-TP) is another alternative that will also give immediate results. Its advantages over darkfield microscopy are that it does not require immediate examination of the specimen and it has higher specificity (Johnson, 1996c; Knodel & Kraynak, 1997).

Serological testing is divided into *nontreponemal* and *treponemal* tests. Nontreponemal tests measure antilipid antibodies that are specific for the treponeme cell surface (Johnson, 1996c; Knodel & Kraynak, 1997). Commonly used nontreponemal tests include the Venereal Disease Research Laboratory (VDRL) test, rapid plasma reagin (RPR) test, reagin screen test (RST), unheated serum reagin (USR) test, automated reagin test (ART), and the toluidine red unheated serum test (TRUST). These tests are used for screening and to assess response to therapy (Knodel & Kraynak, 1997). A titer of 1:16 or greater is indicative of disease progression, and a fourfold decrease demonstrates a successful response to therapy with eventual conversion to seronegativity (Johnson, 1996c; Knodel & Kraynak, 1997). However, patients with latent or tertiary syphilis who have completed a treatment course usually will not become seronegative. These tests may be negative when the chancre first appears and therefore may not be useful tests for early primary syphilis (Johnson, 1996c; Knodel & Kraynak, 1997). These tests have a 1% false-positive rate that is often seen in patients with viral infections and autoimmune disease and in IV drug use and pregnancy (Johnson, 1996c).

Treponemal tests are more sensitive for all stages of syphilis and are used to confirm positive nontreponemal tests (Johnson, 1996c; Knodel & Kraynak, 1997). Examples of treponemal tests include the fluorescent treponemal antibody absorption (FTA-ABS) test, microhemagglutination assay for antibodies to T. pallidum (MHA-TP), and hemagglutination treponemal test for syphilis (HATTS) (Knodel & Kraynak, 1997). Unlike the nontreponemal tests, these can be used to diagnose early primary syphilis. However, because treponemal tests remain reactive for life, they are not useful to assess response to therapy. The false-positive rates for treponemal tests are 1–2% in the healthy population (Johnson, 1996c; Knodel & Kraynak, 1997).

## OUTCOMES MANAGEMENT

### Selecting an Appropriate Agent

Pharmacologic intervention should be initiated as soon as the diagnosis is confirmed to prevent the transmission of disease to others and to prevent potential progression to tertiary syphilis. Despite the development of many new antibiotics, the treatment of choice for the past 50 years has been parenteral penicillin G. In recent years, clinical trials and clinical experience continue to demonstrate and reconfirm the efficacy of penicillin for the treatment of this disease (CDC, 1998). Treatment recommendations from the CDC are presented in Table 36–1.

The usual treatment of primary, secondary, and early latent syphilis in the non-penicillin-allergic patient is a single intramuscular (IM) injection of benzathine penicillin G 2.4 million units. Similarly, the treatment of late latent syphilis is also with benzathine penicillin G 2.4 million units, but given once a week for 3 consecutive weeks. Only neurosyphilis requires treatment with intravenous penicillin G in order to achieve adequate drug levels in the cerebrospinal fluid (CSF) (Hutchinson & Hook, 1990; Johnson, 1996c; Youngkin, 1995).

Although not considered the gold standard, alternative antibiotics have been used for patients allergic to penicillin. Currently, the CDC recommends doxycycline 100 mg b.i.d., or tetracycline 500 mg q.i.d. for 2 weeks to treat syphilis of less than 1 year in duration. Erythromycin 500 mg q.i.d. is another alternative, but is less effective (CDC, 1998). For syphilis greater than 1 year in duration, doxycycline or tetracycline is another good option, and the treatment course is for 4 weeks (Johnson, 1996c; Knodel & Kraynak, 1997). Some experts suggest penicillin

## TABLE 36–1. 1998 CDC TREATMENT RECOMMENDATIONS FOR SYPHILIS

| Stage/Type of Syphilis | Recommended Regimen |
|---|---|
| Primary, secondary, or latent syphilis of less than 1 year's duration (early latent syphilis) | Benzathine penicillin G 2.4 million units IM in a single dose[a] |
| Syphilis of more than 1 year's duration (includes late latent syphilis of unknown duration and late or tertiary syphilis; excludes neurosyphilis) | Benzathine penicillin G 2.4 million units IM once a week for 3 successive weeks |
| Neurosyphilis | Aqueous crystalline penicillin G 12–24 million units IV (2–4 million units every 4 hours) for 10–14 days,[b] or Aqueous procaine penicillin G 2.4 million units IM daily plus probenecid 500 mg PO four times daily, both for 10–14 days[b] |
| Penicillin-allergic patients[c] Primary, secondary, or latent syphilis of less than 1 year's duration | Doxycycline 100 mg PO two times daily for 2 weeks or Tetracycline 500 mg PO four times daily for 2 weeks or Erythromycin 500 mg PO four times daily for 2 weeks |
| Syphilis of more than 1 year's duration (except neurosyphilis) | Doxycycline 100 mg PO two times a day for 4 weeks or Tetracycline 500 mg PO four times daily for 4 weeks |

[a] Some experts recommend multiple doses of benzathine penicillin G or other supplemental antibiotics in addition to benzathine penicillin G in HIV-infected patients with primary or secondary syphilis; HIV-infected patients with early latent syphilis should be treated with the recommended regimen for syphilis of more than 1 year's duration.

[b] Some experts administer benzathine penicillin G 2.4 million units IM after completion of the neurosyphilis regimens to provide a total duration of therapy comparable to that used in late syphilis in the absence of neurosyphilis.

[c] For nonpregnant patients; pregnant patients should be treated with penicillin after desensitization.

*Adapted from Knodel and Kraynak (1997).*

desensitization in penicillin-allergic patients so that penicillin may still be utilized. Although not as cost-effective, this may be advantageous in patients for whom medication compliance is an issue (CDC, 1998; Knodel & Kraynak, 1997).

## Monitoring for Efficacy

Although the failure rate with penicillin is very low, it still can occur. Treatment failure or reinfection should be suspected if symptoms persist, recur, or if non-treponemal titers show a 4-fold increase. These individuals should be retreated with the late latent regimen, unless neurosyphilis is diagnosed. Evaluation for HIV infection is also recommended (CDC, 1998).

## Monitoring for Toxicity

Patients should be informed of the possibility of developing the Jarisch-Herxheimer reaction. The Jarisch-Herxheimer reaction is not an allergic response to penicillin, but can result in myalgias, chills, headache, and rash. This reaction can usually be controlled with antipyretics. Generally, antibiotics should not be discontinued because of the Jarisch-Herxheimer reaction (CDC, 1998).

## Follow-up Recommendations

Follow-up reevaluation, including serology, should be done at 6 months and 12 months (CDC, 1998).

## GONORRHEA

Gonorrhea is a sexually transmitted disease caused by the gram-negative diplococcus *Neisseria gonorrhoeae*. In the United States, approximately 600,000 new cases of gonorrhea are reported by the CDC each year (CDC, 1998). The highest prevalence of gonococcal infection is in individuals 15–29 years of age. Of this group, the majority are women of lower socioeconomic classification, minority race, and unmarried status, living in inner city housing, and who became sexually active at an early age ("Gonorrhea," 1994). Gonorrhea can produce a spectrum of symptoms. The well-known male symptoms of dysuria and urethral discharge cause the patient to seek medical treatment. The symptoms of gonorrhea can be less obvious in women than in men, and in both men and women less recognizable symptoms can present. This can lead to a missed diagnosis by the clinician or a delay or failure to seek medical treatment by the patient. Complications such as pelvic inflammatory disease (PID), ectopic pregnancy, and infertility secondary to tubal scarring can result from unrecognized, untreated gonorrhea (CDC, 1998; "Gonorrhea," 1994; Johnson, 1996b; Sherrard, 1996).

## SPECIFIC CONSIDERATIONS FOR PHARMACOTHERAPY

### When Drug Therapy Is Needed

Pelvic inflammatory disease, infertility from tubal scarring, and ectopic pregnancy are several complications related to gonorrhea. Gonococcal infection during pregnancy can lead to spontaneous abortion, premature rupture of the amniotic membranes, chorioamnionitis, disseminated gonococcal disease, and arthritis. Ophthalmia neonatorum, a conjunctivitis caused by *N. gonorrhoeae* that can lead to blindness, is caused by transmission of the organism to infants during delivery. The goals of therapy and the time for initiating therapy are the same as those for syphilis.

See Drug Tables 102.1–5, 102.11.

### Assessment and History Taking

In women, the endocervical canal is the common site of infection, with extension to involve the urethra in 70–90% of the cases ("Gonorrhea," 1994). In women with hysterectomies, the urethra is the primary site of infection. Frequently reported symptoms caused by gonococcal infection include vaginal discharge, painful urination, abnormal menstrual bleeding, mucopurulent cervical discharge with erythema, and friability of the cervix with swabbing ("Gonorrhea," 1994).

In heterosexual males the urethra is the primary site of infection. Some patients are without symptoms. Nonspecific symptoms of dysuria and discharge, which are also seen in nongonococcal urethritis, are frequently reported (Sherrard, 1996).

Pharyngeal infection occurs in less than 5% of the cases. In the female, the heterosexual male, and the homosexual male, the incidences are 10–20%, 3–7%, and 10–25%, respectively (Sherrard, 1996).

Diagnosis of cervical gonococcal infection can be confirmed with endocervical cultures, Gram's stains, or immunologic assays ("Gonorrhea" 1994). The endocervical culture is the cornerstone of diagnosis and allows for antimicrobial susceptibility. The sensitivity of a single culture is estimated to be 80–90%, with several references reporting values closer to 100% ("Gonorrhea," 1994; Sherrard, 1996). However, this sensitivity is diminished if the specimen is from extragenital sites (ie, pharynx); therefore, positive cultures from these sites should be confirmed by immunologic assays ("Gonorrhea," 1994). Although it is the gold standard, culture diagnosis of gonorrhea requires technical expertise, is expensive, and requires 24–48 h for a full report ("Gonorrhea," 1994).

Unlike endocervical cultures, Gram's stains provide immediate information for complete evaluation of the infection and generally are used in clinical practice. Under a microscope, N. gonorrhoeae appears as a gram-negative intracellular diplococcus ("Gonorrhea," 1994; Sherrard, 1996). The specificity of this method is only 50–70%, but its sensitivity is between 95–100% ("Gonorrhea," 1994; Sherrard, 1996).

Immunoassays are other diagnostic alternatives to the aforementioned methods. Gonozyme is an enzyme-linked immunosorbent assay (ELISA) that is commercially available (Sherrard, 1996). Its advantages are quick results with minimal technical requirements. Although its specificity and sensitivity are high, they appear to be higher in females than males (Sherrard, 1996). Gonozyme should not be used for extragenital specimens or to assess treatment outcomes because of high cross-reactivity with bacterial antigens at those sites; gonococcal antigens still persist despite cure (Sherrard, 1996). Other immunoassays include nucleic acid hybridization, polymerase chain reaction (PCR), and the ligase chain reaction technique. These assays appear to have better sensitivity and specificity compared with more traditional methods; however, cost-effectiveness, cross-reactions and selected yields are issues that must be addressed before the value of these methods can be determined (Sherrard, 1996).

Patients with gonorrhea are often coinfected with other STDs, particularly C. trachomatis. The CDC (1993) recommends that patients re-ceiving treatment for gonococcal infections be concurrently treated for chlamydia. This requires the addition of an antichlamydial antibiotic.

## OUTCOMES MANAGEMENT

### Selecting an Appropriate Agent

The development of antibiotic resistance by N. gonorrhoeae has limited the usefulness of certain antibiotics, particularly penicillin and tetracycline. Emergence of strains resistant to the quinolone antibiotics also has been reported (Tapsall, Phillips, & Schultz, 1996). The occurence rate in the U.S. is currently less than 0.5% (CDC, 1998). Much has been written on the incidence and mechanism of antibiotic resistance in N. gonorrhoeae (Knapp, Wongba, & Limpakarnjanarat, 1997).

For uncomplicated gonococcal infections, the CDC (1993) recommends the regimens outlined in Table 36–2. Cure rates achieved with any of these regimens for anal and genital infection are greater than 95%. For pharyngeal infection, ceftriaxone or ciprofloxacin is recommended. Cure rates with these drugs are greater than 90% (CDC, 1998; Johnson, 1996b).

Currently, there have not been any reports of gonococcal strains resistant to ceftriaxone. Ceftriaxone 125 mg provides sustained bactericidal concentrations in the blood with the same efficacy as higher doses; therefore, higher doses are not necessary (CDC, 1993; Moran & Levine, 1995). Drawbacks to ceftriaxone are higher cost, pain at injection site (some practitioners suggest using a 1% lidocaine solution as a diluent to minimize the pain), and lack of commercially available dosage forms of less than 250 mg (CDC, 1998).

Oral cefixime is a less invasive alternative to ceftriaxone but does not provide the sustained bactericidal concentration in the blood. Therefore, its use should be limited to uncomplicated genital and anal infection (CDC, 1998).

The quinolones ciprofloxacin and ofloxacin have favorable pharmacokinetic properties. Ciprofloxacin 250 mg is effective, but because of reports of resistant strains, the 500-mg dose should be used instead. Like ciprofloxacin, ofloxacin is effective for anal and genital gonorrhea but is not as effective for pharyngeal

## TABLE 36–2. 1998 CDC TREATMENT RECOMMENDATIONS FOR GONORRHEA

| Infection | Recommended Regimen | Alternative Regimen |
|---|---|---|
| Uncomplicated gonococcal infection | Ceftriaxone 125 mg IM single dose<br>or<br>Cefixime 400 mg PO single dose<br>or<br>Ciprofloxacin 500 mg PO single dose<br>or<br>Ofloxacin 400 mg PO single dose<br>plus<br>*C. trachomatis* therapy | Spectinomycin 2 g IM single dose<br>or<br>Ceftizoxime 500 mg IM single dose<br>or<br>Cefotaxime 500 mg IM single dose<br>or<br>Cefotetan 1 g IM single dose<br>or<br>Enoxacin 400 mg PO single dose |
| Gonococcal meningitis and endocarditis | Ceftriaxone 1–2 g IV q12h; meningitis: for 10–14 days; endocarditis: for at least 4 weeks; consultation with expert recommended | |
| Pregnancy | Ceftriaxone 125 mg IM single dose<br>or<br>Cefixime 400 mg PO single dose<br>or<br>Spectinomycin 2 g IM single dose (for cephalosporin allergy)<br>plus<br>*C. trachomatis* therapy | |
| Disseminated gonococcal infection (DGI) | Ceftriaxone 1 g IM or IV q 24h | (see CDC 1998 for alternative initial regimens) |

*Adapted from CDC (1993).*

infection, with a cure rate of only 88% (CDC, 1993).

Patients allergic to penicillin should be treated with a quinolone. Patients who are allergic to both penicillins and quinolones can be treated with spectinomycin 2 g IM (CDC, 1998; Knodel & Kraynak, 1997).

Pregnant women should receive cephalosporins for treatment of gonorrhea because quinolones are contraindicated during pregnancy. Quinolones should also be avoided in nursing mothers and in patients less than 17 years of age. If there is an allergy to the cephalosporin or quinolones, spectinomycin 2 g IM is an effective alternative (CDC, 1998).

All of the above regimens should include a drug regimen effective against possible coinfection with *C. trachomatis*, such as doxycycline 100 mg PO, twice daily for 7 days, or, azithromycin 1 g PO, given as a single dose (CDC, 1998). *Clinicians should be aware that*

*tetracycline and doxycycline are contraindicated in pregnancy.*

Azithromycin given as a single oral dose of 2 g (double the usual dose for treating *C. trachomatis*) has been demonstrated to be an effective treatment for uncomplicated gonorrhea (Handsfield, Dalu, & Martin, 1993) and has the advantage of activity against *C. trachomatis*. At this higher dosage, the increased cost, as well as the higher incidence of GI intolerance, compared to the four regimens recommended by the CDC, limits its usefulness (CDC, 1998).

### Monitoring for Efficacy

All treated patients should be monitored for resolution of symptoms. There is no need to do test-of-cure cultures (CDC, 1998). Some experts suggest that test-of-cure cultures may be useful for patients with pharyngeal involvement or disseminated disease (Moran & Levine, 1995).

## Monitoring for Toxicity

Ceftriaxone can cause pain at the injection site. Toxicities caused by a single 125-mg dose of ceftriaxone are rare. All of the recommended oral medications (ciprofloxacin, ofloxacin, cefixime) may cause diarrhea and nausea in some patients.

## CHLAMYDIA

In 1995, the Centers for Disease Control and Prevention recognized chlamydia as the most common sexually transmitted bacterial infection, with more than 4 million cases occurring annually in the United States. Chlamydia is also the most costly sexually transmitted disease, with an estimated annual total cost in the range of $2.4 billion (Weinstock, Dean, & Bolan, 1994; Youngkin, 1995). It is also the most frequently encountered organism among patients with NGU (nongonococcal urethritis), a condition characterized by inflammation of the urethra with mucoid or purulent discharge, and absence of infection with *N. gonorrhoeae* ("Gonorrhea," 1994; Robinson & Ridgway, 1996; Weinstock et al, 1994). *C. trachomatis* is capable of causing infections within a variety of locations in the body, including cervicitis, PID, epididymitis, proctitis, salpingitis, bartholinitis, conjunctivitis, and systemic infection ("Gonorrhea,", 1994; Robinson & Ridgway, 1996; Weinstock et al, 1994). In this respect, *C. trachomatis* is similar to *N. gonorrhoeae*. Differentiation of infection caused by *C. trachomatis* from infection caused by *N. gonorrhoeae* cannot be accomplished reliably based on signs and symptoms. Simultaneous infection with both *C. trachomatis* and *N. gonorrhoeae* is common among certain patient groups; therefore, treatment regimens for *N. gonorrhoeae* utilize a drug regimen with activity against both organisms (CDC, 1998; "Gonorrhea," 1994; Robinson & Ridgway, 1996).

Individuals at high risk for chlamydia infection are young, sexually active adolescent women. For older women, some demographic characteristics associated with infection are single marital status, nulliparity, black race, and lower socioeconomic status (Weinstock et al, 1994).

## SPECIFIC CONSIDERATIONS FOR PHARMACOTHERAPY

### When Drug Therapy Is Needed

In women, the sequelae of chlamydia are quite severe and include PID, ectopic pregnancy, and infertility (CDC, 1998; Weinstock et al, 1994). However, in men complications are very rare (Weinstock et al, 1994). Pregnant women who are infected with *C. trachomatis* may transmit the disease to infants during birth (CDC, 1998; "Gonorrhea," 1994; Robinson & Ridgway, 1996; Weinstock et al, 1994). Approximately two thirds of infants delivered to mothers infected with endocervical chlamydial infection will become infected; 15–25% will develop conjunctivitis despite prophylaxis, and 3–16% will develop chlamydial pneumonia (Robinson & Ridgway, 1996; Weinstock et al, 1994). If untreated, chlamydial conjunctivitis can lead to corneal scarring. In addition, infants with pneumonia are at an increased risk for future pulmonary complications (Weinstock et al, 1994). Goals of therapy and the time frame for initiating therapy are the same as those for syphilis.

See Drug Tables 102.4, 102.5, 102.11.

### Assessment and History Taking

Approximately 70–80% of women who are infected with *C. trachomatis* are without symptoms (Robinson & Ridgway, 1996; Weinstock et al, 1994). Those with symptoms often report vaginal discharge and dysuria (Robinson & Ridgway, 1996; Weinstock et al, 1994). In addition, the presence of a green or yellow mucous cervical discharge along with polymorphonuclear leukocytes (PMNs) on an oil immersion field, or wet mount, is associated with chlamydial infection (Weinstock et al, 1994). Many practitioners will treat these women without testing because these symptoms are highly predictive and a laboratory workup can be quite expensive.

Approximately 25–50% of men infected with *C. trachomatis* are without symptoms (Robinson & Ridgway, 1996; Weinstock et al, 1994). Urethral infection with *C. trachomatis* can cause dysuria and mucopurulent discharge, or it can be completely asymptomatic. Generally, urethral infection with *C. trachomatis* causes less severe symptoms and is more often asymptomatic than urethral infections caused by *N. gonorrhoeae* (Weinstock et al, 1994).

The gold standard for diagnostic laboratory evaluation of *C. trachomatis* infection is the McCoy cell culture. Cell cultures can be used for endocervical, urethral, eye, and rectal sites of infection (Robinson & Ridgway, 1996). However, this method is fairly cumbersome and expensive and requires special expertise. Its sensitivity is approximately 75–80% and specificity is about

100% (Robinson & Ridgway, 1996). More technically advanced nonculture techniques are currently available that will provide higher specificity and sensitivity, but they may be more expensive. A comparison of these techniques is shown in Table 36–3.

The CDC (1998) continues to recommend annual screening for chlamydia in all sexually active adolescents, as well as for females age 20–24 years with multiple sex partners or who do not use barrier contraceptives. Alternatively, some public health programs screen all sexually active women aged <30 years. The cost-effectiveness of selective screening by criteria versus universal screening is controversial. The CDC recommends screening for high-risk individuals that meet the following criteria: sexually active adolescents, women who do not use contraceptive devices and who have had more than one sexual partner in the last 3 months, pregnant women, women undergoing abortion, women with mucopurulent cervical discharge, and those with rectal pain, tenesmus, or discharge (Mill, 1997). Asymptomatic carriage in men and women may be prolonged for months if treatment is not initiated, thus increasing the potential for transmission (Weinstock et al, 1994).

Patients infected with *C. trachomatis* are often coinfected with other STDs, particularly gonorrhea, and should be tested for other infections. If tests are positive, additional therapies will likely be required.

## OUTCOMES MANAGEMENT

### Selecting an Appropriate Agent

Doxycycline has been widely used for the treatment of *C. trachomatis*. It is inexpensive and is generally well tolerated. Azithromycin has the advantage of being administered as a single oral dose, thus eliminating the potential for poor compliance. However, the cost to health care organizations for azithromycin is considerably higher than for doxycycline. Despite the high cost of purchasing this medication, Haddix, Hillis, & Kassler (1995) have demonstrated azithromycin to be cost-effective compared with doxycycline. Treatment recommendations from the CDC are presented in Table 36–4.

Alternative drug regimens have a limited role in the treatment of *C. trachomatis* because of the superiority of doxycycline and azithromycin in most clinical situations. Ofloxacin is equally effective, but it is more expensive than doxycycline. Like doxycycline, ofloxacin is contraindicated in pregnancy and nursing mothers and in patients less than 17 years of age (CDC, 1998; Robinson & Ridgway, 1996; Weinstock et al, 1994). Erythromycin has been recommended as an alternative medication in the pregnant patient. Erythromycin base and erythromycin ethylsuccinate can cause GI intolerance and require q.i.d. dosing, which may result in poor patient compliance (CDC, 1998).

Very high success rates are obtained with successful completion of either of the two recommended antibiotic treatment regimens (CDC, 1998). If the 7-day doxycycline regimen is utilized, patients should be advised to avoid sexual contact until the treatment regimen is completed (CDC, 1998).

The recommended antibiotic regimens are doxycycline 100 mg PO, b.i.d. for 7 days, or azithromycin 1 g PO, as a single dose. These treatments are both highly effective in eliminating the organism, and are cost-effective as well. So far, no resistance to either of these agents has been reported (Weinstock et al, 1994). In pregnant patients, doxycycline and ofloxacin are contraindicated. Some clinicians do use azithromycin in

**TABLE 36–3. SENSITIVITY AND SPECIFICITY OF VARIOUS DIAGNOSTIC TESTS FOR *C. TRACHOMATIS***

| Test | Sensitivity % | Specificity % |
|------|---------------|---------------|
| Cell culture | 65–80 | 100 |
| Immunofluorescence | 80–85 | >95 |
| Enzyme immunoassay | 60–80 | 99 |
| DNA probe | 75–85 | >99 |
| Amplified DNA probes; LCR/PCR | >95 | >99 |
| Antibody detection | <65 | <65 |

*Adapted from Robinson and Ridgway (1996).*

**TABLE 36–4. 1998 CDC TREATMENT RECOMMENDATIONS FOR CHLAMYDIA**

| Infection or Status | Recommended Regimen | Alternative Regimen |
|---|---|---|
| Adolescents/Adults | Doxycycline 100 mg PO b.i.d. for 7 days<br>or<br>Azithromycin 1 g PO single dose | Ofloxacin 300 mg b.i.d. for 7 days<br>or<br>Erythromycin base 500 mg q.i.d. for 7 days<br>or<br>Erythromycin ethylsuccinate 800 mg q.i.d. for 7 days |
| Pregnancy | Erythromycin base 500 mg q.i.d. for 7 days<br>or<br>Amoxicillin 500 mg t.i.d. for 7 days | Erythromycin base 250 mg q.i.d. for 14 days<br>or<br>Erythromycin ethylsuccinate 800 mg q.i.d. for 7 days<br>or<br>Erythromycin ethylsuccinate 400 mg q.i.d. for 14 days<br>or<br>Azithromycin 1 g PO single dose |

*Adapted from CDC (1998).*

pregnant women, although safety and efficacy in pregnant patients has not been well established.

A single 1-g dose of azithromycin has been shown to be as effective as a 7-day course of doxycycline 100 mg b.i.d. In addition, azithromycin has good tissue concentrations and very high intracellular levels even up to 4 days after administration (Weinstock et al, 1994). Although more expensive than doxycycline, azithromycin may be preferable for patients for whom medication compliance is an issue.

### Monitoring for Efficacy

When the patient is treated with either doxycycline or azithromycin, retesting or test-of-cure cultures are not needed unless symptoms persist or reinfection is suspected. However, if erythromycin is used, a test of cure may be considered 3 weeks after the completion of therapy (CDC, 1998).

### Monitoring for Toxicity

Either doxycycline or azithromycin is capable of causing nausea and/or vomiting. Both agents generally are well tolerated.

## HERPES GENITALIS

Herpes simplex virus (HSV) is a double-stranded DNA surrounded by a glycoprotein envelope (Johnson, 1996a). Herpes simplex virus type 1 (HSV-1) and herpes simplex virus type 2 (HSV-2) are responsible for oral and genital infections, respectively (Johnson, 1996a); the focus of this chapter will be on HSV-2.

Herpes simplex type 2 is responsible for 90% of genital HSV disease, accounts for 200,000–500,000 cases of initial (primary) infection annually (Youngkin, 1995), and is responsible for most cases of recurrent genital herpes (CDC, 1998). The virus is transmitted by direct physical contact with the infected individual (kissing, sexual relations, or delivery of an infant through an infected vagina) (Johnson, 1996a; Youngkin, 1995). The chance of a woman developing genital herpes after exposure to an infected male is 80–90%, whereas the chance of female-to-male transmission is only 50% (Johnson, 1996a; Youngkin, 1995). Upon successful entry into the host, the virus invades the sensory nerve terminals up to the sensory sacral ganglia that innervate the skin and mucosa of the site of entry. The virus will either cause the clinical symptoms or it will remain dormant until "triggered" to reactivate (Johnson, 1996a; Youngkin, 1995).

## SPECIFIC CONSIDERATIONS FOR PHARMACOTHERAPY

### When Drug Therapy Is Needed

Drug therapy helps reduce the duration of symptoms and infectivity. In addition, in immunocompromised individuals, it helps minimize complications such as urethral strictures, neuralgia, hepatitis, meningitis, thrombocytopenia, and monoarticular arthritis (Youngkin, 1995).

The safety of acyclovir and valacyclovir in pregnant women has not been established. Currently, a registry is set up to monitor pregnant women receiving acyclovir or valacyclovir. Women who are prescribed either of these agents should be reported to this registry; telephone (800) 722-9292, ext 38465. Recent analysis of the database does not indicate an increased risk of major birth defects with the use of acyclovir. However, this analysis is still preliminary (CDC, 1998).

Current CDC guidelines suggest treating the first clinical episode of genital herpes with oral acyclovir. For life-threatening maternal HSV infection, intravenous acyclovir is preferred.

See Drug Table 106.

## Assessment and History Taking

Most individuals with primary genital herpes (no previous antibodies to HSV-1 or HSV-2) have no symptoms, but are extremely infectious through viral shedding (Johnson, 1996a; Youngkin, 1995). Approximately two thirds of patients will present with systemic symptoms such as fever, headaches, pharyngitis, malaise, myalgias, or backache. These symptoms usually begin within 1 week of exposure, peak within 4 days, and subside over the next week. Others may present with genital lesions with or without systemic symptoms. These lesions are preceded by a prodromal phase described as itching, erythematous, and painful at the site of viral entry. By the first or second day, small painful vesicles or pustules appear and continue to form and coalesce, forming large wet ulcers, for up to 4–10 days. These large wet ulcers persist for 1–2 weeks, and then crust and heal without scarring. In women, 90% will have cervical involvement (friability and vesiculation) with 75% complaining of vaginal discharge (Johnson, 1996a; Youngkin, 1995).

Recurrent genital herpes is most common after a primary infection with an incidence of 70–90% for HSV-2. Factors such as menses, trauma to the area, emotional stress, or altered immune status are known to trigger these recurrences. Fortunately, symptoms of recurrent disease are generally milder; few have the systemic symptoms; the prodromal phase is less painful and shorter; there are fewer lesions; the eruption period is only 3 days; and everything resolves within 7–10 days (Johnson, 1996a; Youngkin, 1995).

Diagnosis is based primarily on clinical manifestations that are confirmed by one of several tests. The Tzanck smear will provide immediate diagnosis with 85–95% sensitivity and 95% specificity. It requires unroofing the vesicular lesion, scraping the base of the lesion, and transferring the specimen to a glass slide. A positive reading will show multinucleated giant cells with intranuclear bodies. A Papanicolaou (Pap) smear can be taken from the mucous membrane and evaluated in the same manner as the Tzanck smear. Its sensitivity is only 60–70% with a 95% specificity. A culture is the confirmatory test of choice. The specimen is collected similarly to the Tzanck smear. Viruses are detected in 90% of vesicles, 70% of ulcers, and 25% of crusted lesions. Although it is the test of choice, results usually take 3–7 days to return. Test kits using immunologic or DNA hybridization may become the test of choice because of higher specificity and sensitivity and faster results (Johnson, 1996a; Youngkin, 1995).

## OUTCOMES MANAGEMENT

### Selecting an Appropriate Agent

Current therapy for genital herpes does not provide a cure. Instead, therapy helps reduce or suppress symptoms, viral shedding, and recurrent episodes. Until recently, acyclovir was the only agent available to treat genital HSV. Recent availability of valacyclovir and famciclovir has increased the treatment options for genital HSV. Valacyclovir is the prodrug of acyclovir; that is, it will be converted to acyclovir. Acyclovir has a bioavailability of only 15%, whereas valacyclovir has a bioavailability of 54% (Alrabiah & Sacks, 1996). Famciclovir is metabolized to penciclovir, an acyclic, guanosine analog that inhibits HSV DNA synthesis (Alrabiah & Sacks, 1996). Few studies have directly compared valacyclovir or famciclovir with acyclovir. However, results of clinical trials suggest that these two agents are comparable to acyclovir (CDC, 1998).

*First clinical episode of genital HSV.* Management of first episode of genital HSV includes medication and extensive counseling. Either acyclovir, valacyclovir or famciclovir could be used for treatment and the duration of therapy is usually for 7–10 days or until healing is complete. Please refer to Table 36-5 for dosing guideline (CDC, 1998).

**TABLE 36–5.  1998 CDC TREATMENT GUIDELINES FOR GENITAL HERPES SIMPLEX VIRUS**

| Infection or Status | Recommended Regimen |
|---|---|
| First clinical episode of genital herpes | Acyclovir 400 mg orally three times a day for 7–10 days |
| | or |
| | Acyclovir 200 mg five times a day for 7–10 days |
| | or |
| | Famciclovir 250 mg orally three times a day for 7–10 days |
| | or |
| | Valacyclovir 1 g orally twice a day for 7–10 days |
| Episodic recurrent infection | Acyclovir 400 mg orally three times a day for 5 days |
| | or |
| | Acyclovir 200 mg orally five times a day for 5 days |
| | or |
| | Acyclovir 800 mg orally twice a day for 5 days |
| | or |
| | Famciclovir 125 mg orally twice a day for 5 days |
| | or |
| | Valacyclovir 500 mg orally twice a day for 5 days |
| Daily suppressive therapy | Acyclovir 400 mg orally twice a day |
| | or |
| | Famciclovir 250 mg orally twice a day |
| | or |
| | Valacyclovir 250 mg orally twice a day |
| | or |
| | Valacyclovir 500 mg orally once a day |
| | or |
| | Valacyclovir 1,000 mg orally once a day |

*Adapted from CDC (1998).*

Patients should be counseled extensively on the natural history of the disease, recurrent episodes, asymptomatic viral shedding and sexual transmission. Patients should also be advised to notify their partners, abstain from sexual activity when the lesions or prodromal symptoms are present, and the risk of transmission during asymptomatic periods. In addition, the risk of neonatal transmission should be discussed with both partners (CDC, 1998).

**Recurrent episode of genital HSV.** After the first clinical episode, most patients will have recurrent events. Initiating therapy during the prodrom or within 1 day after the formation of lesions, help alleviate symptoms. The recommended regimens for episodic recurrent infection is described in Table 36-5 (CDC, 1998).

Some patients may have frequent recurrences (i.e. greater than six episodes per year). These patient may benefit from daily suppressive ther-apy which has been shown to reduce genital herpes recurrences by >75%. The use of acyclovir for suppressive therapy for as long as 6 years was shown to be safe and effective. The safety and efficacy profile for famciclovir and valacyclovir have been documented for 1 year. After 1 year of suppressive therapy, clinicians and patients should re-evaluate whether therapy should be continued. Table 36-5 list the regimens and their doses for suppressive therapy (CDC, 1998).

**Severe disease.** Intravenous acyclovir 5–10 mg/kg Q8H for 5–7 days or until clinical symptoms improve is recommended for severe genital HSV (CDC, 1998).

## Monitoring for Toxicity

Acyclovir is fairly well tolerated with gastrointestinal side effects being the most common problems.

# LYMPHOGRANULOMA VENEREUM

Lymphogranuloma venereum (LGV) is a sexually transmitted disease caused by one of three serovars (L$_1$, L$_2$, or L$_3$) of *C. trachomatis* (CDC, 1993; Larson, 1996b; Perine & Osoba, 1990). It is a rare and rather sporadic disease throughout North America, Europe, Australia, South America, and Asia. However, in East and West Africa, India, and parts of southeast Asia, the Caribbean, and South America, LGV is endemic (Larson, 1996b; Perine & Osoba, 1990). Similarly to other STDs, LGV is frequently seen in urban areas, lower socioeconomic classes, and individuals with unsafe sexual practices (Perine & Osoba, 1990). Although LGV is not as contagious as gonorrhea, the risk of infection following exposure to an infected individual is not known. It is known, however, that *C. trachomatis* can only gain entry in compromised skin or mucous membranes (Perine & Osoba, 1990). Lymphogranuloma venereum is a chronic disease characterized by three stages of infection. These three stages are the primary, secondary, and tertiary or anorectogenital stage; specific descriptions of these stages will be discussed below (Larson, 1996b; Perine & Osoba, 1990).

## SPECIFIC CONSIDERATIONS FOR PHARMACOTHERAPY

### Short- and Long-Term Goals of Pharmacotherapy

The goals of pharmacotherapy are the same as those for syphilis.

### Time Frame for Initiating Pharmacotherapy

As with other STDs, treatment should be initiated immediately once diagnosis is confirmed to prevent progression to the more severe secondary and tertiary stages.

See Drug Tables 102.5, 102.9, 102.11.

### Assessment and History Taking

Lymphogranuloma venereum is a disease of the lymphatic tissue with extension of the inflammatory process to surrounding tissues (Perine & Osoba, 1990). After an incubation period of about 3–12 days, the primary stage of LGV manifests as one of four types of lesions: papules, nodules, herpetiform coalescent lesions, or urethritis (Larson, 1996b; Perine & Osoba, 1990). Approximately 3–53% of patients are asymptomatic with rather inconspicuous lesions (Larson, 1996b; Perine & Osoba, 1990). In men, these lesions usually occur in the coronal sulcus, frenum prepuce, penis, urethra, glans, and scrotum. These lesions may progress to cord-like lymphangitis of the dorsal penis, forming a lymphangial nodule or "bubonulus." These in turn may progress further and rupture to form draining sinuses, urethral fistulas, or fibrotic scars at the base of the penis.

As the name suggests, the inguinal syndrome (secondary stage) involves inflammation and swelling of the inguinal lymph nodes. The incubation period for this stage is 10–30 days, but may be as long as 4–6 months following the initial infection pain (Larson, 1996b; Perine & Osoba, 1990). Unlike the primary stage, the secondary stage is quite symptomatic, causing patients to seek medical attention.

The inguinal bubo is usually a unilateral, firm, and fairly tender mass that enlarges over 1–2 weeks. The pain increases as the mass enlarges, causing patients to limp and bend over in order to limit the pain. At the end of the second week, the bubo becomes fluctuant, turns a livid color referred to as "blue balls," and shortly thereafter ruptures, relieving pain and fever. The drained fluid is usually thick, yellow, tenacious pus that requires several weeks to months to drain completely without any discomfort. The healing process is fairly lengthy and leaves behind callous and contracted scars in the affected area. The ruptured bubo only occurs in about one third of the remaining cases, the involute bubo forming a firm inguinal mass that does not rupture. Only 20–30% of women present with inguinal syndrome. Most have involvement of the pelvic and lumbar lymph nodes that may form adhesions and fix the pelvic organs together. Patients often complain of lower abdominal and back pain (Larson, 1996b; Perine & Osoba, 1990). As catastrophic as the symptoms may seem, most patients recover without sequelae.

The few patients who do not recover from the secondary stage continue to harbor *C. trachomatis* in the anogenital tissue, leading to the tertiary or anorectogenital stage. The chronic inflammatory response associated with this stage leads to development of genital ulcers, fistulas, perirectal abscesses, and elephantiasis of the genitalia (Larson, 1996b; Perine & Osoba, 1990).

The first laboratory test available for the diagnosis of LGV was the Frei test. However, since the antigen used in this test also reacted with all chlamydia serovars, its diagnostic capability was limited. As a result, it was discontinued in 1974 (Perine & Osoba, 1990). The complement fixation (CF) test is the current recommendation for laboratory diagnosis of LGV. Unfortunately, CF tests also cross-react with other chlamydial infections, but perhaps not to the same degree as the Frei test. For the most part, a CF titer greater than 1:64 is diagnostic for LGV. Unlike the previous aforementioned tests, the microimmunofluorescent (micro-IF) test is much more sensitive, but it is not readily available for general use (Larson, 1996b).

Because most of the diagnostic tests are fraught with cross-reactivity with other chlamydial strains, diagnosis based on clinical presentation is very important. However, some of the clinical presentations of LGV may be similar to other diseases. Inguinal lymphadenitis may be observed in tularemia, tuberculosis, genital herpes, syphilis, chancroid, and Hodgkin's disease. These diseases should be a part of the differential diagnosis (Perine & Osoba, 1990).

## OUTCOMES MANAGEMENT

### Selecting an Appropriate Agent

As with other chlamydial infections, the agent of choice is doxycycline 100 mg twice a day for 21 days. Alternative agents for those who cannot take doxycycline are erythromycin 500 mg four times a day for 21 days or sulfisoxazole (or an equivalent sulfonamide) 500 mg four times a day for 21 days. In the pregnant or lactating female, the recommended agent is erythromycin at the above doses (CDC, 1998).

### Monitoring for Efficacy

As with other STDs, monitor for resolution of symptoms.

### Monitoring for Toxicity

The tetracyclines, macolides, and sulfonamides usually cause gastrointestinal symptoms, but most abate with time.

### Follow-up Recommendation

Treatment is for 21 days or until symptoms resolve (CDC, 1998).

## GRANULOMA INGUINALE

Granuloma inguinale, or donovanosis, is caused by the gram-negative rod *Calymmatobacterium granulomatis*. Although it is a very rare disease in developed countries such as the United States and the United Kingdom, it is more common in tropical or semitropical countries (Hart, 1990; Larson, 1996a). Donovanosis is not a highly contagious disease and appears to require repeated exposure for complete infectivity. Whether sexual transmission is the only mode of infection is controversial because nonsexual transmission, such as repeated trauma of the infected site, has also been demonstrated. It is a genital disease that leads to painless, irregular, and granulomatous ulcers that can be quite disfiguring (Hart, 1990; Larson, 1996a).

## SPECIFIC CONSIDERATIONS FOR PHARMACOTHERAPY

### When Drug Therapy Is Needed

If left untreated, the primary lesion will progress and coalesce with adjacent lesions or form new lesions by autoinoculation (Hart, 1990). In addition, these lesions will erode to form a beefy, exuberant, granulomatous heaped ulcer (Hart, 1990). As the ulcer progresses, lymphatic obstruction is often seen (Larson, 1996a). Finally, hematogenous spread to the bones, joints, and liver has also been reported. The goals of therapy and the time for initiating therapy are the same as those for syphilis.

See Drug Table 102.

### Assessment and History Taking

Ninety percent of cases involve the genitalia, followed by 10% in the inguinal region, 5–10% in the anal region, and 1–5% in distant sites. The incubation period ranges from 8–80 days, after which single or multiple subcutaneous nodules will erode through the skin to form clean, granulomatous, and sharply defined lesions. These lesions are usually painless, bleed easily, and will slowly enlarge to form beefy-red granulomatous tissue (Hart, 1990).

Aside from the clinical presentation, the diagnosis is confirmed by Giemsa or Wright's stain. A positive stain will reveal Donovan bodies as clusters of safety-pin-shaped organisms in the cytoplasm of mononuclear cells (Hart, 1990; Larson, 1996a). Other methods include serum complement–fixing antibodies or a positive skin test to intradermal Donovan antigen.

Other differential diagnoses include carcinoma, secondary syphilis, and amebiasis. Gonorrhea or syphilis are possible concurrent infections that should be part of the diagnostic evaluation (Hart, 1990).

## OUTCOMES MANAGEMENT

### Selecting an Appropriate Agent

The agent of choice for donovanosis is doxycycline 100 mg orally twice a day (Larson, 1996a), or trimethoprim-sulfamethoxazole 160/80 mg orally twice a day for at least 3 weeks or until lesions heal (Larson, 1996a). Ciprofloxacin 750 mg orally twice a day for a minimum of 3 weeks is another alternative (Hart, 1990; Larson, 1996a). Erythromycin 500 mg orally four times a day for at least 3 weeks is the agent of choice for the pregnant or lactating female (CDC, 1998). One reference suggests that erythromycin is not as effective when used alone (Hart, 1990). Regardless, medications should be continued until the lesions heal to prevent recurrence (Hart, 1990). Gentamicin (1 mg/kg IV Q 8 hours) should be considered if lesions do not respond within the first few days of therapy.

### Monitoring for Efficacy

With effective therapy the lesions become paler, less friable, and less exuberant within a few days. By day 7 the lesions begin to shrink in size, but total healing takes up to 3–5 weeks (Hart, 1990).

### Monitoring for Toxicity

The most common side effects with these agents are gastrointestinal in nature and should resolve with continued therapy. If gentamicin is part of the treatment regimen, monitor for renal toxicity.

### Follow-up Recommendations

Treatment should continue until the lesions fully resolve. If a Giemsa or Wright's stain is performed at this time, the specimen should be negative for Donovan Bodies (Hart, 1990).

## HUMAN PAPILLOMAVIRUS

Human papillomavirus (HPV) is the etiologic agent of genital warts, also known as condylomata acuminata, and HPV DNA is found in most carcinomas of the cervix and precursor lesions (NIH Expert Panel, 1996). The virus is transmitted sexually and may produce small exophytic lesions (warts), or the infection may be subclinical. HPV is classified by DNA hybridization into more than 70 different types (NIH Expert Panel, 1996). The different HPV types have been associated with different manifestations of the infection and different propensities to progress to dysplasia. Twenty-three HPV types infect the cervix; about half are associated with squamous intraepithelial lesions (SIL) or invasive carcinoma (NIH Expert Panel, 1996). Types that may progress to severe dysplasia are HPV 16, 18, 31, 33, 35, and 45 (CDC, 1998; NIH Expert Panel, 1996). The typical exophytic lesions, condylomata acuminata, in the anogenital region are associated with HPV types 6, 11, 42, 43, and 44; are generally benign; and are less likely to become dysplastic (Eron, 1992).

HPV infection can be completely asymptomatic and undetectable to the patient, or there can be mild symptoms such as itching, local pain, and friability of the lesion. The goal of treatment is the removal of symptomatic visible warts. Wart removal does not eradicate HPV infection, and recurrence is likely. Similarly, there is no evidence that wart removal by any of the currently used modalities effectively reduces infectivity. Sex partners of patients with HPV infection are very likely to be infected. Treated patients and their partners should be counseled that the patient continues to be infective even though the warts have been removed.

## SPECIFIC CONSIDERATIONS FOR PHARMACOTHERAPY

### When Drug Therapy Is Needed

Topical drug therapies aimed at removal of symptomatic warts are among the local therapies available. There are no effective systemic drug therapies for HPV available. Local removal of warts does not eliminate HPV infection, and it is unclear if it decreases infectivity. "Debulking" of anogenital warts is thought by some experts to reduce the likelihood of transmission of the disease. The development of cervical dysplasia associated with HPV types 16, 18, 31, 33, 35, and 45 probably is not affected by wart removal.

### Short- and Long-Term Goals of Pharmacotherapy

Refer to the syphilis section for general guidelines for all STDs, including the time frame for initiating pharmacotherapy. Since pharmacotherapy does not lead to eradication of HPV, treatment goals are to reduce symptoms, if present, and prevent the transmission of the organism to new partners.

### Nonpharmacologic Therapy

Both nonpharmacologic and pharmacologic therapies are used for "debulking" or wart removal. Efficacy is similar between pharmacologic and nonpharmacologic therapies, and the treatment goals are the same. Currently used nonpharmacologic therapies include:

- Cryotherapy with liquid nitrogen or a cryoprobe
- Electrocoagulation
- Laser ablation
- Surgical excision

Each of these has similar efficacy and recurrence rates. There are some advantages and disadvantages of each of these, depending upon the clinical situation and available resources.

For most exophytic genital and anal warts, cryotherapy with liquid nitrogen or a cryoprobe is the preferred treatment. Cryotherapy is widely available, simple for the provider to administer to the patient, and relatively inexpensive. Cryotherapy has no systemic toxicities and usually does not produce scarring.

Electrocoagulation requires local anesthesia (lidocaine), which is usually painful to administer. Large amounts of wart can be removed quickly. Scarring is common.

Laser ablation requires expensive equipment, general or local anesthesia, and a practitioner skilled in the technique. Precise control of the depth of tissue penetration can be accomplished with this modality. Laser ablation is probably the method of choice for treating flat cervical warts (Ferenczy, 1985).

See Drug Table 809.

### Assessment and History Taking

There are a number of skin growths that can occur in the anogenital region that may be simi-

lar in appearance to HPV infection. These include moles, skin tags, molluscum contagiosum, and condylomata lata keratoses. Differentiation can be difficult and may require consultation with an expert. DNA hybridization tests are useful for identifying the HPV type, but this test is not recommended for screening purposes. Patients can be simultaneously infected with multiple HPV types.

## OUTCOMES MANAGEMENT

### Selecting an Appropriate Agent

The choice of therapy will depend on several factors, including individual provider experience; available treatment modalities and resources; the potential for treatment toxicity; the size, number, and anatomic location of the warts; and patient preference and convenience (CDC, 1998). Warts that are easily visible and anatomically accessible to the patient may be treated with a patient-applied topical therapy, if desired. Patient-applied therapies require the provider to instruct the patient on which specific wart(s) to treat and ensure that the patient understands how to properly apply the medication. Other warts must be treated with provider-administered therapies. Lesions on moist surfaces and in intertriginous areas generally should be treated with a topical agent (CDC, 1998). Drier area warts respond least to cryotherapy. Wart size, number, site, patient preference, cost, convenience, and adverse effects are factors influencing choice of therapy.

Podophyllin resin is a popular topical therapy for genital warts, but it is less effective than cryotherapy (Bashi, 1985). Podophyllin is most effective in mucosal areas, but has diminished effectiveness in dry, highly keratinized areas. Podophyllin should not be used for cervical warts. The principal active ingredient in podophyllin, podophyllotoxin, is a naturally occurring substance extracted from dried plants, and as such, may vary in potency from one batch to the next (McEvoy et al, 1997). The variation in potency may cause decreased efficacy at one extreme, and undesired toxicity at the other. Podophyllin can cause significant local irritation, especially to the eyes and mucous membranes. Systemic absorption of podophyllin can cause a variety of unwanted toxicities including bone marrow suppression and severe gastrointestinal disturbances. Because of the potential for toxicity, the CDC recommends that no more than 0.5 mL be applied per session, and that no more than 10 cm² of wart be treated. Removing the drug by thorough washing 1–4 h after application is also suggested. Treatment sessions should be at least 7–10 days apart. Patient self-administration is not recommended, for obvious reasons. The CDC (1998) advises that the safe use of podophyllin resin in pregnancy has not been established.

Imiquimod (Aldara) is available as a 5% cream. It is given as a patient-applied therapy. Patients should be instructed to apply imiquimod cream to the wart with a finger, at bedtime, three times a week for up to 16 weeks (CDC, 1998). The treated area should be washed with soap and water 6–10 h following application. Mild to moderate skin reactions (erythema, erosion, excoriation/flaking, and edema) are common (*Drug Facts and Comparisons,* 1997, p. 631b). More frequent application is associated with an increase in adverse reactions. Like other topically applied drugs, imiquimod is more effective on mucosal surfaces and intertriginous areas, and is less effective when applied to dry, highly keratinized skin.

As with other topical therapies for HPV, patients should be advised that the organism persists in their body despite the clearance of lesions. Patients should avoid sexual contact while on imiquimod therapy. Patients should be advised that imiquimod may weaken condoms and diaphragms, and that concurrent use of imiquimod and condoms or diaphragms is not recommended. The safety of imiquimod in pregnancy is unknown (CDC, 1998).

Podofilox (Condylox) is a topical antimitotic agent available in a 0.5% solution or gel. This agent, like imiquimod, is designed for patient self-application. Podofilox is indicated for the treatment of external genital or perianal warts, but is not approved for treatment of warts on mucous membranes (*Drug Facts and Comparisons,* 1997, p. 627a). The patient should be instructed to apply podofilox solution or gel with a cotton-tipped applicator to specifically identified warts, twice daily, in the morning and in the evening, for 3 days. The minimum amount of drug necessary to cover the lesion should be applied. In areas where the treated wart comes in contact with opposing skin, the opposing skin should be held apart until the applied medication dries. For podofilox 0.5% gel, the patient may apply the drug with a finger, if desired. When using podofilox solution, application must

be with a cotton-tipped applicator (supplied with the product). The patient should be instructed to discard the cotton-tipped applicator and wash hands after applying the medication. After the drug has been applied for 3 consecutive days, the drug should be withheld for the next 4 consecutive days. The 1-week cycle can be repeated up to 4 times. If the response to therapy after 4 weeks is incomplete, consider an alternative therapy. Like podophyllin, the amount of treated wart should be limited to no more than 10 cm², and no more than 0.5 mL of the drug should be applied in a 24-h period. The CDC (1998) advises that the safety of podofilox during pregnancy is unknown.

Trichloroacetic acid (TCA) and bichloroacetic acid (BCA) are strong acids that require careful application by the provider. The acid is carefully applied to the wart and allowed to dry, with great care taken to use a minimal amount so as not to get the product on surrounding tissue. The application can be reapplied every 1–3 weeks, if necessary. The acid liquid is thin and flows easily, like water. Wherever the acid has contacted tissue, a white frosty-appearing crust will form. In the case of a spill or overapplication, unreacted acid can be neutralized with sodium bicarbonate powder or talc. This must be done very quickly, or the acid will spread, coagulating the skin proteins that the acid comes in contact with. Alternatively, the affected area can be flushed with water, utilizing soap to neutralize the acid. Powdered sodium bicarbonate or talc may also be used to treat painful reactions to the acid treatment.

TCA and BCA have the advantage of low potential systemic toxicity, and can be used safely on pregnant patients (Eron, 1992). As with the other topically applied drugs (podophyllin, imiquimod, and podofilox), efficacy is decreased when treating warts in highly keratinized areas.

Two other drug therapies for HPV should be mentioned. Intralesional injections of interferons have been used with some success (Friedman-Kien et al, 1988; Kirby et al, 1988). Interferons are expensive, have systemic side effects, and have not been demonstrated to be any more effective than available therapies that are less expensive and less potentially toxic. The CDC (1998) does not recommend intralesional interferon for routine use.

5-fluorouracil (5-FU) has good efficacy (Rosemberg, Greenberg, & Reid, 1987), but it is very irritating (Krebs, 1987) and there is potential for systemic toxicity.

# PELVIC INFLAMMATORY DISEASE

Pelvic inflammatory disease (PID) is an infection of the female genital tract characterized by pelvic or lower abdominal pain, often following the onset or cessation of menses. PID encompasses a spectrum of symptoms caused by a variety of circumstances. The causative microorganisms are predominantly sexually transmitted but may include other microorganisms, particularly normal vaginal flora. PID is the major medical and economic consequence of sexually transmitted diseases in women of reproductive age (Washington, Arno, & Brooks, 1986). PID can be caused by trauma, surgery, or ascending infection. PID may be undetected or asymptomatic, or there may be severe symptomatology requiring hospitalization. A variety of sequelae may result from PID, especially impaired reproductive health. Some practitioners use the term PID interchangeably with acute salpingitis.

## SPECIFIC CONSIDERATIONS FOR PHARMACOTHERAPY

### When Drug Therapy Is Needed

PID is a systemic infection that may be associated with severe acute symptoms. As with other systemic infections, there is the possibility of bacteremia with septic shock, peritonitis, or abscess formation. Appropriate antibiotic therapy is essential to eradicate the organism, relieve acute symptoms, prevent the development of sequelae, and prevent the transmission of the disease to others. Less severe cases can be managed on an outpatient basis but also require appropriate antibiotic therapy.

### Short- and Long-Term Goals of Pharmacotherapy

See the syphilis section for general goals. Avoiding or minimizing the impairment of the patient's reproductive health is an important goal.

### Time Frame for Initiating Pharmacotherapy

See the syphilis section for general guidelines. Severe cases of pelvic inflammatory disease may require hospitalization and prompt initiation of parenteral antibiotics. See the CDC 1998 guidelines for hospitalization criteria.

See Drug Tables 102.1–5, 102.11.

## Assessment and History Taking

The clinical diagnosis of PID is difficult because of the broad range and variable intensity of the symptoms. At one extreme, the patient with acute PID may present with minimal or unimpressive symptoms. At the other extreme, the patient may present with septic shock. Many patients have mild to moderate symptoms that are nonspecific for PID or may mimic other conditions.

The following three findings must be present to make a diagnosis of PID (Braodnax, 1993; CDC, 1998). These three findings are referred to as the "minimum" criteria by the CDC:

- Lower abdominal tenderness
- Adnexal tenderness
- Cervical motion tenderness

The following findings may be present and can be used to increase the specificity of the diagnosis (CDC, 1998):

- Oral temperature >38.3°C
- Abnormal cervical or vaginal discharge
- Elevated erythrocyte sedimentation rate
- Elevated C-reactive protein
- Laboratory documentation of cervical infection with *N. gonorrhoeae* or *C. trachomatis*

The CDC has also listed the following "definitive" criteria for diagnosing PID:

- Histopathologic evidence of endometritis on endometrial biopsy
- Radiologic abnormalities (thickened fluid-filled tubes with or without free pelvic fluid or tubo-ovarian complex) on transvaginal sonography or other radiologic tests
- Laparoscopic abnormalities consistent with PID

Clinicians should culture for *C. trachomatis* and *N. gonorrhoeae;* however, the abundance of normal flora in the lower genital tract, as well as potential differences in the flora of the upper versus the lower genital tract can complicate the use of cultures for diagnosis. Any confirmed cases of *C. trachomatis* or *N. gonorrhoeae* will require treatment of sex partners. As is the case with most suspected or confirmed sexually transmitted diseases, the clinician would be prudent to test for HIV. Finally, the CDC recommends a low threshold of diagnosis because of the difficulty of diagnosis, and awareness of the potential for reproductive health impairment with even mild cases of PID.

## OUTCOMES MANAGEMENT

### Selecting an Appropriate Agent

A variety of organisms are capable of causing PID. Frequently encountered organisms include *N. gonorrhoeae, C. trachomatis*, gram-negative facultative bacteria, anaerobes, and streptococci. Since no single antibiotic has a spectrum of activity that can cover all of the most likely causative organisms of PID, empiric therapy is broad-spectrum and is achieved with a combination of antibiotics. The most popular antibiotic combinations for treating PID are listed in Table 36–6. Note that all of the listed regimens have gonococcal, anaerobic, gram-negative, and chlamydial coverage.

A diagnosis of PID is not synonymous with hospitalization in many cases. Parenteral antibiotic therapy can be given in either an inpatient or an outpatient setting. The clinician should consider the severity of the illness, availability of resources and therapies, costs, patient compliance and acceptance, and antibiotic resistance patterns when considering hospitalization versus outpatient treatment and multidose continuous parenteral therapy versus oral or single-dose parenteral therapy. Some clinicians believe that

**TABLE 36–6. 1998 CDC TREATMENT GUIDELINES FOR PELVIC INFLAMMATORY DISEASE**

| Recommended Regimen | Alternative Regimen |
|---|---|
| **Parenteral** | |
| *Regimen A* | Ofloxacin 400 mg IV every 12 h |
| | plus |
| Cefotetan 2 g IV every 12 h | Metronidazole 500 mg IV every 8 h |
| or | or |
| Cefoxitin 2 g IV every 6 h | Ampicillin/sulbactam 3 g IV every 6 h |
| plus | plus |
| Doxycycline 100 mg IV or PO q 12 h | Doxycycline 100 mg IV or PO q 12 h |
| | or |
| *Regimen B* | Ciprofloxacin 200 mg IV every 12 h |
| | plus |
| Clindamycin 900 mg IV every 8 h | Doxycycline 100 mg IV or PO q 12 h |
| plus | plus |
| Gentamicin 2 mg/kg loading dose followed by maintenance dose 1.5 mg/kg every 8 h (IV or IM) (single daily dosing of gentamicin may be substituted for q 8 h dosing) | Metronidazole 500 mg IV or PO q 8 h |
| **Oral** | |
| *Regimen A* | |
| Ofloxacin 400 mg PO b.i.d. for 14 days | |
| plus | |
| Metronidazole 500 mg PO t.i.d. for 14 days | |
| *Regimen B* | |
| Ceftriaxone 250 mg IM single dose | Other parenteral third generation |
| or | cephalosporin |
| Cefoxitin 2 g IM + probenecid 1 g PO single dose | |
| plus | |
| Doxycycline 100 mg PO b.i.d. for 14 days | |

*Adapted from CDC (1998).*

all adolescent patients should be hospitalized for treatment because of the potential for poor compliance with oral antibiotic therapy, likelihood of engaging in risky sexual behaviors prior to completion of therapy, and potential for not returning for follow-up (Ivey, 1997).

The reader is referred to Table 36–6 for a listing of the antibiotic regimens recommended by the CDC. Other antibiotic regimens may work equally as well but have not been studied as extensively as the ones listed in the table. Note that even in the inpatient setting, the preferred route of administration of doxycycline is oral because of the potential for pain on infusion. Azithromycin has been shown to be highly effective against C. trachomatis in lower genital tract infections and has the advantage of single-dose oral therapy. Some clinicians endorse the use of azithromycin for compliance reasons, but because of the expense, it may not be cost-effective (Haddix et al, 1995); azithromycin is not endorsed by the CDC in the 1998 guidelines for the treatment of PID because of a lack of data on the use of azithromycin in treating upper genital tract infections.

The choice of antibiotic regimen to use in the treatment of PID is not straightforward. The reader is referred to the discussion in the treatment section for PID of the 1998 CDC guidelines. The choice of antibiotic regimen should be guided by clinical experience and local antibiotic resistance patterns.

## Monitoring for Efficacy

The patient should respond to therapy and improve clinically, as described by the CDC, within 72 h, whether oral or parenteral therapy is utilized. The CDC 1998 STD guidelines describe clinical improvement as defervescence, reduction in direct or rebound abdominal tenderness and reduction in uterine, adnexal, and cervical motion tenderness. Patients who are on oral therapy and do not improve within 72 h should be reevaluated and placed on parenteral therapy. Patients who are on parenteral therapy and do not improve within 72 h should be reevaluated and considered for surgical intervention. The CDC recommends microbiological reexamination 7–10 days after completion of the antibiotic regimen.

## Monitoring for Toxicity

If the patient receives parenteral regimen B (see Table 36–6), then the clinician may want to monitor gentamicin levels if this therapy is continued for more than 2–3 days, or if the patient has a condition that could complicate aminoglycoside dosing, such as renal impairment.

## Follow-up Recommendations

Rescreening for C. trachomatis and N. gonorrhoeae 4 to 6 weeks after completion of therapy has been recommended by some experts (CDC, 1998). Follow-up to prevent or detect reinfection is important. PID is a disease primarily of young women. The clinician needs to be sensitive to the living situation and circumstances of the patient in order to maximize follow-up and secondary prevention efforts.

# INFESTATIONS

Scabies and pediculosis pubis are sexually transmitted insect infestations primarily seen in young adults, but they may be transmitted by nonsexual skin-to-skin contact and to a lesser degree by fomites (Long, 1996). The distinctive symptoms and clinical findings usually lead to correct diagnosis with little delay.

Scabies infestation by the human itch mite Sarcoptes scabiei usually causes intense pruritis, which tends to be worse at night and after bathing in hot water (Faber, 1996). The itching occurs first on the webs and sides of the fingers, wrists, and elbows, and eventually spreads to other parts of the body. Many patients report similar symptoms in other household members or sexual partners (Long, 1996).

Pediculosis pubis, often called "crabs," is an infestation of pubic hair with the louse Phthirus pubis, a member of the same family as the head louse and the body louse (Faber, 1996). The intense pubic itching and the sensation of insects crawling over the skin that is characteristic of the infestation leads to self-diagnosis by many patients (Rasmussen, 1996). Patients may notice several rust-colored spots on their underwear, a result of blood stains from the bites of the louse (Long, 1996).

## SPECIFIC CONSIDERATIONS FOR PHARMACOTHERAPY

## When Drug Therapy Is Needed

Neither the itch mite nor the pubic louse is known to transmit any other type of disease

(Rasmussen, 1996). Both infestations cause intense itching and discomfort for the patient, and the scratching that accompanies the itching breaks the skin barrier, which can become secondarily infected.

## Short- and Long-Term Goals of Pharmacotherapy

Short-term goals are to kill the insects on the patient, treat associated problems such as itching and secondary skin infection, treat personal contacts, and eradicate the mite from the physical environment (Rasmussen, 1996). The long-term goal is to teach the patient safer intimacy practices to decrease the likelihood of future infections and the risk for other STDs.

## Time Frame for Initiating Pharmacotherapy

Treatment should be initiated as soon as the diagnosis is confirmed.
    See Drug Table 806.

## Assessment and History Taking

The diagnosis is aided by a history of itching in household contacts and/or sexual partners. The physical examination and simple laboratory findings confirm the diagnosis.
    Scabies should be considered in any patient who presents with itching. Using bright light and magnification, a thorough examination for the classic burrow or small, erythematous papules with surrounding erythema should be made (Long, 1996). Once a suspicious lesion is found, a drop of mineral oil is placed on the skin and the lesion vigorously scraped. The material is placed on a slide, covered with a cover slip, and examined under low-power light microscopy. Diagnostic findings include the mite, eggs, egg cases, or fecal pellets (Rasmussen, 1996).
    Pubic lice can be identified with careful examination of the pubic hair or other sites where itching is present using bright light and magnification. Diagnostic findings include the louse itself or nits (egg casings) on the hair shafts.
    Scabies and pubic lice often coexist with other STDs. A thorough search for other infections discussed in this chapter should be made (CDC, 1998).

## Patient/Caregiver Information

To help prevent absorption of toxic levels through the skin, patients should not bathe before using lindane; if a bath is taken, the skin should be dry and cool before application. If applying lindane to more than one person the caregiver should wear rubber gloves (*Physician's Desk Reference* [PDR], 1997, p. 2173). Lindane should not be used by pregnant or nursing women or children younger than 2 years of age (CDC, 1998).
    When applying any of the topical medications, special attention should be paid to the nails and cuticles and intertriginous areas to ensure adequate penetration of the medication. A clean toothbrush may aid in applying medication to nail and cuticle areas. The toothbrush must be thrown away after use (*PDR,* 1997, p. 2173). In addition, the medication should be applied to all crusts and scabs.
    The itching that accompanies parasitic insect infestations is the result of the immune response to the insect. Once the insect is killed, the itching subsides gradually over a period of 2–4 weeks (Faber, 1996) or rarely several months (Rasmussen, 1996). Continued itching does not indicate treatment failure, and retreatment should only be instituted with health care provider approval. Unnecessary retreatment with lindane can lead to severe toxicity such as seizures or less serious problems such as contact dermatitis. Because symptoms can take up to 1 month to become apparent after infestation with scabies, all household and sexual partners should be treated whether symptomatic or not. Only sexual partners of people with pubic lice need to be treated.
    Fomites play a minor role in transmission of scabies and pubic lice, and fumigation of the entire house is not necessary. Even so, patients should be instructed to decontaminate their environment by machine laundering in hot water or machine drying on hot cycles all bed linens, sleeping bags, clothes, and personal articles like bath towels (CDC, 1998; Rasmussen, 1996). Articles that cannot be washed should be dry-cleaned (Faber, 1996).

## OUTCOMES MANAGEMENT

### Selecting an Appropriate Agent

For scabies, the recommended treatment is permethrin cream (5%) applied to all areas of the body from the neck to the soles of the feet and washed off after 8–14 h (Brown, Becher, & Brady, 1995; CDC, 1998). Permethrin is more expensive than lindane but is equally effective and has no known systemic side effects (Faber, 1996). Alternative regimens include:

1. Lindane (1%): 1 oz of lotion or 30 g of cream. Apply to all areas of the body from the neck to the soles of the feet and wash off after 8 h.
2. Sulfur (6%) precipitated in ointment: Apply to all areas of the body each night for three nights. Wash off all medication before applying the next dose and 24 h after the last dose.
3. Ivermectin 200 µg/kg in one single oral dose or 0.8% topical solution: This is a new drug that has shown promise, especially for difficult cases, but studies comparing it to current therapies are not yet available (CDC, 1998).

In addition to treatment for the infestation, patients may require a medication to control itching such as diphenhydramine 25–50 mg by mouth every 6 h or topical hydrocortisone. Appropriate antibiotics for secondary infections are dicloxacillin 250–500 mg q.i.d., or erythromycin 250–500 mg q.i.d. (Faber, 1996).

For pubic lice, the CDC-recommended treatment (CDC, 1998) is:

1. Permethrin, 1% cream rinse applied to the affected area and washed off after 10 min.
2. Lindane 1% shampoo applied to the affected area and thoroughly washed off after 4 min.
3. Pyrethrins with piperonyl butoxide applied to affected area and washed off after 10 min.

For pubic lice infestation of the eyelashes, the only recommended treatment is occlusive ophthalmic ointment to the eyelid margins twice a day for 10 days. The other regimens should not be used near the eyes (CDC, 1998).

Lindane should not be used by pregnant or lactating women, by children less than 2 years of age, or by people with extensive dermatitis. In addition, lindane should not be used by people with seizure disorders (CDC, 1998; Faber, 1996).

## Monitoring for Efficacy

The itching from scabies should decrease gradually over 2–4 weeks. If symptoms persist unchanged or if live mites are seen, patients can be retreated with an alternative regimen in 1 week (CDC, 1998; Rasmussen, 1996). Patients with crusted scabies may require multiple applications of medication over several weeks (Long, 1996) or a combination of oral and topical treatments (Meinking, Taplin, Herminda, Pardo, & Kerdel, 1995).

For pubic lice, follow-up is required only if symptoms do not resolve. If lice continue to be present or nits are present at the skin-hair junction, patients should be retreated (CDC, 1998).

The most common causes of treatment failure for infestation include incorrect use of medication, failure to treat all infected body sites, or exposure to an untreated sexual partner (Long, 1996).

## Monitoring for Toxicity

Lindane is a moderately toxic insecticide with seizures being the most common neurologic adverse event. Most lindane toxicity comes from inappropriate use of the drug, leading to increased absorption in adults or when used in the pediatric or geriatric populations (Fischer, 1994). Symptoms of lindane toxicity include nausea, vomiting, respiratory failure, aplastic anemia, and rarely death (Faber, 1996). Patients should report any adverse events to the health care provider. Adverse events related to other recommended treatments are limited to local burning or stinging (Long, 1996).

## Follow-up Recommendations

Patients may experience feelings of continued infestation even after successful therapy and need emotional support to completely resolve the psychological impact of infestation. If these issues are not addressed, patients may overuse medications and experience toxic reactions.

# VAGINITIS

Vaginitis is one of the most prevalent problems of women in primary care and gynecologic practice settings and may be the result of either a sexually transmitted pathogen or an alteration in the normal vaginal flora. The healthy vaginal milieu is a delicate ecosystem with colonies of multiple organisms existing in dynamic balance. A variety of common activities such as douching, coitus, and hormonal fluctuations can disrupt this balance and result in vaginitis. Vulvovaginal candidiasis, bacterial vaginosis, and trichomonas vaginitis are the specific conditions that will be addressed. The diagnosis and treatment of atrophic vaginitis are discussed in Chap. 19. There are noninfectious causes of vaginal discharge such as vaginal or cervical cancer or discharge from a retained vaginal foreign body that are not addressed in this chapter, but they should be considered in the differential diagnosis of any vaginal discharge, especially one that does not respond to standard therapy.

## VULVOVAGINAL CANDIDIASIS

Vulvovaginal candidiasis (VVC) is a common fungal vaginal infection of reproductive-aged women. Most cases are the result of overgrowth of *Candida albicans,* but the incidence of non-*albicans* infections is increasing. VVC is estimated to affect 20% of women annually (Geiger, Foxman, & Gillespie, 1996). In addition, 75% of women will experience at least one episode of VVC during their lifetime, with 40–45% of women experiencing two or more symptomatic episodes (CDC, 1993). Hypoestrogenic, postmenopausal women seldom experience symptomatic VVC until started on estrogen replacement.

Women typically present with acute onset of pruritus and discharge; often, these symptoms are first noticed during the late luteal phase of the menstrual cycle (Hillier & Arko, 1996). Other symptoms include external dysuria, vulvar burning, and external dyspareunia.

Several studies have identified a variety of risk factors for VVC. These include receptive oral sex, high-dose estrogen oral contraceptive use, spermacide use, sex during menses, pregnancy, diabetes, steroid use, systemic antibiotic use, and African-American ethnicity (Geiger & Foxman, 1996; Geiger et al, 1996; Hellberg, Zdolsek, Nilsson, & Mardh, 1995; Hillier & Arko, 1996).

Recurrent VVC (four or more episodes per year) occurs in <5% of women (CDC, 1993). Recurrent VVC is more often associated with infection with non-*albicans* species such as *C. glabrata* or *C. tropicalis* than are initial acute infections (Spinillo, Capuzzo, Egbe, Nicola, & Piazzi, 1995; Spinillo et al, 1997).

### Specific Considerations for Pharmacotherapy

***When drug therapy is needed.*** Neither asymptomatic vaginal colonization nor acute symptomatic VVC is associated with postsurgical infections, salpingitis, or adverse pregnancy events (Sweet & Gibbs, 1995). Although not life-threatening, the symptoms of VVC are distressing and disruptive to affected women. Prompt treatment is indicated to restore a healthy vaginal environment and improve the quality of life.

***Short- and long-term goals of pharmacotherapy.*** The short- and long-term goals of therapy for all types of vaginitis are very similar. The short-term goal for therapy is to resolve signs and symptoms of infection. Long-term goals are to restore the vaginal ecology and manage risk factors to prevent recurrent infection.

***Nonpharmacologic therapy.*** Although not known to be effective for treatment of acute symptomatic VVC, nonpharmacologic therapy is a mainstay in prevention of recurrent episodes. The following measures should be kept in mind:

1. The daily ingestion of yogurt enriched with live Lactobacillus acidophilus bacteria has been associated with preventing the recurrence of yeast vaginitis (Elmer, Surawicz, & McFarland, 1996; Shalev, Battino, Weiner, Colodner, & Keness, 1996) and bacterial vaginosis.

2. Cotton underwear absorbs the normal vaginal secretions and allows air circulation to prevent continual moisture on the vulva.

3. Women with recurrent VVC should be encouraged to avoid occlusive clothing such as panty hose and tight jeans that prevent air flow and contribute to alterations of the vaginal environment, including overgrowth of yeast organisms.

4. Women should be encouraged to avoid douching. Douching alters the normal vaginal environment and encourages the overgrowth of a variety of organisms, increasing the incidence of yeast vaginitis, bacterial vaginosis, and pelvic inflammatory disease.

***Time frame for initiating pharmacotherapy.*** Therapy should be initiated as soon as the diagnosis is confirmed. There is no benefit from delay. A variety of therapeutic schedules are available to treat VVC including topical and systemic medications. If symptoms resolve, follow-up evaluation is not required.

See Drug Tables 103, 805.

***Assessment and history taking.*** Assessment for vaginal symptoms is usually straightforward and leads to a definitive diagnosis. The assessment includes a targeted history, physical examination, and simple office laboratory studies. Ideally, women should not be menstruating and should avoid intravaginal medications and sexual intercourse for 2–3 days before an examination for vaginitis (Secor, 1997).

The targeted history identifies events that may have altered the delicate balance of organisms that normally colonize the vagina. Factors reported to affect the vaginal ecosystem are broad-spectrum antibiotics, exogenous estrogen (menopausal replacements or high-dose oral contraceptives), contraceptives such as spermacides and latex devices, douches, vaginal medications, sexual intercourse, stress, and a change of sexual partners (ACOG, 1996). It is important to determine if the patient has initiated self-treatment for the presenting symptoms. Ferris, Dekle, and Litaker (1996) noted that only a minority of women were able to correctly diagnose VVC from signs and symptoms. Use of nonprescription antifungals may mask the signs and symptoms of other causes of vaginitis and may select for resistant yeast organisms (ACOG, 1996). As with any skin surface, the vulvar and vaginal epithelia are susceptible to allergic and chemical irritation. Accordingly, the history should include a search for common chemical sources of irritation such as perfumed and medicated soaps and shampoos, laundry detergents, bath oils, perfumed or dyed toilet paper, and chemicals in swimming pools and hot tubs (ACOG, 1996).

The physical examination begins with a careful inspection of the external genitalia, noting any erythema or pallor, edema, excoriation, or lesion such as blisters, fissures, or warts. The femoral and inguinal lymph nodes should be palpated and the findings documented. The presence of vaginal discharge at the introitus should be noted. If the woman reports external symptoms and no obvious abnormalities are noted, it is helpful to ask the woman to point to the area causing discomfort.

Next the clinician inserts the speculum, being careful to not traumatize the cervix. The color, amount, and consistency of the vaginal discharge as well as any cervical ectopy, friability, or mucus in the os are noted. The appearance of the vaginal walls and cervix should be noted. There are no controlled studies documenting the best method for collecting and preparing wet-mount slides of vaginal specimens for microscopic examination. Gant and Cunningham (1993) suggest that specimens for microscopic examination and pH determination of the vaginal discharge be collected from the lateral vaginal walls close to the cervix (between the speculum blades) with a cotton swab. Secor (1997) suggests a wooden or plastic spatula to avoid fiber artifacts. The posterior vaginal pool should be avoided since this contains discharge of cervical rather than vaginal origin. The specimen is then placed in a small test tube (for example a 5-cc red-top tube) with ½ in of fresh normal saline. The solution should be opaque with suspended cells and exudate. The pH of the discharge is best determined with narrow-range (4–5.5) pH paper (Hillier & Arko, 1996). A strip of the paper may be held with ring forceps and placed against the lateral vaginal wall, or placed on the anterior lip of the withdrawn speculum. The history or physical findings may indicate a need for cervical cultures for gonorrhea and chlamydia or a Pap smear. Although not commonly needed in the work-up of vaginal discharge, a colposcopy and biopsy may be indicated if cervical or vaginal lesions are found. The speculum is removed and a bimanual examination performed checking for evidence of upper-level involvement such as uterine, adnexal, or cervical motion tenderness.

Laboratory studies to identify the etiology of a vaginal discharge include ascertaining the pH, as described earlier, as well as microscopic evaluation. Vaginal cultures are rarely necessary except in recurrent infection or those recalcitrant to standard therapy. A saline wet-prep slide is examined for "clue" cells (epithelial cells stippled with bacteria), motile protozoa, white blood cells, epithelial cells, red blood cells, lactobacilli, and background bacteria.

A 10% potassium hydroxide (KOH) slide is examined to identify yeast organisms. A foul "fishy" odor immediately after applying KOH is a "positive whiff" test and suggests bacterial vaginosis or trichomoniasis (CDC, 1993). The KOH slide provides higher sensitivity for identifying yeast organisms than the saline slide.

The examination findings that indicate yeast vaginitis include erythema of the vulva and vagina with possible excoriations or discrete fine pustules. The vagina often has a thick curd-like discharge that adheres to the vaginal wall. Vaginal pH is most often normal. Under microscopy, C. albicans and tropicalis are dimorphic organisms and can be found as both hyphae and buds. In contrast, C. glabrata and other non-C. albicans species are monomorphic and exist only in bud form (Secor, 1997). The differentiation of Candida species is difficult without culture and is not necessary for treatment of simple yeast vaginitis.

***Patient/caregiver information.*** Patients should be counseled to complete the full course of therapy even if symptoms resolve sooner. Many intravaginal medications contain mineral oil and may weaken latex condoms and diaphragms if used concurrently with or within 72 h of using oil-based intravaginal products (*PDR,* 1997). Clinicians should take care to prescribe a non-oil-based product for women using latex condoms or diaphragms. The other option is for the woman to use nonlatex contraceptive devices.

Women should be discouraged from self-diagnosis and treatment with nonprescription antifungals. The use of nonprescription antifungals may have contributed to the increase in non-*albicans* species causing VVC. These non-*albicans* species are less sensitive to the nonprescription antifungals as well as the oral agent fluconazole (Tobin, 1995).

Oral azoles are contraindicated in pregnancy and during breastfeeding and should be prescribed to women only after the possibility of pregnancy has been excluded (*PDR,* 1997). The topical azoles can be used safely after the first trimester. Pregnant women should be counseled to insert only a small portion of the applicator very gently into the vagina to avoid trauma to the cervix. It is probably unwise for women with premature cervical dilatation to use vaginal applicators.

## Outcomes Management

***Selecting an appropriate agent.*** Faro et al (1997) recommend topical azoles as a first-line treatment for VVC because of the high mycological and clinical cure rates, minimal systemic effects, and low side-effect profile. Sobel et al (1995) found similar efficacy rates for oral fluconazole and topical clotrimazole. When compared to the oral preparations, the topical azoles are thought to provide quicker relief of symptoms. The oral agents, although more convenient for some women, have a greater risk of side effects and drug interactions (O-Prasertsawat & Bourlert, 1995). In addition, several non-*albicans* organisms are resistant to oral agents.

The topical agents are available in doses for a variety of treatment schedules from 1-day to 7-day intravaginal therapy. For mild, short-duration, or first-episode VVC the short-course treatments of any product will usually result in high cure rates. It would seem prudent to select a topical agent with broad-spectrum activity to discourage the selection for non-*albicans* treat-

ment failures. For more severe symptomatology (extensive inflammation, severe excoriation, etc.), for symptoms of long duration, or after multiple episodes of self-treatment, the longer course of therapy is recommended (Faro et al, 1997). Terconazole (a topical antifungal in 3- or 7-day dose regimens) appears to have the broadest spectrum of antifungal activity (Tobin, 1995), although clinical cure rates are comparable with all topical and oral agents.

Fluconazole 150 mg in a single dose is the only oral medication that is FDA-approved for the treatment of symptomatic VVC (Desai & Johnson, 1996). Ketoconazole, although not FDA-approved, has been used to treat chronic, recurrent symptomatic VVC.

***Monitoring for efficacy.*** A typical course of therapy for acute VVC is one oral dose of fluconazole or a 3–7 day course of terconazole. Signs and symptoms should start to improve within 2 days and be resolved within 4–6 days with oral therapy. Signs and symptoms should start to resolve within 1–1½ days and be resolved within 4–6 days with topical therapy (Slavin, Benrubi, Parker, Griffin, & Magee, 1992). Continuing symptoms are commonly related to incomplete treatment adherence or a mixed infection that was missed at diagnosis and rarely to resistance.

If short-course treatment does not resolve symptoms, consideration should be given to the 7-day topical treatment. The clinician should consider a mixed etiology for the vaginitis and reevaluate for other pathogens if the 7-day treatment does not relieve symptoms. Treatment failure and recurrent infections should be evaluated with yeast cultures.

Although rarely indicated now that broad-spectrum topical antifungals are available, gentian violet solution painted on the cervix, vagina, and vulva provides almost immediate symptomatic relief. The deep purple solution stains fabrics, and the woman should be counseled to protect her clothing.

Chronic recurrent VVC is a therapeutic challenge, and is best managed by an expert. Women with chronic recurrent infections have often endured repeated symptomatic episodes with the accompanying workup and treatment, only to become symptomatic again. Treatment must be in the context of a partnership of the woman and clinician to determine the regime that balances the woman's needs and desires with the best options for cure or long-term remission. Treatment of the asymptomatic male partner is controversial, since it has not been shown to significantly reduce the recurrence rate in women. Chronic recurrent VVC requires long-term topical or oral treatment until symptoms resolve followed by either intermittent or long-term continuous maintenance. Sobel & Chaim (1997) demonstrated high cure rates for non-*albicans* recurrent VVC infection using boric acid vaginal suppositories (600 mg/day in 0 size gelatin capsules for 14 days). All these women had failed repeated courses of antimycotic therapy with azoles.

*Monitoring for toxicity.* Toxicity is rare with topical therapy. The most common side effects are vaginal burning or itching, although the incidence of these complaints was similar in the treatment and placebo groups (*PDR*, 1997). In addition to symptoms in treated women, the male sexual partners may experience penile irritation (Bennett, 1995).

The oral agent fluconazole has been associated with a variety of side effects such as GI symptoms and adverse events including drug interactions, liver function abnormalities, congenital anomalies (Lee, Feinberg, Abraham, & Murphy, 1992), and rarely angioedema (Abbot, Hughes, Patel, & Kinghorn, 1991) and anaphylaxis (Neuhaus, Pavic, & Pletscher, 1991). Significant drug interactions with oral fluconazole include serious arrhythmias when coadministered with nonsedating antihistamines. In addition, elevated serum levels of cyclosporine, anticoagulants, anticonvulsants, oral hypoglycemic agents, and theophylline can occur when these drugs are coadministered with oral antifungal agents (Faro et al, 1997). More research is required to document whether these interactions are a problem with single-dose oral azoles.

*Follow-up recommendations.* If symptoms resolve with treatment, no follow-up is required. Women who remain symptomatic after a full 7-day course of a broad-spectrum antifungal should be reexamined for mixed infection and vaginal cultures should be performed.

## BACTERIAL VAGINOSIS

Bacterial vaginosis (BV) is the most common cause of abnormal vaginal discharge. BV develops when the normal balance of organisms in the vagina changes with loss of the normally pre-

dominant $H_2O_2$-producing lactobacilli and exuberant growth of a variety of strict and facultative anaerobes, including *Bacteroides, Peptococcus, Mobiluncus, Gardnerella, Streptococcus,* and *Mycoplasma* (Eschenbach, 1993, Hawes et al, 1996). The factors that cause this shift in vaginal flora are unknown. There are no established risk factors for BV, but it is more common in women who have multiple sex partners and is rare in women who have never been sexually active (CDC, 1998). A prominent feature of this condition is the lack of an inflammatory response to the infection; hence the name vaginosis rather than vaginitis (Sweet & Gibbs, 1995, p. 357). However, one recent study (Rein, Shih, Miller, & Guerrant, 1996) suggested that the lack of leukocytes in the vaginal discharge of women with BV was the result of destruction of these cells rather than the absence of a primary inflammatory response.

The most common presenting symptom of women with BV is a copious vaginal discharge, possibly with a foul odor that is more noticeable after coitus. A large portion of affected women (up to 50%) are asymptomatic (CDC, 1998).

### Specific Considerations for Pharmacotherapy

*When drug therapy is needed.* It was once accepted that asymptomatic women should not be treated (CDC, 1998), but recent studies have identified significant morbidity associated with untreated BV (Morales, Schorr, & Albritton, 1994; Newton, Piper, & Peairs, 1997). Untreated BV has been associated with pelvic inflammatory disease, cervicitis, postoperative infection, abnormal cytology in the nonpregnant woman, and with preterm labor and low birth weight when untreated during pregnancy (Hillier et al, 1995, 1996; Platz-Christensen, Sundstrom, & Larsson, 1994; Sweet, 1995). There is growing consensus that at the very least, routine screening and treatment would benefit women undergoing gynecologic surgery, elective abortion, or other invasive procedures and possibly those with abnormal Pap results. During pregnancy, screening and treatment are appropriate for all symptomatic women and should be considered for those women considered at high risk for preterm delivery either by history or physical findings (Sweet, 1996). Although conflicting results have been reported by others, Hauth, Goldenberg, Andrews, DuBard, and Copper (1995) reported a reduced incidence of preterm delivery with systemic treatment of women with BV. Until the risks and benefits of treating low-risk and asymptomatic pregnant women are known, this group deserves special caution.

***Short- and long-term goals of pharmacotherapy.*** As with VVC, the short-term goal is to resolve symptoms and restore the vaginal ecosystem. There are no proven strategies for preventing recurrence, so the long-term goal should be to maintain the normal vaginal flora and a balanced vaginal ecosystem.

***Nonpharmacologic therapy.*** Nonpharmacologic therapy for BV is the same as for VVC. It is focused on restoring and maintaining a healthy vaginal ecosystem.

***Time frame for initiating therapy.*** Therapy should be initiated as soon as the diagnosis is confirmed in symptomatic women. A variety of therapeutic schedules are available to treat BV, including topical and systemic medications. If symptoms resolve, follow-up evaluation is not required.

See Drug Table 101.

***Assessment and history taking.*** The assessment for vaginal discharge is the same as for VVC. The laboratory findings that are diagnostic for BV include finding at least three of the following:

1. "Clue" cells on wet prep or gram stain
2. Fishy odor of vaginal discharge before or after KOH (positive "whiff" test)
3. pH >4.5
4. A thin, adherent, homogenous vaginal discharge

The wet prep usually demonstrates few lactobacilli, few WBCs, and a large number of background bacteria. Cultures are not recommended because the bacteria responsible for BV are normal inhabitants of the vagina and can be cultured from at least 50% of normal women (CDC, 1998).

***Patient/caregiver information.*** In addition to the general caregiver guidelines discussed for VVC, the woman with BV requires the following information. With oral administration of metronidazole, the most common side effects are mild nausea, dry mouth, a metallic taste, or mild headache (*PDR*, 1997; Tracy & Webster, 1995). Patients can minimize these side effects by tak-

ing the medication in divided doses with food. Patients should be warned that metronidazole can cause abdominal distress, vomiting, flushing, or headache if alcohol is consumed during or for 24 h after completion of therapy. Although serum levels are much lower with intravaginal administration than with oral dosing, sensitive individuals could experience the same disulfiram-like reactions when intravaginal metronidazole is used concomitantly with alcohol. Patients should be advised to discontinue the medication and call their health care provider if numbness, tingling, or weakness develops in any extremity or if any other abnormal neurologic symptoms occur. Anyone taking antibacterial agents, including oral and intravaginal clindamycin, should be counseled to report diarrhea, especially bloody diarrhea.

Metronidazole is secreted in breastmilk. To minimize effects on the newborn, breast-feeding should be discontinued for 24 h after maternal ingestion of a single 2-g dose (Knodel & Kraynak, 1997, p. 2216). Expressed milk should be discarded.

## Outcomes Management

***Selecting an appropriate agent.*** Bacterial vaginosis can be effectively treated with oral or topical agents (Ferris, Litaker, Woodward, Mathis, & Hendrich, 1995). The selection should be guided by patient preference, clinician experience, and cost considerations. CDC (1993) guidelines recommend metronidazole 500 mg b.i.d. for 7 days. Alternative treatments include metronidazole 2 g orally in a single dose, or clindamycin 300 mg orally b.i.d. for 7 days. In addition, if a nonoral route is preferred, two treatment options are given: clindamycin cream 2%, one applicator (5 g) intravaginally at bedtime for 7 days, or metronidazole gel 0.75%, one applicator (5 g) intravaginally b.i.d. for 5 days. The nonoral routes are associated with a lack of systemic side effects but significantly higher costs (Mikamo et al, 1997).

Although a recent meta-analysis of the safety of metronidazole in pregnancy found no apparent increase in teratogenic risk (Burtin, Taddio, Ariburnu, Einarsoon, & Koren, 1995), many clinicians remain concerned about the possible adverse effect of metronidazole use during pregnancy. For this reason, metronidazole is not used during the first trimester of pregnancy (CDC, 1998). There is growing consensus but not complete agreement that to decrease the risk of preterm birth, screening and treatment of BV in high-risk women should be conducted early in the second trimester of pregnancy. Appropriate treatment regimens for high-risk pregnant women include metronidazole 250 mg t.i.d. for 7 days, metronidazole 2 g in a single dose, or clindamycin 300 mg b.i.d. for 7 days. If they are symptomatic with BV, pregnant women at low risk for preterm delivery should be treated with one of the above therapies or metronidazole gel 0.75%, one applicator b.i.d. for 5 days (CDC, 1998). Because of reports from two randomized clinical trials of increased rates of preterm birth after treatment with clindamycin vaginal cream, the CDC does not recommend its use in pregnancy (CDC, 1998).

**Monitoring for efficacy.** Women who become asymptomatic during treatment need no further evaluation. For women who remain symptomatic or have symptoms return very shortly after completing treatment, one of the alternative treatment regimens should be used. For women with recurrent BV, Winceslaus and Calver (1996) achieved cure rates equal to current drug therapy and with no side effects using a single vaginal washout with 3% hydrogen peroxide. The hydrogen peroxide was retained in the vagina for 3 min before being drained. Some women may prefer this inexpensive treatment to repeated doses of costly intravaginal drugs or the side effects associated with repeated courses of oral medication.

**Monitoring for toxicity.** Metronidazole has a low side-effect profile in the doses used to treat BV. The most consistent findings include mild nausea and diarrhea and a metallic taste in the mouth. More serious side effects can occur with higher doses or prolonged therapy, including neutropenia, paresthesias and peripheral neuropathies, confusion, hallucinations, and seizures (Simms-Cendan, 1996). Corey, Doebbeling, DeJong, and Britigan (1991) reported metronidazole-induced pancreatitis in three patients treated for bacterial vaginosis. All signs and symptoms of pancreatitis resolved promptly after discontinuation of metronidazole. If administered concomitantly, metronidazole has been shown to increase the serum levels of warfarin, phenytoin, and lithium. In addition, phenobarbital, cimetidine, prednisone, phenazone, and rifampin have been shown to increase the metabolic clearance of metronidazole and may

decrease its effectiveness (Simms-Cendan, 1996). If repeated courses of metronidazole are required, it is recommended that an interval of at least 4 weeks occur between courses of therapy and a total and differential leucocyte count be performed before and after therapy (PDR, 1997).

Metronidazole treatment has been associated with acute onset of *Candida* superinfection. Metronidazole is not effective in treating yeast vaginitis, so appropriate antimycotic therapy should be instituted (PDR, 1997).

As with nearly all antibacterial agents, the use of oral or topical clindamycin has been associated with the development of pseudomembranous colitis (PDR, 1997). The onset of diarrhea during or after antimicrobial treatment should be thoroughly investigated and appropriate treatment instituted.

**Follow-up recommendations.** Bacterial vaginosis is a common condition with frequent recurrences in susceptible women. Treatment of male partners has not been shown to improve the woman's response to therapy or decrease recurrence rates. At this time, treatment of male partners is not recommended (CDC, 1993).

## TRICHOMONAS VAGINITIS

*Trichomonas vaginalis* is a protozoan parasite that can infect the urogenital tract in women and men. Worldwide, trichomonas vaginitis (TV) is thought to be the most common nonviral, nonbacterial sexually transmitted disease (Zhang, 1996). In symptomatic women, *T. vaginalis* infection is characterized by a copious, frothy, vaginal discharge and vulvar irritation. In addition to vaginal infection, trichomonads have been found in the urethra, Skene's glands, and Bartholin's gland. Women often become symptomatic during or shortly after menses when the pH of the vagina is raised by menstrual blood. This produces a favorable environment for trichomonad proliferation (Goode, Grauer, & Gums, 1994). In men, *T. vaginalis* can cause urethral discharge, but symptoms are often mild, if present at all (Kreiger, 1995). The vast majority of cases of trichomonas infection are sexually transmitted, but the organism can survive for several hours on wet towels, bathing suits, toilet seats, and other fomites. The nonsexual transmission of trichomonads, although theoretically possible, has not been conclusively documented (Sobel,

1992). *Trichomonas vaginalis* often coexists with other sexually transmitted pathogens; therefore, infected women should be screened for other sexually transmitted infections (Reynolds & Wilson, 1996).

## Specific Considerations for Pharmacotherapy

*When drug therapy is needed.* Although most men are asymptomatic, trichomonas vaginitis causes acute symptoms in most women and treatment should be instituted to provide relief and prevent transmission to sexual partners. In addition to acute local symptoms and discomfort, trichomonas vaginitis during pregnancy has been associated with preterm rupture of membranes and preterm delivery (CDC, 1998). Women coinfected with *Trichomonas* and *Chlamydia* have an increased risk of developing pelvic inflammatory disease when compared to women infected with *Chlamydia* alone (Paisarntantiwong et al, 1995). Treating TV prevents the transmission to new sexual partners.

*Short- and long-term goals of pharmacotherapy.* Short-term goals are to eliminate the organism from the genital tract, resolve the symptoms of infection, and prevent the transmission to sexual partners. Long-term goals are to prevent adverse events in pregnancy and prevent recurrence through education on the use of barrier contraception and safer sex practices.

*Time frame for initiating pharmacotherapy.* As with all STDs, pharmacotherapy should be instituted as soon as the diagnosis is confirmed. Treatment should be arranged for all sexual partners of the infected woman.

*Assessment and history taking.* The basic history, physical examination, and office laboratory studies for all types of vaginitis, including TV, are the same as those for VVC.

Specific examination findings consistent with TV infection include any or all of the following: diffuse vulvar erythema, copious, sometimes frothy, vaginal discharge, inflamed vagina and cervix, and punctate hemorrhages (strawberry spots). Because the clinical features of TV are nonspecific, diagnosis relies upon the combination of clinical findings and laboratory results. Vaginal pH is almost always >5.0 and many times approaches 6.0. A positive "whiff" test is often present. The wet prep reveals many WBCs and motile, flagellated protozoa. The presence of trichomonads on a Pap smear result is neither sensitive nor specific for infection, and treatment of asymptomatic women based on Pap findings alone could result in unnecessary treatment of up to 30% of cases (Weinberger & Harger, 1993).

*Patient/caregiver information.* TV is a sexually transmitted infection in almost all cases. Infected individuals should be counseled to inform all sex partners of the need for treatment regardless of the presence of symptoms. They should abstain from intercourse or have their male partners use condoms until all medication has been completed and all partners are asymptomatic. In addition, health promotion teaching should stress the importance of barrier contraception and safer sex practices at all times to reduce the risk of reinfection with TV or of acquiring other sexually transmitted infections.

## Outcomes Management

*Selecting an appropriate agent.* Metronidazole is the only recommended treatment for TV in the United States. The recommended treatment for pregnant women after the first trimester, nonpregnant women, and all male sexual partners whether symptomatic or not is 2 g orally, given as a single dose. Alternatively, metronidazole can be given as 500 mg orally, twice daily for 7 days (CDC, 1998). The 1998 CDC treatment recommendations are in conflict with the 1997 PDR which advises against the single 2-g dose in pregnancy in favor of 250 mg t.i.d. for 7 days. When all of a woman's sexual partners cannot be treated, the 7-day course of therapy provides higher long-term cure rates, probably because many men will self-cure over the course of 7 days (*PDR*, 1997). Abstinence or condom use must be practiced faithfully.

Because trichomonads infect the urethra, Skene's glands, and Bartholins's gland as well as the vagina, intravaginal metronidazole gel is not effective for treating TV (Tidwell, Lushbaugh, Laughlin, Cleary, & Finley, 1994). During the first trimester of pregnancy, symptomatic relief but not reliable mycologic cure can sometimes be obtained by using clotrimazole vaginal suppositories, 100 mg at bedtime for 6–8 days (Knodel & Kraynak, 1997, p. 2216). A recent study in nonpregnant women demonstrated similar results using two 100-mg clotrimazole vaginal tablets once a day for 7 days (duBouchet, Spence, Rein, Danzig, & McCormack, 1997).

***Monitoring for efficacy.*** Resolution of symptoms indicates effective therapy, and no further follow-up is needed. Even organisms with diminished susceptibility to metronidazole usually respond to higher doses (CDC, 1993; Pearlman, Yashar, Ernst, & Solomon, 1996). If treatment failure occurs and symptoms remain, and reinfection is excluded, the diagnosis should be reconfirmed and the patient retreated with metronidazole 500 mg b.i.d. for 7 days. Patients who have had treatment failures may respond to a single 2-g dose of metronidazole for 3–5 days. Houang, Ahmet, and Lawrence (1997) reported successful treatment of four patients with culture-positive symptomatic resistant trichomonas vaginitis with a combination of oral metronidazole (200–400 mg t.i.d.), and 1% zinc sulfate douche followed by metronidazole vaginal suppositories (500 mg) b.i.d. This regime included prophylactic douching and suppositories after menses for several months. The lower dose of oral medication resulted in fewer side effects than the standard therapy. Any patient in whom reinfection has been excluded, who fails to respond to standard therapy, or who is allergic to metronidazole should be managed in consultation with an expert (CDC, 1998).

***Monitoring for toxicity.*** Metronidazole side effects and toxicity are the same as those discussed for BV.

***Follow-up recommendations.*** Trichomonas vaginitis is a sexually transmitted infection in almost all cases. Because most men are asymptomatic and there is a high transmission rate of infection between partners, all sexual partners of women with trichomonas vaginitis should be treated. *Trichomonas* often coexists with other sexually transmitted pathogens, and infected individuals should be screened for other conditions (Reynolds & Wilson, 1996).

## SUMMARY

The diagnosis and treatment of vaginitis in women is usually straightforward and involves correlating the findings from history, physical examination, and simple laboratory studies. It is also evident that environmental factors as well as pathogens affect the vaginal milieu and that a clear understanding of normal vaginal flora has not been definitively established. In a recent observational study of the composition of the vaginal flora of healthy women over time, only 4 women out of the 26 in the study had "normal" vaginal microbiology throughout the study period (Priestly, Jones, Dhar, & Goodwin, 1997). A variety of conditions including candidiasis, BV, and *Ureaplasma urealyticum* were found intermittently throughout the study, and symptoms correlated poorly with microbiological findings. More research is required to define the "normal" vaginal environment, establish clear guidelines for screening pregnant and nonpregnant asymptomatic women, and determine the most appropriate treatment for the variety of conditions that affect the reproductive tract of women.

## REFERENCES

Abbott, M., Hughes, D. L., Patel, R., & Kinghorn, G. R. (1991). Angiooedema after fluconazole. *Lancet, 338*(8767), 633.

Alrabiah, F. A., & Sacks, S. L. (1996). New antiherpesvirus agents: Their targets and therapeutic potential. *Drugs, 52*(1), 17–32.

American College of Obstetricians and Gynecologists. (1995). *Condom availability for adolescents.* ACOG Technical Bulletin no. 154. Washington, DC: ACOG.

American College of Obstetricians and Gynecologists. (1996). *Vaginitis.* ACOG Technical Bulletin no. 226. Washington, DC: ACOG.

Bashi, S. A. (1985). Cryotherapy versus podophyllin in the treatment of genital warts. *International Journal of Dermatology, 24*, 535–536.

Bennett, J. E. (1995). Antimicrobial agents: Antifungal agents. In J. G. Hardman, A. G. Silman, & L. E. Limbird (Eds.), *Goodman & Gilman's The pharmacological basis of therapeutics* (9th ed.) (pp. 1175–1190). New York: McGraw-Hill.

Braodnax, J. (1993). Pelvic inflammatory disease. In R. A. Dershewitz (Ed.), *Ambulatory pediatric care* (2nd ed.) (pp. 471–475). Philadelphia: J. B. Lippincott.

Brown, S., Becher, J., & Brady, W. (1995). Treatment of ectoparasitic infections: Review of the English-language literature, 1982–1992. *Clinical Infectious Diseases, 20*(Suppl. 1), S104–S109.

Burtin, P., Taddio, A., Ariburnu, O., Einarsoon, T. R., & Koren, G. (1995). Safety of metronidazole in pregnancy: A meta-analysis. *Obstetrics and Gynecology, 172*, 525–529.

Centers for Disease Control and Prevention. (1993). 1993 sexually transmitted diseases treatment guidelines. *MMWR, 42* (RR-14), i–102.

Centers for Disease Control and Prevention. (1998). 1998 Guidelines for treatment of sexually transmitted diseases. *MMWR, 47* (No. RR-1), 1–4, 18, 20–48, 70–78, 79–85, 88–94, 105–107. Atlanta, GA: U.S. Department of Health and Human Services.

Corey, W. A., Doebbeling, B. N., DeJong, K. J., & Britigan, B. E. (1991). Metronidazole-induced pancreatitis. *Reviews of Infectious Diseases, 13,* 1213–1215.

Desai, P. C., & Johnson, B. A. (1996). Oral fluconazole for vaginal candidiasis. *American Family Physician, 54*(4), 1337–1340, 1345–1346.

*Drugs facts and comparisons.* (1997). St. Louis, MO: Facts and Comparisons.

duBouchet, L., Spence, M. R., Rein, M. F., Danzig, M. R., & McCormack, W. M. (1997). Multicenter comparison of clotrimazole vaginal tablets, oral metronidazole, and vaginal suppositories containing sulfanilamide, aminacrine hydrochloride, and allantoin in the treatment of symptomatic trichomoniasis. *Sexually Transmitted Diseases, 24*(3), 156–160.

Elmer, G. W., Surawicz, C. M., & McFarland, L. V. (1996). Biotherapeutic agents: A neglected modality for the treatment and prevention of selected intestinal and vaginal infections. *JAMA, 275*(11), 870–876.

Eron, L. J. (1992). Human papillomaviruses and anogenital disease. In S. L. Gorbach, J. G. Bartlett, & N. R. Blacklow (Eds.), *Infectious Diseases* (pp. 852–857). Philadelphia: W. B. Saunders.

Eschenbach, D. A. (1993). History and review of bacterial vaginosis. *American Journal of Obstetrics and Gynecology, 169*(2S), 441–445.

Faber, F. M. (1996). The diagnosis and treatment of scabies and pubic lice. *Primary Care Update for OB/Gyns, 3*(1), 20–24.

Faro, S., Apuzzio, J., Bohannon, N., Elliott, K., Martens, M. G., Mou, S. M., Phillips-Smith, L. E., Soper, D. E., Strayer, A., & Young, R. L. (1997). Treatment considerations in vulvovaginal candidiasis. *Female Patient, 22,* 21–38.

Ferenczy, A. (1985). Comparison of 5-fluorouracil and $CO_2$ laser for treatment of vaginal condylomas. *Obstetrics and Gynecology, 64,* 773–778.

Ferris, D. G., Dekle, C., & Litaker, M. S. (1996). Women's use of over-the-counter antifungal medications for gynecologic symptoms. *Journal of Family Practice, 42*(6), 595–600.

Ferris, D. G., Litaker, M. S., Woodward, L., Mathis, D., & Hendrich, J. (1995). Treatment of bacterial vaginosis: A comparison of oral metronidazole, metronidazole vaginal gel, and clindamycin vaginal cream. *Journal of Family Practice, 41*(5), 443–449.

Fischer, T. F. (1994). Lindane toxicity in a 24-year-old woman. *Annals of Emergency Medicine, 24*(5), 972–974.

Friedman-Kien, A. E., Eron, L. J., Conant, M., Growdon, W., Bradiak, H., Bradstreet, P. W., Fedorczyk, D., Trout, J. R., & Plasse, T. F. (1988). Natural interferon-α for treatment of chondylomata acuminata. *JAMA, 259*(4), 533–538.

Gant, N. F., & Cunningham, F. G. (Eds.). (1993). *Basic gynecology and obstetrics* (pp. 43–53). Norwalk, CT: Appleton & Lange.

Geiger, A. M., & Foxman, B. (1996). Risk factors for vulvovaginal candidiasis: A case-control study among university students. *Epidemiology, 7*(2), 182–187.

Geiger, A. M., Foxman, B., & Gillespie, B. W. (1996). The epidemiology of vulvovaginal candidiasis among university students. *American Journal of Public Health, 85*(8, Pt. 1), 1146–1148.

Gonorrhea and chlamydial infections. (1994). *International Journal of Gynaecology and Obstetrics, 45,* 169–174.

Goode, M. A., Grauer, K., & Gums, J. G. (1994). Infectious vaginitis: Selecting therapy and preventing recurrence. *Postgraduate Medical Journal, 96*(6), 85–98.

Haddix, A. C., Hillis, S. D., & Kassler, W. J. (1995). The cost effectiveness of azithromycin for *Chlamydia trachomatis* infections in women. *Sexually Transmitted Diseases, 22*(5), 274–280.

Handsfield, H. H., Dalu, Z. A., & Martin, D. A. (1993). Multicenter trial of single-dose azithromycin vs. ceftriaxone in the treatment of uncomplicated gonorrhea. *Sexually Transmitted Diseases, 21*(2), 107–111.

Hart, G. (1990). Donovanosis. In K. K. Holmes, P. A. Mardh, P. F. Sparling, P. J. Wiesner, W. Cates, S. M. Lemon, & W. E. Stamm, *Sexually transmitted diseases* (2nd ed.) (pp. 273–277). New York: McGraw-Hill.

Hauth, J. C., Goldenberg, R. L., Andrews, W. W., DuBard, M. B., & Copper, R. L. (1995). Reduced incidence of preterm delivery with metronidazole and erythromycin in women with bacterial vaginosis. *New England Journal of Medicine, 33,* 1732–1736.

Hawes, S. E., Hillier, S. L., Benedetti, J., Stevens, C. E., Koutsky, L. A., Wolner-Hanssen, P., & Holmes, K. K. (1996). Hydrogen peroxide-producing lactobacilli and acquisition of vaginal infections. *Journal of Infectious Diseases, 174*(5), 1058–1063.

Hellberg, D., Zdolsek, B., Nilsson, S., & Mardh, P. A. (1995). Sexual behavior of women with repeated episodes of vulvovaginal candidiasis. *European Journal of Epidemiology, 11*(5), 575–579.

Hillier, S., & Arko, R. J. (1996). Vaginal infections. In S. A. Morse, A. A. Moreland, & K. K. Holmes (Eds.), *Atlas of sexually transmitted diseases and AIDS* (2nd ed.) (pp. 149–164). Baltimore: Mosby-Wolfe.

Hillier, S. L., Kiviat, N. B., Hawes, S. E., Hasselquist, M. B., Hanssen, P. W., Eschenbach, D. A., & Holmes, K. K. (1996). Gynecology: Role of bacterial vaginosis-associated microorganisms in endometritis. *American Journal of Obstetrics and Gynecology, 175*(2), 435–441.

Hillier, S. L., Nugent, R. P., Eschenbach, D. A., Krohn, M. A., Gibbs, R. S., Martin, D. H., Cotch, M. F., Edelman, R., Pastorek, J. G., II, Rao, A. V., McNellis, D., Regan, J. A., Carey, J. C., Klebanoff, M. A., & the Vaginal Infections and Prematurity Study Group. (1995). Association between bacterial vaginosis and preterm delivery of a low-birth-weight infant. *New England Journal of Medicine, 333*(26), 1737–1742.

Hook, W. E., III, & Mara, C. M. (1992). Acquired syphilis in adults. *New England Journal of Medicine, 326,* 1060–1069.

Houang, E. T., Ahmet, Z., & Lawrence, A. G. (1997). Successful treatment of four patients with recalcitrant vaginal trichomoniasis with a combination of zinc sulfate douche and metronidazole therapy. *Sexually Transmitted Diseases, 24*(2), 116–119.

Howley, P. M., & Schlegel, R. (1988). The human papillomaviruses: An overview. *American Journal of Medicine, 85,* 155.

Hutchinson, C. M., & Hook, E. W., III. (1990). Syphilis in adults. *Medical Clinics of North America, 74,* 1389–1416.

Ivey, J. B. (1997). The adolescent with pelvic inflammatory disease: Assessment and management. *The Nurse Practitioner, 22*(2), 78–91.

Johnson, C. A. (1996a). Genital herpes. In C. A. Johnson, B. E. Johnson, J. L. Murray, & B. S. Apgar (Eds.), *Women's health care handbook* (pp. 222–225). Philadelphia: C. V. Mosby.

Johnson, C. A. (1996b). Gonorrhea. In C. A. Johnson, B. E. Johnson, J. L. Murray, & B. S. Apgar (Eds.), *Women's health care handbook* (pp. 218–221). Philadelphia: C. V. Mosby.

Johnson, C. A. (1996c). Syphilis. In C. A. Johnson, B. E. Johnson, J. L. Murray, & B. S. Apgar (Eds.), *Women's health care handbook* (pp. 213–217). Philadelphia: C. V. Mosby.

Kirby, P. K., Kiviat, N., Beckman, A., Wells, D., Sherwin, S., & Corey, L. (1988). Tolerance and efficacy of recombinant human interferon-γ in the treatment of refractory genital warts. *American Journal of Medicine, 85,* 183–188.

Knapp, J. S., Wongba, C., & Limpakarnjanarat, K. (1997). Antimicrobial susceptibilities of strains of *Neisseria gonorrhoeae* in Bangkok, Thailand: 1994–1995. *Sexually Transmitted Diseases, 24*(3), 142–148.

Knodel, L. C., & Kraynak, M. A. (1997). Sexually transmitted diseases. In J. T. DiPiro, R. L. Talbert, G. C. Yee, G. R. Matzke, B. G. Wells, & L. M. Posey (Eds.), *Pharmacotherapy: A pathophysiologic approach* (pp. 2195–2219). Stamford, CT: Appleton & Lange.

Krebs, H. B. (1987). The use of topical 5-fluorouracil in the treatment of genital condylomas. *Obstetrics and Gynecology Clinics of North America, 14,* 559–568.

Krieger, J. N. (1995). Trichomoniasis in men: Old issues and new data. *Sexually Transmitted Diseases, 22*(2), 83–96.

Larson, M. (1996a). Granuloma inguinale. In C. A. Johnson, B. E. Johnson, J. L. Murray, & B. S. Apgar (Eds.), *Women's health care handbook* (pp. 235–237). Philadelphia: C. V. Mosby.

Larson, M. (1996b). Lymphogranuloma venereum. In C. A. Johnson, B. E. Johnson, J. L. Murray, & B. S. Apgar (Eds.), *Women's health care handbook* (pp. 233–234). Philadelphia: C. V. Mosby.

Lee, B., Feinberg, M., Abraham, J., & Murphy, A. (1992). Congenital malformations in an infant born to a woman treated with fluconazole. *Pediatric Infectious Disease Journal, 11,* 1062–1064.

Long, J. G. (1996). Vaginal infections. In S. A. Morse, A. A. Moreland, & K. K. Holmes (Eds.), *Atlas of sexually transmitted diseases and AIDS* (2nd ed.) (pp. 306–318). Baltimore: Mosby-Wolfe.

McEvoy, G. K., Litvak, K., & Welsh, O. H. (Eds.). (1997). *American Hospital Formulary Service 97 Drug Information.* Bethesda, MD: The American Society of Health-System Pharmacists, Inc.

Meinking, T. L., Taplin, D., Herminda, J. L., Pardo, R., & Kerdel, F. A. (1995). The treatment of scabies with Invermectin. *New England Journal of Medicine, 333*(1), 26–30.

Mikamo, H., Kawazoe, K., Izumi, K., Watanabe, K., Ueno, K., & Tamaya, T. (1997). Comparative study on vaginal or oral treatment of bacterial vaginosis. *Chemotherapy, 43*(1), 60–68.

Mill, K. E. (1997). Sexually transmitted diseases. *Primary Care, 24*(1), 179–193.

Morales, W. J., Schorr, S., & Albritton, J. (1994). Effect of metronidazole in patients with preterm birth in preceding pregnancy and bacterial vaginosis: A placebo-controlled, double-blind study. *American Journal of Obstetrics and Gynecology, 171*(2), 345–347.

Moran, J. S., & Levine, W. C. (1995). Drugs of choice for the treatment of uncomplicated gonococcal infections. *Clinical Infectious Diseases, 20*(Suppl. 1), S47–S65.

Neuhaus, G., Pavic, N., & Pletscher, M. (1991). Ana-phylactic reaction after oral fluconazole. *BMJ, 302,* 1341.

Newton, E. R., Piper, J., & Peairs, W. (1997). Bac-terial vaginosis and intraamniotic infection. *American Journal of Obstetrics and Gynecology,* 176(3), 672–677.

NIH Expert Panel. (1996). NIH Consensus Devel-opment Conference on Cervical Cancer. National Institutes of Health, April 1–3, 1996.

O-Prasertsawat, P., & Bourlert, A. (1995). Compar-ative study of fluconazole and clotrimazole for the treatment of vulvovaginal candidiasis. *Sexually Transmitted Diseases,* 22(4), 228–230.

Paisarntantiwong, R., Brockmann, S., Clarke, L., Landesman, S., Feldman, J., & Minkoff, H. (1995). The relationship of vaginal trichomoniasis and pelvic inflammatory disease among women colonized with *Chlamydia trachomatis. Sexually Transmitted Diseases,* 22(6), 344–347.

Pearlman, M. D., Yashar, C., Ernst, S., & Solomon, W. (1996). An incremental dosing protocol for women with severe vaginal trichomoniasis and ad-verse reaction to metronidazole. *American Journal of Obstetrics and Gynecology,* 174(3), 934–936.

Perine, P. L., & Osoba, A. O. (1990). Lympho-granuloma venereum. In K. K. Holmes, P. A. Mardh, P. F. Sparling, P. J. Wiesner, W. Cates, S. M. Lemon, & W. E. Stamm, *Sexually transmitted diseases* (2nd ed.) (pp. 195–211). New York: McGraw-Hill.

*Physician's desk reference* (51st ed.). (1997). Oradell, NJ: Medical Economics Data.

Platz-Christensen, J. J., Sundstrom, E., & Larsson, P-G. (1994). Bacterial vaginosis and cervical intra-epithelial neoplasia. *Acta Obstetrica et Gyne-cologica Scandinavica,* 73, 586–588.

Priestley, C. J., Jones, B. M., Dhar, J., & Goodwin, L. (1997). What is normal vaginal flora? *Genito-urinary Medicine,* 73(1), 23–28.

Rasmussen, J. E. (1996). Body lice, head lice, pubic lice and scabies. In K. A. Arndt, P. E. LeBoit, J. K. Robinson, & B. U. Wintroub (Eds.), *Cutaneous medicine and surgery: An integrated program in dermatology* (Vol. 2) (pp. 1190–1200). Phila-delphia: W. B. Saunders.

Rein, M. F., Shih, L. M., Miller, J. R., & Guerrant, R. L. (1996). Use of lactoferrin assay in the differen-tial diagnosis of female genital tract infections and implications for the pathophysiology of bacterial vaginosis. *Sexually Transmitted Diseases,* 23(6), 517–521.

Reynolds, M., & Wilson, J. (1996). Is trichomonas vaginalis still a market for other sexually transmit-ted infections in women? *International Journal of STD and AIDS,* 7(2), 131–132.

Robinson, A. J., & Ridgway, G. L. (1996). Modern di-agnosis and management of genital *Chlamydia trachomatis* infections. *British Journal of Hospital Medicine,* 55(7), 388–393.

Rosemberg, S. K., Greenberg, M. D., & Reid, R. (1987). Sexually transmitted papillomaviral infec-tion in men. *Obstetrics and Gynecology Clinics of North America,* 14, 495–512.

Secor, R. M. C. (1997). Vaginal microscopy: Refining the nurse practitioner's technique. *Clinical Excellence for Nurse Practitioners,* 1(1), 29–34.

Shalev, E., Battino, S., Weiner, E., Colodner, R., & Keness, Y. (1996). Ingestion of yogurt containing *Lactobacillus acidophilus* compared with pasteur-ized yogurt as prophylaxis for recurrent candidal vaginitis and bacterial vaginosis. *Archives of Family Medicine,* 5(1), 593–596.

Sherrard, J. (1996). Modern diagnosis and manage-ment of gonorrhoea. *British Journal of Hospital Medicine,* 55(7), 394–398.

Simms-Cendan, J. S. (1996). Metronidazole: In-fectious diseases update. *Primary Care Update for OB/Gyns,* 3(5), 153–156.

Slavin, M. B., Benrubi, G. I., Parker, R., Griffin, C. R., & Magee, M. J. (1992). Single dose oral flu-conazole vs. intravaginal terconazole in treatment of candida vaginitis. *Journal of the Florida Medical Association,* 79(10), 693–696.

Sobel, J. D. (1992). Vulvovaginitis. *Dermatologic Clinics,* 10(2), 339–359.

Sobel, J. D., Brooker, D., Stein, G. E., Thomason, J. L., Wermeling, D. P., Bradley, B., & Weinstein, L. (1995). Single oral dose fluconazole compared with conventional clotrimazole topical therapy of Candida vaginitis: Fluconazole Vaginitis Study Group. *American Journal of Obstetrics and Gynecology,* 172(4, Pt. 1), 1263–1268.

Sobel, J. D., & Chaim, W. (1997). Treatment of Torulopsis glabrata vaginitis: Retrospective review of boric acid therapy. *Clinical Infectious Diseases,* 24(4), 649–652.

Spinillo, A., Capuzzo, E., Egbe, T. O., Nicola, S., & Piazzi, G. (1995). Torulopsis glabrata vaginitis. *Obstetrics and Gynecology,* 85(6), 993–998.

Spinillo, A., Capuzzo, E., Gulminetti, R., Marone, P., Colonna, L., & Piazzi, G. (1997). Prevalence of and risk factors for fungal vaginitis caused by non-albicans species. *American Journal of Obstetrics and Gynecology,* 176(1), 138–141.

Sweet, R. (Ed.). (1996). *The vaginitis report.* Barrington, IL: National Vaginitis Association.

Sweet, R. L. (1995). Role of bacterial vaginosis in pelvic inflammatory disease. *Clinical Infectious Diseases,* 20(Suppl. 2), S271–S275.

Sweet, R. L., & Gibbs, R. S. (1995). *Infectious dis-eases of the female genital tract* (3rd ed.) (pp. 341–362). Baltimore: Williams & Wilkins.

Tapsall, J. W., Phillips, E. A., & Schultz, T. R. (1996). Quinolone-resistant Neisseria gonorrhoeae isolated in Sydney, Australia, 1991 to 1995. *Sexually Transmitted Diseases, 23*(5), 425–428.

Tartaglione, T. A., & Celum, C. L. (1995). Sexually transmitted diseases. In M. A. Koda-Kimble & L. Y. Young (Eds.), *Applied Therapeutics: The clinical use of drugs* (6th ed.) (Chapter 64, page 10).

Tidwell, B. H., Lushbaugh, W. B., Laughlin, M. D., Cleary, J. D., & Finley, R. W. (1994). A double-blind placebo-controlled trial of single-dose intravaginal versus single-dose oral metronidazole in the treatment of trichomonal vaginitis. *Journal of Infectious Diseases, 170*(1), 242–246.

Tobin, M. J. (1995). Vulvovaginal candidiasis: Topical vs. oral therapy. *American Family Physician, 51*(7), 1715–1720.

Tracy, J. W., & Webster, L. T., Jr. (1995). Drugs used in the chemotherapy of protozoal infections: Trypanosomiasis, leishmaniasis, amebiasis, giardiasis, trichomoniasis, and other protozoal infections. In J. G. Hardman, A. G. Gilman, & L. E. Limbird (Eds.), *Goodman & Gilman's The pharmacological basis of therapeutics* (9th ed.) (pp. 987–1008). New York: McGraw-Hill.

Washington, A. E., Arno, P. S., & Brooks, M. A. (1986). The economic cost of pelvic inflammatory disease. *JAMA, 255*(13), 1735–1738.

Weinberger, M. W., & Harger, J. H. (1993). Accuracy of the Papanicolaou smear in the diagnosis of asymptomatic infection with *Trichomonas vaginalis*. *Obstetrics and Gynecology, 82*(3), 425–429.

Weinstock, H., Dean, D., & Bolan, G. (1994). *Chlamydia trachomatis* infections. *Infectious Disease Clinics of North America, 8*(4), 797–819.

Winceslaus, S. J., & Calver, G. (1996). Recurrent bacterial vaginosis—an old approach to a new problem. *International Journal of STD and AIDS, 7*(4), 284–287.

Youngkin, E. Q. (1995). Sexually transmitted diseases: Current and emerging concerns. *Journal of Obstetric, Gynecologic and Neonatal Nursing, 24*(8), 743–758.

Zhang, Z. (1996, September–October). Epidemiology of *Trichomonas vaginalis*. *Sexually Transmitted Diseases, 23*(5), 415–424.

# 37

## IMMUNE SYSTEM DISORDERS: HIV/AIDS, MONONUCLEOSIS, AND ALLERGIC RESPONSES

*C. Fay Parpart, Mary S. Peery, and Kathleen J. Sawin*

Immune system disorders occur when the immune system responds distressingly to certain specific, foreign substances and when infectious agents, allergens, or the immune system itself causes dysfunction or dysregulation. This chapter addresses in depth two conditions commonly encountered by primary care providers, human immunodeficiency virus (HIV)/acquired immune deficiency syndrome (AIDS) and allergic reactions. A short discussion of the treatment of a very common but usually self-limiting viral infection, infectious mononucleosis, is also included.*

## HIV/AIDS

Although the highest frequency of this infection occurs in adolescents and adults, HIV is found to be steadily increasing in the pediatric population, secondary to the increasing incidence of infected women (Centers for Disease Control and Prevention [CDC], 1994; Wiese, 1997). This section addresses the treatment of HIV in the adult and adolescent population. The next section addresses the treatment of HIV in the pediatric population.

HIV is a retrovirus of the *Lentivirus* genus. Retroviruses are RNA viruses that replicate via DNA intermediates using the viral enzyme reverse transcriptase. After a long incubation period, HIV causes clinical syndromes, which are

characterized by a protracted symptomatic phase. There are two types of HIV, 1 and 2. Although both types are known to cause AIDS, infection with HIV-1 is more common in the United States (Boucher & Larder, 1994; Hecht & Soloway, 1994).

HIV infections most often affect activated cells of the immune system, and particularly T-cell lymphocytes (often referred to as CD4 cells or T4 cells). HIV can also infect other cells such as glial cells in the brain, macrophages, Langerhans' cells (dendritic cells) in the skin, and chromaffin cells in the intestine (Boucher & Larder, 1994).

The overall effect of HIV infection is a severely compromised immune system. Recent findings suggest that the spread of the virus to organs other than lymphoid tissue occurs late in HIV disease, with the onset of AIDS-defining illnesses (Boucher & Larder, 1994). See Table 37–1.

### HIV/AIDS—ADULT AND ADOLESCENT POPULATION

#### Specific Considerations for Pharmacotherapy

***Need for drug therapy and rationale.*** Antiretroviral treatment of HIV infection has undergone great changes in recent years. Theoretically, the multiple steps in the replication of HIV provide many opportunities for antiviral action as noted in Table 37–2 (Lipsky, 1996). Although these multiple steps have inspired the development of

---

* See also section on postexposure prophylaxis on page 920.

## TABLE 37–1. SPECTRUM OF HIV INFECTION

|  | Acute | Asymptomatic | Early Symptoms | AIDS |
|---|---|---|---|---|
| Time frame | 4–6 weeks | Averages 10 years | Months to years | Months to years |
| Antibody status | (−) | (+) | (+) | (+/−) |

At 3 months 90% of HIV-infected persons will have a (+) antibody test; at 6 months >95% of HIV-infected persons will have a (+) antibody test. *From Miralles (1996).*

various drugs, agents that affect only step 2, inhibition of reverse transcriptase, and step 6, inhibition of protein (viral subunits) processing, have been approved as therapies in the treatment of HIV infection. These agents are recommended to be utilized as combination therapies. The combination antiretroviral therapies have improved many patients' overall prognosis by inhibiting viral replication, as noted by significant changes in subsequent viral load testing. In addition, many patients also improve clinically when treated with combination antiretroviral therapies (Boucher and Larder, 1994; Goldschmidt & Dong, 1997).

***Short-term and long-term goals of pharmacotherapy.*** The short-term goals of treatment for HIV/AIDS are to decrease the viral load (burden), obtained by direct quantification of the virus (HIV RNA testing) in the patient's blood; to improve the immune status as indicated by the CD4 cell count; and to reduce or eliminate the constitutional symptoms, eg, malaise, weight loss, and fever.

## TABLE 37–2. OPPORTUNITIES FOR ANTIVIRAL ACTION ON THE PATHOGENESIS OF HIV

1. Attachment of virus to the cell
2. Inhibition of reverse transcriptase, which creates DNA from viral RNA
3. Inhibition of Rnase H, which degrades viral RNA after viral DNA has been synthesized
4. Inhibition of viral integrase, which is used to integrate viral DNA into the cell's DNA
5. Inhibition of expression of the HIV gene once it is integrated into the host cell DNA, including the processes of transcription of more viral RNA and the translation to viral proteins
6. Inhibition of processing and post-translational modification to protein products of the virus

*From Lipsky (1996, p. 800).*

Long-term goals of treatment for HIV/AIDS include the prevention of HIV-related clinical symptoms and opportunistic infections and the maintenance of a stable immune system.

### *Prevention and nonpharmacologic therapy for HIV/AIDS and opportunistic infections*

**PREVENTION.** Inclusion of a nonjudgemental risk assessment about sexual behaviors and drug use into the clinician's history provides an opportunity for discussion about the patient's perception of risk and his or her plans for harm reduction.

Sexual behavior harm reduction includes the following:

1. Abstinence
2. Monogamous relationship with noninfected individual
3. Sexual behavior that does not involve an exchange of body fluids, eg, hugging, erotic massage, self-masturbation while lying next to the partner, and showering together
4. Safer sex, including latex condom use from start to finish of anal or vaginal intercourse, use of latex barrier protection for oral sex, and providing educational materials about the choices involving sexual behavior and safer sex including instruction on proper condom use

Needle-sharing harm reduction includes the following:

1. Providing resources for drug treatment if the client is willing and ready
2. Providing patient educational material and instruction about transmission via blood exposure (American Medical Association [AMA], 1996; Coates, 1994; Makadon & Silian, 1995; Marks, 1994; Report of the NIH Panel to Define Principles of Therapy of HIV Infection, 1997; Stryker et al, 1995).

**NONPHARMACOLOGIC THERAPY.** Many patients utilize a combination of traditional and alternative methodologies. Some of the complementary or supplemental therapies are noted in Table 37–3.

## TABLE 37–3. COMPLEMENTARY OR SUPPLEMENTAL THERAPIES

| | |
|---|---|
| Meditation | Acupuncture; acupressure |
| Counseling | Lymphatic massage |
| Reiki | Natural nutritional |
| Homeopathic remedies | supplements |
| Color and light therapy | Aromatherapy |
| Sound therapy | Healing touch; therapeutic |
| Feng shui | touch |
| Massage therapy | Biofeedback |
| Herbals | |

*From Burroughs (1993); Moon (1997).*

***Time frame for initiating pharmacotherapy.*** Some primary care providers seek specialty consultation or refer clients out for management shortly after the HIV diagnosis. Others choose to work with patients with HIV infection throughout the course of the disease. This is a decision for the provider and patient to make together (Hecht & Soloway, 1994). The Panel on Clinical Practices for Treatment of HIV Infection, convened by the Department of Health and Human Services (DHHS) and the Henry J. Kaiser Family Foundation, recommended that when possible a physician with extensive HIV experience should direct the treatment of patients with HIV infection. When this is not possible, the panel felt it is important that the provider have access to consultations with HIV experts (CDC, 1998a; CDC, 1998b; CDC, 1998c).

When making decisions about initiation of pharmacotherapy, the CD4 cell count and viral load measurement should be performed on two occasions, ideally 1 week apart in the symptomatic patient and 1 month apart in the asymptomatic patient, to ensure accuracy of measurement and to determine whether these parameters are stable or changing (Japour, 1996, Johns Hopkins University AIDS Service, 1997).

It has been estimated that 50% of HIV-infected persons will experience at least some symptoms associated with the acute retroviral syndrome or primary HIV infection (Table 37–4). Therefore, early diagnosis and potential intervention are contingent on providers maintaining a high level of suspicion for HIV infection in patients presenting with this spectrum of symptoms and obtaining an appropriate history (Carpenter et al, 1996; Goldschmidt &

Dong, 1997; Moore & Bartlett, 1996). The benefits and risks associated with initiation of pharmacotherapy during the acute phase and asymptomatic phase of HIV infection are noted in Table 37–5.

The HIV viral load and the CD4 T-cell count in conjunction with the clinical category are used as indicators for the initiation of antiretroviral therapy (Table 37–6). Initiation of antiretroviral therapy for the asymptomatic HIV-infected patient has demonstrated benefit for individuals with less than 500 CD4 T-cells/mm$^3$. No long-term clinical benefit of antiretroviral therapy has yet been demonstrated for patients with CD4 T-cells greater than 500/mm$^3$, although there is theoretical benefit from pharmacotherapy (Carpenter, 1997; Goldschmidt & Dong, 1997; Johns Hopkins University AIDS Service, 1997; CDC, 1998c; Wiese, 1997).

All patients diagnosed clinically or immunologically with advanced HIV disease (AIDS) as defined by the 1993 CDC HIV Classification System are recommended to initiate antiretroviral therapy (Goldschmidt & Dong, 1997; Johns Hopkins University AIDS Service, 1997; CDC, 1998c).

## TABLE 37–4. ACUTE RETROVIRAL SYNDROME: ASSOCIATED SIGNS AND SYMPTOMS

- Fever
- Lymphadenopathy
- Pharyngitis
- Rash
- Erythematous maculopapular rash with 5–10-mm lesions on face and trunk and sometimes extremities including palms and soles; mucocutaneous ulceration involving mouth, esophagus, or genitals
- Myalgia or arthralgia
- Diarrhea
- Headache
- Nausea and vomiting
- Hepatosplenomegaly
- Thrush
- Neurologic symptoms:
  Meningoencephalitis or aseptic meningitis
  Peripheral neuropathy or radiculopathy
  Facial palsy
  Guillain-Barré syndrome
  Brachial neuritis
  Cognitive impairment or psychosis

*From Johns Hopkins University AIDS Service (1997).*

## TABLE 37–5. BENEFITS AND RISKS ASSOCIATED WITH INITIATION OF PHARMACOTHERAPY DURING ACUTE PHASE OF HIV INFECTION OR IN THE ASYMPTOMATIC PHASE OF HIV INFECTION

| Benefits | Risks |
|---|---|
| Suppress viral replication | Adverse effects associated with drugs |
| Improve symptoms of acute infection | Potential for drug resistance |
| Alter the viral "set point" | Potential for indefinite use of drugs |
| Reduce the potential for viral mutations | Poor long-term prognosis in symptomatic |
| Better tolerance, fewer side effects | patients |
| Decreased immunosuppression | |

*Adapted from Perrin and Kinloch-de Loes (1995); Fisher, E. J. (personal communication, March 1997).*

**Assessment needed prior to therapy.** The initial assessment following diagnosis of HIV infection includes a complete history and physical examination (Tables 37–7 and 37–8) and baseline laboratory and diagnostic workup (Table 37–9) (Hecht & Soloway, 1994).

Many patients are diagnosed with HIV infection secondary to the diagnosis of an AIDS-defining illness. Therefore, initiation of antiretroviral therapy may be delayed until the therapy for the acute illness is completed. In addition, a careful review of the history and physical examination and laboratory results for indications of underlying illness or increased potential for drug toxicities is recommended (CDC, 1998c).

**Patient/caregiver information.** Patient education is paramount for successful antiretroviral therapy. Adherence to medication plan is critical. Patient education materials are available from regional AIDS Education and Training Centers [national office—(301) 443-6364], national and state AIDS hotlines [United States, (800) 342-AIDS], AIDS service organizations, pharmaceutical companies, state and local health departments, and the National Institutes of Health [(301) 496-5717)]. The Internet offers chat rooms, educational forums, and access to the CDC (web site: http://www.cdcnac.org), National Institutes of Health, and the U.S. Department of Health and Human Services, Public Health Service's HIV/AIDS Treatment Informa-

## TABLE 37–6. INDICATIONS FOR THE INITIATION OF ANTIRETROVIRAL THERAPY IN THE CHRONICALLY HIV-INFECTED PATIENT

| Clinical Category | CD4+ T Cell Count and HIV RNA | Recommendation |
|---|---|---|
| Symptomatic (AIDS, thrush, unexplained fever) | All | Treat |
| Asymptomatic | CD4+ T Cells <500/mm³ or HIV RNA >10,000 (bDNA) or >20,000 (RT-PCR) | Treatment should be offered. Strength of recommendation is based on prognosis for disease-free survival and willingness of the patient to accept therapy.* |
| Asymptomatic | CD4+ T Cells >500/mm³ and HIV RNA <10,000 (bDNA) or <20,000 (RT-PCR) | Some experts would delay therapy and observe; however, some experts would treat. |

*Some experts would observe patients with CD4+T cell counts between 350–500/mm³ and HIV RNA levels <10,000 (bDNA) or <20,000 (RT-PCR)
*From Johns Hopkins University AIDS Service (1997).*

## TABLE 37–7.  REVIEW OF SYSTEMS

| Symptom | Possible Associated Condition(s) |
|---|---|
| **Constitutional** | |
| • Weight loss, fever, night sweats, fatigue | • Wasting syndrome,[a] opportunistic infection,[a] lymphoma[a]; acute HIV infection, tuberculosis[a] |
| **Lymphatic** | |
| • Lymphadenopathy | • HIV, Kaposi's sarcoma,[a] lymphoma,[a] mycobacteria[a]; acute HIV infection |
| **HEENT** | |
| • Sore/dry mouth<br>White patches in mouth | • Thrush, oral hairy leukoplakia |
| • Acute unilateral vision loss or ↑ floaters | • Cytomegalovirus retinitis[a] |
| • Sinus/ear congestion | • Sinusitis |
| **Respiratory** | |
| • Dyspnea with or without exertion<br>Cough<br>Chest tightness or pain | • Pneumocystis pneumonia,[a] ordinary bacterial pneumonias,[b] tuberculosis[a] |
| **Gastrointestinal** | |
| • Dysphagia/odynophagia | • Candida esophagitis,[a] herpes or CMV esophagitis[a] |
| • Anorexia<br>Nausea and vomiting<br>Abdominal pain<br>Constipation, diarrhea | • Cytomegalovirus,[a] cryptosporidium[a] +/ or microsporidium enteritis, or cholangitis; lymphoma,[a] *Mycobacterium avium,*[a] wasting syndrome |
| • Anorectal pain/sores | • Chronic herpes simplex[a] |
| **Genitourinary** | |
| • Hx abnormal Pap smear | • Cervical carcinoma[b] |
| • Painful sores | • Chronic herpes simplex[a] |
| • Vulvovaginal itch/discharge<br>Symptoms of STD (VD) | • Candidiasis, other vaginitis/urethritis, STD |
| • Decreased libido | |
| **Musculoskeletal** | |
| • Myalgias, arthralgias | • HIV or zidovudine myopathy |
| **Neurologic** | |
| • Headache<br>Seizure<br>Focal symptoms<br>Ataxia<br>Decreased cognition (poor memory, trouble finding words) | • HIV encephalopathy (dementia),[a] CNS opportunistic infection,[a] lymphoma[a]; other HIV neurologic, acute HIV infection |
| • Pain, paresthesias, numbness | • Peripheral neuropathy |
| **Skin** | |
| • Rash | • Acute HIV infection, zoster, syphilis |
| • New lesion | • Kaposi's sarcoma[a] |
| • New or worsening dermatoses | • Dryness, seborrheic dermatitis, folliculitis, tineas, *Candida,* molluscum, psoriasis |
| • Bruising, petechiae | • HIV immune thrombocytopenia |

[a] AIDS-defining condition.
[b] Possible AIDS-defining condition.
*From Fisher (1995).*

## TABLE 37–8.  HIV-DIRECTED PHYSICAL EXAMINATION

| Physical Finding | Possible Associated Condition(s) |
| --- | --- |
| **Skin** | |
| • Purplish lesion | • Kaposi's sarcoma[a] |
| • Common dermatoses | • Dryness, seborrheic dermatitis, folliculitis, tineas, *Candida,* molluscum, psoriasis |
| • Rash | • Zoster; acute HIV infection; syphilis |
| **Eye (retina) (exam indicated if symptoms or very low immune function)** | |
| • Exudates/hemorrhages | |
| • Smaller than disc, do not progress or affect vision | • Cotton wool spots (HIV retinopathy) |
| • Larger, progressive, often affect vision | • Cytomegalovirus retinitis[a] |
| **Mouth** | |
| • Redness, patchy or diffuse | • Thrush |
| • White exudates | |
| • Can be scraped off | • Thrush |
| • Cannot be scraped off | • Oral hairy leukoplakia |
| • Ulcer | • Herpes simplex,[b] aphthous or medication-induced ulcers, acute HIV infection |
| • Red or purple lesion | • Kaposi's sarcoma[a] |
| **Lymphatic** | |
| • Adenopathy | |
| • Relatively symmetric; axillary usually largest | • HIV lymphadenopathy; acute HIV infection |
| • Hard, fixed or disproportionately large | • Lymphoma,[a] Kaposi's sarcoma,[a] mycobacteria[a] |
| **Lungs** | |
| • Rales/wheezes Tachypnea | • Pneumocystis[a] or TB[a] (Note: lungs often clear), bacterial pneumonia,[b] pulmonary Kaposi's[a] |
| **Abdomen** | |
| • Hepatomegaly/splenomegaly | • *Mycobacteria,*[a] lymphoma[a] (Note: organomegaly usually of other cause) |
| • Mass | • Lymphoma[a] |
| • Tenderness | • Cytomegalovirus enterocolitis[a]; AIDS cholangiopathy/cholecystitis[a] |
| **Anogenital** | |
| • Cervical abnormality | • Dysplasia/carcinoma of cervix[b] |
| • Vulvovaginitis | • Candidiasis |
| • Ulcer | • Herpes simplex,[b] syphilis |
| • Rectal mass | • Lymphoma[a] |
| **Neurologic** | |
| • Decreased cognition Psychomotor slowing Ataxia Hypo- or hyperreflexia Hypesthesia/paresthesia Focal deficit | • HIV encephalopathy,[a] CNS opportunistic infection,[a] CNS lymphoma[a]; HIV myelopathy or neuropathy; acute HIV infection |

Low immune function can be suspected from any one of the following physical findings: cachexia, thrush, oral hairy leukoplakia, retinal cotton wool spots, marked new facial seborrhea, or extragenital molluscum.
[a] AIDS-defining condition.
[b] Possible AIDS-defining condition.
*From Fisher (1995).*

## TABLE 37–9.  LABORATORY, SKIN TEST, AND X-RAY EVALUATION SCHEDULE

| Baseline Tests | Routine Follow-up |
|---|---|
| CBC, diff, plt | Repeat every 3–6 months |
| Viral load and T-cell subsets<br>CD4/CD8 ratio | Repeat VL & T-cell subsets every 3–4 months if VL <400 copies/mL; or VL 4–6 weeks after change or initiation of anti-retroviral treatment plan |
| Creatinine, ALT or AST | Repeat every 6–12 months |
| RPR (or VDRL) and FTA-ABS (or MHA-TP) | Repeat RPR every year, or for any STD, or every 6 months if multipartnered unprotected coitus |
| Toxoplasma IgG serology | Repeat every year if negative and CD4 <200 |
| CMV IgG serology | Repeat every year if negative and CD4 <200 |
| Hep B serology: HbsAg, sAb, and cAb IgG | Repeat every year if negative; offer Hep B vaccine if negative |
| Hep C serology | Repeat every year if negative |
| UA | Repeat every year |
| PPD with ≥2 control skin tests (± histoplasmin + coccidiodin) Note: +PPD = 5 mm | Repeat every year if PPD negative |
| Pap smear | Repeat every 6 months |
| GC and *Chlamydia* screen | Repeat prn or every 6 months if multipartnered unprotected coitus |
| Chest x-ray | Repeat prn symptoms |

*Adapted from Fisher (1995, p. 12).*

tion Service (ATIS) (Email: ATIS@CDCNAC. ASPENSYS.COM).

## Outcomes Management

### *Selection of an agent and pharmacoeconomic issues*

REVERSE TRANSCRIPTASE INHIBITORS. *Nucleoside analogues* interfere with DNA synthesis by inhibiting reverse transcriptase. Termination of DNA synthesis prevents the virus from replicating and therefore causes viral stasis. In the time since the development of zidovudine (ZDV, AZT), four other drugs in this class have been approved for human use: zalcitabine (ddC), didanosine (ddI), stavudine (d4T), and lamivudine (3TC). The reason for the continued development of drugs in this class is that all have limitations due to various toxicities and that they lack long-term efficacy, which may partly be due to development of resistance (American Foundation for AIDS Research [AmFAR], 1997).

NONNUCLEOSIDE TRANSCRIPTASE INHIBITORS. Reverse transcriptase can be inhibited by agents that are

not nucleoside analogues (Lipsky, 1996). The principal limitation of non-nucleoside reverse transcriptase inhibitors (NNRTIs) is the rapid development of viral resistance, which is seen both in cell culture systems and in patients on therapy. Combination therapy with a nucleoside analogue tends to slow down the development of resistance. The two FDA-approved NNRTIs are nevirapine (Viramune) and delavirdine (Rescriptor) (AmFAR, 1997).

PROTEASE INHIBITORS. Inhibition of the virally produced protease known as "HIV proteinase" provides another therapeutic category for the treatment of HIV infection. Two of the protein products of HIV are precursors that are cleaved to mature protein products. This cleavage is catalyzed by HIV proteinase. The released proteins are crucial for viral replication and include the protease itself as well as RT, integrase, and structural proteins. If these proteins are not cleaved from the precursor proteins, then HIV is noninfectious. Because the protease inhibitors (PIs) act at an entirely different site in the viral life cycle than the reverse transcriptase inhibitors, the PIs in combination with the nucleoside analogues demonstrate at least additive and often synergistic activity against HIV. The principal limitations of PIs are poor bioavailability with gastrointestinal distress (saquinavir [second generation with improved bioavailability, 1998]), gastrointestinal intolerance (ritonavir), nephrolithiasis (indinavir), and diarrhea (nelfinavir) (AmFAR, 1997; Lipsky, 1996). Because the PIs are metabolized in the liver and some are potent inhibitors of an important hepatic enzyme system (cytochrome P-450), there is the potential for drug-drug interactions with other compounds metabolized by or affecting this system. Cross-resistance between reverse transcriptase inhibitors and PIs does not appear to exist but cross-resistance between PIs may exist (AmFAR, 1997).

**Treatment options.**    The initial medication regimen (adapted from Johns Hopkins University AIDS Service, 1997, and CDC, 1998c) is described in Table 37–10.

Combinations of antiretroviral medications require an understanding of the side effects and possible drug interactions as well as the combinations that have had favorable experience.

A change in pharmacotherapy should be recommended when a therapeutic failure, as defined by provider and patient, occurs. The *preferred goal of treatment* is no detectable virus as indicated by the plasma viral load test. *Modified goals of treatment* are a significant decrease in viral load, a stable CD4 cell count, or no new AIDS-defining illness. When making changes in therapy, consultation with a provider who has significant experience in HIV-related care is recommended (Johns Hopkins University AIDS Service, 1997).

**Opportunistic diseases.**    Prophylaxis and treatment of opportunistic infections remain important elements in managing HIV disease. See Table 37–11. The Centers for Disease Control and Prevention (CDC) guidelines for prevention of opportunistic infections are an excellent source of information about prophylaxis. Recommendations for treating specific opportunistic diseases and the major symptoms of HIV/AIDS are available from sources such as Fisher (1995), Goldschmidt and Dong (1997), AmFAR (1997), AIDS Clinical Trials Information Service (1-800-TRIALS-A; web site: http://www.actis.org), and Johns Hopkins University AIDS Service (1997).

---

**TABLE 37–10. RECOMMENDED ANTIRETROVIRAL AGENTS FOR TREATMENT OF ESTABLISHED HIV INFECTION**

- Preferred: Strong evidence of clinical benefit and sustained suppression of plasma viral load: One choice each from Column A and Column B. Drugs are listed in random, not priority, order.

| Column A | Column B |
|---|---|
| Indinavir | ZDV + ddI |
| Nelfinavir | d4T + ddI |
| Ritonavir | ZDV + ddC |
| Ritonavir + Saquinavir | ZDV + 3TC |
|  | d4T + 3TC |

- Alternative: Less likely to provide sustained virus suppression:
  1 NNRTI (Nevirapine) + 2 NRTIs (Column B above)
  Saquinavir (hard gel capsule) + 2 NRTIs (Column B above)

- Not generally recommended: Clinical benefit demonstrated but initial virus suppression is not sustained in most patients:
  2 NRTIs (Column B)

- Not recommended: Evidence against use, virologically undesirable, or overlapping toxicity:
  All monotherapies, d4T + ZDV, ddC + ddI, ddC + d4T, ddC + 3TC

*From Johns Hopkins University AIDS Service (1997) and CDC (1998c).*

## TABLE 37–11. PROPHYLAXIS OF OPPORTUNISTIC INFECTIONS

| Pathogen | Indication | First Choice | Alternative |
|---|---|---|---|
| *Pneumocystis carinii* pneumonia (PCP) | • CD4 count <200/mm³<br>• Unexplained fever >2 weeks<br>• Thrush | • TMP-SMX, 1 DS q.d. | • TMP-SMX, 1 SS q.d. or 1 DS 3×/week<br>• Dapsone, 100 mg/d<br>• Aerosolized pentamidine 300 mg q month<br>• Regimen for toxoplasmosis |
| *Mycobacterium tuberculosis* | • PPD with >5-mm induration<br>• Prior positive PPD without treatment<br>• Contact with active TB | • INH, 300 mg/d + pyridoxine 50 mg/d × 12 months<br>• INH, 900 mg + pyridoxine, 50 mg 2× weekly × 12 months | • Rifampin, 600 mg/d × 12 months |
| *Toxoplasma gondii* | • IgG antibody to *T. gondii* + CD4 count <100/mm³ | • TMP-SMX, 1 DS q.d. | • TMP-SMX, 1 SS q.d. or 1 DS 3 × week<br>• Dapsone, 50 mg/d + pyrimethamine, 50 mg/week + leucovorin, 25 mg/week<br>• Dapsone, 200 mg/week + pyrimethamine 75 mg/week + leucovorin, 25 mg/week |
| *Mycobacterium avium* | • CD4 count <50/mm³ | • Clarithromycin, 500 mg q.d. or b.i.d.<br>• Azithromycin, 1000–1200 mg/week | • Rifabutin, 300 mg/d |
| *Streptococcus pneumoniae* | • All patients with CD4 count >200/mm³ | • Pneumovax, 0.1 mL IM q 6 years | |

Adapted from Johns Hopkins University AIDS Service (1997).

Dr. Anthony Japour (1996) and other experts suggest that treatment decisions should be based on a mutual agreement between the patient and the provider. The challenges of managing HIV disease include selection of antiretroviral drugs, offering prophylaxis against opportunistic diseases, treating the major complications of advanced HIV disease (AIDS), and providing comprehensive primary care. 1997 recommendations from DHHS support utilization of triple-drug antiretroviral therapy early in the course of HIV infection.

Antiretroviral and prophylactic/suppressive agents' costs range from $10,000 to $20,000/year. Some clients have a third-party payor, but others do not. Resources for financial assistance include the local health department's drug assistance program, community-based AIDS service organizations, research protocols, pharmaceutical companies' compassionate care programs, and local social service departments (Commonwealth of Virginia Department of Health, 1997; Wiese, 1997).

***Monitoring for efficacy.*** HIV-infected patients with CD4 cell counts greater than 500 do not appear to be at any greater risk than other immunocompetent patients of developing unusual or serious illness. As HIV begins to weaken the immune system, patients develop innocuous, self-limited problems, eg, more frequent outbreaks of herpes simplex and skin changes such as exacerbations of eczema, psoriasis, and seborrhea. Education can help patients distinguish these symptoms from the more potentially serious ones listed in Table 37–12.

When an immunocompromised patient with potentially serious symptoms presents, the primary care provider needs to determine the differential diagnosis, appropriate workup, and

## TABLE 37–12. SYMPTOMS REQUIRING MEDICAL ATTENTION

Fever greater than 103°F
Fever greater than 101°F for 3 days or more
Shortness of breath
Productive cough
Persistent headache
Seizures or loss of consciousness
Visual changes
Change in mental status
Localized weakness, paralysis, or change in balance or sensation
Persistent diarrhea
Unusual bleeding

*Adapted from Hecht and Soloway (1994, p. 53).*

therapeutic interventions discussed earlier in this chapter (Hecht & Soloway, 1994).

Ongoing studies are being performed to help determine the optimal guidelines for monitoring viral load and CD4 cell count. Currently, the viral load and CD4 cell count should be monitored every 3–4 months if the CD4 cell count is less than 400 or every 4–6 weeks following initiation of treatment or changes in treatment regimen. Decreases in viral load measurements by threefold or 0.5 log can be interpreted as beneficial effects of therapies, whereas rises of threefold or 0.5 log or more can indicate progressive disease and possible pharmacotherapeutic failure (Goldsmith & Dong, 1997).

***Follow-up recommendations.*** The follow-up recommendations for clients with HIV infection are based on the clinical picture. Follow-up is needed every 3–6 months when the patient is asymptomatic, every 2–3 months when symptomatic and stable, and monthly when symptomatic with ongoing problems (Fisher, E. J., personal communication, March 1997).

## HIV/AIDS IN CHILDREN

HIV infections in children and adults have several common physiologic mechanisms and several unique ones. Readers are encouraged to review the section in this chapter on adults with HIV infection for a general orientation to the condition.

In the United States, pediatric HIV infection has become the seventh leading cause of death in children 1–14 years old. In just a short few years it has become the leading cause of death in preschool children 2–5 years old (Butz, Joyner, Friedman, & Hutton, 1998). Children's unique physiology changes the consideration for drug treatment. This section of the chapter addresses those differences. The majority of children with HIV infection and AIDS are managed by specialty providers because of their complex treatment needs. However, primary care providers are involved in the ongoing primary care of almost all children and need to be aware of the treatment, the unique acute care issues of this population, and the current state of knowledge regarding the presentations and treatment approaches for children with this condition. In addition, fewer than half of the parents or caregivers of these children reveal the nature of the illness to the child (Funck-Brentano et al, 1997). The psychologic treatment and coping issues of both family and child play a central role in the treatment of children with HIV/AIDS. The primary care provider, working closely with a specialty provider, can be a central team member in the care of these children.

HIV is transmitted to children in several ways. The most prevalent is perinatal, or vertical, transmission. This mechanism is suspected to include transmission transplacentally in utero, during delivery by exposure to blood and vaginal secretions, and after delivery if there is ingestion of infected breast milk (Fahrner & Benson, 1996). Maternal, fetal, placental, obstetric, neonatal, and viral factors influence this mother-to-infant transmission. The second most common transmission is from contaminated blood and blood products and factors given between 1978 and 1985. The safeguards instituted in 1985 have eliminated almost all transmission caused by this mechanism. For a small number of children sexual abuse is the overlooked cause of HIV transmission (Butz, Joyner, Friedman, & Hutton, 1998).

The current CDC HIV classification system for children has two components: immunologic categories based on age-specific CD4 lymphocyte counts and percentages as delineated in Table 37–13 and clinical categories as delineated in Table 37–14. Thus, children are classified into different categories based on a matrix of their symptoms and their immune status. Symptoms are classified as none (N), mild (A), moderate (B), or severe (C), and immune status is classified as no evidence of suppression (1), evidence of moderate immune suppression (2), and evi-

**TABLE 37–13. 1994 REVISED PEDIATRIC HIV CLASSIFICATION SYSTEM: IMMUNOLOGIC CATEGORIES BASED ON AGE-SPECIFIC CD4+ LYMPHOCYTE COUNT AND PERCENTAGE**

| | Age of Child | | | | | |
|---|---|---|---|---|---|---|
| | <12 months | | 1–5 years | | 6–12 years | |
| Immune Category | Number/µL | (%) | Number/µL | (%) | Number/µL | (%) |
| Category 1: no suppression | ≥1,500 | (≥25%) | ≥1,000 | (≥25%) | ≥500 | (≥25%) |
| Category 2: moderate suppression | 750–1,499 | (15–24%) | 500–999 | (15–24%) | 200–499 | (15–24%) |
| Category 3: severe suppression | <750 | (<15%) | <500 | (<15%) | <200 | (<15%) |

*Modified from CDC (1998b).*

dence of severe immune suppression (3). Thus, a child with moderate symptoms and evidence of moderate immune suppression would be classified B2 (Fahrner & Benson, 1996; CDC, 1998b).

The vertically infected fetus has an immature immune system. Although the T-cell immune system is relatively well developed, their B-cell system is immature. This causes the infant to have trouble forming adequate antibodies, which can become problematic for some infants early in life. This mechanism puts them at higher susceptibility to bacterial infections than adults with HIV infection. Opportunistic infections such as *Pneumocystis carinii* pneumonia (PCP) are common.

### Specific Considerations for Pharmacotherapy

***Need for drug therapy and rationale.*** HIV is now being seen by many experts as a chronic disease that (though at times life-threatening) is also treatable (Fahrner & Benson, 1996). Since the majority of children with HIV have vertically transmitted conditions, their demographics parallel those of their mothers. Their care is often complicated by the treatment of one or more of their parents. A national study in 1994 (CDC, 1994) dramatically changed the fabric of the HIV quilt for children. The double-blind clinical trial found zidovudine (AZT) given to the mother prenatally dramatically reduced the incidence of children born with HIV. The transmission rate for those who took the placebo was 26% and for those who took zidovudine was 8% (CDC, 1994). Studies are now underway to test altered dose and length of treatment patterns. The current data do suggest that even treatment late in pregnancy has some beneficial effect. Thus, treatment can be initiated at any time in pregnancy that an HIV-positive mother seeks prenatal care (CDC, 1998a). However, prenatal treatment is also a complex issue with unknown effects of prenatal AZT on mother, fetus, or newborn. Although data on children now 2 years old who were treated in the prenatal period show no untoward effects, the long-term effects are unknown. The current guidelines caution that the discussion of treatment options and recommendations should be noncoercive and that the final decision is the responsibility of the woman. A decision not to choose prenatal treatment should not result in punitive action or denial of care. On the other hand, the decision of the mother previously on multitherapy who chooses only to use AZT to avoid exposure of the fetus to other antiviral drugs during pregnancy should also be respected (CDC, 1998a).

Treatment of HIV/AIDS in children has the same goals as in adults: to control the replication of the HIV virus, thus slowing the progression of the condition, and to treat the opportunistic infections and other associated problems that accompany this condition. In addition, most children need supportive therapy to control other complications of the condition.

***Short-term and long-term goals of pharmacotherapy.*** As in adults the short-term goals are to control the viral load (HIV RNA) and to improve immune status (CD4 count). The long-term goals are to delay disease progression, prevent opportunistic infections, and make a positive impact on the quality and length of life.

## TABLE 37–14. 1994 REVISED HIV PEDIATRIC CLASSIFICATION SYSTEM: CLINICAL CATEGORIES

**Category N: Not Symptomatic**
Children who have no signs or symptoms considered to be the result of HIV infection or who have only one of the conditions listed in Category A

**Category A: Mildly Symptomatic**
Children with two or more of the conditions listed below but none of the conditions listed in Categories B and C:
Lymphadenopathy (≥0.5 cm at more than two sites; bilateral = one site)
Hepatomegaly
Splenomegaly
Dermatitis
Parotitis
Recurrent or persistent upper respiratory infection, sinusitis, or otitis media

**Category B: Moderately Symptomatic**
Children who have symptomatic conditions other than those listed for Category A or C that are attributed to HIV infection. Examples of conditions in clinical Category B include but are not limited to:
Anemia (<8 gm/dL), neutropenia (<1,000/mm$^3$), or thrombocytopenia (<100,000/mm$^3$) persisting ≥30 days
Bacterial meningitis, pneumonia, or sepsis (single episode)
Candidiasis, oropharyngeal (thrush) persisting (>2 months) in children >6 months of age
Cardiomyopathy
Cytomegalovirus infection, with onset before 1 month of age
Diarrhea, recurrent or chronic
Hepatitis
Herpes simplex virus (HSV) stomatitis, recurrent (more than two episodes within 1 year)
HSV bronchitis, pneumonitis, or esophagitis with onset before 1 month of age
Herpes zoster (shingles) involving at least two distinct episodes or more than one dermatome
Leiomyosarcoma
Lymphoid interstitial pneumonia (LIP) or pulmonary lymphoid hyperplasia complex
Nephropathy
Nocardiosis
Persistent fever (lasting >1 month)
Toxoplasmosis, onset before 1 month of age
Varicella, disseminated (complicated chickenpox)

**Category C: Severely Symptomatic**
Children who have any condition listed in the 1987 surveillance case definition for acquired immunodeficiency syndrome, with the exception of LIP (which is a Category B condition)

*Modified from CDC (1998b).*

## Prevention and nonpharmacologic therapy for HIV/ AIDS and opportunistic infections

**PREVENTION.** Prevention of this condition can be accomplished by (1) prevention of spread of the disease in the mother (see adult section), (2) prenatal screening and treatment of HIV-positive mothers, (3) education regarding the need for HIV-positive mothers to refrain from breastfeeding, and (4) continual efforts to assure the quality of blood products. In addition, there are many barriers to early initiation of prenatal care by at-risk mothers. Programs that address barriers to obtaining this care such as access, transportation, child care, and the stigma of being HIV-positive need to be implemented to facilitate women receiving early prenatal care.

Prevention of opportunistic infections should be a major focus of anticipatory guidance for families with HIV-positive children. Adults and older children in the home need to understand the details of prevention. The infant's formula needs to be prepared and stored with aseptic technique. At each feeding unused formula should be discarded. Older children are at risk from undercooked food and cross-contamination of foods. Fresh fruits and vegetables need to be thoroughly washed, and raw or uncooked eggs should be avoided. Family members need to be taught to use frequent hand washing and to frequently clean kitchen surfaces where food is prepared. Exposure to pets and farm animals may also pose a risk. At the least, HIV-positive children should not care for pets in the home or farm animals, and some families may decide to remove pets or animals from their environment (Butz et al, 1998).

In addition, the child needs to be taught to avoid contact with the bodily fluids of others and to use good hand-washing techniques. Prevention issues addressed in the section on adults of this chapter relative to sexuality need to be discussed with young adolescents. Many families are still struggling with informing the school-age child of his or her HIV status (Funck-Brentano et al, 1997). Regardless of the child's knowledge of HIV status, the child and others in the family can be taught effective preventive strategies. Primary care providers need to problem-solve with the adults in the family to achieve the optimal environment to prevent secondary infections.

It is extremely important in this population to prevent the development of drug resistance. Lack of adherence to prescribed regimens or subtherapeutic levels of the medication could cause resistance. There are some data to the effect that development of resistance to one protease inhibitor may reduce the effectiveness of other protease inhibitors. Parents and adult caregivers need to realistically discuss the ability to carry out the proposed regimen. Liquid formulations of these drugs can be distasteful. Absorption of some drugs can be affected by food, and attempting to create a schedule for infants and young children may be very challenging. Other barriers such as family stressors may also challenge these families. In addition, if there are

disclosure issues either to the child or the community, there may be consequences for drug schedules. Families may be hesitant to fill the prescription at the local pharmacy, may hide or relabel the medication in an attempt to maintain secrecy at home, or may skip the midday dose in order not to have to take the medication to school (CDC, 1998b). In addition, some families may be struggling with survival issues such as obtaining adequate food or housing or creating a safe environment. These issues may take priority over medication administration. The assessment of each family's stressors and support issues may be most effectively done by the primary care provider if a long-term relationship exists. Communication with the interdisciplinary team managing the HIV treatment is crucial.

Immunizations, a preventive strategy, should be aggressively used with HIV-positive children. Most of the routine childhood immunizations are given on schedule (see Table 11–1, Chap. 11). Primary care providers should also make the substitutions and additions outlined in Table 37–15. Inactivated polio vaccine (IPV) should be used instead of oral polio vaccine (OPV) for the HIV-positive child and all other household contacts to protect both the child and other HIV-positive persons in the home. The other potential substitution is the use of TIG in case of injury.

Several additions to the routine immunization schedule are important for HIV-positive children. Influenza virus vaccines should be added. The first should be at or just after 6 months of age, with a second influenza vaccine given 1 month after the first and annual immunizations on the anniversary of the first influenza vaccine. The pneumococcal vaccine should be added at 2 years, and the varicella vaccine is currently being studied in HIV-positive children (Butz et al, 1998; Fahrner & Benson, 1996; Gershon et al, 1997).

**NONPHARMACOLOGIC THERAPY FOR HIV/AIDS AND OPPORTUNISTIC INFECTIONS.** Either mother or child may need nutritional support for associated problems such as failure to thrive. Each visit is an opportunity to monitor the child's growth and development. Growth charts need to be monitored closely for any sign of the child falling out of his or her growth curve. Nutritional support is an important intervention that can impact immune function, quality of life, and bioactivity of antiretroviral drugs.

The child will need neurodevelopmental testing to address the neurologic impacts of the

**TABLE 37–15. CHANGES IN IMMUNIZATION SCHEDULE FOR HIV-POSITIVE CHILDREN**

| Type of Change | Immunization | Recommendation |
|---|---|---|
| Substitutions | Polio | Substitute IPV for oral polio for all scheduled immunizations |
| Substitutions | DTP | Consider giving tetanus immunoglobulin (TIG) to child at risk of infection due to injury |
| Additions | Influenza | Give influenza virus vaccine 1 at or just after 6 months of age |
| | | Give influenza virus vaccine 2 at 1 month after first influenza virus vaccine |
| | | Give influenza virus annually in 12-month intervals (ie, at 1½, 2½, 3½, and each subsequent year) |
| Additions | Pneumococcal vaccine | Administer after age 2 years |
| Additions | Varicella-zoster vaccine | Vaccine use is controversial and under study but currently not recommended[a,b]; varicella-zoster immune globulin is recommended within 72 h of exposure[c] |
| No change | HBV, DPT, HIB, MMR, DTaP | As scheduled unless changed by above; see Chap. 11 (immunizations) |

The following sources were used for this table: [a] Butz et al (1998), [b] Gershon et al (1997), and [c] Fahrner and Benson (1996).

disease and may need special services in school for developmental delay or learning disability. An interdisciplinary team will be needed to address the physical, financial, and psychosocial issues common in families with a member who is HIV-positive. Close collaboration with the primary care provider will yield optimal care for the family.

***Time frame for initiation of therapy.*** The current protocol for treatment of known HIV-positive mothers is as follows:

• Oral prenatal treatment of the mother at 14–34 weeks' gestation with 100 mg of zidovudine five times a day continued throughout pregnancy. If compliance is an issue, treatment with 200 mg t.i.d. or 300 mg b.i.d. should be considered (Mulder et al., 1994). Comparable clinical response with twice daily dosing has also been seen in clinical trials (Cooper et al, 1993; Mulder et al, 1994). Recent studies in developing countries have shown responses to even a shorter course

of treatment. However, optimal recommendations in our country support the longer treatment, five times a day if possible (CDC, 1998c).

• IV zidovudine during labor, with a 1-h loading dose of 2 mg/kg given IV over 1 h followed by 1 mg/kg per hour IV infusion until delivery. The infant is treated as soon as possible, optimally within the first 8–12 h of life with zidovudine 2 mg/kg every 6 h until 6 weeks of age. Small-for-gestational-age babies and others who might be NPO can be treated by IV infusion of 1.5 mg/kg of zidovudine infused every 6 h (Fahrner & Benson, 1996; CDC, 1998b).

• If infants are definitely identified as HIV-positive while on zidovudine prophylaxis, they are candidates to be changed to a combination antiretroviral drug (see Table 37–16).

Since opportunistic infections are the major threat to the HIV-exposed infant and young child, early initiation of prophylaxis is indicated. The CDC (1994 and 1998b) has indicated that no prophylaxis of HIV-exposed infants is needed

## TABLE 37–16. RECOMMENDED ANTIRETROVIRAL REGIMENS FOR INITIAL THERAPY FOR HUMAN IMMUNODEFICIENCY VIRUS (HIV) INFECTION IN CHILDREN

**Preferred Regimen**

Evidence of clinical benefit and sustained suppression of HIV RNA in clinical trials in HIV-infected adults; clinical trials in HIV-infected children are ongoing.

- One highly active protease inhibitor plus two nucleoside analogue reverse transcriptase inhibitors (NRTIs)
  - Preferred protease inhibitor for infants and children who cannot swallow pills or capsules: nelfinavir or ritonavir. Alternative for children who can swallow pills or capsules: indinavir.
  - Recommended dual NRTI combinations: the most data on use in children are available for the combinations of zidovudine (ZDV) and didanosine (ddI) and for ZDV and lamivudine (3TC). More limited data are available for the combinations of stavudine (d4T) and ddI, d4T and 3TC, and ZDV and zalcitabine (ddC)[a]

**Alternative Regimen**

Less likely to produce sustained HIV RNA suppression in infected adults; the combination of nevirapine, ZDV, and ddI produced substantial and sustained suppression of viral replication in two of six infants first treated at age <4 months.

- Nevirapine[b] and two NRTIs

**Secondary Alternative Regimen**

Clinical benefit demonstrated in clinical trials involving infected adults and/or children, but initial viral suppression may not be sustained.

- Two NRTIs

**Not Recommended**

Evidence against use because of overlapping toxicity and/or because use may be virologically undesirable.

- Any monotherapy[c]
- d4T and ZDV
- ddC and ddI
- ddC and d4T
- ddC and 3TC

[a] ddC is not available in a liquid preparation commercially, although a liquid formulation is available through a compassionate use program of the manufacturer (Hoffman-LaRoche Inc., Nutley, New Jersey). ZDV and ddC is a less preferred choice for use in combination with a protease inhibitor.
[b] A liquid preparation of nevirapine is not available commercially, but is available through a compassionate use program of the manufacturer (Boehringer Ingelheim Pharmaceuticals, Inc., Ridgefield, Connecticut).
[c] Except for ZDV chemoprophylaxis administered to HIV-exposed infants during the first 6 weeks of life to prevent perinatal HIV transmission; if an infant is identified as HIV-infected while receiving ZDV prophylaxis, therapy should be changed to a combination antiretroviral drug regimen.
*From CDC (1998b).*

in the first 6 weeks of life due to the low incidence of the major opportunistic infection (PCP), the well-established adverse side effects of sulfa drugs in infants under 6 weeks, and the unknown interactions for infants on zidovudine during the first 6 weeks of life. Prophylaxis should be initiated at 6 weeks of life. If the HIV-exposed infant is determined to be HIV-infected or if the laboratory tests are inconclusive, prophylaxis with sulfa should be continued until 1 year (see the assessment section). After one year of age the continuation of sulfa will be determined by the CD4 count. From 1–5 years old, prophylaxis is continued if the CD4 count is less than 500 or the CD4% is less than 15%. From 6–12 years of age prophylaxis is continued if the CD4 count is less than 200 or CD4% less than 15%.

***Assessment needed prior to therapy.*** A complete history and physical examination (see Tables 37–7 and 37–8) using the systems appropriate for newborns, infants, children, and young adolescents should be done on each visit. Laboratory tests are crucial to the optimal treatment of this condition. HIV can be definitively diagnosed in most infants at 1 month of age, and for virtually all infants by 6 months of age. Positive HIV culture or DNA or RNA polymerase chain reactions (PCR) indicate HIV infection. HIV DNA PCR is the preferred test. HIV RNA may be more sensitive in HIV-exposed infants, but data are limited. HIV culture is more complex and expensive and may take 2–4 weeks to get results. Repeat testing should be done as soon as possible to confirm the diagnosis. In children of HIV-positive mothers testing should be done by 48 h of age. For those who test negative, repeat testing needs to be done at 1–2 months of age and 3–6 months of age. Testing at 14 days of age is also common. Testing is done at 48 h since 40% of infants can be identified at this time. Cord blood samples should not be used. A child is diagnosed with HIV if two virologic tests done on separate blood samples are positive (CDC, 1998b). A child with no symptoms and two or more negative HIV tests done a month apart after 6 months of life can reasonably exclude HIV. Negative testing in an asymptomatic child at 18 months of life can definitely rule out HIV. The testing pattern used at Virginia Commonwealth University's HIV/AIDS Center is typical, testing at birth, 6 weeks, and 6 months with PCR DNA, and at 15–18 months with the HIV antibody test.

***Patient/caregiver information.*** See the section on adults for a discussion of resources. The National Pediatric HIV Resource Center (800-362-0071) has useful resources for families. Families and caregivers with HIV-positive children will need continual and repeated instruction and support. Often families are dealing with the illness or death of the child's mother simultaneously. The primary care provider must know the ever-changing treatment picture for these children. Most providers accomplish this by keeping in close contact with the HIV center.

## Outcomes Management

***Selection of an agent and pharmacoeconomic issues.*** See the section on adults for an introductory discussion of the current approaches to treatment

of HIV, the categories of drugs (reverse transcriptase inhibitors including nucleoside analogues and non-nucleoside analogues as well as protease inhibitors) and an overview of treatment using these drugs.

INITIAL TREATMENT. Antiviral therapy is recommended for HIV-infected children with any clinical symptoms or any evidence of immune suppression (see Tables 37–12, 37–13, and 37–14). The consensus guidelines indicate most members would recommend starting treatment in HIV-positive children under 12 months of age as soon as the diagnosis is confirmed, regardless of clinical or immunologic status (CDC, 1998b). It is felt that the sooner the treatment is started, the sooner the suppression can "get started." Frequently children are symptomatic at a young age and the majority of those not symptomatic over 1 year of age have a CD4 lymphocyte percentage of 25%, which is indicative of immunosuppression (see Table 37–12) (Butz et al, 1998; CDC, 1998b). If therapy is deferred, the laboratory and clinical values should be monitored closely and treatment initiated with increasing HIV RNA levels, declining CD4 lymphocyte count, or clinical deterioration.

Until recently, children were treated only with monotherapy. Recently pediatric trials have demonstrated that combination therapy with either zidovudine (ZDV) and lamivudine (3TC) or ZDV and didanosine (ddI) are superior to monotherapy with either ddI or ZDV. In addition, there is evidence that combination therapy that includes a protease inhibitor is superior to just dual nucleoside combination therapy (Butz et al, 1998; CDC, 1998b). If the families are able to consistently implement the complex treatment plan using a three-drug combination, a better outcome is achieved. It is felt the combination therapy slows the progress of the disease, results in a larger and sustained virologic change, and delays the development of resistant mutations. Most clinicians would recommend aggressive antiretroviral therapy using a three-drug combination (see Table 37–16). The Working Group (CDC, 1998b) has recommended that all antiviral drugs approved for treatment of HIV in adults may be used in children, when indicated, irrespective of labeling notations.

CHANGES IN TREATMENT. The Working Group (CDC, 1998b) identified three main reasons to change therapy: First, if there is a failure of the current regimen evidenced by virologic, immunologic or clinical parameters; second, if toxicity or intolerance develops; or third, if new data suggest a superior drug regimen. Assessing the failure of treatment is complex (CDC, 1998b).

Virologic response issues suggesting change include the following:

- When the virologic response after 8–12 weeks of therapy is not acceptable, a change in combination treatment should be considered. For children on aggressive therapy taking two NRTIs and a PI, this is defined as less than a tenfold ($1.0 \log_{10}$) decrease from the pretreatment viral load or HIV RNA levels.

- For children on less potent therapy such as two NRTIs the criteria for unacceptable response is less than a fivefold ($0.7 \log_{10}$) decrease in viral load. It should be noted that all measurements should be done at least twice, a week apart, before considering a change.

- Treatment change should also be considered if HIV RNA levels are not optimal at 4–6 months. The HIV RNA should be suppressed to an undetectable level after 4–6 months of an antiviral therapy and most would recommend change if that was not achieved. However, the panel also indicated that the pretreatment HIV RNA had to be taken into account. If the HIV RNA is at a relatively low level and it had fallen 1.5 to 2.0 $\log_{10}$, close observation might be considered. A careful assessment of the barriers to full adherence to the treatment plan should also be conducted.

- Treatment change should also be considered in children who had repeated detection of HIV RNA but a history of initial response to medication with undetectable levels.

Immunologic and clinical issues suggesting change include:

- Worsening of immunologic or clinical classification
- Rapid decline in absolute CD4 count (>30% in less than 6 months)
- Worsening of clinical symptoms including growth failure

Changing of antiretroviral therapy is a complex decision. For some children there may be unique considerations even when they meet the above criteria. Consultation with HIV specialists and reviewing the most recent recommendations for therapy is recommended before initiating such a change (CDC, 1998b).

**TREATMENT OF OPPORTUNISTIC INFECTIONS.** Numerous opportunistic infections need to be treated. The clinician needs to assess all illness of HIV-positive children quickly and treat it aggressively. The antibiotic choice for infections such as otitis media, sinusitis, or urinary tract infection needs to be based on cultures or the most likely organism. It is not appropriate to have a "wait and see" approach for any signs of infections such as fever, increased WBC, tachypnea, or malaise. *Candida* infections of the mouth or diaper area are common and should be treated appropriately (see Chapter 27). Signs of herpes simplex warrant the use of oral or intravenous acyclovir, depending on the severity of the infection, and cytomegalovirus can be treated with oral or intravenous gancyclovir. Whatever the condition, the HIV-positive child needs prompt treatment and close monitoring (Butz et al, 1998).

Trimethoprim-sulfamethoxazole is the first line PCP prophylaxis in children. It can be started at 6 weeks and continued throughout childhood. The major problem with the drug is the frequent IgE-mediated reactions among HIV-positive children. Most studies report a 40% adverse reaction rate (Rieder, King, & Read, 1997). Recent studies have investigated the effect of oral desensitization in both adults and children. Desensitization using a rapid oral protocol was safe in both pediatric and adult populations. However, it was effective in desensitizing non-life-threatening reactions to trimethoprim-sulfamethoxazole in many of the adults (Belchi-Hernandez & Espinosa-Parra, 1996) but in only some of the children (Palusci, Kaul, Lawrence, Haines, & Kwittken, 1996). Currently, the use of atovaquone and azithromycin is being studied as an antiprotozoal drug for mild to moderate PCP in patients unable to tolerate trimethoprim-sulfamethoxazole. Azithromycin is a promising drug because of its extended half-life, relative safety, and once-a-day dosing. The combination of these two drugs may offer useful coverage against the pathogens associated with pediatric diseases (Butz et al, 1998).

### Monitoring for efficacy
**SIGNS AND SYMPTOMS.** Clinical status, growth patterns, and neurodevelopmental status need to be evaluated routinely. Maintaining cognition and growth in the presence of stable laboratory values indicates effective treatment.

**PHYSICAL EXAMINATION FINDINGS.** The continuing development and maturation of organ systems that metabolize and distribute drugs and the impact of the disease in multiple body systems mandate repeated physical examination. The absence of any clinical findings supports the effectiveness of treatment. Any deterioration in clinical status can be assumed to be a potential sign of ineffective treatment.

LABORATORY FINDINGS. The HIV-positive child needs close monitoring for any changes in virologic laboratory tests and any illnesses. Results substantiated by two repeated virologic tests may suggest treatment changes. CD4 counts should improve, or in some cases cease falling. The viral load (DNA HIV) should be undetectable or dramatically reduced. CD4 counts and HIV RNA testing (in children over 3 years) need to be done every 3 months.

In addition, all opportunistic infection indicators need to be followed closely. This may mean obtaining a wide variety of laboratory values. For example, complete blood counts, urine analysis and urine culture, blood or wound cultures, and respiratory function testing may all be indicated to monitor the specific clinical manifestations of a child.

*Monitoring for toxicity.* See the Drug Table 106 for toxicity information. Each drug has a wide range of adverse effects. This is particularly true for drugs administered in the neonatal and early infancy period when there is limited information on pharmacokinetics, doses, and safety of these medications. If the child is responding to the treatment regimen and has mild to moderate adverse reactions, it will be up to the family (and in some instances the child) working with the professionals to determine when or if to change medications. Assess all other medications taken by the child for drug interactions. The Working Group (CDC, 1998b) recommends that all efforts need to be made to continue therapy in the presence of non-life-threatening toxicities. Adjunctive therapies such as granulocyte colony-simulating factor to combat neutropenia and erythropoietin or transfusions to combat anemia can be employed. If the child and family have been able to fully implement the prescribed dosing, assume that drug resistance has developed and change to at least two new antiretroviral agents. If treatment needs to be stopped to reduce the risk of drug resistance, many members of this panel would recommend stopping all antiretroviral drugs at the same time rather than continuing with one or two agents. The issue of quality of life in children with advanced disease needs to be considered by the caregiver and provider in formulating a plan (CDC, 1998b).

*Follow-up recommendations.* It is recommended that children with HIV be followed up at least every 3 months when asymptomatic and more often when there are ongoing problems. In practice, asymptomatic children and adolescents are often followed every 2 months, with symptomatic and young children followed monthly. There may be a "mixed follow-up" model, where the child sees both the primary care provider and the specialists. Providers offering primary care to these families need to be prepared to respond quickly to an ever-changing picture.

# ALLERGIC REACTIONS

## ALLERGIC RESPONSES

An allergy is defined as an adverse physiological reaction of immunologic origin. An allergic reaction must be associated with an antigen relationship between exposure to the antigen and the reaction. Two causes of allergic reactions that will be discussed in this section are (1) drugs and (2) insects. Food allergies will not be discussed, but treatment of food allergic reactions is the same as the treatment of drug and insect reactions. For information pertaining to atopic dermatitis, see Chapter 27 (Dermatologic Disorders); information about latex allergies may be found in Chapter 14.

## ALLERGIC REACTIONS TO DRUGS

Allergic drug reactions account for approximately 6–10% of all observed adverse drug reactions. These data were obtained from hospital and insurance-provider records and therefore do not represent those reactions that are unreported. Because of the limited availability of in vitro and in vivo tests necessary for defining the immune mechanisms of drug reactions, many patients are incorrectly labeled as being allergic to one or more drugs (Bernstein, 1995; Guill, 1991). Therefore, it is important for the primary care provider to better understand the factors that predispose a patient to drug allergies and, in the case of a reaction, the steps to best manage the reaction.

A number of factors may increase the possibility of a patient developing an allergic drug reaction. Such factors include (1) age, (2) atopy, (3) prior drug reactions, and (4) underlying disease. Treatment factors may also increase the chance of a patient developing a drug reaction. These include (1) a drug's molecular weight, (2) its metabolic breakdown products, (3) its ability to form haptens, (4) the route of administration (topical > oral), (5) the frequency of treatment (ie, high doses over a long period of time), and (6) cross-sensitization between structurally homologous drugs (ie, penicillins and cephalosporins) (Bernstein, 1995; Guill, 1991).

When a drug reaction does occur, some criteria that may be helpful in diagnosing such allergies are the following:

1. A reaction unlike any known pharmacologic reaction of the drug in question

2. A latent period of 7–10 days after the first administration of the drug

3. A recurrence of a similar reaction after a rechallenge of the same or a related drug (Breathnach, 1995; Guill, 1991).

Some signs and symptoms include urticaria, angioedema, cardiovascular or respiratory compromise, rhinitis, and nausea and vomiting. The eosinophilia may occur, but it is not necessary in the diagnosis of an immunologically mediated reaction (Guill, 1991).

Allergic drug reactions may involve either one organ system (ie, dermatologic, renal, hematologic, hepatic, or lymphoid systems) or may be multisystem (ie, anaphylaxis, serum sickness, drug fever, or vasculitis). Anaphylaxis is the most feared and most life-threatening of all allergic reactions (Guill, 1991).

The drugs that are the most common cause of allergic reactions include penicillins and their derivatives, sulfonamides, nonsteroidal antiinflammatory drugs (NSAIDs), and aspirin. Other examples of drugs that may cause allergic reactions include hydralazine, procainamide, isoniazid, antineoplastic agents, phenytoin, and allopurinol (Adkinson, 1992; Bernstein, 1995; Breathnach, 1995; Guill, 1991).

Allergic reactions to insect stings or snake bites may also vary in intensity and type, depending on the location and number of cells degranulating their mediators. They may range from local irritation, which resolves in a day, to anaphylaxis. They can also range in presentation time of the reactions (ie, minutes to several days). Other miscellaneous causes of allergic reactions, specifically anaphylaxis, include foods, such as nuts and seafood, exercise, and cold temperatures (Zieve, 1995).

## SPECIFIC CONSIDERATIONS FOR PHARMACOTHERAPY

### Need for Drug Therapy and Rationale

The approach to treatment of an established or presumed drug or insect allergic reaction depends on the severity of the reaction. In minor reactions, symptomatic relief is the main goal. Therapy may be delayed for hours to days, depending on the patient's discomfort. For patients who experience more severe reactions, such as anaphylaxis, immediate attention to managing the complication is necessary, since it may be fatal. In these cases, treatment with epinephrine should be initiated while the patient is still in the primary care provider's office (see Table 37–17). If at home, the patient should be instructed to contact EMS in order to be immediately transported to the nearest emergency department.

Patients with a past history of anaphylaxis must have epinephrine available for emergencies at all times: at home, school, camp, on the ball field, or on the parade route if the patient is in a marching band. Anaphylactic reactions can occur at any time. A convenient way to be prepared is with epinephrine autoinjectors (EpiPen). Patients or parents accompanying children are strongly recommended to carry these devices with them. EpiPen is available for adults and children (see Table 37–18). Do not assume that all children need the EpiPen Jr. The dose in the EpiPen Jr. may not be sufficient for older children. All children over 44 lb need to use the adult EpiPen. It is preferable to give a slightly higher dose than an

---

### TABLE 37–17. EPINEPHRINE DOSING

| | Epinephrine Dose |
|---|---|
| Children | 0.01 mg/kg (0.1 mL/kg of 1:10,000) SC—may repeat every 15–20 min as needed |
| Adults | 0.2–0.5 mg (0.2–0.5 mL of 1:1000) IM or SC—may repeat every 15–20 min as needed |

| TABLE 37-18.  EPIPEN AND EPIPEN JR. DOSING | | |
|---|---|---|
| EpiPen | Delivers 0.3 mg IM of epinephrine 1:1000 (2 mL) | May repeat every 20 min to 4 h |
| EpiPen Jr. | Delivers 0.15 mg IM of epinephrine 1:2000 (2 mL) | May repeat every 15 min for two doses, then every 4 h as needed |

insufficiently low dose (Wood, 1997). Two other brands, Ana-Kit and AnaGuard, are also available, but some experts suggest that the EpiPens are easier to administer (Wood, 1997). The Ana-Kits come in a box and have to be assembled. However, they contain more than one dose of epinephrine. These products usually have an expiration date of 1 year. The clinician needs to reassess the patient's plan and review the expiration date annually. The cost of these products vary from $40–$60. For families without insurance coverage where cost prohibits the family from obtaining these products, sponsorships from church or other community organizations should be sought.

After the first dose of any of these products, the patient should be immediately transported to the emergency department, in case the reaction worsens and the patient requires intravenous therapy with epinephrine, aminophylline, dopamine, norepinephrine, and fluids.

## Short-Term and Long-Term Goals of Pharmacotherapy

The short-term goal of treatment for an allergic reaction is the management of the signs and symptoms. The long-term goal is the consideration of immunotherapy in a patient with a known drug or insect sting allergy. An example of when this may be considered is in an HIV-infected patient who may require treatment or prophylaxis with trimethoprim-sulfamethoxazole and has a known allergic reaction to trimethoprim-sulfamethoxazole.

## Nonpharmacologic Therapy for Allergic Reaction Therapy and Prevention

The following measures should be taken for allergic drug reaction therapy and prevention:

- Discontinue the drug immediately.
- Avoid rough clothing over affected areas.
- Bathe in cool water.

- Avoid scratching affected areas.

  Preventive measures for individuals allergic to insect stings include the following:

- Outdoor activities that involve food should be engaged in cautiously.
- Keep garbage and food covered.
- Always wear long pants tucked into socks and shoes when in grass and field areas.
- Perfumes and brightly colored clothes should not be worn outdoors.
- Always apply insect repellant sprays.

## Time Frame for Initiating Pharmacotherapy

For minor reactions, pharmacologic therapy may be deferred for hours to days, depending on the discomfort of the patient. In the case of severe reactions, the patient should be sent immediately to the emergency room for care, since intravenous drug therapy will probably be necessary.

## Assessment Needed Prior to Therapy

The skin is the organ most commonly affected by allergic reactions; therefore, it should be examined carefully before determining an appropriate treatment. Exanthems, urticaria, angioedema, and contact dermatitis are the most common cutaneous reactions. The first signs of anaphylaxis are often flushing and pruritus. The cutaneous manifestations are most marked on the face, palms, and soles of the feet. Itching is most intense on the head, palms, and soles. Progression to hives and angioedema usually occurs (Wood, 1997). Respiratory symptoms can involve both the upper and lower airways.

Pulmonary manifestations, such as coughing, wheezing, dyspnea, and cyanosis, may also be the result of an allergic reaction. Patients with underlying airway disease may be at the highest risk due to lower airway complications (Wood, 1997). Given the possible seriousness of this type of manifestation, a lung examination should be immediately performed when an allergic reaction is suspected.

Other organ systems that may also be affected include the renal, hepatic, and hematologic systems, but this occurs more infrequently. Depending on the suspected drug, the provider may consider some blood tests, including a complete blood count (CBC), serum creatinine, BUN, or liver function tests.

There are no disease states that would preclude the treatment of an allergic reaction. If a patient is steroid-dependent secondary to asthma or an immunological disease (ie, SLE, rheumatoid arthritis), the provider will need to consider a longer taper of corticosteroid therapy secondary to the adrenal suppression caused by chronic steroid therapy. Also, if the patient has a history of diabetes mellitus, steroid therapy may temporarily affect the patient's blood glucose control.

A thorough drug history is necessary before prescribing an antihistamine. Terfenadine and astemizole, two nonsedating antihistamines, have been associated with serious cardiac arrhythmias when they have been used in combination with drugs that inhibit the cytochrome P-450 system (ie, erythromycin, cisapride, cimetidine).

### Patient/Caregiver Information

When a patient is prescribed an antihistamine, the provider should always inform the patient of possible effects of the sedating antihistamines. If the patient has never taken a sedating antihistamine, the provider should recommend that the patient abstain from driving after the initial dose to allow for adequate assessment of the full sedating effect. Nonsedating antihistamines may also be considered, but they are also more expensive than the sedating antihistamines. Table 37–19 lists some of the more commonly used sedating and nonsedating antihistamines. See Drug Table 705 for more specific information regarding side effects and dosing.

Patients with a past history of anaphylaxis must be reminded to have epinephrine available for emergencies at all times, especially on recreational outings. Anaphylatic reactions can occur at any time. Each year the provider needs to discuss with the patient and parents the different types of epinephrine available for self-administration, reassess the patient's plan for self-administration, and review the expiration date of any products the patient may have for emergency self-administration.

Advise all patients with a history of anaphylaxis to wear a medical alert identification. Provide a detailed plan for management of anaphylaxis to parents of an allergic child, and assess their ability to implement it. In addition, teach patients to identify early symptoms of a reaction and to seek medical attention early.

### OUTCOMES MANAGEMENT

### Selection of an Agent

Antihistamines are the mainstay of therapy for the palliative care of pruritis associated with al-

### TABLE 37–19. COMMONLY USED ANTIHISTAMINES

| Generic Name | Brand Name | Relative Cost (Based on Average Wholesale Price) |
|---|---|---|
| **Sedating Antihistamines** | | |
| Chlorpheniramine | Chlor-Trimeton | $ |
| Brompheniramine | Dimetane | $ |
| Diphenhydramine | Benadryl | $ |
| Hydroxyzine | Atarax, Vistaril | $$ |
| Cetirizine | Zyrtec | $$$$ |
| **Nonsedating Antihistamines** | | |
| Terfenadine | Seldane | $$$$ |
| Astemizole | Hismanal | $$$$ |
| Loratidine | Claritin | $$$$ |
| Fexofenadine | Allegra | $$$$ |

lergic reactions. The main thing to consider is the patient's tolerance for a sedating antihistamine. If the patient cannot tolerate one of the sedating antihistamines, the health care provider may consider one of the available nonsedating formulations, which are more expensive (see Table 37–18).

For those cases in which the reactions do not warrant intravenous therapy, but are severe enough that antihistamines are not effective, the provider may consider an oral corticosteroid, such as prednisone, for a short course. Dosing may vary, but a suggested dose would be prednisone 40 mg daily for 5–7 days. A corticosteroid may also block the late phase response of the allergic reaction.

### Monitoring for Efficacy

If the patient is experiencing a minor allergic reaction, he or she should be considered to monitor the efficacy of treatment with antihistamines and/or corticosteroid therapy. The patient should watch for improvement or worsening of dermatologic manifestations, as well as any change in breathing ability. If no improvement or worsening of symptoms occurs, the patient should contact the provider immediately.

### Monitoring for Toxicity

Patients using sedating antihistamines should monitor for any unacceptable amount of sedation, which may lead to decreased alertness. As stated previously, terfenadine and astemizole are associated with cardiac arrhythmias, which may occur if the patient is taking a higher than recommended dose or is taking it with a drug that may inhibit its metabolism. Because the arrhythmia is potentially fatal, the best thing a provider can do is to complete a thorough medication history before making any prescribing decisions.

### Follow-up Recommendations

Once a drug allergic reaction has occurred, the primary care provider should emphasize to the patient the importance of informing potential prescribers (ie, other health care providers, dentists) or pharmacists of the allergy. This information is critical in order to prevent the reaction from recurring.

As previously stated, a patient with a previous history of anaphylaxis should have an Epi-Pen or similar device available in case the patient is reexposed to whatever had initially caused the reaction (ie, food, drug, insect). The patient may also consider some type of alert bracelet, which would be helpful if the patient is not conscious and requires immediate care. Avoidance is the key to the management of allergic reactions, but in the case of an allergic reaction, rapid assessment and management are necessary.

## INFECTIOUS MONONUCLEOSIS

Infectious mononucleosis is a common acute, relatively benign, self-limited viral infection caused by the Epstein-Barr virus. The condition is uncommon in children under 5, rare before age 2, and seen often in adolescents (Schwartz et al, 1996). This infection is thought to manifest with clinical symptoms only 50% of the time. It is hypothesized that persons who get the symptomatic disease have not been exposed prior to the second decade of life. This illness is characterized by nausea, pharyngitis, and often high fevers. Rapid onset of these symptoms is thought to be related to prolonged recovery (Dornbrand, Hoole, & Pickard, 1992). In most cases the acute symptoms last 7–10 days, but the fatigue can persist for several months. Persons who are immunosuppressed are particularly susceptible to this condition. The symptoms are thought to be caused by the changes in the B-lymphocytes. A rapid and sustained response results in the adenopathy and the atypical lymphocytosis characteristic of this condition.

## SPECIFIC CONSIDERATIONS FOR PHARMACOTHERAPY

### Need for Drug Therapy and Rationale

In most cases there is no need for specific drug treatment. Symptomatic treatment of fever or sore throat with acetaminophen or aspirin (in adults only) and local treatments such as throat gargles or lozenges are recommended. Antibiotics are needed only if there is a documented coexisting streptococcal pharyngitis (see Chapter 21). Avoidance of contact sports should be stressed (Cozad, 1996).

There are several controversial issues in the treatment of this condition. Although there is universal agreement that pharyngeal edema threatening respiratory function needs to be treated with corticosteroids and potentially hospitalization, the treatment of less severe symptoms with corticosteroids is not universally supported. Dornbrand et al (1992) cite controlled studies that indicate corticosteroids lessen fever and pharyngitis, may result in an improved sense of well-being, and shorten the course of the condition but stop short of recommending use of this medication routinely. In addition, Ganzel, Goldman & Padya (1996) in a retrospective review of 109 patients admitted to a hospital with severe airway obstruction concluded that severe pharyngotonsilitis is more common than reported in the literature and recommended parental steroids in these cases.

The other controversy is the use of acyclovir. Dornbrand et al (1992) indicate that it is ineffective, even in high doses. And Boynton, Dunn, and Stephens (1994) concur, indicating even though acyclovir has good in vitro effects on EBV, it has not been shown to modify the course of uncomplicated infectious mononucleosis. However, Avery and First (1994), although indicating that antiviral treatment is not recommended under most circumstances, do indicate that high-dose intravenous treatment has a symptomatic effect in a subset of patients. In addition, Tynell et al (1996) found the combination of acyclovir and prednisone of limited use in patients with mild to moderate symptoms. The use of Zantac was also found ineffective in the treatment of mononucleosis but likely to elevate liver enzymes in 27% of those studied (Vendelbo-Johnson et al, 1997).

## Short-Term and Long-Term Goals of Pharmacotherapy

The short-term goal depends on the severity of the condition. For most it is the control of symptoms. For the severely ill patient it would be to maintain a functional airway. The long-term goal of treatment is return to normal functioning with no sequelae.

## Time Frame for Initiating Treatment

Treatment for any compromised airway should be immediate. Initiation of any other treatment is based on symptoms.

## Assessment Prior to Therapy

In addition to the history and physical examination routinely done with individuals presenting with upper respiratory symptoms, the provider needs to ask about immunosuppressed status, fever, and abdominal pain. In addition, the physical needs to include a thorough evaluation of the abdomen and close inspection of the skin. Lymphadenopathy is usually generalized.

Although a complete blood count is usually done and atypical lymphocytes are common, the definitive diagnosis is usually dependent on a positive "monospot." This laboratory test responds to the rise in heterophile antibodies which occurs in the acute stage of this infection. The "monospot" can be negative in the first few days of the condition. Other specific serologic tests are possible but not used clinically (Avery & First, 1994).

## Patient/Caregiver Information

See Chapter 21. Explain the course of the infection. The residual fatigue and malaise may be frustrating to the patient, especially the adolescent. They may need assistance in understanding their potentially slow recovery.

## OUTCOMES MANAGEMENT

### Selecting an Agent

**Corticosteroids.** Emergency treatment of patients at risk for airway obstruction is 1 mg/kg of prednisone daily for 3 days and tapered over 10 days. No other medication is common in the primary care setting. If antibiotics are used for co-existing streptococcal pharyngitis, penicillin or erythromycin is the drug of choice. Ampicillin should be avoided since it is thought to cause a "monorash."

### Monitoring for Efficacy

The reduction of symptoms can be used to evaluate therapy, especially the enlarged tonsils and spleen. Laboratory work is usually not used to monitor efficiency since the monospot can be positive for an extended time.

### Monitoring for Toxicity

The course of corticosteroids is short, and the normal side effects associated with a longer course usually are not a problem. Any untoward effects are unexpected and should be investigated.

## Follow-up Recommendations

Monitor weekly until the patient is recovered and no splenomegaly exists. Refer for any toxicity, jaundice, or unexpected symptoms.

## POSTEXPOSURE PROPHYLAXIS

Although the risk of HIV infection to health care workers is small even when there is a known exposure to body fluids of patient known to be HIV positive, postexposure prophylaxis (PEP) management has been shown to reduce the risk even more. The critical factor is timing of the prophylaxis, with most programs calling for initiation of treatment in high risk situations within an hour of exposure. Although PEP is common in some hospitals, health care providers in primary care settings may not be aware of the necessity for such a program. The risk of HIV infection due to percutaneous (needle stick) exposure to HIV-infected blood is 0.3%. If the volume of blood is large or the HIV titer is high, risk may be elevated. Mucous membrane and skin exposure to HIV-infected blood carries a risk of 0.1% or less. Zidovudine (ZDV) prophylaxis has been shown to reduce the risk by 79% after percutaneous exposure in a case-controlled study (CDC, 1996). Universal precautions remain the best defense against transmission of a variety of infectious agents. However, PEP programs can offer counseling to assist and inform health care providers exposed to body fluids from a patient of their options and risks. The highest risk is percutaneous (needle stick), and prophylaxis with ZDV plus lamivudine (3TC) and indinavir (IDV) antiretroviral regimen are indicated. The PEP is initiated, the subject is treated, and if the source patient subsequently tests HIV negative, the medications can be terminated. Prophylaxis is given for four weeks and usually is ZDV 200 mg t.i.d., 3TC 150 mg b.i.d., and IDV 800 mg t.i.d. (CDC, 1996). It is best if any health care worker exposed to body fluids is thoroughly counseled by a PEP team member so that all options can be discussed. In some instances the support provided by the team is just as important as the drug therapy. CDC Prevention Guidelines address exposure to body fluids via percutaneous, mucous membrane and skin/blood exposure, and they rank options as "recommend PEP," "offer PEP," and "not offer PEP." Most PEP programs have team members on 24-hour call to respond to emerging problems immediately (CDC, 1996).

## Acknowledgment

The authors would like to acknowledge Denese Goehle, MS, CPNP, Pediatric Infectious Disease Clinic, Medical College of Virginia Hospitals of Virginia Commonwealth University, for her review of the pediatric HIV/AIDS section of an earlier draft of this chapter.

## REFERENCES

Adkinson, N. F. (1992). Drug allergy. *JAMA, 268,* 771–773.

American Foundation for AIDS Research (AmFAR) (1997). *AIDS/HIV treatment directory.* New York: AmFAR.

American Medical Association (AMA). (1996). *A physician guide to HIV prevention.* Chicago: AMA.

Avery, M. E., & First, L. R. (1994). *Pediatric medicine* (2nd ed.). Baltimore: Williams & Wilkins.

Belchi-Hernandez, J., & Espinosa-Parra, F. J. (1996). Management of adverse reactions to prophylactic trimethoprim-sulfamethoxazole in patients with human immunodeficiency virus infection. *Annals of Allergy and Asthma Immunology, 76(4),* 355–358.

Bernstein, J. A. (1995). Allergic drug reactions. *Postgraduate Medicine, 98,* 159–166.

Boucher, C. A., & Larder, B. A. (1994). *Viral variation and therapeutic strategies in HIV infection.* London: MediTech Media.

Boynton, R. W., Dunn, E. S., & Stephens, G. R. (1994). *Manual of ambulatory pediatrics* (3rd ed.). Philadelphia. J. B. Lippincott.

Breathnach, S. M. (1995). Management of drug eruptions: Part II. *Australian Journal of Dermatology, 36,* 187–191.

Burroughs, C. (1993). Alternative therapies for AIDS: An historical review. *The Gay Men's Health Crisis Newsletter of Experimental AIDS Therapies, 7, 11/12,* 2–4.

Butz, A. M., Joyner, M., Friedman, D. G., & Hutton, N. (1998). Primary care for children with Human Immunodeficiency Virus infection. *Journal of Pediatric Health Care, 12(1),* 10–19.

Carpenter, C. C., Fischel, M. A., Hammer, S. M., Hirsch, M. S., Jacobsen, D. M., Katzenstein, D. A., Montaner, J. S., Richman, D. D., Saag, M. S., Schooley, R. T., Thompson, M. A., Vella, S., Yeni, P. G., & Volberding, P. A., for the International AIDS Society–USA. (1996). Antiretroviral therapy for HIV infection in 1996: Recommendations of an international panel. *JAMA, 276(2),* 146–154.

Carpenter, C. C., Fischel, M., Hammer, S. M., Hirsch, M. S., Jacobsen, D. M., Katzenstein, D. A., Montaner, J. S., Richman, D. D., Saag, M. S., Schooley, R. T., Thompson, M. A., Vella, S., Yeni, P. G., & Volberding, P. A. (1997). Antiretroviral therapy for HIV infection in 1997. *JAMA, 277,* 1962–1969.

Centers for Disease Control. (1994). Recommendations of the U.S. Public Health Service Task Force on the use of zidovudine to reduce perinatal transmission of human immunodeficiency virus. *MMWR, 43*(RR-12), 1–19.

Centers for Disease Control. (1996). Update: Provisional Public Health Service recommendation for chemoprophylaxis after occupational exposure to HIV. *MMWR, 45*(22), 468–472.

Centers for Disease Control. (1998a). U.S. Public Health Service Task Force recommendations for use of antiretroviral drugs in pregnant women infected with HIV-1 for maternal health and reducing perinatal HIV-1 transmission in the United States. *MMWR, 47*(RR-2), 1–39.

Centers for Disease Control. (1998b). Guidelines for the use of antiretroviral agents in pediatric HIV infection. *MMWR 47*(RR-4), 1–38.

Centers for Disease Control. (1998c, in press). *Guidelines for the use of antiretroviral agents in HIV-infected adults and adolescents.* Federal Register, June 20, 1997.

Coates, T. (1994). Report from the AIDS Conference. Care and prevention: Hand in hand. *Focus: A Guide to AIDS Research and Counseling, 9*(12), 1–4.

Commonwealth of Virginia Department of Health. (1997). *Division of STD/AIDS Quarterly Surveillance Report, 5*(2), 39–48.

Cooper, D. A., Gatel, J. M., Kroon, S., Clumeck, N., Millard, J., Goebel, F. D., Bruun, J. N., Stingel, G., Melville, R. L., Gonzalez-Lohoz, J., et al. (1993). Zidovudine in persons with asymptomatic HIV infection and CD4 cells count greater than 400 per cubic millimeter. *New England Journal of Medicine, 329,* 297–303.

Cozad, J. (1996). Infectious mononucleosis. *Nurse Practitioner, 21*(3), 14–16.

Dornbrand, L., Hoole, A. J., & Pickard, C. G. (1992). *Manual of clinical problems in adult ambulatory care* (2nd ed.). Boston: Little, Brown.

Fahrner, R., & Benson, M. (1996). HIV infection and AIDS. In P. L. Jackson & J. A. Vessey, *Primary care of the child with a chronic condition* (2nd ed.). St. Louis: Mosby.

Fisher, E. J. (1995). *Clinician's guide to therapy of adults with HIV/AIDS.* Richmond: Virginia Commonwealth University HIV/AIDS Center.

Funck-Brentano, I., Costagliola, D., Seibel, N., Straub, E., Tardieu, M., & Blanche, S. (1997). Patterns of disclosure and perceptions of the human immunodeficiency virus in infected elementary school-age children. *Archives of Pediatric and Adolescent Medicine, 151*(10), 978–985.

Ganzel, T. M., Goldman, J. L., & Padhya, T. A. (1996). Otolaryngologic clinical patterns in pediatric infectious mononucleosis. *American Journal of Otolaryngology, 17*(6), 397–400.

Gershon, A. A., Mervish, N., LaRussa, P., Steinberg, S., Lo, S. H., Hodes, D., Fikrig, S., Bonagura, V., & Bakshi, S. (1997). Varicella-zoster virus infection in children with underlying human immunodeficiency virus infection. *Journal of Infectious Diseases, 176*(6), 1496–1500.

Goldschmidt, R. H., & Dong, B. J. (1997). Current report—HIV. Treatment of AIDS and HIV-related conditions—1997. *JABEFP, 10*(2), 144–167.

Guill, M. F. (1991). Allergic drug reactions: Identification and management. *Hospital Formulary, 26,* 582–589.

Hecht, F. M., & Soloway, B. (1994). *HIV infection: A primary care approach.* Waltham: Massachusetts Medical Society.

Japour, A. J. (1996). Measurement of HIV-1 RNA in clinical practice: An initial management algorithm. *Journal of the International Association of Physicians in AIDS Care, 2,* 16–19.

Johns Hopkins University AIDS Service (1997). Department of HHS Guidelines on use of antiretroviral agents in HIV-infected adults and USPHS & IDSA: 1997 Guidelines for the prevention of opportunistic infections in persons infected with HIV. *The Hopkins HIV Report, 9*(6a), 1–8.

Lipsky, J. J. (1996). Antiretroviral drugs for AIDS. *Lancet, 348,* 800–803.

Makadon, H. J., & Silian, J. G. (1995). Prevention of HIV infection in primary care: Current practices, future possibilities. *Annals of Internal Medicine, 123*(9), 715–719.

Marks, R. (1994). The Brighton Conference and HIV prevention. *Focus: A Guide to Aids Research and Counseling, 9*(12), 5–8.

Miralles, G. D. (1996). Virology and pathogenesis of HIV. In J. A. Bartlett (Ed.), *Care and management of patients with HIV infection* (pp. 14–17). Durham, NC: Glaxo Wellcome.

Moon, J. E. (1997). Collective for Environmental Design, POB 12161, Richmond, VA 23241.

Moore, R. D., & Bartlett, J. G. (1996). Combination antiretroviral therapy in HIV infection: An economic perspective. *PharmacoEconomics, 10*(2), 109–113.

Mulder, J. W., Cooper, D. A., Mathisen, L., Sandstrom, E., Clumeck, N., Gatell, J. M., French, M., Donovan, B., Gray, F., Yeo, J. M., et al. (1994). Zidovudine twice daily in asymptomatic subjects with HIV infection and a high risk of progression to AIDS: A randomized double blind placebo controlled study. *AIDS, 8,* 313–322.

Palusci, V. J., Kaul, A., Lawrence, R. M., Haines, K. A., & Kwittken, P. L. (1996). Rapid oral desensitization to trimethoprim-sulfamethoxazole in infants and children. *Pediatric Infectious Disease Journal, 15*(5), 456–460.

Perrin, L., & Kinloch-de Loes, S. (1995). Rationale for treatment at the time of primary infection with HIV-1. *Transcript, 43,* 7–10.

Rieder, M. J., King, S. M., & Read, S. (1997). Adverse reactions to trimethoprim-sulfamethoxazole among children with human immunodeficiency virus infection. *Pediatric Infectious Disease Journal, 16*(11), 1028–1031.

Schwartz, W. M., Bell, L. M., Brown, L., Clark, B. J., Kim, S. C., & Manno, C. S. (Eds.) (1996). *Clinical handbook of pediatrics.* Baltimore: Williams & Wilkins.

Stryker, J., Coates, T. J., DeCarlo, P., Haynes-Sanstad, K., Shriver, M., & Makadon, H. J. (1995). Prevention of HIV Infection. *JAMA, 272*(14), 1143–1148.

Tynell, E., Aurelius, E., Brazell, A., Jalander, I., Wood, M., Yao, Q. Y., Rickinson, A., Akerlund, B., & Anderson, J. (1996). Acyclovir and prednisolone treatment of acute infectious mononucleosis: A multicenter, double-blind, placebo-controlled study. *Journal of Infectious Diseases, 174*(2), 324–331.

Vendebo-Johnson, L., Lildholdt, T., Bende, M., Toft, A., Brahe-Pederson, C., & Danielsson, G. P. (1997). Infectious mononucleosis treated by antihistamine: A comparison of efficacy of ranitidine (Zantac) vs. placebo in the treatment of infectious mononucleosis. *Clinical Otolaryngology, 22*(2), 123–125.

Virginia Commonwealth University HIV/HIVS Center. (1998). *Update in HIV Care: The Use of Antiretroviral Agents in HIV-Infected Adolescents and Adults.* Richmond, Va., Mid-Atlantic AIDS Education and Training Center.

Wiese, W. (1997). Developments in antiretroviral therapy for AIDS patients. *Internal Medicine,* April, 72–85.

Wood, R. (1997). Anaphylaxis in children. *Patient Care,* 161–183.

Zieve, P. D. (1995). *Handbook of ambulatory care.* Baltimore: Williams & Wilkins.

# V

# TABLES OF PHARMACOTHERAPEUTIC AGENTS

# TABLES OF PHARMACOTHERAPEUTIC AGENTS

**100. ANTI-INFECTIVE AGENTS** . . . . . . . . . . . . . . . . . . . . . . . . . . . .931

    101. AMEBICIDES . . . . . . . . . . . . . . . . . . . . . . . . . . . . . . . . .931

    102. ANTIBIOTICS . . . . . . . . . . . . . . . . . . . . . . . . . . . . . . . . .932

        102.1  Cephalosporins: First Generation . . . . . . . . . . . . . .932

        102.2  Cephalosporins: Second Generation . . . . . . . . . . . . .935

        102.3  Cephalosporins: Third Generation . . . . . . . . . . . . . .939

        102.4  Fluoroquinolones . . . . . . . . . . . . . . . . . . . . . . . . .943

        102.5  Macrolides . . . . . . . . . . . . . . . . . . . . . . . . . . . . .951

        102.6  Penicillins . . . . . . . . . . . . . . . . . . . . . . . . . . . . . .958

        102.7  Aminopenicillins . . . . . . . . . . . . . . . . . . . . . . . . .962

        102.8  Penicillinase-Resistant Penicillins . . . . . . . . . . . . . .966

        102.9  Sulfonamides . . . . . . . . . . . . . . . . . . . . . . . . . . . .969

        102.10 Sulfonamide Combinations . . . . . . . . . . . . . . . . . .973

        102.11 Tetracyclines . . . . . . . . . . . . . . . . . . . . . . . . . . . .976

    103. ANTIFUNGALS . . . . . . . . . . . . . . . . . . . . . . . . . . . . . . . . .979

    104. ANTIMALARIALS . . . . . . . . . . . . . . . . . . . . . . . . . . . . . . . .985

    105. ANTITUBERCULOSIS AGENTS . . . . . . . . . . . . . . . . . . . . . . .994

    106. ANTIVIRAL AGENTS . . . . . . . . . . . . . . . . . . . . . . . . . . . . .1002

        106.1  Agents for Herpes Simplex and Herpes Zoster . . . . .1002

        106.2  Nucleoside Reverse Transcriptase Inhibitors . . . . . .1005

        106.3  Non-nucleoside Reverse Transcriptase Inhibitors . .1009

        106.4  Protease Inhibitors . . . . . . . . . . . . . . . . . . . . . . .1011

        106.5  Agents for Cytomegalovirus . . . . . . . . . . . . . . . . .1015

        106.6  Miscellaneous Antiviral Agents . . . . . . . . . . . . . . .1016

    107. URINARY ANTI-INFECTIVES . . . . . . . . . . . . . . . . . . . . . . .1017

    108. DRUGS FOR PARASITIC INFECTIONS . . . . . . . . . . . . . . . .1023

    109. MISCELLANEOUS ANTIMICROBIAL AGENTS . . . . . . . . .1027

**200. CARDIOVASCULAR AGENTS** . . . . . . . . . . . . . . . . . . . . . . . . .1034

    201. ANTIANGINAL AGENTS . . . . . . . . . . . . . . . . . . . . . . . . . .1034

    202. ANTIARRHYTHMIC AGENTS . . . . . . . . . . . . . . . . . . . . . .1037

    203. ANTICOAGULANTS . . . . . . . . . . . . . . . . . . . . . . . . . . . . .1043

    204. ANTIHYPERLIPIDEMIC AGENTS . . . . . . . . . . . . . . . . . . .1044

        204.1  Bile Acid Sequestrants . . . . . . . . . . . . . . . . . . . . .1044

        204.2  HMG-CoA Reductase Inhibitors . . . . . . . . . . . . . .1045

        204.3  Miscellaneous Antihyperlipidemic Agents . . . . . . .1047

    205. ANTIHYPERTENSIVE AGENTS . . . . . . . . . . . . . . . . . . . . .1049

        205.1  Angiotensin Converting Enzyme Inhibitors . . . . . .1049

        205.2  Angiotensin II Antagonists . . . . . . . . . . . . . . . . . .1054

        205.3  Central and Peripherally Acting

                   Antiadrenergic Agents . . . . . . . . . . . . . . . . . . .1055

| | | |
|---|---|---|
| 205.4 | Alpha/Beta Adrenergic Blocking Agents . . . . . . . . . . | 1059 |
| 205.5 | Beta-Adrenergic Blocking Agents . . . . . . . . . . . . . . . | 1060 |
| 205.6 | Calcium Channel Blockers . . . . . . . . . . . . . . . . . | 1067 |
| 205.7 | Vasodilators . . . . . . . . . . . . . . . . . . . . . . . . . . . . . . . | 1071 |

206. ANTIPLATELET AGENTS . . . . . . . . . . . . . . . . . . . . . . . . 1072
207. CARDIAC GLYCOSIDES . . . . . . . . . . . . . . . . . . . . . . . . . . 1073
208. DIURETICS . . . . . . . . . . . . . . . . . . . . . . . . . . . . . . . . . . . 1075

| | | |
|---|---|---|
| 208.1 | Carbonic Anhydrase Inhibitors . . . . . . . . . . . . . . . | 1075 |
| 208.2 | Loop Diuretics . . . . . . . . . . . . . . . . . . . . . . . . . . . . | 1077 |
| 208.3 | Potassium-Sparing Diuretics . . . . . . . . . . . . . . . . . | 1079 |
| 208.4 | Thiazide and Thiazide-Like Diuretics . . . . . . . . . . | 1081 |

**300. CENTRAL NERVOUS SYSTEM (CNS) AGENTS . . . . . . . . . . . . 1088**

301. ACETAMINOPHEN . . . . . . . . . . . . . . . . . . . . . . . . . . . . . . 1088
302. NARCOTIC AGONISTS . . . . . . . . . . . . . . . . . . . . . . . . . . 1089

| | | |
|---|---|---|
| 302.1 | Phenanthrenes . . . . . . . . . . . . . . . . . . . . . . . . . . . . | 1089 |
| 302.2 | Phenylpiperidines . . . . . . . . . . . . . . . . . . . . . . . . . | 1094 |
| 302.3 | Diphenylheptanes . . . . . . . . . . . . . . . . . . . . . . . . . | 1095 |
| 302.4 | Agonists-Antagonists Combinations . . . . . . . . . . . | 1097 |

303. NARCOTIC COMBINATIONS . . . . . . . . . . . . . . . . . . . . . . 1100
304. NONNARCOTIC ANALGESIC COMBINATIONS . . . . . . . . 1113
305. NONNARCOTIC ANALGESIC COMBINATIONS
     WITH BARBITURATE . . . . . . . . . . . . . . . . . . . . . . . . . 1119
306. NONSTEROIDAL ANTI-INFLAMMATORY
     DRUGS . . . . . . . . . . . . . . . . . . . . . . . . . . . . . . . . . . . . 1122

| | | |
|---|---|---|
| 306.1 | Propionic Acids . . . . . . . . . . . . . . . . . . . . . . . . . . . | 1122 |
| 306.2 | Acetic Acids . . . . . . . . . . . . . . . . . . . . . . . . . . . . . . | 1127 |
| 306.3 | Fenamates and Oxicams . . . . . . . . . . . . . . . . . . . . | 1132 |
| 306.4 | Central Analgesics . . . . . . . . . . . . . . . . . . . . . . . . . | 1134 |

307. SALICYLATES . . . . . . . . . . . . . . . . . . . . . . . . . . . . . . . . . 1135
308. ANTICONVULSANTS . . . . . . . . . . . . . . . . . . . . . . . . . . . . 1141

| | | |
|---|---|---|
| 308.1 | Barbiturates . . . . . . . . . . . . . . . . . . . . . . . . . . . . . . | 1141 |
| 308.2 | Benzodiazepines . . . . . . . . . . . . . . . . . . . . . . . . . . . | 1143 |
| 308.3 | Hydantoins . . . . . . . . . . . . . . . . . . . . . . . . . . . . . . . | 1146 |
| 308.4 | Oxazolidinediones . . . . . . . . . . . . . . . . . . . . . . . . . | 1150 |
| 308.5 | Succinimides . . . . . . . . . . . . . . . . . . . . . . . . . . . . . . | 1151 |
| 308.6 | Miscellaneous Anticonvulsants . . . . . . . . . . . . . . . | 1153 |

309. ANXIOLYTICS . . . . . . . . . . . . . . . . . . . . . . . . . . . . . . . . . 1159

| | | |
|---|---|---|
| 309.1 | Benzodiazepines . . . . . . . . . . . . . . . . . . . . . . . . . . . | 1159 |
| 309.2 | Miscellaneous Anxiolytics . . . . . . . . . . . . . . . . . . . | 1165 |

310. SEDATIVES/HYPNOTICS . . . . . . . . . . . . . . . . . . . . . . . . . 1169

| | | |
|---|---|---|
| 310.1 | Barbiturates . . . . . . . . . . . . . . . . . . . . . . . . . . . . . . | 1169 |
| 310.2 | Benzodiazepines . . . . . . . . . . . . . . . . . . . . . . . . . . . | 1174 |
| 310.3 | Miscellaneous Nonbarbiturates . . . . . . . . . . . . . . . | 1178 |
| 310.4 | Nonprescription Sleep Aids . . . . . . . . . . . . . . . . . . | 1182 |

311. ANTIDEPRESSANTS . . . . . . . . . . . . . . . . . . . . . . . . . . . . . .1185
    311.1  Tricyclic Antidepressants . . . . . . . . . . . . . . . . . . . . .1185
    311.2  Miscellaneous Antidepressants . . . . . . . . . . . . . . . .1194
    311.3  Monoamine Oxidase Inhibitors . . . . . . . . . . .1198
    311.4  Selective Serotonin Reuptake Inhibitors . . . . . . . .1199
312. ANTIPSYCHOTIC AGENTS . . . . . . . . . . . . . . . . . . . . . . . . .1203
    312.1  Phenothiazines . . . . . . . . . . . . . . . . . . . . . . . . .1203
    312.2  Other Typical Antipsychotic Agents . . . . . . . . . . . . .1211
    312.3  Atypical Antipsychotics . . . . . . . . . . . . . . . . . . . . .1216
    312.4  Psychotherapeutic Combinations . . . . . . . . . . . . . .1219
313. MISCELLANEOUS PSYCHOTHERAPEUTIC AGENTS . . . .1221
314. SKELETAL MUSCLE RELAXANTS . . . . . . . . . . . . . . . . .1224
    314.1  Combinations . . . . . . . . . . . . . . . . . . . . . . . . . . .1229
315. AGENTS FOR ALZHEIMER DEMENTIA . . . . . . . . . . . . . .1234
316. AGENTS FOR GOUT . . . . . . . . . . . . . . . . . . . . . . . . . . . .1235
317. AGENTS FOR MIGRAINE . . . . . . . . . . . . . . . . . . . . . . . . .1239
    317.1  Combination Agents for Migraines . . . . . . . . . . . . .1241
318. AGENTS FOR PARKINSON'S DISEASE . . . . . . . . . . . . . . .1243
319. AGENTS FOR RHEUMATISM . . . . . . . . . . . . . . . . . . . . .1252

400. EYE AND EAR PREPARATIONS . . . . . . . . . . . . . . . . . . . . . . . .1257
401. OPHTHALMIC PREPARATIONS . . . . . . . . . . . . . . . . . .1257
    401.1  Agents for Glaucoma . . . . . . . . . . . . . . . . . . . . . .1257
    401.2  Ophthalmic Antibiotic Agents . . . . . . . . . . . . . . . .1264
    401.3  Ophthalmic Antifungal Agents . . . . . . . . . . . . . . .1270
    401.4  Ophthalmic Antiviral Agents . . . . . . . . . . . . . . . . .1271
    401.5  Ophthalmic Antiallergic Agents . . . . . . . . . . . . . . .1273
    401.6  Ophthalmic Nonsteroidal Anti-Inflammatory
            Agents . . . . . . . . . . . . . . . . . . . . . . . . . . . . . . . .1274
    401.7  Ophthalmic Steroidal Agents . . . . . . . . . . . . . . . .1276
402. OTIC PREPARATIONS . . . . . . . . . . . . . . . . . . . . . . . . . .1279
    402.1  Antibiotics . . . . . . . . . . . . . . . . . . . . . . . . . . . . . .1279
    402.2  Miscellaneous Preparations . . . . . . . . . . . . . . . . .1280

500. GASTROINTESTINAL AGENTS . . . . . . . . . . . . . . . . . . . . . . . .1286
501. GASTROINTESTINAL AGENTS . . . . . . . . . . . . . . . . . . .1286
    501.1  Antacids . . . . . . . . . . . . . . . . . . . . . . . . . . . . . . .1286
    501.2  Antacid Combination Products . . . . . . . . . . . . . . .1290
    501.3  Gastrointestinal Anticholinergics/Antispasmodics . . .1291
    501.4  Gastrointestinal Anticholinergic Combinations . . . .1296
    501.5  Agents for Ulcers and GERD . . . . . . . . . . . . . . . . .1297
    501.6  GI Stimulants . . . . . . . . . . . . . . . . . . . . . . . . . . .1302
    501.7  Digestive Enzymes . . . . . . . . . . . . . . . . . . . . . . . .1303
    501.8  Antidiarrheals . . . . . . . . . . . . . . . . . . . . . . . . . . .1306
    501.9  Laxatives . . . . . . . . . . . . . . . . . . . . . . . . . . . . . . .1309

501.10 Laxative Combinations . . . . . . . . . . . . . . . . . . . . . . .1315

501.11 Enemas . . . . . . . . . . . . . . . . . . . . . . . . . . . . . . . . . .1316

501.12 Agents for Ulcerative Colitis and Crohn's Disease . .1318

501.13 Antiflatulent Agents . . . . . . . . . . . . . . . . . . . . . . . .1320

502. ANTIEMETIC/ANTIVERTIGO AGENTS . . . . . . . . . . . . . . .1322

502.1 Anticholinergics . . . . . . . . . . . . . . . . . . . . . . . . . . . .1322

502.2 Antidopaminergics . . . . . . . . . . . . . . . . . . . . . . . . . .1325

502.3 Miscellaneous Agents . . . . . . . . . . . . . . . . . . . . . . . .1325

**600. HORMONES AND SYNTHETIC SUBSTANCES** . . . . . . . . . . . . . . .**1327**

601. ADRENAL CORTICAL STEROIDS . . . . . . . . . . . . . . . . .1327

601.1 Glucocorticoids . . . . . . . . . . . . . . . . . . . . . . . . . . . .1327

601.2 Mineralcorticoids . . . . . . . . . . . . . . . . . . . . . . . . . .1334

602. ANDROGENS AND ANDROGEN INHIBITORS . . . . . . . . .1335

602.1 Androgens . . . . . . . . . . . . . . . . . . . . . . . . . . . . . . . .1335

602.2 Androgen Hormone Inhibitors . . . . . . . . . . . . . . . . .1337

603. CONTRACEPTIVES . . . . . . . . . . . . . . . . . . . . . . . . . . . . .1338

603.1 Oral Contraceptives—Monophasic . . . . . . . . . . . . . .1338

603.2 Oral Contraceptives—Biphasic . . . . . . . . . . . . . . . . .1345

603.3 Oral Contraceptives—Triphasic . . . . . . . . . . . . . . . .1346

603.4 Oral Contraceptives—Progestin Only . . . . . . . . . . . .1349

603.5 Contraceptive Implants . . . . . . . . . . . . . . . . . . . . . .1350

603.6 Contraceptive Injections . . . . . . . . . . . . . . . . . . . . . .1351

604. ANTIDIABETIC AGENTS . . . . . . . . . . . . . . . . . . . . . . . . .1352

604.1 Sulfonylureas . . . . . . . . . . . . . . . . . . . . . . . . . . . . . .1352

604.2 Miscellaneous Antidiabetic Agents . . . . . . . . . . . . . .1357

604.3 Insulin . . . . . . . . . . . . . . . . . . . . . . . . . . . . . . . . . . .1360

605. ESTROGENS AND PROGESTINS . . . . . . . . . . . . . . . . . . .1366

605.1 Estrogens . . . . . . . . . . . . . . . . . . . . . . . . . . . . . . . . .1366

605.2 Progestins . . . . . . . . . . . . . . . . . . . . . . . . . . . . . . . .1372

605.3 Estrogen/Progestin Combinations . . . . . . . . . . . . . . .1373

605.4 Estrogens/Androgen Combinations . . . . . . . . . . . . . .1376

605.5 Selective Estrogen Receptor Modulators . . . . . . . . . .1377

606. DRUGS FOR OSTEOPOROSIS . . . . . . . . . . . . . . . . . . . .1378

606.1 Bisphosphonates . . . . . . . . . . . . . . . . . . . . . . . . . . . .1378

606.2 Miscellaneous Agents for Osteoporosis . . . . . . . . . . .1380

607. THYROID AGENTS . . . . . . . . . . . . . . . . . . . . . . . . . . . . .1381

607.1 Antithyroid Agents . . . . . . . . . . . . . . . . . . . . . . . . . .1381

607.2 Iodine Products . . . . . . . . . . . . . . . . . . . . . . . . . . . .1383

607.3 Thyroid Hormones . . . . . . . . . . . . . . . . . . . . . . . . . .1384

608. GONADOTROPIN RELEASING HORMONES . . . . . . . . . .1388

**700. RESPIRATORY AGENTS** . . . . . . . . . . . . . . . . . . . . . . . . . . . .**1389**

701. RESPIRATORY INHALANTS . . . . . . . . . . . . . . . . . . . . . . .1389

701.1 Anticholinergics . . . . . . . . . . . . . . . . . . . . . . . . . . . .1389

701.2  Corticosteroids . . . . . . . . . . . . . . . . . . . . . . . . . . . .1390

701.3  Miscellaneous Inhalents . . . . . . . . . . . . . . . . . . . . .1393

702. BRONCHODILATORS . . . . . . . . . . . . . . . . . . . . . . . . . . . .1395

702.1  Sympathomimetics . . . . . . . . . . . . . . . . . . . . . . . .1395

702.2  Xanthine Derivatives . . . . . . . . . . . . . . . . . . . . . .1399

703. NASAL DECONGESTANTS . . . . . . . . . . . . . . . . . . . . . . . .1402

704. ANTITUSSIVES . . . . . . . . . . . . . . . . . . . . . . . . . . . . . . .1408

705. ANTIHISTAMINES . . . . . . . . . . . . . . . . . . . . . . . . . . . . .1410

705.1  Antihistamines—First Generation . . . . . . . . . . . . . .1410

705.2  Antihistamines—Second Generation . . . . . . . . . . . .1419

706. INTRANASAL STEROIDS . . . . . . . . . . . . . . . . . . . . . . . .1422

707. EXPECTORANTS . . . . . . . . . . . . . . . . . . . . . . . . . . . . . .1424

708. LEUKOTRIENE RECEPTOR ANTAGONISTS . . . . . . . . . .1425

709. LEUKOTRIENE RECEPTOR INHIBITORS . . . . . . . . . . . .1426


800. TOPICAL PREPARATIONS . . . . . . . . . . . . . . . . . . . . . . . . .1427

801. ACNE PRODUCTS . . . . . . . . . . . . . . . . . . . . . . . . . . . .1427

802. ANTIPSORIATIC PRODUCTS . . . . . . . . . . . . . . . . . . . . .1430

803. ANTISEBORRHEIC PRODUCTS . . . . . . . . . . . . . . . . . . .1433

804. ANTIHISTAMINE-CONTAINING PRODUCTS . . . . . . . . . .1437

805. ANTI-INFECTIVE PRODUCTS (TOPICAL
AND VAGINAL) . . . . . . . . . . . . . . . . . . . . . . . . . . . . . .1438

806. SCABICIDES/PEDICULICIDES . . . . . . . . . . . . . . . . . . . .1450

807. CORTICOSTEROID PRODUCTS . . . . . . . . . . . . . . . . . . .1453

808. CORTICOSTEROID COMBINATIONS . . . . . . . . . . . . . . .1470

809. MISCELLANEOUS TOPICAL PRODUCTS . . . . . . . . . . . .1474


900. URINARY TRACT PRODUCTS . . . . . . . . . . . . . . . . . . . . . .1476

901. ANTISPASMODICS . . . . . . . . . . . . . . . . . . . . . . . . . . . .1476

902. CHOLINERGIC STIMULANTS . . . . . . . . . . . . . . . . . . . .1477

903. URINARY ANALGESICS . . . . . . . . . . . . . . . . . . . . . . . .1478


1000. MISCELLANEOUS AGENTS . . . . . . . . . . . . . . . . . . . . . . . .1479

1001. AGENTS FOR IMPOTENCE . . . . . . . . . . . . . . . . . . . . .1479

1002. AGENTS FOR OBESITY . . . . . . . . . . . . . . . . . . . . . . . .1481

1003. AGENTS FOR NICOTINE WITHDRAWAL . . . . . . . . . . . .1486


1100. VITAMINS, MINERALS, AND TRACE ELEMENTS . . . . . . . . . .1488

1101. FAT-SOLUBLE VITAMINS . . . . . . . . . . . . . . . . . . . . . .1488

1102. WATER-SOLUBLE VITAMINS . . . . . . . . . . . . . . . . . . .1489

1103. MAJOR MINERALS . . . . . . . . . . . . . . . . . . . . . . . . . . .1492

1104. TRACE ELEMENTS . . . . . . . . . . . . . . . . . . . . . . . . . . .1495


BIBLIOGRAPHY . . . . . . . . . . . . . . . . . . . . . . . . . . . . . . . . . . . .1498

# 100. ANTI-INFECTIVE AGENTS
## 101. Amebicides

| Drug and Dosage Forms | Spectrum of Activity and Usual Dosage Range | Administration Issues and Drug–Drug & Drug–Food Interactions | Common Adverse Drug Reactions (ADRs) and Pharmacokinetics | Contraindications, Pregnancy Category, and Lactation Issues |
|---|---|---|---|---|
| **Iodoquinol**<br>Yodoxin<br><br>Tablet:<br>210 mg, 650 mg | **Spectrum of Activity**<br>*Entamoeba histolytica*<br><br>Treatment of intestinal amebiasis<br>**Adults:** 650 mg tid pc for 20 d<br><br>**Children:** 40 mg/kg/d up to max of 650 mg/dose tid 20 days | Administration Issues<br>Complete full course of therapy<br><br>Drug–Drug Interactions<br>Iodoquinol may interfere with the effect of **levothyroxine** by increasing protein bound iodine levels | ADRs<br>skin eruptions, nausea, vomiting, GI upset, blurred vision<br><br>Pharmacokinetics<br>poorly absorbed, metabolized in the liver, excreted in the feces | Contraindications<br>Hypersensitivity to iodine containing products<br><br>Pregnancy Category: C<br><br>Lactation Issues<br>Safety for use during breast feeding has not been established |
| **Paromomycin**<br>Humatin<br><br>Capsule:<br>250 mg | **Spectrum of Activity**<br>*Entamoeba histolytica*<br>*Cryptosporidium* diarrhea<br><br>Treatment of intestinal amebiasis<br>**Adult and children**<br>25–35 mg/kg/d tid for 5–10 days<br><br>*Cryptosporidium* (adults with AIDS): 1.5–2.25 g/d in 3–6 divided doses for 10 to 14 d (courses of up to 4–6 weeks may be needed) | Administration Issues<br>Complete full course of therapy; administer after meals to prevent gastric distress<br><br>Drug–Drug Interactions<br>Rare due to lack of systemic absorption | ADRs<br>skin eruptions, nausea, vomiting, GI upset<br><br>Pharmacokinetics<br>not absorbed systemically; excreted 100% unchanged in feces | Contraindications<br>Hypersensitivity to paromomycin; intestinal obstruction<br><br>Pregnancy Category: C<br><br>Lactation Issues<br>Safety for use during breast feeding has not been established |

# 102. Antibiotics

## 102.1 Cephalosporins: First Generation

| Drug and Dosage Forms | Spectrum of Activity and Usual Dosage Range | Administration Issues and Drug–Drug & Drug–Food Interactions | Common Adverse Drug Reactions (ADRs) and Pharmacokinetics | Contraindications, Pregnancy Category, and Lactation Issues |
|---|---|---|---|---|
| **Cephalexin**<br><br>Tablet:<br>Keftab<br>250 mg, 500 mg<br><br>Keflet<br>250 mg, 500 mg, 1 gm<br><br>Capsule:<br>Keflex<br>250 mg, 500 mg<br><br>Powder for Oral Suspension:<br>100 mg/ml<br>125 mg/5 ml<br>250 mg/5 ml | **Antibacterial Spectrum**<br>Active against *S. aureus*, *S. pneumoniae* and *S. pyogenes*. Majority of urinary isolates of community-acquired *E. coli*, *Klebsiella species* and *P. mirabilis* are susceptible; not very active against *H. influenzae*; inactive against enterococci.<br><br>**General indications**<br>**Adults:** 250–500 mg q 6 h for 10 to 14 d<br>**If oral dose is > 4 gm/day, use parenteral drug**<br><br>**Children:** 25–50 mg/kg/d divided qid for 10 to 14 d<br><br>Otitis media: 75–100 mg/kg/d divided qid for 10 to 14 d<br><br>**Prevention of bacterial endocarditis**<br>Adults 2 gm (children 50 mg/kg) orally 1 hr before procedure | Administration Issues<br>Complete full course of therapy; shake suspension well before administration; store suspension in the refrigerator; discard unused suspension after 14 d<br><br>Drug–Drug Interactions<br>Cephalosporins may decrease the effectiveness of **oral contraceptives**; **probenecid** may increase cephalosporin plasma levels by competitively inhibiting renal excretion of cephalosporins | ADRs<br>hypersensitivity reactions, urticarial rash, nausea, vomiting, diarrhea, superinfections<br><br>Pharmacokinetics<br>well absorbed from GI tract; does not readily enter CSF; use decreased dose with renal failure | Contraindications<br>Use with caution in patients with true penicillin allergy; 5–7% cross-sensitivity between penicillins and cephalosporins in allergic patients<br><br>Pregnancy Category: B<br><br>Lactation Issues<br>Excreted in breast milk in small quantities; use with caution in nursing mothers; modification & alteration of bowel flora in infants may cause side effects such as diarrhea |

# Cefadroxil

Duricef, various generics

Tablet: 1 gm

Capsule: 500 mg

Powder for Oral Suspension:
125 mg/5 ml
250 mg/5 ml
500 mg/5 ml

**Antibacterial Spectrum**
Active against *S. aureus*, *S. pneumoniae* and *S. pyogenes*. Majority of urinary isolates of community-acquired *E. coli*, *Klebsiella species* and *P. mirabilis* are susceptible; not very active against *H. influenzae*; inactive against enterococci.

**Uncomplicated urinary tract infection**
**Adults:** 1–2 gm/d qd or divided bid for 7 to 10 d

**Children:** 30 mg/kg/d divided bid for 7 to 10 d

**Pharyngitis, tonsillitis, skin and soft tissue infections**
**Adults:** 1 gm/d divided bid for 10 d

**Children:** 30 mg/kg/d divided bid for 10 d

**Prevention of bacterial endocarditis**
Adults 2 gm (children 50 mg/kg) orally 1 hr before procedure

Administration Issues
Complete full course of therapy; shake suspension well before administration; store suspension in the refrigerator; discard unused suspension after 14 d

Drug–Drug Interactions
Cephalosporins may decrease the effectiveness of **oral contraceptives**; **probenecid** may increase cephalosporin plasma levels by competitively inhibiting renal excretion of cephalosporins

ADRs
hypersensitivity reactions, urticarial rash, nausea, vomiting, diarrhea, superinfections

Pharmacokinetics
well absorbed from GI tract; does not readily enter CSF; use decreased dose with renal failure

Contraindications
Use with caution in patients with true penicillin allergy; 5–7% cross-sensitivity between penicillins and cephalosporins in allergic patients

Pregnancy Category: B

Lactation Issues
Excreted in breast milk in small quantities; use with caution in nursing mothers; modification & alteration of bowel flora in infants may cause side effects such as diarrhea

# Cephradine

Velosef, various generics

Capsule:
250 mg, 500 mg

**Antibacterial Spectrum**
Active against *S. aureus*, *S. pneumoniae* and *S. pyogenes*. Majority of urinary isolates of community-acquired *E. coli*,

Administration Issues
Complete full course of therapy; shake suspension well before administration; suspension stable for 7 days at room temperature and 14 days if refrigerated

ADRs
hypersensitivity reactions, urticarial rash, nausea, vomiting, diarrhea, superinfections

Contraindications
Use with caution in patients with true penicillin allergy; 5–7% cross-sensitivity between penicillins and cephalosporins in allergic patients

(continues on next page)

## 102.1 Cephalosporins: First Generation  *continued from previous page*

| Drug and Dosage Forms | Spectrum of Activity and Usual Dosage Range | Administration Issues and Drug–Drug & Drug–Food Interactions | Common Adverse Drug Reactions (ADRs) and Pharmacokinetics | Contraindications, Pregnancy Category, and Lactation Issues |
|---|---|---|---|---|
| **Cephradine *cont.*** <br><br> Powder for Oral Suspension: <br> 125 mg/5 ml <br> 250 mg/5 ml | *Klebsiella species* and *P. mirabilis* are susceptible; not very active against *H. influenzae*, inactive against enterococci. <br><br> **General indications** <br> **Adults:** 250–500 mg q 6 h or 500–1000 mg q 12 h for 10 to 14 d <br><br> **Children:** 25–50 mg/kg/d divided q 6 to 12 h for 10 to 14 d <br><br> Otitis media: 75–100 mg/kg/d divided q 6 to 12 h for 10 to 14 d | Drug–Drug Interactions <br> Cephalosporins may decrease the effectiveness of **oral contraceptives**; **probenecid** may increase cephalosporin plasma levels by competitively inhibiting renal excretion of cephalosporins | Pharmacokinetics <br> well absorbed from GI tract; does not readily enter CSF; use decreased dose with renal failure | Pregnancy Category: B <br><br> Lactation Issues <br> Excreted in breast milk in small quantities; use with caution in nursing mothers; modification & alteration of bowel flora in infants may cause side effects such as diarrhea |

## 102.2 Cephalosporins: Second Generation

| Drug and Dosage Forms | Spectrum of Activity and Usual Dosage Range | Administration Issues and Drug–Drug & Drug–Food Interactions | Common Adverse Drug Reactions (ADRs) and Pharmacokinetics | Contraindications, Pregnancy Category, and Lactation Issues |
|---|---|---|---|---|
| **Cefaclor**<br>Ceclor, various generics<br><br>Capsule:<br>250 mg, 500 mg<br><br>Tablets, extended release (Ceclor CD):<br>375 mg, 500 mg<br><br>Powder for Oral Suspension:<br>125 mg/5 ml<br>187 mg/5 ml<br>250 mg/5 ml<br>375 mg/5 ml | **Spectrum of activity**<br>Active against S. aureus, S. pneumoniae, S. pyogenes, E. coli, Klebsiella species, M. catarrhalis and P. mirabilis. More active against ampicillin-susceptible H. influenzae than first generation cephalosporins but variable susceptibility against ampicillin-resistant strain of H. influenzae. Inactive against enterococci, B fragilis and many other gram-negative bacteria such as Pseudomonas, Serratia and Enterobacter species.<br><br>**General indications**<br>250–500 mg q 8 h for 10 to 14 d<br><br>**Acute bronchitis or exacerbations of chronic bronchitis**<br>500 mg q12 h for 7 d<br><br>**Pharyngitis: uncomplicated skin infections**<br>375 mg q 12h for 7 to 10 d<br><br>**Children**<br>20–40 mg/kg/d divided q 8 h for 10 to 14 d<br>**Maximum children's dose is 1 gm/d** | Administration Issues<br>Complete full course of therapy; shake suspension well before administration; store suspension in the refrigerator; discard unused suspension 14 days after reconstitution. Administer tablets with food; do not crush, chew or cut tablets.<br><br>Drug–Drug Interactions<br>Cephalosporins may decrease the effectiveness of **oral contraceptives**; **probenecid** may increase cephalosporin plasma levels by competitively inhibiting renal excretion of cephalosporins | ADRs<br>hypersensitivity reactions, urticarial rash, nausea, vomiting, diarrhea, superinfections<br><br>Pharmacokinetics<br>does not readily enter CSF; use decreased dose with renal failure | Contraindications<br>Use with caution in patients with true penicillin allergy; 5–7% cross-sensitivity between penicillins and cephalosporins in allergic patients<br><br>Pregnancy Category:  B<br><br>Lactation Issues<br>Excreted in breast milk in small quantities; use with caution in nursing mothers; modification/alteration of bowel flora in infants may cause side effects such as diarrhea |

*(continues on next page)*

935

| Drug and Dosage Forms | Spectrum of Activity and Usual Dosage Range | Administration Issues and Drug–Drug & Drug–Food Interactions | Common Adverse Drug Reactions (ADRs) and Pharmacokinetics | Contraindications, Pregnancy Category, and Lactation Issues |
|---|---|---|---|---|
| **Cefuroxime Axetil**<br>Ceftin<br><br>Tablet:<br>125 mg, 250 mg, 500 mg<br><br>Powder for Oral Suspension:<br>125 mg/5 ml | **Spectrum of activity**<br>Active against *S. aureus,*<br>*S. pneumoniae* and *S. pyogenes.*<br>Active against *E. coli, Klebsiella species, M. catarrhalis* and<br>*P. mirabilis.* Active against beta-lactamase positive and beta-lactamase negative *H. influenzae.*<br>Inactive against enterococci, *B fragilis* and many other gram-negative bacteria such as *Pseudomonas* and *Serratia.*<br><br>**Pharyngitis/tonsillitis, bronchitis, and uncomplicated skin and skin structure infections**<br>**Adults and children ≥ 13 yr.**<br>250–500 mg q12 h for 10 d<br><br>**Uncomplicated urinary tract infections**<br>**Adults and children ≥ 13 yr.**<br>125–250 mg q 12 h for 7 to 10 d<br><br>**Uncomplicated gonococcal infections**<br>**Adults and children ≥ 13 yr.**<br>1000 mg as a single dose | Administration Issues<br>Tablets and suspension are not bioequivalent and cannot be substituted on a mg/kg basis; tablets can be taken without regard to meals; suspension must be taken with food; suspension may be stored at room temperature or in the refrigerator; discard unused suspension 10 days after reconstitution<br><br>Drug–Drug Interactions<br>Cephalosporins may decrease the effectiveness of **oral contraceptives; probenecid** may increase cephalosporin plasma levels by competitively inhibiting renal excretion of cephalosporins | ADRs<br>hypersensitivity reactions, urticarial rash, nausea, vomiting, diarrhea, superinfections<br><br>Pharmacokinetics<br>does not readily enter CSF; use decreased dose with renal failure; absorption increased with food | Contraindications<br>Use with caution in patients with true penicillin allergy; 5–7% cross-sensitivity between penicillins and cephalosporins in allergic patients<br><br>Pregnancy Category:  B<br><br>Lactation Issues<br>Excreted in breast milk in small quantities; use with caution in nursing mothers; modification/ alteration of bowel flora in infants may cause side effects such as diarrhea |

| | | | |
|---|---|---|---|
| | **Pharyngitis/tonsillitis**<br>**Children 3 months to 12 yr.**<br>(dosage for suspension)<br>20 mg/kg/d divided q 12 h for 10 d<br>(max: 500mg/d)<br><br>**Uncomplicated skin infections**<br>**and otitis media**<br>**Children 3 months to 12 yr.**<br>(dosage for suspension)<br>30 mg/kg/d divided q 12 h for 10 d<br>(max: 1000mg/d) | | | **Contraindications**<br>Use with caution in patients with true penicillin allergy; 5–7% cross-sensitivity between penicillins and cephalosporins in allergic patients<br><br>**Pregnancy Category:** B<br><br>**Lactation Issues**<br>Excreted in breast milk in small quantities; use with caution in nursing mothers; modification/alteration of bowel flora in infants may cause side effects such as diarrhea |
| **Cefprozil**<br>Cefzil<br><br>Tablet:<br>250 mg, 500 mg<br><br>Powder for Oral Suspension:<br>125 mg/5 ml<br>250 mg/5 ml | **Spectrum of Activity**<br>Active against *S. aureus*, *S. pneumoniae*, *S. pyogenes*, *E. coli*, *Klebsiella species*, *M. catarrhalis* and *P. mirabilis*. Active against beta-lactamase positive and beta-lactamase negative *H. influenzae*. Inactive against enterococci, *B fragilis* and many other gram-negative bacteria such as *Pseudomonas* and *Serratia*.<br><br>**Pharyngitis/tonsillitis and**<br>**bronchitis**<br>**Adults:** 500 mg q12 to 24 h for 10 d<br><br>**Children 2 to 12 yr.**<br>15 mg/kg/d divided q 12 h for 10 d<br><br>**Uncomplicated skin and skin**<br>**structure infections**<br>**Adults:** 250 mg q 12 h for 10 d <u>or</u> 500 mg q 12 to 24 h for 10 d | **Administration Issues**<br>Complete full course of therapy; shake suspension well before administration; store suspension in the refrigerator; discard unused suspension 14 days after reconstitution<br><br>**Drug–Drug Interactions**<br>Cephalosporins may decrease the effectiveness of **oral contraceptives**; **probenecid** may increase cephalosporin plasma levels by competitively inhibiting renal excretion of cephalosporins | **ADRs**<br>hypersensitivity reactions, urticarial rash, nausea, vomiting, diarrhea, superinfections<br><br>**Pharmacokinetics**<br>does not readily enter CSF; use decreased dose with renal failure; absorption increased with food | |

*(continues on next page)*

937

| Drug and Dosage Forms | Spectrum of Activity and Usual Dosage Range | Administration Issues and Drug–Drug & Drug–Food Interactions | Common Adverse Drug Reactions (ADRs) and Pharmacokinetics | Contraindications, Pregnancy Category, and Lactation Issues |
|---|---|---|---|---|
| **Cefprozil** *cont.* | **Children:** 20 mg/kg q 24 h for 10 d<br><br>**Otitis media (Children 6 months to 12 yr.)**<br>30 mg/kg/d divided q 12 h for 10 d | | | |
| **Loracarbef**<br>Lorabid<br><br>Capsule: 200 mg<br><br>Powder for Oral Suspension: 100 mg/5 ml | **Spectrum of Activity**<br>Active against *S. aureus, S. pneumoniae, S. pyogenes, E. coli, Klebsiella species, M. catarrhalis* and *P. mirabilis*. Active against beta-lactamase positive and beta-lactamase negative *H. influenzae.* Inactive against enterococci, *B fragilis* and many other gram-negative bacteria such as *Pseudomonas* and *Serratia*<br><br>**Upper and lower respiratory tract infections, skin and soft tissue infections, uncomplicated UTI**<br>**Adults and children ≥ 13 yr.**<br>200–400 mg q 12 h for 7 to 14 d<br><br>**Pharyngitis, tonsillitis, skin and soft tissue infections**<br>**Children 6 months to 12 yr.**<br>15 mg/kg/d divided q 12 h for 7 to 10 d<br><br>**Acute Otitis Media (use suspension)**<br>30mg/kg/d divided q12 h for 10 d | Administration Issues<br>Complete full course of therapy; shake suspension well before administration; suspension may be kept at room temperature; discard unused suspension after 14 days; suspension is more rapidly absorbed than the capsules<br><br>Drug–Drug Interactions<br>Cephalosporins may decrease the effectiveness of **oral contraceptives; probenecid** may increase cephalosporin plasma levels by competitively inhibiting renal excretion of cephalosporins | ADRs<br>hypersensitivity reactions, urticarial rash, nausea, vomiting, diarrhea, superinfections<br><br>Pharmacokinetics<br>does not readily enter CSF; use decreased dose with renal failure; absorption increased with food | Contraindications<br>Use with caution in patients with true penicillin allergy; 5–7% cross-sensitivity between penicillins and cephalosporins in allergic patients<br><br>Pregnancy Category: B<br><br>Lactation Issues<br>Excreted in breast milk in small quantities; use with caution in nursing mothers; modification/ alteration of bowel flora in infants may cause side effects such as diarrhea |

102.2 Cephalosporins: Second Generation *continued from previous page*

938

## 102.3 Cephalosporins: Third Generation

| Drug and Dosage Forms | Spectrum of Activity and Usual Dosage Range | Administration Issues and Drug–Drug & Drug–Food Interactions | Common Adverse Drug Reactions (ADRs) and Pharmacokinetics | Contraindications, Pregnancy Category, and Lactation Issues |
|---|---|---|---|---|
| **Cefixime**<br>Suprax<br><br><u>Tablet:</u><br>200 mg, 400 mg<br><br><u>Powder for Oral Suspension:</u><br>100 mg/5 ml | **Spectrum of Activity**<br>Active against group A streptococci, S. pneumoniae, H. influenzae, M. catarrhalis, N. gonorrhoeae including beta-lactamase producers. Active against E coli, Klebsiella sp., P. mirabilis and S. marcescens. No activity against staphylococci, Pseudomonas species or anaerobes.<br><br>**Pharyngitis/tonsillitis, bronchitis, uncomplicated UTI**<br>**Adults and children > 12 yr.**<br>400 mg qd or 200 mg q 12 for 7 to 10 d<br><br>**Children < 12 yr.**<br>8 mg/kg/d divided q12 h for 7 to 10 d<br>(Treat otitis media with suspension)<br><br>**Uncomplicated gonococcal infections**<br>**Adults and children > 12 yr.**<br>4900 mg as a single dose<br><br>**Children < 12 yr.**<br>8 mg/kg as a single dose | <u>Administration Issues</u><br>Complete full course of therapy; shake suspension well before administration; give suspension with food; store suspension at room temperature; discard unused suspension 14 days after reconstitution; swallow tablet whole, do not crush; suspension should be use in the treatment of otitis media.<br><br><u>Drug–Drug Interactions</u><br>Cephalosporins may decrease the effectiveness of **oral contraceptives; probenecid** may increase cephalosporin plasma levels by competitively inhibiting renal excretion of cephalosporins | <u>ADRs</u><br>hypersensitivity reactions, urticarial rash. nausea, vomiting, diarrhea, superinfections<br><br><u>Pharmacokinetics</u><br>use decreased dose with renal failure; absorption increased with food | <u>Contraindications</u><br>Use with caution in patients with true penicillin allergy; 5–7% cross-sensitivity between penicillins and cephalosporins in allergic patients<br><br><u>Pregnancy Category:</u> B<br><br><u>Lactation Issues</u><br>Excreted in breast milk in small quantities; use with caution in nursing mothers; modification/ alteration of bowel flora in infants may cause side effects such as diarrhea |

(continues on next page)

| Drug and Dosage Forms | Spectrum of Activity and Usual Dosage Range | Administration Issues and Drug–Drug & Drug–Food Interactions | Common Adverse Drug Reactions (ADRs) and Pharmacokinetics | Contraindications, Pregnancy Category, and Lactation Issues |
|---|---|---|---|---|
| **Cefpodoxime Proxetil**<br>Vantin<br><br>Tablet:<br>100 mg, 200 mg<br><br>Granules for Oral Suspension:<br>50 mg/5 ml<br>100 mg/5 ml | **Spectrum of Activity**<br>Active against *S. pyogenes, S. agalactiae, S. pneumoniae*, beta-lactamase–positive and –negative *H. influenzae, M. catarrhalis, N. gonorrhoeae* and many Enterobacteriaceae (not *Enterobacter, Serratia* or *Morganella*). Modest activity against *S. aureus* with no activity for enterococci or MRSA.<br><br>**Community-acquired pneumonia and bronchitis**<br>**Adults and children ≥ 13 yr.**<br>200 mg q 12 h for 10 to 14 d<br><br>**Uncomplicated gonococcal infection**<br>**Adults and children ≥ 13 yr.**<br>200 mg as a single dose<br><br>**Skin and skin structure infection**<br>**Adults and children ≥ 13 yr.**<br>400 mg q 12 h for 7 to 14 d<br><br>**Pharyngitis/tonsillitis**<br>**Adults and children ≥ 13 yr.**<br>100 mg q 12 h for 10 d<br><br>**Children 6 months to 12 yr.**<br>10 mg/kg/d divided q 12 h for 10 d | Administration Issues<br>Complete full course of therapy; give with food; administer with food to enhance absorption; shake suspension well before administration; store suspension in the refrigerator; discard unused suspension 14 days after reconstitution<br><br>Drug–Drug Interactions<br>Cephalosporins may decrease the effectiveness of **oral contraceptives**; **probenecid** may increase cephalosporin plasma levels by competitively inhibiting renal excretion of cephalosporins | ADRs<br>hypersensitivity reactions, urticarial rash. nausea, vomiting, diarrhea, superinfections<br><br>Pharmacokinetics<br>use decreased dose with renal failure | Contraindications<br>Use with caution in patients with true penicillin allergy; 5–7% cross-sensitivity between penicillins and cephalosporins in allergic patients<br><br>Pregnancy Category: B<br><br>Lactation Issues<br>Excreted in breast milk in small quantities; use with caution in nursing mothers; modification/alteration of bowel flora in infants may cause side effects such as diarrhea |

| | | | | |
|---|---|---|---|---|
| | **Uncomplicated UTI**<br>**Adults and children ≥ 13 yr.**<br>100 mg q 12 h for 10 d<br><br>**Acute otitis media**<br>**Children 6 months to 12 yr.**<br>10 mg/kg /d divided q 12 h for 10 d | | | |
| **Ceftibutin**<br>Cedax<br><br>Capsule: 400 mg<br><br>Powder for Oral Suspension:<br>90 mg/5 ml<br>180 mg/5 ml | **Spectrum of Activity**<br>Active against *S. pneumoniae*<br>(penicillin-susceptible strains only),<br>*S. pyogenes*, beta-lactamase<br>producing strains of *H. influenzae* and<br>*M catarrhalis*.<br><br>**Pharyngitis/tonsillitis,**<br>**bronchitis, and otitis media**<br>**Adults and children ≥ 12 yr.**<br>400 mg qd for 10 d<br><br>**Children ≤ 12 yr.:** 9 mg/kg qd<br>for 10 d<br><br>**Maximum children's dose is**<br>**400 mg/day** | Administration Issues<br>Complete full course of therapy; shake<br>suspension well before administration;<br>store suspension in the refrigerator;<br>discard unused suspension 14 days after<br>reconstitution; give oral suspension at<br>least 2 h before or 1 hour after a meal<br><br>Drug–Drug Interactions<br>Cephalosporins may decrease the<br>effectiveness of **oral contraceptives;**<br>**probenecid** may increase<br>cephalosporin plasma levels by<br>competitively inhibiting renal excretion<br>of cephalosporins | ADRs<br>hypersensitivity reactions,<br>urticarial rash. nausea,<br>vomiting, diarrhea,<br>superinfections<br><br>Pharmacokinetics<br>use decreased dose with renal<br>failure | Contraindications<br>Use with caution in patients with<br>true penicillin allergy; 5–7%<br>cross-sensitivity between<br>penicillins and cephalosporins<br>in allergic patients<br><br>Pregnancy Category: B<br><br>Lactation Issues<br>Excreted in breast milk in small<br>quantities; use with caution in<br>nursing mothers; modification/<br>alteration of bowel flora in<br>infants may cause side effects<br>such as diarrhea |
| **Ceftriaxone**<br>Rocephin<br><br>Powder for Injection:<br>250 mg, 500 mg, 1 gm, 2 gm | **Spectrum of Activity**<br>Ceftriaxone has activity as a single<br>dose for uncomplicated gonococcal<br>infections, chancroid, PID and as a<br>one-time dose for the treatment of<br>otitis media in children. | Administration Issues<br>IM solutions reconstituted to<br>250 mg/ml concentration remain<br>stable for 24 h at room temperature<br>and 3 days refrigerated when<br>reconstituted with sterile water<br>for injection, 0.9% NaCl, dextrose<br>5%, bacteriostatic water, or 1%<br>lidocaine solution without<br>epinephrine | ADRs<br>hypersensitivity reactions,<br>urticarial rash. nausea,<br>vomiting, diarrhea,<br>superinfections; may cause<br>pain upon injection | Contraindications<br>Use with caution in patients with<br>true penicillin allergy; 5–7%<br>cross-sensitivity between<br>penicillins and cephalosporins<br>in allergic patients<br><br>Pregnancy Category: B |

(continues on next page)

| Drug and Dosage Forms | Spectrum of Activity and Usual Dosage Range | Administration Issues and Drug–Drug & Drug–Food Interactions | Common Adverse Drug Reactions (ADRs) and Pharmacokinetics | Contraindications, Pregnancy Category, and Lactation Issues |
|---|---|---|---|---|
| **Ceftriaxone** *cont.* | **Uncomplicated gonococcal infections** **Adults and children** 125 mg IM as a single dose with doxycycline 100 mg q 12 h for 7 days **Children < 8 yr. should not receive doxycycline or any tetracycline antibiotic** **Gonococcal conjunctivitis** **Adults:** 1 gm IM as a single dose with saline irrigation **Neonates:** 25–50 mg/kg (max = 125 mg) IV/IM as a single dose **Chancroid infection** **Adults:** 250 mg IM as a single dose **Pelvic inflammatory disease (outpatient treatment)** 250 mg IM as a single dose with doxycycline 100 mg q 12 h for 14 d **Otitis Media** **Children:** 50 mg/kg (max dose = 1 g) IM one time | <u>Drug–Drug Interactions</u> Cephalosporins may decrease the effectiveness of **oral contraceptives**; **probenecid** may increase cephalosporin plasma levels by competitively inhibiting renal excretion of cephalosporins | | <u>Lactation Issues</u> Excreted in breast milk in small quantities; use with caution in nursing mothers; modification/alteration of bowel flora in infants may cause side effects such as diarrhea |

# 102.4 Fluoroquinolones

| Drug and Dosage Forms | Spectrum of Activity and Usual Dosage Range | Administration Issues and Drug–Drug & Drug–Food Interactions | Common Adverse Drug Reactions (ADRs) and Pharmacokinetics | Contraindications, Pregnancy Category, and Lactation Issues |
|---|---|---|---|---|
| **Ciprofloxacin**<br>Cipro<br><br>Tablet:<br>100 mg, 250 mg, 500 mg, 750 mg | **Spectrum of Activity**<br>Active against Enterobacteriaceae, *Enterobacter* sp., *Morganella morganii*, *N. gonorrhoeae*, *P. aeruginosa*, Proteus sp., *Serratia* sp.; also effective against *Mycobacterium avium*; less active against gram-positive organisms<br><br>**Mild to moderate urinary tract infections**<br>250 mg q 12 h for 7 to 14 d<br><br>**Severe urinary tract infections**<br>500 mg q 12 h for 7 to 14 d<br><br>**Mild to moderate lower respiratory tract infections, bone and joint infections, skin/skin structure infections, infectious diarrhea, and typhoid fever**<br>500 mg q 12 h for 7 to 14 d<br><br>**Severe lower respiratory tract infections, bone/joint infections, skin/skin structure infections**<br>750 mg q 12 h for 7 to 14 d | Administration Issues<br>May be taken without regard to meals; do not take with antacids or products containing iron or zinc or take 2 h before or 2 h after taking such products; give with a full glass of water<br><br>Drug–Drug/Drug–Food Interactions<br>Ciprofloxacin may increase blood levels of **theophylline, cyclosporine, caffeine** and **warfarin. Antacids and products containing calcium, magnesium, aluminum, dairy products, didanosine, iron salts, sucralfate,** and **zinc salts** interfere with the absorption of fluoroquinolones resulting in decreased serum levels. **Cimetidine** may interfere with the elimination of fluoroquinolones | ADRs<br>nausea, abdominal discomfort, diarrhea, dizziness, photosensitivity, superinfections<br><br>**Use with caution in children < 18 yr. due to potential for cartilage damage and erosion**<br><br>Pharmacokinetics<br>well absorbed from GI tract; consider decreased dosage with renal impairment | Contraindications<br>Hypersensitivity to fluoroquinolones<br><br>Pregnancy Category: C<br><br>Lactation Issues<br>Excreted in breast milk with amount ingested by infant low |

*(continues on next page)*

| Drug and Dosage Forms | Spectrum of Activity and Usual Dosage Range | Administration Issues and Drug–Drug & Drug–Food Interactions | Common Adverse Drug Reactions (ADRs) and Pharmacokinetics | Contraindications, Pregnancy Category, and Lactation Issues |
|---|---|---|---|---|
| **Ciprofloxacin** *cont.* | Bone/joint infections may require treatment for 4 to 6 weeks<br><br>**Uncomplicated gonococcal infections**<br>500 mg as a single dose<br><br>**Treatment of *Mycobacterium avium* complex (unlabeled indication)**<br>750 mg q 12 h as part of a multi-drug regimen | | | |
| **Enoxacin**<br>Penetrex<br><br>Tablet:<br>200 mg, 400 mg | **Spectrum of Activity**<br>Same as for ciprofloxacin for organisms confined to the urinary tract plus uncomplicated gonorrhea; no activity vs. *M. avium.*<br><br>**Uncomplicated urinary tract infections**<br>200 mg q 12 h for 7 d<br><br>**Complicated urinary tract infections**<br>400 mg q 12 h for 14 d<br><br>**Uncomplicated gonococcal infections**<br>400 mg as a single dose | Administration Issues<br>Take 1 hour before or 2 h after meals; do not take with antacids or products containing iron or zinc; or take 2 h before or 2 h after product; give with a full glass of water<br><br>Drug–Drug/Drug–Food Interactions<br>Enoxacin may increase blood levels of **theophylline, cyclosporine, caffeine** and **warfarin. Antacids and products containing calcium, magnesium, aluminum, dairy products, didanosine, iron salts, sucralfate,** and **zinc salts** interfere with the absorption of fluoroquinolones resulting in decreased serum levels. | ADRs<br>nausea, abdominal discomfort, diarrhea, dizziness, photosensitivity, superinfections<br><br>**Use with caution in children < 18 yr. due to potential for cartilage damage and erosion**<br><br>Pharmacokinetics<br>well absorbed from GI tract; consider decreased dosage with renal impairment | Contraindications<br>Hypersensitivity to fluoroquinolones<br><br>Pregnancy Category: C<br><br>Lactation Issues<br>Excretion in breast milk is unknown; use with caution, decide whether to discontinue nursing or discontinue the drug |

| | **Spectrum of Activity** | Administration Issues | ADRs | Contraindications |
|---|---|---|---|---|
| | | **Cimetidine** may interfere with the elimination of fluoroquinolones | | |
| **Grepafloxacin**<br>Raxar<br><br>Tablets:<br>200 mg | **Spectrum of Activity**<br>Active against S. aureus, S. pneumoniae, pneumococci, H. influenzae, M. catarrhalis, L. pneumophila, C. pneumophila, M. pneumoniae, N. gonorrhoeae and C. trachomatis. Less active than ciprofloxacin against P. aeruginosa but more active against anaerobes.<br><br>**Acute exacerbations of chronic bronchitis**<br>400 mg or 600 mg qd for 10 d<br><br>**Community-acquired pneumonia**<br>600 mg qd for 10 d<br><br>**Uncomplicated gonococcal infections**<br>400 mg as a single dose<br><br>**Nongonococcal urethritis**<br>400 mg qd for 7 d | Administration Issues<br>Do not take with antacids or products containing iron or zinc or take 4 h before or 4 h after taking such products; give with a full glass of water<br><br>Drug–Drug /Drug–Food Interactions<br>Grepafloxacin may increase blood levels of **theophylline, cyclosporine, caffeine** and **warfarin. Antacids and products containing calcium, magnesium, aluminum, dairy products, didanosine, iron salts, sucralfate,** and **zinc salts** interfere with the absorption of fluoroquinolones resulting in decreased serum levels. **Cimetidine** may interfere with the elimination of fluoroquinolones | ADRs<br>nausea, abdominal discomfort, diarrhea, dizziness, taste disturbances (rare), photosensitivity, superinfections<br><br>**Use with caution in children < 18 yr. due to potential for cartilage damage and erosion**<br><br>Pharmacokinetics<br>well absorbed from GI tract; no dosage adjustment required in patients with impaired renal function. | Contraindications<br>Hypersensitivity to fluoroquinolones<br><br>Pregnancy Category: C<br><br>Lactation Issues<br>Excretion in breast milk is unknown; use with caution, decide whether to discontinue nursing or discontinue the drug |
| **Levofloxacin**<br>Levaquin<br><br>Tablet: 250mg, 500mg | **Spectrum of Activity**<br>Active against S. pneumoniae, H. influenzae, M. catarrhalis, S. aureus, K. pneumoniae, C. pneumoniae, L. pneumophila and urinary tract infections due to | Administration Issues<br>May be taken without regard to meals; do not take with antacids or products containing iron or zinc or take 2 h before or 2 h after taking such products; give with a full glass of water | ADRs<br>nausea, abdominal discomfort, diarrhea, dizziness, photosensitivity, superinfections | Contraindications<br>Hypersensitivity to fluoroquinolones<br><br>Pregnancy Category: C |

(continues on next page)

| Drug and Dosage Forms | Spectrum of Activity and Usual Dosage Range | Administration Issues and Drug–Drug & Drug–Food Interactions | Common Adverse Drug Reactions (ADRs) and Pharmacokinetics | Contraindications, Pregnancy Category, and Lactation Issues |
|---|---|---|---|---|
| **Levofloxacin *cont.*** | *E. cloacae, E. coli, P. mirabilis* and *P. aeruginosa*.<br><br>**Acute exacerbations of chronic bronchitis, community-acquired pneumonia, acute sinusitis**<br>500 mg q 24 h for 7–14 d<br><br>**Complicated UTI/Acute pyelonephritis**<br>250 mg q 24 h for 10 d | <u>Drug–Drug /Drug–Food Interactions</u><br>Levofloxacin may increase blood levels of **theophylline, cyclosporine, caffeine** and **warfarin. Antacids and products containing calcium, magnesium, aluminum, dairy products, didanosine, iron salts, sucralfate,** and **zinc salts** interfere with the absorption of fluoroquinolones resulting in decreased serum levels. **Cimetidine** may interfere with the elimination of fluoroquinolones | **Use with caution in children < 18 yr. due to potential for cartilage damage and erosion**<br><br>Pharmacokinetics<br>well absorbed from GI tract; decrease dosage with renal impairment | <u>Lactation Issues</u><br>Excreted in breast milk with amount ingested by infant low |
| **Lomefloxacin**<br>Maxaquin<br><br><u>Tablet:</u> 400 mg | **Spectrum of Activity**<br>Active against *H. influenzae, M. catarrhalis,* and urinary tract infections caused by *E. coli, K. pneumoniae, P. aeruginosa* and *S. saprophyticus.* Lomefloxacin is not indicated for empiric therapy of acute bacterial exacerbations of chronic bronchitis when *S. pneumoniae* may be a causative pathogen.<br><br>**Uncomplicated urinary tract infections**<br>400 mg qd for 10 d | <u>Administration Issues</u><br>Do not take with antacids or products containing iron or zinc or take 2 h before or 2 h after taking such products; give with a full glass of water<br><br><u>Drug–Drug /Drug–Food Interactions</u><br>Lomefloxacin may increase blood levels of **cyclosporine, caffeine** and **warfarin. Antacids and products containing calcium, magnesium, aluminum, dairy products, didanosine, iron salts, sucralfate,** and **zinc salts** interfere with the absorption of fluoroquinolones | <u>ADRs</u><br>nausea, abdominal discomfort, diarrhea, dizziness, photosensitivity, superinfections<br><br>**Use with caution in children < 18 yr. due to potential for cartilage damage and erosion**<br><br>Pharmacokinetics<br>well absorbed from GI tract; consider decreased dosage with renal impairment | <u>Contraindications</u><br>Hypersensitivity to fluoroquinolones<br><br><u>Pregnancy Category:</u> C<br><br><u>Lactation Issues</u><br>Excretion in breast milk is unknown; use with caution, decide whether to discontinue nursing or discontinue the drug |

| | | | | |
|---|---|---|---|---|
| | **Complicated urinary tract infections**<br>400 mg qd for 14 d<br><br>**Lower respiratory tract infections**<br>400 mg qd for 10 d<br><br>**Uncomplicated gonococcal infections**<br>400 mg as a single dose | resulting in decreased serum levels. **Cimetidine** may interfere with the elimination of fluoroquinolones. Lomefloxacin does **not** appear to alter theophylline or caffeine levels. | | <u>Contraindications</u><br>Hypersensitivity to fluoroquinolones<br><br><u>Pregnancy Category:</u> C<br><br><u>Lactation Issues</u><br>Not detected in breast milk after a 20 mg dose |
| **Norfloxacin**<br>Noroxin<br><br><u>Tablet:</u> 400 mg | **Spectrum of Activity**<br>Active against the following organisms found in urinary tract infections: *E. faecalis, E. coli, K. pneumoniae, P. mirabilis, P. aeruginosa, S. epidermidis, S. saprophyticus, E. aerogenes, E. cloacae, S. aureus, S. agalactiae.* Active against *N. gonorrhoeae* and prostatitis due to *E. coli.*<br><br>**Treatment of uncomplicated urinary tract infections due to *E. coli, Klebsiella pneumonia, or Proteus mirabilis***<br>400 mg q 12 h for 3 d<br><br>Use 400 mg q 12 h for 7 to 10 d for UTI caused by other gram negative organisms<br><br>**Uncomplicated gonococcal infections**<br>800 mg as a single dose<br><br>**Prostatitis due to *E. coli***<br>400 mg q 12 h for 28 d | <u>Administration Issues</u><br>Take 1 hour before or 2 h after meals; do not take with antacids or products containing iron or zinc; give with a full glass of water<br><br><u>Drug–Drug–Food Interactions</u><br>Norfloxacin may increase blood levels of **theophylline, cyclosporine, caffeine** and **warfarin. Antacids and products containing calcium, magnesium, aluminum, dairy products, didanosine, iron salts, sucralfate,** and **zinc salts** interfere with the absorption of fluoroquinolones resulting in decreased serum levels. **Cimetidine** may interfere with the elimination of fluoroquinolones | <u>ADRs</u><br>nausea, abdominal discomfort, diarrhea, dizziness, photosensitivity, superinfections<br><br>**Use with caution in children < 18 yr. due to potential for cartilage damage and erosion**<br><br><u>Pharmacokinetics</u><br>consider decreased dosage with renal impairment | |

*(continues on next page)*

## 102.4 Fluoroquinolones continued from previous page

| Drug and Dosage Forms | Spectrum of Activity and Usual Dosage Range | Administration Issues and Drug–Drug & Drug–Food Interactions | Common Adverse Drug Reactions (ADRs) and Pharmacokinetics | Contraindications, Pregnancy Category, and Lactation Issues |
|---|---|---|---|---|
| **Ofloxacin**<br>Floxin<br><u>Tablet:</u><br>200 mg, 300 mg, 400 mg | **Spectrum of Activity**<br>Active against *H. influenzae, S. pneumoniae, N. gonorrhoeae, C. trachomatis* and against urinary tract infections due to the following organisms: *E. coli, E. aerogenes, K. pneumoniae, P. mirabilis, P. aeruginosa* and prostatitis due to *E. coli.*<br><br><u>**Uncomplicated urinary tract infections due to** *E. coli, Klebsiella pneumonia, Proteus mirabilis*</u><br>200 mg q 12 h for 3 days<br><br>Use 200 mg q 12 h for 7 days for UTI caused by other gram–negative organisms<br><br><u>**Complicated urinary tract infections**</u><br>200 mg q 12 h for 10 days<br><br><u>**Prostatitis**</u><br>300 mg q 12 h for 6 weeks<br><br><u>**Mild to moderate lower respiratory tract infections, bone/joint infections, skin/skin structure infections**</u><br>400 mg q 12 h for 10 days | <u>Administration Issues</u><br>Do not take with food; do not take with antacids or products containing iron or zinc; give with a full glass of water<br><br><u>Drug–Drug Interactions</u><br>Ofloxacin may increase blood levels of **cyclosporine, caffeine** and **warfarin. Antacids and products containing calcium, magnesium, aluminum, dairy products, didanosine, iron salts, sucralfate,** and **zinc salts** interfere with the absorption of fluoroquinolones resulting in decreased serum levels. **Cimetidine** may interfere with the elimination of fluoroquinolones. Ofloxacin may not interfere with theophylline levels but data is inconclusive. | <u>ADRs</u><br>nausea, abdominal discomfort, diarrhea, dizziness, photosensitivity, superinfections<br><br>**Use with caution in children < 18 yr. due to potential for cartilage damage and erosion**<br><br><u>Pharmacokinetics</u><br>well absorbed from GI tract; consider decreased dosage with renal impairment | <u>Contraindications</u><br>Hypersensitivity to fluoroquinolones<br><br><u>Pregnancy Category:</u>  C<br><br><u>Lactation Issues</u><br>Breast milk concentrations have been found that are similar to plasma concentrations |

| | | | |
|---|---|---|---|
| **Sparfloxacin**<br>Zagam<br><br><u>Tablet:</u><br>200 mg | **Uncomplicated gonococcal infections**<br>400 mg as a single dose<br><br>**Spectrum of Activity**<br>Active against S. pneumoniae, S. aureus, H. influenzae, M. catarrhalis, S. aureus, K. pneumoniae, C. pneumoniae, M. pneumoniae<br><br><u>Community-acquired pneumonia</u><br>400 mg day 1, followed by 200 mg qd for 9 d<br><br>**Acute Bacterial Exacerbations of Chronic Bronchitis:** 400 mg day 1, followed by 200 mg qd for 9 d<br><br>**Avoid exposure to direct or indirect sunlight and UV light during therapy and for 5 days after therapy; discontinue sparfloxacin at first sign or symptom of phototoxicity reaction** | <u>Administration Issues</u><br>Can be taken without regards to meals; vitamins and minerals containing iron, antacids products and sucralfate should be taken at least 4 hr before or 4 hr after sparfloxacin; give with a full glass of water; sparfloxacin may cause lightheadedness or dizziness<br><br><u>Drug–Drug Interactions</u><br>**Antacids and products containing calcium, magnesium, aluminum, dairy products, didanosine, iron salts, sucralfate, and zinc salts** interfere with the absorption of fluoroquinolones resulting in decreased serum levels. | <u>ADRs</u><br>photosensitivity, nausea, headache, abdominal discomfort, diarrhea, dizziness, insomnia, superinfections, taste perversion<br><br>**Use with caution in children < 18 yr. due to potential for cartilage damage and erosion**<br><br><u>Pharmacokinetics</u><br>well absorbed from GI tract; consider decreased dosage with renal impairment | <u>Contraindications</u><br>Hypersensitivity to fluoroquinolones<br><br><u>Pregnancy Category:</u>  C<br><br><u>Lactation Issues</u><br>Breast milk concentrations have been found that are similar to plasma concentrations |
| **Trovafloxacin**<br>Trovan<br><br><u>Tablets:</u><br>100 mg, 200 mg | **Spectrum of Activity**<br>Active against S. pneumoniae, S. aureus, H. influenzae, M. catarrhalis, S. aureus, K. pneumoniae, C. pneumoniae, C. trachomatis, N. gonorrhoeae, L. pneumophila, M. pneumoniae, B. fragilis, Peptostreptococcus species, viridans group streptococci, E. faecalis, and urinary tract infections due to E. coli. | <u>Administration Issues</u><br>Can be taken without regards to meals; vitamins and minerals containing iron, antacids products and sucralfate should be taken at least 2 hr before or 2 hr after trovan; give with a full glass of water; trovan may cause lightheadedness or dizziness | <u>ADRs</u><br>dizziness, lightheadedness, nausea, abdominal discomfort, diarrhea, photosensitivity, headache, superinfections<br><br>**Use with caution in children < 18 yr. due to potential for cartilage damage and erosion** | <u>Contraindications</u><br>Hypersensitivity to fluoroquinolones<br><br><u>Pregnancy Category:</u>  C<br><br><u>Lactation Issues</u><br>Breast milk concentrations have been found that are similar to plasma concentrations |

*(continues on next page)*

| Drug and Dosage Forms | Spectrum of Activity and Usual Dosage Range | Administration Issues and Drug–Drug & Drug–Food Interactions | Common Adverse Drug Reactions (ADRs) and Pharmacokinetics | Contraindications, Pregnancy Category, and Lactation Issues |
|---|---|---|---|---|
| **Trovafloxacin *cont.*** | **Community-acquired pneumonia:** 200 mg qd for 7–14 d<br><br>**Acute Bacterial Exacerbations of Chronic Bronchitis:** 100 mg qd for 7–10 d<br><br>**Acute Sinusitis:** 200 mg qd for 10 d<br><br>**Skin/Skin Structure Infections** 100 mg qd for 7–10 d<br><br>**Uncomplicated UTIs** 100 mg qd for 3 d<br><br>**Chronic Bacterial Prostatitis** 200 mg qd for 28 d<br><br>**Uncomplicated Urethral Gonorrhea in Males/ Endocervical & Rectal Gonorrhea in Females** 100 mg as a single dose<br><br>**C. trachomatis cervicitis** 200 mg qd for 5 d<br><br>**PID (mild to moderate)** 200 mg qd for 14 d | Drug–Drug Interactions<br>**Antacids and products containing calcium, magnesium, aluminum, dairy products, didanosine, iron salts, sucralfate, and zinc salts** interfere with the absorption of fluoroquinolones resulting in decreased serum levels. | Pharmacokinetics<br>well absorbed from GI tract; no dosage adjustment necessary in patients with renal impairment | |

| Drug and Dosage Forms | Spectrum of Activity and Usual Dosage Range | Administration Issues and Drug–Drug & Drug–Food Interactions | Common Adverse Drug Reactions (ADRs) and Pharmacokinetics | Contraindications, Pregnancy Category, and Lactation Issues |
|---|---|---|---|---|
| **Azithromycin**<br>Zithromax<br><br>Capsule:  250 mg<br><br>Suspension:<br>100 mg/5 ml<br>200 mg/5 ml | **Antibacterial Spectrum**<br>Gram-positive organisms including S. aureus, Streptococcus sp., Listeria monocytogenes and Corynebacterium sp.; gram-negative organisms including M. catarrhalis, N. gonorrhoeae, and L. pneumophila; other organism such as C. trachomatis, T. pallidum, M. pneumoniae, U. urealyticum, and E. histolytica. Azithromycin is more active than erythromycin against H. influenzae, M. catarrhalis and Neisseria species.<br><br>**General Indications**<br>**Adults**<br>500 mg as a single dose on Day 1 followed by 250 mg once daily on days 2 through 5<br><br>**Children**<br>10 mg/kg (not to exceed 500 mg/d) as a single dose on Day 1 followed by 5 mg/kg (not to exceed 250 mg/d) on days 2 through 5<br><br>**Chlamydial Infection in Adults/Adolescents**<br>1 gm po as a single dose | Administration Issues<br>Complete full course of therapy; take at least 1 hour before or 2 h after meals; shake suspension well prior to administration; store suspension in the refrigerator and use within 10 days of reconstitution<br><br>Drug–Drug Interactions<br>Less drug interactions compared to clarithromycin and erythromycin due to decreased hepatic metabolism.<br><br>Concomitant use of **antacids** may decrease peak serum concentration of azithromycin | ADRs<br>nausea, abdominal discomfort, diarrhea, superinfection<br><br>Pharmacokinetics<br>decreased absorption with food; distributes well into body tissues; poor penetration into the CNS; T $_{1/2}$ approximately 65 h; biliary excretion primarily as unchanged drug | Contraindications<br>Hypersensitivity to azithromycin or other macrolide antibiotics<br><br>Pregnancy Category:  B<br><br>Lactation Issues<br>Excretion in breast milk is unknown; use with caution in nursing mothers |

(continues on next page)

| Drug and Dosage Forms | Spectrum of Activity and Usual Dosage Range | Administration Issues and Drug–Drug & Drug–Food Interactions | Common Adverse Drug Reactions (ADRs) and Pharmacokinetics | Contraindications, Pregnancy Category, and Lactation Issues |
|---|---|---|---|---|
| **Azithromycin** *cont.* | **Prevention of bacterial endocarditis**<br>Adults 500 mg (children 15 mg/kg) orally 1 hr before procedure | | | |
| **Clarithromycin**<br>Biaxin<br><br>Tablet:<br>250 mg, 500 mg<br><br>Granules for Oral Suspension:<br>125 mg/5 ml<br>250 mg/5 ml | **Spectrum of Activity**<br>similar to azithromycin except clarithromycin has limited activity against *H. influenzae*<br><br>**General indications**<br>**Adults:** 250–500 mg q 12 h for 7 to 14 days<br><br>**Children**<br>15 mg/kg/d in divided doses q 12 h for 10 days<br><br>**Prevention of bacterial endocarditis**<br>Adults 500 mg (children 15 mg/kg) orally 1 hr before procedure<br><br>**Treatment of *Mycobacterium avium complex***<br>500 mg q 12 h for 26 weeks in combination with ethambutol, clofazimine, or ciprofloxacin | Administration Issues<br>Complete full course of therapy; may be taken without regard to meals; shake suspension well prior to administration; store suspension at room temperature and use within 14 days from reconstitution<br><br>Drug–Drug Interactions<br>Concomitant use of clarithromycin with the following drugs may result in increased pharmacologic and toxic effects of: **astemizole, carbamazepine, cisapride, cyclosporine, digoxin, disopyramide, ergot alkaloids, methylprednisolone, tacrolimus, terfenadine, theophylline, triazolam, warfarin** | ADRs<br>nausea, abdominal discomfort, diarrhea, superinfection, abnormal taste<br><br>Pharmacokinetics<br>distributes into body tissues; hepatic metabolism; renal excretion | Contraindications<br>Hypersensitivity to clarithromycin or other macrolide antibiotics; patients receiving terfenadine with preexisting cardiac abnormalities<br><br>Pregnancy Category: C<br><br>Lactation Issues<br>Excretion in breast milk is unknown; use with caution in nursing mothers |

| | | | | |
|---|---|---|---|---|
| **Dirithromycin**<br><br>Dynabec<br><br>Tablet, enteric coated:<br>250 mg | **Prophylaxis of *Mycobacterium avium* complex in HIV infected patients**<br>500 mg q 12 h in combination with ethambutol, clofazimine, or rifampin<br><br>**Antibacterial Spectrum**<br>Gram-positive organisms including S. aureus, *Streptococcus* sp. and *Listeria monocytogenes*; gram negative organisms including *M. catarrhalis* and *L. pneumophila*; other organisms such as *M. pneumoniae*<br><br>**General indications**<br>**Adults and children ≥ 12 yr.**<br>500 mg once daily for 7 to 14 days | **Administration Issues**<br>Complete full course of therapy; take with food or within 1 hour of having eaten to decrease abdominal discomfort; do not cut, crush, or chew tablets<br><br>**Drug–Drug Interactions**<br>The following interactions do not appear to occur or occur rarely, **however,** patients should be monitored appropriately. Dirithromycin may inhibit the metabolism of **terfenadine** and **astemizole** leading to serious cardiac dysrhythmias. Dirithromycin may inhibit the metabolism of **theophylline** leading to toxic adverse effects | <u>ADRs</u><br>nausea, abdominal discomfort, diarrhea, superinfection<br><br><u>Pharmacokinetics</u><br>achieves high tissue/plasma ratios; primarily excreted in the bile/feces with little hepatic metabolism | <u>Contraindications</u><br>Hypersensitivity to dirithromycin or other macrolide antibiotics<br><br><u>Pregnancy Category:</u> C<br><br><u>Lactation Issues</u><br>Excretion in breast milk is unknown; use with caution in nursing mothers |
| **Erythromycin Base**<br><br>Tablet, enteric coated:<br>E-Mycin 250 mg, 333 mg<br><br>Ery-Tab: 250 mg, 333 mg, 500 mg<br><br>Tablet, coated particles: PCE<br>Dispertab: 333 mg, 500 mg<br><br>Tablet, delayed release:<br>generics 333 mg | **Spectrum of Activity**<br>similar to azithromycin except erythromycin has limited activity against *H. influenzae*<br><br>**General indications**<br>**Adults:** 250–500 mg q 6 h for 10 days <u>or</u> 333 mg q 8 h for 10 days<br><br>**Children:** 30–50 mg/kg/d in divided doses q 6 h for 10 days | **Administration Issues**<br>Complete full course of therapy; take on empty stomach, however, may be taken with food if GI upset occurs; swallow tablets and capsules whole, do not crush tablets or enteric-coated pellets<br><br>**Drug–Drug Interactions**<br>Concomitant use of erythromycin with the following drugs may result in increased pharmacologic and toxic effects of: **astemizole, carbamazepine, cisapride, cyclosporine, digoxin,** | <u>ADRs</u><br>nausea, abdominal discomfort, diarrhea, superinfection<br><br><u>Pharmacokinetics</u><br>diffuses into body fluids including prostatic fluid, low concentrations found in cerebrospinal fluid; hepatic metabolism; biliary excretion | <u>Contraindications</u><br>Hypersensitivity to erythromycin; preexisting liver disease<br><br><u>Pregnancy Category:</u> B<br><br><u>Lactation Issues</u><br>Excreted in breast milk; erythromycin use is considered compatible with breastfeeding by the American Academy of Pediatrics |

*(continues on next page)*

| Drug and Dosage Forms | Spectrum of Activity and Usual Dosage Range | Administration Issues and Drug–Drug & Drug–Food Interactions | Common Adverse Drug Reactions (ADRs) and Pharmacokinetics | Contraindications, Pregnancy Category, and Lactation Issues |
|---|---|---|---|---|
| **Erythromycin Base cont.**<br><br>Tablet, film coated:<br>Erythromycin Filmtabs 250 mg, 500 mg<br><br>Capsule, delayed release, enteric coated pellets:<br>Eryc 250 mg<br><br>Capsule, delayed release:<br>generics 250 mg | **Prophylaxis of rheumatic heart disease**<br>250 mg twice daily<br><br>**Alternative drug in penicillin and tetracycline hypersensitivity for primary syphilis**<br>500 mg q 6 h for 14 days<br><br>**Chlamydial infection**<br>**Adults**<br>500 mg qid for 7 days or 250 mg qid for 14 days or 666 mg q 8 h for 7 days or 333 mg q 8 h for 14 days<br><br>**Children:** 50 mg/kg/d in divided doses q 6 h for 14 days (conjunctivitis) or 21 days (pneumonia)<br><br>**Legionnaire's disease:** 1–4 gm in divided doses q 6 h for 21 days alone or combined with rifampin | disopyramide, ergot alkaloids, methylprednisolone, tacrolimus, terfenadine, theophylline, triazolam, warfarin | | |
| **Erythromycin Estolate**<br><br>Tablet:<br>Ilosone 500 mg | **Spectrum of Activity**<br>see erythromycin<br><br>**General indications**<br>**Adults**<br>250–500 mg q 6 h for 10 days | Administration Issues<br>Complete full course of therapy; take on empty stomach, however, may be taken with food if GI upset occurs; shake suspension well prior to administration; store suspension in the refrigerator | ADRs<br>nausea, abdominal discomfort, diarrhea, superinfection, abnormal taste | Contraindications<br>Hypersensitivity to erythromycin; preexisting liver disease |

(continues on next page)

Capsule:
Ilosone, generics
250 mg

Suspension:
Ilosone, various generics
125 mg/5 ml
250 mg/5 ml

**Children**
30–50 mg/kg/d in divided doses
q 6 h for 10 days

**Prophylaxis of rheumatic heart disease**
250 mg twice daily

**Chlamydial infection**
**Adults:** 500 mg q 6 h for 7 days **or** 250 mg q 6 h for 14 days

**Children:** 50 mg/kg/d divided q 6 h for 14 days (conjunctivitis) or 21 days (pneumonia)

**Legionnaire's disease**
1–4 gm in divided doses q 6 h for 21 days alone or in combination with rifampin

Drug–Drug Interactions
Concomitant use of erythromycin with the following drugs may result in increased pharmacologic and toxic effects of: **astemizole, carbamazepine, cisapride, cyclosporine, digoxin, disopyramide, ergot alkaloids, methylprednisolone, tacrolimus, terfenadine, theophylline, triazolam, warfarin**

**Do not use erythromycin estolate in pregnant patients**

Pharmacokinetics
diffuses into body fluids including prostatic fluid, low concentrations found in cerebrospinal fluid; hepatic metabolism; biliary excretion

Pregnancy Category: B

Lactation Issues
Excreted in breast milk; erythromycin use is considered compatible with breastfeeding by the American Academy of Pediatrics

---

# Erythromycin Stearate

Erythrocin Stearate, Wyamycin S, various generics

Tablet, film coated:
250 mg, 500 mg

**Spectrum of Activity**
see erythromycin base

**General indications**
**Adults:** 250–500 mg q 6 h for 10 days

**Children:** 30–50 mg/kg/ divided q 6 h for 10 days

**Prophylaxis of rheumatic heart disease**
250 mg twice daily

Administration Issues
Complete full course of therapy; take on empty stomach, however, may be taken with food if GI upset occurs

Drug–Drug Interactions
Concomitant use of erythromycin with the following drugs may result in increased pharmacologic and toxic effects of: **astemizole, carbamazepine, cisapride, cyclosporine, digoxin, disopyramide, ergot alkaloids, methylprednisolone, tacrolimus, terfenadine, theophylline, triazolam, warfarin**

ADRs
nausea, abdominal discomfort, diarrhea, superinfection, abnormal taste

Pharmacokinetics
diffuses into body fluids including prostatic fluid, low concentrations found in cerebrospinal fluid; hepatic metabolism; biliary excretion

Contraindications
Hypersensitivity to erythromycin

Pregnancy Category: B

Lactation Issues
Excreted in breast milk; erythromycin use is considered compatible with breastfeeding by the American Academy of Pediatrics

| Drug and Dosage Forms | Spectrum of Activity and Usual Dosage Range | Administration Issues and Drug–Drug & Drug–Food Interactions | Common Adverse Drug Reactions (ADRs) and Pharmacokinetics | Contraindications, Pregnancy Category, and Lactation Issues |
|---|---|---|---|---|
| **Erythromycin Stearate** *cont.* | **Chlamydial infection**<br>**Adults:** 500 mg q 6 h for 7 d or 250 mg q 6 h for 14 d<br><br>**Children:** 50 mg/kg/d divided q 6 h for 14 d (conjunctivitis) or 21 d (pneumonia)<br><br>**Legionnaire's disease**<br>1–4 gm in divided doses q 6 h for 21 days alone or in combination with rifampin | | | |
| **Erythromycin Ethylsuccinate**<br><br>Tablet, chewable:<br>EryPed 200 mg<br><br>Tablet:<br>E.E.S., generics 400 mg<br><br>Suspension:<br>EryPed: 100 mg/2.5 ml, 200 mg/5 ml, 400 mg/5 ml<br><br>E.E.S., generics:<br>200 mg/5 ml<br>400 mg/5 ml | **Spectrum of Activity**<br>see erythromycin base<br><br>**General indications**<br>**Adults:** 400 mg q 6 h for 10 days<br><br>**Children:** 30–50 mg/kg/d divided q 6 h for 10 d<br><br>**Prophylaxis of rheumatic heart disease**<br>400 mg twice daily<br><br>**Chlamydial infection**<br>**Adults:** 800 mg q 6 h for 7 d or 400 mg q 6 h for 14 days | Administration Issues<br>Complete full course of therapy; take on empty stomach, however, may be taken with food if GI upset occurs; shake suspension well prior to administration; store suspension in the refrigerator<br><br>Drug–Drug Interactions<br>Concomitant use of erythromycin with the following drugs may result in increased pharmacologic and toxic effects of: **astemizole, carbamazepine, cisapride, cyclosporine, digoxin, disopyramide, ergot alkaloids, methylprednisolone, tacrolimus, terfenadine, theophylline, triazolam, warfarin** | ADRs<br>nausea, abdominal discomfort, diarrhea, superinfection, abnormal taste<br><br>Pharmacokinetics<br>diffuses into body fluids including prostatic fluid, low concentrations found in cerebrospinal fluid; hepatic metabolism; biliary excretion | Contraindications<br>Hypersensitivity to erythromycin; preexisting liver disease<br><br>Pregnancy Category: B<br><br>Lactation Issues<br>Excreted in breast milk; erythromycin use is considered compatible with breastfeeding by the American Academy of Pediatrics |

| | | | |
|---|---|---|---|
| Powder for Oral Suspension: E.E.S. 200 mg/5 ml<br><br>EryPed 400 mg/5 ml | **Children:** 50 mg/kg/d divided q 6 h for 14 d (conjunctivitis) or 21 d (pneumonia)<br><br>**Legionnaire's disease**<br>1.6–4 gm in divided doses q 6 h for 21 days alone or in combination with rifampin | | |
| **Troleandomycin**<br>Tao<br><br>Capsule: 250 mg | **Spectrum of Activity**<br>*Streptococcus pyogenes* and *Streptococcus pneumoniae*<br><br>**Streptococcal infections**<br>**Adults:** 250–500 mg q 6 h for 10 days<br><br>**Children:** 125–250 mg q 6 h for 10 days | Administration Issues<br>Complete full course of therapy; take on empty stomach<br><br>Drug–Drug Interactions<br>Troleandomycin may increase the effects of the following drugs by inhibiting their metabolism: **carbamazepine, ergot alkaloids, methylprednisolone, theophylline, triazolam**<br><br>Hepatotoxicity may occur with concomitant use of troleandomycin and **oral contraceptives** | ADRs<br>nausea, abdominal discomfort, diarrhea, superinfection<br><br>Pharmacokinetics<br>acetylated ester of oleandomycin; biliary and renal excretion | Contraindications<br>Hypersensitivity to troleandomycin<br><br>Safety for use during pregnancy has not been established |

957

| Drug and Dosage Forms | Spectrum of Activity and Usual Dosage Range | Administration Issues and Drug–Drug & Drug–Food Interactions | Common Adverse Drug Reactions (ADRs) and Pharmacokinetics | Contraindications, Pregnancy Category, and Lactation Issues |
|---|---|---|---|---|
| **Penicillin G Potassium**<br>Pentids, generics<br><br>Tablet:<br>200,000 units<br>250,000 units<br>400,000 units<br>500,000 units<br>800,000 units<br><br>Powder for Oral Solution:<br>400,000 units/5 ml | **Antibacterial Spectrum**<br>Gram-positive staphylococcal and streptococcal organisms; inactive alone against serious *Streptococcus* group D (enterococcus)<br><br>**General Indications**<br>**Adults**<br>200,000–500,000 units q 6 to 8 h for 10 days<br><br>**Children < 12 yr.**<br>25,000–90,000 units/kg/d in 3 to 6 divided doses for 10 days | Administration Issues<br>Give 1 hour before or 2 h after meals; complete full course of therapy; store reconstituted liquid in the refrigerator, discard unused portion after 14 days<br><br>Drug–Drug Interactions<br>Penicillins may decrease the effectiveness of **oral contraceptives;** the bacteriostatic action of **tetracyclines** may interfere with the bactericidal effects of penicillins | ADRs:<br>hypersensitivity reactions, urticarial rash, nausea, diarrhea, superinfections<br><br>Pharmacokinetics:<br>$T_{1/2}$ 30 min; 35% protein binding; renal excretion mostly unchanged | Contraindications<br>True penicillin allergy<br><br>Pregnancy Category: B<br><br>Lactation Issues<br>Penicillins are excreted in breast milk in low concentrations; nursing infants may develop diarrhea, candidiasis, or an allergic reaction |
| **Penicillin G Procaine**<br>Wycillin<br><br>Injection:<br>600,000 units/ml<br>1,200,000 units/2 ml<br>2,400,000 units/4 ml | **Antibacterial Spectrum**<br>Gram-positive staphylococcal and streptococcal organisms; *treponema pallidum* associated with syphilis<br><br>**Streptococcal and Staphylococcal infections**<br>**Adults and children**<br>600,000–1,200,000 units daily IM for 10 to 14 days<br><br>**Newborns:** 50,000 units/kg IM once daily for 10 to 14 days | Administration Issues<br>Give by deep IM injection into the upper, outer quadrant of the buttocks; for infants and children the midlateral aspect of the thigh may be preferable; rotate injection site for repeated doses<br><br>Drug–Drug Interactions<br>Penicillins may decrease the effectiveness of **oral contraceptives;** the bacteriostatic action of **tetracyclines** may interfere with the bactericidal effects of penicillins | ADRs:<br>hypersensitivity reactions, urticarial rash, nausea, diarrhea, superinfections<br><br>Pharmacokinetics:<br>IM: provides more prolonged but lower penicillin G concentrations than equivalent IM penicillin G potassium; peak serum concentrations in 1–4 h and detectable for 1–2 days; renal excretion mostly unchanged | Contraindications<br>True penicillin allergy<br><br>Pregnancy Category: B<br><br>Lactation Issues<br>Penicillins are excreted in breast milk in low concentrations; nursing infants may develop diarrhea, candidiasis, or an allergic reaction |

| | | | |
|---|---|---|---|
| | | | **Contraindications**<br>True penicillin allergy<br><br>**Pregnancy Category:** B<br><br>**Lactation Issues**<br>Penicillins are excreted in breast milk in low concentrations; nursing infants may develop diarrhea, candidiasis, or an allergic reaction |
| | **Bacterial endocarditis-extremely sensitive infections (_S. viridans, S. bovis_):**<br>1,200,000 units qid IM for 2 to 4 weeks plus streptomycin 500 mg bid IM for the first 2 weeks | | **ADRs:**<br>hypersensitivity reactions, urticarial rash, nausea, diarrhea, superinfections<br><br>**Pharmacokinetics:**<br>IM; provides more prolonged but lower penicillin G concentrations than equivalent IM procaine penicillin G or penicillin G potassium; peak serum concentrations in 13–24 h and detectable for 1–4 weeks; renal excretion mostly unchanged |
| **Penicillin G Benzathine**<br>Bicillin L-A<br><br>Injection:<br>300,000 units/ml<br>600,000 units/ml<br>1,200,000 units/2 ml<br>2,400,000 units/4 ml | **Antibacterial Spectrum**<br>Gram-positive staphylococcal and streptococcal organisms; _treponema pallidum_ associated with syphilis<br><br>**Prevention of recurrent rheumatic fever (_Streptococcal_ group A infection)**<br>**Adult and children:** 1.2 million units IM 4 wk.<br><br>**Early syphilis–primary, secondary, or latent of <1 year's duration**<br>**Adults:** 2,400,000 units IM for one dose<br><br>**Children and neonates**<br>50,000 units/Kg (up to 2.4 million units) IM for one dose<br><br>**Syphilis of >1 year's duration, latent syphilis or cardiovascular syphilis**<br>**Adults:** 2.4 million units IM once weekly for 3 successive wk.<br><br>**Children and neonates**<br>50,000 units/Kg (up to 2.4 million units) IM weekly for 3 successive wk. | **Administration Issues**<br>Give by deep IM injection into the upper, outer quadrant of the buttocks, for infants and children the midlateral aspect of the thigh may be preferable; rotate injection site for repeated doses<br><br>**Drug–Drug Interactions**<br>Penicillins may decrease the effectiveness of **oral contraceptives;** the bacteriostatic action of **tetracyclines** may interfere with the bactericidal effects of penicillins | |

(continues on next page)

| Drug and Dosage Forms | Spectrum of Activity and Usual Dosage Range | Administration Issues and Drug–Drug & Drug–Food Interactions | Common Adverse Drug Reactions (ADRs) and Pharmacokinetics | Contraindications, Pregnancy Category, and Lactation Issues |
|---|---|---|---|---|
| **Penicillin G Benzathine**  *cont.* | **Neurosyphilis:** Following aqueous penicillin G therapy or aqueous procaine penicillin G, benzathine penicillin G 2,400,000 units IM once weekly for 3 successive wk. | | | |
| **Penicillin G Benzathine and Procaine** Bicillin C-R  Injection: 150,000 units/ml penicillin G benzathine and 150,000 units/ml penicillin G procaine  300,000 units/ml penicillin G benzathine and 300,000 units/ml penicillin G procaine  600,000 units/ml penicillin G benzathine and 600,000 units/ml penicillin G procaine  1,200,000 units/ml penicillin G benzathine and 1,200,000 units/ml penicillin G procaine | **Antibacterial Spectrum** Gram-positive streptococcal organisms; *treponema pallidum* associated with syphilis  **Moderately severe to severe streptococcal infections** (*Streptococci* A, C, G, H, L, and M) of the upper respiratory tract, skin, and soft tissue **Adult and children > 60 lbs. or 27 kg:** 2.4 million units IM as a single dose  **Children 30–60 lbs. or 14 to 27 kg:** 900,000–1,200,000 units IM as a single dose  **Infants and children < 30 lbs. or 14 kg:** 600,000 units IM  *Streptococcus pneumoniae* **infections (except meningitis) Adults:** 1.2 million units IM as a single dose | Administration Issues Give by deep IM injection into the upper, outer quadrant of the buttocks, for infants and children the midlateral aspect of the thigh may be preferable; rotate injection site for repeated doses  Drug–Drug Interactions Penicillins may decrease the effectiveness of **oral contraceptives;** the bacteriostatic action of **tetracyclines** may interfere with the bactericidal effects of penicillins | ADRs: hypersensitivity reactions, urticarial rash, nausea, diarrhea, superinfections  Pharmacokinetics: renal excretion mostly unchanged | Contraindications True penicillin allergy; hypersensitivity to procaine  Pregnancy Category:  B  Lactation Issues Penicillins are excreted in breast milk in low concentrations; nursing infants may develop diarrhea, candidiasis, or an allergic reaction |

| | | | | |
|---|---|---|---|---|
| 900,000 units penicillin G benzathine and 300,000 units penicillin G procaine | **Children:** 600,000 units IM as a single dose; repeat q 2 to 3 days until patient has been afebrile for 48 h<br><br>**Congenital syphilis:**<br>**Newborns:** 50,000 U/kg IM qd for 10 d | | | <u>Contraindications</u><br>True penicillin allergy<br><br><u>Pregnancy Category:</u> B<br><br><u>Lactation Issues</u><br>Penicillins are excreted in breast milk in low concentrations; nursing infants may develop diarrhea, candidiasis, or an allergic reaction |
| **Penicillin V Potassium**<br><br><u>Tablets:</u><br>V-Cillin K 125 mg<br><br>Beepen VK, Veetids, Pen-Vee K, generics 250 mg, 500 mg<br><br><u>Powder for Oral Solution:</u><br>Beepen VK, Pen-Vee K, generics 125 mg/5 ml, 250 mg/5 ml | **Antibacterial Spectrum**<br>Gram-positive organisms including non-penicillinase-producing *S. aureus, S. epidermidis, Streptococcus* sp. Coverage also includes gram-positive anaerobes such as *Clostridium* sp. and *Peptostreptococcus* sp.; inactive against gram-negative organisms<br><br>**General indications**<br>**Adults:** 250–500 mg q 6 to 8 h for 10 days<br><br>**Children:** 25–50 mg/kg/d in divided doses q 6 to 8 h for 10 days | <u>Administration Issues</u><br>May be given without regard to meals; complete full course of therapy; store reconstituted liquid in the refrigerator, discard unused portion after 14 days<br><br><u>Drug–Drug Interactions</u><br>Penicillins may decrease the effectiveness of **oral contraceptives;** the bacteriostatic action of **tetracyclines** may interfere with the bactericidal effects of penicillins | <u>ADRs:</u><br>hypersensitivity reactions, urticarial rash, nausea, diarrhea, superinfections<br><br><u>Pharmacokinetics:</u><br>$T_{1/2}$ 60 min; 85% protein binding; renal excretion mostly unchanged | |

## 102.7 Aminopenicillins

| Drug and Dosage Forms | Spectrum of Activity and Usual Dosage Range | Administration Issues and Drug–Drug & Drug–Food Interactions | Common Adverse Drug Reactions (ADRs) and Pharmacokinetics | Contraindications, Pregnancy Category, and Lactation Issues |
|---|---|---|---|---|
| **Amoxicillin**<br><br>Tablet, chewable:<br>Amoxil, generics: 125 mg, 250 mg<br><br>Capsule:<br>Amoxil, Polymox, Trimox, Wymox, generics: 250 mg, 500 mg<br><br>Powder for Oral Suspension:<br>Amoxil, Polymox: 50 mg/ml<br><br>Amoxil, Polymox, Trimox, Wymox, generics: 125 mg/ 5 ml; 250 mg/5 ml | **Antibacterial Spectrum**<br>Gram-positive coverage is the same as penicillin G; gram-negative includes *E. Coli, P. mirabilis, N. gonorrhoeae,* and *H. influenzae* (beta-lactamase negative)<br><br><u>General indications</u><br>**Adults and children > 20 kg:**<br>250–500 mg q 8 h for 10 days<br><br>**Children < 20 kg:** 20–40 mg/kg/d divided q 8 h for 10 days<br><br>**Prevention of bacterial endocarditis**<br>Adults, 2 gm (children 50 mg/kg) given orally 1 hr before procedure. No follow-up dose recommended. | <u>Administration Issues</u><br>May be given without regards to meals; complete full course of therapy; discard any liquid form after 10 days if at room temperature and after 14 days if refrigerated<br><br><u>Drug–Drug Interactions</u><br>Penicillins may decrease the effectiveness of **oral contraceptives;** the bacteriostatic action of **tetracyclines** may interfere with the bactericidal effects of penicillins | <u>ADRs:</u><br>hypersensitivity reactions, urticarial rash, nausea, diarrhea, superinfections<br><br><u>Pharmacokinetics:</u><br>$T_{1/2}$ 60 min; 20% protein binding; renal excretion mostly unchanged | <u>Contraindications</u><br>True penicillin allergy<br><br><u>Pregnancy Category:</u> B<br><br><u>Lactation Issues</u><br>Penicillins are excreted in breast milk in low concentrations; nursing infants may develop diarrhea, candidiasis, or an allergic reaction |
| **Amoxicillin and Potassium Clavulanate**<br>Augmentin<br><br>Tablet, chewable:<br>125 mg amoxicillin/ 31.25 mg clavulanic acid | **Antibacterial Spectrum**<br>Similar to amoxicillin, but addition of clavulanate confers penicillinase resistance, thereby extending the spectrum to include *Klebsiella sp.,* beta lactamase producing strains of *H. influenzae, E. coli,* and methicillin-sensitive *S. aureus* | <u>Administration Issues</u><br>Give with food to decrease nausea and diarrhea; complete full course of therapy; store reconstituted liquid in the refrigerator, discard unused portion after 10 days<br><br><u>Drug–Drug Interactions</u><br>Penicillins may decrease the effectiveness of **oral contraceptives;** | <u>ADRs:</u><br>hypersensitivity reactions, urticarial rash, nausea, diarrhea, superinfections<br><br><u>Pharmacokinetics:</u><br>$T_{1/2}$ 60 min; 20% protein binding; renal excretion mostly unchanged | <u>Contraindications</u><br>True penicillin allergy<br><br><u>Pregnancy Category:</u> B<br><br><u>Lactation Issues</u><br>Penicillins are excreted in breast milk in low concentrations; nursing infants may develop diarrhea, candidiasis, or an allergic reaction |

| | | |
|---|---|---|
| 200 mg amoxicillin/ 28.55 mg clavulanic acid<br><br>250 mg amoxicillin/ 125 mg clavulanic acid<br><br>400 mg amoxicillin/ 57 mg clavulanic acid<br><br><u>Tablet:</u><br>250 mg amoxicillin/ 125 mg clavulanic acid<br><br>500 mg amoxicillin/ 125 mg clavulanic acid<br><br>875 mg amoxicillin/ 125 mg clavulanic acid<br><br><u>Powder for Oral Suspension:</u><br>125 mg amoxicillin/ 31.25 mg clavulanic acid per 5 ml<br><br>200 mg amoxicillin/ 28.55 mg clavulanic acid per 5 ml<br><br>250 mg amoxicillin/ 62.5 mg clavulanic acid per 5 ml<br><br>400 mg amoxicillin/ 57 mg clavulanic acid per 5 ml | Dosage is given as amoxicillin equivalent. Both the 250 mg and 500 mg tablets contain the same amount of clavulanic acid, so two, 250 mg tablets **are not** equivalent to one, 500 mg tablet<br><br>**Adults**<br>250–500 mg q 8 h <u>or</u> 875 mg q 12 h for 10 d<br><br>**<u>Otitis media, sinusitis, lower respiratory tract infections (Children > 3 months old)</u>**<br><u>BID Dosing</u><br>45 mg/kg/d divided bid (use 200 mg/ 5ml or 400 mg/5ml suspension)<br>**or**<br><u>TID Dosing</u><br>40 mg/kg/d divided tid (use 125 mg/ 5ml or 250 mg/5 ml suspension)<br><br>**<u>Less Severe Infections (Children > 3 months old)</u>**<br><u>BID Dosing</u><br>25 mg/kg/d divided bid (use 200 mg/ 5ml or 400 mg/5ml suspension)<br>**or**<br><u>TID Dosing</u><br>20 mg/kg/d divided tid (use 125 mg/ 5ml or 250 mg/5 ml suspension)<br><br>**<u>Pelvic inflammatory disease</u>**<br>500 mg tid with doxycycline 100 mg twice daily for 10 days | the bacteriostatic action of **tetracyclines** may interfere with the bactericidal effects of penicillins |

(continues on next page)

| Drug and Dosage Forms | Spectrum of Activity and Usual Dosage Range | Administration Issues and Drug–Drug & Drug–Food Interactions | Common Adverse Drug Reactions (ADRs) and Pharmacokinetics | Contraindications, Pregnancy Category, and Lactation Issues |
|---|---|---|---|---|
| **Ampicillin**<br>Polycillin, Principen, Totacillin, Omnipen, various generics<br><br>Capsule:<br>250 mg, 500 mg<br><br>Powder for Oral Suspension:<br>125 mg/5 ml<br>250 mg/5 ml<br><br>Polycillin 500 mg/5 ml | **Antibacterial Spectrum**<br>Gram-positive coverage is the same as penicillin G; gram-negative includes *E. Coli, P. mirabilis, N. gonorrhoeae, Shigella* sp., *H. influenzae*<br><br>**General indications**<br>**Adults and children ≥ 20 kg**<br>250–500 mg q 6 h for 10 to 14 days<br><br>**Children**<br>50 mg/kg/d divided q 6 to 8 h for 10 to 14 days | Administration Issues<br>For optimal absorption, give on empty stomach; complete full course of therapy; store reconstituted liquid in the refrigerator, discard unused portion after 14 days<br><br>Drug–Drug Interactions<br>Penicillins may decrease the effectiveness of **oral contraceptives**; the bacteriostatic action of **tetracyclines** may interfere with the bactericidal effects of penicillins; concomitant use of **allopurinol** may increase the risk of an ampicillin-induced rash | ADRs:<br>hypersensitivity reactions, urticarial rash, nausea, diarrhea, superinfections<br><br>Pharmacokinetics:<br>40% absorbed in GI tract; T$_{1/2}$ 60 min; 20% protein binding; renal excretion mostly unchanged | Contraindications<br>True penicillin allergy<br><br>Pregnancy Category: B<br><br>Lactation Issues<br>Penicillins are excreted in breast milk in low concentrations; nursing infants may develop diarrhea, candidiasis, or an allergic reaction |
| **Bacampicillin**<br>Spectrobid<br><br>Tablet:<br>400 mg (chemically equivalent to 280 mg ampicillin)<br><br>Powder for Oral Suspension:<br>125 mg/5 ml (chemically equivalent to 87.5 mg ampicillin) | **Antibacterial Spectrum**<br>Similar to ampicillin<br><br>**General indications**<br>**Adults and children ≥ 25 kg**<br>400–800 mg q 12 h for 10 to 14 days<br><br>**Children**<br>25 mg/kg/d in divided doses q 12 h for 10 to 14 days | Administration Issues<br>For optimal absorption, give on empty stomach; complete full course of therapy; store reconstituted liquid in the refrigerator, discard unused portion after 14 days<br><br>Drug–Drug Interactions<br>Penicillins may decrease the effectiveness of **oral contraceptives**; the bacteriostatic action of **tetracyclines** may interfere with the bactericidal effects of penicillins; | ADRs:<br>hypersensitivity reactions, urticarial rash, nausea, diarrhea, superinfections<br><br>Pharmacokinetics<br>metabolized to ampicillin during GI absorption; more completely absorbed than ampicillin; renal excretion | Contraindications<br>True penicillin allergy<br><br>Pregnancy Category: B<br><br>Lactation Issues<br>Penicillins are excreted in breast milk in low concentrations; nursing infants may develop diarrhea, candidiasis, or an allergic reaction |

| | | | |
|---|---|---|---|
| | | concomitant use of **allopurinol** may increase the risk of an ampicillin-induced rash | Contraindications<br>True penicillin allergy<br><br>Pregnancy Category: B<br><br>Lactation Issues<br>Penicillins are excreted in breast milk in low concentrations; nursing infants may develop diarrhea, candidiasis, or an allergic reaction |
| **Carbenicillin Indanyl Sodium**<br>Geocillin<br><br>Tablet:<br>382 mg | **Antibacterial Spectrum**<br>*E. coli, P. mirabilis, Morganella morganii, Providencia rettgeri, Pseudomonas, Enterobacter,* and enterococcus<br><br>**Urinary tract infection**<br>*E. coli, Proteus mirabilis,* and *Enterobacter* sp. 382–764 mg qid for 10 d<br><br>*Pseudomonas* and enterococci 764 mg qid for 10 d<br><br>**Prostatitis**<br>764 mg qid | Administration Issues<br>For optimal absorption, give on empty stomach; complete full course of therapy<br><br>Drug–Drug Interactions<br>Penicillins may decrease the effectiveness of **oral contraceptives;** the bacteriostatic action of **tetracyclines** may interfere with the bactericidal effects of penicillins | ADRs:<br>Hypersensitivity reactions, urticarial rash, nausea, diarrhea, superinfection<br><br>Pharmacokinetics:<br>$T_{1/2}$ 60 min; 50% protein binding; renal excretion mostly as unchanged drug |

| Drug and Dosage Forms | Spectrum of Activity and Usual Dosage Range | Administration Issues and Drug–Drug & Drug–Food Interactions | Common Adverse Drug Reactions (ADRs) and Pharmacokinetics | Contraindications, Pregnancy Category, and Lactation Issues |
|---|---|---|---|---|
| **Cloxacillin Sodium**<br><br><u>Capsule:</u><br>Cloxapen, Tegopen, generics:  250 mg, 500 mg<br><br><u>Powder for Oral Solution:</u><br>Tegopen, generics:<br>125 mg/5 ml | **Antibacterial Spectrum**<br>Penicillinase-producing *Staphylococcus* sp.; less effective than penicillin G against non-penicillinase-producing staphylococci and other gram positive organisms; inactive against gram-negative organisms<br><br>**Mild to moderate upper respiratory and localized skin and soft tissue infections**<br>**Adults and children > 20 kg**<br>250 mg–1 gm q 6 h for 10 to 14 days<br><br>**Children**<br>50 mg/kg/d divided q 6 h for 10 to 14 days<br><br>**Severe infections (lower respiratory tract or disseminated infections)**<br>**Adults and children > 20 kg**<br>500 mg–1 gm q 6 h for 10 to 14 days<br><br>**Children**<br>50–100 mg/kg/d divided q 6 h for 10 to 14 days | <u>Administration Issues</u><br>For optimal absorption, give on empty stomach; complete full course of therapy; store reconstituted liquid in the refrigerator, discard unused portion after 14 days<br><br><u>Drug–Drug Interactions</u><br>Penicillins may decrease the effectiveness of **oral contraceptives;** the bacteriostatic action of **tetracyclines** may interfere with the bactericidal effects of penicillins | <u>ADRs:</u><br>hypersensitivity reactions. urticarial rash, nausea, diarrhea, superinfections<br><br><u>Pharmacokinetics:</u><br>$T_{1/2}$ 30–60 min; 95% protein binding; renal excretion mostly unchanged | <u>Contraindications</u><br>True penicillin allergy<br><br><u>Pregnancy Category:</u>  B<br><br><u>Lactation Issues</u><br>Penicillins are excreted in breast milk in low concentrations; nursing infants may develop diarrhea, candidiasis, or an allergic reaction |

| Drug | Administration Issues | ADRs / Pharmacokinetics | Contraindications / Lactation |
|---|---|---|---|
| **Dicloxacillin Sodium**<br><br>Capsules:<br>Dynapen 125 mg<br><br>Dynapen, Dycill, generics 250 mg, 500 mg<br><br>Powder for Oral Suspension:<br>Dynapen, Pathocil 62.5 mg/5 ml<br><br>**Antibacterial Spectrum**<br>Penicillinase-producing *Staphylococcus* sp.; less effective than penicillin G against non-penicillinase-producing staphylococci and other gram-positive organisms; inactive against gram-negative organisms<br><br>**Mild to moderate upper respiratory and localized skin and soft tissue infections**<br>**Adults and children > 40 kg** 125–250 mg q 6 h for 10 to 14 d<br><br>**Children:** 12.5–25 mg/kg/d divided q 6 h for 10 to 14 d<br><br>**Severe infections (lower respiratory tract or disseminated infections)**<br>**Adults and children > 40 kg** 250 mg q 6 h for 10 to 14 d<br><br>**Children:** 12.5–25 mg/kg/d divided q 6 h for 10 to 14 d<br><br>**Use in newborns is not recommended** | Administration Issues<br>For optimal absorption, give on empty stomach; complete full course of therapy; store reconstituted liquid in the refrigerator, discard unused portion after 14 days<br><br>Drug–Drug Interactions<br>Penicillins may decrease the effectiveness of **oral contraceptives;** the bacteriostatic action of **tetracyclines** may interfere with the bactericidal effects of penicillins | ADRs:<br>hypersensitivity reactions, urticarial rash, nausea, diarrhea, superinfections<br><br>Pharmacokinetics:<br>$T_{1/2}$ 30–60 min; 95% protein binding; renal excretion mostly unchanged | Contraindications<br>True penicillin allergy<br><br>Pregnancy Category: B<br><br>Lactation Issues<br>Penicillins are excreted in breast milk in low concentrations; nursing infants may develop diarrhea, candidiasis, or an allergic reaction |
| **Nafcillin Sodium**<br>Unipen<br><br>Tablet: 500 mg<br><br>Capsule: 250 mg<br><br>**Antibacterial Spectrum**<br>Penicillinase-producing *Staphylococcus* sp.; less effective than penicillin G against non-penicillinase-producing staphylococci and | Administration Issues<br>For optimal absorption, give on empty stomach; complete full course of therapy | ADRs:<br>hypersensitivity reactions, urticarial rash, nausea, diarrhea, superinfections | Contraindications<br>True penicillin allergy<br><br>Pregnancy Category: B |

(continues on next page)

| 102.8 Penicillinase-Resistant Penicillins | *continued from previous page* | | | |
|---|---|---|---|---|

| Drug and Dosage Forms | Spectrum of Activity and Usual Dosage Range | Administration Issues and Drug–Drug & Drug–Food Interactions | Common Adverse Drug Reactions (ADRs) and Pharmacokinetics | Contraindications, Pregnancy Category, and Lactation Issues |
|---|---|---|---|---|
| **Nafcillin Sodium** *cont.* | other gram-positive organisms; inactive against gram-negative organisms<br><br>**Mild to moderate upper respiratory and localized skin and soft tissue infections**<br>**Adults:** 250–500 mg q 4 to 6 h for 10 to 14 d<br><br>**Children:** 50 mg/kg/d divided q 6 h for 10 to 14 d<br><br>**Neonates:** 10 mg/kg 3 to 4 times daily for 10 to 14 d<br><br>**Use parenteral therapy initially for severe infections** | <u>Drug–Drug Interactions</u><br>Penicillins may decrease the effectiveness of **oral contraceptives;** the bacteriostatic action of **tetracyclines** may interfere with the bactericidal effects of penicillins | <u>Pharmacokinetics:</u><br>$T_{1/2}$ 30–60 min; 95% protein binding; renal excretion mostly unchanged; serum levels of nafcillin after oral administration are low and unpredictable | <u>Lactation Issues</u><br>Penicillins are excreted in breast milk in low concentrations; nursing infants may develop diarrhea, candidiasis, or an allergic reaction |
| **Oxacillin Sodium**<br><br><u>Capsule:</u><br>Bactocill, Prostaphlin, generics: 250 mg, 500 mg<br><br><u>Powder for Oral Solution:</u><br>Prostaphlin 250 mg/5 ml | **Antibacterial Spectrum**<br>Penicillinase-producing *Staphylococcus* sp.; less effective than penicillin G against non-penicillinase-producing staphylococci and other gram-positive organisms; inactive against gram negative organisms<br><br>**Mild to moderate upper respiratory and localized skin and soft tissue infections** | <u>Administration Issues</u><br>For optimal absorption, give on empty stomach; complete full course of therapy; store reconstituted liquid in the refrigerator, discard unused portion after 14 days<br><br><u>Drug–Drug Interactions</u><br>Penicillins may decrease the effectiveness of **oral contraceptives;** the bacteriostatic action of **tetracyclines** may interfere with the bactericidal effects of penicillins | <u>ADRs:</u><br>hypersensitivity reactions, urticarial rash, nausea, diarrhea, superinfections<br><br><u>Pharmacokinetics:</u><br>$T_{1/2}$ 30–60 min; 95% protein binding; renal excretion mostly unchanged | <u>Contraindications</u><br>True penicillin allergy<br><br><u>Pregnancy Category:</u> B<br><br><u>Lactation Issues</u><br>Penicillins are excreted in breast milk in low concentrations; nursing infants may develop diarrhea, candidiasis, or an allergic reaction |

**Adults and children > 20 kg**
500 mg–1 gm q 4 to 6 h for a minimum of 7 days depending on severity of infection

**Children:** 50–100 mg/kg/d divided q 6 h for a minimum of 7 days depending on severity of infection

---

## 102.9 Sulfonamides

| Drug and Dosage Forms | Spectrum of Activity and Usual Dosage Range | Administration Issues and Drug–Drug & Drug–Food Interactions | Common Adverse Drug Reactions (ADRs) and Pharmacokinetics | Contraindications, Pregnancy Category, and Lactation Issues |
|---|---|---|---|---|
| **Sulfadiazine**<br>Various generics<br><br>Tablet: 500 mg | **Antibacterial Spectrum**<br>Gram-negative organisms (E. coli, Klebsiella sp., Enterobacter sp., P. mirabilis, P. vulgaris) and S. aureus in the urine; Nocardia sp., C. trachomatis; H. ducreyi<br><br>**General indications**<br>**Adults:** 2–4 gm loading dose, followed by 4–8 gm/day in 4 to 6 divided doses for 7 to 14 days<br><br>**Children > 2 months:** 75 mg/kg loading dose, followed by 120–150 mg/kg/d in 4 to 6 divided doses for 7 to 14 days; maximum, 6 gm/day | Administration Issues<br>Complete full course of therapy; take on an empty stomach with a full glass of water; avoid prolonged exposure to sunlight, wear protective clothing, and apply sunscreen<br><br>Drug–Drug Interactions<br>Sulfonamides may increase the pharmacological and toxic effects of the following drugs:<br>**methotrexate, phenytoin, sulfonylureas, warfarin** | ADRs:<br>nausea, abdominal discomfort, headache, photosensitivity<br><br>Pharmacokinetics:<br>good GI absorption; readily penetrates into CSF; hepatic metabolism; renal excretion | Contraindications<br>Hypersensitivity to sulfonamides or chemically related drugs such as sulfonylureas, thiazide diuretics, and sunscreens containing PABA<br><br>Pregnancy<br>Safety for use during pregnancy has not been established; sulfonamides do cross the placenta achieving fetal levels approximately 70%–90% of maternal serum levels; do not use during pregnancy at term<br><br>Lactation Issues<br>Sulfonamides are excreted in breast milk; according to the |

(continues on next page)

| Drug and Dosage Forms | Spectrum of Activity and Usual Dosage Range | Administration Issues and Drug–Drug & Drug–Food Interactions | Common Adverse Drug Reactions (ADRs) and Pharmacokinetics | Contraindications, Pregnancy Category, and Lactation Issues |
|---|---|---|---|---|
| **Sulfadiazine** *cont.* | | | | American Academy of Pediatrics, breast feeding and sulfonamides are compatible; avoid sulfonamides and nursing in premature infants, infants with hyperbilirubinemia, and infants with G-6-PD deficiency |
| **Sulfamethoxazole** <br><br> Tablet: <br> Gantanol, various generics <br> 500 mg <br><br> Suspension: <br> Gantanol <br> 500 mg/5 ml | **Antibacterial Spectrum** <br> Gram-negative organisms (*E. coli*, *Klebsiella* sp., *Enterobacter* sp., *P. mirabilis*, *P. vulgaris*) and *S. aureus* in the urine; *Nocardia* sp., *C. trachomatis*; *H. ducreyi* <br><br> **General indications** <br> **Adults:** 2 gm initially, followed by 1 gm 2 to 3 times daily for 7 to 14 days <br><br> **Children > 2 months** <br> 50–60 mg/kg initially, followed by 25–30 mg/kg q 12 h for 7 to 14 d; maximum = 75 mg/kg/d | Administration Issues <br> Complete full course of therapy; take on an empty stomach with a full glass of water; avoid prolonged exposure to sunlight, wear protective clothing, and apply sunscreen; shake suspension well prior to administration <br><br> Drug–Drug Interactions <br> Sulfonamides may increase the pharmacological and toxic effects of the following drugs: **methotrexate, phenytoin, sulfonylureas, warfarin** | ADRs: <br> nausea, abdominal discomfort, headache, photosensitivity <br><br> Pharmacokinetics: <br> good GI absorption; readily penetrates into CSF; hepatic metabolism; renal excretion | Contraindications <br> Hypersensitivity to sulfonamides or chemically related drugs such as sulfonylureas, thiazide diuretics, and sunscreens containing PABA <br><br> Pregnancy <br> Safety for use during pregnancy has not been established; sulfonamides do cross the placenta achieving fetal levels approximately 70%–90% of maternal serum levels; do not use during pregnancy at term <br><br> Lactation Issues <br> Sulfonamides are excreted in breast milk; according to the American Academy of |

| Sulfisoxazole | Antibacterial Spectrum | Administration Issues | ADRs: | |
|---|---|---|---|---|

**Sulfisoxazole**

Tablet:
Gantrisin, various generics 500 mg

Syrup/Suspension:
Gantrisin 500 mg/5 ml

**Antibacterial Spectrum**
Gram-negative organisms (E. coli, Klebsiella sp., Enterobacter sp., P. mirabilis, P. vulgaris) and S. aureus in the urine; Nocardia sp., C. trachomatis; H. ducreyi

**General indications**
**Adults:** 4–8 gm/d in 4 to 6 divided doses for 7 to 14 days

**Children > 2 months**
120–150 mg/kg/d in 4 to 6 divided doses for 7 to 14 days; maximum = 6 gm/d

Administration Issues
Complete full course of therapy; take on an empty stomach with a full glass of water; avoid prolonged exposure to sunlight, wear protective clothing, and apply sunscreen; shake suspension well prior to administration

Drug–Drug Interactions
Sulfonamides may increase the pharmacological and toxic effects of the following drugs:
**methotrexate, phenytoin, sulfonylureas, warfarin**

ADRs:
nausea, abdominal discomfort, headache, photosensitivity

Pharmacokinetics:
good GI absorption; readily penetrates into CSF; hepatic metabolism; renal excretion

Pediatrics, breast feeding and sulfonamides are compatible; avoid sulfonamides and nursing in premature infants, infants with hyperbilirubinemia, and infants with G-6-PD deficiency

Contraindications
Hypersensitivity to sulfonamides or chemically related drugs such as sulfonylureas, thiazide diuretics, and sunscreens containing PABA

Pregnancy
Safety for use during pregnancy has not been established; sulfonamides do cross the placenta achieving fetal levels approximately 70%–90% of maternal serum levels; do not use during pregnancy at term

Lactation Issues
Sulfonamides are excreted in breast milk; according to the American Academy of Pediatrics, breast feeding and sulfonamides are compatible; avoid sulfonamides and nursing in premature infants, infants with hyperbilirubinemia, and infants with G-6-PD deficiency

(continues on next page)

| Drug and Dosage Forms | Spectrum of Activity and Usual Dosage Range | Administration Issues and Drug–Drug & Drug–Food Interactions | Common Adverse Drug Reactions (ADRs) and Pharmacokinetics | Contraindications, Pregnancy Category, and Lactation Issues |
|---|---|---|---|---|
| **Multiple Sulfonamides** Triple Sulfa No. 2 Tablet: 167 mg sulfadiazine/ 167 mg sulfamerazine/ 167 mg sulfamethazine | **Antibacterial Spectrum** Gram-negative organisms (*E. coli, Klebsiella* sp., *Enterobacter* sp., *P. mirabilis, P. vulgaris*) and *S. aureus* in the urine; *Nocardia* sp., *C. trachomatis; H. ducreyi* **General indications** Adults: 2–4 gm initially, followed by 2–4 gm daily in 3 to 6 divided doses for 7 to 14 days **Children > 2 months** 75 mg/kg initially, followed by 120–150 mg/kg/d in 4 to 6 divided doses for 7 to 14 days; maximum = 6 gm daily | Administration Issues Complete full course of therapy; take on an empty stomach with a full glass of water; avoid prolonged exposure to sunlight, wear protective clothing, and apply sunscreen Drug–Drug Interactions Sulfonamides may increase the pharmacological and toxic effects of the following drugs: **methotrexate, phenytoin, sulfonylureas, warfarin** | ADRs: nausea, abdominal discomfort, headache, photosensitivity Pharmacokinetics: good GI absorption; readily penetrates into CSF; hepatic metabolism; renal excretion | Contraindications Hypersensitivity to sulfonamides or chemically related drugs such as sulfonylureas, thiazide diuretics, and sunscreens containing PABA Pregnancy Safety for use during pregnancy has not been established; sulfonamides do cross the placenta achieving fetal levels approximately 70%–90% of maternal serum levels; do not use during pregnancy at term Lactation Issues Sulfonamides are excreted in breast milk; according to the American Academy of Pediatrics, breast feeding and sulfonamides are compatible; avoid sulfonamides and nursing in premature infants, infants with hyperbilirubinemia, and infants with G-6-PD deficiency |

## 102.10 Sulfonamide Combinations

| Drug and Dosage Forms | Spectrum of Activity and Usual Dosage Range | Administration Issues and Drug–Drug & Drug–Food Interactions | Common Adverse Drug Reactions (ADRs) and Pharmacokinetics | Contraindications, Pregnancy Category, and Lactation Issues |
|---|---|---|---|---|
| **Erythromycin Ethylsuccinate and Sulfisoxazole**<br>Pediazole, Eryzole, various generics<br><br><u>Granules for Oral Suspension:</u><br>200 mg erythromycin ethylsuccinate<br>600 mg sulfisoxazole per 5 ml | **Antibacterial Spectrum**<br>Susceptible strains of *H. influenzae*<br><br>**Treatment of otitis media in children**<br>50 mg/kg/d erythromycin and 150 mg/kg/d of sulfisoxazole divided doses qid for 10 d<br><br><u>Recommended Dosage:</u><br><8 kg (<18 lb.): adjust dosage by body weight, qid<br>8 kg (18 lb.): 2.5 ml qid<br>16 kg (35 lb.): 5 ml qid<br>24 kg (53 lb.): 7.5 ml qid<br>>45 kg (>100 lb.): 10 ml qid | <u>Administration Issues</u><br>Complete full course of therapy; may be given without regard to meals; take with a full glass of water; store in the refrigerator; discard unused portion after 14 days; avoid prolonged exposure to sunlight, wear protective clothing, and apply sunscreen<br><br><u>Drug–Drug Interactions</u><br>see monographs for erythromycin ethylsuccinate and sulfisoxazole for potential drug interactions | <u>ADRs:</u><br>nausea, abdominal distress, diarrhea, abnormal taste, photosensitivity<br><br><u>Pharmacokinetics:</u><br>see monographs for erythromycin ethylsuccinate and sulfisoxazole | <u>Contraindications</u><br>Hypersensitivity to sulfonamides or chemically related drugs such as sulfonylureas, thiazide diuretics, and sunscreens containing PABA; hypersensitivity to erythromycin; preexisting liver disease<br><br><u>Pregnancy</u><br>Safety for use during pregnancy has not been established; sulfonamides do cross the placenta achieving fetal levels approximately 70%–90% of maternal serum levels; do not use during pregnancy at term<br><br><u>Lactation Issues</u><br>Sulfonamides are excreted in breast milk; according to the American Academy of Pediatrics, breast feeding and sulfonamides and erythromycin are compatible; avoid sulfonamides and nursing in premature infants, infants with hyperbilirubinemia, and infants with G-6-PD deficiency |

*(continues on next page)*

**102.10 Sulfonamide Combinations** *continued from previous page*

| Drug and Dosage Forms | Spectrum of Activity and Usual Dosage Range | Administration Issues and Drug–Drug & Drug–Food Interactions | Common Adverse Drug Reactions (ADRs) and Pharmacokinetics | Contraindications, Pregnancy Category, and Lactation Issues |
|---|---|---|---|---|
| **Trimethoprim and Sulfamethoxazole (TMP-SMZ)**<br><br>Tablet:<br>Bactrim, Septra, generics<br>80 mg trim/400 mg sulfa<br><br>Bactrim DS, Septra DS, generics<br>160 mg trim/ 800 mg sulfa<br><br>Suspension:<br>Bactrim Pediatric, Septra, generics<br>40 mg trim/ 200 mg sulfa/ 5 ml | **Antibacterial Spectrum**<br>Urinary infections caused by *E. coli*, *Proteus* sp., *K. pneumoniae*, *Enterobacter* sp., and coagulase-negative *Staphylococcus* sp.; *H. influenzae*, *M. catarrhalis*, *S. pneumoniae*, *Shigella* sp., *Salmonella* sp., *Pneumocystis carinii*<br><br>**Treatment of urinary tract infection and otitis media**<br><br>**Adults:** 1 DS tablet bid for 10 to 14 d<br><br>**Children:** 8 mg/kg TMP/40 mg/kg SMZ per day divided q 12 h for 10 d<br><br>**Treatment of travelers' diarrhea in adults**<br><br>1 DS tablet bid for 5 days<br><br>**Acute exacerbation of chronic bronchitis in adults:** 1 DS tablet bid for 14 days<br><br>**Treatment of Pneumocystis carinii pneumonia**<br>**Adults:** 15–20 mg/kg TMP/ 100 mg/kg SMZ/d divided q 6 h for 21 d | Administration Issues<br>Complete full course of therapy; take each oral dose with a full glass of water<br><br>Drug–Drug Interactions<br>TMP-SMZ may increase the pharmacological effect of the following drugs leading to toxicity: **dapsone, methotrexate, phenytoin, sulfonylureas, warfarin.**<br>TMP-SMZ may decrease the effect of **cyclosporine.** Use of **zidovudine, azathioprine,** or **ganciclovir** and TMP-SMZ may have additive bone marrow depressant effects in patients with HIV | ADRs:<br>abdominal distress, nausea, rash, neutropenia<br><br>Pharmacokinetics:<br>rapidly absorbed; $T_{1/2}$ is approximately 10 hours; SMZ undergoes hepatic metabolism; renal excretion | Contraindications<br>Hypersensitivity to trimethoprim or sulfonamides; megaloblastic anemia due to folate deficiency; pregnancy at term and lactation; infants <2 months old<br><br>Pregnancy Category: C<br><br>Lactation Issues<br>Not recommended for use in nursing infants due to possibility of sulfonamide associated kernicterus |

**Children:** (give for 21 days)
8 kg: 5 ml suspension/dose q 6 h
16 kg: 10 ml suspension/dose q 6 h
24 kg: 15 ml suspension/dose q 6 h
32 kg: 20 ml suspension/dose q 6 h

**Follow treatment with prophylactic regimen**

**Prophylaxis of Pneumocystis carinii pneumonia**
**Adults:** 1 DS tablet daily or 1 DS tablet 3 times per week on Mon, Wed, Fri

**Children:** 150 mg/m² TMP/ 750 mg/m² SMZ/d divided bid on 3 consecutive days per week; do not exceed 320 mg TMP/1600 mg SMZ per day

**Dosage reduction is recommended for patients with renal insufficiency**

| Drug and Dosage Forms | Spectrum of Activity and Usual Dosage Range | Administration Issues and Drug–Drug & Drug–Food Interactions | Common Adverse Drug Reactions (ADRs) and Pharmacokinetics | Contraindications, Pregnancy Category, and Lactation Issues |
|---|---|---|---|---|
| **Demeclocycline**<br>Declomycin<br><br><u>Tablet:</u><br>150 mg, 300 mg<br><br><u>Capsule:</u><br>150 mg | **Antibacterial Spectrum**<br>*S. pneumonia*, some gram-negative organisms including *E. coli*, *Klebsiella* sp., *E. aerogenes*, *Acinetobacter* sp., Rickettsiae (Rocky Mountain spotted fever), *M. pneumoniae*, *Bacteriodes* sp., *C. trachomatis*, *Brucella* sp., *Ureaplasma urealyticum*, *Borrelia burgdorferi* (Lyme disease)<br><br>**Second line agent in treating bacterial infections**<br>**Adults:** 150 mg q 6 h <u>or</u> 300 mg q 12 h for 10 to 14 d<br><br>**Children > 8 yr.:** 6–12 mg/kg divided q 6 to 12 h for 10 to 14 d<br><br>**Hyponatremia associated with SIADH**<br>600–1200 mg divided q 6 to 12 h | <u>Administration Issues</u><br>Complete full course of therapy; take on empty stomach at least 1 hour before or 2 h after meals; avoid simultaneous dairy products, antacids, laxatives, or iron-containing products; avoid prolonged exposure to the sun or sunlamps<br><br><u>Drug–Drug Interactions</u><br>**Antacids** containing calcium, magnesium, aluminum, zinc, and bismuth salts, **sucralfate**, and iron-containing products may decrease the absorption of tetracyclines. Tetracyclines may increase serum **digoxin** levels. Tetracyclines may decrease the effectiveness of **oral contraceptives.** Concomitant use of **penicillins** may decrease the effectiveness of tetracyclines | <u>ADRs:</u><br>photosensitivity, nausea, vomiting, dizziness, superinfection, polyuria, polydipsia<br><br><u>Pharmacokinetics:</u><br>65–90% protein binding; 40% excreted unchanged in the urine | <u>Contraindications</u><br>Hypersensitivity to tetracyclines<br><br><u>Pregnancy Category:</u> D<br><br><u>Lactation Issues</u><br>Excreted in breast milk; due to potential, serious adverse effects in nursing infants decide whether to discontinue the drug or nursing |
| **Doxycycline**<br><br><u>Tablets:</u><br>Vibra-Tabs 100 mg<br><br><u>Capsule:</u><br>Vibramycin, generics 50 mg, 100 mg | **Antibacterial Spectrum**<br>*S. pneumonia*, some gram-negative organisms including *E. coli*, *Klebsiella* sp., *E. aerogenes*, *Acinetobacter* sp., Rickettsiae (Rocky Mountain spotted fever), *M. pneumoniae*, *Bacteriodes* sp., *C. trachomatis*, *Brucella* sp., | <u>Administration Issues</u><br>Complete full course of therapy; shake suspension well before administration; may take without regards to meals; avoid simultaneous dairy products, antacids, laxatives, or iron-containing products; avoid prolonged exposure to the sun or sunlamps | <u>ADRs:</u><br>nausea, vomiting, diarrhea, photosensitivity, dizziness, superinfection<br><br><u>Pharmacokinetics:</u><br>increased absorption with food; high lipid solubility and | <u>Contraindications</u><br>Hypersensitivity to tetracyclines<br><br><u>Pregnancy Category:</u> D<br><br><u>Lactation Issues</u><br>Excreted in breast milk; due to potential, serious adverse |

| | | | |
|---|---|---|---|
| Capsule, coated pellets:<br>Doryx 100 mg<br><br>Powder for Oral Suspension:<br>Vibramycin<br>25 mg/5 ml<br><br>Syrup:<br>Vibramycin<br>50 mg/5 ml | *Ureaplasma urealyticum, Borrelia burgdorferi* (Lyme disease), *Plasmodium* sp. (malaria)<br><br>**General indications**<br>**Adults and children > 8 yr. and > 45 kg:**<br>100 mg q 12 h for 7 to 14 d<br><br>**Children > 8 yr. and < 45 kg:**<br>4.4 mg/kg/d divided q 12 h for 7 to 14 d<br><br>**Malaria prophylaxis**<br>**Adults:** 100 mg qd starting 1 to 2 days before travel to malarious area and continue daily during travel and for 4 weeks after leaving malarious area<br><br>**Children > 8 yr.:** 2 mg/kg/d up to 100 mg qd starting 1 to 2 days before travel to malarious area and continue daily during travel and for 4 weeks after leaving malarious area | <u>Drug–Drug Interactions</u><br>**Antacids** containing calcium, magnesium, aluminum, zinc, and bismuth salts, **sucralfate**, and iron-containing products may decrease the absorption of tetracyclines. Tetracyclines may increase serum **digoxin** levels. Tetracyclines may decrease the effectiveness of **oral contraceptives**. Concomitant use of **penicillins** may decrease the effectiveness of tetracyclines. Concomitant use of **carbamazepine, phenytoin,** and **barbiturates** may increase the metabolism of doxycycline. | penetration into cerebrospinal fluid; 90% protein binding; fecal elimination |
| **Minocycline**<br>Minocin<br><br>Tablet:<br>50 mg, 100 mg<br><br>Capsule:<br>50 mg, 100 mg<br><br>Suspension:<br>50 mg/5 ml | **Antibacterial Spectrum**<br>*S. pneumonia,* some gram-negative organisms including *E. coli, Klebsiella* sp., *E. aerogenes, Acinetobacter* sp., Rickettsiae (Rocky Mountain spotted fever), *M. pneumoniae, Bacteriodes* sp., *C. trachomatis, Brucella* sp., *Ureaplasma urealyticum, Borrelia burgdorferi* (Lyme disease)<br><br>**General Indications**<br>**Adults:** 100 mg q 12 h <u>or</u> 50 mg q 6 h for 7 to 14 d | <u>Administration Issues</u><br>Complete full course of therapy; shake suspension well before administration; may take without regards to meals; avoid simultaneous dairy products, antacids, laxatives, or iron-containing products; avoid prolonged exposure to the sun or sunlamps<br><br><u>Drug–Drug Interactions</u><br>**Antacids** containing calcium, magnesium, aluminum, zinc, and bismuth salts, **sucralfate**, and iron- | <u>ADRs:</u><br>nausea, vomiting, diarrhea, photosensitivity, dizziness, superinfection<br><br><u>Pharmacokinetics:</u><br>high lipid solubility and penetration into cerebrospinal fluid; 75% protein binding; biliary excretion |

(top right continuation of previous row): effects in nursing infants decide whether to discontinue the drug or nursing

(bottom right for Minocycline): <u>Contraindications</u><br>Hypersensitivity to tetracyclines<br><br><u>Pregnancy Category:</u> D<br><br><u>Lactation Issues</u><br>Excreted in breast milk; due to potential, serious adverse effects in nursing infants decide whether to discontinue the drug or nursing

*(continues on next page)*

| Drug and Dosage Forms | Spectrum of Activity and Usual Dosage Range | Administration Issues and Drug–Drug & Drug–Food Interactions | Common Adverse Drug Reactions (ADRs) and Pharmacokinetics | Contraindications, Pregnancy Category, and Lactation Issues |
|---|---|---|---|---|
| **Minocycline *cont.*** | **Children > 8 yr.:** 2 mg/kg q 12 h for 7 to 14 d | containing products may decrease the absorption of tetracyclines. Tetracyclines may increase serum **digoxin** levels. Tetracyclines may decrease the effectiveness of **oral contraceptives.** Concomitant use of **penicillins** may decrease the effectiveness of tetracyclines | | |
| **Tetracycline**<br><br>Tablet:<br>Sumycin<br>250 mg, 500 mg<br><br>Capsule:<br>Achromycin V, Sumycin, various generic<br>250 mg, 500 mg<br><br>Suspension:<br>Achromycin V, Sumycin, various generic<br>125 mg/5 ml | **Antibacterial Spectrum**<br>*S. pneumonia*, some gram-negative organisms including *E. coli*, *Klebsiella* sp., *E. aerogenes*, *Acinetobacter* sp., Rickettsiae (Rocky Mountain spotted fever), *M. pneumoniae*, *Bacteriodes* sp., *C. trachomatis*, *Brucella* sp., *Ureaplasma urealyticum*, *Borrelia burgdorferi* (Lyme disease)<br><br>**General Indications**<br>**Adults:** 1–2 gm daily in 2 to 4 divided doses for 7 to 14 d<br><br>**Children > 8 yr.:** 25–50 mg/kg divided qid for 7 to 14 d<br><br>**Severe acne:** 500 mg bid initially, then 125–500 mg daily as a maintenance dose | Administration Issues<br>Complete full course of therapy; shake suspension well before administration; take on empty stomach at least 1 hour before or 2 h after meals; avoid simultaneous dairy products, antacids, laxatives, or iron-containing products; avoid prolonged exposure to the sun or sunlamps<br><br>Drug–Drug Interactions<br>**Antacids** containing calcium, magnesium, aluminum, zinc, and bismuth salts, **sucralfate,** and iron-containing products may decrease the absorption of tetracyclines. Tetracyclines may increase serum **digoxin** levels. Tetracyclines may decrease the effectiveness of **oral contraceptives.** Concomitant use of **penicillins** may decrease the effectiveness of tetracyclines | ADRs:<br>nausea, vomiting, diarrhea, photosensitivity, dizziness, superinfection<br><br>Pharmacokinetics:<br>decreased absorption with food; less CNS penetration than doxycycline; 65% protein binding; 60% excreted unchanged in the urine | Contraindications<br>Hypersensitivity to tetracyclines<br><br>Pregnancy Category: D<br><br>Lactation Issues<br>Excreted in breast milk; due to potential, serious adverse effects in nursing infants decide whether to discontinue the drug or nursing |

# 103. Antifungals

| Drug and Dosage Forms | Spectrum of Activity and Usual Dosage Range | Administration Issues and Drug–Drug & Drug–Food Interactions | Common Adverse Drug Reactions (ADRs) and Pharmacokinetics | Contraindications, Pregnancy Category, and Lactation Issues |
|---|---|---|---|---|
| **Clotrimazole** Mycelex  Troches: 10 mg | **Antifungal Spectrum** C. albicans  **Local treatment of oropharyngeal candidiasis** 1 troche 5 times/d for 14 d.  **Prophylaxis in immunocompromised patients:** 1 troche tid | Administration Issues Dissolve troche slowly in mouth to achieve maximal effect. | ADRs: abnormal LFTs, nausea, vomiting, unpleasant taste in mouth, pruritus  Pharmacokinetics: dosing every 3 h maintains effective salivary levels for most strains of Candida | Contraindications Hypersensitivity to clotrimazole  Pregnancy Category: C  Lactation Issues Fluconazole is excreted in breast milk; use in nursing mothers is not recommended |
| **Fluconazole** Diflucan  Tablet: 50 mg, 100 mg, 150 mg, 200 mg  Powder for Oral Suspension: 10 mg/ml 40 mg/ml | **Antifungal Spectrum** Various fungal infections including: C. neoformans; Candida sp., Aspergillus sp., Coccidioides immitis  **Treatment of vaginal candidiasis:** 150 mg as a single dose  **Oropharyngeal candidiasis** **Adults:** 200 mg on first day, followed by 100 mg once daily, continue treatment for 2 weeks to decrease likelihood of relapse  **Children:** 6 mg/kg on first day, followed by 3 mg/kg once daily; continue treatment for 2 weeks to decrease likelihood of relapse | Administration Issues Complete full course of therapy; shake suspension well prior to administration; store suspension in the refrigerator or at room temperature; discard unused suspension after 2 weeks  Drug–Drug Interactions **Cimetidine** and **rifampin** may decrease the serum level of fluconazole. **Hydrochlorothiazide** may increase the serum level of fluconazole. Fluconazole may increase or decrease the effect of **oral contraceptives.** Fluconazole may cause an increase in the pharmacological and toxic effects of the following drugs: **terfenadine, astemizole, loratadine, cyclosporine,** | ADRs: headache, nausea, abdominal pain, diarrhea  **Adverse effects are reported to occur more frequently in HIV infected patients compared to non-HIV infected patients**  Pharmacokinetics: excellent GI absorption; $T_{1/2}$ is approximately 30 h; good CSF penetration; hepatic metabolism; approximately 80% of a dose is excreted unchanged in the urine | Contraindications Hypersensitivity to fluconazole; use with caution in patients allergic to other azole antifungals  Pregnancy Category: C  Lactation Issues Fluconazole is excreted in breast milk; use in nursing mothers is not recommended |

(continues on next page)

| Drug and Dosage Forms | Spectrum of Activity and Usual Dosage Range | Administration Issues and Drug–Drug & Drug–Food Interactions | Common Adverse Drug Reactions (ADRs) and Pharmacokinetics | Contraindications, Pregnancy Category, and Lactation Issues |
|---|---|---|---|---|
| **Fluconazole** *cont.* | **Esophageal candidiasis**<br>**Adults:** 200 mg on first day, followed by 100 mg once daily, continue treatment for a minimum of 3 weeks and for at least 2 weeks following resolution of symptoms; doses up to 400 mg/day may be used<br><br>**Children:** 6 mg/kg on first day, followed by 3 mg/kg once daily, continue treatment for a minimum of 3 weeks and for at least 2 weeks following resolution of symptoms; doses up to 12 mg/kg/d may be used<br><br>**Candidal UTI:** 50–200 mg/d<br><br>**Systemic Candidal infections**<br>**Adults:** 100–400 mg/day<br><br>**Children:** 6–12 mg/kg/d (based on an open, noncomparative study of a small number of children)<br><br>**Cryptococcal meningitis**<br>**Adults:** 400 mg on first day, followed by 200 mg once daily, continue treatment for 10–12 weeks after CSF cultures are negative; doses up to 400 mg/day may be used | **tacrolimus, phenytoin, theophylline, sulfonylureas, warfarin, zidovudine, cisapride** | | |

| | | |
|---|---|---|
| **Children:** 12 mg/kg on first day, followed by 6 mg/kg qd; continue treatment for 10–12 weeks after CSF cultures are negative; doses up to 12 mg/kg/d may be used<br><br>**Suppression of relapse of cryptococcal meningitis**<br>**Adults:** 200 mg qd<br><br>**Children:** 6 mg/kg qd | | <u>Contraindications</u><br>Hypersensitivity to griseofulvin; porphyria; hepatocellular failure<br><br><u>Pregnancy Category:</u> C |
| **Griseofulvin Microsize**<br><br><u>Tablet:</u><br>Fulvicin U/F<br>Grifulvin V<br>250 mg, 500 mg<br><br><u>Capsule:</u><br>Grisactin<br>125 mg, 250 mg<br><br><u>Oral Suspension:</u><br>Grifulvin V<br>125 mg/5 ml | **Antifungal Spectrum**<br>Limited antifungal spectrum including: *Microsporidium* sp., *Epidermophyton* sp., and *Trichophyton* sp.<br><br><u>Treatment of *tinea corporis*, *tinea cruris*, and *tinea capitis*</u><br>**Adults:** 500 mg microsize or 330–375 mg ultramicrosize daily in a single or divided doses<br><br>**Children > 2 yr.:** 11 mg microsize/kg/d or 7.3 mg ultramicrosize/kg/d<br><br><u>Treatment of *tinea pedis* and *tinea ungulum*</u><br>**Adults:** 0.75 mg–1 gm microsize or 660–750 mg ultramicrosize daily in divided doses<br><br>**Children > 2 yr.:** 11 mg microsize/kg/d or 7.3 mg ultramicrosize/kg/d | <u>Administration Issues</u><br>Complete full course of therapy; avoid prolonged exposure to the sun; shake suspension well prior to administration; store suspension at room temperature. Serum levels may be increased with a high fat content meal. Avoid alcohol.<br><br><u>Drug–Drug Interactions</u><br>Griseofulvin may decrease the effect of the following drugs: **warfarin, oral contraceptives, cyclosporine, and salicylates. Barbiturates** may decrease serum levels of griseofulvin. Disulfuram-type reaction may occur with alcohol. | <u>ADRs:</u><br>rash, urticaria, nausea, headache, abdominal discomfort, dizziness, photosensitivity<br><br><u>Pharmacokinetics:</u><br>poor and inconsistent GI absorption |

(continues on next page)

# 103. Antifungals  *continued from previous page*

| Drug and Dosage Forms | Spectrum of Activity and Usual Dosage Range | Administration Issues and Drug–Drug & Drug–Food Interactions | Common Adverse Drug Reactions (ADRs) and Pharmacokinetics | Contraindications, Pregnancy Category, and Lactation Issues |
|---|---|---|---|---|
| **Griseofulvin Ultramicrosize** <br><br> Tablet: <br> Fulvicin P/G <br> 125 mg, 165 mg, 250 mg, 330 mg <br><br> Grisactin Ultra <br> 125 mg, 250 mg, 330 mg <br><br> Gris-PEG <br> 125 mg, 250 mg | **Antifungal Spectrum** <br> Limited antifungal spectrum including: *Microsporidium* sp., *Epidermophyton* sp., and *Trichophyton* sp. <br><br> **Treatment of *tinea corporis, tinea cruris,* and *tinea capitis*** <br> **Adults:** 500 mg microsize or 330–375 mg ultramicrosize daily in a single or divided doses <br><br> **Children > 2 yr.:** 11 mg microsize/kg/d or 7.3 mg ultramicrosize/kg/d <br><br> **Treatment of *tinea pedis* and *tinea ungulum*** <br> **Adults:** 0.75 mg–1 gm microsize or 660–750 mg ultramicrosize daily in divided doses <br><br> **Children > 2 yr.:** 11 mg microsize/kg/d or 7.3 mg ultramicrosize/kg/d | <u>Administration Issues</u> <br> Complete full course of therapy; avoid prolonged exposure to the sun; shake suspension well prior to administration; store suspension at room temperature. Avoid alcohol. <br><br> <u>Drug–Drug Interactions</u> <br> Griseofulvin may decrease the effect of the following drugs: **warfarin, oral contraceptives, cyclosporine, and salicylates. Barbiturates** may decrease serum levels of griseofulvin. Disulfuram-type reaction may occur with alcohol. | <u>ADRs:</u> <br> rash, urticaria, nausea, headache, abdominal discomfort, dizziness, photosensitivity <br><br> <u>Pharmacokinetics:</u> <br> enhanced GI absorption compared to microsize formulation | <u>Contraindications</u> <br> Hypersensitivity to griseofulvin; porphyria; hepatocellular failure <br><br> <u>Pregnancy Category:</u> C |
| **Itraconazole** <br> Sporanox | **Antifungal Spectrum** <br> Various fungal infections including *Blastomycosis, Histomycosis, Aspergillosis,* and *Onychomycosis* | <u>Administration Issues</u> <br> Complete full course of therapy; do not take with antacids; administer with a cola drink in HIV patients; take with a full meal | <u>ADRs:</u> <br> nausea, vomiting, diarrhea, rash, headache | <u>Contraindications</u> <br> Concomitant use of terfenadine, astemizole, cisapride, triazolam, or |

982

| | | | | |
|---|---|---|---|---|
| **Capsule:** 100 mg | ***Blastomycosis and Histoplasmosis* infections** 200 mg qd; may increase to 400 mg/d if needed for a minimum of 3 months<br><br>Give doses > 200 mg/day in two divided doses<br><br>***Aspergillosis* infection** 200–400 mg/d. Give doses > 200 mg/day in two divided doses for a minimum of 3 months<br><br>***Onychomycosis* infection** 200 mg qd for 12 consecutive weeks | <u>Drug–Drug Interactions</u><br>Itraconazole may increase the pharmacological and toxic effects of the following drugs: **astemizole, loratadine, terfenadine, cyclosporine, quinidine, tacrolimus, warfarin, cisapride, phenytoin, sulfonylureas, triazolam, midazolam**<br><br>The following drugs may decrease the effect of itraconazole: **rifampin, phenytoin, H₂ antagonist (cimetidine, ranitidine), antacids, didanosine** | <u>Pharmacokinetics:</u><br>absorption is dependent on an acidic environment; long T₁/₂ approximately 20 h; extensive hepatic metabolism; renal excretion of inactive metabolites | midazolam; hypersensitivity to itraconazole or other azole antifungals; treatment of onychomycosis in pregnant women<br><br><u>Pregnancy Category:</u> C<br><br><u>Lactation Issues</u><br>Excreted in breast milk; do not use in nursing mothers |
| **Ketoconazole**<br>Nizoral<br><br><u>Tablet:</u><br>200 mg | **Antifungal Spectrum**<br>Various fungal infections including: *Blastomyces dermatitidis, Candida* sp., *Coccidioides immitis, Histoplasma capsulatum, Paracoccidioides brasiliensis, Phialophora* sp., *Trichophyton* sp., *Epidermophyton* sp., and *Microsporidium* sp.<br><br>**General indications**<br>**Adults:** 200 mg qd, for serious infections or if clinical response is insufficient, 400 mg qd may be used<br><br>**Children > 2 yr.:** 3.3–6.6 mg/kg/d as a single dose | <u>Administration Issues</u><br>Complete full course of therapy; do not give within two hours of antacids. take with food to decrease GI disturbances.<br><br><u>Drug–Drug Interactions</u><br>**Antacids, H₂ antagonists,** and **anticholinergics** may increase gastric pH and decrease ketoconazole absorption. Ketoconazole may increase the pharmacological and toxic effects of the following drugs: **warfarin, astemizole, loratadine, terfenadine, corticosteroids, cyclosporine, tacrolimus, sulfonylureas, midazolam.** Ketoconazole may decrease the effect of **theophylline. Isoniazid** and **rifampin** may decrease the serum concentration of ketoconazole | <u>ADRs:</u><br>nausea, vomiting, abdominal discomfort, headache, dizziness. Hepatotoxicity has occurred, including rare fatalities. Frequent measurement of LFTs is recommended.<br><br><u>Pharmacokinetics:</u><br>acidic pH required for dissolution and absorption; negligible CSF penetration; hepatic metabolism; biliary and fecal elimination | <u>Contraindications</u><br>Hypersensitivity to ketoconazole<br><br><u>Pregnancy Category:</u> C<br><br><u>Lactation Issues</u><br>Ketoconazole is probably excreted in breast milk; avoid use in nursing mothers |

*(continues on next page)*

| Drug and Dosage Forms | Spectrum of Activity and Usual Dosage Range | Administration Issues and Drug–Drug & Drug–Food Interactions | Common Adverse Drug Reactions (ADRs) and Pharmacokinetics | Contraindications, Pregnancy Category, and Lactation Issues |
|---|---|---|---|---|
| **Ketoconazole** *cont.* | **Minimum treatment for candidiasis is 1 to 2 weeks. Minimum treatment for other systemic mycoses is 6 months. Chronic mucocutaneous candidiasis usually requires maintenance therapy. Minimum treatment for recalcitrant dermatophyte infections is 4 weeks** | | | |
| **Nystatin**<br>Mycostatin, Nilstat, various generics<br><br>Tablet, film coated:<br>500,000 units<br><br>Oral Suspension:<br>100,000 units/ml<br><br>Troches:<br>Mycostatin Pastilles<br>200,000 units<br><br>Bulk Powder: (million units): 50, 100, 500<br><br>Bulk Powder: (billion units): 1, 2, 5 | **Antifungal Spectrum**<br>*Candida* sp. including *Candida albicans*<br><br>**Intestinal *Candida* infections**<br>**Adults:** 500,000–1 million units tid, continue for 48 h after clinical cure<br><br>**Children:** 100,000 units qid, continue for 48 h after clinical cure<br><br>**Oral *Candida* infections:**<br>**Adults and children:**<br>Suspension: 400,000 to 600,000 units qid<br>Troches: 200,000 to 400,000 units 4–5 times/d; for as long as 14 d, if necessary<br>Powder: Add 1/8 tsp (500,000 units) to ½ cup water and stir well. | Administration Issues<br>Complete full course of therapy; continue therapy for at least two days after symptoms disappear. When using suspension for oral candidiasis, retain drug in mouth as long as possible before swallowing. For the troches, do not chew or swallow whole. Allow troches to dissolve slowly in mouth. Do not store the powder after reconstitution. | ADRs:<br>nausea, vomiting<br><br>Pharmacokinetics:<br>minimal oral absorption; fecal elimination | Contraindications<br>Hypersensitivity to nystatin<br><br>Pregnancy<br>No adverse effects or complications have been attributed to nystatin in infants born to women treated with nystatin<br><br>Lactation Issues<br>Excretion in human breast milk is unknown; use with caution in nursing mothers |

## Terbinafine (continued)

| Drug and Dosage Forms | Spectrum of Activity and Usual Dosage Range | Administration Issues and Drug–Drug & Drug–Food Interactions | Common Adverse Drug Reactions (ADRs) and Pharmacokinetics | Contraindications, Pregnancy Category, and Lactation Issues |
|---|---|---|---|---|
| | | Administer qid; use immediately and do not store. Continue for 48 h after clinical cure. | | |
| **Terbinafine**<br>Lamisil<br><br>Tablet:<br>250 mg | **Antifungal Spectrum:**<br>*Trichophyton mentagrophytes* and *T. rubrum*<br><br>**Treatment of onychomycosis of the toenail/fingernail due to dermatophytes:**<br>Fingernail: 250 mg/d for 6 wk<br>Toenail: 250 mg/d for 12 wk<br><br>Optimal clinical cure is seen months after mycological cure and cessation of treatment. | Administration Issues<br>Use medication for recommended treatment time. Safety and efficacy in children is not established.<br><br>Drug Interactions:<br>Terbinafine clearance is decreased by **cimetidine, terfenadine.** Terbinafine clearance is increased by **rifampin.** Terbinafine increases the clearance of **cyclosporine** and decreases the clearance of **caffeine.** | ADRs:<br>diarrhea, dyspepsia, abdominal pain, nausea, rash, pruritus, LFT abnormalities, headache, taste and visual disturbances.<br><br>Pharmacokinetics:<br>terbinafine is well absorbed | Contraindications<br>Hypersensitivity to terbinafine; pre-existing liver disease or renal impairment (CrCl <50 ml/min)<br><br>Pregnancy:  B<br><br>Lactation Issues<br>Terbinafine is excreted in human breast milk; avoid in nursing mothers |

## 104. Antimalarials

| Drug and Dosage Forms | Spectrum of Activity and Usual Dosage Range | Administration Issues and Drug–Drug & Drug–Food Interactions | Common Adverse Drug Reactions (ADRs) and Pharmacokinetics | Contraindications, Pregnancy Category, and Lactation Issues |
|---|---|---|---|---|
| **Chloroquine Phosphate**<br><br>Tablet: Various generics<br>250 mg<br><br>Tablet:<br>Aralen 500 mg | **Antimalarial Spectrum**<br>*P. falciparum, P. malariae,* and *P. vivax*<br><br>**Treatment of acute malaria**<br>**Adults:**  600 mg on day 1, followed by 300 mg 6 h later, 300 mg on day 2, and 300 mg on day 3<br><br>**Children:**  10 mg/kg on day 1, followed by 5 mg/kg 6 h later, 5 mg/kg on day 2, and 5 mg/kg on day 3 | Administration Issues<br>Complete full course of therapy; take tablets on the same day each week for malaria suppression; do not take on an empty stomach<br><br>Drug–Drug Interactions<br>**Cimetidine** may decrease the elimination of chloroquine. **Kaolin** may decrease the absorption of chloroquine | ADRs:<br>nausea, vomiting, headache, GI upset, visual disturbances (possibly leading to irreversible retinal damage with long term administration)<br><br>Pharmacokinetics:<br>readily absorbed from GI tract; 55% protein bound; long elimination half-life; renal excretion | Contraindications<br>Retinal or visual field changes; hypersensitivity to chloroquine or related compounds<br><br>Pregnancy<br>Use only when clearly needed and potential benefit outweighs the potential hazards to the fetus |

*(continues on next page)*

| Drug and Dosage Forms | Spectrum of Activity and Usual Dosage Range | Administration Issues and Drug–Drug & Drug–Food Interactions | Common Adverse Drug Reactions (ADRs) and Pharmacokinetics | Contraindications, Pregnancy Category, and Lactation Issues |
|---|---|---|---|---|
| **Chloroquine Phosphate** *cont.* | <u>Suppression of malaria</u><br>**Adults:** 300 mg once weekly starting one week prior to travel, continue weekly during travel, and for 4 weeks after leaving areas<br><br>**Children:** 5 mg/kg (max 300 mg) once weekly starting one week prior to travel, continue weekly during travel, and for 4 weeks after leaving such areas<br><br><u>Treatment of extraintestinal amebiasis</u><br>**Adults:** 1 gm qd for 2 days, followed by 500 mg qd for 2 to 3 weeks<br><br>**Combination therapy with an effective intestinal amebicide (paromomycin, metronidazole) should be used** | | | <u>Lactation Issues</u><br>Excreted in breast milk in low concentrations; use with caution in nursing mothers |
| **Chloroquine Phosphate and Primaquine Phosphate**<br>Aralen Phosphate with Primaquine Phosphate | **Antimalarial Spectrum**<br>*Plasmodium* sp.<br><br>**Prophylaxis of malaria**<br>**Adults and children > 45.5 kg:** 1 tablet at least one day prior to entering endemic area, followed by 1 tablet weekly, continuing for | <u>Administration Issues</u><br>Complete full course of therapy; take with food or after meals to decrease GI upset<br><br><u>Drug–Drug Interactions</u><br>**Cimetidine** may decrease the elimination of chloroquine, **Kaolin** may decrease the absorption of chloroquine. | <u>ADRs:</u><br>nausea, vomiting, headache, GI upset, visual disturbances (possibly leading to irreversible retinal damage with long term administration) | <u>Contraindications</u><br>Retinal or visual field changes; hypersensitivity to chloroquine or related compounds; concomitant use of quinacrine and primaquine; patients predisposed to granulocytopenia (rheumatoid |

| Drug / Formulation | Dosing | Administration / Interactions | Pharmacokinetics / ADRs | Contraindications / Pregnancy / Lactation |
|---|---|---|---|---|
| **Tablet:** 500 mg chloroquine phosphate/ 79 mg primaquine phosphate | 8 weeks after leaving the endemic area<br>**Children 25.5–45.5 kg:** ½ tablet at least one day prior to entering endemic area, followed by ½ tablet weekly, continuing for 8 weeks after leaving the endemic area<br>**Children < 25.5 kg use an extemporaneously prepared liquid: (crush 1 tablet in 40 mls fluid)**<br>**20.9–25 kg:** 12.5 ml/dose<br>**16.4–20.5 kg:** 10 ml/dose<br>**11.8–15.9 kg:** 7.5 ml/dose<br>**7.3–11.4 kg:** 5 ml/dose<br>**4.5–6.8 kg:** 2.5 ml/dose<br>**Give one dose weekly, continuing for 8 weeks after leaving the endemic area** | Concomitant use of **quinacrine** and primaquine may lead to toxicities related to primaquine | Pharmacokinetics: combination product provides rapid elimination of both erythrocytic and exoerythrocytic parasites | arthritis and lupus erythematosus)<br><br>Pregnancy<br>Use only when clearly needed and potential benefit outweighs the potential hazards to the fetus<br><br>Lactation Issues<br>Excreted in breast milk in low concentrations; use with caution in nursing mothers |
| **Hydroxychloroquine Sulfate**<br>Plaquenil<br><br>Tablet:<br>200 mg (equivalent to 155 mg hydroxychloroquine) | **Antimalarial Spectrum**<br>P. falciparum, P. malariae, and P. vivax.<br><br>**Hydroxychloroquine is not effective against chloroquine-resistant strains of Plasmodium falciparum**<br><br>**Treatment of acute malaria**<br>**Adults:** 620 mg on day 1, followed by 310 mg 6 h later, 310 mg on day 2, and 310 mg on day 3<br><br>**Children:** 10 mg/kg on day 1, followed by 5 mg/kg 6 h later, 5 mg/kg on day 2, and 5 mg/kg on day 3 | Administration Issues<br>Complete full course of therapy; take tablets on the same day each week for malaria suppression; do not take on an empty stomach<br><br>Drug–Drug Interactions<br>**Cimetidine** may decrease the elimination of chloroquine. **Kaolin** may decrease the absorption of chloroquine | ADRs:<br>nausea, vomiting, headache, GI upset, visual disturbances (possibly leading to irreversible retinal damage with long term administration)<br><br>Pharmacokinetics:<br>readily absorbed from GI tract; 55% protein bound; long elimination half-life; renal excretion | Contraindications<br>Retinal or visual field changes; hypersensitivity to chloroquine or related compounds; long term use in children<br><br>Pregnancy<br>Use only when clearly needed and potential benefit outweighs the potential hazards to the fetus<br><br>Lactation Issues<br>Excreted in breast milk in low concentrations; use with caution in nursing mothers |

(continues on next page)

| Drug and Dosage Forms | Spectrum of Activity and Usual Dosage Range | Administration Issues and Drug–Drug & Drug–Food Interactions | Common Adverse Drug Reactions (ADRs) and Pharmacokinetics | Contraindications, Pregnancy Category, and Lactation Issues |
|---|---|---|---|---|
| **Hydroxychloroquine Sulfate** *cont.* | Suppression of malaria<br>**Adults:** 310 mg once weekly starting one week prior to travel, continue weekly during travel, and for 4 weeks after leaving such areas<br><br>**Children:** 5 mg/kg (max 300 mg) once weekly starting one week prior to travel, continue weekly during travel, and for 4 weeks after leaving such areas | | | |
| **Mefloquine HCl**<br>Larium<br><br>Tablet: 250 mg | **Antimalarial Spectrum**<br>*P. falciparum* (both chloroquine-sensitive and resistant strains) and *P. vivax*<br><br>**Treatment of mild to moderate malaria in adults**<br>Five tablets (1250 mg) as a single dose<br><br>**Patients with acute *P vivax* malaria treated with mefloquine are at high risk of relapse because mefloquine does not eliminate exoerythrocytic (hepatic phase) parasites. To avoid relapse** | Administration Issues<br>Complete full course of therapy; take tablets on the same day each week for malaria suppression; do not take on an empty stomach; take with a full glass of water<br><br>Drug–Drug Interactions<br>Concomitant use of mefloquine and **beta-adrenergic blockers (propranolol, atenolol), calcium channel antagonist (verapamil, diltiazem), quinidine, and quinine** may lead to abnormal cardiac conduction and arrhythmias. Mefloquine may decrease **valproic acid** serum levels increasing the risk of | ADRs:<br>nausea, vomiting, dizziness, headache, visual disturbances<br><br>Pharmacokinetics:<br>long T$_{1/2}$ approximately 21 days; highly protein bound, >95%; concentrates in blood erythrocytes; primarily cleared by the liver | Contraindications<br>Hypersensitivity to mefloquine and related compounds<br><br>Pregnancy Category: C<br><br>Lactation Issues<br>Excreted in breast milk in low concentrations; use with caution in nursing mothers |

| | | | |
|---|---|---|---|
| | **after treatment with mefloquine, subsequently treat with primaquine**<br><br>**Supression of malaria**<br>**Adults:** 250 mg once weekly starting one week prior to travel, continue weekly during travel, and for 4 weeks after leaving such areas<br><br>**Children:**<br>15–19 kg, ¼ tablet; 20–30 kg, ½ tablet; 31–45 kg, ¾ tablet; > 45 kg, 1 tablet. Take appropriate dose once weekly starting one week prior to travel, continue weekly during travel, and for 4 weeks after leaving such areas | seizures. Concomitant mefloquine and **chloroquine** use may lead to increased risk of convulsions | |
| **Primaquine Phosphate**<br><br>Tablet:<br>26.3 mg (15 mg base) | **Antimalarial Spectrum**<br>*P. vivax, P. ovale* and gametocytial forms of *P. falciparum*<br><br>**Treatment of malaria in combination with chloroquine phosphate**<br>**Adults:** 26.3 mg (15 mg base) qd for 14 days during the last 2 weeks of chloroquine therapy<br><br>**Children:** 0.5 mg/kg/d (0.3 mg base/kg/d max 15 mg base/dose) qd for 14 d during the last 2 weeks of chloroquine therapy | Administration Issues<br>Complete full course of therapy; take with food or after meals to decrease GI upset<br><br>Drug–Drug Interactions<br>Concomitant use of **quinacrine** and primaquine may lead to toxicities related to primaquine | ADRs:<br>nausea, vomiting, GI upset, anemia<br><br>Pharmacokinetics:<br>elimination T$_{1/2}$ is approximately 4 h; low concentration in the tissues; reaches high concentrations in the liver, lungs, brain, and heart; excreted primarily as metabolites in the urine<br><br>Contraindications<br>Concomitant use of quinacrine and primaquine; patients predisposed to granulocytopenia (rheumatoid arthritis and lupus erythematosus); patients with G-6-PD deficiency<br><br>Pregnancy<br>Use only when clearly needed and potential benefit outweighs the potential hazards to the fetus |

*(continues on next page)*

| Drug and Dosage Forms | Spectrum of Activity and Usual Dosage Range | Administration Issues and Drug–Drug & Drug–Food Interactions | Common Adverse Drug Reactions (ADRs) and Pharmacokinetics | Contraindications, Pregnancy Category, and Lactation Issues |
|---|---|---|---|---|
| **Pyrimethamine**<br>Daraprim<br><br>Tablet:<br>25 mg | **Antimalarial Spectrum**<br>Susceptible strains of *Plasmodium* sp.<br><br>**Treatment of malaria in combination with chloroquine or quinacrine**<br>**Adults and children > 10 yr.**<br>50 mg qd for 2 days<br><br>**Children 4 to 10 yr.:** 25 mg qd for 2 days<br><br>**After clinical cure, follow with suppressive regimen for 6 to 10 weeks**<br><br>**Suppression of malaria**<br>**Adults and children > 10 yr.**<br>25 mg once weekly for 6 to 10 weeks<br><br>**Children 4 to 10 yr.::** 12.5 mg once weekly for 6 to 10 weeks<br><br>**Infants and children < 4 yr.**<br>6.25 mg once weekly for 6 to 10 weeks<br><br>**Treatment of Toxoplasmosis**<br>**Adults:** Initially, 50–75 mg qd with 1–4 gm of a sulfapyrimidine; continue for 1 to 3 weeks, depending on | Administration Issues<br>Complete full course of therapy; take with food to avoid GI upset<br><br>Drug–Drug Interactions<br>Concomitant use of pyrimethamine and **methotrexate, sulfonamides, or TMP-SMZ** may increase risk of folate deficiency and bone marrow suppression | ADRs:<br>nausea, vomiting, anemia<br><br>Pharmacokinetics:<br>well absorbed orally, $T_{1/2}$ approximately 4 days; 87% protein bound; hepatically metabolized; some renal excretion | Contraindications<br>Hypersensitivity to pyrimethamine; documented megaloblastic anemia<br><br>Pregnancy Category:  C<br><br>Lactation Issues<br>Excreted in breast milk; safety for use has not been established; decide whether to discontinue nursing or discontinue the drug |

| | | |
|---|---|---|
| response and tolerance; dosage of each drug may then be decreased by ½ and continued for an additional 4 to 5 wk.<br><br>**Children:** 1 mg/kg/d divided bid with a sulfapyrimidine; after 2 to 4 days, decrease dose by ½ and continue for 1 month | | |
| **Quinacrine HCl**<br>Atabrine<br><br>Tablet: 100 mg | **Antimalarial Spectrum**<br>Susceptible organisms of the *Plasmodium* sp., *Giardia lamblia*<br><br>**Treatment of malaria**<br>**Adults and children > 8 yr.**: 200 mg with 1 gm sodium bicarbonate q 6 h for 5 doses, then 100 mg 3 times daily for 6 days; total dosage is 2.8 gm in 7 days<br><br>**Children 4–8 yr.:** 200 mg 3 times daily the first day; then 100 mg q 12 h for 6 days<br><br>**Children 1–4 yr.:** 100 mg 3 times daily the first day; then 100 mg once daily for 6 days<br><br>**Suppression of malaria**<br>**Adults:** 100 mg qd for 1 to 3 months<br><br>**Children:** 50 mg daily for 1 to 3 months<br><br>**Use of quinacrine in the treatment of malaria has become obsolete and has been replaced by other therapies** | <u>Administration Issues</u><br>Complete full course of therapy; take tablets on the same day each week for malaria suppression; do not take on an empty stomach; take with a full glass of water<br><br><u>Drug–Drug Interactions</u><br>Concomitant use of quinacrine and **primaquine** may lead to toxicities related to primaquine | <u>ADRs:</u><br>discoloration of the urine and skin, headache, dizziness, GI upset, diarrhea<br><br><u>Pharmacokinetics:</u><br>T₁/₂ is approximately 5 days; metabolism is unknown; renal excretion | <u>Contraindications</u><br>Concomitant use of primaquine<br><br><u>Pregnancy</u><br>Use only when clearly needed and potential benefit outweighs the potential hazards to the fetus |

*(continues on next page)*

| Drug and Dosage Forms | Spectrum of Activity and Usual Dosage Range | Administration Issues and Drug–Drug & Drug–Food Interactions | Common Adverse Drug Reactions (ADRs) and Pharmacokinetics | Contraindications, Pregnancy Category, and Lactation Issues |
|---|---|---|---|---|
| **Quinacrine HCl** *cont.* | <u>Treatment of giardiasis</u><br>**Adults:** 100 mg tid for 5 to 7 d<br>**Children:** 7 mg/kg/d divided tid after meals for 5 days; maximum daily dose is 300 mg | | | |
| **Quinine Sulfate**<br><br><u>Tablet:</u><br>Legatrin 162.5 mg<br><br>Quinamm, various generics: 260 mg<br><br><u>Capsule:</u> Q-vel 64.8 mg<br><br>Various generics 200 mg, 300 mg, 325 mg | <u>Antimalarial Spectrum</u><br>*P. falciparum, P. malariae, P. ovale,* and *P. vivax*<br><br><u>Chloroquine-resistant malaria</u><br>**Adults:** 650 mg q 8 h for 5 to 7 d<br>**Children:** 25 mg/kg/d divided q 8 h for 5 to 7 days<br><br><u>Chloroquine-sensitive malaria</u><br>**Adults:** 600 mg q 8 h for 5 to 7 d<br>**Children:** 10 mg/kg/d divided q 8 h for 5 to 7 d<br><br><u>Treatment of nocturnal leg cramps</u><br>260–300 mg at bedtime; if needed, may be taken after the evening meal and at bedtime | <u>Administration Issues</u><br>Complete full course of therapy; take with food or after meals to decrease GI upset<br><br><u>Drug–Drug Interactions</u><br>**Aluminum containing antacids** may decrease the absorption of quinine. Quinine may enhance the effect of **warfarin.** Quinine may enhance the effect of **digoxin** leading to toxicity. Concomitant use of quinine and **mefloquine** may lead to abnormal cardiac conduction and arrhythmias. **Acetazolamide** and **sodium bicarbonate** may decrease urinary excretion of quinine leading to quinine accumulation | <u>ADRs:</u><br>nausea, vomiting, GI upset, ringing in the ears (tinnitus), headache, vertigo, visual disturbances<br><br><u>Pharmacokinetics:</u><br>readily absorbed orally; approximately 75% protein bound; hepatic metabolism; renal excretion | <u>Contraindications</u><br>Hypersensitivity to quinine; glucose-6-phosphate dehydrogenase (G-6-PD) deficiency; optic neuritis; tinnitus; pregnancy<br><br><u>Pregnancy Category:</u> X<br><br><u>Lactation Issues</u><br>Excreted in small amounts in breast milk; rule out G-6-PD deficiency in infant prior to quinine use in nursing mother |
| **Sulfadoxine and Pyrimethamine**<br>Fansidar | <u>Antimalarial Spectrum</u><br>Chloroquine-resistant strains of *P. falciparum* | <u>Administration Issues</u><br>Complete full course of therapy; take with food to avoid GI upset | <u>ADRs:</u><br>nausea, vomiting, anemia, photosensitivity | <u>Contraindications</u><br>Hypersensitivity to sulfonamides or pyrimethamine; documented |

| | | | |
|---|---|---|---|
| Tablet: 500 mg sulfadoxine 25 mg pyrimethamine | **Treatment of malaria** **Adults and children > 45 kg** 3 tablets orally as a single dose **Children:** **31–45 kg** - 2 tablets as a single dose **21–30 kg** - 1 and ½ tablet as a single dose **11–20 kg** - 1 tablet as a single dose **5–10 kg** - ½ tablet as a single dose **Continue weekly chloroquine prophylaxis after treatment with sulfadoxine/pyrimethamine** **Suppression of malaria** **Adults:** 1 tablet at least 1–2 days prior to entering endemic area, followed by 1 tablet weekly, continuing for 4–6 weeks after leaving the endemic area **Children 9–14 yr.:** ¾ tablet at least 1–2 days prior to entering endemic area, followed by ¾ tablet weekly, continuing for 4–6 weeks after leaving the endemic area **Children 4–8 yr.:** ½ tablet at least 1–2 days prior to entering endemic area, followed by ½ tablet weekly, continuing for 4–6 weeks after leaving the endemic area **Children < 4 yr.:** ¼ tablet at least 1–2 days prior to entering endemic area, followed by ¼ tablet weekly, continuing for 4–6 weeks after leaving the endemic area | Drug–Drug Interactions Concomitant use of pyrimethamine and **methotrexate, sulfonamides, or TMP-SMZ** may increase risk of folate deficiency and bone marrow suppression. Sulfadoxine/pyrimethamine may decrease the effectiveness of **oral contraceptives** | Pharmacokinetics: $T_{1/2}$ mean for sulfadoxine is 169 h and pyrimethamine is 111 h; renal excretion |
| | | | megaloblastic anemia; infants < 2 yr.; pregnancy at term and nursing Pregnancy Category: C Lactation Issues Both drugs are excreted in breast milk; discontinue use during nursing |

| Drug and Dosage Forms | Spectrum of Activity and Usual Dosage Range | Administration Issues and Drug–Drug & Drug–Food Interactions | Common Adverse Drug Reactions (ADRs) and Pharmacokinetics | Contraindications, Pregnancy Category, and Lactation Issues |
|---|---|---|---|---|
| **Aminosalicylate Sodium**<br>Sodium P.A.S.<br><u>Tablet:</u> 0.5 gm | **Antimycobacterial Spectrum**<br>*Mycobacterium tuberculosis*<br>**Treatment of tuberculosis in combination with other agents**<br>**Adults:** 14–16 gm/day in 2 to 3 divided doses<br>**Children:** 275–420 mg/kg/d in 3 to 4 divided doses daily<br>**For multi-drug resistant tuberculosis, continue combination drug therapy for 9 months or 6 months after sputum cultures are negative, whichever is longer** | <u>Administration Issues</u><br>Complete full course of therapy with strict compliance; may take with food if GI upset occurs; do not use tablets that are brown or purple in color, aminosalicylate will not work if it becomes wet or is left in extreme heat or direct sunlight<br><u>Drug–Drug Interactions</u><br>Aminosalicylate sodium may decrease the GI absorption of **vitamin B$_{12}$** | <u>ADRs:</u><br>nausea, vomiting, GI upset, diarrhea<br><u>Pharmacokinetics:</u><br>T$_{1/2}$ is approximately 1 h; widely distributes into body tissues with low concentrations in cerebrospinal fluid; hepatic metabolism; > 80% excreted by the kidneys | <u>Contraindications</u><br>Hypersensitivity to aminosalicylate sodium and related compounds |
| **Clofazimine**<br>Lamprene<br>50 mg, 100 mg | **Antibacterial Spectrum**<br>*Mycobacterium avium-intracellulare (MAC)*<br>**Treatment of MAC**<br>100 mg qd to tid | <u>Administration Issues</u><br>Complete full course of therapy; take with food; reversible red to brownish black skin discoloration may occur | <u>ADRs:</u><br>pigmentation changes, rash, dryness, abdominal distress, diarrhea, nausea<br><u>Pharmacokinetics:</u><br>highly lipophilic and deposits in fatty tissue; T$_{1/2}$ after repeated dosing is 70 days; | <u>Pregnancy Category:</u> C<br><u>Lactation Issues</u><br>Excreted in breast milk, do not use in nursing mothers unless clearly indicated |
| **Cycloserine**<br>Seromycin Pulvules<br><u>Capsule:</u><br>250 mg | **Antimycobacterial Spectrum**<br>*Mycobacterium tuberculosis*<br>**Treatment of tuberculosis in combination with other agents** | <u>Administration Issues</u><br>Complete full course of therapy with strict compliance; avoid concurrent alcohol use; may cause drowsiness. **Administration of pyridoxine** | <u>ADRs:</u><br>drowsiness, headache, depression, seizures | <u>Contraindications</u><br>Hypersensitivity to cycloserine; epilepsy; depression; severe anxiety or psychosis; severe renal |

*(continues on next page)*

| Drug | Dosage | Administration Issues / Drug–Drug Interactions | Pharmacokinetics / ADRs | Contraindications / Pregnancy |
|---|---|---|---|---|
| | **Adults:** Initially, 250 mg q 12 h for 2 weeks increasing up to 1 gm/day in 1 to 3 divided doses; maintain blood concentrations < 30 mcg/ml<br><br>**Children:** 10–20 mg/kg/d up to max of 1 gm/day in 2 divided doses<br><br>**For multi-drug resistant tuberculosis, continue combination drug therapy for 9 months or 6 months after sputum cultures are negative, whichever is longer** | **(Vit B$_6$) 100–300 mg/day is recommended to avoid neurotoxic side effects.**<br><br><u>Drug–Drug Interactions</u><br>Concurrent **alcohol** use with cycloserine may increase the potential for epileptic episodes. **Isoniazid** may increase cycloserine CNS side effects, such as dizziness. Cycloserine may increase the effect of **phenytoin** leading to toxicity | <u>Pharmacokinetics:</u><br>widely distributes into body fluids with cerebrospinal fluids similar to plasma concentrations; 35% of dose is metabolized hepatically; renal excretion | insufficiency; excessive concurrent alcohol use<br><br><u>Pregnancy Category:</u> C<br><br><u>Lactation Issues</u><br>Because of potential for serious adverse events in infants, decided whether to discontinue nursing or discontinue the drug |
| **Ethambutol**<br>Myambutol<br><br><u>Tablet:</u><br>100 mg, 400 mg | **Antimycobacterial Spectrum**<br>*Mycobacterium tuberculosis*<br><br>**Initial treatment of tuberculosis in combination with other agents**<br>**Adults:** 15–25 mg/kg/d as a single dose (max. 2.5 gm)<br>**Children:** 15–25 mg/kg/d as a single dose (max 2.5 gm)<br><br>**Twice weekly TB regimen**<br>**Adults:** 50 mg/kg, max 2.5 gm/dose<br>**Children:** 50 mg/kg, max 2.5 gm/dose<br><br>**Three times/week TB regimen**<br>**Adults:** 25–30 mg/kg; max 2.5 gm/dose<br>**Children:** 25–30 mg/kg; max 2.5 gm/dose<br><br>**Not recommended for use in children < 13 yr.**<br><br>**Retreatment of tuberculosis in combination with other agents** | <u>Administration Issues</u><br>Complete full course of therapy with strict compliance; take with food if GI upset occurs; notify your physician, nurse, or pharmacist if visual changes occur. Ethambutol not recommended for children whose visual acuity cannot be monitored (<6 yr).<br><br>**Monthly eye exams are recommended with a 25 mg/kg/d dose**<br><br><u>Drug–Drug Interactions</u><br>**Aluminum salts (antacids, sucralfate)** may decrease the absorption of ethambutol | <u>ADRs:</u><br>visual changes, rash, nausea, vomiting, headache, dizziness<br><br><u>Pharmacokinetics:</u><br>absorption unaffected by food; cerebrospinal fluid concentrations are 10%–50% of serum concentrations; approximately 20% of a dose is metabolized in the liver; predominantly excreted renally, some fecal excretion | <u>Contraindications</u><br>Hypersensitivity to ethambutol; known optic neuritis, unless clinical judgment determines that it may be used<br><br><u>Pregnancy</u><br>The effect of ethambutol in combination with other agents on the fetus is unknown; administration to pregnant women has produced no detectable effect upon the fetus; use only when clearly needed and when the potential benefits outweigh potential hazards to the fetus |

| Drug and Dosage Forms | Spectrum of Activity and Usual Dosage Range | Administration Issues and Drug–Drug & Drug–Food Interactions | Common Adverse Drug Reactions (ADRs) and Pharmacokinetics | Contraindications, Pregnancy Category, and Lactation Issues |
|---|---|---|---|---|
| **Ethambutol** *cont.* | **Adults:** 25 mg/kg/d as a single dose, after 60 days, decrease dose to 15 mg/kg/d as a single dose<br><br>**For multi-drug resistant tuberculosis, continue combination drug therapy for 9 months or 6 months after sputum cultures are negative, whichever is longer.** | | | |
| **Ethionamide**<br>Trecator-SC<br><br>Tablet: 250 mg | **Antimycobacterial Spectrum**<br>*Mycobacterium tuberculosis*<br><br>**Treatment of tuberculosis in combination with other agents**<br>**Adults:** 0.5–1 gm/d in 1 to 3 divided doses<br><br>**Children:** 15–20 mg/kg/d up to max of 1 gm<br><br>**For multi-drug resistant tuberculosis, continue combination drug therapy for 9 months or 6 months after sputum cultures are negative, whichever is longer** | Administration Issues<br>Complete full course of therapy with strict compliance; may take with food if GI upset occurs; metallic taste may occur. **Administration of pyridoxine (Vit B₆)** 25–50 mg daily is recommended to avoid ethionamide-associated peripheral neuropathy | ADRs:<br>nausea, vomiting, GI upset, diarrhea, depression, drowsiness, asthenia<br><br>Pharmacokinetics:<br>$T_{1/2}$ is approximately 3 h; widely distributes into body fluids including cerebrospinal fluid; hepatic metabolism; renal excretion | Contraindications<br>Hypersensitivity to ethionamide; severe hepatic disease<br><br>Pregnancy<br>Teratogenic effects have been demonstrated in animals receiving doses in excess of recommended human doses; use only when clearly needed and when the potential benefits outweigh potential hazards to the fetus<br><br>Lactation Issues<br>Excretion in breast milk is unknown; use with caution in nursing mothers |
| **Isoniazid**<br>Laniazid, various generics | **Antimycobacterial Spectrum**<br>*Mycobacterium tuberculosis* | Administration Issues<br>Complete full course of therapy with strict compliance; take on an empty stomach; minimize daily alcohol use | ADRs:<br>peripheral neuropathy, (numbness and tingling of extremities), nausea, vomiting, | Contraindications<br>Patients with previous isoniazid-associated hepatic injury; hypersensitivity to isoniazid |

<table>
<tr><td>

**Tablet:**
50 mg, 100 mg, 300 mg

</td><td>

**Treatment of tuberculosis in combination with other agents**
**Adults:** 5 mg/kg/d as a single dose (max. 300 mg/day)

**Children and infants**
10–20 mg/kg/d as a single dose (max. of 300 mg/day)

**Twice weekly TB regimen**
**Adults:** 15 mg/kg, max 900 mg/dose
**Children:** 20–40 mg/kg; max 900 mg/dose

**Three times/week TB regimen:**
**Adults:** 15 mg/kg; max 900 mg/dose
**Children:** 20–40 mg/kg; max 900 mg/dose

**Prevention of tuberculosis**
**Adults:** 300 mg/day as a single dose

**Children and infants:** 10 mg/kg/d as a single dose up to a max of 300 mg/day

**Continue isoniazid therapy in combination with rifampin for 6 months with pyrazinamide for the first 2 months only. For multi-drug resistant tuberculosis, continue combination drug therapy for 9 months or 6 months after sputum cultures are negative, whichever is longer**

</td><td>

with isoniazid. **Administration of pyridoxine (Vit B$_6$) 25–50 mg daily is recommended to avoid isoniazid-associated peripheral neuropathy**

Drug–Drug Interactions
**Alcohol** increases the risk of isoniazid-induced hepatitis. Isoniazid may increase the effect of the following drugs leading to toxicity:
**carbamazepine, phenytoin, warfarin, benzodiazepines.**
Concomitant use of isoniazid and **ketoconazole** may lead to decreased serum levels of ketoconazole and antifungal treatment failure.
Concomitant use of isoniazid and **cycloserine** may lead to increased cycloserine associated CNS toxicity

</td></tr>
<tr><td></td><td></td><td>

GI upset, severe and sometimes fatal hepatitis

Pharmacokinetics:
decreased oral absorption with food; distributes readily into cerebrospinal fluid; metabolized hepatic by acetylation; renal excretion

</td></tr>
</table>

Pregnancy Category: C

Lactation Issues
Excreted in breast milk; use with caution in nursing mothers

*(continues on next page)*

| Drug and Dosage Forms | Spectrum of Activity and Usual Dosage Range | Administration Issues and Drug–Drug & Drug–Food Interactions | Common Adverse Drug Reactions (ADRs) and Pharmacokinetics | Contraindications, Pregnancy Category, and Lactation Issues |
|---|---|---|---|---|
| **Isoniazid and Rifampin Combination**<br><br>Capsule:<br>Rifamate (150 mg isoniazid/300 mg rifampin)<br><br>Tablets/Capsules<br>Rimactane/INH Dual Pack (300 mg isoniazid tablets and 300 mg rifampin capsules) | **Antimicrobial Spectrum**<br>Isoniazid: *M. tuberculosis*<br><br>Rifampin: *M. tuberculosis, N. meningitidis, H. influenzae, S. aureus, S. epidermidis*<br><br>**Treatment of tuberculosis in combination with other agents**<br>2 Rifamate capsules daily as a single dose or 300 mg isoniazid tablet with two 300 mg rifampin capsules once daily as a single dose<br><br>**Continue combination therapy for 6 months with pyrazinamide for the first 2 months only. For multi-drug resistant tuberculosis, continue combination drug therapy for 9 months or 6 months after sputum cultures are negative, whichever is longer** | Administration Issues<br>Complete full course of therapy with strict compliance; take on an empty stomach; may cause reddish-orange discoloration of the urine, stool, sweat, and tears; may permanently discolor contact lenses; minimize daily alcohol use with isoniazid<br><br>Drug–Drug Interactions<br>see isoniazid and rifampin | ADRs:<br>see adverse events for isoniazid and rifampin<br><br>Pharmacokinetics:<br>distributes readily into cerebrospinal fluid; extensive hepatic metabolism; renal excretion | Contraindications<br>Patients with previous isoniazid-associated hepatic injury; hypersensitivity to isoniazid; hypersensitivity to rifampin<br><br>Pregnancy Category: C<br><br>Lactation Issues<br>Excreted in breast milk; decide whether to discontinue nursing or discontinue the drug |
| **Pyrazinamide**<br><br>Tablet:<br>500 mg | **Antimycobacterial Spectrum**<br>*M. tuberculosis*<br><br>**Treatment of tuberculosis in combination with other agents**<br>**Adults:** 15–30 mg/kg once daily, (max. 2 gm/day) | Administration Issues<br>Complete full course of therapy with strict compliance | ADRs:<br>fever, gout attack, nausea, vomiting, arthralgia<br><br>Pharmacokinetics:<br>$T_{1/2}$ is approximately 10 h; widely distributes into body | Contraindications<br>Severe hepatic damage; hypersensitivity to pyrazinamide; acute gout<br><br>Pregnancy Category: C |

| Drug | Administration / Spectrum | ADRs / Pharmacokinetics / Administration Issues | Contraindications / Lactation / Pregnancy |
|---|---|---|---|
| | **Children:** 15–30 mg/kg once daily (max. 2 gm/day)<br><br>**Twice weekly TB regimen**<br>**Adults:** 50–70 mg/kg; max 4 gm/d<br>**Children:** 50–70 mg/kg; max 4 gm/d<br><br>**Three times/week TB regimen:**<br>**Adults:** 50–70 mg/kg; max 3 gm/d<br>**Children:** 50–70 mg/kg; max 3 gm/d<br><br>**Continue isoniazid/rifampin combination therapy for 6 months with pyrazinamide for the first 2 months only** | tissues including cerebrospinal fluid | <u>Lactation Issues</u><br>Excreted in breast milk; use with caution in nursing mothers |
| **Rifabutin**<br>Mycobutin<br><br><u>Capsule:</u><br>150 mg | **Antimycobacterial Spectrum**<br>*M. avium, M. intracellulare, and M. tuberculosis*<br><br><u>**Prevention of disseminated Mycobacterium avium complex disease in HIV affected patients**</u><br>300 mg once daily or 150 mg bid with food if GI upset occurs | <u>ADRs:</u><br>rash, GI upset, anemia, leukopenia, neutropenia<br><br><u>Pharmacokinetics:</u><br>$T_{1/2}$ approximately 45 h; distributes readily into body tissues; hepatic metabolism; fecal and renal excretion; pharmacokinetic parameters may be variable in symptomatic HIV patients compared to healthy volunteers<br><br><u>Administration Issues</u><br>Complete full course of therapy; administer with food if GI upset occurs; may cause reddish-orange discoloration of the urine, stool, sweat, and tears; may permanently discolor contact lenses<br><br><u>Drug–Drug Interactions</u><br>Rifabutin has less hepatic enzyme inducing capabilities compared to rifampin. The significance of potential drug interactions similar to rifampin is unknown. Rifabutin may decrease the serum level of **zidovudine.** Rifabutin may decrease the effectiveness of **oral contraceptives** | <u>Contraindications</u><br>Hypersensitivity to rifabutin or rifampin<br><br><u>Pregnancy Category:</u> B<br><br><u>Lactation Issues</u><br>Excretion in breast milk is unknown; because of potential for serious adverse events in infants, decide whether to discontinue nursing or discontinue the drug |
| **Rifampin**<br><br><u>Capsule:</u><br>Rifadin 150 mg, 300 mg | **Antimicrobial Spectrum**<br>*M. tuberculosis, N. meningitidis, H. influenzae, S. aureus, S. epidermidis* | <u>ADRs:</u><br>flu-like symptoms (fever, chills, malaise), nausea, vomiting, GI upset, rash<br><br><u>Administration Issues</u><br>Complete full course of therapy with strict compliance; take on an empty stomach; may cause reddish-orange | <u>Contraindications</u><br>Hypersensitivity to rifampin<br><br><u>Pregnancy Category:</u> C |

*(continues on next page)*

# 105. Antituberculosis Agents *continued from previous page*

| Drug and Dosage Forms | Spectrum of Activity and Usual Dosage Range | Administration Issues and Drug–Drug & Drug–Food Interactions | Common Adverse Drug Reactions (ADRs) and Pharmacokinetics | Contraindications, Pregnancy Category, and Lactation Issues |
|---|---|---|---|---|
| **Rifampin** *cont.*<br><br>Rimactane 300 mg | **Treatment of tuberculosis in combination with other agents**<br>**Adults:** 10 mg/kg/d as a single dose (max. 600 mg/day)<br>**Children/infants:** 10–20 mg/kg/d as a single dose (max. 600 mg/day)<br><br>**Twice weekly TB regimen**<br>**Adults:** 10 mg/kg, max 600 mg/d<br>**Children:** 10–20 mg/kg; max 600 mg/d<br><br>**Three times/week TB regimen**<br>**Adults:** 10 mg/kg; max 600 mg/d<br>**Children:** 10–20 mg/kg; max 600 mg/d<br><br>**Continue rifampin therapy in combination with isoniazid for 6 months with pyrazinamide for the first 2 months only**<br><br>**For multi-drug resistant tuberculosis, continue combination drug therapy for 9 months or 6 months after sputum cultures are negative, whichever is longer**<br><br>**Contact with invasive Haemophilus influenzae**<br>**Adults:** 600 mg qd as a single dose for 4 consecutive days | discoloration of the urine, stool, sweat, and tears; may permanently discolor contact lenses<br><br>Drug–Drug Interactions<br>Rifampin is a potent inducer of hepatic metabolism and may decrease the effectiveness of the following drugs: **benzodiazepines, beta-blockers, oral contraceptives, corticosteroids, cyclosporine, phenytoin, carbamazepine, quinidine, sulfonylureas, theophylline, digoxin, ketoconazole, warfarin**<br><br>An extemporaneous oral suspension may be prepared by:<br>1. emptying the contents of 4 rifampin 300 mg capsules into a 4 oz. amber bottle,<br>2. adding 20 ml of simple syrup,<br>3. shake vigorously,<br>4. add 100 ml simple syrup, shake again<br>The suspension is stable for 4 weeks at room temperature or in the refrigerator | Pharmacokinetics:<br>food decreases oral absorption; distributes readily into cerebrospinal fluid; metabolized hepatically by deacetylation; renal excretion | Lactation Issues<br>Excreted in breast milk; decide whether to discontinue nursing or discontinue the drug |

| | | | |
|---|---|---|---|
| | **Children:** 10–20 mg/kg/d as a single dose to a max of 600 mg/day for 4 consecutive days<br><br>**Close contact - meningococcal exposure**<br>**Adults:** 600 mg q 12 h for 4 doses<br>**Children:** 10 mg/kg q 12 h for 4 doses<br><br>**Eradicate nasal carriage of _S. aureus_:** 600 mg once daily with dicloxacillin 500 mg four times daily or SMZ-TMP DS one tablet twice daily for 10 days | | |
| **Streptomycin**<br><br>Injection: 400 mg/mL | **Antimicrobial Spectrum**<br>_M. tuberculosis, N. meningitidis, H. influenzae, S. aureus, S. epidermidis_<br><br>**Treatment of tuberculosis in combination with other agents**<br>**Adults:** 1 g IM streptomycin combined with appropriate additional antitubercular drugs<br><br>**Children:** 20–40 mg/kg/d (max. 1 g)<br><br>**Twice weekly TB regimen**<br>**Adults:** 25–30 mg/kg, max 1.5 gm IM<br>**Children:** 25–30 mg/kg; max 1.5 gm IM<br><br>**Three times/week TB regimen**<br>**Adults:** 25–30 mg/kg, max 1 gm IM<br>**Children:** 25–30 mg/kg; max 1 gm IM | Administration Issues<br>Complete full course of therapy with strict compliance. Elderly patients should have a smaller daily dose of streptomycin. Drug is usually administered as a single daily IM dose. Patient should report any unusual symptoms of hearing loss, dizziness, roaring noises or fullness in ear.<br><br>Drug Interactions<br>**Streptomycin** may increase or prolong the effects of depolarizing and nondepolarizing neuromuscular blocking agents. Increased nephrotoxicity may occur with concurrent use of **amphotericin and loop diuretics** | ADRs:<br>ototoxicity (auditory and vestibular), nephrotoxicity, nausea, vomiting, headache, tremor, weakness<br><br>Pharmacokinetics:<br>almost completely excreted as unchanged drug in urine; no metabolism<br><br>Contraindications<br>Hypersensitivity to aminoglycosides<br><br>Use with Caution: in patients with pre-existing vertigo, hearing loss, neuromuscular disorders<br><br>Pregnancy Category: There are reports of total irreversible bilateral congenital deafness in children whose mother received streptomycin during pregnancy.<br><br>Lactation Issues<br>Excreted in breast milk; decide whether to discontinue nursing or discontinue the drug |

# 106. Antiviral Agents

106.1 Agents for Herpes simplex and Zoster

| Drug and Dosage Forms | Spectrum of Activity and Usual Dosage Range | Administration Issues and Drug–Drug & Drug–Food Interactions | Common Adverse Drug Reactions (ADRs) and Pharmacokinetics | Contraindications, Pregnancy Category, and Lactation Issues |
|---|---|---|---|---|
| **Acyclovir**<br>Zovirax<br><br>Tablet:<br>400 mg, 800 mg<br><br>Capsule:<br>200 mg<br><br>Suspension:<br>200 mg/5 ml | **Antiviral Spectrum**<br>Herpes simplex virus type 1 (HSV-1), herpes simplex virus type 2 (HSV-2), varicella-zoster virus (VZV), Epstein-Barr virus, and cytomegalovirus (CMV)<br><br>**Treatment of initial genital herpes episode:** 200 mg q 4 h while awake for 5 doses/day for 10 days **or** 400 mg tid for 10 d<br><br>**Chronic suppressive therapy for recurrent genital herpes:** 400 mg bid for up to 12 months followed by reevaluation; alternative regimens include 200 mg 3 to 5 times daily<br><br>**Intermittent therapy for genital herpes**<br>200 mg q 4 h while awake for 5 doses/d for 5 d **or** 400 mg tid for 5 d **or** 800 mg bid for 5 d; initiate therapy at the earliest sign or symptom of recurrence<br><br>**Treatment of acute herpes zoster attack:** 800 mg q 4 h for 5 doses/d for 7 to 10 d | Administration Issues<br>Complete full course of therapy; acyclovir is not a cure for HSV; may take without regard to meals; avoid sexual intercourse when visible herpes lesions are present<br><br>Drug–Drug Interactions<br>Concurrent acyclovir and **zidovudine** use may increase the potential for severe drowsiness and lethargy. The clearance of acyclovir may be decreased and half-life increased by **probenecid.** | ADRs:<br>nausea, vomiting<br><br>Pharmacokinetics:<br>low oral bioavailability which decreases with increasing doses; absorption unaffected by food; widely distributes into body fluids and tissues including cerebrospinal fluid; primarily eliminated as unchanged drug by the kidneys | Contraindications<br>Hypersensitivity to acyclovir<br><br>Pregnancy Category: C<br><br>Lactation Issues<br>Excreted in breast milk, use with caution in nursing mothers |

| | | | | |
|---|---|---|---|---|
| | **Treatment of chickenpox** 20 mg/kg (not to exceed 800 mg) qid for 5 days<br><br>**Dosage reduction is recommended for patients with renal insufficiency** | | | **Contraindications** Hypersensitivity to famciclovir<br><br>**Pregnancy Category:** B<br><br>**Lactation Issues** Excreted in breast milk of lactating rats in concentrations higher than serum famciclovir concentrations; excretion in human breast milk is unknown; because of potential for tumorigenicity in rats, one must decide whether to discontinue the drug or discontinue nursing, taking into account the drug's importance to the mother |
| **Famciclovir** Famvir<br><br>Tablet: 125 mg, 250 mg, 500 mg | **Antiviral Spectrum** Herpes simplex virus type 1 (HSV-1), herpes simplex virus type 2 (HSV-2), varicella–zoster virus (VZV)<br><br>**Treatment of acute herpes zoster (shingles)** 500 mg q 8 h for 7 days; begin treatment promptly as soon as herpes zoster is diagnosed; most effective when therapy is started within 48 h of the onset of zoster rash<br><br>**Treatment of initial genital herpes episode:** 250 mg tid for 7–10 d<br><br>**Chronic suppressive therapy for recurrent genital herpes** 250 mg bid for up to 12 months followed by reevaluation<br><br>**Genital Herpes (recurrent episodes):** 125 mg bid for 5 days. Initiate therapy at first signs/symptoms<br><br>**Dosage reduction is recommended for patients with renal insufficiency** | Administration Issues Complete full course of therapy; may take without regard to meals. Patients should begin therapy as soon as herpes zoster is diagnosed.<br><br>Drug–Drug Interactions **Probenecid** may decrease the renal excretion of famciclovir. **Digoxin** plasma levels may be increased by famciclovir | ADRs: headache, nausea, fatigue<br><br>Pharmacokinetics: transformed to active compound penciclovir; $T_{1/2}$ is approximately 2 h; metabolism is extrahepatic; 70%–90% renal excreted | |

| Drug and Dosage Forms | Spectrum of Activity and Usual Dosage Range | Administration Issues and Drug–Drug & Drug–Food Interactions | Common Adverse Drug Reactions (ADRs) and Pharmacokinetics | Contraindications, Pregnancy Category, and Lactation Issues |
|---|---|---|---|---|
| **Valacyclovir**<br>Valtrex<br><u>Tablet:</u> 500 mg | **Antiviral Spectrum**<br>Herpes simplex virus type 1 (HSV-1), herpes simplex virus type 2 (HSV-2), varicella–zoster virus (VZV)<br><br>**Treatment of acute herpes zoster (shingles)**<br>1 gm q 8 h for 7 days; begin treatment promptly as soon as herpes zoster is diagnosed; most effective when therapy is started within 48 h of the onset of zoster rash<br><br>**Treatment of initial genital herpes episode:** 1 gm bid for 7–10 d<br><br>**Chronic suppressive therapy for recurrent genital herpes:** 250 mg bid for up to 12 months followed by reevaluation; alternative regimens include 500 mg qd **or** 1 gm qd<br><br>**Recurrent genital herpes**<br>500 mg bid for 5 days; initiate therapy at the first signs/symptoms of herpes.<br><br>**Dosage reduction is recommended for patients with renal insufficiency** | <u>Administration Issues</u><br>Complete full course of therapy; may take without regard to meals<br><br><u>Drug–Drug Interactions</u><br>**Probenecid and cimetidine** may decrease the renal excretion of valacyclovir | <u>ADRs:</u><br>nausea<br><br><u>Pharmacokinetics:</u><br>transformed to active compound acyclovir; $T_{1/2}$ is approximately 2 to 3 h; limited hepatic metabolism; primarily excreted renally with some fecal excretion | <u>Contraindications</u><br>Hypersensitivity to valacyclovir or acyclovir<br><br><u>Pregnancy Category:</u> B<br><br><u>Lactation Issues</u><br>Excretion of valacyclovir in human breast milk is unknown; use with caution in nursing mothers; consider temporary discontinuation of breast feeding |

## 106.2 Nucleoside Reverse Transcriptase Inhibitors

| Drug and Dosage Forms | Spectrum of Activity and Usual Dosage Range | Administration Issues and Drug–Drug & Drug–Food Interactions | Common Adverse Drug Reactions (ADRs) and Pharmacokinetics | Contraindications, Pregnancy Category, and Lactation Issues |
|---|---|---|---|---|
| **Didanosine (ddI)**<br>Videx<br><br>Tablet, buffered, chewable:<br>25 mg, 50 mg, 100 mg,<br>150 mg<br><br>Powder for Oral solution,<br>buffered<br>100 mg, 167 mg, 250 mg,<br>375 mg<br><br>Powder for Oral solution,<br>Pediatric<br>must be mixed with an<br>antacid before dispensing;<br>final concentration =<br>10 mg/ml | **Treatment of advanced HIV infection**<br><br>Chewable Tablets:<br>**Adults/Adolescents ≥ 60 kg**<br>200 mg bid<br><br>**Adults/Adolescents < 60 kg**<br>125 mg bid<br><br>**Children:**<br>**1.1–1.4 m²** – 100 mg bid<br>**0.8–1 m²** – 75 mg bid<br>**0.5–0.7 m²** – 50 mg bid<br>**< 0.4 m²** – 25 mg bid<br><br>**Take 2 tablets at each dose to ensure adequate gastric pH buffering; children < 1 year may use 1 tablet at each dose**<br><br>Powder:<br>**Adults/Adolescents ≥ 60 kg**<br>250 mg bid<br><br>**Adults/Adolescents < 60 kg**<br>167 mg bid<br><br>**Children**<br>**1.1–1.4 m²** – 125 mg bid<br>**0.8–1 m²** – 94 mg bid<br>**0.5–0.7 m²** – 62 mg bid<br>**< 0.4 m²** – 31 mg bid | <u>Administration Issues</u><br>take on an empty stomach; do not share medication; do not exceed recommended dose; take 2 tablets at each dose; chew tablets thoroughly; tablets may be manually crushed prior to administration or dispersed in at least 1 ounce of water; after mixing oral solution, drink entire liquid immediately; shake pediatric solution well prior to administration; pediatric solution is stable for 30 days in the refrigerator<br><br><u>Drug–Drug Interactions</u><br>Didanosine may decrease GI absorption of **itraconazole, ketoconazole, dapsone, fluoroquinolones,** and **tetracyclines**; separate dosing by at least 2 h. Separate the dosing of ddI and **delavirdine** and **protease inhibitors** by at least 2 h.<br>Concomitant use of ddI with the following drugs may increase the risk of peripheral neuropathy: **dapsone, zalcitabine, ethionamide, hydralazine, isoniazid, metronidazole, nitrofurantoin, phenytoin.** | <u>ADRs:</u><br>peripheral neuropathy, pancreatitis, diarrhea, nausea<br><br><u>Pharmacokinetics:</u><br>rapidly degraded at acidic pH, all oral formulations contain buffering agents to increase gastric pH; food decreases oral absorption; renal elimination by filtration and secretion | <u>Contraindications</u><br>Hypersensitivity to didanosine or other components of the product<br><br><u>Pregnancy Category:</u> B<br><br><u>Lactation Issues</u><br>Excretion in breast milk is unknown; HIV infected females should not breast feed to avoid postnatal transmission of HIV to a child who may not be infected |

(continues on next page)

## 106.2 Nucleoside Reverse Transcriptase Inhibitors *continued from previous page*

| Drug and Dosage Forms | Spectrum of Activity and Usual Dosage Range | Administration Issues and Drug–Drug & Drug–Food Interactions | Common Adverse Drug Reactions (ADRs) and Pharmacokinetics | Contraindications, Pregnancy Category, and Lactation Issues |
|---|---|---|---|---|
| **Didanosine (ddl)** *cont.* | | Drug–Food Interactions: Administration with food decreases ddl absorption by as much as 50%; take ddl on an empty stomach (1 h before or 2 h after meal) | | |
| **Lamivudine (3TC)** Epivir<br><br>Tablet: 150 mg<br><br>Solution: 10 mg/ml<br><br>Combination tablet: Combivir: 150 mg lamivudine plus 300 mg zidovudine | **Treatment of HIV infection in combination with zidovudine** **Adults/children > 12 yr.** 150 mg bid with zidovudine<br><br>For adults with low body weight (<50 kg), use 2 mg/kg bid with zidovudine<br><br>**Children 3 months to 12 yr.** 4 mg/kg bid with zidovudine<br><br>**Combivir:** 1 tablet bid | Administration Issues may take without regard to meals; do not share medication; do not exceed recommended dose; oral solution may be stored in the refrigerator or at room temperature<br><br>Pharmacokinetics: **TMP/SMX** may increase lamivudine blood levels. Lamivudine may increase **zidovudine** blood levels. | ADRs: headache, pancreatitis (higher incidence in children), rash, abdominal pain, increased LFTs<br><br>Pharmacokinetics: rapid GI absorption; limited metabolism; primarily excreted renally as unchanged drug<br><br>**Dosage reduction is recommended for patients with renal insufficiency** | Contraindications Hypersensitivity to lamivudine<br><br>Pregnancy Category: C<br><br>Lactation Issues Excretion in breast milk is unknown; HIV infected females should not breast feed to avoid postnatal transmission of HIV to a child who may not be infected |
| **Stavudine (d4T)** Zerit<br><br>Capsule: 15 mg, 20 mg, 30 mg, 40 mg<br><br>Solution: 1 mg/ml | **Treatment of advanced HIV infection** **Adults/Adolescents ≥ 60 kg** 40 mg bid<br><br>**Adults/Adolescents < 60 kg** 30 mg bid<br><br>**Pediatric Dose:** 1 mg/kg bid (up to 30 kg) | Administration Issues may take without regard to meals<br><br>**Temporarily discontinue stavudine therapy if peripheral neuropathy (tingling, numbness, pain of hands or feet) develops; if symptoms resolve completely, resume therapy at one-half the** | ADRs: peripheral neuropathy (dose related), headache, diarrhea, skin rash<br><br>**Dosage reduction is recommended for patients with renal insufficiency** | Contraindications Hypersensitivity to stavudine<br><br>Pregnancy Category: C<br><br>Lactation Issues Excretion in human breast milk is unknown; HIV infected females should not breast |

| | | | | |
|---|---|---|---|---|
| **Zalcitabine (ddC)**<br>Hivid<br><br><u>Tablet:</u><br>0.375 mg, 0.75 mg<br><br><u>Syrup:</u><br>0.1 mg/ml (investigational) | **Treatment of advanced HIV infection**<br>0.75 mg tid<br><br>**Treatment of HIV infection in combination with zidovudine**<br>0.75 mg tid<br><br><u>Pediatric Usual Dose</u><br>0.01 mg/kg q 8h (dosage range 0.005 to 0.01 mg/kg q 8h)<br><br>**Temporarily discontinue zalcitabine therapy if peripheral neuropathy (tingling, numbness, pain of hands or feet) develops; if symptoms resolve completely, resume therapy at one-half the treatment dose based on patient kg weight** | **treatment dose based on patient kg weight**<br><br><u>Administration Issues</u><br>take on an empty stomach; do not share medication; do not exceed recommended dose<br><br><u>Drug–Drug Interactions</u><br>Concomitant administration of **aluminum/magnesium containing antacids** and **sucralfate** may decrease oral absorption of zalcitabine. Concomitant use of zalcitabine with the following drugs may increase the risk of peripheral neuropathy: **dapsone, didanosine, ethionamide, hydralazine, isoniazid, metronidazole, nitrofurantoin, phenytoin.** Clearance of zalcitabine may be decreased by: **probenecid, cimetidine, amphotericin, foscarnet and aminoglycosides.** Concomitant zalcitabine and **pentamidine** use may increase the risk of pancreatitis. | <u>Pharmacokinetics:</u><br>rapid absorption; T$_{1/2}$ is approximately 1 to 1.5 h<br><br><u>ADRs:</u><br>peripheral neuropathy, fatigue, rash, stomatitis<br><br>**Dosage reduction is recommended for patients with renal insufficiency**<br><br><u>Pharmacokinetics:</u><br>good GI tract absorption; food decreases oral absorption; no significant hepatic metabolism | feed to avoid postnatal transmission of HIV to a child who may not be infected<br><br><u>Contraindications</u><br>Hypersensitivity to zalcitabine<br><br><u>Pregnancy Category:</u> C<br><br><u>Lactation Issues</u><br>Excretion in breast milk is unknown; HIV infected females should not breast feed to avoid postnatal transmission of HIV to a child who may not be infected |
| **Zidovudine (AZT, ZDV)**<br>Retrovir<br><br><u>Capsule:</u> 100 mg<br><br><u>Tablet:</u> 300 mg | **Treatment of symptomatic HIV infection**<br>**Adults/Adolescents**<br>200 mg tid or 300 mg bid<br><br>**Children 3 months–12 yr.**<br>180 mg/m$^2$ q 6 h, not to exceed 200 mg q 6 h | <u>Administration Issues</u><br>may take without regard to meals; do not share medication; do not exceed recommended dose<br><br><u>Drug–Drug Interactions</u><br>The following drugs may decrease zidovudine serum levels: **APAP,** | <u>ADRs:</u><br>anemia, granulocytopenia, nausea, headache, fatigue confusion<br><br>**Monitor hematologic indices (WBC, hemoglobin) q 2 weeks,** | <u>Contraindications</u><br>Hypersensitivity to zidovudine<br><br><u>Pregnancy Category:</u> C<br><br><u>Lactation Issues</u><br>Excretion in breast milk is unknown; HIV infected |

*(continues on next page)*

1007

## 106.2 Nucleoside Reverse Transcriptase Inhibitors *continued from previous page*

| Drug and Dosage Forms | Spectrum of Activity and Usual Dosage Range | Administration Issues and Drug–Drug & Drug–Food Interactions | Common Adverse Drug Reactions (ADRs) and Pharmacokinetics | Contraindications, Pregnancy Category, and Lactation Issues |
|---|---|---|---|---|
| **Zidovudine (AZT, ZDV)** *cont.*<br><br>Syrup: 50 mg/5 ml<br><br>Combination tablet:<br>Combivir: 150 mg lamivudine plus 300 mg zidovudine (see lamivudine for dosing) | **Treatment of asymptomatic HIV infection**<br>**Adults**<br>100 mg q 4 h while awake for 5 doses/day<br><br>**Infants born to mothers with HIV infection**<br>2 mg/kg orally q 6 h starting within 12 h of birth and continuing through 6 weeks of age<br><br>**Maternal-fetal HIV transmission ≥ 14 weeks of pregnancy**<br>100 mg q 4 h for 5 doses/day until the start of labor, during labor and delivery, administer IV zidovudine at 2 mg/kg over 1 hour followed by a continuous IV infusion of 1 mg/kg/hr until clamping of the umbilical cord | **clarithromycin, rifampin.** The following drugs may increase zidovudine serum levels: **fluconazole, interferon beta-1b, probenecid, trimethoprim, phenytoin.** Concurrent use of zidovudine and **TMP-SMZ, ganciclovir, flucytosine,** and **interferon alfa** may increase the risk of hematological toxicities such as anemia. **Ribavirin** may inhibit the activation of zidovudine. Concurrent zidovudine and **acyclovir** or **valacyclovir** use may increase the potential for severe drowsiness and lethargy | **discontinue therapy for severe anemia**<br>**hemoglobin < 7.5 gm/dl or granulocytopenia WBC < 750/mm³ or reduction of > 50% from baseline**<br><br><u>Pharmacokinetics:</u><br>rapid absorption in GI tract; hepatic metabolism; renal excretion | females should not breast feed to avoid postnatal transmission of HIV to a child who may not be infected |

1008

| Drug and Dosage Forms | Spectrum of Activity and Usual Dosage Range | Administration Issues and Drug–Drug & Drug–Food Interactions | Common Adverse Drug Reactions (ADRs) and Pharmacokinetics | Contraindications, Pregnancy Category, and Lactation Issues |
|---|---|---|---|---|
| **Delavirdine (DLV)** Rescriptor Tablets: 100 mg | **Treatment of HIV infection in combination with appropriate antiviral therapy** **Adults/Adolescents:** 400 mg tid | Administration Issues may take with food; take 1 h before or 1 hr after ddI or antacids; tablets can be dissolved in water and the resulting dispersion taken promptly; patients with achlorhydria should take delavirdine with an acidic beverage. Drug–Drug Interactions Coadministration of delavirdine with the following agents may result in potentially serious or life-threatening adverse events due to delavirdine being an inhibitor of CYP3A and CYP2C9 hepatic metabolism: **terfenadine, astemizole, clarithromycin, dapsone, rifabutin, benzodiazepines, cisapride, calcium channel blockers, ergot derivatives, protease inhibitors, quinidine, warfarin.** Delavirdine concentrations may be increased by the following drugs: fluoxetine, ketoconazole, The following drugs may decrease delavirdine concentrations: **antacids, anticonvulsants, rifampin, rifabutin, ddI.** | ADRs: headache, fatigue, GI complaints, rash (may be severe) Pharmacokinetics: rapidly absorbed | Contraindications Hypersensitivity to delavirdine or other components of the product Pregnancy Category: C Lactation Issues: HIV infected females should not breast feed to avoid postnatal transmission of HIV to a child who may not be infected |

**106.3** Non-nucleoside Reverse Transcriptase Inhibitors

(continues on next page)

## 106.3 Non-nucleoside Reverse Transcriptase Inhibitors *continued from previous page*

| Drug and Dosage Forms | Spectrum of Activity and Usual Dosage Range | Administration Issues and Drug–Drug & Drug–Food Interactions | Common Adverse Drug Reactions (ADRs) and Pharmacokinetics | Contraindications, Pregnancy Category, and Lactation Issues |
|---|---|---|---|---|
| **Nevirapine (NPV)**<br>Viramune<br><br>Tablets: 200 mg<br><br>Suspension: 10 mg/ml | **Treatment of HIV infection in combination with appropriate antiviral therapy**<br><br>**Adults/Adolescents**<br>Initial therapy: 200 mg qd for 14 days. If no rash or untoward effects increase to maintenance therapy<br><br>Maintenance: 200 mg bid in combination with nucleoside analog antiretroviral agents<br><br>**Pediatric Dose**<br>Initial therapy: 120 mg/m² qd for 14 days. If no rash or untoward effects increase to maintenance dose<br><br>Maintenance: 120 to 200 mg/m² bid | Administration Issues<br>may be administered with food; may be given concurrently with ddI<br><br>Drug Interactions:<br>Nevirapine concentrations may be decreased by **rifampin** and **rifabutin.** Nevirapine may decrease the concentrations of **protease inhibitors** and **oral contraceptives** | ADRs:<br>skin rash (may be severe), sedative effects, headache, diarrhea, nausea<br><br>Pharmacokinetics:<br>well absorbed; extensively metabolized by the cytochrome P-450 system; half-life decreases over a 2–4 week period with chronic dosing due to autoinduction (i.e. T$_{1/2}$ initially 45 h and decreases to 23 h). | Contraindications<br>Hypersensitivity to nevirapine<br><br>Pregnancy Category: C<br><br>Lactation Issues:<br>HIV infected females should not breast feed to avoid postnatal transmission of HIV to a child who may not be infected |

## 106.4 Protease Inhibitors

| Drug and Dosage Forms | Spectrum of Activity and Usual Dosage Range | Administration Issues and Drug–Drug & Drug–Food Interactions | Common Adverse Drug Reactions (ADRs) and Pharmacokinetics | Contraindications, Pregnancy Category, and Lactation Issues |
|---|---|---|---|---|
| **Indinavir**<br>Crixivan<br><u>Capsule:</u><br>200 mg, 400 mg | **Treatment of HIV infection in combination with a nucleoside agent (zidovudine, didanosine) or as monotherapy**<br><br>**Adults/Adolescents**<br>800 mg q 8 h<br><br><u>Cirrhosis</u><br>Reduce dose to 600 mg q 8 h in patients with mild-moderate hepatic insufficiency | <u>Administration Issues</u><br>do not take with food, take with water 1 hour before or 2 h after a meal, or can take with a light meal; do not share medication; do not exceed recommended dose; store capsules in the original container and keep desiccant in the bottle; adequate hydration required to minimize risk of nephrolithiasis; if co-administered with ddI give at least 2 h apart on an empty stomach<br><br><u>Drug–Drug Interactions</u><br>Indinavir may decrease the hepatic metabolism of the following drugs leading to toxicity: **astemizole, terfenadine, cisapride, triazolam, midazolam, clarithromycin, isoniazid, corticosteroids, rifabutin, zidovudine, stavudine.** The following drugs may decrease serum levels of indinavir: **ddI, fluconazole, itraconazole, rifampin, rifabutin.** The following drugs may increase serum levels of indinavir: **ketoconazole, clarithromycin, quinidine, zidovudine** | <u>ADRs:</u><br>abdominal discomfort, nausea, diarrhea, headache, asymptomatic hyperbilirubinemia (10%), nephrolithiasis (4%)<br><br><u>Pharmacokinetics:</u><br>food, especially high fat and protein, decreases oral absorption; extensively metabolized by the cytochrome P-450 system | <u>Contraindications</u><br>Hypersensitivity to indinavir<br><br><u>Pregnancy Category:</u> C<br><br><u>Lactation Issues</u><br>Excretion in breast milk is unknown; HIV infected females should not breast feed to avoid postnatal transmission of HIV to a child who may not be infected |

*(continues on next page)*

| Drug and Dosage Forms | Spectrum of Activity and Usual Dosage Range | Administration Issues and Drug–Drug & Drug–Food Interactions | Common Adverse Drug Reactions (ADRs) and Pharmacokinetics | Contraindications, Pregnancy Category, and Lactation Issues |
|---|---|---|---|---|
| **Nelfinavir** Viracept  Tablets: 250 mg  Powder for oral suspension: 50 mg/level scoop (200 mg/level tsp) | **Adults/Adolescents** 750 mg tid  **Pediatric Dose** 20 to 30 mg/kg/dose tid | Administration Issues: Give with meal or light snack. For oral solution: powder may be mixed with water, milk, pudding, ice cream or formula (for up to 6 h), do not mix with any acidic food or juice because of resulting poor taste. Do not add water to bottles of oral powder—use special scoop provided for measuring purposes. Tablets readily dissolve in water and produce a dispersion that can be mixed with milk, chocolate milk. Tablets can also be crushed and administered with pudding.  Drug–Drug Interactions: Nelfinavir concentrations may be decreased by **anticonvulsants, rifabutin, rifampin.** The following drugs may increase concentrations of nelfinavir: **Indinavir** and **ritonavir.** Nelfinavir may increase the concentrations of **rifabutin** (significantly), **terfenadine, astemizole.** Nelfinavir may decrease the concentrations of oral contraceptives, zidovudine and lamivudine. | ADRs: diarrhea, rash, abdominal pain, asthenia  Pharmacokinetics: extensively metabolized by the cytochrome P-450 system | Contraindications Hypersensitivity to nelfinavir  Pregnancy Category: B  Lactation Issues HIV infected females should not breast feed to avoid postnatal transmission of HIV to a child who may not be infected |

| **Ritonavir**<br>Norvir<br><br>Capsule:<br>100 mg<br><br>Solution:<br>80 mg/ml | **Treatment of HIV infection in combination with a nucleoside agent (zidovudine, didanosine) or as monotherapy**<br><br>**Adults/Adolescents**<br>600 mg bid with food; therapy may be initiated slowly beginning with 300 mg twice daily to avoid GI upset<br><br>**Pediatric Dose**<br>400 mg/m² bid; to minimize GI effects start therapy at 250 mg/m² bid and increase stepwise to full dose over 5 days as tolerated. | Administration Issues<br>take with food; do not share medication; do not exceed recommended dose; store capsules and solution in the refrigerator; solution stored outside the refrigerator should be used within 30 days; the solution may be mixed with chocolate milk or Ensure within 1 hour of administration to improve taste<br><br>Drug–Drug Interactions<br>Ritonavir may decrease the metabolism of the following drugs leading to toxicity: **tricyclic antidepressants, fluconazole, itraconazole, corticosteroids, erythromycin, warfarin, calcium channel blockers, astemizole, terfenadine, cisapride, benzodiazepines, antiarrhythmics, rifabutin, saquinavir.** Ritonavir may decrease serum levels of the following drugs: **ddI, clarithromycin, sulfamethoxazole, theophylline, zidovudine, atovaquone, metoclopramide.** Serum levels of ritonavir may be increased by **fluconazole, clarithromycin, and fluoxetine. Rifampin** may decrease serum levels of ritonavir. | ADRs:<br>nausea, diarrhea, vomiting, anorexia, abdominal discomfort, numbness and tingling of hands and feet<br><br>Pharmacokinetics:<br>extensively metabolized by the cytochrome P-450 system | Contraindications<br>Hypersensitivity to ritonavir; do not coadminister ritonavir with benzodiazepines, astemizole, terfenadine, cisapride, and amiodarone as toxicity may occur due to decreased hepatic metabolism of the drug by ritonavir<br><br>Pregnancy Category:  B<br><br>Lactation Issues<br>Excretion in breast milk is unknown; HIV infected females should not breast feed to avoid postnatal transmission of HIV to a child who may not be infected |
| **Saquinavir***<br>Invirase, Fortovase<br><br>Capsule:<br>200 mg | **Treatment of HIV infection in combination with zidovudine or zalcitabine** | Administration Issues<br>Invirase: may take without regard to meals; do not share medication; do not exceed recommended dose; take within 2 h after a full meal | ADRs:<br>diarrhea, GI upset, nausea, fatigue, photosensitization | Contraindications<br>Hypersensitivity to saquinavir; photosensitization may occur<br><br>Pregnancy Category:  B |

*(continues on next page)*

**106.4** Protease Inhibitors  *continued from previous page*

| Drug and Dosage Forms | Spectrum of Activity and Usual Dosage Range | Administration Issues and Drug–Drug & Drug–Food Interactions | Common Adverse Drug Reactions (ADRs) and Pharmacokinetics | Contraindications, Pregnancy Category, and Lactation Issues |
|---|---|---|---|---|
| **Saquinavir** *cont.*<br><br>*Invirase will be phased out over time and replaced by Fortovase. | **Invirase**<br>**Adults/Adolescents**<br>600 mg tid with zidovudine or zalcitabine<br><br>**Fortovase**<br>Six of the 200 mg capsules (1200 mg) tid with meals or up to 2 hours after meal. Should be given with other antiretroviral agents. | Fortovase:<br>take with meals or up to 2 hours after meal<br><br>Drug–Drug Interactions<br>Saquinavir concentrations may be decreased by the following drugs: **rifampin, rifabutin, phenytoin, carbamazepine, phenobarbital** and **nevirapine.** Saquinavir may inhibit the metabolism of **terfenadine** and **astemizole** leading to drug accumulation and potential arrhythmias. Saquinavir may inhibit the metabolism of the following drugs leading to toxicity: **calcium channel blockers, quinidine, benzodiazepines.** Serum levels of saquinavir may be increased by **ketoconazole, clarithromycin.** | Pharmacokinetics:<br>enhanced bioavailability in HIV patients when given with food; hepatic metabolism via cytochrome P-450 system | Lactation Issues<br>Excretion in breast milk is unknown; HIV infected females should not breast feed to avoid postnatal transmission of HIV to a child who may not be infected |

| | | 106.5 Agents for Cytomegalovirus | | |
|---|---|---|---|---|
| **Drug and Dosage Forms** | **Spectrum of Activity and Usual Dosage Range** | **Administration Issues and Drug–Drug & Drug–Food Interactions** | **Common Adverse Drug Reactions (ADRs) and Pharmacokinetics** | **Contraindications, Pregnancy Category, and Lactation Issues** |
| **Ganciclovir**<br>Cytovene<br><br>Capsule:<br>250 mg | **Antiviral Spectrum**<br>Cytomegalovirus (CMV), herpes simplex virus type 1 (HSV-1), herpes simplex virus type 2 (HSV-2), varicella-zoster virus (VZV), Epstein-Barr virus, and hepatitis B virus<br><br>**Maintenance therapy following induction treatment of CMV retinitis**<br>1000 mg tid with food or 500 mg q 3 h while awake for 6 doses/day<br><br>Dose should be modified in patients with renal impairment.<br><br>**Intravenous therapy should be used for initial (induction) therapy of CMV retinitis; if retinitis progresses during oral therapy, then reinduction therapy with the intravenous product is recommended** | Administration Issues<br>Complete full course of therapy; ganciclovir is not a cure for CMV retinitis and disease may progress during or after therapy; regular ophthalmologic exams are necessary; effective contraception should be used for males and females during ganciclovir therapy<br><br>Drug–Drug Interactions<br>Concomitant use of ganciclovir with the following drugs may increase the potential for hematological disorders: **zidovudine, dapsone, flucytosine, amphotericin B, TMP-SMZ, chemotherapy agents**<br><br>Concomitant use of ganciclovir and **imipenemcilastatin** may increase the risk for seizures. Concomitant use of ganciclovir and **cyclosporine** or **amphotericin B** may increase the risk of nephrotoxicity. **Probenecid** may decrease renal excretion of ganciclovir. Concomitant use of ganciclovir with **zidovudine** or **didanosine** may increase serum levels of zidovudine and didanosine while decreasing serum levels of ganciclovir | ADRs:<br>asthenia, headache, hematological disorders (anemia, neutropenia), photosensitization, infertility<br><br>Pharmacokinetics:<br>poor GI tract absorption with and without food; cerebrospinal fluid concentrations ranged from 25%–70% of plasma concentrations | Contraindications<br>Hypersensitivity to ganciclovir or acyclovir<br><br>Pregnancy Category: C<br><br>Lactation Issues<br>Excreted in breast milk; due to possible carcinogenic and teratogenic effects to infants, discontinue nursing while receiving ganciclovir |

## 106.6 Miscellaneous Antiviral Agents

| Drug and Dosage Forms | Spectrum of Activity and Usual Dosage Range | Administration Issues and Drug–Drug & Drug–Food Interactions | Common Adverse Drug Reactions (ADRs) and Pharmacokinetics | Contraindications, Pregnancy Category, and Lactation Issues |
|---|---|---|---|---|
| **Amantadine**<br>Flumadine<br><br>Capsule:<br>Symmetrel, generics 100 mg<br><br>Syrup:<br>Symmetrel 50 mg/5 ml | **Antiviral Spectrum**<br>Influenza A virus<br><br>**Prophylaxis of Influenza A virus**<br>**Adults and children > 9 yr.**<br>200 mg qd or 100 mg bid for at least 10 days following a known exposure<br><br>**Children 1 to 9 yr.:** 4.4–8.8 mg/kg/d qd or in two divided doses, do not exceed 150 mg/day for at least 10 days following a known exposure<br><br>**Begin therapy in anticipation of contact or as soon as possible after exposure. For symptomatic management, start as soon as possible after onset of symptoms and continue for 24–48 h after symptoms resolve. Dosage reduction is recommended for patients with renal insufficiency.** | Administration Issues<br>Complete full course of therapy<br><br>Drug–Drug Interactions<br>Concomitant use of amantadine and **anticholinergic drugs** may predispose to certain side effects (confusion, dry mouth, constipation, decreased urination, blurred vision) | ADRs:<br>nausea, dizziness, insomnia, confusion, dry mouth, constipation, decreased urination, blurred vision<br><br>Pharmacokinetics:<br>readily absorbed in GI tract; no metabolism occurs; renal excretion as unchanged drug | Contraindications<br>Hypersensitivity to amantidine<br><br>Pregnancy Category: C<br><br>Lactation Issues<br>Amantadine is excreted in breast milk; use with caution in nursing mothers |
| **Rimantadine**<br>Flumadine<br><br>Tablet: 100 mg<br><br>Syrup:<br>50 mg/5 ml | **Antiviral Spectrum**<br>Influenza A virus<br><br>**Prophylaxis of Influenza A virus**<br>**Adults and children ≥ 10 yr.**<br>100 mg bid | Administration Issues<br>Complete full course of therapy<br><br>Drug–Drug Interactions<br>**Aspirin** and **acetaminophen** may decrease rimantadine serum concentrations. **Cimetidine** | ADRs:<br>insomnia, dizziness, nausea, vomiting<br><br>Pharmacokinetics:<br>$T_{1/2}$ is approximately 32 h; extensive hepatic metabolism; | Contraindications<br>Hypersensitivity to amantidine or rimantadine<br><br>Pregnancy Category: C |

1016

| | Lactation Issues |
|---|---|
| | rimantadine should not be used in nursing mothers; adverse events were noted in offspring of rats during the nursing period |

| | |
|---|---|
| may decrease hepatic metabolism of rimantadine | <25% of dose excreted renally as unchanged drug |

| **Children 1 to 9 yr.:** 5 mg/kg/d qd, do not exceed 150 mg/d<br><br>**Treatment of Influenza A virus**<br>**Adults:** 100 mg bid for 7 to 10 days from the initial onset of symptoms<br><br>**In patients with severe hepatic disease, renal failure, or elderly nursing home residents, a dose reduction to 100 mg daily is recommended** | |
|---|---|

## 107. Urinary Anti-Infectives

| Drug and Dosage Forms | Spectrum of Activity and Usual Dosage Range | Administration Issues and Drug–Drug & Drug–Food Interactions | Common Adverse Drug Reactions (ADRs) and Pharmacokinetics | Contraindications, Pregnancy Category, and Lactation Issues |
|---|---|---|---|---|
| **Cinoxacin**<br>Cinobac<br><br>Capsule:<br>250 mg, 500 mg | **Antibacterial Spectrum**<br>Gram-negative organisms including *E. coli, Proteus* sp., *Providencia rettgeri, Klebsiella* sp., and *Enterobacter* sp.<br><br>**Treatment of urinary tract infections by susceptible gram-negative organisms**<br>**Adults:** 1 gm/d in 2 to 4 divided doses for 7 to 14 d<br><br>**Prophylaxis of urinary tract infection**<br>250 mg at bedtime for up to 5 months in women with a history of recurrent urinary tract infections | Administration Issues<br>Complete full course of therapy; may take without regard to meals; take with fluids liberally; avoid prolonged exposure to sunlight, wear protective clothing, and apply sunscreen<br><br>Drug–Drug Interactions<br>**Probenecid** inhibits renal excretion of cinoxacin. Consider possible drug interactions of other **quinolone** and **fluoroquinolone** antibiotics when using cinoxacin | ADRs:<br>nausea, vomiting, headache, dizziness, rash, photosensitivity<br><br>Pharmacokinetics:<br>rapid absorption; concentrates in the urine where approximately 97% of an oral dose is excreted in 24 hours<br><br>**Dosage reduction is recommended for patients with renal insufficiency** | Contraindications<br>Hypersensitivity to cinoxacin or other quinolones<br><br>Pregnancy Category: B<br><br>Lactation Issues<br>due to the potential for adverse effects in infants, decide whether to discontinue nursing or discontinue the drug |

*(continues on next page)*

| Drug and Dosage Forms | Spectrum of Activity and Usual Dosage Range | Administration Issues and Drug–Drug & Drug–Food Interactions | Common Adverse Drug Reactions (ADRs) and Pharmacokinetics | Contraindications, Pregnancy Category, and Lactation Issues |
|---|---|---|---|---|
| **Methenamine Hippurate**<br>Hiprex, Urex<br><br>Tablet:<br>1 gm | **Antibacterial Spectrum**<br>*E. coli*, enterococcal sp., and staphylococcal sp.<br><br>**Prophylaxis or suppression/elimination of frequently recurring urinary tract infections**<br><br>**Adults and children > 12 years**<br>1 gm bid<br><br>**Children 6 to 12 years**<br>0.5 to 1 gm bid | Administration Issues<br>Complete full course of therapy; cranberry juice or vitamin C may be used to acidify the urine and increase the efficacy of methenamine; take with food to decrease GI upset; drink fluids liberally to ensure adequate urine flow<br><br>Drug–Drug Interactions<br>Concurrent use of methenamine and **sulfonamides** may cause the formation of an insoluble precipitate in the urine. **Urinary alkalinizers (milk products, sodium bicarbonate, acetazolamide)** may decrease the efficacy of methenamine by inhibiting its conversion to formaldehyde | ADRs:<br>nausea, vomiting, abdominal discomfort, bladder irritation<br><br>Pharmacokinetics:<br>rapid absorption; 10% to 25% hepatic metabolism; concentrates in the urine; 90% excreted in the urine in 24 hours | Contraindications<br>Hypersensitivity to methenamine; renal insufficiency; concurrent sulfonamide use; severe dehydration; severe hepatic insufficiency<br><br>Pregnancy Category: C<br><br>Lactation Issues<br>Excreted in breast milk; no adverse effects in nursing infants have been reported; use with caution in nursing mothers |
| **Methenamine Mandelate**<br><br>Tablet, enteric coated:<br>Mandelamine, various generics<br>0.5 gm, 1 gm<br><br>Suspension:<br>Various generics<br>0.5 gm/5 ml | **Antibacterial Spectrum**<br>*E. coli*, enterococcal sp., and staphylococcal sp.<br><br>**Prophylaxis or suppression/elimination of frequently recurring urinary tract infections**<br><br>**Adults:** 1 gm qid with meals and at bedtime | Administration Issues<br>Complete full course of therapy; cranberry juice or vitamin C may be used to acidify the urine and increase the efficacy of methenamine; take with food to decrease GI upset; drink fluids liberally to ensure adequate urine flow<br><br>Drug–Drug Interactions<br>Concurrent use of methenamine and **sulfonamides** may cause the formation of an insoluble precipitate in the urine. | ADRs:<br>nausea, vomiting, abdominal discomfort, bladder irritation<br><br>Pharmacokinetics:<br>rapid absorption; 10% to 25% hepatic metabolism; concentrates in the urine; 90% excreted in the urine in 24 hours | Contraindications<br>Hypersensitivity to methenamine; renal insufficiency; concurrent sulfonamide use; severe dehydration; severe hepatic insufficiency<br><br>Pregnancy Category: C<br><br>Lactation Issues<br>Excreted in breast milk; no adverse effects in nursing |

| Drug | Antibacterial Spectrum / Dosing | Administration Issues / Drug–Drug Interactions | ADRs / Pharmacokinetics / Contraindications |
|---|---|---|---|
| | | **Urinary alkalinizers (milk products, sodium bicarbonate, acetazolamide)** may decrease the efficacy of methenamine by inhibiting its conversion to formaldehyde | infants have been reported; use with caution in nursing |
| **Nalidixic Acid**<br>NegGram<br><u>Caplet:</u><br>250 mg, 500 mg, 1 gm<br><u>Suspension:</u><br>250 mg/5 ml | **Children 6 to 12 years:** 0.5 gm qid with meals and at bedtime<br><br>**Children ≤ 6 years:** 0.25 gm/14 kg four times daily with meals and at bedtime<br><br>**Antibacterial Spectrum**<br>Gram-negative organisms including *E. coli, Proteus* sp., *Providencia rettgeri, Klebsiella* sp., and *Enterobacter* sp.<br><br>**Treatment of urinary tract infections by susceptible gram-negative organisms**<br><br>**Adults:** Initial therapy at 1 gm qid for 7 to 14 days; a maintenance therapy of 2 gm/day may be used after the initial treatment period<br><br>**Children 3 months to ≤ 12 years** Initial therapy at 55 mg/kg/d divided qid doses for 7 to 14 days; a maintenance therapy of 33 mg/kg/d may be used after the initial treatment period | <u>Administration Issues</u><br>Complete full course of therapy; take with food to avoid GI upset; avoid prolonged exposure to sunlight, wear protective clothing, and apply sunscreen<br><br>**Nalidixic acid has been shown to cause erosion of cartilage in weight-bearing joints in animals, no joint lesions have been reported in humans, use with caution in prepubertal children**<br><br><u>Drug–Drug Interactions</u><br>Nalidixic acid may displace **warfarin** from protein binding sites increasing the therapeutic effect of warfarin. **Nitrofurantoin** may antagonize the antibiotic effect of nalidixic acid | <u>ADRs:</u><br>photosensitivity, drowsiness, headache, abdominal discomfort, nausea<br><br><u>Pharmacokinetics:</u><br>well absorbed in GI tract; 95% protein bound; T$_{1/2}$ in urine is 6 hours; hepatic metabolism; renal excretion<br><br><u>Contraindications</u><br>Hypersensitivity to nalidixic acid; history of convulsive disorders<br><br><u>Pregnancy Category:</u> B<br><br><u>Lactation Issues</u><br>Data is scant, however nalidixic acid is excreted in breast milk; one report of hemolytic anemia in nursing infant; use with caution in nursing mothers |
| **Nitrofurantoin**<br>Furadantin<br><u>Suspension:</u><br>25 mg/5 ml | **Antibacterial Spectrum**<br>Gram-positive organisms including *S. aureus* and *S. saprophyticus*; gram-negative organisms including *E. coli, Klebsiella* sp., and *Enterobacter* sp., *Enterococcus faecalis* | <u>Administration Issues</u><br>Complete full course of therapy; take with food or milk to decrease upset stomach; may cause brownish discoloration of the urine | <u>ADRs:</u><br>nausea, vomiting, anorexia, abdominal discomfort<br><br><u>Pharmacokinetics:</u><br>food enhanced absorption from GI tract; metabolized by<br><br><u>Contraindications</u><br>Hypersensitivity to nitrofurantoin; renal function impairment, anuria, or oliguria; pregnant women at term, during labor and delivery, or when onset of |

(continues on next page)

## 107. Urinary Anti-Infectives  *continued from previous page*

| Drug and Dosage Forms | Spectrum of Activity and Usual Dosage Range | Administration Issues and Drug–Drug & Drug–Food Interactions | Common Adverse Drug Reactions (ADRs) and Pharmacokinetics | Contraindications, Pregnancy Category, and Lactation Issues |
|---|---|---|---|---|
| **Nitrofurantoin *cont.*** | **Treatment of urinary tract infections** <br><br> **Adults:** 50–100 mg qid with meals and at bedtime for 7 to 10 d <br><br> **Children:** 5–7 mg/kg/ d divided qid for 7 to 10 d <br><br> **Suppressive of urinary tract infections** <br><br> **Adults:** 50–100 mg q hs <br><br> **Children:** 1 mg/kg/d qd or divided bid | <u>Drug–Drug Interactions</u> <br> **Antacids** and **magnesium salts** may decrease the absorption of nitrofurantoin. <br> **Probenecid** may decrease the elimination of nitrofurantoin | body tissues; concentrates in the urine; renal excretion | labor is imminent; infants < 1 month of age <br><br> <u>Pregnancy Category:</u>  B <br><br> <u>Lactation Issues</u> <br> safety for use in nursing mothers not established |
| **Nitrofurantoin Macrocrystals** <br><br> <u>Capsule:</u> <br> Macrodantin 25 mg <br><br> <u>Capsule:</u> <br> Macrodantin, generics 50 mg, 100 mg <br><br> <u>Capsule:</u> <br> Macrobid 100 mg (as 25 mg macrocrystals, 75 mg monohydrate) | **Antibacterial Spectrum** <br> Gram-positive organisms including *S. aureus* and *S. saprophyticus;* gram-negative organisms including *E. coli, Klebsiella* sp., and *Enterobacter* sp., *Enterococcus faecalis* <br><br> **Treatment of urinary tract infections** <br><br> **Adults:** 50–100 mg qid with meals and at bedtime or Macrobid 100 mg bid with meals for 7 to 10 d <br><br> **Children:** 5–7 mg/kg/d divided quid for 7 to 10 d | <u>Administration Issues</u> <br> Complete full course of therapy; take with food or milk to decrease upset stomach; may cause brownish discoloration of the urine <br><br> <u>Drug–Drug Interactions</u> <br> **Antacids** and **magnesium salts** may decrease the absorption of nitrofurantoin. <br> **Probenecid** may decrease the elimination of nitrofurantoin | <u>ADRs:</u> <br> nausea, vomiting, anorexia, abdominal discomfort <br><br> <u>Pharmacokinetics:</u> <br> slower dissolution and absorption compared to nitrofurantoin; food enhances absorption from GI tract; metabolized by body tissues; concentrates in the urine; renal excretion | <u>Contraindications</u> <br> Hypersensitivity to nitrofurantoin; renal function impairment, anuria, or oliguria; pregnant women at term, during labor and delivery, or when onset of labor is imminent; infants < 1 month of age <br><br> <u>Pregnancy Category:</u>  B <br><br> <u>Lactation Issues</u> <br> Excreted in breast milk; safety for use in nursing mothers has not been established |

*(continues on next page)*

| | | |
|---|---|---|
| | **Suppressive of urinary tract infections**<br>**Adults:** 50–100 mg q hs<br><br>**Children:** 1 mg/kg/d qd or divided bid | | |

| | | | |
|---|---|---|---|
| **Sulfamethoxazole and Phenazopyridine**<br>Azo Gantanol<br><br>**NOTE: Drug taken off the market in summer 1998.**<br><br>Tablet:<br>500 mg sulfamethoxazole<br>100 mg phenazopyridine | **Treatment of urinary tract infections**<br><br>**Adults:** 4 tablets initially, then 2 tablets in the morning and evening for up to 2 days; if further treatment is needed, use sulfamethoxazole only | Administration Issues<br>May cause reddish-orange discoloration of the urine and may stain fabric. Staining of contact lenses has also occurred. Combination therapy may mask the symptoms associated with ineffective or inappropriate therapy. Avoid prolonged exposure to sunlight, wear protective clothing, and apply sunscreen<br><br>Drug–Drug Interactions<br>Sulfonamides may increase the pharmacological and toxic effects of the following drugs: **methotrexate, phenytoin, sulfonylureas, warfarin** | ADRs:<br>nausea, abdominal discomfort, headache, photosensitivity<br><br>Pharmacokinetics:<br>good GI absorption; readily penetrates into CSF; hepatic metabolism; renal excretion |

| |
|---|
| Contraindications<br>Hypersensitivity to sulfonamides or chemically related drugs such as sulfonylureas, thiazide diuretics, and sunscreens containing PABA<br><br>Pregnancy<br>Sulfonamides: Safety for use during pregnancy has not been established; sulfonamides do cross the placenta; do not use during pregnancy at term<br><br>Phenazopyridine: C<br><br>Lactation Issues<br>Sulfonamides are excreted in breast milk; according to the American Academy of Pediatrics, breast feeding and sulfonamides are compatible; avoid sulfonamides and nursing in premature infants, infants with hyperbilirubinemia, and infants with G-6-PD deficiency |

# 107. Urinary Anti-Infectives  *continued from previous page*

| Drug and Dosage Forms | Spectrum of Activity and Usual Dosage Range | Administration Issues and Drug–Drug & Drug–Food Interactions | Common Adverse Drug Reactions (ADRs) and Pharmacokinetics | Contraindications, Pregnancy Category, and Lactation Issues |
|---|---|---|---|---|
| **Sulfisoxazole and Phenazopyridine** Azo Gantrisin, various generics **NOTE: Drug taken off the market in summer 1998.** Tablet: 500 mg sulfisoxazole 50 mg phenazopyridine | **Treatment of urinary tract infections** **Adults:** 4 tablets initially, then 2 tablets four times daily for up to 2 days; if further treatment is needed, use sulfamethoxazole only | Administration Issues May cause reddish-orange discoloration of the urine and may stain fabric. Staining of contact lenses has also occurred. Combination therapy may mask the symptoms associated with ineffective or inappropriate therapy. Avoid prolonged exposure to sunlight; wear protective clothing, and apply sunscreen Drug–Drug Interactions Sulfonamides may increase the pharmacological and toxic effects of the following drugs: **methotrexate, phenytoin, sulfonylureas, warfarin** | ADRs: nausea, abdominal discomfort, headache, photosensitivity Pharmacokinetics: good GI absorption; readily penetrates into CSF; hepatic metabolism; renal excretion | Contraindications Hypersensitivity to sulfonamides or chemically related drugs such as sulfonylureas, thiazide diuretics, and sunscreens containing PABA Pregnancy Sulfonamides: Safety for use during pregnancy has not been established; sulfonamides do cross the placenta; do not use during pregnancy at term Phenazopyridine: C Lactation Issues Sulfonamides are excreted in breast milk; according to the American Academy of Pediatrics, breast feeding and sulfonamides are compatible; avoid sulfonamides and nursing in premature infants, infants with hyperbilirubinemia, and infants with G-6-PD deficiency |

## Trimethoprim

**Tablet:**
Proloprim, Trimpex, various generics
100 mg

Proloprim, various generics
200 mg

**Antibacterial Spectrum**
Urinary infections caused by *E. coli*, *P. mirabilis*, *K. pneumoniae*, *Enterobacter* sp., and coagulase-negative *Staphylococcus* sp.

**Treatment of urinary tract infection**
100 mg q 12 hours or 200 mg q 24 hours for 10 days

**Dosage reduction is recommended for patients with renal insufficiency**

Administration Issues
Complete full course of therapy

Drug–Drug Interactions
Trimethoprim may increase the pharmacological effects of **phenytoin** leading to toxicity

ADRs:
rash, pruritus, abdominal distress, superinfection, photosensitivity

Pharmacokinetics:
rapidly absorbed; $T_{1/2}$ is approximately 10 hours; minimal hepatic metabolism; renal excretion

Contraindications
Hypersensitivity to trimethoprim; megaloblastic anemia due to folate deficiency

Pregnancy Category: C

Lactation Issues
Excreted in breast milk; use with caution

---

## 108. Drugs for Parasitic Infections

| Drug and Dosage Forms | Spectrum of Activity and Usual Dosage Range | Administration Issues and Drug–Drug & Drug–Food Interactions | Common Adverse Drug Reactions (ADRs) and Pharmacokinetics | Contraindications, Pregnancy Category, and Lactation Issues |
|---|---|---|---|---|
| **Mebendazole**<br>Vermox<br><br>Tablet, chewable:<br>100 mg | **Antibacterial Spectrum**<br>*Trichuris trichiura* (whipworm), *Enterobius vermicularis* (pinworm), *Ascaris lumbricoides* (roundworm), *Ancylostoma duodenale* (common hookworm), *Necator americanus* (American hookworm)<br><br>**General indications**<br>**Adults and children:** 100 mg each morning and evening for 3 consecutive days | Administration Issues<br>Complete full course of therapy; chew or crush tablet and mix with food; if one family member has a pinworm infection, treat all family members in close contact with the patient; to prevent reinfection, disinfect toilet facilities daily, change and launder undergarments, bed linens, towels, and nightclothes daily<br><br>**If the patient is not cured 3 weeks after treatment, a second treatment course is recommended** | ADRs:<br>abdominal discomfort, diarrhea<br><br>Pharmacokinetics:<br>poorly absorbed; minimal metabolism; fecal excretion | Contraindications<br>Hypersensitivity to mebendazole<br><br>Pregnancy Category: C<br><br>Lactation Issues<br>Safety for use in nursing mothers has not been established |

(continues on next page)

## 108. Drugs for Parasitic Infections  *continued from previous page*

| Drug and Dosage Forms | Spectrum of Activity and Usual Dosage Range | Administration Issues and Drug–Drug & Drug–Food Interactions | Common Adverse Drug Reactions (ADRs) and Pharmacokinetics | Contraindications, Pregnancy Category, and Lactation Issues |
|---|---|---|---|---|
| **Mebendazole** *cont.* | <u>Treatment of Enterobiasis (pinworm) infection</u><br>100 mg given as a single dose | | | |
| **Niclosamide**<br>Niclocide<br><br><u>Tablet, chewable:</u><br>500 mg | **Antibacterial Spectrum**<br>*Taenia saginata* (beef tapeworm), *Diphyllobothrium latum* (fish tapeworm), *Hymenolepis nana* (dwarf tapeworm)<br><br>**Treatment of *Taenia saginata* (beef tapeworm), *Diphyllobothrium latum* (fish tapeworm) infections**<br>**Adults:** 4 tablets as a single dose<br><br>**Children > 34 kg:** 3 tablets as a single dose<br><br>**Children 11–34 kg:** 2 tablets as a single dose<br><br>**Treatment of *Hymenolepis nana* (dwarf tapeworm) infections**<br>**Adults:** 4 tablets qd for 7 d<br><br>**Children > 34 kg:** 3 tablets on the first day, then 2 tablets qd for the next 6 d<br><br>**Children 11–34 kg:** 2 tablets on the first day, then 1 tablet qd for the next 6 d | <u>Administration Issues</u><br>Complete full course of therapy; take after a light meal; chew tablet, then swallow with a small amount of water<br><br>**Detection of tapeworm segments in the stool on the 7th day of treatment indicates treatment failure; give a second course of treatment; a patient is not considered cured unless the stool is negative for a minimum of 3 months** | <u>ADRs:</u><br>nausea, vomiting, abdominal discomfort, diarrhea, dizziness | <u>Contraindications</u><br>Hypersensitivity to niclosamide<br><br><u>Pregnancy Category:</u>  B<br><br><u>Lactation Issues</u><br>Safety for use in nursing mothers has not been established |

## Piperazine
Various generics

Tablet:
250 mg

Syrup:
500 mg/5 ml

**Antibacterial Spectrum**
*Enterobius vermicularis* (pinworm),
*Ascaris lumbricoides* (roundworm)

**Treatment of Ascariasis
(roundworm infection)**
**Adults:** 3.5 gm once daily for
2 consecutive days

**Children:** 75 mg/kg once daily for
2 consecutive days; maximum daily
dose is 3.5 gm

**Treatment of Enterobiasis
(pinworm infection)**
**Adults and children:**
65 mg/kg once daily for
7 consecutive days; maximum
daily dose is 2.5 gm

Administration Issues
Complete full course of therapy; take on
an empty stomach, at least 1 hour
before or 2 hours after meals; if one
family member has a pinworm infection,
treat all family members in close contact
with the patient; to prevent reinfection,
disinfect toilet facilities daily, change
and launder undergarments, bed linens,
towels, and nightclothes daily

**For severe infections, repeat
treatment course after a 1 week
interval**

ADRs:
nausea, vomiting, diarrhea,
abdominal discomfort,
headache, dizziness

Pharmacokinetics:
readily absorbed from GI tract;
approximately 25% is
metabolized; renal excretion

Contraindications
Hypersensitivity to piperazine;
renal or hepatic function
impairment; convulsive
disorders

Pregnancy:
Safety for use in pregnancy
has not been established

Lactation Issues
due to the potential for
adverse effects in infants,
decide whether to discontinue
nursing or discontinue drug

## Praziquantel
Biltricide

Tablet:
600 mg

**Antibacterial Spectrum**
*Schistosoma* sp., *Clonorchis
sinensis* and *Opisthorchis viverrini*
(liver flukes)

**Treatment of Schistosomiasis**
20 mg/kg for 3 doses given on
the same day; the interval between
doses should not be < 4 and not
> 6 hours

**Treatment of liver flukes**
25 mg/kg for 3 doses given on
the same day; the interval between
doses should not be < 4 and not
> 6 hours

Administration Issues
Complete full course of therapy; take
with liquids during meals; do not chew
tablets

ADRs:
headache, dizziness,
abdominal discomfort

Pharmacokinetics:
rapid absorption; undergoes
first-pass hepatic metabolism,
renal excretion

Contraindications
Hypersensitivity to
praziquantel; do not treat
ocular cysticercosis with
praziquantel

Pregnancy Category: B

Lactation Issues
Excreted in breast milk; do not
nurse on the day of treatment
and for 72 hours thereafter

*(continues on next page)*

| Drug and Dosage Forms | Spectrum of Activity and Usual Dosage Range | Administration Issues and Drug–Drug & Drug–Food Interactions | Common Adverse Drug Reactions (ADRs) and Pharmacokinetics | Contraindications, Pregnancy Category, and Lactation Issues |
|---|---|---|---|---|
| **Pyrantel**<br>Antiminth, Pin-Rid<br><br>Capsule: 180 mg<br><br>Suspension:<br>50 mg/ml | **Antibacterial Spectrum**<br>*Enterobius vermicularis* (pinworm),<br>*Ascaris lumbricoides* (roundworm)<br><br>**Treatment of Enterobius vermicularis (pinworm) and Ascaris lumbricoides (roundworm) infections**<br>11 mg/kg as a single dose; maximum total dose is 1 gm | Administration Issues<br>May take with food, milk, juice, or on an empty stomach anytime during the day; if one family member has a pinworm infection, treat all family members in close contact with the patient; to prevent reinfection, disinfect toilet facilities daily, change and launder undergarments, bed linens, towels, and nightclothes daily | ADRs:<br>anorexia, nausea, vomiting, abdominal discomfort, diarrhea<br><br>Pharmacokinetics:<br>poorly absorbed; minimal metabolism | Contraindications<br>Hepatic disease; pregnancy<br><br>Pregnancy:<br>Do not use during pregnancy unless otherwise directed by a physician |
| **Thiabendazole**<br>Mintezol<br><br>Tablet chewable:<br>500 mg<br><br>Suspension:<br>500 mg/5 ml | **Antibacterial Spectrum**<br>*Trichuris trichura* (whipworm),<br>*Enterobius vermicularis* (pinworm),<br>*Ascaris lumbricoides* (roundworm),<br>*Ancylostoma duodenale* (common hookworm), *Necator americanus* (American hookworm), *Strongyloides stercoralis* (threadworm),<br>*Ancylostoma braziliense* (dog and cat hookworm), *Toxocara* sp. (ascarids)<br><br>**Treatment of Strongyloidiasis**<br>**Adults and children < 68kg**<br>22 mg/kg/dose bid for 2 consecutive days<br><br>**Adults and children ≥ 68 kg**<br>1.5 gm/dose bid for 2 consecutive days | Administration Issues<br>Complete full course of therapy; take with food; chew tablets thoroughly before swallowing; if one family member has a pinworm infection, treat all family members in close contact with the patient; to prevent reinfection, disinfect toilet facilities daily, change and launder undergarments, bed linens, towels, and nightclothes daily<br><br>**Thiabendazole is considered second line therapy when other agents are not available for treatment of hookworm, round worm, and whipworm infections** | ADRs:<br>dizziness, headache, drowsiness, anorexia, nausea, vomiting, diarrhea<br><br>Pharmacokinetics:<br>rapid absorbtion; almost completely metabolized; renal excretion mostly as metabolites | Contraindications<br>Hypersensitivity to thiabendazole<br><br>Pregnancy Category: C<br><br>Lactation Issues<br>Excretion in breast milk is unknown; due to the potential for adverse effects in infants, decide whether to discontinue nursing or discontinue the drug |

| | | | |
|---|---|---|---|
| | **Treatment of cutaneous larva migrans (creeping eruption)**<br>**Adults and children < 68 kg:** 22 mg/kg/dose bid for 5 consecutive days, repeat in 2 days if active lesions persist<br><br>**Adults and children ≥ 68 kg**<br>1.5 gm/dose bid for 5 consecutive days, repeat in 2 days if active lesions persist<br><br>Maximum daily dose is 3 gm | | |

## 109. Miscellaneous Antimicrobial Agents

| Drug and Dosage Forms | Spectrum of Activity and Usual Dosage Range | Administration Issues and Drug–Drug & Drug–Food Interactions | Common Adverse Drug Reactions (ADRs) and Pharmacokinetics | Contraindications, Pregnancy Category, and Lactation Issues |
|---|---|---|---|---|
| **Atovaquone**<br>Mepron<br><br><u>Suspension:</u><br>750 mg/5 ml | **Antibacterial Spectrum**<br>*Pneumocystis carinii*<br><br><u>Treatment of mild to moderate Pneumocystis carinii pneumonia in patients who are intolerant to TMP-SMZ</u><br>750 mg bid with food for 21 days | <u>Administration Issues</u><br>Complete full course of therapy; take with food; do not exceed recommended dose<br><br><u>Drug–Drug Interactions</u><br>**Rifampin** and **rifabutin** may decrease serum levels of atovaquone.<br>Atovaquone may decrease protein binding of other highly bound drugs (**warfarin**) leading to toxicity | <u>ADRs:</u><br>rash, nausea, diarrhea, headache<br><br><u>Pharmacokinetics:</u><br>bioavailability increases with food; highly protein bound; $T_{1/2}$ is approximately 65 hours; fecal elimination | <u>Contraindications</u><br>Hypersensitivity to atovaquone<br><br><u>Pregnancy Category:</u> C<br><br><u>Lactation Issues</u><br>Excretion in breast milk is unknown; HIV infected females should not breast feed to avoid postnatal transmission of HIV to a child who may not be infected |
| **Dapsone**<br><br><u>Tablet:</u><br>25 mg, 100 mg | **Antibacterial Spectrum**<br>*Mycobacterium leprae*,<br>*Pneumocystis carinii*<br><br>**Treatment of dermatitis herpetiformis**<br>**Adults:** Initiate with 50 mg qd, increase dose upward to achieve resolution of skin | <u>Administration Issues</u><br>Complete full course of therapy; avoid prolonged exposure to sunlight, wear protective clothing, and apply sunscreen | <u>ADRs:</u><br>photosensitivity, hemolytic anemia, drug-induced lupus, erythematosus, nausea, vomiting, albuminuria | <u>Contraindications</u><br>Hypersensitivity to dapsone<br><br><u>Pregnancy Category:</u> C |

*(continues on next page)*

1027

| Drug and Dosage Forms | Spectrum of Activity and Usual Dosage Range | Administration Issues and Drug–Drug & Drug–Food Interactions | Common Adverse Drug Reactions (ADRs) and Pharmacokinetics | Contraindications, Pregnancy Category, and Lactation Issues |
|---|---|---|---|---|
| **Dapsone** *cont.* | lesions, usual dosage range is 50–300 mg qd; use minimal dose that achieves desired effect, the average time for dosage reduction is 8 months; therapy may be discontinued with the average time for dosage elimination being 29 months<br><br>**Children:** Initiate with 1–2 mg/kg/d, increasing to desired response, maximum daily dose is 100 mg/d; continue therapy for a minimum of 3 years | Drug–Drug Interactions<br>The following drugs may decrease the effect of dapsone leading to treatment failure: **didanosine, para-aminobenzoic acid, rifampin, rifabutin.** The toxicity of dapsone may be increased by **folic acid antagonists (pyrimethamine, methotrexate), probenecid, and trimethoprim** | Pharmacokinetics:<br>rapid absorption; highly protein bound; $T_{1/2}$ is approximately 28 hours; appreciable tissue levels found 3 weeks after therapy is completed; hepatic metabolism; renal excretion | Lactation Issues<br>Excreted in breast milk in substantial amounts; due to the potential for adverse effects in infants, decide whether to discontinue nursing or discontinue the drug |
| **Chloramphenicol**<br>Chloromycetin<br><br>Capsule: 250 mg<br><br>Suspension:<br>150 mg/5 ml | **Antibacterial Spectrum**<br>Effective against a wide range of gram positive and negative organisms particularly *Salmonella typhi* (typhoid fever) and *H. influenzae;* active in vitro against rickettsia; effective against anaerobic infections caused by *B. fragilis*<br><br>**Serious infections where less potentially dangerous antibiotics are ineffective or contraindicated**<br>**Adults:** 50 mg/kg/d divided q 6 h for 10 to 14 days | Administration Issues<br>Complete full course of therapy; shake suspension well before administration; take on empty stomach at least 1 hour before or 2 hours after meals; report symptoms of aplastic anemia (fever, sore throat, tiredness, unusual bleeding, or bruising) to your health care professional<br><br>Drug–Drug Interactions<br>Chloramphenicol may increase the effect of **barbiturates** and **barbiturates** may decrease chloramphenicol serum levels. **Rifampin** may decrease chloramphenicol serum levels. Chloramphenicol may increase the effect of **warfarin** and **phenytoin.** | ADRs:<br>nausea, vomiting, mental confusion, headache<br><br>**Serious and fatal blood dyscrasias have occurred after chloramphenicol administration. Decreased hepatic and renal function in newborns and adults can increase chloramphenicol accumulation and predispose to toxic side effects - carefully monitor the concentration of the drug in the blood** | Contraindications/Warnings<br>Use with caution in premature newborns, fatalities have occurred due to symptoms associated with "gray syndrome", blood dyscrasias, aplastic anemia, optic and peripheral neuritis have been reported with chloramphenicol use<br><br>Pregnancy<br>Safety in pregnancy is unknown; use with caution as potential toxic effects to the fetus may occur (gray syndrome) |

| | | | | |
|---|---|---|---|---|
| | For severe infections (meningitis), doses up to 100 mg/kg/d may be required<br><br>**Children:** 50–75 mg/kg/d divided q 6 h for 10 to 14 d<br><br>For severe infections (meningitis), 50–100 mg/kg/d may be required | Chloramphenicol may enhance the effect of **sulfonylureas** causing hypoglycemia. Chloramphenicol may increase serum levels of **iron salts.** Chloramphenicol may decrease the effects of **vitamin B$_{12}$** in patients with pernicious anemia. | Pharmacokinetics:<br>well absorbed from GI tract; 60% protein binding; enters cerebrospinal fluid; hepatic metabolism<br><br>**Therapeutic range: peak - 10–20 mcg/ml and trough - 5–10 mcg/ml** | Lactation Issues<br>Excreted in breast milk; use with caution due to potential toxic effects to nursing infant (gray syndrome) |
| **Clindamycin**<br>Cleocin, various generics<br><br>Capsules (as the hydrochloride salt):<br>75 mg, 150 mg, 300 mg<br><br>Granules for Oral Solution (as the palmitate salt):<br>75 mg/5 ml | **Antibacterial Spectrum**<br>*S. aureus, S. epidermidis, S. pneumoniae, C. diphtheriae;* Anaerobic organisms including *Bacteriodes* sp., *Fusobacterium, Propionibacterium* (C acnes) and *Clostridium perfringens*<br><br>**General indications (use higher doses for more severe infections)**<br><br>**Adults:** 150–450 mg q 6 h for 10 to 14 d<br><br>**Children:**<br><br>8–20 mg/kg/d (as the hydrochloride salt) divided q 6 to 8 h for 10 to 14 d<br><br>8–25 mg/kg/d (as the palmitate salt) divided q 6 to 8 h for 10 to 14 d<br><br>In children ≤10 kg, give 37.5 mg tid as the minimum dose | Administration Issues<br>Complete full course of therapy; may be taken without regard to meals; notify your health care professional if diarrhea develops<br><br>**Limit clindamycin use to serious infections to avoid pseudomembranous colitis**<br><br>Drug–Drug Interactions<br>**Erythromycin** may antagonize the antibiotic effect of clindamycin. The effect of **nondepolarizing, neuromuscular blocking agents** may be enhanced by clindamycin | ADRs:<br>nausea, vomiting, diarrhea (3.4%–30%), potentially pseudomembranous colitis<br><br>Pharmacokinetics:<br>poor CNS penetration; 85% hepatic elimination with increased half-life in hepatic disease | Contraindications<br>Hypersensitivity to clindamycin; treatment of minor bacterial or viral infections<br><br>Pregnancy Category: Safety has not been established<br><br>Lactation Issues<br>Excreted in breast milk; nursing is probably best discontinued when taking clindamycin |
| **Furazolidone**<br>Furoxone<br><br>Tablet:<br>100 mg | **Antibacterial Spectrum**<br>GI tract organisms including *E. coli, Staphylococcus* sp., *Salmonella* sp., *Proteus* sp., *Aerobacter aerogenes, Vibrio cholerae, Giardia lamblia* | Administration Issues<br>Complete full course of therapy; avoid ingestion of alcohol during and 4 days after treatment; avoid tyramine containing foods (cheese, wine) during treatment; may discolor urine | ADRs:<br>hypotension, rash, urticaria, nausea, headache, hypoglycemia | Contraindications<br>Hypersensitivity to furazolidone; infants <1 month |

*(continues on next page)*

# 109. Miscellaneous Antimicrobial Agents  *continued from previous page*

| Drug and Dosage Forms | Spectrum of Activity and Usual Dosage Range | Administration Issues and Drug–Drug & Drug–Food Interactions | Common Adverse Drug Reactions (ADRs) and Pharmacokinetics | Contraindications, Pregnancy Category, and Lactation Issues |
|---|---|---|---|---|
| **Furazolidone** *cont.* <br><br> Liquid: <br> 50 mg/15 ml | **Treatment of diarrhea and enteritis caused by susceptible organisms** <br> **Adults:** 100 mg qid for 7 d <br><br> **Children** <br> ≥ **5 years** - 25–50 mg qid <br> **1 to 4 years** - 17–25 mg qid <br> **1 month to 1 year** - 8–17 mg qid <br> Continue treatment for 7 d | Drug–Drug Interactions <br> Furazolidine may increase the potential for a hypertensive reaction with the following drugs: <br> **monoamine oxidase inhibitors, amphetamines, sympathomimetics, tricyclic antidepressants, levodopa.** <br> Furazolidine may increase the toxic effects of **meperidine** leading to agitation, seizures, and coma. Furazolidine and **alcohol** may cause a disulfiram-like reaction with vomiting | Pharmacokinetics: <br> extensive metabolism believed to be through the intestines; urinary excretion | Pregnancy Category:  C <br><br> Lactation Issues <br> Excretion in breast milk is unknown; safety for use in nursing mothers has not been established |
| **Kanamycin Sulfate** <br> Kantrex <br><br> Capsule:  500 mg | **Antibacterial Spectrum** <br> bacteria of the intestinal tract <br><br> **Suppression of intestinal bacteria** <br> 1 gm every hour for 4 hours, followed by 1 gm every 6 hours for 36 to 72 hours | Administration Issues <br> Complete full course of therapy; notify your health care professional if ringing of the ears occurs <br><br> Drug–Drug Interactions <br> Oral aminoglycosides may decrease the absorption of the following drugs: **digoxin, methotrexate, vitamin A.** Oral aminoglycosides may increase the effect of **warfarin** by decreasing the absorption of dietary vitamin K | ADRs: <br> nausea, vomiting, diarrhea, ototoxicity, muscle weakness, superinfection <br><br> Pharmacokinetics: <br> poor systemic absorption; elimination of intestinal bacteria persists for 48–72 hours; fecal elimination | Contraindications <br> Presence of intestinal obstruction; hypersensitivity to aminoglycosides <br><br> Pregnancy Category:  D <br><br> Lactation Issues <br> Aminoglycosides are excreted in breast milk; potentially serious adverse reactions may occur in nursing infants; decide whether to discontinue nursing or to discontinue the drug |
| **Methylene Blue** <br> Urolene Blue | **Antibacterial Spectrum** <br> Mild genitourinary antiseptic | Administration Issues <br> Complete full course of therapy; take with meals and a glass of water | ADRs: <br> blue-green urine, stool, and possible skin discoloration, | Contraindications <br> Renal insufficiency; hypersensitivity to methylene |

| | | | | |
|---|---|---|---|---|
| **Tablet:**<br>65 mg | <u>**Genitourinary antiseptic or treatment of chronic urolithiasis**</u><br>65–100 mg tid<br><br><u>**Maintenance therapy in chronic methemoglobinemia**</u><br>100–300 mg daily | | nausea, vomiting, diarrhea, bladder irritation<br><br><u>Pharmacokinetics</u><br>well absorbed from GI tract; reduced to leukomethylene blue in tissues; renal excretion | blue; G-6-PD deficient patients<br><br><u>Pregnancy:</u><br>Safety of methylene blue in pregnancy has not been established |
| **Metronidazole**<br>Flagyl, Protostat<br><br><u>Tablet:</u><br>250 mg, 500 mg<br><br><u>Gel, vaginal:</u><br>0.75% | <u>**Antibacterial Spectrum**</u><br>Anaerobic organisms including *Bacteroides* sp., *Clostridium* sp., *Peptostreptococcus* sp., and *Fusobacterium* sp.; *C. difficile* colitis; adjunct therapy in the treatment of *Helicobacter pylori*; bacterial vaginosis and giardiasis<br><br><u>**General indications**</u><br>250 mg tid or 500 mg bid for 7 to 14 days<br><br><u>**Trichomoniasis**</u><br>**Adults:** 2 gm as a single dose or 500 mg tid for 7 d<br><br>**Children:** 15 mg/kg/d divided q 8 h for 7 d<br><br><u>**Bacterial vaginosis**</u><br>500 mg bid for 7 days or 2 gm as a single dose or vaginal gel 5 gm intravaginally bid for 5 d<br><br><u>**Giardiasis**</u><br>**Adults:** 250 mg tid for 7 d<br><br>**Children:** 15 mg/kg/d divided q 8 h for 7 d | <u>Administration Issues</u><br>Complete full course of therapy; may take with food if GI upset occurs; avoid alcoholic beverages including beer; refrain from sexual intercourse during treatment of trichomoniasis to avoid reinfection<br><br><u>Drug–Drug Interactions</u><br>**Barbiturates** may decrease the effectiveness of metronidazole. **Cimetidine** may increase metronidazole serum concentrations. Metronidazole may increase the pharmacological and toxic effects of the following drugs: **warfarin, phenytoin, lithium.** Concomitant use of **ethanol** and metronidazole may produce flushing, nausea, vomiting, palpitations, and tachycardia | <u>ADRs:</u><br>dizziness, nausea, abdominal discomfort, diarrhea, metallic taste, superinfection<br><br><u>Pharmacokinetics:</u><br>achieves therapeutic levels in cerebrospinal fluid (50% of serum concentration); hepatic metabolism; renal excretion | <u>Contraindications</u><br>Hypersensitivity to metronidazole; pregnancy during first trimester<br><br><u>Pregnancy Category:</u> B<br>**Avoid metronidazole use during the first trimester of pregnancy**<br><br><u>Lactation Issues</u><br>Excreted in breast milk; nursing mothers should express and discard any breast milk produced while on the drug and resume nursing 24 to 48 hours after the drug is discontinued |

*(continues on next page)*

## 109. Miscellaneous Antimicrobial Agents *continued from previous page*

| Drug and Dosage Forms | Spectrum of Activity and Usual Dosage Range | Administration Issues and Drug–Drug & Drug–Food Interactions | Common Adverse Drug Reactions (ADRs) and Pharmacokinetics | Contraindications, Pregnancy Category, and Lactation Issues |
|---|---|---|---|---|
| **Metronidazole** *cont.* | **Treatment of *Helicobacter pylori***<br>250 mg tid for 14 d with bismuth subsalicylate 525 mg qid for 14 d and tetracycline 500 mg qid or amoxicillin 500 mg bid for 14 d<br><br>**Antibiotic-associated pseudomembranous colitis produced by *C. difficile***<br>250 mg qid or 500 mg tid for 7 to 14 d<br><br>**Treatment of intestinal amebiasis**<br>**Adults:** 750 mg q 8 h for 5 to 10 d<br><br>**Children:** 35–50 mg/kg/d up to max of 750 mg/dose divided q 8 h for 5 to 10 d | | | |
| **Neomycin Sulfate**<br><br>Tablet:<br>Various generics<br>500 mg<br><br>Oral Solution:<br>Mycifradin<br>125 mg/5 ml | **Antibacterial Spectrum**<br>bacteria of the intestinal tract<br><br>**Preoperative prophylaxis for elective colorectal surgery**<br>1 gm given in combination with erythromycin 1 gm at 19 hours, 18 hours, and 9 hours prior to procedure | Administration Issues<br>Complete full course of therapy; notify your physician, nurse, or pharmacist if ringing of the ears occurs<br><br>Drug–Drug Interactions<br>Oral aminoglycosides may decrease the absorption of the following drugs: **digoxin, methotrexate, vitamin A.** Oral aminoglycosides may increase effect of **warfarin** by decreasing absorption of dietary vitamin K | ADRs:<br>nausea, vomiting, diarrhea, ototoxicity, muscle weakness, superinfection<br><br>Pharmacokinetics:<br>poor systemic absorption; elimination of intestinal bacteria persists for 48–72 hours; fecal elimination | Contraindications<br>Presence of intestinal obstruction; hypersensitivity to aminoglycosides<br><br>Pregnancy Category: D<br><br>Lactation Issues<br>Aminoglycosides are excreted in breast milk; potential serious adverse reactions may occur in nursing infants; decide whether to discontinue nursing or to discontinue the drug |

| Pentamidine Isethionate | | | |
|---|---|---|---|
| NebuPent | | | |
| **Antibacterial Spectrum**<br>*Pneumocystis carinii*<br><br>**Prophylaxis of *Pneumocystis carinii* pneumonia**<br>300 mg once q 4 weeks via nebulization in the Respirgard® II nebulizer | Administration Issues<br>Reconstitute one vial with 6 ml Sterile Water for Injection, USP only; use of saline solution will cause the drug to precipitate; do not mix pentamidine solution with any other drugs for nebulization; the reconstituted solution is stable for 48 hours in the original vial | ADRs:<br>fatigue, metallic taste, shortness of breath, decreased appetite, dizziness, hypotension, hypoglycemia, hyperglycemia<br><br>Pharmacokinetics:<br>plasma concentrations via nebulization are substantially lower compared to intravenous dosing; renal excretion | Contraindications<br>Anaphylactic reaction to inhaled or intravenous pentamidine<br><br>Pregnancy Category: C<br><br>Lactation Issues<br>HIV infected females should not breast feed to avoid postnatal transmission of HIV to a child who may not be infected |
| Aerosol:<br>300 mg | | | |
| Vancomycin | | | |
| Vancocin | | | |
| **Antibacterial Spectrum**<br>*C. difficile*<br><br>**Antibiotic-associated pseudomembranous colitis produced by *C. difficile* or *Staphylococcus sp.*<br>Adults:** 125 mg qid for 7 to 14 d<br><br>**Children:** 40 mg/kg/d divided qid for 7 to 10 days. Do not exceed 2 gm/day<br><br>**Neonates:** 10 mg/kg/d divided qid for 7 to 10 d | Administration Issues<br>Complete full course of therapy<br><br>**Oral vancomycin is not effective for other types of infection. Metronidazole is the preferred agent for mild to moderate cases of *C difficile* colitis**<br><br>Drug–Drug Interactions<br>Rare due to lack of systemic absorption | ADRs:<br>Rare due to lack of systemic absorption, superinfection<br><br>Pharmacokinetics:<br>very poor systemic absorption; fecal elimination | Contraindications<br>Hypersensitivity of vancomycin<br><br>Pregnancy Category: C<br><br>Lactation Issues<br>Limited systemic absorption with orally administered vancomycin, however, use with caution in nursing mothers |
| Capsule:<br>125 mg, 250 mg | | | |
| Powder for Oral Solution:<br>1 gm bottle<br>10 gm bottle | | | |
| **The parenteral product may be given orally** | | | |

| Drug and Dosage Forms | Usual Dosage Range | Administration Issues and Drug–Drug & Drug–Food Interactions | Common Adverse Drug Reactions (ADRs) and Pharmacokinetics | Contraindications, Pregnancy Category, and Lactation Issues |
|---|---|---|---|---|
| **Isosorbide Dinitrate**<br>Dilatrate-SR, Isordil, Sorbitrate<br><br>Sublingual Tablets:<br>2.5 mg, 5 mg, 10 mg<br><br>Chewable Tablets:<br>5 mg, 10 mg<br><br>Tablets:<br>5 mg, 10 mg, 20 mg, 30 mg, 40 mg<br><br>Sustained Release Tablets:<br>40 mg<br><br>Sustained Release Capsules:<br>40 mg | **Prevention and treatment of angina pectoris:**<br><br>sublingual tablets:<br>2.5–5 mg initially and titrate to relief of angina<br><br>chewable tablets:<br>5–10 mg initially and titrate to relief of angina<br><br>oral tablets:<br>initial dose: 5–20 mg tid<br>maintenance dose: 10–40 mg tid<br><br>SR tablets/capsules:<br>40–80 mg qd, bid or tid as needed | Administration Issues:<br>safety and efficacy have not been established in children; tolerance may develop—adjust dosing schedule to allow a "nitrate-free" period; do not crush or chew sustained release or sublingual tablets; do not crush chewable tablets before administering<br><br>Drug–Drug Interactions:<br>severe hypotension may occur in patients who drink **alcohol**; orthostatic hypotension may occur in patients taking **calcium channel blockers** | ADRs<br>headache, GI upset, flushing, hypotension, rash<br><br>Pharmacokinetics<br>absorption = 100%; SR onset = 4 hours, duration = 6–8 hours; sublingual onset = 2–5 minutes, duration = 1–3 hours; regular release onset = 20–40 minutes, duration = 4–6 hours; hepatically metabolized; 60% protein binding | Contraindications:<br>hypersensitivity to nitrates; severe anemia; closed angle glaucoma; orthostatic hypotension; head trauma or cerebral hemorrhage<br><br>Pregnancy Category: C<br><br>Lactation Issues:<br>it is not known whether nitrates are excreted in breast milk |
| **Isosorbide Mononitrate**<br>Imdur, ISMO, Monoket<br><br>Tablets:<br>10 mg, 20 mg | **Prevention of angina pectoris**<br><br>regular release tablets:<br>20 mg twice daily given 7 hours apart<br><br>extended release tablets:<br>30–120 mg daily | Administration Issues:<br>safety and efficacy have not been established in children; tolerance may develop—adjust dosing schedule to allow a "nitrate-free" period; do not crush or chew extended release tablets but may break tablets | ADRs<br>headache, GI upset, flushing, hypotension, rash<br><br>Pharmacokinetics<br>absorption = 100%; hepatically metabolized; 60% protein binding; onset 30–60 min | Contraindications:<br>hypersensitivity to nitrates; severe anemia; closed angle glaucoma; orthostatic hypotension; head trauma or cerebral hemorrhage<br><br>Pregnancy Category: C |

| | | | |
|---|---|---|---|
| Extended Release Tablets:<br>60 mg | | | Lactation Issues:<br>it is not known whether nitrates are excreted in breast milk |
| **Nitroglycerin Sublingual**<br>Nitrostat<br><br>Tablets:<br>0.15 mg, 0.3 mg, 0.4 mg, 0.6 mg | **prophylaxis of angina pectoris**<br>1 tablet under tongue or between cheek and gum 5–10 minutes before activities which may precipitate an anginal attack<br><br>**treatment of acute anginal attack**<br>1 tablet immediately—may repeat every 5 minutes up to 3 tablets in 15 minutes; if no relief, call physician or EMS | Drug–Drug Interactions:<br>severe hypotension may occur in patients who drink **alcohol;** orthostatic hypotension may occur in patients taking **calcium channel blockers**<br><br>Administration Issues:<br>safety and efficacy have not been established in children; decreased absorption may occur in patients with a dry mouth<br><br>Drug–Drug Interactions:<br>severe hypotension may occur in patients who drink **alcohol;** orthostatic hypotension may occur in patients taking **calcium channel blockers** | ADRs<br>headache, flushing, hypotension, rash, local burning or tingling sensation<br><br>Pharmacokinetics<br>absorption = 100%; onset = 1–3 minutes; duration = 30–60 minutes | Contraindications:<br>hypersensitivity to nitrates; severe anemia; closed angle glaucoma; orthostatic hypotension; head trauma or cerebral hemorrhage<br><br>Pregnancy Category: C<br><br>Lactation Issues:<br>it is not known whether nitrates are excreted in breast milk |
| **Nitroglycerin, Sustained-Release**<br>Nitrong, Nitro-Bid, Nitrocine Timecaps, Nitroglyn<br><br>Sustained Release Tablets:<br>2.6 mg, 6.5 mg, 9 mg<br><br>Sustained Release Capsules:<br>2.5 mg, 6.5 mg, 9 mg, 13 mg | **prevention of angina pectoris:**<br><br>maintenance dose:<br>2.5–13 mg bid<br><br>maximum dose:<br>26 mg bid | Administration Issues:<br>safety and efficacy have not been established in children; tolerance may develop—adjust dosing schedule to allow a "nitrate-free" period; do not crush or chew extended release tablets<br><br>Drug–Drug Interactions:<br>severe hypotension may occur in patients who drink **alcohol;** orthostatic hypotension may occur in patients taking **calcium channel blockers** | ADRs<br>headache, GI upset; flushing; hypotension; rash<br><br>Pharmacokinetics<br>absorption = 100%; onset = 20–45 minutes; duration = 3–8 hours | Contraindications:<br>hypersensitivity to nitrates; severe anemia; closed angle glaucoma; orthostatic hypotension; head trauma or cerebral hemorrhage<br><br>Pregnancy Category: C<br><br>Lactation Issues:<br>it is not known whether nitrates are excreted in breast milk |
| **Nitroglycerin, Topical**<br>Nitro-Bid, Nitrol | **prevention and treatment of angina pectoris:**<br><br>initial dose:<br>1/2 inch q 6–8 hours | Administration Issues:<br>safety and efficacy have not been established in children; tolerance may develop—adjust dosing schedule to allow to | ADRs<br>headache, flushing, hypotension, rash, topical allergic reactions, erythematous, vesicular and pruritic lesions | Contraindications:<br>hypersensitivity to nitrates; severe anemia; closed angle glaucoma; orthostatic hypotension |

(continues on next page)

## 201. Antianginal Agents *continued from previous page*

| Drug and Dosage Forms | Usual Dosage Range | Administration Issues and Drug–Drug & Drug–Food Interactions | Common Adverse Drug Reactions (ADRs) and Pharmacokinetics | Contraindications, Pregnancy Category, and Lactation Issues |
|---|---|---|---|---|
| **Nitroglycerin, Topical cont.**<br>Ointment:<br>2% | maximum dose:<br>2 inches q 6–8 hours<br><br>"wipe off" (or do not give) at midnight to allow a "nitrate-free" period | non-hairy area; do not apply to distal parts of extremities; avoid areas with cuts or irritations<br><br>Drug–Drug Interactions:<br>severe hypotension may occur in patients who drink **alcohol;** orthostatic hypotension may occur in patients taking **calcium channel blockers** | Pharmacokinetics<br>absorption = 100%; onset = 30–60 minutes; duration = 2–12 hours | Pregnancy Category:  C<br><br>Lactation Issues:<br>it is not known whether nitrates are excreted in breast milk |
| **Nitroglycerin, Transdermal**<br>Deponit, Minitran, Nitro-Dur, Nitrodisc, Transderm-Nitro<br><br>Patches:<br>0.1 mg/hr, 0.2 mg/hr,<br>0.3 mg/hr, 0.4 mg/hr,<br>0.6 mg/hr, 0.8 mg/hr | **prevention of angina pectoris:**<br><br>initial dose:<br>0.2–0.4 mg/hr daily<br><br>maximum dose:<br>0.8 mg/hr daily<br><br>remove for at least 12–14 hr to allow a "nitrate-free" period | Administration Issues:<br>safety and efficacy have not been established in children; tolerance may develop—adjust dosing schedule to allow a "nitrate-free" period; apply to non-hairy area; do not apply to distal parts of extremities; avoid areas with cuts or irritations; should not be used for acute anginal attacks<br><br>Drug–Drug Interactions:<br>severe hypotension may occur in patients who drink **alcohol;** orthostatic hypotension may occur in patients taking **calcium channel blockers** | ADRs<br>headache, flushing, hypotension, rash, contact dermatitis<br><br>Pharmacokinetics<br>absorption = 100%; onset = 30–60 minutes; duration is up to 24 hours | Contraindications:<br>hypersensitivity to nitrates; severe anemia; closed angle glaucoma; orthostatic hypotension; allergy to adhesives<br><br>Pregnancy Category:  C<br><br>Lactation Issues:<br>it is not known whether nitrates are excreted in breast milk |
| **Nitroglycerin, Translingual**<br>Nitrolingual | **prophylaxis of angina pectoris:**<br>1–2 sprays onto or under tongue 5–10 minutes before activities which may precipitate an anginal attack | Administration Issues:<br>safety and efficacy have not been established in children; should not be inhaled | ADRs<br>headache, flushing, hypotension, rash, local burning or tingling sensation | Contraindications:<br>hypersensitivity to nitrates; severe anemia; closed angle glaucoma; orthostatic hypotension |

1036

| Drug and Dosage Forms | Usual Dosage Range | Administration Issues and Drug–Drug & Drug–Food Interactions | Pharmacokinetics | Contraindications |
|---|---|---|---|---|
| Spray:<br>0.4 mg per metered dose | treatment of an acute anginal attack:<br>1–2 sprays onto or under tongue q 5 minutes up to 3 doses in 15 minutes; if no relief, call physician or EMS | Drug–Drug Interactions:<br>severe hypotension may occur in patients who drink **alcohol**; orthostatic hypotension may occur in patients taking **calcium channel blockers** | Pharmacokinetics<br>absorption = 100%; onset = 2 minutes; duration = 30–60 minutes | Pregnancy Category: C<br><br>Lactation Issues:<br>it is not known whether nitrates are excreted in breast milk |
| **Nitroglycerin, Transmucosal**<br>Nitrogard<br><br>Controlled Release Buccal Tablets:<br>1 mg, 2 mg, 3 mg | **prevention of angina pectoris:**<br>1 mg q 3–5 hours while awake<br><br>Place tablet between lip and gum above incisors or between cheek and gum | Administration Issues:<br>safety and efficacy have not been established in children; tolerance may develop—adjust dosing schedule to allow a "nitrate-free" period; do not crush or chew extended release tablets<br><br>Drug–Drug Interactions:<br>severe hypotension may occur in patients who drink **alcohol**; orthostatic hypotension may occur in patients taking **calcium channel blockers** | ADRs<br>headache; flushing; hypotension; rash; local burning or tingling sensation<br><br>Pharmacokinetics<br>absorption = 100%; onset = 1–2 minutes; duration = 3–5 hours | Contraindications:<br>hypersensitivity to nitrates; severe anemia; closed angle glaucoma; orthostatic hypotension<br><br>Pregnancy Category: C<br><br>Lactation Issues:<br>it is not known whether nitrates are excreted in breast milk |

## 202. Antiarrhythmic Agents

| Drug and Dosage Forms | Usual Dosage Range | Administration Issues and Drug–Drug & Drug–Food Interactions | Common Adverse Drug Reactions (ADRs) and Pharmacokinetics | Contraindications, Pregnancy Category, and Lactation Issues |
|---|---|---|---|---|
| **Amiodarone**<br>Cordarone<br><br>Tablets:<br>200 mg | **life-threatening recurrent ventricular fibrillation or hemodynamically unstable ventricular tachycardia**<br><br>Loading dose<br>800–1600 mg/d in divided doses for 1–3 weeks | Administration Issues: Safety and efficacy in children have not been established; administer with meals to minimized GI upset<br><br>Drug–Drug Interactions: amiodarone may potentiate the effect of **warfarin;** amiodarone may increase **digoxin, theophylline, phenytoin,** | ADRs<br>Proarrhythmia, corneal microdeposits, pulmonary toxicity, hypothyroidism or hyperthyroidism, photosensitivity, pulmonary fibrosis, worsening congestive heart failure, elevated liver enzymes (AST, ALT), blue discoloration of the skin, GI | Contraindications:<br>severe sinus node dysfunction; second or third degree heart block in the absence of a pacemaker; hypersensitivity to amiodarone<br><br>Pregnancy Category: D |

(continues on next page)

| Drug and Dosage Forms | Usual Dosage Range | Administration Issues and Drug–Drug & Drug–Food Interactions | Common Adverse Drug Reactions (ADRs) and Pharmacokinetics | Contraindications, Pregnancy Category, and Lactation Issues |
|---|---|---|---|---|
| **Amiodarone** *cont.* | Maintenance dose 200–600 mg/d (use lowest effective dose) | **methotrexate, procainamide, quinidine, flecainide and cyclosporine concentrations** | upset, dizziness, ataxia, tremor, fatigue, paresthesias<br><br>Pharmacokinetics<br>absorption = 50%; $v_d$ = 60 l/kg; 96% protein binding; hepatically metabolized; $T_{1/2}$ = 40–55 d | Lactation Issues:<br>amiodarone is excreted in breast milk; either the drug or nursing should be discontinued |
| **Disopyramide**<br>Norpace<br><br>Capsules:<br>100 mg, 150 mg<br><br>Capsules, Extended Release:<br>100 mg, 150 mg | **life-threatening ventricular arrhythmias**<br><br>Patients with moderate renal insufficiency, hepatic insufficiency or adults < 50 kg<br>400 mg/day (q 6 h with regular release capsules and q 12 h with extended release capsules)<br><br>**Adults > 50 kg**<br>400–800 mg/day in divided doses<br><br>**Children (in divided doses):**<br><1 year: 10–30 mg/kg/d<br>1–4 years: 10–20 mg/kg/d<br>4–12 years: 10–15 mg/kg/d<br>12–18 years: 6–15 mg/kg/d | Administration issues:<br>correct hypokalemia or hyperkalemia before instituting therapy<br><br>Drug–Drug Interactions:<br>disopyramide may increase **digoxin** concentrations; **erythromycin** may increase disopyramide levels; **phenytoin** and **rifampin** may decrease disopyramide levels; disopyramide may decrease the effect of **warfarin** | ADRs<br>Dry mouth, urinary hesitancy and retention, constipation, blurred vision, hypotension, congestive heart failure, dizziness, fatigue, headache, GI upset, rash, muscle pain or weakness<br><br>Pharmacokinetics<br>absorption = 90%; 50% excreted in urine as unchanged drug; $T_{1/2}$ = 4–10 hours; $T_{1/2}$ prolonged with impaired renal function ($T_{1/2}$ = 8–18 hours) | Contraindications:<br>hypersensitivity to disopyramide; pre-existing second or third degree heart block (if no pacemaker present); congenital QT prolongation; sick sinus syndrome<br><br>Pregnancy Category: C<br><br>Lactation Issues:<br>disopyramide is present in breast milk; either the drug or nursing should be discontinued |
| **Encainide**<br>Enkaid | **life-threatening ventricular arrhythmias** | Administration issues:<br>Safety and efficacy in children < 18 years of age have not been established | ADRs<br>Proarrhythmia, dizziness, blurred vision, headache, worsening | Contraindications:<br>hypersensitivity to encainide; symptomatic non-sustained |

| | | | | |
|---|---|---|---|---|
| Capsules: 25 mg, 35 mg, 50 mg **Encainide has been voluntarily withdrawn from the market by the manufacturer; available on a limited basis** | Initial dose: 25 mg q 8 h Maintenance dose: 25–50 mg q 8 h Allow 3–5 days before dosage adjustments; patients with renal or hepatic impairment may be controlled with lower doses | Drug–Drug Interactions: cimetidine increases the concentration of encainide and its metabolites | congestive heart failure, palpitations Pharmacokinetics absorption = 100%; absorption rate but not extent is decreased when administered with food; 75–80% protein binding; hepatically metabolized to two active metabolites | ventricular arrhythmias and frequent premature ventricular complexes; pre-existing second or third degree heart block unless a pacemaker is present Pregnancy Category: B Lactation Issues: encainide is excreted in breast milk; either the drug or nursing should be discontinued |
| **Flecainide** Tambocor Tablets: 50 mg, 100 mg, 150 mg | **prevention of paroxysmal atrial flutter, atrial fibrillation or supraventricular tachycardia with disabling symptoms without structural heart disease** Initial dose: 50 mg q 12 h Maintenance dose: 50–100 mg q 12 h maximum dose = 300 mg/d **life threatening ventricular arrhythmias (use lower doses in renal impairment)** Initial dose: 100 mg q 12 h Maintenance dose: 100–150 mg q 12 h maximum dose = 400 mg/d | Administration issues: Safety and efficacy in children <18 years of age have not been established Drug–Drug Interactions: **phenytoin** and **rifampin** may decrease tocainide concentrations; flecainide may increase **digoxin** concentrations; smoking increases flecainide clearance; **cimetidine** may increase flecainide concentrations; additive effects occur when given with other negative inotropic agents (**beta blockers, verapamil**); **amiodarone** may increase plasma levels; use caution in coadministration of disopyramide | ADRs: Proarrhythmia; dizziness; dyspnea; headache; nausea; fatigue; palpitations; chest pain; tremor; asthenia; constipation; edema; GI upset; worsening congestive heart failure Pharmacokinetics absorption = 100%; 40% protein binding; $T_{1/2}$ = 12–27 hours; accumulation may occur with renal or hepatic impairment | Contraindications: hypersensitivity to flecainide; pre-existing second or third degree heart block in the absence of a pacemaker; cardiogenic shock Pregnancy Category: C Lactation Issues: flecainide is excreted in breast milk; either the drug or nursing should be discontinued |

(continues on next page)

| Drug and Dosage Forms | Usual Dosage Range | Administration Issues and Drug–Drug & Drug–Food Interactions | Common Adverse Drug Reactions (ADRs) and Pharmacokinetics | Contraindications, Pregnancy Category, and Lactation Issues |
|---|---|---|---|---|
| **Mexiletine**<br>Mexitil<br><br>Capsules:<br>150 mg, 200 mg, 250 mg | **life-threatening ventricular arrhythmias**<br><br>Initial dose:<br>200 mg q 8 h<br><br>Maintenance dose:<br>200–400 mg q 8 h<br>maximum dose = 1200 mg/d<br><br>Patients with hepatic impairment may be controlled with lower dosages | Administration issues:<br>take with food or an antacid to minimize GI upset<br><br>safety and efficacy in children have not been established<br><br>Drug–Drug Interactions:<br>mexiletine may increase theophylline concentration; rifampin and phenytoin may lower mexiletine concentrations | ADRs<br>Proarrhythmia, GI upset, tremor, lightheadedness, headache, coordination difficulties, palpitations, chest pain, worsening congestive heart failure, diarrhea, constipation, dry mouth, tremor<br><br>Pharmacokinetics<br>absorption = 90%; 50–60% protein binding; hepatically metabolized; $T_{1/2}$ = 10–12 hours (prolonged with hepatic impairment) | Contraindications:<br>hypersensitivity to mexiletine; pre-existing second or third degree heart block in the absence of a pacemaker; cardiogenic shock<br><br>Pregnancy Category: C<br><br>Lactation Issues:<br>mexiletine is excreted in breast milk; either the drug or nursing should be discontinued |
| **Moricizine**<br>Ethmozine<br><br>Tablets:<br>200 mg, 250 mg, 300 mg | **life-threatening ventricular arrhythmias**<br><br>600–900 mg/d divided q 8 h<br><br>In patients with hepatic or renal impairment, start with doses ≤ 600 mg/d | Administration issues:<br>administering after meals slows the rate of absorption but does not decrease the extent of absorption; safety and efficacy in children < 18 years of age have not been established<br><br>Drug–Drug Interactions:<br>cimetidine increases moricizine concentrations; moricizine decreases theophylline concentrations 44–66% | ADRs<br>Proarrhythmia, palpitations, dizziness, headache, fatigue, nausea, dyspnea<br><br>Pharmacokinetics<br>significant first-pass metabolism; large $V_d$ (≥ 300L); 95% protein binding; mainly hepatically metabolized; < 1% excreted unchanged in urine; induces its own metabolism; $T_{1/2}$ = 1.5–3.5 hours | Contraindications:<br>hypersensitivity to moricizine; pre-existing second or third degree heart block; bifasicular block unless a pacemaker is present<br><br>Pregnancy Category: B<br><br>Lactation Issues:<br>moricizine is present in breast milk; because of the potential for serious adverse effects, either the drug or nursing should be discontinued |

| Drug | Dosing | Administration issues | ADRs / Pharmacokinetics | Contraindications / Pregnancy / Lactation |
|---|---|---|---|---|
| **Procainamide**<br>Pronestyl, Procan SR<br><br>Regular release tablet:<br>250 mg, 375 mg, 500 mg<br><br>Regular release capsules:<br>250 mg, 375 mg, 500 mg<br><br>Sustained release tablets:<br>250 mg, 500 mg, 750 mg, 1000 mg | **life-threatening ventricular arrhythmias**<br><br>50 mg/kg/d (q 3 h with regular release products and q 6 h with SR products)<br><br>**Children (suggested dosing):**<br>15–50 mg/kg/d in divided doses q 3–6 h (maximum 4 grams/d) | Administration issues:<br>patients > 50 years of age, or patients with renal, hepatic or cardiac insufficiency may require lower doses or longer dosing intervals; safety and efficacy in children have not been established<br><br>Drug–Drug Interactions:<br>**beta blockers, cimetidine, ranitidine,** and trimethoprim may increase procainamide concentrations.<br><br>**Therapeutic range = 4–8 mcg/ml** | ADRs<br>Proarrhythmia, lupus erythematosus, neutropenia, thrombocytopenia, rash, GI upset, dizziness<br><br>Pharmacokinetics<br>well absorbed; $T_{1/2} \approx$ 1–3 hours; metabolized to N-acetyl procainamide (NAPA) which is renally eliminated | Contraindications:<br>hypersensitivity to procainamide; complete heart block; lupus erythematosus; torsades de pointes<br><br>Pregnancy Category: C<br><br>Lactation Issues:<br>procainamide and NAPA are present in breast milk; either the drug or nursing should be discontinued |
| **Propafenone**<br>Rythmol<br><br>Tablets:<br>150 mg, 300 mg | **life-threatening ventricular arrhythmias**<br><br>Initial dose:<br>150 mg q 8 h<br><br>Maintenance dose:<br>150–300 mg q 8 h<br><br>Usual max dose 900 mg/d<br><br>allow 3–4 days between dosage adjustments | Administration issues:<br>Safety and efficacy in children have not been established<br><br>Drug–Drug Interactions:<br>**Cimetidine** may increase propafenone concentrations; **rifampin** may decrease propafenone concentrations; propafenone may potentiate the effects of **warfarin; propafenone** may increase **digoxin** and **cyclosporine** concentrations and may increase plasma levels and pharmacologic effects of **beta blockers** | ADRS<br>Proarrhythmia, dizziness, unusual taste, first degree AV block, intraventricular conduction delay, nausea, vomiting, constipation, headache, worsening congestive heart failure, palpitations<br><br>Pharmacokinetics<br>absorption = 100%; undergoes extensive first-pass metabolism; absolute bioavailability = 3–20%; hepatically metabolized; $T_{1/2}$ = 2–10 hours; metabolites renally eliminated | Contraindications:<br>hypersensitivity to propafenone; uncontrolled congestive heart failure; pre-existing second or third degree heart block or sick sinus syndrome in the absence of a pacemaker; bradycardia; marked hypotension; bronchospastic disease; electrolyte imbalance<br><br>Pregnancy Category: C<br><br>Lactation Issues:<br>it is not known whether propafenone is excreted in breast milk; either the drug or nursing should be discontinued |
| **Quinidine**<br>Quinidex, Quinaglute<br>Dura-Tabs, Cardioquin | **paroxysmal supraventricular tachycardia (PSVT): atrial flutter; atrial fibrillation; ventricular tachycardia** | Administration issues:<br>take with food to minimize GI upset; safety and efficacy in children have not been established | ADRS<br>proarrhythmia, QRS prolongation (torsades de pointes), GI upset, diarrhea, drug fever, rash, | Contraindications:<br>hypersensitivity to quinidine, myasthenia gravis, complete heart block or severe |

(continues on next page)

**202. Antiarrhythmic Agents**  *continued from previous page*

| Drug and Dosage Forms | Usual Dosage Range | Administration Issues and Drug–Drug & Drug–Food Interactions | Common Adverse Drug Reactions (ADRs) and Pharmacokinetics | Contraindications, Pregnancy Category, and Lactation Issues |
|---|---|---|---|---|
| **Quinidine** *cont.*<br><br>Regular release tablets:<br>quinidine sulfate 200 mg, 300 mg<br><br>quinidine polygalacturonate 275 mg<br><br>Sustained release tablets:<br>quinidine sulfate 300 mg<br>quinidine gluconate 324 mg | regular release tablets<br>200–300 mg tid to qid<br><br>sustained release tablets<br>300–600 mg q 8–12 h<br><br>**children (suggested dosing):**<br>30 mg/kg/d or 900 mg/m²/d in divided doses | Drug–Drug Interactions:<br>hepatic enzyme inducers (**phenytoin, rifampin, phenobarbital**) may decrease quinidine concentrations; hepatic enzyme inhibitors (**cimetidine**) may increase quinidine concentrations; quinidine increases **digoxin** concentrations; **verapamil** increases quinidine concentrations; quinidine may potentiate the anticoagulant effect of **warfarin**<br><br>**Therapeutic range: 2–6 mcg/mL** | photosensitivity, drug-induced lupus erythematosus, ringing in the ears<br><br>Pharmacokinetics<br>absorption = 70%; 80–90% protein binding; 60–80% hepatically metabolized; T$_{1/2}$ = 4–10 hours | intraventricular conduction defects, history of drug induced torsades de pointes or long QT syndrome; thrombocytopenia purpura<br><br>Pregnancy Category:  C<br><br>Lactation Issues:<br>quinidine is excreted in breast milk; use with caution; the American Academy of Pediatrics considers quinidine to be compatible with breast feeding |
| **Tocainide**<br>Tonocard<br><br>Tablets:<br>400 mg, 600 mg | **life-threatening ventricular arrhythmias**<br><br>initial dose: 400 mg q 8 h<br><br>maintenance dose:<br>400–600 mg q 8 h<br><br>patients with renal or hepatic impairment may be controlled with lower doses | Administration issues:<br>hypokalemia should be corrected prior to initiating tocainide<br><br>Drug–Drug Interactions:<br>**cimetidine** and **rifampin** may decrease tocainide concentrations | ADRS<br>proarrhythmia, dizziness, vertigo, nausea, paresthesia, tremor, drowsiness, worsening congestive heart failure, blood dyscrasias; pulmonary fibrosis<br><br>Pharmacokinetics<br>absorption = 100%; T$_{1/2}$ = 15 hours (prolonged in severe renal impairment) | Contraindications:<br>hypersensitivity to tocainide or amide-type local anesthetics; second or third degree heart block in the absence of a pacemaker<br><br>Pregnancy Category: C<br><br>Lactation Issues:<br>tocainide is excreted into breast milk; either the drug or nursing should be discontinued |

## 203. Anticoagulants

| Drug and Dosage Forms | Usual Dosage Range | Administration Issues and Drug–Drug & Drug–Food Interactions | Common Adverse Drug Reactions (ADRs) and Pharmacokinetics | Contraindications, Pregnancy Category, and Lactation Issues |
|---|---|---|---|---|
| **Warfarin**<br>Coumadin, Panwarfarin, Sofarin<br><br>Tablets:<br>1 mg, 2 mg, 2.5 mg, 3 mg, 4 mg, 5 mg, 6 mg, 7.5 mg, 10 mg | **prophylaxis and treatment of deep venous thrombosis (DVT) or pulmonary embolism (PE) and atrial fibrillation with embolization; prophylaxis of systemic embolism after myocardial infarction (MI):** titrate dose to international normalized ratio (INR) between 2–3<br><br>**prophylaxis of systemic embolism in valves:** titrate dose to international normalized ratio (INR) between 2.5–3.5<br><br>Usual dosage range: 1–15 mg/d | Administration Issues:<br>safety and efficacy have not been established in children <18 years of age<br><br>Drug–Drug Interactions:<br>**NSAIDs** and **salicylates** may increase the risk of bleeding; hepatic enzyme inducers (**phenytoin, carbamazepine, rifampin, phenobarbital**) may decrease the anticoagulant effect; **amiodarone, TMP/SMZ, erythromycin, ciprofloxacin, metronidazole, fluconazole, ketoconazole, quinidine, omeprazole, gemfibrozil** and **acetaminophen** may potentiate the anticoagulant effect | ADRs<br>bleeding (major and minor); GI upset, rash<br><br>Pharmacokinetics<br>absorption = 100%; 95% protein binding; hepatically metabolized to inactive metabolites that are renally eliminated; $T_{1/2}$ = 1–2.5 d | Contraindications:<br>pregnancy; hemorrhagic tendencies; active bleeding; uncontrolled, malignant hypertension; history of warfarin-induced necrosis<br><br>Pregnancy Category: X<br><br>Lactation Issues:<br>warfarin is excreted in breast milk in an inactive form; infants nursed by warfarin-treated mothers had no change in prothrombin time (PT) |

## 204. Antihyperlipidemic Agents
### 204.1 Bile Acid Sequestrants

| Drug and Dosage Forms | Usual Dosage Range | Administration Issues and Drug–Drug & Drug–Food Interactions | Common Adverse Drug Reactions (ADRs) and Pharmacokinetics | Contraindications, Pregnancy Category, and Lactation Issues |
|---|---|---|---|---|
| **Cholestyramine**<br>Questran, Questran Light, Prevalite<br><br>Questran powder:<br>49 grams/9 grams of powder<br><br>Questran Light powder:<br>4 grams/5 grams of powder | **hyperlipidemia:**<br><br>powder<br>4 grams 1–6 times daily<br><br>tablets<br>initial dose: 4 grams qd to bid<br><br>maintenance dose: 8–16 grams bid | Administration Issues:<br>take before meals; powder form should be mixed with fluid; other medications should be taken 1 hour before or 4–6 hours after taking cholestyramine; swallow tablets whole–do not crush or chew<br><br>Drug–Drug Interactions:<br>bile acid resins may interfere with the absorption of **warfarin, digoxin, gemfibrozil, glipizide, propranolol, tetracyclines; thiazide diuretics, thyroid hormone** and **vitamins A, D, E and K, aspirin, penicillin** | ADRs<br>constipation; abdominal pain, bloating or cramping; transient increases in AST, ALT and alkaline phosphatase; increased triglycerides<br><br>Pharmacokinetics<br>not significantly absorbed from the GI tract | Contraindications:<br>hypersensitivity to bile acid resins; complete biliary obstruction<br><br>Pregnancy Category: safety for use during pregnancy has not been established<br><br>Lactation Issues:<br>use caution when nursing—the potential lack of proper vitamin absorption may have an effect on nursing infants |
| **Colestipol**<br>Colestid<br><br>Granules<br>5 gm colestipol/7.5 gm powder<br><br>Tablets:<br>1 gram | **hyperlipidemia**<br><br>**granules**<br>initial dose: 5 grams qd to bid<br><br>maintenance dose: 5–30 grams qd or in divided doses<br><br>**tablets:**<br>initial dose: 2 grams qd to bid<br><br>maintenance dose: 2–16 grams qd or in divided doses | Administration Issues:<br>take before meals; powder form should be mixed with fluid; other medications should be taken 1 hour before or 4–6 hours after taking colestipol; swallow tablets whole—do not crush or chew<br><br>Drug–Drug Interactions:<br>bile acid resins may interfere with the absorption of **warfarin, digoxin, gemfibrozil, glipizide, propranolol, tetracyclines; thiazide diuretics, thyroid hormone** and **vitamins A, D, E and K** | ADRs<br>constipation, abdominal pain, bloating or cramping; transient increases in AST, ALT and alkaline phosphatase, increased triglycerides<br><br>Pharmacokinetics<br>not significantly absorbed from the GI tract | Contraindications:<br>hypersensitivity to bile acid resins; complete biliary obstruction<br><br>Pregnancy Category: safety for use during pregnancy has not been established<br><br>Lactation Issues:<br>use caution when nursing—the potential lack of proper vitamin absorption may have an effect on nursing infants |

## 204.2  HMG-CoA Reductase Inhibitors

| Drug and Dosage Forms | Usual Dosage Range | Administration Issues and Drug–Drug & Drug–Food Interactions | Common Adverse Drug Reactions (ADRs) and Pharmacokinetics | Contraindications, Pregnancy Category, and Lactation Issues |
|---|---|---|---|---|
| **Atorvastatin**<br>Lipitor<br><br><u>Tablets</u><br>10 mg, 20 mg 40 mg | **hypercholesterolemia**<br><u>Initial Dose:</u>  10 mg/d<br><br><u>Dose Range:</u>  10–80  mg/d | <u>Administration Issues:</u><br>May be given without regards to food<br><br><u>Drug–Drug Interactions:</u><br>atorvastatin may potentiate the anticoagulant effects of **warfarin;** concurrent use with **erythromycin, gemfibrozil** or **niacin** may lead to severe myopathy or rhabdomyolysis; coadministration with **Maalox TC** may decrease atorvastatin levels | <u>ADRs:</u><br>increased serum transaminases (AST, ALT), headache, myalgia, rash, flatulence, dyspepsia<br><br><u>Pharmacokinetics:</u><br>98% protein binding, undergoes hepatic recycling, $T_{1/2}$ = 14 h | <u>Contraindications:</u><br>hypersensitivity to HMG-CoA reductase inhibitors; active liver disease or unexplained persistent elevated liver function tests; pregnancy; lactation; use with caution in patients who consume excessive amounts of alcohol<br><br><u>Pregnancy Category:</u>  X<br><br><u>Lactation Issues:</u><br>women taking HMG-CoA reductase inhibitors should not nurse while taking these agents |
| **Fluvastatin**<br>Lescol<br><br><u>Capsules:</u><br>20 mg, 40 mg | **hypercholesterolemia**<br>20–40 mg/day as a single dose in the evening | <u>Administration Issues:</u><br>safety and efficacy in children < 18 years of age have not been established; dose should be taken in the evening<br><br><u>Drug–Drug Interactions:</u><br>fluvastatin may potentiate the anticoagulant effects of **warfarin;** concurrent use with **gemfibrozil** may lead to severe myopathy or rhabdomyolysis; **rifampin** may decrease fluvastatin levels | <u>ADRs</u><br>increased serum transaminases (AST, ALT), GI upset, muscle pain, headache, rash, photosensitivity, lens opacities (association unknown)<br><br><u>Pharmacokinetics:</u><br>extensive first pass metabolism; $T_{1/2}$ = 1.2 hours; 98% protein binding | <u>Contraindications:</u><br>hypersensitivity to HMG-CoA reductase inhibitors; active liver disease or unexplained persistent elevated liver function tests; pregnancy; lactation<br><br><u>Pregnancy Category:</u>  X<br><br><u>Lactation Issues:</u><br>women taking HMG-CoA reductase inhibitors should not nurse while taking these agents |

(continues on next page)

## 204.2 HMG-CoA Reductase Inhibitors *continued from previous page*

| Drug and Dosage Forms | Usual Dosage Range | Administration Issues and Drug–Drug & Drug–Food Interactions | Common Adverse Drug Reactions (ADRs) and Pharmacokinetics | Contraindications, Pregnancy Category, and Lactation Issues |
|---|---|---|---|---|
| **Lovastatin**<br>Mevacor<br><u>Tablets:</u><br>10 mg, 20 mg, 40 mg | **hypercholesterolemia; atherosclerosis:**<br><br>20–80 mg/day in single or divided doses<br><br>maximum recommended dose in patients taking immunosuppressive agents: 20 mg/d | <u>Administration Issues:</u><br>safety and efficacy in children < 18 years of age have not been established; dose should be taken with the evening meal<br><br><u>Drug–Drug Interactions:</u><br>lovastatin may potentiate the anticoagulant effects of **warfarin**; concurrent use with **gemfibrozil, cyclosporine, erythromycin** or **niacin** may lead to severe myopathy or rhabdomyolysis<br><br><u>Drug–Food Interactions:</u><br>administering lovastatin with food increases its bioavailability | <u>ADRs:</u><br>increased serum transaminases (AST, ALT), GI upset, muscle pain, headache, rash, photosensitivity, lens opacities (association unknown)<br><br><u>Pharmacokinetics</u><br>extensive first pass metabolism, 95% protein binding | <u>Contraindications:</u><br>hypersensitivity to HMG-CoA reductase inhibitors; active liver disease or unexplained persistent elevated liver function tests; pregnancy; lactation<br><br><u>Pregnancy Category:</u>  X<br><br><u>Lactation Issues:</u><br>women taking HMG-CoA reductase inhibitors should not nurse while taking these agents |
| **Pravastatin**<br>Pravachol<br><u>Tablets:</u><br>10 mg, 20 mg, 40 mg | **hypercholesterolemia:**<br><br>10–40 mg/day as a single dose in the evening | <u>Administration Issues:</u><br>May be taken without regards to meals; safety and efficacy in children < 18 years of age have not been established; dose should be taken in the evening<br><br><u>Drug–Drug Interactions:</u><br>pravastatin may potentiate the anticoagulant effects of **warfarin**; **bile acid resins** decrease the absorption of pravastatin; concurrent use with **gemfibrozil** may lead to severe myopathy or rhabdomyolysis | <u>ADRs</u><br>increased serum transaminases (AST, ALT); GI upset; muscle pain; headache; rash; photosensitivity; lens opacities (association unknown)<br><br><u>Pharmacokinetics</u><br>extensive first pass metabolism; 50% protein binding | <u>Contraindications:</u><br>hypersensitivity to HMG-CoA reductase inhibitors; active liver disease or unexplained persistent elevated liver function tests; pregnancy; lactation<br><br><u>Pregnancy Category:</u>  X<br><br><u>Lactation Issues:</u><br>women taking HMG-CoA reductase inhibitors should not nurse while taking these agents |

| Drug and Dosage Forms | Usual Dosage Range | Administration Issues and Drug–Drug & Drug–Food Interactions | Common Adverse Drug Reactions (ADRs) and Pharmacokinetics | Contraindications, Pregnancy Category, and Lactation Issues |
|---|---|---|---|---|
| **Simvastatin**<br>Zocor<br><br>Tablets:<br>5 mg, 10 mg, 20 mg, 40 mg | **hypercholesterolemia:**<br><br>5–40 mg/day as a single dose in the evening | Administration Issues:<br>safety and efficacy in children < 18 years of age have not been established; dose should be taken in the evening<br><br>Drug–Drug Interactions:<br>simvastatin may potentiate the anticoagulant effects of **warfarin**; concurrent use with **gemfibrozil** may lead to severe myopathy or rhabdomyolysis | ADRs<br>increased serum transaminases (AST, ALT); GI upset; muscle pain; headache; rash; photosensitivity; lens opacities (association unknown)<br><br>Pharmacokinetics<br>extensive first pass metabolism; 95% protein binding | Contraindications:<br>hypersensitivity to HMG-CoA reductase inhibitors; active liver disease or unexplained persistent elevated liver function tests; pregnancy; lactation<br><br>Pregnancy Category: X<br><br>Lactation Issues:<br>women taking HMG-CoA reductase inhibitors should not nurse while taking these agents |

### 204.3  Miscellaneous Antihyperlipidemic Agents

| Drug and Dosage Forms | Usual Dosage Range | Administration Issues and Drug–Drug & Drug–Food Interactions | Common Adverse Drug Reactions (ADRs) and Pharmacokinetics | Contraindications, Pregnancy Category, and Lactation Issues |
|---|---|---|---|---|
| **Gemfibrozil**<br>Lopid<br><br>Capsules:<br>300 mg<br><br>Tablets:<br>600 mg | **hypertriglyceridemia**<br><br>600 mg bid given 30 minutes before the morning and evening meals | Administration Issues:<br>safety and efficacy in children have not been established<br><br>Drug–Drug Interactions:<br>gemfibrozil may potentiate the anticoagulant effects of **warfarin**; concurrent use with **HMG-CoA reductase inhibitors** may lead to severe myopathy or rhabdomyolysis | ADRs<br>GI upset; fatigue; increased liver function tests (AST, ALT, LDH, bilirubin, alkaline phosphatase); increased risk of cholelithiasis<br><br>Pharmacokinetics:<br>99% protein binding, metabolized by the liver, $T_{1/2} = 1.4$ hrs | Contraindications:<br>hypersensitivity to gemfibrozil; hepatic or severe renal insufficiency; preexisting gallbladder disease<br><br>Pregnancy Category: B<br><br>Lactation Issues:<br>due to the potential for tumorigenicity, either the drug or nursing should be discontinued |

(continues on next page)

## 204.3 Miscellaneous Antihyperlipidemic Agents *continued from previous page*

| Drug and Dosage Forms | Usual Dosage Range | Administration Issues and Drug–Drug & Drug–Food Interactions | Common Adverse Drug Reactions (ADRs) and Pharmacokinetics | Contraindications, Pregnancy Category, and Lactation Issues |
|---|---|---|---|---|
| **Nicotinic Acid (Niacin)**<br>Slo-Niacin, Nicobid Tempules, Nicotinex<br><br>Tablets:<br>25 mg, 50 mg, 100 mg, 250 mg, 500 mg<br><br>Tablets, timed release:<br>250 mg, 500 mg, 750 mg<br><br>Capsules, timed release:<br>125 mg, 250 mg, 300 mg, 400 mg, 500 mg<br><br>Elixir:  50 mg/ 5 mL | **hyperlipidemia:**<br><br>initial dose:<br>50 mg bid (titrate slowly to decrease the incidence of adverse effects)<br><br>maintenance dose:<br>3–6 grams/day given in 2–3 divided doses<br><br>maximum dose:  8 grams/day | Administration Issues:<br>take with meals to minimize GI upset; aspirin taken 30–60 minutes before niacin may decrease cutaneous flushing<br><br>Drug–Drug Interactions:<br>concurrent use with **lovastatin** may lead to severe myopathy or rhabdomyolysis | ADRS<br>cutaneous flushing; GI upset; glucose intolerance; hyperuricemia; doses >2 g/d may result in hepatotoxicity—this is more common with SR products with severe cases resulting in fulminant hepatic failure and liver transplantation<br><br>Pharmacokinetics<br>completely absorbed from GI tract; mainly excreted in urine | Contraindications:<br>active peptic ulcer disease; use with caution in patients predisposed to gout, those with gallbladder disease, hepatic dysfunction or diabetes; severe hypotension<br><br>Pregnancy Category:  C<br><br>Lactation Issues:<br>niacin is excreted in breast milk |

# 205. Antihypertensive Agents

205.1 Angiotensin Converting Enzyme Inhibitors

| Drug and Dosage Forms | Usual Dosage Range | Administration Issues and Drug–Drug & Drug–Food Interactions | Common Adverse Drug Reactions (ADRs) and Pharmacokinetics | Contraindications, Pregnancy Category, and Lactation Issues |
|---|---|---|---|---|
| **Benazepril**<br>Lotensin<br><br>Tablets:<br>5 mg, 10 mg, 20 mg, 40 mg<br><br>Combinations:<br>w/ varying strengths of HCTZ and benazepril (combinations should not be used as initial therapy for HTN) | **hypertension:**<br><br>initial dose: 10 mg qd<br>max dose: 40 mg qd<br><br>patients taking diuretics<br>initial dose: 5 mg qd<br><br>CrCl <30 ml/min<br>initial dose: 5 mg qd | Administration Issues:<br>discontinue as soon as possible if pregnancy is detected; safety and efficacy have not been established in children<br><br>Drug–Drug Interactions:<br>concomitant use of **potassium sparing diuretics** or **potassium supplements** may result in hyperkalemia; may increase **lithium** concentrations; increased risk of hypersensitivity reactions when given with **allopurinol; may increase digoxin** concentrations; **phenothiazine** may increase the effects of ACEIs; **indomethacin** may decrease the effects of ACEIs | ADRs:<br>hypotension; hyperkalemia; cough; rash; dysgeusia; renal insufficiency; bone marrow suppression; angioedema (rare)<br><br>Pharmacokinetics:<br>onset = 1 h; duration = 24 hours; >95% protein bound; $T_{1/2}$ = 10–11 hours (prolonged in renal insufficiency | Contraindications:<br>hypersensitivity to angiotensin converting enzyme inhibitors<br><br>Pregnancy Category: C (first trimester); D (second and third trimester)<br><br>Lactation Issues:<br>benazepril is excreted in breast milk; either the drug or nursing should be discontinued |
| **Captopril**<br>Capoten<br><br>Tablets:<br>12.5 mg, 25 mg, 50 mg, 100 mg<br><br>Combinations:<br>w/ varying strengths of HCTZ and captopril (combinations should not be used as initial therapy for HTN) | **hypertension:**<br>initial dose: 12.5 mg tid<br>maximum dose: 50 mg tid<br><br>**congestive heart failure and left ventricular dysfunction after myocardial infarction:**<br>initial dose: 6.25 mg tid<br>max dose: 50 mg tid | Administration Issues:<br>food decreases the absorption of captopril—take on an empty stomach; discontinue as soon as possible if pregnancy is detected; safety and efficacy have not been established in children<br><br>Drug–Drug Interactions:<br>concomitant use of **potassium sparing diuretics** or **potassium supplements** may result in hyperkalemia; may increase **lithium** concentrations; increased risk of | ADRs:<br>hypotension; hyperkalemia; cough; rash; dysgeusia; renal insufficiency; bone marrow suppression; angioedema (rare)<br><br>Pharmacokinetics:<br>onset = 15 minutes; food decreases absorption; protein binding = 25–30%; $T_{1/2}$ <2 hours (prolonged in renal insufficiency) | Contraindications:<br>hypersensitivity to angiotensin converting enzyme inhibitors<br><br>Pregnancy Category: C (first trimester); D (second and third trimester)<br><br>Lactation Issues:<br>captopril is excreted in breast milk; either the drug or nursing should be discontinued |

(continues on next page)

| Drug and Dosage Forms | Usual Dosage Range | Administration Issues and Drug–Drug & Drug–Food Interactions | Common Adverse Drug Reactions (ADRs) and Pharmacokinetics | Contraindications, Pregnancy Category, and Lactation Issues |
|---|---|---|---|---|
| **Captopril** *cont.* | **diabetic nephropathy:** <br> initial dose: 12.5 mg tid <br> max dose: 25 mg tid | hypersensitivity reactions when given with **allopurinol;** may increase **digoxin** concentrations; **phenothiazine** may increase the effects of ACEIs; **indomethacin** may decrease the effects of ACEIs; **antacids** may decrease the absorption of captopril | | |
| **Enalapril** <br> Vasotec <br><br> Tablets: <br> 2.5 mg, 5 mg, 10 mg, 20 mg <br><br> Combinations: <br> 25 mg HCTZ/10 mg enalapril <br> (do not use combination as initial therapy for HTN) | **hypertension:** <br> initial dose: 5 mg qd <br> maximum dose: 40 mg qd <br><br> patients taking diuretics <br> initial dose: 2.5 mg qd <br><br> CrCl <30 ml/min or hyponatremia <br> initial dose: 2.5 mg qd <br><br> **congestive heart failure:** <br> initial dose: 2.5 mg bid <br> max dose: 20 mg bid <br><br> **asymptomatic left ventricular dysfunction:** <br> initial dose: 2.5 mg bid <br> max dose: 10 mg bid | Administration Issues: <br> discontinue as soon as possible if pregnancy is detected; safety and efficacy have not been established in children <br><br> Drug–Drug Interactions: <br> concomitant use of **potassium sparing diuretics** or **potassium supplements** may result in hyperkalemia; may increase **lithium** concentrations; increased risk of hypersensitivity reactions when given with **allopurinol;** may increase **digoxin** concentrations; **phenothiazine** may increase the effects of ACEIs; **indomethacin** may decrease the effects of ACEIs | ADRs: hypotension; hyperkalemia; cough; rash; dysgeusia; renal insufficiency; bone marrow suppression; angioedema (rare) <br><br> Pharmacokinetics: <br> onset = 1 hour; duration = 24 hours; $T_{1/2}$ = 1.3 hours | Contraindications: <br> hypersensitivity to angiotensin converting enzyme inhibitors <br><br> Pregnancy Category: C (first trimester); D (second and third trimester) <br><br> Lactation Issues: <br> enalapril is excreted in breast milk; either the drug or nursing should be discontinued |
| **Fosinopril** <br> Monopril | **hypertension:** <br> initial dose: 10 mg qd <br> max dose: 80 mg qd | Administration Issues: <br> discontinue as soon as possible if pregnancy is detected; safety and | ADRs: <br> hypotension; hyperkalemia; cough; rash; dysgeusia; renal | Contraindications: <br> hypersensitivity to angiotensin converting enzyme inhibitors |

| | | | | |
|---|---|---|---|---|
| **Tablets:** 10 mg, 20 mg | **patients taking diuretics:** initial dose: 5 mg qd<br><br>**congestive heart failure:** initial dose: 5 mg qd<br>max dose: 40 mg qd | efficacy have not been established in children<br><br>Drug–Drug Interactions: concomitant use of **potassium sparing diuretics** or **potassium supplements** may result in hyperkalemia; may increase **lithium** concentrations; increased risk of hypersensitivity reactions when given with **allopurinol;** may increase **digoxin** concentrations; **phenothiazine** may increase the effects of ACEIs; **indomethacin** may decrease the effects of ACEIs | insufficiency; bone marrow suppression; angioedema (rare)<br><br>Pharmacokinetics: onset = 1 hour; duration = 24 hours; protein binding = 95%; $T_{1/2}$ = 12 hours (prolonged in renal insufficiency) | Pregnancy Category: C (first trimester); D (second and third trimester)<br><br>Lactation Issues: fosinopril is excreted in breast milk; either the drug or nursing should be discontinued |
| **Lisinopril**<br>Prinivil, Zestril<br><br>Tablets:<br>2.5 mg, 5 mg, 10 mg, 20 mg, 40 mg<br><br>Combinations:<br>w/ varying strengths of HCTZ and 20 mg lisinopril (combinations should not be used as initial therapy for HTN) | **hypertension:** initial dose: 10 mg qd<br>max dose: 40 mg qd<br><br>patients taking diuretics: initial dose: 5 mg qd<br><br>patients with renal insufficiency: CrCl 10–30 ml/min: 5 mg qd<br>CrCl <10 ml/min: 2.5 mg qd<br><br>**congestive heart failure:** initial dose: 5 mg qd<br>max dose: 20 mg qd<br><br>patients with hyponatremia or CrCl <30 ml/min initial dose: 2.5 mg qd<br><br>**acute myocardial infarction:** initial dose: 5 mg qd<br>max dose: 10 mg qd for 6 weeks | Administration Issues: discontinue as soon as possible if pregnancy is detected; safety and efficacy have not been established in children<br><br>Drug–Drug Interactions: concomitant use of **potassium sparing diuretics** or **potassium supplements** may result in hyperkalemia; may increase **lithium** concentrations; increased risk of hypersensitivity reactions when given with **allopurinol;** may increase **digoxin** concentrations; **phenothiazine** may increase the effects of ACEIs; **indomethacin** may decrease the effects of ACEIs | ADRs: hypotension; hyperkalemia; cough; rash; dysgeusia; renal insufficiency; bone marrow suppression; angioedema (rare)<br><br>Pharmacokinetics: onset = 1 hour; duration = 24 hours; 100% excreted in urine; $T_{1/2}$ = 12 hours (prolonged in renal insufficiency) | Contraindications: hypersensitivity to angiotensin converting enzyme inhibitors<br><br>Pregnancy Category: C (first trimester); D (second and third trimester)<br><br>Lactation Issues: it is not known if lisinopril is excreted in breast milk; either the drug or nursing should be discontinued |

**205.1 Angiotensin Converting Enzyme Inhibitors** *continued from previous page*

| Drug and Dosage Forms | Usual Dosage Range | Administration Issues and Drug–Drug & Drug–Food Interactions | Common Adverse Drug Reactions (ADRs) and Pharmacokinetics | Contraindications, Pregnancy Category, and Lactation Issues |
|---|---|---|---|---|
| **Moexipril**<br>Univasc<br><br>Tablets:<br>7.5 mg, 15 mg | **hypertension:**<br>initial dose: 7.5 mg qd<br>max dose: 30 mg qd<br><br>patients taking diuretics<br>initial dose: 3.75 mg qd<br><br>CrCl < 40 ml/min:<br>initial dose: 3.75 mg qd<br>max dose: 15 mg qd | Administration Issues:<br>food decreases the absorption of moexipril—take on an empty stomach; discontinue as soon as possible if pregnancy is detected; safety and efficacy have not been established in children<br><br>Drug–Drug Interactions:<br>concomitant use of **potassium sparing diuretics** or **potassium supplements** may result in hyperkalemia; may increase **lithium** concentrations; increased risk of hypersensitivity reactions when given with **allopurinol;** may increase **digoxin** concentrations; **phenothiazine** may increase the effects of ACEIs; **indomethacin** may decrease the effects of ACEIs | ADRs:<br>hypotension; hyperkalemia; cough; rash; dysgeusia; renal insufficiency; bone marrow suppression; angioedema (rare)<br><br>Pharmacokinetics:<br>onset = 1 hour; duration = 24 hours; protein binding = 50%; $T_{1/2}$ = 2–9 hours (prolonged in renal insufficiency) | Contraindications:<br>hypersensitivity to angiotensin converting enzyme inhibitors<br><br>Pregnancy Category: C (first trimester); D (second and third trimester)<br><br>Lactation Issues:<br>it is not known if moexipril is excreted in breast milk; either the drug or nursing should be discontinued |
| **Quinapril**<br>Accupril<br><br>Tablets:<br>5 mg, 10 mg, 20 mg, 40 mg | **hypertension:**<br>initial dose: 10 mg qd<br>max dose: 80 mg/d<br><br>patients taking diuretics:<br>initial dose: 5 mg qd<br><br>patients with renal insufficiency:<br>CrCl 30–60 ml/min: 5 mg qd<br>CrCl 10–30 ml/min: 2.5 mg qd | Administration Issues:<br>discontinue as soon as possible if pregnancy is detected; safety and efficacy have not been established in children<br><br>Drug–Drug Interactions:<br>concomitant use of **potassium sparing diuretics** or **potassium supplements** may result in hyperkalemia; may increase **lithium** concentrations; increased risk of hypersensitivity reactions when given with | ADRs:<br>hypotension; hyperkalemia; cough; rash; dysgeusia; renal insufficiency; bone marrow suppression; angioedema (rare)<br><br>Pharmacokinetics:<br>onset = 1 hour; duration = 24 hours; protein binding = 97%; $T_{1/2}$ = 2 hours (prolonged in renal insufficiency) | Contraindications:<br>hypersensitivity to angiotensin converting enzyme inhibitors<br><br>Pregnancy Category: C (first trimester); D (second and third trimester)<br><br>Lactation Issues:<br>it is not known if quinapril is excreted in breast milk; either |

| | Dosage | | |
|---|---|---|---|
| | **congestive heart failure:**<br>initial dose: 5 mg bid<br>max dose: 40 mg/d, divided bid<br><br>patients with hyponatremia or CrCl 10–30 ml/min initial dose: 2.5 mg bid | | **allopurinol;** may increase **digoxin** concentrations; **phenothiazine** may increase the effects of ACEIs; **indomethacin** may decrease the effects of ACEIs | the drug or nursing should be discontinued |
| **Ramipril**<br>Altace<br><br>Capsules:<br>1.25 mg, 2.5 mg, 5 mg, 10 mg | **hypertension:**<br>initial dose: 2.5 mg qd<br>max dose: 20 mg/d<br><br>CrCl < 40 ml/min:<br>initial dose: 1.25 mg qd<br><br>**congestive heart failure:**<br>initial dose: 2.5 mg bid<br>max dose: 5 mg bid<br><br>CrCl < 40 ml/min<br>initial dose: 1.25 mg qd<br>max dose: 2.5 mg bid<br><br>patients taking diuretics<br>initial dose: 1.25 mg qd | Administration Issues:<br>discontinue as soon as possible if pregnancy is detected; safety and efficacy have not been established in children<br><br>Drug–Drug Interactions:<br>concomitant use of **potassium sparing diuretics** or **potassium supplements** may result in hyperkalemia; may increase **lithium** concentrations; increased risk of hypersensitivity reactions when given with **allopurinol;** may increase **digoxin** concentrations; **phenothiazine** may increase the effects of ACEIs; **indomethacin** may decrease the effects of ACEIs | ADRs:<br>hypotension; hyperkalemia; cough; rash; dysgeusia; renal insufficiency; bone marrow suppression; angioedema (rare)<br><br>Pharmacokinetics:<br>onset = 1–2 hours; duration = 24 hours; protein binding = 73%; $T_{1/2}$ = 13–17 hours (prolonged in renal insufficiency) | Contraindications:<br>hypersensitivity to angiotensin converting enzyme inhibitors<br><br>Pregnancy Category: C (first trimester); D (second and third trimester)<br><br>Lactation Issues:<br>it is not known if ramipril is excreted in breast milk; either the drug or nursing should be discontinued |

## 205.2 Angiotensin II Antagonists

| Drug and Dosage Forms | Usual Dosage Range | Administration Issues and Drug–Drug & Drug–Food Interactions | Common Adverse Drug Reactions (ADRs) and Pharmacokinetics | Contraindications, Pregnancy Category, and Lactation Issues |
|---|---|---|---|---|
| **Losartan**<br>Cozaar<br><br>Tablets:<br>25 mg, 50 mg | **hypertension:**<br>initial dose: 50 mg qd<br>maintenance dose: 50–100 mg qd<br><br>patients taking diuretics or with hepatic failure: initial dose: 25 mg qd | Administration Issues:<br>discontinue losartan as soon as possible if pregnancy is detected; safety and efficacy have not been established in children<br><br>Drug–Drug Interactions:<br>**cimetidine** increases losartan concentrations; **phenobarbital** decreases losartan concentrations | ADRs:<br>dizziness; cough; diarrhea; GI upset; insomnia; nasal congestion<br><br>Pharmacokinetics:<br>well absorbed; extensive first pass metabolism to an active metabolite; both losartan and its active metabolite are highly protein bound (>98%) | Contraindications:<br>hypersensitivity to losartan<br><br>Pregnancy Category: C (first trimester); D (second and third trimester)<br><br>Lactation Issues:<br>it is not known if losartan is excreted in breast milk; either the drug or nursing should be discontinued |
| **Valsartan**<br>Diovan<br><br>Capsules:<br>80 mg, 160 mg | **hypertension:**<br>initial dose: 80 mg qd<br>maintenance dose: 80 to 320 mg qd | Administration Issues:<br>discontinue valsartan as soon as possible if pregnancy is detected; safety and efficacy have not been established in children<br><br>Drug–Drug Interactions:<br>none reported | ADRs:<br>dizziness; cough; diarrhea; GI upset; insomnia; nasal congestion | Contraindications:<br>hypersensitivity to losartan<br><br>Pregnancy Category: C (first trimester); D (second and third trimester)<br><br>Lactation Issues:<br>it is not known if losartan is excreted in breast milk; either the drug or nursing should be discontinued |

## 205.3 Centrally and Peripherally Acting Antiadrenergic Agents

| Drug and Dosage Forms | Usual Dosage Range | Administration Issues and Drug–Drug & Drug–Food Interactions | Common Adverse Drug Reactions (ADRs) and Pharmacokinetics | Contraindications, Pregnancy Category, and Lactation Issues |
|---|---|---|---|---|
| **Clonidine**<br>Catapres<br><br><u>Tablets:</u><br>0.1 mg, 0.2 mg, 0.3 mg<br><br>Combinations:<br>15 mg chlorthalidone and varying strengths of clonidine (do not use combinations as initial therapy for HTN)<br><br><u>Transdermal Patch:</u><br>TTS-1 (0.1 mg/day), TTS-2 (0.2 mg/day), TTS-3 (0.3 mg/day) | **hypertension:**<br>**adults (oral):**<br>initial dose: 0.1 mg bid<br>maintenance dose: 0.2–0.8 mg daily in divided doses<br>max dose: 2.4 mg/d<br><br>**children (oral):**<br>5–25 mcg/kg/d, divided q 6 h<br><br>**adults (transdermal patch):**<br>0.1–0.6 mg/d reapplied q 7 d<br><br>**alcohol withdrawal:**<br>0.3–0.6 mg q 6 h<br><br>**smoking cessation:**<br>oral: 0.15–0.4 mg qd<br>transdermal patch: 0.2 mg/d | <u>Administration Issues:</u><br>abrupt discontinuation may result in rebound hypertension—clonidine should be tapered gradually; safety and efficacy have not been established in children<br><br><u>Drug–Drug Interactions:</u><br>concomitant use of **beta blockers** may result in paradoxical hypertension; **tricyclic antidepressants** may block the antihypertensive effects of clonidine | <u>ADRs:</u><br>dry mouth; drowsiness; dizziness; sedation; constipation; impotence; contact dermatitis (with transdermal patch)<br><br><u>Pharmacokinetics:</u><br><br><u>oral:</u><br>onset = 30–60 minutes; 50% metabolized by the liver; $T_{1/2}$ = 12–16 hours (prolonged in renal insufficiency); minimal amount removed by dialysis<br><br><u>transdermal patch:</u><br>therapeutic levels are reached in 2–3 days; $T_{1/2}$ = 19 hours | <u>Contraindications:</u><br>hypersensitivity to clonidine or any component of transdermal system<br><br><u>Pregnancy Category:</u> C<br><br><u>Lactation Issues:</u><br>clonidine is excreted in breast milk; use with caution in nursing mothers |
| **Guanabenz**<br>Wytensin<br><br><u>Tablets:</u><br>4 mg, 8 mg | **hypertension:**<br>initial dose: 4 mg bid<br><br>max dose: 32 mg bid | <u>Administration Issues:</u><br>allow 1–2 weeks before adjusting dose; rebound hypertension rarely occurs with abrupt discontinuation; safety and efficacy have not been established in children < 12 years of age | <u>ADRs:</u><br>dry mouth; drowsiness; dizziness; sedation; headache; constipation; impotence<br><br><u>Pharmacokinetics:</u><br>$T_{1/2}$ = 6 hours (prolonged in hepatic and renal insufficiency) | <u>Contraindications:</u><br>hypersensitivity to guanabenz<br><br><u>Pregnancy Category:</u> C<br><br><u>Lactation Issues:</u><br>it is not known if guanabenz is excreted in breast milk; either the drug or nursing should be discontinued |

*(continues on next page)*

1055

| Drug and Dosage Forms | Usual Dosage Range | Administration Issues and Drug–Drug & Drug–Food Interactions | Common Adverse Drug Reactions (ADRs) and Pharmacokinetics | Contraindications, Pregnancy Category, and Lactation Issues |
|---|---|---|---|---|
| **Guanfacine**<br>Tenex<br><br>Tablets:<br>1 mg, 2 mg | **hypertension:**<br><br>initial dose: 1 mg q hs<br><br>maintenance dose: 1–2 mg q hs | Administration Issues:<br>administer at bedtime to minimize daytime somnolence; allow 3–4 weeks before adjusting dose; rebound HTN rarely occurs with abrupt discontinuation—when it does occur, it does so after 2–4 days, which is delayed compared to clonidine; safety and efficacy have not been established in children < 12 years of age | ADRs:<br>dry mouth; drowsiness; dizziness; sedation; headache; constipation; impotence<br><br>Pharmacokinetics:<br>protein binding = 70%; 50% excreted unchanged in urine; $T_{1/2}$ = 17 hours | Contraindications:<br>hypersensitivity to guanfacine<br><br>Pregnancy Category: B<br><br>Lactation Issues:<br>guanfacine is excreted in breast milk; use with caution in nursing mothers |
| **Methyldopa**<br>Aldomet<br><br>Tablets:<br>125 mg, 250 mg<br>500 mg<br><br>Oral Suspension:<br>250 mg/5 mL | **hypertension:**<br><br>**adults:**<br>initial dose: 250 mg bid to tid<br>maintenance dose: 500 mg–3000 mg in 2–4 divided doses<br><br>**children:**<br>initial dose: 10 mg/kg daily in 2–4 divided doses<br><br>max dose: 65 mg/kg up to 3000 mg | Administration Issues:<br>allow two days for maximum response before adjusting dosage<br><br>Drug–Drug Interactions:<br>methyldopa may potentiate the effects of **levodopa, lithium, haloperidon, MAO inhibitors** and **sympathomimetics;** paradoxical hypertension may occur with concomitant administration of **propranolol;** methyldopa may decrease the metabolism of **tolbutamide** | ADRs:<br>sedation; orthostatic hypotension; edema; GI upset; dry mouth; abnormal LFTs; hemolytic anemia; rash; lupus-like syndrome; amenorrhea; gynecomastia; impotence; nasal stuffiness<br><br>Pharmacokinetics:<br>$T_{1/2}$ = 105 minutes (prolonged in renal insufficiency) | Contraindications:<br>hypersensitivity to methyldopa; active hepatitis or cirrhosis; coadministration with MAO inhibitors<br><br>Pregnancy Category: B<br><br>Lactation Issues:<br>methyldopa is excreted in breast milk |
| **Guanadrel**<br>Hylorel<br><br>Tablets:<br>10 mg, 25 mg | **hypertension:**<br><br>initial dose: 5 mg bid<br>maintenance dose: 20–75 mg/d in 2–4 divided doses | Administration Issues:<br>safety and efficacy have not been established in children<br><br>Drug–Drug Interactions:<br>**beta blockers** and **vasodilators** may potentiate the effects of guanadrel; | ADRs:<br>orthostatic hypotension; dizziness; GI upset; impotence; fluid retention; congestive heart failure; asthma in susceptible individuals | Contraindications:<br>hypersensitivity to guanadrel; pheochromocytoma; congestive heart failure; use of MAO inhibitors<br><br>Pregnancy Category: B |

# Guanethidine

Ismelin

Tablets:
10 mg, 25 mg

Combinations:
25 mg HCTZ/ 10 mg guanethidine (do not use combination as initial therapy in HTN)

---

renal impairment (initial dose):
CrCl = 30–60 ml/min: 5 mg qd
CrCl < 30 ml/min: 5 mg qod

hypertension:

adults:
initial dose: 10 mg qd
maintenance dose: 10–50 mg qd

children:
initial dose: 0.2 mg/kg/d
max dose: 3 mg/kg/d

---

**phenothiazines, sympathomimetics** and **tricyclic antidepressants** may inhibit the antihypertensive effects of guanadrel

Administration Issues:
allow 1–2 weeks before adjusting dose; safety and efficacy have not been established in children

Drug–Drug Interactions:
the antihypertensive effect of guanethidine may be inhibited by **haloperidol, methylphenidate, MAO inhibitors, phenothiazines, sympathomimetics, thioxanthenes,** and **tricyclic antidepressants;** concomitant use with **minoxidil** may result in profound orthostatic hypotension

---

Pharmacokinetics:
$T_{1/2}$ = 10 hours

ADRs:
orthostatic hypotension; dizziness; GI upset; impotence; fluid retention; congestive heart failure; asthma in susceptible individuals

Pharmacokinetics:
$T_{1/2}$ = 4–8 days

---

Lactation Issues:
it is not known if guanadrel is excreted in breast milk; either the drug or nursing should be discontinued

Contraindications:
hypersensitivity to guanethidine; pheochromocytoma; congestive heart failure; use of MAO inhibitors

Pregnancy Category: C

Lactation Issues:
guanethidine is excreted in breast milk; either the drug or nursing should be discontinued

---

# Reserpine

Tablets:
0.1 mg, 0.25 mg

Combinations:
w/ varying strengths of HCTZ, polythiazide, chlorothiazide, hydroxyflumethazide, chlorthalidone, methyclothiazide and reserpine (do not use combinations as initial therapy for HTN)

---

hypertension:

adults:
0.1–0.25 mg qd

children:
initial dose: 20 mcg/kg qd
max dose: 0.25 mg qd

---

Administration Issues:
safety and efficacy have not been established in children < 12 years of age (use in children is not recommended)

Drug–Drug Interactions:
**tricyclic antidepressants** may block the antihypertensive effect of reserpine; concomitant use of **MAO inhibitors** may cause excitation and hypertension; concomitant use with **digitalis glycosides** may predispose patients to arrhythmias

---

ADRs:
GI upset; increased gastric acid secretion; depression; drowsiness; nasal congestion; impotence

Pharmacokinetics:
protein binding = 96%;
$T_{1/2}$ = 33 hours

---

Contraindications:
hypersensitivity to reserpine; history of mental depression; active peptic ulcer disease; ulcerative colitis

Pregnancy Category: C

Lactation Issues:
reserpine is excreted in breast milk; either the drug or nursing should be discontinued

(continues on next page)

**205.3 Centrally and Peripherally Acting Antiadrenergic Agents** *continued from previous page*

| Drug and Dosage Forms | Usual Dosage Range | Administration Issues and Drug–Drug & Drug–Food Interactions | Common Adverse Drug Reactions (ADRs) and Pharmacokinetics | Contraindications, Pregnancy Category, and Lactation Issues |
|---|---|---|---|---|
| **Doxazosin**<br>Cardura<br><br>Tablets:<br>1 mg, 2 mg, 4 mg, 8 mg | **hypertension:**<br>initial dose: 1 mg q hs<br>max dose: 16 mg/d<br><br>**benign prostatic hypertrophy (BPH):**<br>initial dose: 1 mg q hs<br>max dose: 8 mg/d | Administration Issues:<br>safety and efficacy have not been established in children; administer at bedtime to minimize adverse effects<br><br>Drug–Drug Interactions:<br>the antihypertensive effect of **clonidine** may be decreased | ADRs:<br>orthostatic hypotension; palpitations; GI upset; headache; peripheral edema; impotence<br><br>Pharmacokinetics:<br>protein binding = 98%;<br>$T_{1/2}$ = 22 h | Contraindications:<br>hypersensitivity to prazosin, terazosin or doxazosin<br><br>Pregnancy Category: C<br><br>Lactation Issues:<br>doxazosin is excreted in breast milk; use caution in nursing mothers |
| **Prazosin**<br>Minipress<br><br>Capsules:<br>1 mg, 2 mg, 5 mg<br><br>Combinations:<br>0.5 mg polythiazide and varying strengths of prazosin (do not use combinations as initial therapy in HTN) | **hypertension:**<br><br>**adults:**<br>initial dose: 1 mg bid to tid<br>max dose: 20 mg/d<br><br>**children:**<br>0.5–7 mg tid | Administration Issues:<br>take the first dose at bedtime; safety and efficacy not established in children<br><br>Drug–Drug Interactions:<br>the antihypertensive effect of **clonidine** may be decreased; **indomethacin** may decrease the antihypertensive effect of prazosin; **verapamil** may increase serum prazosin concentrations; **beta blockers** may enhance the first dose syncope effect of prazosin | ADRs:<br>"first dose syncope", orthostatic hypotension; palpitations; GI upset; headache; peripheral edema; impotence<br><br>Pharmacokinetics:<br>protein binding = 92–97%; extensively metabolized;<br>$T_{1/2}$ = 2–3 h (prolonged in renal insufficiency) | Contraindications:<br>hypersensitivity to prazosin, terazosin or doxazosin<br><br>Pregnancy Category: C<br><br>Lactation Issues:<br>prazosin is excreted in breast milk; use caution in nursing mothers |
| **Terazosin**<br>Hytrin<br><br>Tablets:<br>1 mg, 2 mg, 5 mg, 10 mg | **hypertension:**<br>initial dose: 1 mg q hs<br>maintenance dose: 1–5 mg/d<br>max dose: 20 mg/d | Administration Issues:<br>take the first dose at bedtime; safety and efficacy have not been established in children | ADRs:<br>orthostatic hypotension; palpitations; GI upset; headache; peripheral edema; impotence | Contraindications:<br>hypersensitivity to prazosin, terazosin or doxazosin<br><br>Pregnancy Category: C |

| | | | |
|---|---|---|---|
| Capsules:<br>1 mg, 2 mg, 5 mg, 10 mg | benign prostatic hypertrophy (BPH):<br>initial dose: 1 mg q hs<br>max dose: 20 mg/d | Drug–Drug Interactions:<br>the antihypertensive effect of **clonidine** may be decreased | Lactation Issues:<br>it is not known if terazosin is excreted in breast milk; use caution in nursing mothers |

## 205.4 Alpha/Beta Adrenergic Blocking Agents

| Drug and Dosage Forms | Usual Dosage Range | Administration Issues and Drug–Drug & Drug–Food Interactions | Common Adverse Drug Reactions (ADRs) and Pharmacokinetics | Contraindications, Pregnancy Category, and Lactation Issues |
|---|---|---|---|---|
| **Carvedilol**<br>Coreg<br><br>Tablets:<br>3.125 mg, 6.25 mg, 12.5 mg, 25 mg | hypertension:<br>initial dose: 6.25 mg bid<br><br>max dose: 50 mg/d | Administration Issues:<br>take with food; therapy should not be abruptly discontinued; use with caution in patients with hepatic impairment<br><br>Drug–Drug Interactions:<br>additive effects when given with other **negative inotropes** or **antihypertensive agents;** carvedilol may increase **digoxin** levels; **cimetidine** increases carvedilol levels; **rifampin** decreases carvedilol levels | ADRs:<br>bradycardia; hypotension; worsening congestive heart failure (CHF); worsening peripheral vascular disease (PVD); bronchospasm (in susceptible individuals); impotence; mask the signs of hypoglycemia; GI upset; dizziness; fatigue; increased cholesterol levels; increased liver function tests<br><br>Pharmacokinetics:<br>protein binding > 98%;<br>$T_{1/2} = 5$–11 h | Contraindications:<br>hypersensitivity to carvedilol; symptomatic bradycardia; greater than first degree heart block; NYHA Class IV heart failure; asthma<br><br>Pregnancy Category: C<br><br>Lactation Issues:<br>it is not known if carvedilol is excreted in breast milk; either the drug or nursing should be discontinued |
| **Labetalol**<br>Normodyne, Trandate<br><br>Tablets:<br>100 mg, 200 mg, 300 mg | hypertension:<br>initial dose: 100 mg bid<br><br>maintenance dose: 200–400 mg bid<br><br>max dose: 2400 mg/d | Administration Issues:<br>therapy should not be abruptly discontinued; safety and efficacy have not been established in children | ADRs:<br>bradycardia; hypotension; worsening congestive heart failure (CHF); worsening peripheral vascular disease (PVD); bronchospasm (in susceptible individuals); impotence; mask the | Contraindications:<br>hypersensitivity to beta blocking agents; symptomatic bradycardia; greater than first degree heart block; CHF (relative); asthma |

*(continues on next page)*

1059

## 205.4  Alpha/Beta Adrenergic Blocking Agents  *continued from previous page*

| Drug and Dosage Forms | Usual Dosage Range | Administration Issues and Drug–Drug & Drug–Food Interactions | Common Adverse Drug Reactions (ADRs) and Pharmacokinetics | Contraindications, Pregnancy Category, and Lactation Issues |
|---|---|---|---|---|
| **Labetalol** *cont.* | | Drug–Drug Interactions:<br>additive effects when given with other **negative inotropes** or **antihypertensive agents; cimetidine** may increase the bioavailability of labetalol | signs of hypoglycemia; GI upset; dizziness; fatigue<br><br>Pharmacokinetics:<br>protein binding = 50%; $T_{1/2}$ = 5–8 hours | Pregnancy Category:  C<br><br>Lactation Issues:<br>labetalol is excreted in breast milk; use with caution in nursing mothers |

## 205.5  Beta-Adrenergic Blocking Agents

| Drug and Dosage Forms | Usual Dosage Range | Administration Issues and Drug–Drug & Drug–Food Interactions | Common Adverse Drug Reactions (ADRs) and Pharmacokinetics | Contraindications, Pregnancy Category, and Lactation Issues |
|---|---|---|---|---|
| **Acebutolol**<br>Sectral<br><br>Capsules:<br>200 mg, 400 mg | **hypertension:**<br>initial dose:  400 mg qd<br>max dose:  1200 mg/d<br><br>renal insufficiency:<br>CrCl < 50 mL/min:  reduce dose by 50%<br>CrCl < 25 mL/min:  reduce dose by 75%<br><br>elderly patients may require lower maintenance doses | Administration Issues:<br>therapy should not be abruptly discontinued; safety and efficacy have not been established in children<br><br>Drug–Drug Interactions:<br>additive effects when given with other **negative inotropes** or **antihypertensive agents** | ADRs<br>bradycardia; hypotension; worsening CHF; worsening PVD; bronchospasm (in susceptible individuals); impotence; mask the signs of hypoglycemia; GI upset; dizziness; fatigue; sleep disturbance<br><br>Pharmacokinetics:<br>protein binding = 26%; does not enter the CNS; $T_{1/2}$ = 3–4 h | Contraindications:<br>hypersensitivity to beta blocking agents; symptomatic bradycardia; greater than first degree heart block; CHF (relative); asthma<br><br>Pregnancy Category:  B<br><br>Lactation Issues:<br>acebutolol is excreted in breast milk; either the drug or nursing should be discontinued |

| Drug | Dosing | Administration Issues / Drug–Drug Interactions | ADRs / Pharmacokinetics | Contraindications / Pregnancy / Lactation |
|---|---|---|---|---|
| **Atenolol**<br>Tenormin<br><br>Tablets:<br>25 mg, 50 mg, 100 mg<br><br>Combinations:<br>25 mg chlorthalidone w/varying strengths of atenolol (do not use combinations as initial therapy for HTN) | **hypertension:**<br>50–100 mg qd<br><br>**angina:**<br>50–200 mg qd<br><br>renal insufficiency:<br>CrCl 15–35 mL/min: max dose = 50 mg qd<br>CrCl < 15 mL/min: max dose = 50 mg qod<br><br>hemodialysis: 50 mg after dialysis | Administration Issues:<br>therapy should not be abruptly discontinued; safety and efficacy have not been established in children<br><br>Drug–Drug Interactions:<br>additive effects when given with other **negative inotropes** or **antihypertensive agents** | ADRs:<br>bradycardia; hypotension; worsening CHF, worsening PVD; bronchospasm (in susceptible individuals); impotence; mask the signs of hypoglycemia; GI upset; dizziness; fatigue; sleep disturbance; increased triglycerides, total and LDL cholesterol; decreased HDL cholesterol<br><br>Pharmacokinetics:<br>protein binding = 6–16%; does not enter the CNS; $T_{1/2}$ = 6–9 h | Contraindications:<br>hypersensitivity to beta blocking agents; symptomatic bradycardia; greater than first degree heart block; CHF (relative); bronchospastic lung disease (asthma)<br><br>Pregnancy Category: C<br><br>Lactation Issues:<br>atenolol is excreted in breast milk; either the drug or nursing should be discontinued |
| **Betaxolol**<br>Kerlone<br><br>Tablets:<br>10 mg, 20 mg | **hypertension:**<br>10–20 mg qd<br><br>consider starting with 5 mg QD in elderly patients | Administration Issues:<br>therapy should not be abruptly discontinued; safety and efficacy have not been established in children<br><br>Drug–Drug Interactions:<br>additive effects when given with other **negative inotropes** or **antihypertensive agents** | ADRs:<br>bradycardia; hypotension; worsening CHF; worsening PVD; bronchospasm (in susceptible individuals); impotence; mask the signs of hypoglycemia; GI upset; dizziness; fatigue; sleep disturbance; increased triglycerides, total and LDL cholesterol; decreased HDL cholesterol<br><br>Pharmacokinetics:<br>protein binding = 50%; $T_{1/2}$ = 14–22 h | Contraindications:<br>hypersensitivity to beta blocking agents; symptomatic bradycardia; greater than first degree heart block; CHF (relative); asthma<br><br>Pregnancy Category: C<br><br>Lactation Issues:<br>betaxolol is excreted in breast milk; either the drug or nursing should be discontinued |
| **Bisoprolol**<br>Zebeta | **hypertension:**<br>5–20 mg qd | Administration Issues:<br>therapy should not be abruptly discontinued; safety and efficacy have not been established in children | ADRs:<br>bradycardia; hypotension; worsening CHF; worsening PVD; bronchospasm (in susceptible | Contraindications:<br>hypersensitivity to beta blocking agents; symptomatic bradycardia; greater than first |

(continues on next page)

## 205.5 Beta-Adrenergic Blocking Agents *continued from previous page*

| Drug and Dosage Forms | Usual Dosage Range | Administration Issues and Drug–Drug & Drug–Food Interactions | Common Adverse Drug Reactions (ADRs) and Pharmacokinetics | Contraindications, Pregnancy Category, and Lactation Issues |
|---|---|---|---|---|
| **Bisoprolol** *cont.* <br><br>Tablets: <br>5 mg, 10 mg <br><br>Combinations: <br>6.25 mg HCTZ w/varying strengths of bisoprolol (do not use combinations as initial therapy for HTN) | renal insufficiency: <br>CrCl < 40 mL/min:  initial dose = 2.5 mg qd | Drug–Drug Interactions: <br>additive effects when given with other **negative inotropes** or **antihypertensive agents** | individuals); impotence; mask the signs of hypoglycemia; GI upset; dizziness; fatigue; sleep disturbance <br><br>Pharmacokinetics: <br>protein binding = 30%; $T_{1/2}$ = 9–12 h | degree heart block; CHF (relative); asthma <br><br>Pregnancy Category:  C <br><br>Lactation Issues: <br>bisoprolol is excreted in breast milk; either the drug or nursing should be discontinued |
| **Carteolol** <br>Cartrol <br><br>Tablets: <br>2.5 mg, 5 mg | hypertension: <br>2.5–10 mg qd <br><br>renal insufficiency: <br>CrCl 20–60 mL/min:  dosing interval = qod <br>CrCl < 20 mL/min:  dosing interval = q 3 d | Administration Issues: <br>therapy should not be abruptly discontinued; safety and efficacy have not been established in children <br><br>Drug–Drug Interactions: <br>additive effects when given with other **negative inotropes** or **antihypertensive agents** | ADRs: <br>bradycardia; hypotension; worsening CHF; worsening PVD; bronchospasm (in susceptible individuals); impotence; mask the signs of hypoglycemia; GI upset; dizziness; fatigue; sleep disturbance <br><br>Pharmacokinetics: <br>protein binding = 23–30%; does not enter the CNS; $T_{1/2}$ = 6 h | Contraindications: <br>hypersensitivity to beta blocking agents; symptomatic bradycardia; greater than first degree heart block; CHF (relative); asthma <br><br>Pregnancy Category:  C <br><br>Lactation Issues: <br>it is not known if carteolol is excreted in breast milk; either the drug or nursing should be discontinued |
| **Metoprolol** <br>Lopressor, Toprol XL <br><br>Tablets: <br>50 mg, 100 mg | **hypertension, angina and myocardial infarction:** <br><br>immediate release tablets: <br>initial dose:  50 mg bid <br>max dose:  400 mg/d | Administration Issues: <br>food increases the absorption of metoprolol; therapy should not be abruptly discontinued; safety and efficacy have not been established in children | ADRs: <br>bradycardia; hypotension; worsening CHF; worsening PVD; bronchospasm (in susceptible individuals); impotence; mask the signs of hypoglycemia; GI upset; | Contraindications: <br>hypersensitivity to beta blocking agents; symptomatic bradycardia; greater than first degree heart block; CHF (relative); asthma |

| | | | | |
|---|---|---|---|---|
| **Extended Release Tablets:** 50 mg, 100 mg, 200 mg | extended release tablets: initial dose: 50 mg qd max dose: 400 mg/d | Drug–Drug Interactions: additive effects when given with other **negative inotropes** or **antihypertensive agents; cimetidine** may decrease the metabolism of metoprolol | dizziness; fatigue; sleep disturbance; increased triglycerides, total and LDL cholesterol; decreased HDL cholesterol. Pharmacokinetics: protein binding = 12%; readily enters into the CNS; $T_{1/2}$ = 3–7 h | Pregnancy Category: C. Lactation Issues: metoprolol is excreted in breast milk; either the drug or nursing should be discontinued |
| **Nadolol** Corgard. Tablets: 20mg, 40 mg, 80 mg, 120 mg, 160 mg. Combinations: w/ varying strengths of nadolol and 5 mg bendroflumethiazide (combinations should not be used as initial therapy for HTN) | **hypertension:** initial dose: 40 mg qd max dose: 320 mg/d. **angina:** initial dose: 40 mg qd max dose: 240 mg/d. renal insufficiency: CrCl 31–50 mL/min: dosing interval = 24–36 h; CrCl 10–30 mL/min: dosing interval = 24–48 h; CrCl < 10 mL/min: 40–60 h | Administration Issues: therapy should not be abruptly discontinued; safety and efficacy have not been established in children. Drug–Drug Interactions: additive effects when given with other **negative inotropes** or **antihypertensive agents** | ADRs: bradycardia; hypotension; worsening CHF; worsening PVD; bronchospasm (in susceptible individuals); impotence; mask the signs of hypoglycemia; GI upset; dizziness; fatigue; sleep disturbance; increased triglycerides, total and LDL cholesterol; decreased HDL cholesterol. Pharmacokinetics: protein binding = 30%; does not enter the CNS; $T_{1/2}$ = 20–24 h | Contraindications: hypersensitivity to beta blocking agents; symptomatic bradycardia; greater than first degree heart block; CHF (relative); asthma. Pregnancy Category: C. Lactation Issues: nadolol is excreted in breast milk; either the drug or nursing should be discontinued |
| **Penbutolol** Levatol. Tablets: 20 mg | **hypertension:** 20 mg qd. Max dose = 80 mg | Administration Issues: therapy should not be abruptly discontinued; safety and efficacy have not been established in children. Drug–Drug Interactions: additive effects when given with other **negative inotropes** or **antihypertensive agents** | ADRs: bradycardia; hypotension; worsening CHF; worsening PVD; bronchospasm (in susceptible individuals); impotence; mask the signs of hypoglycemia; GI upset; dizziness; fatigue; sleep disturbance; increased triglycerides, total and LDL | Contraindications: hypersensitivity to beta blocking agents; symptomatic bradycardia; greater than first degree heart block; CHF (relative); asthma. Pregnancy Category: C |

(continues on next page)

## 205.5 Beta-Adrenergic Blocking Agents *continued from previous page*

| Drug and Dosage Forms | Usual Dosage Range | Administration Issues and Drug–Drug & Drug–Food Interactions | Common Adverse Drug Reactions (ADRs) and Pharmacokinetics | Contraindications, Pregnancy Category, and Lactation Issues |
|---|---|---|---|---|
| **Penbutolol** *cont.* | | | cholesterol; decreased HDL cholesterol<br><br>Pharmacokinetics:<br>protein binding = 80–98%;<br>$T_{1/2}$ = 5 h | Lactation Issues:<br>it is not known if penbutolol is excreted in breast milk; either the drug or nursing should be discontinued |
| **Pindolol**<br>Visken<br><br>Tablets:<br>5 mg, 10 mg | **hypertension:**<br><br>initial dose: 5 mg bid<br><br>max dose: 60 mg/d | Administration Issues:<br>therapy should not be abruptly discontinued; safety and efficacy have not been established in children<br><br>Drug–Drug Interactions:<br>additive effects when given with other **negative inotropes** or **antihypertensive agents** | ADRs<br>bradycardia; hypotension; worsening CHF, worsening PVD; bronchospasm (in susceptible individuals); impotence; mask the signs of hypoglycemia; GI upset; dizziness; fatigue; sleep disturbance<br><br>Pharmacokinetics:<br>protein binding = 40%;<br>$T_{1/2}$ = 3–4 h | Contraindications:<br>hypersensitivity to beta blocking agents; symptomatic bradycardia; greater than first degree heart block; CHF (relative); asthma<br><br>Pregnancy Category: B<br><br>Lactation Issues:<br>pindolol is excreted in breast milk; either the drug or nursing should be discontinued |
| **Propranolol**<br>Inderal<br><br>Tablets:<br>10 mg, 20 mg, 40 mg, 60 mg, 80 mg, 90 mg | **hypertension:**<br>immediate release tablets:<br>initial dose: 40 mg bid<br><br>sustained release capsules:<br>initial dose: 80 mg qd<br>maximum dose: 640 mg/d | Administration Issues:<br>food increases the absorption of propranolol; therapy should not be abruptly discontinued; safety and efficacy have not been established in children<br><br>Drug–Drug Interactions:<br>additive effects when given with other **negative inotropes** or | ADRs<br>bradycardia; hypotension; worsening CHF; worsening PVD; bronchospasm (in susceptible individuals); impotence; mask the signs of hypoglycemia; GI upset; dizziness; fatigue; sleep disturbance; increased triglycerides, total and LDL | Contraindications:<br>hypersensitivity to beta blocking agents; symptomatic bradycardia; greater than first degree heart block; CHF (relative); asthma<br><br>Pregnancy Category: C |

| | | | |
|---|---|---|---|
| **Sustained Release Capsules:** 60 mg, 80 mg, 120 mg, 160 mg<br><br>**Solution:** 4 mg/ml, 8 mg/ml, 80 mg/ml<br><br>**Combinations:** w/ varying strengths of HCTZ and propranolol (combinations should not be used as initial therapy for HTN) | **angina/myocardial infarction:** initial dose: 80 mg bid (immediate release tablets)<br><br>160 mg qd (SR capsules)<br><br>max dose: 320 mg/d<br><br>**migraine prophylaxis:** initial dose: 40 mg bid (immediate release tablets)<br><br>initial dose: 80 mg qd (sustained release capsules)<br><br>max dose: 240 mg/d<br><br>**essential tremor:** initial dose: 40 mg bid max dose: 320 mg/d<br><br>**Traumatic Brain Injury** 5 mg bid, increase 5 mg q 5 d up to 45 mg | **antihypertensive agents; cimetidine** may decrease the metabolism of propranolol; **bile acid resins** may decrease the absorption of propranolol | cholesterol; decreased HDL cholesterol<br><br>Pharmacokinetics: protein binding = 90%; readily enters the CNS; $T_{1/2} = 3–5$ h | Lactation Issues: propranolol is excreted in breast milk; either the drug or nursing should be discontinued |

| | | | |
|---|---|---|---|
| **Sotalol**<br>Betapace<br><br>Tablets: 80 mg, 160 mg, 240 mg | **ventricular arrhythmias:** initial dose: 80 mg bid max dose: 320 mg/d<br><br>renal insufficiency: CrCl 30–60 mL/min: dosing interval = q 24 h<br>CrCl 10–30 mL/min: dosing interval = q 36–48 h<br>CrCl < 10 mL/min: individual dose | Administration Issues: food decreases the absorption of sotalol approximately 20%; therapy should not be abruptly discontinued; safety and efficacy have not been established in children<br><br>Drug–Drug Interactions: additive effects when given with other **negative inotropes** or **antihypertensive agents** | ADRs proarrhythmia; bradycardia; hypotension; worsening CHF; PVD; bronchospasm (in susceptible individuals); impotence; mask the signs of hypoglycemia; GI upset; dizziness; fatigue; sleep disturbance; increased triglycerides, total and LDL cholesterol; decreased HDL cholesterol<br><br>Pharmacokinetics: no protein binding; $T_{1/2} = 12$ h | Contraindications: hypersensitivity to beta blocking agents; symptomatic bradycardia; greater than first degree heart block; CHF (relative); asthma<br><br>Pregnancy Category: B<br><br>Lactation Issues: sotalol is excreted in breast milk; either the drug or nursing should be discontinued |

(continues on next page)

## 205.5 Beta-Adrenergic Blocking Agents   *continued from previous page*

| Drug and Dosage Forms | Usual Dosage Range | Administration Issues and Drug–Drug & Drug–Food Interactions | Common Adverse Drug Reactions (ADRs) and Pharmacokinetics | Contraindications, Pregnancy Category, and Lactation Issues |
|---|---|---|---|---|
| **Timolol**<br>Blocadren<br><br><u>Tablets:</u> 5 mg, 10 mg, 20 mg | **hypertension:**<br>initial dose: 10 mg bid<br>max dose: 60 mg/d<br><br>**myocardial infarction:**<br>10 mg bid<br><br>**migraine prophylaxis:**<br>initial dose: 10 mg bid<br>max dose: 30 mg/d | <u>Administration Issues:</u><br>therapy should not be abruptly discontinued; safety and efficacy have not been established in children<br><br><u>Drug–Drug Interactions:</u><br>additive effects when given with other **negative inotropes** or **antihypertensive agents** | <u>ADRs:</u><br>bradycardia; hypotension; worsening congestive heart failure (CHF); worsening peripheral vascular disease (PVD); bronchospasm (in susceptible individuals); impotence; mask the signs of hypoglycemia; GI upset; dizziness; fatigue; sleep disturbance; increased triglycerides, total and LDL cholesterol; decreased HDL cholesterol<br><br><u>Pharmacokinetics:</u><br>protein binding = 10%; $T_{1/2}$ = 4 h | <u>Contraindications:</u><br>hypersensitivity to beta blocking agents; symptomatic bradycardia; greater than first degree heart block; CHF (relative); asthma<br><br><u>Pregnancy Category:</u> C<br><br><u>Lactation Issues:</u><br>timolol is excreted in breast milk; either the drug or nursing should be discontinued |

## 205.6 Calcium Channel Blockers

| Drug and Dosage Forms | Usual Dosage Range | Administration Issues and Drug–Drug & Drug–Food Interactions | Common Adverse Drug Reactions (ADRs) and Pharmacokinetics | Contraindications, Pregnancy Category, and Lactation Issues |
|---|---|---|---|---|
| **Amlodipine**<br>Norvasc<br><br>Tablets:<br>2.5 mg, 5 mg, 10 mg | **hypertension:**<br>2.5–10 mg qd<br><br>**chronic stable and vasospastic angina:**<br>5–10 mg qd | Administration Issues:<br>safety and efficacy have not been established in children<br><br>Drug–Drug Interactions:<br>additive myocardial depression may occur in patients taking beta blockers | ADRs<br>hypotension, peripheral edema, tachycardia, flushing, headache, GI upset<br><br>Pharmacokinetics:<br>absorption = 80–90%; extensive first pass metabolism; hepatically metabolized; 93% protein bound; half-life = 30–50 hours | Contraindications:<br>hypersensitivity to amlodipine; hypotension; sick sinus syndrome; second or third degree AV block<br><br>Pregnancy Category: C<br><br>Lactation Issues:<br>it is not known if amlodipine is excreted in breast milk |
| **Bepridil**<br>Vascor<br><br>Tablets:<br>200 mg, 300 mg, 400 mg | **chronic stable angina:**<br>200–400 mg qd<br><br>Max dose = 400 mg/day | Administration Issues:<br>due to the risk of serious ventricular arrhythmias, use should be reserved to patients who fail to respond to or who are intolerant of other anti-anginals; safety and efficacy have not been established in children<br><br>Drug–Drug Interactions:<br>additive myocardial depression may occur in patients taking beta blockers | ADRs<br>hypotension, flushing, headache, GI upset, drowsiness, arrhythmias, prolonged QT interval<br><br>Pharmacokinetics:<br>absorption = 100%; onset = 60 minutes; hepatically metabolized; >99% protein bound; half-life = 24 hours | Contraindications:<br>hypersensitivity to bepridil; hypotension; sick sinus syndrome; second or third degree AV block; ventricular arrhythmias; prolonged QT interval; uncompensated heart failure<br><br>Pregnancy Category: C<br><br>Lactation Issues:<br>bepridil is excreted in breast milk |
| **Diltiazem**<br>Cardizem, Dilacor XR<br><br>Tablets:<br>30 mg, 60 mg, 90 mg, 120 mg | **hypertension, chronic stable and vasospastic angina:**<br>regular release tablets:<br>30–120 mg tid or qid | Administration Issues:<br>do not crush or chew extended release capsules; Dilacor XR should be taken on an empty stomach; safety and efficacy have not been established in children | ADRs<br>hypotension, peripheral edema, bradycardia, flushing, headache, GI upset, congestive heart failure | Contraindications:<br>hypersensitivity to diltiazem; hypotension; sick sinus syndrome; second or third degree AV block; acute MI; CHF |

(continues on next page)

**205.6 Calcium Channel Blockers** *continued from previous page*

| Drug and Dosage Forms | Usual Dosage Range | Administration Issues and Drug–Drug & Drug–Food Interactions | Common Adverse Drug Reactions (ADRs) and Pharmacokinetics | Contraindications, Pregnancy Category, and Lactation Issues |
|---|---|---|---|---|
| **Diltiazem** *cont.*<br><br>Sustained Release Capsules:<br>60 mg, 90 mg, 120 mg, 180 mg, 240 mg, 300 mg | sustained release capsules (Cardizem SR):<br>60–240 mg bid<br><br>sustained release capsules (Cardizem CD, Dilacor XR):<br>120–480 mg qd | Drug–Drug Interactions:<br>additive myocardial depression may occur in patients taking beta blockers; **cimetidine** and **ranitidine** may increase diltiazem levels | Pharmacokinetics:<br>absorption = 80–90%; onset = 30–60 minutes; hepatically metabolized; 70–80% protein bound; half-life = 3.5–7 hours | Pregnancy Category: C<br><br>Lactation Issues:<br>diltiazem is excreted in breast milk |
| **Felodipine**<br>Plendil<br><br>Extended Release Tablets:<br>2.5 mg, 5 mg, 10 mg | **hypertension:**<br>2.5–10 mg qd | Administration Issues:<br>avoid grapefruit products before and after dosing; do not crush or chew extended release tablets; safety and efficacy have not been established in children<br><br>Drug–Drug Interactions:<br>additive myocardial depression may occur in patients taking **beta blockers**; **cimetidine** and **ranitidine** may increase felodipine levels | ADRs<br>hypotension, peripheral edema, tachycardia, flushing, headache, GI upset<br><br>Pharmacokinetics:<br>absorption = 100%; onset = 2–5 hours; hepatically metabolized; >99% protein bound; half-life = 11–16 hours | Contraindications:<br>hypersensitivity to felodipine; hypotension; sick sinus syndrome; second or third degree AV block<br><br>Pregnancy Category: C<br><br>Lactation Issues:<br>it is not known if felodipine is excreted in breast milk |
| **Isradipine**<br>Dynacirc<br><br>Capsules:<br>2.5 mg, 5 mg | **hypertension:**<br>2.5–10 mg bid | Administration Issues:<br>safety and efficacy have not been established in children<br><br>Drug–Drug Interactions:<br>additive myocardial depression may occur in patients taking **beta blockers** | ADRs<br>hypotension, peripheral edema, tachycardia, flushing, headache, GI upset<br><br>Pharmacokinetics:<br>absorption = 90–95%; onset = 2 hours; hepatically metabolized; 95% protein bound; half-life = 8 hours | Contraindications:<br>hypersensitivity to isradipine; hypotension; sick sinus syndrome; second or third degree AV block<br><br>Pregnancy Category: C<br><br>Lactation Issues:<br>it is not known if isradipine is excreted in breast milk |

| | | | |
|---|---|---|---|
| **Mibefradil**<br>Posicor<br><br>Tablets:<br>50 mg, 100 mg | **hypertension and chronic stable angina:**<br>50–100 mg qd | Administration Issues:<br>has been safely administered with diuretics, ACE inhibitors, beta blockers and nitrates<br><br>Drug–Drug Interactions:<br>mibefradil inhibits the metabolism of **tricyclic antidepressants, terfenadine, astemizole, cisapride, cyclosporine, quinidine, metoprolol, lovastatin and simvastatin, atorvastatin** and **cerivistatin** | ADRs<br>dizziness, hypotension, peripheral edema, bradycardia, flushing, headache, GI upset<br><br>Pharmacokinetics:<br>absorption = 70%; hepatically metabolized; >99% protein bound; duration = 24 hours | Contraindications:<br>hypersensitivity to mibefradil; hypotension; sick sinus syndrome; second or third degree AV block; co-administration with terfenadine, astemizole, cisapride, lovastatin and simvastatin<br><br>Pregnancy Category: C<br><br>Lactation Issues:<br>it is not known if mibefradil is excreted in breast milk |
| **Nicardipine**<br>Cardene<br><br>Capsules:<br>20 mg, 30 mg<br><br>Sustained Release Capsules:<br>45 mg, 60 mg | **hypertension:**<br><br>regular release capsules:<br>20–40 mg tid<br><br>sustained release capsules:<br>30–60 mg bid<br><br>**angina:**<br>20–40 mg tid | Administration Issues:<br>do not crush or chew extended release capsules; lower doses may be required in patients with hepatic insufficiency<br><br>Drug–Drug Interactions:<br>additive myocardial depression may occur in patients taking **beta blockers** | ADRs<br>hypotension, peripheral edema, tachycardia, flushing, headache, GI upset<br><br>Pharmacokinetics:<br>absorption = 100%; onset = 20 minutes; hepatically metabolized; >95% protein bound; half-life = 2–4 hours | Contraindications:<br>hypersensitivity to nicardipine; hypotension; sick sinus syndrome; second or third degree AV block; advanced aortic stenosis<br><br>Pregnancy Category: C<br><br>Lactation Issues:<br>nicardipine is excreted in breast milk |
| **Nifedipine**<br>Adalat, Procardia<br><br>Capsules:<br>10 mg, 20 mg<br><br>Sustained Release Tablets:<br>30 mg, 60 mg, 90 mg | **hypertension:**<br><br>regular release capsules:<br>10–20 mg tid or qid<br><br>sustained release tablets:<br>30–120 mg qd | Administration Issues:<br>do not crush or chew extended release tablets<br><br>Drug–Drug Interactions:<br>additive myocardial depression may occur in patients taking **beta blockers** | ADRs<br>hypotension, peripheral edema, tachycardia, flushing, headache, GI upset<br><br>Pharmacokinetics:<br>absorption = 90%; onset = 20 minutes; hepatically | Contraindications:<br>hypersensitivity to nifedipine; hypotension; sick sinus syndrome; second or third degree AV block<br><br>Pregnancy Category: C |

(continues on next page)

**205.6 Calcium Channel Blockers** *continued from previous page*

| Drug and Dosage Forms | Usual Dosage Range | Administration Issues and Drug–Drug & Drug–Food Interactions | Common Adverse Drug Reactions (ADRs) and Pharmacokinetics | Contraindications, Pregnancy Category, and Lactation Issues |
|---|---|---|---|---|
| **Nifedipine** *cont.* | **chronic stable and vasospastic angina:**<br><br>regular release capsules:<br>10–20 mg tid or qid<br><br>sustained release tablets:<br>30–90 mg qd | | metabolized; 92–98% protein bound; half-life = 2–5 hours | Lactation Issues:<br>an insignificant amount of nifedipine is excreted in breast milk |
| **Nisoldipine**<br>Sular<br><br>Extended Release Tablets:<br>10 mg, 20 mg, 30 mg, 40 mg | **hypertension:**<br>10–60 mg qd | Administration Issues:<br>avoid administration with a high fat meal; avoid grapefruit products before and after dosing; do not crush or chew extended release tablets; lower doses may be required in patients > 65 years or in patients with hepatic insufficiency<br><br>Drug–Drug Interactions:<br>additive myocardial depression may occur in patients taking **beta blockers** | ADRs<br>hypotension, peripheral edema, tachycardia, flushing, headache, GI upset<br><br>Pharmacokinetics:<br>absorption = 80–90%; extensive first pass metabolism; hepatically metabolized; >99% protein bound; half-life = 7–12 hours | Contraindications:<br>hypersensitivity to nisoldipine; hypotension; sick sinus syndrome; second or third degree AV block<br><br>Pregnancy Category: C<br><br>Lactation Issues:<br>it is not known if nisoldipine is excreted in breast milk |
| **Verapamil**<br>Calan, Covera-HS, Isoptin, Verelan<br><br>Tablets:<br>40 mg, 80 mg, 120 mg<br><br>Sustained Release Tablets:<br>120 mg, 180 mg, 240 mg | **hypertension:**<br><br>regular release tablets: 40–160 mg tid<br><br>SR tablets and capsules:<br>120–480 mg qd (doses > 240 mg should be given divided bid) | Administration Issues:<br>do not crush or chew extended release tablets and capsules<br><br>Drug–Drug Interactions:<br>additive myocardial depression may occur in patients taking **beta blockers**; increased **digoxin** and **quinidine** levels may occur with concomitant administration | ADRs<br>hypotension, peripheral edema, bradycardia, flushing, headache, GI upset, congestive heart failure, constipation<br><br>Pharmacokinetics:<br>absorption = 90%; onset = 30 minutes; hepatically | Contraindications:<br>hypersensitivity to verapamil; hypotension; sick sinus syndrome; second or third degree AV block; uncompensated heart failure<br><br>Pregnancy Category: C |

| Drug and Dosage Forms | Usual Dosage Range | | Contraindications, Pregnancy Category, and Lactation Issues |
|---|---|---|---|
| Extended Release Tablets: 180 mg, 240 mg<br><br>Sustained Release Capsules: 180 mg, 240 mg, 360 mg | angina: 40–120 mg tid<br><br>atrial fibrillation, atrial flutter, supraventricular tachycardia: 240–480 mg, divided, tid or qid | metabolized; 83–92% protein bound; half-life = 3–7 hours | Lactation Issues: verapamil is excreted in breast milk |

## 205.7 Vasodilators

| Drug and Dosage Forms | Usual Dosage Range | Administration Issues and Drug–Drug & Drug–Food Interactions | Common Adverse Drug Reactions (ADRs) and Pharmacokinetics | Contraindications, Pregnancy Category, and Lactation Issues |
|---|---|---|---|---|
| **Hydralazine**<br>Apresoline<br><br>Tablets: 10 mg, 25 mg, 50 mg, 100 mg<br><br>Combinations: w/ varying strengths of HCTZ, hydralazine and reserpine (do not use combinations as initial therapy for HTN) | hypertension:<br><br>adults: initial dose: 10 mg qid<br>max dose: 300 mg/d, divided<br><br>children: initial dose: 0.75 mg/kg/d qid<br>max dose: 7.5 mg/kg/d or 200 mg/d | Administration Issues: taking hydralazine with food increases absorption; take with meals; safety and efficacy have not been established in children<br><br>Drug–Drug Interactions: **metoprolol and propranolol** may increase hydralazine concentrations; hydralazine may increase **metoprolol** and **propranolol** concentrations; **indomethacin** may decrease the effects of hydralazine | ADRs: reflex tachycardia; peripheral edema; headache; GI upset; palpitations; lupus-like syndrome<br><br>Pharmacokinetics: protein binding = 87%; extensive hepatic metabolism; $T_{1/2}$ = 3–7 h | Contraindications: hypersensitivity to hydralazine; coronary artery disease; rheumatic mitral valve disease<br><br>Pregnancy Category: C<br><br>Lactation Issues: hydralazine is excreted in breast milk; according to the American Academy of Pediatrics, hydralazine is compatible with breast feeding |
| **Minoxidil**<br>Loniten<br><br>Tablets: 2.5 mg, 10 mg | hypertension:<br><br>adults: initial dose: 2.5 mg qd<br>maximum dose: 100 mg/d | Administration Issues: allow at least 3 days before titrating dosage; safety and efficacy have not been established in children | ADRs: reflex tachycardia; peripheral edema; GI upset; headache; hirsutism; pericardial effusion | Contraindications: hypersensitivity to minoxidil; coronary artery disease; pheochromocytoma; acute myocardial infarction |

(continues on next page)

| Drug and Dosage Forms | Usual Dosage Range | Administration Issues and Drug–Drug & Drug–Food Interactions | Common Adverse Drug Reactions (ADRs) and Pharmacokinetics | Contraindications, Pregnancy Category, and Lactation Issues |
|---|---|---|---|---|
| **Minoxidil** *cont.* | **children:** initial dose: 0.2 mg/kg/d maximum dose: 50 mg/day | Drug–Drug Interactions: concomitant use with **guanethidine** may result in profound orthostatic hypotension | Pharmacokinetics: no protein binding; metabolites are renally eliminated; $T_{1/2}$ = 4.2 h | Pregnancy Category: C  Lactation Issues: minoxidil is excreted in breast milk; either the drug or nursing should be discontinued |

## 206. Antiplatelet Agents

| Drug and Dosage Forms | Usual Dosage Range | Administration Issues and Drug–Drug & Drug–Food Interactions | Common Adverse Drug Reactions (ADRs) and Pharmacokinetics | Contraindications, Pregnancy Category, and Lactation Issues |
|---|---|---|---|---|
| **Dipyridamole** Persantine  Tablets: 25 mg, 50 mg, 75 mg | **Adjunct to warfarin in the prevention of post-operative thromboembolic complications of cardiac valve replacement**  75–100 mg qid along with warfarin therapy | Administration Issues: Safety and efficacy in children < 12 years has not been established | ADRs Hypotension; dizziness; GI upset; headache; rash; flushing  Pharmacokinetics $T_{1/2}$ = 10 hours; highly protein bound; metabolized by the liver and excreted in bile | Contraindications: Hypersensitivity to dipyridamole  Pregnancy Category: B  Lactation issues: Dipyridamole is excreted in breast milk; use with caution in nursing women |
| **Ticlopidine** Ticlid | **To reduce the risk of stroke in patients who are intolerant of aspirin, who have experienced** | Administration Issues: Safety and efficacy in patients < 18 years of age have not been established; take with | ADRs GI upset; diarrhea; rash; vomiting; **neutropenia;** increased risk of | Contraindications: Hypersensitivity to ticlopidine; neutropenia; thrombocytopenia; |

| Drug and Dosage Forms | Usual Dosage Range | Administration Issues and Drug–Drug & Drug–Food Interactions | Common Aderse Drug Reactions (ADRs) and Pharmacokinetics | Contraindications, Pregnancy Category, and Lactation Issues |
|---|---|---|---|---|
| Tablets:<br>250 mg | **stroke precursors or have had a completed thrombotic stroke.**<br><br>250 mg bid with food | food to minimized GI upset. **CBCs should be done every 2 weeks through the third month of treatment.**<br><br>Drug–Drug Interactions:<br>Administering ticlopidine with **antacids** may decrease its absorption; **cimetidine** may increase the concentration of ticlopidine; **aspirin** may potentiate the effects of ticlopidine; ticlopidine increases **theophylline** levels and decreases **digoxin** levels<br><br>Drug–Food Interactions:<br>Administering with food increases the bioavailability approximately 20% | bleeding, increased liver function tests (AST, ALT, alkaline phosphatase)<br><br>Pharmacokinetics:<br>absorption = 80%; $T_{1/2}$ = 4–5 days; protein binding = 98%; extensively metabolized by the liver to inactive metabolites | active bleeding; severe liver impairment<br><br>Pregnancy Category: B<br><br>Lactation issues:<br>Due to the potential risk for serious adverse effects, either the drug or nursing should be discontinued |

## 207. Cardiac Glycosides

| Drug and Dosage Forms | Usual Dosage Range | Administration Issues and Drug–Drug & Drug–Food Interactions | Common Aderse Drug Reactions (ADRs) and Pharmacokinetics | Contraindications, Pregnancy Category, and Lactation Issues |
|---|---|---|---|---|
| **Digoxin**<br>Lanoxin, Lanoxicaps<br><br>Tablets:<br>0.125 mg, 0.25 mg, 0.5 mg<br><br>Capsules:<br>0.05 mg, 0.1 mg, 0.2 mg<br><br>Pediatric Elixir:<br>0.05 mg per ml | **Congestive Heart Failure, Atrial Fibrillation, Atrial Flutter, Paroxysmal Atrial Tachycardia**<br><br>Oral Loading Dose:<br>0.01–0.02 mg/kg (using lean body weight). Give 50% to start. Give remaining 50% in two equal doses at 6–8 hour intervals.<br><br>Assess for toxicity before each dose. | Administration Issues:<br>Bioavailability may vary among products.<br><br>Drug–Drug Interactions:<br>The following drugs may increase digoxin levels:<br>**amiodarone, quinidine, verapamil, antibiotics, propafenone, omeprazole, ibuprofen, indomethacin, captopril, itraconazle** | ADRs<br>anorexia, nausea, vomiting, diarrhea, headache, visual disturbances (blurred, green or yellow vision or halo effect), altered mental status, cardiac arrhythmias, gynecomastia, rash, eosinophilia, thrombocytopenia<br><br>**hypokalemia, hypomagnesesemia and** | Contraindications:<br>ventricular fibrillation, ventricular tachycardia, presence of digoxin toxicity, beriberi heart disease, hypersensitivity to digoxin, hypersensitive carotid sinus syndrome<br><br>Pregnancy Category: C |

(continues on next page)

| Drug and Dosage Forms | Usual Dosage Range | Administration Issues and Drug–Drug & Drug–Food Interactions | Common Adverse Drug Reactions (ADRs) and Pharmacokinetics | Contraindications, Pregnancy Category, and Lactation Issues |
|---|---|---|---|---|
| **Digoxin** *cont.* | Maintenance Dose: Tablets: 0.625 mg to 0.5 mg daily based on size and renal function Capsules: 0.05 to 0.2 mg daily based on size and renal function | The following drugs may decrease digoxin levels: **cholestyramine, colestipol, antacids, rifampin, sucralfate, hydantoins, barbiturates** **Therapeutic range: 0.5 to 2 ng/ml** | **hypercalcemia may predispose to cardiac arrhythmias** Pharmacokinetics absorption: tablets 60%–80%; elixir 70%–85%; capsules 90%–100%; distributed into myocardium, skeletal muscle, liver and kidney; crosses blood brain barrier and placenta; correlates with lean body weight; primarily excreted by the kidney; not removed by dialysis | Lactation Issues: digoxin is excreted in breast milk; safety has not been established |
| **Digitoxin** Crystodigin Tablets: 0.05 mg, 0.1 mg, | **Congestive Heart Failure, Atrial Fibrillation, Atrial Flutter, Paroxysmal Atrial Tachycardia** Rapid Loading: 0.6 mg followed by 0.4 mg followed by 0.2 mg separated by 4–6 hours Slow Loading: 0.2 mg bid for 4 d Maintenance Dose: 0.05–0.3 mg daily **Children** Loading Dose: <1 year: 0.045 mg/kg 1–2 years: 0.04 mg/kg >2 years: 0.03 mg/kg Maintenance Dose: one-tenth of loading dose | Drug–Drug Interactions: The following drugs may increase digitoxin levels: **amiodarone, quinidine, verapamil, antibiotics, propafenone, omeprazole, ibuprofen, indomethacin, captopril, itraconazle** The following drugs may decrease digitoxin levels: **cholestyramine, colestipol, antacids, rifampin, sucralfate, hydantoins, barbiturates** **Therapeutic range: 14–26 ng/ml** | ADRs anorexia, nausea, vomiting, diarrhea, headache, visual disturbances (blurred, green or yellow vision or halo effect), altered mental status, cardiac arrhythmias, gynecomastia, rash, eosinophilia, thrombocytopenia Pharmacokinetics almost completely absorbed; distributed into myocardium, skeletal muscle, liver and kidney; metabolized by the liver primarily to inactive metabolites; not removed by dialysis | Contraindications: ventricular fibrillation, ventricular tachycardia, presence of digitoxin toxicity; beriberi heart disease, hypersensitivity to digitoxin, hypersensitive carotid sinus syndrome Pregnancy Category: C Lactation Issues: it is not known whether digitoxin is excreted in breast milk |

| Drug and Dosage Forms | Usual Dosage Range | Administration Issues and Drug–Drug & Drug–Food Interactions | Common Adverse Drug Reactions (ADRs) and Pharmacokinetics | Contraindications, Pregnancy Category, and Lactation Issues |
|---|---|---|---|---|
| **Acetazolamide**<br>Diamox<br><br>Tablets:<br>125 mg, 250 mg<br><br>Sustained-Released Capsules:<br>500 mg | **open angle glaucoma:**<br>250–1000 mg in divided doses<br><br>**closed angle glaucoma:**<br>(short term) 250 mg q 4 hours<br><br>**children** 10–15 mg/kg/d divided, q 6–8 h<br><br>**diuresis:**<br>5 mg/kg (usually 250–375 mg) daily<br><br>**epilepsy:**<br>8–30 mg/kg/d (375–1000 mg daily), divided<br><br>**acute mountain sickness:**<br>500–1000 mg, divided; should initiate 24–48 h before ascent and continue for 48 h while at high altitude or longer to control symptoms | Administration Issues:<br>increasing the dose does not appear to increase diuresis<br><br>Drug–Drug Interactions:<br>Acetazolamide may increase **cyclosporine** levels; may decrease **primidone** levels; concurrent use with **salicylates** may result in accumulation and toxicity of acetazolamide | ADRs:<br>hypokalemia, GI upset, paresthesias, bone marrow suppression, urticaria, rash, photosensitivity, metabolic acidosis<br><br>Pharmacokinetics:<br>Tablets:<br>onset = 1–1.5 hours;<br>peak = 1–4 hours;<br>duration = 8–12 hours<br><br>SR Capsules:<br>onset = 2 hours;<br>peak = 3–6 hours;<br>duration = 18–24 hours | Contraindications:<br>hypersensitivity to acetazolamide<br><br>Pregnancy Category: C<br><br>Lactation Issues:<br>safety has not been established |
| **Dichlorphenamide**<br>Daranide<br><br>Tablets:<br>50 mg | **glaucoma:**<br><br>initial dose:<br>100–200 mg followed by 100 mg q 12 h<br><br>maintenance dose: 25–50 mg qd to tid | Drug–Drug Interactions:<br>concurrent use with **salicylates** may result in accumulation and toxicity of dichlorphenamide | ADRs:<br>hypokalemia, GI upset, paresthesias, bone marrow suppression, urticaria, rash, photosensitivity, metabolic acidosis | Contraindications:<br>use caution in patients with severe respiratory acidosis, pulmonary obstruction or emphysema (may impair ventilation)<br><br>Pregnancy Category: C |

(continues on next page)

**208.1 Carbonic Anhydrase Inhibitors** *continued from previous page*

| Drug and Dosage Forms | Usual Dosage Range | Administration Issues and Drug–Drug & Drug–Food Interactions | Common Adverse Drug Reactions (ADRs) and Pharmacokinetics | Contraindications, Pregnancy Category, and Lactation Issues |
|---|---|---|---|---|
| **Dichlorphenamide** *cont.* | | | Pharmacokinetics: onset = 1 hour; peak = 2–4 hours; duration = 6–12 hours | Lactation Issues: safety has not been established |
| **Methazolamide** Neptazane  Tablets: 25 mg, 50 mg | **glaucoma:** 50–100 mg 2 to 3 times daily | Drug–Drug Interactions: concurrent use with **salicylates** may result in accumulation and toxicity of methazolamide | ADRs: hypokalemia, GI upset, paresthesias, bone marrow suppression, urticaria, rash, photosensitivity, metabolic acidosis  Pharmacokinetics: onset = 2–4 hours; peak = 6–8 hours; duration = 10–18 hours | Contraindications: use in patients with hepatic dysfunction may precipitate hepatic coma  Pregnancy Category: C  Lactation Issues: safety has not been established |

## 208.2 Loop Diuretics

| Drug and Dosage Forms | Usual Dosage Range | Administration Issues and Drug–Drug & Drug–Food Interactions | Common Adverse Drug Reactions (ADRs) and Pharmacokinetics | Contraindications, Pregnancy Category, and Lactation Issues |
|---|---|---|---|---|
| **Bumetanide**<br>Bumex<br><br>Tablets:<br>0.5 mg, 1 mg, 2 mg | **edema:**<br>initial dose: 0.5–2 mg/d<br>maximum dose: 10 mg/d | Administration Issues:<br>take early in the day to avoid nocturia<br><br>Drug–Drug Interactions:<br>additive effect with **thiazide** and **thiazide-like diuretics; salicylates** and **NSAIDs** may decrease efficacy of loop diuretics; may increase **lithium** levels | ADRs:<br>dehydration; hyponatremic, hypochloremic; hypokalemia; hypomagnesemia; hypocalcemia; hyperuricemia; increased triglycerides, LDL and total cholesterol; decreased HDL cholesterol; photosensitivity; hypotension; GI upset; pancreatitis; thrombocytopenia<br><br>Pharmacokinetics:<br>$T_{1/2}$ = 60–90 minutes; onset = 30 minutes; duration = 4–6 hours | Contraindications: severe electrolyte depletion until improved or corrected; anuria; hypersensitivity to bumetanide or sulfonylureas<br><br>Pregnancy Category: C<br><br>Lactation Issues: it is unknown if bumetanide is excreted in breast milk |
| **Ethacrynic Acid**<br>Edecrin<br><br>Tablets:<br>25 mg, 50 mg | **ascites, CHF, nephrotic syndrome, acute pulmonary edema:**<br>initial dose: 50–200 mg/d<br>maximum dose: 200 mg bid<br><br>**children:**<br>initial dose: 25 mg/d then titrate to response | Administration Issues:<br>take early in the day to avoid nocturia<br><br>Drug–Drug Interactions:<br>additive effect with **thiazide** and **thiazide-like diuretics; salicylates** and **NSAIDs** may decrease efficacy of loop diuretics; may increase **lithium** levels | ADRs:<br>severe, watery diarrhea; dehydration; hyponatremia; hypokalemia; hypochloremic alkalosis, hypomagnesemia; hypocalcemia; hyperuricemia; ototoxicity; increased triglycerides, LDL and total cholesterol; decreased HDL cholesterol; photosensitivity; hypotension; GI upset; pancreatitis;<br><br>Pharmacokinetics:<br>absorption = 100%; $T_{1/2}$ = 60 minutes; onset = 30 minutes; duration = 6–8 hours | Contraindications:<br>anuria; hypersensitivity to ethacrynic acid; not recommended for use in children<br><br>Pregnancy Category: B<br><br>Lactation Issues: it is unknown if ethacrynic acid is excreted in breast milk |

(continues on next page)

| Drug and Dosage Forms | Usual Dosage Range | Administration Issues and Drug–Drug & Drug–Food Interactions | Common Adverse Drug Reactions (ADRs) and Pharmacokinetics | Contraindications, Pregnancy Category, and Lactation Issues |
|---|---|---|---|---|
| **Furosemide**<br>Lasix<br><br><u>Tablets:</u><br>20 mg, 40 mg, 80 mg<br><br><u>Oral Solution:</u><br>10 mg/ml, 40 mg/5 ml | **edema:**<br>initial dose: 20–40 mg/d<br>maximum dose: 600 mg/d<br><br>**hypertension:**<br>initial dose: 20–40 mg/d<br><br>**children:**<br>initial dose: 2 mg/kg/d<br>maintenance dose: 0.5–2 mg/kg bid<br>maximum dose: 6 mg/kg/d | <u>Administration Issues:</u><br>take early in the day to avoid nocturia<br><br><u>Drug–Drug Interactions:</u><br>additive effect with **thiazide** and **thiazide-like diuretics; salicylates** and **NSAIDs** may decrease efficacy of loop diuretics; may increase **lithium** levels | <u>ADRs:</u><br>dehydration; ototoxicity; hyponatremic, hypokalemia; hypomagnesemia; alkalosis, hypocalcemia; hyperuricemia; glucose intolerance; increased triglycerides, LDL and total cholesterol; decreased HDL cholesterol; photosensitivity; hypotension; GI upset; pancreatitis<br><br><u>Pharmacokinetics</u><br>$T_{1/2}$ = 120 minutes; onset = 60 minutes; duration = 6–8 hours | <u>Contraindications:</u><br>anuria; hypersensitivity to furosemide or sulfonylureas<br><br><u>Pregnancy Category:</u> C<br><br><u>Lactation Issues:</u> furosemide is excreted in breast milk |
| **Torsemide**<br>Demadex<br><br><u>Tablets:</u><br>5 mg, 10 mg, 20 mg, 100 mg | **CHF:**<br>initial dose: 10–20 mg/d<br>maximum dose: 200 mg/d<br><br>**chronic renal failure:**<br>initial dose: 20 mg/d<br>maximum dose: 200 mg/d<br><br>**hepatic cirrhosis:**<br>initial dose: 5–10 mg/d<br>maximum dose: 40 mg/d<br><br>**hypertension:**<br>initial dose: 5 mg/d<br>maximum dose: 10 mg/d | <u>Administration Issues:</u><br>take early in the day to avoid nocturia; may be taken without regards to meals<br><br><u>Drug–Drug Interactions:</u><br>additive effect with **thiazide** and **thiazide-like diuretics; salicylates** and **NSAIDs** may decrease efficacy of loop diuretics; may increase **lithium** levels | <u>ADRs</u><br>dehydration; ototoxicity; hyponatremic alkalosis; hypokalemia; hypomagnesemia; hypocalcemia; hyperuricemia; increased triglycerides, LDL and total cholesterol; decreased HDL cholesterol; photosensitivity; hypotension; GI upset<br><br><u>Pharmacokinetics:</u><br>$T_{1/2}$ = 210 minutes; onset = 60 minutes; duration = 6–8 hours | <u>Contraindications:</u><br>anuria; hypersensitivity to torsemide or sulfonylureas<br><br><u>Pregnancy Category:</u> B<br><br><u>Lactation Issues:</u> it is unknown if torsemide is excreted in breast milk |

| Drug and Dosage Forms | Usual Dosage Range | Administration Issues and Drug–Drug & Drug–Food Interactions | Common Adverse Drug Reactions (ADRs) and Pharmacokinetics | Contraindications, Pregnancy Category, and Lactation Issues |
|---|---|---|---|---|
| **Amiloride**<br>Midamor<br><br>Tablets:<br>5 mg<br><br>Combinations<br>5 mg amiloride and 50 mg HCTZ (do not use combinations as initial therapy of edema or HTN) | **Adjunctive therapy with a thiazide or loop diuretic in CHF and HTN; maintain normal potassium level in patients who develop hypokalemia with diuretic therapy**<br><br>Initial dose:  5 mg<br>Maximum dose:  20 mg/d | Administration Issues<br>Take with food or milk; avoid salt substitutes and excessive ingestion of foods high in potassium<br><br>Drug–Drug Interactions:<br>**potassium supplements, other potassium sparing diuretics,** and **ACE inhibitors** may potentiate hyperkalemia; **NSAIDs** may decrease the effectiveness of amiloride; may decrease **digoxin** concentrations | ADRs:<br>hyperkalemia; dehydration; headache; GI upset; dizziness; impotence; weakness; hypotension; cough; dyspnea; may reactivate peptic ulcer disease<br><br>Pharmacokinetics:<br>onset = 2 hours; duration = 24 hours; T$_{1/2}$ = 6–9 hours | Contraindications:<br>hypersensitivity to amiloride; potassium > 5.5, renal impairment; patients receiving spironolactone or triamterene<br><br>Pregnancy Category:  B<br><br>Lactation Issues:<br>it is not known whether amiloride is excreted in breast milk |
| **Spironolactone**<br>Aldactone<br><br>Tablets:<br>25 mg, 50 mg, 100 mg<br><br>Combinations<br>w/varying strengths of spironolactone and HCTZ (do not use combinations as initial therapy of edema or HTN) | **Hyperaldosteronism:**<br>100–400 mg/d<br><br>**Edema:**<br>25–200 mg/d (continue therapy at least 5 days before making a dosage adjustment)<br><br>**Children:**<br>3.3 mg/kg/d qd or in divided doses<br><br>**Hypertension:**<br>Initial Dose:  50–100 mg/d in single or divided doses (continue for 2 weeks before making a dosage adjustment)<br><br>**Hypokalemia:**<br>25–100 mg/d | Administration Issues<br>Take with food or milk; avoid salt substitutes and excessive ingestion of foods high in potassium<br><br>Drug–Drug Interactions:<br>spironolactone may increase **digoxin** levels; **potassium supplements, ACE inhibitors,** and **other potassium sparing diuretics** may result in hyperkalemia; **salicylates** may decrease the diuretic effect of spironolactone<br><br>Drug–Food Interaction:<br>administering spironolactone with food appears to increase its absorption | ADRs<br>hyperkalemia; gynecomastia; irregular menses or amenorrhea; postmenopausal bleeding; hirsutism; hyperchloremic metabolic acidosis in decompensated hepatic cirrhosis; hyponatremia; drowsiness<br><br>Pharmacokinetics:<br>onset = 24–48 hours; 98% protein binding; T$_{1/2}$ = 20 hours; active metabolite (canrenone) has T$_{1/2}$ = 10–35 hours | Contraindications:<br>anuria; potassium > 5.5; renal impairment<br><br>Pregnancy Category:  D<br><br>Lactation Issues:<br>The American Academy of Pediatricians considers spironolactone safe for use during breast feeding |

(continues on next page)

## 208.3 Potassium-Sparing Diuretics *continued from previous page*

| Drug and Dosage Forms | Usual Dosage Range | Administration Issues and Drug–Drug & Drug–Food Interactions | Common Adverse Drug Reactions (ADRs) and Pharmacokinetics | Contraindications, Pregnancy Category, and Lactation Issues |
|---|---|---|---|---|
| **Spironolactone** *cont.* | | Drug–Laboratory Interaction: spironolactone and its metabolites may falsely elevate **digoxin** levels when measured using radioimmunoassay | | |
| **Triamterene** Dyrenium Capsules: 50 mg, 100 mg Combinations w/varying strengths of triamterene and HCTZ (do not use combinations as initial therapy of edema or HTN) | **edema:** usual starting dose: 100 mg bid pc maximum dose: 300 mg per day | Administration Issues Take with food or milk; avoid salt substitutes and excessive ingestion of foods high in potassium Drug–Drug Interactions **indomethacin** may increase risk of acute renal failure; may increase **amantadine** levels; increase potassium with **potassium supplements** and **angiotensin converting enzyme inhibitors; cimetidine** may increase triamterene levels | ADRs: hyperkalemia, thrombocytopenia, megaloblastic anemia, rash, photosensitivity, GI upset, fatigue, weakness, dizziness, headache, dry mouth, metabolic acidosis, glucose intolerance, renal stones Pharmacokinetics: onset = 2–4 hours; duration = 12–16 hours; $T_{1/2}$ = 3 hours | Contraindications: potassium > 5.5; renal impairment; severe hepatic disease Pregnancy Category: B Lactation Issues: appears in breast milk in animals; if the drug is essential, patient should stop nursing |

| 208.4 Thiazide and Thiazide–Like Diuretics | | | | |
|---|---|---|---|---|
| **Drug and Dosage Forms** | **Usual Dosage Range** | **Administration Issues and Drug–Drug & Drug–Food Interactions** | **Common Adverse Drug Reactions (ADRs) and Pharmacokinetics** | **Contraindications, Pregnancy Category, and Lactation Issues** |
| **Bendroflumethiazide**<br>Naturetin<br><br>Tablets:<br>5 mg, 10 mg<br><br>Combinations<br>reserpine, nadolol<br>(combinations should not be used as initial therapy for edema or HTN) | **edema:**<br>initially: up to 20 mg daily or divided bid<br><br>maintenance: 2.5–5.0 mg qd<br><br>**hypertension:**<br>initially: 5–20 mg daily<br><br>maintenance: 2.5–15 mg/d | Administration Issues:<br>safety /efficacy not established in children; take early in the day to avoid nocturia; ineffective if CrCl <30 mL/min; allow 2–4 weeks for maximum antihypertensive effect<br><br>Drug–Drug Interactions:<br>may increase **lithium** levels; may decrease effectiveness of **anti-gout agents, sulfonylureas** and **insulin;** additive effects with **loop diuretics; NSAIDs** may decrease the effectiveness of thiazide diuretics; may increase hypersensitivity reactions to **allopurinol; bile acid resins** may decrease the absorption of thiazide diuretics | ADRs:<br>dehydration; hypotension; hypokalemia; hypomagnesemia; hypercalcemia; hyponatremic, alkalosis; hyperuricemia; glucose intolerance; transient negative effects on lipids, photosensitivity; impotence; GI upset<br><br>Pharmacokinetics:<br>absorption = 100%; excreted unchanged in urine within 24 hours | Contraindications:<br>hypersensitivity to thiazide diuretics or sulfonamide derivatives; anuria; pregnancy<br><br>Pregnancy Category: C<br><br>Lactation Issues:<br>it is not known whether bendroflumethiazide is excreted in breast milk; some manufacturers state that women receiving thiazide diuretics should not nurse |
| **Benzthiazide**<br>Exna<br><br>Tablets:<br>50 mg | **edema:**<br>initially: 50–200 mg daily<br>maintenance: 50–150 mg qd<br><br>if dose > 100 mg, give bid following morning and evening meal<br><br>**hypertension:**<br>initially: 50 mg bid<br>maximum: 200 mg daily | Administration Issues:<br>safety /efficacy not established in children; take early in the day to avoid nocturia; ineffective if CrCl <30 mL/min; allow 2–4 weeks for maximum antihypertensive effect<br><br>Drug–Drug Interactions:<br>may increase **lithium** levels; may decrease effectiveness of **anti-gout agents, sulfonylureas** and **insulin;** additive effects with **loop diuretics; NSAIDs** may decrease the effectiveness of thiazide | ADRs<br>dehydration; hypotension; hypokalemia; hypomagnesemia; hypercalcemia; hyponatremic, alkalosis; hyperuricemia; glucose intolerance; transient negative effects on lipids, photosensitivity; impotence; GI upset<br><br>Pharmacokinetics<br>absorption = 100%; excreted unchanged in urine within 24 hours | Contraindications:<br>hypersensitivity to thiazide diuretics or sulfonamide derivatives; anuria; pregnancy<br><br>Pregnancy Category: C<br><br>Lactation Issues:<br>it is not known whether benzthiazide is excreted in breast milk; some manufacturers state that women receiving thiazide diuretics should not nurse |

(continues on next page)

| Drug and Dosage Forms | Usual Dosage Range | Administration Issues and Drug–Drug & Drug–Food Interactions | Common Adverse Drug Reactions (ADRs) and Pharmacokinetics | Contraindications, Pregnancy Category, and Lactation Issues |
|---|---|---|---|---|
| **Benzthiazide** *cont.* | | diuretics; may increase hypersensitivity reactions to **allopurinol; bile acid resins** may decrease the absorption of thiazide diuretics | | |
| **Chlorothiazide**<br>Diuril<br><br>Tablets:<br>250 mg, 500 mg<br><br>Oral Suspension:<br>250 mg/5 ml<br><br>Combinations<br>reserpine, methyldopa<br>(combinations should not be used as initial therapy for edema or HTN) | **edema:**<br>500–1000 mg qd to bid<br><br>**hypertension:**<br>initially: 500–1000 mg daily<br>maximum: 2000 mg daily<br><br>**children:**<br>22 mg/kg/d<br><br>**infants < 6 months:**<br>33 mg/kg/d in divided doses | Administration Issues:<br>take early in the day to avoid nocturia; ineffective if CrCl <30 mL/min; allow 2–4 weeks for maximum antihypertensive effect<br><br>Drug–Drug Interactions:<br>may increase **lithium** levels; may decrease effectiveness of **anti-gout agents, sulfonylureas** and **insulin;** additive effects with **loop diuretics; NSAIDs** may decrease the effectiveness of thiazide diuretics; may increase hypersensitivity reactions to **allopurinol; bile acid resins** may decrease the absorption of thiazide diuretics | ADRs:<br>dehydration; hypotension; hypokalemia; hypomagnesemia; hypercalcemia; hyponatremic, alkalosis; hyperuricemia; glucose intolerance; transient negative effects on lipids; photosensitivity; impotence; GI upset<br><br>Pharmacokinetics<br>$T_{1/2}$ = 45–120 minutes | Contraindications:<br>hypersensitivity to thiazide diuretics or sulfonamide derivatives; anuria; pregnancy<br><br>Pregnancy Category: B<br><br>Lactation Issues:<br>it is not known whether chlorothiazide is excreted in breast milk; some manufacturers state that women receiving thiazide diuretics should not nurse |
| **Chlorthalidone**<br>Hygroton, Thalitone<br><br>Tablets:<br>15 mg, 25 mg, 50 mg, 100 mg<br><br>Combinations<br>reserpine, clonidine atenolol<br>(do not use combinations | **edema:**<br>50–100 mg daily<br>maximum: 200 mg daily<br><br>**hypertension:**<br>25–100 mg daily | Administration Issues:<br>safety/efficacy not established in children; take early in the day to avoid nocturia; ineffective if CrCl <30 mL/min; allow 2–4 weeks for maximum antihypertensive effect | ADRs:<br>hypokalemia; hypomagnesemia; hypercalcemia; alkalosis; hyperuricemia; glucose intolerance; transient negative effects on lipids; photosensitivity; impotence; GI upset | Contraindications:<br>hypersensitivity to thiazide diuretics or sulfonamide derivatives; anuria; pregnancy<br><br>Pregnancy Category: B |

| | | | |
|---|---|---|---|
| as initial therapy for edema or HTN) | | **Drug–Drug Interactions:** may increase **lithium** levels; may decrease effectiveness of **anti-gout agents, sulfonylureas** and **insulin;** additive effects with **loop diuretics; NSAIDs** may decrease the effectiveness of thiazide diuretics; may increase hypersensitivity reactions to **allopurinol; bile acid resins** may decrease the absorption of thiazide diuretics | **Pharmacokinetics:** T$_{1/2}$ = 54 hours | **Lactation Issues:** it is not known whether chlorthalidone is excreted in breast milk; some manufacturers state that women receiving thiazide diuretics should not nurse |
| **Hydrochlorothiazide** Esidrix, Hydrodiuril, Oretic <br><br> Tablets: 25 mg, 50 mg, 100 mg <br><br> Solution: 50 mg/5 ml <br><br> Intensol Solution: 100 mg/ml <br><br> Combinations amiloride, benazapril, bisoprolol, captopril, enalapril, hydralazine, guanethidine, lisinopril, methyldopa, nadolol, metoprolol, reserpine, spironolactone, triamterene (do not use combinations as initial therapy for edema or HTN) | **edema:** initially: 25 mg daily maximum: 50 mg daily <br><br> **hypertension:** 12.5–50 mg daily <br><br> **infants < 6 months:** 3.3 mg/kg divided bid <br><br> **children 6 months to 2 yr:** 12.5–37.5 mg divided bid <br><br> **children 2 to 12 yr:** 37.5–50 mg divided bid | **Administration Issues:** take early in the day to avoid nocturia; ineffective if CrCl <30 mL/min; allow 2–4 weeks for maximum antihypertensive effect <br><br> **Drug–Drug Interactions:** may increase **lithium** levels; may decrease effectiveness of **anti-gout agents, sulfonylureas** and **insulin;** additive effects with **loop diuretics; NSAIDs** may decrease the effectiveness of thiazide diuretics; may increase hypersensitivity reactions to **allopurinol; bile acid resins** may decrease the absorption of thiazide diuretics | **ADRs:** dehydration; hypotension; hypokalemia; hypomagnesemia; hypercalcemia; alkalosis; hyperuricemia; glucose intolerance; transient negative effects on lipids; photosensitivity; impotence; GI upset <br><br> **Pharmacokinetics:** absorption = 65–75%; excreted unchanged in urine; T$_{1/2}$ = 5.5–14.5 hours | **Contraindications:** hypersensitivity to thiazide diuretics or sulfonamide derivatives; anuria; pregnancy <br><br> **Pregnancy Category:** B <br><br> **Lactation Issues:** hydrochlorothiazide is excreted in breast milk; some manufacturers state that women receiving thiazide diuretics should not nurse |
| **Hydroflumethiazide** Diucardin, Saluron <br><br> Tablets: 50 mg | **edema:** initially: 50 mg qd or bid maintenance: 25–200 mg qd <br><br> if dose > 100 mg, divide doses | **Administration Issues:** safety/efficacy not established in children; take early in the day to avoid nocturia; ineffective if CrCl <30 mL/min; allow 2–4 weeks for maximum antihypertensive effect | **ADRs:** dehydration; hypotension; hypokalemia; hypomagnesemia; hypercalcemia; alkalosis; | **Contraindications:** hypersensitivity to thiazide diuretics or sulfonamide derivatives; anuria; pregnancy <br><br> **Pregnancy Category:** C |

(continues on next page)

| Drug and Dosage Forms | Usual Dosage Range | Administration Issues and Drug–Drug & Drug–Food Interactions | Common Adverse Drug Reactions (ADRs) and Pharmacokinetics | Contraindications, Pregnancy Category, and Lactation Issues |
|---|---|---|---|---|
| **Hydroflumethiazide cont.**<br><br>Combinations:<br>reserpine (do not use combinations as initial therapy for edema or HTN) | **hypertension:**<br>initially: 50 mg bid<br>maintenance: 50–100 mg qd<br>maximum dose: 200 mg daily | Drug–Drug Interactions:<br>may increase **lithium** levels; may decrease effectiveness of **anti-gout agents, sulfonylureas** and **insulin;** additive effects with **loop diuretics; NSAIDs** may decrease the effectiveness of thiazide diuretics; may increase hypersensitivity reactions to **allopurinol; bile acid resins** may decrease the absorption of thiazide diuretics | hyperuricemia; glucose intolerance; transient negative effects on lipids; photosensitivity; impotence; GI upset<br><br>Pharmacokinetics:<br>$T_{1/2}$ = 17 hours | Lactation Issues:<br>it is not known whether hydroflumethiazide is excreted in breast milk; some manufacturers state that women receiving thiazide diuretics should not nurse |
| **Indapamide**<br>Lozol<br><br>Tablets:<br>1.25 mg, 2.5 mg | **edema:**<br>2.5–5 mg daily<br><br>**hypertension:**<br>1.25–5 mg daily | Administration Issues:<br>take early in the day to avoid nocturia; allow 2–4 weeks for maximum antihypertensive effect<br><br>Drug–Drug Interactions:<br>may increase **lithium** levels; may decrease effectiveness of **anti-gout agents, sulfonylureas** and **insulin;** additive effects with **loop diuretics; NSAIDs** may decrease the effectiveness of thiazide diuretics; may increase hypersensitivity reactions to **allopurinol; bile acid resins** may decrease the absorption of thiazide diuretics | ADRs:<br>dehydration; hypotension; hypokalemia; hypomagnesemia; hypercalcemia; alkalosis; hyperuricemia; glucose intolerance; transient negative effects on lipids; photosensitivity; impotence; GI upset<br><br>Pharmacokinetics:<br>$T_{1/2}$ = 14–18 hours | Contraindications:<br>hypersensitivity to thiazide diuretics or sulfonamide derivatives; anuria; pregnancy<br><br>Pregnancy Category: B<br><br>Lactation Issues:<br>it is not known whether indapamide is excreted in breast milk; some manufacturers state that women receiving thiazide diuretics should not nurse |
| **Methyclothiazide**<br>Enduron, Aquatensen | **edema:**<br>2.5–10 mg daily | Administration Issues:<br>safety/efficacy not established in children; take early in the day to avoid nocturia; | ADRs:<br>dehydration; hypotension; hypokalemia; hypomagnesemia; | Contraindications:<br>hypersensitivity to thiazide diuretics or sulfonamide |

| | Dosage | Administration / Drug–Drug Interactions | ADRs / Pharmacokinetics | Contraindications / Pregnancy / Lactation |
|---|---|---|---|---|
| **Tablets:** 2.5 mg, 5 mg<br><br>Combinations: reserpine (do not use combinations as initial therapy for edema or HTN) | **hypertension:** 2.5–5 mg daily | ineffective if CrCl <30 mL/min; allow 2–4 weeks for maximum antihypertensive effect<br><br>Drug–Drug Interactions: may increase **lithium** levels; may decrease effectiveness of **anti-gout agents, sulfonylureas** and **insulin;** additive effects with **loop diuretics; NSAIDs** may decrease the effectiveness of thiazide diuretics; may increase hypersensitivity reactions to **allopurinol; bile acid resins** may decrease the absorption of thiazide diuretics | hypercalcemia; alkalosis; hyperuricemia; glucose intolerance; transient negative effects on lipids; photosensitivity; impotence; GI upset<br><br>Pharmacokinetics: absorption = 100%; excreted unchanged in urine within 24 hours | derivatives; anuria; pregnancy<br><br>Pregnancy Category: C<br><br>Lactation Issues: it is not known whether methyclothiazide is excreted in breast milk; some manufacturers state that women receiving thiazide diuretics should not nurse |
| **Metolazone**<br>Zaroxolyn, Mykrox<br><br>Tablets:<br>0.5 mg, 2.5 mg, 5 mg, 10 mg | **edema:**<br>zaroxolyn: 5–20 mg daily<br><br>**hypertension:**<br>zaroxolyn: 2.5–5 mg daily<br>mykrox: 0.5–1 mg daily | Administration Issues: not recommended for use in children; take early in the day to avoid nocturia; allow 2–4 weeks for maximum antihypertensive effect; **mykrox** and **zaroxolyn** are not bioequivalent<br><br>Drug–Drug Interactions: may increase **lithium** levels; may decrease effectiveness of **anti-gout agents, sulfonylureas** and **insulin;** additive effects with **loop diuretics; NSAIDs** may decrease the effectiveness of thiazide diuretics; may increase hypersensitivity reactions to **allopurinol; bile acid resins** may decrease the absorption of thiazide diuretics | ADRs:<br>dehydration; hypotension; hypokalemia; hypomagnesemia; hypercalcemia; alkalosis; hyperuricemia; glucose intolerance; photosensitivity; impotence; GI upset<br><br>Pharmacokinetics: absorption = 65% (**mykrox** is more completely and rapidly absorbed than **zaroxolyn** and should not be considered bioequivalent); $T_{1/2}$ = 14 h | Contraindications: hypersensitivity to thiazide diuretics or sulfonamide derivatives; anuria; pregnancy<br><br>Pregnancy Category: B<br><br>Lactation Issues: metolazone is excreted in breast milk; some manufacturers state that women receiving thiazide diuretics should not nurse |

(continues on next page)

| Drug and Dosage Forms | Usual Dosage Range | Administration Issues and Drug–Drug & Drug–Food Interactions | Common Adverse Drug Reactions (ADRs) and Pharmacokinetics | Contraindications, Pregnancy Category, and Lactation Issues |
|---|---|---|---|---|
| **Polythiazide**<br>Renese<br><br>Tablets:<br>1 mg, 2 mg, 4 mg<br><br>Combinations:<br>reserpine, polythiazide (combinations should not be used as initial therapy for edema or HTN) | edema:<br>1–4 mg daily<br><br>hypertension:<br>2–4 mg daily | Administration Issues:<br>take early in the day to avoid nocturia; ineffective if CrCl <30 mL/min; allow 2–4 weeks for maximum antihypertensive effect<br><br>Drug–Drug Interactions:<br>may increase **lithium** levels; may decrease effectiveness of **anti-gout agents, sulfonylureas** and **insulin;** additive effects with **loop diuretics; NSAIDs** may decrease the effectiveness of thiazide diuretics; may increase hypersensitivity reactions to **allopurinol; bile acid resins** may decrease the absorption of thiazide diuretics | ADRs:<br>dehydration; hypotension; hypokalemia; hypomagnesemia; hypercalcemia; alkalosis; hyperuricemia; glucose intolerance; transient negative effects on lipids; photosensitivity; impotence; GI upset<br><br>Pharmacokinetics:<br>absorption = 100% | Contraindications:<br>hypersensitivity to thiazide diuretics or sulfonamide derivatives; anuria; pregnancy<br><br>Pregnancy Category:  D<br><br>Lactation Issues:<br>it is not known whether polythiazide is excreted in breast milk; some manufacturers state that women receiving thiazide diuretics should not nurse |
| **Quinethazone**<br>Hydromox<br><br>Tablets:<br>50 mg | **edema and hypertension:**<br>50–100 mg daily<br>maximum dose:  200 mg daily | Administration Issues:<br>take early in the day to avoid nocturia; ineffective if CrCl <30 mL/min; allow 2–4 weeks for maximum antihypertensive effect<br><br>Drug–Drug Interactions:<br>may increase **lithium** levels; may decrease effectiveness of **anti-gout agents, sulfonylureas** and **insulin;** additive effects with **loop diuretics;** | ADRs:<br>dehydration; hypotension; hypokalemia; hypomagnesemia; hypercalcemia; alkalosis; hyperuricemia; glucose intolerance; transient negative effects on lipids; photosensitivity; impotence; GI upset | Contraindications:<br>hypersensitivity to thiazide diuretics or sulfonamide derivatives; anuria; pregnancy<br><br>Pregnancy Category:  D<br><br>Lactation Issues:<br>it is not known whether quinethazone is excreted in breast milk; some manufacturers state |

| | | | | |
|---|---|---|---|---|
| | | **NSAIDs** may decrease the effectiveness of thiazide diuretics; may increase hypersensitivity reactions to **allopurinol; bile acid resins** may decrease the absorption of thiazide diuretics | Pharmacokinetics: absorption = 100%; excreted unchanged in urine within 24 hours | that women receiving thiazide diuretics should not nurse |
| **Trichlormethiazide** Metahydrin, Naqua, Diurese Tablets: 2 mg, 4 mg | **edema and hypertension:** 2–4 mg daily (may give in divided doses) | Administration Issues: safety/ efficacy not established in children; take early in the day to avoid nocturia; ineffective if CrCl <30 mL/min; allow 2–4 weeks for maximum antihypertensive effect Drug–Drug Interactions: may increase **lithium** levels; may decrease effectiveness of **anti-gout agents, sulfonylureas** and **insulin;** additive effects with **loop diuretics; NSAIDs** may decrease the effectiveness of thiazide diuretics; may increase hypersensitivity reactions to **allopurinol; bile acid resins** may decrease the absorption of thiazide diuretics | ADRs: dehydration; hypotension; hypokalemia; hypomagnesemia; hypercalcemia; alkalosis; hyperuricemia; glucose intolerance; transient negative effects on lipids; photosensitivity; impotence; GI upset Pharmacokinetics: absorption = 100%; excreted unchanged in urine within 24 hours | Contraindications: hypersensitivity to thiazide diuretics or sulfonamide derivatives; anuria; pregnancy Pregnancy Category: C Lactation Issues: it is not known whether trichlormethiazide is excreted in breast milk; some manufacturers state that women receiving thiazide diuretics should not nurse |

# 300. CENTRAL NERVOUS SYSTEM (CNS) AGENTS

## 301. Acetaminophen

| Drug and Dosage Forms | Usual Dosage Range | Administration Issues and Drug–Drug & Drug–Food Interactions | Common Adverse Drug Reactions (ADRs) and Pharmacokinetics | Contraindications, Pregnancy Category, and Lactation Issues |
|---|---|---|---|---|
| **Acetaminophen (APAP)**<br><br>Acephen, Anacin-3, Panadol, Tempra, Tylenol, various generics<br><br>Tablets, chewable:<br>80 mg, 160 mg<br><br>Tablets:<br>325 mg, 500 mg, 650 mg<br><br>Caplets<br>160 mg, 500 mg, 650 mg<br><br>Capsules:<br>325 mg, 500 mg<br><br>Capsules, sprinkle<br>80 mg, 160 mg<br><br>Gelcaps: 500 mg<br><br>Elixir:<br>80 mg/2.5 mL, 80 mg/5 mL, 120 mg/5 mL, 160 mg/5 mL<br><br>Liquid:<br>160 mg/5 mL; 500 mg/15 mL | **Analgesic/antipyretic:**<br><br>Oral<br>**Adults:** 325–650 mg q 4–6 h or 1 g 3–4 times daily. Do not exceed 4 g/d<br>**Pediatrics** (dose given 4–5 times daily, max of 5 doses): 10 mg/kg or the following:<br>0–3 months: 40 mg<br>4–11 months: 80 mg<br>1–2 years: 120 mg<br>2–3 years: 160 mg<br>4–5 years: 240 mg<br>6–8 years: 320 mg<br>9–10 years: 400 mg<br>11 years: 480 mg<br><br>**Warning: when prescribing liquid/solution/ suspension for pediatric patients, write the dose based on "mgs/dose" and NOT "mLs/dose."**<br>**Hepatotoxicity has occurred due to accidental overdosing of infants/children**<br><br>Suppositories:<br>**Adults:** 650 mg q 4–6 h.<br>Max of 6 suppositories daily. | Administration Issues:<br>If pain persists longer than 5 days, consult physician.<br><br>Drug–Drug Interactions:<br>**increased toxic or pharmacologic effects of APAP:**<br>alcohol (chronic); barbiturates, carbamazepine, hydantoins, propranolol, rifampin, sulfinpyrazone<br><br>**decreased effect of APAP:**<br>charcoal<br>**increased effect on** warfarin (possible increase in the INR) | ADRs:<br>Very few adverse reactions<br>Infrequent: hemolytic anemia, neutropenia, leukopenia, pancytopenia, thrombocytopenia, skin rash, fever, hypoglycemia, jaundice<br><br>Overdose: nausea, vomiting, drowsiness, confusion, liver tenderness, low blood pressure, cardiac arrhythmias, jaundice, acute hepatic and renal failure<br><br>Pharmacokinetics<br>rapid onset (0.5–2 h); hepatically metabolized (toxic metabolite is metabolized by conjugation with hepatic glutathione); $T_{1/2} = 1–3$ h or 2.2–5 h in patients with cirrhosis | Contraindications:<br>Hypersensitivity to APAP<br><br>Precautions: Use cautiously in those with hepatic dysfunction, chronic alcohol use<br><br>Pregnancy/Lactation Issues:<br>Used in all trimesters of pregnancy with no known harm to fetus. Excreted in breast milk, but no known harm to infant |

(continues on next page)

| | |
|---|---|
| Solution (drops)<br>80 mg/1.66 mL, 100 mg/mL<br><br>Suspension<br>32 mg/mL; 80 mg/mL<br><br>Syrup: 16 mg/mL<br><br>Suppositories:<br>80 mg, 120 mg, 125 mg,<br>300 mg, 325 mg, 650 mg | **Pediatrics:**<br>3–6 years: 120 mg q 4–6 h.<br>Max of 720 mg/d<br>6–12 years: 325 mg q 4–6 h.<br>Max of 2.6 g/d<br><br>**Unlabeled Use:** prophylactic use in children receiving DTP vaccination |

## 302. Narcotic Agonists
### 302.1 Phenanthrenes

| Drug and Dosage Forms | Usual Dosage Range | Administration Issues and Drug–Drug & Drug–Food Interactions | Common Adverse Drug Reactions (ADRs) and Pharmacokinetics | Contraindications, Pregnancy Category, and Lactation Issues |
|---|---|---|---|---|
| **Codeine Sulfate**<br>various generics<br><br>Tablets:<br>15 mg, 30 mg, 60 mg<br><br>Soluble Tablets:<br>15 mg, 30 mg, 60 mg<br>(30 mg, 60 mg—also available as codeine phosphate) | **Moderate to severe pain:**<br>15–60 mg every 4–6 h prn<br>Max dose is 360 mg/d<br><br>**Pediatrics** (>1 yr old): 0.5 mg/kg q 4–6 h prn<br><br>Antitussive:<br>10–20 mg q 4–6 h prn<br>Max dose is 120 mg/d<br><br>**Pediatrics** (2–6 yrs): 2.5–5 mg q 4–6 h (Max dose is 30 mg/d)<br><br>**Pediatrics** (6–12 yrs): 5–10 mg q 4–6 h (Max dose is 60 mg/d) | Administration Issues:<br>Take with food if GI upset occurs.<br><br>Drug–Drug Interactions:<br>**increased level/effect of:** warfarin; barbiturates, alcohol, other CNS depressants (increased respiratory/CNS depressant effect); chlorpromazine (increased toxic effects); cimetidine (increased CNS toxicity)<br><br>**Drug Dependence, Tolerance:**<br>Narcotics have abuse potential although this potential is low if used for medical | ADRs<br>lightheadedness, dizziness, sedation, nausea, vomiting, sweating, constipation, drowsiness<br><br>Pharmacokinetics<br>onset of action = 10–30 min; duration of action = 4–6 h; extensive hepatic metabolism; $T_{1/2} = 3$ h; renal elimination of metabolites | Contraindications:<br>Hypersensitivity to codeine, diarrhea caused by poisoning, acute bronchial asthma, upper airway obstruction.<br><br>Precautions: Use cautiously in patients with hepatic or renal dysfunction, acute abdominal conditions, in elderly or debilitated patients, patients with respiratory conditions, cardiovascular or seizure disorders, hypothyroidism, |

| Drug and Dosage Forms | Usual Dosage Range | Administration Issues and Drug–Drug & Drug–Food Interactions | Common Adverse Drug Reactions (ADRs) and Pharmacokinetics | Contraindications, Pregnancy Category, and Lactation Issues |
|---|---|---|---|---|
| **Codeine Sulfate** *cont.* | | reasons. Prolonged use of these agents can lead to tolerance, thereby requiring increased doses. If medication is to be withdrawn, it should be tapered to prevent withdrawal symptoms. | | Addisons Disease, acute alcoholism, DT's, prostatic hypertrophy. <br><br> Pregnancy Category: C <br><br> Lactation Issues: Use cautiously. Excreted in breast milk although no significant effects on infant seen. |
| **Hydromorphone** <br> Dilaudid, various generics <br><br> Tablets: <br> 1 mg, 2 mg, 3 mg, 4 mg <br><br> Suppositories: 3 mg | **Moderate to severe pain:** <br> Oral: 2 mg q 4–6 h. May use 4 mg q 4–6 h for severe pain. <br><br> Rectal: 3 mg every 6–8 h | Administration Issues: <br> Take with food if GI upset occurs. Safety/efficacy in children is not established <br><br> Drug–Drug Interactions: <br> **increased level/effect of:** warfarin; barbiturates, alcohol, other CNS depressants (increased respiratory/CNS depressant effect); chlorpromazine (increased toxic effects); cimetidine (increased CNS toxicity) <br><br> **Drug Dependence, Tolerance:** Narcotics have abuse potential although this potential is low if used for medical reasons. Prolonged use of these agents can lead to tolerance, thereby requiring increased doses. If medication is to be withdrawn, it should be tapered to prevent withdrawal symptoms. | ADRs <br> lightheadedness, dizziness, sedation, nausea, vomiting, sweating, constipation, drowsiness <br><br> Pharmacokinetics <br> onset of action = 15–30 min; duration of action = 4–5 h; extensive hepatic metabolism; $T_{1/2}$ = 2–3 h; renal elimination of metabolites | Contraindications: <br> Hypersensitivity to hydrocodone, diarrhea caused by poisoning, acute bronchial asthma, upper airway obstruction <br><br> Precautions: Use cautiously in patients with hepatic or renal dysfunction, acute abdominal conditions, in elderly or debilitated patients, patients with respiratory conditions, cardiovascular or seizure disorders, hypothyroidism, Addisons Disease, acute alcoholism, DT's, prostatic hypertrophy. |

| | | | |
|---|---|---|---|
| | | | Pregnancy Category: C<br><br>Lactation Issues: Use cautiously. Excreted in breast milk although no significant effects on infant seen. |
| **Levorphanol**<br>Levo-Dromoran<br><br>Tablets: 2 mg | **Moderate to severe pain:**<br>2 mg q 8–12 h prn | Administration Issues:<br>Take with food if GI upset occurs.<br><br>Drug–Drug Interactions:<br>**increased level/effect of:** warfarin; barbiturates, alcohol, other CNS depressants (increased respiratory/CNS depressant effect); chlorpromazine (increased toxic effects); cimetidine (increased CNS toxicity)<br><br>**Drug Dependence, Tolerance:**<br>Narcotics have abuse potential although this potential is low if used for medical reasons. Prolonged use of these agents can lead to tolerance, thereby requiring increased doses. If medication is to be withdrawn, it should be tapered to prevent withdrawal symptoms. | ADRs<br>lightheadedness, dizziness, sedation, nausea, vomiting, sweating, constipation, drowsiness<br><br>Pharmacokinetics<br>onset of action = 30–90 min; duration of action = 6–8 h; extensive hepatic metabolism; $T_{1/2}$ = 12–16 h; renal elimination of metabolites | Contraindications:<br>Hypersensitivity to levorphanol, diarrhea caused by poisoning, acute bronchial asthma, upper airway obstruction<br><br>Precautions: Use cautiously in patients with hepatic or renal dysfunction, acute abdominal conditions, in elderly or debilitated patients, patients with respiratory conditions, cardiovascular or seizure disorders, hypothyroidism, Addisons Disease, acute alcoholism, DT's, prostatic hypertrophy.<br><br>Pregnancy Category: C<br><br>Lactation Issues: Use cautiously. Excreted in breast milk although no significant effects on infant seen. |
| **Morphine**<br>MSIR, Roxanol, RMS, various generics | **Moderate to severe acute or chronic pain:**<br>Oral: 10–30 mg q 4 h | Administration Issues:<br>Take with food if GI upset occurs. Do not crush or chew controlled release products. | ADRs<br>lightheadedness, dizziness, sedation, nausea, vomiting, sweating, constipation, drowsiness | Contraindications:<br>Hypersensitivity to morphine, diarrhea caused by poisoning, acute bronchial asthma, upper airway obstruction |

*(continues on next page)*

| Drug and Dosage Forms | Usual Dosage Range | Administration Issues and Drug–Drug & Drug–Food Interactions | Common Adverse Drug Reactions (ADRs) and Pharmacokinetics | Contraindications, Pregnancy Category, and Lactation Issues |
|---|---|---|---|---|
| **Morphine** *cont.*<br><u>Soluble tablets:</u><br>10 mg, 15 mg, 30 mg<br><br><u>Tablets:</u> 15 mg, 30 mg<br><br><u>Tablets, controlled-release</u><br>30 mg, 60 mg<br><br><u>Solution:</u><br>10 mg/5 mL<br>20 mg/5 mL<br>20 mg/1 mL<br>100 mg/5 mL<br><br><u>Suppositories:</u> 5 mg, 10 mg, 20 mg, 30 mg | <u>Controlled Release:</u><br>30 mg q 8–12 h<br><br><u>Rectal:</u> 10–20 mg q 4 h<br><br>**Pediatric:** 0.1–0.2 mg/kg q 4 h<br><br>**Elderly or debilitated:** use smaller initial doses to prevent respiratory depression. | <u>Drug–Drug Interactions:</u><br>**increased level/effect of:** warfarin, barbiturates, alcohol, other CNS depressants (increased respiratory/CNS depressant effect); chlorpromazine (increased toxic effects), cimetidine (increased CNS toxicity)<br><br>**Drug Dependence. Tolerance:**<br>Narcotics have abuse potential although this potential is low if used for medical reasons. Prolonged use of these agents can lead to tolerance, thereby requiring increased doses. If medication is to be withdrawn, it should be tapered to prevent withdrawal symptoms. | <u>Pharmacokinetics</u><br>onset of action = 15–60 min; duration of action = 3–7 h; extensive hepatic metabolism; $T_{1/2}$ = 1.5–2 h; renal elimination of metabolites | <u>Precautions:</u> Use cautiously in patients with hepatic or renal dysfunction, acute abdominal conditions, in elderly or debilitated patients, patients with respiratory conditions, cardiovascular or seizure disorders, hypothyroidism, Addisons Disease, acute alcoholism, DT's, prostatic hypertrophy.<br><br><u>Pregnancy Category:</u> C<br><br><u>Lactation Issues:</u> Use cautiously. Excreted in breast milk although no significant effects on infant seen. |
| **Oxycodone**<br>Roxicodone, OxyContin, Roxicodone intensol<br><br><u>Capsule:</u> 5 mg<br><br><u>Tablets:</u> 5 mg<br><br><u>Tablets, extended release:</u><br>10 mg, 20 mg, 40 mg, 80 mg | **Moderate to severe pain:**<br>5 mg q 4–6 h prn. May titrate dose as needed/tolerated.<br><br><u>Extended Release:</u> After an established dose is made with the immediate release product, may switch to the extended-release product and use q 12 hr prn. May titrate dose as needed/tolerated | <u>Administration Issues:</u><br>Take with food if GI upset occurs. Not recommended for children<br><br><u>Drug–Drug Interactions:</u><br>**increased level/effect of:** warfarin, barbiturates, alcohol, other CNS depressants (increased respiratory/CNS depressant effect); chlorpromazine (increased toxic effects), cimetidine (increased CNS toxicity) | <u>ADRs</u><br>lightheadedness, dizziness, sedation, nausea, vomiting, sweating, constipation, drowsiness<br><br><u>Pharmacokinetics</u><br>onset of action = 15–30 min; duration of action = 4–6 h; extensive hepatic metabolism; $T_{1/2}$— no data available; renal elimination of metabolites | <u>Contraindications:</u><br>Hypersensitivity to oxycodone, diarrhea caused by poisoning, acute bronchial asthma, upper airway obstruction<br><br><u>Precautions:</u> Use cautiously in patients with hepatic or renal dysfunction, acute abdominal conditions, in elderly or debilitated patients, patients |

with respiratory conditions, cardiovascular or seizure disorders, hypothyroidism, Addisons Disease, acute alcoholism, DT's, prostatic hypertrophy.

Pregnancy Category:  C

Lactation Issues:  Use cautiously. Excreted in breast milk although no significant effects on infant seen.

---

**Drug Dependence, Tolerance:**
Narcotics have abuse potential although this potential is low if used for medical reasons. Prolonged use of these agents can lead to tolerance, thereby requiring increased doses. If medication is to be withdrawn, it should be tapered to prevent withdrawal symptoms.

---

Solution: 5 mg/5 mL

Concentrate:
20 mg/1 mL

---

Contraindications:
Hypersensitivity to oxymorphone, diarrhea caused by poisoning, acute bronchial asthma, upper airway obstruction

Precautions:  Use cautiously in patients with hepatic or renal dysfunction, acute abdominal conditions, in elderly or debilitated patients, patients with respiratory conditions, cardiovascular or seizure disorders, hypothyroidism, Addisons Disease, acute alcoholism, DT's, prostatic hypertrophy.

Pregnancy Category:  C

Lactation Issues:  Use cautiously. Excreted in breast milk although no significant effects on infant seen.

ADRs
lightheadedness, dizziness, sedation, nausea, vomiting, sweating, constipation, drowsiness

Pharmacokinetics
onset of action = 5–10 min; duration of action = 3–6 h; extensive hepatic metabolism; $T_{1/2}$ —no data available; renal elimination of metabolites

---

Administration Issues:
Take with food if GI upset occurs. Refrigerate suppositories. Safety/efficacy not established in children <12 yrs.

Drug–Drug Interactions:
**increased level/effect of:** warfarin; barbiturates, alcohol, other CNS depressants (increased respiratory/CNS depressant effect); chlorpromazine (increased toxic effects); cimetidine (increased CNS toxicity)

**Drug Dependence, Tolerance:**
Narcotics have abuse potential although this potential is low if used for medical reasons. Prolonged use of these agents can lead to tolerance, thereby requiring increased doses. If medication is to be withdrawn, it should be tapered to prevent withdrawal symptoms.

---

# Oxymorphone
Numorphan
Suppositories:  5 mg

**Moderate to severe pain:**
5 mg q 4–6 h. May titrate dose in nondebilitated patients if pain not relieved.

| Drug and Dosage Forms | Usual Dosage Range | Administration Issues and Drug–Drug & Drug–Food Interactions | Common Adverse Drug Reactions (ADRs) and Pharmacokinetics | Contraindications, Pregnancy Category, and Lactation Issues |
|---|---|---|---|---|
| **Fentanyl**<br>Duragesic<br><br><u>Transdermal System</u>:<br>25 mcg/hr,<br>50 mcg/hr,<br>75 mcg/hr,<br>100 mcg/hr | **Moderate to severe chronic pain:**<br>Individualize dose. Apply patch every 72 hrs. If switching from another narcotic analgesic, convert daily dose to oral morphine equivalent and choose transdermal dose as follows:<br><br>45–134 mg/d:  25 mcg/hr<br>135–224 mg/d:  50 mcg/hr<br>225–314 mg/d:  75 mcg/hr<br>315–404 mg/d:  100 mcg/hr<br>405–494 mg/d:  125 mcg/hr<br>495–584 mg/d:  150 mcg/hr<br>585–674 mg/d:  175 mcg/hr<br>675–764 mg/d:  200 mcg/hr<br>765–854 mg/d:  225 mcg/hr<br>etc | <u>Administration Issues:</u><br>Apply patch to nonirritated clean, dry portion of skin. Clip hair at site of application (do not shave). To cleanse the site use clear water (avoid irritating the skin prior to application)<br><br><u>Drug–Drug Interactions:</u><br>**increased level/effect of:**  warfarin; barbiturates, alcohol, other CNS depressants (increased respiratory/CNS depressant effect); chlorpromazine (increased toxic effects); cimetidine (increased CNS toxicity)<br><br>**Drug Dependence, Tolerance:**<br>Narcotics have abuse potential although this potential is low if used for medical reasons. Prolonged use of these agents can lead to tolerance, thereby requiring increased doses. If medication is to be withdrawn, it should be tapered to prevent withdrawal symptoms | <u>ADRs</u><br>lightheadedness, dizziness, sedation, nausea, vomiting, sweating, constipation, drowsiness<br><br><u>Pharmacokinetics:</u><br>duration of action = 72 hr. (transdermal system); extensive hepatic metabolism; $T_{1/2}$ = 1.5–6 hr.; renal elimination of metabolites | <u>Contraindications:</u><br>Hypersensitivity to fentanyl, diarrhea caused by poisoning, acute bronchial asthma, upper airway obstruction<br><br><u>Precautions:</u>  Use cautiously in patients with hepatic or renal dysfunction, acute abdominal conditions, in elderly or debilitated patients, patients with respiratory conditions, cardiovascular or seizure disorders, hypothyroidism, Addisons Disease, acute alcoholism, DT's, prostatic hypertrophy.<br><br><u>Pregnancy Category:</u>  C<br><br><u>Lactation Issues:</u>  Use cautiously. Excreted in breast milk although no significant effects on infant seen. |
| **Meperidine**<br>Demerol, various generics<br><u>Tablets</u>:  50 mg, 100 mg<br><u>Syrup</u>: 50 mg/5 mL | **Moderate to severe pain:**<br>50–150 mg q 3–4 h prn<br><br>**Pediatrics:**  1–1.8 mg/kg up to an adult dose q 3–4 h prn | <u>Administration Issues:</u><br>Take with food if GI upset occurs.<br><br><u>Drug–Drug Interactions:</u><br>increased level/effect of:  warfarin; | <u>ADRs:</u><br>lightheadedness, dizziness, sedation, nausea, vomiting, sweating, constipation, drowsiness | <u>Contraindications:</u><br>Hypersensitivity, diarrhea caused by poisoning, acute bronchial asthma, upper airway obstruction |

| Drug and Dosage Forms | Usual Dosage Range | Administration Issues and Drug–Drug & Drug–Food Interactions | Common Adverse Drug Reactions (ADRs) and Pharmacokinetics | Contraindications, Pregnancy Category, and Lactation Issues |
|---|---|---|---|---|
| | | barbiturates, alcohol, other CNS depressants (increased respiratory/CNS depressant effect); chlorpromazine (increased toxic effects); cimetidine (increased CNS toxicity); MAO inhibitors (increased risk of hypertensive crisis)<br><br>**Drug Dependence, Tolerance:**<br>Narcotics have abuse potential although this potential is low if used for medical reasons. Prolonged use of these agents can lead to tolerance, thereby requiring increased doses. If medication is to be withdrawn, it should be tapered to prevent withdrawal symptoms. | Pharmacokinetics:<br>onset of action = 10–45 min; duration of action = 2–4 hr.; extensive hepatic metabolism (active metabolite: normeperidine); $T_{1/2}$ = 3–4 hr. ($T_{1/2}$ of metabolite = 15–30 hr.); renal elimination of metabolite | Precautions: Use cautiously in patients with hepatic or renal dysfunction, acute abdominal conditions, in elderly or debilitated patients, patients with respiratory conditions, cardiovascular or seizure disorders, hypothyroidism, Addisons Disease, acute alcoholism, DT's, prostatic hypertrophy.<br><br>Pregnancy Category: C<br><br>Lactation Issues: Use cautiously. Excreted in breast milk although no significant effects on infant seen. |

## 302.3 Diphenylheptanes

| Drug and Dosage Forms | Usual Dosage Range | Administration Issues and Drug–Drug & Drug–Food Interactions | Common Adverse Drug Reactions (ADRs) and Pharmacokinetics | Contraindications, Pregnancy Category, and Lactation Issues |
|---|---|---|---|---|
| **Methadone**<br>Dolophine, various generics<br><br>Tablets:<br>5 mg, 10 mg<br><br>Dispersible Tablets:<br>40 mg | Severe pain:<br>2.5–10 mg q 3–4 h prn<br><br>**Heroin Detoxification treatment:**<br>15–20 mg daily for not more than 21 days. Repeated courses may not start earlier than 4 weeks after completion of previous course. May titrate to | Administration Issues:<br>Take with food if GI upset occurs. Not recommended for children.<br><br>Drug–Drug Interactions:<br>increased level/effect of: warfarin; barbiturates, alcohol, other CNS depressants (increased respiratory/CNS depressant effect); chlorpromazine | ADRs:<br>lightheadedness, dizziness, sedation, nausea, vomiting, sweating, constipation, drowsiness<br><br>Pharmacokinetics:<br>onset of action = 30–60 min; duration of action = 4–6 hr.; | Contraindications:<br>Hypersensitivity, diarrhea caused by poisoning, acute bronchial asthma, upper airway obstruction<br><br>Precautions: Use cautiously in patients with hepatic or renal dysfunction, acute abdominal |

(continues on next page)

| Drug and Dosage Forms | Usual Dosage Range | Administration Issues and Drug–Drug & Drug–Food Interactions | Common Adverse Drug Reactions (ADRs) and Pharmacokinetics | Contraindications, Pregnancy Category, and Lactation Issues |
|---|---|---|---|---|
| **Methadone** *cont.* <br><br> Solution: <br> 5 mg/5 mL <br> 10 mg/5 mL <br> 10 mg/10 mL <br><br> Concentrate: <br> 10 mg/mL | higher dose if withdrawal symptoms are not suppressed. Maintain dose to suppress withdrawal symptoms for 2–3 days, then gradually decrease dose on a daily or every 2 day schedule. | (increased toxic effects); cimetidine (increased CNS toxicity) <br><br> **Drug Dependence, Tolerance:** <br> Narcotics have abuse potential although this potential is low if used for medical reasons. Prolonged use of these agents can lead to tolerance, thereby requiring increased doses. If medication is to be withdrawn, it should be tapered to prevent withdrawal symptoms. | extensive hepatic metabolism; $T_{1/2}$ = 15–30 hr.; renal elimination of metabolites | conditions, in elderly or debilitated patients, patients with respiratory conditions, cardiovascular or seizure disorders, hypothyroidism, Addisons Disease, acute alcoholism, DT's, prostatic hypertrophy. <br><br> Pregnancy Category:  C <br><br> Lactation Issues:  Use cautiously. Excreted in breast milk although no significant effects on infant seen. |
| **Propoxyphene** <br> Darvon, Dolene, various generics <br><br> Capsules:  32 mg, 65 mg <br><br> Propoxyphene napsylate Darvon-N <br><br> Tablets:  100 mg <br><br> Suspension: <br> 10 mg/1 mL | **Mild to moderate pain:** <br> Propoxyphene <br> 65 mg q 4 h prn. Max dose is 390 mg/d. <br><br> Propoxyphene Napsylate <br> 100 mg (equivalent to 65 mg propoxyphene) q 4 h prn. Max dose is 600 mg/d. <br><br> **Elderly or debilitated patients** <br> (renal or hepatic dysfunction):  use smaller daily doses. | Administration Issues: <br> Take with food if GI upset occurs. Not recommended for children. <br><br> Drug–Drug Interactions: <br> **increased level/effect of:**  warfarin; barbiturates, alcohol, other CNS depressants (inc respiratory/CNS depressant effect); chlorpromazine (inc CNS toxic effects); cimetidine (inc CNS toxicity); carbamazepine (inc toxicity) <br> decreased level/effect of propoxyphene: charcoal, smoking | ADRs: <br> dizziness, sedation, nausea, vomiting <br><br> Pharmacokinetics: <br> onset of action = 30–60 min; duration of action = 4–6 hrs; extensive hepatic metabolism; $T_{1/2}$ = 6–12 hrs; renal elimination of metabolites | Contraindications: <br> Hypersensitivity to ingredients <br><br> Precautions:  Use cautiously in patients with hepatic or renal dysfunction, in elderly or debilitated patients, patients with respiratory conditions. <br><br> Pregnancy Issues:  Safety not established. Use cautiously. <br><br> Lactation Issues:  Use cautiously. Excreted in breast |

| | | Drug Dependence, Tolerance: <br> Narcotics have abuse potential although this potential is low if used for medical reasons. Prolonged use of these agents can lead to tolerance, thereby requiring increased doses. If medication is to be withdrawn, it should be tapered to prevent withdrawal symptoms. | milk although no significant effects on infant seen. |

## 302.4 Narcotic Agonists-Antagonists Combinations

| Drug and Dosage Forms | Usual Dosage Range | Administration Issues and Drug–Drug & Drug–Food Interactions | Common Adverse Drug Reactions (ADRs) and Pharmacokinetics | Contraindications, Pregnancy Category, and Lactation Issues |
|---|---|---|---|---|
| **Pentazocine & Naloxone** <br> Talwin NX <br><br> Tablets: <br> 50 mg/0.5 mg | **Moderate to Severe Pain:** <br><br> 50 mg of pentazocine q 3–4 h, initially. May titrate to 100 mg if necessary. Max dose is 600 mg/d. | Administration Issues: <br> Avoid alcohol use. Safety/efficacy not established for children <12 yrs. <br><br> Drug–Drug Interactions: <br> **increased effect of:** alcohol, other CNS depressants. <br><br> **Dependence, Tolerance:** <br> Psychological and physical dependence have occurred with prolonged use of this agent. Withdrawal symptoms have been associated with abrupt discontinuation. | ADRs: <br> nausea, dizziness, lightheadedness, vomiting, euphoria, sedation, constipation. <br><br> Pharmacokinetics: <br> extensively hepatically metabolized | Contraindications: <br> Hypersensitivity <br><br> Precautions: Use cautiously in patients with severe renal or hepatic dysfunction, or respiratory dysfunction. Use cautiously in patients previously receiving narcotic agonist — this may precipitate withdrawal. <br><br> Pregnancy Category: C <br><br> Lactation Issues: safety not established. |

(continues on next page)

## 302.4 Narcotic Agonists-Antagonists Combinations continued from previous page

| Drug and Dosage Forms | Usual Dosage Range | Administration Issues and Drug–Drug & Drug–Food Interactions | Common Adverse Drug Reactions (ADRs) and Pharmacokinetics | Contraindications, Pregnancy Category, and Lactation Issues |
|---|---|---|---|---|
| **Pentazocine & Aspirin**<br>Talwin Compound Caplets<br><br>Tablets:<br>12.5 mg/325 mg | **Moderate to Severe Pain:**<br>2 tablets tid to qid | Administration Issues:<br>Avoid alcohol use. Safety/efficacy not established for children <12 yrs. Aspirin use in children with fever has been associated with Reye's syndrome.<br><br>Drug–Drug Interactions:<br>**increased effect of:** alcohol, other CNS depressants.<br><br>Aspirin<br>**increased level/effect of:** alcohol (GI effects); anticoagulants (bleeding effects); methotrexate, valproic acid, sulfonylureas (inc hypoglycemic effect)<br>**decreased level/effect of:** ACE inhibitors, beta blockers, diuretics (decreased antihypertensive effect); probenecid & sulfinpyrazone (decreased uricosuric effect)<br><br>Drug–Lab Interactions:<br>**Aspirin:** false negative or positive urine glucose tests, uric acid levels (inc with salicylate levels <10 mg/dL; decreased with salicylate levels >10 mg/dL), falsely elevated urine vanillymandelic acid tests.<br><br>**Dependence, Tolerance:**<br>Psychological & physical dependence have occurred with prolonged use of this agent. Withdrawal symptoms have been associated with abrupt discontinuation | ADRs:<br>nausea, dizziness, lightheadedness, vomiting, euphoria, sedation, constipation.<br><br>**Aspirin:**<br>Most frequent: nausea, dyspepsia, heartburn, GI bleeding, hives, rash, prolonged bleeding time, thrombocytopenia, aspirin intolerance (bronchospasm, rhinitis), "Salicylism": dizziness, tinnitus, difficulty hearing, nausea, vomiting, diarrhea, confusion, CNS depression, headache, sweating, hyperventilation, lassitude<br><br>Pharmacokinetics:<br>Aspirin: hepatically metabolized | Contraindications:<br>Hypersensitivity<br>Aspirin: hemophilia, bleeding ulcers, hemorrhagic states<br><br>Precautions: Use cautiously in patients with severe renal or hepatic dysfunction, or respiratory dysfunction. Use cautiously in patients previously receiving narcotic agonist — this may precipitate withdrawal. Aspirin: Use cautiously in patients with asthma, nasal polyposis, chronic urticaria (inc risk of hypersensitivity); chronic renal insufficiency, PUD, bleeding disorders.<br><br>Pregnancy Category: C<br>Aspirin: Category D<br><br>Lactation Issues: safety not established. |

## Pentazocine & Acetaminophen

Talacen Caplets

Tablets:
25 mg/650 mg

**Moderate to Severe Pain:**
1 tablet q 4 h up to 6 tablets daily.

Administration Issues:
Avoid alcohol use. Safety/efficacy not established for children <12 yrs.

Drug–Drug Interactions:
**increased effect of:** alcohol, other CNS depressants.

Acetaminophen:
**increased toxic effect of APAP:** alcohol (chronic); barbiturates, carbamazepine, hydantoins, rifampin, sulfinpyrazone

**decreased effect of APAP:** charcoal

**Dependence, Tolerance:**
Psychological & physical dependence have occurred with prolonged use of this agent. Withdrawal symptoms have been associated with abrupt discontinuation

ADRs:
nausea, dizziness, lightheadedness, vomiting, euphoria, sedation, constipation.

Acetaminophen:
Very few adverse reactions

Pharmacokinetics:
APAP: rapid onset (0.5–2 hrs); hepatically metabolized (toxic metabolite is metabolized by conjugation with hepatic glutathione); T$_{1/2}$ = 1–3 hrs or 2.2–5 hrs in patients with cirrhosis

Contraindications:
Hypersensitivity

Precautions: Use cautiously in patients with severe renal or hepatic dysfunction, or respiratory dysfunction. Use cautiously in patients previously receiving narcotic agonist — this may precipitate withdrawal.

Pregnancy Category: C

Lactation Issues: safety not established.

## Butorphanol

Stadol NS

Nasal Spray:
10 mg/mL

**Moderate to Severe Pain:**
1–2 mg q 3–4 h prn. Give 1 mg then wait 60 minutes before the next 1 mg if full pain relief not achieved.

**Elderly or debilitated:** 1 mg may repeat in 90–120 min if full effect not reached. Give q 6–8 h prn.

**Unlabeled Use:** pain associated with migraine headache

Administration Issues:
Avoid alcohol use. Safety/efficacy in those <18 yrs not established. Half-life is prolonged in the elderly. These patients may be more prone to adverse effects.

Drug–Drug Interactions:
**increased effect of:** barbiturates, alcohol, other CNS depressants

ADRs: vasodilatation, palpitations, hypertension, anorexia, constipation, insomnia, tremor, convulsion, delusions, depression, nasal congestion, dyspnea, epistaxis, nasal irritation, pharyngitis, rhinitis, cough.

Pharmacokinetics:
onset of action = 15 min; duration of action = 4–5 hrs; T$_{1/2}$ = 2.9–9.2 hrs; extensively metabolized; renal or fecal elimination of metabolites

Contraindications:
Hypersensitivity

Precautions: Use cautiously in patients with severe respiratory, cardiovascular, hepatic or renal dysfunction.

Pregnancy Category: C

Lactation Issues: Use cautiously, excreted in breast milk; however amount to infant may be negligible.

| Drug and Dosage Forms | Usual Dosage Range | Administration Issues and Drug–Drug & Drug–Food Interactions | Common Adverse Drug Reactions (ADRs) and Pharmacokinetics | Contraindications, Pregnancy Category, and Lactation Issues |
|---|---|---|---|---|
| **Acetaminophen w/Codeine**<br><br>Capital w/Codeine, Tylenol w/Codeine No. 2, No. 3, No. 4; Phenaphen w/Codeine No. 3, Margesic No. 3, various generics<br><br>Solution:<br>120 mg/ 12 mg (15 mL)<br><br>Tablets:<br>300 mg/15 mg,<br>325 mg/30 mg,<br>300 mg/30 mg,<br>650 mg/30 mg,<br>300 mg/60 mg,<br>325 mg/60 mg | **Moderate to Severe Pain:**<br><br>1–4 tablets q 4 h prn (codeine content 15 mg)<br><br>0.5–2 tablets q 4 h prn (codeine content 30 mg)<br><br>1 tablet q 4 h prn (codeine content 60 mg or APAP content 650 mg)<br><br>15 mL q 4 h prn (for solution) | Administration Issues:<br>Take with food if GI upset occurs.<br><br>Drug–Drug Interactions:<br>**increased level/effect of:** warfarin; barbiturates, alcohol, other CNS depressants (inc respiratory/CNS depressant effect); chlorpromazine (inc toxic effects); cimetidine (inc CNS toxicity)<br><br>Acetaminophen:<br>**increased toxic effect of APAP:** alcohol (chronic); barbiturates, carbamazepine, hydantoins, rifampin, sulfinpyrazone<br><br>**decreased effect of APAP:** charcoal<br><br>**Drug Dependence, Tolerance:** Narcotics have abuse potential although this potential is low if used for medical reasons. Prolonged use of these agents can lead to tolerance, thereby requiring increased doses. If medication is to be withdrawn, it should be tapered to prevent withdrawal symptoms. | ADRs:<br>lightheadedness, dizziness, sedation, GI effects, sweating, constipation, drowsiness<br><br>Acetaminophen:<br>Very few adverse reactions<br><br>Pharmacokinetics:<br>see individual agents | Contraindications:<br>Hypersensitivity, diarrhea caused by poisoning, acute bronchial asthma, upper airway obstruction<br><br>Precautions: Use cautiously in patients with hepatic or renal dysfunction, acute abdominal conditions, in elderly or debilitated patients, patients with respiratory conditions, cardiovascular or seizure disorders, hypothyroidism, Addisons Disease, acute alcoholism, DT's, prostatic hypertrophy.<br><br>Pregnancy Category: C<br><br>Lactation Issues: Use cautiously. Excreted in breast milk although no significant effects on infant seen. |

## Aspirin w/Codeine

Empirin w/Codeine No. 3 or No. 4, various generics

Tablets:
325 mg/30 mg
325 mg/60 mg

---

**Moderate to severe pain:**

1–2 tablets q 4 h prn (codeine content 30 mg)

1 tablet q 4 h prn (codeine content 60 mg)

---

Administration Issues:
Take with food if GI upset occurs. Aspirin use in children with fever has been associated with Reye's syndrome.

Drug–Drug Interactions:
**increased level/effect of:** warfarin; barbiturates, alcohol, other CNS depressants (inc respiratory/CNS depressant effect); chlorpromazine (inc toxic effects); cimetidine (inc CNS toxicity)

Aspirin
**increased level/effect of:** alcohol (GI effects), anticoagulants (bleeding effects); methotrexate, valproic acid, sulfonylureas (inc hypoglycemic effect) **decreased level/effect of:** ACE inhibitors, beta blockers, diuretics (decreased antihypertensive effect); probenecid & sulfinpyrazone (decreased uricosuric effect)

Drug–Lab Interactions:
Aspirin: see table 307

**Drug Dependence, Tolerance:**
Narcotics have abuse potential although this potential is low if used for medical reasons. Prolonged use can lead to tolerance, thereby requiring increased doses. If medication is to be withdrawn, it should be tapered to prevent withdrawal symptoms.

---

ADRs:
lightheadedness, dizziness, sedation, GI effects, sweating, constipation, drowsiness

Aspirin: nausea, dyspepsia, heartburn, GI bleeding, hives, rash, prolonged bleeding time, thrombocytopenia, aspirin intolerance (bronchospasm, rhinitis), "Salicylism"; dizziness, tinnitus, difficulty hearing, nausea, vomiting, diarrhea, confusion, CNS depression, headache, sweating, hyperventilation, lassitude

Pharmacokinetics:
see individual agents

---

Contraindications:
Hypersensitivity, diarrhea caused by poisoning, acute bronchial asthma, upper airway obstruction

Aspirin: hemophilia, bleeding ulcers, hemorrhagic states

Precautions: Use cautiously in patients with hepatic or renal dysfunction, acute abdominal conditions, in elderly or debilitated patients, patients with respiratory conditions, cardiovascular or seizure disorders, hypothyroidism, Addisons Disease, acute alcoholism, DT's, prostatic hypertrophy.

Aspirin: Use cautiously in patients with asthma, nasal polyposis, chronic urticaria (inc risk of hypersensitivity); chronic renal insufficiency, PUD, bleeding disorders.

Pregnancy Category: C

Aspirin: Category D

Lactation Issues: Use cautiously. Excreted in breast milk although no significant effects on infant seen.

*(continues on next page)*

**303. Narcotic Combinations** *continued from previous page*

| Drug and Dosage Forms | Usual Dosage Range | Administration Issues and Drug–Drug & Drug–Food Interactions | Common Adverse Drug Reactions (ADRs) and Pharmacokinetics | Contraindications, Pregnancy Category, and Lactation Issues |
|---|---|---|---|---|
| **Acetaminophen, Codeine, Caffeine, Butalbital**<br>Fioricet w/Codeine<br><br>Tablet:<br>325 mg APAP plus<br>30 mg Codeine plus<br>40 mg Caffeine plus<br>50 mg Butalbital | **Moderate to severe pain**<br><br>1–2 tablets q 4 h prn (up to 6 tablets a day) | Administration Issues:<br>Take with food if GI upset occurs.<br><br>Drug–Drug Interactions:<br>**increased level/effect of:** warfarin; barbiturates, alcohol, other CNS depressants (inc respiratory/CNS depressant effect); chlorpromazine (inc toxic effects); cimetidine (inc CNS toxicity)<br><br>Acetaminophen:<br>**increased toxic effect of APAP:** alcohol (chronic); barbiturates, carbamazepine, hydantoins, rifampin, sulfinpyrazone<br>**decreased effect of APAP:** charcoal<br><br>Caffeine:<br>**decreased effect/levels of caffeine:** smoking<br>**increased effect/levels of caffeine:** cimetidine, oral contraceptives, disulfiram, fluoroquinolones<br><br>**Drug Dependence, Tolerance:**<br>Narcotics have abuse potential although this potential is low if used for medical reasons. Prolonged use can lead to tolerance, thereby requiring increased doses. If medication is to be withdrawn, it should be tapered to prevent withdrawal symptoms. | ADRs:<br>lightheadedness, dizziness, sedation, GI effects, sweating, constipation, drowsiness<br><br>Acetaminophen:<br>Very few adverse reactions<br><br>Caffeine:<br>insomnia, restlessness, tremor, excitement, anxiety, headaches, GI effects, palpitations, diuresis, withdrawal headaches after abrupt discontinuation (500–600 mg/d of caffeine)<br><br>Pharmacokinetics:<br>see individual agents | Contraindications:<br>Hypersensitivity, diarrhea caused by poisoning, acute bronchial asthma, upper airway obstruction<br><br>Precautions: Use cautiously in patients with hepatic or renal dysfunction, acute abdominal conditions, in elderly or debilitated patients, patients with respiratory conditions, cardiovascular or seizure disorders, hypothyroidism, Addisons Disease, acute alcoholism, DT's, prostatic hypertrophy.<br><br>Pregnancy Category: C<br><br>Lactation Issues: Use cautiously. Excreted in breast milk although no significant effects on infant seen. |

## Aspirin, Codeine, Caffeine, Butalbital

Fiorinal w/Codeine

### Tablets:
325 mg aspirin plus
30 mg codeine plus
40 mg caffeine plus
50 mg butalbital

### Moderate to severe pain:

1–2 tablets q 4 h prn (up to 6 tablets a day)

### Administration Issues:
Take with food if GI upset occurs. Aspirin use in children with fever has been associated with Reye's syndrome

### Drug–Drug Interactions:
**increased level/effect of:** warfarin; barbiturates, alcohol, other CNS depressants (inc respiratory/CNS depressant effect); chlorpromazine (inc toxic effects); cimetidine (inc CNS toxicity)

### Aspirin
**increased level/effect of:** alcohol (GI effects), anticoagulants (bleeding effects); methotrexate, valproic acid, sulfonylureas (inc hypoglycemic effect)
**decreased level/effect of:** ACE inhibitors, beta blockers, diuretics (decreased antihypertensive effect); probenecid & sulfinpyrazone (decreased uricosuric effect)

### Caffeine:
**decreased effect/levels of caffeine:** smoking
**increased effect/levels of caffeine:** cimetidine, oral contraceptives, disulfiram, fluoroquinolones

### Drug Dependence, Tolerance:
Narcotics have abuse potential although this potential is low if used for medical reasons. Prolonged use can lead to tolerance, thereby requiring increased doses. If medication is to be withdrawn, it should be tapered to prevent withdrawal symptoms.

### ADRs:
lightheadedness, dizziness, sedation, nausea, vomiting, sweating, constipation, drowsiness

Aspirin: nausea, dyspepsia, heartburn, GI bleeding, hives, rash, prolonged bleeding time, thrombocytopenia, aspirin intolerance (bronchospasm, rhinitis), "Salicylism": dizziness, tinnitus, difficulty hearing, nausea, vomiting, diarrhea, confusion, CNS depression, headache, sweating, hyperventilation, lassitude

Caffeine: insomnia, restlessness, tremor, excitement, anxiety, headaches, GI effects, palpitations, diuresis, withdrawal headaches after abrupt discontinuation (500–600 mg/d of caffeine)

### Pharmacokinetics:
see individual agents

### Contraindications:
Hypersensitivity, diarrhea caused by poisoning, acute bronchial asthma, upper airway obstruction

Aspirin: hemophilia, bleeding ulcers, hemorrhagic states

Precautions: Use cautiously in patients with hepatic or renal dysfunction, acute abdominal conditions, in elderly or debilitated patients, patients with respiratory conditions, cardiovascular or seizure disorders, hypothyroidism, Addisons Disease, acute alcoholism, DT's, prostatic hypertrophy.

Aspirin: Use cautiously in patients with asthma, nasal polyposis, chronic urticaria (inc risk of hypersensitivity); chronic renal insufficiency; PUD, bleeding disorders.

### Pregnancy Category: C
Aspirin: Category D

### Lactation Issues: Use cautiously. Excreted in breast milk although no significant effects on infant seen.

(continues on next page)

## 303. Narcotic Combinations continued from previous page

| Drug and Dosage Forms | Usual Dosage Range | Administration Issues and Drug–Drug & Drug–Food Interactions | Common Adverse Drug Reactions (ADRs) and Pharmacokinetics | Contraindications, Pregnancy Category, and Lactation Issues |
|---|---|---|---|---|
| **Acetaminophen, Hydrocodone**<br><br>Lortab, Bancap, Ceta-Plus, Co-Gesic, Duocet, Dolacte, Hydrocet, Vicodin, Lorcet, various generics, others<br><br>Tablets:<br>500 mg/2.5 mg,<br>500 mg/5 mg<br>500 mg/7.5 mg<br>650 mg/7.5 mg<br>750 mg/7.5 mg<br>650 mg/10 mg<br><br>Elixir:<br>167 mg/2.5 mg (15 mL) | **Moderate to severe pain:**<br>15 mL q4–6 h prn (solution)<br><br>1–2 tablets q 4–6 h prn (up to 8 tablets a day)<br><br>1 tablet q 4–6 h prn (hydrocodone content 7.5 mg or higher)<br><br>Max dose of 5 tablets a day if APAP content is 750 mg | Administration Issues:<br>Take with food if GI upset occurs.<br><br>Drug–Drug Interactions:<br>**increased level/effect of:** warfarin; barbiturates, alcohol, other CNS depressants (inc respiratory/CNS depressant effect); chlorpromazine (inc toxic effects); cimetidine (inc CNS toxicity)<br><br>Acetaminophen:<br>**increased toxic effect of APAP:** alcohol (chronic); barbiturates, carbamazepine, hydantoins, rifampin, sulfinpyrazone<br><br>**decreased effect of APAP:** charcoal<br><br>**Drug Dependence, Tolerance:**<br>Narcotics have abuse potential although this potential is low if used for medical reasons. Prolonged use can lead to tolerance, thereby requiring increased doses. If medication is to be withdrawn, it should be tapered to prevent withdrawal symptoms. | ADRs:<br>lightheadedness, dizziness, sedation, nausea, vomiting, sweating, constipation, drowsiness<br><br>Acetaminophen:<br>Very few adverse reactions<br><br>Pharmacokinetics:<br>see individual agents | Contraindications:<br>Hypersensitivity, diarrhea caused by poisoning, acute bronchial asthma, upper airway obstruction<br><br>Precautions:  Use cautiously in patients with hepatic or renal dysfunction, acute abdominal conditions, in elderly or debilitated patients, patients with respiratory conditions, cardiovascular or seizure disorders, hypothyroidism, Addisons Disease, acute alcoholism, DT's, prostatic hypertrophy.<br><br>Pregnancy Category:  C<br><br>Lactation Issues:  Use cautiously. Excreted in breast milk although no significant effects on infant seen. |

# Aspirin, Hydrocodone

Azdone, Damason, Lortab ASA, Panasal

Tablets:
500 mg/5 mg

| | | | |
|---|---|---|---|

**Moderate to severe pain:**

1–2 tablets q 4–6 h prn; up to 8 tablets a day.

Administration Issues:
Take with food if GI upset occurs. Aspirin use in children with fever has been associated with Reye's syndrome

Drug–Drug Interactions:
**increased level/effect of:** warfarin; barbiturates, alcohol, other CNS depressants (inc respiratory/CNS depressant effect); chlorpromazine (inc toxic effects); cimetidine (inc CNS toxicity)

Aspirin
**increased level/effect of:** alcohol (GI effects), anticoagulants (bleeding effects); methotrexate, valproic acid, sulfonylureas (inc hypoglycemic effect)

**decreased level/effect of:** ACE inhibitors, beta blockers, diuretics (decreased antihypertensive effect); probenecid & sulfinpyrazone (decreased uricosuric effect)

Drug–Lab Interactions:
Aspirin: see table 307

**Drug Dependence, Tolerance:**
Narcotics have abuse potential although this potential is low if used for medical reasons. Prolonged use can lead to tolerance, thereby requiring increased doses. If medication is to be withdrawn, it should be tapered to prevent withdrawal symptoms.

ADRs:
lightheadedness, dizziness, sedation, nausea, vomiting, sweating, constipation, drowsiness

Aspirin:
nausea, dyspepsia, heartburn, GI bleeding, hives, rash, prolonged bleeding time, thrombocytopenia, aspirin intolerance (bronchospasm, rhinitis), "Salicylism"; dizziness, tinnitus, difficulty hearing, nausea, vomiting, diarrhea, confusion, CNS depression, headache, sweating, hyperventilation, lassitude

Pharmacokinetics:
see individual agents

Contraindications:
Hypersensitivity, diarrhea caused by poisoning, acute bronchial asthma, upper airway obstruction

Aspirin: hemophilia, bleeding ulcers, hemorrhagic states

Precautions: Use cautiously in patients with hepatic or renal dysfunction, acute abdominal conditions, in elderly or debilitated patients, patients with respiratory conditions, cardiovascular or seizure disorders, hypothyroidism, Addisons Disease, acute alcoholism, DT's, prostatic hypertrophy.

Aspirin: Use cautiously in patients with asthma, nasal polyposis, chronic urticaria (inc risk of hypersensitivity); chronic renal insufficiency, PUD, bleeding disorders.

Pregnancy Category: C
Aspirin: Category D

Lactation Issues: Use cautiously. Excreted in breast milk although no significant effects on infant seen.

(continues on next page)

| Drug and Dosage Forms | Usual Dosage Range | Administration Issues and Drug–Drug & Drug–Food Interactions | Common Adverse Drug Reactions (ADRs) and Pharmacokinetics | Contraindications, Pregnancy Category, and Lactation Issues |
|---|---|---|---|---|
| **Acetaminophen, Dihydrocodeine, Caffeine**<br>DHC Plus Capsules<br><br>Capsules:<br>356.4 mg APAP plus 16 mg dihydrocodeine plus 30 mg caffeine | **Moderate to severe pain:**<br><br>2 capsules q 4 h prn | Administration Issues:<br>Take with food if GI upset occurs.<br><br>Drug–Drug Interactions:<br>**increased level/effect of:** warfarin; barbiturates, alcohol, other CNS depressants (inc respiratory/CNS depressant effect); chlorpromazine (inc toxic effects); cimetidine (inc CNS toxicity)<br><br>Acetaminophen:<br>**increased toxic effect of APAP:** alcohol (chronic); barbiturates, carbamazepine, hydantoins, rifampin, sulfinpyrazone<br>**decreased effect of APAP:** charcoal<br><br>Caffeine:<br>**decreased effect/levels of caffeine:** smoking<br>**increased effect/levels of caffeine:** cimetidine, oral contraceptives, disulfiram, fluoroquinolones<br><br>**Drug Dependence, Tolerance:**<br>Narcotics have abuse potential although this potential is low if used for medical reasons. Prolonged use can lead to tolerance, thereby requiring increased doses. If medication is to be withdrawn, it should be tapered to prevent withdrawal symptoms. | ADRs:<br>lightheadedness, dizziness, sedation, nausea, vomiting, sweating, constipation, drowsiness<br><br>Acetaminophen:<br>Very few adverse reactions<br><br>Caffeine:<br>insomnia, restlessness, tremor, excitement, anxiety, headaches, GI effects, palpitations, diuresis, withdrawal headaches after abrupt discontinuation (500–600 mg/d of caffeine)<br><br>Pharmacokinetics:<br>see individual agents | Contraindications:<br>Hypersensitivity, diarrhea caused by poisoning, acute bronchial asthma, upper airway obstruction<br><br>Precautions: Use cautiously in patients with hepatic or renal dysfunction, acute abdominal conditions, in elderly or debilitated patients, patients with respiratory conditions, cardiovascular or seizure disorders, hypothyroidism, Addisons Disease, acute alcoholism, DT's, prostatic hypertrophy.<br><br>Pregnancy Category: C<br><br>Lactation Issues: Use cautiously. Excreted in breast milk although no significant effects on infant seen. |

## Aspirin, Dihydrocodeine, Caffeine
Synalogos-DC

Capsules:
356.4 mg aspirin plus 16 mg dihydrocodeine plus 30 mg caffeine

**Moderate to severe pain:**

2 capsules q 4 h prn

Administration Issues:
Take with food if GI upset occurs. Aspirin use in children with fever has been associated with Reye's syndrome.

Drug–Drug Interactions:

**increased level/effect of:** warfarin; barbiturates, alcohol, other CNS depressants (inc respiratory/CNS depressant effect); chlorpromazine (inc toxic effects); cimetidine (inc CNS toxicity)

Aspirin

**increased level/effect of:** alcohol (GI effects); anticoagulants (bleeding effects); methotrexate, valproic acid, sulfonylureas (inc hypoglycemic effect) **decreased level/effect of:** ACE inhibitors, beta blockers, diuretics (decreased antihypertensive effect); probenecid & sulfinpyrazone (decreased uricosuric effect)

Caffeine:

**decreased effect/levels of caffeine:** smoking
**increased effect/levels of caffeine:** cimetidine, oral contraceptives, disulfiram, fluoroquinolones

Drug–Lab Interactions:
Aspirin: see table 307

**Drug Dependence, Tolerance:**
Narcotics have abuse potential although this potential is low if used for medical

ADRs:
lightheadedness, dizziness, sedation, nausea, vomiting, sweating, constipation, drowsiness

Aspirin:
nausea, dyspepsia, heartburn, GI bleeding, hives, rash, prolonged bleeding time, thrombocytopenia, aspirin intolerance (bronchospasm, rhinitis), "Salicylism":
dizziness, tinnitus, difficulty hearing, nausea, vomiting, diarrhea, confusion, CNS depression, headache, sweating, hyperventilation, lassitude

Caffeine:
insomnia, restlessness, tremor, excitement, anxiety, headaches, GI effects, palpitations, diuresis, withdrawal headaches after abrupt discontinuation (500–600 mg/d of caffeine)

Pharmacokinetics:
see individual agents

Contraindications:
Hypersensitivity, diarrhea caused by poisoning, acute bronchial asthma, upper airway obstruction

Aspirin: hemophilia, bleeding ulcers, hemorrhagic states

Precautions: Use cautiously in patients with hepatic or renal dysfunction, acute abdominal conditions, in elderly or debilitated patients, patients with respiratory conditions, cardiovascular or seizure disorders, hypothyroidism, Addisons Disease, acute alcoholism, DT's, prostatic hypertrophy.

Aspirin: Use cautiously in patients with asthma, nasal polyposis, chronic urticaria (inc risk of hypersensitivity); chronic renal insufficiency; PUD, bleeding disorders.

Pregnancy Category: C
Aspirin: Category D

Lactation Issues: Use cautiously. Excreted in breast milk although no significant effects on infant seen.

(continues on next page)

| Drug and Dosage Forms | Usual Dosage Range | Administration Issues and Drug–Drug & Drug–Food Interactions | Common Adverse Drug Reactions (ADRs) and Pharmacokinetics | Contraindications, Pregnancy Category, and Lactation Issues |
|---|---|---|---|---|
| **Aspirin, Dihydrocodeine, Caffeine** | | reasons. Prolonged use can lead to tolerance, thereby requiring increased doses. If medication is to be withdrawn, it should be tapered to prevent withdrawal symptoms. | | |
| **Acetaminophen, Oxycodone** Percocet, Roxicet, Tylox, various generics <u>Tablets:</u> 325 mg/5 mg <u>Capsules:</u> 500 mg/5 mg <u>Solution:</u> 325 mg/5 mg (5 mL) | <u>**Moderate to severe pain:**</u> 1 tablet or capsule q 6 h prn 5 mL every 6 hrs prn | <u>Administration Issues:</u> Take with food if GI upset occurs. <u>Drug–Drug Interactions:</u> **increased level/effect of:** warfarin; barbiturates, alcohol, other CNS depressants (inc respiratory/CNS depressant effect); chlorpromazine (inc toxic effects); cimetidine (inc CNS toxicity) <u>Acetaminophen:</u> **increased toxic effect of APAP:** alcohol (chronic); barbiturates, carbamazepine, hydantoins, rifampin, sulfinpyrazone **decreased effect of APAP:** charcoal **<u>Drug Dependence, Tolerance:</u>** Narcotics have abuse potential although this potential is low if used for medical reasons. Prolonged use can lead to tolerance, thereby requiring increased doses. If medication is to be withdrawn, it should be tapered to prevent withdrawal symptoms. | <u>ADRs:</u> lightheadedness, dizziness, sedation, nausea, vomiting, sweating, constipation, drowsiness <u>Acetaminophen:</u> Very few adverse reactions <u>Pharmacokinetics:</u> see individual agents | <u>Contraindications:</u> Hypersensitivity, diarrhea caused by poisoning, acute bronchial asthma, upper airway obstruction <u>Precautions:</u> Use cautiously in patients with hepatic or renal dysfunction, acute abdominal conditions, in elderly or debilitated patients, patients with respiratory conditions, cardiovascular or seizure disorders, hypothyroidism, Addisons Disease, acute alcoholism, DT's, prostatic hypertrophy. <u>Pregnancy Category:</u> C <u>Lactation Issues:</u> Use cautiously. Excreted in breast milk although no significant effects on infant seen. |

## Aspirin, Oxycodone

Percodan, Percodan-Demi, Roxiprin, various generics

Tablets:
325 mg/2.25 mg oxycodone HCL/ 0.19 mg oxycodone terephthalate,
325 mg/4.5 mg oxycodone HCL/0.38 mg oxycodone terephthalate

| Moderate to severe pain: | Administration Issues: | ADRs: | Contraindications: |
|---|---|---|---|
| 1–2 tablets q 6 h prn | Take with food if GI upset occurs. Aspirin use in children with fever has been associated with Reye's syndrome. | lightheadedness, dizziness, sedation, nausea, vomiting, sweating, constipation, drowsiness | Hypersensitivity, diarrhea caused by poisoning, acute bronchial asthma, upper airway obstruction |
| | Drug–Drug Interactions: **increased level/effect of:** warfarin; barbiturates, alcohol, other CNS depressants (inc respiratory/CNS depressant effect); chlorpromazine (inc toxic effects); cimetidine (inc CNS toxicity) | Aspirin nausea, dyspepsia, heartburn, GI bleeding, hives, rash, prolonged bleeding time, thrombocytopenia, aspirin intolerance (bronchospasm, rhinitis), "Salicylism": dizziness, tinnitus, difficulty hearing, nausea, vomiting, diarrhea, confusion, CNS depression, headache, sweating, hyperventilation, lassitude | Aspirin: hemophilia, bleeding ulcers; hemorrhagic states |
| | | | Precautions: Use cautiously in patients with hepatic or renal dysfunction, acute abdominal conditions, in elderly or debilitated patients, patients with respiratory conditions, cardiovascular or seizure disorders, hypothyroidism, Addisons Disease, acute alcoholism, DT's, prostatic hypertrophy. |
| | Aspirin **increased level/effect of:** alcohol (GI effects); anticoagulants (bleeding effects); methotrexate, valproic acid, sulfonylureas (inc hypoglycemic effect) **decreased level/effect of:** ACE inhibitors, beta blockers, diuretics (decreased antihypertensive effect); probenecid & sulfinpyrazone (decreased uricosuric effect) | Pharmacokinetics: see individual agents | Aspirin: Use cautiously in patients with asthma, nasal polyposis, chronic urticaria (inc risk of hypersensitivity); chronic renal insufficiency, PUD, bleeding disorders. |
| | Drug–Lab Interactions: Aspirin: see table 307 | | Pregnancy Category: C Aspirin: Category D |
| | **Drug Dependence. Tolerance:** Narcotics have abuse potential although this potential is low if used for medical reasons. Prolonged use can lead to tolerance, thereby requiring increased doses. If medication is to be withdrawn, it should be tapered to prevent withdrawal symptoms. | | Lactation Issues: Use cautiously. Excreted in breast milk although no significant effects on infant seen. |

(continues on next page)

| Drug and Dosage Forms | Usual Dosage Range | Administration Issues and Drug–Drug & Drug–Food Interactions | Common Adverse Drug Reactions (ADRs) and Pharmacokinetics | Contraindications, Pregnancy Category, and Lactation Issues |
|---|---|---|---|---|
| **Meperidine, Promethazine** Mepergan Fortis <br><br> Capsules: 50 mg/25 mg | **Moderate to severe pain:** 1 capsule q 4–6 h prn | Administration Issues: Take with food if GI upset occurs. Limit use in children because of the possibility of extrapyramidal reactions. <br><br> Meperidine Drug–Drug Interactions: **increased level/effect of:** warfarin; barbiturates, alcohol, other CNS depressants (inc respiratory/CNS depressant effect); chlorpromazine (inc toxic effects); cimetidine (inc CNS toxicity); **MAO inhibitors (hypertensive crisis)** <br><br> Promethazine Drug–Drug Interactions: **increased effect:** CNS effects (alcohol); EPS effect (fluoxetine, lithium); sedation/hypotension (meperidine); **increased level of:** TCAs, valproic acid, phenytoin (or decreased level), propranolol (also increases level of antipsychotic) **decreased level of antipsychotic:** aluminum antacids, barbiturates, carbamazepine, charcoal **decreased effect of antipsychotic:** anticholinergics | ADRs: lightheadedness, dizziness, sedation, nausea, vomiting, sweating, constipation, drowsiness <br><br> Promethazine ADRs: sedation, anticholinergic effects (dry mouth, constipation, urinary retention, blurred vision, miosis), pseudoparkinsonism, dystonias, orthostatic hypotension. (For other ADRs see table 312.1) <br><br> Pharmacokinetics: see individual agents | Contraindications: Hypersensitivity, diarrhea caused by poisoning, acute bronchial asthma, upper airway obstruction <br><br> Promethazine: comatose or severely depressed states, concomitant use of large amounts of other CNS depressants; bone marrow depression, liver damage, cerebral arteriosclerosis, coronary artery disease <br><br> Precautions: Use cautiously in patients with hepatic or renal dysfunction, acute abdominal conditions, in elderly or debilitated patients, patients with respiratory conditions, cardiovascular or seizure disorders, hypothyroidism, Addisons Disease, acute alcoholism, DT's, prostatic hypertrophy. Promethazine: use cautiously in patients with hyperthyroidism; do not use 48 hrs prior to myelography; do not abruptly withdraw therapy |

| Acetaminophen, Propoxyphene | | |
|---|---|---|
| **Acetaminophen, Propoxyphene**<br>Darvocet-N, Propacet, various generics<br><br>Tablets:<br>325 mg/50 mg (as napsylate)<br>650 mg/100 mg (as napsylate)<br>650 mg/65 mg | **Mild to Moderate pain:**<br><br>2 tablets q 4 h prn<br><br>1 tablet q 4 h prn (propoxyphene napsylate content 100 mg, or propoxyphene content 65 mg) | ADRs:<br>lightheadedness, dizziness, sedation, nausea, vomiting, sweating, constipation, drowsiness<br><br>Acetaminophen:<br>Very few adverse reactions<br><br>Pharmacokinetics:<br>see individual agents |
| | **Drug Dependence, Tolerance:**<br>Narcotics have abuse potential although this potential is low if used for medical reasons. Prolonged use can lead to tolerance, thereby requiring increased doses. If medication is to be withdrawn, it should be tapered to prevent withdrawal symptoms. | Pregnancy Category: C.<br>Safety not established for promethazine.<br><br>Lactation Issues: Use cautiously. Excreted in breast milk although no significant effects on infant seen. |
| | Administration Issues:<br>Take with food if GI upset occurs.<br><br>Drug–Drug Interactions:<br>**increased level/effect of:** warfarin; barbiturates, alcohol, other CNS depressants (inc respiratory/CNS depressant effect); chlorpromazine (inc CNS effects); cimetidine (inc CNS toxicity)<br><br>Acetaminophen:<br>**increased toxic effect of APAP:** alcohol (chronic); barbiturates, carbamazepine, hydantoins, rifampin, sulfinpyrazone<br>**decreased effect of APAP:** charcoal<br><br>**Drug Dependence, Tolerance:**<br>Narcotics have abuse potential although this potential is low if used for medical reasons. Prolonged use can lead to tolerance, thereby requiring increased doses.<br>If medication is to be withdrawn, it should be tapered to prevent withdrawal symptoms. | Contraindications:<br>Hypersensitivity, diarrhea caused by poisoning, acute bronchial asthma, upper airway obstruction<br><br>Precautions: Use cautiously in patients with hepatic or renal dysfunction, acute abdominal conditions, in elderly or debilitated patients, patients with respiratory conditions, cardiovascular or seizure disorders, hypothyroidism, Addisons Disease, acute alcoholism, DT's, prostatic hypertrophy.<br><br>Pregnancy Category: C<br><br>Lactation Issues: Use cautiously. Excreted in breast milk although no significant effects on infant seen. |

1111

| Drug and Dosage Forms | Usual Dosage Range | Administration Issues and Drug–Drug & Drug–Food Interactions | Common Adverse Drug Reactions (ADRs) and Pharmacokinetics | Contraindications, Pregnancy Category, and Lactation Issues |
|---|---|---|---|---|
| **Aspirin, Propoxyphene, Caffeine**<br>Darvon, various generics<br><br>Capsules:<br>389 mg aspirin plus 65 mg proproxyphene plus 32.4 mg caffeine | **Mild to Moderate pain:**<br>1 capsule q 4 h prn | Administration Issues:<br>Take with food if GI upset occurs. Aspirin use in children with fever has been associated with Reye's syndrome.<br><br>Drug–Drug Interactions:<br>**increased level/effect of:** warfarin; barbiturates, alcohol, other CNS depressants (inc respiratory/CNS depressant effect); chlorpromazine (inc toxic effects); cimetidine (inc CNS toxicity)<br><br>Aspirin<br>**increased level/effect of:** alcohol (GI effects); anticoagulants (bleeding effects); methotrexate, valproic acid, sulfonylureas (inc hypoglycemic effect) **decreased level/effect of:** ACE inhibitors, beta blockers, diuretics (decreased antihypertensive effect); probenecid & sulfinpyrazone (decreased uricosuric effect)<br><br>Drug–Lab Interactions:<br>Aspirin: see table 307<br><br>**Drug Dependence, Tolerance:**<br>Narcotics have abuse potential although this potential is low if used for medical | ADRs:<br>lightheadedness, dizziness, sedation, nausea, vomiting, sweating, constipation, drowsiness<br><br>Aspirin:<br>nausea, dyspepsia, heartburn, GI bleeding, hives, rash, prolonged bleeding time, thrombocytopenia, aspirin intolerance (bronchospasm, rhinitis), "Salicylism": dizziness, tinnitus, difficulty hearing, nausea, vomiting, diarrhea, confusion, CNS depression, headache, sweating, hyperventilation, lassitude | Contraindications:<br>Hypersensitivity, diarrhea caused by poisoning, acute bronchial asthma, upper airway obstruction<br><br>Aspirin: hemophilia, bleeding ulcers, hemorrhagic states<br><br>Precautions: Use cautiously in patients with hepatic or renal dysfunction, acute abdominal conditions, in elderly or debilitated patients, patients with respiratory conditions, cardiovascular or seizure disorders, hypothyroidism, Addisons Disease, acute alcoholism, DTs, prostatic hypertrophy.<br><br>Aspirin: Use cautiously in patients with asthma, nasal polyposis, chronic urticaria (inc risk of hypersensitivity); chronic renal insufficiency; PUD, bleeding disorders.<br><br>Pregnancy Category: C<br>Aspirin: Category D |

| | Lactation Issues: Use cautiously. Excreted in breast milk although no significant effects on infant seen. |
|---|---|
| reasons. Prolonged use can lead to tolerance, thereby requiring increased doses. If medication is to be withdrawn, it should be tapered to prevent withdrawal symptoms. | |

## 304. Nonnarcotic Analgesic Combinations

| Drug and Dosage Forms | Usual Dosage Range | Administration Issues and Drug–Drug & Drug–Food Interactions | Common Adverse Drug Reactions (ADRs) and Pharmacokinetics | Contraindications, Pregnancy Category, and Lactation Issues |
|---|---|---|---|---|
| **Acetaminophen, Aspirin, Caffeine**<br>Saleto (with salicylamide), Gelpirin, Excedrin, Goody's Extra Strength Powders, various generics<br><br>*With antacids* (to minimize GI effects):<br>Supac, Buffets, Vanquish<br><br>Tablets:<br>115 mg/210 mg/16 mg;<br>125 mg/240 mg/32 mg<br>160 mg/230 mg/33 mg;<br>162 mg/227 mg/32.4 mg<br>194 mg/227 mg/33 mg;<br>250 mg/250 mg/65 mg<br><br>Powders:<br>260 mg/520 mg/32.5 mg | **Minor Aches/Pains:**<br>Adults: 1–2 tablets or 1 powder packet every 2–6 hrs as needed. | Administration Issues:<br>If pain persists longer than 5 days, consult physician. Take with food. Safety/efficacy not established in those <12 yrs old. Aspirin use in children with fever has been associated with Reye's syndrome.<br><br>Drug–Drug Interactions:<br>see individual agents | ADRs and Pharmacokinetics:<br>see individual agents | Contraindications:<br>Hypersensitivity; hemophilia, bleeding ulcers, hemorrhagic states<br><br>Precautions: Use cautiously in those with hepatic dysfunction, chronic alcohol use. Use cautiously in patients with asthma, nasal polyposis, chronic urticaria (inc risk of hypersensitivity); chronic renal or hepatic dysfunction, PUD, bleeding disorders.<br><br>Pregnancy Category: D<br><br>Lactation Issues: safety not established. |

*(continues on next page)*

# 304. Nonnarcotic Analgesic Combinations   *continued from previous page*

| Drug and Dosage Forms | Usual Dosage Range | Administration Issues and Drug–Drug & Drug–Food Interactions | Common Adverse Drug Reactions (ADRs) and Pharmacokinetics | Contraindications, Pregnancy Category, and Lactation Issues |
|---|---|---|---|---|
| **Acetaminophen, Magnesium salicylate, Pamabrom (used as a diuretic)** <br> Maximum Pain Relief Pampin <br><br> Tablets: <br> 250 mg/250 mg/25 mg | **Minor Aches/Pains:** <br> Adults:  1–2 tablets every 2–6 hrs as needed. | Administration Issues: <br> If pain persists longer than 5 days, consult physician. Take with food. Safety/efficacy not established in children. <br><br> Drug–Drug Interactions: <br> see individual agents | ADRs and Pharmacokinetics: <br> see individual agents | Contraindications: <br> Hypersensitivity; hemophilia, bleeding ulcers, hemorrhagic states <br><br> Precautions:  Use cautiously in those with hepatic dysfunction, chronic alcohol use. Use cautiously in patients with asthma, nasal polyposis, chronic urticaria (inc risk of hypersensitivity); chronic renal or hepatic dysfunction, PUD, bleeding disorders. <br><br> Pregnancy Category:  D <br><br> Lactation Issues: safety not established. |
| **Acetaminophen, Caffeine** <br> Aspirin-Free Excedrin, Bayer Select *With pyrilamine* (an antihistamine for sedation): Midol Maximum Strength <br><br> Caplets:  500 mg/65 mg; 500 mg/60 mg | **Minor Aches/Pains:** <br> Adults:  1–2 caplets every 2–6 hrs as needed. | Administration Issues: <br> If pain persists longer than 5 days, consult physician. <br><br> Drug–Drug Interactions: <br> see individual agents | ADRs and Pharmacokinetics: <br> see individual agents | Contraindications: <br> Hypersensitivity <br><br> Precautions:  Use cautiously in those with hepatic dysfunction, chronic alcohol use <br><br> Pregnancy/Lactation Issues: <br> Used in all trimesters of pregnancy with no known harm to fetus. Excreted in breast milk, but no known harm to infant |

| | **Minor Aches/Pains:** | Administration Issues: | ADRs and Pharmacokinetics: | Contraindications: |
|---|---|---|---|---|
| **Acetaminophen, Pamabrom (used as a diuretic)** | Adults: 1–2 tablets or caplets every 2–6 hrs as needed. | If pain persists longer than 5 days, consult physician. | see individual agents | Hypersensitivity |
| Premsyn PMS, Bayer Select Maximum Strength Menstrual Caplets | | Drug–Drug Interactions: see individual agents | | Precautions: Use cautiously in those with hepatic dysfunction, chronic alcohol use |
| *With pyridoxine:* Lurline | | | | Pregnancy/Lactation Issues: Used in all trimesters of pregnancy with no known harm to fetus. Excreted in breast milk, but no known harm to infant |
| *With pyrilamine* (an antihistamine for sedation): Multi-Symptom Pamprin, Maximum Strength Midol | | | | |
| Caplets: 500 mg/25 mg | | | | |
| Tablets: 500 mg/25 mg | | | | |
| **Acetaminophen, antacid combinations (to minimize GI effects)** | **Minor Aches/Pains:** Adults: 1–2 caplets every 2–6 hrs as needed. | Administration Issues: If pain persists longer than 5 days, consult physician. | ADRs and Pharmacokinetics: see individual agents | Contraindications: Hypersensitivity |
| Aspirin Free Excedrin, Extra Strength Tylenol Headache Plus Caplets | | Drug–Drug Interactions: see individual agents | | Precautions: Use cautiously in those with hepatic dysfunction, chronic alcohol use |
| Caplets: 500 mg | | | | Pregnancy/Lactation Issues: Used in all trimesters of pregnancy with no known harm to fetus. Excreted in breast milk, but no known harm to infant |
| **Aspirin, Caffeine** | **Minor Aches/Pains:** Adults: 1–2 tablets or 1 powder packet every 2–6 hrs as needed. | Administration Issues: Take with food. Safety/efficacy not established in those <12 yrs old. Aspirin use in children with fever has been associated with Reye's syndrome. | ADRs and Pharmacokinetics: see individual agents | Contraindications: Hypersensitivity, hemophilia, bleeding ulcers, hemorrhagic states |
| Anacin or Maximum Strength Anacin, Gensan | | | | |
| *With salicylamide* (added analgesia): BC | | | | |

(continues on next page)

| Drug and Dosage Forms | Usual Dosage Range | Administration Issues and Drug–Drug & Drug–Food Interactions | Common Adverse Drug Reactions (ADRs) and Pharmacokinetics | Contraindications, Pregnancy Category, and Lactation Issues |
|---|---|---|---|---|
| **Aspirin, Caffeine** *cont.*<br><br>Tablets or Powder<br>*With antacids* (to minimize GI effects):<br>Cope Tablets<br><br>Tablets:<br>325 mg/16 mg; 400 mg/32 mg; 421 mg/32 mg; 500 mg/32 mg; 650 mg/32 mg; 742 mg/36 mg | | Drug–Drug Interactions: see individual agents | | Precautions: Use cautiously in patients with asthma, nasal polyposis, chronic urticaria (inc risk of hypersensitivity); chronic renal or hepatic dysfunction, PUD, bleeding disorders.<br><br>Pregnancy Category: D<br><br>Lactation Issues: safety not established. |
| **Aspirin, Meprobamate (for sedative properties)**<br>Equagesic Tablets<br><br>Tablets:<br>325 mg/200 mg | **Minor Aches/Pains:**<br>Adults: 1–2 tablets every 2–6 hrs as needed. | Administration Issues:<br>Take with food. Safety/efficacy not established in those <12 yrs old. Aspirin use in children with fever has been associated with Reye's syndrome.<br><br>Drug–Drug Interactions:<br>see individual agents | ADRs and Pharmacokinetics: see individual agents | Contraindications:<br>Hypersensitivity, hemophilia, bleeding ulcers, hemorrhagic states, acute intermittent porphyria<br><br>Precautions: Use cautiously in patients with asthma, nasal polyposis, chronic urticaria (inc risk of hypersensitivity); chronic renal or hepatic dysfunction, PUD, bleeding disorders. Meprobamate: Drug dependency is observed (avoid prolonged use); abrupt discontinuation may precipitate |

| | | | | |
|---|---|---|---|---|
| | | | | withdrawal. Use cautiously in patients with seizure disorders. Use cautiously in patients with severe renal or hepatic dysfunction.<br><br>Pregnancy Category: D. Meprobamate should not be used in pregnant women – increased risk of congenital malformations during the first trimester.<br><br>Lactation Issues: safety not established. |
| **Sodium Salicylate, Aminobenzoate (to prolong action of salicylate)**<br>Pabalate Enteric Coated Tablets<br><br>Tablets:<br>300 mg/300 mg | | **Minor Aches/Pains:**<br>Adults: 1–2 tablets every 2–6 hrs as needed. | Administration Issues:<br>Take with food. Safety/efficacy not established in those <12 yrs old. Aspirin use in children with fever has been associated with Reye's syndrome.<br><br>Drug–Drug Interactions:<br>see individual agents | ADRs and Pharmacokinetics:<br>see individual agents | Contraindications:<br>Hypersensitivity, hemophilia, bleeding ulcers, hemorrhagic states<br><br>Precautions: Use cautiously in patients with asthma, nasal polyposis, chronic urticaria (inc risk of hypersensitivity); chronic renal or hepatic dysfunction, PUD, bleeding disorders.<br><br>Pregnancy Category: D<br><br>Lactation Issues: safety not established. |

(continues on next page)

## 304. Nonnarcotic Analgesic Combinations continued from previous page

| Drug and Dosage Forms | Usual Dosage Range | Administration Issues and Drug–Drug & Drug–Food Interactions | Common Adverse Drug Reactions (ADRs) and Pharmacokinetics | Contraindications, Pregnancy Category, and Lactation Issues |
|---|---|---|---|---|
| **Magnesium Salicylate, Phenyltoloxamine (an antihistamine for sedation)** Mobigesic, Magsal Tablets: 325 mg/30 mg 600 mg/25 mg | **Minor Aches/Pains:** Adults: 1–2 tablets every 2–6 hrs as needed. | Administration Issues: Take with food. Safety/efficacy not established in children Drug–Drug Interactions: see individual agents | ADRs and Pharmacokinetics: see individual agents | Contraindications: Hypersensitivity, hemophilia, bleeding ulcers, hemorrhagic states Precautions: Use cautiously in patients with asthma, nasal polyposis, chronic urticaria (inc risk of hypersensitivity); chronic renal or hepatic dysfunction, PUD, bleeding disorders. Pregnancy Category: D Lactation Issues: safety not established. |

## 305. Nonnarcotic Analgesic Combinations with Barbiturates

| Drug and Dosage Forms | Usual Dosage Range | Administration Issues and Drug–Drug & Drug–Food Interactions | Common Adverse Drug Reactions (ADRs) and Pharmacokinetics | Contraindications, Pregnancy Category, and Lactation Issues |
|---|---|---|---|---|
| **Acetaminophen, Caffeine, Butalbital (a barbiturate for sedation)** <br><br> Esgic, Fioricet, Repan, Anoquan, Amaphen, Butace, Endolor, Femcet, various generics <br><br> Tablets: <br> 325 mg/40 mg/50 mg <br><br> Capsules: <br> 325 mg/40 mg/50 mg | **Mild to Moderate Pain:** <br> Adults: 1–2 every 4 hrs as needed. | Administration Issues: <br> May produce irritability, excitability or aggression in children. Safety/efficacy not established for <6 yrs old <br><br> Drug–Drug Interactions: <br> see individual agents | ADRs and Pharmacokinetics: <br> see individual agents <br><br> Elderly: may observe paradoxical excitement <br><br> Precautions: <br> **Drug Abuse & Dependence:** <br> Prolonged use at high doses leads to physical dependence. If dependent on barbiturate, slowly withdraw over several weeks. May use long-acting barbiturate (phenobarbital) at dose of 30 mg per every 100–200 mg of butalbital to help prevent withdrawal symptoms | Contraindications: <br> Hypersensitivity <br><br> Precautions: Use cautiously in those with hepatic dysfunction, chronic alcohol use <br><br> **Barbiturate** <br> Contraindications: <br> Hypersensitivity; manifest or latent porphyria, severe hepatic, renal, or respiratory dysfunction; previous addiction to sedative/hypnotic <br><br> Pregnancy Category: D <br><br> Lactation Issues: use cautiously in nursing mothers, sedation has been reported in infants |
| **Acetaminophen, Butalbital (a barbiturate for sedation)** <br><br> Phrenilin, Bancap, Triaprin, Sedapap-10, Phrenilin Forte | **Mild to Moderate Pain:** <br> Adults: 1–2 every 4 hrs as needed. | Administration Issues <br> May produce irritability, excitability or aggression in children. Safety/efficacy not established for <6 yrs old <br><br> Drug–Drug Interactions: <br> see individual agents | ADRs and Pharmacokinetics: <br> see individual agents <br><br> Elderly: may observe paradoxical excitement | Contraindications: <br> Hypersensitivity <br><br> Precautions: Use cautiously in those with hepatic dysfunction, chronic alcohol use |

(continues on next page)

# 305. Nonnarcotic Analgesic Combinations with Barbiturates *continued from previous page*

| Drug and Dosage Forms | Usual Dosage Range | Administration Issues and Drug–Drug & Drug–Food Interactions | Common Adverse Drug Reactions (ADRs) and Pharmacokinetics | Contraindications, Pregnancy Category, and Lactation Issues |
|---|---|---|---|---|
| **Acetaminophen, Butalbital (a barbiturate for sedation)** *cont.* <br><br> Tablets: <br> 325 mg/50 mg <br> 650 mg/50 mg <br><br> Capsules: <br> 325 mg/50 mg <br> 650 mg/50 mg | | | Precautions: <br> **Drug Abuse & Dependence:** Prolonged use at high doses leads to physical dependence. If dependent on barbiturate, slowly withdraw over several weeks. May use long-acting barbiturate (phenobarbital) at dose of 30 mg per every 100–200 mg of butalbital to help prevent withdrawal symptoms | **Barbiturate** <br> Contraindications: <br> Hypersensitivity; manifest or latent porphyria; severe hepatic, renal, or respiratory dysfunction; previous addiction to sedative/hypnotic <br><br> Pregnancy Category: D <br><br> Lactation Issues: use cautiously in nursing mothers, sedation has been reported in infants |
| **Aspirin, Caffeine, Butalbital (a barbiturate for sedation)** <br> Fiorinal, Fiorgen PF, Lanorinal, various generics <br><br> Tablets: <br> 325 mg/40 mg/50 mg <br> 650 mg/40 mg/50 mg <br><br> Capsules: <br> 325 mg/40 mg/50 mg | **Mild to Moderate Pain:** <br> Adults: 1–2 every 4 hrs as needed. | Administration Issues: <br> Take with food. May produce irritability, excitability or aggression in children. Safety/efficacy not established in those <6 yrs old. Aspirin use in children with fever has been associated with Reye's syndrome. <br><br> Drug–Drug Interactions: <br> see individual agents | ADRs and Pharmacokinetics: <br> see individual agents <br><br> Elderly: may observe paradoxical excitement <br><br> Precautions: <br> **Drug Abuse & Dependence:** Prolonged use at high doses leads to physical dependence. If dependent on barbiturate, slowly withdraw over several weeks. May use | Contraindications: <br> Hypersensitivity, hemophilia, bleeding ulcers, hemorrhagic states <br><br> Precautions: Use cautiously in patients with asthma, nasal polyposis, chronic urticaria (inc risk of hypersensitivity); chronic renal or hepatic dysfunction, PUD, bleeding disorders. <br><br> Pregnancy Category: D <br><br> Lactation Issues: safety not established. Use cautiously if at all. |

| Aspirin, Butalbital (a barbiturate for sedation)<br>BAC, Axotal<br><br>Tablets:<br>650 mg/50 mg | Mild to Moderate Pain:<br>Adults: 1–2 every 4 hrs as needed. | Administration Issues:<br>Take with food. May produce irritability, excitability or aggression in children. Safety/efficacy not established for <6 yrs old. Aspirin use in children with fever has been associated with Reye's syndrome.<br><br>Drug-Drug Interactions:<br>see individual agents | ADRs and Pharmacokinetics:<br>see individual agents<br><br>Elderly: may observe paradoxical excitement<br><br>Precautions:<br>Drug Abuse & Dependence: Prolonged use at high doses leads to physical dependence. If dependent on barbiturate, slowly withdraw over several weeks. May use long-acting barbiturate (phenobarbital) at dose of 30 mg per every 100–200 mg of butalbital to help prevent withdrawal symptoms | Contraindications:<br>Hypersensitivity, hemophilia, bleeding ulcers, hemorrhagic states<br><br>Precautions: Use cautiously in patients with asthma, nasal polyposis, chronic urticaria (inc risk of hypersensitivity); chronic renal or hepatic dysfunction, PUD, bleeding disorders.<br><br>Pregnancy Category: D<br><br>Lactation Issues: safety not established. Use cautiously if at all. |
|  |  |  | long-acting barbiturate (phenobarbital) at dose of 30 mg per every 100–200 mg of butalbital to help prevent withdrawal symptoms |  |

# 306 Nonsteroidal Anti-Inflammatory Agents

306.1 Propionic Acids

| Drug and Dosage Forms | Usual Dosage Range | Administration Issues and Drug–Drug & Drug–Food Interactions | Common Adverse Drug Reactions (ADRs) and Pharmacokinetics | Contraindications, Pregnancy Category, and Lactation Issues |
|---|---|---|---|---|
| **Fenoprofen**<br>Nalfon, various generics<br><br><u>Capsules:</u><br>200 mg, 300 mg<br><br><u>Tablets:</u> 600 mg | **Rheumatoid Arthritis or Osteoarthritis:**<br>300–600 mg tid to qid<br><br>**Mild to moderate pain:**<br>200 mg q 4–6 h prn<br><br>**Maximum adult daily dose: 3200mg** | <u>Administration Issues:</u><br>Take with food; avoid alcohol and aspirin use. Safety/efficacy in children not established.<br><br><u>Drug–Drug Interactions:</u><br>**increased levels/effects of:**<br>anticoagulants, cyclosporine (inc renal toxic effects), digoxin, dipyridamole, hydantoins, lithium<br><br>**decreased levels/effects of:** ACE inhibitors, beta blocker, diuretics, (antihypertensive effect)<br><br>**increased levels/effects of NSAID:** probenecid | <u>ADRs:</u><br>nausea, vomiting, diarrhea, constipation, abdominal distress, dyspepsia, dizziness, headache, drowsiness, rash<br><br><u>Less Frequent:</u> GI ulceration, cholestatic hepatitis, pancreatitis, hematuria, proteinuria, elevated BUN, increased serum creatinine, renal insufficiency/failure<br><br><u>Elderly patients:</u> May be more prone to adverse effects.<br><br><u>Pharmacokinetics:</u><br>antirheumatic action onset = 2 days; hepatically metabolized; $T_{1/2}$ = 2–3 hrs; renal elimination of metabolites | <u>Contraindications:</u><br>Hypersensitivity to this or aspirin; preexisting renal disease<br><br><u>Precautions:</u><br>use cautiously in patients with PUD, severe renal or hepatic dysfunction, bleeding disorders<br><br><u>Pregnancy Category:</u> B<br><br><u>Lactation Issues:</u> Excreted in breast milk—do not use in nursing mothers |
| **Flurbiprofen**<br>Ansaid<br><br><u>Tablets:</u><br>50 mg, 100 mg | **Rheumatoid Arthritis or Osteoarthritis:**<br>200–300 mg/d in 2–4 divided doses, initially. | <u>Administration Issues:</u><br>Take with food; avoid alcohol and aspirin use. Safety/efficacy in children is not established. | <u>Most Frequent:</u> nausea, vomiting, diarrhea, constipation, abdominal distress, dyspepsia, dizziness, headache, drowsiness, rash | <u>Contraindications:</u><br>Hypersensitivity to this or aspirin; preexisting renal disease |

| | | | | |
|---|---|---|---|---|
| | **Max single dose is 100 mg and max daily dose is 300mg** | Drug–Drug Interactions: **increased levels/effects of:** anticoagulants, cyclosporine (inc renal toxic effects), digoxin, dipyridamole, hydantoins, lithium **decreased levels/effects of:** ACE inhibitors, beta blocker, diuretics, (antihypertensive effect) **increased levels/effects of NSAID:** probenecid | Less Frequent: see Fenoprofen<br><br>Elderly patients: May be more prone to adverse effects<br><br>Pharmacokinetics: hepatically metabolized; $T_{1/2}$ = 5.7 hrs; renal elimination of metabolites | Precautions: Use cautiously in patients with PUD, severe renal or hepatic dysfunction, bleeding disorders<br><br>Pregnancy Category: B<br><br>Lactation Issues: Excreted in breast milk—do not use in nursing mothers |
| **Ibuprofen**<br>Motrin, Advil, Bayer Select, Genpril, Haltran, Menadol, Midol IB, Nuprin, various generics<br><br>Tablets:<br>100 mg, 200 mg, 300 mg, 400 mg, 600 mg, 800 mg<br><br>Tablets, chewable:<br>50 mg, 100 mg<br><br>Suspension:<br>100 mg/5 mL<br><br>Oral Drops:<br>40 mg/mL | **Rheumatoid Arthritis or Osteoarthritis:**<br>300 mg qid or 400–800 mg tid to qid<br><br>Pediatrics: 30–70 mg/kg/d tid to qid<br><br>**Mild to Moderate Pain:**<br>400 mg q 4–6 h prn<br><br>**Primary Dysmenorrhea:**<br>400 mg q 4 h prn<br><br>**OTC use (mild pain, dysmenorrhea, fever reduction):**<br>200 mg q 4–6 h prn (May increase to 400 mg q 4–6 h prn)<br><br>**Max adult dose is 3200mg**<br><br>**Pediatrics** (fever reduction in 6 months to 12 yrs old): Temp ≤102.5F: 5 mg/kg q 6–8 hrs prn Temp >102.5F: 10 mg/kg q 6–8 h prn **Max Pediatric dose : 40mg/kg/d** | Administration Issues: Take with food; avoid alcohol and aspirin use; OTC use: Do not use for >3 days for fever or >10 days for pain—consult physician if those symptoms last longer<br><br>Drug–Drug Interactions: **increased levels/effects of:** anticoagulants, cyclosporine (inc renal toxic effects), digoxin, dipyridamole, hydantoins, lithium<br><br>**decreased levels/effects of:** ACE inhibitors, beta blocker, diuretics, (antihypertensive effect)<br><br>**increased levels/effects of NSAID:** probenecid | ADRs: nausea, vomiting, diarrhea, constipation, abdominal distress, dyspepsia, dizziness, headache, drowsiness, rash<br><br>Less Frequent: see Fenoprofen<br><br>Elderly patients: May be more prone to adverse effects<br><br>Pharmacokinetics: analgesic onset of action = 0.5 hrs; analgesic duration of action = 4–6 hrs; antirheumatic onset of action = within 7 days; hepatically metabolized; $T_{1/2}$ = 1.8 – 2.5 hrs; renal elimination of metabolites | Contraindications: Hypersensitivity to this or aspirin; preexisting renal disease<br><br>Precautions: Use cautiously in patients with PUD, severe renal or hepatic dysfunction, bleeding disorders<br><br>Pregnancy Category: B<br><br>Lactation Issues: Excreted in breast milk—do not use in nursing mothers |

(continues on next page)

| Drug and Dosage Forms | Usual Dosage Range | Administration Issues and Drug–Drug & Drug–Food Interactions | Common Adverse Drug Reactions (ADRs) and Pharmacokinetics | Contraindications, Pregnancy Category, and Lactation Issues |
|---|---|---|---|---|
| **Ketoprofen** Orudis KT, Actron, Orudis, Oruvail, various generics<br><br>Tablets: 12.5 mg<br><br>Capsules: 25 mg, 50 mg, 75 mg<br><br>Capsules, extended release: 100 mg, 150 mg, 200 mg | **Rheumatoid Arthritis or Osteoarthritis:** 150–300 mg/d divided tid to qid<br><br>Extended Release formulation: 200 mg qd<br><br>**Elderly, debilitated patients, or those with renal dysfunction:** 75–150 mg/d divided tid to qid. May titrate slowly if needed. **Max adult dose is 300 mg/d**<br><br>**Mild to Moderate Pain or Primary Dysmenorrhea:** 25–50 mg q 6–8 h prn. Use smaller doses for elderly, debilitated or small patients, and those with renal or hepatic disease.<br><br>**OTC use (mild pain, fever reduction):** 12.5 mg q 4–6 h prn. May repeat dose after 1 hr if pain or fever persists. Do not exceed 25 mg in 4–6 h | <u>Administration Issues:</u> Take with food, avoid alcohol and aspirin use. Not recommended for those <16 yrs old.<br><br><u>Drug–Drug Interactions:</u> **increased levels/effects of:** anticoagulants, cyclosporine (inc renal toxic effects), digoxin, dipyridamole, hydantoins, lithium<br><br>**decreased levels/effects of:** ACE inhibitors, beta blocker, diuretics, (antihypertensive effect)<br><br>**decreased levels/effects of NSAID:** probenecid | <u>ADRs:</u> nausea, vomiting, diarrhea, constipation, abdominal distress, dyspepsia, dizziness, headache, drowsiness, rash<br><br><u>Less Frequent:</u> see Fenoprofen<br><br><u>Elderly patients:</u> May be more prone to adverse effects.<br><br><u>Pharmacokinetics:</u> hepatically metabolized; $T_{1/2}$ = 2–4 hrs; renal elimination of metabolites | <u>Contraindications:</u> Hypersensitivity to this or aspirin; preexisting renal disease<br><br><u>Precautions:</u> Use cautiously in patients with PUD, severe renal or hepatic dysfunction, bleeding disorders<br><br><u>Pregnancy Category:</u> B<br><br><u>Lactation Issues:</u> Excreted in breast milk—do not use in nursing mothers |
| **Naproxen** Naprosyn, Napron X, EC-Naprosyn, Naprelan, various generics | **Rheumatoid Arthritis, Osteoarthritis, Ankylosing spondylitis:** | <u>Administration Issues:</u> Take with food, avoid alcohol and aspirin use. Do not break, crush, or chew extended release products. Safety | ADRs: nausea, vomiting, diarrhea, constipation, abdominal distress, dyspepsia, dizziness, headache, drowsiness, rash | <u>Contraindications:</u> Hypersensitivity to this or aspirin; preexisting renal disease |

| Preparations / Dosage | Drug–Drug Interactions | Adverse Effects / Pharmacokinetics |
|---|---|---|
| **Tablets:** 250 mg, 375 mg, 500 mg<br><br>**Tablets, delayed release:** 375 mg, 500 mg<br><br>**Suspension:** 125 mg/5 mL<br><br>**Naproxen Sodium**<br>Anaprox, Aleve, various generics<br><br>**Tablets:** 220 mg (200 mg of naproxen), 275 mg (250 mg naproxen), 550 mg (500 mg naproxen)<br><br>**Tablets, controlled release:** 421.5 mg (375 mg naproxen), 550 mg (500 mg naproxen)<br><br>**Naproxen:** 250–500 mg bid. May titrate to 1.5 g/d if needed for a limited period of time.<br><br>**Delayed-release:** 375–500 mg bid<br><br>**Controlled-release:** 750–1000 mg qd Max dose is 1000 mg/d<br><br>**Naproxen Sodium:** 275–550 mg bid. May titrate to 1.65 g/d for limited periods of time.<br>Pediatrics: 10 mg/kg divided bid. For the suspension:<br>13 kg: 2.5 mL twice daily<br>25 kg: 5 mL twice daily<br>38 kg: 7.5 mL twice daily<br><br>**Acute Gout:**<br>Naproxen: 750 mg followed by 250 mg q 8 h until attack is over.<br><br>Naproxen Sodium: 825 mg followed by 275 mg q 8 hrs until attack is over.<br><br>Controlled Release: 1000–1500 mg once daily on first day, then 1000 mg daily until attack is over.<br><br>**Mild to Moderate pain, dysmenorrhea, acute tendinitis, and bursitis:**<br>Naproxen: 500 mg followed by 250 mg q 6–8 hrs. MAX DOSE IS 1.25 g/d<br><br>Naproxen Sodium: 550 mg followed by 275 mg q 6–8 h. MAX DOSE IS 1.375 g/d | and efficacy in children <12 years of age has not been established.<br><br><u>Drug–Drug Interactions:</u><br>**increased levels/effects of:** anticoagulants, cyclosporine (inc renal toxic effects), digoxin, dipyridamole, hydantoins, lithium<br><br>**decreased levels/effects of:** ACE inhibitors, beta blocker, diuretics, (antihypertensive effect)<br><br>**increased levels/effects of NSAID:** probenecid | <u>Less Frequent:</u> see Fenoprofen<br><br><u>Elderly patients:</u> May be more prone to adverse effects.<br><br><u>Pharmacokinetics:</u><br>analgesic onset of action = 1 hr; analgesic duration of action = 7 hrs; antirheumatic onset of action = within 14 days; hepatically metabolized; $T_{1/2}$ = 12–15 hrs; renal elimination of metabolites<br><br><u>Precautions:</u> Use cautiously in patients with PUD, severe renal or hepatic dysfunction, bleeding disorders<br><br><u>Pregnancy Category:</u> B<br><br><u>Lactation Issues:</u> Excreted in breast milk—do not use in nursing mothers |

(continues on next page)

| Drug and Dosage Forms | Usual Dosage Range | Administration Issues and Drug–Drug & Drug–Food Interactions | Common Adverse Drug Reactions (ADRs) and Pharmacokinetics | Contraindications, Pregnancy Category, and Lactation Issues |
|---|---|---|---|---|
| **Naproxen Sodium** *cont.* | <u>Controlled Release:</u> 1000 mg once daily. May titrate to 1500 mg/d for limited period of time as needed.<br><br>**OTC analgesic use:** 200 mg q 8–12 h prn. May initiate therapy with 400 mg then follow with above schedule. MAX DOSE IS 600 mg/d unless otherwise directed by a health-care professional.<br><br>**Elderly:** Max = 200 mg q 12 h | | | |
| **Oxaprozin**<br>Daypro<br><br><u>Caplets:</u> 600 mg | **Rheumatoid Arthritis or Osteoarthritis:**<br><br>1200 mg qd. May initiate with 600 mg qd for smaller, elderly, or debilitated patients.<br><br>**Max dose is 1800 mg/d, divided** | <u>Administration Issues:</u><br>Take with food, avoid alcohol and aspirin use. Safety/efficacy in children is not established<br><br><u>Drug–Drug Interactions:</u><br>**increased levels/effects of:**<br>anticoagulants, cyclosporine (inc renal toxic effects), digoxin, dipyridamole, hydantoins, lithium<br><br>**decreased levels/effects of:** ACE inhibitors, beta blocker, diuretics, (antihypertensive effect)<br><br>**increased levels/effects of NSAID:** probenecid | <u>ADRs:</u><br>nausea, vomiting, diarrhea, constipation, abdominal distress, dyspepsia, dizziness, headache, drowsiness, rash<br><br><u>Less Frequent:</u> see Fenoprofen<br><br><u>Elderly patients:</u> May be more prone to adverse effects<br><br><u>Pharmacokinetics:</u><br>antirheumatic onset of action = within 7 days; hepatically metabolized; $T_{1/2}$ = 42–50 hrs; renal elimination of metabolites | <u>Contraindications:</u><br>Hypersensitivity to this or aspirin; preexisting renal disease<br><br><u>Precautions:</u> Use cautiously in patients with PUD, severe renal or hepatic dysfunction, bleeding disorders<br><br><u>Pregnancy Category:</u> B<br><br><u>Lactation Issues:</u> Excreted in breast milk—do not use in nursing mothers. |

| Drug and Dosage Forms | Usual Dosage Range | Administration Issues and Drug–Drug & Drug–Food Interactions | Common Adverse Drug Reactions (ADRs) and Pharmacokinetics | Contraindications, Pregnancy Category, and Lactation Issues |
|---|---|---|---|---|
| **Diclofenac Sodium**<br>Voltaren, Cataflam<br><br>Tablets:  50 mg<br><br>Tablets, delayed release<br>(enteric coated):  25 mg,<br>50 mg, 75 mg | **Osteoarthritis:**<br>100–150 mg/d bid to tid<br><br>**Rheumatoid Arthritis:**<br>150–200 mg/d tid to qid<br><br>**Ankylosing Spondylitis:**<br>100–125 mg/d in 4–5 divided doses.<br><br>**Moderate pain or Primary Dysmenorrhea:**<br>50 mg tid. May initiate therapy with 100 mg followed by 50 mg tid<br><br>**Max dose is 200 mg/d.** | Administration Issues:<br>Take with food, avoid alcohol and aspirin use. Safety/efficacy in children is not established.<br><br>Drug–Drug Interactions:<br>**increased levels/effects of:**<br>anticoagulants, cyclosporine (inc renal toxic effects), digoxin, dipyridamole, hydantoins, lithium<br><br>**decreased levels/effects of:**  ACE inhibitors, beta blocker, diuretics, (antihypertensive effect)<br><br>**increased levels/effects of NSAID:**<br>probenecid | ADRs:  nausea, vomiting, diarrhea, constipation, abdominal distress, dyspepsia, dizziness, headache, drowsiness, rash<br><br>Less Frequent:  GI ulceration, cholestatic hepatitis, pancreatitis, hematuria, proteinuria, elevated BUN, increased serum creatinine, renal insufficiency/failure<br><br>Elderly patients:  May be more prone to adverse effects<br><br>Pharmacokinetics:<br>hepatically metabolized;<br>$T_{1/2}$ = 1–2 hrs; renal elimination of metabolites | Contraindications:<br>Hypersensitivity to this or aspirin; preexisting renal disease<br><br>Precautions:  Use cautiously in patients with PUD, severe renal or hepatic dysfunction, bleeding disorders<br><br>Pregnancy Category:  B<br><br>Lactation Issues:  Excreted in breast milk—do not use in nursing mothers |
| **Etodolac**<br>Lodine<br><br>Capsules:<br>200 mg, 300 mg | **Osteoarthritis:**<br>800–1200 mg/d in bid to tid<br><br>**Moderate Pain:**<br>200–400 mg q 6–8 h prn<br><br>**Max dose is 1200 mg/d**<br><br>Patients ≤60 kg: Do not exceed 20 mg/kg. | Administration Issues:<br>Take with food, avoid alcohol and aspirin use. Safety/efficacy in children is not established.<br><br>Drug–Drug Interactions:<br>**increased levels/effects of:**<br>anticoagulants, cyclosporine (inc renal toxic effects), digoxin, dipyridamole, hydantoins, lithium | Most Frequent:  nausea, vomiting, diarrhea, constipation, abdominal distress, dyspepsia, dizziness, headache, drowsiness, rash<br><br>Less Frequent:  see Diclofenac | Contraindications:<br>Hypersensitivity to this or aspirin; preexisting renal disease<br><br>Precautions:  Use cautiously in patients with PUD, severe renal or hepatic dysfunction, bleeding disorders |

(continues on next page)

| Drug and Dosage Forms | Usual Dosage Range | Administration Issues and Drug–Drug & Drug–Food Interactions | Common Adverse Drug Reactions (ADRs) and Pharmacokinetics | Contraindications, Pregnancy Category, and Lactation Issues |
|---|---|---|---|---|
| **Etodolac** *cont.* | | **decreased levels/effects of:** ACE inhibitors, beta blocker, diuretics, (antihypertensive effect)<br><br>**increased levels/effects of NSAID:** probenecid | Elderly patients: May be more prone to adverse effects<br><br>Pharmacokinetics: analgesic onset of action = 0.5 hrs; analgesic duration of action = 4–12 hrs; hepatically metabolized; $T_{1/2}$ = 7.3 hrs; renal elimination of metabolites | Pregnancy Category: B<br><br>Lactation Issues: Excreted in breast milk—do not use in nursing mothers |
| **Indomethacin**<br>Indocin, Indochron E-R, various generics<br><br>Capsules: 25 mg, 50 mg<br><br>Capsules, sustained release: 75 mg<br><br>Suspension: 25 mg/5 mL<br><br>Suppositories: 50 mg | **Rheumatoid Arthritis, osteoarthritis, ankylosing spondylitis:**<br>25 mg bid to tid. Titrate by 25–50 mg/d q 7 d prn up to 200 mg/d<br><br>Sustained Release: 75 mg qd to bid<br><br>**Acute bursitis or tendinitis:**<br>75–150 mg daily in 3–4 divided doses for 7–14 d<br><br>**Acute Gout:** 50 mg tid until attack is over (3–5 days).<br><br>**Unlabeled uses:** to prevent premature labor (not for long periods of time); topical eye drops 0.5% and 1% used to treat cystoid macular edema.<br><br>**Max dose is 200 mg/d (150 mg of SR capsules)** | Administration Issues:<br>Take with food, avoid alcohol and aspirin use. Not recommended for those <14 yrs except when need outweighs risk.<br><br>Drug–Drug Interactions:<br>**increased levels/effects of:** anticoagulants, cyclosporine (inc renal toxic effects), digoxin, dipyridamole, hydantoins, lithium<br><br>**decreased levels/effects of:** ACE inhibitors, beta blocker, diuretics, (antihypertensive effect)<br><br>**increased levels/effects of NSAID:** probenecid | Most Frequent: nausea, vomiting, diarrhea, constipation, abdominal distress, dyspepsia, dizziness, headache, drowsiness, rash<br><br>Less Frequent: see Diclofenac<br><br>Elderly patients: May be more prone to adverse effects.<br><br>Pharmacokinetics:<br>90% protein bound; analgesic onset of action = 0.5 hrs; analgesic duration of action = 4–6 hrs; antirheumatic onset of action = within 7 days; $T_{1/2}$ = 4.5 hrs; renal elimination of metabolites | Contraindications:<br>Hypersensitivity to this or aspirin; preexisting renal disease<br><br>Precautions: Use cautiously in patients with PUD, severe renal or hepatic dysfunction, bleeding disorders<br><br>Pregnancy Category: B<br><br>Lactation Issues: Excreted in breast milk—do not use in nursing mothers |

| Drug | Dosing | Administration/Drug Interactions | Adverse Effects/Pharmacokinetics | Contraindications/Precautions |
|---|---|---|---|---|
| **Ketorolac**<br>Toradol<br><br><u>Tablets:</u> 10 mg<br><br><u>Injection:</u><br>15 mg/mL; 30 mg/mL | **Short-term (<5d) management of pain:**<br>Oral: 10 mg q 4–6 h prn<br>Max oral = 40mg/d<br><br>**Continuation treatment to IM therapy for the management of moderately severe pain that requires analgesia at the opioid level:** 20 mg as first dose, followed by 10 mg every 4–6 hrs for those patients who received 60 mg IM, 30 mg IV or multiple 30 mg IM doses.<br>**MAX DOSE IS 40 mg/d (oral) or 120 mg/d (IM). DO NOT EXCEED 5 DAYS OF THERAPY.**<br><br>**Elderly, debilitated (those with renal dysfunction), or small patients:** 10 mg first dose followed by 10 mg q 4–6 h for those who received 30 mg IM, 15 mg IV, or 15 mg IM multiple dosing. | <u>Administration Issues:</u><br>Take with food, avoid alcohol and aspirin use. Safety/efficacy in children is not established.<br><br><u>Drug–Drug Interactions:</u><br>**increased levels/effects of:** anticoagulants, cyclosporine (inc renal toxic effects), digoxin, dipyridamole, hydantoins, lithium<br><br>**decreased levels/effects of:** ACE inhibitors, beta blocker, diuretics, (antihypertensive effect)<br><br>**increased levels/effects of NSAID:** probenecid | <u>Most Frequent:</u> **serious GI bleeding and ulceration may occur,** nausea, vomiting, diarrhea, constipation, abdominal distress, dyspepsia, dizziness, headache, drowsiness, rash<br><br><u>Less Frequent:</u> see Diclofenac<br><br><u>Elderly patients:</u> May be more prone to adverse effects.<br><br><u>Pharmacokinetics:</u><br>90% protein bound;<br>$T_{1/2} = 2.4–8.6$ hrs; renal elimination of metabolites | <u>Contraindications:</u><br>Hypersensitivity to this or aspirin; preexisting renal disease<br><br><u>Precautions:</u> Use cautiously in patients with PUD, severe renal or hepatic dysfunction, bleeding disorders<br><br><u>Pregnancy Category:</u> B<br><br><u>Lactation Issues:</u> Excreted in breast milk—do not use in nursing mothers |
| **Nabumetone**<br>Relafen<br><br><u>Tablets:</u> 500 mg, 750 mg | **Rheumatoid Arthritis or Osteoarthritis:**<br><br>1000 mg qd. May titrate to 1500–2000 mg/d in 1–2 divided doses<br><br>**Max dose is 2000 mg/d** | <u>Administration Issues:</u><br>Take with food, avoid alcohol and aspirin use. Safety/efficacy in children not established.<br><br><u>Drug–Drug Interactions:</u><br>**increased levels/effects of:** anticoagulants, cyclosporine (inc renal toxic effects), digoxin, dipyridamole, hydantoins, lithium | <u>Most Frequent:</u> nausea, vomiting, diarrhea, constipation, abdominal distress, dyspepsia, dizziness, headache, drowsiness, rash<br><br><u>Less Frequent:</u> see Diclofenac<br><br><u>Elderly patients:</u> May be more prone to adverse effects. | <u>Contraindications:</u><br>Hypersensitivity to this or aspirin; preexisting renal disease<br><br><u>Precautions:</u> Use cautiously in patients with PUD, severe renal or hepatic dysfunction, bleeding disorders |

| Drug and Dosage Forms | Usual Dosage Range | Administration Issues and Drug–Drug & Drug–Food Interactions | Common Adverse Drug Reactions (ADRs) and Pharmacokinetics | Contraindications, Pregnancy Category, and Lactation Issues |
|---|---|---|---|---|
| **Nabumetone** *cont.* | | **decreased levels/effects of:** ACE inhibitors, beta blocker, diuretics, (antihypertensive effect)<br><br>**increased levels/effects of NSAID:** probenecid | Pharmacokinetics: 90% protein bound; inactive prodrug that must be converted to an active metabolite; $T_{1/2}$ = 22.5–30 hrs (active metabolite); renal elimination of metabolites | Pregnancy Category: B<br><br>Lactation Issues: Excreted in breast milk—do not use in nursing mothers |
| **Sulindac**<br>Clinoril, various generics<br><br>Tablets: 150 mg, 200 mg | **Rheumatoid Arthritis, Osteoarthritis or Ankylosing Spondylitis:**<br>150 mg bid<br><br>**Acute subacromial bursitis, tendinitis, or acute gouty arthritis:**<br>200 mg bid for 7–14 d (bursitis or tendinitis) or 7 d (for gout).<br><br>**Max dose is 400 mg/d** | Administration Issues:<br>Take with food<br>Avoid alcohol and aspirin use<br><br>Drug–Drug Interactions:<br>**increased levels/effects of:**<br>anticoagulants, cyclosporine (inc renal toxic effects), digoxin, dipyridamole, hydantoins, lithium<br><br>**decreased levels/effects of:** ACE inhibitors, beta blocker, diuretics, (antihypertensive effect)<br><br>**increased levels/effects of NSAID:** probenecid | Most Frequent: nausea, vomiting, diarrhea, constipation, abdominal distress, dyspepsia, dizziness, headache, drowsiness, rash<br><br>Less Frequent: see Diclofenac<br><br>Elderly patients: May be more prone to adverse effects<br><br>Pharmacokinetics:<br>antirheumatic onset of action = within 7 days; $T_{1/2}$ = 7.8 h | Contraindications:<br>Hypersensitivity to this or aspirin; preexisting renal disease<br><br>Precautions: Use cautiously in patients with PUD, severe renal or hepatic dysfunction, bleeding disorders<br><br>Pregnancy Category: B<br><br>Lactation Issues: Excreted in breast milk—do not use in nursing mothers<br><br>Pediatrics: Safety/efficacy not established. |

# Tolmetin
Tolectin

Tablets: 200 mg, 600 mg

Capsules: 400 mg

| | | | |
|---|---|---|---|
| **Rheumatoid Arthritis or Osteoarthritis:** | Administration Issues: Take with food; avoid alcohol and aspirin use | Most Frequent: nausea, vomiting, diarrhea, constipation, abdominal distress, dyspepsia, dizziness, headache, drowsiness, rash | Contraindications: Hypersensitivity to this or aspirin; preexisting renal disease |
| 400 mg tid/ May titrate up to 1800 mg/d divided tid | Drug–Drug Interactions: **increased levels/effects of:** anticoagulants, cyclosporine (inc renal toxic effects), digoxin, dipyridamole, hydantoins, lithium | Less Frequent: see Diclofenac | Precautions: Use cautiously in patients with PUD, severe renal or hepatic dysfunction, bleeding disorders |
| **Pediatrics (≥2 yrs):** 20 mg/kg/d in 3–4 divided doses. May titrate up to 30 mg/kg/d if needed | | Elderly patients: May be more prone to adverse effects. | Pregnancy Category: B |
| **Max dose is 2000 mg/d** | **decreased levels/effects of:** ACE inhibitors, beta blocker, diuretics, (antihypertensive effect) **increased levels/effects of NSAID:** probenecid | Pharmacokinetics: 90% protein bound; antirheumatic onset of action = within 7 days; $T_{1/2}$ = 1–1.5 hrs; renal elimination of metabolites | Lactation Issues: Excreted in breast milk—do not use in nursing mothers |

| Drug and Dosage Forms | Usual Dosage Range | Administration Issues and Drug–Drug & Drug–Food Interactions | Common Adverse Drug Reactions (ADRs) and Pharmacokinetics | Contraindications, Pregnancy Category, and Lactation Issues |
|---|---|---|---|---|
| **Meclofenamate**<br>Meclomen, various generics<br><br><u>Capsules:</u> 50 mg, 100 mg | **Rheumatoid Arthritis or Osteoarthritis:**<br>200–400 mg/d in 3–4 divided doses.<br><br>**Mild to Moderate Pain:**<br>50 mg q 4–6 h. May titrate to 100 mg q 4–6 h prn<br><br>**Primary Dysmenorrhea, excessive menstrual blood loss:**<br>100 mg tid for up to 6 days. Start with onset of bleeding.<br><br>**Max dose is 400 mg/d** | <u>Administration Issues:</u><br>Take with food; avoid alcohol and aspirin use; not recommended for those <14 yrs old.<br><br><u>Drug–Drug Interactions:</u><br>**increased levels/effects of:**<br>anticoagulants, cyclosporine (inc renal toxic effects), digoxin, dipyridamole, hydantoins, lithium<br><br>**decreased levels/effects of:** ACE inhibitors, beta blocker, diuretics, (antihypertensive effect)<br><br>**increased levels/effects of NSAID:** probenecid | <u>ADRs:</u><br>Most Frequent: nausea, vomiting, diarrhea, constipation, abdominal distress, dyspepsia, dizziness, headache, drowsiness, rash<br><br>Less Frequent: GI ulceration, cholestatic hepatitis, pancreatitis, hematuria, proteinuria, elevated BUN, increased serum creatinine, renal insufficiency/failure<br><br>Elderly patients: May be more prone to adverse effects<br><br><u>Pharmacokinetics:</u><br>antirheumatic onset of action = within a few days; hepatically metabolized; $T_{1/2}$ = 2–3.3 hrs; renal elimination of metabolites | <u>Contraindications:</u><br>Hypersensitivity to this or aspirin; preexisting renal disease<br><br><u>Precautions:</u> Use cautiously in patients with PUD, severe renal or hepatic dysfunction, bleeding disorders<br><br><u>Pregnancy Category:</u> B<br><br><u>Lactation Issues:</u> Excreted in breast milk—do not use in nursing mothers |
| **Mefenamic acid**<br>Ponstel<br><br><u>Capsules:</u> 250 mg | **Moderate Pain (≤1 week duration):** 500 mg initially, then 250 mg every 6 hrs as needed. | <u>Administration Issues:</u><br>Take with food; avoid alcohol and aspirin use; not recommended for those <14 yrs old. | Most Frequent: nausea, vomiting, diarrhea, constipation, abdominal distress, dyspepsia, dizziness, headache, drowsiness, rash | <u>Contraindications:</u><br>Hypersensitivity to this or aspirin; preexisting renal disease |

| | | | | |
|---|---|---|---|---|
| | **Primary Dysmenorrhea:** 500 mg initially, then 250 mg every 6 hrs for 2–3 days. Start with onset of bleeding.<br><br>**Max dose is 1000 mg/d** | Drug–Drug Interactions:<br>**increased levels/effects of:** anticoagulants, cyclosporine (inc renal toxic effects), digoxin, dipyridamole, hydantoins, lithium<br><br>**decreased levels/effects of:** ACE inhibitors, beta blocker, diuretics, (antihypertensive effect)<br><br>**increased levels/effects of NSAID:** probenecid | Less Frequent: GI ulceration, cholestatic hepatitis, pancreatitis, hematuria, proteinuria, elevated BUN, increased serum creatinine, renal insufficiency/failure, **autoimmune hemolytic anemia associated with >12 months of therapy**<br><br>Elderly patients: May be more prone to adverse effects.<br><br>Pharmacokinetics:<br>$T_{1/2} = 2$–4 hrs; renal elimination of metabolites | Precautions: Use cautiously in patients with PUD, severe renal or hepatic dysfunction, bleeding disorders<br><br>Pregnancy Category: B<br><br>Lactation Issues: Excreted in breast milk—do not use in nursing mothers |
| **Piroxicam**<br>Feldene, various generics<br>Capsules 10 mg, 20 mg | **Osteoarthritis and Rheumatoid Arthritis:**<br>Initial and maintenance dose is 10 to 20 mg/d; may divide bid<br><br>**Max dose is 20mg/d** | Administration Issues:<br>Take with food; avoid alcohol and aspirin use; safety/efficacy in children is not established<br><br>Drug–Drug Interactions:<br>**increased levels/effects of:** anticoagulants, cyclosporine (inc renal toxic effects), digoxin, dipyridamole, hydantoins, lithium<br><br>**decreased levels/effects of:** ACE inhibitors, beta blocker, diuretics, (antihypertensive effect)<br><br>**increased levels/effects of NSAID:** probenecid | Most Frequent: nausea, vomiting, diarrhea, constipation, abdominal distress, dyspepsia, dizziness, headache, drowsiness, rash<br><br>Less Frequent: GI ulceration, cholestatic hepatitis, pancreatitis, hematuria, proteinuria, elevated BUN, increased serum creatinine, renal insufficiency/failure, **autoimmune hemolytic anemia associated with >12 months of therapy**<br><br>Elderly patients: May be more prone to adverse effects.<br><br>Pharmacokinetics: onset of antirheumatic action is 7–12 days; $T_{1/2} = 30$–86 hrs; renal elimination of metabolites | Contraindications:<br>Hypersensitivity to this or aspirin; preexisting renal disease<br><br>Precautions: Use cautiously in patients with PUD, severe renal or hepatic dysfunction, bleeding disorders<br><br>Pregnancy Category: C<br><br>Lactation Issues: Excreted in breast milk—do not use in nursing mothers |

| Drug and Dosage Forms | Usual Dosage Range | Administration Issues and Drug–Drug & Drug–Food Interactions | Common Adverse Drug Reactions (ADRs) and Pharmacokinetics | Contraindications, Pregnancy Category, and Lactation Issues |
|---|---|---|---|---|
| **Tramadol**<br>Ultram<br><br>Tablets: 50 mg | **Moderate to moderately severe pain:**<br>50–100 mg q 4–6 h<br><br>**Elderly patients** (>75 yrs):<br>300 mg/d divided in 4–6 doses.<br><br>**Renal Impairment**<br>(CrCl <30 mL/min): 100 mg q 12 h<br><br>**Hepatic dysfunction**<br>(cirrhosis): 50 mg q 12 h<br><br>**Max dose is 400 mg/d.** | Administration Issues:<br>Safety/efficacy not established in those <16 yrs old; tramadol may impair physical or mental abilities<br><br>**Use in Opioid Dependence: Do not use in patients dependent on opioids —will precipitate opioid withdrawal.**<br><br>Drug–Drug Interactions:<br>**increased level/effect of tramadol:** MAO inhibitors (increased toxicity)<br>**decreased level/effect of tramadol:** carbamazepine | ADRs:<br>dizziness, vertigo, nausea, constipation, headache, somnolence, vomiting, pruritus, CNS stimulation, asthenia, sweating, dyspepsia, dry mouth, diarrhea<br><br>Pharmacokinetics:<br>20% protein bound; renal elimination of metabolites; $T_{1/2}$ = 6–7 hrs | Contraindications:<br>Hypersensitivity; acute alcohol, hypnotic, centrally acting analgesic, opioid, or psychotropic intoxication<br><br>Precautions: Use cautiously in patients with seizure disorders, severe renal or hepatic dysfunction.<br><br>Pregnancy Category: C<br><br>Lactation Issues: Use cautiously, safety not established. |

# 307. Salicylates

| Drug and Dosage Forms | Usual Dosage Range | Administration Issues and Drug–Drug & Drug–Food Interactions | Common Adverse Drug Reactions (ADRs) and Pharmacokinetics | Contraindications, Pregnancy Category, and Lactation Issues |
|---|---|---|---|---|
| **Aspirin**<br>Bayer, Aspergum, Empirin, Genprin, Ecotrin, Easprin, various generics<br><br>Tablets, chewable:<br>81 mg<br><br>Tablets, enteric coated:<br>165 mg, 325 mg, 500 mg, 650 mg, 975 mg<br><br>Tablets: 325 mg, 500 mg<br><br>Gum Tablets:<br>227.5 mg<br><br>Tablets, controlled release:<br>650 mg, 800 mg<br><br>Suppositories:<br>120 mg, 200 mg, 300 mg, 600 mg<br><br>**Aspirin, buffered**<br>Bufferin, Buffex, Wesprin Buffered, Ascriptin, Alka Seltzer with Aspirin, various generics | **Minor aches/pains:** 325–650 mg every 4 hrs as needed. Extra strength products: 500 mg every 3 hrs or 1000 mg every 6 hrs as needed.<br><br>**Arthritis/other rheumatic conditions:**<br>3.2–6 g/d in divided doses<br><br>**Pediatrics:** 60–110 mg/kg/d in divided doses (q 6–8 h). Start at 60 mg/kg/d and titrate by 20 mg/kg/d after 5–7 days prn by 10 mg/kg/d after another 5–7 days prn<br><br>**Acute rheumatic fever:**<br>5–8 g/d in divided doses<br><br>**Pediatrics:** 100 mg/kg/d for 2 weeks, then decrease to 75 mg/kg/d for 4–6 weeks.<br><br>**Transient Ischemic Attacks:**<br>1300 mg/d in divided doses. May use smaller doses if not tolerated.<br><br>**Myocardial Infarction Prophylaxis:** 81–325 mg/d (optimal dose has not been established; individualize) | Administration Issues:<br>Take with food; Safety/efficacy not established in those <12 yrs old.<br>**Aspirin use in children with fever has been associated with Reye's syndrome.**<br><br>Drug–Drug Interactions:<br>**increased level/effect of:** alcohol (GI effects); anticoagulants (bleeding effects); methotrexate, valproic acid, sulfonylureas (inc hypoglycemic effect)<br>**decreased level/effect of:** ACE inhibitors, beta blockers, diuretics (decreased antihypertensive effect); probenecid & sulfinpyrazone (decreased uricosuric effect)<br><br>Drug–Lab Interactions:<br>False negative or positive urine glucose tests, uric acid levels (inc with salicylate levels <10 mg/dL; decreased with salicylate levels >10 mg/dL), falsely elevated urine vanillylmandelic acid tests. | ADRs:<br>nausea, dyspepsia, heartburn, GI bleeding, hives, rash, prolonged bleeding time, thrombocytopenia, aspirin intolerance (rhinitis, (bronchospasm) "Salicylism". dizziness, tinnitus, difficulty hearing, nausea, vomiting, diarrhea, confusion, CNS depression, headache, sweating, hyperventilation, lassitude<br><br>Pharmacokinetics:<br>90% protein bound; hepatically metabolized; renal elimination of metabolites; $T_{1/2}$ of aspirin = 15–20 min; $T_{1/2}$ of salicylic acid = 2–3 h at low doses (may exceed 20 h at antiinflammatory doses) | Contraindications:<br>Hypersensitivity, hemophilia, bleeding ulcers, hemorrhagic states<br><br>Precautions: Use cautiously in patients with asthma, nasal polyposis, chronic urticaria (inc risk of hypersensitivity); chronic renal or hepatic dysfunction, PUD, bleeding disorders.<br><br>Pregnancy Category: D<br><br>Lactation Issues: safety not established. Use cautiously if at all. |

*(continues on next page)*

1135

| Drug and Dosage Forms | Usual Dosage Range | Administration Issues and Drug–Drug & Drug–Food Interactions | Common Adverse Drug Reactions (ADRs) and Pharmacokinetics | Contraindications, Pregnancy Category, and Lactation Issues |
|---|---|---|---|---|
| **Aspirin, buffered** *cont.* Contain small amounts of antacids (calcium carbonate, magnesium oxide, magnesium carbonate, aluminum glycinate, magnesium carbonate, magnesium or aluminum hydroxides) Tablets: 325 mg, 500 mg Tablets, coated: 325 mg, 500 mg Tablets, effervescent: 325 mg, 500 mg | **Pediatric Analgesic or Antipyretic:** 10–15 mg/kg/dose every 4 hrs up to 60–80 mg/kg/d. **DO NOT USE IN CHILDREN WITH CHICKEN POX OR FLU SYMPTOMS DUE TO POSSIBILITY OF REYE'S SYNDROME.** **Kawasaki Disease:** 80–180 mg/kg/d for acute febrile period, then reduce to 10 mg/kg/d | | | |
| **Choline Salicylate** Arthropan Liquid: 870 mg/5 mL | **Minor Aches/Pains:** Adults or children (>12 yrs): 870 mg q 3–4 h. Max is 6 doses/day. **Rheumatoid Arthritis:** Adults or children (>12 yrs): 5–10 mL up to 4 times per day. | Administration Issues: Take with food; Safety/ efficacy not established in those <12 yrs old. **Aspirin use in children with fever has been associated with Reye's syndrome.** Drug–Drug Interactions: **increased level/effect of:** alcohol (GI effects); anticoagulants (bleeding effects); methotrexate, valproic acid, sulfonylureas (inc hypoglycemic effect) | ADRs: (less GI effects than Aspirin): nausea, dyspepsia, heartburn, GI bleeding, hives, rash, prolonged bleeding time, thrombocytopenia, aspirin intolerance (rhinitis bronchospasm), "Salicylism": dizziness, tinnitus, difficulty hearing, nausea, vomiting, diarrhea, confusion, CNS depression, headache, sweating, hyperventilation, lassitude | Contraindications: Hypersensitivity, hemophilia, bleeding ulcers, hemorrhagic states Precautions: Use cautiously in patients with asthma, nasal polyposis, chronic urticaria (inc risk of hypersensitivity); chronic renal or hepatic dysfunction, PUD, bleeding disorders. |

| | | | | |
|---|---|---|---|---|
| | | **decreased level/effect of:** ACE inhibitors, beta blockers, diuretics (decreased antihypertensive effect); probenecid & sulfinpyrazone (decreased uricosuric effect)<br><br>Drug–Lab Interactions: see aspirin | Pharmacokinetics: 90% protein bound; renal elimination of metabolites; $T_{1/2}$ of salicylic acid = 2–3 hrs at low doses (may exceed 20 hrs at antiinflammatory doses) | Pregnancy Category: D<br><br>Lactation Issues: safety not established. Use cautiously if at all. |
| **Diflunisal**<br>Dolobid<br><br>Tablets: 250 mg, 500 mg | **Mild to Moderate Pain:**<br>1 g initially, followed by 500 mg q 8–12 h.<br><br>**Elderly or debilitated patients:** 500 mg initially, followed by 250 mg q 8–12 h<br><br>**Osteoarthritis/Rheumatoid Arthritis:**<br>500–1000 mg daily in 2 divided doses. **Max of 1500 mg daily.** | Administration Issues: Take with food; do not crush or chew tablets; do not take with aspirin or acetaminophen; Safety/efficacy in children <12 yrs not established. **Use in children with fever has been associated with Reye's syndrome.**<br><br>Drug–Drug Interactions:<br>**increased levels/effects of:** acetaminophen, oral anticoagulants, indomethacin, hydrochlorothiazide<br><br>**decreased levels/effects of:** sulindac | ADRs: nausea, dyspepsia, diarrhea, headache, insomnia, rash, tinnitus.<br><br>Pharmacokinetics: onset of action = 1 hr; 99% protein bound; renal elimination of metabolites; $T_{1/2}$ = 8–12 hrs. | Contraindications: Hypersensitivity to this or aspirin<br><br>Precautions: Use cautiously in those with asthma, nasal polyposis, chronic urticaria (inc risk of hypersensitivity); severe cardiac, renal, or hepatic dysfunction, PUD, bleeding disorders.<br><br>Pregnancy Category: C<br><br>Lactation Issues: Use cautiously if at all; it is excreted in breast milk |
| **Magnesium salicylate**<br>Doan's, Magan, Mobidin<br><br>Caplets: 325 mg, 500 mg<br><br>Tablets: 545 mg, 600 mg | **Minor Aches/Pains:**<br>650 mg q 4 h or 1090 mg tid. May increase to 3.6–4.8 g/d in 3–4 divided doses. | Administration Issues: Take with food; Safety/ efficacy not established in children.<br><br>Drug–Drug Interactions:<br>**increased level/effect of:** alcohol (GI effects); anticoagulants (bleeding effects); methotrexate, valproic acid, sulfonylureas (inc hypoglycemic effect) | (less GI effects than Aspirin): nausea, dyspepsia, heartburn, GI bleeding, hives, rash, prolonged bleeding time, thrombocytopenia, aspirin intolerance (rhinitis, bronchospasm). | Contraindications: Hypersensitivity, hemophilia, bleeding ulcers, hemorrhagic states<br><br>Precautions: Use cautiously in patients with asthma, nasal polyposis, chronic urticaria (inc risk of hypersensitivity); |

(continues on next page)

| Drug and Dosage Forms | Usual Dosage Range | Administration Issues and Drug–Drug & Drug–Food Interactions | Common Adverse Drug Reactions (ADRs) and Pharmacokinetics | Contraindications, Pregnancy Category, and Lactation Issues |
|---|---|---|---|---|
| **Magnesium salicylate** *cont.* | | **decreased level/effect of:** ACE inhibitors, beta blockers, diuretics (decreased antihypertensive effect); probenecid & sulfinpyrazone (decreased uricosuric effect)<br><br>Drug–Lab Interactions:<br>see aspirin | "Salicylism": dizziness, tinnitus, difficulty hearing, nausea, vomiting, diarrhea, confusion, CNS depression, headache, sweating, hyperventilation, lassitude<br><br>Pharmacokinetics:<br>90% protein bound; renal elimination of metabolites; $T_{1/2}$ of salicylic acid = 2–3 hrs at low doses (may exceed 20 hrs at antiinflammatory doses) | chronic renal or hepatic dysfunction, PUD, bleeding disorders.<br><br>Pregnancy Category: D<br><br>Lactation Issues: safety not established. Use cautiously if at all. |
| **Salicylate Combinations (choline salicylate & magnesium salicylate)**<br>Trilisate<br><br>Tablets: 500 mg, 750 mg, 1000 mg<br><br>Liquid: 500 mg/5 mL | **Minor Aches/Pains**:<br>500–750 mg q 3 h or 1000 mg q 6 h prn | Administration Issues:<br>Take with food; Safety/ efficacy not established in those <12 yrs old. **Aspirin use in children with fever has been associated with Reye's syndrome.**<br><br>Drug–Drug Interactions: **increased level/effect of:** alcohol (GI effects); anticoagulants (bleeding effects); methotrexate, valproic acid, sulfonylureas (inc hypoglycemic effect)<br><br>**decreased level/effect of:** ACE inhibitors, beta blockers, diuretics (decreased antihypertensive effect); | (less GI effects than aspirin): nausea, dyspepsia, heartburn, GI bleeding, hives, rash, prolonged bleeding time, thrombocytopenia, aspirin intolerance (rhinitis, bronchospasm), "Salicylism": dizziness, tinnitus, difficulty hearing, nausea, vomiting, diarrhea, confusion, CNS depression, headache, sweating, hyperventilation, lassitude | Contraindications:<br>Hypersensitivity, hemophilia, bleeding ulcers, hemorrhagic states<br><br>Precautions: Use cautiously in patients with asthma, nasal polyposis, chronic urticaria (inc risk of hypersensitivity); chronic renal or hepatic dysfunction, PUD, bleeding disorders.<br><br>Pregnancy Category: D<br><br>Lactation Issues: safety not established. Use cautiously if at all. |

| | | | |
|---|---|---|---|
| | | Pharmacokinetics: Oral; 90% protein bound; renal elimination of metabolites; $T_{1/2}$ of salicylic acid = 2–3 hrs at low doses (may exceed 20 hrs at antiinflammatory doses) | |
| | probenecid & sulfinpyrazone (decreased uricosuric effect)<br><br>Drug–Lab Interactions:<br>see aspirin | | Contraindications:<br>Hypersensitivity, hemophilia, bleeding ulcers, hemorrhagic states<br><br>Precautions: Use cautiously in patients with asthma, nasal polyposis, chronic urticaria (inc risk of hypersensitivity); chronic renal or hepatic dysfunction, PUD, bleeding disorders.<br><br>Pregnancy Category: C<br><br>Lactation Issues: safety not established. Use cautiously if at all. |
| **Salsalate**<br>Disalcid, Amigesic, Argesic-SA, Salflex, Salsitab, Artha-G, various generics<br><br>Capsules: 500 mg<br><br>Tablets: 500 mg, 750 mg | **Minor aches/pains, arthritis**<br><br>3000 mg/d in divided doses (2–4 times daily).<br><br>Administration Issues:<br>Take with food; Safety/efficacy not established in children.<br><br>Drug–Drug Interactions:<br>**increased level/effect of:** alcohol (GI effects); anticoagulants (bleeding effects); methotrexate, valproic acid, sulfonylureas (inc hypoglycemic effect)<br><br>**decreased level/effect of:** ACE inhibitors, beta blockers, diuretics (decreased antihypertensive effect); probenecid & sulfinpyrazone (decreased uricosuric effect)<br><br>Drug–Lab Interactions:<br>see aspirin | ADRs:<br>(less GI effects than Aspirin): nausea, dyspepsia, heartburn, GI bleeding, hives, rash, prolonged bleeding time, thrombocytopenia, aspirin intolerance (rhinitis, bronchospasm), "Salicylism": dizziness, tinnitus, difficulty hearing, nausea, vomiting, diarrhea, confusion, CNS depression, headache, sweating, hyperventilation, lassitude<br><br>Pharmacokinetics:<br>insoluble in gastric secretions, not absorbed until it reaches small intestine; 90% protein bound; renal elimination of metabolites; $T_{1/2}$ of salicylic acid = 2–3 hrs at low doses (may exceed 20 hrs at antiinflammatory doses) | |
| **Sodium Salicylate**<br>various generics | **Minor Aches/Pains:**<br>325–650 mg q 4 hr<br><br>Administration Issues:<br>Take with food; Safety/ efficacy not established in children. **Salicylate use in children with fever has been** | ADRs:<br>(less GI effects than Aspirin): nausea, dyspepsia, heartburn, GI bleeding, hives, rash, | Contraindications:<br>Hypersensitivity, hemophilia, bleeding ulcers, hemorrhagic states |

(continues on next page)

## 307. Salicylates
continued from previous page

| Drug and Dosage Forms | Usual Dosage Range | Administration Issues and Drug–Drug & Drug–Food Interactions | Common Adverse Drug Reactions (ADRs) and Pharmacokinetics | Contraindications, Pregnancy Category, and Lactation Issues |
|---|---|---|---|---|
| **Sodium Salicylate** *cont.*<br><br>Tablets, enteric coated: 325 mg, 650 mg | | **associated with Reye's syndrome.**<br><br>Drug–Drug Interactions:<br>**increased level/effect of:** alcohol (GI effects); anticoagulants (bleeding effects); methotrexate, valproic acid, sulfonylureas (inc hypoglycemic effect)<br><br>**decreased level/effect of:** ACE inhibitors, beta blockers, diuretics (decreased antihypertensive effect); probenecid & sulfinpyrazone (decreased uricosuric effect)<br><br>Drug–Lab Interactions:<br>see aspirin | prolonged bleeding time, thrombocytopenia, aspirin intolerance (rhinitis, bronchospasm). "Salicylism": dizziness, tinnitus, difficulty hearing, nausea, vomiting, diarrhea, confusion, CNS depression, headache, sweating, hyperventilation, lassitude<br><br>Pharmacokinetics:<br>90% protein bound; renal elimination of metabolites; $T_{1/2}$ of salicylic acid = 2–3 hrs at low doses (may exceed 20 hrs at antiinflammatory doses) | Precautions: Use cautiously in patients with asthma, nasal polyposis, chronic urticaria (inc risk of hypersensitivity); chronic renal or hepatic dysfunction, PUD, bleeding disorders.<br><br>Pregnancy Category: D<br><br>Lactation Issues: safety not established. Use cautiously if at all. |

## 308. Anticonvulsants

308.1 Barbiturates

| Drug and Dosage Forms | Usual Dosage Range | Administration Issues and Drug–Drug & Drug–Food Interactions | Common Adverse Drug Reactions (ADRs) and Pharmacokinetics | Contraindications, Pregnancy Category, and Lactation Issues |
|---|---|---|---|---|
| **Mephobarbital**<br>Mebaral<br><br>Tablets: 32 mg, 50 mg, 100 mg | **Tonic/Clonic, cortical focal:**<br>400–600 mg/d in 3–4 divided doses<br><br>**Pediatrics:** <5 yrs: 16–32 mg 3–4 times daily; >5 yrs: 32–64 mg 3–4 times daily<br><br>**Elderly or debilitated patients (hepatic/renal dysfunction):** 16–32 mg 2–3 times daily. Titrate to higher doses as needed/tolerated | Administration Issues:<br>When replacing another anticonvulsant, slowly titrate this agent, while decreasing the other agent; may produce irritability, excitability or aggression in children<br><br>Drug–Drug Interactions:<br>**decreased levels of:** anticoagulants, beta blockers, carbamazepine, clonazepam, oral contraceptives, corticosteroids, doxycycline, doxorubicin, felodipine, quinidine, verapamil, theophylline<br><br>**increased effect of:** alcohol & possibly narcotics (CNS effects), acetaminophen (liver toxicity)<br><br>**increased effect of barbiturates:** MAO inhibitors, valproic acid<br><br>**Unknown effects (monitor patient closely):** hydantoins | ADRs:<br>somnolence, agitation, confusion, ataxia, nightmares, nervousness, hallucinations, bradycardia, hypotension, nausea, vomiting, skin rash, angioedema, exfoliative dermatitis<br><br>Elderly: may observe paradoxical excitement<br><br>Pharmacokinetics:<br>onset of action = 30–60 min; hepatically metabolized; $T_{1/2}$ = 11–67 hrs; duration of action = 10–16 hrs | Contraindications:<br>Hypersensitivity; manifest or latent porphyria, severe hepatic, renal, or respiratory dysfunction; previous addiction to sedative/hypnotic<br><br>Precautions:<br>**Drug Abuse & Dependence:** Prolonged use at high doses leads to physical dependence. If dependent on barbiturate, slowly withdraw over several weeks. May use long-acting barbiturate (phenobarbital) at dose of 30 mg per every 100-200 mg of mephobarbital to help prevent withdrawal symptoms.<br><br>Pregnancy Category: D<br><br>Lactation Issues: use cautiously in nursing mothers, sedation has been reported in infants |

*(continues on next page)*

| Drug and Dosage Forms | Usual Dosage Range | Administration Issues and Drug–Drug & Drug–Food Interactions | Common Adverse Drug Reactions (ADRs) and Pharmacokinetics | Contraindications, Pregnancy Category, and Lactation Issues |
|---|---|---|---|---|
| **Phenobarbital**<br>Solfoton, various generics<br><br>Tablets: 15 mg, 16 mg, 30 mg, 60 mg, 100 mg<br><br>Capsules: 16 mg<br><br>Elixir: 15 mg/5 mL, 20 mg/5 mL | **Tonic/Clonic, cortical focal:**<br><br>60–100 mg/d in 2–3 divided doses<br><br>**Pediatrics:** 3–6 mg/kg/d in 2–3 divided doses<br><br>**Elderly or debilitated patients (hepatic/renal dysfunction):** Use lower initial dose and greater dosing intervals. Titrate to higher doses as needed/tolerated<br><br>**Traumatic Brain Injury**<br>60–200 mg qd | Administration Issues:<br>When replacing another anticonvulsant, slowly titrate this agent, while decreasing the other agent; may produce irritability, excitability or aggression in children<br><br>Drug–Drug Interactions:<br>**decreased levels of:** anticoagulants, beta blockers, carbamazepine, clonazepam, oral contraceptives, corticosteroids, doxycycline, doxorubicin, felodipine, quinidine, verapamil, theophylline<br><br>**increased effect of:** alcohol & possibly narcotics (CNS effects), acetaminophen (liver toxicity)<br><br>**increased effect of barbiturates:** MAO inhibitors, valproic acid<br><br>**Unknown effects (monitor patient closely):** hydantoins | ADRs:<br>somnolence, agitation, confusion, ataxia, nightmares, nervousness, hallucinations, bradycardia, hypotension, nausea, vomiting, skin rashes, angioedema, exfoliative dermatitis<br><br>Elderly: may observe paradoxical excitement<br><br>Pharmacokinetics:<br>onset of action = 30–60 min; hepatically metabolized; T$_{1/2}$ = 53–118 hrs; duration of action = 10–16 hrs<br><br>**Therapeutic plasma levels = 15–40 mcg/mL** | Contraindications:<br>Hypersensitivity; manifest or latent porphyria, severe hepatic, renal, or respiratory dysfunction; previous addiction to sedative/hypnotic<br><br>Precautions:<br><u>Drug Abuse & Dependence:</u><br>Prolonged use at high doses leads to physical dependence. If dependent on barbiturate, slowly withdraw over several weeks.<br><br>Pregnancy Category: D<br><br>Lactation Issues: use cautiously in nursing mothers, sedation has been reported in infants |
| **Primidone**<br>Mysoline, various generics<br><br>Tablets: 50 mg, 250 mg | **Tonic/Clonic, psychomotor, focal:**<br><br>Initially, 100–125 mg at bedtime. Titrate by 100–125 mg/d q 3 days up to max of 500 mg qid | Administration Issues:<br>When replacing another anticonvulsant, slowly titrate this agent, while decreasing the other agent. | ADRs:<br>drowsiness, dizziness, ataxia, vertigo, nystagmus, nausea, vomiting, anorexia, thrombocytopenia, | Contraindications:<br>Hypersensitivity to primidone or phenobarbital; acute intermittent porphyria |

| | | | |
|---|---|---|---|
| **Pediatrics (<8 yrs):** Initially, 50 mg at bedtime. Titrate by 50 mg/d q 3 days up to 125–250 mg tid or 10–25 mg/kg/d in divided doses.<br><br>*Full therapeutic effect may not be seen for several weeks | May take with food if GI upset occurs **Due to bioequivalence differences, brand interchange is not recommended**<br><br>Drug–Drug Interactions:<br>**decreased levels of primidone:** acetazolamide, carbamazepine, succinimides<br><br>**increased levels of primidone:** hydantoins, isoniazid<br><br>**increased levels of:** carbamazepine | megaloblastic anemia (responsive to folic acid), impotence, skin rash<br><br>Pharmacokinetics:<br>hepatically metabolized to PEMA and phenobarbital (both active metabolites); $T_{1/2}$ = 5–15 hrs (primidone); $T_{1/2}$ = 10–18 hrs (PEMA); $T_{1/2}$ = 53–140 hrs (phenobarbital)<br><br>**Therapeutic concentrations: 5–12 mcg/mL (primidone), 15–40 mcg/mL (phenobarbital)** | Precautions:<br>Abrupt withdrawal may precipitate status epilepticus<br><br>Pregnancy Issues: reports of fetal malformation; greater risk to fetus if medication is discontinued during pregnancy<br><br>Lactation Issues: women should not nurse |

## 308.2 Benzodiazepines

| Drug, and Dosage Forms | Usual Dosage Range | Administration Issues and Drug–Drug & Drug–Food Interactions | Common Adverse Drug Reactions (ADRs) and Pharmacokinetics | Contraindications, Pregnancy Category, and Lactation Issues |
|---|---|---|---|---|
| **Clonazepam (CIV)** Klonopin<br><br>Tablets: 0.5 mg, 1 mg, 2 mg | **Absence, myoclonic, akinetic:** 0.5 mg tid. Titrate by 0.5–1 mg/d every 3 days as needed to max dose of 20 mg/d.<br><br>**Pediatrics (<10 yrs):** 0.01–0.03 mg/kg/d in 2–3 divided doses. Titrate by 0.25–0.5 mg/d q 3 days as needed to max dose of 0.1–0.2 mg/kg/d | Administration Issues: When replacing another anticonvulsant, slowly titrate this agent, while decreasing the other agent; not recommended for children <9 yrs old<br><br>Drug–Drug Interactions:<br>**increased level of BZ:** cimetidine, oral contraceptives, disulfiram, | ADRs:<br>Drowsiness, ataxia, confusion (especially in elderly)<br><br>Dependence: abrupt discontinuation can precipitate withdrawal symptoms (e.g., anxiety, flu-like illness, concentration difficulties, | Contraindications:<br>Hypersensitivity, psychoses, acute narrow-angle glaucoma, clinical or biochemical evidence of significant liver disease<br><br>Pregnancy Category: none, but avoid in pregnant women |

(continues on next page)

| Drug and Dosage Forms | Usual Dosage Range | Administration Issues and Drug–Drug & Drug–Food Interactions | Common Adverse Drug Reactions (ADRs) and Pharmacokinetics | Contraindications, Pregnancy Category, and Lactation Issues |
|---|---|---|---|---|
| **Clonazepam (CIV)** *cont.* | **Unlabeled uses:** leg movements during sleep (0.5–2 mg/night); Parkinsonian dysarthria (0.25–0.5 mg/d); acute manic episodes of bipolar disorder (0.75–16 mg/d); multifocal tic disorders (1.5–12 mg/d); adjunctive treatment for schizophrenia (0.5–2 mg/d); neuralgias (2–4 mg/d) <br><br> **Traumatic Brain Injury** <br> 0.5–20 mg/d | fluoxetine, isoniazid, ketoconazole, metoprolol, propoxyphene, propranolol, valproic acid. <br><br> **increased CNS effects:** alcohol, barbiturates, narcotics <br><br> **increased levels of:** digoxin, phenytoin (possibly) <br><br> **decreased level or effect of BZ:** rifampin (decreased level); theophylline (decreased effect) | fatigue, anorexia, restlessness, confusion, psychosis, paranoid delusions, grand mal seizures). Withdrawal can occur after as little as 4–6 weeks of therapy. Clonidine, propranolol, carbamazepine have been used as adjuncts in withdrawal. <u>Drug</u> <u>Discontinuation:</u> gradual decrease over 4–8 weeks <br><br> <u>Pharmacokinetics:</u> $T_{1/2}$ = 18–50 hrs; speed of onset = intermediate; renal elimination | <u>Lactation Issues:</u> excreted in breast milk—do not give to nursing mothers |
| **Clorazepate dipotassium (CIV)** <br> Tranxene, Tranxene-SD, Tranxene-SD- Half, Gen-Xene, various generics <br><br> <u>Capsules:</u> 3.75 mg 7.5 mg, 15 mg <br><br> <u>Tablets:</u> 3.75 mg, 7.5 mg, 15 mg <br><br> <u>Tablet, single dose:</u> 11.25 mg, 22.5 mg | **Adjunctive therapy for partial** <br> **seizures:** <br> 7.5 mg tid. Titrate by 7.5 mg/d every week to max dose of 90 mg/d. <br><br> **Pediatrics** (<12 yrs): 7.5 mg bid. Titrate by ≤ 7.5 mg/d each week to max of 60 mg/d. | <u>Administration Issues:</u> <br> When replacing another anticonvulsant, slowly titrate this agent, while decreasing the other agent; not recommended for children <9 yrs old <br><br> <u>Drug–Drug Interactions:</u> <br> **increased level of BZ:** cimetidine, oral contraceptives, disulfiram, fluoxetine, isoniazid, ketoconazole, metoprolol, propoxyphene, propranolol, valproic acid. | <u>ADRs:</u> <br> drowsiness, ataxia, confusion (especially in elderly) <br><br> <u>Dependence:</u> abrupt discontinuation can precipitate withdrawal symptoms (e.g., anxiety, flu-like illness, concentration difficulties, fatigue, anorexia, restlessness, confusion, psychosis, paranoid delusions, grand mal seizures). Withdrawal can | <u>Contraindications:</u> <br> Hypersensitivity, psychoses, acute narrow-angle glaucoma, clinical or biochemical evidence of significant liver disease <br><br> <u>Pregnancy Category:</u> <br> none, but avoid in pregnant women <br><br> <u>Lactation Issues:</u> excreted in breast milk—do not give to nursing mothers |

| | | | | |
|---|---|---|---|---|
| | | **increased CNS effects:** alcohol, barbiturates, narcotics<br><br>**increased levels of:** digoxin, phenytoin (possibly)<br><br>**decreased level or effect of BZ:** rifampin (decreased level); theophylline (decreased effect) | occur after as little as 4–6 weeks of therapy. Clonidine, propranolol, carbamazepine have been used as adjuncts in withdrawal. <u>Drug Discontinuation:</u> gradual decrease over 4–8 weeks<br><br><u>Pharmacokinetics:</u> $T_{1/2}$ = 30–100 hrs (includes $T_{1/2}$ of metabolite); speed of onset = fast | <u>Contraindications:</u> Hypersensitivity, psychoses, acute narrow-angle glaucoma<br><br><u>Pregnancy Category:</u> D<br><br><u>Lactation Issues:</u> excreted in breast milk—do not give to nursing mothers |
| **Diazepam (CIV)**<br>Valium, Valrelease, Zetran, various generics<br><br><u>Tablets:</u> 2 mg, 5 mg, 10 mg<br><br><u>Capsule sustained release:</u> 15 mg<br><br><u>Oral Solution:</u> 5 mg/5 mL, 5 mg/mL | **Adjunctive therapy in convulsive disorders:**<br>2–10 mg 2–4 times daily (sustained release preparation: 15–30 mg qd)<br><br>**Pediatrics** (>6 mos): 1–2.5 mg 3–4 times daily. Titrate as needed/tolerated<br><br>**Elderly or debilitated patients:** 2–2.5 mg 1–2 times daily. Titrate slowly as needed/tolerated | <u>Administration Issues:</u><br>Do not crush or chew sustained release products. Concentrated solution (5 mg/mL) should be diluted in liquid or semi-solid foods. When replacing another anticonvulsant, slowly titrate this agent, while decreasing the other agent; not recommended for <6 mos old.<br><br><u>Drug–Drug Interactions:</u><br>**increased level of BZ:** cimetidine, oral contraceptives, disulfiram, fluoxetine, isoniazid, ketoconazole, metoprolol, propoxyphene, propranolol, valproic acid.<br><br>**increased CNS effects:** alcohol, barbiturates, narcotics<br><br>**increased levels of:** digoxin, phenytoin (possibly)<br><br>**decreased level or effect of BZ:** rifampin (decreased level); theophylline (decreased effect) | <u>ADRs:</u><br>Drowsiness, ataxia, confusion (especially in elderly)<br><br><u>Dependence:</u> abrupt discontinuation can precipitate withdrawal symptoms (e.g., anxiety, flu-like illness, concentration difficulties, fatigue, anorexia, restlessness, confusion, psychosis, paranoid delusions, grand mal seizures). Withdrawal can occur after as little as 4–6 weeks of therapy. Clonidine, propranolol, carbamazepine have been used as adjuncts in withdrawal.<br><br><u>Drug Discontinuation:</u> gradual decrease over 4–8 weeks<br><br><u>Pharmacokinetics:</u><br>$T_{1/2}$ = 20–80 hrs; speed of onset = very fast | |

| Drug and Dosage Forms | Usual Dosage Range | Administration Issues and Drug–Drug & Drug–Food Interactions | Common Adverse Drug Reactions (ADRs) and Pharmacokinetics | Contraindications, Pregnancy Category, and Lactation Issues |
|---|---|---|---|---|
| **Ethotoin**<br>Peganone<br><br>Tablets:<br>250 mg, 500 mg | **Tonic/Clonic or psychomotor:**<br>250 mg 3–4 times daily, initially. Titrate to 2–3 g/d over several days.<br><br>**Pediatrics:** 250 mg 1–3 times daily. Titrate to 500–1000 mg/d (some may require 2–3 g/d) | Administration Issues: May take with food to avoid GI upset. Draw serum levels just prior to next dose. Maintain good oral hygiene. When replacing another anticonvulsant, slowly titrate this agent, while decreasing the other agent.<br><br>Drug–Drug Interactions:<br>**increased levels and/or effects of hydantoin:**<br>allopurinol, amiodarone, benzodiazepines, cimetidine, ethanol (acute), fluconazole, isoniazid, metronidazole, miconazole, omeprazole, sulfonamides & trimethoprim, valproic acid, TCAs, salicylates, chlorpheniramine, ibuprofen, phenothiazines<br><br>**decreased levels and/or effects of hydantoin:**<br>barbiturates, carbamazepine, ethanol (chronic), rifampin, theophylline, antacids, sucralfate, charcoal, antineoplastics, folic acid, loxapine, pyridoxine, nitrofurantoin, influenza virus vaccine | ADRs:<br>nystagmus, ataxia, confusion, slurred speech, fatigue, drowsiness, tremor, headache, nervousness, diplopia, irritability, nausea, vomiting, diarrhea, constipation, thrombocytopenia, leukopenia, granulocytopenia, anemias, gingival hyperplasia, hepatitis, dermatologic reactions, osteomalacia<br><br>Overdose: far-lateral nystagmus (>20 mcg/mL), ataxia (>30 mcg/mL), dysarthria, decreased level of consciousness (>40 mcg/mL).<br><br>Pharmacokinetics:<br>saturable hepatic metabolism to inactive metabolites;<br>$T_{1/2} = 3$–9 hrs when level is < 8 mcg/mL.<br><br>**Therapeutic plasma levels = 15–50 mcg/mL** | Contraindications:<br>hypersensitivity; hepatic abnormalities; hematologic disorders<br><br>Precautions: abrupt withdrawal of medication may precipitate status epilepticus; some patients are genetically predisposed to slowed metabolism, monitor carefully; use cautiously in patients with hepatic dysfunction<br><br>Pregnancy Issues: reports of fetal malformation; greater risk to fetus if medication is discontinued during pregnancy<br><br>Lactation Issues: women should not nurse |

| | | | |
|---|---|---|---|
| | | **decreased levels and/or effects of:** amiodarone, acetaminophen (leads to inc risk of hepatotoxicity), carbamazepine, digoxin, corticosteroids, disopyramide, doxycycline, estrogens & oral contraceptives, haloperidol, mexiletine, quinidine, theophylline, valproic acid, cyclosporine, furosemide, levodopa, phenothiazines, sulfonylureas <br><br> **increased effect (toxicity) of:** lithium, meperidine, primidone, warfarin <br><br> Drug–Food Interaction: **decreased effect of hydantoin:** enteral feedings | Contraindications: hypersensitivity <br><br> Precautions: abrupt withdrawal of medication may precipitate status epilepticus; some patients are genetically predisposed to slowed metabolism, monitor carefully; use cautiously in patients with hepatic dysfunction <br><br> Pregnancy Issues: reports of fetal malformation; greater risk to fetus if medication is discontinued during pregnancy <br><br> Lactation Issues: women should not nurse |
| **Mephenytoin** <br> Mesantoin <br><br> Tablets: 100 mg | **Tonic/Clonic or psychomotor (refractory to other agents); focal: Jacksonian:** 50–100 mg/d, initially. Titrate each week by 50 or 100 mg/d to a range of 200–600 mg/d. <br><br> **Pediatrics:** initiate therapy as above. Titrate to range of 100–400 mg/d | Administration Issues: May take with food to avoid GI upset. Draw serum levels just prior to next dose. Maintain good oral hygiene. When replacing another anticonvulsant, slowly titrate this agent, while decreasing the other agent. <br><br> Drug–Drug Interactions: **increased levels and/or effects of hydantoin:** allopurinol, amiodarone, benzodiazepines, cimetidine, ethanol (acute), fluconazole, isoniazid, metronidazole, miconazole, omeprazole, sulfonamides & trimethoprim, valproic acid, TCAs, salicylates, chlorpheniramine, ibuprofen, phenothiazines | ADRs: nystagmus, ataxia, confusion, slurred speech, fatigue, drowsiness, tremor, headache, nervousness, diplopia, irritability, nausea, vomiting, diarrhea, constipation, thrombocytopenia, leukopenia, granulocytopenia, anemias, gingival hyperplasia, hepatitis, dermatologic reactions, osteomalacia <br><br> Overdose: far-lateral nystagmus (>20 mcg/mL), ataxia (>30 mcg/mL), dysarthria, decreased level of consciousness (>40 mcg/mL). |

(continues on next page)

| Drug and Dosage Forms | Usual Dosage Range | Administration Issues and Drug–Drug & Drug–Food Interactions | Common Adverse Drug Reactions (ADRs) and Pharmacokinetics | Contraindications, Pregnancy Category, and Lactation Issues |
|---|---|---|---|---|
| **Mephenytoin** *cont.* | | **decreased levels and/or effects of hydantoin:** barbiturates, carbamazepine, ethanol (chronic), rifampin, theophylline, antacids, sucralfate, charcoal, antineoplastics, folic acid, loxapine, pyridoxine, nitrofurantoin, influenza virus vaccine<br><br>**decreased levels and/or effects of:** amiodarone, acetaminophen (inc risk of hepatotoxicity), carbamazepine, digoxin, corticosteroids, disopyramide, doxycycline, estrogens & oral contraceptives, haloperidol, mexiletine, quinidine, theophylline, valproic acid, cyclosporine, furosemide, levodopa, phenothiazines, sulfonylureas<br><br>**increased effect (toxicity) of:** lithium, meperidine, primidone, warfarin<br><br>Drug–Food Interaction:<br>**decreased effect of hydantoin:** enteral feedings | Pharmacokinetics:<br>absorption varies depending on formulation; saturable hepatic metabolism to inactive metabolites; $T_{1/2}$ = 6–24 hrs when level is <10 mcg/mL.<br><br>**Therapeutic plasma levels = 10–20 mcg/mL; at these levels, time to eliminate 50% of the drug is extended (20–60 hrs)** | |
| **Phenytoin**<br>Dilantin, Diphenylan, various generics | **Tonic/Clonic or psychomotor:** 100 mg tid initially. Titrate 100 mg/week as needed (some need 600 mg/d) | Administration Issues: May take with food to avoid GI upset. Draw serum levels just prior to next dose. Maintain | ADRs:<br>nystagmus, ataxia, confusion, slurred speech, fatigue, | Contraindications:<br>hypersensitivity; sinus bradycardia; second/third |

degree AV block; Adams–Stokes syndrome

**Precautions:** abrupt withdrawal of medication may precipitate status epilepticus; some patients are genetically predisposed to slowed metabolism, monitor carefully; use cautiously in patients with hepatic dysfunction, hypotension, or severe myocardial insufficiency

**Pregnancy Issues:** reports of fetal malformation; greater risk to fetus if medication is discontinued during pregnancy

**Lactation Issues:** women should not nurse

drowsiness, tremor, headache, nervousness, diplopia, irritability, nausea, vomiting, diarrhea, constipation, thrombocytopenia, leukopenia, granulocytopenia, anemias, gingival hyperplasia, hepatitis, dermatologic reactions, osteomalacia

Overdose: far-lateral nystagmus (>20 mcg/mL), ataxia (>30 mcg/mL), dysarthria, decreased level of consciousness (>40 mcg/mL).

Pharmacokinetics: absorption varies depending on formulation; saturable hepatic metabolism to inactive metabolites; $T_{1/2}$ = 6–24 hrs when level is <10 mcg/mL.

**Therapeutic plasma levels = 10–20 mcg/mL; at these levels, time to eliminate 50% of the drug is extended (20–60 hrs)**

good oral hygiene. When replacing another anticonvulsant, slowly titrate this agent, while decreasing the other agent. **Due to bioequivalence differences, brand interchange is not recommended**

Drug–Drug Interactions:
**increased levels and/or effects of hydantoin:** allopurinol, amiodarone, benzodiazepines, cimetidine, ethanol (acute), fluconazole, isoniazid, metronidazole, miconazole, omeprazole, sulfonamides & trimethoprim, valproic acid, TCAs, salicylates, chlorpheniramine, ibuprofen, phenothiazines

**decreased levels and/or effects of hydantoin:** barbiturates, carbamazepine, ethanol (chronic), rifampin, theophylline, antacids, sucralfate, charcoal, antineoplastics, folic acid, loxapine, pyridoxine, nitrofurantoin, influenza virus vaccine

**decreased levels and/or effects of:** amiodarone, acetaminophen (leads to inc risk of hepatotoxicity), carbamazepine, digoxin, corticosteroids, disopyramide, doxycycline, estrogens & oral contraceptives, haloperidol, mexiletine, quinidine, theophylline, valproic acid, cyclosporine, furosemide, levodopa, phenothiazines, sulfonylureas
**increased effect (toxicity) of:** lithium, meperidine, primidone, warfarin

Drug–Food Interaction:
**decreased effect of hydantoin:** enteral feedings

**Phenytoin:**
Chewable tablets: 50 mg

Suspension: 30 mg/5 mL, 125 mg/5 mL

**Phenytoin Sodium:**
Capsules: 30 mg (27.6 mg phenytoin), 100 mg (92 mg phenytoin)

Extended-release Capsules: 30 mg (27.6 mg phenytoin), 100 mg (92 mg phenytoin)

**Phenytoin Sodium with Phenobarbital:**
Capsules: 100 mg/16 mg (respectively), 100 mg/32 mg (respectively)

**Pediatrics:** 5 mg/kg/d in 2–3 divided doses. Titrate to max of 300 mg/d as needed

Single daily dose: once the patient is controlled on 100 mg tid, 300 mg may be given as a single dose (must use extended-release capsules).

**Unlabeled Use:** trigeminal neuralgia (tic douloureux)

**Traumatic Brain Injury**
100–600 mg qd

**308.4 Oxazolidinediones**

| Drug and Dosage Forms | Usual Dosage Range | Administration Issues and Drug–Drug & Drug–Food Interactions | Common Adverse Drug Reactions (ADRs) and Pharmacokinetics | Contraindications, Pregnancy Category, and Lactation Issues |
|---|---|---|---|---|
| **Paramethadione**<br>Paradione<br><br>Capsules: 150 mg, 300 mg | **Absence:**<br>300 mg tid initially. Titrate by 300 mg/d each week as needed to range of 900–2400 mg/d<br><br>**Pediatrics:** 300–900 mg/d in 3–4 divided doses | Administration Issues:<br>When replacing another anticonvulsant, slowly titrate this agent, while decreasing the other agent. May take with food to decrease GI upset<br><br>Drug–Drug Interactions:<br>None known | ADRs:<br>drowsiness, headache, irritability, myasthenia-like syndrome, personality changes, nausea, vomiting, anorexia, rash, erythema multiforme, exfoliative dermatitis, photosensitivity, aplastic anemia, pancytopenia, hypoplastic anemia, proteinuria, hepatitis, lupus erythematosus<br><br>Pharmacokinetics:<br>hepatically metabolized to active metabolite (renal elimination of metabolite; $T_{1/2}$ = 16–24 hrs | Contraindications:<br>Hypersensitivity<br><br>Precautions: Use cautiously in patients with hepatic or renal dysfunction, acute intermittent porphyria.<br><br>Pregnancy Category: D.<br><br>Lactation Issues: women should not nurse |
| **Trimethadione**<br>Tridione<br><br>Chewable tablets:<br>150 mg<br><br>Capsules: 300 mg<br><br>Solution: 40 mg/mL | **Absence:**<br>300 mg tid initially. Titrate by 300 mg/d each week as needed to range of 900–2400 mg/d<br><br>**Pediatrics:** 300–900 mg/d in 3–4 divided doses | Administration Issues:<br>When replacing another anticonvulsant, slowly titrate this agent, while decreasing the other agent. May take with food to decrease GI upset<br><br>Drug–Drug Interactions:<br>None known | ADRs:<br>drowsiness, headache, irritability, myasthenia-like syndrome, personality changes, nausea, vomiting, anorexia, rash, erythema multiforme, exfoliative dermatitis, photosensitivity, aplastic anemia, pancytopenia, hypoplastic anemia, proteinuria, hepatitis, lupus erythematosus<br><br>Pharmacokinetics:<br>renal elimination of metabolite; $T_{1/2}$ = 16–24 hrs | Contraindications:<br>Hypersensitivity<br><br>Precautions: Use cautiously in patients with hepatic or renal dysfunction, acute intermittent porphyria.<br><br>Pregnancy Issues: reports of fetal malformation; greater risk to fetus if medication is discontinued during pregnancy<br><br>Lactation Issues: women should not nurse |

## 308.5 Succinimides

| Drug and Dosage Forms | Usual Dosage Range | Administration Issues and Drug–Drug & Drug–Food Interactions | Common Adverse Drug Reactions (ADRs) and Pharmacokinetics | Contraindications, Pregnancy Category, and Lactation Issues |
|---|---|---|---|---|
| **Ethosuximide**<br>Zarontin<br><br>Capsules: 250 mg<br><br>Syrup: 250 mg/5 mL | **Absence:**<br><br>**Adults/pediatrics** (>6 yrs): 500 mg/d, initially. Titrate by 250 mg/d every 4–7 days as needed. Doses >1.5 g/d require strict supervision<br><br>**Pediatrics** (3–6 yrs): 250 mg/d initially. Titrate as above. | Administration Issues:<br>When replacing another anticonvulsant, slowly titrate this agent, while decreasing the other agent. May take with food to decrease GI upset<br><br>Drug–Drug Interactions:<br>**increased levels of:** hydantoins<br><br>**decreased levels of:** barbiturates, primidone<br><br>**increased & decreased levels (both) of:** valproic acid | ADRs:<br>drowsiness, ataxia, dizziness, confusion, nervousness, other psychological changes, nausea, vomiting, cramps, anorexia, diarrhea, weight loss, abdominal pain, constipation, eosinophilia, granulocytopenia, leukopenia, agranulocytosis (monitor blood counts during therapy), rash, gum hypertrophy<br><br>Pharmacokinetics:<br>extensively metabolized; $T_{1/2}$ = 2.6–4 h<br><br>**Therapeutic serum levels = 40–100 mcg/mL** | Contraindications:<br>hypersensitivity<br><br>Precautions: use cautiously in patients with renal or hepatic dysfunction (monitor renal and hepatic function); if used alone in mixed epilepsy—may increase frequency of grand mal seizures<br><br>Pregnancy Issues: reports of fetal malformation; greater risk to fetus if medication is discontinued during pregnancy<br><br>Lactation Issues: women should not nurse |
| **Methsuximide**<br>Celontin Kapseals<br><br>Capsules: 150 mg, 300 mg | **Absence (refractory to other agents):**<br>300 mg/d initially. Titrate by 300 mg/d each week as needed to max of 1.2 g/d<br><br>**Pediatrics:** 150 mg/d initially. Titrate as above. | Administration Issues:<br>When replacing another anticonvulsant, slowly titrate this agent, while decreasing the other agent. May take with food to decrease GI upset<br><br>Drug–Drug Interactions:<br>**increased levels of:** hydantoins | ADRs:<br>drowsiness, ataxia, dizziness, confusion, nervousness, other psychological changes, nausea, vomiting, cramps, anorexia, diarrhea, weight loss, abdominal pain, constipation, eosinophilia, granulocytopenia, leukopenia, agranulocytosis (monitor | Contraindications:<br>hypersensitivity<br><br>Precautions: use cautiously in patients with renal or hepatic dysfunction (monitor renal and hepatic function); if used alone in mixed epilepsy—may increase frequency of grand mal seizures |

*(continues on next page)*

| Drug and Dosage Forms | Usual Dosage Range | Administration Issues and Drug–Drug & Drug–Food Interactions | Common Adverse Drug Reactions (ADRs) and Pharmacokinetics | Contraindications, Pregnancy Category, and Lactation Issues |
|---|---|---|---|---|
| **Methsuximide *cont.*** | | **decreased levels of:** barbiturates, primidone<br><br>**increased & decreased levels (both) of:** valproic acid | blood counts during therapy), rash, gum hypertrophy<br><br>Pharmacokinetics:<br>extensively metabolized;<br>$T_{1/2} = 2.6$–4 h | Pregnancy Issues: reports of fetal malformation; greater risk to fetus if medication is discontinued during pregnancy<br><br>Lactation Issues: women should not nurse |
| **Phensuximide**<br>Milontin Kapseals<br><br>Capsules: 500 mg | **Absence:**<br>500–1000 mg 2–3 times daily, initially. Titrate by 500 mg/d every few days to range of 1–3 g/d | Administration Issues:<br>When replacing another anticonvulsant, slowly titrate this agent, while decreasing the other agent. May take with food to decrease GI upset May change urine color to pink, red, or red-brown (not harmful)<br><br>Drug–Drug Interactions:<br>**increased levels of:** hydantoins<br><br>**decreased levels of:** barbiturates, primidone<br><br>**increased and decreased levels (both) of:** valproic acid | ADRs:<br>drowsiness, ataxia, dizziness, confusion, nervousness, other psychological changes, nausea, vomiting, cramps, anorexia, diarrhea, weight loss, abdominal pain, constipation, eosinophilia, granulocytopenia, leukopenia, agranulocytosis (monitor blood counts during therapy), rash, gum hypertrophy<br><br>Pharmacokinetics:<br>$T_{1/2} = 4$ hrs; renal and bile elimination of drug unchanged | Contraindications:<br>hypersensitivity<br><br>Precautions: use cautiously in patients with renal or hepatic dysfunction (monitor renal and hepatic function); if used alone in mixed epilepsy—may increase frequency of grand mal seizures; use cautiously in patients with acute intermittent porphyria<br><br>Pregnancy Issues: reports of fetal malformation; greater risk to fetus if medication is discontinued during pregnancy<br><br>Lactation Issues: women should not nurse |

| Drug and Dosage Forms | Usual Dosage Range | Administration Issues and Drug–Drug & Drug–Food Interactions | Common Adverse Drug Reactions (ADRs) and Pharmacokinetics | Contraindications, Pregnancy Category, and Lactation Issues |
|---|---|---|---|---|
| **Acetazolamide**<br>Diamox, AK-Zol, various generics<br><br>Tablets: 125 mg, 250 mg | **Centraencephalic petit mal, unlocalized seizures:**<br>8–30 mg/kg/d in 2 divided doses (range: 375–1000 mg/d) | Administration Issues:<br>When replacing another anticonvulsant, slowly titrate this agent, while decreasing the other agent. Do not use sustained-release product<br><br>Drug–Drug Interactions:<br>**increased levels/effects of:**<br>cyclosporine, salicylates<br><br>**increased levels/effects of acetazolamide:**<br>salicylates, diflunisal<br><br>**decreased levels/effects of:**<br>primidone | ADRs:<br>anorexia, nausea, vomiting, constipation, melena, diarrhea, hematuria, glycosuria, urinary frequency, renal colic, renal calculi, polyuria, weakness, malaise, fatigue, nervousness, drowsiness, ataxia, disorientation, rash (including Stevens Johnson Syndrome), urticaria, pruritus, photosensitivity, bone marrow suppression, thrombocytopenia, hemolytic anemia, thrombocytopenic purpura, weight loss, fever, acidosis, decreased libido, impotence, electrolyte imbalance, hepatic insufficiency<br><br>Pharmacokinetics<br>peak effect 1–4 hrs; duration 8–12 hrs | Contraindications:<br>hypersensitivity to sulfonamides;<br>↓ sodium/potassium levels; severe renal or hepatic dysfunction.<br><br>Pregnancy Issues:<br>reports of fetal malformation; greater risk to fetus if medication is discontinued during pregnancy<br><br>Lactation Issues: women should not nurse |
| **Carbamazepine**<br>Tegretol, Atretol, Epitol, Depitol, various generics | **Tonic/Clonic, mixed, psychomotor:**<br>200 mg bid initially. Titrate by 200 mg/d each week (use 3–4 times daily regimen) up to 1200 mg/d (>15 yrs old), or 1000 mg/d (12–15 yrs) | Administration Issues: When replacing another anticonvulsant, slowly titrate this agent, while decreasing the other agent, safety/efficacy not established in those <6 yrs old | ADRs:<br>dizziness, drowsiness, unsteadiness, nausea, vomiting, aplastic anemia, leukopenia, agranulocytosis, | Contraindications:<br>Hypersensitivity to this or TCAs, history of bone marrow suppression, concomitant use of MAO inhibitors |

(continues on next page)

| Drug and Dosage Forms | Usual Dosage Range | Administration Issues and Drug–Drug & Drug–Food Interactions | Common Adverse Drug Reactions (ADRs) and Pharmacokinetics | Contraindications, Pregnancy Category, and Lactation Issues |
|---|---|---|---|---|
| **Carbamazepine** *cont.*<br><br>Tablets, chewable:<br>100 mg<br><br>Tablets: 200 mg<br><br>Suspension:<br>100 mg/5 mL | **Pediatrics** (6–12 yrs): 100 mg twice daily, initially. Titrate by 100 mg/d each week (use 3–4 times daily regimen) up to 1000 mg/d or 20–30 mg/kg/d<br><br>**Trigeminal neuralgia:** 100 mg twice daily, initially. Titrate by 200 mg/d as needed.<br><br>**Suspension:** daily dose (including initial dose) is given in 4 divided doses.<br><br>**Unlabeled uses:**<br>bipolar disorder, unipolar depression, schizoaffective illness, alcohol or cocaine or benzodiazepine withdrawal, restless leg syndrome<br><br>**Traumatic Brain Injury**<br>Initially, 200 mg bid titrate up to 2 gm/d as needed for seizures | Drug–Drug Interactions:<br>**decreased levels/effects of:** TCAs, felbamate, valproic acid, anticoagulants, oral contraceptives, haloperidol, succinimides<br><br>**decreased levels/effects of carbamazepine:** theophylline, hydantoins, barbiturates, charcoal<br><br>**increased levels/effects of:** theophylline (possibly)<br><br>**increased levels/effects of carbamazepine:** cimetidine, diltiazem, isoniazid, macrolides (not azithromycin), propoxyphene, verapamil, terfenadine, fluoxetine, fluvoxamine, valproic acid | other hematologic effects, abnormal LFTs, hepatitis, rash, Stevens-Johnson syndrome, SIADH, congestive heart failure, hypotension, arrhythmias<br><br>Pharmacokinetics:<br>76% protein bound; hepatically metabolized to carbamazepine epoxide; $T_{1/2}$ = 12–17 hrs (after continued dosing); renal elimination of metabolites<br><br>**Therapeutic plasma concentrations = 4–12 mcg/mL** | Precautions: closely monitor CBC and LFTs; use cautiously in patients with cardiac, hepatic, or renal dysfunction<br><br>Pregnancy Issues:<br>reports of fetal malformation; greater risk to fetus if medication is discontinued during pregnancy<br><br>Lactation Issues: women should not nurse |
| **Felbamate**<br>Felbatol<br><br>Tablets: 400 mg, 600 mg<br><br>Suspension:<br>600 mg/5 mL | **Partial with/without secondary generalization or Lennox-Gastaut syndrome:** (>14 yrs old):<br><br>Monotherapy: 1200 mg/d in 3–4 divided doses. Titrate by 600 mg/d q 2 weeks up to 3600 mg/d as needed/tolerated | Administration Issues: Patients should wear protective clothing to prevent photosensitivity. When replacing another anticonvulsant, slowly titrate this agent, while decreasing the other agent. Do not abruptly discontinue this medication. | ADRs:<br>fatigue, headache, somnolence, dizziness, insomnia, nausea, dyspepsia, vomiting, anorexia, aplastic anemia, hepatic failure | Contraindications:<br>Hypersensitivity to this or other carbamates<br><br>Precautions: use cautiously in patients with severe hepatic or renal dysfunction; monitor blood levels of other |

| Drug | Dosing | Drug–Drug Interactions / Administration | Pharmacokinetics / ADRs | Contraindications / Pregnancy / Lactation |
|---|---|---|---|---|
| | Conversion to monotherapy: 1200 mg/d divided tid to qid; reduce current AEDs by 1/3. Titrate felbamate to 2400 mg/d after 1 week; reduce current AEDs by 1/3. Titrate felbamate to 3600 mg/d after 1 week; reduce other AEDs as clinically indicated<br><br>Adjunctive therapy: Follow above directions, except reduce current AEDs by 20% initially, then as clinically indicated.<br><br>Elderly or debilitated patients: Use lower doses and greater dosage intervals; titrate more slowly<br><br>Pediatrics with Lennox-Gastaut Syndrome: (2–14 yrs old) 15 mg/kg/d divided tid to qid. Reduce present antiepileptics by 20%. Titrate felbamate by 15 mg/kg/d q week up to 45 mg/kg/d | Drug–Drug Interactions:<br>increased levels of: phenytoin, valproic acid, carbamazepine epoxide, warfarin<br><br>decreased levels of: carbamazepine<br><br>decreased levels of felbamate: phenytoin, carbamazepine | Pharmacokinetics:<br>22–25% protein bound;<br>$T_{1/2}$ = 20–23 hrs<br><br>Therapeutic plasma levels have not been established<br><br>**BECAUSE OF THE REPORTS OF APLASTIC ANEMIA, THE FDA HAS RECOMMENDED THAT FELBAMATE BE DISCONTINUED IN ALL PATIENTS UNLESS DISCONTINUATION WOULD POSE A SERIOUS THREAT TO THE PATIENT | concomitant anticonvulsants due to drug interactions; monitor closely for signs of aplastic anemia, hepatic failure<br><br>Pregnancy Category: C<br><br>Lactation Issues:<br>felbamate is found in breast milk although effects unknown; women should not nurse |
| **Gabapentin**<br>Neurontin<br><br>Capsules: 100 mg, 300 mg, 400 mg | Add-on therapy for partial seizures with/without secondary generalization: 300 mg day 1, 300 mg twice daily on day 2, 300 mg 3 times daily on day 3. Titrate further by 300–400 mg a day up to 1800 mg/d. Higher doses (2400–3600 mg) have been used and well-tolerated.<br><br>Renal Impairment: CrCl:<br>>60 ml/min: 400 mg TID<br>30–60 ml/min: 300 mg BID | Administration Issues:<br>When replacing another anticonvulsant, slowly titrate this agent, while decreasing the other agent.<br><br>Drug–Drug Interactions:<br>decreased levels of gabapentin: antacids | ADRs<br>somnolence, dizziness, ataxia, fatigue, nystagmus.<br>Other (<1%): leukopenia, anemia, purpura<br><br>Pharmacokinetics:<br>bioavailability is decreased with increasing doses; not protein bound; primarily RENALLY ELIMINATED as unchanged drug; $T_{1/2}$ = 5–7 hrs (prolonged by renal insufficiency) | Contraindications:<br>Hypersensitivity<br><br>Pregnancy Category: C.<br><br>Lactation Issues: women should not nurse<br><br>Pediatrics: safety/efficacy not established in <12 yrs old |

(continues on next page)

| Drug and Dosage Forms | Usual Dosage Range | Administration Issues and Drug–Drug & Drug–Food Interactions | Common Adverse Drug Reactions (ADRs) and Pharmacokinetics | Contraindications, Pregnancy Category, and Lactation Issues |
|---|---|---|---|---|
| **Gabapentin** *cont.* | 15–30 ml/min: 300 mg QD<br><15 ml/min: 300 mg QOD<br>Hemodialysis: 200–300 mg following each hemodialysis session | | Therapeutic plasma levels have not been established | |
| **Lamotrigine**<br>Lamictal<br><br>Tablets: 25 mg, 100 mg, 150 mg, 200 mg | **Adjunctive therapy for partial seizures:**<br>On enzyme inducing anti-epileptics (but not valproate): 50 mg once daily for 2 weeks, then 50 mg twice daily for 2 weeks. Usual maintenance dose is 300–500 mg/d in 2 divided doses<br><br>On valproic acid: 25 mg every other day for 2 weeks, then 25 mg once daily for 2 weeks. Titrate after this to max of 150 mg/d | Administration Issues:<br>When replacing another anticonvulsant, slowly titrate this agent, while decreasing the other agent. Advise patients to wear protective clothing against UV light to prevent photosensitivity reactions, safety/efficacy in <16 yrs old not established<br><br>Drug–Drug Interactions:<br>**decreased levels/effect of lamotrigine:** carbamazepine, phenobarbital, primidone, phenytoin; **increased levels/effect of:** carbamazepine;<br>**increased levels of lamotrigine:** valproic acid; **decreased levels/effect of:** valproic acid | ADRs:<br>somnolence, dizziness, diplopia, ataxia, blurred vision, headache, nausea, vomiting, **rash (severe, potentially life-threatening, including Stevens-Johnson syndrome)**<br><br>Pharmacokinetics:<br>55% protein bound; hepatically metabolized; $T_{1/2}$ = 25–33 hrs (on no other antiepileptics); $T_{1/2}$ = 12–14 hrs (on enzyme inducing antiepileptics); $T_{1/2}$ = 48–70 hrs (on valproic acid) | Contraindications: Hypersensitivity<br><br>Precautions: use cautiously in patients with severe renal or hepatic dysfunction.<br><br>Pregnancy Category: C.<br><br>Lactation Issues: women should not nurse |
| **Phenacemide**<br>Phenurone<br><br>Tablets: 500 mg | **Severe mixed psychomotor:**<br>500 mg tid initially. Titrate by 500 mg/d each week as needed up to 5 g/d. | Administration Issues: When replacing another anticonvulsant, slowly titrate this agent, while decreasing the other agent, safety/efficacy not established in those <5 yrs old. | Therapeutic plasma levels have not been established<br><br>ADRs:<br>nausea, anorexia, drowsiness, headache, nephritis, psychic changes, rash, hepatitis, blood dyscrasias (e.g., fatal aplastic anemia) | Contraindications: hypersensitivity<br><br>Precautions: abrupt withdrawal of medication may precipitate status epilepticus; use |

| | | | | |
|---|---|---|---|---|
| | **Pediatrics** (5–10yrs): 250 mg tid initially. Titrate by 250 mg/d each week as needed | Drug–Drug Interactions: **increased levels/effect of:** hydantoins | Pharmacokinetics: hepatic metabolism | cautiously in patients with hepatic dysfunction<br><br>Pregnancy Category: D.<br><br>Lactation Issues: women should not nurse |
| **Tiagabine**<br>Gabatril<br><br>Filmtabs: 4 mg, 12 mg, 16 mg, 20 mg | **Adjunctive therapy for partial seizures**<br><br>**Adults (>18 years):** Initiate at 4 mg qd; Total daily dose may be increased by 4 to 8 mg at weekly intervals until clinical response or max of 56 mg/d achieved. Give total daily dose in 2 to 4 divided doses<br><br>**Children (12–18 years):**<br>Initiate at 4 mg qd. The total daily dose may be increased by 4 mg at beginning of week 2; thereafter, weekly increases of 4 to 8 mg up to a max of 32 mg/d may be done. Give total daily dose in 2 to 4 divided doses. | Administration Issues:<br>Tiagabine should be taken with food. Tiagabine may cause dizziness or somnolence.<br><br>Drug–Drug Interactions<br>Tiagabine clearance is 60% **greater** when give with valproate, carbamazepine, phenytoin and phenobarbital<br><br>Tiagabine causes a **slight decrease** in valproate concentrations | ADRs<br>dizziness, somnolence, confusion, asthenia, nervousness, tremor, nausea, diarrhea, pharyngitis, rash<br><br>Pharmacokinetics:<br>$T_{1/2}$ = 7–9 hr; hepatic metabolism | Contraindications:<br>hypersensitivity<br><br>Precautions: abrupt withdrawal of medication may precipitate status epilepticus<br><br>Pregnancy Category: C<br><br>Lactation Issues:<br>Tiagabine is excreted in breast milk; use cautiously |
| **Topiramate**<br>Topamax<br><br>Tablets:<br>25 mg, 100 mg, 200 mg | **Adjunctive therapy for partial seizures in adults:**<br>Recommended dose is 200 mg bid; use the following titration schedule:<br><br>Week  AM dose  PM dose<br>1   none     50 mg<br>2   50 mg    50 mg<br>3   50 mg    100 mg<br>4   100 mg   100 mg | Administration Issues:<br>Do not break tablets; can be taken without regards to meals; safety/efficacy in children not established<br><br>Drug–Drug Interactions:<br>topiramate may **increase** phenytoin concentrations and may **increase** the CNS effect of alcohol/ CNS depressants; | ADRs<br>asthenia, back pain, chest pain, ataxia, somnolence, dizziness, psychomotor slowing, speech disorders, nervousness, nystagmus, paresthesia, depression, rash, nausea, breast pain, dysmenorrhea, diplopia, weight decrease, fatigue | Contraindications:<br>Hypersensitivity<br><br>Pregnancy Category: C.<br><br>Lactation Issues: it is not known if topiramate is excreted in breast milk |

(continues on next page)

| Drug and Dosage Forms | Usual Dosage Range | Administration Issues and Drug–Drug & Drug–Food Interactions | Common Adverse Drug Reactions (ADRs) and Pharmacokinetics | Contraindications, Pregnancy Category, and Lactation Issues |
|---|---|---|---|---|
| **Topiramate** *cont.* | 5   100 mg   150 mg<br>6   150 mg   150 mg<br>7   150 mg   200 mg<br>8   200 mg   200 mg | **decreased levels/effects of topiramate** may occur with phenytoin, carbamazepine, valproic acid; topiramate may **decrease effectiveness** of oral contraceptives and digoxin; avoid use with carbonic anhydrase inhibitors | Pharmacokinetics:<br>$T_{1/2}$ = 18–27 hr; decrease dose for moderate to severe renal impairment | |
| **Valproic Acid**<br>Depakene, various generics<br><br>Capsules: 250 mg<br><br>Syrup: 250 mg/5 mL (sodium valproate)<br><br>**Divalproex Sodium**<br>Depakote<br><br>Tablets, delayed release: 125 mg, 250 mg, 500 mg<br><br>Capsules, sprinkle: 125 mg | **Absence:** 15 mg/kg/d. Titrate by 5–10 mg/kg/d as needed/tolerated to max of 60 mg/kg/d. Doses >250 mg should be divided.<br><br>**Mania (Bipolar Disorder):** 750 mg in divided doses. Titrate as needed/tolerated to max of 60 mg/kg/d<br><br>**Elderly or debilitated patients (hepatic/renal dysfunction):** Use lower initial doses and greater dosing intervals. Titrate to higher doses as needed/tolerated<br><br>**Prophylaxis of migraine headache:** 250 mg bid. Some patients may benefit from doses up to 1000 mg/d<br><br>**Traumatic Brain Injury**<br>250–500 mg tid to qid | Administration Issues:<br>When replacing another anticonvulsant, slowly titrate this agent, while decreasing the other agent. May take with food to decrease GI upset.<br>Do not chew tablets or capsules; May sprinkle contents of capsule on soft food. May take dose (<250 mg/d) at bedtime to minimize daytime sedation<br><br>Drug–Drug Interactions:<br>**increased levels/effects of valproic acid:** cimetidine, felbamate, chlorpromazine, salicylates<br><br>**increased levels/effects of:** zidovudine, warfarin, phenobarbital, primidone, lamotrigine, ethosuximide, clozapine, phenytoin, benzodiazepines, alcohol, other CNS depressants<br><br>**decreased levels/effects of valproic acid:** charcoal, rifampin, | ADRs:<br>nausea, vomiting, indigestion, diarrhea, anorexia, sedation, tremor, ataxia, headache, nystagmus, diplopia, dizziness, incoordination, depression, aggression, psychosis, hyperactivity, rash, photosensitivity, transient hair loss, Stevens-Johnson syndrome, thrombocytopenia, leukopenia, anemia, bone marrow suppression, acute intermittent porphyria, increased LFTs, hepatotoxicity, irregular menses, breast enlargement, abnormal thyroid function tests, hyperammonemia, hyponatremia, SIADH, pancreatitis, lupus erythematosus, fever, hearing loss | Contraindications:<br>Hypersensitivity; severe hepatic dysfunction<br><br>Precautions:<br>monitor closely for hepatotoxicity, thrombocytopenia. Use cautiously in patients with severe hepatic/renal dysfunction<br><br>Pregnancy Category: D<br><br>Lactation Issues: women should not nurse |

carbamazepine, clonazepam, lamotrigine, phenytoin

**decreased levels/effects of:**
ethosuximide

Pharmacokinetics:
equivalent doses of divalproex sodium and valproic acid deliver equivalent quantities of valproate ion; 90% protein bound; hepatically metabolized; $T_{1/2}$ = 9–16 hrs (up to 18 hrs in patients with cirrhosis; 10–67 hrs for children <10 days old)

**Therapeutic plasma concentrations = 50–100 mcg/mL**

## 309. Anxiolytics
### 309.1 Benzodiazepines

| Drug and Dosage Forms | Usual Dosage Range | Administration Issues and Drug–Drug & Drug–Food Interactions | Common Adverse Drug Reactions (ADRs) and Pharmacokinetics | Contraindications, Pregnancy Category, and Lactation Issues |
|---|---|---|---|---|
| **Alprazolam (CIV)**<br>Xanax<br><br>Tablets: 0.25 mg, 0.5 mg, 1 mg, 2 mg | **Anxiety disorders:** starting dose of 0.25–0.5 mg tid. Slowly titrate up to maximum of 4 mg/d<br><br>**Elderly patients:** starting dose of 0.25 mg 2–3 times daily.<br><br>**Panic disorder with or without agoraphobia:** Initially 0.5 mg tid. Titrate by ≤1mg/d q 3–4 days up to 10 mg/d if needed | Administration Issues:<br>Safety/efficacy in children <18 yrs old not established<br><br>Drug–Drug Interactions:<br>**increased level of BZ:** cimetidine, oral contraceptives, disulfiram, fluoxetine, isoniazid, ketoconazole, metoprolol, propoxyphene, propranolol, valproic acid.<br><br>**increased CNS effects:** alcohol, barbiturates, narcotics | ADRs:<br>drowsiness, ataxia, confusion<br><br>Dependence: prolonged use can lead to dependence; abrupt discontinuation can precipitate withdrawal symptoms (e.g., anxiety, flu-like illness, concentration difficulties, fatigue, anorexia, restlessness, confusion, psychosis, paranoid delusions, grand mal | Contraindications:<br>Hypersensitivity, psychoses, acute narrow-angle glaucoma<br><br>Pregnancy Category: D<br><br>Lactation Issues: excreted in breast milk—do not give to nursing mothers |

(continues on next page)

| Drug and Dosage Forms | Usual Dosage Range | Administration Issues and Drug–Drug & Drug–Food Interactions | Common Adverse Drug Reactions (ADRs) and Pharmacokinetics | Contraindications, Pregnancy Category, and Lactation Issues |
|---|---|---|---|---|
| **Alprazolam (CIV)** *cont.* | **Elderly patients:** starting dose of 0.25 mg 2–3 times daily.<br><br>**Unlabeled uses:** agoraphobia & social phobia (2–8 mg/d), depression (0.25–3 mg/d), premenstrual syndrome (0.25–3 mg/d). | **increased levels of:** digoxin, phenytoin (possibly)<br><br>**decreased level or effect of BZ:** rifampin (decreased level); theophylline (decreased effect) | seizures). Withdrawal can occur after as little as 4–6 weeks of therapy.<br><br>Drug Discontinuation: Slow taper by 0.5 mg/d at most every 3 days or as tolerated. May take weeks or months to fully discontinue drug<br><br>Pharmacokinetics:<br>$T_{1/2}$ = 12–15 hrs; renal elimination | |
| **Chlordiazepoxide (CIV)**<br>Librium, Mitran, Reposans-10, Libritabs, various generics<br><br>Capsules: 5 mg, 10 mg, 25 mg<br><br>Tablets: 5 mg, 10 mg, 25 mg | **Anxiety Disorders:** Oral:<br>Mild/moderate: 5 or 10 mg tid to qid<br>Severe: 20 or 25 mg 3–4 times daily<br>Elderly patients: 5 mg 2–4 times daily<br>Children (>6 yrs old): 5 mg 2–4 times daily or 0.5 mg/kg/d q 6–8 hours<br><br>**Acute Alcohol Withdrawal Syndrome:**<br>50–100 mg followed by repeated doses as needed (up to 300 mg/d). Reduce to maintenance dose as soon as possible. | Administration Issues:<br>Not recommended for children <6 yrs old<br><br>Drug–Drug Interactions:<br><br>**increased level of BZ:** cimetidine, oral contraceptives, disulfiram, fluoxetine, isoniazid, ketoconazole, metoprolol, propoxyphene, propranolol, valproic acid.<br><br>**increased CNS effects:** alcohol, barbiturates, narcotics<br><br>**increased levels of:** digoxin, phenytoin (possibly) | ADRs:<br>drowsiness, ataxia, confusion<br><br>Dependence: prolonged use can lead to dependence; abrupt discontinuation can precipitate withdrawal symptoms (e.g., anxiety, flu-like illness, concentration difficulties, fatigue, anorexia, restlessness, confusion, psychosis, paranoid delusions, grand mal seizures). Withdrawal can occur after as little as 4–6 weeks of therapy. | Contraindications:<br>Hypersensitivity, psychoses, acute narrow-angle glaucoma<br><br>Pregnancy Category: D<br><br>Lactation Issues: excreted in breast milk—do not give to nursing mothers |

| Drug | Dosage | Administration Issues / Drug-Drug Interactions | Pharmacokinetics / Discontinuation | Contraindications / Pregnancy |
|---|---|---|---|---|
| | Elderly patients: 25–50 mg initially.<br><br>Unlabeled uses: Also used for irritable bowel syndrome | decreased level or effect of BZ: rifampin (decreased level); theophylline (decreased effect) | Drug Discontinuation: gradual decrease over 4–8 weeks<br><br>Pharmacokinetics: $T_{1/2}$ = 5–30 hrs; renal elimination | Contraindications: Hypersensitivity, psychoses, acute narrow-angle glaucoma, clinical or biochemical evidence of significant liver disease<br><br>Pregnancy Category: none, but avoid in pregnant women<br><br>Lactation Issues: excreted in breast milk—do not give to nursing mothers |
| **Clorazepate dipotassium (CIV)**<br>Tranxene, Tranxene-SD, Tranxene-SD-Half, Gen-Xene, various generics<br><br>Capsules: 3.75 mg, 7.5 mg, 15 mg<br><br>Tablets: 3.75 mg, 7.5 mg, 15 mg<br><br>Tablet, single dose: 11.25 mg, 22.5 mg | **Anxiety disorders:**<br>initially: 15 mg bid; titrate to 60 mg/d if needed<br><br>Elderly patients: 3.75–7.5 mg bid initially; titrate based on response<br><br>**Acute Alcohol Withdrawal:**<br>Day 1: 30 mg followed by 30–60 mg, divided<br>Day 2: 45–90 mg, divided<br>Day 3: 22.5–45 mg, divided<br>Day 4: 15–30 mg, divided<br>Then reduce dose to 7.5–15 mg daily; discontinue drug when patient stable<br><br>Unlabeled uses: also used in irritable bowel syndrome | Administration Issues: May give daily dose at bedtime; not recommended for children <9 yrs old<br><br>Drug–Drug Interactions:<br>increased level of BZ: cimetidine, oral contraceptives, disulfiram, fluoxetine, isoniazid, ketoconazole, metoprolol, propoxyphene, propranolol, valproic acid.<br><br>increased CNS effects: alcohol, barbiturates, narcotics<br><br>increased levels of: digoxin, phenytoin (possibly)<br><br>decreased level or effect of BZ: rifampin (decreased level); theophylline (decreased effect) | ADRs: drowsiness, ataxia, confusion<br><br>Dependence: prolonged use can lead to dependence; abrupt discontinuation can precipitate withdrawal symptoms (e.g., anxiety, flu-like illness, concentration difficulties, fatigue, anorexia, restlessness, confusion, psychosis, paranoid delusions, grand mal seizures). Withdrawal can occur after as little as 4–6 weeks of therapy.<br><br>Drug Discontinuation: gradual decrease over 4–8 weeks<br><br>Pharmacokinetics: $T_{1/2}$ = 30–100 hrs; renal elimination | |
| **Diazepam (CIV)**<br>Valium, Valrelease, Zetran, various generics<br><br>Tablets: 2 mg, 5 mg, 10 mg<br><br>Capsule sustained release: 15 mg | **Anxiety disorders or short-term relief of anxiety symptoms:**<br>2–10 mg 2–4 times daily (individualize dose);<br>15–30 mg/d of sustained release product | Administration Issues: Do not crush or chew sustained release products. Concentrated solution (5 mg/mL) should be diluted in liquid or semi-solid foods, not recommended for children <6 mos old. | ADRs: drowsiness, ataxia, confusion<br><br>Dependence: prolonged use can lead to dependence; abrupt discontinuation can precipitate withdrawal symptoms (e.g., anxiety, flu-like illness, | Contraindications: Hypersensitivity, psychoses, acute narrow-angle glaucoma<br><br>Pregnancy Category: D |

(continues on next page)

| Drug and Dosage Forms | Usual Dosage Range | Administration Issues and Drug–Drug & Drug–Food Interactions | Common Adverse Drug Reactions (ADRs) and Pharmacokinetics | Contraindications, Pregnancy Category, and Lactation Issues |
|---|---|---|---|---|
| **Diazepam (CIV)** *cont.*<br><br>Oral Solution:<br>5 mg/5 mL, 5 mg/mL | **Acute Alcohol Withdrawal:** 10 mg 3–4 times during first 24 hours, decrease to 5 mg 3–4 times daily prn<br><br>**Muscle Relaxant:** 2–10 mg tid to qid<br><br>**Elderly or debilitated patients:** 2–2.5 mg 1–2 times daily initially. Titrate slowly to avoid adverse effects<br><br>**Pediatrics:** 1–2.5 mg tid to qid initially. Titrate slowly prn. As a muscle relaxant: 0.12–0.8 mg/kg/d divided in 3–4 doses.<br><br>**Unlabeled uses:** panic attacks, irritable bowel syndrome. | Drug Interactions<br>**increased level of BZ:** cimetidine, oral contraceptives, disulfiram, fluoxetine, isoniazid, ketoconazole, metoprolol, propoxyphene, propranolol, valproic acid.<br><br>**increased CNS effects:** alcohol, barbiturates, narcotics<br><br>**increased levels of:** digoxin, phenytoin (possibly)<br><br>**decreased level or effect of BZ:** rifampin (decreased level); theophylline (decreased effect) | concentration difficulties, fatigue, anorexia, restlessness, confusion, psychosis, paranoid delusions, grand mal seizures). Withdrawal can occur after as little as 4–6 weeks of therapy.<br><br>Drug Discontinuation:<br>gradual decrease over 4–8 weeks<br><br>Pharmacokinetics:<br>$T_{1/2}$ = 20–80 hrs; renal elimination | Lactation Issues: excreted in breast milk—do not give to nursing mothers |
| **Halazepam (CIV)**<br>Paxipam<br><br>Tablets: 20 mg, 40 mg | **Anxiety Disorders:** 20–40 mg 3–4 times daily<br><br>**Elderly patients:** 20 mg 1–2 times daily | Administration Issues: should not be used in children <6 mos old<br><br>Drug Interactions<br>**increased level of BZ:** cimetidine, oral contraceptives, disulfiram, fluoxetine, isoniazid, ketoconazole, metoprolol, propoxyphene, propranolol, valproic acid.<br><br>**increased CNS effects:** alcohol, barbiturates, narcotics | ADRs:<br>drowsiness, ataxia, confusion<br><br>Dependence: prolonged use can lead to dependence; abrupt discontinuation can precipitate withdrawal symptoms (e.g., anxiety, flu-like illness, concentration difficulties, fatigue, anorexia, restlessness, confusion, psychosis, | Contraindications:<br>Hypersensitivity, psychoses, acute narrow-angle glaucoma<br><br>Pregnancy Category: D<br><br>Lactation Issues: excreted in breast milk. Contraindicated in nursing mothers |

| | | | | |
|---|---|---|---|---|
| | | **increased levels of:** digoxin, phenytoin (possibly)<br><br>**decreased level or effect of BZ:** rifampin (decreased level); theophylline (decreased effect) | paranoid delusions, grand mal seizures). Withdrawal can occur after as little as 4–6 weeks of therapy.<br><br>Drug Discontinuation: gradual decrease over 4–8 weeks<br><br>Pharmacokinetics: $T_{1/2}$ = 14 hrs; renal elimination | Contraindications: Hypersensitivity, psychoses, acute narrow-angle glaucoma<br><br>Pregnancy Category: D<br><br>Lactation Issues: excreted in breast milk—do not give to nursing mothers |
| **Lorazepam (CIV)**<br>Ativan, various generics<br><br>Tablets: 0.5 mg, 1 mg, 2 mg | **Anxiety disorders, short-term relief of symptoms of anxiety, or anxiety associated with depressive symptoms:**<br>2–3 mg given 2–3 times daily (dose range is 1–10 mg/d)<br><br>**Elderly or debilitated patients:** 1–2 mg/d in divided doses. Titrate slowly and as needed.<br><br>**Unlabeled uses:** acute alcohol withdrawal syndrome, irritable bowel syndrome. | Administration Issues<br>Safety/efficacy in children <18 yrs old not established<br><br>Drug Interactions<br>**increased level of BZ:** cimetidine, oral contraceptives, disulfiram, fluoxetine, isoniazid, ketoconazole, metoprolol, propoxyphene, propranolol, valproic acid.<br><br>**increased CNS effects:** alcohol, barbiturates, narcotics<br><br>**increased levels of:** digoxin, phenytoin (possibly)<br><br>**decreased level or effect of BZ:** rifampin (decreased level); theophylline (decreased effect) | ADRs:<br>drowsiness, ataxia, confusion<br><br>Dependence: prolonged use can lead to dependence; abrupt discontinuation can precipitate withdrawal symptoms (e.g., anxiety, flu-like illness, concentration difficulties, fatigue, anorexia, restlessness, confusion, psychosis, paranoid delusions, grand mal seizures). Withdrawal can occur after as little as 4–6 weeks of therapy.<br><br>Drug Discontinuation: gradual decrease over 4–8 weeks<br><br>Pharmacokinetics: $T_{1/2}$ = 10–20 hrs; renal elimination | |

| 309.1 Benzodiazepines *continued from previous page* | | | |
|---|---|---|---|
| **Drug and Dosage Forms** | **Usual Dosage Range** | **Administration Issues and Drug–Drug & Drug–Food Interactions** | **Common Adverse Drug Reactions (ADRs) and Pharmacokinetics** | **Contraindications, Pregnancy Category, Lactation Issues** |
| **Oxazepam (CIV)**<br>Serax, various generics<br><br>Capsules: 10 mg, 15 mg, 30 mg<br><br>Tablets: 15 mg | **Anxiety Disorders:**<br>Mild/Moderate: 10–15 mg 3–4 times daily<br>Severe anxiety, agitation or anxiety associated with depression: 15–30 mg 3–4 times daily<br><br>**Alcoholics with acute inebriation, tremulousness or anxiety on withdrawal:** 15 mg 3–4 times daily<br><br>**Anxiety, tension, irritability, and agitation in elderly patients:** 10 mg tid. May increase to 15–30 mg 3–4 times daily if needed—do so cautiously.<br><br>**Unlabeled uses:** Also used for irritable bowel syndrome. | Administration Issues<br>safety/efficacy for <12 yrs old not established<br><br>Drug Interactions<br>**increased level of BZ:** cimetidine, oral contraceptives, disulfiram, fluoxetine, isoniazid, ketoconazole, metoprolol, propoxyphene, propranolol, valproic acid.<br><br>**increased CNS effects:** alcohol, barbiturates, narcotics<br><br>**increased levels of:** digoxin, phenytoin (possibly)<br><br>**decreased level or effect of BZ:** rifampin (decreased level); theophylline (decreased effect) | ADRs:<br>drowsiness, ataxia, confusion (especially in elderly)<br><br>Dependence: prolonged use can lead to dependence; abrupt discontinuation can precipitate withdrawal symptoms (e.g., anxiety, flu-like illness, concentration difficulties, fatigue, anorexia, restlessness, confusion, psychosis, paranoid delusions, grand mal seizures). Withdrawal can occur after as little as 4–6 weeks of therapy.<br><br>Drug Discontinuation:<br>gradual decrease over 4–8 weeks<br><br>Pharmacokinetics:<br>$T_{1/2}$ = 5–20 hrs; renal elimination | Contraindications:<br>Hypersensitivity, psychoses, acute narrow-angle glaucoma<br><br>Pregnancy Category: D<br><br>Lactation Issues: excreted in breast milk—do not give to nursing mothers |
| **Prazepam (CIV)**<br>Centrax<br><br>Capsules: 5 mg, 10 mg, 20 mg<br><br>Tablets: 10 mg | **Anxiety disorders:**<br>initial dose of 10 mg tid. Slowly titrate to 60 mg/d as needed.<br><br>**Elderly patients:** 5 mg 2–3 times daily | Administration Issues: Can give daily dose at bedtime. Start with 20 mg and titrate up as needed, safety/efficacy in children <18 yrs old not established<br><br>Drug Interactions<br>**increased level of BZ:** cimetidine, oral contraceptives, disulfiram, | ADRs:<br>drowsiness, ataxia, confusion<br><br>Dependence: prolonged use can lead to dependence; abrupt discontinuation can precipitate withdrawal symptoms (e.g., anxiety, flu-like illness, | Contraindications:<br>Hypersensitivity, psychoses, acute narrow-angle glaucoma<br><br>Pregnancy Category: D<br><br>Lactation Issues: excreted in breast milk—do not give to nursing mothers |

concentration difficulties, fatigue, anorexia, restlessness, confusion, psychosis, paranoid delusions, grand mal seizures). Withdrawal can occur after as little as 4–6 weeks of therapy.

Drug Discontinuation:
gradual decrease over 4–8 weeks

Pharmacokinetics:
$T_{1/2}$ = 30–100 hrs; renal elimination

fluoxetine, isoniazid, ketoconazole, metoprolol, propoxyphene, propranolol, valproic acid.

**increased CNS effects:** alcohol, barbiturates, narcotics

**increased levels of:** digoxin, phenytoin (possibly)

**decreased level or effect of BZ:** rifampin (decreased level); theophylline (decreased effect)

## 309.2 Miscellaneous Anxiolytics

| Drug and Dosage Forms | Usual Dosage Range | Administration Issues and Drug–Drug Interactions | Common Adverse Drug Reactions (ADRs) and Pharmacokinetics | Contraindications, Pregnancy Category, and Lactation Issues |
|---|---|---|---|---|
| **Buspirone** BuSpar Tablets: 5 mg, 10 mg | **Anxiety disorders or short term relief of symptoms of anxiety.** Initial dose: 5 mg tid. Titrate by 5 mg/d every 2–3 days as needed. Max dose is 60 mg/d Elderly patients: 5 mg bid. Titrate as above, as needed. **Unlabeled use:** 25 mg/d used in decreasing the symptoms of premenstrual syndrome **Traumatic Brain Injury:** 5 mg bid; increase by 5 mg q 5 d up to 45 mg | Drug–Drug Interactions: **increased level of:** haloperidol **Hypertensive crisis:** MAOIs. | ADRs: dizziness, lightheadedness, excitement, drowsiness, nervousness, nausea. headache Pharmacokinetics: 95% protein bound; $T_{1/2}$ = 2–11 hrs; optimal therapeutic effect seen 3–4 weeks. | Contraindications: Hypersensitivity Pregnancy Category: B Lactation Issues: Unknown extent of excretion in breast milk. Use cautiously in nursing mothers Other Precautions: May bind to dopamine receptors, monitor for extrapyramidal symptoms, tardive dyskinesia. |

(continues on next page)

| Drug and Dosage Forms | Usual Dosage Range | Administration Issues and Drug–Drug Interactions | Common Adverse Drug Reactions (ADRs) and Pharmacokinetics | Contraindications, Pregnancy Category, and Lactation Issues |
|---|---|---|---|---|
| **Chlormezanone** Trancopal Caplets <br><br> Tablets: 100 mg, 200 mg | **Mild anxiety and tension states:** 200 mg 3–4 times daily; some patients respond to 100 mg 3–4 times daily <br><br> **Pediatrics** (5–12 yrs): 50–100 mg 3–4 times daily; titrate as needed. | Drug–Drug Interactions: additive CNS effects with alcohol, barbiturates, narcotics, other CNS depressants. | ADRs: drowsiness, depression, excitement, tremor, confusion, nausea, dry mouth, rash, edema, inability to void <br><br> Pharmacokinetics speed of onset: 15–30 minutes; $T_{1/2} = 24$ h | Contraindications: hypersensitivity <br><br> Pregnancy and Lactation Issues: safety not established—use cautiously |
| **Doxepin** Adapin, Sinequan, various generics <br><br> Capsules: 10 mg, 25 mg, 50 mg, 75 mg, 100 mg, 150 mg <br><br> Liquid concentrate: 10 mg/1 mL | **Anxiety:** 75 mg/d at bedtime starting dose. Titrate up to 300 mg/d in 2–3 divided doses. Single dose ≤ 150 mg <br><br> **Elderly patients:** 10–25 mg at bedtime starting dose. Titrate by 10–25 mg every 3–5 days to 75 mg/d. <br><br> **Unlabeled uses:** 50–300 mg/d used for chronic pain (migraine, chronic tension headache, diabetic neuropathy, tic douloureux, cancer pain, peripheral neuropathy with pain, postherpetic neuralgia, arthritic pain) 10–30 mg/d used in chronic urticaria and angioedema, nocturnal pruritis in atopic eczema Also used in peptic ulcer disease. | Administration issues: Maintenance doses may be given once daily at bedtime to reduce daytime sedation. Concentrate: protect from light, dilute in juice or other liquid prior to administration; Not recommended for children <12 yrs old <br><br> Drug–Drug Interactions **Hypertensive crisis:** clonidine, MAO inhibitors; can occur weeks after MAO inhibitor discontinued. <br><br> **increased TCA level:** cimetidine, ethanol, fluoxetine, haloperidol, oral contraceptives, phenothiazines <br><br> **decreased TCA level:** barbiturates, phenytoin, chronic ethanol ingestion | ADRs: dry mouth, urinary retention, blurred vision, constipation, orthostatic hypotension, tachycardia, palpitations, arrhythmias, sedation, seizures, confusion (esp. elderly), hallucinations, anxiety, nervousness, agitation, panic, hypomania, mania, nausea, vomiting, anorexia, constipation or diarrhea, flatulence, abdominal cramps, sexual dysfunction (increased or decreased libido; impotence, painful ejaculation) <br><br> Pharmacokinetics: >90% protein bound, lipid soluble, $T_{1/2} = 8$–24 hrs; time | Contraindications: any hypersensitivity to a TCA, concomitant use of MAO inhibitors, patients with glaucoma or tendency to urinary retention. <br><br> Precautions: use with caution in patients with severe cardiovascular disease, seizure disorders. Patients with schizophrenia may experience worsening psychosis; patients with bipolar disorder may experience a switch to mania. Dosage reductions necessary in patients with hepatic or severe renal dysfunction. |

| | | | | |
|---|---|---|---|---|
| | **increased level of:** phenytoin, warfarin<br><br>**increased effect:** anticholinergic agents, ethanol or sedatives (increased CNS effects), thyroid hormones (increased effect of both drugs)<br><br>**decreased effect of:** guanethidine, methyldopa | to maximal clinical benefit = 2–4 weeks<br><br>**Therapeutic plasma level = 100–200 ng/mL** (plasma levels and therapeutic effect are subject to wide interpatient variability) | | Pregnancy Category: C<br><br>Lactation issues: TCA's are excreted into breast milk. Use with caution in nursing mothers. |
| **Hydroxyzine**<br>Atarax, Anaxinal, Vistaril<br><br>Tablets: 10 mg, 25 mg, 50 mg, 100 mg<br><br>Capsules: 25 mg, 50 mg, 100 mg<br><br>Syrup: 10 mg/5 mL<br><br>Suspension: 25 mg/5 mL | **Symptomatic relief of anxiety/tension associated with psychoneurosis or organic disease states:** 50–100 mg qid<br><br>**Pediatrics (>6 yrs):** 50–100 mg/d in divided doses<br>**Pediatrics (<6 yrs):** 50 mg/d divided<br><br>**Pruritus due to allergic conditions (chronic urticaria, atopic/contact dermatoses, histamine-mediated pruritus):** 25 mg 3–4 times daily<br><br>**Pediatrics (>6 yrs):** 50–100 mg/d in divided doses<br>**Pediatrics (<6 yrs):** 50 mg/d in divided doses<br><br>**Elderly patients:** 10 mg tid to qid | Drug–Drug Interactions:<br>**increased CNS depressant effects:** alcohol, narcotics, barbiturates | ADRs:<br>drowsiness, dry mouth<br><br>Pharmacokinetics:<br>$T_{1/2}$ = 3 hrs; hepatic metabolism | Contraindications:<br>Hypersensitivity<br><br>Pregnancy Category: C<br><br>Lactation Issues: Safety not established—do not use in lactating women |

(continues on next page)

## 309.2 Miscellaneous Anxiolytics *continued from previous page*

| Drug and Dosage Forms | Usual Dosage Range | Administration Issues and Drug–Drug Interactions | Common Adverse Drug Reactions (ADRs) and Pharmacokinetics | Contraindications, Pregnancy Category, and Lactation Issues |
|---|---|---|---|---|
| **Meprobamate (CIV)** Equanil, Miltown, Neuramate, Miltown 600, Meprospan, various generics <br><br> Tablets: 200 mg, 400 mg, 600 mg <br><br> Capsules, sustained release: 200 mg, 400 mg | **Anxiety disorders or short term relief of symptoms of anxiety:** 400 mg 3–4 times daily; max dose is 2400 mg/d (using SR capsules: 400–800 mg twice daily). <br><br> Elderly or pediatric (6–12 yrs) patients: 100–200 mg 2–3 times daily | Administration Issues: Safety/efficacy not established in children <6 years old. <br><br> Drug–Drug Interactions: **increased CNS depressant effects:** alcohol, barbiturates, narcotics, and others. | ADRs: itching, urticarial erythematous maculopapular rash, drowsiness, ataxia, dizziness, slurred speech, headache, nausea, vomiting, diarrhea <br><br> Pharmacokinetics: 15% protein binding; $T_{1/2}$ = 24–48 hrs during chronic administration; extensive hepatic metabolism | Contraindications: hypersensitivity, acute intermittent porphyria <br><br> Other Precautions: Drug dependency is observed (avoid prolonged use); abrupt discontinuation may precipitate withdrawal. Use cautiously in patients with seizure disorders. Use cautiously in patients with severe renal or hepatic dysfunction. <br><br> Pregnancy Category: D <br><br> Lactation Issues: Meprobamate is excreted in breast milk—use cautiously in nursing mothers |

# 310. Sedatives/Hypnotics

310.1 Barbiturates

| Drug and Dosage Forms | Usual Dosage Range | Administration Issues and Drug–Drug & Drug–Food Interactions | Common Adverse Drug Reactions (ADRs) and Pharmacokinetics | Contraindications, Pregnancy Category, and Lactation Issues |
|---|---|---|---|---|
| **Aprobarbital (CII)** Alurate  <u>Elixir:</u>  40 mg/5 mL | **Short-term (<2 weeks) treatment of insomnia:** 40–80 mg at bedtime  **Elderly or debilitated patients (hepatic/renal dysfunction):** 20–40 mg at bedtime. Titrate to higher dose if needed/tolerated  **Sedative:** 40 mg tid  **Elderly or debilitated patients (hepatic/renal dysfunction):** 20 mg 1–2 times daily. Titrate to higher doses if needed/tolerated. | <u>Administration Issues:</u> May produce irritability, excitability or aggression in children. Safety/efficacy not established for children <6 yrs old  <u>Drug–Drug Interactions:</u> **decreased levels of:** anticoagulants, beta blockers, carbamazepine, clonazepam, oral contraceptives, corticosteroids, doxycycline, doxorubicin, felodipine, quinidine, verapamil, theophylline  **increased effect of:** alcohol & possibly narcotics (CNS effects), acetaminophen (liver toxicity)  **increased effect of barbiturates:** MAO inhibitors, valproic acid  **Unknown effects (monitor patient closely):** hydantoins | <u>ADRs:</u> somnolence, agitation, confusion, ataxia, nightmares, nervousness, hallucinations, bradycardia, hypotension, nausea, vomiting, skin rash  <u>Elderly:</u> may observe paradoxical excitement  <u>Precautions:</u> **Drug Abuse & Dependence:** Prolonged use at high doses leads to physical dependence. If dependent on barbiturate, slowly withdraw over several weeks. May use long-acting barbiturate (phenobarbital) at dose of 30 mg per every 100–200 mg of aprobarbital to help prevent withdrawal symptoms.  <u>Pharmacokinetics</u> onset of action = 45–60 min; $T_{1/2}$ = 14–34 hrs; duration of action = 6–8 hrs | <u>Contraindications:</u> Hypersensitivity; manifest or latent porphyria, severe hepatic, renal, or respiratory dysfunction; previous addiction to sedative/hypnotic  <u>Pregnancy Category:</u>  D  <u>Lactation Issues:</u>  use cautiously in nursing mothers; sedation has been reported in infants |

*(continues on next page)*

| Drug and Dosage Forms | Usual Dosage Range | Administration Issues and Drug–Drug & Drug–Food Interactions | Common Adverse Drug Reactions (ADRs) and Pharmacokinetics | Contraindications, Pregnancy Category, and Lactation Issues |
|---|---|---|---|---|
| **Butabarbital (CII)**<br>Butisol Sodium, various generics<br><br>Tablets: 15 mg, 30 mg, 50 mg, 100 mg<br><br>Elixir: 30 mg/5 mL | **Short-term (<2 weeks) treatment of insomnia:** 50–100 mg at bedtime<br><br>**Elderly or debilitated patients (hepatic/renal dysfunction):** 30–50 mg at bedtime. Titrate to higher dose as needed/tolerated<br><br>**Sedation:** 15–30 mg 3–4 times daily (use smaller dose in elderly or debilitated patients) | Administration Issues:<br>May produce irritability, excitability or aggression in children<br><br>Drug–Drug Interactions:<br>**decreased levels of:** anticoagulants, beta blockers, carbamazepine, clonazepam, oral contraceptives, corticosteroids, doxycycline, doxorubicin, felodipine, quinidine, verapamil, theophylline<br><br>**increased effect of:** alcohol & possibly narcotics (CNS effects), acetaminophen (liver toxicity)<br><br>**increased effect of barbiturates:** MAO inhibitors, valproic acid<br><br>**Unknown effects (monitor patient closely):** hydantoins | ADRs:<br>somnolence, agitation, confusion, ataxia, nightmares, nervousness, hallucinations, bradycardia, hypotension, nausea, vomiting, skin rash<br><br>Elderly: may observe paradoxical excitement<br><br>Precautions:<br>**Drug Abuse & Dependence:** Prolonged use at high doses leads to physical dependence. If dependent on barbiturate, slowly withdraw over several weeks. May use long-acting barbiturate (phenobarbital) at dose of 30 mg per every 100–200 mg of butabarbital to help prevent withdrawal symptoms.<br><br>Pharmacokinetics<br>onset of action = 45–60 min; T½ = 66–140 hrs; duration of action = 6–8 hrs | Contraindications:<br>Hypersensitivity; manifest or latent porphyria, severe hepatic, renal, or respiratory dysfunction; previous addiction to sedative/hypnotic<br><br>Pregnancy Category: D<br><br>Lactation Issues: use cautiously in nursing mothers; sedation has been reported in infants |

## Mephobarbital (CII)
Mebaral

Tablets: 32 mg, 50 mg, 100 mg

**Sedative:** 32–100 mg 3–4 times daily

**Pediatrics:** 16–32 mg 3–4 times daily

**Elderly or debilitated patients (hepatic/renal dysfunction):** 16–32 mg 2–3 times daily. Titrate to higher doses as needed/tolerated.

Administration Issues: may produce irritability, excitability or aggression in children

Drug–Drug Interactions:
**decreased levels of:** anticoagulants, beta blockers, carbamazepine, clonazepam, oral contraceptives, corticosteroids, doxycycline, doxorubicin, felodipine, quinidine, verapamil, theophylline

**increased effect of:** alcohol & possibly narcotics (CNS effects), acetaminophen (liver toxicity)

**increased effect of barbiturates:** MAO inhibitors, valproic acid

**Unknown effects (monitor patient closely):** hydantoins

ADRs:
somnolence, agitation, confusion, ataxia, nightmares, nervousness, hallucinations, bradycardia, hypotension, nausea, vomiting, skin rash

Elderly: may observe paradoxical excitement

Precautions:
**Drug Abuse & Dependence:** Prolonged use at high doses leads to physical dependence. If dependent on barbiturate, slowly withdraw over several weeks. May use long-acting barbiturate (phenobarbital) at dose of 30 mg per every 100–200 mg of mephobarbital to help prevent withdrawal symptoms.

Pharmacokinetics
onset of action = 30–>60 min; $T_{1/2}$ = 11–67 hrs; duration of action = 10–16 hrs

Contraindications:
Hypersensitivity; manifest or latent porphyria, severe hepatic, renal, or respiratory dysfunction; previous addiction to sedative/hypnotic

Pregnancy Category: D

Lactation Issues: use cautiously in nursing mothers; sedation has been reported in infants

## Pentobarbital (CII)
Nembutal Sodium, various generics

Capsules: 50 mg, 100 mg

Suppositories: 30 mg, 60 mg, 120 mg, 200 mg

**Short-term (<2 weeks) treatment of insomnia:** 100 mg at bedtime (120–200 mg by suppository)

**Sedative:** 20 mg tid to qid

Administration Issues: may produce irritability, excitability or aggression in children

Drug–Drug Interactions:
**decreased levels of:** anticoagulants, beta blockers, carbamazepine,

ADRs:
somnolence, agitation, confusion, ataxia, nightmares, nervousness, hallucinations, bradycardia, hypotension, nausea, vomiting, skin rash

Contraindications:
Hypersensitivity; manifest or latent porphyria, severe hepatic, renal, or respiratory dysfunction; previous addiction to sedative/hypnotic

(continues on next page)

| Drug and Dosage Forms | Usual Dosage Range | Administration Issues and Drug–Drug & Drug–Food Interactions | Common Adverse Drug Reactions (ADRs) and Pharmacokinetics | Contraindications, Pregnancy Category, and Lactation Issues |
|---|---|---|---|---|
| **Pentobarbital (CII)** *cont.* | **Pediatrics:** 2–6 mg/kg/d orally for sedative dose or hypnotic dose) Rectal administration: 12–14 yrs: 60–120 mg 5–12 yrs: 60 mg 1–4 yrs: 30–60 mg 2 months–1 yr: 30 mg **Elderly or debilitated patients (hepatic/renal dysfunction):** Use smaller doses and greater dosing intervals (for sedative dose). Titrate dose as needed/tolerated | clonazepam, oral contraceptives, corticosteroids, doxycycline, doxorubicin, felodipine, quinidine, verapamil, theophylline **increased effect of:** alcohol & possibly narcotics (CNS effects), acetaminophen (liver toxicity) **increased effect of barbiturates:** MAO inhibitors, valproic acid **Unknown effects (monitor patient closely):** hydantoins | Elderly: may observe paradoxical excitement Precautions: **Drug Abuse & Dependence:** Prolonged use at high doses leads to physical dependence. If dependent on barbiturate, slowly withdraw over several weeks. May use long-acting barbiturate (phenobarbital) at dose of 30 mg per every 100–200 mg of pentobarbital to help prevent withdrawal symptoms. Pharmacokinetics onset of action = 10–15 min; $T_{1/2}$ = 15–50 hrs; duration of action = 3–4 hrs | Pregnancy Category: D Lactation Issues: use cautiously in nursing mothers; sedation has been reported in infants |
| **Phenobarbital (CIV)** Solfoton, various generics Tablets: 15 mg, 16 mg, 30 mg, 60 mg, 100 mg Capsules: 16 mg Elixir: 15 mg/5 mL, 20 mg/5 mL | **Short-term (<2 weeks) treatment of insomnia:** 100–200 mg at bedtime **Pediatrics:** 3–6 mg/kg/d **Sedative:** 15–40 mg 2–3 times daily. Titrate as needed (max dose is 400 mg/d) | Administration Issues: may produce irritability, excitability or aggression in children Drug–Drug Interactions: **decreased levels of:** anticoagulants, beta blockers, carbamazepine, clonazepam, oral contraceptives, corticosteroids, doxycycline, | ADRs: somnolence, agitation, confusion, ataxia, nightmares, nervousness, hallucinations, bradycardia, hypotension, nausea, vomiting, skin rash Elderly: may observe paradoxical excitement | Contraindications: Hypersensitivity; manifest or latent porphyria, severe hepatic, renal, or respiratory dysfunction; previous addiction to sedative/hypnotic Pregnancy Category: D |

| Dosing | Drug Interactions | Precautions / ADRs / Pharmacokinetics | Contraindications / Lactation |
|---|---|---|---|
| **Pediatrics:** 8–32 mg/d<br><br>**Elderly or debilitated patients (hepatic/renal dysfunction):** Use smaller doses and greater dosing intervals (for sedative dose). Titrate dose prn | doxorubicin, felodipine, quinidine, verapamil, theophylline<br><br>**increased effect of:** alcohol & possibly narcotics (CNS effects), acetaminophen (liver toxicity)<br><br>**increased effect of barbiturates:** MAO inhibitors, valproic acid<br><br>**Unknown effects (monitor patient closely):** hydantoins | Precautions:<br>**Drug Abuse & Dependence:** Prolonged use at high doses leads to physical dependence. If dependent on barbiturate, slowly withdraw over several weeks.<br><br>Pharmacokinetics<br>onset of action = 30–>60 min; $T_{1/2}$ = 53–118 hrs; duration of action = 10–16 hrs | Lactation Issues: use cautiously in nursing mothers; sedation has been reported in infants |
| **Secobarbital (CII)**<br>Seconal Sodium Pulvules, various generics<br><br>Capsules: 100 mg<br><br>**Short-term (<2 weeks) treatment of insomnia:** 100 mg at bedtime<br><br>**Elderly or debilitated patients (hepatic/renal dysfunction):** Use smaller doses and greater dosing intervals (for sedative dose). Titrate dose as needed/tolerated | Administration Issues: may produce irritability, excitability or aggression in children<br><br>Drug–Drug Interactions:<br>**decreased levels of:** anticoagulants, beta blockers, carbamazepine, clonazepam, oral contraceptives, corticosteroids, doxycycline, doxorubicin, felodipine, quinidine, verapamil, theophylline<br><br>**increased effect of:** alcohol & possibly narcotics (CNS effects), acetaminophen (liver toxicity)<br><br>**increased effect of barbiturates:** MAO inhibitors, valproic acid<br><br>**Unknown effects (monitor patient closely):** hydantoins | ADRs:<br>somnolence, agitation, confusion, ataxia, nightmares, nervousness, hallucinations, bradycardia, hypotension, nausea, vomiting, skin rash<br><br>Elderly: may observe paradoxical excitement<br><br>Precautions:<br>**Drug Abuse & Dependence:** Prolonged use at high doses leads to physical dependence. If dependent on barbiturate, slowly withdraw over several weeks. May use long-acting barbiturate (phenobarbital) at dose of 30 mg per every 100–200 mg of secobarbital to help prevent withdrawal symptoms.<br><br>Pharmacokinetics<br>onset of action = 10–15 min; $T_{1/2}$ = 15–40 hrs; duration of action = 3–4 hrs | Contraindications:<br>Hypersensitivity; manifest or latent porphyria, severe hepatic, renal, or respiratory dysfunction; previous addiction to sedative/hypnotic<br><br>Pregnancy Category: D<br><br>Lactation Issues: use cautiously in nursing mothers; sedation has been reported in infants |

| Drug and Dosage Forms | Usual Dosage Range | Administration Issues and Drug–Drug & Drug–Food Interactions | Common Adverse Drug Reactions (ADRs) and Pharmacokinetics | Contraindications, Pregnancy Category, and Lactation Issues |
|---|---|---|---|---|
| **Estazolam (CIV)**<br>Pro Som<br><br>Tablets: 1 mg, 2 mg | Insomnia:<br>1 mg at bedtime; some require 2 mg<br><br>**Debilitated or small elderly patients:** 0.5 mg at bedtime; titrate slowly | Administration Issues:<br>Safety/efficacy in children <18 yrs old not established<br><br>Drug–Drug Interactions:<br>**increased level of BZ:** cimetidine, oral contraceptives, disulfiram, fluoxetine, isoniazid, ketoconazole, metoprolol, propoxyphene, propranolol, valproic acid.<br><br>**increased CNS effects:** alcohol, barbiturates, narcotics<br><br>**increased levels of:** digoxin, phenytoin (possibly)<br><br>**decreased level or effect of BZ:** rifampin (decreased level); theophylline (decreased effect) | ADRs:<br>drowsiness, ataxia, confusion (especially in elderly), nervousness<br><br>Dependence: prolonged use can lead to dependence; abrupt discontinuation can precipitate withdrawal symptoms (e.g., anxiety, flu-like illness, concentration difficulties, fatigue, anorexia, restlessness, confusion, psychosis, paranoid delusions, grand mal seizures). Withdrawal can occur after as little as 4–6 weeks of therapy.<br><br>Drug Discontinuation:<br>Slow taper of drug suggested if patient has received long course of therapy.<br><br>Pharmacokinetics:<br>>90% protein bound; time to peak levels: 2 hrs; $T_{1/2}$ = 10–24 hrs; renal elimination | Contraindications:<br>Hypersensitivity<br><br>Pregnancy Category: X<br><br>Lactation Issues: excreted in breast milk—do not give to nursing mothers |

| Flurazepam (CIV)<br>Dalmane, various generics<br><br>Capsules: 15 mg, 30 mg | Insomnia:<br>30 mg at bedtime<br><br>Elderly or debilitated patients:<br>15 mg at bedtime; titrate as needed | Administration Issues:<br>Safety/efficacy in children <15 yrs old not established<br><br>Drug–Drug Interactions:<br>increased level of BZ: cimetidine, oral contraceptives, disulfiram, fluoxetine, isoniazid, ketoconazole, metoprolol, propoxyphene, propranolol, valproic acid.<br><br>increased CNS effects: alcohol, barbiturates, narcotics<br><br>increased levels of: digoxin, phenytoin (possibly)<br><br>decreased level or effect of BZ: rifampin (decreased level); theophylline (decreased effect) | ADRs:<br>drowsiness, ataxia, confusion (especially in elderly), nervousness<br><br>Dependence: prolonged use can lead to dependence; abrupt discontinuation can precipitate withdrawal symptoms (e.g., anxiety, flu-like illness, concentration difficulties, fatigue, anorexia, restlessness, confusion, psychosis, paranoid delusions, grand mal seizures). Withdrawal can occur after as little as 4–6 weeks of therapy.<br><br>Drug Discontinuation: Slow taper of drug suggested if patient has received long course of therapy.<br><br>Pharmacokinetics:<br>>90% protein bound; time to peak levels: 0.5-1 hr; $T_{1/2}$ = 50–100 hrs; renal elimination | Contraindications:<br>Hypersensitivity<br><br>Pregnancy Category: X<br>Contraindicated in pregnancy<br><br>Lactation Issues: excreted in breast milk—do not give to nursing mothers |
| Quazepam (CIV)<br>Doral<br><br>Tablets: 7.5 mg, 15 mg | Insomnia:<br>15 mg at bedtime; some only require 7.5 mg at bedtime<br><br>Elderly or debilitated patients:<br>may initiate at 15 mg at bedtime; attempt to reduce dose after first 2–3 nights | Administration Issues:<br>Safety/efficacy in children <18 yrs old not established<br><br>Drug–Drug Interactions:<br>increased level of BZ: cimetidine, oral contraceptives, disulfiram, fluoxetine, isoniazid, ketoconazole, | ADRs:<br>drowsiness, ataxia, confusion (especially in elderly), nervousness<br><br>Dependence: prolonged use can lead to dependence; abrupt discontinuation can precipitate | Contraindications:<br>Hypersensitivity, suspected or established sleep apnea<br><br>Pregnancy Category: X<br><br>Lactation Issues: excreted in breast milk—do not give to nursing mothers |

(continues on next page)

| Drug and Dosage Forms | Usual Dosage Range | Administration Issues and Drug–Drug & Drug–Food Interactions | Common Adverse Drug Reactions (ADRs) and Pharmacokinetics | Contraindications, Pregnancy Category, and Lactation Issues |
|---|---|---|---|---|
| **Quazepam (CIV)** *cont.* | | metoprolol, propoxyphene, propranolol, valproic acid.<br><br>**increased CNS effects:** alcohol, barbiturates, narcotics<br><br>**increased levels of:** digoxin, phenytoin (possibly)<br><br>**decreased level or effect of BZ:** rifampin (decreased level); theophylline (decreased effect) | withdrawal symptoms (e.g., anxiety, flu-like illness, concentration difficulties, fatigue, anorexia, restlessness, confusion, psychosis, paranoid delusions, grand mal seizures). Withdrawal can occur after as little as 4–6 weeks of therapy.<br><br>Drug Discontinuation:  Slow taper of drug suggested if patient has received long course of therapy.<br><br>Pharmacokinetics:<br>>90% protein bound; time to peak levels: 2 hrs; $T_{1/2}$ = 25–41 hrs; renal elimination | |
| **Temazepam (CIV)**<br>Restoril, various generics<br><br>Capsules:  15 mg, 30 mg | **Insomnia:**<br>15 mg at bedtime; titrate to 30 mg if needed<br><br>**Elderly or debilitated patients:**<br>15 mg at bedtime | Administration Issues:<br>Safety/efficacy in children <18 yrs old not established<br><br>Drug–Drug Interactions:<br>**increased level of BZ:**  cimetidine, oral contraceptives, disulfiram, fluoxetine, isoniazid, ketoconazole, metoprolol, propoxyphene, propranolol, valproic acid. | ADRs:<br>drowsiness, ataxia, confusion (especially in elderly), nervousness<br><br>Dependence:  prolonged use can lead to dependence; abrupt discontinuation can precipitate withdrawal symptoms (e.g., anxiety, flu-like illness, concentration difficulties, | Contraindications:<br>Hypersensitivity<br><br>Pregnancy Category:  X<br><br>Lactation Issues:  excreted in breast milk—do not give to nursing mothers |

| | | Drug–Drug Interactions | ADRs / Pharmacokinetics | Contraindications |
|---|---|---|---|---|
| | | **increased CNS effects:** alcohol, barbiturates, narcotics<br><br>**increased levels of:** digoxin, phenytoin (possibly)<br><br>**decreased level or effect of BZ:** rifampin (decreased level); theophylline (decreased effect) | fatigue, anorexia, restlessness, confusion, psychosis, paranoid delusions, grand mal seizures). Withdrawal can occur after as little as 4–6 weeks of therapy.<br><br><u>Drug Discontinuation:</u> Slow taper of drug suggested if patient has received long course of therapy.<br><br><u>Pharmacokinetics:</u> >90% protein bound; time to peak levels: 2–4 hrs; $T_{1/2}$ = 10–17 hrs; renal elimination | <u>Contraindications:</u> Hypersensitivity<br><br><u>Pregnancy Category:</u> X<br><br><u>Lactation Issues:</u> excreted in breast milk—do not give to nursing mothers |
| **Triazolam (CIV)**<br>Halcion<br><br><u>Tablets:</u> 0.125 mg, 0.25 mg | <u>Insomnia:</u><br>0.125–0.5 mg at bedtime<br><br>**Elderly or debilitated patients:** 0.125 mg at bedtime initially; titrate slowly by 0.125 mg/d if needed | <u>Administration Issues:</u><br>Safety/efficacy in children <18 yrs old not established<br><br><u>Drug–Drug Interactions:</u><br>**increased level of BZ:** cimetidine, oral contraceptives, disulfiram, fluoxetine, isoniazid, ketoconazole, metoprolol, propoxyphene, propranolol, valproic acid.<br><br>**increased CNS effects:** alcohol, barbiturates, narcotics<br><br>**increased levels of:** digoxin, phenytoin (possibly)<br><br>**decreased level or effect of BZ:** rifampin (decreased level); theophylline (decreased effect) | <u>ADRs:</u><br>drowsiness, ataxia, confusion (especially in elderly), nervousness, anterograde amnesia<br><br><u>Dependence:</u> prolonged use can lead to dependence; abrupt discontinuation can precipitate withdrawal symptoms (e.g., anxiety, flu-like illness, concentration difficulties, fatigue, anorexia, restlessness, confusion, psychosis, paranoid delusions, grand mal seizures). Withdrawal can occur after as little as 4–6 weeks of therapy. | |

(continues on next page)

## 310.2 Benzodiazepines  *continued from previous page*

| Drug and Dosage Forms | Usual Dosage Range | Administration Issues and Drug–Drug & Drug–Food Interactions | Common Adverse Drug Reactions (ADRs) and Pharmacokinetics | Contraindications, Pregnancy Category, and Lactation Issues |
|---|---|---|---|---|
| **Triazolam (CIV)** *cont.* | | | Drug Discontinuation: Slow taper of drug suggested if patient has received long course of therapy.<br><br>Pharmacokinetics:<br>>90% protein bound; time to peak levels: 0.5–2 hrs; $T_{1/2}$ = 1.5–5.5 hrs; renal elimination | |

## 310.3 Miscellaneous Nonbarbiturates

| Drug and Dosage Forms | Usual Dosage Range | Administration Issues and Drug–Drug Interactions | Common Adverse Drug Reactions (ADRs) and Pharmacokinetics | Cotraindications, Pregnancy Category, and Lactation Issues |
|---|---|---|---|---|
| **Acetylcarbromal**<br>Paxarel<br><br>Tablets: 250 mg | Sedative:<br>250–500 mg 2–3 times daily<br><br>**Pediatrics:** no specific recommendations; give smaller doses proportionally based on age and weight. | Administration Issues: Avoid alcohol use | ADRs<br>drowsiness (particularly with high doses)<br><br>Overdose: result from bromide accumulation and its displacement of chloride in body fluids. Symptoms: narcosis, respiratory | Contraindications:<br>Hypersensitivity to bromides<br><br>Precautions:<br>may be habit forming<br><br>Pregnancy Category: Unknown |

| Drug / Forms | Indications & Dosage | Administration & Interactions | Adverse Reactions / Pharmacokinetics | Contraindications / Precautions / Lactation |
|---|---|---|---|---|
| *(continued from previous page)* | | | depression, mental disturbances, dizziness, irritability, dermatitis, headache, constipation, others<br><br>Pharmacokinetics<br>No Data | Lactation Issues:<br>Excreted in breast milk—women should not nurse |
| **Chloral Hydrate**<br>Noctec, Aquachloral Supprettes, various generics<br><br>Capsules: 250 mg, 500 mg<br><br>Syrup: 250 mg/5 mL, 500 mg/5 mL<br><br>Suppositories:<br>324 mg, 500 mg, 648 mg | **Nocturnal sedation:**<br>**postoperative adjunct to opiates & analgesics for control of pain. alcohol withdrawal syndrome:**<br><br>Hypnotic: 500–1000 mg at bedtime (15–30 min prior)<br>Sedative: 250 mg tid pc<br><br>**Max dose = 2g/d**<br><br>**Pediatrics:**<br>Hypnotic: 50 mg/kg/d up to 1g/dose; may use divided doses<br>Sedative: 25 mg/kg/d up to 500 mg/dose; may use divided doses | Administration Issues: Give with a full glass of liquid. Syrup should be mixed in 1/2 glass of water, fruit juice, or ginger ale<br><br>Drug–Drug Interactions:<br>**increased levels/effects of:** alcohol, CNS depressants, oral anticoagulants, furosemide<br><br>**decreased levels/effects of:** phenytoin | ADRs: somnambulism, disorientation, excitement, delirium, ataxia, dizziness, nightmares, malaise, headache, mental confusion, rash, hives, erythema, urticaria, nausea, vomiting, flatulence, diarrhea, unpleasant taste in mouth<br><br>Drug Abuse & Dependence: may be habit forming if taken at high doses and prolonged intervals; withdrawal symptoms have occurred with acute discontinuation of this medication. Discontinue medication in manner similar to barbiturate withdrawal<br><br>Pharmacokinetics:<br>onset of action is 30 min; $T_{1/2}$ = 7–10 hrs; renal elimination of metabolites | Contraindications:<br>Hypersensitivity; severe hepatic, renal, cardiac dysfunction; gastritis<br><br>Precautions: Use cautiously in patients with acute intermittent porphyria<br><br>Pregnancy Category: C<br><br>Lactation Issues: excreted in breast milk; use cautiously |

(continues on next page)

| Drug and Dosage Forms | Usual Dosage Range | Administration Issues and Drug–Drug Interactions | Common Adverse Drug Reactions (ADRs) and Pharmacokinetics | Cotraindications, Pregnancy Category, and Lactation Issues |
|---|---|---|---|---|
| **Ethchlorvynol**<br>Placidyl<br><br>Capsules: 200 mg, 500 mg, 750 mg | **Short-term relief of insomnia:**<br>500 mg at bedtime. May titrate to 750 mg if needed/tolerated. Max dose is 1000 mg at bedtime<br><br>**Unlabeled Use: Sedative:**<br>100–200 mg 2–3 times daily | Administration Issues:<br>Do not give for longer than 7 days; safety/efficacy not established in children<br><br>Drug–Drug Interactions:<br>**increased levels/effects of:** alcohol, CNS depressants<br><br>**decreased levels/effects of:** oral anticoagulants | ADRs:<br>dizziness, facial numbness, giddiness, ataxia, vomiting, gastric upset, nausea, rash, thrombocytopenia, urticaria<br><br>Drug Abuse & Dependence:<br>may be habit forming if taken at high doses at prolonged intervals. Withdrawal symptoms have occurred after abrupt discontinuation.<br><br>Pharmacokinetics:<br>onset of action is 15–60 min; duration of action = 5 hrs; $T_{1/2}$ = 10–20 h | Contraindications:<br>Hypersensitivity; porphyria<br><br>Precautions: Use cautiously in elderly patients, severe hepatic, renal dysfunction<br><br>Pregnancy Category: C<br><br>Lactation Issues: unknown if excreted in breast milk—use cautiously |
| **Ethanimate**<br>Valmid Pulvules<br><br>Capsules: 500 mg | **Short-term relief of insomnia:**<br>500–1000 mg 20 min before bedtime | Administration Issues:<br>Not effective after 7 days; safety/efficacy not established in those <15 yrs old<br><br>Drug–Drug Interactions:<br>**increased levels/effects of:** alcohol, CNS depressants | ADRs:<br>thrombocytopenic purpura, idiosyncrasy with fever, skin rash, mild GI symptoms<br><br>Drug Abuse & Dependence:<br>may be habit forming if taken at high doses at prolonged intervals. | Contraindications:<br>Hypersensitivity<br><br>Pregnancy Category: C<br><br>Lactation Issues: unknown if excreted in breast milk. Use cautiously |

| Drug | Dosing | Administration/Interactions | ADRs/Pharmacokinetics | Contraindications/Precautions |
|---|---|---|---|---|
| | | | Withdrawal symptoms have occurred after abrupt discontinuation.<br><br>Pharmacokinetics:<br>onset of action is 20 min; duration of action = 3–5 hrs; $T_{1/2}$ = 2.5 h | Contraindications:<br>Hypersensitivity; porphyria<br><br>Pregnancy Category: C<br><br>Lactation Issues: do not nurse while taking this drug |
| **Glutethimide**<br>Doriden, various generics<br><br>Tablets: 250 mg, 500 mg | **Short-term relief of insomnia:**<br>250–500 mg at bedtime<br><br>**Elderly or debilitated patients:**<br>do not exceed 500 mg/d | Administration Issues: Do not administer for longer than 3–7 days; safety/ efficacy not established in children<br><br>Drug–Drug Interactions:<br>**decreased levels/effects of:** oral anticoagulants<br><br>**increased levels/effects of:** alcohol, CNS depressants | ADRs:<br>drowsiness, hangover, rash, nausea<br><br>Drug Abuse & Dependence:<br>may be habit forming if taken at high doses and prolonged intervals. Withdrawal symptoms have occurred after abrupt discontinuation.<br><br>Pharmacokinetics:<br>50% protein bound; onset of action is 30 min; duration of action = 4–8 hrs; $T_{1/2}$ = 10–12 hrs; renal elimination | |
| **Zolpidem**<br>Ambien<br><br>Tablets: 5 mg, 10 mg | **Short-term treatment of insomnia:** 10 mg at bedtime (max dose is 10 mg/d)<br><br>**Elderly or debilitated patients:**<br>5 mg at bedtime | Administration Issues:<br>For faster onset of sleep, do not administer with food. Use only for 7–10 days; safety/efficacy not established in those <18 yrs<br><br>Drug–Drug Interactions:<br>Additive CNS effects with alcohol or other CNS depressants | ADRs:<br>daytime drowsiness, amnesia, dizziness, headache, nausea, vomiting, diarrhea<br><br>Elderly: closely monitor these patients for excessive sedation or impairment of motor or cognitive performance | Contraindications: None<br><br>Precautions: Use cautiously in those with respiratory or severe hepatic dysfunction, or those with depression<br><br>Pregnancy Category: B |

(continues on next page)

## 310.3 Miscellaneous Nonbarbiturates *continued from previous page*

| Drug and Dosage Forms | Usual Dosage Range | Administration Issues and Drug–Drug Interactions | Common Adverse Drug Reactions (ADRs) and Pharmacokinetics | Cotraindications, Pregnancy Category, and Lactation Issues |
|---|---|---|---|---|
| **Zolpidem *cont.*** | | Drug–Food Interaction: Food decreases the absorption of zolpidem | Drug Abuse & Dependence: Withdrawal symptoms may occur following abrupt discontinuation  Pharmacokinetics: 92.5% protein bound; rapid onset of action; $T_{1/2}$ = 1.0–5.5 hrs; renal elimination | Lactation Issues: not appreciably excreted in breast milk, however use cautiously in nursing mothers |

## 310.4 Nonprescription Sleep Aids

| Drug and Dosage Forms | Usual Dosage Range | Administration Issues and Drug–Drug & Drug–Food Interactions | Common Adverse Drug Reactions (ADRs) and Pharmacokinetics | Contraindications, Pregnancy Category, and Lactation Issues |
|---|---|---|---|---|
| **Doxylamine** Unisom Nighttime Sleep-Aid  Tablets: 25 mg | **Aid in relief of insomnia:** 25 mg at bedtime | Administration Issues: Do not use for >2 weeks; safety/efficacy in children <12 yrs not established  Drug–Drug Interactions: **increased effect of antihistamine:** MAO inhibitors (anticholinergic effects) | ADRs: urinary retention, blurred vision, dry mouth, drowsiness, irritability, thickening of bronchial secretions | Contraindications: Hypersensitivity, asthma, glaucoma, prostate gland enlargement  Precautions: use carefully if operating heavy machinery, |

| | | | | |
|---|---|---|---|---|
| | | **increased effect of:** MAO inhibitors, alcohol, CNS depressants | Pharmacokinetics: rapid onset (15–30 minutes); duration of action 4–6 hrs; renal elimination of metabolites | history of sleep apnea, hepatic dysfunction<br><br>Pregnancy Category: X.<br><br>Lactation Issues: women should not nurse |
| **Diphenhydramine**<br>Dormin Caplets, Nytol, Sleep-eze 3, Sominex, Sleep Aid, Twilite, various generics<br><br>Tablets: 25 mg, 50 mg<br><br>Capsules: 25 mg, 50 mg | **Aid in relief of insomnia:**<br>25–50 mg at bedtime | Administration Issues: Do not use for >2 weeks; safety/efficacy in children <12 yrs not established<br><br>Drug–Drug Interactions<br>**increased effect of antihistamine:** MAO inhibitors (anticholinergic effects)<br><br>**increased effect of:** MAO inhibitors, alcohol, CNS depressants | ADRs:<br>urinary retention, blurred vision, dry mouth, drowsiness, irritability, thickening of bronchial secretions<br><br>Elderly (>60yrs): more likely to experience confusion, dizziness, hypotension<br><br>Pharmacokinetics<br>rapid onset (15–30 minutes); duration of 4–6 hrs; renal elimination of metabolites | Contraindications:<br>Hypersensitivity, asthma, glaucoma, prostate gland enlargement<br><br>Precautions: use carefully if operating heavy machinery, history of sleep apnea, hepatic dysfunction<br><br>Pregnancy Category: B.<br><br>Lactation Issues: women should not nurse |
| **Diphenhydramine & Acetaminophen**<br>Extra-Strength<br>Tylenol PM, Aspirin Free Anacin PM<br>Caplets, Excedrin PM, others | **Aid in relief of insomnia and minor pain:**<br>25–50 mg diphenhydramine and 500–650 mg acetaminophen at bedtime | Administration Issues: Do not use for >2 weeks; safety/efficacy in children <12 yrs not established<br><br>Drug–Drug Interactions:<br>Antihistamine:<br>**increased effect of antihistamine:** MAO inhibitors (anticholinergic effects) | ADRs:<br>Antihistamine: urinary retention, blurred vision, dry mouth, drowsiness, irritability, thickening of bronchial secretions | Contraindications:<br>Hypersensitivity, asthma, glaucoma, prostate gland enlargement |

(continues on next page)

## 310.4 Nonprescription Sleep Aids  *continued from previous page*

| Drug and Dosage Forms | Usual Dosage Range | Administration Issues and Drug–Drug & Drug–Food Interactions | Common Adverse Drug Reactions (ADRs) and Pharmacokinetics | Contraindications, Pregnancy Category, and Lactation Issues |
|---|---|---|---|---|
| **Diphenhydramine & Acetaminophen** *cont.*<br><br>Tablets:<br>25 mg/500 mg, 38 mg/ 500 mg, 50 mg/650 mg,<br><br>Powder:<br>50 mg/650 mg<br><br>Liquid:<br>8.3 mg/167 mg/ 5 mL | | **increased effect of:** MAO inhibitors, alcohol, CNS depressants<br><br>Acetaminophen:<br>**increased toxic effect of acetaminophen:** alcohol (chronic); barbiturates, carbamazepine, hydantoins, rifampin, sulfinpyrazone | Elderly (>60yrs): more likely to experience confusion, dizziness, hypotension<br><br>Acetaminophen:<br>Very few adverse reactions<br><br>Pharmacokinetics:<br>see individual ingredients | Precautions: use carefully if operating heavy machinery, history of sleep apnea, hepatic dysfunction<br><br>Pregnancy Category: B. Consult physician before taking<br><br>Lactation Issues: women should not nurse |

# 311. Antidepressants

## 311.1 Tricyclic Antidepressants (TCAs)

| Drug and Dosage Forms | Usual Dosage Range | Administration Issues and Drug–Drug Interactions | Common Adverse Drug Reactions (ADRs) and Pharmacokinetics | Contraindications, Pregnancy Category, and Lactation Issues |
|---|---|---|---|---|
| **Amitriptyline**<br>Elavil, Endep, various generic forms<br><br>Tablets: 10 mg, 25 mg, 50 mg, 75 mg, 100 mg, 150 mg. | **Major Depression:**<br>starting dose of 50–100 mg/d at bedtime. Titrate by 25–50 mg q week to 150 mg/d. For severely depressed patients increase dose to 200–300 mg/d<br><br>**Adolescent or Elderly patients:**<br>starting dose of 10–25 mg q hs. Titrate dose by 10–25 mg q week to 150 mg/d<br><br>**Unlabeled uses:**<br>50–100 mg/d used for chronic pain. Also used in Bulimia nervosa. | Administration issues:<br>Maintenance doses may be given once daily at bedtime to reduce daytime sedation.<br><br>Drug–Drug Interactions:<br>**Hypertensive crisis:**<br>clonidine, MAO inhibitors (can occur weeks after MAOI discontinued)<br><br>**increased TCA level:**<br>cimetidine, ethanol, fluoxetine, haloperidol, oral contraceptives, phenothiazines<br><br>**decreased TCA level:**<br>barbiturates, phenytoin, chronic ethanol ingestion<br><br>**increased level of:**<br>phenytoin, warfarin<br><br>**increased effect:**<br>anticholinergic agents, ethanol or sedatives (increased CNS effects), | ADRs:<br>dry mouth, urinary retention, blurred vision, constipation, orthostatic hypotension, tachycardia, sedation, confusion (esp. elderly), anxiety, nervousness, agitation, nausea, vomiting, anorexia, constipation or diarrhea, flatulence, abdominal cramps, sexual dysfunction (increased or decreased libido; impotence, painful ejaculation)<br><br>Pharmacokinetics:<br>$T_{1/2}$ = 31–46 hrs; time to maximal clinical benefit = 2–4 weeks; hepatic elimination (active metabolite = nortriptyline)<br><br>**Therapeutic plasma level = 110–250 ng/mL** (plasma levels and therapeutic effect are subject to wide interpatient variability) | Contraindications:<br>any hypersensitivity to a TCA, concomitant use of MAO inhibitors<br><br>Precautions:<br>use with caution in patients with severe cardiovascular disease, seizure disorders. Patients with schizophrenia may experience worsening psychosis; patients with bipolar disorder may experience a switch to mania. Dosage reductions necessary in patients with hepatic or severe renal dysfunction.<br><br>Pregnancy Category: C<br><br>Lactation issues:<br>TCA's are excreted into breast milk. Use with caution. |

(continues on next page)

| | | | |
|---|---|---|---|
| 311.1 Tricyclic Antidepressants (TCAs) *continued from previous page* | | | |
| **Drug and Dosage Forms** | **Usual Dosage Range** | **Administration Issues and Drug–Drug Interactions** | **Common Adverse Drug Reactions (ADRs) and Pharmacokinetics** | **Contraindications, Pregnancy Category, and Lactation Issues** |

| **Drug and Dosage Forms** | **Usual Dosage Range** | **Administration Issues and Drug–Drug Interactions** | **Common Adverse Drug Reactions (ADRs) and Pharmacokinetics** | **Contraindications, Pregnancy Category, and Lactation Issues** |
|---|---|---|---|---|
| **Amitriptyline** *cont.* | | thyroid hormones (increased effect of both drugs) <br><br> **decreased effect of:** guanethidine, methyldopa | | |
| **Amoxapine** <br> Asendin, various generics <br><br> <u>Tablets:</u> 25 mg, 50 mg, 100 mg, 150 mg | **Major Depression:** <br> 50 mg 2–3 times daily starting dose. Titrate to 100 mg 2–3 times daily within 1 week. If no effect with 300 mg/d for 2 weeks, increase dose to 400 mg/d in divided doses. <br><br> **Elderly patients:** <br> 25 mg 2–3 times daily starting dose. Titrate to 50 mg 2–3 times daily within 1 week. If required, may titrate to 300 mg/d after 2 weeks. | <u>Administration issues:</u> <br> Maintenance doses may be given once daily at bedtime to reduce daytime sedation. Not recommended for children < 16 yrs old <br><br> <u>Drug–Drug Interactions:</u> <br> **Hypertensive crisis:** <br> clonidine, MAO inhibitors (can occur weeks after MAOI discontinued) <br><br> **increased TCA level:** <br> cimetidine, ethanol, fluoxetine, haloperidol, oral contraceptives, phenothiazines <br><br> **decreased TCA level:** <br> barbiturates, phenytoin, chronic ethanol ingestion <br><br> **increased level of:** <br> phenytoin, warfarin <br><br> **increased effect:** <br> anticholinergic agents, ethanol or | <u>ADRs:</u> <br> dry mouth, urinary retention, blurred vision, constipation, orthostatic hypotension, tachycardia, sedation, confusion (esp. elderly), anxiety, nervousness, agitation, nausea, vomiting, anorexia, constipation or diarrhea, flatulence, abdominal cramps, sexual dysfunction (increased or decreased libido; impotence, painful ejaculation) <br><br> <u>Pharmacokinetics:</u> <br> $T_{1/2}$ = 8 hrs; time to maximal clinical benefit = 2–4 weeks <br><br> **Therapeutic plasma level = 200–500 ng/mL** (plasma levels and therapeutic effect are subject to wide interpatient variability) | <u>Contraindications:</u> <br> any hypersensitivity to a TCA, concomitant use of MAO inhibitors <br><br> <u>Precautions:</u> <br> Due to its dopamine effects, patients may develop **neuroleptic malignant syndrome or tardive dyskinesia.** Use with caution in patients with severe cardiovascular disease, seizure disorders. Patients with schizophrenia may experience worsening psychosis; patients with bipolar disorder may experience a switch to mania. Dosage reductions necessary in patients with hepatic or severe renal dysfunction. <br><br> <u>Pregnancy Category:</u>  C |

|  | | | |
|---|---|---|---|
| **Clomipramine**<br>Anafranil<br><br>Capsules:<br>25 mg, 50 mg, 75 mg | | sedatives (increased CNS effects), thyroid hormones (increased effect of both drugs)<br><br>**decreased effect of:**<br>guanethidine, methyldopa | Lactation issues:<br>TCA's are excreted into breast milk. Use with caution. |
| | **Obsessive–Compulsive Disorder:**<br>25 mg/d starting dose. Titrate by 25 mg/d to 200 mg/d within 2 weeks. Max dose of 250 mg/d.<br><br>**Children & Adolescents:**<br>25 mg/d at bedtime starting dose. Titrate within 2 weeks by 25 mg/d to the smaller of 3 mg/kg or 100 mg/d. Max dose of 3 mg/kg or 200 mg/d.<br><br>**Unlabeled uses:**<br>25–200 mg/d used for chronic pain | Administration issues:<br>Maintenance doses may be given once daily at bedtime to reduce daytime sedation; Not recommended for children <10 yrs old<br><br>Drug–Drug Interactions:<br>**Hypertensive crisis:**<br>clonidine, MAO inhibitors (can occur weeks after MAOI discontinued)<br><br>**increased TCA level:**<br>cimetidine, ethanol, fluoxetine, haloperidol, oral contraceptives, phenothiazines<br><br>**decreased TCA level:**<br>barbiturates, phenytoin, chronic ethanol ingestion<br><br>**increased level of:**<br>phenytoin, warfarin<br><br>**increased effect:**<br>anticholinergic agents, ethanol or sedatives (increased CNS effects), thyroid hormones (increased effect of both drugs)<br><br>**decreased effect of:**<br>guanethidine, methyldopa | ADRs:<br>dry mouth, urinary retention, blurred vision, constipation, orthostatic hypotension, tachycardia, sedation, confusion (esp. elderly), anxiety, nervousness, agitation, nausea, vomiting, anorexia, constipation or diarrhea, flatulence, abdominal cramps, sexual dysfunction (increased or decreased libido; impotence, painful ejaculation)<br><br>Pharmacokinetics:<br>$T_{1/2}$=19–37 hrs; time to maximal clinical benefit = 2–4 weeks<br><br>**Therapeutic plasma level = 80–100 ng/mL** (plasma levels and therapeutic effect are subject to wide interpatient variability) | Contraindications:<br>any hypersensitivity to a TCA, concomitant use of MAO inhibitors<br><br>Precautions:<br>use with caution in patients with severe cardiovascular disease, seizure disorders. Patients with schizophrenia may experience worsening psychosis; patients with bipolar disorder may experience a switch to mania. Dosage reductions necessary in patients with hepatic or severe renal dysfunction.<br><br>Pregnancy Category: C<br><br>Lactation issues:<br>TCA's are excreted into breast milk. Use with caution in nursing mothers. |

(continues on next page)

(continues on next page)

## 311.1 Tricyclic Antidepressants (TCAs) *continued from previous page*

| Drug and Dosage Forms | Usual Dosage Range | Administration Issues and Drug–Drug Interactions | Common Adverse Drug Reactions (ADRs) and Pharmacokinetics | Contraindications, Pregnancy Category, and Lactation Issues |
|---|---|---|---|---|
| **Desipramine**<br>Norpramin, various generics<br><br>Tablets: 10 mg, 25 mg, 50 mg, 75 mg, 100 mg, 150 mg<br><br>Capsules: 25 mg, 50 mg | **Major Depression:**<br>75 mg/d at bedtime starting dose. Titrate by 50 mg/d every 3–4 days to 150–200 mg/d. Max dose is 300 mg/d.<br><br>**Adolescent & Elderly patients:**<br>10–25 mg at bedtime starting dose. Titrate by 10–25 mg every 3–4 days to 100–150 mg/d.<br><br>**Unlabeled uses:**<br>50–200 mg/d for facilitation of cocaine withdrawal. Has also been used in bulimia nervosa.<br><br>**Traumatic Brain Injury:**<br>10 mg tid; up to 150 mg/d | Administration issues:<br>Maintenance doses may be given once daily at bedtime to reduce daytime sedation. Not recommended for children <12 yrs old<br><br>Drug–Drug Interactions:<br>**Hypertensive crisis:**<br>clonidine, MAO inhibitors; can occur weeks after MAOI discontinued.<br><br>**increased TCA level:**<br>cimetidine, ethanol, fluoxetine, haloperidol, oral contraceptives, phenothiazines<br><br>**decreased TCA level:**<br>barbiturates, phenytoin, chronic ethanol ingestion<br><br>**increased level of:**<br>phenytoin, warfarin<br><br>**increased effect:**<br>anticholinergic agents, ethanol or sedatives (increased CNS effects), thyroid hormones (increased effect of both drugs)<br><br>**decreased effect of:**<br>guanethidine, methyldopa | ADRs:<br>dry mouth, urinary retention, blurred vision, constipation, orthostatic hypotension, tachycardia, sedation, confusion (esp. elderly), anxiety, nervousness, agitation, nausea, vomiting, anorexia, constipation or diarrhea, flatulence, abdominal cramps, sexual dysfunction (increased or decreased libido; impotence, painful ejaculation)<br><br>Pharmacokinetics:<br>$T_{1/2}$ = 12–24 hrs; time to maximal clinical benefit = 2–4 weeks<br><br>**Therapeutic plasma level = 125–300 ng/mL** (plasma levels and therapeutic effect are subject to wide interpatient variability) | Contraindications:<br>any hypersensitivity to a TCA, concomitant use of MAO inhibitors<br><br>Precautions:<br>use with caution in patients with severe cardiovascular disease, seizure disorders. Patients with schizophrenia may experience worsening psychosis; patients with bipolar disorder may experience a switch to mania. Dosage reductions necessary in patients with hepatic or severe renal dysfunction.<br><br>Pregnancy Category:  C<br><br>Lactation issues:<br>TCA's are excreted into breast milk. Use with caution. |

## Doxepin

Adapin, Sinequan, various generics

Capsules: 10 mg, 25 mg, 50 mg, 75 mg, 100 mg, 150 mg

Liquid concentrate: 10 mg/1 mL

---

**Major Depression or anxiety:** 75 mg/d at bedtime starting dose. Titrate up to 300 mg/d in 2–3 divided doses. Single dose ≤150 mg.

**Elderly patients:** 10–25 mg at bedtime starting dose. Titrate by 10–25 mg every 3–5 days to 75 mg/d.

**Unlabeled uses:** 50–300 mg/d used for chronic pain; 10–30 mg/d used in chronic urticaria and angioedema, nocturnal pruritis in atopic eczema. Also used in peptic ulcer disease.

---

Administration issues:
Maintenance doses may be given once daily at bedtime to reduce daytime sedation. Concentrate: protect from light, dilute in juice or other liquid; Not recommended for children <12 yrs old

Drug–Drug Interactions:
**Hypertensive crisis:** clonidine, MAO inhibitors; can occur weeks after MAOI discontinued.

**increased TCA level:** cimetidine, ethanol, fluoxetine, haloperidol, oral contraceptives, phenothiazines

**decreased TCA level:** barbiturates, phenytoin, chronic ethanol ingestion

**increased level of:** phenytoin, warfarin

**increased effect:** anticholinergic agents, ethanol or sedatives (increased CNS effects), thyroid hormones (increased effect of both drugs)

**decreased effect of:** guanethidine, methyldopa

---

ADRs:
dry mouth, urinary retention, blurred vision, constipation, orthostatic hypotension, tachycardia, sedation, confusion (esp. elderly), anxiety, nervousness, agitation, nausea, vomiting, anorexia, constipation or diarrhea, flatulence, abdominal cramps, sexual dysfunction (increased or decreased libido; impotence, painful ejaculation)

Pharmacokinetics:
$T_{1/2}$ = 8–24 hrs; time to maximal clinical benefit = 2–4 weeks

**Therapeutic plasma level = 100–200 ng/mL** (plasma levels and therapeutic effect are subject to wide interpatient variability.)

---

Contraindications:
any hypersensitivity to a TCA, concomitant use of MAO inhibitors, patients with glaucoma or tendency to urinary retention.

Precautions: use with caution in patients with severe cardiovascular disease, seizure disorders. Patients with schizophrenia may experience worsening psychosis; patients with bipolar disorder may experience a switch to mania. Dosage reductions necessary in patients with hepatic or severe renal dysfunction.

Pregnancy Category: C

Lactation issues: TCA's are excreted into breast milk. Use with caution.

(continues on next page)

## 311.1 Tricyclic Antidepressants (TCAs) *continued from previous page*

| Drug and Dosage Forms | Usual Dosage Range | Administration Issues and Drug–Drug Interactions | Common Adverse Drug Reactions (ADRs) and Pharmacokinetics | Contraindications, Pregnancy Category, and Lactation Issues |
|---|---|---|---|---|
| **Imipramine** Tofranil, Janimine, various generics<br><br>Tablets: 10 mg, 25 mg, 50 mg<br><br>Capsules (imipramine pamoate–Tofranil PM): 75 mg, 100 mg, 125 mg, 150 mg | **Major Depression:** starting dose of 75 mg/d in divided doses or at bedtime. Titrate by 25 mg every 3–4 days up to 300 mg/d<br><br>**Adolescent or elderly patients:** starting dose of 10–40 mg at bedtime. Titrate by 10–25 mg every 3–4 days up to 100 mg/d<br><br>**Children:** starting dose of 1.5 mg/kg divided tid. Titrate by 1–1.5 mg/kg/d every 3–5 days to maximum of 5 mg/kg/d<br><br>**Childhood enuresis >6yrs old:** 25 mg 1 hour before bedtime. Titrate by 25 mg/d each week up to 50 mg for children <12 yr and 75 mg for children >12<br><br>**Unlabeled uses:** 75–150 mg/d used in chronic pain; 25–75 mg/d used in panic disorder. Also used in bulimia nervosa. | Administration issues: Maintenance doses may be given once daily at bedtime to reduce daytime sedation.<br><br>Drug–Drug Interactions: **Hypertensive crisis:** clonidine, MAO inhibitors; can occur weeks after MAOI discontinued.<br><br>**increased TCA level:** cimetidine, ethanol, fluoxetine, haloperidol, oral contraceptives, phenothiazines<br><br>**decreased TCA level:** barbiturates, phenytoin, chronic ethanol ingestion<br><br>**increased level of:** phenytoin, warfarin<br><br>**increased effect:** anticholinergic agents, ethanol or sedatives (increased CNS effects), thyroid hormones (increased effect of both drugs)<br><br>**decreased effect of:** guanethidine, methyldopa | ADRs: dry mouth, urinary retention, blurred vision, constipation, orthostatic hypotension, tachycardia, sedation, confusion (esp. elderly), anxiety, nervousness, agitation, nausea, vomiting, anorexia, constipation or diarrhea, flatulence, abdominal cramps, sexual dysfunction (increased or decreased libido; impotence, painful ejaculation)<br><br>Pharmacokinetics: $T_{1/2}$ = 11–25 hrs; time to maximal clinical benefit = 2–4 weeks; hepatic elimination (active metabolite = desipramine)<br><br>**Therapeutic plasma level = 200–350 ng/mL** (plasma levels and therapeutic effect are subject to wide interpatient variability) | Contraindications: any hypersensitivity to a TCA, concomitant use of MAO inhibitors<br><br>Precautions: use with caution in patients with severe cardiovascular disease, seizure disorders. Patients with schizophrenia may experience worsening psychosis; patients with bipolar disorder may experience a switch to mania. Dosage reductions necessary in patients with hepatic or severe renal dysfunction.<br><br>Pregnancy Category: B<br><br>Lactation issues: TCA's are excreted into breast milk. Use with caution in nursing mothers. |

## Nortriptyline

Aventyl, Pamelor

Capsules: 10 mg, 25 mg, 50 mg, 75 mg

Liquid: 10 mg/5 mL

**Major Depression:**
starting dose of 25 mg 3–4 times daily. Titrate every 3–4 days to 100–150 mg/d

**Elderly patients:**
starting dose of 10–25 mg at bedtime. Titrate by 25 mg/d every 3–4 days up to 75 mg/d

**Unlabeled uses:**
25–75 mg/d used in panic disorder. 50–125 mg/d used in premenstrual depression. 75 mg/d used in chronic urticaria and angioedema, nocturnal pruritis in atopic eczema

**Traumatic Brain Injury:**
25 mg q hs; up to 150 mg/d

Administration issues:
Maintenance doses may be given once daily at bedtime to reduce daytime sedation. Not recommended for children

Drug–Drug Interactions:
**Hypertensive crisis:** clonidine, MAO inhibitors; can occur weeks after MAOI discontinued.

**increased TCA level:** cimetidine, ethanol, fluoxetine, haloperidol, oral contraceptives, phenothiazines

**decreased TCA level:** barbiturates, phenytoin, chronic ethanol ingestion

**increased level of:** phenytoin, warfarin

**increased effect:** anticholinergic agents, ethanol or sedatives (increased CNS effects), thyroid hormones (increased effect of both drugs)

**decreased effect of:** guanethidine, methyldopa

ADRs:
dry mouth, urinary retention, blurred vision, constipation, orthostatic hypotension, tachycardia, sedation, confusion (esp. elderly), anxiety, nervousness, agitation, nausea, vomiting, anorexia, constipation or diarrhea, flatulence, abdominal cramps, sexual dysfunction (increased or decreased libido; impotence, painful ejaculation)

Pharmacokinetics:
$T_{1/2}$ = 18–44 hrs; time to maximal clinical benefit = 2–4 weeks

**Therapeutic plasma level = 50–150 ng/mL** (plasma levels and therapeutic effect are subject to wide interpatient variability)

Contraindications:
any hypersensitivity to a TCA, concomitant use of MAO inhibitors

Precautions:
use with caution in patients with severe cardiovascular disease, seizure disorders. Patients with schizophrenia may experience worsening psychosis; patients with bipolar disorder may experience a switch to mania. Dosage reductions necessary in patients with hepatic or severe renal dysfunction.

Pregnancy Category: C

Lactation issues:
TCA's are excreted into breast milk. Use with caution.

## Protriptyline

Vivactil

Tablets: 5 mg, 10 mg

**Major Depression:**
15–40 mg/d in 3–4 divided doses starting dose. Titrate by 15 mg every 3–4 days to 60 mg/d

Administration issues:
Maintenance doses may be given once daily at bedtime to reduce daytime sedation. Not recommended for children

ADRs:
dry mouth, urinary retention, blurred vision, constipation, orthostatic hypotension, tachycardia, sedation,

Contraindications:
any hypersensitivity to a TCA, concomitant use of MAO inhibitors

(continues on next page)

# 311.1 Tricyclic Antidepressants (TCAs) *continued from previous page*

| Drug and Dosage Forms | Usual Dosage Range | Administration Issues and Drug–Drug Interactions | Common Adverse Drug Reactions (ADRs) and Pharmacokinetics | Contraindications, Pregnancy Category, and Lactation Issues |
|---|---|---|---|---|
| **Protriptyline** *cont.* | **Adolescent & Elderly patients:** 5 mg 1–3 times daily starting dose. Titrate by 5 mg/d every 3–7 days to 15–20 mg/d<br><br>**Unlabeled use:** obstructive sleep apnea | Drug–Drug Interactions<br>**Hypertensive crisis:** clonidine, MAO inhibitors; can occur weeks after MAOI discontinued.<br><br>**increased TCA level:** cimetidine, ethanol, fluoxetine, haloperidol, oral contraceptives, phenothiazines<br><br>**decreased TCA level:** barbiturates, phenytoin, chronic ethanol ingestion<br><br>**increased level of:** phenytoin, warfarin<br><br>**increased effect:** anticholinergic agents, ethanol or sedatives (increased CNS effects), thyroid hormones (increased effect of both drugs)<br><br>**decreased effect of:** guanethidine, methyldopa | confusion (esp. elderly), anxiety, nervousness, agitation, nausea, vomiting, anorexia, constipation or diarrhea, flatulence, abdominal cramps, sexual dysfunction (increased or decreased libido; impotence, painful ejaculation)<br><br>Pharmacokinetics:<br>$T_{1/2}$ = 67–89 hrs; time to maximal clinical benefit = 2–4 weeks;<br><br>**Therapeutic plasma level = 100–200 ng/mL** (plasma levels and therapeutic effect are subject to wide interpatient variability) | Precautions:<br>use with caution in patients with severe cardiovascular disease, seizure disorders. Patients with schizophrenia may experience worsening psychosis; patients with bipolar disorder may experience a switch to mania. Dosage reductions necessary in patients with hepatic or severe renal dysfunction.<br><br>Pregnancy Category: C<br><br>Lactation issues:<br>TCA's are excreted into breast milk. Use with caution. |
| **Trimipramine**<br>Surmontil<br><u>Capsules:</u> 25 mg, 50 mg, 100 mg | **Major Depression:** 75 mg/d at bedtime starting dose. Titrate by 25–50 mg q 3 days to max dose of 200 mg/d. | Administration issues:<br>Maintenance doses may be given once daily at bedtime to reduce daytime sedation. Not recommended for children | ADRs:<br>dry mouth, urinary retention, blurred vision, constipation, orthostatic hypotension, tachycardia, sedation, | Contraindications:<br>any hypersensitivity to a TCA, concomitant use of MAO inhibitors |

For severe depression, max dose of 300 mg/d

**Adolescent & Elderly patients:**
50 mg/d at bedtime starting dose. Titrate by 25 mg every 3 days to 100 mg/d

**Unlabeled use:**
50 mg/d used in chronic urticaria and angioedema, nocturnal pruritis in atopic eczema. Also, has been used in peptic ulcer disease.

Drug–Drug Interactions:
**Hypertensive crisis:**
clonidine, MAO inhibitors; can occur weeks after MAOI discontinued.

**increased TCA level:**
cimetidine, ethanol, fluoxetine, haloperidol, oral contraceptives, phenothiazines

**decreased TCA level:**
barbiturates, phenytoin, chronic ethanol ingestion

**increased level of:**
phenytoin, warfarin

**increased effect:**
anticholinergic agents, ethanol or sedatives (increased CNS effects), thyroid hormones (increased effect of both drugs)

**decreased effect of:**
guanethidine, methyldopa

confusion (esp. elderly), anxiety, nervousness, agitation, nausea, vomiting, anorexia, constipation or diarrhea, flatulence, abdominal cramps, sexual dysfunction (increased or decreased libido; impotence, painful ejaculation)

Pharmacokinetics:
$T_{1/2}$ = 7–30 hrs; time to maximal clinical benefit = 2–4 weeks

**Therapeutic plasma level = 180 ng/mL** (plasma levels and therapeutic effect are subject to wide interpatient variability)

Precautions:
use with caution in patients with severe cardiovascular disease, seizure disorders. Patients with schizophrenia may experience worsening psychosis; patients with bipolar disorder may experience a switch to mania. Dosage reductions necessary in patients with hepatic or severe renal dysfunction.

Pregnancy Category: C

Lactation issues:
TCA's are excreted into breast milk. Use with caution.

| Drug and Dosage Forms | Usual Dosage Range | Administration Issues and Drug–Drug Interactions | Common Adverse Drug Reactions (ADRs) and Pharmacokinetics | Contraindications, Pregnancy Category, and Lactation Issues |
|---|---|---|---|---|
| **Buproprion**<br>Wellbutrin<br><br>Tablets: 75 mg, 100 mg<br><br>Sustained Release:<br>100 mg, 150 mg | **Major Depression:**<br>starting dose of 100 mg bid. Titrate by 100 mg/d after 3 days to dose of 300 mg/d. Max dose is 450 mg/d; max single dose is 150 mg<br><br>**Elderly patients:**<br>starting dose of 50–100 mg/d. Titrate dose by 50–100 mg/d every 3–4 days as tolerated. | Administration Issues:<br>Safety/efficacy not yet established in those <18 years old<br><br>Drug–Drug Interactions:<br>buproprion induces metabolism<br><br>**increased toxicity of:**<br>levodopa; buproprion (with concurrent use of MAOIs)<br><br>**increased seizure potential:**<br>other agents that decrease seizure threshold. | ADRs:<br>dizziness, tachycardia, dry mouth, headache, sweating, tremor, sedation, insomnia, auditory disturbances, nausea, vomiting, constipation, weight loss, anorexia<br><br>Pharmacokinetics<br>$T_{1/2}$ = 8–24 hrs; time to maximal clinical benefit = 2–4 weeks; hepatic elimination | Contraindications:<br>Hypersensitivity; seizure disorder; current or prior diagnosis of bulimia or anorexia; concurrent use of MAOI within 14 days of stopping the MAOI.<br><br>Pregnancy Category: B<br><br>Lactation Issues:<br>Women should not nurse while receiving buproprion. |
| **Maprotiline**<br>Ludiomil, various generics<br><br>Tablets: 25 mg, 50 mg, 75 mg | **Depressive illness associated with dysthymic disorder, manic-depression, and major depressive disorder:**<br>75 mg/d at bedtime starting dose. Titrate after 2 weeks by 25 mg/d to 150 mg/d. Max dose 225 mg/d.<br><br>**Elderly patients:**<br>25 mg/d at bedtime starting dose. Titrate by 25 mg/d every week to 50–75 mg/d. | Administration issues:<br>Maintenance doses may be given once daily at bedtime to reduce daytime sedation. Not recommended for children.<br><br>Drug–Drug Interactions:<br>**Hypertensive crisis:**<br>clonidine, MAO inhibitors; can occur weeks after MAO inhibitor discontinued.<br><br>**increased maprotiline level:**<br>cimetidine, ethanol, fluoxetine, haloperidol, oral contraceptives, phenothiazines | ADRs:<br>dry mouth, urinary retention, blurred vision, orthostatic hypotension, tachycardia, sedation, confusion (esp. elderly), hallucinations, anxiety, nervousness, agitation, nausea, vomiting, anorexia, constipation or diarrhea, flatulence, abdominal cramps, sexual dysfunction (increased or decreased libido; impotence; painful ejaculation) | Contraindications:<br>any hypersensitivity to tetracyclic; concomitant use of MAO inhibitors, known or suspected seizure disorder<br><br>Precautions:<br>use with caution in patients with severe cardiovascular disease. Patients with schizophrenia may experience worsening psychosis; patients with bipolar disorder may experience a switch to mania. Dosage reductions necessary in patients with hepatic or severe renal dysfunction. |

| Drug | Dosage | Drug Interactions / Administration | Pharmacokinetics / ADRs | Contraindications / Precautions |
|---|---|---|---|---|
| | | **decreased maprotiline level:** barbiturates, phenytoin, chronic ethanol ingestion<br><br>**increased level of:** phenytoin, warfarin<br><br>**increased effect:** anticholinergic agents, ethanol or sedatives (increased CNS effects), thyroid hormones (increased effect of both drugs)<br><br>**decreased effect of:** guanethidine, methyldopa | Pharmacokinetics<br>$T_{1/2}$ = 21–25 hrs; time to maximal clinical benefit = 2–4 weeks<br><br>**Therapeutic plasma level = 200–300 ng/mL** (plasma levels and therapeutic effect are subject to wide interpatient variability.) | Pregnancy Category: B<br><br>Lactation issues:<br>Maprotiline is excreted into breast milk. Use with caution. |
| **Mirtazapine**<br>Remeron<br><br>Tablets: 15 mg, 30 mg | **Treatment of Depression:**<br>Initial: 15 mg/d as a single dose<br><br>May increase every 1–2 wk to max 45 mg/d. Use lower doses in geriatric patients. | Administration Issues:<br>Take in the evening, prior to sleep.<br><br>Drug–Drug Interactions:<br>**Additive CNS effects** when taken with alcohol and benzodiazepines | ADRs:<br>somnolence, dry mouth, constipation, increased appetite, weight gain, abnormal dreams, dizziness<br><br>Pharmacokinetics:<br>$T_{1/2}$ = 20–40 h; extensively metabolized | Contraindications:<br>any hypersensitivity to drug, concomitant use of MAO inhibitors<br><br>Precautions:<br>use with caution in patients with severe cardiovascular disease. Patients with schizophrenia may experience worsening psychosis; patients with bipolar disorder may experience a switch to mania. Dosage reductions necessary in patients with hepatic or severe renal dysfunction.<br><br>Pregnancy Category: C |

(continues on next page)

# 311.2 Miscellaneous Antidepressants continued from previous page

| Drug and Dosage Forms | Usual Dosage Range | Administration Issues and Drug–Drug Interactions | Common Adverse Drug Reactions (ADRs) and Pharmacokinetics | Contraindications, Pregnancy Category, and Lactation Issues |
|---|---|---|---|---|
| **Mirtazapine** *cont.* | | | | Lactation issues:<br>It is not known if mirtazapine is excreted in breast milk. Use with caution. |
| **Nefazodone**<br>Serzone<br><br>Tablets: 100 mg, 150 mg, 200 mg, 250 mg | **Major Depression:**<br>starting dose of 100 mg twice daily. Titrate dose by 100–200 mg/d each week up to 600 mg/d.<br><br>**Elderly patients:**<br>start with 50 mg twice daily. Titrate by 50–100 mg/d each week. | Administration Issues:<br>Safety/efficacy not established for those <18 years old<br><br>Drug–Drug Interactions:<br>**Hypertensive crisis:** with MAOIs<br><br>**increased levels of: astemizole,** terfenadine, benzodiazepines, digoxin due to inhibition of metabolism.<br><br>**decreased levels of** propranolol and **increased levels of** nefazodone during concurrent use. | ADRs:<br>postural hypotension, dizziness, drowsiness, insomnia, agitation, nausea, dry mouth, constipation, headache<br><br>Pharmacokinetics:<br>rapidly absorbed but bioavailability is 20% due to first-pass metabolism; $T_{1/2}$ = 2–4 hours but with active metabolites $T_{1/2}$ = 11–24 hours; time to maximal benefit is 2–4 weeks | Contraindications:<br>hypersensitivity; coadministration with terfenadine or astemizole.<br><br>Pregnancy Category: C<br><br>Lactation Issues:<br>It is unknown if nefazodone and metabolites are excreted in breast milk. Use caution in nursing mothers. |
| **Trazodone**<br>Desyrel, Desyrel Dividose, various generic forms<br><br>Tablets: 50 mg, 100 mg, 150 mg<br><br>Tablet dividose:<br>150 mg, 300 mg | **Major Depression:**<br>starting dose of 50 mg tid. Titrate dose by 50 mg/d q 3–4 days. Max dose is 600 mg/d in 2 divided doses.<br><br>**Elderly patients:** start at 25–50 mg at bedtime. Titrate dose by 25–50 mg q 3–4 d to 75–150 mg/d | Administration Issues<br>Safety/efficacy not established in children <18 yrs old.<br><br>Drug–Drug Interactions:<br>**increased CNS depressant activity:** alcohol, barbiturates, other CNS depressants | ADRs:<br>orthostatic tension, tachycardia, palpitations, drowsiness, fatigue, dizziness, tremors, anger, hostility, nightmares, confusion, nervousness, dry mouth, nausea, vomiting, constipation, bad taste in | Contraindications:<br>Hypersensitivity<br><br>Other Precautions:<br>Use cautiously in patients with preexisting cardiac disease—patients may be predisposed to cardiac arrhythmias. |

| | Dosing | Administrative/Drug–Drug Interactions | ADRs/Pharmacokinetics | Contraindications/Pregnancy/Lactation |
|---|---|---|---|---|
| | **Traumatic Brain Injury:** 50 mg, up to 150 mg q hs | **increased levels of:** digoxin, phenytoin. | mouth, priapism, decreased libido, impotence, malaise, weight gain or loss musculoskeletal aches/pains<br><br>Pharmacokinetics:<br>$T_{1/2}$ = 4–9 hrs; time to maximal clinical benefit = 1–4 weeks;<br><br>**Therapeutic plasma level = 800–1600 ng/mL** (plasma levels and therapeutic effect are subject to wide interpatient variability.) | Pregnancy Category: C<br><br>Lactation Issues:<br>Trazodone and metabolites have been found in breast milk - use cautiously in nursing mothers. |
| **Venlafaxine**<br>Effexor<br><br>Tablets: 25 mg, 37.5 mg, 50 mg, 75 mg, 100 mg<br><br>Extended Release:<br>37.5 mg, 75 mg, 150 mg | **Major Depression:**<br>Regular Release Tablets:<br>starting dose of 75 mg/d in 2–3 divided doses. Titrate by 75 mg/d q 4d up to 225 mg/d or, for severely depressed patients, up to 350 mg/d. Max dose is 375 mg/d generally divided tid<br><br>Extended Release Tablets:<br>37.5 or 75 mg qd initially; increase at dosages of 75 mg/d at intervals of at least 4 d; max XR = 225 mg/d<br><br>**Elderly patients:** 12.5–25 mg bid. Titrate by 25 mg/d as needed.<br><br>**Hepatic dysfunction:** 50% dose reduction recommended.<br>**Renal dysfunction:** 25% dose reduction with 50% dose reduction in patients undergoing hemodialysis | Administrative Issues:<br>Safety/efficacy in those <18 years old not established. Extended release tablets can be taken in the morning or evening, but patients should consistently take venlafaxine at the same time every day. Patients stabilized on the regular release tablets can be converted to the nearest equivalent dose of the XR tablets.<br><br>Drug–Drug Interactions:<br>**Hypertensive crisis:** with concurrent use of MAOIs<br><br>**increased levels of venlafaxine by:** cimetidine (but does not appear to affect metabolite) | ADRs:<br>hypertension, drowsiness, dry mouth, dizziness, insomnia, nervousness, anxiety, nausea, constipation, anorexia, abnormal ejaculation/orgasm, impotence, headache, asthenia<br><br>Pharmacokinetics:<br>$T_{1/2}$ = 5 hours and for active metabolite it is 11 hours; Time to maximal benefit is 2–4 weeks. | Contraindications:<br>hypersensitivity<br><br>Pregnancy Category: C<br><br>Lactation Issues:<br>Unknown whether venlafaxine is excreted in breast milk. Use caution in nursing mothers. |

| Drug and Dosage Forms | Usual Dosage Range | Administration Issues and Drug–Drug & Drug–Food Interactions | Common Adverse Drug Reactions (ADRs) and Pharmacokinetics | Contraindications, Pregnancy Category, and Lactation Issues |
|---|---|---|---|---|
| **Phenelzine**<br>Nardil<br><br>Tablets: 15 mg | **Atypical Major Depression:**<br>15 mg tid. Titrate to 60 mg/d within a few days as tolerated. Max dose is 90 mg/d<br><br>**Elderly patients:**<br>7.5 mg/d starting dose. Titrate by 7.5–15 mg/d every 3–4 days to 60 mg/d<br><br>**Unlabeled uses:**<br>bulimia nervosa, panic disorder with agoraphobia and treatment of cocaine addiction | Drug–Drug Interactions:<br>**increased effect of:**<br>beta-blockers (bradycardia); antidiabetic agents (hypoglycemia); meperidine (agitation, seizures, diaphoresis, fever, coma, death).<br><br>**Hypertensive crisis:**<br>antidepressants (SSRIs, TCAs); levodopa, sympathomimetics, ʟ-tryptophan.<br><br>Drug–Food Interactions:<br>Tyramine-containing foods in combination with MAOI may result in hypertensive crisis: Cheeses (camembert, cheddar, others); Meat/Fish (fermented sausages - bologna, pepperoni; pickled or spoiled herring; others); Alcoholic beverages; Fruit/Vegetables (yeast extracts, others); Other foods containing vasopressors (e.g., caffeine, chocolate) | ADRs:<br>orthostatic hypotension, disturbances in cardiac rate and rhythm, dizziness, vertigo, headache, overactivity, hyperreflexia, tremors, jitteriness, confusion, memory impairment, insomnia, weakness, fatigue, drowsiness, agitation, constipation, nausea, diarrhea, abdominal pain, edema, dry mouth, blurred vision, rash, anorexia, weight gain<br><br>Pharmacokinetics:<br>onset of activity 3–4 weeks; effects continue for up to 2 weeks after discontinuation; primarily renal route of elimination | Contraindications:<br>Hypersensitivity, pheochromocytoma, congestive heart failure, history of liver disease or abnormal LFTs, severe renal impairment, cardiovascular disease, cerebrovascular disease.<br><br>Other Precautions:<br>Use with caution in elderly due to increased morbidity from adverse effects<br><br>Pregnancy Category:<br>Effects have not been established; use only when benefits far outweigh risks.<br><br>Lactation issues:<br>Effects not well established, use with caution. |
| **Tranylcypromine**<br>Parnate<br><br>Tablets: 10 mg | **Atypical Reactive Depression:**<br>30 mg/d in divided doses. Titrate after 2 weeks by 10 mg/d to 60 mg/d.<br><br>**Unlabeled uses:**<br>bulimia nervosa, panic disorder with agoraphobia and treatment of cocaine addiction | Drug–Drug Interactions:<br>**increased effect of:**<br>beta-blockers (bradycardia); antidiabetic agents (hypoglycemia); meperidine (agitation, seizures, diaphoresis, fever, coma, death). | ADRs:<br>orthostatic hypotension, disturbances in cardiac rate and rhythm, dizziness, vertigo, headache, overactivity, hyperreflexia, tremors, jitteriness, confusion, memory impairment, insomnia, | Contraindications:<br>Hypersensitivity, pheochromocytoma, congestive heart failure, history of liver disease or abnormal LFTs, severe renal impairment, cardiovascular disease, cerebrovascular disease. |

**(continuation of previous table)**

| Administration Issues and Drug–Drug Interactions | Common Adverse Drug Reactions (ADRs) and Pharmacokinetics | Contraindications, Pregnancy Category and Lactation Issues |
|---|---|---|
| **Hypertensive crisis:** antidepressants (SSRIs, TCAs); levodopa, sympathomimetics, L-tryptophan.<br><br>Drug–Food Interactions:<br>Tyramine-containing foods in combination with MAOI may result in hypertensive crisis: Cheeses (camembert, cheddar, others); Meat/Fish (fermented sausages – bologna, pepperoni; pickled or spoiled herring; others); Alcoholic beverages; Fruit/Vegetables (yeast extracts, others); Other foods containing vasopressors (e.g., caffeine, chocolate) | weakness, fatigue, drowsiness, agitation, constipation, nausea, diarrhea, abdominal pain, edema, dry mouth, blurred vision, rash, anorexia, weight gain<br><br>Pharmacokinetics:<br>onset of activity 10 days; effects continue for up to 10 days after discontinuation; $T_{1/2}$ = 90–190 minutes; primarily renal route of elimination | Other Precautions:<br>Use with caution in elderly due to increased morbidity from adverse effects<br><br>Pregnancy Category:<br>Effects have not been established; use only when benefits far outweigh risks.<br><br>Lactation issues:<br>Effects not well established, use with caution. Tranylcypromine is excreted in breast milk. |

## 311.4 Selective Serotonin Reuptake Inhibitors

| Drug and Dosage Forms | Usual Dosage Range | Administration Issues and Drug–Drug Interactions | Common Adverse Drug Reactions (ADRs) and Pharmacokinetics | Contraindications, Pregnancy Category and Lactation Issues |
|---|---|---|---|---|
| **Fluoxetine**<br>Prozac<br><br>Pulvules: 10 mg, 20 mg<br><br>Liquid: 20 mg/5 mL | **Major Depression:**<br>20 mg/d q am.<br>Max dose: 80 mg/d<br><br>**Obsessive–Compulsive Disorder:**<br>20 mg/d to 60 mg/d q m<br>Max dose: 80 mg/d<br><br>**Traumatic Brain Injury:**<br>Initial dose: 5–10 mg qd<br>Maintenance dose: 10–20 mg qd | Administration Issues:<br>Administer dose in the morning to decrease nighttime insomnia<br><br>Drug–Drug Interactions:<br>**Hypertensive Crisis:**<br>MAO inhibitors (may be fatal). Avoid use within 14 days of stopping an MAOI; avoid starting MAOI within 5 weeks of stopping the SSRI<br><br>**increased levels of:**<br>carbamazepine, phenytoin, lithium | ADRs:<br>nervousness, insomnia, anxiety, asthenia, tremor, increased sweating, dizziness; decreased libido; drowsiness, fatigue, anorexia, weight loss, nausea, diarrhea, dyspepsia, constipation<br><br>Pharmacokinetics:<br>$T_{1/2}$ = 48–96 hrs; $T_{1/2}$ of active metabolite 48–216 hrs | Contraindications:<br>Hypersensitivity, in combination with MAOI, coadministration with astemizole or terfenadine<br><br>Other precautions:<br>Watch for precipitation of mania in bipolar patients. SSRIs may precipitate seizures in patients with seizure disorder<br><br>Pregnancy Category: B |

*(continues on next page)*

| Drug and Dosage Forms | Usual Dosage Range | Administration Issues and Drug–Drug Interactions | Common Adverse Drug Reactions (ADRs) and Pharmacokinetics | Contraindications, Pregnancy Category and Lactation Issues |
|---|---|---|---|---|
| **Fluoxetine** *cont.* | Dose titration if needed is done after several weeks of therapy.<br><br>**Hepatic dysfunction or elderly:**<br>Initiate at lower dose (i.e., 10 mg q am) | **increased effect:**<br>dextromethorphan (hallucinations occurred), L-tryptophan (headache, sweating, dizziness, agitation, nausea, vomiting)<br><br>**decreased effect of SSRI:**<br>cyproheptadine | | **Lactation Issues:**<br>SSRIs are secreted in breast milk although no adverse effects have been noted in infants. Use caution in nursing women. |
| **Fluvoxamine**<br>Luvox<br><u>Tablets:</u> 50 mg, 100 mg | **Obsessive–Compulsive Disorder:**<br>Initiate at 50 mg q hs (range 100–300 mg/d). Increase dose in 50 mg increments q 4 to 7 days as needed. Doses >100 mg/d should be divided in two doses<br><br>**Hepatic dysfunction or elderly:**<br>Initiate at lower dose (i.e., 25 mg q hs—50 mg tablets are scored) | **Administration Issues:**<br>safety and efficacy in children <18 years old not established<br><br><u>Drug–Drug Interactions:</u><br>**Hypertensive Crisis:**<br>MAO inhibitors (may be fatal) Avoid use within 14 days of stopping an MAOI; avoid starting MAOI within 5 weeks of stopping the SSRI<br><br>**increased levels of:**<br>theophylline, carbamazepine, warfarin<br><br>**increased effect:**<br>diltiazem (bradycardia), L-tryptophan (headache, sweating, dizziness, agitation, nausea, vomiting) | <u>ADRs:</u><br>nervousness, anxiety, asthenia, tremor, increased sweating, dizziness; decreased libido; drowsiness or fatigue, anorexia, nausea, diarrhea, dyspepsia, constipation<br><br><u>Pharmacokinetics:</u><br>$T_{1/2}$ = 14–16 hrs; 80% protein binding; renal route of elimination | <u>Contraindications:</u><br>Hypersensitivity, in combination with MAOI, coadministration with astemizole or terfenadine<br><br><u>Other precautions:</u><br>Watch for precipitation of mania in bipolar patients. SSRIs may precipitate seizures in patients with seizure disorder.<br><br><u>Pregnancy Category:</u> C<br><br><u>Lactation Issues:</u><br>SSRIs are secreted in breast milk although no adverse effects have been noted in infants. Use caution in nursing women |

| Paroxetine<br>Paxil<br><br>Tablets: 10 mg, 20 mg, 30 mg, 40 mg | | | | |
|---|---|---|---|---|
| | **Major Depression:**<br>Initiate at 20 mg q am (range 20–50 mg/d). Dose titration of 10 mg/d every week as needed.<br><br>**Traumatic Brain Injury:**<br>5 mg/d; may titrate up to 20–30 mg/d<br><br>**Renal / hepatic dysfunction or elderly:**<br>Initiate at 10 mg/d (range 10–40 mg/d) | **increased effect of SSRI:** lithium, TCAs<br><br>**decreased effect of SSRI:** smoking<br><br>**increased risk of cardiac arrhythmias:** astemizole and terfenadine<br><br>Administration Issues:<br>Administer dose in the morning to decrease nighttime insomnia.<br><br>Drug–Drug Interactions:<br>**Hypertensive Crisis:** MAO inhibitors (may be fatal) Avoid use within 14 days of stopping an MAOI; avoid starting MAOI within 5 weeks of stopping the SSRI<br><br>**increased levels of:** phenytoin, warfarin<br><br>**increased SSRI plasma levels:** cimetidine<br><br>**increased effect:** L-tryptophan (headache, sweating, dizziness, agitation, nausea, vomiting)<br><br>**decreased effect of SSRI:** barbiturates, phenytoin | ADRs:<br>nervousness, insomnia, anxiety, asthenia, tremor, increased sweating, dizziness; decreased libido; drowsiness or fatigue may occur, anorexia, nausea, diarrhea, dyspepsia, constipation<br><br>Pharmacokinetics:<br>$T_{1/2}$ = 21 hrs | Contraindications:<br>Hypersensitivity, in combination with MAOI, coadministration with astemizole or terfenadine<br><br>Other precautions:<br>Watch for precipitation of mania in bipolar patients.<br>SSRIs may precipitate seizures in patients with seizure disorder.<br><br>Pregnancy Category: B<br><br>Lactation Issues:<br>SSRIs are secreted in breast milk although no adverse effects have been noted in infants. Use caution in nursing women |

(continues on next page)

# 311.4 Selective Serotonin Reuptake Inhibitors *continued from previous page*

| Drug and Dosage Forms | Usual Dosage Range | Administration Issues and Drug–Drug Interactions | Common Adverse Drug Reactions (ADRs) and Pharmacokinetics | Contraindications, Pregnancy Category and Lactation Issues |
|---|---|---|---|---|
| **Sertraline**<br>Zoloft<br><br>Tablets: 50 mg, 100 mg | **Major Depression:**<br>Initiate at 50 mg qd (range 50–200 mg/d). Dose titration of 50 mg/d every week as needed.<br><br>**Traumatic Brain Injury:**<br>25 mg/d; may titrate up to 100 mg/d<br><br>**Renal/hepatic dysfunction:**<br>Initiate at 25 mg/d (50 mg tablets are scored) | Administration Issues:<br>Administer dose in the morning to decrease nighttime insomnia.<br><br>Drug–Drug Interactions:<br>**Hypertensive Crisis:**<br>MAO inhibitors (may be fatal). Avoid use within 14 days of stopping an MAOI; avoid starting MAOI within 5 weeks of stopping the SSRI<br><br>**increased levels of:**<br>tolbutamide, lithium, warfarin | ADRs:<br>nervousness, insomnia, anxiety, asthenia, tremor, increased sweating, dizziness; decreased libido; drowsiness or fatigue may occur, Male sexual dysfunction: primary ejaculatory delay, anorexia, nausea, diarrhea, dyspepsia, constipation<br><br>Pharmacokinetics:<br>$T_{1/2}$ = 26–65 hrs | Contraindications:<br>Hypersensitivity, in combination with MAOI, coadministration with astemizole or terfenadine<br><br>Other precautions:<br>Watch for precipitation of mania in bipolar patients. SSRIs may precipitate seizures in patients with seizure disorder.<br><br>Pregnancy Category: B<br><br>Lactation Issues:<br>SSRIs are secreted in breast milk although no adverse effects have been noted in infants. Use caution in nursing women |

# 312. Antipsychotic Agents

312.1 Phenothiazines

| Drug and Dosage Forms | Usual Dosage Range | Administration Issues, Drug–Drug & Drug–Food Interactions | Common Adverse Drug Reactions (ADRs) and Pharmacokinetics | Contraindications, Pregnancy Category, and Lactation Issues |
|---|---|---|---|---|
| **Acetophenazine**<br>Tindal<br><br>Tablets: 20 mg | **Psychotic Disorders:**<br>20 mg tid up to 60–120 mg/d.<br><br>**Elderly patients:**<br>initial dose: 20 mg qd and slowly titrate prn<br><br>**Unlabeled uses:**<br>Torero's syndrome, acute agitation in elderly, symptoms of dementia (agitation, hyperactivity, hallucinations, suspiciousness, hostility) | Administration Issues:<br>To decrease daytime sedation, the daily dose may be given as a single dose at bedtime once appropriate dose has been established. Titrate oral doses to response; once psychosis is controlled, decrease dose to lowest dose required by patient; not generally recommended for children <12 yrs old<br><br>Drug–Drug Interactions:<br>**increased effect:** CNS effects (alcohol); EPS effect (fluoxetine, lithium); sedation/ hypotension (meperidine)<br><br>**increased level of:** TCAs, valproic acid, phenytoin (or decreased level), propranolol (also increases level of antipsychotic)<br><br>**decreased level of antipsychotic:** aluminum antacids, barbiturates, carbamazepine, charcoal<br><br>**decreased effect of antipsychotic:** anticholinergics | **ADRs:**<br>Sedation: Moderate<br>Anticholinergic Effects (dry mouth, blurred vision, constipation, urinary retention): Low<br>Extrapyramidal Effects (pseudoparkinsonism, akathisia, dystonias): High<br>Orthostatic hypotension: Low<br><br>**Other ADRs:**<br>arrhythmias, myocardial depression, headache, hypertension, lethargy, restlessness, weight gain, hyperactivity, breast enlargement, galactorrhea, menstrual irregularities, changes in libido, Tardive Dyskinesia (after prolonged therapy—may be irreversible), Neuroleptic Malignant Syndrome<br><br>Pharmacokinetics:<br>$T_{1/2}$ = 10–20 hrs; full therapeutic effect may not be seen for 6 weeks | Contraindications:<br>Hypersensitivity, comatose or severely depressed states, concomitant use of large amounts of other CNS depressants; bone marrow depression, liver damage, cerebral arteriosclerosis, coronary artery disease<br><br>Precautions:<br>Use cautiously in patients with: seizure disorders, impaired renal or hepatic dysfunction, hyperthyroidism; do not use 48 hrs prior to myelography; do not abruptly withdraw therapy<br><br>Pregnancy/Lactation Issues:<br>Safety not established. Use only when benefits clearly outweigh risks to fetus/neonate. |

(continues on next page)

| Drug and Dosage Forms | Usual Dosage Range | Administration Issues, Drug–Drug & Drug–Food Interactions | Common Adverse Drug Reactions (ADRs) and Pharmacokinetics | Contraindications, Pregnancy Category, and Lactation Issues |
|---|---|---|---|---|
| **Chlorpromazine**<br>Thorazine, various generics<br><br>Tablets: 10 mg, 25 mg, 50 mg, 100 mg, 200 mg<br><br>Capsules (sustained release): 30 mg, 75 mg, 150 mg, 200 mg, 300 mg<br><br>Syrup: 10 mg/5 mL<br><br>Concentrate: 30 mg/mL, 100 mg/mL<br><br>Suppositories: 25 mg, 100 mg | **Psychotic Disorders:**<br>10 mg tid to qid or 25 mg bid to tid. Titrate by 20–50 mg/d biweekly until desired response. Doses of 800 mg/d not unusual.<br><br>**Elderly or debilitated:**<br>10–25 mg 1–2 times daily; slowly titrate as needed by 10–25 mg/d every 4–7 days<br><br>**Pediatrics:**<br>Oral dose: 0.5 mg/kg q 4–6 hrs<br>rectal dose: 1 mg/kg q 6–8 hrs<br><br>**Unlabeled uses:**<br>see Acetophenazine | Administration Issues:<br>To decrease daytime sedation, the daily dose may be given as a single dose at bedtime once appropriate dose has been established. Concentrates: protect from light, dilute in juices or other liquid. Titrate oral doses to patient response; once psychosis is controlled, decrease dose to lowest dose required by patient; not recommended for those <6 mos old<br><br>Drug–Drug Interactions:<br>**increased effect:** CNS effects (alcohol); EPS effect (fluoxetine, lithium); sedation/ hypotension (meperidine)<br><br>**increased level of:** TCAs, valproic acid, phenytoin (or decreased level), propranolol (also increases level of antipsychotic)<br><br>**decreased level of antipsychotic:** aluminum antacids, barbiturates, carbamazepine, charcoal<br><br>**decreased effect of antipsychotic:** anticholinergics | **ADRs:**<br>Sedation: High<br>Anticholinergic Effects (dry mouth, constipation, urinary retention, blurred vision): Moderate<br>Extrapyramidal Effects (pseudoparkinsonism, akathisia, dystonias): Moderate<br>Orthostatic hypotension: High<br><br>**Other ADRs:**<br>arrhythmias, myocardial depression, headache, hypertension, lethargy, restlessness, weight gain, hyperactivity, breast enlargement, galactorrhea, menstrual irregularities, changes in libido, Tardive Dyskinesia (after prolonged therapy—may be irreversible); Neuroleptic Malignant Syndrome<br><br>Pharmacokinetics:<br>T$_{1/2}$ = 10–20 hrs; full therapeutic effect may not be seen for 6 weeks | Contraindications:<br>Hypersensitivity, comatose or severely depressed states; concomitant use of large amounts of other CNS depressants; bone marrow depression, liver damage, cerebral arteriosclerosis, coronary artery disease<br><br>Precautions:<br>Use cautiously in patients with: seizure disorders, impaired renal or hepatic dysfunction, hyperthyroidism; do not use 48 hrs prior to myelography; do not abruptly withdraw therapy<br><br>Pregnancy/Lactation issues:<br>Safety not establishes. Use only when benefits clearly outweigh risks to fetus/neonate. |
| **Fluphenazine**<br>Prolixin, Permitil, various generics | **Psychotic Disorders:**<br>0.5–10 mg/d tid to qid (daily doses >3 mg not usually necessary) | Administration Issues: To decrease daytime sedation, the daily dose may be given as a single dose at bedtime once appropriate | **ADRs:**<br>Sedation: Low<br>Anticholinergic Effects (dry | Contraindications:<br>Hypersensitivity, comatose or severely depressed states, |

| Forms | Dosage | Administration & Interactions | ADRs, Precautions & Contraindications |
|---|---|---|---|
| **Tables:** 1 mg, 2.5 mg, 5 mg, 10 mg<br><br>**Elixir:** 2.5 mg/5 mL<br><br>**Concentrate:** 5 mg/mL<br><br>**Fluphenazine Enanthate or Deconate**<br>Prolixin Enanthate, Prolixin Deconate, various generics<br><br>**Injection:** 25 mg/mL | **Elderly or debilitated:**<br>1–2.5 mg daily; slowly titrate as needed<br><br>Deconate or Ethanate injection:<br>12.5–25 mg initially q 3–4 weeks. Subsequent dose and interval based on response. Max dose is 100 mg. One study showed 20 mg/d of short acting agent is approximately equal to 25 mg of deconate q 3 weeks.<br><br>**Unlabeled uses:**<br>see Acetophenazine<br><br>**Traumatic Brain Injury**<br>start at 0.5 mg bid | dose has been established. Concentrates: protect from light, dilute in juices or other liquid; Titrate oral doses to patient response; once psychosis is controlled, decrease dose to lowest dose required by patient; not generally recommended in children <12 yrs old<br><br>Drug–Drug Interactions:<br>**increased effect:** CNS effects (alcohol); EPS effect (fluoxetine, lithium); sedation/hypotension (meperidine)<br><br>**increased level of:** TCAs, valproic acid, phenytoin (or decreased level), propranolol (also increases level of antipsychotic)<br><br>**decreased level of antipsychotic:** aluminum antacids, barbiturates, carbamazepine, charcoal<br><br>**decreased effect of antipsychotic:** anticholinergics | mouth, constipation, urinary retention, blurred vision): Low<br>Extrapyramidal Effects (pseudoparkinsonism, akathisia, dystonias): High<br>Orthostatic hypotension: Low<br><br>**Other ADRs:**<br>arrhythmias, myocardial depression, headache, hypertension, lethargy, restlessness, weight gain, hyperactivity, breast enlargement, galactorrhea, menstrual irregularities, changes in libido, Tardive Dyskinesia (after prolonged therapy—may be irreversible): Neuroleptic Malignant Syndrome<br><br>Pharmacokinetics:<br>$T_{1/2}$ = 10–20 hrs; full therapeutic effect may not be seen for 6 weeks<br><br>concomitant use of large amounts of other CNS depressants; bone marrow depression, liver damage, cerebral arteriosclerosis, coronary artery disease<br><br>Precautions:<br>Use cautiously in patients with: seizure disorders, impaired renal or hepatic dysfunction, hyperthyroidism; do not use 48 hrs prior to myelography; do not abruptly withdraw therapy<br><br>Pregnancy/Lactation issues:<br>Safety not established. Use only when benefits clearly outweigh risks to fetus/neonate. |
| **Mesoridazine**<br>Serentil<br><br>**Tables:**<br>10 mg, 25 mg, 50 mg, 100 mg<br><br>**Concentrate:**<br>25 mg/mL | **Psychotic Disorders:**<br>50 mg tid; titrate based on response to 100–400 mg/d<br><br>**Elderly or debilitated patients:**<br>10 mg qd to bid; slow titration to max dose of 250 mg/d<br><br>**Behavior problems in mental deficiency and chronic brain syndrome:** 25 mg tid; titrate to 75–300 mg/d | Administration Issues:<br>To decrease daytime sedation, the daily dose may be given as a single dose at bedtime once appropriate dose has been established; Concentrates: protect from light, dilute in juices or other liquid. Titrate oral doses to patient response; once psychosis is controlled, decrease dose to lowest dose required by patient; not generally recommended for children <12 yrs old | **ADRs:**<br>Sedation: High<br>Anticholinergic Effects (dry mouth, constipation, urinary retention, blurred vision): High<br>Extrapyramidal Effects (pseudoparkinsonism, akathisia, dystonias): Low<br>Orthostatic hypotension: Moderate<br><br>Contraindications:<br>Hypersensitivity, comatose or severely depressed states, concomitant use of large amounts of other CNS depressants; bone marrow depression, liver damage, cerebral arteriosclerosis, coronary artery disease |

(continues on next page)

| Drug and Dosage Forms | Usual Dosage Range | Administration Issues, Drug–Drug & Drug–Food Interactions | Common Adverse Drug Reactions (ADRs) and Pharmacokinetics | Contraindications, Pregnancy Category, and Lactation Issues |
|---|---|---|---|---|
| **Mesoridazine** *cont.* | **Psychoneurotic manifestations:** 10 mg tid; titrate to 30–150 mg/d  **Unlabeled uses:** see Acetophenazine | Drug–Drug Interactions: **increased effect:** CNS effects (alcohol); EPS effect (fluoxetine, lithium); sedation/hypotension (meperidine);  **increased level of:** TCAs, valproic acid, phenytoin (or decreased level), propranolol (also increases level of antipsychotic)  **decreased level of antipsychotic:** aluminum antacids, barbiturates, carbamazepine, charcoal  **decreased effect of antipsychotic:** anticholinergics | **Other ADRs:** arrhythmias, myocardial depression, headache, hypertension, lethargy, restlessness, weight gain, hyperactivity, breast enlargement, galactorrhea, menstrual irregularities, changes in libido, Tardive Dyskinesia (after prolonged therapy—may be irreversible); Neuroleptic Malignant Syndrome  Pharmacokinetics: $T_{1/2} = 10$–20 hrs; full therapeutic effect may not be seen for 6 weeks | Precautions: Use cautiously in patients with: seizure disorders, impaired renal or hepatic dysfunction, hyperthyroidism; do not use 48 hrs prior to myelography; do not abruptly withdraw therapy  Pregnancy/Lactation issues: Safety not established. Use only when benefits clearly outweigh risks to fetus/neonate. |
| **Perphenazine** Trilafon, various generics  Tablets: 2 mg, 4 mg, 8 mg, 16 mg  Concentrate: 16 mg/5 mL | **Psychotic Disorders:** 4–16 mg tid  **Elderly or debilitated patients:** 2–4 mg qd to bid; slowly titrate to max dose of 32 mg/d  **Pediatrics:** (>12 yrs old) 4 mg tid; slowly titrate as needed  **Unlabeled uses:** see Acetophenazine | Administration Issues: To decrease daytime sedation, the daily dose may be given as a single dose at bedtime once appropriate dose has been established. Concentrates: protect from light, dilute in juices or other liquid; titrate oral doses to patient response; once psychosis is controlled, decrease dose to lowest dose required by patient; not generally recommended for children <12 yrs old  Drug–Drug Interactions: **increased effect:** CNS effects (alcohol); | **ADRs:** Sedation: Low Anticholinergic Effects (dry mouth, constipation, urinary retention, blurred vision): Low Extrapyramidal Effects (pseudoparkinsonism, akathisia, dystonias): High Orthostatic hypotension: Low  **Other ADRs:** arrhythmias, myocardial depression, headache, | Contraindications: Hypersensitivity, comatose or severely depressed states, concomitant use of large amounts of other CNS depressants; bone marrow depression, liver damage, cerebral arteriosclerosis, coronary artery disease  Precautions: use cautiously in patients with: seizure disorders, impaired renal or hepatic disease |

| Drug | Dosage | Drug Interactions | ADRs | Contraindications/Precautions |
|---|---|---|---|---|
| **Prochlorperazine**<br>Compazine, various generics<br><br><u>Tablets:</u> 5 mg, 10 mg, 25 mg<br><br><u>Capsules sustained release:</u><br>10 mg, 15 mg, 30 mg<br><br><u>Suppositories:</u><br>2.5 mg, 5 mg, 25 mg<br><br><u>Syrup:</u> 5 mg/5 mL | **Psychotic Disorders:**<br>5–10 mg tid to qid; slowly titrate to 50–75 mg/d for less severe conditions; slowly titrate to 100–150 mg/d for more severe conditions.<br><br>**Elderly or debilitated patients:**<br>2.5–5 mg qd to bid; slowly titrate to max dose of 75 mg/d<br><br>**Pediatrics:** (2–12 yrs old) 2.5 mg bid to tid; slowly titrate to max dose of 20 mg/d (for 2–5 yrs old) or 25 mg/d (for 6–12 yrs old)<br><br>**Nonpsychotic anxiety:**<br>5 mg tid to qid; max dose is 20 mg/d; max length of therapy is 12 weeks. | <u>Administration Issues:</u><br>To decrease daytime sedation, the daily dose may be given as a single dose at bedtime once appropriate dose has been established<br><br>Titrate oral doses to patient response; once psychosis is controlled, decrease dose to lowest dose required by patient; not recommended for children <2 yrs old.<br><br><u>Drug–Drug Interactions:</u><br>**increased effect:** CNS effects (alcohol); EPS effect (fluoxetine, lithium); sedation/hypotension (meperidine)<br><br>**increased level of:** TCAs, valproic acid, phenytoin (or decreased level), propranolol (also increases level of antipsychotic) | **ADRs:**<br>Sedation: Moderate<br>Anticholinergic Effects (dry mouth, constipation, urinary retention, blurred vision): Low<br>Extrapyramidal Effects (pseudoparkinsonism, akathisia, dystonias): High<br>Orthostatic hypotension: Low<br><br>**Other ADRs:**<br>arrhythmias, myocardial depression, headache, hypertension, lethargy, restlessness, weight gain, hyperactivity, breast enlargement, galactorrhea, menstrual irregularities, changes in libido, <u>Tardive</u> | <u>Contraindications:</u><br>Hypersensitivity, comatose or severely depressed states; concomitant use of large amounts of other CNS depressants; bone marrow depression, liver damage, cerebral arteriosclerosis, coronary artery disease<br><br><u>Precautions:</u><br>Use cautiously in patients with: seizure disorders, impaired renal or hepatic dysfunction, hyperthyroidism; do not use 48 hrs prior to myelography; do not abruptly withdraw therapy |
| | | **increased level of:** TCAs, valproic acid, phenytoin (or decreased level), propranolol (also increases level of antipsychotic)<br><br>**decreased level of antipsychotic:**<br>aluminum antacids, barbiturates, carbamazepine, charcoal<br><br>**decreased effect of antipsychotic:**<br>anticholinergics | EPS effect (fluoxetine, lithium); sedation/hypotension (meperidine)<br><br>hypertension, lethargy, restlessness, weight gain, hyperactivity, breast enlargement, galactorrhea, menstrual irregularities, changes in libido, <u>Tardive Dyskinesia (after prolonged therapy—may be irreversible)</u>; <u>Neuroleptic Malignant Syndrome</u><br><br><u>Pharmacokinetics:</u><br>$T_{1/2}$ = 10–20 hrs; full therapeutic effect may not be seen for 6 weeks | dysfunction, hyperthyroidism; do not use 48 hrs prior to myelography; do not abruptly withdraw therapy<br><br><u>Pregnancy/Lactation issues:</u> safety not established. Use only when benefits clearly outweigh risks to fetus/neonate. |

(continues on next page)

**312.1 Phenothiazines** *continued from previous page*

| Drug and Dosage Forms | Usual Dosage Range | Administration Issues, Drug–Drug & Drug–Food Interactions | Common Adverse Drug Reactions (ADRs) and Pharmacokinetics | Contraindications, Pregnancy Category, and Lactation Issues |
|---|---|---|---|---|
| **Prochlorperazine cont.** | **Unlabeled uses:** see Acetophenazine | **decreased level of antipsychotic:** aluminum antacids, barbiturates, carbamazepine, charcoal <br><br> **decreased effect of antipsychotic:** anticholinergics | Dyskinesia (after prolonged therapy—may be irreversible); Neuroleptic Malignant Syndrome <br><br> Pharmacokinetics: $T_{1/2}$ = 10–20 hrs; full therapeutic effect may not be seen for 6 weeks | Pregnancy/Lactation issues: safety not established. Use only when benefits clearly outweigh risks to fetus/neonate. |
| **Promazine** <br> Sparine, various generics <br><br> Tablets: 25 mg, 50 mg, 100 mg | **Psychotic Disorders:** 10–200 mg q 4–6 h <br><br> **Elderly or debilitated patients:** 25 mg qd to bid; slowly titrate as needed. <br><br> **Pediatrics:** (>12 yrs old) 10–25 mg q 4–6 h <br><br> **Unlabeled uses:** see Acetophenazine | Administration Issues: To decrease daytime sedation, the daily dose may be given as a single dose at bedtime once appropriate dose has been established. Titrate oral doses to patient response; once psychosis is controlled, decrease dose to lowest dose required by patient; not generally recommended for children <12 yrs old <br><br> Drug–Drug Interactions: **increased effect:** CNS effects (alcohol); EPS effect (fluoxetine, lithium); sedation/ hypotension (meperidine) <br><br> **increased level of:** TCAs, valproic acid, phenytoin (or decreased level), propranolol (also increases level of antipsychotic) <br><br> **decreased level of antipsychotic:** aluminum antacids, barbiturates, carbamazepine, charcoal | **ADRs:** <br> Sedation: Moderate <br> Anticholinergic Effects (dry mouth, constipation, urinary retention, blurred vision, miosis): High <br> Extrapyramidal Effects (pseudoparkinsonism, akathisia, dystonias): Moderate <br> Orthostatic hypotension: Moderate <br><br> **Other ADRs:** <br> arrhythmias, myocardial depression, headache, hypertension, lethargy, restlessness, weight gain, hyperactivity, breast enlargement, galactorrhea, menstrual irregularities, changes in libido, Tardive Dyskinesia (after prolonged therapy—may be irreversible); Neuroleptic Malignant Syndrome | Contraindications: <br> Hypersensitivity, comatose or severely depressed states, concomitant use of large amounts of other CNS depressants; bone marrow depression, liver damage, cerebral arteriosclerosis, coronary artery disease <br><br> Precautions: <br> Use cautiously in patients with: seizure disorders, impaired renal or hepatic dysfunction, hyperthyroidism; do not use 48 hrs prior to myelography; do not abruptly withdraw therapy <br><br> Pregnancy/Lactation issues: Safety not established. Use only when benefits clearly outweigh risks to fetus/neonate. |

| Drug | Dosing | Interactions / Administration | Pharmacokinetics / ADRs | Contraindications / Precautions |
|---|---|---|---|---|
| **Thioridazine**<br>Mellaril, various generics<br><br><u>Tablets:</u> 10 mg, 15 mg, 25 mg, 50 mg, 100 mg, 150 mg, 200 mg<br><br><u>Concentrate (either alcohol or water base):</u><br>30 mg/mL, 100 mg/mL<br><br><u>Suspension:</u><br>25 mg/5 mL, 100 mg/5 mL | **Psychotic Disorders:**<br>50–100 mg tid; slowly titrate to max dose of 800 mg/d<br><br>**Elderly or debilitated patients:**<br>25 mg tid; slowly titrate to max dose of 200 mg/d<br><br>**Pediatrics:** (2–12 yrs old) 10 mg 2–3 times daily; slowly titrate to doses of 0.5–3 mg/kg/d<br><br>**Unlabeled uses:**<br>see Acetophenazine | **decreased effect of antipsychotic:** anticholinergics<br><br><u>Administration Issues:</u><br>To decrease daytime sedation, the daily dose may be given as a single dose at bedtime once appropriate dose has been established. Concentrates: protect from light, dilute in juices or other liquid. Titrate oral doses to patient response; once psychosis is controlled, decrease dose to lowest dose required by patient; not recommended for children <2 yrs old.<br><br><u>Drug–Drug Interactions:</u><br>**increased effect:** CNS effects (alcohol); EPS effect (fluoxetine, lithium); sedation/hypotension (meperidine)<br><br>**increased level of:** TCAs, valproic acid, phenytoin (or decreased level); propranolol (also increases level of antipsychotic) | <u>Pharmacokinetics:</u><br>$T_{1/2}$ = 10–20 hrs; full therapeutic effect may not be seen for 6 weeks<br><br>**ADRs:**<br><u>Sedation:</u> High<br><u>Anticholinergic Effects</u> (dry mouth, constipation, urinary retention, blurred vision): High<br><u>Extrapyramidal Effects</u> (pseudoparkinsonism, akathisia, dystonias): Low<br><u>Orthostatic hypotension:</u> Moderate | <u>Contraindications:</u><br>Hypersensitivity, comatose or severely depressed states, concomitant use of large amounts of other CNS depressants; bone marrow depression, liver damage, cerebral arteriosclerosis, coronary artery disease<br><br><u>Precautions:</u><br>Use cautiously in patients with: seizure disorders, impaired renal or hepatic dysfunction, hyperthyroidism; do not use 48 hrs prior to myelography; do not abruptly withdraw therapy<br><br><u>Pregnancy/Lactation issues:</u><br>Safety not established. Use only when benefits clearly outweigh risks to fetus/neonate. |
| **Trifluoperazine**<br>Stelazine, various generics<br><u>Tablets:</u> 1 mg, 2 mg, 5 mg, 10 mg | **Psychotic Disorders:**<br>2–5 mg bid; slowly titrate to max dose of 40 mg/d as needed | **decreased level of antipsychotic:** aluminum antacids, barbiturates, carbamazepine, charcoal<br><br>**decreased effect of antipsychotic:** anticholinergics<br><br><u>Administration Issues:</u><br>To decrease daytime sedation, the daily dose may be given as a single dose at bedtime once appropriate dose has been established | **Other ADRs:**<br>arrhythmias, myocardial depression, headache, hypertension, lethargy, restlessness, weight gain, hyperactivity, breast enlargement, galactorrhea, menstrual irregularities, changes in libido, <u>Tardive Dyskinesia (after prolonged therapy—may be irreversible)</u>; <u>Neuroleptic Malignant Syndrome</u><br><br><u>Pharmacokinetics:</u><br>$T_{1/2}$ = 10–20 hrs; full therapeutic effect may not be seen for 6 weeks<br><br>**ADRs:**<br><u>Sedation:</u> Low<br><u>Anticholinergic Effects</u> (dry mouth, constipation, urinary retention, blurred vision): Low | <u>Contraindications:</u><br>Hypersensitivity, comatose or severely depressed states, concomitant use of large amounts of other CNS depressants; bone |

(continues on next page)

| Drug and Dosage Forms | Usual Dosage Range | Administration Issues, Drug–Drug & Drug–Food Interactions | Common Adverse Drug Reactions (ADRs) and Pharmacokinetics | Contraindications, Pregnancy Category, and Lactation Issues |
|---|---|---|---|---|
| **Trifluoperazine** *cont.* <br><br> <u>Concentrate</u>: 10 mg/mL | **Elderly or debilitated patients:** 0.5–1 mg qd to bid; slowly titrate to max dose of 40 mg/d <br><br> **Pediatrics:** (6–12 yrs old –usually should be hospitalized) 1 mg qd to bid; slowly titrate to 15 mg/d as needed <br><br> **Nonpsychotic Anxiety:** 1–2 mg bid. Max dose is 6 mg/d; max length of therapy is 12 weeks. <br><br> <u>Unlabeled uses:</u> see Acetophenazine | Concentrates: protect from light, dilute in juices or other liquid. Titrate oral doses to patient response; once psychosis is controlled, decrease dose to lowest dose required by patient; not recommended for children <6 yrs old <br><br> <u>Drug–Drug Interactions:</u> **increased effect:** CNS effects (alcohol); EPS effect (fluoxetine, lithium); sedation/ hypotension (meperidine) <br><br> **increased level of:** TCAs, valproic acid, phenytoin (or decreased level), propranolol (also increases level of antipsychotic) <br><br> **decreased level of antipsychotic:** aluminum antacids, barbiturates, carbamazepine, charcoal <br><br> **decreased effect of antipsychotic:** anticholinergics | <u>Extrapyramidal Effects</u> (pseudoparkinsonism, akathisia, dystonias): High <br> <u>Orthostatic hypotension:</u> Low <br><br> **Other ADRs:** arrhythmias, myocardial depression, headache, hypertension, lethargy, restlessness, weight gain, hyperactivity, breast enlargement, galactorrhea, menstrual irregularities, changes in libido, <u>Tardive Dyskinesia</u> (after prolonged therapy—may be irreversible); Neuroleptic Malignant Syndrome <br><br> <u>Pharmacokinetics:</u> $T_{1/2}$= 10–20 hrs; full therapeutic effect may not be seen for 6 weeks | marrow depression, liver damage, cerebral arteriosclerosis, coronary artery disease <br><br> <u>Precautions:</u> Use cautiously in patients with: seizure disorders, impaired renal or hepatic dysfunction, hyperthyroidism; do not use 48 hrs prior to myelography; do not abruptly withdraw therapy <br><br> <u>Pregnancy/Lactation issues:</u> Safety not established. Use only when benefits clearly outweigh risks to fetus/neonate. |

| Drug and Dosage Forms | Usual Dosage Range | Administration Issues and Drug–Drug Interactions | Common Adverse Drug Reactions (ADRs) and Pharmacokinetics | Contraindications, Pregnancy Category, and Lactation Issues |
|---|---|---|---|---|
| **Chlorprothixene**<br>Taractan<br><br>Tablets (contain tartrazine):<br>10 mg, 25 mg, 50 mg, 100 mg<br><br>Concentrate:<br>100 mg/5 mL | **Psychotic Disorders:**<br>25–50 mg tid to qid times daily; slowly titrate to 600 mg/d as needed<br><br>**Elderly or debilitated patients:**<br>10–25 mg qd to bid; slowly titrate as needed<br><br>**Pediatrics:** (6–12 yrs old) 10–25 mg tid to qid; slowly titrate as needed.<br><br>**Unlabeled uses:**<br>Tourette's syndrome, acute agitation in elderly, symptoms of dementia (agitation, hyperactivity, hallucinations, suspiciousness, hostility) | Administration Issues:<br>To decrease daytime sedation, the daily dose may be given as a single dose at bedtime once appropriate dose has been established. Concentrates: protect from light, dilute in juices or other liquid. Titrate oral doses to patient response; once psychosis is controlled, decrease dose to lowest dose required by patient; not recommended for children <12 yrs old.<br><br>Drug–Drug Interactions:<br>**increased effect:** CNS effects (alcohol); EPS effect (fluoxetine, lithium); sedation/ hypotension (meperidine)<br><br>**increased level of:** TCAs, valproic acid, phenytoin (or decreased level), propranolol (also increases level of antipsychotic)<br><br>**decreased level of antipsychotic:** aluminum antacids, barbiturates, carbamazepine, charcoal<br><br>**decreased effect of antipsychotic:** anticholinergics | **ADRs:**<br>Sedation: High<br>Anticholinergic Effects (dry mouth, blurred vision, constipation, urinary retention): Moderate<br>Extrapyramidal Effects (pseudoparkinsonism, akathisia, dystonias): Moderate<br>Orthostatic hypotension: Moderate<br><br>**Other ADRs:**<br>arrhythmias, myocardial depression, headache, hypertension, lethargy, restlessness, weight gain, hyperactivity, breast enlargement, galactorrhea, menstrual irregularities, changes in libido, Tardive Dyskinesia (after prolonged therapy—may be irreversible), Neuroleptic Malignant Syndrome<br><br>Pharmacokinetics:<br>$T_{1/2}$ = 10–20 hrs; full therapeutic effect may not be seen for 6 weeks | Contraindications:<br>Hypersensitivity, comatose or severely depressed states, concomitant use of large amounts of other CNS depressants; bone marrow depression, liver damage, cerebral arteriosclerosis, coronary artery disease<br><br>Precautions:<br>Use cautiously in patients with: seizure disorders, impaired renal or hepatic dysfunction, hyperthyroidism; do not use 48 hrs prior to myelography; do not abruptly withdraw therapy<br><br>Pregnancy/Lactation issues:<br>Safety not established. Use only when benefits clearly outweigh risks to fetus/neonate. |

(continues on next page)

312.2 Other Typical Antipsychotics *continued from previous page*

| Drug and Dosage Forms | Usual Dosage Range | Administration Issues and Drug–Drug Interactions | Common Adverse Drug Reactions (ADRs) and Pharmacokinetics | Contraindications, Pregnancy Category, and Lactation Issues |
|---|---|---|---|---|
| **Haloperidol**<br>Haldol, Haldol Deconate, various generics<br><br><u>Tablets:</u> 0.5 mg, 1 mg, 2 mg, 5 mg, 10 mg, 20 mg<br><br><u>Concentrate:</u><br>2 mg/mL<br><br><u>Injection (deconate):</u><br>50 mg/mL, 100 mg/mL | **Psychotic Disorders:**<br>**Mild conditions, elderly or debilitated patients:**<br>0.5–2 mg bid to tid; slowly titrate to max dose of 100 mg/d as needed.<br><br>**Severe psychoses:** 3–5 mg bid to tid; slowly titrate to 100 mg/d as needed.<br><br>**Pediatrics:** (3–12 yrs old) 0.5 mg/d in 2–3 divided doses; slowly titrate as needed (range is 0.05–0.15 mg/kg/d)<br><br><u>Deconate injection (IM):</u><br>No more than 100 mg initially (equivalent to 10 mg/d oral haloperidol) q 4 weeks<br><br>**Tourette's Syndrome**<br>Pediatrics: 0.05–0.75 mg/kg/d divided bid to tid<br><br>**Hyperactive Children**<br>dose range is 0.05–0.15 mg/kg/d divided bid to tid<br><br><u>Unlabeled uses:</u><br>see Chlorprothixene<br><br>**Traumatic Brain Injury**<br>start at 0.5 mg bid | <u>Administration Issues:</u><br>To decrease daytime sedation, the daily dose may be given as a single dose at bedtime once appropriate dose has been established.<br>Concentrates: protect from light, dilute in juices or other liquid. Titrate oral doses to patient response; once psychosis is controlled, decrease dose to lowest dose required by patient; not recommended for children <3 yrs old<br><br><u>Drug–Drug Interactions:</u><br>**increased effect:** CNS effects (alcohol); EPS effect (fluoxetine, lithium); sedation/ hypotension (meperidine)<br><br>**increased level of:** TCAs, valproic acid, phenytoin (or decreased level), propranolol (also increases level of antipsychotic)<br><br>**decreased level of antipsychotic:** aluminum antacids, barbiturates, carbamazepine, charcoal<br><br>**decreased effect of antipsychotic:** anticholinergics | **Rate of most common:**<br><u>Sedation:</u> Low<br><u>Anticholinergic Effects</u> (dry mouth, blurred vision, constipation, urinary retention): Low<br><u>Extrapyramidal Effects</u> (pseudoparkinsonism, akathisia, dystonias): High<br><u>Orthostatic hypotension:</u> Low<br><br><u>**Other ADRs:**</u><br>arrhythmias, myocardial depression, headache, hypertension, lethargy, restlessness, weight gain, hyperactivity, breast enlargement, galactorrhea, menstrual irregularities, changes in libido, <u>Tardive Dyskinesia</u> (after prolonged therapy—may be irreversible); <u>Neuroleptic Malignant Syndrome</u><br><br><u>Pharmacokinetics:</u><br>$T_{1/2}$ = 24 hrs; full therapeutic effect may not be seen for 6 weeks | <u>Contraindications:</u><br>Hypersensitivity, comatose or severely depressed states, concomitant use of large amounts of other CNS depressants; bone marrow depression, liver damage, cerebral arteriosclerosis, coronary artery disease<br><br><u>Precautions:</u><br>Use cautiously in patients with: seizure disorders, impaired renal or hepatic dysfunction, hyperthyroidism; do not use 48 hrs prior to myelography; do not abruptly withdraw therapy<br><br><u>Pregnancy/Lactation issues:</u><br>Safety not established. Use only when benefits clearly outweigh risks to fetus/neonate. |

## Loxapine
Loxitane

Capsules: 5 mg, 10 mg, 25 mg, 50 mg

Concentrate:
25 mg/mL

**Psychotic Disorders:**
10 mg bid; titrate fairly rapidly over first 7–10 days until psychotic symptoms are controlled. Max dose is 250 mg/d

**Elderly or debilitated patients:**
5–10 mg 1–2 times daily; slowly titrate to max dose of 125 mg/d as needed

Unlabeled uses:
see Chlorprothixene

Administration Issues:
To decrease daytime sedation, the daily dose may be given as a single dose at bedtime once appropriate dose has been established. Concentrates: protect from light, dilute in juices or other liquid. Titrate oral doses to patient response; once psychosis is controlled, decrease dose to lowest dose required by patient; not recommended for children <16 yrs old.

Drug–Drug Interactions:

**increased effect:** CNS effects (alcohol); EPS effect (fluoxetine, lithium); sedation/ hypotension (meperidine)

**increased level of:** TCAs, valproic acid, phenytoin (or decreased level), propranolol (also increases level of antipsychotic)

**decreased level of antipsychotic:** aluminum antacids, barbiturates, carbamazepine, charcoal

**decreased effect of antipsychotic:** anticholinergics

ADRs:
Sedation: Moderate
Anticholinergic Effects
(dry mouth, blurred vision, constipation, urinary retention): Low
Extrapyramidal Effects
(pseudoparkinsonism, akathisia, dystonias): High
Orthostatic hypotension:
Moderate

**Other ADRs:**
arrhythmias, myocardial depression, headache, hypertension, lethargy, restlessness, weight gain, hyperactivity, breast enlargement, galactorrhea, menstrual irregularities, changes in libido, Tardive Dyskinesia (after prolonged therapy—may be irreversible), Neuroleptic Malignant Syndrome

Pharmacokinetics:
$T_{1/2}$ = 10–20 hrs; full therapeutic effect may not be seen for 6 weeks

Contraindications:
Hypersensitivity, comatose or severely depressed states, concomitant use of large amounts of other CNS depressants; bone marrow depression, liver damage, cerebral arteriosclerosis, coronary artery disease

Precautions:
Use cautiously in patients with: seizure disorders, impaired renal or hepatic dysfunction, hyperthyroidism; do not use 48 hrs prior to myelography; do not abruptly withdraw therapy

Pregnancy/Lactation issues:
Safety not established. Use only when benefits clearly outweigh risks to fetus/neonate.

## Molindone
Moban

Tablets: 5 mg, 10 mg, 25 mg, 50 mg, 100 mg

**Psychotic Disorders:**
50–75 mg/d; titrate to 225 mg/d as needed

Administration Issues:
To decrease daytime sedation, the daily dose may be given as a single dose at bedtime once appropriate dose has been established. Concentrates: protect from light, dilute in juices or other liquid. Titrate

ADRs:
Sedation: Low
Anticholinergic Effects (dry mouth, blurred vision, constipation, urinary retention): Low
Extrapyramidal Effects

Contraindications:
Hypersensitivity, comatose or severely depressed states, concomitant use of large amounts of other CNS depressants; bone marrow

*(continues on next page)*

| Drug and Dosage Forms | Usual Dosage Range | Administration Issues and Drug–Drug Interactions | Common Adverse Drug Reactions (ADRs) and Pharmacokinetics | Contraindications, Pregnancy Category, and Lactation Issues |
|---|---|---|---|---|
| **Molindone** *cont.*<br><br><u>Concentrate:</u><br>20 mg/mL | **Elderly or debilitated patients:**<br>5–10 mg 1–2 times daily; slowly titrate to max dose of 112 mg/d as needed.<br><br>**Unlabeled uses:**<br>see Chlorprothixene | oral doses to patient response; once psychosis is controlled, decrease dose to lowest dose required by patient; not recommended for children <12 yrs old.<br><br><u>Drug–Drug Interactions:</u><br>**increased effect:** CNS effects (alcohol); EPS effect (fluoxetine, lithium); sedation/ hypotension (meperidine)<br><br>**increased level of:** TCAs, valproic acid, phenytoin (or decreased level), propranolol (also increases level of antipsychotic)<br><br>**decreased level of antipsychotic:** aluminum antacids, barbiturates, carbamazepine, charcoal<br><br>**decreased effect of antipsychotic:** anticholinergics | (pseudoparkinsonism, akathisia, dystonias): High<br>Orthostatic hypotension: Low<br><br>**Other ADRs:**<br>arrhythmias, myocardial depression, headache, hypertension, lethargy, restlessness, weight gain, hyperactivity, breast enlargement, galactorrhea, menstrual irregularities, changes in libido, <u>Tardive Dyskinesia</u> (after prolonged therapy—may be irreversible); <u>Neuroleptic Malignant Syndrome</u><br><br><u>Pharmacokinetics:</u><br>$T_{1/2}$ = 10–20 hrs; full therapeutic effect may not be seen for 6 weeks | depression, liver damage, cerebral arteriosclerosis, coronary artery disease<br><br><u>Precautions:</u><br>Use cautiously in patients with: seizure disorders, impaired renal or hepatic dysfunction, hyperthyroidism; do not use 48 hrs prior to myelography; do not abruptly withdraw therapy<br><br><u>Pregnancy/Lactation issues:</u><br>Safety not established. Use only when benefits clearly outweigh risks to fetus/neonate |
| **Pimozide**<br>Orap<br><u>Tablets:</u> 2 mg | **Tourette's Syndrome refractory to traditional treatment:**<br>1–2 mg/d bid. Titrate dose every other day to 10 mg/d or 0.2 mg/kg (whichever is less) | <u>Administration Issues:</u><br>Perform baseline ECG and periodically through treatment. Titrate oral doses to patient response; once psychosis is controlled, decrease dose to lowest dose required by patient; efficacy/safety in <12 yrs old not established | **ADRs:**<br>Sedation: Moderate<br>Anticholinergic Effects (dry mouth, blurred vision, constipation, urinary retention): Moderate<br>Extrapyramidal Effects (pseudoparkinsonism, akathisia, | <u>Contraindications:</u><br>Hypersensitivity; treatment of simple tics or tics other than those associated with Tourette's; drug-induced tics; long QT syndrome; history of cardiac arrhythmias; severe toxic CNS depression or comatose states |

| Drug / Dosage | Administration / Drug–Drug Interactions | ADRs | Contraindications / Precautions / Pregnancy |
|---|---|---|---|
| | Drug–Drug Interactions: **increased effect (additive):** phenothiazines, TCAs or Type 1 antiarrhythmics (additive prolongation of QT interval); CNS depressants | dystonias): High<br>Orthostatic hypotension: Low<br><br>**Other ADRs:** arrhythmias, myocardial depression, headache, hypertension, lethargy, restlessness, weight gain, hyperactivity, breast enlargement, galactorrhea, menstrual irregularities, changes in libido, Tardive Dyskinesia (after prolonged therapy—may be irreversible); Neuroleptic Malignant Syndrome<br><br>Pharmacokinetics:<br>T$_{1/2}$ = 55 hrs | Pregnancy Category: C<br>Lactation Issues: Should not be used in nursing mothers |
| **Thiothixene**<br>Navane, various generics<br><br>Capsules: 1 mg, 2 mg, 5 mg, 10 mg, 20 mg<br><br>Concentrate:<br>5 mg/mL<br><br>**Psychotic Disorders:** 2 mg tid; slowly titrate to 15 mg/d as needed.<br><br>**Severe psychoses:** 5 mg bid; slowly titrate to 60 mg/d as needed<br><br>**Elderly or debilitated patients:** 1–2 mg qd to bid; slowly titrate to max dose of 30 mg/d as needed.<br><br>**Pediatrics:** (>12 yrs old) 2 mg tid; slowly titrate to 15 mg/d as needed.<br><br>**Unlabeled uses:** see Chlorprothixene | Administration Issues: To decrease daytime sedation, the daily dose may be given as a single dose at bedtime once appropriate dose has been established. Concentrates: protect from light, dilute in juices or other liquid. Titrate oral doses to patient response; once psychosis is controlled, decrease dose to lowest dose required by patient; not recommended for children <12 yrs old.<br><br>Drug–Drug Interactions:<br>**increased effect:** CNS effects (alcohol); EPS effect (fluoxetine, lithium); sedation/hypotension (meperidine)<br><br>**increased level of:** TCAs, valproic acid, phenytoin (or decreased level), | **ADRs:**<br>Sedation: Low<br>Anticholinergic Effects (dry mouth, blurred vision, constipation, urinary retention): Low<br>Extrapyramidal Effects (pseudoparkinsonism, akathisia, dystonias): High<br>Orthostatic hypotension: Low<br><br>**Other ADRs:** arrhythmias, myocardial depression, headache, hypertension, lethargy, restlessness, weight gain, hyperactivity, breast enlargement, galactorrhea, | Contraindications:<br>Hypersensitivity, comatose or severely depressed states, concomitant use of large amounts of other CNS depressants; bone marrow depression, liver damage, cerebral arteriosclerosis, coronary artery disease<br><br>Precautions:<br>Use cautiously in patients with: seizure disorders, impaired renal or hepatic dysfunction, hyperthyroidism; do not use 48 hrs prior to myelography; do not abruptly withdraw therapy |

(continues on next page)

| Drug and Dosage Forms | Usual Dosage Range | Administration Issues and Drug–Drug Interactions | Common Adverse Drug Reactions (ADRs) and Pharmacokinetics | Contraindications, Pregnancy Category, and Lactation Issues |
|---|---|---|---|---|
| **Thiothixene** *cont.* | | propranolol (also increases level of antipsychotic)<br><br>**decreased level of antipsychotic:** aluminum antacids, barbiturates, carbamazepine, charcoal<br><br>**decreased effect of antipsychotic:** anticholinergics | menstrual irregularities, changes in libido, Tardive Dyskinesia (after prolonged therapy—may be irreversible); Neuroleptic Malignant Syndrome<br><br>Pharmacokinetics:<br>$T_{1/2}$ = 10–20 hrs; full therapeutic effect may not be seen for 6 weeks | Pregnancy/Lactation issues: Safety not established. Use only when benefits clearly outweigh risks to fetus/neonate. |

312.3 Atypical Antipsychotics

| Drug and Dosage Forms | Usual Dosage Range | Administration Issues and Drug–Drug Interactions | Common Adverse Drug Reactions (ADRs) and Pharmacokinetics | Contraindications, Pregnancy Category, and Lactation Issues |
|---|---|---|---|---|
| **Clozapine** Clozaril<br><br>Tablets: 25 mg, 100 mg | **Severely Ill schizophrenia; refractory to traditional therapy:** 25 mg 1–2 times daily. Titrate by 25–50 mg/d each day as tolerated to 300–450 mg/d.<br><br>Further dosage adjustments: ≤100 mg/d, no more frequently than 1–2 times each week. Max dose is 900 mg/d | Administration Issues: Due to potential for agranulocytosis, monitor WBC and granulocyte count weekly: WBC <3500 at baseline: do not start therapy. WBC <3500 or >3500 with substantial drop after starting therapy: repeat WBC and monitor. WBC 3000–3500, granulocyte count >1500: monitor WBC twice weekly. WBC <3000 and gran <1500: stop therapy, monitor for infection, restart therapy when WBC returns to baseline. WBC <2000, gran | **ADRs:**<br>Sedation: High<br>Anticholinergic Effects (dry mouth, constipation, urinary retention, blurred vision, miosis): High<br>Extrapyramidal Effects (pseudoparkinsonism, akathisia, dystonias): Low<br>Orthostatic hypotension: High | Contraindications: Hypersensitivity; myeloproliferative disorders; history of severe granulocytopenia; concomitant administration of other bone-marrow suppressing agents; severe CNS depression or comatose states<br><br>Pregnancy Category: B |

| Drug | Dosing / Administration | ADRs / Pharmacokinetics | Contraindications / Pregnancy / Lactation |
|---|---|---|---|
| | **Traumatic Brain Injury:** Start 25 mg qd; may titrate up to 300–400 mg/d divided qd or bid | **Others ADRs:** tachycardia, hypertension, dizziness, headache, tremor, syncope, nightmares, restlessness, agitation, seizures, constipation, nausea, agranulocytosis<br><br>Pharmacokinetics: $T_{1/2}$ = 12 hrs (at steady-state dosing) | Lactation Issues: Should not be used in nursing mothers |
| | <1000: stop therapy, monitor closely, do not rechallenge. Dispense medication for 1 week at a time. Titrate oral doses to patient response; once psychosis is controlled, decrease dose to lowest dose required by patient; safety/efficacy not established for those <16 yrs old.<br><br>Drug–Drug Interactions: **increased effect (additive effects):** anticholinergics; antihypertensives; CNS agents; bone marrow suppressing agents | | |
| **Olanzapine**<br>Zyprexa<br><br>Tablets<br>5 mg, 7.5 mg, 10 mg | **Psychotic Disorders**<br>5–10 mg qd, initially. Target dose = 10 mg within several days.<br><br>**Debilitated patients**<br>starting dose = 5 mg; increase with caution<br><br>Administration Issues: Dose increases should be done at an interval of not less than 1 week, though doses >10 mg did not show an increase in efficacy. Give without regards to meals. Avoid alcohol.<br><br>Drug Interactions: olanzapine concentrations are **decreased** by carbamazepine; olanzapine may have additive effect with **antihypertensive agents** and may cause **increased CNS effects** when given with other CNS drugs and alcohol. Olanzapine may **decrease** the effectiveness of levodopa and dopamine agonists | ADRs: orthostatic hypotension, weight gain, somnolence, dizziness, headache, agitation, insomnia, rhinitis, constipation, nervousness, hostility, akathisia,<br><br>Pharmacokinetics: $T_{1/2}$ = 21–54 hrs | Contraindications: Hypersensitivity<br><br>Pregnancy Category: C<br><br>Lactation Issues: Should not be used in nursing mothers |
| **Quetiapine**<br>Seroquel<br><br>Tablets: 25 mg, 100 mg, 200 mg | **Psychotic Disorders**<br>25 mg bid, initially, with increases in increments of 25–50 mg bid or tid on the second and third day, as tolerated. Target dose range of 300–400 mg/d divided bid or tid by day 4. Further<br><br>Administration Issues: Patients should be advised of the risk of orthostatic hypotension during drug initiation and following any dose increase. Drug may cause somnolence and avoid the use of alcohol while taking this medication. | ADRs: headache, somnolence, dizziness, constipation, dry mouth, dyspepsia, postural hypotension, tachycardia, rash, asthenia | Contraindications: Hypersensitivity to drug<br><br>Pregnancy Category: C<br><br>Lactation Issues: Should not be used in nursing mothers |

(continues on next page)

| Drug and Dosage Forms | Usual Dosage Range | Administration Issues and Drug–Drug Interactions | Common Adverse Drug Reactions (ADRs) and Pharmacokinetics | Contraindications, Pregnancy Category, and Lactation Issues |
|---|---|---|---|---|
| **Quetiapine** *cont.* | dosage increments should be done at intervals of ≥2 d<br><br>**Elderly, debilitated, hepatic impairment:**<br>consider slower rate of dose escalation | Drug Interactions:<br>Phenytoin and thioridazine may increase the clearance of quetiapine. Cimetidine may **decrease** quetiapine clearance. Quetiapine may antagonize the effects of levodopa and dopamine agonists and may **decrease** clearance of lorazepam. | Pharmacokinetics<br>T$_{1/2}$ = 6 h; extensively metabolized | |
| **Risperidone**<br>Risperdal<br><br>Tablets: 1 mg, 2 mg, 3 mg, 4 mg | **Psychotic Disorders:**<br>1 mg bid initially.<br>Titrate by 1–2 mg/d every 2–3 days to target of 3 mg twice daily. Continued dose adjustments made each week. Max dose is 16 mg/d<br><br>**Elderly or debilitated patients:**<br>0.5 mg twice daily initially. Titrate by 0.5 mg twice daily every 3–5 days as tolerated. | Administration Issues:<br>Titrate oral doses to patient response; once psychosis is controlled, decrease dose to lowest dose required by patient; safety and efficacy in children is not established.<br><br>Drug–Drug Interactions:<br>**increased level of risperidone:**<br>SSRIs, quinidine, others that inhibit P450IID6<br><br>**decreased effect of:** levodopa<br><br>**decreased level of risperidone:**<br>carbamazepine | **ADRs:**<br>Sedation: Low<br>Anticholinergic Effects (dry mouth, constipation, urinary retention, blurred vision, miosis): Low<br>Extrapyramidal Effects (pseudoparkinsonism, akathisia, dystonias): Low or none<br>Orthostatic hypotension: Low<br><br>**Other ADRs:**<br>tachycardia; potential for QT prolongation and arrhythmias at high doses (12–16 mg/d), headache, agitation, anxiety, insomnia, constipation, dyspepsia, nausea/vomiting, rash, dry skin, rhinitis<br>Tardive Dyskinesia (after prolonged therapy—may be irreversible); Neuroleptic Malignant Syndrome | Contraindications:<br>Hypersensitivity<br><br>Precautions: use caution in patients with: seizure disorder. Reduce dose in patients with severe renal or hepatic dysfunction, or those predisposed to orthostatic hypotension<br><br>Pregnancy Category: C<br><br>Lactation Issues:<br>Safety is not established; women should not nurse |

Pharmacokinetics:
$T_{1/2}$ = 3 hrs (risperidone) &
21 hrs (metabolite); $T_{1/2}$ (in poor
metabolizers) = 20 hrs & 30 hrs,
respectively

## 312.4  Psychotherapeutic Combinations

| Drug and Dosage Forms | Usual Dosage Range | Administration Issues and Drug–Drug Interactions | Common Adverse Drug Reactions (ADRs) and Pharmacokinetics | Contraindications, Pregnancy Category, and Lactation Issues |
|---|---|---|---|---|
| **Chlordiazepoxide/ Amitriptyline**<br>Limbitrol DS, various generics<br><br>Tablets:<br>Chlordiazep/amitrip<br>5 mg/12.5 mg<br>10 mg/25 mg | **Moderate/severe depression associated with moderate/severe anxiety:**<br>10 mg chlordiazepoxide and 25 mg amitriptyline 3–4 times daily. May titrate to 6 times daily.<br><br>**Elderly or debilitated patients:**<br>5 mg/12.5 mg 1–2 times daily. Titrate as tolerated and as needed. | Administration Issues:<br>Once symptoms are controlled, slowly decrease dose to find lowest effective dose. Give largest dose at bedtime; in some patients, may give total daily dose at bedtime; not recommended for <6 yrs old<br><br>Drug–Drug Interactions<br>see individual agents | ADRs:<br>TCA: dry mouth, orthostatic hypotension, sedation, others Chlordiazepoxide: Drowsiness, ataxia, confusion (especially in elderly)<br><br>Dependence:  Prolonged use can lead to dependence; abrupt discontinuation can precipitate withdrawal symptoms (e.g., anxiety, flu-like illness, concentration difficulties, fatigue, anorexia, restlessness, confusion, psychosis, paranoid delusions, grand mal seizures). Withdrawal can occur after as little as 4–6 weeks of therapy.<br><br>Drug Discontinuation: gradual decrease over 4–8 weeks<br><br>Pharmacokinetics:<br>see individual agents | Contraindications:<br>Any hypersensitivity to a TCA or benzodiazepine, concomitant use of MAO inhibitors<br><br>Other Precautions:<br>Use with caution in patients with severe cardiovascular disease, seizure disorders. Patients with schizophrenia may experience worsening psychosis; patients with bipolar disorder may experience a switch to mania. Dosage reductions necessary in patients with hepatic or severe renal dysfunction.<br><br>Pregnancy Category:  D<br><br>Lactation Issues:  excreted in breast milk—women should not nurse |

(continues on next page)

## 312.4 Psychotherapeutic Combinations _continued from previous page_

| Drug and Dosage Forms | Usual Dosage Range | Administration Issues and Drug–Drug Interactions | Common Adverse Drug Reactions (ADRs) and Pharmacokinetics | Contraindications, Pregnancy Category, and Lactation Issues |
|---|---|---|---|---|
| **Perphenazine/ Amitriptyline**<br>Etrafon, Triavil, various generics<br><br>Tablets:<br>2 mg/10 mg, 2 mg/25 mg, 4 mg/10 mg, 4 mg/25 mg, 4 mg/50 mg | **Moderate/severe anxiety or agitation and depressed mood; schizophrenic patients with symptoms of depression; anxiety and depression associated with chronic physical disease; anxiety and depression that are not clearly differentiated:**<br><br>2–4 mg perphenazine with 10–50 mg amitriptyline 3–4 times daily | Administration Issues:<br>Once symptoms are controlled, slowly decrease dose to find lowest effective dose; not generally recommended for children <12 yrs old.<br><br>Drug–Drug Interactions:<br>see individual agents | ADRs:<br>Amitriptyline: dry mouth, orthostatic hypotension, sedation, others<br><br>Perphenazine:<br>Sedation, anticholinergic effects (dry mouth, constipation, urinary retention, blurred vision, miosis), extrapyramidal effects (pseudoparkinsonism, akathisia, dystonias), orthostatic hypotension, Tardive Dyskinesia (after prolonged therapy—may be irreversible); Neuroleptic Malignant Syndrome<br><br>Pharmacokinetics:<br>see individual agents | Contraindications:<br>Any hypersensitivity to a TCA or perphenazine, concomitant use of MAO inhibitors, comatose or severely depressed states, concomitant use of large amounts of other CNS depressants; bone marrow depression, liver damage, cerebral arteriosclerosis, coronary artery disease<br><br>Precautions:<br>Use with caution in patients with severe cardiovascular disease, seizure disorders, hyperthyroidism. Dosage reductions necessary in patients with hepatic or severe renal dysfunction. Do not use 48 hrs prior to myelography; do not abruptly withdraw therapy<br><br>Pregnancy issues:<br>Safety not established. Use only when benefits clearly outweigh risks to fetus/neonate.<br><br>Lactation issues:<br>TCA's are excreted into breast milk. Use with caution in nursing mothers. |

## 313. Miscellaneous Psychotherapeutic Agents

| Drug and Dosage Forms | Usual Dosage Range | Administration Issues and Drug–Drug Interactions | Common Adverse Drug Reactions (ADRs) and Pharmacokinetics | Contraindications, Pregnancy Category, and Lactation Issues |
|---|---|---|---|---|
| **Lithium**<br><br>Eskalith, Lithane, Lithotabs, Lithobid, Eskalith CR, Cibalith-S, various generics<br><br>Tablets: 300 mg (8.12 mEq lithium)<br><br>Capsules: 150 mg (4.06 mEq Li), 300 mg (8.12 mEq Li), 600 mg (16.24 mEq Li)<br><br>Tablets, slow release or controlled release: 300 mg (8.12 mEq Li), 450 mg (12.18 mEq Li)<br><br>Syrup: 300 mg/5 mL (8.12 mEq Li) | **Acute Manic Episodes:** 600 mg tid or 900 mg bid of the extended release form or until reach target serum levels of 0.8 to 1.4 mg/L<br><br>**Maintenance Therapy:** 300 mg tid to qid or until reach target serum levels of 0.4 to 1.0 mg/L<br><br>**Elderly patients:** 300 mg bid. Titrate by 300 mg/d each week until reach target clinical and/or serum level<br><br>**Renal impairment:**<br>CrCl=10–50 mL/min: give 50–75% of dose<br>CrCl<10 mL/min: give 25–50% of dose. Monitor levels closely<br><br>**Unlabeled uses:** improves neutrophil count in cancer-chemotherapy induced neutropenia and in AIDS patients taking zidovudine; prophylaxis of cluster headaches, premenstrual tension, bulimia, alcoholism, SIADH, tardive dyskinesia, hyperthyroidism, postpartum affective psychosis, corticosteroid-induced psychosis.<br><br>**Traumatic Brain Injury**<br>start 300 mg qd to bid; monitor levels | Administration Issues: Give with food to decrease GI upset. Drink 8–12 glasses of water while taking medication and maintain normal diet (including sodium). Draw serum levels 8–12 hours after the last dose at steady-state (reached in 5–7 days). Evaluate clinical response when interpreting serum levels; do not rely on serum levels alone; safety/efficacy not established in children <12 yrs old<br><br>Other Monitoring Parameters:<br>Serum levels, electrolytes, renal function, hydration status<br><br>Drug–Drug Interactions:<br>**decreased Li levels:** Acetazolamide, urinary alkalinizers, osmotic diuretics<br><br>**increased Li levels:** Fluoxetine, loop & thiazide diuretics, NSAIDs<br><br>**increased Li toxicity/effect:** Carbamazepine, haloperidol, methyldopa.<br><br>**Li increases the effect of:** tricyclic antidepressants, iodide salts, neuromuscular blocking agents<br><br>**Li decreased the effect of:** sympathomimetics. | **Dose related adverse effects are decreased when serum levels are maintained less than 1.5 mEq/L. Mild to moderate toxicity may occur at levels of 1.5–2.5 mEq/L; moderate to severe reactions may occur at levels >2 mEq/L**<br><br>ADRs: Fine hand tremor, polyuria, mild thirst, and nausea can occur during initial therapy but may persist throughout treatment.<br><br>Others ADRs: hypotension, arrhythmias, headache, blackouts, seizures, slurred speech, dizziness, drowsiness, blurred vision, cog wheel rigidity, impaired cognition, hallucinations, anorexia, nausea, vomiting, diarrhea, dry mouth, dehydration, impotence, oliguria, glycosuria, albuminuria, polyuria, symptoms of nephrogenic diabetes, euthyroid goiter or hypothyroidism | Contraindications: None<br><br>Precautions/Warnings:<br>Lithium toxicity is increased in patients with significant renal or cardiovascular disease, severe debilitation, dehydration or sodium depletion or in patients receiving diuretics. Monitor patients closely<br><br>Pregnancy Category: D<br><br>Lactation Issues:<br>40% of Li dose is excreted in breast milk. Patients should not nurse while taking Lithium |

*(continues on next page)*

1221

| Drug and Dosage Forms | Usual Dosage Range | Administration Issues and Drug–Drug Interactions | Common Adverse Drug Reactions (ADRs) and Pharmacokinetics | Contraindications, Pregnancy Category, and Lactation Issues |
|---|---|---|---|---|
| **Lithium** *cont.* | | | Overdose: **Levels <2mEq/L:** diarrhea, vomiting, nausea, drowsiness, muscular weakness, lack of coordination. **Levels 2–3mEq/L:** giddiness, ataxia, blurred vision, tinnitus, vertigo, confusion, slurred speech, blackouts, muscle twitching of entire limbs, agitation **Levels >3mEq/L:** seizures, arrhythmias, hypotension, peripheral vascular collapse, stupor, muscle twitching, spasticity, coma<br><br>Pharmacokinetics:<br>$T_{1/2}$ = 24 hrs (range 17–36 hrs); onset of action 5 to 14 days; sodium and lithium compete for reabsorption in the kidney—sodium depletion will make kidney reabsorb lithium causing lithium levels to rise. | |
| **Methylphenidate (CII)** Ritalin, various generics<br><br>Tablets: 5 mg, 10 mg, 20 mg<br><br>Sustained-release tablets: 20 mg | **Attention Deficit Disorder or Narcolepsy:**<br>**Adults:** 10 mg bid to tid<br>Titrate to range of 10–60 mg/d as needed by patient | Administration Issues:<br>Give medication before breakfast and lunch (30–45 minutes prior to meals). Discontinue medication occasionally to assess need for continued therapy; safety/efficacy in <6 yrs old not established | ADRs:<br>nervousness, insomnia, dizziness, headache, dyskinesia, tachycardia, palpitations, hyper- or hypotension, anorexia, nausea, weight loss | Contraindications:<br>Hypersensitivity; glaucoma; marked anxiety, tension, or agitation; motor tics or family history or diagnosis of Tourette's Syndrome |

| | Dosing / Uses | Drug–Drug Interactions | ADRs / Pharmacokinetics | Pregnancy / Lactation |
|---|---|---|---|---|
| | **Pediatrics:** 5 mg bid. Titrate by 5–10 mg/d each week as needed and tolerated. Max dose is 60 mg/d<br><br>Sustained release: May use when dose for 8 hours is established using regular release tablets.<br><br>**Unlabeled uses:** treatment of depression in elderly, cancer, and post-stroke patients<br><br>**Traumatic Brain Injury**<br>5–15 mg up to 4 times/d (60 mg/d max) | Drug–Drug Interactions:<br>**increases effect of methylphenidate:** monoamine oxidase inhibitors (headache, hypertension, nausea, etc)<br><br>**decreased effect of:** guanethidine | ADRs Common among Pediatrics:<br>anorexia, weight loss, insomnia, tachycardia. Other effects may occur (listed above).<br><br>Drug dependence: chronic use/abuse can lead to drug dependence. Carefully supervise withdrawal of medication.<br><br>Pharmacokinetics:<br>$T_{1/2}$ = 1–3 h (pharmacological effect is 4–6 h) | Pregnancy Category:<br>Use only when benefits far outweigh risks to fetus<br><br>Lactation Issues:<br>methylphenidate is excreted in breast milk; safety not established |
| **Pemoline (CIV)**<br>Cylert<br><br>Tablets: 18.75 mg, 37.5 mg, 75 mg<br><br>Chewable tablets: 37.5 mg | **Attention Deficit Disorder**<br>37.5 mg/d each morning. Titrate each week by 18.75 mg/d as needed. Max dose is 112.5 mg/d<br><br>**Unlabeled use:** 50–200 mg used for narcolepsy and excessive daytime sleepiness | Administration Issues:<br>Interrupt therapy occasionally to assess need for continued therapy. Gradual onset of action—full clinical benefit may not be seen for 3–4 weeks; safety/efficacy in <6 yrs old not established<br><br>Drug–Drug Interactions: None | ADRs:<br>Insomnia, headache, dizziness, dyskinetic movements, abnormal oculomotor function, anorexia, nausea, asymptomatic elevated LFTs, hepatitis, jaundice, rash, growth suppression with prolonged use<br><br>Drug dependence: chronic use/abuse can lead to drug dependence. Carefully supervise withdrawal of medication.<br><br>Pharmacokinetics:<br>$T_{1/2}$ = 7–12 hrs. | Contraindications:<br>Hypersensitivity; hepatic insufficiency. Use cautiously in renal insufficiency<br><br>Pregnancy Category: B<br><br>Lactation Issues:<br>Safety not established. Use cautiously |

| Drug and Dosage Forms | Usual Dosage Range | Administration Issues and Drug–Drug Interactions | Common Adverse Drug Reactions (ADRs) and Pharmacokinetics | Contraindications, Pregnancy Category, and Lactation Issues |
|---|---|---|---|---|
| **Baclofen**<br>Lioresal, various generics<br><br>Tablets: 10 mg, 20 mg | **Spasticity resulting from multiple sclerosis (flexor spasms, clonus, muscular rigidity):**<br>5 mg tid for 3 days; 10 mg tid for 3 days; 15 mg tid for 3 days; 20 mg tid for 3 days. May further titrate but do not exceed 80 mg/d<br><br>**Elderly or debilitated patients:**<br>5 mg 2–3 times daily. Titrate as needed/tolerated<br><br>**Unlabeled uses:** 40 mg/d for tic douloureux or tardive dyskinesia | Administration Issues:<br>Avoid alcohol use; safety/efficacy not established in those <12 yrs old<br><br>Drug–Drug Interactions:<br>**increased effect of:** alcohol, other CNS depressants | ADRs:<br>drowsiness, depression, excitement, euphoria, hallucinations, tinnitus, ataxia, nystagmus, diplopia, dry mouth, anorexia, taste disorder, diarrhea, urinary retention, dysuria, impotence, rash, edema, weight gain, increased perspiration, elevated blood sugar, elevated AST<br><br>Pharmacokinetics:<br>absorption may be dose-dependent (may decrease with increasing doses);<br>$T_{1/2}$ = 3–4 hrs | Contraindications:<br>Hypersensitivity; skeletal muscle spasm resulting from rheumatic disorders, stroke, cerebral palsy, or Parkinson's disease.<br><br>Precautions: taper drug upon discontinuation to decrease risk of withdrawal symptoms (hallucinations, psychosis); use cautiously in those with seizure disorders, psychotic disorders, autonomic dysreflexia<br><br>Pregnancy Category: C<br><br>Lactation Issues: may be excreted in breast milk. Use cautiously. |
| **Carisoprodol**<br>Soma, various generics<br><br>Tablets: 350 mg | **As an adjunct to rest, physical therapy and other measures for the relief of discomfort associated with acute, painful musculoskeletal conditions:**<br><br>350 mg 3–4 times a day. Take last dose at bedtime. | Administration Issues: may take with food; not recommended for children <12 yrs old.<br><br>Drug–Drug Interactions:<br>None known | ADRs:<br>drowsiness, dizziness, vertigo, ataxia, tremor, agitation, irritability, headache, insomnia, syncope, depression, tachycardia, postural hypotension, flushing, nausea, vomiting, hiccoughs, epigastric distress, allergic reactions, rash, erythema | Contraindications:<br>Hypersensitivity to this or meprobamate; acute intermittent porphyria<br><br>Precautions: Use cautiously in patients with severe renal or hepatic dysfunction. |

| Drug | Indications/Dose | Administration/Interactions | ADRs/Pharmacokinetics | Contraindications/Precautions |
|---|---|---|---|---|
| **Chlorphenesin Carbamate**<br>Maolate<br><br>Tablets: 400 mg | **As an adjunct to rest, physical therapy and other measures for the relief of discomfort associated with acute, painful musculoskeletal conditions:**<br>800 mg tid. Maintenance dose: 400 mg qid. Not recommended for use longer than 8 weeks. | Administration Issues: May take with food. Safety not established in children.<br><br>Drug–Drug Interactions: **increased effect of:** alcohol, other CNS depressants | multiforme, cross reaction with meprobamate<br><br>Pharmacokinetics: onset of action = 30 min; duration of action = 4–6 hrs | Pregnancy/lactation issues: safety not established. Use cautiously. It is excreted in breast milk. |
| **Chlorzoxazone**<br>Paraflex, Remular-S, Parafon Forte DSC, various generics<br><br>Tablets: 250 mg, 500 mg<br>Caplets: 250 mg, 500 mg | **As an adjunct to rest, physical therapy and other measures for the relief of discomfort associated with acute, painful musculoskeletal conditions:**<br>250 mg 3–4 times daily. May increase to 500 mg 3–4 times daily or 750 mg 3–4 times daily. | Administration Issues: May take with food. Avoid alcohol or other CNS depressants.<br><br>Drug–Drug Interactions: **increased effect of:** alcohol, other CNS depressants | ADRs: drowsiness, dizziness, confusion, nervousness, headache, insomnia, stimulation, nausea, epigastric distress, hypersensitivity reactions, leukopenia, thrombocytopenia, agranulocytosis, pancytopenia<br><br>Pharmacokinetics: rapidly absorbed; $T_{1/2}$ = 3.5 hrs | Contraindications: Hypersensitivity<br><br>Precautions: Use cautiously in patients with severe hepatic dysfunction; not recommended for use longer than 8 weeks<br><br>Pregnancy/lactation issues: safety not established. Use cautiously or not at all. |
| **Cyclobenzaprine**<br>Flexeril, various generics<br><br>Tablets: 10 mg | **As an adjunct to rest, physical therapy and other measures for the relief of discomfort associated with acute, painful musculoskeletal conditions:** | Administration Issues: Avoid alcohol or other CNS depressants; safety/efficacy in children <15 yrs old not established. | ADRs: drowsiness, dizziness, lightheadedness, malaise, overstimulation, minor GI upset, rash, hypersensitivity reactions, liver toxicity (drug-induced hepatitis), urine discoloration<br><br>Pharmacokinetics: onset = 1 hr; duration of action = 3–4 h<br><br>ADRs: drowsiness, dizziness, fatigue, tiredness, asthenia, blurred vision, headache, nervousness, convulsions, | Contraindications: Hypersensitivity<br><br>Precautions: Use cautiously in patients with hepatic dysfunction; if signs of liver toxicity are observed; discontinue use<br><br>Pregnancy/lactation issues: safety not established.<br><br>Contraindications: Hypersensitivity; concomitant use of MAO inhibitors; acute recovery phase of myocardial infarction, other cardiac |

(continues on next page)

## 314. Skeletal Muscle Relaxants *continued from previous page*

| Drug and Dosage Forms | Usual Dosage Range | Administration Issues and Drug–Drug Interactions | Common Adverse Drug Reactions (ADRs) and Pharmacokinetics | Contraindications, Pregnancy Category, and Lactation Issues |
|---|---|---|---|---|
| **Cyclobenzaprine** *cont.* | 10 mg tid. Do not exceed 60 mg/d. Do not give for longer than 2–3 weeks.<br><br>**Unlabeled Use:** 10–40 mg/d useful adjunct in fibrositis syndrome | Drug–Drug Interactions:<br>**increased levels/effects of:** anticholinergics, barbiturates (CNS effects), clonidine (hypertensive crisis), oral anticoagulants<br><br>**decreased levels/effects of:** guanethidine, levodopa<br><br>**increased levels/effects of cyclobenzaprine:** cimetidine, fluoxetine, oral contraceptives, phenothiazines<br><br>**decreased levels/effects of cyclobenzaprine:** barbiturates (drug levels), charcoal, smoking | ataxia, vertigo, dysarthria, tremors, decreased/increased libido, extrapyramidal reactions, tachycardia, vasodilatation, hypotension, dry mouth, nausea, constipation, dyspepsia, vomiting, anorexia, gastritis, urinary retention, impotence, gynecomastia, hepatitis, jaundice, rash, photosensitivity<br><br>Pharmacokinetics:<br>onset of action = 1 hr; duration of 12–24 hrs; $T_{1/2}$ = 1–3 days | problems (CHF, arrhythmias, heart block); hyperthyroidism<br><br>Precautions: Use cautiously in patients with urinary retention, angle-closure glaucoma, intraocular pressure; use only for short (2–3 weeks) periods of time<br><br>Pregnancy Category: B<br><br>Lactation Issues: Not known if excreted in breast milk. Use cautiously. |
| **Dantrolene Sodium**<br>Dantrium<br><br>Capsules: 25 mg, 50 mg, 100 mg | **Spasticity from upper motor neuron disorders (e.g., spinal cord injury, stroke, cerebral palsy, multiple sclerosis):** 25 mg once daily, initially. Titrate by 25 mg/d up to 100 mg 2–4 times daily every 4–7 days as needed/tolerated.<br><br>**Pediatrics:** 0.5 mg/kg bid. Titrate by 0.5 mg/kg/d up to 3 mg/kg 2–4 times daily if needed. Do not exceed 100 mg 4 times daily. | Administration Issues: Avoid alcohol or CNS depressant use. Safety/efficacy not established in those <5 yrs old.<br><br>Drug–Drug Interactions:<br>**increased effect/levels of dantrolene:** estrogens (potential for hepatotoxicity)<br><br>**decreased effect/levels of dantrolene:** clofibrate, warfarin | ADRs:<br>drowsiness, dizziness, diarrhea, tachycardia, weakness, general malaise, fatigue<br><br>Pharmacokinetics<br>incomplete absorption; $T_{1/2}$ = 9 hrs | Contraindications:<br>Hypersensitivity, active hepatic disease, where spasticity is utilized to sustain upright posture and balance in locomotion or to obtain or maintain increased function, treatment of skeletal muscle spasm resulting from rheumatic disorders<br><br>Precautions: Use cautiously in patients with impaired |

(continues on next page)

| Drug | Indications / Dosing | Administration / Interactions | ADRs | Contraindications / Pregnancy |
|---|---|---|---|---|
| **Diazepam (CIV)**<br>Valium, Valrelease, Zetran, various generics<br><br>Tablets: 2 mg, 5 mg, 10 mg<br><br>Capsule sustained release: 15 mg<br><br>Oral Solution: 1 mg/mL, 5 mg/mL | **As an adjunct to rest, physical therapy and other measures for the relief of discomfort associated with acute, painful musculoskeletal conditions:**<br>2–10 mg 3–4 times daily. 15–30 mg daily of the sustained release product<br><br>**Elderly or debilitated patients:**<br>2–2.5 mg 1–2 times daily. Titrate as needed/tolerated<br><br>**Pediatrics (>6 months old):**<br>1–2.5 mg 3–4 times daily. Titrate as needed/tolerated | **increased effect/levels of:** verapamil, alcohol, CNS depressants<br><br>Administration Issues:<br>Do not crush or chew sustained release products. Concentrated solution (5 mg/mL) should be diluted in liquid or semi-solid foods; not recommended for <6 mos old.<br><br>Drug–Drug Interactions:<br>**increased level of BZ:** cimetidine, oral contraceptives, disulfiram, fluoxetine, isoniazid, ketoconazole, metoprolol, propoxyphene, propranolol, valproic acid.<br><br>**increased CNS effects:** alcohol, barbiturates, narcotics<br><br>**increased levels of:** digoxin, phenytoin (possibly)<br><br>**decreased level or effect of BZ:** rifampin (decreased level); theophylline (decreased effect) | ADRs:<br>drowsiness, ataxia, confusion (especially in elderly)<br><br>Dependence: prolonged use can lead to dependence; abrupt discontinuation can precipitate withdrawal symptoms (anxiety, flu-like illness, concentration difficulties, fatigue, anorexia, restlessness, confusion, psychosis, paranoid delusions, grand mal seizures). Withdrawal can occur after as little as 4–6 weeks of therapy. Clonidine, propranolol, carbamazepine have been used as adjuncts in withdrawal.<br><br>Drug Discontinuation: gradual decrease over 4–8 weeks<br><br>Pharmacokinetics:<br>$T_{1/2}$ = 20–80 hrs; speed of onset = very fast | pulmonary, cardiac, or hepatic function.<br><br>Pregnancy/Lactation Issues: safety not established<br><br>Contraindications:<br>Hypersensitivity, psychoses, acute narrow-angle glaucoma<br><br>Pregnancy Category: D<br><br>Lactation Issues: excreted in breast milk—do not give to nursing mothers |
| **Metaxalone**<br>Skelaxin<br><br>Tablets: 400 mg | **As an adjunct to rest, physical therapy and other measures for the relief of discomfort associated with acute, painful** | Administration Issues:<br>Avoid alcohol or CNS depressants; Safety/efficacy not established for those <12 yrs old | ADRs:<br>drowsiness, dizziness, headache, nervousness, irritability, nausea, vomiting, | Contraindications:<br>Hypersensitivity; drug-induced hemolytic or other anemias; |

## 314. Skeletal Muscle Relaxants *continued from previous page*

| Drug and Dosage Forms | Usual Dosage Range | Administration Issues and Drug–Drug Interactions | Common Adverse Drug Reactions (ADRs) and Pharmacokinetics | Contraindications, Pregnancy Category, and Lactation Issues |
|---|---|---|---|---|
| **Metaxalone** *cont.* | **musculoskeletal conditions:** 800 mg 3–4 times daily | Drug–Drug Interactions: **increased effect of:** alcohol or other CNS depressants | hypersensitivity (rash); leukopenia, hemolytic anemia, jaundice<br><br>Pharmacokinetics: onset = 1 hr; duration = 4–6 hrs; $T_{1/2}$ = 2–3 h | severe renal or hepatic dysfunction<br><br>Pregnancy/lactation Issues: Safety has not been established; use cautiously if at all. |
| **Methocarbamol**<br>Robaxin, various generics<br><br>Tablets: 500 mg, 750 mg | **As an adjunct to rest, physical therapy and other measures for the relief of discomfort associated with acute, painful musculoskeletal conditions:** 1.5 g qid, initially (first 48–72 hrs). Maintenance doses include: 1 g qid or 750 mg q 4 h | Administration Issues: Avoid alcohol or CNS depressants; safety/efficacy not established in those <12 yrs old.<br><br>Drug–Drug Interactions: **increased effect of:** alcohol or other CNS depressants | ADRs: lightheadedness, dizziness, drowsiness, headache, blurred vision, nausea, fever, rash, conjunctivitis, urticaria, pruritis, urine discoloration (brown, black, green)<br><br>Pharmacokinetics: onset of action = 30 min; $T_{1/2}$ = 1–2 h | Contraindications: Hypersensitivity<br><br>Pregnancy/lactation Issues: safety not established. Use cautiously if at all. |
| **Orphenadrine Citrate**<br>Norflex, various generics<br><br>Tablets: 100 mg<br><br>Tablets, sustained release: 100 mg | **As an adjunct to rest, physical therapy and other measures for the relief of discomfort associated with acute, painful musculoskeletal conditions:** 100 mg bid<br><br>**Unlabeled Use:** 100 mg at bedtime is useful for quinine-resistant leg cramps | Administration Issues: Do not crush or chew sustained release preparations; safety/efficacy not established for children.<br><br>Drug–Drug Interactions: **increased effects of orphenadrine:** amantadine (increased anticholinergic effects) | ADRs: dry mouth, tachycardia, constipation, urinary hesitancy, blurred vision, weakness, headache, dizziness, agitation, tremor, drowsiness, confusion, nausea, vomiting, urticaria | Contraindications: Hypersensitivity; glaucoma; pyloric/duodenal obstruction; peptic ulcers; prostatic hypertrophy; bladder obstruction; cardiospasm; myasthenia gravis.<br><br>Precautions: Use cautiously in those with cardiac disease. |

|  |  | increased effects of: haloperidol (tardive dyskinesia)<br><br>decreased effects of: phenothiazines, haloperidol | Pharmacokinetics: duration of action is 4–6 hrs; $T_{1/2}$ = 2–25 hrs | Long-term safety has not been established.<br><br>Pregnancy Category: C<br><br>Lactation Issues: Use cautiously, unknown if excreted in breast milk. |

## 314.1 Skeletal Muscle Relaxant Combinations

| Drug and Dosage Forms | Usual Dosage Range | Administration Issues and Drug–Drug Interactions | Common Adverse Drug Reactions (ADRs) and Pharmacokinetics | Contraindications, Pregnancy Category, and Lactation Issues |
|---|---|---|---|---|
| **Methocarbamol/ Aspirin**<br>Robaxisal, various generics<br><br>Tablets:<br>400 mg/325 mg | **Adjunct to rest, physical therapy, and other therapy for relief of discomfort associated with acute, painful musculoskeletal conditions:**<br>2 tabs 4 times daily | Administration Issues:<br>Take with food. Avoid alcohol or CNS depressants. Safety/efficacy not established in those <12 yrs old. Aspirin use in children with fever has been associated with Reye's syndrome.<br><br>Drug–Drug Interactions:<br>see individual agents | ADRs:<br>Methocarbamol<br>lightheadedness, dizziness, drowsiness, headache, blurred vision, nausea, fever, rash, conjunctivitis, urticaria, pruritis, urine discoloration (brown, black, green)<br><br>Aspirin:<br>nausea, dyspepsia, heartburn, GI bleeding, hives, rash, prolonged bleeding time, thrombocytopenia, aspirin intolerance (bronchospasm, rhinitis), "Salicylism": dizziness, tinnitus, difficulty hearing, nausea, vomiting, diarrhea, | Contraindications:<br>Hypersensitivity<br>Aspirin: hemophilia, bleeding ulcers, hemorrhagic states<br><br>Precautions:<br>Aspirin: Use cautiously in patients with asthma, nasal polyposis, chronic urticaria (inc risk of hypersensitivity); chronic renal insufficiency, PUD, bleeding disorders.<br><br>Pregnancy/lactation Issues:<br>safety not established. Use cautiously if at all.<br><br>Aspirin: Category D |

*(continues on next page)*

| Drug and Dosage Forms | Usual Dosage Range | Administration Issues and Drug–Drug Interactions | Common Adverse Drug Reactions (ADRs) and Pharmacokinetics | Contraindications, Pregnancy Category, and Lactation Issues |
|---|---|---|---|---|
| **Methocarbamol/ Aspirin** *cont.* | | | confusion, CNS depression, headache, sweating, hyperventilation, lassitude<br><br>Pharmacokinetics:<br>see individual agents | |
| **Carisoprodol/Aspirin**<br>Sodol Compound, Soma Compound, various generics<br><br>Tablets:<br>200 mg/325 mg | **Adjunct to rest, physical therapy, and other therapy for relief of discomfort associated with acute, painful musculoskeletal conditions:**<br>1–2 tabs 4 times daily | Administration Issues:<br>Take with food. Not recommended for children <12 yrs old. Aspirin use in children with fever has been associated with Reye's syndrome<br><br>Drug–Drug Interactions:<br>see individual agents | ADRs:<br>Carisoprodol<br>drowsiness, dizziness, vertigo, ataxia, tremor, agitation, irritability, headache, insomnia, syncope, depression, tachycardia, postural hypotension, flushing, nausea, vomiting, hiccoughs, epigastric distress, allergic reactions, rash, erythema multiforme, cross reaction with meprobamate<br><br>Aspirin:<br>nausea, dyspepsia, heartburn, GI bleeding, hives, rash, prolonged bleeding time, thrombocytopenia, aspirin intolerance (bronchospasm, rhinitis), "Salicylism": dizziness, tinnitus, difficulty hearing, nausea, vomiting, | Contraindications:<br>Hypersensitivity to this or meprobamate; acute intermittent porphyria<br>Aspirin: hemophilia, bleeding ulcers, hemorrhagic states<br><br>Precautions: Use cautiously in patients with severe renal or hepatic dysfunction. Aspirin: Use cautiously in patients with asthma, nasal polyposis, chronic urticaria (inc risk of hypersensitivity); chronic renal insufficiency; PUD, bleeding disorders.<br><br>Pregnancy/lactation issues:<br>safety not established. Use cautiously. It is excreted in breast milk.<br><br>Aspirin: Category D |

|  | | | | | |
|---|---|---|---|---|---|
| **Carisoprodol/ Aspirin/Codeine** Soma Compound w/ Codeine _Tablets:_ 200 mg/325 mg/16 mg | **Adjunct to rest, physical therapy, and other therapy for relief of discomfort associated with acute, painful musculoskeletal conditions:** 1–2 tabs 4 times daily | Administration Issues: Take with food; Carisoprodol not recommended for children <12 yrs old. Aspirin use in children with fever has been associated with Reye's syndrome. Drug–Drug Interactions: see individual agents | ADRs: Carisoprodol: ataxia, tremor, agitation, irritability, headache, insomnia, syncope, depression, tachycardia, postural hypotension, flushing, nausea, vomiting, hiccoughs, epigastric distress, allergic reactions, rash, erythema multiforme, cross reaction with meprobamate Codeine: lightheadedness, dizziness, sedation, nausea, vomiting, sweating, constipation, drowsiness Aspirin: nausea, dyspepsia, heartburn, GI bleeding, hives, rash, prolonged bleeding time, thrombocytopenia, aspirin intolerance (bronchospasm, rhinitis), "Salicylism": dizziness, tinnitus, difficulty hearing, nausea, vomiting, diarrhea, confusion, CNS depression, headache, sweating, hyperventilation, lassitude Pharmacokinetics: see individual agents | Contraindications: Hypersensitivity to any ingredients or meprobamate; acute intermittent porphyria Codeine: diarrhea caused by poisoning, acute bronchial asthma, upper airway obstruction Aspirin: hemophilia, bleeding ulcers, hemorrhagic states Precautions: Use cautiously in patients with severe renal or hepatic dysfunction. Codeine: Use cautiously in patients with acute abdominal conditions, in elderly or debilitated patients, patients with respiratory conditions, cardiovascular or seizure disorders, hypothyroidism, Addisons Disease, acute alcoholism, prostatic hypertrophy. Narcotics can lead to physical dependence when used for prolonged periods of time; withdrawal symptoms can occur following abrupt withdrawal. |

(continues on next page)

| Drug and Dosage Forms | Usual Dosage Range | Administration Issues and Drug–Drug Interactions | Common Adverse Drug Reactions (ADRs) and Pharmacokinetics | Contraindications, Pregnancy Category, and Lactation Issues |
|---|---|---|---|---|
| **Carisoprodol/ Aspirin/Codeine** *cont.* | | | depression, headache, sweating, hyperventilation, lassitude<br><br>Pharmacokinetics:<br>see individual agents | Aspirin: Use cautiously in patients with asthma, nasal polyposis, chronic urticaria (inc risk of hypersensitivity); chronic renal insufficiency, PUD, bleeding disorders.<br><br>Pregnancy/lactation issues: safety not established. Use cautiously. It is excreted in breast milk.<br>Codeine: Category C<br>Aspirin: Category D |
| **Chlorzoxazone/ Acetaminophen**<br>Chlorofon-F, Chlorzone Forte, Pargen Fortified, Flexaphen, Lobac, Mus-Lax, Skelex, various generics<br><br>Tablets:<br>250 mg/300 mg | **Adjunct to rest, physical therapy, and other therapy for relief of discomfort associated with acute, painful musculoskeletal conditions:**<br>2 tabs 4 times daily | Administration Issues: May take with food. Avoid alcohol or other CNS depressants.<br><br>Drug–Drug Interactions:<br>see individual agents | ADRs:<br>Chlorzoxazone:<br>drowsiness, dizziness, lightheadedness, malaise, overstimulation, minor GI upset, rash, hypersensitivity reactions, liver toxicity (drug-induced hepatitis), urine discoloration<br><br>Acetaminophen:<br>Very few adverse reactions<br><br>Pharmacokinetics:<br>see individual agents | Contraindications:<br>Hypersensitivity<br><br>Precautions: Use cautiously in patients with hepatic dysfunction; if signs of liver toxicity are observed; discontinue use<br><br>Pregnancy/lactation issues:<br>safety not established. |

# Orphenadrine citrate/Aspirin/Caffeine

Orphengesic, Norgesic, Orphengesic Forte, Norgesic Forte

**Tablets:**
25 mg/385 mg/30 mg
50 mg/770 mg/60 mg

**Adjunct to rest, physical therapy, and other therapy for relief of discomfort associated with acute, painful musculoskeletal conditions:**

1–2 tabs 3–4 times daily (of the smaller dose); ½–1 tab 3–4 times daily (of the larger dose)

---

Administration Issues: Do not crush or chew sustained release preparations. Safety/efficacy not established for children. Use not recommended. Aspirin use in children with fever has been associated with Reye's syndrome.

Drug–Drug Interactions:
Caffeine:
**decreased effect/levels of caffeine:**
smoking

**increased effect/levels of caffeine:**
cimetidine, oral contraceptives, disulfiram, fluoroquinolones

Aspirin and Orphenadrine
see individual agents

---

ADRs:
Orphenadrine:
dry mouth, tachycardia, constipation, urinary hesitancy, blurred vision, weakness, headache, dizziness, agitation, tremor, drowsiness, confusion, nausea, vomiting, urticaria

Caffeine:
insomnia, restlessness, excitement, nervousness, tremor, headaches, anxiety, nausea, vomiting, diarrhea, tachycardia, palpitations, diuresis; withdrawal headaches after abrupt discontinuation (500–600 mg/d of caffeine)

Aspirin:
nausea, dyspepsia, heartburn, GI bleeding, hives, rash, prolonged bleeding time, thrombocytopenia, aspirin intolerance (bronchospasm, rhinitis)

"Salicylism":
dizziness, tinnitus, difficulty hearing, nausea, vomiting, diarrhea, confusion, CNS depression, headache, sweating, hyperventilation, lassitude

Pharmacokinetics:
see individual agents

---

Contraindications:
Hypersensitivity; glaucoma; pyloric/duodenal obstruction; peptic ulcers; prostatic hypertrophy; bladder obstruction; cardiospasm; myasthenia gravis. Aspirin: hemophilia, bleeding ulcers, hemorrhagic states

Precautions:  Use cautiously in those with cardiac disease. Long-term safety has not been established.
Aspirin:  Use cautiously in patients with asthma, nasal polyposis, chronic urticaria (inc risk of hypersensitivity); chronic renal insufficiency, PUD, bleeding disorders.

Pregnancy Category:  C
Aspirin:  Category D

Lactation Issues:  Use cautiously, unknown if excreted in breast milk.

## 315. Agents for Alzheimer's Dementia

| Drug and Dosage Forms | Usual Dosage Range | Administration Issues and Drug–Drug & Drug–Food Interactions | Common Adverse Drug Reactions (ADRs) and Pharmacokinetics | Contraindications, Pregnancy Category, and Lactation Issues |
|---|---|---|---|---|
| **Donepezil**<br>Aricept<br><br><u>Tablets:</u><br>5 mg, 10 mg | **Mild/Moderate Alzheimer's dementia:**<br>Usual dose is 5–10 mg qd. Some evidence exists that doses >10mg may be beneficial in some patients. Do not increase to 10 mg until patients have been on daily dose of 5 mg for 4–6 weeks. | <u>Administration Issues:</u><br>Take in evening, just prior to going to bed. May be taken without regards to food.<br><br><u>Drug–Drug Interactions:</u><br>Donepezil may **decrease** the effectiveness of anticholinergics; ketoconazole and quinidine may inhibit the metabolism of donepezil | <u>ADRs:</u><br>headache, fatigue, nausea, diarrhea, muscle cramps, insomnia, dizziness<br><br><u>Pharmacokinetics:</u><br>$T_{1/2} = 70$ hrs | <u>Contraindications:</u><br>Hypersensitivity to donepezil or to piperidine derivative<br><br><u>Pregnancy Category:</u> C<br><br><u>Lactation Issues:</u> it is not known whether donepezil is excreted in breast milk |
| **Ergoloid Mesylates**<br>Hydergine, various generics<br><br><u>Tablets, sublingual:</u><br>0.5 mg, 1 mg<br><br><u>Tablets:</u> 0.5 mg, 1 mg<br><br><u>Capsules:</u> 1 mg<br><br><u>Liquid:</u> 1 mg/mL | **Age-related mental capacity decline (primary progressive Alzheimer's, senile onset, or multi-infarct dementia):**<br>1 mg tid (alleviation of symptoms may take 3–4 weeks). Titrate dose based on clinical response and tolerance (range: 4.5–12 mg/d). | <u>Administration Issues:</u><br>Do not crush or chew sublingual forms.<br><br>Drug–Drug Interactions: None known | <u>ADRs:</u><br>sublingual irritation, nausea, other GI disturbances<br><br><u>Pharmacokinetics:</u><br>extensive first-pass metabolism (bioavailablity is 6%–25%; capsule has 12% higher bioavailability);<br>$T_{1/2} = 2.6$–5.1 hrs | <u>Contraindications:</u><br>hypersensitivity; acute or chronic psychosis<br><br><u>Other Considerations:</u><br>Rule out delirium and dementiform illness secondary to systemic disease, primary neurological disease, or primary disturbance of mood.<br>Periodically reassess patient for continued benefit. |
| **Tacrine**<br>Cognex<br><br><u>Capsules:</u> 10 mg, 20 mg, 30 mg, 40 mg | **Mild/Moderate Alzheimer's dementia:**<br>10 mg tid for 6 weeks, initially. Titrate by 40 mg/d every 6 weeks based on tolerance. Max dose is 160 mg/d.<br><br>Rechallenging: If drug was stopped due to elevated transaminases | <u>Administration Issues:</u> must monitor transaminases weekly ($\leq 3 \times$ upper limit of normal): continue treatment; >3 but $\leq 5 \times$ upper limit of normal: decrease dose by 40 mg/d then increase dose once normal; >5 × upper limit of normal: discontinue medication); | <u>ADRs:</u><br>nausea, vomiting, diarrhea, dyspepsia, anorexia, increased transaminase levels, myalgia, ataxia | <u>Contraindications:</u><br>Hypersensitivity, previous treatment with tacrine that resulted in jaundice (total bilirubin >3 mg/dL) |

| | | | Pharmacokinetics: $T_{1/2}$ = 2–4 hrs; levels are higher in women (50%) due to lower activity of liver enzyme responsible for metabolism of tacrine | Pregnancy Category: C<br><br>Lactation Issues: should not be used in nursing mothers |
|---|---|---|---|---|
| (>5 × upper limit of normal), may be rechallenged once LFTs have returned to normal. Follow titration as above | | safety/efficacy not established in any dementing disease found in children.<br><br>Drug–Drug Interactions:<br>increased effect: cholinergic agents; decreased effect: anticholinergic agents; increased level of: theophylline; increased tacrine level: cimetidine; decreased tacrine level: smoking<br><br>Drug–Food Interaction: food decreases levels of tacrine (take on empty stomach if possible) | | |

## 316. Agents for Gout

| Drug and Dosage Forms | Usual Dosage Range | Administration Issues and Drug–Drug & Drug–Food Interactions | Common Adverse Drug Reactions (ADRs) and Pharmacokinetics | Contraindications, Pregnancy Category, and Lactation Issues |
|---|---|---|---|---|
| **Allopurinol**<br>Zyloprim, various generics<br><br>Tablets: 100 mg, 300 mg | **Control of gout and hyperuricemia:**<br>to reduce incidence of gout flare-up: Initially, 100 mg/d, titrate q week by 100 mg/d.<br><br>**Maintenance therapy:**<br>200–300 mg/d for mild gout; 400–600 mg/d for moderately severe tophaceous gout. Divide daily doses >300 mg into 2 doses. Max dose is 800 mg/d. | Administration Issues:<br>Drink 10–12 glasses of water daily. May take with food if GI upset occurs. When replacing a uricosuric, gradually reduce the uricosuric dose over several weeks while increasing allopurinol dose. Rarely indicated for children except in malignancies.<br><br>Drug–Drug Interactions:<br>**increased levels/effects of:** ampicillin, cyclophosphamide, theophylline, thiopurines | ADRS:<br>rash, dermatitis, urticaria, pruritus, nausea, vomiting, diarrhea, intermittent abdominal pain, gastritis, dyspepsia, increased liver function tests, leukopenia, leukocytosis, eosinophilia, thrombocytopenia, headache, somnolence, arthralgia, acute attacks of gout, fever myopathy, epistaxis, renal failure, alopecia | Contraindications:<br>Hypersensitivity; prior severe reactions to this agent.<br><br>Precautions: Use cautiously in those with severe renal impairment. Do not use to treat asymptomatic hyperuricemia. Monitor closely for signs of acute gout. Monitor liver and kidney function periodically.<br><br>Pregnancy Category: C |

(continues on next page)

| Drug and Dosage Forms | Usual Dosage Range | Administration Issues and Drug–Drug & Drug–Food Interactions | Common Adverse Drug Reactions (ADRs) and Pharmacokinetics | Contraindications, Pregnancy Category, and Lactation Issues |
|---|---|---|---|---|
| **Allopurinol** *cont.* | **Prevention of uric acid nephropathy during vigorous therapy of neoplastic disease:** 600–800 mg/d for 2–3 days<br><br>**Pediatrics:** 300 mg/d (6–10 yrs old) or 150 mg/d (<6 yrs old). May also use 10 mg/kg/d divided q 6 h to max of 600 mg/d. Titrate dose after 48 hrs to minimum effective dose to maintain uric acid levels in normal range.<br><br>**Recurrent calcium oxalate stones:** 200–300 mg/d divided qd to bid<br><br>**Renal Impairment:**<br>CrCl = 60 mL/min: 200 mg/d<br>CrCl = 40 mL/min: 150 mg/d<br>CrCl = 20 mL/min: 100 mg/d<br>CrCl = 10 mL/min: 100 mg on alternate days.<br>CrCl<10 mL/min: 100 mg 3 times weekly. | **increased levels/effects of allopurinol:** ACE inhibitors, thiazide diuretics.<br><br>**decreased levels/effects of allopurinol:** uricosuric agents, aluminum salts | Pharmacokinetics<br>$T_{1/2}$ = 1–2 hrs for allopurinol | Lactation Issues: excreted in breast milk—use cautiously. |
| **Colchicine** various generics<br><br>Tablets: 0.5 mg, 0.6 mg | **Acute Gout:** 1–1.2 mg at onset of symptoms, followed by 0.5–1.2 mg q 1–2 hrs until pain is relieved or nausea, vomiting or diarrhea occurs. Usual dose is 4–8 mg/attack. | Drug–Drug Interactions: None known. | Most Frequent: bone marrow depression, aplastic anemia, agranulocytosis, thrombocytopenia, peripheral neuritis, purpura, myopathy, alopecia, reversible | Contraindications: Hypersensitivity; serious GI, renal, hepatic, or cardiac disorders; blood dyscrasias.<br><br>Precautions: Use cautiously in the elderly or debilitated |

| | | | | |
|---|---|---|---|---|
| | **Prevention of gouty arthritis:** <1 attack/year: 0.5–0.6 mg/d for 3–4 days/week. >1 attack/year: 0.5–0.6 mg/d. More severe cases may require 1–1.8 mg/d Prior to surgery: 0.5–0.6 mg 3 times daily for 3 days prior to surgical procedure. | | azoospermia, dermatoses, hypersensitivity, vomiting, diarrhea, abdominal pain, nausea. <br><br> Pharmacokinetics: <br> $T_{1/2}$ = 12–30 min. | patients (severe hepatic or renal dysfunction); monitor blood counts periodically. <br><br> Pregnancy Category: C <br><br> Lactation Issues: Use cautiously, not known if excreted in breast milk. |
| **Probenecid** <br> Benemid, Probalan, various generics <br><br> Tablets: 500 mg | **Hyperuricemia associated with gout and gouty arthritis:** 250 mg bid for 1 week, followed by 500 mg twice daily thereafter. <br><br> **Renal Impairment:** may need to titrate to 1500–2000 mg/d to achieve good uric acid excretion. If CrCl <30 mL/min, probenecid likely to be ineffective. <br><br> **Maintenance doses:** when no attacks for 6 months, may decrease dose by 500 mg/d every 6 months. Monitor serum uric acid levels | Administration Issues: <br> May take with food if GI upset occurs. Drink 6–8 glasses of water daily. Consider 3–7.5 g/d of sodium bicarbonate or potassium citrate to alkalinize the urine. <br><br> Drug–Drug Interactions: <br> **increased levels/effects of:** acyclovir, allopurinol, benzodiazepines, dapsone, methotrexate, NSAIDs, penicillamine, sulfonylureas, zidovudine <br> **decreased levels/effects of probenecid:** salicylates | ADRs: <br> headache, anorexia, nausea, vomiting, urinary frequency, hypersensitivity, sore gums, flushing dizziness, anemia, hemolytic anemia, nephrotic syndrome, hepatic necrosis, aplastic anemia, exacerbation of gout, uric acid stones with or without hematuria, renal colic or costovertebral pain. <br><br> Pharmacokinetics: <br> $T_{1/2}$ = 5–8 hrs (dose dependent and could be <5 and >8 hrs | Contraindications: <br> Hypersensitivity; children <2 yrs; blood dyscrasias, uric acid kidney stones. **DO NOT START THERAPY UNTIL ACUTE GOUT ATTACK IS OVER.** <br><br> Precautions: Some renal adverse effects may be reduced by alkalinizing the urine. Use cautiously in those with PUD, severe renal or hepatic dysfunction. <br><br> Pregnancy Issues: Does cross placental barrier—use cautiously. |
| **Probenecid & Colchicine** <br> ColBenemid, Proben-C, Col-Probenecid, various generics <br><br> Tablets: <br> 500 mg/0.5 mg | **Chronic gouty arthritis:** 1 tablet daily for 1 week followed by 1 tablet twice daily thereafter. <br><br> **Renal Impairment:** may need to titrate to 4 tablets/d to achieve good uric acid excretion. If CrCl <30 mL/min, probenecid likely to be ineffective. | Administration Issues: <br> May take with food if GI upset occurs. Drink 6–8 glasses of water daily. Consider 3–7.5 g/d of sodium bicarbonate or potassium citrate to alkalinize the urine. Do not use in those <2 yrs old. | ADRs: <br> Probenecid: <br> headache, anorexia, nausea, vomiting, urinary frequency, hypersensitivity, sore gums, flushing, exacerbation of gout, uric acid stones with or without hematuria, renal colic or costovertebral pain. | Contraindications: <br> Hypersensitivity; children <2 yrs; blood dyscrasias, uric acid kidney stones, serious GI, renal, hepatic, or cardiac disorders <br><br> Precautions: Some renal adverse effects may be reduced by alkalinizing the urine. Use |

(continues on next page)

| Drug and Dosage Forms | Usual Dosage Range | Administration Issues and Drug–Drug & Drug–Food Interactions | Common Adverse Drug Reactions (ADRs) and Pharmacokinetics | Contraindications, Pregnancy Category, and Lactation Issues |
|---|---|---|---|---|
| **Probenecid & Colchicine *cont.*** | | Drug–Drug Interactions: **increased levels/effects of:** acyclovir, allopurinol, benzodiazepines, dapsone, methotrexate, NSAIDs, penicillamine, sulfonylureas, zidovudine <br><br> **decreased levels/effects of probenecid:** salicylates <br><br> **Colchicine** <br> Drug–Drug Interactions: None known. | Colchicine <br> bone marrow depression, aplastic anemia, agranulocytosis, thrombocytopenia, peripheral neuritis, purpura, myopathy, alopecia, reversible azoospermia, dermatoses, hypersensitivity, vomiting, diarrhea, abdominal pain, nausea <br><br> Pharmacokinetics: see individual agents | cautiously in those with PUD, severe renal or hepatic dysfunction. Use cautiously in the elderly; monitor blood counts periodically. <br><br> Pregnancy Issues: Does cross placental barrier—use cautiously. <br><br> Lactation Issues: Not known if excreted in breast milk. |
| **Sulfinpyrazone** <br> Anturane, various generics <br><br> Tablets: 100 mg, 200 mg | **Chronic & intermittent gouty arthritis:** <br> Initially, 200–400 mg/d in 2 divided doses. <br> Titrate to full maintenance dose within 1 week: 400 mg daily in 2 divided doses. May titrate further to 800 mg/d if needed. | Administration Issues: <br> May take with food if GI upset occurs. Drink 10–12 glasses of water daily. Consider 3–7.5 g/d of sodium bicarbonate or potassium citrate to alkalinize the urine. <br><br> Drug–Drug Interactions: **increased levels/effects of:** acetaminophen (toxic effects), anticoagulants, tolbutamide <br><br> **decreased levels/effects of:** acetaminophen (therapeutic effects), theophylline, verapamil <br><br> **decreased levels/effects of sulfinpyrazone:** niacin, salicylates | ADRs: <br> upper GI disturbances <br><br> Less Frequent: blood dyscrasias, rash, bronchoconstriction (in those intolerant to aspirin) <br><br> Pharmacokinetics: <br> $T_{1/2}$ = 2.2–3 hrs | Contraindications: <br> Hypersensitivity; active peptic ulcer or symptoms of GI inflammation or ulceration; blood dyscrasias <br><br> Precautions: Use cautiously in those with history of PUD. Monitor blood counts and renal function periodically. <br><br> Pregnancy Issues: use cautiously—only when benefits clearly outweigh risks |

# 317. Agents for Migraine

Note: Additional agents used for migraine and/or tension headaches include: ASA (table 307), APAP (table 301), Analgesics with Butalbital (table 305), Narcotic analgesics (tables 302 & 303) and NSAIDs (table 306). For additional agents for migraine prophylaxis see: valproic acid (table 308.6), propranolol and timolol (table 205.5).

| Drug and Dosage Forms | Usual Dosage Range | Administration Issues and Drug–Drug & Drug–Food Interactions | Common Adverse Drug Reactions (ADRs) and Pharmacokinetics | Contraindications, Pregnancy Category, and Lactation Issues |
|---|---|---|---|---|
| **Ergotamine Tartrate**<br>Ergostat, Medihaler, Ergotamine<br><br>Tablets, sublingual: 2 mg<br><br>Aerosol: 9 mg/mL | **To abort vascular headaches (migraine, migraine variant, cluster headache):**<br>**Sublingual:**<br>1 tablet at onset of symptoms, take subsequent doses at 30 min intervals. Max of 3 tablets/d and 10 tablets/week<br><br>**Inhalation:** 1 inhalation, may repeat in 5 minutes if not relieved. Max of 6 inhalations/d or 15 inhalations/week. | Administration Issues:<br>Take with food. Continuous administration should not exceed 6 months. Need a drug free period every 6 months for 3–4 weeks. Taper medication – do not abruptly discontinue medication. Not recommended for use in children.<br><br>Drug–Drug Interactions:<br>**increased vasoconstrictive effects in periphery:** beta-blockers<br><br>**increased effects of ergot derivatives:** macrolides | ADRs: nausea, vomiting, numbness and tingling of fingers/toes, muscle pain in extremities, weakness in legs, edema, itching, transient tachycardia or bradycardia<br><br>Pharmacokinetics:<br>$T_{1/2}$ = 2 hrs | Contraindications:<br>Hypersensitivity; pregnancy; peripheral vascular disease, hepatic or renal impairment; severe pruritus, coronary artery disease, hypertension, sepsis, malnutrition<br><br>Precautions: Do not use for long periods of time (leads to ergotism, gangrene, drug dependence)<br><br>Pregnancy Category: X<br><br>Lactation Issues: Do not use in nursing mothers - symptoms of ergotism (vomiting, diarrhea) have occurred in infants. |
| **Methysergide Maleate**<br>Sansert<br><br>Tablets: 2 mg | **Prophylaxis of vascular headaches:**<br>4–8 mg daily. If no response after 3 weeks of therapy, discontinue treatment. | Administration Issues:<br>Take with food. Continuous administration should not exceed 6 months. Need a drug free period every 6 months for 3–4 weeks. Taper medication—do not abruptly | ADRs:<br>vasoconstriction of large and small arteries; postural hypotension, tachycardia, nausea, vomiting, diarrhea, heartburn, abdominal pain. insomnia, drowsiness, | Contraindications:<br>Hypersensitivity; pregnancy; peripheral vascular disease; severe arteriosclerosis, hypertension, coronary artery disease; phlebitis or cellulitis of the lower limbs; pulmonary |

*(continues on next page)*

| Drug and Dosage Forms | Usual Dosage Range | Administration Issues and Drug–Drug & Drug–Food Interactions | Common Adverse Drug Reactions (ADRs) and Pharmacokinetics | Contraindications, Pregnancy Category, and Lactation Issues |
|---|---|---|---|---|
| **Methysergide Maleate *cont.*** | | discontinue medication. Not recommended for use in children<br><br>Drug–Drug Interactions:<br>**increased vasoconstrictive effects in periphery:** beta-blockers | euphoria, dizziness, ataxia, weakness, lightheadedness, facial flush, telangiectasia, rash, hair loss, retroperitoneal fibrosis, peripheral edema, neutropenia, arthralgia, myalgia, weight gain<br><br>Pharmacokinetics:<br>Oral. No other data available | disease; collagen diseases; impaired liver or renal function; valvular heart disease; debilitated states; serious infections.<br><br>Precautions: Prolonged uninterrupted use is not recommended.<br><br>Pregnancy Category:<br>Contraindicated.<br><br>Lactation Issues: Do not use in nursing mothers—symptoms of ergotism (vomiting, diarrhea) have occurred in infants. |
| **Sumatriptan**<br>Imitrex<br><br>Tablets: 25 mg, 50 mg<br><br>Injection: 12 mg/mL | **Acute Migraine with or without aura:**<br>Injection:<br>6 mg SC one time dose. Max of 12 mg/d (separate 2 doses by at least 1 hr).<br><br>Oral:<br>25 mg per dose. Max of 100 mg per dose. May repeat dose after 2 hrs if no response. Max dose is 300 mg/d. | Administration Issues:<br>Use the autoinjector for injections into SC area. Protect injection from light. Take medication as soon as symptoms appear. Safety/efficacy not established in children.<br><br>Drug–Drug Interactions:<br>**increased levels/effects of sumatriptan:** MAO inhibitors, ergot-containing drugs | ADRs:<br>SC reactions:<br>dizziness, drowsiness, headache, anxiety, malaise, chest tightness, hypertension, hypotension, bradycardia, tachycardia, palpitations, transient ECG changes, weakness, neck pain, myalgia, muscle cramps, tingling, warm, feeling of heaviness, numbness, injection site reaction, flushing, jaw discomfort | Contraindications:<br>Hypersensitivity; IV use; patients with ischemic heart disease, uncontrolled hypertension; concurrent use of MAO inhibitors or ergotamine derivatives; management of hemiplegic or basilar migraine.<br><br>Precautions: Use cautiously in patients with severe renal or hepatic dysfunction. |

| | | | Oral Reactions: | Pregnancy Category: C |
|---|---|---|---|---|
| | | | confusion, photophobia, convulsions, drowsiness; dizziness, fatigue, chest discomfort, hypertension, hypotension, arrhythmia, angina, cerebral ischemia, diarrhea, dysphagia, GERD, constipation, feeling of heaviness, tightness, tingling, warm sensation, weakness | Lactation Issues: Excreted in breast milk—use cautiously in nursing mothers. |
| | | | Pharmacokinetics: SC; $T_{1/2}$ = 1.5–2 hrs Oral; $T_{1/2}$ = 2.5 hrs | |

## 317.1 Combination Agents for Migraines

| Drug and Dosage Forms | Usual Dosage Range | Administration Issues and Drug–Drug Interactions | Common Adverse Drug Reactions (ADRs) and Pharmacokinetics | Contraindications, Pregnancy Category, and Lactation Issues |
|---|---|---|---|---|
| **Ergotamine & Caffeine** Cafergot, Ercaf, Wigraine, Cafatine With belladona alkaloids and pentobarbital: Cafatine-PB Tablets: 1 mg/100 mg with belladona alkaloids and pentobarbital (used as antiemetic and | **For relief of vascular headaches:** 2 tablets at first sign of symptoms, follow with 1 tablet every 1/2 hr as needed. Max dose is 6 tablets/attack or 10 tablets/week. For the 2 mg/100 mg dose: Follow above directions except the Max Dose is 2 tablets/attack | Administration Issues: Take with food. Continuous administration should not exceed 6 months. Need a drug free period every 6 months for 3–4 weeks. Taper medication—do not abruptly discontinue medication. Not recommended for use in children. Drug–Drug Interactions: see individual agents | ADRs: Ergotamine nausea, vomiting, numbness and tingling of fingers/toes, muscle pain in extremities, weakness in legs, edema, itching, transient tachycardia or bradycardia Caffeine: insomnia, restlessness, excitement, nervousness, | Contraindications: Hypersensitivity; pregnancy; peripheral vascular disease, hepatic or renal impairment, severe pruritus, coronary artery disease, hypertension, sepsis, malnutrition Precautions: Do not use for long periods of time (leads to ergotism, gangrene, drug dependence) |

(continues on next page)

## 317.1 Combination Agents for Migraines *continued from previous page*

| Drug and Dosage Forms | Usual Dosage Range | Administration Issues and Drug–Drug Interactions | Common Adverse Drug Reactions (ADRs) and Pharmacokinetics | Contraindications, Pregnancy Category, and Lactation Issues |
|---|---|---|---|---|
| **Ergotamine & Caffeine** *cont.* <br> sedative, respectively): 1 mg/100 mg/0.125 mg/30 mg <br><br> Suppositories: <br> 2 mg/100 mg | | | tremor, headaches, anxiety, nausea, vomiting, diarrhea, tachycardia, palpitations, diuresis, withdrawal headaches after abrupt discontinuation (500–600 mg/d of caffeine) <br><br> Pharmacokinetics: <br> see individual agents | Pregnancy Category: <br> Contraindicated <br><br> Lactation Issues: Do not use in nursing mothers—symptoms of ergotism (vomiting, diarrhea) have occurred in infants. |
| **Isometheptene Mucate/ Dichloralphenazone/ Acetaminophen** <br> Midrin, Isocom, Isopap, Migratine, various generics <br><br> Capsules: <br> 65 mg/100 mg/325 mg | **For relief of vascular headaches:** <br> 2 capsules at onset of symptoms, followed by 1 capsule q hr until relieved. Max of 5 capsules/12 hrs. <br><br> **For relief of tension headaches:** <br> 1–2 capsules q 4 h up to 8 capsules/d | Drug–Drug Interactions: <br> **increased effects of:** MAO inhibitors (hypertensive crisis) <br><br> **increased toxic effect of acetaminophen:** alcohol (chronic); barbiturates, carbamazepine, hydantoins, rifampin, sulfinpyrazone <br><br> **decreased effect of acetaminophen:** charcoal | ADRS: <br> Isometheptene/ Dichloralphenazone: dizziness, rash <br><br> Acetaminophen: <br> Very few adverse reactions <br><br> Pharmacokinetics: <br> **Data only available for acetaminophen** (see table 301) | Contraindications: <br> Hypersensitivity; glaucoma, severe renal disease, hypertension, organic heart disease, hepatic disease, concurrent MAO inhibitor use. <br><br> Precautions: Use cautiously in those with peripheral vascular disease and after recent cardiovascular attacks. |

## 318. Agents for Parkinson's Disease

| Drug and Dosage Forms | Usual Dosage Range | Administration Issues and Drug–Drug & Drug–Food Interactions | Common Adverse Drug Reactions (ADRs) and Pharmacokinetics | Contraindications, Pregnancy Category, and Lactation Issues |
|---|---|---|---|---|
| **Amantadine**<br>Symadine, Symmetrel, various generics<br><br>Capsules: 100 mg<br><br>Syrup: 50 mg/5 mL | **Parkinson's:**<br>100 mg bid when used alone. May titrate to 400 mg/d if needed/tolerated<br><br>**Concurrent therapy with levodopa:**<br>100 mg qd to bid while titrating levodopa dose.<br><br>**Elderly /debilitated:** 100 mg qd<br><br>**Renal dysfunction (CrCl):**<br>80–100 ml/min:  100 mg bid<br>60 ml/min:  200 mg qod + 100 mg qod<br>40–50 ml/min:  100 mg/d<br>30 ml/min:  200 mg 2/week<br>20 ml/min:  100 mg 3/week<br>≤10 ml/min:  200 mg/week alternating with 10/week<br><br>**Drug-induced extrapyramidal reactions:**  100 mg bid. May titrate to 100 mg tid if needed<br><br>**Traumatic Brain Injury**<br>50 mg bid up to 400 mg/d | Administration Issues:<br>Safety/efficacy not established in those <1 yr old.<br><br>Drug–Drug Interactions:<br>**increased effects of:**  anticholinergic agents<br><br>**increased levels of amantadine:**<br>hydrochlorthiazide/ triamterene combination | ADRs:<br>nausea, dizziness, lightheadedness, insomnia, depression, anxiety, irritability, hallucinations, confusion, anorexia, dry mouth, constipation, ataxia, orthostatic hypotension, headache, livedo reticularis, peripheral edema<br><br>Elderly:  Use smaller doses<br><br>Pharmacokinetics:<br>$T_{1/2}$ = 15 hrs (prolonged in elderly and those with renal dysfunction) | Contraindications:<br>Hypersensitivity<br><br>Precautions:  Do not abruptly discontinue medication due to precipitation of Parkinsonian crisis<br><br>Pregnancy Category:  C<br><br>Lactation Issues:  excreted in breast milk. Use cautiously |
| **Benztropine**<br>Cogentin, various generics | **Adjunct in therapy of all forms of parkinsonism:**<br>0.5–1 mg at bedtime. Titrate as needed/tolerated to 4–6 mg/d. May take | Administration Issues:<br>May take with food if GI upset occurs. If substituting another anticholinergic: gradually reduce other agent while | ADRs:<br>disorientation, confusion, memory loss, agitation, euphoria, excitement, dizziness, | Contraindications:<br>Hypersensitivity; angle-closure glaucoma; pyloric/duodenal obstruction; peptic ulcers; |

(continues on next page)

| Drug and Dosage Forms | Usual Dosage Range | Administration Issues and Drug–Drug & Drug–Food Interactions | Common Adverse Drug Reactions (ADRs) and Pharmacokinetics | Contraindications, Pregnancy Category, and Lactation Issues |
|---|---|---|---|---|
| **Benztropine *cont.*** <br><br> <u>Tablets</u>: 0.5 mg, 1 mg, 2 mg | as one daily dose or divide into 2–4 daily doses. <br><br> **Drug-induced extrapyramidal reactions:** 1–2 mg 2–3 times daily initially for 1–2 weeks. Slowly withdraw medication to determine its continued need. If EPS recurs, reinstitute medication. | gradually increasing this agent. Safety/efficacy not established in children. DO NOT USE IN THOSE <3 YRS <br><br> <u>Drug–Drug Interactions:</u> **decreased levels/effects of:** haloperidol, phenothiazines, levodopa <br><br> **increased levels/effects of:** amantadine, digoxin, cannabinoids, barbiturates, alcohol | headache, drowsiness, dry mouth, acute suppurative parotitis, nausea, constipation, tachycardia, hypotension, blurred vision, mydriasis, urinary retention, muscle weakness, cramping, flushing, decreased sweating, impotence, skin rash <br><br> <u>Elderly (≥60 yrs):</u> More sensitive to CNS adverse effects. Use smaller doses <br><br> <u>Pharmacokinetics:</u> **No data available** | prostatic hypertrophy or bladder neck obstructions; achalasia; myasthenia gravis; megacolon <br><br> <u>Precautions:</u> Use cautiously in those with arrhythmias, hypertension, hypotension, GI/GU obstructions. Not useful in patients with tardive dyskinesia—may actually aggravate symptoms. These agents may be abused—for the production of mood elevation or psychedelic experiences <br><br> <u>Pregnancy Category:</u> C <br><br> <u>Lactation Issues:</u> Use cautiously; effects on infant not known |
| **Biperiden** <br> Akineton <br><br> <u>Tablets</u>: 2 mg | **<u>Adjunct in therapy of all forms of parkinsonism:</u>** <br> 2 mg 3–4 times daily. May titrate to max of 16 mg/d as needed <br><br> **Drug-induced extrapyramidal reactions:** 2 mg 1–3 times daily | <u>Administration Issues:</u> May take with food if GI upset occurs. If substituting another anticholinergic: gradually reduce other agent while gradually increasing this agent; safety/efficacy not established in children. <br><br> <u>Drug–Drug Interactions:</u> **decreased levels/effects of:** haloperidol, phenothiazines, levodopa | <u>ADRs:</u> disorientation, confusion, memory loss, hallucinations, nervousness, euphoria, excitement, dizziness, headache, drowsiness, dry mouth, acute suppurative parotitis, nausea, vomiting, constipation, tachycardia, hypotension, blurred vision, mydriasis, | <u>Contraindications:</u> Hypersensitivity; angle-closure glaucoma; pyloric/duodenal obstruction; peptic ulcers; prostatic hypertrophy or bladder neck obstructions; achalasia; myasthenia gravis; megacolon <br><br> <u>Precautions:</u> Use cautiously in those with arrhythmias, |

| Drug | Indications & Dosing | Administration / Drug–Drug Interactions | ADRs / Pharmacokinetics | Contraindications / Precautions / Pregnancy / Lactation |
|---|---|---|---|---|
| | | **increased levels/effects of:** amantadine, digoxin, cannabinoids, barbiturates, alcohol | urinary retention, muscle weakness, cramping, elevated temperature, flushing, decreased sweating, impotence, skin rash<br><br>Elderly (>60 yrs): More sensitive to CNS adverse effects. Use smaller doses<br><br>Pharmacokinetics: $T_{1/2}$ = 18.4–24.3 hrs | hypertension, hypotension, GI/GU obstructions. Not useful in patients with tardive dyskinesia—may actually aggravate symptoms. These agents may be abused—for the production of mood elevation or psychedelic experiences<br><br>Pregnancy Category: C<br><br>Lactation Issues: Use cautiously; effects on infant not known |
| **Bromocriptine**<br>Parlodel Snap tabs, Parlodel<br><br>Tablets: 2.5 mg<br><br>Capsules: 5 mg | **Parkinsonism:**<br>1.25 mg bid with meals. Titrate every 2–4 weeks by 2.5 mg/d to 10–40 mg/d<br><br>**Traumatic Brain Injury**<br>2.5 mg/d up to 30 mg/d | Administration Issues:<br>Take with food<br>Take first dose lying down due to possibility of dizziness/fainting; safety/efficacy in children <15 yrs not established<br><br>Drug–Drug Interactions:<br>**increased levels/effects of bromocriptine:** erythromycin, sympathomimetics<br><br>**decreased levels/effects of bromocriptine:** phenothiazines | ADRs:<br>nausea, headache, dizziness, fatigue, lightheadedness, vomiting, nasal congestion, constipation, diarrhea, drowsiness, psychosis, hypotension, abdominal cramps<br><br>Pharmacokinetics:<br>$T_{1/2}$ = 6–8 hrs | Contraindications:<br>Hypersensitivity to this or ergot derivatives; severe ischemic heart disease or peripheral vascular disease<br><br>Precautions: digital vasospasm has occurred in patients with acromegaly. Long-term treatment (20–100 mg/d) has resulted in pulmonary infiltrates, pleural effusion, pleural thickening (slowly reversible upon drug discontinuation)<br><br>Pregnancy Category: B. Should discontinue medication once pregnancy is confirmed<br><br>Lactation Issues: prevents lactation—mothers should not nurse. |

*(continues on next page)*

# 318. Agents for Parkinson's Disease *continued from previous page*

| Drug and Dosage Forms | Usual Dosage Range | Administration Issues and Drug–Drug & Drug–Food Interactions | Common Adverse Drug Reactions (ADRs) and Pharmacokinetics | Contraindications, Pregnancy Category, and Lactation Issues |
|---|---|---|---|---|
| **Carbidopa/Levodopa**<br>Sinemet, Sinemet CR<br><br>Tablets: 10/100 mg, 25/100 mg, 25/250 mg<br><br>Tablets, sustained release: 50/200 mg<br><br>**Levodopa**<br>Larodopa, Dopar<br><br>Tablets: 100 mg, 250 mg, 500 mg<br><br>Capsules: 100 mg, 250 mg, 500 mg<br><br>**Carbidopa**<br>Lodosyn<br><br>Tablets: 25 mg | **Levodopa:**<br>**Treatment of all forms of parkinsonism:** 0.5–1 g daily divided into 2 or more doses. Titrate by 0.75 g every 3–7 days as tolerated. Max dose is 8 g/d<br><br>**Carbidopa:**<br>**For use with levodopa:**<br>Titrate carefully. Usually require 70–100 mg/d to saturate peripheral dopa decarboxylase.<br><br>**Combination Product:**<br>If currently treated with levodopa, discontinue at least 8 days prior to initiation of combination product and reduce levodopa dose by 25%. Give 25 mg/100 mg (carbidopa/levodopa) tid or 10 mg/100 mg (carbidopa/levodopa) tid to qid. Titrate by 1 tablet daily every day or every other day as tolerated/needed. Max of 8 tablets daily.<br>* When more carbidopa is required: use the 25 mg/100 mg tablet<br>* When more levodopa is required: use the 25 mg/250 mg tablet | _Administration Issues:_<br>Combination of carbidopa/levodopa is the preferred method, but some patients require individual drug titration. Peripheral dopa decarboxylase is saturated by carbidopa at approximately 70–100 mg/d. May take a few weeks to months to see full effects<br>Give with food. Safety/ efficacy not established for those <12 yrs old<br><br>_Drug–Drug Interactions:_<br>**decreased levels/effects of levodopa:** anticholinergics, benzodiazepines, hydantoins, papaverine, pyridoxine, TCAs, methionine<br><br>**increased levels/effects of levodopa:** antacids, MAO inhibitors<br><br>**increased adverse effects of:** TCAs (by carbidopa)<br><br>_Drug–Food Interaction:_ Protein-rich food reduces and delays peak plasma concentrations—causing fluctuations in response to levodopa | _ADRs:_<br>adventitious movements (choreiform, dystonic), anorexia, nausea, vomiting, dry mouth, abdominal pain, headache, dizziness, numbness, weakness, faintness, confusion, insomnia, nightmares, hallucinations, delusions, agitation, anxiety, malaise, fatigue, euphoria<br><br>_Elderly:_ often require smaller doses due to decrease in peripheral dopa decarboxylase<br><br>_Pharmacokinetics:_<br>**Levodopa:**<br>$T_{1/2}$ = 1–3 hrs<br><br>**Carbidopa:** only given with levodopa to prolong $T_{1/2}$ of levodopa. Also increases urinary excretion of levodopa as unchanged drug | _Contraindications:_<br>Hypersensitivity; narrow-angle glaucoma; concomitant use of MAO inhibitors (not selegiline); history of or suspected melanoma<br><br>_Precautions:_ Use cautiously in those with wide-angle glaucoma; use carefully to prevent "on–off" phenomenon by using lowest dose, reserving drug for severe cases, using drug holidays (5–14 days)<br><br>_Pregnancy/lactation Issues:_ safety not established. Use only when benefit far outweighs risk |

| Drug | Indications/Dosage | Administration/Drug Interactions | ADRs/Pharmacokinetics | Contraindications/Precautions |
|---|---|---|---|---|
| | **Sustained Release Combination:** 1 tablet bid at intervals not less than 6 hrs. Titrate q 3 days to 2–8 tablets/d at intervals of 4–8 hrs while awake.<br><br>**Traumatic Brain Injury** 10/100 mg tid to 25/250 mg qid | | | Contraindications: Hypersensitivity, asthma, glaucoma, prostate gland enlargement<br><br>Precautions: use carefully if operating heavy machinery, history of sleep apnea, hepatic dysfunction<br><br>Pregnancy Category: B.<br><br>Lactation Issues: women should not nurse |
| **Diphenhydramine**<br>Benadryl, various generics<br><br>Tablets: 25 mg, 50 mg<br><br>Capsules: 25 mg, 50 mg<br><br>Syrup: 12.5 mg/ml | **Mild parkinsonism (e.g. drug induced) in combination with centrally acting anticholinergic agents; drug-induced extrapyramidal reactions in elderly unable to tolerate more potent agents:**<br>25–50 mg 3–4 times daily<br><br>**Pediatrics (>9 kg):**<br>12.5–25 mg 3–4 times daily or 5 mg/kg/d. Max dose is 300 mg/d or 150 mg/m²/day | Administration Issues<br>Safety/efficacy in children <12 yrs not established<br><br>Drug–Drug Interactions<br>increased effect of antihistamine: MAO inhibitors (anticholinergic effects)<br><br>increased effect of: MAO inhibitors, alcohol, CNS depressants<br><br>decreased effect of: levodopa, phenothiazines, haloperidol | ADRs:<br>urinary retention, blurred vision, dry mouth, drowsiness, irritability, thickening of bronchial secretions<br><br>Elderly (>60yrs): more sensitive to CNS adverse effects. Use smaller doses<br><br>Pharmacokinetics:<br>rapid onset (15–30 minutes); duration of action = 4–6 hrs | |
| **Ethopropazine**<br>Parsidol<br><br>Tablets: 10 mg, 50 mg | **Adjunct in therapy of all forms of parkinsonism; drug-induced extrapyramidal reactions:**<br>50 mg 1–2 times daily. May titrate slowly if needed (mild/moderate symptoms: 100–400 mg/d; severe symptoms: 500–600 mg/d) | Administration Issues:<br>May take with food if GI upset occurs. If substituting another anticholinergic: gradually reduce other agent while gradually increasing this agent; safety/efficacy not established in children<br><br>Drug–Drug Interactions:<br>decreased levels/effects of: haloperidol, phenothiazines, levodopa | ADRs:<br>disorientation, confusion, memory loss, hallucinations, nervousness, euphoria, excitement, dizziness, headache, drowsiness, dry mouth, acute suppurative parotitis, nausea, vomiting, constipation, tachycardia, hypotension, blurred vision, mydriasis, urinary retention, | Contraindications: Hypersensitivity; angle-closure glaucoma; pyloric/duodenal obstruction; peptic ulcers; prostatic hypertrophy or bladder neck obstructions; achalasia; myasthenia gravis; megacolon<br><br>Precautions: Use cautiously in those with arrhythmias, hypertension, hypotension, |

(continues on next page)

| Drug and Dosage Forms | Usual Dosage Range | Administration Issues and Drug–Drug & Drug–Food Interactions | Common Adverse Drug Reactions (ADRs) and Pharmacokinetics | Contraindications, Pregnancy Category, and Lactation Issues |
|---|---|---|---|---|
| **Ethopropazine** *cont.* | | **increased levels/effects of:** amantadine, digoxin, cannabinoids, barbiturates, alcohol | muscle weakness, cramping, elevated temperature, flushing, decreased sweating, impotence, skin rash<br><br>Elderly (>60 yrs): More sensitive to CNS adverse effects. Use smaller doses<br><br>Pharmacokinetics: No data available | GI/GU obstructions. Not useful in patients with tardive dyskinesia; may actually aggravate symptoms. These agents may be abused—for the production of mood elevation or psychedelic experiences<br><br>Pregnancy Category: C<br><br>Lactation Issues: Use cautiously; effects on infant not known |
| **Pergolide**<br>Permax<br><br>Tablets: 0.05 mg, 0.25 mg, 1 mg | **Adjunct to carbidopa/levodopa in the management of parkinsonism:**<br>0.05 mg/d for first 2 days. Titrate by 0.1–0.15 mg q 3 days for the next 12 days of therapy. Titrate further by 0.25 mg/d q 3 days as needed/tolerated. Divide daily dose into 3 doses. | Administration Issues: During dose titration, cautiously decrease dose of carbidopa/levodopa; safety/efficacy not established for children<br><br>Drug–Drug Interactions:<br>**decreased effect of pergolide:** neuroleptics, metoclopramide | ADRs:<br>dyskinesia, dizziness, hallucinations, dystonia, confusion, somnolence, insomnia, anxiety, personality disorder, psychosis, orthostatic hypotension, vasodilatation, palpitation, syncope, arrhythmia, nausea, constipation, diarrhea, dyspepsia, anorexia, dry mouth, vomiting<br><br>Pharmacokinetics:<br>no data on $T_{1/2}$ | Contraindications:<br>Hypersensitivity to this or ergot derivatives<br><br>Precautions: Use cautiously in patients with arrhythmias, those who are elderly, very ill, or at high risk for death.<br><br>Pregnancy Category: B<br><br>Lactation Issues: Effects unknown; not recommended for mothers to nurse |

# Pramipexole

Mirapex

<u>Tablets:</u>
0.125 mg, 0.25 mg, 1 mg, 1.5 mg

**Signs and symptoms of Parkinson's disease:**
Suggested dosage schedule:

| Week | Dosage | Total daily dosage |
|------|--------|--------------------|
| 1 | 0.125 mg tid | 0.375 mg |
| 2 | 0.25 mg tid | 0.75 mg |
| 3 | 0.5 mg tid | 1.5 mg |
| 4 | 0.75 mg tid | 2.25 mg |
| 5 | 1 mg tid | 3 mg |
| 6 | 1.25 mg tid | 3.75 mg |
| 7 | 1.5 mg tid | 4.5 mg |

It is recommended that pramipexole be decreased over a 1 week period.

<u>Administration Issues</u>
May be taken with food to decrease nausea; safety/efficacy in children not established; warn patients that they may experience postural hypotension

<u>Drug–Drug Interactions</u>
pramipexole may **increase** levodopa concentrations; pramipexole clearance may be **decreased** by verapamil, ciprofloxacin, cimetidine, diltiazem, quinidine; pramipexole may have **decreased effectiveness** if given with dopamine antagonists (phenothiazines, thioxanthenes, metoclopramide)

<u>ADRs*:</u>
asthenia, dizziness, somnolence, insomnia, postural hypotension, extrapyramidal syndrome, hallucinations, confusion, constipation, dry mouth

*some ADRs seen in patients also taking levodopa

<u>Pharmacokinetics:</u>
$T_{1/2}$ = 6 hrs; decrease dosage moderate to severe renal impairment

<u>Contraindications:</u>
Hypersensitivity

<u>Pregnancy Category:</u> C

<u>Lactation Issues</u>
It is not known whether pramipexole is excreted in breast milk

# Procyclidine

Kemadrin

<u>Tablets:</u> 5 mg

**Adjunct in therapy of all forms of parkinsonism:**
2.5 mg tid. Titrate to 5 mg 3–4 times daily

**Drug-induced extrapyramidal reactions:**
2.5 mg tid. Titrate as needed/tolerated to 10–20 mg/d

<u>Administration Issues:</u>
May take with food if GI upset occurs. If substituting another anticholinergic: gradually reduce other agent while gradually increasing this agent; safety/efficacy not established in children.

<u>Drug–Drug Interactions:</u>

**decreased levels/effects of:**
haloperidol, phenothiazines, levodopa

**increased levels/effects of:**
amantadine, digoxin, cannabinoids, barbiturates, alcohol

<u>ADRs:</u>
disorientation, confusion, memory loss, hallucinations, nervousness, euphoria, excitement, dizziness, headache, drowsiness, dry mouth, acute suppurative parotitis, nausea, vomiting, constipation, tachycardia, hypotension, blurred vision, mydriasis, urinary retention, muscle weakness, cramping, elevated temperature, flushing, decreased sweating, impotence, skin rash

<u>Elderly (≥60 yrs):</u> More sensitive to CNS adverse effects. Use smaller doses

<u>Contraindications:</u>
Hypersensitivity; angle-closure glaucoma; pyloric/duodenal obstruction; peptic ulcers; prostatic hypertrophy or bladder neck obstructions; achalasia; myasthenia gravis; megacolon

<u>Precautions:</u> Use cautiously in those with arrhythmias, hypertension, hypotension, GI/GU obstructions. Not useful in patients with tardive dyskinesia—may actually aggravate symptoms. These agents may be abused—for the production of mood elevation or psychedelic experiences

*(continues on next page)*

## 318. Agents for Parkinson's Disease  *continued from previous page*

| Drug and Dosage Forms | Usual Dosage Range | Administration Issues and Drug–Drug & Drug–Food Interactions | Common Adverse Drug Reactions (ADRs) and Pharmacokinetics | Contraindications, Pregnancy Category, and Lactation Issues |
|---|---|---|---|---|
| **Procyclidine** *cont.* | | | Pharmacokinetics<br>$T_{1/2}$ = 11.5–12.6 hrs | Pregnancy Category: C<br><br>Lactation Issues: Use cautiously; effects on infant not known |
| **Ropinirole**<br>Requip<br><br>Tablets:<br>0.25 mg, 0.5 mg, 1 mg,<br>2 mg, 5 mg | **Signs and symptoms of Parkinson's disease:** 0.25 mg tid initially then follow the titration schedule below:<br><br>Week   Dosage   Total daily dose<br>1   0.25 mg tid   0.75 mg<br>2   0.5 mg tid   1.5 mg<br>3   0.75 mg tid   2.25 mg<br>4   1 mg tid   3 mg<br><br>After week 4, dosage may be increased by 1.5 mg/d on a weekly basis up to a dose of 9 mg/d, and then by ≤ 3 mg/d weekly to total dose of 24 mg/d<br><br>Discontinue ropinirole gradually over a 7–day period. Decrease administration from tid to bid for 4 days then to qd for the remaining 3 days.<br><br>**With levodopa:** concurrent dose of levodopa may be decreased gradually as tolerated | Administration Issues<br>Can be taken without regards to food; administration with food may reduce nausea; safety/efficacy in children not established; warn patients that they may experience postural hypotension<br><br>Drug–Drug Interactions:<br>ropinirole may **increase** levodopa concentrations; ropinirole clearance may be **decreased** by estrogens, tacrine, erythromycin, fluvoxamine, verapamil, ciprofloxacin, enoxacin, cimetidine, diltiazem, quinidine; ropinirole may have **decreased effectiveness** if given with dopamine antagonists (phenothiazines, thioxanthenes, metoclopramide) | ADRs*:<br>fatigue, postural hypotension, syncope, dizziness, somnolence, nausea, vomiting, asthenia<br><br>*some ADRs seen in patients also taking levodopa<br><br>Pharmacokinetics:<br>$T_{1/2}$ = 8 hrs; titrate with caution in patients with impaired hepatic function | Contraindications:<br>Hypersensitivity<br><br>Pregnancy Category: C<br><br>Lactation Issues<br>It is not known whether ropinirole is excreted in breast milk |

| Drug | Indications/Dosing | Administration Issues / Drug–Drug Interactions | ADRs / Pharmacokinetics | Contraindications / Precautions |
|---|---|---|---|---|
| **Selegiline**<br>Eldepryl<br><br><u>Tablets:</u> 5 mg | **Adjunct to carbidopa/levodopa in the management of parkinsonism in patients who have exhibited deterioration in response to carbidopa/levodopa:** 5 mg before breakfast and lunch. Attempt to reduce levodopa/carbidopa dose after 2–3 days of treatment with selegiline. | <u>Administration Issues:</u> Do not exceed 10 mg/d. May need to decrease dose of levodopa by 10–30% due to increased side effects of levodopa after initiating therapy with selegiline; safety/efficacy not established in children<br><br><u>Drug–Drug Interactions:</u> **increased adverse effects of (death has occurred):** fluoxetine, meperidine | <u>ADRs:</u> dizziness, lightheadedness, fainting, confusion, vivid dreams, headache, increased tremor, nausea, vomiting, constipation, weight loss, anorexia, dysphagia, diarrhea, heartburn, orthostatic hypotension, hypertension, palpitations, urinary retention, prostatic hypertrophy, increased sweating, diaphoresis, facial hair, rash, photosensitivity, asthma, diplopia, dry mouth<br><br><u>Pharmacokinetics:</u> extensively metabolized to 3 metabolites | <u>Contraindications:</u> Hypersensitivity; meperidine use<br><br><u>Precautions:</u> Do not use doses >10 mg/d (nonselectivity for MAO inhibition is lost)<br><br><u>Pregnancy Category:</u> C<br><br><u>Lactation Issues:</u> effects unknown, use cautiously |
| **Trihexyphenidyl**<br>Artane, Artane-Sequels, Trihexy-2, Trihexy-5, various generics<br><br><u>Tablets:</u> 2 mg, 5 mg<br><br><u>Capsules, sustained-release:</u> 5 mg<br><br><u>Elixir:</u> 2 mg/5 mL | **Adjunct in therapy of all forms of parkinsonism:** 1–2 mg/d in 3 divided doses; titrate by 2 mg/d every 3–5 days as needed/tolerated up to 6–10 mg/d.<br><br>Some patients may need higher doses (12–15 mg/d)—divide higher doses in 4 equal doses.<br><br>Concurrent use with levodopa: Generally use smaller doses (3–6 mg/d)<br><br>**Drug-induced extrapyramidal reactions:** 1 mg dose initially (determine effect). Titrate to 5–15 mg/d as needed/tolerated | <u>Administration Issues:</u> May take with food if GI upset occurs If substituting another anticholinergic: gradually reduce other agent while gradually increasing this agent; safety/efficacy<br><br><u>Drug–Drug Interactions:</u> **decreased levels and/or effects of:** haloperidol, phenothiazines, levodopa **increased levels and/or effects of:** amantadine, digoxin, cannabinoids, barbiturates, alcohol | <u>ADRs:</u> disorientation, confusion, memory loss, hallucinations, nervousness, euphoria, excitement, dizziness, headache, drowsiness, dry mouth, acute suppurative parotitis, nausea, vomiting, constipation, tachycardia, hypotension, blurred vision, mydriasis, urinary retention, muscle weakness, cramping, elevated temperature, flushing, decreased sweating, impotence, skin rash<br><br><u>Elderly (>60 yrs):</u> More sensitive to CNS adverse effects. Use smaller doses | <u>Contraindications:</u> Hypersensitivity; angle-closure glaucoma; pyloric/duodenal obstruction; peptic ulcers; prostatic hypertrophy or bladder neck obstructions; achalasia; myasthenia gravis; megacolon<br><br><u>Precautions:</u> Use cautiously in those with arrhythmias, hypertension, hypotension, GI/GU obstructions. Not useful in patients with tardive dyskinesia—may actually aggravate symptoms. These agents may be abused—for the production of mood elevation or psychedelic experiences |

*(continues on next page)*

## 318. Agents for Parkinson's Disease *continued from previous page*

| Drug and Dosage Forms | Usual Dosage Range | Administration Issues and Drug–Drug & Drug–Food Interactions | Common Adverse Drug Reactions (ADRs) and Pharmacokinetics | Contraindications, Pregnancy Category, and Lactation Issues |
|---|---|---|---|---|
| **Trihexyphenidyl** *cont.* | **Sustained-Release Preparation:** Use after stabilized on immediate release. Substitute mg per mg. Give sustained release as one daily dose or divide into 2 doses given 12 hrs apart | | Pharmacokinetics $T_{1/2}$ = 5.6–10.2 hrs | Pregnancy Category: C  Lactation Issues: Use cautiously; effects on infant not known |

## 319. Agents for Rheumatism (for additional agents see NSAIDs (table 306))

| Drug and Dosage Forms | Usual Dosage Range | Administration Issues, Drug–Drug & Drug–Food Interactions | Common Adverse Drug Reactions (ADRs) and Pharmacokinetics | Contraindications, Pregnancy Category, and Lactation Issues |
|---|---|---|---|---|
| **Auranofin** Ridaura  Capsules: 3 mg | **Rheumatoid Arthritis:** 6 mg daily in 1–2 divided doses. May titrate to 3 mg 3 times daily after 6 months if needed.  **Pediatrics:** 0.1 mg/kg/d initially. Maintenance doses: 0.15 mg/kg/d. Max dose: 0.2 mg/kg/d  **Unlabeled Uses:** pemphigus, psoriatic arthritis in those not tolerant to NSAIDs. | Administration Issues Safety/efficacy not established in children.  Drug–Drug Interactions: **increased levels/effects of:** phenytoin | ADRs: diarrhea, rash, stomatitis, anemia, elevated liver function test, leukopenia, proteinuria, thrombocytopenia, pulmonary effects  Pharmacokinetics: $T_{1/2}$ = 26 days | Contraindications: Hypersensitivity; uncontrolled diabetes; severe debilitation, renal disease, hepatic dysfunction or history of hepatitis; uncontrolled CHF; systemic lupus erythematosus; agranulocytosis; blood dyscrasias; urticaria; eczema, colitis; pregnancy  Pregnancy Category: C; however it is contraindicated.  Lactation Issues: excreted in breast milk—discontinue nursing. |

| Drug | Administration Issues / Uses | ADRs / Pharmacokinetics | Contraindications |
|---|---|---|---|
| **Aurothioglucose**<br>Solganal<br><br>Injection, suspension:<br>50 mg/mL<br><br>**Rheumatoid Arthritis:**<br>First dose = 10 mg, followed by 25 mg (2nd & 3rd dose), followed by 50 mg (4th and subsequent doses). Continue with 50 mg/week until 0.8–1 g has been given. Then continue 50 mg dose every 3–4 weeks.<br><br>**Pediatrics:** 1/4 of adult dose based on body weight (not to exceed 25 mg/dose).<br><br>**Unlabeled Uses:** pemphigus, psoriatic arthritis in those not tolerant to NSAIDs. | Administration Issues:<br>Given by IM injection weekly in doctor's office. Observe patient (recumbent) for 15 minutes after administration. Safety/efficacy not established for those <6 yrs.<br><br>Drug–Drug Interactions:<br>None known | ADRs:<br>Most Frequent (when cumulative dose is 300–500 mg): diarrhea, rash, stomatitis, anemia, elevated liver function test, leukopenia, proteinuria, thrombocytopenia, pulmonary effects<br><br>Pharmacokinetics:<br>$T_{1/2}$ = 3–27 days (first dose), 14–40 days (3rd dose); up to 168 days (11th dose) | Contraindications:<br>Hypersensitivity; uncontrolled diabetes; severe debilitation, renal disease, hepatic dysfunction or history of hepatitis; uncontrolled CHF; systemic lupus erythematosus; agranulocytosis; blood dyscrasias; urticaria; eczema, colitis; pregnancy<br><br>Pregnancy Category: C; it is contraindicated.<br><br>Lactation Issues: excreted in breast milk—discontinue nursing. |
| **Azathioprine**<br>Imuran<br><br>Tablets: 50 mg<br><br>**Rheumatoid Arthritis:**<br>**Adults:** 1 mg/kg/d for 6–8 wk.; increase by 0.5 mg/kg q 4 wk. until response or up to 2.5 mg/kg/d<br><br>**Elderly or renal impairment:** use a decreased dose | Administration Issues:<br>Response may take up to 3 months; do not have any vaccinations before checking with prescriber; report persistent sore throat, unusual bleeding or bruising or fatigue; take with food if GI upset occurs<br><br>Drug–Drug Interactions<br>**Increased toxicity /effects of azathioprine:** allopurinol (decrease azathioprine dose to 1/3 to 1/4 of normal dose) | ADRs:<br>fever, chills, nausea, vomiting, anorexia, diarrhea, thrombocytopenia, leukopenia, anemia, secondary infections, rash, pancytopenia, hepatotoxicity<br><br>Pharmacokinetics:<br>extensively metabolized; $T_{1/2}$ (parent) = 12 min | Contraindications:<br>Hypersensitivity to drug; pregnancy or lactation<br><br>Pregnancy Category: D; it is contraindicated.<br><br>Lactation Issues: excreted in breast milk—discontinue nursing. |
| **Gold Sodium Thiomalate**<br>Myochrisine, Aurolate<br><br>Injection: 25 mg/mL, 50 mg/mL<br><br>**Rheumatoid Arthritis:**<br>First dose = 10 mg, followed by 25 mg (2nd dose), followed by 25–50 mg (3rd and subsequent doses). Continue with 25–50 mg/week until 1 g has been given. If clinical | Administration Issues:<br>Given by IM injection weekly in doctor's office. Observe patient (recumbent) for 15 minutes after administration. Safety/efficacy not established in children. | ADRs:<br>Most Frequent (when cumulative dose is 400–800 mg): diarrhea, rash, stomatitis, anemia, elevated liver function test, leukopenia, proteinuria, | Contraindications:<br>Hypersensitivity; uncontrolled diabetes; severe debilitation, renal disease, hepatic dysfunction or history of hepatitis; uncontrolled CHF; |

(continues on next page)

## 319. Agents for Rheumatism *continued from previous page*

| Drug and Dosage Forms | Usual Dosage Range | Administration Issues, Drug–Drug & Drug–Food Interactions | Common Adverse Drug Reactions (ADRs) and Pharmacokinetics | Contraindications, Pregnancy Category, and Lactation Issues |
|---|---|---|---|---|
| **Gold Sodium Thiomalate** *cont.* | improvement before 1 g, may give dose q other week for weeks 2–20. Then continue 25–50 mg dose q 3–4 weeks<br><br>**Pediatrics:** Initially, 10 mg, then 1 mg/kg up to 50 mg for a single injection. Follow above schedule.<br><br>**Unlabeled Uses:** pemphigus, psoriatic arthritis in those not tolerant to NSAIDs. | <u>Drug–Drug Interactions:</u> None known | thrombocytopenia, pulmonary effects<br><br><u>Pharmacokinetics:</u><br>T<sub></sub>$T_{1/2}$ = 3–27 days (first dose), 14–40 days (3rd dose); up to 168 days (11th dose) | systemic lupus erythematosus; agranulocytosis; blood dyscrasias; urticaria; eczema, colitis; pregnancy<br><br><u>Pregnancy Category:</u> C; it is contraindicated.<br><br><u>Lactation Issues:</u> excreted in breast milk—discontinue nursing. |
| **Hydroxychloroquine**<br>Plaquenil<br><br><u>Tablets:</u> 200 mg | **Rheumatoid Arthritis:**<br>Initially, 400–600 mg daily. When clinical improvement noted, decrease dose to 200–400 mg/d<br><br>**Systemic Lupus Erythematosus:**<br>400 mg qd to bid<br><br>**Pediatrics (for either indication):**<br>3–5 mg/kg/d up to a max of 400 mg/d in 1–2 divided doses. May titrate to 7 mg/kg/d if needed. | <u>Administration Issues:</u><br>May take with food if GI upset occurs. Use cautiously, in children as they are more sensitive to toxic effects.<br><br><u>Drug–Drug Interactions:</u><br>**increased levels of:** digoxin | <u>ADRs:</u><br>irritability, nervousness, emotional changes, nightmares, psychosis, headache, ataxia, dizziness, nystagmus, blurred vision, edema of cornea or retina, corneal opacities, retinal atrophy, abnormal pigmentation, optic disc atrophy, decreased visual acuity, bleaching of hair, alopecia, pruritus, skin pigmentation; skin eruptions (urticarial, others), non-light sensitive psoriasis, hemolysis in those with G-6-PD deficiency, anorexia, nausea, vomiting, diarrhea, abdominal cramps, skeletal muscle weakness, weight loss, lassitude, exacerbation, precipitation of porphyria, peripheral neuropathy | <u>Contraindications:</u><br>Hypersensitivity; retinal or visual field changes attributable to any 4-aminoquinoline compound; long-term therapy in children.<br><br><u>Precautions:</u> Use cautiously in those with severe renal or hepatic dysfunction, or in alcoholics. Monitor complete blood counts periodically.<br><br><u>Pregnancy Issues:</u> Avoid use.<br><br><u>Lactation Issues:</u> Not significantly excreted in breast milk; however use cautiously. |

| | Rheumatoid Arthritis / Dosage | Administration Issues / Interactions | Pharmacokinetics / ADRs | Contraindications / Precautions |
|---|---|---|---|---|
| **Methotrexate**<br>Rheumatrex Dose Pack, various generics<br><br><u>Tablets:</u> 2.5 mg | **Rheumatoid Arthritis:**<br>2.5 mg every 12 hrs for 3 doses. This schedule is repeated weekly. | <u>Administration Issues:</u><br>Drink plenty of fluid. Safety/efficacy for rheumatoid arthritis not established in children<br><br><u>Drug–Drug Interactions:</u><br>**increased levels/effects of:**<br>etretinate (increased hepatotoxicity)<br><br>**increased levels/effects of methotrexate:** probenecid, salicylates, sulfonamides, NSAIDs (MAY inc toxicity)<br><br>**decreased levels/effects of methotrexate:** folic acid, charcoal<br><br><u>Drug–Food Interaction:</u><br>Food may decrease absorption of MTX. | <u>Pharmacokinetics:</u><br>concentrates in liver, spleen, kidney, heart, and brain and is strongly bound in melanin-containing cells such as those in the eyes and skin; slow elimination<br><br><u>ADRs:</u><br>elevated liver function tests, nausea, vomiting, thrombocytopenia, stomatitis, rash, pruritus, dermatitis, diarrhea, alopecia, leukopenia, pancytopenia, dizziness, anorexia, abdominal cramps, pulmonary toxicity, hepatotoxicity<br><br><u>Pharmacokinetics:</u><br>$T_{1/2}$ = 3–10 hrs | <u>Contraindications:</u><br>Hypersensitivity; pregnant or lactating women; alcoholism; liver disease; immunodeficiency syndromes; preexisting blood dyscrasias<br><br><u>Precautions:</u> Monitor hematology liver and renal function every 1–2 months<br><br><u>Pregnancy Category:</u> X<br><br><u>Lactation Issues:</u><br>Contraindicated |
| **Penicillamine**<br>Cuprimine, Depen<br><br><u>Tablets, titratable:</u> 250 mg<br><br><u>Capsules:</u> 125 mg, 250 mg | **Rheumatoid Arthritis:**<br><br>**Adults:**<br>Initial Therapy: 125–250 mg as a single daily dose; increase at 1–3 month intervals by 125–250 mg/d as patient response and tolerance indicates. If satisfactory remission achieved, continue the dose. If no improvement | <u>Administration Issues:</u><br>Take on an empty stomach, 1 hr before or 2 hr after meals and at least 1 hr apart from any other drug, food or milk; notify prescriber if skin rash, unusual bruising or bleeding, sore throat, unexplained coughing/wheezing, fever or chills occur | <u>ADRs:</u><br>fever, rash, urticaria, hypogeusia, arthralgia; edema of face, feet or lower limbs; chills, weight gain, sore throat, bloody or cloudy urine, aplastic or hemolytic anemia, leukopenia, thrombocytopenia, white spots on lips or mouth, proteinuria | <u>Contraindications:</u><br>Hypersensitivity to drug; history of penicillamine-related aplastic anemia or agranulocytosis; renal insufficiency, pregnancy, breastfeeding<br><br><u>Pregnancy Category:</u> D |

(continues on next page)

| Drug and Dosage Forms | Usual Dosage Range | Administration Issues, Drug–Drug & Drug–Food Interactions | Common Adverse Drug Reactions (ADRs) and Pharmacokinetics | Contraindications, Pregnancy Category, and Lactation Issues |
|---|---|---|---|---|
| **Penicillamine** *cont.* | after 3–4 months with 1–1.5 gm/d, discontinue drug<br><br>**Children:**<br>Initial: 3 mg/kg/d (≤250 mg/d) for 3 months, then 6 mg/kg/d (≤500 mg/d), divided bid for 3 months to a maximum of 10 mg/kg/d divided tid to qid | <u>Drug Interactions:</u><br>The absorption of penicillamine is **decreased** with coadministration with iron salts and antacid.<br><br>Penicillamine may **decrease** digoxin serum levels.<br><br>Penicillamine should not be coadministered with gold therapy, antimalarial or cytotoxic drugs due to similar **serious hematologic and renal reactions.** | <u>Pharmacokinetics:</u><br>$T_{1/2} = 1.7$–3.2 h | <u>Lactation Issues:</u> do not breastfeed |
| **Sulfasalazine**<br>Azulfidine<br><br><u>Tablets:</u><br>500 mg<br><br><u>Tablet, enteric coated:</u> 500 mg<br><br><u>Suspension:</u> 250 mg/5 mL | **Rheumatoid Arthritis:**<br><br>1 g tid to qid, 2g/d maintenance in divided doses; do not exceed 600 gm/d | <u>Administration Issues:</u><br>Maintain adequate fluid intake; take after meals; may cause an orange-yellow discoloration of urine and skin; may permanently stain contact lenses; avoid prolonged exposure to sunlight; do not take with antacids<br><br><u>Drug Interactions:</u><br>**Decreased effect** with iron and digoxin<br><br>**Increased effects/actions of:** oral anticoagulants, methotrexate, oral hypoglycemic agents<br><br>**Increased risk** of folate deficiency | <u>ADRs:</u><br>fever, dizziness, headache, rash, photosensitivity, anorexia, nausea, diarrhea, reversible oligospermia, granulocytopenia, leukopenia, thrombocytopenia, aplastic anemia, hemolytic anemia<br><br><u>Pharmacokinetics:</u><br>10–15% of dose is absorbed as unchanged drug from the small intestine, $T_{1/2} = 6$–10 hr | <u>Contraindications:</u><br>Hypersensitivity to sulfasalazine or sulfa drugs, porphyria, GI or GU obstruction; hypersensitivity to salicylates, pregnancy<br><br><u>Precautions:</u> Use cautiously in those with severe renal or hepatic dysfunction, those with G-6-PD deficiency<br><br><u>Pregnancy Category:</u> B<br>(D at term)<br><br><u>Lactation Issues:</u> use cautiously. |

# 400. EYE AND EAR PREPARATIONS
## 401. Ophthalmic Preparations
401.1 Agents for Glaucoma (for oral treatment see Carbonic Anhydrase Inhibitors, section 208.1)

| Drug, Dosage Forms and *Pharmacologic Action* | Usual Dosage Range | Administration Issues and Drug–Drug Interactions | Common Adverse Drug Reactions (ADRs) | Contraindications, Pregnancy Category, and Lactation Issues |
|---|---|---|---|---|
| **Apraclonidine**<br>Iopidine<br><br>Solution:<br>0.5%<br><br>*Sympathomimetic* | short term adjunctive therapy in patients on maximally tolerated medical therapy who require additional IOP reduction:<br><br>**0.5% solution**<br>1–2 drops in affected eye(s) tid | Administration Issues:<br>do not touch tip of container to any surface; tachyphylaxis occurs in most patients—he benefit for most patients is < 1 month; safety and efficacy have not been established in children | ADRs:<br>hyperemia; pruritus; tearing; eye discomfort; lid edema; dry mouth; foreign body sensation; upper lid elevation; GI upset; bradycardia; insomnia, lethargy, dry nose | Contraindications:<br>hypersensitivity to apraclonidine or clonidine; concurrent monoamine oxidase inhibitor therapy<br><br>Pregnancy Category:  C<br><br>Lactation Issues:  it is not known whether apraclonidine is excreted in breast milk; use caution in nursing women |
| **Betaxolol**<br>Betoptic, Betoptic S<br><br>Solution:<br>0.5%<br><br>Suspension:<br>0.25%<br><br>*Beta Blocker* | chronic open-angle glaucoma/ocular hypertension:<br><br>1–2 drops in affected eye(s) bid | Administration Issues:<br>shake suspension well before use; do not touch tip of container to any surface; safety and efficacy have not been established in children<br><br>Drug–Drug Interactions:<br>additive effects may occur when given with oral **beta blockers** or **verapamil** | ADRs:<br>transient burning/stinging; tearing; bradycardia; hypotension; congestive heart failure; bronchospasm; masked symptoms of hypoglycemia; dizziness | Contraindications:<br>hypersensitivity to beta blockers; asthma; sinus bradycardia; second or third degree AV block; overt CHF<br><br>Pregnancy Category:  C<br><br>Lactation Issues:  it is not known whether betaxolol is excreted in breast milk; either the drug or breast feeding should be discontinued |

*(continues on next page)*

| Drug, Dosage Forms and *Pharmacologic Action* | Usual Dosage Range | Administration Issues and Drug–Drug Interactions | Common Adverse Drug Reactions (ADRs) | Contraindications, Pregnancy Category, and Lactation Issues |
|---|---|---|---|---|
| **Carbachol** Isopto Carbachol, Carboptic  Solution: 0.75%, 1.5%, 2.25%, 3%  *Cholinergic Agent & Miotic, Direct Acting* | glaucoma: 2 drops in affected eye(s) tid | Administration Issues: do not touch tip of container to any surface; safety and efficacy have not been established in children  Drug–Drug Interactions: reports exists that both **topical NSAIDs** and acetylcholine are ineffective when used concurrently | ADRs: transient stinging/burning; corneal clouding; ciliary spasm; headache; salivation; flushing; sweating; GI upset; hypotension; frequent urge to urinate, eye pain | Contraindications: hypersensitivity to acetylcholine; conditions where pupillary constriction is undesirable; acute inflammatory disease of the anterior chamber  Pregnancy Category:  C  Lactation Issues:  it is not known whether carbachol is excreted in breast milk; either the drug or breast milk; either the drug or breast feeding should be discontinued |
| **Carteolol** Ocupress  Solution: 1%  *Beta Blocker* | chronic open-angle glaucoma/ocular hypertension: 1 drop in affected eye(s) bid | Administration Issues: do not touch tip of container to any surface; safety and efficacy have not been established in children  Drug–Drug Interactions: additive effects may occur when given with oral **beta blockers** or **verapamil** | ADRs: transient burning/stinging; tearing; bradycardia; hypotension; congestive heart failure; bronchospasm; masked symptoms of hypoglycemia; dizziness | Contraindications: hypersensitivity to beta blockers; asthma; sinus bradycardia; second or third degree AV block; overt CHF  Pregnancy Category:  C  Lactation Issues:  carteolol is excreted in breast milk; either the drug or breast feeding should be discontinued |

| Drug | Indication/Dosage | Administration Issues | ADRs | Contraindications |
|---|---|---|---|---|
| **Demecarium**<br>Humorsol<br><br>Solution:<br>0.125%, 0.25%<br><br>*Miotic, Cholinesterase Inhibitor* | open-angle glaucoma, when shorter acting miotics have proved inadequate:<br>1–2 drops in affected eye(s) frequency of administration may range from bid to twice weekly | Administration Issues:<br>do not touch tip of container to any surface; wash hands immediately after administration; protect from heat; do not freeze<br><br>Drug–Drug Interactions:<br>additive effects may occur when administered concurrently with systemic anticholinesterases | ADRs:<br>iris cysts (more common in children); burning; lacrimation; lid muscle twitching; browache; headache; blurring; retinal detachment; GI upset; urinary incontinence; sweating; salivation; myopia | Contraindications:<br>hypersensitivity to cholinesterase inhibitors; glaucoma associated with iridocyclitis; inflammatory disease of the iris or ciliary body; pregnancy<br><br>Pregnancy Category: C<br><br>Lactation Issues:<br>it is not known whether demecarium is excreted in breast milk; either the drug or breast feeding should be discontinued |
| **Dipivefrin**<br>Propine<br><br>Solution:<br>0.1%<br><br>*Sympathomimetic* | glaucoma:<br>1 drop q 12 h | Administration Issues:<br>do not touch tip of container to any surface; do not use while wearing soft contact lenses; when used with other miotics, instill the miotic first; safety and efficacy have not been established in children; avoid exposure to light and air; discolored or darkened solutions indicate loss of potency | ADRs:<br>transient stinging/burning; eye pain; browache; headache; watery eyes; ocular congestion, photophobia; blurred vision | Contraindications:<br>hypersensitivity to dipivefrin; narrow angle glaucoma<br><br>Pregnancy Category: B<br><br>Lactation Issues: it is not known whether dipivefrin is excreted in breast milk; use caution in nursing women |
| **Dorzolamide**<br>Trusopt<br><br>Solution:<br>2%<br><br>*Carbonic Anhydrase Inhibitor* | open-angle glaucoma/ocular hypertension:<br>1 drop in affected eye(s) tid | Administration Issues:<br>do not touch tip of container to any surface; if more than one topical ophthalmic drug is being used, administer the drugs at least ten minutes apart; safety and efficacy have not been established in children | ADRs:<br>ocular burning/stinging; bitter taste; superficial punctate keratitis; blurred vision; tearing; dryness; photophobia; headache | Contraindications:<br>hypersensitivity to dorzolamide<br><br>Pregnancy Category: C<br><br>Lactation Issues:<br>it is not known whether dorzolamide is excreted in |

*(continues on next page)*

| Drug, Dosage Forms and *Pharmacologic Action* | Usual Dosage Range | Administration Issues and Drug–Drug Interactions | Common Adverse Drug Reactions (ADRs) | Contraindications, Pregnancy Category, and Lactation Issues |
|---|---|---|---|---|
| **Dorzolamide** *cont.* | | Drug–Drug Interactions: additive effects may occur when administered concurrently with systemic carbonic anhydrase inhibitors | | breast milk; either the drug or breast feeding should be discontinued |
| **Echothiophate** Phospholine Solution: 0.03%, 0.06%, 0.125%, 0.25% *Miotic, Cholinesterase Inhibitor* | open-angle glaucoma; angle-closure glaucoma: 1 drop in affected eye(s) frequency of administration may range from qod to bid | Administration Issues: do not touch tip of container to any surface; administer one of the two daily doses at bedtime to avoid inconvenience due to miosis; store in refrigerator to maintain potency for 6 months; must be reconstituted with diluent<br><br>Drug–Drug Interactions: additive effects may occur when administered concurrently with systemic anticholinesterases | ADRs: iris cysts (more common in children); burning; lacrimation; lid muscle twitching; browache; headache; blurring; retinal detachment; GI upset; urinary incontinence; sweating; salivation | Contraindications: hypersensitivity to cholinesterase inhibitors; glaucoma associated with iridocyclitis; inflammatory disease of the iris or ciliary body; closed-angle glaucoma<br><br>Pregnancy Category: C<br><br>Lactation Issues: it is not known whether phospholine is excreted in breast milk; either the drug or breast feeding should be discontinued |
| **Epinephrine** Epifrin, Glaucon Solution: 0.1%, 0.5%, 1%, 2% | glaucoma: 1 drop into affected eye(s) qd to bid | Administration Issues: do not touch tip of container to any surface; do not use while wearing soft contact lenses; when used with other miotics, instill the miotic first; safety and efficacy have not been established in children | ADRs: transient stinging/burning; eye pain; browache; headache; watery eyes | Contraindications: hypersensitivity to epinephrine; narrow or shallow angle glaucoma; aphakia<br><br>Pregnancy Category: C |

| | | | | |
|---|---|---|---|---|
| | | | | Lactation Issues: it is not known whether epinephrine is excreted in breast milk; use caution in nursing women |
| **Latanoprost** Xalatan Solution 0.005% (50 mcg/ml) *Prostaglandin Analog* | elevated intraocular pressure in patients with open-angle glaucoma and ocular hypertension who have failed other medications: one drop (1.5 mcg) in affected eye(s) qd in the evening. Do not exceed once daily dosage. | Administration Issues inform patient about possibility of iris color change (increasing the amount of brown pigment); do not touch tip of container to any surface; remove contact lenses prior to administration and reinsert 15 minutes after administration; if using concomitantly with another ophthalmic drug, administer drugs at least 5 minutes apart; protect from light; refrigerate unopened bottle; once opened, container may be stored at room temperature for 6 weeks | ADRs: blurred vision, burning; stinging; conjunctival hyperemia, foreign body sensation; itching; increased pigmentation of iris; punctate epithelial keratopathy, dry eye; eye pain; photophobia | Contraindications: hypersensitivity to latanoprost Pregnancy Category: C Lactation Issues: it is not known whether latanoprost is excreted in breast milk; either the drug or breast feeding should be discontinued |
| **Levobunolol** AKBeta, Betagan, Levobunolol Solution: 0.25%, 0.5% *Beta Blocker* | chronic open-angle glaucoma/ocular hypertension: 1 drop in affected eye(s) qd to bid | Administration Issues: do not touch tip of container to any surface; safety and efficacy have not been established in children Drug–Drug Interactions: additive effects may occur when given with oral **beta blocker, quinidine** or **verapamil** | ADRs: transient burning/stinging; tearing; bradycardia; hypotension; congestive heart failure; bronchospasm; masked symptoms of hypoglycemia; dizziness; headache, conjunctivitis; keratitis | Contraindications: hypersensitivity to beta blockers; asthma; sinus bradycardia; second or third degree AV block; overt CHF; severe COPD Pregnancy Category: C Lactation Issues: it is not known whether levobunolol is excreted in breast milk; either the drug or breast feeding should be discontinued |

(continues on next page)

| Drug, Dosage Forms and *Pharmacologic Action* | Usual Dosage Range | Administration Issues and Drug–Drug Interactions | Common Adverse Drug Reactions (ADRs) | Contraindications, Pregnancy Category, and Lactation Issues |
|---|---|---|---|---|
| **Metipranolol** Optipranolol  Solution: 0.3%  *Beta Blocker* | chronic open-angle glaucoma/ocular hypertension: 1 drop in affected eye(s) bid | Administration Issues: do not touch tip of container to any surface; safety and efficacy have not been established in children  Drug–Drug Interactions: additive effects may occur when given with oral **beta blockers** or **verapamil** | ADRs: transient burning/stinging; tearing; bradycardia; hypotension; congestive heart failure; bronchospasm; masked symptoms of hypoglycemia; dizziness | Contraindications: hypersensitivity to beta blockers; asthma; sinus bradycardia; second or third degree AV block; overt CHF  Pregnancy Category: C  Lactation Issues: it is not known whether metipranolol is excreted in breast milk; either the drug or breast feeding should be discontinued |
| **Physostigmine** Eserine  Ointment: 0.25%  *Miotic, Cholinesterase Inhibitor* | open-angle glaucoma: apply small quantity to lower fornix in affected eye(s) up to tid | Administration Issues: do not touch tip of container to any surface; wash hands immediately after administration; safety and efficacy have not been established in children  Drug–Drug Interactions: additive effects may occur when administered concurrently with systemic anticholinesterases | ADRs: iris cysts (more common in children); burning; lacrimation; lid muscle twitching; browache; headache; blurring; retinal detachment; GI upset; urinary incontinence; sweating; salivation; eye pain | Contraindications: hypersensitivity to cholinesterase inhibitors; glaucoma associated with iridocyclitis; inflammatory disease of the iris or ciliary body  Pregnancy Category: C  Lactation Issues: it is not known whether physostigmine is excreted in breast milk; either the drug or breast feeding should be discontinued |

| | | | |
|---|---|---|---|
| **Pilocarpine**<br>Isopto Carpine, Pilocar, Piloptic, Akarpine, Pilostat, Adsorbocarpine<br><br>Solution:<br>0.25%, 0.5%, 1%, 2%, 3%, 4%, 5%, 6%, 8%, 10%<br><br>Gel:<br>4%<br><br>*Cholinergic Agent & Miotic, Direct Acting* | chronic simple glaucoma, chronic angle-closure glaucoma:<br><br>**solution**<br>1–2 drops in affected eye(s) tid to qid<br><br>**gel**<br>1/2 inch in the lower conjunctival sac of affected eye(s) q hs | Administration Issues:<br>do not touch tip of container to any surface; if other glaucoma medication is also used at bedtime, use drops at least 5 minutes before using the gel; safety and efficacy have not been established in children<br><br>Drug–Drug Interactions:<br>reports exists that both **topical NSAIDs** and acetylcholine are ineffective when used concurrently | ADRs:<br>transient stinging/burning; tearing; ciliary spasm; headache; hypertension; tachycardia; salivation; sweating; GI upset<br><br>Contraindications:<br>hypersensitivity to acetylcholine; conditions where pupillary constriction is undesirable<br><br>Pregnancy Category: C<br><br>Lactation Issues:<br>it is not known whether pilocarpine is excreted in breast milk; either the drug or breast feeding should be discontinued |
| **Pilocarpine Ocular Therapeutic System**<br>Ocusert Pilo<br><br>Ocular Therapeutic System:<br>20 mcg/hr; 40 mcg/hr<br><br>*Miotic, Direct Acting* | glaucoma/IOP reduction:<br>initial dose: 20 mcg/hr system every 7 days<br><br>maximum dose: 40 mcg/hr system every 7 days | Administration Issues:<br>wash hands with soap and water before touching the system; discard contaminated systems and replace with a fresh unit; safety and efficacy have not been established in children<br><br>Drug–Drug Interactions:<br>reports exists that both **topical NSAIDs** and acetylcholine are ineffective when used concurrently | ADRs:<br>conjunctival irritation; tearing; ciliary spasm; headache; hypertension; tachycardia; salivation; sweating; GI upset<br><br>Contraindications:<br>hypersensitivity to acetylcholine; conditions where pupillary constriction is undesirable<br><br>Pregnancy Category: C<br><br>Lactation Issues:<br>it is not known whether pilocarpine is excreted in breast milk; either the drug or breast feeding should be discontinued |
| **Timolol**<br>Timoptic<br><br>Solution:<br>0.25%, 0.5%<br><br>Gel:<br>0.25%, 0.5% | chronic open-angle glaucoma/ocular hypertension/aphakic patients with glaucoma:<br><br>**solution**<br>initial dose: 1 drop (0.25%) in affected eye(s) bid | Administration Issues:<br>shake gel once before use; administer other ophthalmics at least 10 minutes before the gel; do not touch tip of container to any surface; safety and efficacy have not been established in children | ADRs:<br>transient burning/stinging; tearing; bradycardia; hypotension; congestive heart failure; bronchospasm; masked symptoms of hypoglycemia; dizziness<br><br>Contraindications:<br>hypersensitivity to beta blockers; asthma; sinus bradycardia; second or third degree AV block; overt CHF; severe COPD<br><br>Pregnancy Category: C |

*(continues on next page)*

## 401.1 Agents for Glaucoma continued from previous page

| Drug, Dosage Forms and *Pharmacologic Action* | Usual Dosage Range | Administration Issues and Drug–Drug Interactions | Common Adverse Drug Reactions (ADRs) | Contraindications, Pregnancy Category, and Lactation Issues |
|---|---|---|---|---|
| **Timolol *cont.***<br><br>*Beta Blocker* | maximum dose: 1 drop (0.5%) in affected eye(s) bid<br><br>some patients may be maintained with qd dosing<br><br>**gel**<br>initial dose: apply (0.25%) to affected eye (s) qd<br><br>maximum dose: apply (0.5%) to affected eye(s) qd | <u>Drug–Drug Interactions:</u><br>additive effects may occur when given with oral **beta blockers** or **verapamil** | | <u>Lactation Issues:</u><br>timolol is excreted in breast milk; either the drug or breast feeding should be discontinued |

## 401.2 Ophthalmic Antibiotic Agents

| Drug and Dosage Forms | Usual Dosage Range | Administration Issues and Drug–Drug Interactions | Common Adverse Drug Reactions (ADRs) | Contraindications, Pregnancy Category, and Lactation Issues |
|---|---|---|---|---|
| **Bacitracin**<br>AK-Tracin<br><br><u>Ointment:</u><br>500 units/g | <u>superficial ocular infection due to strains of microorganisms susceptible to antibiotics:</u><br>1/2 inch in affected eye(s) qd to bid | <u>Administration Issues:</u><br>do not touch tip of container to any surface; do not use while wearing soft contact lenses<br><br><u>Drug–Drug Interactions:</u><br>sensitization from the topical use of an antibiotic may contraindicate the drug's later systemic use in serious infections | <u>ADRs:</u><br>burning/stinging; itching | <u>Contraindications:</u><br>hypersensitivity to bacitracin; vaccinia; varicella; mycobacterial infections of the eye; ocular fungal infection; use of steroid combinations after uncomplicated removal of a corneal foreign body |

| | | | ADRs / Administration | Contraindications / Lactation / Pregnancy |
|---|---|---|---|---|
| | | | | Pregnancy Category: C<br><br>Lactation Issues:<br>it is not known if bacitracin is excreted in breast milk; either the drug or nursing should be discontinued |
| **Chloramphenicol**<br>AK-Chlor, Chloroptic, Chloromycetin<br><br>Solution:<br>0.5% (5 mg/mL)<br><br>Ointment:<br>1% (10 mg/g) | superficial ocular infection due to strains of microorganisms susceptible to antibiotics:<br><br>**solution**<br>1–2 drops in affected eye(s) q 3–4 h<br><br>**ointment**<br>1/2 inch in affected eye(s) q 3–4 h<br><br>the dosing interval may be increased after the first 48 hours; treatment should continue for at least 48 hours after the eye appears normal | Administration Issues:<br>do not touch tip of container to any surface; do not use while wearing soft contact lenses<br><br>Drug–Drug Interactions:<br>sensitization from the topical use of an antibiotic may contraindicate the drug's later systemic use in serious infections | ADRs:<br>burning/stinging; itching; bone marrow suppression (rare); headache, rash | Contraindications:<br>hypersensitivity to chloramphenicol; vaccinia; varicella; mycobacterial infections of the eye; ocular fungal infection; use of steroid combinations after uncomplicated removal of a corneal foreign body<br><br>Pregnancy Category: C<br><br>Lactation Issues:<br>it is not known if chloramphenicol is excreted in breast milk; either the drug or nursing should be discontinued |
| **Ciprofloxacin**<br>Ciloxan<br><br>Solution:<br>3.5 mg/ml | bacterial keratitis:<br>2 drops in the affected eye(s) q 15 minutes for 6 h, then 2 drops in the affected eye(s) q 30 minutes for the remainder of the first day; on day 2, 2 drops in the affected eye(s) q hour; on days 3–14, 2 drops in the affected eye(s) q 4 h | Administration Issues:<br>do not touch tip of container to any surface; do not use while wearing soft contact lenses; safety and efficacy in infants <1 year have not been established<br><br>Drug–Drug Interactions:<br>sensitization from the topical use of an antibiotic may contraindicate the drug's later systemic use in serious infections | ADRs:<br>burning/stinging; itching; white crystalline precipitates; crusting; foreign body sensation; bitter taste; tearing; photophobia | Contraindications:<br>hypersensitivity to fluoroquinolones; vaccinia; varicella; mycobacterial infections of the eye; ocular fungal infection; use of steroid combinations after uncomplicated removal of a corneal foreign body<br><br>Pregnancy Category: C |

(continues on next page)

**401.2 Ophthalmic Antibiotic Agents** *continued from previous page*

| Drug and Dosage Forms | Usual Dosage Range | Administration Issues and Drug–Drug Interactions | Common Adverse Drug Reactions (ADRs) | Contraindications, Pregnancy Category, and Lactation Issues |
|---|---|---|---|---|
| **Ciprofloxacin** *cont.* | <u>bacterial conjunctivitis:</u><br>1–2 drops in the affected eye(s) q 2 h while awake for 2 days, then 1–2 drops in the affected eye(s) q 4 h while awake for the next 5 days | | | <u>Lactation Issues:</u><br>it is not known if ciprofloxacin is excreted in breast milk; either the drug or nursing should be discontinued |
| **Erythromycin**<br>Ilotycin<br><br><u>Ointment:</u><br>5 mg/g | <u>superficial ocular infection due to strains of microorganisms susceptible to antibiotics:</u><br>1/2 inch in affected eye(s) qd to bid<br><br><u>trachoma:</u><br>1/2 inch in the affected eye(s) bid for 2 months or 1/2 inch in the affected eye(s) for the first 5 days of each month for 6 months | <u>Administration Issues:</u><br>do not touch tip of container to any surface; do not use while wearing soft contact lenses<br><br><u>Drug–Drug Interactions:</u><br>sensitization from the topical use of an antibiotic may contraindicate the drug's later systemic use in serious infections | <u>ADRs:</u><br>burning/stinging; itching | <u>Contraindications:</u><br>hypersensitivity to erythromycin; vaccinia; varicella; mycobacterial infections of the eye; ocular fungal infection; use of steroid combinations after uncomplicated removal of a corneal foreign body<br><br><u>Pregnancy Category:</u>  B<br><br><u>Lactation Issues:</u><br>it is not known if erythromycin is excreted in breast milk; either the drug or nursing should be discontinued |
| **Gentamicin**<br>Garamycin, Genoptic, Gentacidin, Gentak<br><br><u>Solution:</u><br>3 mg/ml | <u>superficial ocular infection due to strains of microorganisms susceptible to antibiotics:</u><br><br>**solution**<br>1–2 drops in affected eye(s) q 2–4 h; up to 2 drops q h for severe infections | <u>Administration Issues:</u><br>do not touch tip of container to any surface; do not use while wearing soft contact lenses<br><br><u>Drug–Drug Interactions:</u><br>sensitization from the topical use of an antibiotic may contraindicate | <u>ADRs:</u><br>burning/stinging; itching; conjunctival erythema; corneal ulcers | <u>Contraindications:</u><br>hypersensitivity to gentamicin; vaccinia; varicella; mycobacterial infections of the eye; ocular fungal infection; use of steroid combinations after uncomplicated removal of a corneal foreign body |

| | | | |
|---|---|---|---|
| Ointment:<br>3 mg/g (0.3%) | ointment<br>1/2 inch in affected eye(s) bid to tid | the drug's later systemic use in serious infections | Pregnancy Category: C<br><br>Lactation Issues:<br>it is not known if gentamicin is excreted in breast milk; either the drug or nursing should be discontinued |
| Norfloxacin<br>Chibroxin<br><br>Solution:<br>3 mg/ml (0.3%) | bacterial conjunctivitis:<br>1–2 drops in the affected eye(s) qid for up to 7 days; in severe infections, 1–2 drops in the affected eye(s) q 2 h while awake may be used on the first 2 days of therapy | Administration Issues:<br>do not touch tip of container to any surface; do not use while wearing soft contact lenses; safety and efficacy in infants < 1 year have not been established<br><br>Drug–Drug Interactions:<br>sensitization from the topical use of an antibiotic may contraindicate the drug's later systemic use in serious infections | Contraindications:<br>hypersensitivity to fluoroquinolones; vaccinia; varicella; mycobacterial infections of the eye; ocular fungal infection; use of steroid combinations after uncomplicated removal of a corneal foreign body<br><br>ADRs:<br>burning/stinging; itching; white crystalline precipitates; crusting; foreign body sensation; bitter taste; tearing; photophobia<br><br>Pregnancy Category: C<br><br>Lactation Issues:<br>it is not known if norfloxacin is excreted in breast milk; either the drug or nursing should be discontinued |
| Ofloxacin<br>Ocuflox<br><br>Solution:<br>3 mg/ml (0.3%) | bacterial conjunctivitis; corneal ulcers:<br>1–2 drops in the affected eye(s) q 2–4 h while awake for 2 days, then 1–2 drops in the affected eye(s) qid for up to 5 more days; for more severe infections, more frequent administration may be required | Administration Issues:<br>do not touch tip of container to any surface; do not use while wearing soft contact lenses; safety and efficacy in infants < 1 year have not been established<br><br>Drug–Drug Interactions:<br>sensitization from the topical use of an antibiotic may contraindicate the drug's later systemic use in serious infections | Contraindications:<br>hypersensitivity to fluoroquinolones; vaccinia; varicella; mycobacterial infections of the eye; ocular fungal infection; use of steroid combinations after uncomplicated removal of a corneal foreign body<br><br>ADRs:<br>burning/stinging; itching; white crystalline precipitates; crusting; foreign body sensation; bitter taste; tearing; photophobia<br><br>Pregnancy Category: C |

(continues on next page)

| Drug and Dosage Forms | Usual Dosage Range | Administration Issues and Drug–Drug Interactions | Common Adverse Drug Reactions (ADRs) | Contraindications, Pregnancy Category, and Lactation Issues |
|---|---|---|---|---|
| **Ofloxacin** *cont.* | | | | Lactation Issues:<br>it is not known if ofloxacin is excreted in breast milk; either the drug or nursing should be discontinued |
| **Polymyxin B**<br>Solution:<br>25,000 units/ml | superficial ocular infection due to strains of microorganisms susceptible to antibiotics:<br><br>**solution**<br>1–2 drops in affected eye(s) bid to qid<br><br>**ointment**<br>1/2 inch in affected eye(s) q 3–4 h | Administration Issues:<br>do not touch tip of container to any surface; do not use while wearing soft contact lenses; safety and efficacy in infants < 2 months have not been established<br><br>Drug–Drug Interactions:<br>sensitization from the topical use of an antibiotic may contraindicate the drug's later systemic use in serious infections | ADRs:<br>burning/stinging; itching | Contraindications:<br>hypersensitivity to polymyxin; vaccinia; varicella; mycobacterial infections of the eye; ocular fungal infection; use of steroid combinations after uncomplicated removal of a corneal foreign body<br><br>Pregnancy Category: B<br><br>Lactation Issues:<br>it is not known if polymyxin is excreted in breast milk; either the drug or nursing should be discontinued |
| **Sulfacetamide**<br>AK-Sulf, Bleph-10, Ocusulf-10, Sodium Sulamyd, Sulf-10, Cetamide<br><br>Solution:<br>10%, 15%, 30% | superficial ocular infection due to strains of microorganisms susceptible to antibiotics:<br><br>**solution**<br>1–2 drops in the affected eye(s) q 1–4 h initially according to severity | Administration Issues:<br>do not touch tip of container to any surface; do not use while wearing soft contact lenses; safety and efficacy in children have not been established; protect from light | ADRs:<br>burning/stinging; itching; periorbital edema; rash; photosensitivity; headache; GI upset; bone marrow suppression (rare); rare occurrences of severe | Contraindications:<br>hypersensitivity to sulfonamides; infants < 2 months; epithelial herpes simplex keratitis; vaccinia; viral, mycobacterial or fungal infection of the ocular structures; after uncomplicated |

| Drug | Dosing | Administration Issues / Drug–Drug Interactions | ADRs | Contraindications / Pregnancy / Lactation |
|---|---|---|---|---|
| Ointment: 10% | of infection; taper dose by increasing the time interval between doses<br>**ointment**<br>1/2 inch in affected eye(s) tid to qid and q hs<br>trachoma:<br>**solution**<br>2 drops in affected eye(s) q 2 h | Drug–Drug Interactions:<br>**silver preparations** are incompatible with topical sulfonamides | sensitivity reactions have been reported | removal of a corneal foreign body<br>Pregnancy Category: C<br>Lactation Issues:<br>sulfacetamide is excreted in breast milk |
| **Sulfisoxazole**<br>Gantrisin<br>Solution:<br>4% | superficial ocular infection due to strains of microorganisms susceptible to antibiotics:<br>1–2 drops in affected eye(s) q 1–4 h initially according to severity of infection; taper dose by increasing the time interval between doses<br>trachoma:<br>2 drops in affected eye(s) q 2 h | Administration Issues:<br>do not touch tip of container to any surface; do not use while wearing soft contact lenses; safety and efficacy in children have not been established; protect from light<br>Drug–Drug Interactions:<br>**silver preparations** are incompatible with topical sulfonamides | ADRs:<br>burning/stinging; itching; periorbital edema; photosensitivity; headache; rash; GI upset; bone marrow suppression (rare); rare occurrences of severe sensitivity reactions have been reported | Contraindications:<br>hypersensitivity to sulfonamides; infants < 2 months; epithelial herpes simplex keratitis; vaccinia; viral, mycobacterial or fungal infection of the ocular structures; after uncomplicated removal of a corneal foreign body<br>Pregnancy Category: B (Category D at term)<br>Lactation Issues:<br>sulfisoxazole is excreted in breast milk |
| **Tobramycin**<br>AKTob, Tobrex<br>Solution:<br>0.3%<br>Ointment:<br>3 mg/g | superficial ocular infection due to strains of microorganisms susceptible to antibiotics:<br>**solution**<br>1–2 drops in affected eye(s) q 4 h<br>**ointment**<br>1/2 inch in affected eye(s) bid to tid | Administration Issues:<br>do not touch tip of container to any surface; do not use while wearing soft contact lenses; safe and effective in children<br>Drug–Drug Interactions:<br>sensitization from the topical use of an | ADRs:<br>burning/stinging; itching; conjunctival erythema; corneal ulcers | Contraindications:<br>hypersensitivity to tobramycin; vaccinia; varicella; mycobacterial infections of the eye; ocular fungal infection; use of steroid combinations after uncomplicated removal of a corneal foreign body |

(continues on next page)

## 401.2 Ophthalmic Antibiotic Agents *continued from previous page*

| Drug and Dosage Forms | Usual Dosage Range | Administration Issues and Drug–Drug Interactions | Common Adverse Drug Reactions (ADRs) | Contraindications, Pregnancy Category, and Lactation Issues |
|---|---|---|---|---|
| **Tobramycin** *cont.* | therapy should be continued for at least 48 hours after the infection is controlled | antibiotic may contraindicate the drug's later systemic use in serious infections | | Pregnancy Category: C<br><br>Lactation Issues:<br>it is not known if tobramycin is excreted in breast milk; either the drug or nursing should be discontinued |

## 401.3 Ophthalmic Antifungal Agents

| Drug and Dosage Forms | Usual Dosage Range for Specific Indications | Administration Issues and Drug Interactions | Common Adverse Drug Reactions (ADRs) | Contraindications, Pregnancy Category, and Lactation Issues |
|---|---|---|---|---|
| **Natamycin**<br>Natacyn<br><br>Suspension:<br>5% | fungal blepharitis, conjunctivitis:<br>1 drop in the affected eye(s) 4–6 times daily for up to 7–10 days<br><br>fungal keratitis:<br>1 drop in the affected eye(s) q 1–2 h for 3–4 days followed by 1 drop 6–8 times daily to complete 14–21 days or until resolution | Administration Issues:<br>do not touch tip of container to any surface; shake well before use; safety and efficacy have not been established in children<br><br>Drug Interactions:<br>Increased toxicity with **topical corticosteroids** (concomitant use is contraindicated) | ADRs:<br>blurred vision, eye pain, photophobia, one case of conjunctival chemosis and hyperemia, thought to be allergic in nature, has been reported | Contraindications:<br>hypersensitivity to natamycin<br><br>Pregnancy Category: C<br><br>Lactation Issues:<br>it is not known whether natamycin is excreted in breast milk; use caution in nursing women |

# 401.4 Ophthalmic Antiviral Agents

| Drug and Dosage Forms | Usual Dosage Range | Administration Issues and Drug–Drug Interactions | Common Adverse Drug Reactions (ADRs) | Contraindications, Pregnancy Category, and Lactation Issues |
|---|---|---|---|---|
| **Idoxuridine**<br><br>Herplex<br><br>Solution:<br>0.1% | herpes simplex keratitis:<br>1 drop in the affected eye(s) q h during the day and q 2 h at night until definite improvement (usually within 7 days), then 1 drop in the affected eye(s) q 2 h during the day and q 4 hours at night until 3–7 days after healing appears complete<br><br>maximum treatment period = 21 days | Administration Issues:<br>do not touch tip of container to any surface; corticosteroids are usually contraindicated in herpes simplex virus eye infections—if administered with topical corticosteroid therapy, consider corticosteroid-induced ocular side effects such as glaucoma or cataract formation and progression of bacterial or viral infection; safety and efficacy have not been established in children; solution must be stored in the refrigerator<br><br>Drug–Drug Interactions:<br>coadministration of solutions containing boric acid may result in the formation of a precipitant | ADRs:<br>local irritation, pain, pruritus, inflammation or edema; photophobia; corneal clouding; superficial punctate keratitis | Contraindications:<br>hypersensitivity to idoxuridine<br><br>Pregnancy Category: C<br><br>Lactation Issues:<br>it is not known whether idoxuridine is excreted in breast milk; either the drug or nursing should be discontinued |
| **Trifluridine**<br><br>Viroptic<br><br>Solution:<br>1% | recurrent epithelial keratitis due to herpes simplex virus 1 and 2:<br>superficial keratitis caused by herpes simplex virus which has not responded to topical idoxuridine or when adverse reactions to idoxuridine have occurred:<br><br>1 drop in affected eye(s) q 2 h while awake for a maximum daily dose of 9 drops until the corneal ulcer has | Administration Issues:<br>do not touch tip of container to any surface; corticosteroids are usually contraindicated in herpes simplex virus eye infections—if administered with topical corticosteroid therapy, consider corticosteroid-induced ocular side effects such as glaucoma or cataract formation and progression of bacterial or viral infection; solution must be stored in the refrigerator | ADRs:<br>burning/stinging; palpebral edema; superficial punctate keratitis; stromal edema | Contraindications:<br>hypersensitivity to trifluridine<br><br>Pregnancy Category: C<br><br>Lactation Issues:<br>it is not known whether trifluridine is excreted in breast milk; either the drug or breast feeding should be discontinued |

(continues on next page)

**401.4 Ophthalmic Antiviral Agents** *continued from previous page*

| Drug and Dosage Forms | Usual Dosage Range | Administration Issues and Drug–Drug Interactions | Common Adverse Drug Reactions (ADRs) | Contraindications, Pregnancy Category, and Lactation Issues |
|---|---|---|---|---|
| **Trifluridine** *cont.* | completely re-epithelialized; treat for an additional 7 days with 1 drop in the affected eye(s) q 4 h while awake (minimum 5 drops daily); do not exceed 21 days of treatment | | | |
| **Vidarabine**<br>Vira-A<br><br><u>Ointment:</u><br>3% | acute keratoconjunctivitis and recurrent epithelial keratitis due to herpes simplex virus 1 and 2: superficial keratitis caused by herpes simplex virus which has not responded to topical idoxuridine or when adverse reactions to idoxuridine have occurred:<br>1/2 inch in the affected eye(s) 5 times daily at 3 hour intervals; treat for an additional 7 days after re-epithelialization has occurred with 1/2 inch in the affected eye(s) bid to prevent recurrence | <u>Administration Issues:</u><br>do not touch tip of container to any surface; corticosteroids are usually contraindicated in herpes simplex virus eye infections—if administered with topical corticosteroid therapy, consider corticosteroid-induced ocular side effects such as glaucoma or cataract formation and progression of bacterial or viral infection | <u>ADRs:</u><br>lacrimation; foreign body sensation; conjunctival infection; burning/irritation; superficial punctate keratitis; photophobia | <u>Contraindications:</u><br>hypersensitivity to vidarabine; sterile trophic ulcers<br><br><u>Pregnancy Category:</u> C<br><br><u>Lactation Issues:</u><br>it is not known whether vidarabine is excreted in breast milk; either the drug or breast feeding should be discontinued |

## 401.5 Ophthalmic Antiallergic Agents

| Drug and Dosage Forms | Usual Dosage Ranges | Administration Issues and Drug–Drug Interactions | Common Adverse Drug Reactions (ADRs) | Contraindications, Pregnancy Category, and Lactation Issues |
|---|---|---|---|---|
| **Cromolyn**<br>Crolom<br><br><u>Solution:</u><br>4% | <u>conjunctivitis:</u><br>1–2 drops in each eye 4–6 times daily at regular intervals | <u>Administration Issues:</u><br>do not touch tip of container to any surface; shake well before use; do not wear soft contact lenses during treatment with cromolyn; safety and efficacy have not been established in children < 4 years | <u>ADRs:</u><br>ocular stinging/burning; tearing; itchy eyes | <u>Contraindications:</u><br>hypersensitivity to cromolyn<br><br><u>Pregnancy Category:</u>  B<br><br><u>Lactation Issues:</u><br>it is not known if cromolyn is excreted in breast milk; use caution in nursing women |
| **Levocabastine**<br>Livostin<br><br><u>Suspension:</u><br>0.05% | <u>allergic conjunctivitis:</u><br>1 drop in the affected eye(s) qid for up to 2 weeks | <u>Administration Issues:</u><br>do not touch tip of container to any surface; shake well before use; do not wear soft contact lenses during treatment with levocabastine; safety and efficacy have not been established in children < 12 years | <u>ADRs:</u><br>burning/stinging; headache; blurred vision; dry mouth; lacrimation/discharge | <u>Contraindications:</u><br>hypersensitivity to levocabastine<br><br><u>Pregnancy Category:</u>  B<br><br><u>Lactation Issues:</u><br>levocabastine is excreted in breast milk; use caution in nursing women |
| **Lodoxamide**<br>Alomide<br><br><u>Solution:</u><br>0.1% | <u>vernal keratoconjunctivitis,</u><br><u>conjunctivitis and keratitis:</u><br>**adults and children > 2 years**<br>1–2 drops in the affected eye(s) qid for up to 3 months | <u>Administration Issues:</u><br>do not touch tip of container to any surface; do not wear soft contact lenses during treatment with lodoxamide; safety and efficacy have not been established in children < 2 years | <u>ADRs:</u><br>burning/stinging; ocular pruritus; blurred vision; dry eye; tearing; foreign body sensation; headache | <u>Contraindications:</u><br>hypersensitivity to lodoxamide<br><br><u>Pregnancy Category:</u>  B<br><br><u>Lactation Issues:</u><br>it is not known if lodoxamide is excreted in breast milk; use caution in nursing women |

# 401.6 Ophthalmic Nonsteroidal Anti-Inflammatory Agents

| Drug and Dosage Forms | Usual Dosage Range | Administration Issues | Common Adverse Drug Reactions (ADRs) | Contraindications, Pregnancy Category, and Lactation Issues |
|---|---|---|---|---|
| **Diclofenac**<br>Voltaren<br><br><u>Solution</u><br>0.1% | <u>Postoperative inflammation following cataract extraction:</u><br>One drop into affected eye qid beginning 24 h post cataract surgery and continuing throughout the first 2 weeks of the postoperative period | <u>Administration Issues:</u><br>do not touch tip of container to any surface; safety and efficacy have not been established in children | <u>ADRs:</u><br>burning/stinging, keratitis, ocular allergy, nausea, vomiting | <u>Contraindications:</u><br>hypersensitivity to diclofenac or other NSAIDs; patients wearing soft contacts may experience ocular irritation<br><br><u>Pregnancy Category:</u> B<br><br><u>Lactation Issues:</u><br>it is not known if diclofenac is excreted in breast milk; use caution in nursing women |
| **Flurbiprofen**<br>Ocufen, various generics<br><br><u>Solution</u><br>0.03% | <u>Inhibition of intraoperative miosis:</u><br>instill one drop every 30 minutes beginning 2 h prior to surgery (total of 4 drops) | <u>Administration Issues:</u><br>do not touch tip of container to any surface; safety and efficacy have not been established in children | <u>ADRs:</u><br>burning/stinging; increased bleeding tendency of ocular tissue in conjunction with ocular surgery | <u>Contraindications:</u><br>hypersensitivity to flurbiprofen or other NSAIDs; epithelial herpes simplex keratitis (dendritic keratitis)<br><br><u>Pregnancy Category:</u> C<br><br><u>Lactation Issues:</u><br>it is not known if flurbiprofen is excreted in breast milk; use caution in nursing women |
| **Ketorolac**<br>Acular | <u>Relief of ocular itching caused by seasonal allergic conjunctivitis:</u><br>One drop (0.25 mg) qid | <u>Administration Issues:</u><br>do not touch tip of container to any surface; safety and efficacy have not been established in children | <u>ADRs:</u><br>ocular irritation, allergic reactions, superficial keratitis, superficial ocular infections, | <u>Contraindications:</u><br>hypersensitivity to ketorolac or other NSAIDs |

| Drug | Dosage/Administration | ADRs | Pregnancy/Lactation |
|---|---|---|---|
| Solution 0.5% | Treatment of postoperative inflammation following cataract extraction: One drop into affected eye qid beginning 24 h post cataract surgery and continuing throughout the first 2 weeks of the postoperative period | eye dryness, corneal infiltrates, corneal ulcer, blurry vision | Pregnancy Category: B (Category D in 3rd trimester) Lactation Issues: it is not known if ketorolac is excreted in breast milk; use caution in nursing women |
| **Suprofen** Profenal Solution 1% | Inhibition of intraoperative miosis: On the day of surgery, instill 2 drops into conjunctival sac at 3, 2, and 1 hour(s) prior to surgery. Two drops may be instilled into conjunctival sac q 4 h while awake the day preceding surgery | Administration Issues: do not touch tip of container to any surface; safety and efficacy have not been established in children ADRs: discomfort, itching, redness, allergy, iritis, pain, chemosis, photophobia, irritation | Contraindications: hypersensitivity to suprofen or other NSAIDs; epithelial herpes simplex keratitis (dendritic keratitis) Pregnancy Category: C Lactation Issues: suprofen is excreted in breast milk after oral use and systemic absorption may occur following ocular administration therefore use caution in nursing women |

| Drug and Dosage Forms | Usual Dosage Range | Administration Issues | Common Adverse Drug Reactions (ADRs) | Contraindications, Pregnancy Category, and Lactation Issues |
|---|---|---|---|---|
| **Dexamethasone**<br>AK-Dex, Decadron, Maxidex<br><br>Solution:<br>0.1%<br><br>Suspension:<br>0.1%. 0.5%<br><br>Ointment:<br>0.05% | inflammatory ocular conditions; corneal injury; graft rejection after keratoplasty:<br>**solution and suspension**<br>1–2 drops in the affected eye(s) q hour during the day and q 2 h at night initially; after response, reduce dose to 1 drop in the affected eye(s) q 4 h then tid to qid<br><br>**ointment**<br>1/2 inch in affected eye(s) tid to qid initially; after response, reduce dose to bid then qd<br><br>postoperative inflammation:<br>1–2 drops in the affected eye(s) qid beginning 24 hours after surgery and continue for 2 weeks | Administration Issues:<br>shake suspension well before use; do not touch tip of container to any surface; relapse may occur if therapy is reduced too rapidly—taper over several days; safety and efficacy have not been established in children | ADRs:<br>elevated IOP; posterior subcapsular cataract formation; secondary ocular infection | Contraindications:<br>hypersensitivity to topical steroids; herpes simplex keratitis; ocular fungal or viral infection; ocular tuberculosis; after uncomplicated removal of a superficial corneal foreign body<br><br>Pregnancy Category:  C<br><br>Lactation Issues:<br>it is not known if topical steroids are excreted in breast milk; exercise caution when administering to a nursing woman |
| **Fluorometholone**<br>Fluor-Op, FML, Flarex<br><br>Suspension:<br>0.1%, 0.25%<br><br>Ointment:<br>0.1% | inflammatory ocular conditions; corneal injury; graft rejection after keratoplasty:<br>**suspension**<br>1–2 drops in the affected eye(s) q hour during the day and q 2 h at night initially; after response, reduce dose to 1 drop in the affected eye(s) q 4 hours then tid to qid | Administration Issues:<br>shake suspension well before use; do not touch tip of container to any surface; relapse may occur if therapy is reduced too rapidly—taper over several days; safety and efficacy have not been established in children | ADRs:<br>elevated IOP; posterior subcapsular cataract formation; secondary ocular infection | Contraindications:<br>hypersensitivity to topical steroids; herpes simplex keratitis; ocular fungal or viral infection; ocular tuberculosis; after uncomplicated removal of a superficial corneal foreign body<br><br>Pregnancy Category:  C |

| Drug | Indications / Dosing | Administration Issues / ADRs | Contraindications / Lactation / Pregnancy |
|---|---|---|---|
| | **ointment**<br>1/2 inch in affected eye(s) tid to qid initially; after response, reduce dose to bid then qd<br><br>postoperative inflammation:<br>1–2 drops in the affected eye(s) qid beginning 24 hours after surgery and continue for 2 weeks | | Lactation Issues:<br>it is not known if topical steroids are excreted in breast milk; exercise caution when administering to a nursing woman |
| **Medrysone**<br>HMS<br><br>Suspension:<br>1% | inflammatory ocular conditions; corneal injury; graft rejection after keratoplasty:<br>1–2 drops in the affected eye(s) q hour during the day and q 2 h at night initially; after response, reduce dose to 1 drop in the affected eye(s) q 4 h then tid to qid<br><br>postoperative inflammation:<br>1–2 drops in the affected eye(s) qid beginning 24 hours after surgery and continue for 2 weeks | Administration Issues:<br>shake suspension well before use; do not touch tip of container to any surface; relapse may occur if therapy is reduced too rapidly—taper over several days; safety and efficacy have not been established in children<br><br>ADRs:<br>elevated IOP; posterior subcapsular cataract formation; secondary ocular infection | Contraindications:<br>hypersensitivity to topical steroids; herpes simplex keratitis; ocular fungal or viral infection; ocular tuberculosis; after uncomplicated removal of a superficial corneal foreign body<br><br>Pregnancy Category: C<br><br>Lactation Issues:<br>it is not known if topical steroids are excreted in breast milk; exercise caution when administering to a nursing woman |
| **Prednisolone**<br>AK-Pred, Pred Forte, Econopred Plus, Pred Mild<br><br>Suspension:<br>0.12%, 0.125%, 1% | inflammatory ocular conditions; corneal injury; graft rejection after keratoplasty:<br>1–2 drops in the affected eye(s) q hour during the day and q 2 h at night initially; after response, reduce dose to 1 drop in the affected eye(s) q 4 h then tid to qid | Administration Issues:<br>shake suspension well before use; do not touch tip of container to any surface; relapse may occur if therapy is reduced too rapidly—taper over several days; safety and efficacy have not been established in children<br><br>ADRs:<br>elevated IOP; posterior subcapsular cataract formation; secondary ocular infection | Contraindications:<br>hypersensitivity to topical steroids; herpes simplex keratitis; ocular fungal or viral infection; ocular tuberculosis; after uncomplicated removal of a superficial corneal foreign body<br><br>Pregnancy Category: C |

*(continues on next page)*

## 401.7 Opthalmic Steroidal Agents *continued from previous page*

| Drug and Dosage Forms | Usual Dosage Range | Administration Issues | Common Adverse Drug Reactions (ADRs) | Contraindications, Pregnancy Category, and Lactation Issues |
|---|---|---|---|---|
| **Prednisolone** *cont.* | <u>postoperative inflammation:</u> 1–2 drops in the affected eye(s) qid beginning 24 hours after surgery and continue for 2 weeks | | | <u>Lactation Issues:</u> it is not known if topical steroids are excreted in breast milk; exercise caution when administering to a nursing woman |
| **Rimexolone** Vexol <u>Suspension:</u> 1% | <u>inflammatory ocular conditions:</u> <u>corneal injury; graft rejection after keratoplasty:</u> 1–2 drops in the affected eye(s) q hour during the day and q 2 h at night initially; after response, reduce dose to 1 drop in the affected eye(s) q 4 h then tid to qid  <u>postoperative inflammation:</u> 1–2 drops in the affected eye(s) qid beginning 24 hours after surgery and continue for 2 weeks | <u>Administration Issues:</u> shake suspension well before use; do not touch tip of container to any surface; relapse may occur if therapy is reduced too rapidly—taper over several days; safety and efficacy have not been established in children | <u>ADRs:</u> elevated IOP; posterior subcapsular cataract formation; secondary ocular infection | <u>Contraindications:</u> hypersensitivity to topical steroids; herpes simplex keratitis; ocular fungal or viral infection; ocular tuberculosis; after uncomplicated removal of a superficial corneal foreign body  <u>Pregnancy Category:</u>  C  <u>Lactation Issues:</u> it is not known if topical steroids are excreted in breast milk; exercise caution when administering to a nursing woman |

# 402. Otic Preparations

## 402.1 Antibiotics

| Drug and Dosage Forms | Usual Dosage Range | Administration Issues and Patient Education | Common Adverse Drug Reactions (ADRs) and Contraindications |
|---|---|---|---|
| **Chloramphenicol**<br>Chloromycetin Otic<br><br>Solution<br>0.5% | **Treatment of superficial infections involving the external auditory canal:**<br>2–3 drops tid<br><br>For serious infections, supplement with systemic antibiotics | **FOR OTIC USE ONLY**<br><br>Do not touch dropper to ear; wash hands prior to use<br><br>To allow drops to flow into ear, tilt head to side and:<br>**Adults:** hold earlobe up and back<br>**Children:** hold earlobe down and back | <u>ADRs:</u><br>*Local irritation:* itching, burning, angioneurotic edema, urticaria, vesicular and maculopapular dermatitis indicate a sensitivity to chloramphenicol and constitute discontinuation of medication.<br><br>*Superinfection:* prolonged use may result in overgrowth of nonsusceptible organisms and fungi (e.g., herpes simplex, vaccinia, varicella)<br><br>*Warnings:*<br>Bone marrow hypoplasia has occurred; Ototoxicity more likely if medication enters the middle ear (i.e., perforated tympanic membrane)<br><br><u>Contraindications:</u><br>Hypersensitivity to any component; perforated tympanic membrane |
| **Hydrocortisone 1% plus Neomycin 5 mg/mL plus Polymyxin B 10,000 U/mL**<br>Cortisporin Otic, Otosporin, others (Solution or suspension)<br><br>**Hydrocortisone 0.5% plus Polymyxin B 10,000 U/mL**<br>Otobiotic Otic (Solution)<br><br>**Hydrocortisone 1% plus Neomycin 4.71 mg/mL**<br>Coly-Mycin S Otic (Suspension) | **Treatment of superficial bacterial infections of the external auditory canal:**<br>*Solution or suspension:*<br>4 drops tid to qid<br><br>**Treatment of infections related to mastoidectomy and fenestration cavities:**<br>*Suspension Only:* 4 drops tid to qid | **FOR OTIC USE ONLY**<br><br>For the suspension—shake well for 10 seconds prior to use.<br><br>Do not touch dropper to ear; wash hands prior to use<br><br>To allow drops to flow into ear, tilt head to side and:<br>**Adults:** hold earlobe up and back<br>**Children:** hold earlobe down and back | <u>ADRs:</u><br>*Superinfection:* prolonged use may result in overgrowth of nonsusceptible organisms and fungi (e.g., herpes simplex, vaccinia, varicella).<br><br><u>Contraindications:</u><br>Hypersensitivity to any component<br>Perforated tympanic membrane<br>FOR OTIC USE ONLY |

| Drug and Dosage Forms | Usual Dosage Range | Ingredient Use(s) | Administration Issues & Patient Education | Common Adverse Drug Reactions (ADRs) and Contraindications |
|---|---|---|---|---|
| **Acetic Acid (2%); Propylene Glycol Diacetate (3%); Benzethonium Chloride (0.02%); Sodium Acetate (0.015%)** Acetasol; VoSol; Acetic Acid Otic (Solution) | **Minor Outer Ear Complaints:** Insert saturated wick; keep moist for 24 hrs. Remove wick and instill 5 drops 3–4 times daily. | **Acetic Acid, Acetate, Benzethonium Chloride:** antibacterial or antifungal action | **For Otic Use ONLY** Do not touch dropper to ear; wash hands prior to use To allow drops to flow into ear, tilt head to side and: **Adults:** hold earlobe up and back **Children:** hold earlobe down and back | ADRs: Local reactions (redness, itching) Contraindications: Hypersensitivity to any ingredient. |
| **Acetic Acid (2%); Aluminum Acetate** Burow's Otic; Otic Domeboro; generic (Solution) | **Minor Outer Ear Complaints:** Insert saturate wick; keep moist for 24 hrs. Remove wick and instill 4–6 drops every 2–3 hrs. | **Acetic Acid, Aluminum Acetate:** antibacterial or antifungal action | **For Otic Use ONLY** Do not touch dropper to ear; wash hands prior to use To allow drops to flow into ear, tilt head to side and: **Adults:** hold earlobe up and back **Children:** hold earlobe down and back | ADRs: Local reactions (redness, itching) Contraindications: Hypersensitivity to any ingredient. |
| **Acetic Acid (Nonaqueous); Burow's Solution; Boric Acid; Propylene Glycol** | **Minor Outer Ear Complaints:** 2–3 drops in each ear before and after swimming or showering. | **Acetic Acid, Burow's Solution, Boric Acid:** antibacterial or antifungal activity | **For Otic Use ONLY** Do not touch dropper to ear; wash hands prior to use | ADRs: Local reactions (redness, itching) Contraindications: Hypersensitivity to any ingredient. |

| | | | | |
|---|---|---|---|---|
| Star Otic (Solution) | | | To allow drops to flow into ear, tilt head to side and:<br>**Adults:** hold earlobe up and back<br>**Children:** hold earlobe down and back | <u>ADRs:</u><br>Local reactions (redness, itching)<br><br><u>Contraindications:</u><br>Hypersensitivity to any ingredient. |
| **Benzocaine (1.4%); Antipyrine (5.4%); Glycerin**<br>Allergan Ear Drops; Antipyrine & Benzocaine Otic; Auralgan; Auroto; Otocalm (Solution) | **Benzocaine:** Local anesthetic<br><br>**Antipyrine:** Analgesic<br><br>**Glycerin:** solvent and vehicle. It is an emollient; hygroscopic and humectant | **Minor Outer Ear Complaints:** Fill ear canal with 2–4 drops; insert saturated cotton pledget. Repeat 3–4 times daily or once every 1–2 hrs. | **For Otic Use ONLY**<br><br>Do not touch dropper to ear; wash hands prior to use<br><br>To allow drops to flow into ear, tilt head to side and:<br>**Adults:** hold earlobe up and back<br>**Children:** hold earlobe down and back | <u>ADRs:</u><br>Local reactions (redness, itching)<br><br><u>Contraindications:</u><br>Hypersensitivity to any ingredient. |
| **Benzocaine (5%); Antipyrine (5%); Phenylephrine (0.25%); Propylene Glycol**<br>Tympagesic (Solution) | **Benzocaine:** Local anesthetic<br><br>**Antipyrine:** Analgesic<br><br>**Phenylephrine:** Vasoconstrictor (decongestant) | **Minor Outer Ear Complaints:** Fill ear canal; plug with saturated cotton and repeat every 2–4 hrs. | **For Otic Use ONLY**<br><br>Do not touch dropper to ear; wash hands prior to use<br><br>To allow drops to flow into ear, tilt head to side and:<br>**Adults:** hold earlobe up and back<br>**Children:** hold earlobe down and back | <u>ADRs:</u><br>Local reactions (redness, itching)<br><br><u>Contraindications:</u><br>Hypersensitivity to any ingredient. |
| **Benzocaine (20%); Benzothonium Chloride (0.1%); Glycerin (1%); PEG 300** | **Benzocaine:** Local anesthetic<br><br>**Benzothonium Chloride:** antibacterial or antifungal action | **Minor Outer Ear Complaints:** Fill canal with 4–5 drops; insert a cotton pledget. Repeat every 1–2 hrs. | **For Otic Use ONLY**<br><br>Do not touch dropper to ear; wash hands prior to use | <u>ADRs:</u><br>Local reactions (redness, itching)<br><br><u>Contraindications:</u><br>Hypersensitivity to any ingredient. |

(continues on next page)

**402.2** Miscellaneous Otic Preparations *continued from previous page*

| Drug and Dosage Forms | Usual Dosage Range | Ingredient Use(s) | Administration Issues & Patient Education | Common Adverse Drug Reactions (ADRs) and Contraindications |
|---|---|---|---|---|
| **Benzocaine**<br>Americaine Otic; Otocain (Solution) | | **Glycerin:** solvent and vehicle. It is an emollient; hygroscopic and humectant | To allow drops to flow into ear, tilt head to side and:<br>**Adults:** hold earlobe up and back<br>**Children:** hold earlobe down and back | |
| **Boric Acid (2.75%); Isopropyl alcohol**<br>Auro-Dri; Dri/Ear; Ear-Dry (Solution) | **Minor Outer Ear Complaints:**<br>3–8 drops in each ear. | **Boric Acid:** antibacterial or antifungal activity<br>**Isopropyl Alcohol:** drying agent | **For Otic Use ONLY**<br>Do not touch dropper to ear; wash hands prior to use<br>To allow drops to flow into ear, tilt head to side and:<br>**Adults:** hold earlobe up and back<br>**Children:** hold earlobe down and back | ADRs:<br>Local reactions (redness, itching)<br>Contraindications:<br>Hypersensitivity to any ingredient. |
| **Carbamide Peroxide (6.5%); Glycerin, Propylene Glycol; Sodium Stannate**<br>Debrox (Solution) | **Minor Outer Ear Complaints:**<br>5–10 drops bid for up to 4 d | **Carbamide Peroxide:** emulsify/disperse ear wax<br>**Glycerin:** solvent and vehicle. It is an emollient; hygroscopic and humectant | **For Otic Use ONLY**<br>Do not touch dropper to ear; wash hands prior to use<br>To allow drops to flow into ear, tilt head to side and:<br>**Adults:** hold earlobe up and back<br>**Children:** hold earlobe down and back | ADRs:<br>Local reactions (redness, itching)<br>Contraindications:<br>Hypersensitivity to any ingredient. |

| Drug (Brand) | Minor Outer Ear Complaints | Ingredients | Administration | ADRs / Contraindications |
|---|---|---|---|---|
| **Carbamide Peroxide (6.5%); Alcohol (6.3%); Glycerin, Polysorbate 20**<br>Murine Ear (Solution) | **Minor Outer Ear Complaints:** 5–10 drops bid for up to 4 d | **Carbamide Peroxide:** emulsify/disperse ear wax<br><br>**Alcohol:** drying agent<br><br>**Glycerin:** solvent and vehicle. It is an emollient; hygroscopic and humectant | **For Otic Use ONLY**<br><br>Do not touch dropper to ear; wash hands prior to use<br><br>To allow drops to flow into ear, tilt head to side and:<br>**Adults:** hold earlobe up and back<br>**Children:** hold earlobe down and back | ADRs:<br>Local reactions (redness, itching)<br><br>Contraindications:<br>Hypersensitivity to any ingredient. |
| **Carbamide Peroxide (6.5%); anhydrous glycerin base**<br>Auro Ear Drops (Solution) | **Minor Outer Ear Complaints:** 5–10 drops bid for up to 4 d | **Carbamide Peroxide:** emulsify/disperse ear wax<br><br>**Glycerin:** solvent and vehicle. It is an emollient; hygroscopic and humectant | **For Otic Use ONLY**<br><br>Do not touch dropper to ear; wash hands prior to use<br><br>To allow drops to flow into ear, tilt head to side and:<br>**Adults:** hold earlobe up and back<br>**Children:** hold earlobe down and back | ADRs:<br>Local reactions (redness, itching)<br><br>Contraindications:<br>Hypersensitivity to any ingredient. |
| **Desonide (0.05%); Acetic Acid (2%); Propylene glycol**<br>Otic Tridesilon (Solution) | **Minor Outer Ear Complaints:** 3–4 drops in ear 3–4 times daily. Or insert saturated wick and leave in until relief. | **Desonide:** anti-inflammatory and antipruritic effects<br><br>**Acetic Acid:** antibacterial or antifungal activity | **For Otic Use ONLY**<br><br>Do not touch dropper to ear; wash hands prior to use<br><br>To allow drops to flow into ear, tilt head to side and:<br>**Adults:** hold earlobe up and back<br>**Children:** hold earlobe down and back | ADRs:<br>Local reactions (redness, itching)<br><br>Contraindications:<br>Hypersensitivity to any ingredient. |

(continues on next page)

# 402.2 Miscellaneous Otic Preparations *continued from previous page*

| Drug and Dosage Forms | Usual Dosage Range | Ingredient Use(s) | Administration Issues & Patient Education | Common Adverse Drug Reactions (ADRs) and Contraindications |
|---|---|---|---|---|
| **Hydrocortisone (1%); Acetic Acid (2%); Propylene glycol diacetate (3%); Sodium acetate (0.015%); Benzethonium Chloride (0.02%)** VoSol HC; Acetasol HC (Solution) | **Minor Outer Ear Complaints:** Insert saturated wick into ear; leave in ear for 24 h keeping it moist with 3–5 drops every 4–6 hrs. Remove wick and instill 5 drops 3–4 times daily. | **Hydrocortisone:** anti-inflammatory and antipruritic effects.<br><br>**Acetic Acid, Acetate, Benzethonium Chloride:** antibacterial or antifungal action | **For Otic Use ONLY**<br><br>Do not touch dropper to ear; wash hands prior to use<br><br>To allow drops to flow into ear, tilt head to side and:<br>**Adults:** hold earlobe up and back<br>**Children:** hold earlobe down and back | ADRs:<br>Local reactions (redness, itching)<br><br>Contraindications:<br>Hypersensitivity to any ingredient. |
| **Hydrocortisone (1%); Alcohol (44%); Propylene glycol; Dermprotective Factor yerba santa; Benzyl Benzoate** EarSol HC (Solution) | **Minor Outer Ear Complaints:** 4–6 drops into ear 3–4 times daily | **Hydrocortisone:** anti-inflammatory and antipruritic effects.<br><br>**Alcohol:** drying agent | **For Otic Use ONLY**<br><br>Do not touch dropper to ear; wash hands prior to use<br><br>To allow drops to flow into ear, tilt head to side and:<br>**Adults:** hold earlobe up and back<br>**Children:** hold earlobe down and back | ADRs:<br>Local reactions (redness, itching)<br><br>Contraindications:<br>Hypersensitivity to any ingredient. |
| **Hydrocortisone (1%); Acetic Acid glacial (2%); Propylene Glycol diacetate (3%);** | **Minor Outer Ear Complaints:** Insert saturated wick into ear; leave in ear for 24 h keeping it moist with 3–5 drops every 4–6 hrs. Remove wick and instill 5 drops 3–4 times daily. | **Hydrocortisone:** anti-inflammatory and antipruritic effects.<br><br>**Acetic Acid, Acetate, Benzothonium Chloride, citric acid:** antibacterial or antifungal action | **For Otic Use ONLY**<br><br>Do not touch dropper to ear; wash hands prior to use | ADRs:<br>Local reactions (redness, itching)<br><br>Contraindications:<br>Hypersensitivity to any ingredient. |

| | | |
|---|---|---|
| **Sodium Acetate (0.015%); Benzothonium Chloride (0.02%); Citric Acid (0.2%)** AA-HC (Solution) | | To allow drops to flow into ear, tilt head to side and: **Adults:** hold earlobe up and back **Children:** hold earlobe down and back |
| **M-Cresyl Acetate (25%); Isopropanol (25%); Chlorobutanol (1%); Benzyl alcohol (1%); 5% Castor Oil; Propylene Glycol** Cresylate (Solution) | **Minor Outer Ear Complaints:** 2–4 drops as needed. | **M-Cresyl Acetate:** Antibacterial or antifungal action | **For Otic Use ONLY** Do not touch dropper to ear; wash hands prior to use To allow drops to flow into ear, tilt head to side and: **Adults:** hold earlobe up and back **Children:** hold earlobe down and back | ADRs: Local reactions (redness, itching) Contraindications: Hypersensitivity to any ingredient. |
| **Triethanolamine Polypeptide Oleate-Condensate (10%); Chlorobutanol (0.5%); Propylene glycol** Cerumenex Drops (Solution) | **Minor Outer Ear Complaints:** Fill ear canal; insert cotton plug. Allow to remain for 15–30 min; then flush ear canal. | **Triethanolamine:** emulsify and disperse ear wax | **For Otic Use ONLY** Do not touch dropper to ear; wash hands prior to use To allow drops to flow into ear, tilt head to side and: **Adults:** hold earlobe up and back **Children:** hold earlobe down and back | ADRs: Local reactions (redness, itching) Contraindications: Hypersensitivity to any ingredient. |

# 500. GASTROINTESTINAL AGENTS

501.1  Antacids

| Drug and Dosage Forms | Usual Dosage Range | Administration Issues and Drug–Drug Interactions | Common Adverse Drug Reactions (ADRs) | Contraindications, Pregnancy Category, and Lactation Issues |
|---|---|---|---|---|
| **Aluminum Carbonate Gel, Basic**<br>Basaljel<br><br>Tablets, Capsules:<br>Equivalent to 500 mg of aluminum hydroxide<br><br>Suspension:<br>Equivalent to 400 mg of aluminum hydroxide per 5 ml | **Antacid**<br>Tablets, Capsules:<br>1000 mg as often as q 2 h, up to 12 doses/d<br><br>Suspension:<br>10 ml as often as q 2 hours, up to 12 dose/d<br><br>**Hyperphosphatemia**<br>Tablets, Capsules:<br>1000 mg with meals and at bedtime<br><br>Suspension:<br>15–30 ml in water or juice with meals and at bedtime | Administration issues<br>Antacid dosing should be staggered at least 2 hours from other drugs where a potential drug interaction may occur<br><br>Drug–Drug Interactions<br>Antacids may interfere with drugs by increasing gastric pH, thus decreasing absorption of such drugs as **digoxin, ciprofloxacin, ofloxacin, norfloxacin, phenytoin, iron supplements, isoniazid, ethambutol, and ketoconazole.** Antacids may bind other drugs decreasing the drug's absorption **(tetracycline)** | ADRs:<br>constipation<br><br>Warnings/Precautions<br>Hypophosphatemia (anorexia, malaise, tremors, muscle weakness), aluminum toxicity (dementia) may occur with repeated dosing | Contraindications:<br>prolonged use of high doses in presence of low serum phosphate<br><br>Pregnancy Category:  C<br><br>Lactation Issues<br>Safety not established, do not use in nursing mothers |
| **Aluminum Hydroxide Gel**<br>Amphojel, Alu-Tab, AlternaGEL, various generic<br><br>Tablets:  300 mg, 600 mg<br><br>Capsules:  400 mg<br><br>Suspension:  320 mg/5ml | **Antacid**<br>Tablets, Capsules:<br>500 –1800 mg 3–6 times daily 1 h pc & hs<br><br>Suspension, Liquid:<br>5–30 ml prn between meals and bedtime<br><br>**Hyperphosphatemia**<br>Tablets, Capsules: | Administration issues<br>Antacid dosing should be staggered at least 2 hours from other drugs where a potential drug interaction may occur<br><br>Drug–Drug Interactions<br>Antacids may interfere with drugs by increasing gastric pH, thus decreasing absorption of such drugs as **digoxin, ciprofloxacin, ofloxacin, norfloxacin, phenytoin, iron supplements,** | ADRs:<br>constipation<br><br>Warnings/Precautions<br>Hypophosphatemia (anorexia, malaise, tremors, muscle weakness), aluminum toxicity (dementia) may occur with repeated dosing | Contraindications:<br>prolonged use of high doses in presence of low serum phosphate<br><br>Pregnancy Category:  C<br><br>Lactation Issues<br>Safety not established, do not use in nursing mothers |

| | | | | |
|---|---|---|---|---|
| Suspension, concentrated: 450 mg/5ml<br><br>Liquid: 600 mg/5ml | 500–1800 mg 3 to 6 times daily, with meals and at bedtime<br><br>Suspension, Liquid: 5–30 ml with meals and at bedtime | **isoniazid, ethambutol, and ketoconazole.** Antacids may bind other drugs decreasing the drug's absorption **(tetracycline)** | | |
| **Calcium Carbonate**<br><br>Tablets: Various generics: 500 mg, 600 mg, 650 mg, 1000 mg, 1250 mg<br><br>Tablets, chewable: Tums, Extra Strength Tums, various generics: 500 mg, 750 mg<br><br>Alka-Mints: 850 mg<br><br>Tums Ultra: 1000 mg<br><br>Gum tablets: 500 mg<br><br>Suspension: Various generics: 1250 mg / 5ml<br><br>Lozenges: Mylanta 600 mg | **All doses are in terms of elemental calcium: 1 gm calcium carbonate = 400 mg (20 mEq) elemental calcium**<br><br>Antacid<br>0.5–1.5 gm 3 to 6 times a day as needed<br><br>**Supplement for Osteoporosis**<br>1–2 gm bid or tid | Administration issues<br>Antacid dosing should be staggered at least 2 hours from other drugs where a potential drug interaction may occur<br><br>Drug–Drug Interactions<br>Antacids may interfere with drugs by increasing gastric pH, thus decreasing absorption of such drugs as **ciprofloxacin, ofloxacin, norfloxacin, phenytoin, and iron supplements.** Antacids may bind other drugs decreasing the drug's absorption **(tetracycline)** | ADRs:<br>constipation, flatulence<br><br>Warnings/Precautions<br>Milk-alkali syndrome with hypercalcemia and metabolic alkalosis; acid rebound may occur with repeated dosing | Contraindications:<br>hypercalcemia and hypercalciuria, severe renal disease, renal calculi, GI hemorrhage or obstruction, dehydration<br><br>Pregnancy Category: C<br><br>Lactation Issues<br>Safety not established, do not use in nursing mothers |
| **Dihydroxyaluminum Sodium Carbonate**<br>Rolaids<br><br>Tablets, chewable: 334 mg | Antacid<br>1–2 tablets 3 to 6 times daily prn | Administration issues<br>Antacid dosing should be staggered at least 2 hours from other drugs where a potential drug interaction may occur<br><br>Drug–Drug Interactions<br>Antacids may interfere with drugs by increasing gastric pH, thus decreasing absorption of such drugs as **digoxin,** | ADRs:<br>constipation<br><br>Warnings/Precautions<br>May worsen hypertension and heart failure due to sodium content | Contraindications:<br>aluminum sensitivity, severe renal disease, dehydration, patients on sodium-restricted diets<br><br>Pregnancy Category: C |

(continues on next page)

| Drug and Dosage Forms | Usual Dosage Range | Administration Issues and Drug–Drug Interactions | Common Adverse Drug Reactions (ADRs) and Pharmacokinetics | Contraindications, Pregnancy Category, and Lactation Issues |
|---|---|---|---|---|
| **Dihydroxyaluminum Sodium Carbonate** *cont.* | | **ciprofloxacin, ofloxacin, norfloxacin, phenytoin, iron supplements, isoniazid, ethambutol, and ketoconazole.** Antacids may bind other drugs decreasing the drug's absorption **(tetracycline)** | | Lactation Issues Safety not established, do not use in nursing mothers |
| **Magaldrate (Aluminum Magnesium Hydroxide Sulfate)** Riopan Tablets, chewable: 480 mg Suspension/Liquid: 540 mg / 5ml Liquid, extra-strength: 1080 mg / 5ml | **Antacid** Tablet, chewable: 1–2 between meals and at bedtime Suspension, Liquid: 5–10 ml between meals and at bedtime Liquid, extra-strength: 5 ml between meals and at bedtime | Administration issues Antacid dosing should be staggered at least 2 hours from other drugs where a potential drug interaction may occur Drug–Drug Interactions Antacids may interfere with drugs by increasing gastric pH, thus decreasing absorption of such drugs as **digoxin, ciprofloxacin, ofloxacin, norfloxacin, phenytoin, iron supplements, and ketoconazole.** Antacids may bind other drugs decreasing the drug's absorption **(tetracycline)** | ADRs: diarrhea, constipation | Pregnancy Category: C Lactation Issues Safety not established, do not use in nursing mothers |
| **Magnesium Hydroxide** Phillips' Milk of Magnesia, various generic Tablets, chewable: 311 mg | **Antacid** **Adults and children > 12:** 2–4 tablets up to 4 times daily 5–15 ml liquid up to 4 times daily 2.5–7.5 ml liquid concentrate up to 4 times daily with water | Administration issues Antacid dosing should be staggered at least 2 hours from other drugs where a potential drug interaction may occur; chew tablets thoroughly and follow with glass of water | ADRs diarrhea Warning/Precautions Hypermagnesemia characterized by hypotension, nausea, vomiting may occur with repeated dosing in patients with renal impairment (CrCl <30 mL/min) | Contraindications: abdominal pain, nausea, vomiting, diarrhea, severe renal dysfunction, fecal impaction, rectal bleeding, colostomy, ileostomy Pregnancy Category: B |

| Drug / Forms | Dosing & Administration / Drug–Drug Interactions | ADRs / Warnings/Precautions | Pregnancy / Lactation |
|---|---|---|---|
| **Liquid:** 400 mg/5ml<br><br>**Liquid, concentrated:** 800 mg/5ml | **Laxative**<br>**Adults:**<br>15–30 ml liquid<br>10–20 ml liquid concentrate<br><br>**Children > 2 years:**<br>5–30 ml liquid<br><br>**Drug–Drug Interactions**<br>Antacids may interfere with drugs by increasing gastric pH, thus decreasing absorption of such drugs as **digoxin, ciprofloxacin, ofloxacin, norfloxacin, phenytoin, iron supplements, and ketoconazole.** Antacids may bind other drugs decreasing the drug's absorption **(tetracycline)** | | **Lactation Issues**<br>Safety not established |
| **Magnesium Oxide**<br>Tablets: Mag-Ox 400 mg<br>Various generics: 500 mg<br>Capsules: Uro-Mag 140 m | **Antacid**<br>Tablets:<br>280–1500 mg with water/milk qid, pc and hs<br><br>Capsules:<br>140 mg 3 to 4 times daily<br><br>**Laxative**<br>2–4 gm with water/milk hs<br><br>**Magnesium supplement**<br>400–1200 mg/d in divided doses<br><br>Administration issues<br>Antacid dosing should be staggered at least 2 hours from other drugs where a potential drug interaction may occur<br><br>Drug–Drug Interactions<br>Antacids may interfere with drugs by increasing gastric pH, thus decreasing absorption of such drugs as **digoxin, ciprofloxacin, ofloxacin, norfloxacin, phenytoin, iron supplements, and ketoconazole.** Antacids may bind other drugs decreasing the drug's absorption **(tetracycline)** | ADRs:<br>diarrhea<br><br>Warnings/Precautions<br>Hypermagnesemia characterized by hypotension, nausea, vomiting may occur with repeated dosing in patients with renal impairment | Pregnancy Category: C<br><br>Lactation Issues<br>Safety not established, do not use in nursing mothers |
| **Sodium Bicarbonate**<br>Soda Mint, various generic<br><br>Tablets:<br>325 mg, 520 mg, 650 mg | **Antacid**<br>Tablet:<br>0.3–2 gm 1 to 4 times daily<br><br>Administration issues<br>Antacid dosing should be staggered at least 2 hours from other drugs where a potential drug interaction may occur<br><br>Drug–Drug Interactions<br>Sodium bicarbonate may increase urinary pH inhibiting excretion of basic drugs **(quinidine, amphetamines)** and enhance the excretion of acidic drugs **(salicylates)** | ADRs:<br>belching, gastric distension<br><br>Warnings/Precautions<br>Milk-alkali syndrome with hypercalcemia and metabolic alkalosis; acid rebound may occur with repeat dosing; May worsen hypertension and heart failure due to sodium content | Pregnancy Category: C<br><br>Lactation Issues<br>Safety not established, do not use in nursing mothers |

**501.2 Antacid Combination Products**

Listed below is a representative sample of antacid combination products. Administration and dosage depends on the condition being treated and the agent being used. See individual products (section 501.1) for administration issues, interactions, ADRs, etc.

**Aluminum Hydroxide and Magnesium Hydroxide**
Maalox, RuLox, Extra Strength Maalox (all are chewable tablets)
Maalox Suspension, RuLox Suspension, Maalox Therapeutic Concentrate Suspension

**Calcium Carbonate and Magnesium Carbonate**
Mylanta Gelcaps

**Calcium Carbonate and Simethicone**
Titralac Plus Chewable Tablets, Titralac Plus Liquid

**Aluminum Hydroxide, Alginic Acid, Sodium Bicarbonate, and Magnesium Trisilicate**
Gaviscon, Double Strength Gaviscon-2 (all are chewable tablets)
Gaviscon Liquid, Gaviscon Extra Strength Relief Formula Liquid

**Aluminum Hydroxide, Magnesium Hydroxide, and Simethicone**
Mylanta, Rulox Plus, Gelusil, Maalox Plus, Extra Strength Maalox Plus, Mylanta Double Strength (all are chewable tablets)
Mylanta Liquid, RuLox Plus Suspension, Gelusil Liquid, Di-Gel Liquid, Mylanta Double Strength Liquid, Extra Strength Maalox Plus Suspension

**Aluminum Hydroxide, Magnesium Hydroxide, Calcium Carbonate, and Simethicone**
Tempo Chewable Tablets

**Magnesium Hydroxide, Calcium Carbonate, and Simethicone**
Advanced Formula Di-Gel Chewable Tablets

**Magaldrate and Simethicone**
Riopan Plus, Riopan Plus Double Strength (all are chewable tablets)
Riopan Plus Suspension, Riopan Plus Double Strength Suspension

**Sodium Bicarbonate, Acetaminophen, Citric Acid**

Bromo Seltzer Effervescent Granules

**Sodium Bicarbonate, Citric Acid, Potassium Bicarbonate**

Gold Alka -Seltzer Effervescent Tablets

**Sodium Bicarbonate, Citric Acid, and Aspirin**

Alka-Seltzer, Extra Strength Alka-Seltzer (all are effervescent tablets)

---

501.3  Gastrointestinal Anticholinergics/Antispasmodics

| Drug and Dosage Forms | Usual Dosage Range | Administration Issues and Drug–Drug Interactions | Common Adverse Drug Reactions (ADRs) and Pharmacokinetics | Contraindications, Pregnancy Category, and Lactation Issues |
|---|---|---|---|---|
| **Atropine Sulfate**<br><br>Tablets:<br>0.4 mg<br><br>Tablets, soluble:<br>0.4 mg, 0.6 mg | **Management of peptic ulcer disease; GI hypermotility: control rhinorrhea of acute rhinitis or hay fever; adjunctive therapy in the treatment of sialorrhea and hyperhidrosis associated with parkinsonism**<br><br>**Adults**<br>0.4 mg–0.6 mg q 4 to 6 h<br><br>**Children**<br>0.1 mg/kg q 4 to 6 h; not to exceed 0.4 mg q 4 to 6 h | Administration Issues<br>Take 30–60 minutes before a meal<br><br>Drug–Drug Interactions<br>Administration of atropine with **amantadine, tricyclic antidepressants (amitriptyline, nortriptyline), or phenothiazines** may result in increased anticholinergic side effects<br><br>Atropine may decrease the effect of **phenothiazines** such as **chlorpromazine, thioridazine, and prochlorperazine**<br><br>The pharmacological effects of **atenolol** may be increased by anticholinergic agents such as atropine | ADRs<br>Hypersensitivity reactions, urticarial rash, dry mouth, nausea, vomiting, constipation, urinary hesitancy and retention, impotence, blurred vision, worsening of glaucoma, palpitations, headache, flushing, drowsiness, dizziness, confusion<br><br>Pharmacokinetics:<br>liver metabolism, renal excretion may be prolonged with renal dysfunction | Contraindications<br>Hypersensitivity to anticholinergic agents; narrow-angle glaucoma; obstructive GI disease; paralytic ileus; intestinal atony of the elderly; obstructive uropathy (bladder neck obstruction)<br><br>Pregnancy Category:  C<br><br>Lactation Issues<br>Atropine is excreted in breast milk and may result in infant toxicity and decreased milk production; refrain from use in nursing women |

*(continues on next page)*

| Drug and Dosage Forms | Usual Dosage Range | Administration Issues and Drug–Drug Interactions | Common Adverse Drug Reactions (ADRs) and Pharmacokinetics | Contraindications, Pregnancy Category, and Lactation Issues |
|---|---|---|---|---|
| **Belladonna (alkaloids of hyoscyamine, scopolamine, and others)**<br>Belladonna tincture<br><br>Liquid:<br>0.3 mg alkaloids of belladonna leaf/ ml | **Adjunctive therapy in peptic ulcer disease; motion sickness; GI motility disturbances (irritable bowel syndrome); adjunctive therapy in the treatment of sialorrhea and hyperhidrosis associated with parkinsonism**<br><br>**Adults**<br>0.5–1 ml 3 to 4 times daily<br><br>**Children**<br>0.03 mg/kg 3 times daily | Administration Issues<br>Take 30–60 minutes before a meal<br><br>Drug–Drug Interactions<br>Administration of belladonna liquid with **amantadine, tricyclic antidepressants (amitriptyline, nortriptyline), or phenothiazines** may result in increased anticholinergic side effects<br><br>Belladonna liquid may decrease the effect of **phenothiazines** such as **chlorpromazine, thioridazine, and prochlorperazine**<br><br>Administration of belladonna liquid and **phenothiazines** may result in increased anticholinergic side effects | ADRs<br>Hypersensitivity reactions, urticarial rash, dry mouth, nausea, vomiting, constipation, urinary hesitancy and retention, impotence, blurred vision, worsening of glaucoma, palpitations, headache, flushing, drowsiness, dizziness, confusion<br><br>Pharmacokinetics:<br>little information is available on belladonna distribution, metabolism, and excretion | Contraindications<br>Hypersensitivity to anticholinergic agents; narrow-angle glaucoma; obstructive GI disease; paralytic ileus; intestinal atony of the elderly; obstructive uropathy (bladder neck obstruction)<br><br>Pregnancy Category:  C<br><br>Lactation Issues<br>Belladonna alkaloids are excreted in breast milk and may result in infant toxicity and decreased milk production; refrain from use in nursing women |
| **Clidinium Bromide**<br>Quarzan<br><br>Capsules:<br>2.5 mg, 5 mg | **Adjunctive therapy in the treatment of peptic ulcer disease; GI motility disturbances (irritable bowel syndrome)**<br><br>**Adults**<br>2.5 mg–5 mg 3 to 4 times daily before meals and at bedtime | Administration Issues<br>Take 30–60 minutes before a meal<br><br>Drug–Drug Interactions<br>Administration of clidinium bromide with **amantadine, tricyclic antidepressants (amitriptyline, nortriptyline), or phenothiazines** may result in increased anticholinergic side effects | ADRs<br>Hypersensitivity reactions, urticarial rash, dry mouth, nausea, vomiting, constipation, urinary hesitancy and retention, impotence, blurred vision, worsening of glaucoma, palpitations, headache, flushing, drowsiness, dizziness, confusion | Contraindications<br>Hypersensitivity to anticholinergic agents; narrow-angle glaucoma; obstructive GI disease; paralytic ileus; intestinal atony of the elderly; obstructive uropathy (bladder neck obstruction) |

| | | | |
|---|---|---|---|
| | **Geriatric, debilitated**<br>2.5 mg tid before meals | Clidinium bromide may decrease the effect of **phenothiazines** such as **chlorpromazine, thioridazine, and prochlorperazine** | *Pharmacokinetics:*<br>longer duration of action than alkaloids; hepatic metabolism; renal and fecal excretion | <u>Lactation Issues</u><br>Clidinium bromide is excreted in breast milk and may result in infant toxicity and decreased milk production; refrain from use in nursing women |
| **Dicyclomine**<br>Bentyl, various generics<br><br><u>Tablets:</u><br>20 mg<br><br><u>Capsules:</u><br>10 mg, 20 mg<br><br><u>Syrup:</u><br>10 mg/5 ml | **Treatment of functional bowel/irritable bowel syndrome**<br><br>**Adult**<br>20 mg qid, then increase to 40 mg qid<br><br>**160 mg / day is the only dose shown to be effective; however side effects frequently occur at this dose**<br><br>**Children**<br>5–10 mg 3 to 4 times daily | <u>Administration Issues</u><br>Take 30–60 minutes before a meal | <u>ADRs:</u><br>Hypersensitivity reactions, urticarial rash, dry mouth, nausea, vomiting, constipation, urinary hesitancy and retention, impotence, blurred vision, worsening of glaucoma, palpitations, headache, flushing, drowsiness, dizziness, confusion<br><br><u>Pharmacokinetics:</u><br>Rapid absorption in the GI tract; approximately 80% is renally eliminated and 10% is fecally eliminated | <u>Contraindications</u><br>Dicyclomine use has been associated with respiratory distress, seizures, and syncope in infants < 6 months<br><br><u>Lactation Issues</u><br>Dicyclomine is excreted in breast milk and may result in infant toxicity and decreased milk production; refrain from use in nursing women |
| **Glycopyrrolate**<br>Robinul, Robinul Forte<br><br><u>Tablets:</u><br>Robinul<br>1 mg<br><br>Robinul Forte<br>2 mg | **Adjunctive therapy in the treatment of peptic ulcer disease; GI motility disturbances (irritable bowel syndrome)**<br><br>**Adults, initial dosing**<br>1 mg tid or 2 mg bid to tid<br><br>**maintenance dosing**<br>1 mg bid<br><br>**Use in children < 12 years for the treatment of peptic ulcer disease is not established** | <u>Administration Issues</u><br>Take 30–60 minutes before a meal<br><br><u>Drug–Drug Interactions</u><br>Administration of glycopyrrolate with **amantadine, tricyclic antidepressants (amitriptyline, nortriptyline), or phenothiazines** may result in increased anticholinergic side effects<br><br>Glycopyrrolate may decrease the effect of **phenothiazines** such as **chlorpromazine, thioridazine, and prochlorperazine** | <u>ADRs</u><br>Hypersensitivity reactions, urticarial rash, dry mouth, nausea, vomiting, constipation, urinary hesitancy and retention, impotence, blurred vision, worsening of glaucoma, palpitations, headache, flushing, drowsiness, dizziness, confusion<br><br><u>Pharmacokinetics:</u><br>excreted as unchanged drug in the feces and urine | <u>Contraindications</u><br>Hypersensitivity to anticholinergic agents; narrow-angle glaucoma; obstructive GI disease; paralytic ileus; intestinal atony of the elderly; obstructive uropathy (bladder neck obstruction)<br><br><u>Pregnancy Category:</u>  B<br><br><u>Lactation Issues</u><br>Glycopyrrolate is excreted in breast milk and may result in infant toxicity and decreased milk production; refrain from use in nursing women |

(continues on next page)

| Drug and Dosage Forms | Usual Dosage Range | Administration Issues and Drug–Drug Interactions | Common Adverse Drug Reactions (ADRs) and Pharmacokinetics | Contraindications, Pregnancy Category, and Lactation Issues |
|---|---|---|---|---|
| **L-Hyoscyamine Sulfate**<br><br>Tablets:<br>Anaspaz<br>0.125 mg<br><br>Cystospaz<br>0.15 mg<br><br>Capsules, time released:<br>Cystospaz-M, Levsinex<br>Timecaps<br>0.375 mg<br><br>Solution:<br>Levsinex Drops<br>0.125 mg/ml<br><br>Elixir:<br>Levsin<br>0.125 mg/5 ml | **To control gastric secretions; adjunctive therapy in peptic ulcer disease; GI hypermotility; pylorospasm and associated abdominal cramps; neurogenic bowel disturbances; adjunctive therapy in the treatment of sialorrhea and hyperhidrosis associated with parkinsonism**<br><br>Tablets:<br>0.125 mg–0.25 mg 3 to 4 times daily orally or sublingually<br><br>Capsules, time released:<br>0.375 mg–0.75 mg q 2 h<br><br>Solution:<br>1–2 ml 3 to 4 times daily orally or sublingually<br><br>Elixir:<br>5–10 ml 3 to 4 times daily | Administration Issues<br>Take 30–60 minutes before a meal<br><br>Drug–Drug Interactions<br>Administration of hyoscyamine with **amantadine, tricyclic antidepressants (amitriptyline, nortriptyline), or phenothiazines** may result in increased anticholinergic side effects<br><br>Hyoscyamine may decrease the effect of **phenothiazines** such as **chlorpromazine, thioridazine, and prochlorperazine**<br><br>The pharmacological effects of **atenolol** may be increased by anticholinergic agents such as hyoscyamine | ADRs<br>Hypersensitivity reactions, urticarial rash, dry mouth, nausea, vomiting, constipation, urinary hesitancy and retention, impotence, blurred vision, worsening of glaucoma, palpitations, headache, flushing, drowsiness, dizziness, confusion<br><br>Pharmacokinetics:<br>liver metabolism, renal excretion may be prolonged with renal dysfunction | Contraindications<br>Hypersensitivity to anticholinergic agents; narrow-angle glaucoma; obstructive GI disease; paralytic ileus; intestinal atony of the elderly; obstructive uropathy (bladder neck obstruction)<br><br>Pregnancy Category: C<br><br>Lactation Issues<br>Hyoscyamine is excreted in breast milk and may result in infant toxicity and decreased milk production; refrain from use in nursing women |
| **Methantheline Bromide**<br>Banthine<br><br>Tablets:<br>50 mg | **Adjunctive treatment of peptic ulcer disease; uninhibited hypertonic neurogenic bladder**<br><br>**Adults**<br>50 mg–100 mg q 6 h | Administration Issues<br>Take 30–60 minutes before a meal<br><br>Drug–Drug Interactions<br>Administration of methantheline with **amantadine, tricyclic** | ADRs:<br>Hypersensitivity reactions, urticarial rash, dry mouth, nausea, vomiting, constipation, urinary hesitancy and retention, impotence, blurred vision, | Contraindications<br>Hypersensitivity to anticholinergic agents; narrow-angle glaucoma; obstructive GI disease; paralytic ileus; intestinal atony of the elderly; obstructive |

| Drug/Dosage Forms | Dosage | Administration Issues / Drug–Drug Interactions | ADRs / Pharmacokinetics | Contraindications / Pregnancy / Lactation |
|---|---|---|---|---|
| | **Pediatric, newborns** 12.5 mg bid, then 12.5 mg tid<br><br>**Infants, 1–12 months** 12.5 mg qid, then 25 mg qid<br><br>**Children, > 12 months** 12.5 mg–50 mg qid | **antidepressants (amitriptyline, nortriptyline), or phenothiazines** may result in increased anticholinergic side effects<br><br>Methantheline may decrease the effect of **phenothiazines** such as **chlorpromazine, thioridazine, and prochlorperazine** | worsening of glaucoma, palpitations, headache, flushing, drowsiness, dizziness, confusion<br><br>Pharmacokinetics: little information is available on belladonna distribution, metabolism; fecal excretion of unabsorbed drug | uropathy (bladder neck obstruction)<br><br>Pregnancy Category: C<br><br>Lactation Issues Methantheline is excreted in breast milk and may result in infant toxicity and decreased milk production; refrain from use in nursing women |
| **Propantheline Bromide** Pro-Banthine, various generics<br><br>Tablets: 7.5 mg, 15 mg | **Adjunctive treatment of peptic ulcer disease**<br><br>**Adults** 15 mg tid before meals and 30 mg at bedtime<br><br>**Geriatrics** 7.5 mg tid before meals | Administration Issues Take 30–60 minutes before a meal<br><br>Drug–Drug Interactions Administration of propantheline with **amantadine, tricyclic antidepressants (amitriptyline, nortriptyline), or phenothiazines** may result in increased anticholinergic side effects<br><br>Propantheline may decrease the effect of **phenothiazines** such as **chlorpromazine, thioridazine, and prochlorperazine** | ADRs: Hypersensitivity reactions, urticarial rash, dry mouth, nausea, vomiting, constipation, urinary hesitancy and retention, impotence, blurred vision, worsening of glaucoma, palpitations, headache, flushing, drowsiness, dizziness, confusion<br><br>Pharmacokinetics: GI tract and/or hepatic metabolism; renal excretion of metabolites and unchanged drug | Contraindications Hypersensitivity to anticholinergic agents; narrow-angle glaucoma; obstructive GI disease; paralytic ileus; intestinal atony of the elderly; obstructive uropathy (bladder neck obstruction)<br><br>Pregnancy Category: C<br><br>Lactation Issues Propantheline is excreted in breast milk and may result in infant toxicity and decreased milk production; refrain from use in nursing women |

Listed below are combination anticholinergic GI products and dosage forms available. Refer to the individual drugs for information on ADRs, etc.

## Atropine, Scopolamine, Hyoscyamine, and Phenobarbital
Barbidonna No. 2, Barbidonna, Donnatal, Hyosphen, Donnatal Extentabs

Tablet, Capsule, Sustained release tablet, Elixir

## Belladonna Extract, Butabarbital Sodium
Butibel

Tablet, Elixir

## Belladonna Extract and Phenobarbital
Chardonna -2

Tablet

## Hyoscyamine Sulfate and Phenobarbital
Levsin w/Phenobarbital, Levsin PB Drops

Tablet, Liquid

## Clidinium Bromide and Chlordiazepoxide
Librax, Clindex, various generics

Capsule

## Belladonna, Phenobarbital, and Ergotamine Tartrate
Bellergal-S, Bellacane SR

Tablet, Sustained release Tablet

## 501.5 Agents for Ulcers and GERD

| Drug and Dosage Forms | Usual Dosage Range | Administration Issues and Drug–Drug Interactions | Common Adverse Drug Reactions (ADRs) and Pharmacokinetics | Contraindications, Pregnancy Category, and Lactation Issues |
|---|---|---|---|---|
| **Cimetidine**<br><br>Tablet:<br>Tagamet HB<br>100 mg<br><br>Tagamet<br>200 mg, 300 mg, 400 mg,<br>800 mg<br><br>Liquid:<br>Tagamet<br>300 mg/5 ml | **Duodenal and gastric ulcers, treatment**<br><br>**Adults and children > 12**<br>800 mg q hs OR 300 mg qid with meals and q hs OR 400 mg bid<br>(Continue treatment for 4–8 weeks unless healing is demonstrated by endoscopy)<br><br>**Duodenal and gastric ulcers, maintenance**<br>**Adults and children >12**<br>400 mg q hs<br><br>**Gastroesophageal reflux (GERD)**<br>**Adults and children > 12**<br>800 mg bid OR 400 mg qid (Continue treatment for 12 weeks; use beyond 12 weeks has not been established)<br><br>**Hypersecretory conditions (Zollinger-Ellison syndrome)**<br>**Adults and children > 12**<br>300 mg qid with meals and q hs; may need to give more often than 4 times daily; individualize treatment; do not exceed 2400 mg/d. (Continue treatment as long as clinically indicated) | <u>Administration Issues</u><br>Give antacids as needed for pain relief; separate antacid dosing from cimetidine by 1 hour if possible. Use not recommended for children <12.<br><br><u>Drug–Drug Interactions</u><br>Cimetidine may increase the effect of the following drugs by inhibiting their hepatic metabolism: metoprolol, **labetalol, propranolol, warfarin, carbamazepine, phenytoin, theophylline, terfenadine, tricyclic antidepressants, propafenone, metronidazole, sulfonylureas**<br><br>Cimetidine may decrease the absorption of **ferrous salts, indomethacin, ketoconazole, tetracycline** | <u>ADRs:</u><br>headache, dizziness, somnolence, gynecomastia, diarrhea<br><br><u>Pharmacokinetics:</u><br>Decrease dosage with renal impairment (CrCl < 30 ml/min) | <u>Contraindications</u><br>Patients hypersensitive to $H_2$ antagonists<br><br><u>Pregnancy Category:</u> B<br><br><u>Lactation Issues</u><br>Excreted in breast milk in high concentrations; do not use |

(continues on next page)

| Drug and Dosage Forms | Usual Dosage Range | Administration Issues and Drug–Drug Interactions | Common Adverse Drug Reactions (ADRs) and Pharmacokinetics | Contraindications, Pregnancy Category, and Lactation Issues |
|---|---|---|---|---|
| **Cimetidine** *cont.* | **Heartburn, acid indigestion** <br> **Adults and children > 12** <br> 200 mg (2 tablets) with water as symptoms occur; up to 400 mg (4 tablets) in 24 hours | | | |
| **Famotidine** <br><br> Tablet: <br> Pepcid AC <br> 10 mg <br><br> Pepcid <br> 20 mg, 40 mg <br><br> Powder for Oral Suspension: <br> Pepcid <br> 40 mg/5 ml | **Duodenal and gastric ulcers, treatment** <br> **Adults and children > 12** <br> 40 mg q hs OR 20 mg bid (Continue treatment for 4–8 weeks unless healing is demonstrated by endoscopy) <br><br> **Duodenal and gastric ulcers, maintenance** <br> **Adults and children > 12** <br> 20 mg q hs <br><br> **Gastroesophageal reflux (GERD):** <br> **Adults and children > 12** <br> 20 mg bid (Continue treatment for 12 weeks; use beyond 12 weeks has not been established) <br><br> **Hypersecretory conditions (Zollinger–Ellison syndrome):** <br> **Adults and children > 12** <br> 20 mg q 6 h; may need to give more often than q 6 h; individualize treatment; do not exceed 640 mg/d. | Administration Issues <br> Give antacids as needed for pain relief; reconstituted suspension may be stored at room temperature, keep away from heat, discard unused portion 30 days after reconstitution. Use not recommended for children < 12. | ADRs: <br> headache, dizziness, somnolence, diarrhea, constipation <br><br> Pharmacokinetics: <br> Decrease dosage with renal impairment (CrCl < 30 ml/min) | Contraindications <br> Patients hypersensitive to $H_2$ antagonists <br><br> Pregnancy Category: B <br><br> Lactation Issues <br> Not known if drug is excreted in human breast milk; use caution when administering to nursing mother |

(continues on next page)

| | | | | |
|---|---|---|---|---|
| | (Continue treatment as long as clinically indicated)<br><br>**Heartburn, acid indigestion:**<br>**Adults and children > 12**<br>20 mg (2 tablets) with water as symptoms occur; up to 40 mg (4 tablets) in 24 h | | | |
| **Lansoprazole**<br>Prevacid<br><br><u>Capsule, delayed release:</u><br>15 mg, 30 mg | **Duodenal ulcer, treatment**<br>15 mg qd for 4 weeks<br><br>**Hypersecretory conditions**<br>**(Zollinger-Ellison syndrome)**<br>60 mg qd individualize treatment, doses up to 90 mg bid have been used.<br>(Continue treatment as long as clinically indicated)<br><br>**Erosive esophagitis**<br>20 mg qd for 4 to 8 weeks | <u>Administration Issues</u><br>Do not chew or crush capsule, swallow whole capsule; take capsule before eating. Give lansoprazole at least 30 minutes prior to sucralfate<br><br><u>Drug–Drug Interactions</u><br>Lansoprazole may decrease the absorption of **ketoconazole, iron supplements, and digoxin** by altering gastric pH<br><br>Lansoprazole may decrease the effect of **theophylline** | <u>ADRs:</u><br>diarrhea, abdominal pain, headache<br><br><u>Pharmacokinetics:</u><br>extensive hepatic metabolism; primarily excreted by biliary/fecal route | <u>Contraindications:</u><br>Hypersensitivity<br><br><u>Pregnancy Category:</u> B<br><br><u>Lactation Issues</u><br>It is not known whether lansoprazole is excreted in human breast milk |
| **Misoprostol**<br>Cytotec<br><br><u>Tablet:</u><br>100 mcg, 200 mcg | **Prevention of NSAID-induced**<br>**gastric ulcers**<br>100 mcg qid, pc and hs <u>OR</u> 200 mcg bid or tid<br><br>**Duodenal and gastric ulcer,**<br>**treatment**<br>100–200 mcg qid for 4 to 8 weeks | <u>Administration Issues</u><br>Avoid concomitant use of misoprostol with antacids and food; if GI upset occurs, misoprostol may be given with meals. | <u>ADRs:</u><br>diarrhea, abdominal pain, headache, dizziness<br><br><u>Pharmacokinetics:</u><br>Rapid oral absorption; renal excretion | <u>Contraindications</u><br>Misoprostol is contraindicated in pregnant women because of abortifacent properties; exercise **extreme caution** when misoprostol is used in women of childbearing potential<br><br><u>Pregnancy Category:</u> X<br><br><u>Lactation Issues</u><br>Use in nursing mothers is not recommended due to potential diarrhea in nursing infant |

| Drug and Dosage Forms | Usual Dosage Range | Administration Issues and Drug–Drug Interactions | Common Adverse Drug Reactions (ADRs) and Pharmacokinetics | Contraindications, Pregnancy Category, and Lactation Issues |
|---|---|---|---|---|
| **Nizatidine**<br>Axid<br><br>Tablet:<br>150 mg, 300 mg | **Duodenal and gastric ulcers, treatment**<br>300 mg q hs OR 150 mg bid (Continue treatment for 4–8 weeks unless healing is demonstrated by endoscopy)<br><br>**Duodenal and gastric ulcers, maintenance**<br>150 mg q hs<br><br>**Gastroesophageal reflux (GERD)**<br>150 mg bid (Use beyond 6 weeks not adequately studied) | Administration Issues<br>Give antacids as needed for pain relief; separate antacid dosing from nizatidine by 1 hour if possible | ADRs:<br>headache, dizziness, somnolence, diarrhea, constipation, sweating<br><br>Pharmacokinetics:<br>Decrease dosage with renal impairment (CrCl < 30 ml/min) | Contraindications<br>Patients hypersensitive to $H_2$ antagonists<br><br>Pregnancy Category: C<br><br>Lactation Issues<br>Is excreted in breast milk, use caution |
| **Omeprazole**<br>Prilosec<br><br>Capsule, sustained release:<br>10 mg, 20 mg | **Duodenal ulcer, treatment**<br>20 mg qd for 4 to 8 weeks<br><br>**Gastroesophageal reflux (GERD)**<br>20 mg qd for 4 to 8 weeks<br><br>**Hypersecretory conditions (Zollinger-Ellison syndrome)**<br>60 mg qd; individualize treatment, doses up to 120 mg tid have been used (Continue treatment as long as clinically indicated)<br><br>**Erosive esophagitis**<br>20 mg qd for 4 to 8 weeks | Administration Issues<br>Do not chew or crush capsule, swallow whole capsule; take capsule before eating<br><br>Drug–Drug Interactions<br>Omeprazole may decrease the absorption of **iron supplements, ketoconazole and digoxin** by altering gastric pH. Omeprazole may inhibit the metabolism of **diazepam, phenytoin, and warfarin,** increasing each drug's effect | ADRs:<br>diarrhea, nausea, vomiting, abdominal pain, headache, dizziness<br><br>Pharmacokinetics:<br>hepatic/biliary metabolism; renal excretion | Pregnancy Category: C<br><br>Lactation Issues<br>Use with caution in nursing mothers, excretion in breast milk is unknown |

| Sucralfate | Treatment of Duodenal Ulcer | Administration Issues | ADRs: | Pregnancy Category: B |
|---|---|---|---|---|
| Carafate | **Tablets:** Sucralfate should be taken on an empty | constipation, diarrhea, nausea, | |
| | 1 gm qid 1 hour ac and hs | stomach; do not take antacids 1/2 hour | vomiting, indigestion | Lactation Issues |
| **Tablets:** | | before or after taking sucralfate | | It is not known if sucralfate is |
| 1 gm | Suspension: | | Pharmacokinetics: | excreted in breast milk; use |
| | 10 ml qid 1 hour ac and hs | Drug–Drug Interactions | Minimally absorbed from the GI | caution when sucralfate is |
| Suspension: | | Sucralfate may decrease the effect of | tract (<5%); approximately 90% | administered to nursing |
| 1 gm/10 ml | **Maintenance Therapy of** | **warfarin, digoxin, phenytoin,** | is excreted in the stool | mothers |
| | **Duodenal Ulcer** | **ketoconazole, ciprofloxacin,** | | |
| | Tablets: 1 gm bid | **ofloxacin, and norfloxacin** | | |
| **Ranitidine** | **Duodenal and gastric ulcers,** | Administration Issues | ADRs: | Contraindications |
| | **treatment** | Give antacids as needed for pain relief; | headache, dizziness, | Patients hypersensitive to H$_2$ |
| Zantac, Zantac 75, Zantac | 300 mg q hs OR 150 mg bid (Continue | separate dosing from ranitidine by 1 hour | somnolence, diarrhea | antagonists |
| EFFERdose, Zantac GELdose | treatment for 4–8 weeks unless healing | if possible | constipation | |
| | is demonstrated by endoscopy) | | | Pregnancy Category: B |
| **Tablet:** | | Drug–Drug Interactions | Pharmacokinetics: | |
| 75 mg, 150 mg, 300 mg | **Duodenal and gastric ulcers,** | Ranitidine may increase the effect of the | Decrease dosage with renal | Lactation Issues |
| | **maintenance** | following drugs by inhibiting their hepatic | impairment (CrCl < 30 ml/min) | Excreted in breast milk 1:1 to |
| Tablet, effervescent: | 150 mg q hs | metabolism: **propranolol, warfarin,** | | 6.7:1 milk:plasma ratio; use |
| 150 mg | | **carbamazepine, phenytoin,** | | caution when administering to |
| | **Gastroesophageal reflux (GERD)** | **theophylline, terfenadine, tricyclic** | | nursing mothers |
| Capsules: | 150 mg bid (Use beyond 6 weeks has | **antidepressants, valproic acid.** | | |
| 150 mg, 300 mg | not been adequately studied) | | | |
| | | The hepatic inhibition of other drugs by | | |
| Granules, effervescent: | **Hypersecretory conditions** | ranitidine is approximately 10% of | | |
| 150 mg | **(Zollinger-Ellison syndrome)** | cimetidine's inhibitory potential and may | | |
| | 150 mg bid; may need to give more often; | be of less clinical importance | | |
| Syrup: | individualize treatment; dosages up to | | | |
| 150 mg / 10 ml | 6 gm/day have been used. (Continue | | | |
| | treatment as long as clinically indicated) | | | |
| | | | | |
| | **Erosive esophagitis, treatment:** | | | |
| | 150 mg qid | | | |
| | | | | |
| | **Erosive esophagitis,** | | | |
| | **maintenance:** 150 mg bid | | | |
| | | | | |
| | **Heartburn, acid indigestion:** | | | |
| | 75 mg qd or bid | | | |

| Drug and Dosage Forms | Usual Dosage Range | Administration Issues and Drug–Drug Interactions | Common Adverse Drug Reactions (ADRs) and Pharmacokinetics | Contraindications, Pregnancy Category, and Lactation Issues |
|---|---|---|---|---|
| **Cisapride**<br>Propulsid<br><br>Tablet:<br>10 mg, 20 mg<br><br>Suspension:<br>1 mg/ml | **Heartburn due to gastroesophageal reflux**<br>10 mg 4 times daily at least 15 minutes before meals and at bedtime; increase dose to 20 mg if needed | Administration Issues<br>Take at least 15 minutes before meals. Safety and efficacy in children have not been established.<br><br>Drug–Drug Interactions<br>Cisapride may decrease the absorption of drugs such as **digoxin and cimetidine** by increasing gastric transit time<br><br>**Anticholinergic agents (hyoscyamine, tricyclic antidepressants)** may antagonize the effects of cisapride<br><br>The following drugs have been shown to inhibit the metabolism of cisapride and concurrent use with cisapride is contraindicated: **erythromycin, clarithromycin, fluconazole, itraconazole, ketoconazole, miconazole IV, troleandomycin** | ADRs:<br>diarrhea, abdominal pain, dizziness<br><br>Pharmacokinetics<br>onset of action is 30–60 minutes | Contraindications<br>Concurrent use of cisapride with **ketoconazole, itraconazole, miconazole IV, fluconazole, erythromycin, clarithromycin, and troleandomycin** may cause serious cardiac arrhythmias<br><br>Pregnancy Category: C<br><br>Lactation Issues<br>Cisapride is excreted in breast milk in small amounts; use with caution in nursing mothers |
| **Metoclopramide**<br>Reglan, various generics<br><br>Tablet:<br>5 mg, 10 mg | **Diabetic gastroparesis**<br>10 mg 30 minutes ac and hs for 2 to 8 weeks<br><br>**Gastroesophageal reflux:**<br>10 mg–15 mg up to 4 times daily 30 minutes ac and hs; | Administration Issues<br>Take 30 minutes before meals<br><br>Drug–Drug Interactions<br>Metoclopramide may decrease the absorption of drugs such as **digoxin and** | ADRs:<br>diarrhea, drowsiness, restlessness, fatigue, parkinson-like symptoms (bradykinesia, tremors, cogwheel rigidity) | Contraindications<br>Patients where stimulation of GI motility may be dangerous (mechanical obstruction, perforation) |

| | Usual Dosage Range | Administration Issues and Drug–Drug Interactions | Common Adverse Drug Reactions (ADRs) and Pharmacokinetics | Pregnancy Category, and Lactation Issues |
|---|---|---|---|---|

**Syrup:**
5 mg/5 ml

10 mg–20 mg may be given as a single dose prior to events known to provoke reflux symptoms

**Elderly may require only 5 mg per dose**

**Unlabeled Use in nausea/vomiting of a variety of etiologies:**
Oral: 5–10 mg tid

**cimetidine** by increasing gastric transit time

**Anticholinergic agents (hyoscyamine, tricyclic antidepressants)** may antagonize the effects of metoclopramide

**Levodopa** has opposite effects on dopamine receptors and may antagonize the effects of metoclopramide

Metoclopramide may increase the hypertensive effects of **MAO inhibitors (isocarboxazid, phenelzine, and tranylcypromine)**

**Pharmacokinetics**
onset of action is 30–60 minutes following oral dose; dosage decrease may be needed with renal impairment (CrCl < 40 ml/min)

**Pregnancy Category:** B

**Lactation Issues**
Metoclopramide is excreted in breast milk in small amounts; there appears to be no risk to the nursing infant when the mother's dose is ≤ 45 mg/day; use with caution in nursing mothers

---

## 501.7 Digestive Enzymes

| Drug and Dosage Forms | Usual Dosage Range | Administration Issues and Drug–Drug Interactions | Common Adverse Drug Reactions (ADRs) and Pharmacokinetics | Contraindications, Pregnancy Category, and Lactation Issues |
|---|---|---|---|---|
| **Digestive enzymes**<br>Kutrase, Ku–Zyme<br><br>Capsules:<br>Kutrase (Amylase 30 mg, Protease 6 mg, Lipase 75 mg, Cellulase 2 mg, Hyoscyamine sulfate 0.0625 mg, Phenyltoloxamine citrate 15 mg) | **Enzyme replacement therapy in patients with cystic fibrosis, chronic pancreatitis, ductal obstructions, pancreatic insufficiency**<br><br>Adjust dosage according to the severity of pancreatic enzyme deficiency; estimate dosage by assessing which dose minimizes steatorrhea and maintains good nutritional status<br><br>Take 1–3 capsules with or after meals | Administration Issues<br>Swallow tablets / capsules whole; do not crush microspheres; if swallowing is difficult, give contents of capsule on applesauce or gelatin and swallow without chewing<br><br>Drug–Drug Interactions<br>Administration with **antacids** may cause the enteric coated capsules to dissolve in the stomach and inactivate the product. The effect of oral **iron supplements** may be decreased with concomitant use of pancreatic enzymes | ADRs:<br>nausea, diarrhea, abdominal cramps<br><br>Pharmacokinetics:<br>pancreatic lipase is inactivated at pH ≤ 4; enteric coated products decrease gastric destruction and increase delivery of product to the duodenum for therapeutic effect | Contraindications<br>Hypersensitivity to pork protein or enzymes; acute pancreatitis<br><br>Pregnancy Category: C<br><br>Lactation Issues<br>It is unknown if pancreatin is excreted in breast milk; use with caution |

| Drug and Dosage Forms | Usual Dosage Range | Administration Issues and Drug–Drug Interactions | Common Adverse Drug Reactions (ADRs) and Pharmacokinetics | Contraindications, Pregnancy Category, and Lactation Issues |
|---|---|---|---|---|
| **Pancreatin**<br>Entozyme, Donnazyme, Creon<br><br>Tablet:<br>Entozyme (Pancreatin 300 mg, Lipase 600 units, Protease 7,500 units, Amylase 7,500 units)<br><br>Donnazyme (Pancreatin 500 mg, Lipase 1,000 units, Protease 12,500 units, Amylase 12,500 units)<br><br>Capsules:<br>Creon (Pancreatin strength not known, Lipase 8,000 units, Protease 13,000 units, Amylase 30,000 units) | **Enzyme replacement therapy in patients with cystic fibrosis, chronic pancreatitis, ductal obstructions, pancreatic insufficiency**<br>Adjust dosage according to the severity of pancreatic enzyme deficiency; estimate dosage by assessing which dose minimizes steatorrhea and maintains good nutritional status<br><br>Take 1–2 tablets or capsules with meals or snacks | Administration Issues<br>Swallow tablets / capsules whole; do not crush microspheres; if swallowing is difficult, give contents of capsule on applesauce or gelatin and swallow without chewing<br><br>Drug–Drug Interactions<br>Administration with **antacids** may cause the enteric coated capsules to dissolve in the stomach and inactivate the product. The effect of oral **iron supplements** may be decreased with concomitant use of pancreatic enzymes | ADRs:<br>nausea, diarrhea, abdominal cramps<br><br>Pharmacokinetics:<br>pancreatic lipase is inactivated at pH ≤ 4; enteric coated products decrease gastric destruction and increase delivery of product to the duodenum for therapeutic effect | Contraindications<br>Hypersensitivity to pork protein or enzymes; acute pancreatitis<br><br>Pregnancy Category: C<br><br>Lactation Issues<br>It is unknown if pancreatin is excreted in breast milk; use with caution in nursing mothers |
| **Pancrelipase**<br>Pancrease, Cotazyme, Viokase, plus others<br><br>Tablet:<br>Viokase (Lipase 8,000 units, Protease 30,000 units, Amylase 30,000 units)<br><br>Ilozyme (Lipase 11,000 units, Protease ≥ 30,000 units, Amylase ≥ 30,000 units) | **Enzyme replacement therapy in patients with cystic fibrosis, chronic pancreatitis, ductal obstructions, pancreatic insufficiency**<br>Adjust dosage according to the severity of pancreatic enzyme deficiency; estimate dosage by assessing which dose minimizes steatorrhea and maintains good nutritional status | Administration Issues<br>Swallow tablets / capsules whole; do not crush microspheres; if swallowing is difficult, give contents of capsule on applesauce or gelatin and swallow without chewing. The dosage has not been established for children < 6 months.<br><br>Drug–Drug Interactions<br>Administration with **antacids** may cause the enteric coated capsules to dissolve in | ADRs:<br>nausea, diarrhea, abdominal cramps<br><br>Pharmacokinetics:<br>pancreatic lipase is inactivated at pH ≤ 4; enteric coated products decrease gastric destruction and increase delivery of product to the duodenum for therapeutic effect | Contraindications<br>Hypersensitivity to pork protein or enzymes; acute pancreatitis<br><br>Pregnancy Category: C<br><br>Lactation Issues<br>It is unknown if pancreatin is excreted in breast milk; use with caution in nursing mothers |

| Drug/Preparations | Dosage | Drug–Drug Interactions | ADRs/Pharmacokinetics/Other |
|---|---|---|---|
| Capsules:<br>Pancrease MT 4 (Lipase 4,000 units, Protease 12,000 units, Amylase 12,000 units)<br><br>Pancrease (Lipase 4,000 units, Protease 25,000 units, Amylase 20,000 units)<br><br>Plus others<br><br>Powder:<br>Viokase, 0.7 gm (Lipase 16,800 units, Protease 70,000 units, Amylase 70,000 units) | **Adults**<br>4,000 units–48,000 units lipase with each meal and with snacks<br><br>**Children 7–12 years**<br>4,000 units–12,000 units lipase with each meal and with snacks<br><br>**Children 1–6 years**<br>4,000 units–8,000 units lipase with each meal and with snacks<br><br>**Children 6 months–1 year**<br>2,000 units lipase per meal | the stomach and inactivate the product. The effect of oral **iron supplements** may be decreased with concomitant use of pancreatic enzymes | |
| **Ursodiol**<br>Actigall<br><br>Capsule:<br>300 mg | **Dissolution of gallbladder stones**<br>8–10 mg/kg/d given in 2 to 3 divided doses<br>**Use beyond 24 months has not been established** | Drug–Drug Interactions<br>**Antacids and bile acid sequestrants (cholestyramine, colestipol)** may interfere with the action of ursodiol by decreasing its absorption | ADRs:<br>nausea, vomiting, abdominal pain, constipation<br><br>Pharmacokinetics<br>absorbed in small bowel; secreted into hepatic bile ducts and expelled into the duodenum in response to eating<br><br>Contraindications<br>Patients with calcified cholesterol stones, radiopaque stones, radiolucent bile pigment stones<br><br>Pregnancy Category: B<br><br>Lactation Issues<br>Excretion in breast milk is not known; use with caution |

| Drug and Dosage Forms | Usual Dosage Range | Administration Issues and Drug–Drug Interactions | Common Adverse Drug Reactions (ADRs) and Pharmacokinetics | Contraindications, Pregnancy Category, and Lactation Issues |
|---|---|---|---|---|
| **Bismuth Subsalicylate** Pepto-Bismol Tablet, chewable: 262 mg Liquid: 262 mg/ml, 524 mg/ml | **Indigestion, diarrhea, nausea** **Adults** 2 tablets or 30 ml; repeat dose q 30 min to 1 hour prn; do not exceed 8 doses in 24 hours **Children** 9–12 years: 1 tablet or 15 ml 6–9 years: 2/3 tablet or 10 ml 3–6 years: 1/3 tablet or 5 ml repeat dose q 30 min to 1 hour prn do not exceed 8 doses in 24 hours | Administration Issues Shake liquid well; chew tablets thoroughly; stool may appear gray-black; (may mask GI bleeding), separate dosing from other medication. Do not use in children who have a high fever. Consult health-care professional if diarrhea persists for > 2 days Drug–Drug Interactions Bismuth subsalicylate contains salicylate, concomitant use of **aspirin** may cause toxicity. Bismuth may decrease the GI absorption of **tetracycline** | ADRs: temporary darkening of stools Pharmacokinetics: absorption of bismuth is negligible; salicylate is absorbed, > 90% of salicylate excreted renally | Contraindications hypersensitivity to aspirin or other salicylate Pregnancy Category:  NA Lactation Issues:  NA |
| **Difenoxin and Atropine Sulfate** Motofen Tablet: 1 mg difenoxin 0.025 mg atropine sulfate | **Antidiarrheal** 2 tablets, then 1 tablet after each loose stool; 1 tablet every 3 to 4 hours as needed **Total dosage in 24 hours should not exceed 8 tablets** | Administration Issues Studies in children <12 year are inadequate to evaluate safety and efficacy. Consult health-care professional if diarrhea persists for > 2 days Drug–Drug Interactions **Barbiturates, narcotics, and alcohol** may potentiate the sedative effects of difenoxin. Use of **MAO inhibitors (phenelzine)** and diphenoxylate may precipitate hypertensive crisis | ADRs: vomiting, dry mouth, dizziness, drowsiness, constipation Pharmacokinetics: hepatic metabolism; excreted in urine and feces | Contraindications Diarrhea associated with toxigenic E. coli, Salmonella sp., or Shigella pseudomembranous colitis Pregnancy Category:  C Lactation Issues Serious adverse effects may occur in nursing infants; evaluate need for nursing versus need for antidiarrheal |
| **Diphenoxylate and Atropine Sulfate** Lomotil, various generics | **Antidiarrheal** **Adults** 1–2 tablets qid prn; individualize | Administration Issues Children should receive the liquid form only. Do not use in children <2 years. | ADRs: nausea, vomiting, dry mouth, dizziness, drowsiness, constipation | Contraindications Diarrhea associated with toxigenic E. coli, Salmonella |

| Drug/Forms | Dosage | Administration Issues | ADRs/Pharmacokinetics | Contraindications/Pregnancy/Lactation |
|---|---|---|---|---|
| **Tablet:** 2.5 mg diphenoxylate 0.025 mg atropine sulfate<br><br>**Liquid:** 2.5 mg diphenoxylate 0.025 mg atropine sulfate per 5 ml | dosage to control symptoms; clinical improvement usually occurs within 48 hours<br><br>**Reduce dosage as soon as initial control of symptoms is achieved. Total dosage in 24 hours should not exceed 8 tablets**<br><br>**Children**<br>9–12 years: 3.5–5 ml qid<br>6–8 years: 2.5–5 ml qid<br>5 years: 2.5–4.5 ml qid<br>4 years: 2–4 ml qid<br>3 years: 2–3 ml qid<br>2 years: 1.5–3 ml qid | Consult health-care professional if diarrhea persists for > 2 days.<br><br><u>Drug–Drug Interactions</u><br>**Barbiturates, narcotics, and alcohol** may potentiate the sedative effects of diphenoxylate. Use of **MAO inhibitors (phenelzine)** and diphenoxylate may precipitate hypertensive crisis | <u>Pharmacokinetics:</u> hepatic metabolism; excreted in urine and feces | sp., or Shigella pseudomembranous colitis<br><br><u>Pregnancy Category:</u> C<br><br><u>Lactation Issues</u> Use with caution in nursing mothers |
| **Loperamide**<br>Imodium, Maalox Anti-Diarrheal, Pepto Diarrhea Control<br><br><u>Tablet Capsule:</u> 2 mg<br><br><u>Liquid:</u> 1 mg/5 ml | **Antidiarrheal**<br>**Adults**<br>4 mg followed by 2 mg after each loose stool; do not exceed 16 mg / day<br><br>**Children, first day**<br>8–12 years: 2mg tid<br>6–8 years: 2 mg bid<br>2–5 years: 1 mg tid<br><br>**Children, subsequent dosing**<br>1 mg/10 kg after each loose stool | <u>Administration Issues</u><br>Drink fluids to avoid dehydration. Do not exceed prescribed dosage. Not intended for use in children <6 yrs old. Consult health-care professional if diarrhea persists for > 2 days | <u>ADRs:</u><br>nausea, vomiting, dry mouth, dizziness, drowsiness, constipation | <u>Contraindications</u><br>Diarrhea associated with toxigenic E. coli, Salmonella sp., or Shigella pseudomembranous colitis.<br><br><u>Pregnancy Category:</u> B<br><br><u>Lactation Issues:</u> Excretion in breast milk is unknown; safety in nursing mothers has not been established |
| **Kaolin with Pectin**<br>Kaopectin, various generic<br><br><u>Suspension:</u><br>90 gm kaolin and 2 gm pectin per 30 ml | **Antidiarrheal**<br>**Adults**<br>60–120 ml after each loose stool<br><br>**Children (after each loose stool)**<br>6–12 years: 30–60 ml<br>3–6 years: 15–30 ml | <u>Administration Issues</u><br>Shake suspension well; separate dosing from other medication. Consult health-care professional if diarrhea persists for > 2 days. | <u>ADRs:</u><br>constipation (usually mild and transient) | <u>Contraindications</u><br>suspected obstructive bowel lesion, pseudomembranous colitis, diarrhea associated with bacteria toxins |

(continues on next page)

| Drug and Dosage Forms | Usual Dosage Range | Administration Issues and Drug–Drug Interactions | Common Adverse Drug Reactions (ADRs) and Pharmacokinetics | Contraindications, Pregnancy Category, and Lactation Issues |
|---|---|---|---|---|
| **Kaolin with Pectin** *cont.* | | <u>Drug–Drug Interactions</u> May decrease the absorption of many orally administered medications. | | <u>Pregnancy Category:</u>  C <br><br> <u>Lactation Issues:</u> safety not established |
| **Products with Attapulgite (an adsorbent and protectant agent)** <br><br> <u>Tablet:</u> Diasorb:  750 mg <br><br> <u>Tablet, chewable:</u> Children's Kaopectate 300 mg <br><br> Donnagel:  600 mg <br><br> <u>Caplets:</u>  Kaopectate Maximum Strength 750 mg, generics <br><br> <u>Liquid:</u> Donnagel, Children's Kaopectate, generics: 600 mg/15 ml <br><br> Diasorb: 750 mg/5 ml | **Antidiarrheal** <br> **Adults** <br> 4 tablets (750 mg/tablet) or 20 ml (750 mg/5 ml) or 2 tablets (600 mg/tablet) or 30 ml (600 mg/15 ml) after each loose stool; do not exceed 7 doses per day <br><br> **Children (after each loose stool)** <br> 6–12 years:  2 tablets (750 mg/tablet) or 10 ml (750 mg/5 ml) or 1 tablet (600mg/tablet) or 15 ml (600 mg/15 ml) <br><br> 3–6 years:  1 tablet (750 mg/tablet) or 5 ml (750 mg/5 ml) or 1/2 tablet (600 mg/tablet) or 7.5 ml (600 mg/ 15 ml) | <u>Administration Issues</u> Shake suspension well; separate dosing from other medication. Consult health-care professional if diarrhea persists for > 2 days. <br><br> <u>Drug–Drug Interactions</u> May decrease the absorption of many orally administered medications | | <u>Contraindications</u> suspected obstructive bowel lesion, pseudomembranous colitis, diarrhea associated with bacteria toxins <br><br> <u>Pregnancy Category:</u>  C <br><br> <u>Lactation Issues:</u> safety not established |

| Drug and Dosage Forms | Usual Dosage Range | Administration Issues and Drug–Drug Interactions | Common Adverse Drug Reactions (ADRs) and Pharmacokinetics | Contraindications, Pregnancy Category, and Lactation Issues |
|---|---|---|---|---|
| **Bisacodyl**<br>Dulcolax, various generics<br><br>Tablet, enteric:<br>5 mg<br><br>Suppository:<br>10 mg | **Laxative**<br>**Adult**<br>5–15 mg qd pm<br>10 mg PR pm<br><br>**Children**<br>5–10 mg qd pm | Administration Issues<br>Swallow tablet whole, do not crush; do not take within 1 hour of antacids or milk | ADRs:<br>abdominal discomfort, cramps, nausea, diarrhea, electrolyte disturbances, loss of normal bowel function, and laxative dependence with excessive use<br><br>Pharmacokinetics<br>onset = 6–8 h | Contraindications<br>Intestinal obstruction fecal impaction<br><br>Pregnancy Category: C<br><br>Lactation Issues: NA |
| **Cascara Sagrada**<br>Nature's Remedy<br>various generics<br><br>Tablet:<br>150 mg, 325 mg<br><br>Liquid:<br>approximately 18% alcohol | **Laxative**<br>Tablet:<br>1 tablet at bedtime<br><br>Liquid:<br>5 ml once daily | Administration Issues<br>Administer with a full glass of water on an empty stomach for best results | ADRs:<br>abdominal discomfort, cramps, nausea, diarrhea, electrolyte disturbances, loss of normal bowel function, and laxative dependence with excessive use, may discolor urine<br><br>Pharmacokinetics:<br>onset = 6–12 hr | Contraindications<br>Intestinal obstruction fecal impaction<br><br>Pregnancy Category: C<br><br>Lactation Issues<br>Cascara is excreted in breast milk, use with caution |
| **Castor Oil**<br>Fleet Flavored Castor Oil,<br>Emulsoil, various generics<br><br>Liquid<br><br>Emulsion:<br>Fleet Flavored Castor Oil 67% castor oil | **Used to prepare abdomen for radiographic exam of colon/kidneys and to clear irritants/poisons from GI tract.**<br><br>**Adult**<br>25–60 ml as a single dose 16 h before procedure | Administration Issues<br>Shake emulsion well before use; mix emulsion with 8 oz. of water or fruit juice prior to administration | ADRs:<br>abdominal discomfort, cramps nausea, diarrhea, electrolyte disturbances, loss of normal bowel function, and laxative dependence with excessive use<br><br>Pharmacokinetics:<br>onset = 2–3 h | Contraindications<br>Intestinal obstruction fecal impaction<br><br>Pregnancy Category: X<br>Use during pregnancy may induce premature labor due to irritant effect |

(continues on next page)

| Drug and Dosage Forms | Usual Dosage Range | Administration Issues and Drug–Drug Interactions | Common Adverse Drug Reactions (ADRs) and Pharmacokinetics | Contraindications, Pregnancy Category, and Lactation Issues |
|---|---|---|---|---|
| **Castor Oil** *cont.*<br>Emulsoil 95% castor oil | **Children**<br>2–12 years: 5–15 ml<br><2 yr: 1–5 ml | | | Lactation Issues: NA |
| **Docusate Calcium**<br>Surfak, various generics<br><br>Capsules:<br>50 mg, 240 mg | **Laxative**<br>**Adult**<br>240 mg daily until bowel movements normal<br><br>**Children**<br>≥6 years, 50–150 mg/d | Administration Issues<br>Give each dose with a glass of water<br><br>Drug–Drug Interactions<br>Do not give **mineral oil** with docusate calcium | ADRs:<br>abdominal discomfort, cramps<br><br>Pharmacokinetics:<br>onset = 24–72 h | Contraindications<br>Intestinal obstruction<br>fecal impaction<br><br>Pregnancy Category: C<br><br>Lactation Issues<br>Excretion in breast milk is unknown, use with caution |
| **Docusate Potassium**<br>Dialose<br><br>Capsule:<br>100 mg, 240 mg | **Laxative**<br>**Adult**<br>100–300 mg daily until bowel movements normal<br><br>**Children**<br>≥6 years, 100 mg hs | Administration Issues<br>Give each dose with a glass of water.<br><br>Drug–Drug Interactions<br>Do not give **mineral oil** with docusate potassium | ADRs:<br>abdominal discomfort, cramps<br><br>Pharmacokinetics:<br>onset = 24–72 h | Contraindications<br>Intestinal obstruction<br>fecal impaction<br><br>Pregnancy Category: C<br><br>Lactation Issues<br>Excretion in breast milk is unknown, use with caution |
| **Docusate Sodium**<br>Colace, Regutol, various generics<br><br>Tablet: 100 mg | **Laxative**<br>**Adult**<br>50 mg–500 mg/d<br>PR: 50 mg–100 mg liquid to enema | Administration Issues<br>Give each dose with a glass of water; give liquid preparation in milk, fruit juice, or infant formula to mask taste | ADRs:<br>abdominal discomfort, cramps<br><br>Pharmacokinetics:<br>onset = 24–72 h | Contraindications<br>Intestinal obstruction<br>fecal impaction<br><br>Pregnancy Category: C |

| Drug / Dosage Forms | Dosage | Administration Issues / Drug–Drug Interactions | Clinical Information |
|---|---|---|---|
| Capsules: 50 mg, 100 mg, 240 mg, 250 mg<br><br>Liquid: 50 mg/15 ml, 60 mg/15 ml, 150 mg/15 ml | Children 6–12 yrs: 40 mg–120 mg/d; 3–6 yrs: 20 mg–60 mg/d; <3 yrs: 10 mg–40 mg/d | Drug–Drug Interactions Do not give mineral oil with docusate sodium | Lactation Issues: Excretion in breast milk is unknown, use with caution in nursing mothers |
| Glycerin Sani-Supp, Fleet, generics<br><br>Suppository: glycerin/sodium stearate<br><br>Liquid: 4 ml per applicator | Laxative Adult 1 suppository rectally; 1 liquid applicator in rectum<br><br>Children 1 suppository rectally; 2–5 ml of liquid in rectum | Administration Issues Retain suppository in rectum for 15 min; suppository does not have to melt to produce laxative action; insert applicator stem with tip pointing towards navel and squeeze unit gently; a small portion of liquid will remain in applicator | Contraindications Intestinal obstruction, fecal impaction<br><br>Pregnancy Category: C<br><br>Lactation Issues: safety not established<br><br>ADRs: rectal discomfort, rectal irritation, burning<br><br>Pharmacokinetics onset = 15–30 min |
| Magnesium Citrate Evac-Q-Mag, Citrate of Magnesia<br><br>Dosage Forms Available: Liquid: 300 ml | Laxative Adult 1 glassful as needed<br><br>Children 1/2 glassful as needed | Administration Issues Keep in the refrigerator to maintain potency and palatability | Contraindications Intestinal obstruction, fecal impaction<br><br>Pregnancy Category: B<br><br>Lactation Issues: NA<br><br>ADRs: dehydration, electrolyte imbalance (with repeated use)<br><br>Pharmacokinetics onset = 0.5–3 hr |
| Magnesium Sulfate Epsom Salt<br><br>Granules: 40 mEq magnesium/5 gm | Laxative Adult 10 gm–15 gm in glass of water<br><br>Children 5 gm–10 gm in a glass of water | Administration Issues Dissolve granules in 8 oz. of water or juice before administration; mix with lemon juice to mask bitter taste | Contraindications Intestinal obstruction, fecal impaction<br><br>Pregnancy Category: A<br><br>Lactation Issues: NA<br><br>ADRs: dehydration, electrolyte imbalance (with repeated use)<br><br>Pharmacokinetics onset = 1–2 hr |
| Methylcellulose Citrucel, Citrucel Sugar Free | Laxative Adults 1 heaping tablespoonful in 8 oz. of cold water 1 to 3 times daily | Administration Issues Take with a full glass of water. Use sugar-free preparation with caution in patients with phenylketonuria | Contraindications Intestinal obstruction, fecal impaction<br><br>ADRs: abdominal discomfort, bloating. Esophageal obstruction, swelling, or blockage may |

(continues on next page)

| Drug and Dosage Forms | Usual Dosage Range | Administration Issues and Drug–Drug Interactions | Common Adverse Drug Reactions (ADRs) and Pharmacokinetics | Contraindications, Pregnancy Category, and Lactation Issues |
|---|---|---|---|---|
| **Methylcellulose** *cont.*<br><br><u>Powder:</u><br>Citrucel (2 gm methylcellulose/heaping tablespoon)<br><br>Citrucel Sugar Free (2 gm methylcellulose, 52 mg phenylalanine/heaping tablespoon) | **Children**<br>6–12 years, 1/2 heaping tablespoonful in 4 oz. of cold water 1 to 3 times daily | <u>Drug–Drug Interactions</u><br>The absorption of **digoxin, nitrofurantoin, and salicylates** in the GI tract may be decreased by bulk-forming laxatives | **occur when insufficient liquid is administered with bulk-forming laxatives.**<br><br><u>Pharmacokinetics:</u><br>onset 12–24 h | <u>Pregnancy Category:</u> NA<br><br><u>Lactation Issues:</u> NA |
| **Mineral Oil**<br>Kondremul Plain, Milkinol, various generics<br><br><u>Emulsion:</u><br>Kondrumel Plain<br>2.75 ml/5 ml<br><br>Milkinol<br>4.75 ml/5 ml | **Laxative**<br>**Adults**<br>5 ml–45 ml preferably at bedtime<br><br>**Children**<br>5 ml–20 ml preferably at bedtime | <u>Administration Issues</u><br>Give nonemulsified mineral oil on an empty stomach; shake emulsion well before use; emulsion product may be given with meals<br><br><u>Drug–Drug Interactions</u><br>The absorption of **fat soluble vitamins (Vit A, E, D, K)** may be decreased by mineral oil. The absorption of **oral contraceptives and warfarin** may be decreased by mineral oil. Do not give **docusate products** with mineral oil | <u>ADRs:</u> seepage of mineral oil from rectum following oral and rectal administration<br><br><u>Pharmacokinetics</u><br>onset = 6–8 h | <u>Contraindications</u><br>Use with caution in debilitated or elderly patients, aspiration upon reclining may cause lipid pneumonitis;<br>Intestinal obstruction<br>fecal impaction<br><br><u>Pregnancy Category:</u> C<br><br><u>Lactation Issues:</u> NA |
| **Phenolphthalein**<br>Ex-Lax, Alophen, Feen-a-mint, Evac-U-Lax, Evac-U-Gen<br><br><u>Tablet:</u> 60 mg, 90 mg, 130 mg | **Laxative**<br>60–194 mg at bedtime | | <u>ADRs:</u><br>abdominal discomfort, cramps nausea, diarrhea, electrolyte disturbances, loss of normal bowel function, and laxative | <u>Contraindications</u><br>Hypersensitivity to phenolphthalein<br>intestinal obstruction<br>fecal impaction |

| Drug / Forms | Dosage / Indication | Administration Issues / Drug–Drug Interactions | ADRs / Pharmacokinetics | Contraindications / Pregnancy Category / Lactation Issues |
|---|---|---|---|---|
| Tablet, chewable: 65 mg, 90 mg, 97.2 mg, 120 mg<br><br>Gum: 97.2 mg | | | dependence with excessive use, may discolor urine<br><br>Pharmacokinetics:<br>onset = 6–8 h | Pregnancy Category: C<br><br>Lactation Issues<br>Distributes into breast milk; use with caution in nursing mothers |
| **Polycarbophil**<br>FiberCon, Mitrolan, Fiberall<br><br>Tablet: 500 mg<br><br>Tablet, chewable: 500 mg, 1000 mg | **Laxative**<br>**Adult**<br>1 gm 1 to 4 times daily prn; do not exceed 6 gm in 24 h<br><br>**Children**<br>6–12 years, 500 mg qd to tid prn; do not exceed 3 gm in 24 h<br><br>3–6 years, 500 mg qd to bid prn; do not exceed 1.5 gm in 24 h | Administration Issues<br>Take with a full glass of water.<br><br>Drug–Drug Interactions<br>The absorption of **digoxin, nitrofurantoin, and salicylates** in the GI tract may be decreased by bulk-forming laxatives | ADRs:<br>abdominal discomfort, bloating<br>**Esophageal obstruction, swelling, or blockage may occur when insufficient liquid is administered with bulk-forming laxatives**<br><br>Pharmacokinetics:<br>onset 12–24 h | Contraindications<br>Intestinal obstruction<br>fecal impaction<br><br>Pregnancy Category: NA<br><br>Lactation Issues: NA |
| **Psyllium**<br>Fiberall, Metamucil, Perdiem Fiber, Hydrocil<br><br>Powder, effervescent:<br>Fiberall, Metamucil<br>3.4 gm psyllium/dose<br><br>Granules: Perdiem Fiber 4.03 gm psyllium/tsp<br><br>Wafer:<br>Fiberall (3.4 gm psyllium/dose) | **Laxative**<br>**Adult**<br>1–2 teaspoonful or 1 packet or 1 wafer 1–3 times/d prn<br><br>**Children**<br>7–11 years: 1 teaspoonful 1 to 2 times daily<br><br>**Psyllium has been shown to reduce cholesterol levels as an adjunct to a dietary program** | Administration Issues<br>Take with a full glass of water; do not chew psyllium granules. Use sugar-free preparation with caution in patients with phenylketonuria<br><br>Drug–Drug Interactions<br>The absorption of **digoxin, nitrofurantoin, and salicylates** in the GI tract may be decreased by bulk-forming laxatives | ADRs:<br>abdominal discomfort, bloating<br>**Esophageal obstruction, swelling, or blockage may occur when insufficient liquid is administered with bulk-forming laxatives.**<br><br>Pharmacokinetics:<br>onset 12–24 h | Contraindications<br>Intestinal obstruction<br>fecal impaction<br><br>Pregnancy Category: C<br><br>Lactation Issues: NA |
| **Senna**<br>Senokot, generics | **Laxative**<br>Standard senna concentrate<br>**Adults:** 1–2 tablets or 1/2–1 tsp hs (max 4 tablets or 2 tsp bid) | Administration Issues<br>generally administered at bedtime | ADRs:<br>abdominal discomfort, cramps, nausea, diarrhea, electrolyte disturbances, loss of normal | Contraindications<br>Intestinal obstruction<br>fecal impaction |

(continues on next page)

| Drug and Dosage Forms | Usual Dosage Range | Administration Issues and Drug–Drug Interactions | Common Adverse Drug Reactions (ADRs) and Pharmacokinetics | Contraindications, Pregnancy Category, and Lactation Issues |
|---|---|---|---|---|
| **Senna** *cont.*<br><br>Tablet: Senokot 187 mg<br>Senna-Gen 217 mg<br>Senokotxtra 374 mg<br><br>Liquid:<br>Black-Draught 90 mg/15 ml casanthranol/senna extract<br><br>Senokot (218 mg/5 ml)<br>Fletcher's Castoria (33.3 mg/ml) | **Children**<br>>27 kg: 1 tablet or 1/2 tsp hs<br><br>Syrup/liquid<br>**Adults:** 10–15 ml hs<br><br>**Children**<br>5–10 yrs: 5 ml–10 ml hs<br>1–5 yrs: 2.5 ml–5 ml hs<br>1 month–1 yr: 1.25 ml–2.5 ml hs | | bowel function, and laxative dependence with excessive use, may discolor urine<br><br>Pharmacokinetics:<br>onset = 6–12 h; may take up to 24 h | Pregnancy Category: C<br><br>Lactation Issues<br>Conflicting information concerning senna's excretion in breast milk, use with caution in nursing mothers |
| **Sodium Phosphate and Sodium Biphosphate**<br><br>Fleet Phospha-soda<br><br>Solution:<br>18 gm sodium phosphate and 48 gm sodium biphosphate/100 ml | **Laxative**<br>**Adult**<br>20–30 ml in glass cool water<br><br>**Children**<br>5–15 ml mixed in glass cool water | Administration Issues<br>mix with water before use | ADRs:<br>dehydration, electrolyte imbalance (with repeated use)<br><br>Pharmacokinetics<br>onset = 0.3–3 hr; minimal absorption of phosphate; renally excreted | Contraindications<br>Intestinal obstruction fecal impaction<br><br>Pregnancy Category: NA<br><br>Lactation Issues: NA |

## 501.10 Laxative Combinations

Listed below is a representative sample of laxative combination products. Administration and dosage depends on the condition being treated and the agent being used. See individual products (section 501.9) for administration issues, interactions, ADRs, etc.

### Corrector, Feen-a-mint, Modane Plus

Tablet:
100 mg docusate sodium/65 mg phenolphthalein

### Dialose Plus, various generics

Capsule:
60 mg docusate calcium/30 mg casanthranol

### Doxidan

Capsule:
60 mg docusate calcium/65 mg phenolphthalein

### Ex-Lax Extra Gentle

Tablet:
75 mg docusate sodium/65 mg phenolphthalein

### Peri-Colace, various generics

Capsule:
100 mg docusate calcium/30 mg casanthranol

Liquid:
60 mg docusate calcium/30 mg casanthranol per 15 ml

### Perdiem

Granules:
3.25 mg psyllium/0.74 gm senna per teaspoonful

### Senokot-S

Tablet:
50 mg docusate/187 mg senna

| Drug and Dosage Forms | Usual Dosage Range | Administration Issues and Drug–Drug Interactions | Common Adverse Drug Reactions (ADRs) | Contraindications, Pregnancy Category, and Lactation Issues |
|---|---|---|---|---|
| **Fleet, Therevac**<br>Enema:<br><br>Fleet: 7 gm sodium phosphate, 19 gm sodium biphosphate per 118 ml<br><br>Fleet Bisacodyl 10 mg bisacodyl/30 ml<br><br>Fleet Bisacodyl Prep 10 mg bisacodyl in 10 ml suspension packet<br><br>Fleet Mineral Oil<br><br>Therevac -SB<br>283 mg docusate sodium w/base of soft soap, PEG 400 and glycerin/3.9 gm capsule | **Laxative**<br>**Adults:** 118 ml (1 adult bottle) or 30ml prn<br><br>**Children**<br>≥ 2 years, 59 ml (1/2 adult bottle or 1 pediatric bottle)<br><br>Cleansing enema–1 packet in 1.5 L water<br><br>Barium enema–1 packet in barium suspension | Administration Issues<br>For rectal use only. **Do not use enemas in children < 2 years.** | | |
| **Polyethylene Glycol-Electrolyte Solution**<br>CoLyte, GoLYTELY<br><br>Powder for Oral Suspension:<br>CoLyte<br><br>GoLYTLY | **Bowel cleansing prior to GI exam**<br>Drink 4 liters prior to GI exam, drink 8 oz. every 10 minutes until 4 liters is consumed; the first bowel movement should occur in approximately 1 hour | Administration Issues<br>Patient should fast for 3–4 hours prior to ingesting fluid; no solid foods should be given < 2 hours before solution is given; reconstitute solution with tap water; shake solution well prior to administration; store solution in the refrigerator; use solution within 48 hours after reconstitution; do not add additional flavorings or | ADRs:<br>Nausea, abdominal bloating, cramps | Contraindications<br>GI obstruction<br>gastric retention bowel perforation<br>toxic megacolon or ileus<br><br>Pregnancy Category:  C |

| | Dosing | Administration / Interactions | ADRs / Contraindications |
|---|---|---|---|
| **Oral Solution**<br>OCL | | ingredients to solution before ingestion. **Safe use in children has not been established**<br><br>Drug–Drug Interactions<br>Do not give oral medications within one hour of start of drinking solution, decreased drug absorption may occur due to laxative effect of solution | Contraindications<br>Patients requiring a low galactose diet<br><br>Pregnancy Category: B<br><br>Lactation Issues<br>Excretion in breast milk is unknown; use with caution in nursing mothers |
| **Lactulose**<br>Cephulac, Chronulac, Duphalac, various generics<br><br>Syrup:<br>10 gm / 15 ml | **Laxative**<br>15 ml–30 ml daily, increase to 60 ml / day if necessary<br><br>**Prevention and treatment of encephalopathy**<br>**Adults:** 30 ml–45 ml 3 to 4 times daily, adjust dose to achieve 2 to 3 loose stools daily<br><br>**Children:** 2.5 ml–10 ml 3 to 4 times daily, adjust dose to achieve 2 to 3 loose stools daily<br><br>**Rectal enemas may be extemporaneously compounded by mixing 300 ml of lactulose with 700 ml of water of normal saline, have patient retain enema for 30 to 60 minutes, repeat enema if needed every 4 to 6 hours** | Administration Issues<br>May not see beneficial effects for 24 hours; give with fruit juice, water, or milk to make more palatable<br><br>Drug–Drug Interactions<br>**Neomycin and other antibiotics** may eliminate colonic bacteria necessary for the action of lactulose<br><br>**Antacids** given with lactulose may inhibit the desired lactulose-induced decrease in colonic pH | ADRs:<br>Flatulence, abdominal discomfort, cramps, nausea, vomiting |

## 501.12 Agents for Ulcerative Colitis and Crohn's Disease

| Drug and Dosage Forms | Usual Dosage Range | Administration Issues and Drug–Drug Interactions | Common Adverse Drug Reactions (ADRs) and Pharmacokinetics | Contraindications, Pregnancy Category, and Lactation Issues |
|---|---|---|---|---|
| **Mesalamine**<br>Asacol, Pentasa, Rowasa<br><br>Tablet, delayed release:<br>Asacol 400 mg<br><br>Capsule, controlled release:<br>Pentasa 250 mg<br><br>Suppositories:<br>Rowasa 500 mg<br><br>Rectal suspension:<br>Rowasa 4 gm / 60 ml | **Chronic inflammatory bowel disease, including ulcerative colitis and proctitis**<br><br>800 mg tid for 6 weeks<br><br>1 gm qid for up to 8 weeks<br><br>1 suppository bid for 3 to 6 weeks; retain suppository for 1 to 3 hours<br><br>60 ml rectally at bedtime for 3 to 6 weeks; retain enema for approximately 8 hours | Administration Issues<br>Swallow tablet and capsule whole, do not crush; remove foil from suppository before administration; shake suspension enema well before administration | ADRs:<br>abdominal pain, discomfort, nausea, headache<br><br>Pharmacokinetics:<br>tablet and capsule formulations release mesalamine for topical action throughout the GI tract; converted to active mesalamine by bacteria in the colon; <30 % is absorbed; metabolized in the gut; excreted renally | Contraindications<br>hypersensitivity to salicylates<br><br>Pregnancy Category: B<br><br>Lactation Issues<br>Use with caution in nursing mothers |
| **Olsalazine**<br>Dipentum<br><br>Capsule: 250 mg | **Ulcerative colitis**<br>500 mg bid | Administration Issues<br>Take with food; give daily dose in two divided doses | ADRs:<br>diarrhea, headache, nausea abdominal pain, discomfort<br><br>Pharmacokinetics<br>olsalazine is converted to active mesalamine by bacteria in the colon; mesalamine exerts topical, local action in the colon; highly protein bound; primarily excreted in feces | Contraindications<br>hypersensitivity to salicylates<br><br>Pregnancy Category: C<br><br>Lactation Issues<br>Excretion in breast milk is unknown; use with caution in nursing mothers |
| **Sulfasalazine**<br>Tablet:<br>Azulfidine, generics 500 mg | **Treatment of ulcerative colitis and Crohn's disease**<br>**Adults:** Initially, 3–4 gm daily given in equally divided doses according to | Administration Issues<br>Take with food after meals; orange-yellow discoloration of the urine may occur; avoid prolonged exposure to sunlight, | ADRs:<br>nausea, abdominal discomfort, diarrhea, headache, rash photosensitivity | Contraindications<br>Hypersensitivity to sulfonamides and salicylic acid (aspirin) derivatives; patients |

| | | | |
|---|---|---|---|
| Tablet, enteric coated: Azulfidine EN-tabs, generics: 500 mg<br><br>Suspension: Azulfidine: 250 mg/5 ml<br><br>patient response; doses of 2 gm daily in 4 divided doses may be used for maintenance therapy<br><br>**Children > 2 years** Initially, 40–60 mg/kg daily in 3–6 divided doses according to patient response; doses of 30 mg/kg daily in 4 divided doses may be used for maintenance therapy | wear protective clothing, and apply sunscreen<br><br>Drug–Drug Interactions Sulfasalazine may decrease the absorption of **digoxin** and **folic acid** | Pharmacokinetics: 1/3 of oral dose is absorbed in small intestines; remainder passes to the colon where it is split into 5-aminosalicylic acid and sulfapyridine; some absorption in colon with a predominate local effect; fecal excretion | with intestinal or urinary tract obstruction<br><br>Pregnancy Safety for use during pregnancy has not been established; sulfonamides do cross the placenta achieving fetal levels approximately 70%–90% of maternal serum levels; do not use during pregnancy at term<br><br>Lactation Issues Sulfonamides are excreted in breast milk; according to the American Academy of Pediatrics, breast feeding and sulfonamides are compatible; avoid sulfonamides and nursing in premature infants, infants with hyperbilirubinemia, and infants with G-6-PD |

| Drug and Dosage Forms | Usual Dosage Range | Administration Issues and Drug–Drug Interactions | Pharmacokinetics |
|---|---|---|---|
| **Charcoal**<br>Charco Caps, various generics<br><br>Capsules:<br>260 mg | **Relief of intestinal gas, diarrhea, indigestion**<br>520 mg after meals or at first sign of discomfort; repeat as needed up to 4.16 gm daily | Administration Issues<br>Take charcoal 2 hours before or 1 hour after other medications. **Do not use in children < 3.**<br><br>Drug–Drug Interactions<br>Charcoal may decrease the absorption of the following drugs or remove them from the systemic circulation: **Acetaminophen, barbiturates, carbamazepine, digoxin, phenytoin, salicylates, theophylline, tricyclic antidepressants, valproic acid** | Pharmacokinetics<br>Charcoal is not absorbed or metabolized. |
| **Charcoal and Simethicone**<br><br>Tablet, enteric coated:<br>250 mg charcoal<br>80 mg simethicone<br><br>Tablet:<br>200 mg charcoal<br>40 mg simethicone | **Relief of intestinal gas, diarrhea, indigestion**<br>520 mg after meals or at first sign of discomfort; repeat as needed up to 4.16 gm daily | Administration Issues<br>Take charcoal 2 hours before or 1 hour after other medications; do not crush enteric coated tablet. **Do not use in children < 3.**<br><br>Drug–Drug Interactions<br>Charcoal may decrease the absorption of the following drugs or remove them from the systemic circulation: **Acetaminophen, barbiturates, carbamazepine, digoxin, phenytoin, salicylates, theophylline, tricyclic antidepressants, valproic acid** | Pharmacokinetics<br>Simethicone is physiologically inert and remains in the GI tract after oral administration. Charcoal is not absorbed or metabolized. |

## Simethicone

Mylanta Gas, Gas-X, Maximum Strength
Mylanta Gas, Phazyme, Maximum Strength
Phazyme 125, Mylicon, various generics

Tablet:
60 mg, 95 mg

Tablet, chewable:
40 mg, 80 mg, 125 mg

Capsules: 125 mg

Drops: 40 mg/0.6 ml

### Antiflatulent
**Adult and children > 12**
40 mg–125 mg qid after meals and at bedtime

**Children 2–12 years**
40 mg 4 times daily

Infant colic
**Children < 2**
20 mg (0.3 ml) qid up to 240 mg/d

**Simethicone is not recommended for the treatment of infant colic**

Administration Issues
Ensure that chewable tablets are chewed thoroughly. Shake drops well before use; give drops with meals; drops can be mixed with 30 ml of cool water or infant formula to ease administration

Pharmacokinetics
Simethicone is physiologically inert and remains in the GI tract after oral administration

# 502. Antiemetic/Antivertigo Agents

## 502.1 Anticholinergic Agents

| Drug and Dosage Forms | Usual Dosage Range | Administration Issues and Drug–Drug Interactions | Common Adverse Drug Reactions (ADRs) and Pharmacokinetics | Contraindications, Pregnancy Category, and Lactation Issues |
|---|---|---|---|---|
| **Buclizine**<br>Bucladin-S Softabs<br><br>Tablets: 50 mg | **Motion Sickness:** 50 mg before departure; repeat q 4–6 hrs as needed up to 150 mg/d. | Administration Issues:<br>Give dose 30 minutes prior to motion, then before meals and at bedtime for duration of journey. Tablets can be allowed to dissolve in mouth, can be chewed, or can be swallowed whole; safety/efficacy in children <12 yrs not established<br><br>Drug–Drug Interactions<br>**increased effect of antihistamine:** MAO inhibitors (anticholinergic effects)<br><br>**increased effect of:** MAO inhibitors, alcohol, CNS depressants | ADRs:<br>urinary retention, blurred vision, dry mouth, drowsiness, irritability, thickening of bronchial secretions<br><br>Elderly (>60yrs): more likely to experience confusion, dizziness, hypotension<br><br>**Pharmacokinetics**<br>rapid onset (15–30 minutes); hepatically metabolized; duration of action = 4–6 hrs | Contraindications:<br>Hypersensitivity, asthma, glaucoma, prostate gland enlargement<br><br>Precautions: use carefully if operating heavy machinery, history of sleep apnea, hepatic dysfunction<br><br>Pregnancy Category: B.<br><br>Lactation Issues: women should not nurse |
| **Cyclizine**<br>Marezine<br><br>Tablets: 50 mg | **Motion Sickness:** 50 mg before departure; repeat q 4–6 hrs. Max daily dose is 200 mg.<br><br>Pediatrics (6–12 yrs): 25 mg up to 3 times daily | Administration Issues:<br>Give dose 30 minutes prior to motion, then before meals and at bedtime for duration of journey; safety/efficacy in children <12 yrs not established<br><br>Drug–Drug Interactions<br>**increased effect of antihistamine:** MAO inhibitors (anticholinergic effects)<br><br>**increased effect of:** MAO inhibitors, alcohol, CNS depressants | ADRs:<br>urinary retention, blurred vision, dry mouth, drowsiness, irritability, thickening of bronchial secretions<br><br>Elderly (>60yrs): more likely to experience confusion, dizziness, hypotension<br><br>**Pharmacokinetics**<br>onset = 30–60 minutes; duration of action = 4–6 hrs | Contraindications:<br>Hypersensitivity, asthma, glaucoma, prostate gland enlargement<br><br>Precautions: use carefully if operating heavy machinery, history of sleep apnea, hepatic dysfunction<br><br>Pregnancy Category: B.<br><br>Lactation Issues: women should not nurse |

| Drug | Dosage | Administration Issues / Drug–Drug Interactions | ADRs / Pharmacokinetics | Contraindications / Precautions |
|---|---|---|---|---|
| **Dimenhydrinate** Calm-X, Dimetabs, Dramamine, Marmine, Triptone Caplets, various generics  Tablets: 50 mg  Chewable tablets: 50 mg  Capsules: 50 mg | **Motion Sickness:** 50–100 mg every 4–6 hrs. Max dose is 400 mg/d  Pediatrics (6–12 yrs): 25–50 mg every 6–8 hrs. Max dose is 150 mg/d | Administration Issues: Give dose 30 minutes prior to motion, then before meals and at bedtime for duration of journey; safety/efficacy in children <12 yrs not established  Drug–Drug Interactions **increased effect of antihistamine:** MAO inhibitors (anticholinergic effects)  **increased effect of:** MAO inhibitors, alcohol, CNS depressants | ADRs: urinary retention, blurred vision, dry mouth, drowsiness, irritability, thickening of bronchial secretions  Elderly (>60yrs): more likely to experience confusion, dizziness, hypotension  **Pharmacokinetics** rapid onset (15–30 minutes); duration of action = 4–6 hrs | Contraindications: Hypersensitivity, asthma, glaucoma, prostate gland enlargement  Precautions: use carefully if operating heavy machinery, history of sleep apnea, hepatic dysfunction  Pregnancy Category: B.  Lactation Issues: women should not nurse |
| **Diphenhydramine** Benadryl, various generics  Tablets: 25 mg, 50 mg  Capsules: 25 mg, 50 mg | **Motion sickness:** 25–50 mg 3–4 times daily  **Pediatrics (>9.1 kg):** 12.5–25 mg 3–4 times daily. Do not exceed 300 mg/d | Administration Issues: Give dose 30 minutes prior to motion, then before meals and at bedtime for duration of journey; safety/efficacy in children <12 yrs not established  Drug–Drug Interactions **increased effect of antihistamine:** MAO inhibitors (anticholinergic effects)  **increased effect of:** MAO inhibitors, alcohol, CNS depressants | ADRs: Urinary retention, blurred vision, dry mouth, drowsiness, irritability, thickening of bronchial secretions  Elderly (>60yrs): more likely to experience confusion, dizziness, hypotension  **Pharmacokinetics** rapid onset (15–30 minutes); duration of action = 4–6 hrs | Contraindications: Hypersensitivity, asthma, glaucoma, prostate gland enlargement  Precautions: use carefully if operating heavy machinery, history of sleep apnea, hepatic dysfunction  Pregnancy Category: B.  Lactation Issues: women should not nurse |
| **Meclizine** Antivert, Antrizine, RuVert-M, Bonine, Dizmiss, Meni-D, various generics  Tablets: 12.5 mg, 25 mg, 50 mg | **Motion Sickness:** 25–50 mg before departure; may repeat every 24 hrs for duration of journey  **Vertigo:** 25–100 mg daily in 2–3 divided doses | Administration Issues: Give dose 60 minutes prior to motion; safety/efficacy in children <12 yrs not established | ADRs: urinary retention, blurred vision, dry mouth, drowsiness, irritability, thickening of bronchial secretions | Contraindications: Hypersensitivity, asthma, glaucoma, prostate gland enlargement  Precautions: use carefully if operating heavy machinery, |

(continues on next page)

| Drug and Dosage Forms | Usual Dosage Range | Administration Issues and Drug–Drug Interactions | Common Adverse Drug Reactions (ADRs) and Pharmacokinetics | Contraindications, Pregnancy Category, and Lactation Issues |
|---|---|---|---|---|
| **Meclizine *cont.*** Chewable tablets: 25 mg  Capsules: 25 mg | | Drug–Drug Interactions **increased effect of antihistamine:** MAO inhibitors (anticholinergic effects)  **increased effect of:** MAO inhibitors, alcohol, CNS depressants | Elderly (>60yrs): more likely to experience confusion, dizziness, hypotension  **Pharmacokinetics** Oral; onset = 30–60 minutes; duration of action = 8–24 hrs | history of sleep apnea, hepatic dysfunction  Pregnancy Category: B.  Lactation Issues: women should not nurse |
| **Scopolamine, Transdermal** Transderm-Scop  Transdermal Therapeutic System 1.5 mg | **Control of nausea/vomiting associated with motion sickness:** Apply 1 system behind the ear at least 4 h before antiemetic effect is required. Wear only 1 disk at a time. | Administration Issues: Wash hands thoroughly after handling disk. Temporary dilation of pupils and blurred vision may occur if drug comes in contact with eyes. If therapy longer than 3 days is required, remove old disc and place a new one in hairless area behind ear. Do not use system in children. | ADRs: Dry mouth, blurred vision, drowsiness  Pharmacokinetics System delivers 0.5 mg scopolamine/d over 3 d | Contraindications: Hypersensitivity to scopolamine, glaucoma  Pregnancy Category: C  Lactation Issues: It is not known whether drug is excreted in breast milk. Use caution in nursing women. |
| **Trimethobenzamide** Tigan, Trimazide, Tebamide, generics  Capsules: 100 mg, 250 mg  Suppositories: 100 mg, 200 mg | **Control of nausea/vomiting: Adults:** oral: 250 mg tid to qid rectal: 200 mg tid to qid  Pediatrics (13.6–40.9 kg): oral: 100–200 mg tid to qid rectal: 100–200 mg tid to qid **(<13.6 kg):** 100 mg tid to qid | None known | ADRs: drowsiness, dizziness, headache, disorientation, Parkinson-like symptoms, coma convulsions, depression, diarrhea, hypersensitivity reactions, rash  **Pharmacokinetics** Oral; onset = 10–40 minutes; duration of action = 3–4 hrs | Contraindications: Hypersensitivity to this or benzocaine or other local anesthetics; suppository use in premature infants or neonates  Pregnancy/Lactation Issues: safety has not been established. Use cautiously |

## 502.2 Antipaminergic Agents

See chlorpromazine, perphanazine, prochlorperazine, promethazine, thiethylperazine (Table 312) and metoclopramide (Table 501.6) for doses, ADRs, etc of these agents as antiemetics.

## 502.3 Miscellaneous Agents

| Drug and Dosage Forms | Usual Dosage Range | Administration Issues and Drug–Drug Interactions | Common Adverse Drug Reactions (ADRs) and Pharmacokinetics | Contraindications, Pregnancy Category, and Lactation Issues |
|---|---|---|---|---|
| **Dronabinol**<br>Marinol<br><br>Capsules: 2.5 mg, 5 mg, 10 mg | **Treatment of nausea/vomiting associated with cancer chemotherapy:** 5 mg/m² 1–3 hrs prior to chemotherapy, then every 2–4 hrs after chemotherapy for a total of 4–6 doses/day. May titrate by 2.5 mg/m² to a max of 15 mg/m² per dose if needed.<br><br>**Appetite stimulant in AIDS patients:** 2.5 mg bid before lunch and supper. Titrate to 2.5 mg at lunch and 5 mg at supper if tolerated. Titrate to 10 mg/d if needed/tolerated. Max dose is 20 mg/d | **Administration Issues**<br>not recommended as an appetite stimulant in children with AIDS<br><br>Drug–Drug Interactions:<br>**increased levels/effects of:**<br>amphetamines, sympathomimetics, anticholinergics, antihistamines, TCAs, alcohol, sedatives, hypnotics, psychomimetics, disulfiram, fluoxetine<br><br>**decreased levels/effects of:**<br>theophylline | ADRs:<br>palpitations, tachycardia, vasodilation, nausea, vomiting, diarrhea, euphoria, dizziness, paranoid reaction, somnolence, asthenia, amnesia, ataxia, confusion, hallucination<br><br>Elderly: Use cautiously due to increased sensitivity to psychoactive effects.<br><br>**Pharmacokinetics**<br>onset of action is 0.5–1 hr; duration of action is 4–6 hrs (antiemetic effect) but may exceed 24 hrs (appetite stimulant effect)<br><br>Drug Abuse & Dependence:<br>Highly abusable/addicting. Withdrawal can occur within 12 hrs of abrupt discontinuation of this medication (continues for 96 hrs). Therefore, gradual discontinuation is advised. | Contraindications:<br>Hypersensitivity to this, marijuana or sesame oil<br><br>Precautions: Use cautiously in patients with hypertension, heart disease, or psychiatric disorders<br><br>Pregnancy Category: B<br><br>Lactation Issues: excreted in breast milk—mothers should not nurse |

(continues on next page)

| Drug and Dosage Forms | Usual Dosage Range | Administration Issues and Drug–Drug Interactions | Common Adverse Drug Reactions (ADRs) and Pharmacokinetics | Contraindications, Pregnancy Category, and Lactation Issues |
|---|---|---|---|---|
| **Granisetron**<br>Kytril<br><br>Tablets: 1 mg | **Nausea/vomiting associated with emetogenic chemotherapy (including cisplatin):**<br>1 mg bid only on the days chemotherapy is given | Administration Issues<br>Safety/efficacy not established for those ≤2 yrs.<br><br>Drug–Drug Interactions:<br>Clinically significant interactions are not known | ADRS:<br>headache, asthenia, dizziness, diarrhea, constipation, abdominal pain<br><br>**Pharmacokinetics**<br>T$_{1/2}$ = 6.23 hrs (may be prolonged in cancer patients) | Contraindications:<br>Hypersensitivity<br><br>Pregnancy Category: B<br><br>Lactation Issues: may be excreted in breast milk—use cautiously. |
| **Ondansetron**<br>Zofran<br><br>Tablets: 4 mg, 8 mg | **Nausea/vomiting associated with moderately emetogenic chemotherapy:**<br>8 mg bid for 1–2 days after completion of chemotherapy.<br><br>**Pediatrics (4–11 yrs):** 4 mg tid for 1–2 days after completion of chemotherapy.<br><br>**Hepatic dysfunction:** do not exceed 8 mg/d | Administration Issues<br>Safety/efficacy not established for those ≤3 yrs.<br><br>Drug–Drug Interactions:<br>Clinically significant interactions are not known | ADRs:<br>headache, fatigue, dizziness, diarrhea, constipation, abdominal pain<br><br>**Pharmacokinetics**<br>T$_{1/2}$ = 3 hrs (4.5–6.2 hrs in elderly, but no difference in safety/efficacy) | Contraindications:<br>Hypersensitivity<br><br>Precautions: Use cautiously in patients with severe hepatic dysfunction; those undergoing abdominal surgery<br><br>Pregnancy Category: B<br><br>Lactation Issues: may be excreted in breast milk—use cautiously. |

## 600. HORMONES AND SYNTHETIC SUBSTANCES

### 601. Adrenal Corticosteroids

601.1 Glucocorticoids

| Drug and Dosage Forms | Usual Dosage Range | Administration Issues and Drug–Drug Interactions | Common Adverse Drug Reactions (ADRs) and Pharmacokinetics | Contraindications, Pregnancy Category, and Lactation Issues |
|---|---|---|---|---|
| **Betamethasone**<br>Celestone<br><br>Tablets: 0.6 mg<br><br>Syrup: 0.6 mg/5 mL | **Endocrine disorders (adrenal insufficiency), rheumatic disorders, collagen diseases (systemic lupus erythematosus), dermatologic diseases, allergic states, respiratory disease, hematologic disorders, neoplastic disease, edematous states, GI diseases, neurological diseases: MUST INDIVIDUALIZE DOSE:**<br><br>0.6–7.2 mg/d | Administration Issues:<br>Use lowest possible dose. Take with food if GI upset occurs. Avoid abrupt withdrawal of therapy. Closely monitor growth and development of children who receive long-term corticosteroid therapy<br><br>Drug Interactions<br>**increased toxicity with:**<br>cyclosporine, digoxin, diuretics<br>**decreased levels/effects of:** anticholinesterases, isoniazid, salicylates<br>**decreased levels/effects of corticosteroids:** barbiturates, hydantoins, rifampin<br>**increased levels/effects of corticosteroids:** oral contraceptives, estrogens, ketoconazole | ADRs:<br>insomnia, increased appetite, indigestion, temporary mild blurred vision, erythema, itching, hyperglycemia, skin dryness, headache, impaired wound healing, acne, sodium retention, peptic ulcer<br><br>Elderly: Use cautiously. Use lower doses.<br><br>Pharmacokinetics<br>hepatically metabolized; plasma $T_{1/2}$ = 300+ min; biologic $T_{1/2}$ = 36–54 hrs. | Contraindications:<br>Hypersensitivity; systemic fungal infections; administration of live virus vaccines in patients receiving immunosuppressives<br><br>Precautions: Monitor closely for infection (these agents may mask signs of infection); avoid prolonged therapy (leads to adrenal suppression); monitor electrolytes, blood glucose, weight, and blood pressure. Use cautiously in those with PUD, hypertension, CHF, osteoporosis, convulsive disorders, myasthenia gravis, diabetes mellitus, hypothyroidism, cirrhosis.<br><br>Pregnancy/Lactation Issues:<br>Use cautiously (only when benefits clearly outweigh risks), these do cross placental barrier and are excreted into breast milk. |

(continues on next page)

**601.1 Glucocorticoids** *continued from previous page*

| Drug and Dosage Forms | Usual Dosage Range | Administration Issues and Drug–Drug Interactions | Common Adverse Drug Reactions (ADRs) and Pharmacokinetics | Contraindications, Pregnancy Category, and Lactation Issues |
|---|---|---|---|---|
| **Cortisone**<br>Cortone, various generics<br><br>Tablets: 5 mg, 10 mg, 25 mg | **Endocrine disorders (adrenal insufficiency), rheumatic disorders, collagen diseases (systemic lupus erythematosus), dermatologic diseases, allergic states, respiratory disease, hematologic disorders, neoplastic disease, edematous states, GI diseases, neurological diseases: MUST INDIVIDUALIZE DOSE:**<br><br>25–300 mg/d | Administration Issues:<br>Use lowest possible dose. Take with food if GI upset occurs. Avoid abrupt withdrawal of therapy. Closely monitor growth and development of children who receive long-term corticosteroid therapy<br><br>Drug Interactions<br>**increased toxicity with:** cyclosporine, digoxin, diuretics<br>**decreased levels/effects of:** anticholinesterases, isoniazid, salicylates<br>**decreased levels/effects of corticosteroids:** barbiturates, hydantoins, rifampin<br>**increased levels/effects of corticosteroids:** oral contraceptives, estrogens, ketoconazole | ADRs:<br>insomnia, increased appetite, indigestion, temporary mild blurred vision, erythema, itching, hyperglycemia, skin dryness, headache, impaired wound healing, acne, sodium retention, peptic ulcer<br><br>Pharmacokinetics:<br>hepatically metabolized; plasma $T_{1/2}$ = 30 min; biologic $T_{1/2}$ = 8–12 hrs | Contraindications:<br>Hypersensitivity; systemic fungal infections; administration of live virus vaccines in patients receiving immunosuppressives<br><br>Precautions: Monitor closely for infection (these agents may mask signs of infection); avoid prolonged therapy (leads to adrenal suppression); monitor electrolytes, blood glucose, weight, and blood pressure. Use cautiously in those with PUD, hypertension, CHF, osteoporosis, convulsive disorders, myasthenia gravis, diabetes mellitus, hypothyroidism, cirrhosis.<br><br>Pregnancy/Lactation Issues:<br>Use cautiously (only when benefits clearly outweigh risks), these do cross placental barrier and are excreted into breast milk. |
| **Dexamethasone**<br>Decadron, Hexadrol, various generics | **Endocrine disorders (adrenal insufficiency), rheumatic disorders, collagen diseases (systemic lupus** | Administration Issues:<br>Use lowest possible dose. Take with food if GI upset occurs. Avoid abrupt withdrawal of therapy. Closely monitor | ADRs:<br>insomnia, increased appetite, indigestion, temporary mild blurred vision, erythema, | Contraindications:<br>Hypersensitivity; systemic fungal infections; administration of live virus |

| | | | | |
|---|---|---|---|---|
| Tablets: 0.25 mg, 0.5 mg, 0.75 mg, 1 mg, 1.5 mg, 2 mg, 4 mg, 6 mg<br><br>Elixir: 0.5 mg/5 mL<br><br>Oral Solution: 0.5 mg/5 mL | erythematosus), dermatologic diseases, allergic states, respiratory disease, hematologic disorders, neoplastic disease, edematous states, GI diseases, neurological diseases: MUST INDIVIDUALIZE DOSE:<br><br>0.75–9 mg/d initially.<br><br>Tapering schedule for acute self-limited allergic disorders or exacerbations of chronic allergic disorders:<br>First day: 1–2 mL IM injection; Second day: 4 tablets (0.75 mg) in 2 divided doses; Third day: 4 tablets in 2 divided doses; Fourth day: 2 tablets in 2 divided doses; Fifth day: 1 tablet; Sixth day: 1 tablet.<br><br>Suppression Test: 1 mg at 11 p.m. Draw blood for plasma cortisol determination the following day at 8 a.m. For greater accuracy: give 0.5 mg every 6 hrs for 48 hrs, then measure 17-hydroxycorticosteroid excretion collected in a 24 hr urine sample. | growth and development of children who receive long-term corticosteroid therapy<br><br>Drug Interactions<br>increased toxicity with:<br>cyclosporine, digoxin, diuretics<br>decreased levels/effects of: anticholinesterases, isoniazid, salicylates<br>decreased levels/effects of corticosteroids: barbiturates, hydantoins, rifampin<br>increased levels/effects of corticosteroids: oral contraceptives, estrogens, ketoconazole | itching, hyperglycemia, skin dryness, headache, impaired wound healing, acne, sodium retention, peptic ulcer<br><br>Pharmacokinetics:<br>hepatically metabolized; plasma $T_{1/2}$ = 110–210 min; biologic $T_{1/2}$ = 36–54 hrs. | vaccines in patients receiving immunosuppressives<br><br>Precautions: Monitor closely for infection (these agents may mask signs of infection); avoid prolonged therapy (leads to adrenal suppression); monitor electrolytes, blood glucose, weight, and blood pressure. Use cautiously in those with PUD, hypertension, CHF, osteoporosis, convulsive disorders, myasthenia gravis, diabetes mellitus, hypothyroidism, cirrhosis.<br><br>Pregnancy/Lactation Issues: Use cautiously (only when benefits clearly outweigh risks); these do cross placental barrier and are excreted into breast milk. |
| **Hydrocortisone**<br>Cortef, various generics<br><br>Tablets: 5 mg, 10 mg, 20 mg | Endocrine disorders (adrenal insufficiency), rheumatic disorders, collagen diseases (systemic lupus erythematosus), dermatologic | Administration Issues:<br>Use lowest possible dose.<br>Take with food if GI upset occurs. Avoid abrupt withdrawal of therapy. Closely monitor growth and development of | ADRs:<br>insomnia, increased appetite, indigestion, temporary mild blurred vision, erythema, itching, hyperglycemia, skin | Contraindications:<br>Hypersensitivity; systemic fungal infections; administration of live virus vaccines in patients receiving immunosuppressives |

(continues on next page)

| Drug and Dosage Forms | Usual Dosage Range | Administration Issues and Drug–Drug Interactions | Common Adverse Drug Reactions (ADRs) and Pharmacokinetics | Contraindications, Pregnancy Category, and Lactation Issues |
|---|---|---|---|---|
| **Hydrocortisone *cont.*** Oral Suspension: 10 mg/5 mL (as cypionate) | **diseases, allergic states, respiratory disease, hematologic disorders, neoplastic disease, edematous states, GI diseases, neurological diseases: MUST INDIVIDUALIZE DOSE:** 20–240 mg/d | children who receive long-term corticosteroid therapy Drug Interactions **increased toxicity with:** cyclosporine, digoxin, diuretics **decreased levels/effects of:** anticholinesterases, isoniazid, salicylates **decreased levels/effects of corticosteroids:** barbiturates, hydantoins, rifampin **increased levels/effects of corticosteroids:** oral contraceptives, estrogens, ketoconazole | dryness, headache, impaired wound healing, acne, sodium retention, peptic ulcer Pharmacokinetics: hepatically metabolized; plasma $T_{1/2}$ = 80–118 min; biologic $T_{1/2}$ = 8–12 hrs. | Precautions: Monitor closely for infection (these agents may mask signs of infection); avoid prolonged therapy (leads to adrenal suppression); monitor electrolytes, blood glucose, weight, and blood pressure. Use cautiously in those with PUD, hypertension, CHF, osteoporosis, convulsive disorders, myasthenia gravis, diabetes mellitus, hypothyroidism, cirrhosis. Pregnancy/Lactation Issues: Use cautiously (only when benefits clearly outweigh risks), these do cross placental barrier and are excreted into breast milk. |
| **Methylprednisolone** Medrol, various generics Tablets: 2 mg, 4 mg, 8 mg, 16 mg, 24 mg, 32 mg | **Endocrine disorders (adrenal insufficiency), rheumatic disorders, collagen diseases (systemic lupus erythematosus), dermatologic diseases, allergic states, respiratory disease, hematologic disorders, neoplastic disease, edematous** | Administration Issues: Use lowest possible dose. Take with food if GI upset occurs. Avoid abrupt withdrawal of therapy. Closely monitor growth and development of children who receive long-term corticosteroid therapy | ADRs: insomnia, increased appetite, indigestion, temporary mild blurred vision, erythema, itching, hyperglycemia, skin dryness, headache, impaired wound healing, acne, sodium retention, peptic ulcer | Contraindications: Hypersensitivity; systemic fungal infections; administration of live virus vaccines in patients receiving immunosuppressives Precautions: Monitor closely for infection (these agents may mask signs of infection); avoid |

| | Uses/Dosing | Drug Interactions | Pharmacokinetics / ADRs | Contraindications / Precautions |
|---|---|---|---|---|
| | **states, GI diseases, neurological diseases: MUST INDIVIDUALIZE DOSE:**<br><br>4–48 mg/d<br><br>Tapering schedule for acute self-limited allergic disorders or exacerbations of chronic allergic disorders:<br>Dosepak 21 therapy—follow manufacturer's directions | Drug Interactions<br>**increased toxicity with:**<br>cyclosporine, digoxin, diuretics<br>**decreased levels/effects of:**<br>anticholinesterases, isoniazid, salicylates<br>**decreased levels/effects of corticosteroids:** barbiturates, hydantoins, rifampin<br>**increased levels/effects of corticosteroids:** oral contraceptives, estrogens, ketoconazole | Pharmacokinetics:<br>hepatically metabolized; plasma $T_{1/2}$ = 78–188 min; biologic $T_{1/2}$ = 18–36 hrs | prolonged therapy (leads to adrenal suppression); monitor electrolytes, blood glucose, weight, and blood pressure. Use cautiously in those with PUD, hypertension, CHF, osteoporosis, convulsive disorders, myasthenia gravis, diabetes mellitus, hypothyroidism, cirrhosis.<br><br>Pregnancy/Lactation Issues:<br>Use cautiously (only when benefits clearly outweigh risks); these do cross placental barrier and are excreted into breast milk. |
| **Prednisone**<br>Deltasone, Orasone, various generics<br><br>Tablets: 1 mg, 2.5 mg, 5 mg, 10 mg, 20 mg, 50 mg<br><br>Oral Solution:<br>5 mg/5 mL<br><br>Syrup: 5 mg/5 mL | **Endocrine disorders (adrenal insufficiency), rheumatic disorders, collagen diseases (systemic lupus erythematosus), dermatologic diseases, allergic states, respiratory disease, hematologic disorders, neoplastic disease, edematous states, GI diseases, neurological diseases: MUST INDIVIDUALIZE DOSE:**<br><br>5–60 mg/d | Administration Issues:<br>Use lowest possible dose.<br>Take with food if GI upset occurs. Avoid abrupt withdrawal of therapy. Closely monitor growth and development of children who receive long-term corticosteroid therapy<br><br>Drug Interactions<br>**increased toxicity with:**<br>cyclosporine, digoxin, diuretics<br>**decreased levels/effects of:**<br>anticholinesterases, isoniazid, salicylates<br>**decreased levels/effects of corticosteroids:** barbiturates, hydantoins, rifampin<br>**increased levels/effects of corticosteroids:** oral contraceptives, estrogens, ketoconazole | ADRs:<br>insomnia, increased appetite, indigestion, temporary mild blurred vision, erythema, itching, hyperglycemia, skin dryness, headache, impaired wound healing, acne, sodium retention, peptic ulcer<br><br>Pharmacokinetics:<br>converted to prednisolone; $T_{1/2}$ = 2.5–3.5 h | Contraindications:<br>Hypersensitivity; systemic fungal infections; administration of live virus vaccines in patients receiving immunosuppressives<br><br>Precautions: Monitor closely for infection (these agents may mask signs of infection); avoid prolonged therapy (leads to adrenal suppression); monitor electrolytes, blood glucose, weight, and blood pressure. Use cautiously in those with PUD, hypertension, CHF, osteoporosis, convulsive disorders, myasthenia gravis, diabetes mellitus, hypothyroidism, cirrhosis. |

(continues on next page)

| Drug and Dosage Forms | Usual Dosage Range | Administration Issues and Drug–Drug Interactions | Common Adverse Drug Reactions (ADRs) and Pharmacokinetics | Contraindications, Pregnancy Category, and Lactation Issues |
|---|---|---|---|---|
| **Prednisone** *cont.* | | | | Pregnancy/Lactation Issues: Use cautiously (only when benefits clearly outweigh risks), these do cross placental barrier and are excreted into breast milk. |
| **Prednisolone** Prelone, Delta-Cortef, various generics <br><br> Tablets: 5 mg <br><br> Syrup: 15 mg/5 mL | **Endocrine disorders (adrenal insufficiency), rheumatic disorders, collagen diseases (systemic lupus erythematosus), dermatologic diseases, allergic states, respiratory disease, hematologic disorders, neoplastic disease, edematous states, GI diseases, neurological diseases: MUST INDIVIDUALIZE DOSE:** <br><br> 5–60 mg/d <br><br> Acute exacerbations of multiple sclerosis: 200 mg daily for 1 week followed by 80 mg every other day for 1 month. | Administration Issues: Use lowest possible dose. Take with food if GI upset occurs. Avoid abrupt withdrawal of therapy. Closely monitor growth and development of children who receive long-term corticosteroid therapy <br><br> Drug Interactions **increased toxicity with:** cyclosporine, digoxin, diuretics **decreased levels/effects of:** anticholinesterases, isoniazid, salicylates **decreased levels/effects of corticosteroids:** barbiturates, hydantoins, rifampin **increased levels/effects of corticosteroids:** oral contraceptives, estrogens, ketoconazole | ADRs: insomnia, increased appetite, indigestion, temporary mild blurred vision, erythema, itching, hyperglycemia, skin dryness, headache, impaired wound healing, acne, sodium retention, peptic ulcer <br><br> Pharmacokinetics: $T_{1/2} = 3.6$ h | Contraindications: Hypersensitivity; systemic fungal infections; administration of live virus vaccines in patients receiving immunosuppressives <br><br> Precautions: Monitor closely for infection (these agents may mask signs of infection); avoid prolonged therapy (leads to adrenal suppression); monitor electrolytes, blood glucose, weight, and blood pressure. Use cautiously in those with PUD, hypertension, CHF, osteoporosis, convulsive disorders, myasthenia gravis, diabetes mellitus, hypothyroidism, cirrhosis. <br><br> Pregnancy/Lactation Issues: Use cautiously (only when benefits clearly outweigh risks), these do cross placental barrier and are excreted into breast milk. |

| **Triamcinolone** | **MUST INDIVIDUALIZE DOSE:** | Administration Issues: | ADRs: | Contraindications: |
|---|---|---|---|---|
| Aristocort, Kenacort, various generics | **Endocrine disorders (adrenal insufficiency):** 4–12 mg/d in addition to mineralocorticoid therapy. | Use lowest possible dose. Take with food if GI upset occurs. Avoid abrupt withdrawal of therapy. Closely monitor growth and development of children who receive long-term corticosteroid therapy | insomnia, increased appetite, indigestion, temporary mild blurred vision, erythema, itching, hyperglycemia, skin dryness, headache, impaired wound healing, acne, sodium retention, peptic ulcer | Hypersensitivity; systemic fungal infections; administration of live virus vaccines in patients receiving immunosuppressives |
| Tablets: 1 mg, 2 mg, 4 mg, 8 mg | **Rheumatic disorders, dermatological, and bronchial asthma:** 8–16 mg/d | | Pharmacokinetics: hepatically metabolized; plasma $T_{1/2}$ = 200+ min; biologic $T_{1/2}$ = 18–36 hrs | Precautions:  Monitor closely for infection (these agents may mask signs of infection); avoid prolonged therapy (leads to adrenal suppression); monitor electrolytes, blood glucose, weight, and blood pressure. Use cautiously in those with PUD, hypertension, CHF, osteoporosis, convulsive disorders, myasthenia gravis, diabetes mellitus, hypothyroidism, cirrhosis. |
| Syrup: 4 mg/5 mL | **Collagen diseases (systemic lupus erythematosus):** 20–32 mg/d | **Drug Interactions** **increased toxicity with:** cyclosporine, digoxin, diuretics **decreased levels/effects of:** anticholinesterases, isoniazid, salicylates | | |
| | **Allergic states:** 8–12 mg/d | **decreased levels/effects of corticosteroids:** barbiturates, hydantoins, rifampin | | Pregnancy/Lactation Issues: Use cautiously (only when benefits clearly outweigh risks), these do cross placental barrier and are excreted into breast milk. |
| | **Respiratory diseases:** 16–48 mg/d | **increased levels/effects of corticosteroids:** oral contraceptives, estrogens, ketoconazole | | |
| | **Hematologic disorders:** 16–60 mg/d | | | |
| | **Neoplastic disease:** 16–40 mg/d up to 100 mg/d. Children may need 1–2 mg/kg | | | |
| | **Edematous states:** 16–20 mg/d up to 48 mg/d until diuresis occurs. | | | |
| | **Tuberculous meningitis:** 32–48 mg/d | | | |

## 601.2 Mineralocorticoids

| Drug and Dosage Forms | Usual Dosage Range | Administration Issues and Drug–Drug Interactions | Common Adverse Drug Reactions (ADRs) and Pharmacokinetics | Contraindications, Pregnancy Category, and Lactation Issues |
|---|---|---|---|---|
| **Fludrocortisone**<br>Florinef<br><br>Tablets: 0.1 mg | **Addison's Disease:**<br>0.1 mg/d. May titrate to 0.2 mg/d if needed. If hypertension develops, decrease dose to 0.05 mg/d<br><br>**Pediatrics:** 0.05–0.1 mg/d<br><br>**Infants:** 0.1–0.2 mg/d<br><br>**Salt-losing adrenogenital syndrome:** 0.1–0.2 mg/d | Administration Issues:<br>Use smallest dose.<br>Take with food if GI upset occurs.<br>Avoid abrupt withdrawal of therapy. | ADRs:<br>edema, hypertension, CHF, enlargement of the heart, bruising, increased sweating, hives, allergic skin rash<br><br>Pharmacokinetics:<br>hepatically metabolized; plasma $T_{1/2}$ = 3.5 hrs; biological $T_{1/2}$ = 18–36 hrs | Contraindications:<br>Hypersensitivity; systemic fungal infections<br><br>Precautions: Monitor closely for infection (these agents may mask signs of infection); monitor electrolytes, weight, and blood pressure. Monitor patients with Addison's disease closely for exaggerated side effects.<br><br>Pregnancy Category: C<br><br>Lactation Issues: Use cautiously—is excreted into breast milk. |

# 602. Androgens and Androgen Inhibitors

## 602.1 Androgens

| Drug and Dosage Forms | Usual Dosage Range | Administration Issues and Drug–Drug Interactions | Common Adverse Drug Reactions (ADRs) and Pharmacokinetics | Contraindications, Pregnancy Category, and Lactation Issues |
|---|---|---|---|---|
| **Fluoxymesterone**<br>Halotestin, various generics<br><br>Tablets: 2 mg, 5 mg, 10 mg | Males<br>**Hypogonadism:** 5–20 mg/d<br><br>Females<br>**Breast cancer:** 10–40 mg/d in divided doses.<br><br>**Prevention of postpartum breast pain and engorgement:**<br>2.5 mg shortly after delivery, then 5–10 mg/d in divided doses for 4–5 days. | Administration Issues:<br>Take with food if GI upset occurs. Use very cautiously in children due to the bone maturation effects.<br><br>Drug–Drug Interactions:<br>**increased level/effect of:**<br>anticoagulants, imipramine (increased paranoid symptoms) | **ADRs:**<br>Most Frequent for Males:<br>gynecomastia, excessive frequency and duration of penile erections, decreased ejaculatory volume, oligospermia (at high doses)<br><br>Most Frequent for Females:<br>amenorrhea, other menstrual irregularities, virilization, (deepening of voice, clitoral enlargement)<br><br>Pharmacokinetics:<br>56% bioavailable; 98% protein bound; hepatically metabolized; $T_{1/2}$ = 9.2 hrs | Contraindications:<br>Hypersensitivity; serious cardiac, hepatic or renal disease, men with carcinomas of the breast or prostate, pregnancy, allergy to mercury compounds.<br><br>Precautions: Monitor women for signs of virilization, monitor serum/urine calcium levels. Use cautiously in those with acute intermittent porphyria, hypercholesterolemia, elderly males (increased risk of prostatic hypertrophy and carcinoma).<br><br>Pregnancy Category: X<br><br>Lactation Issues: Unknown if excreted in breast milk. Use cautiously if at all. |
| **Methyltestosterone**<br>Android, Oreton Methyl, Testred, Virilon, various generics | Males<br>**Hypogonadism:** 10–40 mg/d orally.<br>**Androgen deficiency:** 10–50 mg/d orally or 5–25 mg buccally. | Administration Issues:<br>Take with food if GI upset occurs. Buccal tablets should not be chewed or swallowed. They should dissolve | **ADRs:**<br>Most Frequent for Males:<br>gynecomastia, excessive frequency and duration of | Contraindications:<br>Hypersensitivity; serious cardiac, hepatic or renal disease, men with carcinomas |

*(continues on next page)*

| Drug and Dosage Forms | Usual Dosage Range | Administration Issues and Drug–Drug Interactions | Common Adverse Drug Reactions (ADRs) and Pharmacokinetics | Contraindications, Pregnancy Category, and Lactation Issues |
|---|---|---|---|---|
| **Methyltestosterone cont.**<br><br>Tablets:<br>10 mg, 25 mg<br><br>Tablets, buccal:<br>10 mg<br><br>Capsules: 10 mg | **Postpubertal cryptorchidism:**<br>30 mg/d orally<br><br>Females<br>**Postpartum breast pain and engorgement:** 80 mg/d orally for 3–5 days<br>**Breast Cancer:** 50–200 mg/d orally or 25–100 mg/d buccally. | between gum and cheek. Use very cautiously in children due to the bone maturation effects.<br><br>Drug–Drug Interactions:<br>**increased level/effect of:**<br>anticoagulants, imipramine (increased paranoid symptoms) | penile erections, decreased ejaculatory volume, oligospermia (at high doses)<br><br>Most Frequent for Females: amenorrhea, other menstrual irregularities, virilization (deepening of voice, clitoral enlargement)<br><br>Pharmacokinetics:<br>56% bioavailable (more bioavailable if given buccally); 98% protein bound; hepatically metabolized; $T_{1/2}$ = 2.5–3 hrs | of the breast or prostate, pregnancy, allergy to mercury compounds.<br><br>Precautions: Monitor women for signs of virilization, monitor serum/urine calcium levels. Use cautiously in those with acute intermittent porphyria, hypercholesterolemia, elderly males (increased risk of prostatic hypertrophy and carcinoma).<br><br>Pregnancy Category: X<br><br>Lactation Issues: Unknown if excreted in breast milk. Use cautiously if at all. |
| **Testosterone Transdermal System**<br>Testoderm, Androderm<br><br>Testoderm Patch:<br>4 mg/24 hrs<br>6 mg/24 hrs<br><br>Androderm Patch:<br>2.5 mg/24 hrs | **Primary or Secondary Hypogonadism:** Testoderm:<br>6 mg/d. If scrotal area is small, use the 4 mg/d patch.<br><br>**Androderm: 5 mg/d (2 patches worn daily). For non-virilized patient may start with 2.5 mg/d.** | Administration Issues:<br>Use very cautiously in children due to the bone maturation effects.<br><br>Testoderm: apply to scrotal skin. Place on clean, dry portion of scrotal skin. Dry shave the area.<br>Androderm: apply to non-scrotal skin. Place on clean dry area of back, abdomen, upper arms or thighs. | ADRs:<br>Most Frequent for Males: gynecomastia, excessive frequency and duration of penile erections, decreased ejaculatory volume, oligospermia (at high doses)<br><br>Most Frequent for Females: amenorrhea, other menstrual irregularities, virilization | Contraindications:<br>Hypersensitivity; serious cardiac, hepatic or renal disease, men with carcinomas of the breast or prostate, pregnancy, allergy to mercury compounds.<br><br>Precautions: Monitor women for signs of virilization, monitor serum/urine calcium levels. Use cautiously in those with acute |

| | | Drug–Drug Interactions:<br>**increased level/effect of:**<br>anticoagulants, imipramine (increased paranoid symptoms) | (deepening of voice, clitoral enlargement)<br><br>Pharmacokinetics:<br>transdermal; peak levels achieved after 2–4 hrs; serum levels reach plateau after 3–4 weeks of therapy. | intermittent porphyria, hypercholesterolemia, elderly males (increased risk of prostatic hypertrophy and carcinoma).<br><br>Pregnancy Category: X<br><br>Lactation Issues: Unknown if excreted in breast milk. Use cautiously if at all. |

## 602.2 Androgen Inhibitors

| Drug and Dosage Forms | Usual Dosage Range | Administration Issues and Drug–Drug Interactions | Common Adverse Drug Reactions (ADRs) and Pharmacokinetics | Contraindications, Pregnancy Category, and Lactation Issues |
|---|---|---|---|---|
| **Finasteride**<br>Proscar<br><br>Tablets: 5 mg | **Symptomatic Benign Prostatic Hyperplasia (BPH):** 5 mg once daily. | Drug–Drug Interactions:<br>**Increased levels/effects of:**<br>theophylline<br><br>Drug–Lab Interaction:<br>PSA levels are decreased during therapy. | ADRs:<br>impotence, decreased libido, decreased volume of ejaculate<br><br>Pharmacokinetics:<br>hepatically metabolized; $T_{1/2}$ = 6 hrs; renal elimination of metabolites. | Contraindications:<br>Hypersensitivity; pregnancy; lactation; children<br><br>Precautions: Use cautiously in those with liver or severe renal dysfunction. |

| Drug and Dosage Forms | Usual Dosage Range | Administration Issues and Drug–Drug Interactions | Common Adverse Drug Reactions (ADRs) | Contraindications, Pregnancy Category, and Lactation Issues |
|---|---|---|---|---|
| **Norethindrone & Mestranol**<br>Genora 1/50, Nelova 1/50, Norethin 1/50, Norinyl 1+50, Ortho-Novum 1/50<br><br>Tablets: 1 mg/50 mcg | **Contraception:**<br>Sunday start packs: take first tablet on first Sunday after menstruation begins; if menstruation begins on Sunday, take the first tablet on that day.<br><br>21-day regimen: To start—take 1 tablet daily for 21 days starting on the 5th day of the menstruation period. After 7 days with no tablets, begin 21 day cycle again.<br>28-day regimen: Follow same schedule as above. These packs will have 7 inert tablets for the 7-day free period. | Administration Issues:<br>Take exactly as directed. Do not miss doses. If > 2 days are missed, use another means of contraception until 7 days of therapy have been adhered to.<br><br>Follow schedule below for missed doses:<br>If 1 dose is missed: may take 2 tablets the next day. If 2 doses are missed: take 2 tablets as soon as remembered with the next pill or take 2 tablets daily for the next 2 days. If 3 doses are missed: begin a new compact of tablets starting on day one of the cycle after the last pill was taken<br><br>Drug–Drug Interactions:<br>**increased levels/effects of:** TCAs, benzodiazepines (oxidative metabolism); beta blockers, caffeine, corticosteroids, theophyllines<br>**decreased levels/effects of:** benzodiazepines, salicylates, clofibrate<br>**decreased levels/effects of contraceptives:** antibiotics, barbiturates, hydantoins, rifampin | ADRs:<br>breakthrough bleeding, spotting, change in menstrual flow, amenorrhea, vaginal candidiasis, change in cervical secretions, nausea, vomiting, abdominal cramps, bloating, rash, headaches, depression, edema, weight change<br><br>Serious: thrombophlebitis, venous thrombosis, pulmonary embolism, coronary thrombosis, MI, cerebral thrombosis, arterial thromboembolism, cerebral hemorrhage, hypertension, gallbladder disease, hepatic adenomas, hepatocellular carcinoma, mesenteric thrombosis, Budd–Chiari syndrome | Contraindications:<br>Hypersensitivity; thrombophlebitis, thromboembolic disorders, cerebral vascular disease, myocardial infarction, coronary artery disease, breast carcinoma or estrogen dependent neoplasia, carcinoma of endometrium, hepatic adenomas/carcinomas, undiagnosed abnormal genital bleeding, pregnancy, cholestatic jaundice<br><br>Precautions: Monitor cholesterol and glucose levels, blood pressure, for bleeding irregularities, thromboembolic events, development of pregnancy. Use cautiously in those patients with acute intermittent porphyria. Prolonged use (>5 yr.) should be done cautiously.<br><br>Pregnancy Category: X |

| | | | ADRs: | Contraindications: |
|---|---|---|---|---|

**Norethindrone & Ethinyl estradiol**

Ovcon, Genora, NEE, Nelova, Norinyl, Ortho-Novum, Brevicon, Modicon, Loestrin

Tablets:
1 mg/50 mcg
1 mg/35 mcg
0.5 mg/35 mcg
0.4 mg/35 mcg
1.5 mg/30 mcg
1 mg/20 mcg

**Contraception:**
Sunday start packs: take first tablet on first Sunday after menstruation begins; if menstruation begins on Sunday, take the first tablet on that day.

21-day regimen: To start—take 1 tablet daily for 21 days starting on the 5th day of the menstruation period. After 7 days with no tablets, begin 21 day cycle again.

28-day regimen: Follow same schedule as above. These packs will have 7 inert tablets for the 7-day free period.

Administration Issues:
Take exactly as directed. Do not miss doses. If >2 days are missed, use another means of contraception until 7 days of therapy have been adhered to.

Follow schedule below for missed doses:
If 1 dose is missed: may take 2 tablets the next day. If 2 doses are missed: take 2 tablets as soon as remembered with the next pill or take 2 tablets daily for the next 2 days. If 3 doses are missed: begin a new compact of tablets starting on day one of the cycle after the last pill was taken

Drug–Drug Interactions:
**increased levels/effects of:** TCAs, benzodiazepines (oxidative metabolism); beta blockers, caffeine, corticosteroids, theophyllines

**decreased levels/effects of:** benzodiazepines, salicylates, clofibrate

**decreased levels/effects of contraceptives:** antibiotics, barbiturates, hydantoins, rifampin

ADRs:
breakthrough bleeding, spotting, change in menstrual flow, amenorrhea, vaginal candidiasis, change in cervical secretions, nausea, vomiting, abdominal cramps, bloating, rash, headaches, depression, edema, weight change

Serious: thrombophlebitis, venous thrombosis, pulmonary embolism, coronary thrombosis, MI, cerebral thrombosis, arterial thromboembolism, cerebral hemorrhage, hypertension, gallbladder disease, hepatic adenomas, hepatocellular carcinoma, mesenteric thrombosis, Budd-Chiari syndrome

Lactation Issues: some excreted in breast milk. Mother should not nurse or should not take these pills until infant is weaned.

Contraindications:
Hypersensitivity; thrombophlebitis, thromboembolic disorders, cerebral vascular disease, myocardial infarction, coronary artery disease, breast carcinoma or estrogen dependent neoplasia, carcinoma of endometrium, hepatic adenomas/carcinomas, undiagnosed abnormal genital bleeding, pregnancy, cholestatic jaundice

Precautions: Monitor cholesterol and glucose levels, blood pressure, for bleeding irregularities, thromboembolic events, development of pregnancy. Use cautiously in those patients with acute intermittent porphyria. Prolonged use (>5 yr.) should be done cautiously.

Pregnancy Category: X

Lactation Issues: some excreted in breast milk. Mother should not nurse or should not take these pills until infant is weaned.

*(continues on next page)*

| Drug and Dosage Forms | Usual Dosage Range | Administration Issues and Drug–Drug Interactions | Common Adverse Drug Reactions (ADRs) | Contraindications, Pregnancy Category, and Lactation Issues |
|---|---|---|---|---|
| **Ethynodiol diacetate & Ethinyl estradiol**<br>Demulen<br><br><u>Tablets:</u>  1 mg/50 mcg | **Contraception:**<br><u>Sunday start packs:</u>  take first tablet on first Sunday after menstruation begins; if menstruation begins on Sunday, take the first tablet on that day.<br><u>21-day regimen:</u>  To start—take 1 tablet daily for 21 days starting on the 5th day of the menstruation period. After 7 days with no tablets, begin 21 day cycle again.<br><u>28-day regimen:</u>  Follow same schedule as above. These packs will have 7 inert tablets for the 7-day free period. | <u>Administration Issues:</u><br>Take exactly as directed. Do not miss doses. If >2 days are missed, use another means of contraception until 7 days of therapy have been adhered to.<br><br><u>Follow schedule below for missed doses:</u><br>If 1 dose is missed: may take 2 tablets the next day. If 2 doses are missed: take 2 tablets as soon as remembered with the next pill or take 2 tablets daily for the next 2 days. If 3 doses are missed: begin a new compact of tablets starting on day one of the cycle after the last pill was taken<br><br><u>Drug–Drug Interactions:</u><br>**increased levels/effects of:** TCAs, benzodiazepines (oxidative metabolism); beta blockers, caffeine, corticosteroids, theophyllines<br>**decreased levels/effects of:** benzodiazepines, salicylates, clofibrate<br>**decreased levels/effects of contraceptives:** antibiotics, barbiturates, hydantoins, rifampin | <u>ADRs:</u><br>breakthrough bleeding, spotting, change in menstrual flow, amenorrhea, vaginal candidiasis, change in cervical secretions, nausea, vomiting, abdominal cramps, bloating, rash, headaches, depression, edema, weight change<br><br><u>Serious:</u>  thrombophlebitis, venous thrombosis, pulmonary embolism, coronary thrombosis, MI, cerebral thrombosis, arterial thromboembolism, cerebral hemorrhage, hypertension, gallbladder disease, hepatic adenomas, hepatocellular carcinoma, mesenteric thrombosis, Budd-Chiari syndrome | <u>Contraindications:</u><br>Hypersensitivity; thrombophlebitis, thromboembolic disorders, cerebral vascular disease, myocardial infarction, coronary artery disease, breast carcinoma or estrogen dependent neoplasia, carcinoma of endometrium, hepatic adenomas/carcinomas, undiagnosed abnormal genital bleeding, pregnancy, cholestatic jaundice<br><br><u>Precautions:</u>  Monitor cholesterol and glucose levels, blood pressure, for bleeding irregularities, thromboembolic events, development of pregnancy. Use cautiously in those patients with acute intermittent porphyria. Prolonged use (>5 yr.) should be done cautiously.<br><br><u>Pregnancy Category:</u>  X<br><br><u>Lactation Issues:</u>  some excreted in breast milk. Mother should not nurse or should not take these pills until infant is weaned. |

## Norgestrel & Ethinyl estradiol

Ovral, Lo/Ovral

Tablets:
0.5 mg/50 mcg
0.3 mg/30 mcg

**Contraception:**

Sunday start packs: take first tablet on first Sunday after menstruation begins; if menstruation begins on Sunday, take the first tablet on that day.

21-day regimen: To start—take 1 tablet daily for 21 days starting on the 5th day of the menstruation period. After 7 days with no tablets, begin 21 day cycle again.

28-day regimen: Follow same schedule as above. These packs will have 7 inert tablets for the 7-day free period.

Administration Issues:
Take exactly as directed. Do not miss doses. If >2 days are missed, use another means of contraception until 7 days of therapy have been adhered to.

Follow schedule below for missed doses:

If 1 dose is missed: may take 2 tablets the next day. If 2 doses are missed: take 2 tablets as soon as remembered with the next pill or take 2 tablets daily for the next 2 days. If 3 doses are missed: begin a new compact of tablets starting on day one of the cycle after the last pill was taken

Drug–Drug Interactions:

**increased levels/effects of:** TCAs, benzodiazepines (oxidative metabolism); beta blockers, caffeine, corticosteroids, theophyllines

**decreased levels/effects of:** benzodiazepines, salicylates, clofibrate

**decreased levels/effects of contraceptives:** antibiotics, barbiturates, hydantoins, rifampin

ADRs:
breakthrough bleeding, spotting, change in menstrual flow, amenorrhea, vaginal candidiasis, change in cervical secretions, nausea, vomiting, abdominal cramps, bloating, rash, headaches, depression, edema, weight change

Serious: thrombophlebitis, venous thrombosis, pulmonary embolism, coronary thrombosis, MI, cerebral thrombosis, arterial thromboembolism, cerebral hemorrhage, hypertension, gallbladder disease, hepatic adenomas, hepatocellular carcinoma, mesenteric thrombosis, Budd-Chiari syndrome

Contraindications:
Hypersensitivity; thrombophlebitis, thromboembolic disorders, cerebral vascular disease, myocardial infarction, coronary artery disease, breast carcinoma or estrogen dependent neoplasia, carcinoma of endometrium, hepatic adenomas/carcinomas, undiagnosed abnormal genital bleeding, pregnancy, cholestatic jaundice

Precautions: Monitor cholesterol and glucose levels, blood pressure, for bleeding irregularities, thromboembolic events, development of pregnancy. Use cautiously in those patients with acute intermittent porphyria. Prolonged use (>5 yr.) should be done cautiously.

Pregnancy Category: X

Lactation Issues: some excreted in breast milk. Mother should not nurse or should not take these pills until infant is weaned.

(continues on next page)

| Drug and Dosage Forms | Usual Dosage Range | Administration Issues and Drug–Drug Interactions | Common Adverse Drug Reactions (ADRs) | Contraindications, Pregnancy Category, and Lactation Issues |
|---|---|---|---|---|
| **Norgestimate & Ethinyl estradiol**<br>Ortho-Cyclen<br><u>Tablets:</u><br>0.25 mg/35 mcg | **Contraception:**<br><u>Sunday start packs:</u> take first tablet on first Sunday after menstruation begins; if menstruation begins on Sunday, take the first tablet on that day.<br><u>21-day regimen:</u> To start—take 1 tablet daily for 21 days starting on the 5th day of the menstruation period. After 7 days with no tablets, begin 21 day cycle again.<br><u>28-day regimen:</u> Follow same schedule as above. These packs will have 7 inert tablets for the 7-day free period.<br><br>Titrate dose of contraceptives as needed by patient | <u>Administration Issues:</u><br>Take exactly as directed. Do not miss doses. If > 2 days are missed, use another means of contraception until 7 days of therapy have been adhered to.<br><br><u>Follow schedule below for missed doses:</u><br>If 1 dose is missed: may take 2 tablets the next day. If 2 doses are missed: take 2 tablets as soon as remembered with the next pill or take 2 tablets daily for the next 2 days. If 3 doses are missed: begin a new compact of tablets starting on day one of the cycle after the last pill was taken<br><br><u>Drug–Drug Interactions:</u><br>**increased levels/effects of:** TCAs, benzodiazepines (oxidative metabolism); beta blockers, caffeine, corticosteroids, theophyllines<br>**decreased levels/effects of:** benzodiazepines, salicylates, clofibrate<br>**decreased levels/effects of contraceptives:** antibiotics, barbiturates, hydantoins, rifampin | <u>ADRs:</u><br>breakthrough bleeding, spotting, change in menstrual flow, amenorrhea, vaginal candidiasis, change in cervical secretions, nausea, vomiting, abdominal cramps, bloating, rash, headaches, depression, edema, weight change<br><br><u>Serious:</u> thrombophlebitis, venous thrombosis, pulmonary embolism, coronary thrombosis, MI, cerebral thrombosis, arterial thromboembolism, cerebral hemorrhage, hypertension, gallbladder disease, hepatic adenomas, hepatocellular carcinoma, mesenteric thrombosis, Budd-Chiari syndrome | <u>Contraindications:</u><br>Hypersensitivity; thrombophlebitis, thromboembolic disorders, cerebral vascular disease, myocardial infarction, coronary artery disease, breast carcinoma or estrogen dependent neoplasia, carcinoma of endometrium, hepatic adenomas/carcinomas, undiagnosed abnormal genital bleeding, pregnancy, cholestatic jaundice<br><br><u>Precautions:</u> Monitor cholesterol and glucose levels, blood pressure, for bleeding irregularities, thromboembolic events, development of pregnancy. Use cautiously in those patients with acute intermittent porphyria. Prolonged use (>5 yr.) should be done cautiously.<br><br><u>Pregnancy Category:</u> X<br><br><u>Lactation Issues:</u> some excreted in breast milk. Mother should not nurse or should not take these pills until infant is weaned. |

| Desogestrel & Ethinyl estradiol | Contraception: | Administration Issues: | ADRs: | Contraindications: |
|---|---|---|---|---|
| Desogen, Ortho-Cept | Sunday start packs: take first tablet on first Sunday after menstruation begins; if menstruation begins on Sunday, take the first tablet on that day. | Take exactly as directed. Do not miss doses. If >2 days are missed, use another means of contraception until 7 days of therapy have been adhered to. | breakthrough bleeding, spotting, change in menstrual flow, amenorrhea, vaginal candidiasis, change in cervical secretions, nausea, vomiting, abdominal cramps, bloating, rash, headaches, depression, edema, weight change | Hypersensitivity; thrombophlebitis, thromboembolic disorders, cerebral vascular disease, myocardial infarction, coronary artery disease, breast carcinoma or estrogen dependent neoplasia, carcinoma of endometrium, hepatic adenomas/carcinomas, undiagnosed abnormal genital bleeding, pregnancy, cholestatic jaundice |
| Tablets: 0.15 mg/30 mcg | 21-day regimen: To start—take 1 tablet daily for 21 days starting on the 5th day of the menstruation period. After 7 days with no tablets, begin 21 day cycle again. | Follow schedule below for missed doses: If 1 dose is missed: may take 2 tablets the next day. If 2 doses are missed: take 2 tablets as soon as remembered with the next pill or take 2 tablets daily for the next 2 days. If 3 doses are missed: begin a new compact of tablets starting on day one of the cycle after the last pill was taken | Serious: thrombophlebitis, venous thrombosis, pulmonary embolism, coronary thrombosis, MI, cerebral thrombosis, arterial thromboembolism, cerebral hemorrhage, hypertension, gallbladder disease, hepatic adenomas, hepatocellular carcinoma, mesenteric thrombosis, Budd-Chiari syndrome | |
| | 28-day regimen: Follow same schedule as above. These packs will have 7 inert tablets for the 7-day free period. | Drug–Drug Interactions: increased levels/effects of: TCAs, benzodiazepines (oxidative metabolism); beta blockers, caffeine, corticosteroids, theophyllines decreased levels/effects of: benzodiazepines, salicylates, clofibrate decreased levels/effects of contraceptives: antibiotics, barbiturates, hydantoins, rifampin | | Precautions: Monitor cholesterol and glucose levels, blood pressure, for bleeding irregularities, thromboembolic events, development of pregnancy. Use cautiously in those patients with acute intermittent porphyria. Prolonged use (>5 yr.) should be done cautiously.

Pregnancy Category: X

Lactation Issues: some excreted in breast milk. Mother should not nurse or should not take these pills until infant is weaned. |

(continues on next page)

| Drug and Dosage Forms | Usual Dosage Range | Administration Issues and Drug–Drug Interactions | Common Adverse Drug Reactions (ADRs) | Contraindications, Pregnancy Category, and Lactation Issues |
|---|---|---|---|---|
| **Levonorgestrel & Ethinyl estradiol** Levlen, Levora, Nordette Tablets: 0.15 mg/30 mcg | **Contraception:** Sunday start packs:  take first tablet on first Sunday after menstruation begins; if menstruation begins on Sunday, take the first tablet on that day. 21-day regimen:  To start—take 1 tablet daily for 21 days starting on the 5th day of the menstruation period. After 7 days with no tablets, begin 21 day cycle again. 28-day regimen:  Follow same schedule as above. These packs will have 7 inert tablets for the 7-day free period. | Administration Issues: Take exactly as directed. Do not miss doses. If >2 days are missed, use another means of contraception until 7 days of therapy have been adhered to. Follow schedule below for missed doses: If 1 dose is missed: may take 2 tablets the next day. If 2 doses are missed: take 2 tablets as soon as remembered with the next pill or take 2 tablets daily for the next 2 days. If 3 doses are missed: begin a new compact of tablets starting on day one of the cycle after the last pill was taken Drug–Drug Interactions: **increased levels/effects of:**  TCAs, benzodiazepines (oxidative metabolism); beta blockers, caffeine, corticosteroids, theophyllines **decreased levels/effects of:** benzodiazepines, salicylates, clofibrate **decreased levels/effects of contraceptives:**  antibiotics, barbiturates, hydantoins, rifampin | ADRs: breakthrough bleeding, spotting, change in menstrual flow, amenorrhea, vaginal candidiasis, change in cervical secretions, nausea, vomiting, abdominal cramps, bloating, rash, headaches, depression, edema, weight change Serious:  thrombophlebitis, venous thrombosis, pulmonary embolism, coronary thrombosis, MI, cerebral thrombosis, arterial thromboembolism, cerebral hemorrhage, hypertension, gallbladder disease, hepatic adenomas, hepatocellular carcinoma, mesenteric thrombosis, Budd-Chiari syndrome | Contraindications: Hypersensitivity; thrombophlebitis, thromboembolic disorders, cerebral vascular disease, myocardial infarction, coronary artery disease, breast carcinoma or estrogen dependent neoplasia, carcinoma of endometrium, hepatic adenomas/carcinomas, undiagnosed abnormal genital bleeding, pregnancy, cholestatic jaundice Precautions:  Monitor cholesterol and glucose levels, blood pressure, for bleeding irregularities, thromboembolic events, development of pregnancy. Use cautiously in those patients with acute intermittent porphyria. Prolonged use (>5 yr.) should be done cautiously. Pregnancy Category:  X Lactation Issues:  some excreted in breast milk. Mother should not nurse or should not take these pills until infant is weaned. |

603.2  Oral Contraceptives—Biphasic

| Drug and Dosage Forms | Usual Dosage Range | Administration Issues and Drug–Drug Interactions | Common Adverse Drug Reactions (ADRs) | Contraindications, Pregnancy Category, and Lactation Issues |
|---|---|---|---|---|
| **Norethindrone & Ethinyl estradiol**<br>Jenest-28, Nelova 10/11, Ortho-Novum 10/11<br><br>Tablets (1st phase):<br>0.5 mg/35 mcg (7 tabs)<br>0.5 mg/35 mcg (10 tabs)<br><br>Tablets (2nd phase):<br>1 mg/35 mcg (14 tabs)<br>1 mg/35 mcg (11 tabs) | **Contraception:**<br>Follow directions contained in pack describing when cycle should start, etc. | Administration Issues:<br>Take exactly as directed. Do not miss doses. If >2 days are missed, use another means of contraception until 7 days of therapy have been adhered to.<br><br>Follow schedule below for missed doses:<br>If 1 dose is missed: may take 2 tablets the next day. If 2 doses are missed: take 2 tablets as soon as remembered with the next pill or take 2 tablets daily for the next 2 days. If 3 doses are missed: begin a new compact of tablets starting on day one of the cycle after the last pill was taken<br><br>Drug–Drug Interactions:<br>**increased levels/effects of:** TCAs, benzodiazepines (oxidative metabolism); beta blockers, caffeine, corticosteroids, theophyllines<br>**decreased levels/effects of:** benzodiazepines, salicylates, clofibrate<br>**decreased levels/effects of contraceptives:** antibiotics, barbiturates, hydantoins, rifampin | ADRs:<br>breakthrough bleeding, spotting, change in menstrual flow, amenorrhea, vaginal candidiasis, change in cervical secretions, nausea, vomiting, abdominal cramps, bloating, rash, headaches, depression, edema, weight change<br><br>Serious: thrombophlebitis, venous thrombosis, pulmonary embolism, coronary thrombosis, MI, cerebral thrombosis, arterial thromboembolism, cerebral hemorrhage, hypertension, gallbladder disease, hepatic adenomas, hepatocellular carcinoma, mesenteric thrombosis, Budd-Chiari syndrome | Contraindications:<br>Hypersensitivity; thrombophlebitis, thromboembolic disorders, cerebral vascular disease, myocardial infarction, coronary artery disease, breast carcinoma or estrogen dependent neoplasia, carcinoma of endometrium, hepatic adenomas/carcinomas, undiagnosed abnormal genital bleeding, pregnancy, cholestatic jaundice<br><br>Precautions: Monitor cholesterol and glucose levels, blood pressure, for bleeding irregularities, thromboembolic events, development of pregnancy. Use cautiously in those patients with acute intermittent porphyria. Prolonged use (>5 yr.) should be done cautiously.<br><br>Pregnancy Category: X<br><br>Lactation Issues: some excreted in breast milk. Mother should not nurse or should not take these pills until infant is weaned. |

| Drug and Dosage Forms | Usual Dosage Range | Administration Issues and Drug–Drug Interactions | Common Adverse Drug Reactions (ADRs) | Contraindications, Pregnancy Category, and Lactation Issues |
|---|---|---|---|---|
| **Norethindrone & Ethinyl estradiol** Tri-Norinyl, Ortho-Novum 7/7/7  Tablets (1st phase): 0.5 mg/35 mcg (7 tabs)  Tablets (2nd phase): 1 mg/35 mcg (9 tabs) 0.75 mg/35 mcg (7 tabs)  Tablets (3rd phase): 0.5 mg/35 mcg (5 tabs) 1 mg/35 mcg (7 tabs) | **Contraception:** Follow directions contained in pack describing when cycle should start, etc. | Administration Issues: Take exactly as directed. Do not miss doses. If >2 days are missed, use another means of contraception until 7 days of therapy have been adhered to.  Follow schedule below for missed doses: If 1 dose is missed: may take 2 tablets the next day. If 2 doses are missed: take 2 tablets as soon as remembered with the next pill or take 2 tablets daily for the next 2 days. If 3 doses are missed: begin a new compact of tablets starting on day one of the cycle after the last pill was taken  Drug–Drug Interactions: **increased levels/effects of:** TCAs, benzodiazepines (oxidative metabolism); beta blockers, caffeine, corticosteroids, theophyllines **decreased levels/effects of:** benzodiazepines, salicylates, clofibrate **decreased levels/effects of contraceptives:** antibiotics, barbiturates, hydantoins, rifampin | ADRs: breakthrough bleeding, spotting, change in menstrual flow, amenorrhea, vaginal candidiasis, change in cervical secretions, nausea, vomiting, abdominal cramps, bloating, rash, headaches, depression, edema, weight change  Serious: thrombophlebitis, venous thrombosis, pulmonary embolism, coronary thrombosis, MI, cerebral thrombosis, arterial thromboembolism, cerebral hemorrhage, hypertension, gallbladder disease, hepatic adenomas, hepatocellular carcinoma, mesenteric thrombosis, Budd-Chiari syndrome | Contraindications: Hypersensitivity; thrombophlebitis, thromboembolic disorders, cerebral vascular disease, myocardial infarction, coronary artery disease, breast carcinoma or estrogen dependent neoplasia, carcinoma of endometrium, hepatic adenomas/carcinomas, undiagnosed abnormal genital bleeding, pregnancy, cholestatic jaundice  Precautions: Monitor cholesterol and glucose levels, blood pressure, for bleeding irregularities, thromboembolic events, development of pregnancy. Use cautiously in those patients with acute intermittent porphyria. Prolonged use (>5 yr.) should be done cautiously.  Pregnancy Category: X  Lactation Issues: some excreted in breast milk. Mother should not nurse or should not take these pills until infant is weaned. |

## Levonorgestrel & Ethinyl estradiol

Tri-Levlen, Triphasil

Tablets (1st phase):
0.05 mg/30 mcg (6 tabs)

Tablets (2nd phase):
0.075 mg/40 mcg (5 tabs)

Tablets (3rd phase):
0.125 mg/30 mcg (10 tabs)

**Contraception:**
Follow directions contained in pack describing when cycle should start, etc.

Administration Issues:
Take exactly as directed. Do not miss doses. If >2 days are missed, use another means of contraception until 7 days of therapy have been adhered to.

Follow schedule below for missed doses:

If 1 dose is missed: may take 2 tablets the next day. If 2 doses are missed: take 2 tablets as soon as remembered with the next pill or take 2 tablets daily for the next 2 days. If 3 doses are missed: begin a new compact of tablets starting on day one of the cycle after the last pill was taken

Drug–Drug Interactions:
**increased levels/effects of:** TCAs, benzodiazepines (oxidative metabolism); beta blockers, caffeine, corticosteroids, theophyllines
**decreased levels/effects of:** benzodiazepines, salicylates, clofibrate
**decreased levels/effects of contraceptives:** antibiotics, barbiturates, hydantoins, rifampin

ADRs:
breakthrough bleeding, spotting, change in menstrual flow, amenorrhea, vaginal candidiasis, change in cervical secretions, nausea, vomiting, abdominal cramps, bloating, rash, headaches, depression, edema, weight change

Serious: thrombophlebitis, venous thrombosis, pulmonary embolism, coronary thrombosis, MI, cerebral thrombosis, arterial thromboembolism, cerebral hemorrhage, hypertension, gallbladder disease, hepatic adenomas, hepatocellular carcinoma, mesenteric thrombosis, Budd-Chiari syndrome

Contraindications:
Hypersensitivity; thrombophlebitis, thromboembolic disorders, cerebral vascular disease, myocardial infarction, coronary artery disease, breast carcinoma or estrogen dependent neoplasia, carcinoma of endometrium, hepatic adenomas/carcinomas, undiagnosed abnormal genital bleeding, pregnancy, cholestatic jaundice

Precautions: Monitor cholesterol and glucose levels, blood pressure, for bleeding irregularities, thromboembolic events, development of pregnancy. Use cautiously in those patients with acute intermittent porphyria. Prolonged use (>5 yr.) should be done cautiously.

Pregnancy Category: X

Lactation Issues: some excreted in breast milk. Mother should not nurse or should not take these pills until infant is weaned.

(continues on next page)

## 603.3  Oral Contraceptives—Triphasic *continued from previous page*

| Drug and Dosage Forms | Usual Dosage Range | Administration Issues and Drug–Drug Interactions | Common Adverse Drug Reactions (ADRs) | Contraindications, Pregnancy Category, and Lactation Issues |
|---|---|---|---|---|
| **Norgestimate & Ethinyl estradiol**<br>Ortho Tri-Cyclen<br><br>Tablets (1st phase):<br>0.18 mg/35 mcg (7 tabs)<br><br>Tablets (2nd phase):<br>0.215 mg/35 mcg (7 tabs)<br><br>Tablets (3rd phase):<br>0.25 mg/35 mcg (7 tabs) | **Contraception:**<br>Follow directions contained in pack describing when cycle should start, etc. | Administration Issues:<br>Take exactly as directed. Do not miss doses. If >2 days are missed, use another means of contraception until 7 days of therapy have been adhered to.<br><br>Follow schedule below for missed doses:<br>If 1 dose is missed: may take 2 tablets the next day. If 2 doses are missed: take 2 tablets as soon as remembered with the next pill or take 2 tablets daily for the next 2 days. If 3 doses are missed: begin a new compact of tablets starting on day one of the cycle after the last pill was taken<br><br>Drug–Drug Interactions:<br>**increased levels/effects of:** TCAs, benzodiazepines (oxidative metabolism); beta blockers, caffeine, corticosteroids, theophyllines<br>**decreased levels/effects of:** benzodiazepines, salicylates, clofibrate<br>**decreased levels/effects of contraceptives:** antibiotics, barbiturates, hydantoins, rifampin | ADRs:<br>breakthrough bleeding, spotting, change in menstrual flow, amenorrhea, vaginal candidiasis, change in cervical secretions, nausea, vomiting, abdominal cramps, bloating, rash, headaches, depression, edema, weight change<br><br>Serious:  thrombophlebitis, venous thrombosis, pulmonary embolism, coronary thrombosis, MI, cerebral thrombosis, arterial thromboembolism, cerebral hemorrhage, hypertension, gallbladder disease, hepatic adenomas, hepatocellular carcinoma, mesenteric thrombosis, Budd-Chiari syndrome | Contraindications:<br>Hypersensitivity; thrombophlebitis, thromboembolic disorders, cerebral vascular disease, myocardial infarction, coronary artery disease, breast carcinoma or estrogen dependent neoplasia, carcinoma of endometrium, hepatic adenomas/carcinomas, undiagnosed abnormal genital bleeding, pregnancy, cholestatic jaundice<br><br>Precautions:  Monitor cholesterol and glucose levels, blood pressure, for bleeding irregularities, thromboembolic events, development of pregnancy. Use cautiously in those patients with acute intermittent porphyria. Prolonged use (>5 yr.) should be done cautiously.<br><br>Pregnancy Category:  X<br><br>Lactation Issues:  some excreted in breast milk. Mother should not nurse or should not take these pills until infant is weaned. |

| Drug and Dosage Forms | Usual Dosage Range | Administration Issues and Drug–Drug Interactions | Common Adverse Drug Reactions (ADRs) | Contraindications, Pregnancy Category, and Lactation Issues |
|---|---|---|---|---|
| **Norethindrone**<br>Micronor, Nor-QD<br><br><u>Tablets:</u> 0.35 mg | **Contraception:**<br>take 1 tablet daily beginning on the first day of menstruation. Take daily for every day of the year. | <u>Administration Issues:</u><br>Take exactly as directed<br>Do not miss doses. If >2 days are missed, use another means of contraception until 7 days of therapy have been adhered to.<br><br><u>Follow the schedule below for missed doses:</u><br>If 1 dose is missed: take as soon as remembered. If 2 doses are missed: do not make up doses.<br>Discard the 2 tablets and start back on schedule. If 3 doses are missed: discontinue altogether.<br><br><u>Drug–Drug Interactions:</u><br>**decreased levels/effects of progestin:** aminoglutethimide, rifampin, carbamazepine, phenytoin | <u>ADRs:</u><br>headache, nervousness, dizziness, rash, acne, photosensitivity, weight gain, many days of bleeding, breakthrough bleeding, spotting, change in menstrual flow, amenorrhea, changes in cervical secretions, breast changes, mastalgia, scalp hair loss, hypertrichosis, edema, hirsutism. | <u>Contraindications:</u><br>Hypersensitivity, thrombophlebitis, thromboembolic disorders, cerebral hemorrhage, impaired liver function, carcinoma of the breast or genital organs, undiagnosed vaginal bleeding, missed abortion, for use as a diagnostic test for pregnancy.<br><br><u>Pregnancy Category:</u> D<br><br><u>Lactation Issues:</u> small amounts excreted in breast milk—effects on infant not known. |
| **Norgestrel**<br>Ovrette<br><br><u>Tablets:</u> 0.075 mg | **Contraception:**<br>take 1 tablet daily beginning on the first day of menstruation. Take daily for every day of the year. | <u>Administration Issues:</u><br>Take exactly as directed<br>Do not miss doses. If >2 days are missed, use another means of contraception until 7 days of therapy have been adhered to. | <u>ADRs:</u><br>headache, nervousness, dizziness, rash, acne, photosensitivity, weight gain, many days of bleeding, breakthrough bleeding, spotting, change in menstrual flow, amenorrhea, changes in | <u>Contraindications:</u><br>Hypersensitivity, thrombophlebitis, thromboembolic disorders, cerebral hemorrhage, impaired liver function, carcinoma of the breast or genital organs, undiagnosed vaginal bleeding, |

*(continues on next page)*

1349

## 603.4 Oral Contraceptives—Progestin Only *continued from previous page*

| Drug and Dosage Forms | Usual Dosage Range | Administration Issues and Drug–Drug Interactions | Common Adverse Drug Reactions (ADRs) | Contraindications, Pregnancy Category, and Lactation Issues |
|---|---|---|---|---|
| **Norgestrel** *cont.* | | Follow the schedule below for missed doses: If 1 dose is missed: take as soon as remembered. If 2 doses are missed: do not make up doses. Discard the 2 tablets and start back on schedule. If 3 doses are missed: discontinue altogether. <br><br> Drug–Drug Interactions: **decreased levels/effects of progestin:** aminoglutethimide, rifampin, carbamazepine, phenytoin | cervical secretions, breast changes, mastalgia, scalp hair loss, hypertrichosis, edema, hirsutism. | missed abortion, for use as a diagnostic test for pregnancy. <br><br> Pregnancy Category: D <br><br> Lactation Issues: small amounts excreted in breast milk—effects on infant not known. |

## 603.5 Contraceptive Implants

| Drug and Dosage Forms | Usual Dosage Range | Administration Issues and Drug–Drug Interactions | Common Adverse Drug Reactions (ADRs) | Contraindications, Pregnancy Category, and Lactation Issues |
|---|---|---|---|---|
| **Levonorgestrel** <br> Norplant <br><br> Capsules (kit): 6 (each contains 36 mg) | **Contraception:** All 6 capsules should be implanted during the 7 days of the onset of menses. Contraceptive protection should last 5 years. | Administration Issues: Surgically implanted. Implantation is subdermal in the mid-portion of the upper arm. <br><br> Drug–Drug Interactions: **decreased levels/effects of progestin:** | ADRs: fluid retention, headache, nervousness, dizziness, rash, acne, weight gain, many days of bleeding, breakthrough bleeding, spotting, change in menstrual flow, amenorrhea, changes in cervical secretions, | Contraindications: Hypersensitivity, thrombophlebitis, thromboembolic disorders, cerebral hemorrhage, impaired liver function, carcinoma of the breast or genital organs, undiagnosed vaginal bleeding, |

603.6 Contraceptive Injections

| | Administration Issues and Drug–Drug Interactions | Common Adverse Drug Reactions (ADRs) | Contraindications, Pregnancy Category, and Lactation Issues |
|---|---|---|---|
| | aminoglutethimide, rifampin, carbamazepine, phenytoin<br><br>Drug–Lab Interaction:<br>the following tests may be affected by progestins: hepatic function, coagulation, thyroid, metyrapone, and endocrine function. | breast changes, mastalgia, scalp hair loss, hypertrichosis, edema, hirsutism | missed abortion, for use as a diagnostic test for pregnancy.<br><br>Pregnancy Category: Implants should be removed if pregnancy occurs.<br><br>Lactation Issues: small amounts excreted in breast milk—effects on infant not known. |

| Drug and Dosage Forms | Usual Dosage Range | Administration Issues and Drug–Drug Interactions | Common Adverse Drug Reactions (ADRs) | Contraindications, Pregnancy Category, and Lactation Issues |
|---|---|---|---|---|
| **Medroxyprogesterone**<br>Depo-Provera<br><br>Injection (suspension):<br>150 mg/mL | **Contraception:** 150 mg by IM injection every 3 months | Administration Issues:<br>Shake vial prior to administration to ensure complete suspension.<br><br>Drug–Drug Interactions:<br>**decreased levels/effects of progestin:** aminoglutethimide, rifampin, carbamazepine, phenytoin<br><br>Drug–Lab Interaction:<br>the following tests may be affected by progestins: hepatic function, coagulation, thyroid, metyrapone, and endocrine function. | ADRs:<br>headache, nervousness, dizziness, rash, acne, weight gain, many days of bleeding, breakthrough bleeding, spotting, change in menstrual flow, amenorrhea, changes in cervical secretions, breast changes, mastalgia, scalp hair loss, hypertrichosis, edema, hirsutism | Contraindications:<br>Hypersensitivity, thrombophlebitis, thromboembolic disorders, cerebral hemorrhage, impaired liver function, carcinoma of the breast or genital organs, undiagnosed vaginal bleeding, missed abortion, for use as a diagnostic test for pregnancy.<br><br>Pregnancy Category: Implants should be removed if pregnancy occurs.<br><br>Lactation Issues: small amounts excreted in breast milk—effects on infant not known. |

# 604. Antidiabetic Agents

604.1 Sulfonylureas

| Drug and Dosage Forms | Usual Dosage Range | Administration Issues and Drug–Drug Interactions | Common Adverse Drug Reactions (ADRs) and Pharmacokinetics | Contraindications, Pregnancy Category, and Lactation Issues |
|---|---|---|---|---|
| **Chlorpropamide**<br>Diabinese, various generics<br><br>Tablets: 100 mg, 250 mg | **As adjunct to diet/exercise to control blood glucose in NIDDM (Type II):**<br>250 mg/d, initially. May titrate to 500 mg/d if needed. Do not exceed 750 mg/d.<br><br>**Elderly or debilitated patients:**<br>100–125 mg/d initially. | Administration Issues:<br>Take with food if GI upset occurs. Avoid alcohol<br><br>Drug–Drug Interactions:<br>**increased hypoglycemic effect:**<br>androgens, anticoagulants, chloramphenicol, clofibrate, fenfluramine, fluconazole, gemfibrozil, H₂ antagonists, magnesium salts, methyldopa, MAO inhibitors, phenylbutazone, probenecid, salicylates, sulfinpyrazone, sulfonamides, TCAs, urinary acidifiers, alcohol (acute use)<br><br>**increased levels/effects of:** digoxin<br><br>**decreased hypoglycemic effect:**<br>beta blockers, cholestyramine, diazoxide, hydantoins, rifampin, thiazide diuretics, urinary alkalinizers, activated charcoal, alcohol (chronic use) | ADRs:<br>hypoglycemia, nausea, heartburn, epigastric fullness, allergic skin reactions, eczema, pruritus, erythema, disulfiram-like reactions (if taken with alcohol), elevated liver function tests, SIADH. Chlorpropamide has a higher incidence of side-effects than other sulfonylureas.<br><br>Elderly: Use cautiously—particularly susceptible to hypoglycemic effects. Also, elderly patients may not recognize symptoms of hypoglycemia<br><br>Pharmacokinetics:<br>onset of action = 1 hr; duration of action = up to 60 hrs; 80% metabolized in liver; renal elimination of metabolites; $T_{1/2}$ = 36 h (Agents with shorter $T_{1/2}$ are generally better choices for elderly patients). | Contraindications:<br>Hypersensitivity, diabetes complicated by ketoacidosis with or without coma; sole therapy of Type I diabetes; diabetes complicated by pregnancy.<br><br>Precautions: Monitor patients closely during periods of stress (e.g., infection, etc) for poor glucose control. Use cautiously in those with severe hepatic or renal impairment.<br><br>Pregnancy Category: C<br><br>Lactation Issues: excreted in breast milk—do not give to nursing mothers. |

| Glipizide | As adjunct to diet/exercise to control blood glucose in NIDDM (Type II): | Administration Issues: | ADRs: | Contraindications: |
|---|---|---|---|---|
| Glucotrol, various generics | 5 mg each morning, initially. May titrate by 2.5–5 mg/d every several days as needed. Max single daily dose is 15 mg; max daily dose is 40 mg. | Take 30 minutes prior to a meal. Avoid alcohol. | hypoglycemia, nausea, heartburn, epigastric fullness, allergic skin reactions, eczema, pruritus, erythema, disulfiram-like reactions (if taken with alcohol), elevated liver function tests, SIADH | Hypersensitivity, diabetes complicated by ketoacidosis with or without coma; sole therapy of Type I diabetes; diabetes complicated by pregnancy. |
| Tablets: 5 mg, 10 mg | | Drug–Drug Interactions: | | |
| | | increased hypoglycemic effect: | Other effects: increased effects on total cholesterol, total triglycerides, LDL, body weight (3–8 kg). | Precautions: Monitor patients closely during periods of stress (e.g., infection, etc) for poor glucose control. Use cautiously in those with severe hepatic or renal impairment. |
| Tablets, extended release: 5 mg, 10 mg | | androgens, anticoagulants, chloramphenicol, clofibrate, fenfluramine, fluconazole, ketoconazole, gemfibrozil, H₂ antagonists, magnesium salts, methyldopa, MAO inhibitors, phenylbutazone, probenecid, salicylates, sulfinpyrazone, sulfonamides, TCAs, urinary acidifiers, alcohol (acute use) | | |
| | Elderly or debilitated patients: 2.5 mg/d initially. | increased levels/effects of: digoxin | Elderly: Use cautiously—particularly susceptible to hypoglycemic effects. Also, elderly patients may not recognize symptoms of hypoglycemia | Pregnancy Category: C |
| | | decreased hypoglycemic effect: beta blockers, cholestyramine, diazoxide, hydantoins, rifampin, thiazide diuretics, urinary alkalinizers, charcoal, alcohol (chronic use) | | Lactation Issues: excreted in breast milk—do not give to nursing mothers. |
| | | | Pharmacokinetics: onset of action = 1–1.5 hrs; duration of action = 10–16 hrs; hepatically metabolized; renal elimination of metabolites; $T_{1/2}$ = 2–4 hrs | |
| **Glimepiride** | **As adjunct to diet/exercise to control blood glucose in NIDDM (Type II):** | Administration Issues: | ADRs: | Contraindications: |
| Amaryl | 1–2 mg once daily, initially. May titrate by 1–2 mg/d each week up to 4 mg once daily if needed. Max dose is 8 mg/d. Combination therapy with insulin: 8 mg/d with low dose insulin. | Take with food if GI upset occurs. Avoid alcohol | hypoglycemia, nausea, heartburn, epigastric fullness, allergic skin reactions, eczema, pruritus, erythema, disulfiram-like reactions (if taken with alcohol), elevated liver function tests, SIADH, photosensitivity | Hypersensitivity, diabetes complicated by ketoacidosis with or without coma; sole therapy of Type I diabetes; diabetes complicated by pregnancy. |
| Tablets: 1 mg, 2 mg, 4 mg | | Drug–Drug Interactions: | | |
| | | increased hypoglycemic effect: androgens, anticoagulants, chloramphenicol, clofibrate, | | |

(continues on next page)

| Drug and Dosage Forms | Usual Dosage Range | Administration Issues and Drug–Drug Interactions | Common Adverse Drug Reactions (ADRs) and Pharmacokinetics | Contraindications, Pregnancy Category, and Lactation Issues |
|---|---|---|---|---|
| **Glimepiride *cont.*** | | fenfluramine, fluconazole, gemfibrozil, H₂ antagonists, magnesium salts, methyldopa, MAO inhibitors, phenylbutazone, probenecid, salicylates, sulfinpyrazone, sulfonamides, TCAs, urinary acidifiers, alcohol (acute use)<br><br>**increased levels/effects of:** digoxin<br><br>**decreased hypoglycemic effect:** beta blockers, cholestyramine, diazoxide, hydantoins, rifampin, thiazide diuretics, urinary alkalinizers, charcoal, alcohol (chronic use) | Other effects: increased effects on total cholesterol, total triglycerides, LDL, body weight (3–8 kg).<br><br>Elderly: Use cautiously—particularly susceptible to hypoglycemic effects. Also, elderly patients may not recognize symptoms of hypoglycemia<br><br>Pharmacokinetics: onset of action = 2–4 hr; duration of action = 24 hrs; 80% metabolized in liver; renal elimination of metabolites; $T_{1/2}$ = 10 hrs | Precautions: Monitor patients closely during periods of stress (e.g., infection, etc) for poor glucose control. Use cautiously in those with severe hepatic or renal impairment.<br><br>Pregnancy Category: C<br><br>Lactation Issues: excreted in breast milk—do not give to nursing mothers. |
| **Glyburide**<br>Diabeta, Micronase, Glynase Pres Tab, various generics<br><br>Tablets: 1.25 mg, 2.5 mg, 5 mg<br><br>Tablets: micronized: 1.5 mg, 3 mg, 6 mg | **As adjunct to diet/exercise to control blood glucose in NIDDM (Type II):**<br>Non-micronized: 2.5–5 mg/d, initially. May titrate by 2.5–5 mg/d every several days up to 20 mg/d if needed, though doses >10 mg/d rarely provide added glucose lowering.<br><br>**Elderly or debilitated patients:** 1.25 mg/d initially. | Administration Issues:<br>Take with food if GI upset occurs. Avoid alcohol.<br><br>Drug–Drug Interactions:<br>**increased hypoglycemic effect:** androgens, anticoagulants, chloramphenicol, clofibrate, fenfluramine, fluconazole, ketoconazole, gemfibrozil, H₂ antagonists, magnesium salts, methyldopa, MAO inhibitors, | ADRs:<br>hypoglycemia, nausea, heartburn, epigastric fullness, allergic skin reactions, eczema, pruritus, erythema, disulfiram-like reactions (if taken with alcohol), elevated liver function tests, SIADH, photosensitivity | Contraindications:<br>Hypersensitivity, diabetes complicated by ketoacidosis with or without coma; sole therapy of Type I diabetes; diabetes complicated by pregnancy.<br><br>Precautions: Monitor patients closely during periods of stress (e.g., infection, etc) for poor |

| | Dosage | Drug–Drug Interactions | ADRs / Other Effects / Pharmacokinetics | Contraindications / Precautions |
|---|---|---|---|---|
| | Micronized: 1.5–3 mg/d, initially. May titrate by 0.75–1.5 mg/d every several days up to 12 mg/d if needed. Doses >6 mg/d may be divided into 2 doses.<br><br>**Elderly or debilitated patients:** 0.75 mg/d initially. | phenylbutazone, probenecid, salicylates, sulfinpyrazone, sulfonamides, TCAs, urinary acidifiers, alcohol (acute use)<br><br>**increased levels/effects of:** digoxin<br><br>**decreased hypoglycemic effect:** beta blockers, cholestyramine, diazoxide, hydantoins, rifampin, thiazide diuretics, urinary alkalinizers, charcoal, alcohol (chronic use) | Other effects: increased effects on total cholesterol, total triglycerides, LDL, body weight (3–8 kg).<br><br>Elderly: Use cautiously—particularly susceptible to hypoglycemic effects. Also, elderly patients may not recognize symptoms of hypoglycemia<br><br>Pharmacokinetics: onset of action = 2–4 hrs (micronized = 1 hr); duration of action = 24 hrs (for micronized and non-micronized); hepatically metabolized; renal elimination of metabolites; $T_{1/2}$ = 10 hrs (micronized = 4 hrs) | glucose control. Use cautiously in those with severe hepatic or renal impairment.<br><br>Pregnancy Category: C<br><br>Lactation Issues: excreted in breast milk—do not give to nursing mothers. |
| **Tolazamide**<br>Tolinase, various generics<br>Tablets: 100 mg, 250 mg, 500 mg | **As adjunct to diet/exercise to control blood glucose in NIDDM (Type II):**<br>100–250 mg/d, initially. If fasting glucose <200 mg/dL, use 100 mg/d; if >200 mg/dL, use 250 mg/d. May titrate to 1000 mg/d if needed. Doses >500 mg/d should be divided in two daily doses.<br><br>**Elderly or debilitated patients:** 100 mg/d | Administration Issues: Take with food if GI upset occurs. Avoid alcohol<br><br>Drug–Drug Interactions: increased hypoglycemic effect: androgens, anticoagulants, chloramphenicol, clofibrate, fenfluramine, fluconazole, ketoconazole, gemfibrozil, H₂ antagonists, magnesium salts, methyldopa, MAO inhibitors, phenylbutazone, probenecid, salicylates, sulfinpyrazone, sulfonamides, TCAs, urinary acidifiers, alcohol (acute use)<br><br>increased levels/effects of: digoxin | ADRs: hypoglycemia, nausea, heartburn, epigastric fullness, allergic skin reactions, eczema, pruritus, erythema, disulfiram-like reactions (if taken with alcohol), elevated liver function tests, SIADH, photosensitivity<br><br>Other effects: increased effects on total cholesterol, total triglycerides, LDL, body weight (3–8 kg).<br><br>Elderly: Use cautiously—particularly susceptible to | Contraindications: Hypersensitivity, diabetes complicated by ketoacidosis with or without coma; sole therapy of Type I diabetes; diabetes complicated by pregnancy.<br><br>Precautions: Monitor patients closely during periods of stress (e.g., infection, etc) for poor glucose control. Use cautiously in those with severe hepatic or renal impairment.<br><br>Pregnancy Category: C |

(continues on next page)

| Drug and Dosage Forms | Usual Dosage Range | Administration Issues and Drug–Drug Interactions | Common Adverse Drug Reactions (ADRs) and Pharmacokinetics | Contraindications, Pregnancy Category, and Lactation Issues |
|---|---|---|---|---|
| **Tolazamide** *cont.* | | **decreased hypoglycemic effect:** beta blockers, cholestyramine, diazoxide, hydantoins, rifampin, thiazide diuretics, urinary alkalinizers, charcoal, alcohol (chronic use) | hypoglycemic effects. Also, elderly patients may not recognize symptoms of hypoglycemia<br><br>Pharmacokinetics:<br>onset of action = 4–6 hrs; duration of action = 12–24 hrs; hepatically metabolized; renal elimination of metabolites; $T_{1/2}$ = 7 hrs | Lactation Issues: excreted in breast milk—do not give to nursing mothers. |
| **Tolbutamide**<br>Orinase, various generics<br><br>Tablets: 500 mg | **As adjunct to diet/exercise to control blood glucose in NIDDM (Type II):**<br><br>250 mg each morning initially. May titrate to 2 gm/d. Max of 3 gm/d. (Doses >2 gm/d usually not therapeutically beneficial). | Administration Issues:<br>Take with food if GI upset occurs. Avoid alcohol<br><br>Drug–Drug Interactions:<br>**increased hypoglycemic effect:** androgens, anticoagulants, chloramphenicol, clofibrate, fenfluramine, fluconazole, ketoconazole, gemfibrozil, $H_2$ antagonists, magnesium salts, methyldopa, MAO inhibitors, phenylbutazone, probenecid, salicylates, sulfinpyrazone, sulfonamides, TCAs, urinary acidifiers, alcohol (acute use)<br>**increased levels/effects of:** digoxin | ADRs:<br>hypoglycemia, nausea, heartburn, epigastric fullness, allergic skin reactions, eczema, pruritus, erythema, disulfiram-like reactions (if taken with alcohol), elevated liver function tests, SIADH, photosensitivity<br><br>Other effects: increased effects on total cholesterol, total triglycerides, LDL, body weight (3–8 kg).<br><br>Elderly: Use cautiously—particularly susceptible to hypoglycemic effects. Also, elderly patients may not | Contraindications:<br>Hypersensitivity, diabetes complicated by ketoacidosis with or without coma; sole therapy of Type I diabetes; diabetes complicated by pregnancy.<br><br>Precautions: Monitor patients closely during periods of stress (e.g., infection, etc) for poor glucose control. Use cautiously in those with severe hepatic or renal impairment.<br><br>Pregnancy Category: C |

| | |
|---|---|
| **decreased hypoglycemic effect:** beta blockers, cholestyramine, diazoxide, hydantoins, rifampin, thiazide diuretics, urinary alkalinizers, charcoal, alcohol (chronic use) | recognize symptoms of hypoglycemia<br><br>Pharmacokinetics:<br>onset of action = 1 hr;<br>duration of action = 6–12 hrs;<br>hepatically metabolized; renal elimination of metabolites;<br>$T_{1/2}$ = 4.5–6.5 hrs | Lactation Issues: excreted in breast milk—do not give to nursing mothers. |

## 604.2 Miscellaneous Antidiabetic Agents

| Drug and Dosage Forms | Usual Dosage Range | Administration Issues and Drug–Drug Interactions | Common Adverse Drug Reactions (ADRs) and Pharmacokinetics | Contraindications, Pregnancy Category, and Lactation Issues |
|---|---|---|---|---|
| **Acarbose**<br>Precose<br><br>Tablets:<br>25 mg, 50 mg, 100 mg | **As monotherapy as an adjunct to diet to lower blood glucose in patients with NIDDM, or as adjunctive therapy with a sulfonylurea for control of blood glucose:** Initially, 25 mg tid. Titrate the dose by 25 mg 3 times daily every 4–8 week intervals based on 1-hr postprandial glucose levels and tolerance up to 100 mg 3 times daily. Max dose is 100 mg 3 times daily for those >60kg; 50 mg 3 times daily for those <60kg. | Administration Issues:<br>Take with the start of each main meal. Patients must continue to follow regular diet & exercise program<br><br>Drug–Drug Interactions:<br>**decreased effect of acarbose:** digestive enzymes, intestinal absorbents (e.g., charcoal) | ADRs:<br>abdominal pain, diarrhea, flatulence.<br><br>Pharmacokinetics:<br><2% absorbed from GI tract (51% excreted in feces); metabolized within the GI tract (some absorbed then excreted in urine); plasma $T_{1/2}$ = 2 hrs | Contraindications:<br>Hypersensitivity; diabetic ketoacidosis; cirrhosis; inflammatory bowel disease; colonic ulcerations; partial intestinal obstruction; chronic intestinal diseases<br><br>Precautions: Monitor patients closely during periods of stress (e.g., infection, etc) for poor glucose control. Use cautiously in those with severe renal impairment.<br><br>Pregnancy Category: B<br><br>Lactation Issues: May be excreted in breast milk—do not give to nursing mothers. |

(continues on next page)

| Drug and Dosage Forms | Usual Dosage Range | Administration Issues and Drug–Drug Interactions | Common Adverse Drug Reactions (ADRs) and Pharmacokinetics | Contraindications, Pregnancy Category, and Lactation Issues |
|---|---|---|---|---|
| **Metformin**<br>Glucophage<br><br>Tablets:<br>500 mg, 850 mg | **As an adjunct to diet/exercise or sulfonylurea for the control of blood glucose in NIDDM (Type II diabetes):**<br>250 mg or 500 mg qd, initially, increasing over 2 wks to at least 1 gm. Give increased doses bid.<br><br>May also initiate therapy with 425 mg once daily. May titrate in increments of 425 mg/d every other week up to max of 2550 mg/d (in 2–3 divided doses).<br><br>**Elderly or debilitated patients:**<br>Use smaller doses, do not titrate to maximum doses. | Administration Issues:<br>Avoid alcohol. Take with food to help minimize GI effects. **Temporarily hold metformin, if possible, 24 to 48 hr prior to undergoing radiologic studies involving parenteral administration of iodinated contrast materials—can restart metformin 48 h after study if kidney function at baseline**<br><br>Drug–Drug Interactions:<br>**increased effects of metformin:** furosemide, alcohol, cationic drugs (amiloride, digoxin, morphine, etc), cimetidine, iodinated contrast material, nifedipine<br><br>**decreased levels/ effects of:** furosemide, glyburide | ADRs:<br>diarrhea, nausea, vomiting, abdominal bloating, flatulence, anorexia, unpleasant metallic taste, asymptomatic subnormal serum vitamin B12 levels<br>Rare, but potentially fatal: lactic acidosis<br><br>Other effects: increased effects on triglycerides; decreased effects on cholesterol and LDL; no change or decrease in body weight<br><br>Elderly: Use cautiously and use smaller doses, initially. Monitor renal function frequently. Not recommended in those > 80 years f age.<br><br>Pharmacokinetics:<br>50–60% bioavailable; >90% protein bound; renal elimination of unchanged drug (no hepatic metabolism); $T_{1/2}$ = 6.2 hrs | Contraindications:<br>Hypersensitivity; renal disease (SrCr >1.5 mg/dL in men, >1.4 mg/dL in women); acute or chronic metabolic acidosis (including diabetic ketoacidosis), acute MI, septicemia<br><br>Precautions: Monitor patients closely during periods of stress (e.g., infection, etc) for poor glucose control; monitor for signs of lactic acidosis<br><br>Pregnancy Category: B<br><br>Lactation Issues: Excreted in breast milk—use cautiously. |

| Drug | Indications/Dosing | Administration Issues / Drug Interactions | ADRs / Pharmacokinetics | Contraindications / Precautions |
|---|---|---|---|---|
| **Miglitol**<br>Glyset<br><br>Tablets:<br>25 mg, 50 mg, 100 mg | **As monotherapy as an adjunct to diet to lower blood glucose in patients with NIDDM, or as adjunctive therapy with a sulfonylurea for control of blood glucose:**<br>Initially, 25 mg tid. Some may need to start at 25 mg qd to minimize GI effects, then gradually increase administration to tid.<br><br>Maintenance Dose: 50 mg tid (After 4–8 weeks, increases dose to 50 mg tid; some may benefit from doses up to 100 mg tid) | Administration Issues:<br>Take drug with first bite of each main meal.<br><br>Drug Interactions:<br>**decreased effects/levels of:** digoxin, glyburide, metformin, propranolol, ranitidine<br><br>**decreased effects of miglitol by:** digestive enzymes, intestinal adsorbents (charcoal) | ADRs:<br>flatulence, diarrhea, abdominal pain, skin rash<br><br>Pharmacokinetics:<br>$T_{1/2} = 2$ h. Duration of action 4–6 hr. | Contraindications:<br>hypersensitivity to product, diabetic ketoacidosis, inflammatory bowel disease, colonic ulceration, patients predisposed to intestinal obstruction<br><br>Precaution: Not recommended in patients with SrCr >2 mg/dL<br><br>Pregnancy Category: B<br><br>Lactation Issues:<br>Miglitol is excreted in low doses in breast milk; do not administer to nursing mothers |
| **Repaglinide**<br>Prandin<br><br>Tablets: 0.5 mg, 1 mg, 2 mg | **As adjunct to diet/exercise to control blood glucose in NIDDM (Type II) or in combination with metformin:**<br><br>Initially, 0.5 mg before meals up to 4 mg before meals. Max dose = 16 mg/d | Administration Issues:<br>Take before meals. Monitor LFTs frequently and evaluate patients clinically for signs/symptoms of hepatic failure.<br><br>Drug Interactions:<br>**increased effects of repaglinide:** ketoconazole, erythromycin<br>**decreased action/effects of repaglinide:** troglitazone, rifampin, barbiturates, carbamazepine | ADRs:<br>hyperglycemia, hypoglycemia, nausea, diarrhea, arthralgia<br><br>Pharmacokinetics:<br>$T_{1/2} < 1$hr; well absorbed | Contraindications:<br>hypersensitivity to repaglinide, diabetic ketoacidosis, IDDM<br><br>Pregnancy Category: C<br><br>Lactation Issues:<br>It is not known whether repaglinide is excreted in breast milk |
| **Troglitazone**<br>Rezulin<br><br>Tablets: 200 mg, 300 mg, 400 mg | **Management of Type II DM as monotherapy, in combination with other agents and in patients currently receiving insulin but who not controlled** | Administration Issues:<br>Take with food. **Must monitor LFTs frequently. Evaluate LFTs prior to initiating therapy, monthly for the first 6 months, then once every 2 months for 6 months and then** | ADRs:<br>infection, headache, pain, asthenia, dizziness, nausea, rhinitis, diarrhea, elevations in LFTs. Increased risk of | Contraindications:<br>hypersensitivity to troglitazone<br><br>Pregnancy Category: B |

*(continues on next page)*

## 604.2 Miscellaneous Antidiabetic Agents *continued from previous page*

| Drug and Dosage Forms | Usual Dosage Range | Administration Issues and Drug–Drug Interactions | Common Adverse Drug Reactions (ADRs) and Pharmacokinetics | Contraindications, Pregnancy Category, and Lactation Issues |
|---|---|---|---|---|
| **Troglitazone** *cont.* | **(HgA1C>8.5) on >30 units insulin/d**<br><br>Initially, continue current insulin dose and start troglitazone at 200 mg qd. If not response after 2–4 wk then increase to 400 mg/d. Max dose = 600 mg/d. Insulin may be decreased by 10–25% after FBS <120 mg/dL. Individualize all insulin dosage adjustments. | **periodically continue to evaluate patients for signs/symptoms of hepatic failure.**<br><br>Drug Interactions<br>**decreased effects/levels of:** oral contraceptives, terfenadine<br>**decreased effects of troglitazone:** cholestyramine<br>**increased effects of troglitazone:** glyburide | hypoglycemia when combined with insulin.<br><br>Pharmacokinetics:<br>$T_{1/2}$ = 16–34h | Lactation Issues:<br>Do not administer to nursing mothers |

## 604.3 Insulin

| Drug and Dosage Forms | Usual Dosage Range | Administration Issues and Drug–Drug Interactions | Common Adverse Drug Reactions (ADRs) and Pharmacokinetics | Contraindications, Pregnancy Category, and Lactation Issues |
|---|---|---|---|---|
| **Lispro**<br>Humalog<br><br>Injection: 100 U/mL human insulin lispro (rDNA) | **Diabetes mellitus type I.**<br>**Dosage must be individualized**<br><br>One unit of lispro has the same glucose-lowering ability of human regular insulin but the effect is more rapid and of shorter duration | Administration Issues:<br>Use the same type and brand of syringe and insulin(s). Do not change order of mixing insulins (if applicable). When mixing insulins, draw up clear regular insulin first. Rotate injection sites. During periods of stress, monitor glucose (insulin requirements may increase). Store vial or cartridge in | ADRs:<br>Hypoglycemia, insulin allergy: (rarely: either local reactions or systemic reactions), lipoatrophy, breakdown of adipose tissue at the insulin injection site perhaps due to less pure insulins, lipohypertrophy, accumulation | Contraindications:<br>None<br><br>Precautions:  Monitor for insulin resistance (>100 u/d of insulin required).<br><br>Pregnancy:  Monitor these patients closely, blood glucose |

| Drug | Dosage | Administration / Drug–Drug Interactions | ADRs / Pharmacokinetics | Contraindications / Precautions |
|---|---|---|---|---|
| | **Adults:** 5–10 U 0–15 min before meals | refrigerator. Discard unused insulin after 28 days.<br><br>Drug–Drug Interactions:<br>**decreased hypoglycemic effect:** oral contraceptives, corticosteroids, dextrothyroxine, diltiazem, dobutamine, epinephrine, smoking, thiazide diuretics, thyroid hormone<br>**increased hypoglycemic effect:** alcohol, anabolic steroids, beta-blockers, clofibrate, guanethidine, fenfluramine, MAO inhibitors, phenylbutazone, salicylates, sulfinpyrazone, tetracyclines | of SC fat at the injection site if the same site is used continuously.<br><br>Pharmacokinetics<br>Injection SC; onset of action 0.25 hr peak = 0.5–1.5 h; duration = 6–8 h. | may be more difficult to control.<br><br>Lactation Issues: Does not pass into breast milk. Breastfeeding may decrease insulin requirements |
| **Regular Insulin**<br>Regular Iletin, Humulin R, Novolin R, Velosulin Human, various generics<br><br>Injection: 100 U/mL human insulin<br><br>Cartridge for PenFill: 100 U/mL human insulin | **Diabetes mellitus type I, or type II: Dosage must be individualized:**<br><br>**Adults/children:** 0.5–1 u/kg/day<br><br>**Adolescents during a growth phase:** 0.8–1.2 u/kg/day | Administration Issues:<br>Use the same type and brand of syringe and insulin(s). Do not change order of mixing insulins (if applicable). When mixing insulins, draw up clear regular insulin first. Rotate injection sites. During periods of stress, monitor glucose (insulin requirements may increase). Store extra insulin in refrigerator; current "in-use" insulin can be kept at room temperature. Prefilled syringes should be refrigerated and are good for 7–14 days.<br><br>Drug–Drug Interactions:<br>**decreased hypoglycemic effect:** oral contraceptives, corticosteroids, dextrothyroxine, diltiazem, dobutamine, epinephrine, smoking, thiazide diuretics, thyroid hormone | ADRs:<br>Hypoglycemia, insulin allergy: (rarely: either local reactions or systemic reactions), lipoatrophy, breakdown of adipose tissue at the insulin injection site perhaps due to less pure insulins, lipohypertrophy, accumulation of SC fat at the injection site if the same site is used continuously.<br><br>Pharmacokinetics:<br>Injection SC; onset of action = 0.5–1 hr; peak effect = 2–6 hrs; duration of action = 6–8 hrs. | Contraindications:<br>None<br><br>Precautions: Monitor for insulin resistance (>100 u/d of insulin required).<br><br>Pregnancy: Monitor these patients closely, blood glucose may be more difficult to control.<br><br>Lactation Issues: Does not pass into breast milk. Breastfeeding may decrease insulin requirements. |

(continues on next page)

| Drug and Dosage Forms | Usual Dosage Range | Administration Issues and Drug–Drug Interactions | Common Adverse Drug Reactions (ADRs) and Pharmacokinetics | Contraindications, Pregnancy Category, and Lactation Issues |
|---|---|---|---|---|
| **Regular Insulin *cont.*** | | **increased hypoglycemic effect:** alcohol, anabolic steroids, beta-blockers, clofibrate, guanethidine, fenfluramine, MAO inhibitors, phenylbutazone, salicylates, sulfinpyrazone, tetracyclines | | |
| **Isophane Insulin Suspension (NPH)** NPH Iletin, NPH-N, Humulin N, Novolin N, various generics  Injection: 100 U/mL human insulin  Cartridge for PenFill: 100 U/mL human insulin | **Diabetes mellitus type I or type II: Dosage must be individualized:**  **Adults/Children:** 0.5–1 u/kg/day  **Adolescents during a growth phase:** 0.8–1.2 u/kg/day | Administration Issues: Use the same type and brand of syringe and insulin(s). Do not change order of mixing insulins (if applicable). When mixing insulins, draw up clear regular insulin first. Rotate injection sites. During periods of stress, monitor glucose (insulin requirements may increase). Store extra insulin in refrigerator; current "in-use" insulin can be kept at room temperature. Prefilled syringes should be refrigerated and are good for 7–14 days.  Drug–Drug Interactions: **decreased hypoglycemic effect:** oral contraceptives, corticosteroids, dextrothyroxine, diltiazem, dobutamine, epinephrine, smoking, thiazide diuretics, thyroid hormone  **increased hypoglycemic effect:** alcohol, anabolic steroids, beta-blockers, clofibrate, guanethidine, | ADRs: Hypoglycemia, insulin allergy: (rarely: either local reactions or systemic reactions), lipoatrophy, breakdown of adipose tissue at the insulin injection site perhaps due to less pure insulins, lipohypertrophy, accumulation of SC fat at the injection site if the same site is used continuously.  Pharmacokinetics: Injection SC; onset of action = 1–1.5 hr; peak effect = 4–12 hrs; duration of action = 24 hrs. | Contraindications: None  Precautions: Monitor for insulin resistance (>100 u/d of insulin required).  Pregnancy: Monitor these patients closely, blood glucose may be more difficult to control.  Lactation Issues: Does not pass into breast milk. Breastfeeding may decrease insulin requirements. |

| | | | |
|---|---|---|---|
| | | fenfluramine, MAO inhibitors, phenylbutazone, salicylates, sulfinpyrazone, tetracyclines | |
| **Insulin Zinc Suspension (Lente)** Lente Iletin, Lente L, Humulin L, Novolin L Injection: 100 U/mL human, insulin | **Diabetes mellitus type I or type II: Dosage must be individualized:** **Adults/Children:** 0.5–1 u/kg/day **Adolescents during a growth phase:** 0.8–1.2 u/kg/day | Administration Issues: Use the same type and brand of syringe and insulin(s). Do not change order of mixing insulins (if applicable). When mixing insulins, draw up clear regular insulin first. Rotate injection sites. During periods of stress, monitor glucose (insulin requirements may increase). Store extra insulin in refrigerator; current "in-use" insulin can be kept at room temperature. Prefilled syringes should be refrigerated and are good for 7–14 days. Drug–Drug Interactions: **decreased hypoglycemic effect**: oral contraceptives, corticosteroids, dextrothyroxine, diltiazem, dobutamine, epinephrine, smoking, thiazide diuretics, thyroid hormone **increased hypoglycemic effect**: alcohol, anabolic steroids, beta-blockers, clofibrate, guanethidine, fenfluramine, MAO inhibitors, phenylbutazone, salicylates, sulfinpyrazone, tetracyclines | ADRs: Hypoglycemia, insulin allergy: (rarely: either local reactions or systemic reactions), lipoatrophy, breakdown of adipose tissue at the insulin injection site perhaps due to less pure insulins, lipohypertrophy, accumulation of SC fat at the injection site if the same site is used continuously. Pharmacokinetics: Injection SC; onset of action = 1–2.5 hr; peak effect = 7–15 hrs; duration of action = 24 hrs. | Contraindications: None Precautions: Monitor for insulin resistance (>100 u/d of insulin required). Pregnancy: Monitor these patients closely, blood glucose may be more difficult to control. Lactation Issues: Does not pass into breast milk. Breastfeeding may decrease insulin requirements. |
| **Insulin Zinc Suspension, Extended (Ultralente)** Ultralente U, Humulin U Ultralente | **Diabetes mellitus type I or type II: Dosage must be individualized:** **Adults/Children:** 0.5–1 u/kg/day | Administration Issues: Use the same type and brand of syringe and insulin(s). Do not change order of mixing insulins (if applicable). When mixing insulins, draw up clear regular insulin first. Rotate injection sites. During periods of stress, monitor | ADRs: Hypoglycemia, insulin allergy: (rarely: either local reactions or systemic reactions), lipoatrophy, breakdown of adipose tissue at the insulin injection site perhaps due | Contraindications: None Precautions: Monitor for insulin resistance (>100 u/d of insulin required). |

| Drug and Dosage Forms | Usual Dosage Range | Administration Issues and Drug–Drug Interactions | Common Adverse Drug Reactions (ADRs) and Pharmacokinetics | Contraindications, Pregnancy Category, and Lactation Issues |
|---|---|---|---|---|
| **Insulin Zinc Suspension, Extended (Ultralente)** *cont.*<br><br>Injection: 100 U/mL human insulin | **Adolescents during a growth phase:** 0.8–1.2 u/kg/day | glucose (insulin requirements may increase). Store extra insulin in refrigerator; current "in-use" insulin can be kept at room temperature. Prefilled syringes should be refrigerated and are good for 7–14 days.<br><br>Drug–Drug Interactions:<br>**decreased hypoglycemic effect:**<br>oral contraceptives, corticosteroids, dextrothyroxine, diltiazem, dobutamine, epinephrine, smoking, thiazide diuretics, thyroid hormone<br>**increased hypoglycemic effect:**<br>alcohol, anabolic steroids, beta-blockers, clofibrate, guanethidine, fenfluramine, MAO inhibitors, phenylbutazone, salicylates, sulfinpyrazone, tetracyclines | to less pure insulins, lipohypertrophy, accumulation of SC fat at the injection site if the same site is used continuously.<br><br>Pharmacokinetics<br>Injection SC;<br>onset of action = 4–8 hr;<br>peak effect = 10–30 hrs;<br>duration of action = >36 hrs | Pregnancy: Monitor these patients closely, blood glucose may be more difficult to control.<br><br>Lactation Issues: Does not pass into breast milk. Breastfeeding may decrease insulin requirements. |
| **Combination Isophane Insulin Suspension & Regular Insulin (50%/50%)**<br>Humulin 50/50<br><br>Injection: 100 U/mL human insulin | **Diabetes mellitus type I, or type II: Dosage must be individualized:**<br><br>**Adults/Children:** 0.5–1 u/kg/day<br><br>**Adolescents during a growth phase:** 0.8–1.2 u/kg/day | Administration Issues:<br>Use the same type and brand of syringe and insulin(s). Do not change order of mixing insulins (if applicable). When mixing insulins, draw up clear regular insulin first. Rotate injection sites. During periods of stress, monitor glucose (insulin requirements may increase). Store extra insulin in refrigerator; current "in-use" insulin can be kept at room temperature. Prefilled | ADRs:<br>Hypoglycemia, insulin allergy: (rarely: either local reactions or systemic reactions), lipoatrophy, breakdown of adipose tissue at the insulin injection site perhaps due to less pure insulins, lipohypertrophy, accumulation of SC fat at the injection site if the same site is used continuously. | Contraindications:<br>None<br><br>Precautions: Monitor for insulin resistance (>100 u/d of insulin required).<br><br>Pregnancy: Monitor these patients closely, blood glucose may be more difficult to control. |

| | | | Pharmacokinetics: | Lactation Issues: Does not pass |
|---|---|---|---|---|

| Drug | Dosage | Administration / Interactions | Pharmacokinetics | Contraindications / Precautions / Lactation |
|---|---|---|---|---|
| | | syringes should be refrigerated and are good for 7–14 days.<br><br>Drug–Drug Interactions:<br>**decreased hypoglycemic effect**: oral contraceptives, corticosteroids, dextrothyroxine, diltiazem, dobutamine, epinephrine, smoking, thiazide diuretics, thyroid hormone<br>**increased hypoglycemic effect**: alcohol, anabolic steroids, beta-blockers, clofibrate, guanethidine, fenfluramine, MAO inhibitors, phenylbutazone, salicylates, sulfinpyrazone, tetracyclines | Pharmacokinetics:<br>**Regular:** Injection SC; onset of action = 0.5–1 hr; peak effect = 5–10 h; duration of action = 6–8 h<br><br>**NPH:** Injection SC; onset of action = 1–1.5 h; peak effect = 4–12 h; duration of action = 24 h | Lactation Issues: Does not pass into breast milk. Breastfeeding may decrease insulin requirements. |
| **Combination Isophane Insulin Suspension & Regular Insulin (70/30)**<br><br>Humulin 70/30, Novolin 70/30<br><br>Injection: 100 U/mL human insulin<br><br>Cartridge for PenFill: 100 U/mL human insulin | **Diabetes mellitus type I or type II: Dosage must be individualized:**<br><br>**Adults/children:** 0.5–1 u/kg/day<br><br>**Adolescents during a growth phase:** 0.8–1.2 u/kg/day | Administration Issues:<br>Use the same type and brand of syringe and insulin(s). Do not change order of mixing insulins (if applicable). When mixing insulins, draw up clear regular insulin first. Rotate injection sites. During periods of stress, monitor glucose (insulin requirements may increase). Store extra insulin in refrigerator; current "in-use" insulin can be kept at room temperature. Prefilled syringes should be refrigerated and are good for 7–14 days.<br><br>Drug–Drug Interactions:<br>**decreased hypoglycemic effect:** oral contraceptives, corticosteroids, dextrothyroxine, diltiazem, dobutamine, epinephrine, smoking, thiazide diuretics, thyroid hormone | ADRs:<br>Hypoglycemia, insulin allergy: (rarely: either local reactions or systemic reactions), lipoatrophy, breakdown of adipose tissue at the insulin injection site perhaps due to less pure insulins, lipohypertrophy, accumulation of SC fat at the injection site if the same site is used continuously.<br><br>Pharmacokinetics:<br>**Regular:** Injection SC; onset of action = 0.5–1 hr; peak effect = 5–10 h; duration of action = 6–8 h | Contraindications:<br>None<br><br>Precautions: Monitor for insulin resistance (>100 u/d of insulin required).<br><br>Pregnancy: Monitor these patients closely, blood glucose may be more difficult to control.<br><br>Lactation Issues: Does not pass into breast milk. Breastfeeding may decrease insulin requirements. |

*(continues on next page)*

| Drug and Dosage Forms | Usual Dosage Range | Administration Issues and Drug–Drug Interactions | Common Adverse Drug Reactions (ADRs) and Pharmacokinetics | Contraindications, Pregnancy Category, and Lactation Issues |
|---|---|---|---|---|
| **Combination Isophane Insulin Suspension & Regular Insulin (70/30) *cont.*** | | **increased hypoglycemic effect:** alcohol, anabolic steroids, beta-blockers, clofibrate, guanethidine, fenfluramine, MAO inhibitors, phenylbutazone, salicylates, sulfinpyrazone, tetracyclines | **NPH:** Injection SC; onset of action = 1–1.5 hr; peak effect = 4–12 h; duration of action = 24 h | |

## 605. Estrogen and Progestin Products
605.1 Estrogens

| Drug and Dosage Forms | Usual Dosage Range | Administration Issues and Drug–Drug Interactions | Common Adverse Drug Reactions (ADRs) and Pharmacokinetics | Contraindications, Pregnancy Category, and Lactation Issues |
|---|---|---|---|---|
| **Conjugated Estrogens** Premarin <u>Tablets:</u> 0.3 mg, 0.625 mg, 0.9 mg, 1.25 mg, 2.5 mg | **Use cyclical pattern of therapy (3 weeks on, 1 week off) unless otherwise specified.** **Vasomotor symptoms associated with menopause, female castration or primary ovarian failure:** 1.25 mg/d initially. Titrate to patient response **Atrophic vaginitis, kraurosis vulvae:** 0.3–1.25 mg/d. | <u>Administration Issues:</u> Avoid prolonged exposure to sunlight <u>Drug–Drug Interactions:</u> **increased levels/effects of:** corticosteroids **decreased levels/effects of:** anticoagulants, hydantoins **decreased levels/effects of estrogens:** hydantoins, barbiturates, rifampin | <u>ADRs:</u> breakthrough bleeding, spotting, dysmenorrhea, PMS-like syndrome, amenorrhea, vaginal candidiasis, hemolytic uremic syndrome; endometrial cystic hyperplasia, nausea, vomiting, abdominal cramps, bloating, photosensitivity; urticaria, dermatitis, headache, dizziness, depression, edema, changes in libido, breast tenderness or enlargement | <u>Contraindications:</u> Hypersensitivity; breast cancer (some exceptions); active thrombophlebitis; thromboembolic disorders; estrogen-dependent neoplasia; undiagnosed abnormal genital bleeding; pregnancy. <u>Precautions:</u> Use cautiously in those with hepatic or renal dysfunction; monitor serum calcium. |

| Dosage | Administration / Drug Interactions | Pharmacokinetics / ADRs | Contraindications / Pregnancy |
|---|---|---|---|
| **Hypogonadism:** 2.5–7.5 mg/d in divided doses for 20 days, followed by rest period of 10 days.<br><br>**Breast Cancer:** 10 mg tid for 3 months (do not use cyclical therapy).<br><br>**Prostatic carcinoma:** 1.25–2.5 mg tid (do not use cyclical therapy)<br><br>**Osteoporosis:** 0.625 mg/d<br><br>**Stress Urinary Incontinence** 0.3 to 1.25 mg qd continuous or cyclic (days 1–25) | | Pharmacokinetics: Oral or transdermal; 98% protein bound; hepatically metabolized | Pregnancy Category: X<br><br>Lactation Issues: excreted in breast milk. Use only if benefit clearly outweighs risk. |
| **Esterified Estrogens**<br>Estratab, Menest<br><br>Tablets: 0.3 mg, 0.625 mg, 1.25 mg, 2.5 mg<br><br>**Use cyclical pattern of therapy (3 weeks on, 1 week off) unless otherwise specified.**<br><br>**Vasomotor symptoms associated with menopause, atrophic vaginitis, kraurosis vulvae:** 0.3–1.25 mg/d. Titrate to patient response.<br><br>**Hypogonadism:** 2.5–7.5 mg/d in divided doses for 20 days, followed by rest period of 10 days.<br><br>**Female castration or primary ovarian failure:** 1.25 mg/d<br><br>**Breast Cancer:** 10 mg tid for 3 months. (do not use cyclical therapy)<br><br>**Prostatic carcinoma:** 1.25–2.5 mg tid (do not use cyclical therapy) | Administration Issues: Avoid prolonged exposure to sunlight<br><br>Drug–Drug Interactions:<br>**increased levels/effects of:** corticosteroids<br>**decreased levels/effects of:** anticoagulants, hydantoins<br>**decreased levels/effects of estrogens:** hydantoins, barbiturates, rifampin | ADRs:<br>breakthrough bleeding, spotting, dysmenorrhea, PMS-like syndrome, amenorrhea, vaginal candidiasis, hemolytic uremic syndrome; endometrial cystic hyperplasia, nausea, vomiting, abdominal cramps, bloating, photosensitivity; urticaria, dermatitis, headache, dizziness, depression, edema, changes in libido, breast tenderness or enlargement<br><br>Pharmacokinetics: Oral or transdermal; 98% protein bound; hepatically metabolized | Contraindications: Hypersensitivity; breast cancer (some exceptions); active thrombophlebitis; thromboembolic disorders; estrogen-dependent neoplasia; undiagnosed abnormal genital bleeding; pregnancy.<br><br>Precautions: Use cautiously in those with hepatic or renal dysfunction; monitor serum calcium.<br><br>Pregnancy Category: X<br><br>Lactation Issues: excreted in breast milk. Use only if benefit clearly outweighs risk. |

(continues on next page)

| Drug and Dosage Forms | Usual Dosage Range | Administration Issues and Drug–Drug Interactions | Common Adverse Drug Reactions (ADRs) and Pharmacokinetics | Contraindications, Pregnancy Category, and Lactation Issues |
|---|---|---|---|---|
| **Estradiol**<br>Estrace<br><br>Tablets: 0.5 mg, 1 mg, 2 mg<br><br>**Estradiol**<br>**Transdermal System**<br>Vivelle, Climara, Estraderm, Alora, Fempatch<br><br>Patch:<br>0.025 mg/24 hr<br>0.0375 mg/24 hr<br>0.05 mg/24 hr<br>0.075 mg/24 hr<br>0.1 mg/24 hr | **Vasomotor symptoms associated with menopause, atrophic vaginitis, kraurosis vulvae, hypogonadism:**<br>Oral: 1–2 mg/d. Titrate to patient response.<br><br>**Breast Cancer:**<br>Oral: 10 mg tid for at least 3 months.<br><br>**Prostatic carcinoma:** 1–2 mg tid<br><br>**Osteoporosis:** 0.5 mg/d for 23 days, then 5 days off. Continue the cycle.<br><br>Transdermal for all indications:<br>0.05 mg/d system initially. For the Estraderm and Vivelle systems, must apply twice weekly. The Climara patch is applied once weekly. Titrate dose based on patient response. For patients with an intact uterus, therapy is given on a cyclical basis (3 weeks of therapy, 1 week off); if not, therapy is continuous. | Administration Issues:<br>Avoid prolonged exposure to sunlight. Apply patch to clean, dry area on the trunk of the body (including buttocks and abdomen)<br><br>Drug–Drug Interactions:<br>**increased levels/effects of:** corticosteroids<br>**decreased levels/effects of:** anticoagulants, hydantoins<br>**decreased levels/effects of estrogens:** hydantoins, barbiturates, rifampin | ADRs:<br>breakthrough bleeding, spotting, dysmenorrhea, PMS-like syndrome, amenorrhea, vaginal candidiasis, hemolytic uremic syndrome; endometrial cystic hyperplasia, nausea, vomiting, abdominal cramps, bloating, photosensitivity; urticaria, dermatitis, headache, dizziness, depression, edema, changes in libido, breast tenderness or enlargement<br><br>Pharmacokinetics:<br>Oral or transdermal; 98% protein bound; hepatically metabolized | Contraindications:<br>Hypersensitivity; breast cancer (some exceptions); active thrombophlebitis; thromboembolic disorders; estrogen-dependent neoplasia; undiagnosed abnormal genital bleeding; pregnancy.<br><br>Precautions: Use cautiously in those with hepatic or renal dysfunction; monitor serum calcium.<br><br>Pregnancy Category: X<br><br>Lactation Issues: excreted in breast milk. Use only if benefit clearly outweighs risk. |
| **Estropipate**<br>Ortho-Est, Ogen, various generics | **Use cyclical pattern of therapy (3 weeks on, 1 week off) unless otherwise specified.** | Administration Issues:<br>Avoid prolonged exposure to sunlight. | ADRs:<br>breakthrough bleeding, spotting, dysmenorrhea, PMS-like syndrome, amenorrhea, | Contraindications:<br>Hypersensitivity; breast cancer (some exceptions); active thrombophlebitis; |

| | | | | |
|---|---|---|---|---|
| Tablets:<br>0.625 mg (0.75 mg estropipate)<br>1.25 mg (1.5 mg estropipate)<br>2.5 mg (3 mg estropipate) | **Vasomotor symptoms associated with menopause, atrophic vaginitis, kraurosis vulvae:**<br>0.625–5 mg/d given for 25 days of a 31 day cycle.<br><br>**Hypogonadism, female castration, primary ovarian failure:** 1.25–7.5 mg/d given cyclically.<br><br>**Osteoporosis:** 0.625 mg qd for 25 days of a 31 day cycle. | Drug–Drug Interactions:<br>**increased levels/effects of:** corticosteroids<br>**decreased levels/effects of:** anticoagulants, hydantoins<br>**decreased levels/effects of estrogens:** hydantoins, barbiturates, rifampin | vaginal candidiasis, hemolytic uremic syndrome; endometrial cystic hyperplasia, nausea, vomiting, abdominal cramps, bloating, photosensitivity; urticaria, dermatitis, headache, dizziness, depression, edema, changes in libido, breast tenderness or enlargement<br><br>Pharmacokinetics:<br>Oral or transdermal; 98% protein bound; hepatically metabolized | thromboembolic disorders; estrogen-dependent neoplasia; undiagnosed abnormal genital bleeding; pregnancy.<br><br>Precautions: Use cautiously in those with hepatic or renal dysfunction; monitor serum calcium.<br><br>Pregnancy Category: X<br><br>Lactation Issues: excreted in breast milk. Use only if benefit clearly outweighs risk. |
| **Ethinyl Estradiol**<br>Estinyl<br><br>Tablets: 0.02 mg, 0.05 mg, 0.5 mg | **Use cyclical pattern of therapy (3 weeks on, 1 week off) unless otherwise specified.**<br><br>Vasomotor symptoms associated with menopause, atrophic vaginitis, kraurosis vulvae: 0.02–0.05 mg/d.<br><br>**Hypogonadism, female castration, primary ovarian failure:** 0.05 mg 1-tid during 1st 2 weeks of theoretical menstrual cycle followed by progestin during last half of arbitrary cycle. Continue for 3–6 months.<br>**Breast Cancer:** 1 mg tid given chronically.<br><br>**Prostatic Carcinoma:**<br>0.15–2 mg/d given chronically. | Administration Issues:<br>Avoid prolonged exposure to sunlight<br><br>Drug–Drug Interactions:<br>**increased levels/effects of:** corticosteroids<br>**decreased levels/effects of:** anticoagulants, hydantoins<br>**decreased levels/effects of estrogens:** hydantoins, barbiturates, rifampin | ADRs:<br>breakthrough bleeding, spotting, dysmenorrhea, PMS-like syndrome, amenorrhea, vaginal candidiasis, hemolytic uremic syndrome; endometrial cystic hyperplasia, nausea, vomiting, abdominal cramps, bloating, photosensitivity; urticaria, dermatitis, headache, dizziness, depression, edema, changes in libido, breast tenderness or enlargement<br><br>Pharmacokinetics:<br>Oral or transdermal; 98% protein bound; hepatically metabolized | Contraindications:<br>Hypersensitivity; breast cancer (some exceptions); active thrombophlebitis; thromboembolic disorders; estrogen-dependent neoplasia; undiagnosed abnormal genital bleeding; pregnancy.<br><br>Precautions: Use cautiously in those with hepatic or renal dysfunction; monitor serum calcium.<br><br>Pregnancy Category: X<br><br>Lactation Issues: excreted in breast milk. Use only if benefit clearly outweighs risk. |

*(continues on next page)*

| Drug and Dosage Forms | Usual Dosage Range | Administration Issues and Drug–Drug Interactions | Common Adverse Drug Reactions (ADRs) and Pharmacokinetics | Contraindications, Pregnancy Category, and Lactation Issues |
|---|---|---|---|---|
| **Quinestrol**<br>Estrovis<br><br><u>Tablets:</u> 100 mcg | **Vasomotor symptoms associated with menopause, atrophic vaginitis, kraurosis vulvae, hypogonadism, female castration, primary ovarian failure:** 100 mcg daily for 7 days, then 100 mcg once weekly for maintenance starting 2 weeks after treatment begins. Titrate to 200 mcg/week if needed. | <u>Administration Issues:</u><br>Avoid prolonged exposure to sunlight<br><br><u>Drug–Drug Interactions:</u><br>**increased levels/effects of:** corticosteroids<br>**decreased levels/effects of:** anticoagulants, hydantoins<br>**decreased levels/effects of estrogens:** hydantoins, barbiturates, rifampin | <u>ADRs:</u><br>breakthrough bleeding, spotting, dysmenorrhea, PMS-like syndrome, amenorrhea, vaginal candidiasis, hemolytic uremic syndrome; endometrial cystic hyperplasia, nausea, vomiting, abdominal cramps, bloating, photosensitivity; urticaria, dermatitis, headache, dizziness, depression, edema, changes in libido, breast tenderness or enlargement<br><br><u>Pharmacokinetics:</u><br>Oral or transdermal; 98% protein bound; hepatically metabolized | <u>Contraindications:</u><br>Hypersensitivity; breast cancer (some exceptions); active thrombophlebitis; thromboembolic disorders; estrogen-dependent neoplasia; undiagnosed abnormal genital bleeding; pregnancy.<br><br><u>Precautions:</u> Use cautiously in those with hepatic or renal dysfunction; monitor serum calcium.<br><br><u>Pregnancy Category:</u> X<br><br><u>Lactation Issues:</u> excreted in breast milk. Use only if benefit clearly outweighs risk. |
| **Vaginal Estrogens**<br>Vaginal Creams and Ring<br><br><u>Ogen Cream:</u> 1.5 mg estropipate<br><br><u>Premarin Cream:</u> 0.625 mg conj, estrogens/g<br><br><u>Ortho Dienestrol Cream:</u> 0.01% dienestrol | **Atrophic vaginitis, kraurosis vulvae associated with menopause:**<br><br>**Estropipate and conjugated estrogen:**<br>Administer cyclically: 3 wks on and 1 wk off. Give 0.5 to 2 g daily of conjugated and 2 to 4 g daily of estropipate intravaginally | <u>Administration Issues:</u><br>Avoid prolonged exposure to sunlight. Cream: insert high into the vagina (the length of the applicator). Ring: press the ring into an oval and insert into the upper third of the vaginal vault.<br><br><u>Drug–Drug Interactions:</u><br>**increased levels/effects of:** corticosteroids | <u>ADRs:</u><br>breakthrough bleeding, spotting, dysmenorrhea, PMS-like syndrome, amenorrhea, vaginal candidiasis, hemolytic uremic syndrome; endometrial cystic hyperplasia, nausea, vomiting, abdominal cramps, bloating, photosensitivity; urticaria, dermatitis, headache, | <u>Contraindications:</u><br>Hypersensitivity; breast cancer (some exceptions); active thrombophlebitis; thromboembolic disorders; estrogen-dependent neoplasia; undiagnosed abnormal genital bleeding; pregnancy. |

| | | | |
|---|---|---|---|
| Estrace Cream: 0.1 mg estradiol/g<br><br>Estring: 2 mg estradiol/ring | depending on severity of condition.<br><br>**Dienestrol:** 1 applicatorful 1–2 times daily for 1 or 2 wks, then reduce to one-half the inital dose for a similar period. A maintenance dose of 1 applicatorful 1 to 3 times/wk may be used after restoration of vaginal mucosa.<br><br>**Estradiol:**<br>Cream: 2 to 4 g daily for 2 wk. Gradually reduce dose to one-half initial dosage for a similar period. A maintenance dose of 1 g 1 to 3 times/wk may be used after restoration of vaginal mucosa.<br><br>Ring: insert deeply as possible unto the upper one-third of the vaginal vault. The ring should remain in place continuosly for 3 months, then removed and replace by a new ring, if indicated. Assess need for continuation at 3 or 6 month interval. | **decreased levels/effects of:** anticoagulants, hydantoins<br>**decreased levels/effects of estrogens:** hydantoins, barbiturates, rifampin | |
| | | dizziness, depression, edema, changes in libido, breast tenderness or enlargement | **Precautions:** Use cautiously in those with hepatic or renal dysfunction; monitor serum calcium.<br><br>**Pregnancy Category:** X<br><br>**Lactation Issues:** excreted in breast milk. Use only if benefit clearly outweighs risk. |

| Drug and Dosage Forms | Usual Dosage Range | Administration Issues, Drug–Drug & Drug–Lab Interactions | Common Adverse Drug Reactions (ADRs) | Contraindications, Pregnancy Category, and Lactation Issues |
|---|---|---|---|---|
| **Medroxyprogesterone**<br>Cycrin, Provera, Amen, Curretab, various generics<br><br>Tablets: 2.5 mg, 5 mg, 10 mg | **Secondary amenorrhea:**<br>5–10 mg/d for 5–10 days<br><br>**Abnormal uterine bleeding:**<br>5–10 mg/d for 5–10 days beginning on the 16th or 21st day of the cycle<br><br>**Stress Urinary Incontinence:**<br>2.5 to 10 mg qd, continuous or cyclic (days 16–25 if uterus present) | Administration Issues:<br>Take with food if GI upset occurs<br><br>Drug–Drug Interactions:<br>**decreased levels/effects of progestin:**<br>aminoglutethimide, rifampin<br><br>Drug–Lab Interaction:<br>the following tests may be affected by progestins: hepatic function, coagulation, thyroid, metyrapone, and endocrine function. | ADRs:<br>insomnia, somnolence, mental depression, rash, acne, melasma, changes in weight, breakthrough bleeding, spotting, change in menstrual flow, amenorrhea, changes in cervical secretions, breast changes, masculinization of the female fetus, edema, cholestatic jaundice, hirsutism. | Contraindications:<br>Hypersensitivity, thrombophlebitis, thromboembolic disorders, cerebral hemorrhage, impaired liver function, carcinoma of the breast or genital organs, undiagnosed vaginal bleeding, missed abortion, for use as a diagnostic test for pregnancy.<br><br>Pregnancy Category: D<br><br>Lactation Issues: small amounts excreted in breast milk—effects on infant not known. |
| **Megestrol**<br>Megace<br><br>Suspension: 40 mg/mL | **Appetite enhancement in AIDS patients, palliative treatment of advanced breast or endometrium cancer:**<br>800 mg/d. Titrate based on patient response to range of 400–800 mg/d. | Administration Issues:<br>Store at room temperature, protect from heat. Safety/efficacy in children is not established<br><br>Drug–Drug Interactions:<br>**decreased levels/effects of progestin:**<br>aminoglutethimide, rifampin<br><br>Drug–Lab Interaction:<br>the following tests may be affected by progestins: hepatic function, coagulation, thyroid, metyrapone, and endocrine function. | ADRs:<br>impotence, rash, diarrhea, insomnia, fever, headache, hypertension | Contraindications:<br>Hypersensitivity, pregnancy, prophylactic use to avoid weight loss; for use as a diagnostic test for pregnancy.<br><br>Pregnancy Category: D<br><br>Lactation Issues: small amounts excreted in breast milk—effects on infant not known. |

# Norethindrone

| Drug and Dosage Forms | Usual Dosage Range | Administration Issues, Drug–Drug & Drug–Lab Interactions | Common Adverse Drug Reactions (ADRs) and Pharmacokinetics | Contraindications, Pregnancy Category, and Lactation Issues |
|---|---|---|---|---|
| **Norethindrone**<br>Aygestin<br><br><u>Tablets:</u> 5 mg | **Amenorrhea, abnormal uterine bleeding:** 2.5–10 mg/d for 5–10 days during 2nd half of menstrual cycle.<br><br>**Endometriosis:** 5 mg/d for 2 weeks. Titrate by 2.5 mg/d every 2 weeks until 15 mg/d is reached. Continue for 6–9 months. | <u>Administration Issues:</u><br>Take with food if GI upset occurs<br><br><u>Drug–Drug Interactions:</u><br>**decreased levels/effects of progestin:**<br>aminoglutethimide, rifampin<br><br><u>Drug–Lab Interaction:</u><br>the following tests may be affected by progestins: hepatic function, coagulation, thyroid, metyrapone, and endocrine function. | <u>ADRs:</u><br>insomnia, somnolence, mental depression, rash, acne, melasma, changes in weight, breakthrough bleeding, spotting, change in menstrual flow, amenorrhea, changes in cervical secretions, breast changes, masculinization of the female fetus, edema, cholestatic jaundice, hirsutism. | <u>Contraindications:</u><br>Hypersensitivity, thrombophlebitis, thromboembolic disorders, cerebral hemorrhage, impaired liver function, carcinoma of the breast or genital organs, undiagnosed vaginal bleeding, missed abortion, for use as a diagnostic test for pregnancy.<br><br><u>Pregnancy Category:</u> D<br><br><u>Lactation Issues:</u> small amounts excreted in breast milk—effects on infant not known. |

## 605.3 Estrogen/Progestin Combinations

| Drug and Dosage Forms | Usual Dosage Range | Administration Issues, Drug–Drug & Drug–Lab Interactions | Common Adverse Drug Reactions (ADRs) and Pharmacokinetics | Contraindications, Pregnancy Category, and Lactation Issues |
|---|---|---|---|---|
| **Conjugated estrogens & medroxyprogesterone acetate**<br><br>Premphase<br><u>Tablets:</u> 0.625 mg estrogen alone and the combination of 0.625 mg/5 mg | **Symptoms associated with menopause, Vulvar/Vaginal Atrophy, prevention of osteoporosis**<br>combination tablet qd or 0.625 mg estrogen qd days 1–14 & combination 0.625 mg/5 mg qd days 15–28 | <u>Administration Issues:</u><br>Avoid prolonged exposure to sunlight.<br><br><u>Drug–Drug Interactions:</u><br>**increased levels/effects of:**<br>corticosteroids<br>**decreased levels/effects of:**<br>anticoagulants, hydantoins<br>**decreased levels/effects of estrogens:**<br>hydantoins, barbiturates, rifampin | <u>ADRs:</u><br>Estrogen<br>breakthrough bleeding, spotting, dysmenorrhea, PMS-like syndrome, amenorrhea, vaginal candidiasis, hemolytic uremic syndrome; endometrial cystic hyperplasia, nausea, vomiting, abdominal cramps, bloating, photosensitivity, urticaria, dermatitis, headache, | <u>Contraindications:</u><br>Hypersensitivity; breast cancer (some exceptions); active thromboembolic disorders; estrogen-dependent neoplasia; undiagnosed abnormal genital bleeding; pregnancy, for use as a diagnostic test for pregnancy. |

(continues on next page)

| Drug and Dosage Forms | Usual Dosage Range | Administration Issues, Drug–Drug & Drug–Lab Interactions | Common Adverse Drug Reactions (ADRs) and Pharmacokinetics | Contraindications, Pregnancy Category, and Lactation Issues |
|---|---|---|---|---|
| **Conjugated estrogens & medroxyprogesterone acetate** *cont.*<br>Prempro<br><u>Tablets</u>: 0.625 mg/2.5 mg (in combination) | | **decreased levels/effects of progestin:**<br>aminoglutethimide, rifampin<br><br><u>Drug–Lab Interaction:</u><br>the following tests may be affected by progestins: hepatic function, coagulation, thyroid, metyrapone, and endocrine function | dizziness, depression, edema, changes in libido, breast tenderness or enlargement<br><br>**Progestin**<br>insomnia, somnolence, mental depression, rash, acne, melasma, photosensitivity, changes in weight, breakthrough bleeding, spotting, change in menstrual flow, amenorrhea, changes in cervical secretions, breast changes, masculinization of the female fetus, edema, cholestatic jaundice, hirsutism.<br><br><u>Pharmacokinetics:</u><br>see individual drugs | <u>Precautions:</u> Use cautiously in those with hepatic or renal dysfunction; monitor serum calcium.<br><br><u>Pregnancy Category:</u> X<br><br><u>Lactation Issues:</u> excreted in breast milk. Use only if benefit clearly outweighs risk. |
| **Mestranol & Norethynodrel**<br>Enovid<br><br><u>Tablets</u>: 75 mcg/5 mg<br>150 mcg/9.85 mg | **Endometriosis:**<br>5–10 mg/d for 2 weeks beginning on day 5 of the menstrual cycle. Titrate by 5–10 mg/d every 2 weeks up to 20 mg/d (up to 40 mg/d if breakthrough bleeding occurs). Continue dose for 6–9 months.<br><br>**Hypermenorrhea:** 20–30 mg/d until bleeding is controlled, then | <u>Administration Issues:</u><br>Avoid prolonged exposure to sunlight.<br><br><u>Drug–Drug Interactions:</u><br>**increased levels/effects of:**<br>corticosteroids<br>**decreased levels/effects of:**<br>anticoagulants, hydantoins | **ADRs:**<br><u>Estrogen</u><br>breakthrough bleeding, spotting, dysmenorrhea, PMS-like syndrome, amenorrhea, vaginal candidiasis, hemolytic uremic syndrome; endometrial cystic hyperplasia, nausea, vomiting, abdominal cramps, bloating, photosensitivity; | <u>Contraindications:</u><br>Hypersensitivity; breast cancer (some exceptions); active thrombophlebitis; thromboembolic disorders; estrogen-dependent neoplasia; undiagnosed abnormal genital bleeding; pregnancy, for use as a diagnostic test for pregnancy. |

| | | | |
|---|---|---|---|
| reduce to 10 mg/d and continue through day 24 of the cycle. | **decreased levels/effects of estrogens:** hydantoins, barbiturates, rifampin<br><br>**decreased levels/effects of progestin:** aminoglutethimide, rifampin<br><br>Drug–Lab Interaction: the following tests may be affected by progestins: hepatic function, coagulation, thyroid, metyrapone, and endocrine function | urticaria, dermatitis, headache, dizziness, depression, edema, changes in libido, breast tenderness or enlargement<br><br>**Progestin**<br>insomnia, somnolence, mental depression, rash, acne, melasma, photosensitivity, changes in weight, breakthrough bleeding, spotting, change in menstrual flow, amenorrhea, changes in cervical secretions, breast changes, masculinization of the female fetus, edema, cholestatic jaundice, hirsutism.<br><br>Pharmacokinetics: see individual drugs | Precautions: Use cautiously in those with hepatic or renal dysfunction; monitor serum calcium.<br><br>Pregnancy Category: X<br><br>Lactation Issues: excreted in breast milk. Use only if benefit clearly outweighs risk. |

605.4 Estrogen/Androgen Combinations

| Drug and Dosage Forms | Usual Dosage Range | Administration Issues and Drug–Drug Interactions | Common Adverse Drug Reactions (ADRs) and Pharmacokinetics | Contraindications, Pregnancy Category, and Lactation Issues |
|---|---|---|---|---|
| **Estratest**<br><br>Tablets:<br>1.25 mg esterified estrogens/ 2.5 mg methyltestosterone<br><br>**Estratest H.S.**<br><br>Tablets:<br>0.625 mg esterified estrogens/1.25 mg methyltestosterone | **Moderate to severe vasomotor symptoms associated with menopause in those patients not improved by estrogen alone**<br><br>1 tablet Estratest or 1 to 2 tablets Estratest HS | Administration Issues:<br>Administration should be cyclic (e.g. three wk on and one wk off). Attempts to discontinue or taper medication should be done at three to six month intervals.<br><br>Drug–Drug Interactions:<br>**increased levels/effects of:** corticosteroids, imipramine (increased paranoid symptoms)<br>**decreased levels/effects of:** hydantoins<br>**decreased levels/effects of estrogens:** hydantoins, barbiturates, rifampin<br><br>**variable effects:** may increase or decrease effects of anticoagulants | ADRs:<br>Estrogen:<br>breakthrough bleeding, spotting, dysmenorrhea, PMS-like syndrome, amenorrhea, vaginal candidiasis, hemolytic uremic syndrome; endometrial cystic hyperplasia, nausea, vomiting, abdominal cramps, bloating, photosensitivity; urticaria, dermatitis, headache, dizziness, depression, edema, changes in libido, breast tenderness or enlargement<br><br>Methyltestosterone:<br>amenorrhea, other menstrual irregularities, virilization (deepening of voice, clitoral enlargement)<br><br>Pharmacokinetics:<br>hepatically metabolized | Contraindications:<br>Hypersensitivity; breast cancer (some exceptions); active thrombophlebitis; thromboembolic disorders; estrogen-dependent neoplasia; undiagnosed abnormal genital bleeding; pregnancy; breastfeeding; presence of severe liver damage<br><br>Precautions:  Use cautiously in those with hepatic or renal dysfunction; monitor serum calcium.<br><br>Pregnancy Category:  X<br><br>Lactation Issues:  Do not use |

## 605.5 Selective Estrogen Receptor Modulators

| Drug and Dosage Forms | Usual Dosage Range | Administration Issues and Drug–Drug Interactions | Common Adverse Drug Reactions (ADRs) and Pharmacokinetics | Contraindications, Pregnancy Category, and Lactation Issues |
|---|---|---|---|---|
| **Raloxifene**<br>Evista<br><br><u>Tablets:</u> 60 mg | **Prevention of Osteoporosis in Postmenopausal Women:**<br><br>60 mg daily | <u>Administration Issues:</u><br>May be taken any time of day without regards to meals. Discontinue raloxifine at least 72 hr before periods of prolonged immobilization and avoid prolonged restrictions of movement during travel due to increased risk of venous thromboembolic events. Raloxifene is not effective in reducing hot flashed or flushes.<br><br><u>Drug–Drug Interactions:</u><br>**decreased levels/effects of:** warfarin (decreases seen in PT)<br>**decreased levels/effects of raloxifine:** ampicillin (though both can be given concurrently), cholestyramine (avoid coadministration) | <u>ADRs:</u><br>hot flashes, leg cramps, abdominal pain, nausea, weight gain, arthralgia<br><br><u>Pharmacokinetics:</u><br>$T_{1/2} = 32$ hr; undergoes extensive first-pass metabolism | <u>Contraindications:</u><br>Hypersensitivity; women who are or may become pregnant, women with an active history of thromboembolic events (DVT, PE)<br><br><u>Pregnancy Category:</u> X<br><br><u>Lactation Issues:</u> Unknown if excreted in milk; however it is not recommended to give to nursing mothers. |

## 606. Drugs for Osteoporosis

For Selective Estrogen Receptor Modulators see Section 605.5

606.1 Biphosphonates

| Drug and Dosage Forms | Usual Dosage Range | Administration Issues and Drug–Drug Interactions | Common Adverse Drug Reactions (ADRs) and Pharmacokinetics | Contraindications, Pregnancy Category, and Lactation Issues |
|---|---|---|---|---|
| **Alendronate**<br>Fosamax<br><br>Tablets:  10 mg, 40 mg | **Postmenopausal Osteoporosis:**<br>10 mg qd<br>Mild renal impairment or elderly patients: No dosage adjustments necessary.<br><br>**Paget's Disease:**  40 mg once daily for 6 months. May retreat the patient after 6 months of evaluation. | Administration Issues:<br>**Take on an empty stomach, at least 30 minutes before a meal. Drink a full glass of water only. Remain upright after taking medication for at least 30 minutes.**<br><br>Drug–Drug Interactions:<br>**increased levels/effects of:** aspirin (increased toxic effects to GI)<br>**decreased levels/effects of alendronate:** calcium supplements, antacids, vitamins (decrease absorption) | ADRs:<br>flatulence, acid regurgitation, esophageal ulcer, dysphagia, abdominal distention, gastritis, musculoskeletal pain<br><br>Pharmacokinetics:<br>plasma levels decrease by >95% after 6 hrs; bone $T_{1/2}$ >10 yr. | Contraindications:<br>Hypersensitivity; hypocalcemia; severe renal impairment<br><br>Precautions:  Use cautiously in those with active upper GI problems.<br><br>Pregnancy Category:  C<br><br>Lactation Issues:  Unknown if excreted in milk; however it is not recommended to give to nursing mothers. |
| **Etidronate**<br>Didronel<br><br>Tablets:  200 mg, 400 mg | **Paget's Disease:**  5–10 mg/kg/d for not more than 6 months or 11–20 mg/kg/d for not more than 3 months. May retreat patients if needed after etidronate-free period of at least 90 days.<br><br>**Heterotopic ossification:**<br>Spinal Cord Injury: 20 mg/kg/d for 2 weeks followed by 10 mg/kg/d for 10 weeks. | Administration Issues:<br>Take on an empty stomach, 2 hrs before a meal. Drink a full glass of water.<br><br>Drug–Drug Interactions:<br>**increased levels/effects of:** aspirin (increased toxic effects to GI)<br>**decreased levels/effects of etidronate:**  calcium supplements, antacids (decrease absorption) | ADRs:<br>diarrhea, nausea, flatulence, musculoskeletal pain, hypersensitivity reactions (rarely)<br><br>Pharmacokinetics:<br>$T_{1/2}$ = 6 hrs;<br>bone $T_{1/2}$ >90 days. | Contraindications:<br>Hypersensitivity; hypocalcemia; severe renal impairment<br><br>Precautions:  Use cautiously in those with active upper GI problems.<br><br>Pregnancy Category:  B<br><br>Lactation Issues:  Unknown if excreted in milk; however it is |

| | | | |
|---|---|---|---|
| **Total hip replacement:** 20 mg/kg/d for 2 weeks for 1 month preoperatively then 20 mg/kg/d for 3 months postoperatively.<br><br>**Unlabeled use: Postmenopausal Osteoporosis:** 400 mg/d for 1 week followed by several weeks of calcium therapy. This cyclical treatment is repeated every 3 months | | | not recommended to give to nursing mothers.<br><br>Pediatrics: Safety/efficacy not established for children. |
| **Tiludronate Sodium**<br>Skelid<br><br>Tablets:<br>240 mg (contains 200 mg tiludronic acid) | **Paget's Disease**<br>400 mg single daily dose with 6 to 8 ounces plain water for 3 months. Do not remove tablets from foil strips until they are to be used.<br><br>Administration Issues:<br>Drink a full glass of water. Beverages other than plain water (including mineral water), food and some medications may reduce absorption of tiludronate. Do not take within 2 hr of food. Take calcium or mineral supplements at least 2 hr before or after tiludronate. Take antacids at least 2 hr after taking tiludronate. Do not take within 2 hr of indomethacin.<br><br>Drug–Drug Interactions:<br>**increased levels/effects of tiludronate:** indomethacin<br>**decreased levels/effects of tiludronate:** calcium supplements, antacids (decrease absorption), aspirin (due to decreased bioavailability) | ADRs:<br>vertigo, involuntary muscle contractions, anxiety, pruritus, increased sweating, dry mouth, gastritis, asthenia, flushing<br><br>Pharmacokinetics:<br>Bioavailability reduced by food. | Contraindications:<br>Hypersensitivity; hypocalcemia; severe renal impairment<br><br>Precautions: Use cautiously in those with active upper GI problems.<br><br>Pregnancy Category: C<br><br>Lactation Issues: Unknown if excreted in milk; however it is not recommended to give to nursing mothers.<br><br>Pediatrics: Safety/efficacy not established for children. |

## 606.2 Miscellaneous Agents for Osteoporosis

| Drug and Dosage Forms | Usual Dosage Range | Administration Issues and Drug–Drug Interactions | Common Adverse Drug Reactions (ADRs) and Pharmacokinetics | Contraindications, Pregnancy Category, and Lactation Issues |
|---|---|---|---|---|
| **Calcitonin**<br>Calcimar, Salmonine, Osteocalcin, Miacalcin<br><br>Injection:<br>200 IU/mL<br><br>Nasal Spray:<br>200 IU/activation | **Postmenopausal Osteoporosis:**<br>Injection: 100 IU/d SC or IM<br>Nasal: 200 IU/d<br><br>Patients must also receive 1.5 g of calcium daily and 400 U/d of Vitamin D.<br><br>**Paget's Disease:** (Injection only)<br>100 IU/d SC or IM. May decrease to 50 IU/d or 100 IU every other day as a maintenance dose. | Administration Issues:<br>Test dose of 1 IU is given intracutaneously on inner aspect of the forearm. Site is observed for 15 minutes. Injection is given either subcutaneously or intramuscularly. Intranasal administration—alternate nostrils daily. Store both the injection and unopened bottle of nasal spray in the refrigerator. Once the nasal spray is opened, store at room temperature.<br><br>Drug–Drug Interactions:<br>None Known. | ADRs:<br>Nasal spray: rhinitis, nasal irritation, back pain.<br>Injection: flu-like symptoms, polymyalgia, stiffness, dizziness, insomnia, anxiety, migraine, injection site reactions, flushing of face or hands, nausea with or without vomiting<br><br>Pharmacokinetics:<br>Injection or inhalation; metabolized to smaller inactive fragments primarily in the kidneys, blood, peripheral tissues; $T_{1/2}$ = 43 min. | Contraindications:<br>Hypersensitivity<br><br>Precautions:  Monitor closely for acute hypersensitivity reactions. Antibody formation has occurred after 2–18 months of treatment in many patients—monitor for decreasing efficacy.<br><br>Pregnancy Category:  C<br><br>Lactation Issues:  Safety for use is not established |

# 607. Thyroid Agents

607.1 Antithyroid Agents

| Drug and Dosage Forms | Usual Dosage Range | Administration Issues and Drug–Drug Interactions | Common Adverse Drug Reactions (ADRs) and Pharmacokinetics | Contraindications, Pregnancy Category, and Lactation Issues |
|---|---|---|---|---|
| **Methimazole**<br><br>Tapazole<br><br>Tablets: 5 mg, 10 mg | **Hyperthyroidism:**<br>15 mg/d for mild disease; 30–40 mg/d for moderately severe disease; 60 mg/d for severe disease.<br><br>Once Euthyroid: 5–15 mg/d<br><br>Daily doses usually given in 3 divided doses every 8 hrs; single daily doses (i.e. 30 mg qd) produce similar therapeutic results and may be used in noncompliant patients.<br><br>**Pediatrics:** 0.4 mg/kg/d given in 3 divided doses, initially. Reduce to 1/2 dose as a maintenance dose.<br>Another regimen: 0.5–0.7 mg/kg/d in 3 divided doses initially. Reduce to 1/2–2/3 of initial dose when patient is euthyroid. Max dose is 30 mg/d | Drug–Drug Interactions:<br>None known | ADRs: (<1%):<br>agranulocytosis, paresthesias, neuritis, headache, drowsiness, nausea, vomiting, skin rash, urticaria, jaundice, hepatitis, nephritis, abnormal hair loss, arthralgia, myalgia, edema, drug fever.<br><br>Pharmacokinetics:<br>80–95% bioavailable; no protein binding; hepatically metabolized; $T_{1/2}$ = 6–13 hrs; renal elimination of metabolites | Contraindications:<br>Hypersensitivity; nursing mothers.<br><br>Precautions: Monitor closely for signs of agranulocytosis<br><br>Pregnancy Category: D<br><br>Lactation Issues: excreted in breast milk. Nursing is contraindicated. |

*(continues on next page)*

**607.1 Antithyroid Agents** *continued from previous page*

| Drug and Dosage Forms | Usual Dosage Range | Administration Issues and Drug–Drug Interactions | Common Adverse Drug Reactions (ADRs) and Pharmacokinetics | Contraindications, Pregnancy Category, and Lactation Issues |
|---|---|---|---|---|
| **Propylthiouracil (PTU)**<br>various generics<br><br><u>Tablets:</u>  50 mg | **Hyperthyroidism:**<br>300 mg/d in 3 divided doses given every 8 hrs, initially.<br>For severe disease, may use 400–900 mg/d initially.<br>Once Euthyroid:  100–150 mg/d in 3 divided doses.<br><br>**Pediatrics:**<br><u>6–10 yr.:</u>  50–150 mg/d in 3 divided doses given q 8 h<br><u>≥10 yr.:</u>  150–300 mg/d in 3 divided doses q 8 h<br>Once Euthyroid: based on patient response.<br><u>Another regimen:</u>  5–7 mg/kg/d in 3 divided doses q 8 h. Once euthyroid—1/3–2/3 of the initial dose. | <u>Administration Issues:</u><br>Monitor closely for hepatotoxicity in children<br><br><u>Drug–Drug Interactions:</u><br>**increased effect of:**<br>anticoagulants | <u>ADRs (<1%):</u><br>agranulocytosis, paresthesias, neuritis, headache, drowsiness, nausea, vomiting, skin rash, urticaria, jaundice, hepatitis, nephritis, abnormal hair loss, arthralgia, myalgia, edema, drug fever.<br><br><u>Pharmacokinetics:</u><br>80–95% bioavailable;<br>75–80% protein bound;<br>hepatically metabolized;<br>$T_{1/2}$ = 1–2 hrs; 35% renal elimination of unchanged drug | <u>Contraindications:</u><br>Hypersensitivity; nursing mothers.<br><br><u>Precautions:</u>  Monitor closely for signs of agranulocytosis; monitor the prothrombin time and for bleeding.<br><br><u>Pregnancy Category:</u>  D<br><br><u>Lactation Issues:</u>  excreted in breast milk. Nursing is contraindicated. |

## 607.2 Iodine Products

| Drug and Dosage Forms | Usual Dosage Range | Administration Issues and Drug–Drug Interactions | Common Adverse Drug Reactions (ADRs) and Pharmacokinetics | Contraindications, Pregnancy Category, and Lactation Issues |
|---|---|---|---|---|
| **Iodine**<br>Lugol's Solution, Thyro-Block<br><br>Tablets: 130 mg potassium iodide<br><br>Solution: 5% iodine and 10% potassium iodide | **As an adjunct to an antithyroid drug in hyperthyroid patients in preparation for thyroidectomy:** 2–6 drops of solution 3 times daily for 10 days prior to surgery.<br><br>**For thyroid blocking in a radiation emergency:** 130 mg tablet daily.<br>Pediatrics (<1 yr.): 65 mg (1/2 tablet) crushed daily. | Administration Issues:<br>Strong iodide solution should be diluted with water or fruit juice.<br><br>Drug–Drug Interactions:<br>**increased effects:** lithium (increased potential for hypothyroidism) | ADRs:<br>skin rash, swelling of salivary glands, iodism (metallic taste, burning mouth and throat, sore teeth and gums, symptoms of a head cold and sometimes stomach upset and diarrhea), allergic reactions (fever, joint pain, swelling of face/body, severe shortness of breath requiring immediate medical attention)<br><br>Pharmacokinetics:<br>onset of action = 24 hrs; maximum effects attained after 10–15 days of continuous therapy; chronic administration leads to therapeutic effects that may persist for up to 6 weeks after the crisis has abated | Contraindications:<br>Hypersensitivity<br><br>Pregnancy Category: D<br><br>Lactation Issues: It is excreted in breast milk, but breastfeeding is not contraindicated. |

| Drug and Dosage Forms | Usual Dosage Range | Administration Issues and Drug–Drug Interactions | Common Adverse Drug Reactions (ADRs) and Pharmacokinetics | Contraindications, Pregnancy Category, and Lactation Issues |
|---|---|---|---|---|
| **Levothyroxine (T4)**<br>Synthroid, various generics<br><br>Tablets:<br>0.025 mg, 0.05 mg<br>0.075 mg, 0.088 mg<br>0.1 mg, 0.112 mg<br>0.125 mg, 0.137 mg<br>0.15 mg, 0.175 mg<br>0.2 mg, 0.3 mg | **Hypothyroidism: Must individualize dose:**<br>0.025–0.05 mg/d initially. May titrate by 0.025 mg/d every 2–3 weeks up to max of 0.3 mg/d (most do not need more than 0.2 mg/d).<br><br>**Pediatrics:**<br>0–6 mos (8–10 mcg/kg):<br>25–50 mcg/d<br>6–12 mos (6–8 mcg/kg):<br>50–75 mcg/d<br>1–5 yr. (5–6 mcg/kg): 75–100 mcg/d<br>6–12 yr. (4–5 mcg/kg):<br>100–150 mcg/d<br>>12 yr. (2–3 mcg/kg): >150 mcg/d<br><br>**Thyroid suppression therapy:**<br>2.6 mcg/kg/d for 7–10 days. | Administration Issues:<br>Take on an empty stomach (enhances absorption of T4). Do not change from one brand to another.<br><br>Drug–Drug Interactions:<br>**increased levels/effects of:**<br>anticoagulants, theophylline<br>**decreased levels/effects of:**<br>beta-blockers, digoxin<br>**decreased levels/effects of thyroid hormone:**<br>cholestyramine, colestipol, estrogens | ADRs:<br>Very few adverse effects noted unless indicating hyperthyroidism or overdose.<br><br>Pharmacokinetics<br>T4 bioavailability = 48–79%; 99% protein bound; 35% peripheral conversion of T4 to T3; biological potency of T4 = 1; $T_{1/2}$ = 6–7 days | Contraindications:<br>Hypersensitivity; acute myocardial infarction and thyrotoxicosis uncomplicated by hypothyroidism; when hypothyroidism and hypoadrenalism coexist unless hypoadrenalism is treated first.<br><br>Precautions: Use cautiously in those with cardiac disease, other endocrine disorders (unless the other disorders are appropriately treated first). Use smaller doses in those with myxedema. Monitor bone density following long term therapy.<br><br>Pregnancy Category: A<br><br>Lactation Issues: minimally excreted in breast milk. Use cautiously. |
| **Liothyronine (T3)**<br>Cytomel, various generics<br><br>Tablets: 5 mcg, 25 mcg, 50 mcg | **Hypothyroidism: Must individualize dose:**<br>25 mcg/d initially. May titrate by 12.5–25 mcg/d q 1–2 wk. up to 0.1 mg/d prn | Administration Issues:<br>Do not change from one brand to another.<br><br>Drug–Drug Interactions:<br>**increased levels/effects of:** | ADRs:<br>Very few adverse effects noted unless indicating hyperthyroidism or overdose. | Contraindications:<br>Hypersensitivity; acute myocardial infarction and thyrotoxicosis uncomplicated by hypothyroidism; when hypothyroidism and |

| | Dosing | Interactions / Administration | Pharmacokinetics / ADRs | Contraindications / Precautions |
|---|---|---|---|---|
| | **Congenital hypothyroidism:** 5 mcg/d initially. May titrate by 5 mcg/d q 3–4 days prn<br><br>**Simple goiter:** 5 mcg/d initially. May titrate by 5–10 mcg/d q 1–2 wk. up to 75 mcg/d.<br><br>**Myxedema:** 5 mcg/d initially. May titrate by 5–10 mcg/d q 1–2 wk. up to 100 mg/d. When 25 mcg/d is reached, may titrate by 12.5–25 mcg/d q 1–2 wk.<br><br>**Elderly or pediatrics:** 5 mcg/d initially. May titrate by 5 mcg/d q 1–2 wk. as needed/tolerated. | anticoagulants, theophylline<br>**decreased levels/effects of:** beta-blockers, digoxin<br>**decreased levels/effects of thyroid hormone:** cholestyramine, colestipol, estrogens | Pharmacokinetics: T3 bioavailability = 95%; 99% protein bound; peripheral metabolism; biologic potency of T3 = 4; $T_{1/2}$ ≤2 days. | hypoadrenalism coexist unless hypoadrenalism is treated first.<br><br>Precautions: Use cautiously in those with cardiac disease, other endocrine disorders (unless the other disorders are appropriately treated first). Use smaller doses in those with myxedema. Monitor bone density following long term therapy.<br><br>Pregnancy Category: A<br><br>Lactation Issues: minimally excreted in breast milk. Use cautiously. |
| **Liotrix (T4/T3 = 4/1)**<br>Euthyroid, Thyrolar<br><br>Tablets: Thyroid equivalent (T4/T3 content)<br>30 mg (30 mcg/7.5 mcg)<br>60 mg (60 mcg/15 mcg)<br>120 mg (120 mcg/30 mcg)<br>180 mg (180 mcg/45 mcg)<br>15 mg (12.5 mcg/3.1 mcg)<br>30 mg (25 mcg/6.25 mcg)<br>60 mg (50 mcg/12.5 mcg)<br>120 mg (100 mcg/25 mcg)<br>180 mg (150 mcg/37.5 mcg) | **Hypothyroidism:**<br>**Must individualize dose:**<br>30 mg/d of thyroid equivalent initially. May titrate by 15 mg/d q 2–3 wk. Maintenance doses range from 60–120 mg/d, rarely exceed 180 mg/d.<br><br>**Myxedema:** Initially, 15 mg/d.<br><br>**Pediatrics** (dose based on T4):<br>0–6 mos (8–10 mcg/kg): 25–50 mcg/d<br>6–12 mos (6–8 mcg/kg): 50–75 mcg/d<br>1–5 yr. (5–6 mcg/kg): 75–100 mcg/d<br>6–12 yr. (4–5 mcg/kg): 100–150 mcg/d<br>>12 yr. (2-3 mcg/kg): >150 mcg/d | Administration Issues:<br>Take on an empty stomach (enhances absorption of T4).<br>Do not change from one brand to another.<br><br>Drug–Drug Interactions:<br>**increased levels/effects of:** anticoagulants, theophylline<br>**decreased levels/effects of:** beta-blockers, digoxin<br>**decreased levels/effects of thyroid hormone:** cholestyramine, colestipol, estrogens | ADRs:<br>Very few adverse effects noted unless indicating hyperthyroidism or overdose.<br><br>Pharmacokinetics:<br>**T4:** T4 bioavailability = 48–79%; 99% protein bound; 35% peripheral conversion of T4 to T3; biological potency of T4 = 1; $T_{1/2}$ = 6–7 days.<br>**T3:** T3 bioavailability = 95%; 99% protein bound; peripheral metabolism; biologic potency of T3 = 4; $T_{1/2}$ ≤2 days. | Contraindications:<br>Hypersensitivity; acute myocardial infarction and thyrotoxicosis uncomplicated by hypothyroidism; when hypothyroidism and hypoadrenalism coexist unless hypoadrenalism is treated first.<br><br>Precautions: Use cautiously in those with cardiac disease, other endocrine disorders (unless the other disorders are appropriately treated first). Use smaller doses in those with myxedema. Monitor bone density following long term therapy. |

(continues on next page)

| Drug and Dosage Forms | Usual Dosage Range | Administration Issues and Drug–Drug Interactions | Common Adverse Drug Reactions (ADRs) and Pharmacokinetics | Contraindications, Pregnancy Category, and Lactation Issues |
|---|---|---|---|---|
| **Liotrix** *cont.* | | | | Pregnancy Category: A<br><br>Lactation Issues: minimally excreted in breast milk. Use cautiously. |
| **Thyroglobulin (T4/T3 = 2.5/1)**<br>Proloid<br><br>Tablets: 30 mg, 60 mg, 90 mg, 120 mg, 180 mg | **Hypothyroidism: Must individualize dose:**<br>30 mg/d initially. May titrate by 15 mg/d q 2–3 weeks as needed. Maintenance doses range from 60–120 mg/d, rarely exceed 180 mg/d.<br><br>**Myxedema:** Initially, 15 mg/d.<br><br>**Pediatrics:**<br>0–6 mos (4.8–6 mg/kg): 15–30 mg/d<br>6–12 mos (3.6–4.8 mg/kg): 30–45 mg/d<br>1–5 yr. (3–3.6 mg/kg): 45–60 mg/d<br>6–12 yr. (2.4–3 mg/kg): 60–90 mg/d<br>>12 yr. (1.2–1.8 mg/kg): >90 mg/d | Administration Issues:<br>Take on an empty stomach (enhances absorption of T4).<br>Do not change from one brand to another.<br><br>Drug–Drug Interactions:<br>**increased levels/effects of:**<br>anticoagulants, theophylline<br>**decreased levels/effects of:**<br>beta-blockers, digoxin<br>**decreased levels/effects of thyroid hormone:**<br>cholestyramine, colestipol, estrogens | ADRs:<br>Very few adverse effects noted unless indicating hyperthyroidism or overdose.<br><br>Pharmacokinetics:<br>**T4:** T4 bioavailability = 48–79%; 99% protein bound; 35% peripheral conversion of T4 to T3; biological potency of T4 = 1; $T_{1/2}$ = 6–7 days.<br><br>**T3:** T3 bioavailability = 95%; 99% protein bound; peripheral metabolism; biologic potency of T3 = 4; $T_{1/2}$ ≤ 2 days. | Contraindications:<br>Hypersensitivity; acute myocardial infarction and thyrotoxicosis uncomplicated by hypothyroidism; when hypothyroidism and hypoadrenalism coexist unless hypoadrenalism is treated first.<br><br>Precautions: Use cautiously in those with cardiac disease, other endocrine disorders (unless the other disorders are appropriately treated first). Use smaller doses in those with myxedema. Monitor bone density following long term therapy.<br><br>Pregnancy Category: A<br><br>Lactation Issues: minimally excreted in breast milk. Use cautiously. |

| Thyroid Desiccated Thyroid USP (T4/T3 = 2-5/1) | | | | |
| --- | --- | --- | --- | --- |

**Thyroid Desiccated Thyroid USP (T4/T3 = 2-5/1)**

Armour Thyroid, various generics

Tablets: 15 mg, 30 mg, 60 mg, 90 mg, 120 mg, 180 mg, 240 mg, 300 mg

**Thyroid Strong (T4/T3 = 3.1/1) (each 60 mg is equivalent to 90 mg)**

Tablets: 30 mg, 60 mg, 120 mg

Tablets, sugar coated: 30 mg, 60 mg, 120 mg, 180 mg

**Thyrar (T4/T3 = 2-5/1) (Bovine thyroid)**

Tablets: 30 mg, 60 mg, 120 mg

**S-P-T (T4/T3 = 2-5/1) (pork thyroid)**

Capsules: 60 mg, 120 mg, 180 mg, 300 mg

---

**Hypothyroidism: Must individualize dose:**
30 mg/d initially. May titrate by 15 mg/d q 2–3 wk as needed. Maintenance doses range from 60–120 mg/d, rarely exceed 180 mg/d.

**Myxedema:** Initially, 15 mg/d.

**Pediatrics:**
0–6 mos (4.8–6 mg/kg): 15–30 mg/d
6–12 mos (3.6–4.8 mg/kg): 30–45 mg/d
1–5 yr. (3–3.6 mg/kg): 45–60 mg/d
6–12 yr. (2.4–3 mg/kg): 60–90 mg/d
>12 yr. (1.2–1.8 mg/kg): >90 mg/d

---

Administration Issues:
Take on an empty stomach (enhances absorption of T4).
Do not change from one brand to another.

Drug–Drug Interactions:
**increased levels/effects of:** anticoagulants, theophylline
**decreased levels/effects of:** beta-blockers, digoxin
**decreased levels/effects of thyroid hormone:** cholestyramine, colestipol, estrogens

---

ADRs:
Very few adverse effects noted unless indicating hyperthyroidism or overdose.

Pharmacokinetics:
T4 bioavailability = 48–79%; 99% protein bound; 35% peripheral conversion of T4 to T3; biologic potency of T4 = 1; $T_{1/2}$ = 6–7 days

---

Contraindications:
Hypersensitivity; acute myocardial infarction and thyrotoxicosis uncomplicated by hypothyroidism; when hypothyroidism and hypoadrenalism coexist unless hypoadrenalism is treated first.

Precautions: Use cautiously in those with cardiac disease, other endocrine disorders (unless the other disorders are appropriately treated first). Use smaller doses in those with myxedema. Monitor bone density following long term therapy.

Pregnancy Category: A

Lactation Issues: minimally excreted in breast milk. Use cautiously.

## 608. Gonadotropin Releasing Hormones

| Drug and Dosage Forms | Usual Dosage Range | Administration Issues and Drug–Drug Interactions | Common Adverse Drug Reactions (ADRs) and Pharmacokinetics | Contraindications, Pregnancy Category, and Lactation Issues |
|---|---|---|---|---|
| **Gonadorelin acetate**<br>Lutrepulse<br><br>Powder for injection<br>(10 mls vials)<br>0.8 mg, 3.2 mg | **Primary hypothalamic amenorrhea:**<br>IV: 5 mcg q 90 minutes via Lutrepulse pump kit at treatment intervals of 21 days (pump will pulsate every 90 minutes for 7 days) | Administration Issues:<br>Drug should be administered via the Lutrepulse pump. Set pump to deliver 25–50 ml of solution, over a pulse period of 1 minute and a pulse frequency of 90 minutes.<br><br>Drug Interactions:<br>**decreased levels/effects:** oral contraceptives, digoxin, phenothiazines, dopamine antagonists<br>**increased levels/effect:** androgens, estrogens, progestins, glucocorticoids, spironolactone, levodopa | ADRs:<br>pain at site of injection, flushing, headache, rash, nausea, abdominal discomfort<br><br>Pharmacokinetics:<br>maximal LH release occurs w/in 20 minutes, duration = 3–5 hr; $T_{1/2}$ = 4 h | Contraindications:<br>Hypersensitivity; women who have cysts or causes of anovulation other than those of hypothalamic origin.<br><br>Precautions: multiple pregnancy is a possibility<br><br>Pregnancy Category: B |
| **Nafarelin acetate**<br>Synarel<br><br>Nasal solution<br>2 mg/ml | **Treatment of endometriosis:**<br>1 spray (200 mcg) in 1 nostril each morning and the other nostril each evening starting on days 2–4 of menstrual cycle for 6 months | Administration Issues:<br>Begin treatment between days 2–4 of menstrual cycle; usually menstruation will stop (as well as ovulation) but is not a reliable form of contraception and use of a nonhormonal contraceptive is recommended. Full compliance is very important; do not use a nasal decongestant for at least 30 minutes after using nafarelin. | ADRs:<br>headache, emotional lability, acne, hot flashes, decreased libido, decreased breast size, vaginal dryness, myalgia, nasal irritation, insomnia, rash, shortness of breath<br><br>Pharmacokinetics:<br>not absorbed from GI tract | Contraindications:<br>Hypersensitivity to GnRH, GnRH-agonist analogs; undiagnosed abnormal vaginal bleeding, pregnancy, lactation<br><br>Pregnancy Category: X<br><br>Lactation Issues: Nursing is contraindicated. |

# 700. RESPIRATORY AGENTS
## 701. Respiratory Inhalants
701.1 Anticholinergics

| Drug and Dosage Forms | Usual Dosage Range | Administration Issues | Common Adverse Drug Reactions (ADRs) and Pharmacokinetics | Contraindications, Pregnancy Category, and Lactation Issues |
|---|---|---|---|---|
| **Ipratropium**<br>Atrovent<br><br>Aerosol:<br>18 mcg/dose<br><br>Solution for Inhalation:<br>0.02%<br><br>Nasal Spray:<br>0.03%, 0.06% | **Bronchospasm associated with chronic obstructive pulmonary disease:**<br><br>initial dose: 2 inhalations qid<br>maximum dose: 12 inhalations/day<br><br>**perennial rhinitis (0.03% nasal spray):**<br>2 sprays bid to tid<br><br>**rhinorrhea associated with the common cold (0.06% nasal spray):**<br>2 sprays tid to qid | Administration Issues:<br>safety and efficacy have not been established in children <12 years of age; nasal spray pump requires initial priming with 7 actuation's; safety and efficacy beyond 4 days with the common cold have not been established | ADRs:<br>**aerosol/inhalation solution:** cough; dry mouth; nervousness; agitation; dizziness; headache; GI upset; palpitations; urinary retention; constipation; worsening narrow angle glaucoma<br><br>**nasal spray:** headache; epistaxis; pharyngitis; GI upset; nasal dryness/irritation; dry mouth; hoarseness; cough<br><br>Pharmacokinetics:<br>poorly absorbed; protein binding < 9%; metabolized to inactive metabolites; $t_{1/2}$ = 1.6 hours | Contraindications:<br>hypersensitivity to ipratropium, atropine, soya lecithin or related products (soya bean or peanut)<br><br>Pregnancy Category: B<br><br>Lactation Issues:<br>it is not known if ipratropium is excreted in breast milk; use caution when administering to a nursing mother |

| Drug and Dosage Forms | Usual Dosage Range | Administration Issues | Common Adverse Drug Reactions (ADRs) and Pharmacokinetics | Contraindications, Pregnancy Category, and Lactation Issues |
|---|---|---|---|---|
| **Beclomethasone**<br><br>Aerosol:<br>Beclovent, Vanceril<br>42 mcg/dose<br><br>Vanceril Double Strength<br>(84 mcg/dose)<br><br>Becloforte inhaler<br>250 mcg/dose | **Bronchial asthma in patients requiring chronic treatment with corticosteroids**<br><br>**Adults:** 2 inhalations tid to qid or 4 inhalations bid. Maximum dose: 20 inhalations (840 mcg) daily<br><br>**Children 6–12 years:**<br>1–2 inhalations tid to qid or 2–4 inhalations bid. Maximum dose: 10 inhalations (420 mcg) daily | Administration Issues:<br>Use bronchodilator therapy several minutes before using inhaled steroid therapy to enhance penetration; use as preventative therapy only; not to be used to abort an acute attack; safety/efficacy have not been established in children < 6 years | ADRs:<br>throat irritation; hoarseness; coughing; dry mouth; oral thrush; adrenal suppression may occur with large doses over a prolonged period of time; rare cases of immediate and delayed hypersensitivity reactions reported<br><br>Pharmacokinetics:<br>systemic absorption occurs rapidly; principle route of elimination is via feces | Contraindications:<br>hypersensitivity to steroids; systemic fungal infections<br><br>Pregnancy Category: C<br><br>Lactation Issues:<br>it is not known whether inhaled steroids are excreted in breast milk; decide whether to discontinue nursing or the drug |
| **Budesonide**<br>Pulmicort Turbuhaler<br>200 mcg/dose<br><br>Rhinocort Turbuhaler<br>100 mcg/dose | **Bronchial asthma in patients requiring chronic treatment with corticosteroids**<br>For adults and children, starting and maintenance doses depend upon patient's previous therapy (bronchodilators alone, inhaled corticosteroids, oral steroids)<br><br>**Adults:**<br>Starting dose range:<br>200–800 mcg bid<br>Highest recommended dose:<br>400–800 mcg bid | Administration Issues:<br>Use bronchodilator therapy several minutes before using inhaled steroid therapy to enhance penetration; use as preventative therapy only; not to be used to abort an acute attack; safety/efficacy have not been established in children < 6 years | ADRs:<br>throat irritation; hoarseness; coughing; dry mouth; oral thrush; adrenal suppression may occur with large doses over a prolonged period of time; rare cases of immediate and delayed hypersensitivity reactions reported<br><br>Pharmacokinetics:<br>systemic absorption occurs rapidly; principle route of elimination is via feces | Contraindications:<br>hypersensitivity to steroids; systemic fungal infections<br><br>Pregnancy Category: C<br><br>Lactation Issues:<br>it is not known whether inhaled steroids are excreted in breast milk; decide whether to discontinue nursing or the drug |

| Drug | Dosing | ADRs / Pharmacokinetics | Contraindications / Other |
|---|---|---|---|
| | **Children > 6 years of age:**<br>Starting dose range: 200–400 mcg bid<br>Highest recommended dose: 200–400 mcg bid | | Contraindications:<br>hypersensitivity to steroids; systemic fungal infections<br><br>Lactation Issues:<br>it is not known whether inhaled steroids are excreted in breast milk; decide whether to discontinue nursing or the drug |
| **Dexamethasone**<br>Decadron<br><br>Aerosol:<br>84 mcg/dose | Administration Issues:<br>Use bronchodilator therapy several minutes before using inhaled steroid therapy to enhance penetration; use as preventative therapy only; not to be used to abort an acute attack<br><br>**Bronchial asthma in patients requiring chronic treatment with corticosteroids**<br><br>**Adults:** 3 inhalations tid to qid<br>Maximum dose: 12 inhalations daily<br><br>**Children:** 2 inhalations tid to qid<br>Maximum dose: 8 inhalations daily | ADRs:<br>throat irritation; hoarseness; coughing; dry mouth; oral thrush<br><br>Pharmacokinetics:<br>systemic absorption = 40%–60% | |
| **Flunisolide**<br>AeroBid<br><br>Aerosol:<br>250 mcg/dose | Administration Issues:<br>Use bronchodilator therapy several minutes before using inhaled steroid therapy to enhance penetration; use as preventative therapy only; not to be used to abort an acute attack; safety/efficacy have not been established in children < 6 years<br><br>**Bronchial asthma in patients requiring chronic treatment with corticosteroids**<br><br>**Adults:** 2 inhalations bid<br>Maximum dose: 8 inhalations daily<br><br>**Children 6–15 years:**<br>2 inhalations bid<br>Maximum dose: 4 inhalations daily | ADRs:<br>throat irritation; hoarseness; coughing; dry mouth; oral thrush<br><br>Pharmacokinetics:<br>systemic absorption = 40%; rapidly undergoes first pass metabolism; $T_{1/2}$ = 1.8 hours | Contraindications:<br>hypersensitivity to steroids; systemic fungal infections<br><br>Pregnancy Category: C<br><br>Lactation Issues:<br>it is not known whether inhaled steroids are excreted in breast milk; decide whether to discontinue nursing or the drug |
| **Fluticasone**<br>Flovent<br><br>Aerosol:<br>44 mcg/dose, 110 mcg/dose, 220 mcg/dose | Administration Issues:<br>Use bronchodilator therapy several minutes before using inhaled steroid therapy to enhance penetration; use as preventative therapy only; not to be used to abort an acute attack; safety/efficacy have not been established in children < 12 years<br><br>**Bronchial asthma in patients requiring chronic treatment with corticosteroids**<br><br>For adults and children, starting and maintenance doses depend upon patient's previous therapy (bronchodilators alone, inhaled corticosteroids, oral steroids) | ADRs:<br>throat irritation; hoarseness; coughing; dry mouth; oral thrush, nasal congestion, nasal discharge, headache, upper respiratory infection<br><br>Pharmacokinetics:<br>$T_{1/2}$ = 7.8 hours | Contraindications:<br>hypersensitivity to steroids; systemic fungal infections<br><br>Pregnancy Category: C<br><br>Lactation Issues:<br>it is not known whether inhaled steroids are excreted in breast milk; decide whether to discontinue nursing or the drug |

(continues on next page)

| Drug and Dosage Forms | Usual Dosage Range | Administration Issues | Common Adverse Drug Reactions (ADRs) and Pharmacokinetics | Contraindications, Pregnancy Category, and Lactation Issues |
|---|---|---|---|---|
| **Fluticasone** *cont.* | **Adults and Adolescents > 12 yr.:** Previous therapy with Broncho-dilators alone: 88 mcg bid initially, increase prn to a max of 440 mcg bid<br><br>Previous therapy with Inhaled corticosteroids: 88–220 mcg bid initially, increase prn to max of 440 mcg bid<br><br>Previous therapy with oral corticosteroids: 880 mcg bid (initial and max dose) | | | |
| **Triamcinolone**<br>Azmacort<br><br>Aerosol:<br>100 mcg/dose | **Bronchial asthma in patients requiring chronic treatment with corticosteroids**<br><br>**Adults:** 2 inhalations tid to qid Maximum dose: 16 inhalations daily<br><br>**Children 6–12 years:**<br>1–2 inhalations tid to qid. Maximum dose: 12 inhalations daily | Administration Issues:<br>Use bronchodilator therapy several minutes before using inhaled steroid therapy to enhance penetration; use as preventative therapy only; not to be used to abort an acute attack; safety/efficacy have not been established in children < 6 years | ADRs:<br>throat irritation; hoarseness; coughing; dry mouth; oral thrush; adrenal suppression may occur with large doses over a prolonged period of time<br><br>Pharmacokinetics:<br>rapidly absorbed from lung; rapidly metabolized; mainly eliminated via feces | Contraindications:<br>hypersensitivity to steroids; systemic fungal infections<br><br>Pregnancy Category: D<br><br>Lactation Issues:<br>it is not known whether inhaled steroids are excreted in breast milk; decide whether to discontinue nursing or the drug |

**701.3** Miscellaneous Inhalants

| Drug and Dosage Forms | Usual Dosage Range | Administration Issues | Common Adverse Drug Reactions (ADRs) and Pharmacokinetics | Contraindications, Pregnancy Category, and Lactation Issues |
|---|---|---|---|---|
| **Cromolyn**<br>Intal, Gastrocrom, Nasalcrom<br><br>Capsules for Inhalation:<br>20 mg<br><br>Nebulizer Solution:<br>20 mg/amp<br><br>Aerosol:<br>800 mcg/dose<br><br>Nasal Solution:<br>5.2 mg/dose<br><br>Oral Capsules:<br>100 mg | **Severe asthma (nebulizer solution, capsules, aerosol):**<br>20 mg inhaled capsule or nebulizer solution or 2 sprays of aerosol qid<br><br>**Prevention of exercise induced asthma (nebulizer solution, capsules, aerosol):**<br>20 mg inhaled capsule or nebulizer solution or 2 sprays of aerosol no more than 1 hour before exercise<br><br>**Allergic rhinitis (nasal spray):**<br>1 spray in each nostril 3–6 times daily<br><br>**Mastocytosis (oral capsules):**<br>**adults:** 2 capsules qid ac and hs<br><br>**Children:**<br>**2–12 years:** 1 capsule qid ac; maximum dose: 40 mg/kg/day<br><br>**term to 2 years:** 20 mg/kg/day divided qid<br>maximum dose (6 months to two years): 30 mg/kg/day | Administration Issues:<br>must be used regularly to achieve benefit; safety and efficacy have not been established in children <5 years of age (inhalation capsules/aerosol), <2 years of age (nebulizer solution/oral capsule) and <6 years of age (nasal solution) | ADRs:<br>**inhalation capsules/aerosol:** lacrimation; swollen parotid gland; urinary frequency; dizziness; headache; rash<br><br>**nebulizer solution:** cough; wheezing; nasal congestion/ itching; sneezing; epistaxis<br><br>**nasal solution:** sneezing; headache; nasal stinging/ burning/irritation; bad taste in mouth; epistaxis<br><br>**oral capsules:** headache; diarrhea; pruritus; flushing; GI upset; dizziness; myalgia<br><br>Pharmacokinetics:<br>7–8% absorbed from the lung; poorly absorbed from the GI tract | Contraindications:<br>hypersensitivity to cromolyn<br><br>Pregnancy Category: B<br><br>Lactation Issues:<br>it not known if cromolyn is excreted in breast milk; use caution when administering to a nursing mother |
| **Nedocromil**<br>Tilade<br><br>Aerosol:<br>1.75 mg/dose | **Asthma:**<br>2 inhalations qid | Administration Issues:<br>must be used regularly to achieve benefit; safety and efficacy have not been established in children <12 years of age | ADRs:<br>cough; pharyngitis; rhinitis; bronchospasm; dry mouth; unpleasant taste; GI upset; dizziness; headache | Contraindications:<br>hypersensitivity to nedocromil<br><br>Pregnancy Category: B |

*(continues on next page)*

## 701.3 Miscellaneous Inhalants *continued from previous page*

| Drug and Dosage Forms | Usual Dosage Range | Administration Issues | Common Adverse Drug Reactions (ADRs) and Pharmacokinetics | Contraindications, Pregnancy Category, and Lactation Issues |
|---|---|---|---|---|
| **Nedocromil** *cont.* | | | Pharmacokinetics: poorly absorbed; protein binding = 89% | Lactation Issues: it not known if nedocromil is excreted in breast milk; use caution when administering to a nursing mother |
| **Dornase Alfa** Pulmozyme  Solution for Inhalation: 1 mg/mL (2.5 mL) | **Cystic fibrosis:** 2.5 mg inhaled qd to bid | Administration Issues: clinical efficacy documented with the use of the following nebulizers: Hudson T Up-draft II, Marquest Acorn II in conjunction with Pulmo-Aide compressor, Pari LC Jet in conjunction with the PARI PRONEB compressor; safety and efficacy >12 months have not been established | ADRs: voice alteration; pharyngitis; laryngitis; rash; cough  Pharmacokinetics: poorly absorbed | Contraindications: hypersensitivity to domase or Chinese Hamster Ovary cell products  Pregnancy Category: B  Lactation Issues: it not known if domase is excreted in breast milk; use caution when administering to a nursing mother |

## 702. Bronchodilators

702.1 Sympathomimetics

| Drug and Dosage Forms | Usual Dosage Range | Administration Issues and Drug–Drug Interactions | Common Adverse Drug Reactions (ADRs) and Pharmacokinetics | Contraindications, Pregnancy Category, and Lactation Issues |
|---|---|---|---|---|
| **Albuterol**<br>Proventil, Ventolin<br><br>Tablets:<br>2 mg, 4 mg<br><br>Extended Release Tablets:<br>4 mg<br><br>Aerosol: 90 mcg/dose<br><br>Solution for Inhalation:<br>0.083%, 0.5%<br><br>Capsules for Inhalation:<br>200 mcg<br>(Ventolin Rotacaps) | **Asthma/bronchospasm:**<br>aerosol<br>**adults and children > 12 yr.:**<br>1–2 inhalations q 4–6 hours<br><br>solution for inhalation<br>**adults and children > 12 yr.:**<br>2.5 mg tid to qid<br><br>capsules for inhalation<br>**adults and children > 4yr:**<br>200–400 mcg q 4–6 hours<br><br>**tablets and syrup**<br>**adults and children > 12:** 2–4 mg<br>tid to qid; max dose: 32 mg daily<br><br>**children 6–12:** 2 mg tid to qid;<br>max dose: 24 mg daily<br><br>extended release tablets<br>**adults and children > 12:** 4–8 mg<br>q 12 hours; maximum dose: 32 mg daily<br><br>syrup<br>**children 2–6:** 0.1 mg/kg tid;<br>max dose: 12 mg daily | Administration Issues:<br>shake well before using; allow one full minute between inhalations; safety and efficacy have not been established in children < 12 years (inhalation, extended release tablets), < 6 years (tablets), <2 years (syrup)<br><br>Drug–Drug Interactions:<br>albuterol may decrease serum **digoxin** concentrations; increased risk of cardiac toxicity when given with theophylline | ADRs<br>palpitations; tachycardia; anxiety; irritability; tremor; GI upset; cough; dry mouth; hoarseness; flushing; headache<br><br>Pharmacokinetics:<br>(aerosol) onset = 5 minutes; duration = 3–8 hours; (tablets) onset = 30 minutes; duration = 4–8 hours | Contraindications:<br>hypersensitivity to beta adrenergic agents; cardiac arrhythmias; narrow angle glaucoma<br><br>Pregnancy Category: C<br><br>Lactation Issues:<br>it is not known if albuterol is excreted in breast milk; either the drug or the nursing should be discontinued |

(continues on next page)

| Drug and Dosage Forms | Usual Dosage Range | Administration Issues and Drug–Drug Interactions | Common Adverse Drug Reactions (ADRs) and Pharmacokinetics | Contraindications, Pregnancy Category, and Lactation Issues |
|---|---|---|---|---|
| **Albuterol** *cont.* | **Prevention of exercise-induced asthma: adults and children > 12 yr.:** 2 inhalations 15 minutes prior to exercise | | | |
| **Bitolterol** Tornalate  Aerosol: 0.37 mg/dose | **Asthma/bronchospasm: adults and children > 12 yr.:** 2 inhalations q 4–6 hours  maximum dose: 3 inhalations within 6 hours or 2 inhalations within 4 hours | Administration Issues: shake well before using; allow one full minute between inhalations; safety and efficacy have not been established in children < 12 years  Drug–Drug Interactions: increased risk of cardiac toxicity when given with **theophylline** | ADRs: palpitations; tachycardia; anxiety; irritability; tremor; GI upset; cough; dry mouth; hoarseness; flushing; headache  Pharmacokinetics: onset = 3–4 minutes; duration = 5–8 hours | Contraindications: hypersensitivity to beta adrenergic agents; cardiac arrhythmias; narrow angle glaucoma  Pregnancy Category: C  Lactation Issues: it is not known if bitolterol is excreted in breast milk; either the drug or nursing should be discontinued |
| **Ephedrine** Capsules: 25 mg, 50 mg | **Asthma: adults:** 25–50 mg bid to tid  **children:** 3 mg/kg/day in 4–6 divided doses | Administration Issues: Do not exceed prescribed dosage. If GI upset occurs, take with food.  Drug–Drug Interactions: increased risk of cardiac toxicity when given with **theophylline** | ADRs: palpitations; tachycardia; anxiety; irritability; tremor; GI upset; cough; dry mouth; hoarseness; flushing; headache  Pharmacokinetics: onset = 60 minutes; duration = 3–5 hours | Contraindications: hypersensitivity to beta adrenergic agents; cardiac arrhythmias; narrow angle glaucoma  Pregnancy Category: C  Lactation Issues: it is not known if ephedrine is excreted in breast milk; either the drug or nursing should be discontinued |

| Epinephrine | Asthma/bronchospasm: | Administration Issues: | ADRs: | Contraindications: |
|---|---|---|---|---|
| Adrenalin, Primatene Mist, Bronkaid Mist | aerosol<br>1–2 inhalations q 4–6 h<br><br>solution for inhalation<br>1 treatment q 4–6 h | shake well before using; allow one full minute between inhalations<br><br>Drug–Drug Interactions:<br>increased risk of cardiac toxicity when given with **theophylline** | palpitations; tachycardia; anxiety; irritability; tremor; GI upset; cough; dry mouth; hoarseness; flushing; headache<br><br>Pharmacokinetics:<br>onset = 1–5 minutes; duration = 1–3 hours | hypersensitivity to beta adrenergic agents; cardiac arrhythmias; narrow angle glaucoma<br><br>Pregnancy Category: C<br><br>Lactation Issues:<br>epinephrine is excreted in breast milk; either the drug or nursing should be discontinued |
| Solution for Inhalation:<br>2%, 2.25%<br><br>Aerosol:<br>0.2 mg/dose, 0.25 mg/dose, 0.3 mg/dose | | | | |
| Isoetharine | Asthma/bronchospasm: | Administration Issues: | ADRs: | Contraindications: |
| Bronkosol | solution for inhalation<br>1 treatment q 4 h<br><br>aerosol<br>1–2 inhalations q 4 h | shake well before using; allow one full minute between inhalations; safety and efficacy have not been established in children < 12 years<br><br>Drug–Drug Interactions:<br>increased risk of cardiac toxicity when given with **theophylline** | palpitations; tachycardia; anxiety; irritability; tremor; GI upset; cough; dry mouth; hoarseness; flushing; headache<br><br>Pharmacokinetics:<br>onset within 5 minutes; duration = 1–3 hours | hypersensitivity to beta adrenergic agents; cardiac arrhythmias; narrow angle glaucoma<br><br>Pregnancy Category: C<br><br>Lactation Issues:<br>it is not known if isoetharine is excretedin breast milk; either the drug or nursing should be discontinued |
| Solution for Inhalation:<br>0.062%, 0.08%, 0.1%, 0.125%, 0.167%, 0.17%, 0.2%, 0.25%, 1%<br><br>Aerosol:<br>340 mcg/dose | | | | |
| Metaproterenol | Asthma/bronchospasm: | Administration Issues: | ADRs: | Contraindications: |
| Alupent, Metaprel | inhaler: 2–3 inhalation q 3–4 h; maximum dose: 12 inhalations daily<br>solution for inhalation: 1 soln q 4–6 h<br><br>tablets<br>**adults and children > 9 yr.:**<br>20 mg tid to qid<br><br>**children 6–9 yr.:** 10 mg tid to qid<br><br>syrup<br>**children < 6 yr.:** 1.3–2.6 mg/kg/day in divided doses | shake well before using; allow one full minute between inhalations; safety and efficacy have not been established in children < 6 years<br><br>Drug–Drug Interactions:<br>increased risk of cardiac toxicity when given with **theophylline** | palpitations; tachycardia; anxiety; irritability; tremor; GI upset; cough; dry mouth; hoarseness; flushing; headache<br><br>Pharmacokinetics:<br>onset = 5–30 minutes; duration = 2–6 hours | hypersensitivity to beta adrenergic agents; cardiac arrhythmias; narrow angle glaucoma<br><br>Pregnancy Category: C<br><br>Lactation Issues:<br>it is not known if metaproterenol is excreted in breast milk; either the drug or the nursing should be discontinued |
| Tablets:<br>10 mg, 20 mg<br><br>Syrup:<br>10 mg/5 mL<br><br>Aerosol:<br>0.65 mg/dose<br><br>Solution for Inhalation:<br>0.4%, 0.6%, 5% | | | | |

(continues on next page)

| Drug and Dosage Forms | Usual Dosage Range | Administration Issues and Drug–Drug Interactions | Common Adverse Drug Reactions (ADRs) and Pharmacokinetics | Contraindications, Pregnancy Category, and Lactation Issues |
|---|---|---|---|---|
| **Pirbuterol**<br>Maxair<br><br>Aerosol:<br>0.2 mg/dose | **Asthma/bronchospasm adults and children > 12 yr.:**<br>1–2 inhalations q 4–6 h<br><br>maximum dose: 12 inhalations daily | Administration Issues:<br>shake well before using; allow one full minute between inhalations; safety and efficacy have not been established in children < 12 years<br><br>Drug–Drug Interactions:<br>increased risk of cardiac toxicity when given with **theophylline** | ADRs:<br>palpitations; tachycardia; anxiety; irritability; tremor; GI upset; cough; dry mouth; hoarseness; flushing; headache<br><br>Pharmacokinetics:<br>onset within 5 minutes; duration = 5 hours | Contraindications:<br>hypersensitivity to beta adrenergic agents; cardiac arrhythmias; narrow angle glaucoma<br><br>Pregnancy Category: C<br><br>Lactation Issues:<br>it is not known if pirbuterol is excreted in breast milk; either the drug or nursing should be discontinued |
| **Salmeterol**<br>Serevent<br><br>Aerosol:<br>25 mcg/dose<br><br>Diskus<br>50 mcg/dose | **Asthma/bronchospasm:**<br>Aerosol: 1–2 inhalations bid<br><br>Diskus: 1 inhalation bid<br><br>**Exercise-induced bronchospasm:**<br>Aerosol: 2 inhalations 30–60 minutes before exercise<br><br>**COPD:**<br>Aerosol: 1–2 inhalations bid | Administration Issues:<br>shake well before using; allow one full minute between inhalations; should not be used for relief of acute asthmatic symptoms; safety and efficacy have not been established in children < 12 years. Do not exceed 4 inhalations per day of the aerosol product.<br><br>Drug–Drug Interactions:<br>increased risk of cardiac toxicity when given with **theophylline** | ADRs:<br>palpitations; tachycardia; anxiety; irritability; tremor; GI upset; cough; dry mouth; hoarseness; flushing; headache<br><br>Pharmacokinetics:<br>onset = 20 minutes; duration = 12 hours | Contraindications:<br>hypersensitivity to beta adrenergic agents; cardiac arrhythmias; narrow angle glaucoma<br><br>Pregnancy Category: C<br><br>Lactation Issues:<br>it is not known if salmeterol is excreted in breast milk; either the drug or nursing should be discontinued |
| **Terbutaline**<br>Brethine, Bricanyl<br><br>Tablets:<br>2.5 mg, 5 mg | **Asthma/bronchospasm:**<br>aerosol<br>1–2 inhalations q 4–6 h | Administration Issues:<br>shake well before using; allow one full minute between inhalations; safety and efficacy have not been established in children < 12 years | ADRs:<br>palpitations; tachycardia; anxiety; irritability; tremor; GI upset; cough; dry mouth; hoarseness; flushing; headache | Contraindications:<br>hypersensitivity to beta adrenergic agents; cardiac arrhythmias; narrow angle glaucoma |

| Drug and Dosage Forms | Usual Dosage Range | Pharmacokinetics | Drug–Drug Interactions | Pregnancy Category / Lactation Issues |
|---|---|---|---|---|
| Aerosol: 0.2 mg/dose | tablets<br>**adults and children > 15 yr.:** 5 mg tid; maximum dose: 15 mg daily<br><br>**children 12-15 years:** 2.5 mg tid maximum dose: 7.5 mg daily | Pharmacokinetics: (aerosol)<br>onset = 5–30 minutes;<br>duration = 3–6 hours; (tablets)<br>onset = 30 minutes;<br>duration = 4–8 hours | Drug–Drug Interactions:<br>increased risk of cardiac toxicity when given with **theophylline** | Pregnancy Category: B<br><br>Lactation Issues:<br>terbutaline is excreted in breast milk; either the drug or the nursing should be discontinued |

## 702.2 Xanthine Derivatives

| Drug and Dosage Forms | Usual Dosage Range | Common Adverse Drug Reactions (ADRs) and Pharmacokinetics | Administration Issues and Drug–Drug Interactions | Contraindications, Pregnancy Category, and Lactation Issues |
|---|---|---|---|---|
| **Aminophylline**<br><br>Tablets:<br>100 mg, 200 mg<br><br>Controlled Release Tablets:<br>225 mg<br><br>Liquid:<br>105 mg/5 mL<br><br>Suppositories:<br>250 mg, 500 mg | **Asthma/bronchospasm:**<br><br>regular release tablets<br>initial dose: 16 mg/kg (up to 400 mg) in 3–4 divided doses<br><br>controlled release tablets<br>initial dose: 12 mg/kg (up to 450 mg) in 2–3 divided doses<br><br>maximum dose:<br>**adults:** 13 mg/kg/day<br><br>**children 12–16 yr.:** 18 mg/kg/day<br><br>**children 9–12 yr.:** 20 mg/kg/day<br><br>**children 1–9 yr.:** 24 mg/kg/day | ADRs:<br>GI irritation; diarrhea; increased gastroesophageal reflux; palpitations, tachycardia; potentiation of diuresis; toxic levels may result in cardiac arrhythmias, convulsions and death<br><br>**Aminophylline therapeutic range: 5–15 mcg/mL**<br><br>Pharmacokinetics:<br>liquids and regular release tablets are well absorbed; absorption of sustained release preparation may vary; T$_{1/2}$ averages 3–15 h depending on age, smoking status; T$_{1/2}$ prolonged in patients with CHF, liver disease, alcoholism and respiratory infections | Administration Issues:<br>do not chew or crush enteric coated or sustained release capsules or tablets; take at the same time, with or without food each day; do not change from one brand to another without consulting a physician<br><br>Drug–Drug Interactions:<br>agent that may decrease aminophylline concentrations include **phenobarbital, phenytoin, ketoconazole, rifampin** and **smoking**, agents that may increase aminophylline concentrations include **allopurinol, cimetidine, corticosteroids, erythromycin, ciprofloxacin** | Contraindications:<br>hypersensitivity to xanthines or ethylenediamine; peptic ulcer disease; underlying seizure disorder unless well controlled<br><br>Pregnancy Category: C<br><br>Lactation Issues:<br>aminophylline is excreted in breast milk and may cause signs of irritability in the nursing infants; decide whether nursing or the drug should be discontinued |

(continues on next page)

| Drug and Dosage Forms | Usual Dosage Range | Administration Issues and Drug–Drug Interactions | Common Adverse Drug Reactions (ADRs) and Pharmacokinetics | Contraindications, Pregnancy Category, and Lactation Issues |
|---|---|---|---|---|
| **Dyphylline**<br>Dilor, Lufyllin<br><br>Tablets:<br>200 mg, 400 mg<br><br>Elixir:<br>100 mg/15 mL, 160 mg/15 mL<br><br>Combination Products:<br>w/ guaifenesin | **Asthma/bronchospasm:**<br>200 mg–400 mg q 6 h<br><br>maximum dose: 15 mg/kg every 6 hours | Administration Issues:<br>take at the same time, with or without food each day; do not change from one brand to another without consulting a physician<br><br>Drug–Drug Interactions:<br>agents that may decrease theophylline concentrations include **phenobarbital, phenytoin, ketoconazole, rifampin** and **smoking,** agents that may increase theophylline concentrations include **allopurinol, cimetidine, corticosteroids, erythromycin, ciprofloxacin** | ADRs:<br>GI irritation; diarrhea; increased gastroesophageal reflux; palpitations, tachycardia; potentiation of diuresis; toxic levels may result in cardiac arrhythmias, convulsions and death<br><br>**Serum theophylline levels do not measure dyphylline**<br><br>Pharmacokinetics:<br>absorption = 68–82%; 83% excreted unchanged in urine; $T_{1/2}$ = 2 hours; dyphylline is 70% theophylline by molecular weight ratio | Contraindications:<br>hypersensitivity to xanthines; peptic ulcer disease; underlying seizure disorder unless well controlled<br><br>Pregnancy Category: C<br><br>Lactation Issues:<br>theophylline is excreted in breast milk and may cause signs of irritability in the nursing infant; decide whether nursing or the drug should be discontinued |
| **Oxtriphylline**<br>Choledyl<br><br>Tablets:<br>100 mg, 200 mg<br><br>Sustained Release Tablets:<br>400 mg<br><br>Elixir:<br>100 mg/5 mL | **Asthma/bronchospasm:**<br>tablets, elixir, syrup<br>**adults:** 4.7 mg/kg q 8 h<br><br>**children 9–16 yr. and adult smokers:** 4.7 mg/kg q 6 h<br><br>**children 1–9 yr.:** 6.2 mg/kg q 6 h<br><br>sustained release tablets<br>400–800 mg q 12 h | Administration Issues:<br>do not chew or crush enteric coated or sustained release capsules or tablets; take at the same time, with or without food each day; do not change from one brand to another without consulting a physician<br><br>Drug–Drug Interactions:<br>agents that may decrease oxtriphylline concentrations include **phenobarbital,** | ADRs:<br>GI irritation; diarrhea; increased gastroesophageal reflux; palpitations, tachycardia; potentiation of diuresis; toxic levels may result in cardiac arrhythmias, convulsions and death | Contraindications:<br>hypersensitivity to xanthines; peptic ulcer disease; underlying seizure disorder unless well controlled<br><br>Pregnancy Category: C |

| | | |
|---|---|---|
| **Pediatric Syrup:**<br>50 mg/5 mL | **phenytoin, ketoconazole, rifampin** and **smoking**, agents that may increase oxtriphylline concentrations include **allopurinol, cimetidine, corticosteroids, erythromycin, ciprofloxacin** | **Oxtriphylline therapeutic range: 5–15 mcg/mL**<br><br>Pharmacokinetics:<br>liquids and regular release tablets are well absorbed; absorption of sustained release preparation may vary; hepatically metabolized; $T_{1/2}$ averages 3–15 hours depending on age and smoking status; $T_{1/2}$ may be prolonged in patients with CHF, liver disease, alcoholism and respiratory infections | Lactation Issues:<br>oxtriphylline is excreted in breast milk and may cause signs of irritability in the nursing infant; decide whether nursing or the drug should be discontinued |

| | | | |
|---|---|---|---|
| **Theophylline**<br>Elixophyllin, Quibron-T, Slo-bid, Slo-Phyllin, Theo-Dur, Theolair, Uniphyl, plus<br><br>Regular Release Tablets:<br>100 mg, 125 mg, 200 mg, 250 mg, 300 mg<br><br>Regular Release Capsules:<br>100 mg, 200 mg<br><br>Syrup:  80 mg/15 mL, 150 mg/15 mL<br><br>Elixir:  80 mg/15 mL<br><br>Solution:  80 mg/15 mL, 150 mg/15 mL<br><br>Timed Release Capsule:<br>50 mg, 60 mg, 75 mg, 100 mg, 125 mg, 130 mg, 200 mg, 250 mg, 260 mg, 300 mg | **Asthma/bronchospasm:**<br>regular release preparations<br>initial dose:  16 mg/kg (up to 400 mg) in 3–4 divided doses<br><br>time release preparations<br>initial dose:  12 mg/kg (up to 400 mg) in 2–3 divided doses<br><br>**maximum dose:**<br>**adults:**  13 mg/kg/day<br>**children 12–16 yr.:**  18 mg/kg/day<br>**children 9–12 yr.:**  20 mg/kg/day<br>**children 1–9 yr.:**  24 mg/kg/day<br><br>Administration Issues:<br>do not chew or crush enteric coated or sustained release capsules or tablets; take at the same time, with or without food each day; do not change from one brand to another without consulting a physician<br><br>Drug–Drug Interactions:<br>agents that may decrease theophylline concentrations include **phenobarbital, phenytoin, ketoconazole, rifampin** and **smoking**, agents that may increase theophylline concentrations include **allopurinol, cimetidine, corticosteroids, erythromycin, ciprofloxacin** | **Theophylline therapeutic range: 5–15 mcg/mL**<br><br>Pharmacokinetics:<br>liquids and regular release tablets are well absorbed; absorption of sustained release preparation may vary; hepatically metabolized; $T_{1/2}$ averages 3–15 hours depending on age and smoking<br><br>ADRs:<br>GI irritation; diarrhea; increased gastroesophageal reflux; palpitations; tachycardia; potentiation of diuresis; toxic levels may result in cardiac arrhythmias, convulsions and death | Contraindications:<br>hypersensitivity to xanthines; peptic ulcer disease; underlying seizure disorder unless well controlled<br><br>Pregnancy Category:  C<br><br>Lactation Issues:<br>theophylline is excreted in breast milk and may cause signs of irritability in the nursing infant; decide whether nursing or the drug should be discontinued |

1401

## 702.2 Xanthine Derivatives *continued from previous page*

| Drug and Dosage Forms | Usual Dosage Range | Administration Issues and Drug–Drug Interactions | Common Adverse Drug Reactions (ADRs) and Pharmacokinetics | Contraindications, Pregnancy Category, and Lactation Issues |
|---|---|---|---|---|
| **Theophylline *cont.*** <br><br> Timed Release Tablets: <br> 200 mg, 250 mg, 300 mg, 400 mg, 450 mg, 500 mg <br><br> Combination Products: <br> w/ various combinations of guaifenesin, ephedrine, hydroxyzine, potassium iodide, phenobarbital | | | status; $T_{1/2}$ may be prolonged in patients with CHF, liver disease, alcoholism and respiratory infections | |

## 703. Nasal Decongestants

| Drug and Dosage Forms | Usual Dosage Range | Administration Issues and Drug–Drug Interactions | Common Adverse Drug Reactions (ADRs) and Pharmacokinetics | Contraindications, Pregnancy Category, and Lactation Issues |
|---|---|---|---|---|
| **Ephedrine** <br> Kondon's Nasal, Vicks Vatronol, Pretz-D <br><br> Spray: 0.25% <br><br> Drops: 0.5% <br><br> Jelly: 1% | **relief of nasal and nasopharyngeal mucosal congestion due to common cold, hay fever, sinusitis or allergies** <br><br> 1 spray in each nostril no more frequently than every 4 hours | Administration Issues: <br> nasal sprays are preferred to drops because of the lesser risk of swallowing the drug and resultant systemic absorption; dropper and dispensers should not be used by more than one person; tips of the dispensers or droppers should be rinsed with hot water following use; do not use topical nasal sprays longer than 3–5 days | ADRs: <br> burning; stinging; sneezing; dryness; local irritation; rebound congestion <br><br> Pharmacokinetics: <br> onset = 15–30 minutes; duration = 2–4 hours; systemic absorption is minimal | Contraindications: <br> hypersensitivity to decongestants; monoamine oxidase (MAO) inhibitor therapy; severe hypertension or coronary artery disease <br><br> Pregnancy Category: C |

| | | |
|---|---|---|
| | | **Lactation Issues:**<br>it is not known whether topical decongestants are excreted in breast milk; use with caution |
| **Epinephrine**<br>Adrenalin<br><br>Solution:<br>0.1% | **relief of nasal and nasopharyngeal mucosal congestion due to common cold, hay fever, sinusitis or allergies**<br><br>**Adults and children > 6 years:**<br><br>1 spray or drop as needed | **Administration Issues:**<br>nasal sprays are preferred to drops because of the lesser risk of swallowing the drug and resultant systemic absorption; dropper and dispensers should not be used by more than one person; tips of the dispensers or droppers should be rinsed with hot water following use; do not use topical nasal sprays longer than 3–5 days | **ADRs:**<br>burning; stinging; sneezing; dryness; local irritation; rebound congestion<br><br>**Pharmacokinetics:**<br>onset = 5 minutes; systemic absorption is minimal | **Contraindications:**<br>hypersensitivity to decongestants; monoamine oxidase (MAO) inhibitor therapy; severe hypertension or coronary artery disease<br><br>**Pregnancy Category:** C<br><br>**Lactation Issues:**<br>it is not known whether topical decongestants are excreted in breast milk; use with caution |
| **Naphazoline**<br>Privine<br><br>Solution:<br>0.05% | **relief of nasal and nasopharyngeal mucosal congestion due to common cold, hay fever, sinusitis or allergies**<br><br>**Adults and children > 12 years:**<br>1–2 drops or sprays in each nostril as needed—no more frequently than q 6 hours | **Administration Issues:**<br>safety and efficacy have not been established in children < 12 years of age; nasal sprays are preferred to drops because of the lesser risk of swallowing the drug and resultant systemic absorption; dropper and dispensers should not be used by more than one person; tips of the dispensers or droppers should be rinsed with hot water following use; do not use topical nasal sprays longer than 3–5 days | **ADRs:**<br>burning; stinging; sneezing; dryness; local irritation; rebound congestion<br><br>**Pharmacokinetics:**<br>onset = 10 minutes; duration = 2–6 hours; systemic absorption is minimal | **Contraindications:**<br>hypersensitivity to decongestants; monoamine oxidase (MAO) inhibitor therapy; severe hypertension or coronary artery disease; glaucoma<br><br>**Pregnancy Category:** C<br><br>**Lactation Issues:**<br>it is not known whether topical decongestants are excreted in breast milk; use with caution |

*(continues on next page)*

**703.** Nasal Decongestants *continued from previous page*

| Drug and Dosage Forms | Usual Dosage Range | Administration Issues and Drug–Drug Interactions | Common Adverse Drug Reactions (ADRs) and Pharmacokinetics | Contraindications, Pregnancy Category, and Lactation Issues |
|---|---|---|---|---|
| **Oxymetazoline**<br>Afrin, Dristan, Duration, Sinex<br><br>Solution:<br>0.025%, 0.05% | **relief of nasal and nasopharyngeal mucosal congestion due to common cold, hay fever, sinusitis or allergies**<br><br>0.05% solution:<br>**Adults and children > 6 years:**<br>2–3 sprays or drops in each nostril bid<br><br>0.025% solution:<br>**Children 2–5 years:** 2–3 drops in each nostril bid | Administration Issues:<br>nasal sprays are preferred to drops because of the lesser risk of swallowing the drug and resultant systemic absorption; dropper and dispensers should not be used by more than one person; tips of the dispensers or droppers should be rinsed with hot water following use; do not use topical nasal sprays longer than 3–5 days | ADRs:<br>burning; stinging; sneezing; dryness; local irritation; rebound congestion<br><br>Pharmacokinetics:<br>onset = 5–10 minutes; duration = 5–6 hours; systemic absorption is minimal | Contraindications:<br>hypersensitivity to decongestants; monoamine oxidase (MAO) inhibitor therapy; severe hypertension or coronary artery disease<br><br>Pregnancy Category: C<br><br>Lactation Issues:<br>it is not known whether topical decongestants are excreted in breast milk; use with caution |
| **Phenylephrine**<br>Neo-Synephrine, Sinex<br><br>Solution:<br>0.125%, 0.16%, 0.25%, 0.5%, 1% | **relief of nasal and nasopharyngeal mucosal congestion due to common cold, hay fever, sinusitis or allergies**<br><br>**Adults and children > 12 years:**<br>2–3 sprays or drops in each nostril q 3–4 hours (1% solution should not be given more frequently than every 4 hours)<br><br>0.25% solution:<br>**Children 6–12 years:** 2–3 sprays or drops in each nostril q 3–4 hours | Administration Issues:<br>nasal sprays are preferred to drops because of the lesser risk of swallowing the drug and resultant systemic absorption; dropper and dispensers should not be used by more than one person; tips of the dispensers or droppers should be rinsed with hot water following use; do not use topical nasal sprays longer than 3–5 days | ADRs:<br>burning; stinging; sneezing; dryness; local irritation; rebound congestion<br><br>Pharmacokinetics:<br>onset = 30 minutes; systemic absorption is minimal | Contraindications:<br>hypersensitivity to decongestants; monoamine oxidase (MAO) inhibitor therapy; severe hypertension or coronary artery disease<br><br>Pregnancy Category: C<br><br>Lactation Issues:<br>it is not known whether topical decongestants are excreted in breast milk; use with caution |

| Phenylpropanolamine | | | | |
|---|---|---|---|---|
| **Phenylpropanolamine**<br><br>*Nasal congestion products:*<br>Propagest, Rhindecon, others<br><br>*Nonprescription Diet Aids:*<br>Dexatrim Pre-Meal, Acutrim, Phenoxine, others<br><br>Tablets: 25 mg, 50 mg<br><br>Timed Release Capsules:<br>25 mg, 37.5 mg, 75 mg<br><br>Timed Release Tablets:<br>75 mg<br><br>Precision Release Tablets:<br>75 mg<br><br>Combination Products:<br>w/ various combinations of antihistamines, non-narcotic analgesics, narcotic analgesics, expectorants, antitussives | 0.16% solution:<br>**Infants:** 1–2 drops in each nostril q 3 hours<br><br>**Temporary relief of nasal congestion due to common cold, hay fever, allergies and sinusitis; promote nasal and sinus drainage; relief of eustachian tube congestion**<br><br>**Adults and children > 12 years**<br>(Maximum dose: 150 mg daily)<br><br>Tablets: 25 mg q 4 h<br>Sustained release capsules:<br>75 mg q 12 h<br><br>**Children 6–12 years:**<br>(Max dose: 75 mg daily) 12.5 mg q 4 hours<br><br>**Children 2–6 years:** 6.25 mg every 4 hours<br><br>**Stress Urinary Incontinence:**<br>25 to 100 mg bid<br><br>**Short-term (8–12 weeks) adjunct in a regimen of weight loss based on caloric restriction**<br>Immediate release: 25 mg tid, 30 min ac<br>Timed release: 75 mg qd at 9 am<br>Precision release (16 hr duration): 75 mg after breakfast | Administration Issues:<br>safety and efficacy have not been established in children < 12 years of age; do not crush or chew sustained release preparations<br><br>Drug–Drug Interactions:<br>concurrent use with **monoamine oxidase inhibitors** may result in severe headache, hypertension, hyperpyrexia and possibly hypertensive crisis; concomitant administration with **reserpine, tricyclic antidepressants, guanethidine** or **methyldopa** may result in hypertension; additive effects may occur when given with other **sympathomimetic agents** | ADRs:<br>increased blood pressure; anxiousness; restlessness; GI upset<br><br>Pharmacokinetics:<br>rapidly absorbed; onset = 15–30 minutes; duration of action = 3 hours; $T_{1/2}$ = 3–4 hours | Contraindications:<br>hypersensitivity to decongestants; monoamine oxidase (MAO) inhibitor therapy; severe hypertension or coronary artery disease<br><br>Pregnancy Category: C<br><br>Lactation Issues:<br>phenylpropanolamine is contraindicated because of the higher than usual risks to infants from sympathomimetic agents |

(continues on next page)

**703.** Nasal Decongestants *continued from previous page*

| Drug and Dosage Forms | Usual Dosage Range | Administration Issues and Drug–Drug Interactions | Common Adverse Drug Reactions (ADRs) and Pharmacokinetics | Contraindications, Pregnancy Category, and Lactation Issues |
|---|---|---|---|---|
| **Pseudoephedrine**<br>Afrin, Dorcol, Sudafed<br><br>Tablets:<br>30 mg, 60 mg<br><br>Sustained Release Tablets:<br>120 mg<br><br>Capsules: 60 mg<br><br>Sustained Release Capsules:<br>120 mg<br><br>Liquid: 15 mg/5 mL,<br>30 mg/5 mL<br><br>Drops: 7.5 mg/0.8 mL<br><br>Combination Products:<br>w/ various combinations of antihistamines, non-narcotic analgesics, narcotic analgesics, expectorants, antitussives | **Temporary relief of nasal congestion due to common cold, hay fever, allergies and sinusitis: promote nasal and sinus drainage; relief of eustachian tube congestion**<br><br>**Adults and children > 12 years:**<br><br>Tablets: 60 mg q 4–6 h<br><br>Sustained release preparations:<br>120 mg q 12 h<br><br>Maximum dose: 240 mg daily<br><br>**Children 6–12 years:**<br>30 mg q 4–6 h. Maximum dose:<br>120 mg daily<br><br>**Children 2–5 years:**<br>15 mg q 4–6 h. Maximum dose:<br>60 mg daily<br><br>Drops:<br>**Children 1–2 years:** 7 drops/kg<br>q 4–6 h up to 4 doses<br><br>**Children 3–12 months:** 3 drops/kg<br>q 4–6 h up to 4 doses<br><br>**Stress Urinary Incontinence:**<br>15 to 30 mg tid | Administration Issues:<br>safety and efficacy have not been established in children < 12 years of age; do not crush or chew sustained release preparations<br><br>Drug–Drug Interactions:<br>concurrent use with **monoamine oxidase inhibitors** may result in severe headache, hypertension, hyperpyrexia and possibly hypertensive crisis; concomitant administration with **reserpine, tricyclic antidepressants, guanethidine** or **methyldopa** may result in hypertension; additive effects may occur when given with other **sympathomimetic agents** | ADRs:<br>increased blood pressure; anxiousness; restlessness; GI upset<br><br>Pharmacokinetics:<br>onset within 30 minutes; duration = 4–8 hours (12 hours for sustained release formulations) | Contraindications:<br>hypersensitivity to decongestants; monoamine oxidase (MAO) inhibitor therapy; severe hypertension or coronary artery disease<br><br>Pregnancy Category: C<br><br>Lactation Issues:<br>oral pseudoephedrine is contraindicated because of the higher than usual risks to infants from sympathomimetic agents |

| | | | | |
|---|---|---|---|---|
| **Tetrahydrozoline**<br>Tyzine<br><br>Solution:<br>0.05%, 0.1% | **relief of nasal and nasopharyngeal mucosal congestion due to common cold, hay fever, sinusitis or allergies**<br><br>0.1% solution:<br>**Adults and children > 6 years:**<br>2–4 drops in each nostril q 3–4 hours; 3–4 sprays in each nostril q 4 hours as needed<br><br>0.05% solution:<br>**Children 2–6 years:**<br>2–3 drops in each nostril q 4–6 hours as needed | Administration Issues:<br>safety and efficacy have not been established for the 0.1% solution in children < 6 years of age or for the 0.05% solution in infants < 2 years of age; dropper and dispensers should not be used by more than one person; tips of the dispensers or droppers should be rinsed with hot water following use; do not use topical nasal sprays longer than 3–5 days | ADRs:<br>burning; stinging; sneezing; dryness; local irritation; rebound congestion<br><br>Pharmacokinetics:<br>onset = 5–10 minutes; duration = 4–8 hours; systemic absorption is minimal | Contraindications:<br>hypersensitivity to decongestants; monoamine oxidase (MAO) inhibitor therapy; severe hypertension or coronary artery disease<br><br>Pregnancy Category: C<br><br>Lactation Issues:<br>it is not known whether topical decongestants are excreted in breast milk; use with caution |
| **Xylometazoline**<br>Otrivin<br><br>Solution:<br>0.05%, 0.1% | **relief of nasal and nasopharyngeal mucosal congestion due to common cold, hay fever, sinusitis or allergies**<br><br>0.1% solution:<br>**Adults and children > 12 years:**<br>2–3 drops or sprays in each nostril q 8–10 h<br><br>0.05% solution:<br>**Children 2–12 years:** 2–3 drops in q nostril q 8–10 h | Administration Issues:<br>dropper and dispensers should not be used by more than one person; tips of the dispensers or droppers should be rinsed with hot water following use; do not use topical nasal sprays longer than 3–5 days | ADRs:<br>burning; stinging; sneezing; dryness; local irritation; rebound congestion<br><br>Pharmacokinetics:<br>onset = 5–10 minutes; duration = 5–6 hours; systemic absorption is minimal | Contraindications:<br>hypersensitivity to decongestants; monoamine oxidase (MAO) inhibitor therapy; severe hypertension or coronary artery disease<br><br>Pregnancy Category: C<br><br>Lactation Issues:<br>it is not known whether topical decongestants are excreted in breast milk; use with caution |

# 704. Antitussives

| Drug and Dosage Forms | Usual Dosage Range | Administration Issues and Drug–Drug Interactions | Common Adverse Drug Reactions (ADRs) and Pharmacokinetics | Contraindications, Pregnancy Category, and Lactation Issues |
|---|---|---|---|---|
| **Benzonatate**<br>Tessalon Perles<br><br>Capsules:<br>100 mg | **Symptomatic relief of cough**<br><br>**Adults and Children > 10 years:**<br>100 mg tid<br>maximum dose = 600 mg/day | Administration Issues:<br>do not chew or break capsules, swallow whole | ADRs:<br>sedation; headache; dizziness; constipation; GI upset; rash<br><br>Pharmacokinetics:<br>onset = 15–20 minutes; duration = 3–8 hours | Contraindications:<br>hypersensitivity to benzonatate or related compounds (tetracaine)<br><br>Pregnancy Category: C<br><br>Lactation Issues:<br>it is not known whether benzonatate is excreted in breast milk |
| **Codeine (CII)**<br><br>Tablets:<br>15 mg, 30 mg, 60 mg<br><br>Combination Products:<br>w/ various combinations of antihistamines, decongestants, expectorants | **Cough suppression**<br><br>**Adults:**<br>10–20 mg q 4–6 hours; maximum dose = 120 mg/day<br><br>**Children (6–12 years:)**<br>5–10 mg q 4–6 h; maximum dose = 60 mg/day<br><br>**Children (2–6 years):**<br>2.5–5 mg q 4–6 h; maximum dose = 30 mg/day | Administration Issues:<br>safety and efficacy in newborns have not been established; take with food to minimize GI upset; should not be used for the persistent cough associated with smoking, asthma or emphysema or for a cough accompanied by excessive secretions<br><br>Drug–Drug Interactions:<br>additive effects occur with concomitant administration with other CNS depressants **(alcohol, sedatives, hypnotics, phenothiazines, antihistamines, tricyclic antidepressants, tranquilizers)** | ADRs:<br>nausea; vomiting; sedation; dizziness; constipation; orthostatic hypotension; dry mouth<br><br>Pharmacokinetics:<br>absorption = 100%; metabolized in the liver and excreted in the urine; $T_{1/2}$ = 3 hours | Contraindications:<br>hypersensitivity to codeine; premature infants<br><br>Pregnancy Category: C<br><br>Lactation Issues:<br>codeine is excreted in breast, use with caution |
| **Dextromethorphan**<br>St. Josephs Cough Suppressant, Robitussin Pediatric, | **Control of nonproductive cough**<br><br>Lozenges, Liquid, Syrup:<br>**Adults:** | Administration Issues:<br>should not be used for the persistent cough associated with smoking, asthma or emphysema or for a | ADRs:<br>GI upset; drowsiness; dizziness | Contraindications:<br>hypersensitivity to dextromethorphan; patients receiving MAO inhibitors |

| Drug / Formulations | Dosage | Indications / Drug–Drug Interactions | Pharmacokinetics / ADRs / Contraindications |
|---|---|---|---|
| Pertussin CS, Hold, Sucrets, Vicks 44, Benylin DM, Delsym<br><br>Lozenges:<br>2.5 mg, 5 mg, 7.5 mg<br><br>Liquid:<br>3.5 mg/5 mL,<br>7.5 mg/5 mL,<br>15 mg/5 mL<br><br>Syrup: 10 mg/5 mL,<br>15 mg/15 mL<br><br>Sustained Action<br>Liquid: 30 mg/5 mL<br><br>Combination Products:<br>w/ various combinations of antitussive, methylxanthines, decongestants | 10–30 mg q 4–8 h; maximum dose = 120 mg/day<br><br>**Children (6–12 years):**<br>5–10 mg q 4 h or 15 mg q 6–8 h; maximum dose = 60 mg/day<br><br>**Children (2–6 years) Syrup:**<br>2.5–7.5 mg q 4–8 h; maximum dose = 30 mg/day<br><br>Sustained Action Liquid:<br>**Adults:** 60 mg q 12 h<br><br>**Children (6–12 years):** 30 mg q 12 h<br><br>**Children (2–6 years):** 15 mg q 12 h | cough accompanied by excessive secretions<br><br>Drug–Drug Interactions:<br>**MAO inhibitors** in combination with dextromethorphan may lead to hypotension, hyperpyrexia, nausea, myoclonic leg jerks and coma | Pharmacokinetics:<br>rapidly absorbed from GI tract; onset = 15–30 minutes; duration = 3–6 hours |
| **Diphenhydramine**<br>Benylin, Tusstat<br><br>Syrup: 12.5 mg/5 mL<br><br>Combination Products:<br>w/ various combinations of decongestants, analgesics | **Cough due to colds or allergy**<br><br>**Adults:**<br>25 mg q 4 h; maximum dose = 150 mg/day<br><br>**Children (6–12 years):**<br>12.5 mg q 4 h; maximum dose = 75 mg/day<br><br>**Children (2–6 years):**<br>6.25 mg q 4 h; maximum dose = 25 mg/day | Drug–Drug Interactions:<br>**MAO inhibitors** may potentiate the anticholinergic effects of antihistamines; additive CNS depressant effects may occur with concurrent use of **alcohol** or **other CNS depressants** | ADRs:<br>drowsiness; GI upset; dry mouth; thickening of bronchial secretions; urinary retention; constipation<br><br>Pharmacokinetics:<br>well absorbed; onset = 15–30 minutes; duration = 6–8 hours<br><br>Contraindications:<br>hypersensitivity to antihistamines; narrow-angle glaucoma; stenosing peptic ulcer, symptomatic prostatic hypertrophy; bladder neck obstruction; asthmatic attack; concurrent monoamine oxidase inhibitor (MAO) therapy; newborns and premature infants; third trimester of pregnancy<br><br>Pregnancy Category: B<br><br>Lactation Issues:<br>antihistamine therapy is contraindicated in nursing mothers |

# 705. Antihistamines

## 705.1 Antihistamines—First Generation

| Drug and Dosage Forms | Usual Dosage Range | Administration Issues and Drug–Drug Interactions | Common Adverse Drug Reactions (ADRs) and Pharmacokinetics | Contraindications, Pregnancy Category, and Lactation Issues |
|---|---|---|---|---|
| **Azatadine**<br>Optimine<br><br><u>Tablets:</u>  1 mg | **Allergic rhinitis and conjunctivitis: relief of runny nose and sneezing due to the common cold: pruritus and urticaria:**<br><br>**Adults and children > 12 years:**<br>1–2 mg bid | <u>Administration Issues:</u><br>safety and efficacy in children < 12 have not been established<br><br><u>Drug–Drug Interactions:</u><br>**MAO inhibitors** may potentiate the anticholinergic effects of antihistamines; additive CNS depressant effects may occur with concurrent use of **alcohol** or **other CNS depressants** | <u>ADRs:</u><br>drowsiness; GI upset; dry mouth; thickening of bronchial secretions; urinary retention; constipation<br><br><u>Pharmacokinetics:</u><br>well absorbed; onset = 15–30 minutes; duration up to 12 hours | <u>Contraindications:</u><br>hypersensitivity to antihistamines; narrow-angle glaucoma; stenosing peptic ulcer, symptomatic prostatic hypertrophy; bladder neck obstruction; asthmatic attack; concurrent monoamine oxidase inhibitor (MAOI) therapy; newborns and premature infants; third trimester of pregnancy<br><br><u>Pregnancy Category:</u>  B<br><br><u>Lactation Issues:</u><br>antihistamine therapy is contraindicated in nursing mothers |
| **Brompheniramine**<br>Bromphen, Dimetane<br><br><u>Tablets:</u>  4 mg, 8 mg, 12 mg<br><br>**Sustained Release**<br>**Tablets:** 8 mg, 12 mg<br><br><u>Elixir:</u>  2 mg/5 mL | **Allergic rhinitis and conjunctivitis: relief of runny nose and sneezing due to the common cold: pruritus and urticaria**<br><br><u>Tablets and elixir:</u><br>**Adults and children > 12 years:**<br>4 mg q 4–6 h; Maximum dose: 24 mg daily | <u>Drug–Drug Interactions:</u><br>**MAO inhibitors** may potentiate the anticholinergic effects of antihistamines; additive CNS depressant effects may occur with concurrent use of **alcohol** or **other CNS depressants** | <u>ADRs:</u><br>drowsiness; GI upset; dry mouth; thickening of bronchial secretions; urinary retention; constipation<br><br><u>Pharmacokinetics</u><br>well absorbed; onset = 15–30 minutes; duration = 4–6 hours | <u>Contraindications:</u><br>hypersensitivity to antihistamines; narrow-angle glaucoma; stenosing peptic ulcer, symptomatic prostatic hypertrophy; bladder neck obstruction; asthmatic attack; concurrent monoamine oxidase inhibitor (MAOI) therapy; newborns and premature |

| | | | | |
|---|---|---|---|---|
| Combination Products:<br>w/ various combinations of decongestants, analgesics, antitussives | Children 6–12 years: 2 mg q 4–6 h; Maximum dose: 12 mg daily<br><br>Sustained release tablets:<br>Adults and children > 12 years: 8–12 mg q 8–12 h | | | infants; third trimester of pregnancy<br><br>Pregnancy Category: C<br><br>Lactation Issues:<br>antihistamine therapy is contra-indicated in nursing mothers |
| Carbinoxamine<br>Clistin<br><br>Tablets: 4 mg | Allergic rhinitis and conjunctivitis; relief of runny nose and sneezing due to the common cold; pruritus and urticaria<br><br>Adults: 4–8 mg tid to qid<br><br>Children > 6 years: 4–6 mg tid to qid<br><br>Children 3–6 years: 2–4 mg tid to qid<br><br>Children 1–3 years: 2 mg tid to qid | Drug–Drug Interactions:<br>MAO inhibitors may potentiate the anticholinergic effects of antihistamines; additive CNS depressant effects may occur with concurrent use of alcohol or other CNS depressants | ADRs:<br>drowsiness; GI upset; dry mouth; thickening of bronchial secretions; urinary retention; constipation<br><br>Pharmacokinetics:<br>well absorbed; onset = 15–30 minutes; duration = 6–8 hours | Contraindications:<br>hypersensitivity to antihistamines; narrow-angle glaucoma; stenosing peptic ulcer, symptomatic prostatic hypertrophy; bladder neck obstruction; asthmatic attack; concurrent monoamine oxidase inhibitor (MAOI) therapy; newborns and premature infants; third trimester of pregnancy<br><br>Pregnancy Category: C<br><br>Lactation Issues:<br>antihistamine therapy is contra-indicated in nursing mothers |
| Chlorpheniramine<br>Chlor-Trimeton<br><br>Chewable Tablets: 2 mg<br><br>Tablets: 4 mg, 8 mg, 12 mg<br><br>Capsules: 12 mg | Allergic rhinitis and conjunctivitis; relief of runny nose and sneezing due to the common cold; pruritus and urticaria<br><br>Tablets and syrup:<br>Adults and children > 12 years: 4 mg q 4–6 h; Maximum dose: 24 mg daily | Drug–Drug Interactions:<br>MAO inhibitors may potentiate the anticholinergic effects of antihistamines; additive CNS depressant effects may occur with concurrent use of alcohol or other CNS depressants | ADRs:<br>drowsiness; GI upset; dry mouth; thickening of bronchial secretions; urinary retention; constipation<br><br>Pharmacokinetics:<br>well absorbed; onset = 15–30 minutes; duration = 4–6 hours | Contraindications:<br>hypersensitivity to antihistamines; narrow-angle glaucoma; stenosing peptic ulcer, symptomatic prostatic hypertrophy; bladder neck obstruction; asthmatic attack; concurrent monoamine oxidase inhibitor (MAOI) therapy; newborns and premature |

(continues on next page)

| Drug and Dosage Forms | Usual Dosage Range | Administration Issues and Drug–Drug Interactions | Common Adverse Drug Reactions (ADRs) and Pharmacokinetics | Contraindications, Pregnancy Category, and Lactation Issues |
|---|---|---|---|---|
| **Chlorpheniramine cont.**<br><br><u>Sustained Release Tablets:</u><br>8 mg, 12 mg<br><br><u>Sustained Release Capsules:</u><br>8 mg, 12 mg<br><br><u>Syrup:</u> 2 mg/5 mL<br><br><u>Combination Products:</u><br>w/ various combinations of decongestants, analgesics, antitussives | **Children 6–12 years:**<br>2 mg q 4–6 h; Maximum dose: 12 mg daily<br><br>**Children 2–6 years:**<br>1 mg q 4–6 h; Maximum dose: 4 mg daily<br><br><u>Sustained release forms:</u><br>**Adults and children > 12 years:**<br>8–12 mg q 8–12 h<br><br>**Children 6–12 years:** 8 mg q 8–12 h | | | infants; third trimester of pregnancy<br><br><u>Pregnancy Category:</u> B<br><br><u>Lactation Issues:</u><br>antihistamine therapy is contraindicated in nursing mothers |
| **Clemastine**<br>Tavist<br><br><u>Tablets:</u> 1.34 mg, 2.68 mg<br><br><u>Syrup:</u> 0.67 mg/5 mL | **Allergic rhinitis and conjunctivitis; relief of runny nose and sneezing due to the common cold; pruritus and urticaria**<br><br>**Adults and children > 12 years:**<br>1.34 mg bid 2.68 mg tid<br><br>Maximum dose: 8.04 mg daily | <u>Drug–Drug Interactions:</u><br>**MAO inhibitors** may potentiate the anticholinergic effects of antihistamines; additive CNS depressant effects may occur with concurrent use of **alcohol** or **other CNS depressants** | <u>ADRs:</u><br>drowsiness; GI upset; dry mouth; thickening of bronchial secretions; urinary retention; constipation<br><br><u>Pharmacokinetics:</u><br>well absorbed; onset = 15–30 minutes; duration up to 12 hours | <u>Contraindications:</u><br>hypersensitivity to antihistamines; narrow-angle glaucoma; stenosing peptic ulcer, symptomatic prostatic hypertrophy; bladder neck obstruction; asthmatic attack; concurrent monoamine oxidase inhibitor (MAOI) therapy; newborns and premature infants; third trimester of pregnancy<br><br><u>Pregnancy Category:</u> B<br><br><u>Lactation Issues:</u><br>antihistamine therapy is contra-indicated in nursing mothers |

| Cyproheptadine | Allergic rhinitis and conjunctivitis: relief of runny nose and sneezing due to the common cold; pruritus and urticaria | Administration Issues: safety and efficacy in children < 2 have not been established | ADRs: drowsiness; GI upset; dry mouth; thickening of bronchial secretions; urinary retention; constipation | Contraindications: hypersensitivity to antihistamines; narrow-angle glaucoma; stenosing peptic ulcer, symptomatic prostatic hypertrophy; bladder neck obstruction; asthmatic attack; concurrent monoamine oxidase inhibitor (MAOI) therapy; newborns and premature infants; third trimester of pregnancy |
|---|---|---|---|---|
| Periactin | | | | |
| | **Adults:** Initial dose: 4 mg tid. Maintenance dose: 12–32 mg daily in divided doses | Drug–Drug Interactions: **MAO inhibitors** may potentiate the anticholinergic effects of antihistamines; additive CNS depressant effects may occur with concurrent use of **alcohol** or **other CNS depressants** | Pharmacokinetics: well absorbed; onset = 15–30 minutes; duration up to 8 hours | Pregnancy Category:  B |
| Tablets: 4 mg | | | | |
| | **Children 7–14 years:** 4 mg bid to tid; Maximum dose: 16 mg daily | | | Lactation Issues: antihistamine therapy is contra-indicated in nursing mothers |
| Syrup: 2 mg/5 mL | | | | |
| | **Children 2–7 years:** 2 mg bid to tid; Maximum dose: 12 mg daily | | | |
| **Dexchlorpheniramine** | **Allergic rhinitis and conjunctivitis: relief of runny nose and sneezing due to the common cold; pruritus and urticaria** | Administration Issues: safety and efficacy in children < 12 have not been established | ADRs: drowsiness; GI upset; dry mouth; thickening of bronchial secretions; urinary retention; constipation | Contraindications: hypersensitivity to antihistamines; narrow-angle glaucoma; stenosing peptic ulcer, symptomatic prostatic hypertrophy; bladder neck obstruction; asthmatic attack; concurrent monoamine oxidase inhibitor (MAOI) therapy; newborns and premature infants; third trimester of pregnancy |
| Poladex, Polaramine | | | | |
| | Tablets and syrup: **Adults:** 2 mg q 4–6 h | Drug–Drug Interactions: **MAO inhibitors** may potentiate the anticholinergic effects of antihistamines; additive CNS depressant effects may occur with concurrent use of **alcohol** or **other CNS depressants** | Pharmacokinetics: well absorbed; onset = 15–30 minutes; duration = 4–6 hours | Pregnancy Category:  B |
| Tablets: 2 mg | | | | |
| | **Children 6–11 years:** 1 mg q 4–6 h | | | Lactation Issues: antihistamine therapy is contraindicated in nursing mothers |
| Sustained Release Tablets: 4 mg, 6 mg | **Children 2–5 years:** 0.5 mg q 4–6 h | | | |
| | Sustained release tablets: **Adults:** 4–6 mg q 8–10 h | | | |
| Syrup: 2 mg/5 mL | | | | |
| | **Children 6–11 years:** 4 mg q hs | | | |

(continues on next page)

| Drug and Dosage Forms | Usual Dosage Range | Administration Issues and Drug–Drug Interactions | Common Adverse Drug Reactions (ADRs) and Pharmacokinetics | Contraindications, Pregnancy Category, and Lactation Issues |
|---|---|---|---|---|
| **Diphenhydramine** <br> Benadryl <br><br> Capsules: 25 mg, 50 mg <br><br> Tablets: 25 mg, 50 mg <br><br> Elixir: 12.5 mg/5 mL <br><br> Syrup: 12.5 mg/5 mL <br><br> Combination Products: <br> w/ various combinations of decongestants, analgesics, antitussives | **Allergic rhinitis and conjunctivitis: relief of runny nose and sneezing due to the common cold: pruritus and urticaria** <br><br> **Adults:** 25–50 mg q 6–8 h <br><br> **Children > 10 kg:** 12.5–25 mg q 6–8 h <br><br> **Motion sickness:** <br> 25–50 mg given 30 minutes before exposure to motion <br><br> **Nighttime sleep aid for adults:** <br> 50 mg hs <br><br> **Cough Suppression (syrup):** <br> **Adults:** 25–50 mg q 6–8 h <br><br> **Children > 10 kg:** 12.5–25 mg q 6–8 h | Drug–Drug Interactions: <br> **MAO inhibitors** may potentiate the anticholinergic effects of antihistamines; additive CNS depressant effects may occur with concurrent use of **alcohol** or **other CNS depressants** | ADRs: <br> drowsiness; GI upset; dry mouth; thickening of bronchial secretions; urinary retention; constipation <br><br> Pharmacokinetics: <br> well absorbed; onset = 15–30 minutes; duration = 6–8 hours | Contraindications: <br> hypersensitivity to antihistamines; narrow-angle glaucoma; stenosing peptic ulcer, symptomatic prostatic hypertrophy; bladder neck obstruction; asthmatic attack; concurrent monoamine oxidase inhibitor (MAO) therapy; newborns and premature infants; third trimester of pregnancy <br><br> Pregnancy Category: B <br><br> Lactation Issues: <br> antihistamine therapy is contraindicated in nursing mothers |
| **Hydroxyzine** <br> Atarax, Vistaril, generics <br><br> Tablets: 10 mg, 25 mg, 50 mg, 100 mg | **Management of pruritus due to allergic conditions such as chronic urticaria and atopic or chronic dermatitis** <br><br> **Adults:** 25 mg 3–4 times/d | Administration Issues: <br> Avoid alcohol use. <br><br> Drug–Drug Interactions: <br> **MAO inhibitors** may potentiate the anticholinergic effects of antihistamines; additive CNS depressant effects may occur | ADRs: <br> drowsiness; GI upset; dry mouth; thickening of bronchial secretions; urinary retention; constipation; photosensitivity; involuntary muscle movements | Contraindications: <br> hypersensitivity to antihistamines; narrow-angle glaucoma; prostatic hypertrophy <br><br> Pregnancy Category: C |

| | | | | |
|---|---|---|---|---|
| Capsules: 25 mg, 50 mg, 100 mg<br><br>Syrup: 10 mg/5 mL<br><br>Oral Suspension: 25 mg/5 mL | Children:<br>> 6 y: 50 to 100 mg daily in divided doses<br>< 6 y: 50 mg daily in divided doses | with concurrent use of **alcohol** or **other CNS depressants** | Pharmacokinetics:<br>well absorbed; onset = 15–30 minutes; duration = 4–6 hours | Lactation Issues: antihistamine therapy is contraindicated in nursing mothers |
| **Methdilazine**<br>Tacaryl<br><br>Chewable Tablets: 4 mg<br><br>Tablets: 8 mg<br><br>Syrup: 4 mg/5 mL | **Allergic rhinitis and conjunctivitis; relief of runny nose and sneezing due to the common cold; pruritus and urticaria**<br><br>**Adults:** 8 mg bid to qid<br><br>**Children > 3 years:** 4 mg bid to qid | Administration Issues:<br>safety and efficacy in children < 3 have not been established<br><br>Drug–Drug Interactions:<br>**MAO inhibitors** may potentiate the anticholinergic effects of antihistamines; additive CNS depressant effects may occur with concurrent use of **alcohol** or **other CNS depressants** | ADRs:<br>drowsiness; GI upset; dry mouth; thickening of bronchial secretions; urinary retention; constipation; photosensitivity; involuntary muscle movements<br><br>Pharmacokinetics:<br>well absorbed; onset = 15–30 minutes; duration = 6–12 hours | Contraindications:<br>hypersensitivity to antihistamines; narrow-angle glaucoma; stenosing peptic ulcer, symptomatic prostatic hypertrophy; bladder neck obstruction; asthmatic attack; concurrent monoamine oxidase inhibitor (MAO) therapy; hypersensitivity to phenothiazines; newborns and premature infants; third trimester of pregnancy<br><br>Pregnancy Category: B<br><br>Lactation Issues:<br>antihistamine therapy is contra-indicated in nursing mothers |
| **Phenindamine**<br>Nolahist<br><br>Tablets: 25 mg | **Allergic rhinitis and conjunctivitis; relief of runny nose and sneezing due to the common cold; pruritus and urticaria**<br><br>**Adults and children > 12 years:**<br>25 mg q 4–6 h; Maximum dose: 150 mg daily | Drug–Drug Interactions:<br>**MAO inhibitors** may potentiate the anticholinergic effects of antihistamines; additive CNS depressant effects may occur with concurrent use of **alcohol** or **other CNS depressants** | ADRs:<br>drowsiness; GI upset; dry mouth; thickening of bronchial secretions; urinary retention; constipation<br><br>Pharmacokinetics:<br>well absorbed; | Contraindications:<br>hypersensitivity to antihistamines; narrow-angle glaucoma; stenosing peptic ulcer, symptomatic prostatic hypertrophy; bladder neck obstruction; asthmatic attack; concurrent monoamine oxidase inhibitor (MAO) therapy; |

*(continues on next page)*

| Drug and Dosage Forms | Usual Dosage Range | Administration Issues and Drug–Drug Interactions | Common Adverse Drug Reactions (ADRs) and Pharmacokinetics | Contraindications, Pregnancy Category, and Lactation Issues |
|---|---|---|---|---|
| **Phenindamine** *cont.* | **Children 6–12 years:** 12.5 mg q 4–6 h; Maximum dose: 75 mg daily | | onset = 15–30 minutes; duration = 4–6 hours | newborns and premature infants; third trimester of pregnancy<br><br>Pregnancy Category: C<br><br>Lactation Issues: antihistamine therapy is contraindicated in nursing mothers |
| **Pyrilamine**<br>Nisaval<br><br>Tablets: 25 mg<br><br>Combination Products: w/ various combinations antitussives, decongestants | **Allergic rhinitis and conjunctivitis: relief of runny nose and sneezing due to the common cold; pruritus and urticaria**<br><br>**Adults:** 25–50 mg tid to qid | Drug–Drug Interactions:<br>**MAO inhibitors** may potentiate the anticholinergic effects of antihistamines; additive CNS depressant effects may occur with concurrent use of **alcohol** or **other CNS depressants** | ADRs:<br>drowsiness; GI upset; dry mouth; thickening of bronchial secretions; urinary retention; constipation<br><br>Pharmacokinetics:<br>well absorbed; onset = 15–30 minutes; duration = 6–8 hours | Contraindications:<br>hypersensitivity to antihistamines; narrow-angle glaucoma; stenosing peptic ulcer, symptomatic prostatic hypertrophy; bladder neck obstruction; asthmatic attack; concurrent monoamine oxidase inhibitor (MAOI) therapy; newborns and premature infants; third trimester of pregnancy<br><br>Pregnancy Category: C<br><br>Lactation Issues:<br>antihistamine therapy is contra-indicated in nursing mothers |
| **Trimeprazine**<br>Temaril | **Allergic rhinitis and conjunctivitis: relief of runny nose** | Drug–Drug Interactions:<br>**MAO inhibitors** may potentiate the | ADRs:<br>drowsiness; GI upset; dry mouth; | Contraindications:<br>hypersensitivity to |

| | | |
|---|---|---|
| Tablets: 2.5 mg<br><br>Sustained Release Capsules: 5 mg<br><br>Syrup: 2.5 mg/5 mL | **and sneezing due to the common cold; pruritus and urticaria**<br><br>Tablets and syrup:<br>**Adults:** 2.5 mg qid<br><br>**Children > 3 years:** 2.5 mg tid<br><br>**Children 6 months to 3 years:** 1.25 mg tid<br><br>Sustained release capsules:<br>**Adults:** 5 mg q 12 h<br><br>**Children >6 yr.:** 5 mg qd | anticholinergic effects of antihistamines; additive CNS depressant effects may occur with concurrent use of **alcohol** or **other CNS depressants** | thickening of bronchial secretions; urinary retention; constipation; photosensitivity; involuntary muscle movements<br><br>Pharmacokinetics:<br>well absorbed; onset = 15–30 minutes; duration = 4–6 hours | antihistamines; narrow-angle glaucoma; stenosing peptic ulcer, symptomatic prostatic hypertrophy; bladder neck obstruction; asthmatic attack; concurrent monoamine oxidase inhibitor (MAOI) therapy; hypersensitivity to phenothiazines; newborns and premature infants; third trimester of pregnancy<br><br>Pregnancy Category:  C<br><br>Lactation Issues:<br>antihistamine therapy is contraindicated in nursing mothers |
| **Tripelennamine**<br>PBZ, Pelamine<br><br>Tablets: 25 mg, 50 mg<br><br>Sustained Release Tablets: 100 mg | **Allergic rhinitis and conjunctivitis; relief of runny nose and sneezing due to the common cold; pruritus and urticaria**<br><br>Tablets and elixir:<br>**Adults:** 25–50 mg q 4–6 h<br><br>**Children and infants:**<br>5 mg/kg/day in 4–6 divided doses<br><br>Sustained release tablets:<br>**Adults:  100 mg bid to tid** | Drug–Drug Interactions:<br>**MAO inhibitors** may potentiate the anticholinergic effects of antihistamines; additive CNS depressant effects may occur with concurrent use of **alcohol** or **other CNS depressants** | ADRs:<br>drowsiness; GI upset; dry mouth; thickening of bronchial secretions; urinary retention; constipation<br><br>Pharmacokinetics:<br>well absorbed; onset = 15–30 minutes; duration = 4–6 hours | Contraindications:<br>hypersensitivity to antihistamines; narrow-angle glaucoma; stenosing peptic ulcer, symptomatic prostatic hypertrophy; bladder neck obstruction; asthmatic attack; concurrent monoamine oxidase inhibitor (MAOI) therapy; newborns and premature infants; third trimester of pregnancy<br><br>Pregnancy Category:  C<br><br>Lactation Issues:<br>antihistamine therapy is contra-indicated in nursing mothers |

(continues on next page)

| Drug and Dosage Forms | Usual Dosage Range | Administration Issues and Drug–Drug Interactions | Common Adverse Drug Reactions (ADRs) and Pharmacokinetics | Contraindications, Pregnancy Category, and Lactation Issues |
|---|---|---|---|---|
| **Triprolidine**<br>Actidil<br><br>Tablets: 2.5 mg<br><br>Syrup: 1.25 mg/5 mL<br><br>Combination Products:<br>w/ various combinations of<br>decongestants | **Allergic rhinitis and conjunctivitis; relief of runny nose and sneezing due to the common cold; pruritus and urticaria**<br><br>**Adults and children > 12 years:**<br>2.5 mg q 4–6 h; Maximum dose: 10 mg daily<br><br>**Children 6–12 years:**<br>1.25 mg q 4–6 h; Maximum dose: 5 mg daily | Drug–Drug Interactions:<br>**MAO inhibitors** may potentiate the anticholinergic effects of antihistamines; additive CNS depressant effects may occur with concurrent use of **alcohol** or **other CNS depressants** | ADRs:<br>drowsiness; GI upset; dry mouth; thickening of bronchial secretions; urinary retention; constipation<br><br>Pharmacokinetics:<br>well absorbed; onset = 15–30 minutes; duration = 4–6 hours | Contraindications:<br>hypersensitivity to antihistamines; narrow-angle glaucoma; stenosing peptic ulcer, symptomatic prostatic hypertrophy; bladder neck obstruction; asthmatic attack; concurrent monoamine oxidase inhibitor (MAOI) therapy; newborns and premature infants; third trimester of pregnancy<br><br>Pregnancy Category:  C<br><br>Lactation Issues:<br>antihistamine therapy is contra-indicated in nursing mothers |

## 705.2 Antihistamines—Second Generation

| Drug and Dosage Forms | Usual Dosage Range | Administration Issues and Drug–Drug Interactions | Common Adverse Drug Reactions (ADRs) and Pharmacokinetics | Contraindications, Pregnancy Category, and Lactation Issues |
|---|---|---|---|---|
| **Astemizole**<br>Hismanal<br><br><u>Tablets:</u> 10 mg | **Allergic rhinitis and conjunctivitis: relief of runny nose and sneezing due to the common cold: pruritus and urticaria**<br><br>**Adults and children >12 years:**<br>10 mg qd | <u>Administration Issues:</u><br>take at least 1 hour before or 2 hours after eating; use with caution in patients with hepatic dysfunction; safety and efficacy in children < 12 have not been established<br><br><u>Drug–Drug Interactions:</u><br>**fluconazole, itraconazole, ketoconazole, miconazole, erythromycin, azithromycin, clarithromycin, troleandomycin** may increase astemizole levels; **MAO inhibitors** may potentiate the anticholinergic effects of antihistamines; additive CNS depressant effects may occur with concurrent use of **alcohol** or **other CNS depressants**<br><br><u>Drug–Food Interactions:</u><br>food decreases absorption of astemizole by 60% | <u>ADRs:</u><br>GI upset; headache; appetite increase with weight gain; nervousness; dizziness; diarrhea; dry mouth; thickening of bronchial secretions; drowsiness (less frequent)<br><br><u>Pharmacokinetics:</u><br>well absorbed; absorption decreased by 60% when taken with food; slow onset of action secondary to distribution; duration = 24 hours; $T_{1/2}$ = 7–14 days | <u>Contraindications:</u><br>hypersensitivity to antihistamines; narrow-angle glaucoma; stenosing peptic ulcer, symptomatic prostatic hypertrophy; bladder neck obstruction; asthmatic attack; concurrent monoamine oxidase inhibitor (MAO) therapy; newborns and premature infants; third trimester of pregnancy; concurrent use of erythromycin, ketoconazole or itraconazole; significant hepatic dysfunction<br><br><u>Pregnancy Category:</u> C<br><br><u>Lactation Issues:</u><br>antihistamine therapy is contraindicated in nursing mothers |
| **Cetirizine (considered "low-sedating")**<br>Zyrtec<br><br><u>Tablets:</u><br>5 mg, 10 mg | **Allergic rhinitis and conjunctivitis: relief of runny nose and sneezing due to the common cold: pruritus and urticaria**<br><br>**Adults and children > 12 years:**<br>5–10 mg qd | <u>Administration Issues:</u><br>safety and efficacy in children < 12 have not been established<br><br><u>Drug–Drug Interactions:</u><br>**MAO inhibitors** may potentiate the anticholinergic effects of antihistamines; | <u>ADRs:</u><br>headache; dry mouth; GI upset; dizziness; insomnia; nervousness; thickening of bronchial secretions; drowsiness (less frequent) | <u>Contraindications:</u><br>hypersensitivity to antihistamines; narrow-angle glaucoma; stenosing peptic ulcer, symptomatic prostatic hypertrophy; bladder neck obstruction; asthmatic attack; |

(continues on next page)

| Drug and Dosage Forms | Usual Dosage Range | Administration Issues and Drug–Drug Interactions | Common Adverse Drug Reactions (ADRs) and Pharmacokinetics | Contraindications, Pregnancy Category, and Lactation Issues |
|---|---|---|---|---|
| **Cetirizine (considered "low-sedating")** *cont.*<br><br>Syrup: 5 mg/5 mL | **Patients with renal or hepatic dysfunction:**<br>5 mg qd | additive CNS depressant effects may occur with concurrent use of **alcohol** or **other CNS depressants** | Pharmacokinetics:<br>well absorbed; onset = 1 hour; duration = 24 hours | concurrent monoamine oxidase inhibitor (MAOI) therapy; newborns and premature infants; third trimester of pregnancy<br><br>Pregnancy Category: C<br><br>Lactation Issues:<br>antihistamine therapy is contra-indicated in nursing mothers |
| **Fexofenadine**<br>Allegra<br><br>Capsules: 60 mg | **Allergic rhinitis and conjunctivitis: relief of runny nose and sneezing due to the common cold: pruritus and urticaria**<br><br>**Adults and children > 12 years:**<br>60 mg bid<br><br>**Patients with hepatic dysfunction:**<br>60 mg qd (starting dose) | Administration Issues:<br>safety and efficacy in children < 12 have not been established<br><br>Drug–Drug Interactions:<br>**MAO inhibitors** may potentiate the anticholinergic effects of antihistamines; additive CNS depressant effects may occur with concurrent use of **alcohol** or **other CNS depressants** | ADRs:<br>GI upset; headache; appetite increase with weight gain; nervousness; dizziness; diarrhea; dry mouth; thickening of bronchial secretions; drowsiness (less frequent)<br><br>Pharmacokinetics:<br>rapid onset of action | Contraindications:<br>hypersensitivity to antihistamines; narrow-angle glaucoma; stenosing peptic ulcer, symptomatic prostatic hypertrophy; bladder neck obstruction; asthmatic attack; concurrent monoamine oxidase inhibitor (MAOI) therapy; newborns and premature infants; third trimester of pregnancy<br><br>Pregnancy Category: C<br><br>Lactation Issues:<br>antihistamine therapy is contra-indicated in nursing mothers |

| | | | |
|---|---|---|---|
| **Loratadine**<br>Claritin<br><br>Tablets: 10 mg<br><br>Reditabs (rapidly-disintegrating tablets):<br>10 mg<br><br>Syrup: 1 mg/mL<br><br>Combination:<br>w/ 120 mg pseudoephedrine | **Allergic rhinitis and conjunctivitis; relief of runny nose and sneezing due to the common cold; pruritus and urticaria**<br><br>**Adults and children > 12 years:**<br>10 mg qd<br><br>**Children (6–11yr):** 10 mg (10 mL) qd<br><br>**Patients with hepatic or renal dysfunction:**<br>10 mg qod | Administration Issues:<br>take on an empty stomach; safety and efficacy in children < 6 have not been established. If taking rapidly disintegrating tablets: place tablet on tongue and it should disintegrate rapidly (seconds). Dissolved tablet may then be swallowed with or without water.<br><br>Drug–Drug Interactions:<br>**fluconazole, itraconazole, ketoconazole, miconazole, erythromycin, azithromycin, clarithromycin, troleandomycin** may increase loratadine levels. **MAO inhibitors** may potentiate the anticholinergic effects of antihistamines; additive CNS depressant effects may occur with concurrent use of **alcohol** or **other CNS depressants.** | ADRs:<br>GI upset; dry mouth; thickening of bronchial secretions; urinary retention; constipation; drowsiness (less frequent)<br><br>Pharmacokinetics:<br>well absorbed; onset = 1–3 hours; duration = 24 hours<br><br>Contraindications:<br>hypersensitivity to antihistamines; narrow-angle glaucoma; stenosing peptic ulcer, symptomatic prostatic hypertrophy; bladder neck obstruction; asthmatic attack; concurrent monoamine oxidase inhibitor (MAO) therapy; newborns and premature infants; third trimester of pregnancy<br><br>Pregnancy Category: B<br><br>Lactation Issues:<br>antihistamine therapy is contraindicated in nursing mothers |
| **Terfenadine**<br>Seldane | **Taken off the market 2/1/98** | | |

| Drug and Dosage Forms | Usual Dosage Range | Administration Issues and Drug–Drug Interactions | Common Adverse Drug Reactions (ADRs) | Contraindications, Pregnancy Category, and Lactation Issues |
|---|---|---|---|---|
| **Beclomethasone** Beconase, Vancenase _Aerosol:_ 42 mcg/dose _Spray:_ 0.042% | **Symptomatic relief of seasonal or perennial rhinitis; prevention of recurrence of nasal polyps following surgical removal; nonallergic rhinitis (spray)** **Adults and children > 12 years:** 1 inhalation in each nostril bid to qid **Children 6–12 years:** 1 inhalation in each nostril tid | Administration Issues: safety and efficacy have not been established in children < 6 years of age; use smallest maintenance dose possible to control symptoms; discontinue therapy if no improvement is noted within three weeks | ADRs: nasal irritation, burning, stinging and dryness; headache; delayed wound healing | Contraindications: hypersensitivity to steroids; untreated nasal infection Pregnancy Category:  C Lactation Issues: it is not known whether beclomethasone is excreted in breast milk; use caution if nursing |
| **Budesonide** Rhinocort _Aerosol:_ 32 mcg/dose | **Symptomatic relief of seasonal or perennial rhinitis in adults and children; nonallergic perennial rhinitis in adults** **Adults and children > 6 years:** 2 sprays in each nostril bid or 4 sprays in each nostril qd | Administration Issues: not recommended for children < 6 years of age with nonallergic perennial rhinitis; use smallest maintenance dose possible to control symptoms; discontinue therapy if no improvement is noted within three weeks | ADRs: nasal irritation, burning, stinging and dryness; headache; delayed wound healing | Contraindications: hypersensitivity to steroids; untreated nasal infection Pregnancy Category:  C Lactation Issues: it is not known whether budesonide is excreted in breast milk; use caution if nursing |
| **Dexamethasone** Decadron _Aerosol:_ 84 mcg/dose | **Allergic or inflammatory nasal conditions; nasal polyps:** **Adults:** 2 sprays in each nostril bid to tid. Maximum dose: 12 sprays daily | Administration Issues: discontinue therapy as soon as possible; do not exceed recommended dosage | ADRs: nasal irritation, burning, stinging and dryness; headache; delayed wound healing | Contraindications: hypersensitivity to steroids; untreated nasal infection Pregnancy Category:  C Lactation Issues: dexamethasone is excreted in |

| Drug | Dosing | Administration Issues | ADRs | Contraindications / Pregnancy / Lactation |
|---|---|---|---|---|
| *(continued)* | **Children:** 1-2 sprays in each nostril bid. Maximum dose: 8 sprays daily | | | breast milk; may suppress growth or interfere with endogenous corticosteroid production |
| **Flunisolide**<br>Nasalide<br><br><u>Spray:</u><br>25 mcg/dose | **Symptomatic relief of seasonal or perennial rhinitis:**<br><br>**Adults:**<br>Initial dose: 2 sprays in each nostril bid to tid. Maintenance dose: 1 spray in each nostril qd. Maximum dose: 8 sprays daily<br><br>**Children:** 1 spray in each nostril tid or 2 sprays in each nostril bid. Maximum dose: 4 sprays daily | <u>Administration Issues:</u><br>use smallest maintenance dose possible to control symptoms; discontinue therapy if no improvement is noted within three weeks | <u>ADRs</u><br>nasal irritation, burning, stinging and dryness; headache; delayed wound healing | <u>Contraindications:</u><br>hypersensitivity to steroids; untreated nasal infection<br><br><u>Pregnancy Category:</u> C<br><br><u>Lactation Issues:</u><br>it is not known whether flunisolide is excreted in breast milk; use caution if nursing |
| **Fluticasone**<br>Flonase<br><br><u>Spray:</u><br>50 mcg/dose | **Symptomatic relief of seasonal or perennial rhinitis**<br><br>**Adults:**<br>2 sprays in each nostril qd. Maximum dose: 4 sprays daily<br><br>**Adolescents > 12 years:**<br>1 spray in each nostril qd. Maximum dose: 2 sprays daily | <u>Administration Issues:</u><br>not recommended for nonallergic rhinitis in children < 12 years; use smallest maintenance dose possible to control symptoms | <u>ADRs</u><br>nasal irritation, burning, stinging and dryness; headache; delayed wound healing | <u>Contraindications:</u><br>hypersensitivity to steroids; untreated nasal infection<br><br><u>Pregnancy Category:</u> C<br><br><u>Lactation Issues:</u><br>it is not known whether fluticasone is excreted in breast milk; use caution if nursing |
| **Triamcinolone**<br>Nasacort<br><br><u>Spray:</u><br>55 mcg/dose | **Symptomatic relief of seasonal or perennial rhinitis**<br><br>**Adults and children > 12 years:**<br>2 sprays in each nostril qd<br><br>Maximum dose: 4 sprays daily | <u>Administration Issues:</u><br>use smallest maintenance dose possible to control symptoms; discontinue therapy if no improvement is noted within three weeks | <u>ADRs</u><br>nasal irritation, burning, stinging and dryness; headache; delayed wound healing | <u>Contraindications:</u><br>hypersensitivity to steroids; untreated nasal infection<br><br><u>Pregnancy Category:</u> C<br><br><u>Lactation Issues:</u><br>it is not known whether triamcinolone is excreted in breast milk; use caution if nursing |

## 707. Expectorants

| Drug and Dosage Forms | Usual Dosage Range | Administration Issues and Drug–Drug Interactions | Common Adverse Drug Reactions (ADRs) | Contraindications, Pregnancy Category, and Lactation Issues |
|---|---|---|---|---|
| **Guaifenesin**<br>Robitussin, Guiatuss, Halotussin, Humibid, Hytuss<br><br>Syrup: 100 mg/5 mL<br><br>Sustained Release Capsules: 300 mg<br><br>Tablets: 100 mg, 200 mg<br><br>Sustained Release Tablets: 600 mg<br><br>Combination Products: w/ varying combinations of methylxanthines, antihistamines, decongestants, analgesics | **Symptomatic relief of dry, nonproductive cough**<br><br>**Adults:** 100–400 mg q 4 hours. Maximum dose: 2400 mg/day<br><br>**Children (6–12 years):** 100–200 mg q 4 hours; Maximum dose: 1200 mg/day<br><br>**Children (2–6 years):** 50–100 mg q 4 hours. Maximum dose: 600 mg/day | Administration Issues:<br>should not be used for the persistent cough associated with smoking, asthma or emphysema or for a cough accompanied by excessive secretions | ADRs:<br>nausea, vomiting, dizziness, headache, rash | Contraindications:<br>hypersensitivity to guaifenesin<br><br>Pregnancy Category: C<br><br>Lactation Issues:<br>No data available |
| **Terpin Hydrate**<br><br>Elixir: 85 mg/5 mL | **Symptomatic relief of dry, nonproductive cough**<br><br>**Adults:** 85–170 mg tid to qid<br><br>**Children (1–4 yr.):** 20 mg tid to qid<br><br>**Children (5–9 yr.):** 40 mg tid to qid<br><br>**Children (10–12 yr.):** 85 mg tid to qid | Administration Issues:<br>take with food to minimize GI upset; take with plenty of liquids; do not give to children unless directed by a physician; contain alcohol | ADRs:<br>drowsiness, nausea, vomiting, abdominal pain | Contraindications:<br>hypersensitivity to terpin hydrate<br><br>Lactation Issues:<br>terpin hydrate is excreted in breast milk |

## 708. Leukotriene Receptor Antagonists

| Drug and Dosage Forms | Usual Dosage Range | Administration Issues and Drug–Drug Interactions | Common Adverse Drug Reactions (ADRs) and Pharmacokinetics | Contraindications, Pregnancy Category, and Lactation Issues |
|---|---|---|---|---|
| **Montelukast**<br>Singulair<br><br>Chewable Tablets:<br>5 mg<br><br>Film-coated Tablets:<br>10 mg | **Prophylaxis and chronic treatment of asthma in adults and children >6 years:**<br><br>**Adults and children >15 yr.:**<br>10 mg in the evening<br><br>**Children 6-14 years:**<br>5 mg chewable tablet in the evening | Administration Issues:<br>Take regularly as prescribed, even during symptom-free periods. Do not use to treat acute episode of asthma.<br><br>Drug Interactions:<br>none reported | ADRs:<br>headache, dizziness, nausea, diarrhea, abdominal pain<br><br>Pharmacokinetics<br>Food does not effect bioavailability; $T_{1/2}$ = 3–6 hr. | Contraindications:<br>Hypersensitivity to montelukast<br><br>Pregnancy Category: B<br><br>Lactation Issues: It is not known if montelukast is excreted in breast milk |
| **Zafirlukast**<br>Accolate<br><br>Tablets: 20 mg | **Prophylaxis and chronic treatment of asthma in adults and children >12 years:**<br><br>**Adults and children >12 yr.:**<br>20 mg bid | Administration Issues:<br>Take zafirlukast at least 1 hour before or 2 hours after meals. Take regularly as prescribed, even during symptom-free periods. Do not use to treat acute episode of asthma.<br><br>Drug Interactions:<br>Aspirin may increase Zafirlukast levels. **Erythromycin, terfenadine, theophylline** may decrease zafirlukast levels. Zafirlukast may increase the anticoagulant effects of **warfarin.** | ADRs:<br>headache, dizziness, nausea, diarrhea, abdominal pain<br><br>Pharmacokinetics<br>Food reduces bioavailability by 40%; $T_{1/2}$ = 10 hr. | Contraindications:<br>Hypersensitivity to zafirlukast<br><br>Pregnancy Category: B<br><br>Lactation Issues: Nursing women should not take this drug. |

## 709. Leukotriene Receptor Inhibitors

| Drug and Dosage Forms | Usual Dosage Range | Administration Issues and Drug–Drug Interactions | Common Adverse Drug Reactions (ADRs) and Pharmacokinetics | Contraindications, Pregnancy Category, and Lactation Issues |
|---|---|---|---|---|
| **Zileutin**<br>Zyflo<br><u>Tablets:</u> 600 mg | **Prophylaxis and chronic treatment of asthma in adults and children >12 years:**<br><br>**Adults and children >12 yr.:**<br>600 mg qid with meals and hs. | <u>Administration Issues:</u><br>Take regularly as prescribed, even during symptom-free periods. Do not use to treat acute episode of asthma. Zileutin may be taken with food. If patients experience signs or symptoms of liver dysfunction (nausea, fatigue, right upper quadrant pain, lethargy, jaundice, "flu–like" symptoms), contact health-care professional immediately.<br><br><u>Drug Interactions:</u><br>Zileutin may increase levels of **propranolol, terfenadine and theophylline.** Zileutin may increase the anticoagulant effects of **warfarin** | <u>ADRs:</u><br>headache, ALT elevations, chest pain, dizziness, fever, insomnia, malaise, dyspepsia, abdominal pain, constipation, flatulence, weakness, myalgia<br><br><u>Pharmacokinetics:</u><br>rapidly absorbed; $T_{1/2} = 1.7$ hr. | <u>Contraindications:</u><br>Hypersensitivity to zileutin, active liver disease, transaminase elevations $\geq 3$ times upper limits of normal<br><br><u>Pregnancy Category:</u> C<br><br><u>Lactation Issues:</u><br>Nursing women should not take this drug. |

# 800. TOPICAL PREPARATIONS
## 801. Acne Products

| Drug and Dosage Forms | Usual Dosage Range | Administration Issues and Drug–Drug Interactions | Common Adverse Drug Reactions (ADRs) | Contraindications, Pregnancy Category, and Lactation Issues |
|---|---|---|---|---|
| **Benzoyl Peroxide** <br> many products on the market with the following strengths and dosage forms: <br><br> Liquid: 2.5%, 5%, 10% <br><br> Bar: 5%, 10% <br><br> Mask: 5% <br><br> Lotion: 5%, 5.5%, 10% <br><br> Cream: 5%, 10% <br><br> Gel: 2.5%, 4%, 5%, 10%, 20% | **Treatment of mild to moderate acne vulgaris and oily skin** <br> Wash with cleansers once or twice daily <br><br> Apply other dose forms qd, gradually increasing to 2 to 3 times daily as needed | Administration Issues <br> For external use only; keep preparation away from the eyes, mouth, angles of nose, and mucous membranes; wash hands thoroughly after application; avoid excessive exposure to the sunlight or sunlamps; shake lotion well prior to administration; normal use of water-based cosmetics is permissible; avoid contact with hair or colored fabric, bleaching may occur. Safety and efficacy in children < 12 years of age have not been established <br><br> Drug–Drug Interactions <br> Concomitant use of **tretinoin** and benzoyl peroxide may cause significant skin irritation | ADRs: <br> excessive drying, erythema, hypersensitivity | Contraindications <br> Hypersensitivity to benzoyl peroxide, cross-sensitivity may occur with benzoic acid derivatives <br><br> Pregnancy Category:  C <br><br> Lactation Issues <br> Excretion in breast milk is unknown, use with caution in nursing mothers |
| **Clindamycin Phosphate** <br> Gel: Cleocin T, generics: 10 mg/ml <br><br> Lotion: Cleocin T, generics: 10 mg/ml <br><br> Solution: Cleocin T, generics: 10 mg/ml | **Treatment of acne vulgaris** <br> Apply a thin film to affected area twice daily | Administration Issues <br> For external use only; keep preparation away from the eyes, mouth, angles of nose, and mucous membranes; wash hands thoroughly after application; shake lotion well prior to administration; remove pledget from foil wrapper just prior to administration; use pledget only once, then discard. Safety and efficacy in children < 12 years of age have not been established | ADRs: <br> dryness, erythema, burning, peeling, itching, oily skin, diarrhea, abdominal pain and colitis | Contraindications <br> Hypersensitivity to clindamycin or lincomycin; history of antibiotic-associated colitis <br><br> Pregnancy Category:  B <br><br> Lactation Issues <br> due to potential for serious adverse events in infants, |

(continues on next page)

| Drug and Dosage Forms | Usual Dosage Range | Administration Issues and Drug–Drug Interactions | Common Adverse Drug Reactions (ADRs) | Contraindications, Pregnancy Category, and Lactation Issues |
|---|---|---|---|---|
| **Clindamycin Phosphate** *cont.* | | <u>Drug–Drug Interactions</u><br>**Erythromycin** may antagonize the effects of clindamycin | | discontinue nursing or the drug, taking into account the importance of the drug to the mother |
| **Erythromycin**<br><br><u>Solution</u>: 1.5%, 2%<br><br><u>Gel</u>: 2%<br><br>Benzamycin<br>30 mg erythromycin<br>50 mg benzoyl peroxide per gm<br><br><u>Ointment</u>: 2% | **Treatment of acne vulgaris**<br>Apply twice daily to affected area in the morning and evening | <u>Administration Issues</u><br>For external use only; keep preparation away from the eyes, mouth, angles of nose, and mucous membranes; wash hands thoroughly after application; cleanse areas to be treated before applying medication; store Benzamycin gel in the refrigerator and discard unused portion after 3 months. Safety and efficacy in children < 12 years of age have not been established<br><br><u>Drug–Drug Interactions</u><br>Concomitant use of other acne products (**benzoyl peroxide, tretinoin**) with erythromycin may cause increased irritant effects. Erythromycin may antagonize the effects of **clindamycin** | <u>ADRs:</u><br>erythema, burning, dryness | <u>Contraindications</u><br>Hypersensitivity to erythromycin<br><br><u>Pregnancy Category:</u> B (Eryderm 2%, Erygel); C (A/T/S, T-Stat, Staticin)<br><br><u>Lactation Issues</u><br>Erythromycin is excreted in breast milk; use with caution in nursing mothers |
| **Isotretinoin**<br>Accutane<br><br><u>Capsules:</u><br>10 mg, 20 mg, 40 mg | **Treatment of severe recalcitrant cystic acne**<br>Initially, 0.5–1 mg/kg/d divided into 2 doses for 15 to 20 weeks; patients with severe disease or disease primarily manifest on the body may require up to 2 mg/kg/d | <u>Administration Issues</u><br>Patient information leaflet should be discussed with the patient; do not crush capsule; take with meals; women of childbearing potential should practice contraception during therapy and for 1 month before and after therapy; a pregnancy test 2 weeks prior to starting | <u>ADRs:</u><br>dry mouth, nausea, vomiting, abdominal pain, conjunctivitis, decreased night vision, hypertriglyceridemia, arthralgia, hepatotoxicity, photosensitivity | <u>Contraindications</u><br>Pregnancy; hypersensitivity to parabens<br><br><u>Pregnancy Category:</u> X<br><br><u>Lactation Issues</u><br>Excretion in breast milk is |

| Drug | Administration Issues / Drug–Drug Interactions | ADRs | Contraindications / Pregnancy / Lactation |
|---|---|---|---|
| A second course of therapy may be initiated after ≥ 2 months off therapy if severe cystic acne persists or recurs | therapy is advised. Safety and efficacy in children have not been established.<br><br>**Drug–Drug Interactions**<br>Concomitant use of **vitamin A** and isotretinoin may result in additive toxic effects | | unknown; due to potential for adverse effects, do not use in nursing mothers |
| **Metronidazole**<br>MetroGel<br><br><u>Gel:</u><br>0.75% | **Treatment of inflammatory papules, pustules, and erythema of rosacea**<br>Apply and rub into a thin film twice daily in the morning and evening; therapeutic results should be noticed within 3 weeks; studies have shown continuing improvement through 9 weeks of therapy<br><br><u>Administration Issues</u><br>For external use only; keep preparation away from the eyes, mouth, angles of nose, and mucous membranes; wash hands thoroughly after application; cleanse areas to be treated before applying medication. Safety and efficacy in children have not been established | <u>ADRs:</u><br>transient redness<br>dryness<br>burning<br>skin irritation | <u>Contraindications</u><br>Hypersensitivity to metronidazole and parabens<br><br><u>Pregnancy Category:</u> B<br><br><u>Lactation Issues</u><br>Metronidazole is excreted in breast milk; discontinue nursing or the drug, taking into account the importance of the drug to the mother |
| **Tretinoin**<br>Retin-A<br><br><u>Cream:</u><br>0.025%, 0.05%, 0.1%<br><br><u>Gel:</u> 0.025%, 0.01%<br><br><u>Liquid:</u> 0.05% | **Treatment of acne vulgaris**<br>Apply lightly to affected area once daily, before bedtime<br><br>Therapeutic results should be seen after 2 to 3 weeks, but may not be optimal until after 6 weeks<br><br><u>Administration Issues</u><br>For external use only; keep preparation away from the eyes, mouth, angles of nose, and mucous membranes; wash hands thoroughly after application; avoid excessive exposure to the sunlight or sunlamps; apply liquid with the fingertip, gauze pad, or cotton swab, do not oversaturate gauze or cotton; normal use of cosmetics is permissible<br><br><u>Drug–Drug Interactions</u><br>Concomitant use of **sulfur, resorcinol, benzoyl peroxide, medicated soaps,** or **salicylic acid** with tretinoin may cause significant skin irritation | <u>ADRs:</u><br>photosensitivity, skin irritation, hyperpigmentation, hypopigmentation | <u>Contraindications</u><br>Hypersensitivity to tretinoin or any component of the product<br><br><u>Pregnancy Category:</u> C<br><br><u>Lactation Issues</u><br>Excretion in breast milk is unknown; use with caution in nursing mothers |

| Drug and Dosage Forms | Usual Dosage Range | Administration Issues and Drug–Drug Interactions | Common Adverse Drug Reactions (ADRs) | Contraindications, Pregnancy Category, and Lactation Issues |
|---|---|---|---|---|
| **Acitretin** Soriatane <br> <u>Capsules:</u> 10 mg, 25 mg | <u>**Treatment of severe psoriasis, including erythrodermic and generalized pustular types**</u> <br><br> Initiate therapy at 25 or 50 mg/d as a single dose with main meal. Maintenance doses of 25 to 50 mg/d may be given | <u>Administration Issues:</u> <br> Women should **NOT** become pregnant while taking acitretin and should use contraception during treatment and for 3 years after discontinuing therapy; do not consume alcohol during therapy and for 2 months following discontinuation of acitretin since alcohol may interfere with the excretion of acitretin <br><br> <u>Drug Interactions:</u> <br> Acitretin may interfere with the contraceptive effect of **microdose progestin** preparations | <u>ADRs:</u> <br> fatigue, asthenia, headache, dysesthesia, dizziness, dry nose, dry eyes, conjunctivitis, chelitis, alopecia, nail fragility, pruritus, dermatitis, arthralgias, mylagias, chills, diaphoresis, hypertriglyceridemia (monitor lipids monthly × 4 months then q 2–3 months), LFT elevations (monitor monthly × 6 months then q 3 months) <br><br> <u>Pharmacokinetics:</u> <br> $T_{1/2}$ (parent); 50 h; food increases bioavailability | <u>Contraindications</u> <br> Hypersensitivity to acitretin or etretinate, pregnancy, intention to become pregnant during therapy or within 3 yr after discontinuation <br><br> <u>Pregnancy Category:</u> X <br><br> <u>Lactation Issues</u> <br> Excretion in breast milk is unknown |
| **Anthralin** <br> <u>Ointment</u> <br> Anthra-Derm 0.1%, 0.25%, 0.5%, 1% <br><br> Lasan 0.4% <br><br> <u>Cream:</u> Lasan 0.1%, 0.2%, 0.4% <br><br> Lasan HP-1 (1%) | <u>**Treatment of quiescent or chronic psoriasis**</u> <br> Rub gently into skin until absorbed once daily beginning with the lowest strength available; increase strength as needed; the optimal period of contact will vary according to the strength used and the patient's response to treatment; initial contact time is 0.1% to 2% for 15 to 20 minutes, followed by thorough removal of the anthralin with soap or petrolatum; continue treatment until the patient's skin is entirely clear | <u>Administration Issues</u> <br> For external use only; keep preparation away from the eyes, mouth, angles of nose, and mucous membranes; wash hands thoroughly after application; anthralin may stain fabrics, skin, fingernails, or hair. Safety and efficacy in children have not been established. <br><br> <u>Drug–Drug Interactions</u> <br> **Topical corticosteroids** may destabilize psoriasis, allow at least one week between the discontinuation of | <u>ADRs:</u> <br> skin irritation | <u>Contraindications</u> <br> Hypersensitivity to anthralin; use on the face; acutely or actively inflamed psoriatic eruptions <br><br> <u>Pregnancy Category:</u> C <br><br> <u>Lactation Issues</u> <br> Excretion in breast milk is unknown; due to the potential for tumorigenicity in animals, discontinue nursing or the drug, |

| | | | taking into account the importance of the drug to the mother |
|---|---|---|---|
| Drithocreme 0.1%, 0.25%, 0.5% <br><br> Drithocreme HP 1% <br><br> Dritho-Scalp 0.25%, 0.5% | | | topical steroids and the commencement of anthralin therapy |
| **Calcipotriene** <br> Dovonex <br><br> Ointment: <br> 0.005% | **Treatment of moderate plaque psoriasis** <br> Apply a thin layer to the affected area twice daily and rub in gently; improvement in clinical trials was shown after 2 weeks of therapy with 70% of patients showing at least marked improvement after 8 weeks <br><br> Administration Issues <br> For external use only; keep preparation away from the eyes, mouth, angles of nose, and mucous membranes; wash hands thoroughly after application. Safety and efficacy in children have not been established | ADRs: <br> burning, itching, erythema, dry skin <br><br> Absorption Issues <br> approximately 6% of the applied dose is absorbed systemically; most of the absorbed dose is converted to inactive metabolites within 24 hours of application | Contraindications <br> Hypersensitivity to any component of the preparation; patients with demonstrated hypercalcemia or evidence of vitamin D toxicity; use on the face <br><br> Pregnancy Category: C <br><br> Lactation Issues <br> Excretion in breast milk is unknown; use with caution in nursing mothers |
| **Etretinate** <br> Tegison <br><br> Capsule: <br> 10 mg, 25 mg | **Treatment of severe, recalcitrant psoriasis** <br> Initially, 0.75–1 mg/kg/d in divided doses, do not exceed 1.5 mg/kg/d <br><br> Maintenance doses of 0.5–0.75 mg/kg/d generally begin after 8 to 16 weeks of therapy; treatment may be terminated in patients whose lesions have sufficiently resolved <br><br> Administration Issues <br> Women of childbearing potential should practice contraception during therapy and for 1 month before and after therapy; a pregnancy test 2 weeks prior to starting therapy is advised; transient exacerbation of psoriasis may occur during the initial period of therapy; take with food. Ligament and tendon abnormalities have been reported in children receiving etretinate, use only when alternative therapies have failed | ADRs: <br> dry nose, chapped lips, thirst, sore mouth, hair loss, palm & sole & fingertip peeling, dry skin, itching, hyperostosis, bone & joint pain, muscle cramps, eye irritation, decreased visual acuity, abdominal pain, nausea <br><br> Absorption Issues <br> increased absorption when taken with food, especially high lipid diet | Contraindications <br> Pregnancy <br><br> Pregnancy Category: X <br><br> Lactation Issues <br> Excretion in breast milk is unknown, due to the potential for adverse effects, nursing mothers should not receive etretinate |

1431

# 802. Antipsoriatic Products *continued from previous page*

| Drug and Dosage Forms | Usual Dosage Range | Administration Issues and Drug–Drug Interactions | Common Adverse Drug Reactions (ADRs) | Contraindications, Pregnancy Category, and Lactation Issues |
|---|---|---|---|---|
| **Etretinate** *cont.* | | <u>Drug–Drug Interactions</u><br>Concomitant use of **vitamin A** may cause additive toxic effects | | |
| **Nitrofurazone**<br>Furacin, generics<br><br><u>Solution:</u> 0.2%<br><br><u>Ointment, soluble:</u> 0.2%<br><br><u>Cream:</u> 0.2% | **Adjunctive therapy for patients with second and third degree burns when bacterial resistance to other agents is a potential problem and in skin grafting to prevent bacterial contamination**<br>Apply once daily directly to lesion or place on gauze; may reapply every few days, depending on dressing technique | <u>Administration Issues</u><br>For external use only; keep preparation away from the eyes, mouth, angles of nose, and mucous membranes; wash hands thoroughly after application; flush dressing with sterile saline to facilitate removal | <u>ADRS:</u><br>rash, pruritis, superinfection<br><br><u>Antibacterial Spectrum</u><br>*Staphylococcus aureus*, Streptococcal sp., *E. coli*, *Clostridium perfringens*, *Aerobacter aerogenes*, and *Proteus* sp. | <u>Contraindications</u><br>Hypersensitivity to nitrofurazone<br><br><u>Pregnancy Category:</u> C<br><br><u>Lactation Issues</u><br>Excretion in breast milk is unknown; discontinue nursing or the drug, taking into account the importance of the drug to the mother |
| **Tar Containing Products**<br>The following types of products are available in varying strengths of coal tar:<br>**creams, lotions, liquids, gels, soaps, oil** | **Adjunct treatment of psoriasis, seborrheic dermatitis, atopic dermatitis, and eczema**<br>Add to bath water; soak 10 to 20 minutes; pat dry<br><br>**Do not use in children < 2 years** | <u>Administration Issues</u><br>For external use only; keep preparation away from the eyes, mouth, and mucous membranes; avoid prolonged exposure to the sun for 72 hours after use; staining of hair, clothes, and plastic or fiberglass tubs may occur | <u>ADRs:</u><br>irritation, photosensitivity, dermatitis | <u>Contraindications</u><br>Open or infected lesions; acute inflammation<br><br><u>Pregnancy Category:</u> C<br><br><u>Lactation Issues</u><br>Excretion in breast milk is unknown; decide whether to discontinue breast feeding or discontinue the drug, taking into account the importance of coal tar to the mother |

| Usual Dosage Range | Administration Issues | Common Adverse Drug Reactions (ADRs) | Contraindications |
|---|---|---|---|
| **Treatment of scalp psoriasis, eczema, seborrheic dermatitis, dandruff, cradle-cap, and other oily, itchy conditions of the body and scalp**<br>Rub shampoo liberally into wet hair and scalp; rinse thoroughly; repeat and leave on for 5 minutes; rinse thoroughly<br><br>Depending on product, use from once daily to at least twice a week; use daily for severe scalp problems | Administration Issues<br>For external use only; keep preparation away from the eyes, mouth, angles of nose, and mucous membranes; wash hands thoroughly after application; do not use on acutely inflamed skin; avoid prolonged exposure to sunlight for 24 hours after application | ADRs:<br>rash, burning, photosensitivity, skin discoloration | Contraindications<br>Acute inflammation; open or infected lesions |

## 803. Antiseborrheic Products

| Drug and Dosage Forms | Usual Dosage Range | Administration Issues | Common Adverse Drug Reactions (ADRs) | Contraindications, Pregnancy Category, and Lactation Issues |
|---|---|---|---|---|
| **Chloroxine**<br>Capitrol<br><br>Shampoo:<br>2% | **Treatment of dandruff and mild to moderate seborrheic dermatitis of the scalp**<br>Massage into wet hair, lather for 3 minutes, rinse, repeat, rinse thoroughly<br><br>Apply twice weekly | Administration Issues<br>For external use only; keep preparation away from the eyes, mouth, angles of nose, and mucous membranes; wash hands thoroughly after application | ADRs:<br>irritation, burning, discoloration of light colored hair | Contraindications<br>Hypersensitivity to any of the ingredients<br><br>Pregnancy Category: C<br><br>Lactation Issues<br>Excretion in breast milk is unknown; use with caution in nursing mothers |
| **Povidone-Iodine**<br>Betadine | **Temporary relief of scaling and itching due to dandruff** | Administration Issues<br>For external use only; keep preparation | ADRs:<br>rash, burning, irritation | |

*(continues on next page)*

1433

**803.** Antiseborrheic Products *continued from previous page*

| Drug and Dosage Forms | Usual Dosage Range | Administration Issues | Common Adverse Drug Reactions (ADRs) | Contraindications, Pregnancy Category, and Lactation Issues |
|---|---|---|---|---|
| **Povidone-Iodine cont.**<br><br>Shampoo: 7.5% | Apply 2 teaspoonful to hair and scalp, lather with warm water, rinse, repeat application, massage gently into scalp, allow to remain on scalp for 5 minutes, rinse scalp thoroughly; repeat twice weekly until improvement is noticed, thereafter use once weekly | away from the eyes, mouth, angles of nose, and mucous membranes; wash hands thoroughly after application; do not use on acutely inflamed skin | | |
| **Pyrithione Zinc**<br><br>Shampoo:<br>Zincon, Head & Shoulders, Head & Shoulders Dry Scalp 1%<br><br>Sebulon 2%<br>Soap: ZNP Bar 2% | **Control dandruff and seborrheic dermatitis of the body (ZNP Bar) and scalp**<br>Apply shampoo, lather, rinse, and repeat; use once or twice weekly | Administration Issues<br>For external use only; keep preparation away from the eyes, mouth, angles of nose, and mucous membranes; wash hands thoroughly after application; do not use on acutely inflamed skin | ADRs<br>rash, burning | |
| **Selenium Sulfide**<br><br>Lotion-Shampoo:<br>Selsun Blue, Head & Shoulders Intensive Treatment Dandruff Shampoo, various 1% | **Treatment of dandruff and seborrheic dermatitis of the scalp**<br>Massage 5 to 10 ml into wet scalp; allow to remain on the scalp for 2 to 3 minutes; rinse thoroughly<br><br>Usually 2 applications per week for 2 weeks will afford control; for maintenance therapy, it may be used | Administration Issues<br>For external use only; keep preparation away from the eyes, mouth, angles of nose, and mucous membranes; wash hands thoroughly after application; do not use on acutely inflamed skin; may damage jewelry. Safety and efficacy in children have not been established | ADRs:<br>skin irritation<br>dryness of hair and scalp | Contraindications<br>Hypersensitivity to components of the product<br><br>Pregnancy Category: C<br>(tinea versicolor) |

| | | |
|---|---|---|
| Selsun, Exsel, various generics 2.5% | once weekly, once every 2 weeks, or once every 3 to 4 weeks in some cases<br><br>**Treatment of tinea versicolor**<br>Apply to affected areas and lather with a small amount of water; allow to remain on skin for 10 minutes, rinse body thoroughly; repeat once daily for 7 days | |
| **Sulfacetamide Sodium**<br>Sebizon<br><br>Lotion: 10% | **Treatment of dandruff and seborrheic dermatitis**<br>Apply at bedtime and allow to remain overnight; precede application by a shampoo if the hair and scalp are oily or greasy or if there is considerable debris; in severe cases with crusting, heavy scaling, and inflammation of the scalp, apply twice daily<br><br>The following morning wash the hair and scalp if desired, wash hair at least once weekly, continue treatment for 8 to 10 nights; increase the interval between applications as improvement occurs, once or twice weekly or every other week applications may prevent recurrence<br><br>**Treatment of secondary bacterial infection of the skin:** Apply 2 to 4 times daily until infection clears | Administration Issues<br>For external use only; keep preparation away from the eyes, mouth, angles of nose, and mucous membranes; wash hands thoroughly after application; completely moisten scalp and gently rub in with fingertips, brush hair thoroughly for 2 to 3 minutes after application. Safety and efficacy in children < 12 years have not been established.<br><br>ADRs:<br>rash, burning, irritation, superinfection<br><br>Antibacterial Spectrum<br>Bacteriostatic effect against gram-positive and gram-negative organisms | Contraindications<br>Hypersensitivity to sulfonamides<br><br>Pregnancy Category: C<br><br>Lactation Issues<br>Excretion in breast milk is unknown; use with caution in nursing mothers |
| **Sulfur Preparations**<br>Adne lotion 10, others | **Treatment of seborrheic dermatitis. May also be useful in the treatment of acne vulgaris.** | Administration Issues<br>For external use only. For best results, wash skin thoroughly with a mild<br><br>ADRs:<br>skin irritation | Contraindications<br>Hypersensitivity to sulfur or any component of the product |

(continues on next page)

## 803. Antiseborrheic Products *continued from previous page*

| Drug and Dosage Forms | Usual Dosage Range | Administration Issues | Common Adverse Drug Reactions (ADRs) | Contraindications, Pregnancy Category, and Lactation Issues |
|---|---|---|---|---|
| **Sulfur Preparations** *cont.* <br> Cream: 5% <br> Lotion: 4%, 10% <br> Soap: 5% <br> Mask: 6.4% | **oily skin, rosacea and tinea versicolor** <br> Apply a thin layer. Use qd to tid. | cleanser prior to application. Keep away from eyes. If undue irritation develops discontinue use. Preferred treatment for infants, small children, patients with seizures or other neurologic disorders and pregnant or lactating women | | |
| **Antiseborrheic Combinations** <br><br> Shampoo: <br> Fostex Medicated Cleansing, plus | **Treatment of dandruff and mild to moderate seborrheic dermatitis of the scalp** <br> Massage into wet hair, lather for 3 minutes, rinse, repeat, rinse thoroughly | Administration Issues <br> For external use only; keep preparation away from the eyes, mouth, angles of nose, and mucous membranes; wash hands thoroughly after application | ADRs: <br> irritation, burning | |

## 804. Antihistamine-Containing Products

| Drug and Dosage Forms | Usual Dosage Range | Administration Issues and Drug–Drug Interactions | Common Adverse Drug Reactions (ADRs) |
|---|---|---|---|
| **Diphenhydramine**<br><br>Cream:<br>Benadryl (1% diphenhydramine)<br><br>Maximum Strength Benadryl (2% diphenhydramine)<br><br>Caladryl (1% diphenhydramine, 8% calamine)<br><br>Lotion:<br>Caladryl (1% diphenhydramine)<br><br>Ziradryl (1% diphenhydramine, 2% zinc oxide)<br><br>Spray:<br>Benadryl (1% diphenhydramine, 85% alcohol)<br><br>Caladryl (1% diphenhydramine, 8% calamine) | **Temporary relief of itching due to minor skin disorders, sunburn, insect bites and stings, and poison ivy, sumac, and oak**<br>Apply to affected area 3 to 4 times daily as needed | Administration Issues<br>For external use only; keep preparation away from the eyes, mouth, angles of nose, and mucous membranes; wash hands thoroughly after application; do not apply to blistered, raw, or oozing areas of the skin; avoid prolonged use (> 7 days) | ADRs:<br>irritation, burning |
| **Doxepin**<br>Zonalon<br><br>Cream:<br>5% | **Short-term management of moderate pruritis in adults**<br>Apply to affected area 4 times daily with at least a 3 to 4 hour interval between applications<br><br>No safety or efficacy data for use > 8 days | Administration Issues<br>For external use only; keep preparation away from the eyes, mouth, angles of nose, and mucous membranes; wash hands thoroughly after application; do not use occlusive dressings which may increase the absorption of doxepin; apply a thin coat<br><br>Drug–Drug Interactions<br>**Alcohol** ingestion may increase the potential for sedative effects of doxepin; **Cimetidine** may inhibit the metabolism of doxepin leading to increased toxic effects; Concurrent use of doxepin and **monoamine oxidase inhibitors** may lead to serious toxic adverse effects | ADRs:<br>drowsiness, dry mouth, headache, burning, stinging<br><br>Absorption Issues:<br>Topical: plasma concentrations ranged from 0–47 ng/ml; target therapeutic level following oral dosing is 30–150 ng/ml |

# 805. Anti-Infective Products (Topical and Vaginal)

| Drug and Dosage Forms | Usual Dosage Range | Administration Issues | Adverse Drug Reaction (ADRs) Spectrum (If listed) and Absorption issues | Contraindications, Pregnancy Category, and Lactation Issues |
|---|---|---|---|---|
| **Acyclovir**<br>Zovirax<br><br>Ointment:<br>5% | **Treatment of initial episodes of herpes genitalis and in limited mucocutaneous herpes simplex virus infections**<br>Apply to affected areas q 3 to 6 hours for 7 days | Administration Issues<br>For external use only; keep preparation away from the eyes, mouth, angles of nose, and mucous membranes; initiate therapy as early as possible following onset of symptoms; apply using a finger cot or rubber glove to avoid autoinoculation of other body sites; acyclovir is not a cure for HSV infections | ADRs:<br>mild pain, burning, stinging<br><br>Antiviral Spectrum<br>Herpes simplex virus types 1 (HSV-1) and type 2 (HSV-2) | Contraindications<br>Hypersensitivity or intolerance to components of the preparation<br><br>Pregnancy Category: C<br><br>Lactation Issues<br>Excretion in breast milk is unknown; use with caution in nursing mothers |
| **Amphotericin B**<br>Fungizone<br><br>Cream: 3%<br><br>Lotion: 3%<br><br>Ointment: 3% | **Treatment of cutaneous and mucocutaneous infections caused by _Candida sp._**<br>Apply liberally to affected area 2 to 4 times daily for 1 to 3 weeks | Administration Issues<br>For external use only; keep preparation away from the eyes, mouth, and mucous membranes; cleanse the affected area with soap and water and dry thoroughly prior to application; wash hands thoroughly after application | ADRs:<br>skin discoloration, burning, itching | Contraindications<br>Hypersensitivity to any component of the product |
| **Bacitracin**<br>Baciguent, generics<br><br>Ointment:<br>500 units per gm | **Aid to healing and prophylaxis of infection in minor cuts, wounds, burns, and skin abrasions**<br>Apply to affected area 1 to 4 times daily | Administration Issues<br>For external use only; keep preparation away from the eyes, mouth, and mucous membranes; wash hands thoroughly after application; area to be treated may be covered with a gauze dressing if desired | ADRs:<br>skin irritation<br>superinfection | Contraindications<br>Hypersensitivity to any ingredients in the preparation |
| **Butoconazole**<br>Femstat | **Treatment of vulvovaginal candidiasis** | Administration Issues<br>For external use only. Follow patient information sheet. | ADRs:<br>irritation, burning, discharge, swelling, itchy fingers (0.2%) | Contraindications<br>Hypersensitivity to buconazole |

| Drug / Formulation | Indications / Dosing | Administration Issues | ADRs | Contraindications / Pregnancy / Lactation |
|---|---|---|---|---|
| Vaginal Cream: 2% | Pregnant patients (2nd/3rd trimesters only): 1 applicatorful × 6 d<br><br>Nonpregnant patients: 1 applicatorful × 3 d; may be extended to 6 d if needed | | | Pregnancy Category: C<br><br>Lactation Issues: use with caution |
| **Ciclopirox Olamine**<br>Loprox<br><br>Cream: 1%<br><br>Lotion: 1% | **Treatment of athlete's foot, jock itch, ringworm, cutaneous candidiasis, and tinea versicolor**<br>Apply to affected area twice daily, morning and evening; improvement should occur within 7 days | Administration Issues<br>For external use only; keep preparation away from the eyes, mouth, and mucous membranes; cleanse the affected area with soap and water and dry thoroughly prior to application; wash hands thoroughly after application; for athlete's foot, wear well-fitting, ventilated shoes and change shoes and socks at least once daily; reevaluate therapy if no improvement occurs in 4 weeks | ADRs:<br>irritation, pruritis, burning | Contraindications<br>Hypersensitivity to ciclopirox olamine<br><br>Pregnancy Category: B<br><br>Lactation Issues<br>Excretion in breast milk is unknown; use with caution in nursing mothers |
| **Clioquinol**<br>Vioform<br><br>Cream: 3%<br><br>Ointment: 3% | **Treatment of inflamed conditions of the skin such as eczema, athlete's foot, and other fungal infections**<br>Apply to affected area 2 to 3 times daily<br><br>Avoid use for > 7 days | Administration Issues<br>For external use only; keep preparation away from the eyes, mouth, and mucous membranes; cleanse the affected area with soap and water and dry thoroughly prior to application; wash hands thoroughly after application; for athlete's foot, wear well-fitting, ventilated shoes and change shoes and socks at least once daily; reevaluate therapy if no improvement occurs in 4 weeks | ADRs:<br>irritation, stinging; may have systemic reactions (if applied on large area of skin): iodism, hair loss, agranulocytosis | Contraindications<br>Hypersensitivity to chloroxine, iodine or iodine-containing preparations; severe renal or hepatic disease; thyroid disorder<br><br>Pregnancy Category: C<br><br>Lactation Issues: Safety not established |
| **Clotrimazole**<br>Topical Cream: 1% | **Treatment of athlete's foot, jock itch, ringworm, cutaneous candidiasis, and tinea versicolor** | Administration Issues<br>Topical:<br>For external use only; keep preparation | ADRs:<br>Topical:<br>irritation, pruritis, burning | Contraindications<br>Hypersensitivity to clotrimazole |

(continues on next page)

## 805. Anti–Infective Products (Topical and Vaginal) *continued from previous page*

| Drug and Dosage Forms | Usual Dosage Range | Administration Issues | Adverse Drug Reaction (ADRs) Spectrum (If listed) and Absorption issues | Contraindications, Pregnancy Category, and Lactation Issues |
|---|---|---|---|---|
| **Clotrimazole** *cont.*<br>Lotrimin, Lotrimin AF<br>Mycelex, Mycelex OTC<br><br>Topical Solution: 1%<br>Lotrimin, Lotrimin AF<br>Mycelex, Mycelex OTC<br><br>Topical Lotion: Lotrimin 1%<br><br>Vaginal Tablets: Mycelex,<br>Gyne–Lotrimin<br>100 mg, 500 mg<br><br>Vaginal Cream: 1% | Topical: Apply to affected area twice daily, morning and evening; improvement should occur within 7 days<br><br>**Treatment of vulvovaginal candidiasis**<br>Vaginal Tablets:<br>100 mg tablet q hs × 7 d or<br>100 mg tablet, 2 tabs × 3 d or<br>500 mg tablet × 1 dose<br>Vaginal Cream: 1 applicatorful intravaginally × 7–14 d | away from the eyes, mouth, and mucous membranes; cleanse the affected area with soap and water and dry thoroughly prior to application; wash hands thoroughly after application; for athlete's foot, wear well-fitting, ventilated shoes and change shoes and socks at least once daily; reevaluate therapy if no improvement occurs in 4 weeks<br><br>Vaginal:<br>For vaginal use only. Follow instructions carefully. Refrain from sexual intercourse during therapy. | Vaginal:<br>skin rash, lower abdominal cramps, vulval irritation, vaginal irritation, itching, burning | Pregnancy Category: B<br><br>Lactation Issues<br>Excretion in breast milk is unknown; use with caution in nursing mothers |
| **Combination Anti-infectives**<br><br>Ointment:<br>Polysporin (10,000 units/gm polymyxin, 500 units/gm bacitracin)<br><br>Maximum Strength Neosporin (10,000 units/gm polymyxin, 3.5 mg/gm neomycin, 500 units/gm bacitracin)<br><br>Neosporin, Triple Antibiotic (5,000 units/gm polymyxin, | **Aid to healing and prophylaxis of infection in minor cuts, wounds, burns, and skin abrasions**<br>Apply to affected area 1 to 4 times daily | Administration Issues<br>For external use only; keep preparation away from the eyes, mouth, and mucous membranes; wash hands thoroughly after application; area to be treated may be covered with a gauze dressing if desired | ADRs:<br>skin irritation, superinfection | Contraindications<br>Hypersensitivity to any ingredients in the preparation |

| | | | |
|---|---|---|---|
| 3.5 mg/gm neomycin, 400 units/gm bacitracin)<br><br>Maximum Strength Mycitracin Triple Antibiotic (5,000 units/gm polymyxin, 3.5 mg/gm neomycin, 500 units/gm bacitracin)<br><br>Mycitracin Plus (5,000 units/gm polymyxin, 3.5 mg/gm neomycin, 500 units/gm bacitracin, 40 mg/gm lidocaine)<br><br>Cream:<br>Neosporin (10,000 units/gm polymyxin B sulfate, 3.5 mg/gm neomycin)<br><br>Powder:<br>Polysporin (10,000 units/gm polymyxin, 500 units/gm bacitracin)<br><br>Spray:<br>Polysporin (2222 units/ml polymyxin, 111 units/ml bacitracin) | | | |
| **Econazole Nitrate**<br>Spectazole<br><br><u>Cream:</u> 1% | **Treatment of athlete's foot, jock itch, ringworm, and tinea versicolor**<br>Apply to affected area once daily; treat for 2 weeks, except athlete's foot treat for 4 weeks | <u>Administration Issues</u><br>For external use only; keep preparation away from the eyes, mouth, and mucous membranes; cleanse the affected area with soap and water and dry thoroughly prior to application; wash hands | <u>ADRs:</u><br>irritation, burning, itching, erythema | <u>Contraindications</u><br>Hypersensitivity to econazole nitrate<br><br><u>Pregnancy Category:</u> C |

(continues on next page)

| Drug and Dosage Forms | Usual Dosage Range | Administration Issues | Adverse Drug Reaction (ADRs) Spectrum (if listed) and Absorption issues | Contraindications, Pregnancy Category, and Lactation Issues |
|---|---|---|---|---|
| **Econazole Nitrate cont.** | **Treatment of cutaneous candidiasis** Apply to affected area twice daily for 2 weeks | thoroughly after application; for athlete's foot, wear well-fitting, ventilated shoes and change shoes and socks at least once daily; reevaluate therapy if no improvement occurs in 4 weeks | | <u>Lactation Issues</u> Excretion in breast milk is unknown; use with caution in nursing mothers |
| **Erythromycin** <u>Ointment</u>: Akne-mycin 2% <u>Gel</u>: Erygel 2% | **Aid to healing and prophylaxis of infection in minor cuts, wounds, burns, and skin abrasions** Apply to affected area 1 to 4 times daily | <u>Administration Issues</u> For external use only; keep preparation away from the eyes, mouth, and mucous membranes; wash hands thoroughly after application; area to be treated may be covered with a gauze dressing if desired | <u>ADRs:</u> skin irritation, superinfection | <u>Contraindications</u> Hypersensitivity to any ingredients in the preparation |
| **Gentamicin** Garamycin, generics <u>Ointment</u>: 0.1% <u>Cream</u>: 0.1% | **Aid to healing and prophylaxis of infection in minor cuts, wounds, burns, and skin abrasions** Apply to affected area 1 to 4 times daily | <u>Administration Issues</u> For external use only; keep preparation away from the eyes, mouth, and mucous membranes; wash hands thoroughly after application; area to be treated may be covered with a gauze dressing if desired | <u>ADRs:</u> skin irritation, superinfection | <u>Contraindications</u> Hypersensitivity to any ingredients in the preparation |
| **Haloprogin** Halotex <u>Cream</u>: 1% <u>Solution</u>: 1% | **Treatment of athlete's foot, jock itch, ringworm, and tinea versicolor** Apply liberally to the affected area twice daily for 2 to 3 weeks | <u>Administration Issues</u> For external use only; keep preparation away from the eyes, mouth, and mucous membranes; cleanse the affected area with soap and water and dry thoroughly prior to application; wash hands thoroughly after application | <u>ADRs:</u> irritation, burning, erythema | <u>Contraindications</u> Hypersensitivity to any component of the product <u>Pregnancy Category</u>: B <u>Lactation Issues</u> Excretion in breast milk is unknown; use with caution in nursing mothers |

| | | | Contraindications |
|---|---|---|---|
| **Imiquimod**<br>Aldara<br><br><u>Cream:</u> 5% | **Treatment of genital and perianal warts**<br>Apply 3 times/wk, prior to normal sleeping hours and leave on skin for 6 to 10 h. Wash with soap and water after treatment period. | <u>Administration Issues</u><br>For external use only; keep preparation away from the eyes, mouth, and mucous membranes. Do not occlude area with bandages, covers or wraps. Imiquimod may weaken condoms and vaginal diaphragms.<br><br><u>ADRs:</u><br>erythema, itching, erosion, burning, pain, excoriation, flaking, edema, induration, ulceration | <u>Contraindications</u><br>Hypersensitivity to any component of the product<br><br><u>Pregnancy Category:</u>  do not use in pregnant women<br><br><u>Lactation Issues</u><br>Excretion in breast milk is unknown |
| **Ketoconazole**<br>Nizoral<br><br><u>Cream:</u> 2%<br><br><u>Shampoo:</u> 2% | **Treatment of athlete's foot, jock itch, ringworm, cutaneous candidiasis, and tinea versicolor**<br>Apply to affected area once daily for 2 weeks; treat athlete's foot for 6 weeks<br><br>**Treatment of seborrheic dermatitis**<br>Apply to affected area twice daily for 4 weeks<br><br>**Treatment of dandruff and scaling**<br>Apply to hair and scalp; lather and wash for 1 minute; rinse thoroughly; repeat, leaving shampoo on scalp for 3 minutes; rinse thoroughly; dry hair. Shampoo twice weekly for 4 weeks with at least 3 days between each shampooing; may shampoo intermittently as needed to maintain control | <u>Administration Issues</u><br>For external use only; keep preparation away from the eyes, mouth, and mucous membranes; cleanse the affected area with soap and water and dry thoroughly prior to application; moisten hair and scalp thoroughly prior to application; wash hands thoroughly after application<br><br><u>ADRs:</u><br>irritation, pruritis, stinging, mild dryness of skin | <u>Contraindications</u><br>Hypersensitivity to any component of the product<br><br><u>Pregnancy Category:</u>  C<br><br><u>Lactation Issues</u><br>Safety for use in nursing mothers has not been established; use with caution |
| **Miconazole Nitrate**<br><u>Cream:</u><br>Micatin, Monistat-Derm 2% | **Treatment of athlete's foot, jock itch, ringworm, and cutaneous candidiasis** | <u>Administration Issues</u><br>For external use only; keep preparation away from the eyes, mouth, and mucous<br><br><u>ADRs:</u><br><u>Topical:</u><br>irritation, burning | <u>Contraindications</u><br>Hypersensitivity to any component of the product |

(continues on next page)

## 805. Anti–Infective Products (Topical and Vaginal) *continued from previous page*

| Drug and Dosage Forms | Usual Dosage Range | Administration Issues | Adverse Drug Reaction (ADRs) Spectrum (If listed) and Absorption issues | Contraindications, Pregnancy Category, and Lactation Issues |
|---|---|---|---|---|
| **Miconazole Nitrate *cont.*** Powder: Micatin 2% Spray: Micatin Liquid 2% Vaginal Suppositories: 100 mg, 200 mg Vaginal Cream: 2% | Apply to affected area twice daily, morning and evening; treat for 2 weeks, except athlete's foot treat for 4 weeks **Treatment of tinea versicolor** Apply to affected area once daily; clinical improvement should be seen in 2 weeks **Treatment of vulvovaginal candidiasis** Vaginal Suppository: 200 mg, 1 dose × 3 d or 100 mg, 1 dose × 7 d Vaginal Cream: 1 applicatorful q hs × 7 d Cream: Apply to affected areas bid × 7 d | membranes; cleanse the affected area with soap and water and dry thoroughly prior to application; wash hands thoroughly after application; for athlete's foot, wear well-fitting, ventilated shoes and change shoes and socks at least once daily; reevaluate therapy if no improvement occurs in 4 weeks | Vaginal: vulvovaginal burning, itching, irritation, headache, pelvic cramps, contact dermatitis | Pregnancy Category: topical safe in pregnancy Lactation Issues Safety for use in nursing mothers has not been established; use with caution |
| **Mupirocin** Bactroban Ointment: 2% | **Treatment of impetigo** Apply a small amount to affected area 3 times daily; reevaluate patients not showing clinical response in 3 to 5 days | Administration Issues For external use only; keep preparation away from the eyes, mouth, and mucous membranes; wash hands thoroughly after application; area to be treated may be covered with a gauze dressing if desired | ADRs: burning, stinging, local pain Antibacterial Spectrum *Staphylococcus aureus* (methicillin-resistant and beta lactamase producing strains), *S. saprophyticus, S. epidermidis* and *pyogenes* | Contraindications Hypersensitivity to any components of the product Pregnancy Category: B Lactation Issues Excretion in breast milk is unknown; temporarily discontinue nursing while using mupirocin |

| | Administration Issues | | Contraindications / Pregnancy / Lactation |
|---|---|---|---|
| **Naftifine**<br>Naftin<br><br><u>Cream:</u> 1%<br><br><u>Gel:</u> 1% | **Treatment of athlete's foot, jock itch, and ringworm**<br>Apply to affected area once daily with cream or twice daily with gel | <u>ADRs:</u><br>burning, stinging, dryness, irritation<br><br><u>Absorption Issues:</u><br>systemic absorption was approximately 6% of administered dose following topical administration | <u>Contraindications</u><br>Hypersensitivity to naftifine<br><br><u>Pregnancy Category:</u> B<br><br><u>Lactation Issues</u><br>Excretion in breast milk is unknown; use with caution in nursing mothers |
| **Neomycin Sulfate**<br><br><u>Ointment:</u><br>Myciguent, generics: 3.5 mg/gm<br><br><u>Cream:</u><br>Myciguent 3.5 mg/gm | **Aid to healing and prophylaxis of infection in minor cuts, wounds, burns, and skin abrasions**<br>Apply to affected area 1 to 4 times daily<br><br>For external use only; keep preparation away from the eyes, mouth, and mucous membranes; wash hands thoroughly after application; area to be treated may be covered with a gauze dressing if desired | <u>ADRs:</u><br>skin irritation, superinfection | <u>Contraindications</u><br>Hypersensitivity to any ingredients in the preparation |
| **Nystatin**<br>Mycostatin, Nilstat, various generics<br><br><u>Cream:</u> 100,000 units/gm<br><br><u>Ointment:</u> 100,000 units/gm<br><br><u>Powder:</u> Mycostatin 100,000 units/gm<br><br><u>Vaginal Tablets:</u> 100,000 units | **Treatment of cutaneous and mucocutaneous infections caused by _Candida sp._**<br>Apply to affected area 2 to 3 times daily until healing is complete<br><br>For fungal infections of the feet, dust powder freely on the feet as well as the shoes and socks<br><br>**Treatment of vulvovaginal candidiasis**<br>1 tablet intravaginally qd × 2 wk | <u>Topical:</u><br>For external use only; keep preparation away from the eyes, mouth, and mucous membranes; cleanse the affected area with soap and water and dry thoroughly prior to application; massage a small amount into affected area; wash hands thoroughly after application; use the cream for infections involving the intertriginous areas; reevaluate therapy if no improvement occurs in 4 weeks<br><br><u>Vaginal:</u> Symptomatic relief may occur in a few days; continue for full course of therapy | <u>Contraindications</u><br>Hypersensitivity to any components of the product<br><br><u>Pregnancy Category:</u> A<br><br><u>Lactation Issues</u><br>Excretion in breast milk is unknown; use with caution in nursing mothers |

Note: The Administration Issues for Naftifine also include: "For external use only; keep preparation away from the eyes, mouth, and mucous membranes; cleanse the affected area with soap and water and dry thoroughly prior to application; wash hands thoroughly after application; reevaluate therapy if no improvement occurs in 4 weeks"

(continues on next page)

**805. Anti-Infective Products (Topical and Vaginal)** *continued from previous page*

| Drug and Dosage Forms | Usual Dosage Range | Administration Issues | Adverse Drug Reaction (ADRs) Spectrum (If listed) and Absorption issues | Contraindications, Pregnancy Category, and Lactation Issues |
|---|---|---|---|---|
| **Oxiconazole Nitrate** Oxistat <br><br> <u>Cream</u>: 1% <br><br> <u>Lotion</u>: 1% | **Treatment of athlete's foot, jock itch, and ringworm** <br> Apply to affected area twice daily for 2 weeks; treat athlete's foot for 4 weeks to decrease possibility of recurrence | <u>Administration Issues</u> <br> For external use only; keep preparation away from the eyes, mouth, and mucous membranes; cleanse the affected area with soap and water and dry thoroughly prior to application; wash hands thoroughly after application; for athlete's foot, wear well-fitting, ventilated shoes and change shoes and socks at least once daily; reevaluate therapy if no improvement occurs in 4 weeks | <u>ADRs:</u> <br> pruritis, burning, stinging, irritation <br><br> <u>Absorption Issues:</u> <br> systemic absorption is very low; < 0.3% of applied dose is recovered in urine 5 days after application | <u>Contraindications</u> <br> Hypersensitivity to oxiconazole nitrate <br><br> <u>Pregnancy Category:</u> B <br><br> <u>Lactation Issues</u> <br> Excretion in breast milk is unknown; use with caution in nursing mothers |
| **Podofilox** Condylox <br><br> <u>Topical Gel:</u> 0.5% <br><br> <u>Topical Solution:</u> 0.5% | **Topical treatment of anogenital warts (gel) and topical treatment of external warts (solution) due to HPV** <br> Apply solution or gel bid × 3 days, then off for 4 days. May repeat cycle total of 4 times. Minimize application on surrounding normal tissue. Allow to dry before allowing the return of the opposing skin surfaces to normal positions. | <u>Administration Issues</u> <br> Instruct patient to wash hands thoroughly before using and after each application. For external use only. Avoid contact with eyes. If no improvement after 4 weeks of treatment have patient consult health-care provider. | <u>ADRs:</u> <br> burning, pain, inflammation, erosion, itching, bleeding <br> Side-effects more common in patients treated with the solution than with the gel | <u>Contraindications</u> <br> Hypersensitivity to product <br><br> <u>Pregnancy Category:</u> Do not use on pregnant patients <br><br> <u>Lactation Issues</u> <br> Weight risk to infant versus benefit to nursing mother |
| **Podophyllum Resin** Podcon-25, Podofin <br><br> <u>Liquid:</u> 25% podophyllum resin in tincture of benzoin | **Treatment of soft genital (venereal) warts (condylomata acuminata) and other papillomas: CDC recommends podophyllum as an alternative treatment of HPV** | <u>Administration Issues</u> <br> To be applied only by a trained health-care professional. For external use only. Avoid contact with eyes. | <u>ADRs:</u> <br> paresthesia, polyneuritis, pyrexia, leukopenia, diarrhea, abdominal pain, confusion, dizziness | <u>Contraindications</u> <br> Hypersensitivity to product; diabetics, patients using steroids or with poor blood circulation, bleeding warts |

| Drug | Dosage/Indications | Administration Issues | ADRs | Contraindications / Pregnancy / Lactation |
|------|--------------------|-----------------------|------|--------------------------------------------|
| | Apply no more than 0.5 mL to the lesion per visit. Wash in 1–4 h. Retreat in 7 to 10 days. If no improvement after 3–4 treatments, refer to specialist | | | **Pregnancy Category:** Do not use on pregnant patients<br><br>**Lactation Issues**<br>Do not use in nursing mothers |
| **Sulconazole Nitrate**<br>Exelderm<br><br>Cream: 1%<br><br>Solution: 1% | **Treatment of athlete's foot, jock itch, ringworm, and tinea versicolor**<br>Apply to affected area 1 to 2 times daily for 3 to 4 weeks; athlete's foot should be treated twice daily for 4 weeks | Administration Issues<br>For external use only; keep preparation away from the eyes, mouth, and mucous membranes; cleanse the affected area with soap and water and dry thoroughly prior to application; massage a small amount into affected area; wash hands thoroughly after application; for athlete's foot, wear well-fitting, ventilated shoes and change shoes and socks at least once daily; reevaluate therapy if no improvement occurs in 4 to 6 weeks | ADRs:<br>itching, burning, stinging | Contraindications<br>Hypersensitivity to sulconazole nitrate<br><br>Pregnancy Category: C<br><br>Lactation Issues<br>Excretion in breast milk is unknown; use with caution in nursing mothers |
| **Terbinafine**<br>Lamisil<br><br>Cream: 1% | **Treatment of athlete's foot, jock itch, ringworm, cutaneous candidiasis, and tinea versicolor**<br>Apply to affected area once or twice daily for 1 to 4 weeks | Administration Issues<br>For external use only; keep preparation away from the eyes, mouth, and mucous membranes; cleanse the affected area with soap and water and dry thoroughly prior to application; wash hands thoroughly after application; avoid the use of occlusive dressings; reevaluate therapy if no improvement occurs in 4 weeks | ADRs:<br>irritation, itching, dryness<br><br>Absorption Issues:<br>approximately 3.5% of a topical dose is recovered in the urine | Contraindications<br>Hypersensitivity to terbinafine<br><br>Pregnancy Category: B<br><br>Lactation Issues<br>Excreted in breast milk in small concentrations; due to potential for adverse events in nursing infants, discontinue nursing or the drug, taking into account the importance of the drug to the mother |
| **Terconazole**<br>Terazol 7, Terazol 3 | **Treatment of vulvovaginal candidiasis**<br>Suppositories: | Administration Issues<br>Before prescribing another course of therapy, reconfirm diagnosis by smears | ADRs:<br>headache, body pain, dysmenorrhea, itching, pruritus | Contraindications<br>Hypersensitivity to terconazole |

*(continues on next page)*

| Drug and Dosage Forms | Usual Dosage Range | Administration Issues | Adverse Drug Reaction (ADRs) Spectrum (If listed) and Absorption issues | Contraindications, Pregnancy Category, and Lactation Issues |
|---|---|---|---|---|
| **Terconazole** *cont.*<br><br>Vaginal Cream: 0.4%, 0.8%<br><br>Vaginal Suppositories: 80 mg | Insert 1 dose (80 mg) × 3 d<br><br><u>Cream:</u><br>0.4%: 1 applicatorful q hs × 7 d or<br>0.8%: 1 applicatorful q hs × 3 d | or culture to rule out other pathogens. The therapeutic effect of Terconazole is not affected by menstruation | | <u>Pregnancy Category:</u> C<br><br><u>Lactation Issues:</u> use with caution |
| **Tetracycline**<br>Achromycin<br><br><u>Ointment:</u> 3% | **Aid to healing and prophylaxis of infection in minor cuts, wounds, burns, and skin abrasions**<br>Apply to affected area 1 to 4 times daily | <u>Administration Issues</u><br>For external use only; keep preparation away from the eyes, mouth, and mucous membranes; wash hands thoroughly after application; area to be treated may be covered with a gauze dressing if desired | <u>ADRs:</u><br>skin irritation, superinfection | <u>Contraindications</u><br>Hypersensitivity to any ingredients in the preparation |
| **Tioconazole**<br>Vagistat-1<br><br><u>Vaginal Ointment:</u> 6.5% | **Treatment of vulvovaginal candidiasis**<br>1 applicatorful intravaginally × 1 dose | <u>Administration Issues</u><br>For external use only. Follow patient instruction information sheet. | <u>ADRs:</u><br>irritation, burning, discharge, vulvar edema | <u>Contraindications</u><br>Hypersensitivity to tioconazole<br><br><u>Pregnancy Category:</u> C<br><br><u>Lactation Issues:</u> use with caution |
| **Tolnaftate**<br>Cream: Tinactin, generics 1%<br><br>Solution: Tinactin, generics 1%<br><br>Gel: Aftate 1% | **Treatment of athlete's foot, jock itch, ringworm, and tinea versicolor**<br>Apply to affected area twice daily for 2 to 3 weeks | <u>Administration Issues</u><br>For external use only; keep preparation away from the eyes, mouth, and mucous membranes; cleanse the affected area with soap and water and dry thoroughly prior to application; powders are used mainly as adjunctive therapy; use a small quantity; wash hands thoroughly after application; for athlete's foot, wear well-fitting, | <u>ADRs:</u><br>irritation | |

| | | |
|---|---|---|
| Powder: Tinactin, generics: 1%<br><br>Spray Powder: Tinactin, generics 1%<br><br>Spray Liquid: Aftate, Desenex, Tinactin | ventilated shoes and change shoes and socks at least once daily; reevaluate therapy if no improvement occurs after 10 days | Contraindications<br>Sensitivity to any components of the product |
| **Triacetin**<br>Solution: Fungoid Tincture 30 ml<br><br>Fungoid 15 ml<br><br>Cream: Fungoid Creme 30 gm | **Treatment of athlete's foot, jock itch, ringworm, and monilial impetigo**<br>Apply cream or solution to affected area 3 times daily; improvement should occur within 7 days; reevaluate therapy if no improvement occurs in 4 weeks<br><br>**Treatment of nail fungus**<br>Apply tincture to nail surface, beds, edges, and under surface of nail 3 times daily; continued treatment for several months may be necessary to see results<br><br>Administration Issues<br>For external use only; keep preparation away from the eyes, mouth, and mucous membranes; cleanse the affected area with soap and water and dry thoroughly prior to application; wash hands thoroughly after application; for athlete's foot, wear well-fitting, ventilated shoes and change shoes and socks at least once daily. | ADRs:<br>irritation; Use with caution in diabetic or patients with impaired blood circulation |
| **Trichloroacetic Acid**<br>Tri-Chlor<br><br>Liquid: 80% | **Treatment of genital and perianal warts**<br>Apply once or twice weekly depending on patient's tolerance. Apply baking soda and water paste after treatment to the area to neutralize acid. If no improvement after 3 treatments, refer to specialist<br><br>Administration Issues<br>For external use only; keep preparation away from the eyes, mouth, and mucous membranes. Can pretreat with topical anesthetic to lessen burning. | ADRs:<br>burning, irritation, pain<br><br>Contraindications<br>Sensitivity to any components of the product; severely irritated tissue<br><br>Pregnancy: safe to use in pregnancy |

| Drug and Dosage Forms | Usual Dosage Range | Administration Issues | Adverse Drug Reactions (ADRs) | Contraindications, Pregnancy Category, and Lactation Issues |
|---|---|---|---|---|
| **Crotamiton**<br>Eurax<br><br>Cream: 10%<br><br>Lotion: 10% | **Treatment of scabies**<br>Apply a thin layer to dry skin from neck down and rub in thoroughly over entire body; a second application is advisable 24 hours later; remove medication with a cleansing bath 48 hours after the second application | Administration Issues<br>For external use only; keep preparation away from the eyes, mouth, and mucous membranes; avoid use on the face; apply with rubber gloves; flush eyes well with water several minutes if contact occurs; avoid use on cuts; shake lotion and cream well prior to administration; change clothing and bed linen the next day, contaminated clothing and linen may be dry cleaned or washed in the hot cycle and machine dried in the hot cycle for 20 minutes; consider treatment in other family members and close personal contacts | ADRs:<br>irritation | Contraindications<br>Hypersensitivity to crotamiton<br><br>Pregnancy Category: C |
| **Lindane**<br><br>Cream:<br>Kwell 1%<br><br>Lotion:<br>Kwell, generics 1%<br><br>Shampoo:<br>Kwell, generics 1% | **Treatment of head lice and pubic lice**<br>Apply lotion thinly to cover the dry hair and skin of affected area and rub in thoroughly; leave on for 12 hours; remove thoroughly with washing; one application is usually curative.<br><br>Apply shampoo to dry hair; lather with a small quantity of water; work thoroughly into hair for 4 minutes; rinse thoroughly and towel dry; one application is usually curative | Administration Issues<br>For external use only; keep preparation away from the eyes, mouth, and mucous membranes; avoid use on the face; apply with rubber gloves; flush eyes well with water several minutes if contact occurs; avoid use on cuts; treat sexual contacts simultaneously; shake lotion and cream well prior to administration; a fine toothed comb may be used to comb hair to remove any remaining nit shells; reapply if there are demonstrable nits after 7 days; change clothing and bed linen the next day, contaminated clothing and linen may be dry cleaned or washed in the hot cycle and | ADRs:<br>dizziness, irritation | Contraindications<br>Hypersensitivity to lindane; use in premature neonates; patients with known seizure disorders<br><br>Pregnancy Category: B<br><br>Lactation Issues<br>Excreted in breast milk; due to potential for serious adverse events in infants, use an alternate method of feeding while using lindane |

| Drug | Treatment | Administration Issues | ADRs | Contraindications / Pregnancy / Lactation |
|---|---|---|---|---|
| | **Treatment of scabies**<br>Apply a thin layer of cream or lotion to dry skin from neck down and rub in thoroughly over entire body (generally 2 oz. of medication is adequate for adults); leave on for 8 to 12 hours; remove thoroughly with washing; one application is usually curative | machine dried in the hot cycle for 20 minutes; consider treatment in other family members and close personal contacts. **Use with caution in children, potential toxic effects are greater in the young due to enhanced topical absorption** | | Contraindications<br>Hypersensitivity to synthetic pyrethroid or pyrethrin, chrysanthemums, or any component of the product<br><br>Pregnancy Category: B<br><br>Lactation Issues<br>Excretion in breast milk is unknown; use an alternate method of feeding while using permethrin |
| **Permethrin**<br><br>Cream:<br>Elimite 5%<br><br>Liquid:<br>Nix 1% | **Treatment of scabies**<br>Apply a thin layer to dry skin from neck down and rub in thoroughly over entire body (usually 30 gm is sufficient for adults); leave on for 8 to 14 hours; remove thoroughly with washing; one application is usually curative<br><br>**Treatment of head lice**<br>Apply shampoo to dry hair; lather; leave on hair for 10 minutes; rinse thoroughly and towel dry; one application is usually curative | Administration Issues<br>For external use only; keep preparation away from the eyes, mouth, and mucous membranes; avoid use on the face; apply with rubber gloves; flush eyes well with water several minutes if contact occurs; avoid use on cuts; shake lotion and cream well prior to administration; wash hair with shampoo, rinse with water, and towel dry prior to apply medication; a fine toothed comb may be used to comb hair to remove any remaining nit shells; reapply if there are demonstrable nits after 7 days; change clothing and bed linen the next day, contaminated clothing and linen may be dry cleaned or washed in the hot cycle and machine dried in the hot cycle for 20 minutes; consider treatment in other family members and close personal contacts | ADRs:<br>pruritis. burning, stinging | |
| **Malathion**<br>Ovide<br><br>Lotion: 0.5% | **Treatment of head lice and their ova**<br>Sprinkle lotion on dry hair and rub gently until the scalp is thoroughly moistened. Allow to dry naturally; use no heat and leave uncovered. After 8–12 hours, wash the hair with | Administration Issues<br>For external use only; keep preparation away from the eyes, mouth, and mucous membranes; avoid use on the face; apply with rubber gloves; flush eyes well with water several minutes if contact occurs; avoid use on cuts | ADRs:<br>irritation | Contraindications<br>Hypersensitivity to product<br><br>Pregnancy Category: B<br><br>Lactation Issues<br>Excretion in breast milk is |

(continues on next page)

| Drug and Dosage Forms | Usual Dosage Range | Administration Issues | Adverse Drug Reactions (ADRs) | Contraindications, Pregnancy Category, and Lactation Issues |
|---|---|---|---|---|
| **Malathion *cont.*** | a nonmedicated shampoo. Rinse and use a fine toothed comb to remove dead lice and eggs. If required, repeat with second application in 7 to 9 days. | | | unknown; use caution in nursing mothers |
| **Miscellaneous Pediculicides**<br><br>Liquid: Control–L, End Lice (0.3% pyrethrin, 3% piperonyl butoxide)<br><br>Shampoo: A-200, R&C, RID (0.3% pyrethrin, 3% piperonyl butoxide) | **Treatment of head lice, body lice, and pubic lice**<br>Apply to affected hairy and surrounding area, lather hair; allow to remain for 10 minutes; wash hair and surrounding area thoroughly and dry with a clean towel<br><br>A second treatment after 7–10 days is recommended to kill any newly hatched lice | Administration Issues<br>For external use only; keep preparation away from the eyes, mouth, and mucous membranes; avoid use on the face; apply with rubber gloves; flush eyes well with water several minutes if contact occurs; avoid use on cuts; treat sexual contacts simultaneously; a fine toothed comb may be used to comb hair to remove any remaining nit shells; change clothing and bed linen the next day, contaminated clothing and linen may be dry cleaned or washed in the hot cycle and machine dried in the hot cycle for 20 minutes; consider treatment in other family members and close personal contacts | ADRs:<br>irritation | Contraindications<br>Hypersensitivity to pyrethrins, permethrins, or any component of the product |

## 807. Corticosteroid Products

**Warnings about topical steroid products:** Topical corticosteroids have a repository effect; with continuous use, 1 to 2 applications per day may be as effective as 3 or more applications. Short term or intermittent therapy with high potency agents (i.e. every other day, 3 to 4 consecutive days per week) may be more effective and cause fewer adverse effects than continuous regimens using lower potency products. After long-term use or after using a potent agent, in order to prevent a rebound effect, switch to a less potent agent or alternative use of topical corticosteroids and emollient products. Treatment with very high potency topical corticosteroids should not exceed 2 consecutive weeks

| Drug and Dosage Forms | Usual Dosage Range | Administration Issues | Adverse Drug Reactions (ADRs) and Pharmacokinetics | Contraindications, Pregnancy Category, and Lactation Issues |
|---|---|---|---|---|
| **Alclometasone Dipropionate** Aclovate Ointment: 0.05% Cream: 0.05% | **Relief of inflammation associated with contact dermatitis, poison ivy, poison sumac, poison oak, eczema, insect bites, sunburn, and second-degree localized burns; adjunctive therapy in the treatment of psoriasis, seborrheic dermatitis, severe diaper rash, and chronic discoid lupus erythematosus** Apply to affected area 2 to 4 times daily  Topical corticosteroids have a repository effect; with continuous use, 1 to 2 applications per day may be as effective as 3 or more applications  Short term or intermittent therapy with high potency agents (i.e. every other day, 3 to 4 consecutive days per week) may be more effective and cause fewer adverse effects than continuous regimens using lower potency products After long-term use or after using a potent agent, in order to prevent a | Administration Issues: For external use only; keep preparation away from the eyes, mouth, and mucous membranes; apply sparingly in a light film and rub in gently; do not use tight-fitting diapers or plastic pants on children treated with corticosteroids in the diaper area; do not use occlusive dressings with very potent agents such as augmented betamethasone dipropionate, clobetasol, halobetasol propionate, and mometasone | ADRS: Burning, itching, irritation, erythema, dryness, skin atrophy (especially with potent preparations), HPA axis suppression (especially with potent preparations)  Pharmacokinetics: Systemic absorption through the skin depends on intrinsic properties of the drug itself, the vehicle used, the duration of exposure, and the surface area and condition of the skin involved; occlusive dressings greatly enhance skin penetration and drug absorption | Contraindications: Hypersensitivity to any component of the product; monotherapy in primary bacterial infections (i.e. impetigo)  Pregnancy Category: C  Lactation Issues: Excretion in breast milk is unknown; use with caution in nursing mothers |

(continues on next page)

| Drug and Dosage Forms | Usual Dosage Range | Administration Issues | Adverse Drug Reactions (ADRs) and Pharmacokinetics | Contraindications, Pregnancy Category, and Lactation Issues |
|---|---|---|---|---|
| | rebound effect, switch to a less potent agent or alternative use of topical corticosteroids and emollient products<br><br>Treatment with very high potency topical corticosteroids should not exceed 2 consecutive weeks | | | |
| **Amcinonide**<br>Cyclocort<br><br>Ointment: 0.1%<br><br>Cream: 0.1%<br><br>Lotion: 0.1% | See page 1453 for specific indications<br>Apply to affected area 2 to 4 times daily | Administration Issues:<br>For external use only; keep preparation away from the eyes, mouth, and mucous membranes; apply sparingly in a light film and rub in gently; shake lotion and spray preparations prior to administration; do not use tight-fitting diapers or plastic pants on children treated with corticosteroids in the diaper area | ADRS:<br>Burning, itching, irritation, erythema, dryness, skin atrophy (especially with potent preparations), HPA axis suppression (especially with potent preparations)<br><br>Pharmacokinetics:<br>Systemic absorption through the skin depends on intrinsic properties of the drug itself, the vehicle used, the duration of exposure, and the surface area and condition of the skin involved; occlusive dressings greatly enhance skin penetration and drug absorption | Contraindications:<br>Hypersensitivity to any component of the product; monotherapy in primary bacterial infections (i.e. impetigo)<br><br>Pregnancy Category:  C<br><br>Lactation Issues:<br>Excretion in breast milk is unknown; use with caution in nursing mothers |
| **Augmented Betamethasone Dipropionate** | See page 1453 for specific indications<br>Apply to affected area 2 to 4 times daily | Administration Issues:<br>For external use only; keep preparation away from the eyes, mouth, and mucous | ADRS:<br>Burning, itching, irritation, erythema, dryness, skin atrophy | Contraindications:<br>Hypersensitivity to any component of the product; |

| Formulations | Usual Dosage | Administration Issues / ADRs / Pharmacokinetics | Contraindications / Pregnancy / Lactation |
|---|---|---|---|
| Ointment: Diprolene 0.05%<br><br>Cream: Diprolene AF 0.05%<br><br>Gel: Diprolene 0.05%<br><br>Lotion: Diprolene 0.05% | | membranes; apply sparingly in a light film and rub in gently; shake lotion and spray preparations prior to administration; do not use tight-fitting diapers or plastic pants on children treated with corticosteroids in the diaper area; do not use occlusive dressings with very potent agents such as augmented betamethasone dipropionate, clobetasol, halobetasol propionate, and mometasone<br><br>(especially with potent preparations), HPA axis suppression (especially with potent preparations)<br><br>Pharmacokinetics:<br>Systemic absorption through the skin depends on intrinsic properties of the drug itself, the vehicle used, the duration of exposure, and the surface area and condition of the skin involved; occlusive dressings greatly enhance skin penetration and drug absorption | monotherapy in primary bacterial infections (i.e. impetigo)<br><br>Pregnancy Category: C<br><br>Lactation Issues:<br>Excretion in breast milk is unknown; use with caution in nursing mothers |
| **Betamethasone Benzoate**<br>Uticort<br><br>Cream: 0.025%<br><br>Lotion: 0.025%<br><br>Gel: 0.025% | See page 1453 for specific indications<br>Apply to affected area 2 to 4 times daily | Administration Issues:<br>For external use only; keep preparation away from the eyes, mouth, and mucous membranes; apply sparingly in a light film and rub in gently; shake lotion and spray preparations prior to administration; do not use tight-fitting diapers or plastic pants on children treated with corticosteroids in the diaper area<br><br>ADRS:<br>Burning, itching, irritation, erythema, dryness, skin atrophy (especially with potent preparations), HPA axis suppression (especially with potent preparations)<br><br>Pharmacokinetics:<br>Systemic absorption through the skin depends on intrinsic properties of the drug itself, the vehicle used, the duration of exposure, and the surface area and condition of the skin involved; occlusive dressings greatly enhance skin penetration and drug absorption | Contraindications:<br>Hypersensitivity to any component of the product; monotherapy in primary bacterial infections (i.e. impetigo)<br><br>Pregnancy Category: C<br><br>Lactation Issues:<br>Excretion in breast milk is unknown; use with caution in nursing mothers |

(continues on next page)

| Drug and Dosage Forms | Usual Dosage Range | Administration Issues | Adverse Drug Reactions (ADRs) and Pharmacokinetics | Contraindications, Pregnancy Category, and Lactation Issues |
|---|---|---|---|---|
| **Betamethasone Dipropionate** Diprosone, Maxivate, various generics<br><br>Ointment: 0.05%<br><br>Cream: 0.05%<br><br>Lotion: 0.05%<br><br>Aerosol: Diprosone 0.1% | See page 1453 for specific indications Apply to affected area 2 to 4 times daily | Administration Issues: For external use only; keep preparation away from the eyes, mouth, and mucous membranes; apply sparingly in a light film and rub in gently; shake lotion and spray preparations prior to administration; hold spray 3 to 6 inches away from affected area while in use, spray for about 2 seconds to cover an area the size of your hand; do not use tight-fitting diapers or plastic pants on children treated with corticosteroids in the diaper area | ADRS: Burning, itching, irritation, erythema, dryness, skin atrophy (especially with potent preparations), HPA axis suppression (especially with potent preparations)<br><br>Pharmacokinetics: Systemic absorption through the skin depends on intrinsic properties of the drug itself, the vehicle used, the duration of exposure, and the surface area and condition of the skin involved; occlusive dressings greatly enhance skin penetration and drug absorption. In some cases, generic "equivalents" have less vasoconstrictive activity compared to the name brand medication | Contraindications: Hypersensitivity to any component of the product; monotherapy in primary bacterial infections (i.e. impetigo)<br><br>Pregnancy Category: C<br><br>Lactation Issues: Excretion in breast milk is unknown; use with caution in nursing mothers |
| **Betamethasone Valerate** Valisone, various generics<br><br>Ointment: 0.1% | See page 1453 for specific indications Apply to affected area 2 to 4 times daily | Administration Issues: For external use only; keep preparation away from the eyes, mouth, and mucous membranes; apply sparingly in a light film and rub in gently; shake lotion and spray preparations prior to administration; do not use tight-fitting diapers or plastic | ADRS: Burning, itching, irritation, erythema, dryness, skin atrophy (especially with potent preparations), HPA axis suppression (especially with potent preparations) | Contraindications: Hypersensitivity to any component of the product; monotherapy in primary bacterial infections (i.e. impetigo)<br><br>Pregnancy Category: C |

(continues on next page)

| | Administration Issues | Pharmacokinetics / ADRS / Contraindications | Lactation Issues |
|---|---|---|---|
| Cream: 0.01%, 0.1%<br><br>Lotion: 0.1% | pants on children treated with corticosteroids in the diaper area; do not use occlusive dressings with very potent agents such as augmented betamethasone dipropionate, clobetasol, halobetasol propionate, and mometasone | Pharmacokinetics:<br>Systemic absorption through the skin depends on intrinsic properties of the drug itself, the vehicle used, the duration of exposure, and the surface area and condition of the skin involved; occlusive dressings greatly enhance skin penetration and drug absorption. In some cases, generic "equivalents" have less vasoconstrictive activity compared to the name brand medication | Lactation Issues:<br>Excretion in breast milk is unknown; use with caution in nursing mothers |
| **Clobetasol Propionate**<br>Temovate<br><br>Ointment: 0.05%<br><br>Cream: 0.05%<br><br>Scalp application: 0.05% | See page 1453 for specific indications<br>Apply to affected area 2 to 4 times daily<br><br>Administration Issues:<br>For external use only; keep preparation away from the eyes, mouth, and mucous membranes; apply sparingly in a light film and rub in gently; do not use tight-fitting diapers or plastic pants on children treated with corticosteroids in the diaper area; do not use occlusive dressings with very potent agents such as augmented betamethasone dipropionate, clobetasol, halobetasol propionate, and mometasone | ADRS:<br>Burning, itching, irritation, erythema, dryness, skin atrophy (especially with potent preparations), HPA axis suppression (especially with potent preparations)<br><br>Pharmacokinetics:<br>Systemic absorption through the skin depends on intrinsic properties of the drug itself, the vehicle used, the duration of exposure, and the surface area and condition of the skin involved; occlusive dressings greatly enhance skin penetration and drug absorption. | Contraindications:<br>Hypersensitivity to any component of the product; monotherapy in primary bacterial infections (i.e. impetigo)<br><br>Pregnancy Category: C<br><br>Lactation Issues:<br>Excretion in breast milk is unknown; use with caution in nursing mothers |

| Drug and Dosage Forms | Usual Dosage Range | Administration Issues | Adverse Drug Reactions (ADRs) and Pharmacokinetics | Contraindications, Pregnancy Category, and Lactation Issues |
|---|---|---|---|---|
| **Clocortolone Pivalate**<br>Cloderm<br><br><u>Cream:</u> 0.1% | <u>See page 1453 for specific indications</u><br>Apply to affected area 2 to 4 times daily | <u>Administration Issues:</u><br>For external use only; keep preparation away from the eyes, mouth, and mucous membranes; apply sparingly in a light film and rub in gently; do not use tight-fitting diapers or plastic pants on children treated with corticosteroids in the diaper area | <u>ADRS:</u><br>Burning, itching, irritation, erythema, dryness, skin atrophy (especially with potent preparations), HPA axis suppression (especially with potent preparations)<br><br><u>Pharmacokinetics:</u><br>Systemic absorption through the skin depends on intrinsic properties of the drug itself, the vehicle used, the duration of exposure, and the surface area and condition of the skin involved; occlusive dressings greatly enhance skin penetration and drug absorption. In some cases, generic "equivalents" have less vasoconstrictive activity compared to the name brand medication | <u>Contraindications:</u><br>Hypersensitivity to any component of the product; monotherapy in primary bacterial infections (i.e. impetigo)<br><br><u>Pregnancy Category:</u> C<br><br><u>Lactation Issues:</u><br>Excretion in breast milk is unknown; use with caution in nursing mothers |
| **Desonide**<br><u>Ointment:</u><br>DesOwen, Tridesilon 0.05%<br><br><u>Cream:</u><br>DesOwen, Tridesilon, various generics 0.05% | <u>See page 1453 for specific indications</u><br>Apply to affected area 2 to 4 times daily | <u>Administration Issues:</u><br>For external use only; keep preparation away from the eyes, mouth, and mucous membranes; apply sparingly in a light film and rub in gently; shake lotion and spray preparations prior to administration; do not use tight-fitting diapers or plastic pants on | <u>ADRS:</u><br>Burning, itching, irritation, erythema, dryness, skin atrophy (especially with potent preparations), HPA axis suppression (especially with potent preparations) | <u>Contraindications:</u><br>Hypersensitivity to any component of the product; monotherapy in primary bacterial infections (i.e. impetigo)<br><br><u>Pregnancy Category:</u> C |

| | | | |
|---|---|---|---|
| | | **Pharmacokinetics:** Systemic absorption through the skin depends on intrinsic properties of the drug itself, the vehicle used, the duration of exposure, and the surface area and condition of the skin involved; occlusive dressings greatly enhance skin penetration and drug absorption. In some cases, generic "equivalents" have less vasoconstrictive activity compared to the name brand medication | **Lactation Issues:** Excretion in breast milk is unknown; use with caution in nursing mothers |
| **Lotion:** DesOwen 0.05% | children treated with corticosteroids in the diaper area | | |
| **Desoximetasone** **Ointment:** Topicort 0.25% **Cream:** Topicort, various generics 0.05%, 0.25% **Gel:** Topicort 0.05% | **Administration Issues:** For external use only; keep preparation away from the eyes, mouth, and mucous membranes; apply sparingly in a light film and rub in gently; do not use tight-fitting diapers or plastic pants on children treated with corticosteroids in the diaper area | **ADRS:** Burning, itching, irritation, erythema, dryness, skin atrophy (especially with potent preparations), HPA axis suppression (especially with potent preparations) **Pharmacokinetics:** Systemic absorption through the skin depends on intrinsic properties of the drug itself, the vehicle used, the duration of exposure, and the surface area and condition of the skin involved; occlusive dressings greatly enhance skin penetration and drug absorption. In some cases, generic "equivalents" have less vasoconstrictive activity compared to the name brand medication | **Contraindications:** Hypersensitivity to any component of the product; monotherapy in primary bacterial infections (i.e. impetigo) **Pregnancy Category:** C **Lactation Issues:** Excretion in breast milk is unknown; use with caution in nursing mothers |

See page 1453 for specific indications
Apply to affected area 2 to 4 times daily

(continues on next page)

# 807. Corticosteroid Products continued from previous page

| Drug and Dosage Forms | Usual Dosage Range | Administration Issues | Adverse Drug Reactions (ADRs) and Pharmacokinetics | Contraindications, Pregnancy Category, and Lactation Issues |
|---|---|---|---|---|
| **Dexamethasone**<br><br>Aerosol:<br>Aeroseb–Dex 0.01%<br><br>Decaspray 0.04% | See page 1453 for specific indications<br>Apply to affected area 2 to 4 times daily | Administration Issues:<br>For external use only; keep preparation away from the eyes, mouth, and mucous membranes; apply sparingly in a light film and rub in gently; shake lotion and spray preparations prior to administration; hold spray 3 to 6 inches away from affected area while in use, spray for about 2 seconds to cover an area the size of your hand; do not use tight-fitting diapers or plastic pants on children treated with corticosteroids in the diaper area | ADRS:<br>Burning, itching, irritation, erythema, dryness, skin atrophy (especially with potent preparations), HPA axis suppression (especially with potent preparations)<br><br>Pharmacokinetics:<br>Systemic absorption through the skin depends on intrinsic properties of the drug itself, the vehicle used, the duration of exposure, and the surface area and condition of the skin involved; occlusive dressings greatly enhance skin penetration and drug absorption. In some cases, generic "equivalents" have less vasoconstrictive activity compared to the name brand medication | Contraindications:<br>Hypersensitivity to any component of the product; monotherapy in primary bacterial infections (i.e. impetigo)<br><br>Pregnancy Category:  C<br><br>Lactation Issues:<br>Excretion in breast milk is unknown; use with caution in nursing mothers |
| **Dexamethasone Sodium Phosphate**<br>Decadron Phosphate<br><br>Cream:  0.1% | See page 1453 for specific indications<br>Apply to affected area 2 to 4 times daily | Administration Issues:<br>For external use only; keep preparation away from the eyes, mouth, and mucous membranes; apply sparingly in a light film and rub in gently; do not use  tight-fitting diapers or plastic pants on children | ADRS:<br>Burning, itching, irritation, erythema, dryness, skin atrophy (especially with potent preparations), HPA axis suppression (especially with potent preparations) | Contraindications:<br>Hypersensitivity to any component of the product; monotherapy in primary bacterial infections (i.e. impetigo)<br><br>Pregnancy Category:  C |

| | | | |
|---|---|---|---|
| | treated with corticosteroids in the diaper area | Pharmacokinetics: Systemic absorption through the skin depends on intrinsic properties of the drug itself, the vehicle used, the duration of exposure, and the surface area and condition of the skin involved; occlusive dressings greatly enhance skin penetration and drug absorption. | Lactation Issues: Excretion in breast milk is unknown; use with caution in nursing mothers |
| **Diflorasone Diacetate**<br><br>Ointment: 0.05%<br>Florone, Maxiflor, Psorcon<br><br>Cream: 0.05%<br>Florone, Florone E, Maxiflor | See page 1453 for specific indications<br>Apply to affected area 2 to 4 times daily | Administration Issues: For external use only; keep preparation away from the eyes, mouth, and mucous membranes; apply sparingly in a light film and rub in gently; do not use tight-fitting diapers or plastic pants on children treated with corticosteroids in the diaper area | Contraindications: Hypersensitivity to any component of the product; monotherapy in primary bacterial infections (i.e. impetigo)<br><br>Pregnancy Category: C<br><br>Lactation Issues: Excretion in breast milk is unknown; use with caution in nursing mothers |
| | | ADRs: Burning, itching, irritation, erythema, dryness, skin atrophy (especially with potent preparations), HPA axis suppression (especially with potent preparations)<br><br>Pharmacokinetics: Systemic absorption through the skin depends on intrinsic properties of the drug itself, the vehicle used, the duration of exposure, and the surface area and condition of the skin involved; occlusive dressings greatly enhance skin penetration and drug absorption. | |
| **Fluocinolone Acetonide**<br><br>Ointment: 0.025%<br>Synalar, generics | See page 1453 for specific indications<br>Apply to affected area 2 to 4 times daily | Administration Issues: For external use only; keep preparation away from the eyes, mouth, and mucous membranes; apply sparingly in a light film and rub in gently; do not use tight-<br><br>ADRs: Burning, itching, irritation, erythema, dryness, skin atrophy (especially with potent preparations), HPA axis | Contraindications: Hypersensitivity to any component of the product; monotherapy in primary bacterial infections (i.e. impetigo) |

*(continues on next page)*

*continued from previous page*

| Drug and Dosage Forms | Usual Dosage Range | Administration Issues | Adverse Drug Reactions (ADRs) and Pharmacokinetics | Contraindications, Pregnancy Category, and Lactation Issues |
|---|---|---|---|---|
| **Fluocinolone Acetonide** *cont.* <br><br> Cream: <br> Synalar, Synalar HP, various generics <br> 0.01%, 0.025%, 0.2% <br><br> Solution: 0.01% <br> Synalar, Fluonid, various generics <br><br> Shampoo: <br> FS Shampoo 0.01% <br><br> Oil: 0.01% <br> Derma-Smoothe/FS | | fitting diapers or plastic pants on children treated with corticosteroids in the diaper area | suppression (especially with potent preparations) <br><br> Pharmacokinetics: <br> Systemic absorption through the skin depends on intrinsic properties of the drug itself, the vehicle used, the duration of exposure, and the surface area and condition of the skin involved; occlusive dressings greatly enhance skin penetration and drug absorption. In some cases, generic "equivalents" have less vasoconstrictive activity compared to the name brand medication | Pregnancy Category: C <br><br> Lactation Issues: <br> Excretion in breast milk is unknown; use with caution in nursing mothers |
| **Fluocinonide** <br><br> Ointment: 0.05% <br> Lidex, generics <br><br> Cream: 0.05% <br> Lidex, Lidex E, Fluonex, generics <br><br> Solution: 0.05% <br> Lidex, generics | See page 1453 for specific indications <br> Apply to affected area 2 to 4 times daily | Administration Issues: <br> For external use only; keep preparation away from the eyes, mouth, and mucous membranes; apply sparingly in a light film and rub in gently; do not use tight-fitting diapers or plastic pants on children treated with corticosteroids in the diaper area | ADRs: <br> Burning, itching, irritation, erythema, dryness, skin atrophy (especially with potent preparations), HPA axis suppression (especially with potent preparations) <br><br> Pharmacokinetics: <br> Systemic absorption through the skin depends on intrinsic properties of the drug itself, the | Contraindications: <br> Hypersensitivity to any component of the product; monotherapy in primary bacterial infections (i.e. impetigo) <br><br> Pregnancy Category: C <br><br> Lactation Issues: <br> Excretion in breast milk is unknown; use with caution in nursing mothers |

| | | | | |
|---|---|---|---|---|
| **Gel:** 0.05%<br>Lidex, generics | | | vehicle used, the duration of exposure, and the surface area and condition of the skin involved; occlusive dressings greatly enhance skin penetration and drug absorption. In some cases, generic "equivalents" have less vasoconstrictive activity compared to the name brand medication) | **Contraindications:**<br>Hypersensitivity to any component of the product; monotherapy in primary bacterial infections (i.e. impetigo)<br><br>**Pregnancy Category:** C<br><br>**Lactation Issues:**<br>Excretion in breast milk is unknown; use with caution in nursing mothers |
| **Flurandrenolide**<br><br>**Ointment:**<br>Cordran<br>0.025%, 0.05%<br><br>**Cream:**<br>Cordran SP<br>0.025%, 0.05%<br><br>**Lotion:** (0.05%)<br>Cordran, generics<br><br>**Tape:**<br>Cordran 4 mcg/cm$^2$ | **See page 1453 for specific indications**<br>Apply to affected area 2 to 4 times daily | **Administration Issues:**<br>For external use only; keep preparation away from the eyes, mouth, and mucous membranes; apply sparingly in a light film and rub in gently; shake lotion and spray preparations prior to administration; do not use tight-fitting diapers or plastic pants on children treated with corticosteroids in the diaper area | **ADRS:**<br>Burning, itching, irritation, erythema, dryness, skin atrophy (especially with potent preparations), HPA axis suppression (especially with potent preparations)<br><br>**Pharmacokinetics:**<br>Systemic absorption through the skin depends on intrinsic properties of the drug itself, the vehicle used, the duration of exposure, and the surface area and condition of the skin involved; occlusive dressings greatly enhance skin penetration and drug absorption. | |
| **Fluticasone Propionate**<br>Cutivate<br><br>**Ointment:** 0.05% | **See page 1453 for specific indications**<br>Apply to affected area 2 to 4 times daily | **Administration Issues:**<br>For external use only; keep preparation away from the eyes, mouth, and mucous membranes; apply sparingly in a light film and rub in gently; do not use tight-fitting diapers or plastic pants on | **ADRS:**<br>Burning, itching, irritation, erythema, dryness, skin atrophy (especially with potent preparations), HPA axis suppression | **Contraindications:**<br>Hypersensitivity to any component of the product; monotherapy in primary bacterial infections (i.e. impetigo) |

(continues on next page)

| Drug and Dosage Forms | Usual Dosage Range | Administration Issues | Adverse Drug Reactions (ADRs) and Pharmacokinetics | Contraindications, Pregnancy Category, and Lactation Issues |
|---|---|---|---|---|
| **Fluticasone Propionate** *cont.*<br><br>Cream: 0.05% | | children treated with corticosteroids in the diaper area | (especially with potent preparations)<br><br>Pharmacokinetics:<br>Systemic absorption through the skin depends on intrinsic properties of the drug itself, the vehicle used, the duration of exposure, and the surface area and condition of the skin involved; occlusive dressings greatly enhance skin penetration and drug absorption. | Pregnancy Category: C<br><br>Lactation Issues:<br>Excretion in breast milk is unknown; use with caution in nursing mothers |
| **Halcinonide**<br>Halog<br><br>Ointment: 0.1%<br><br>Cream:<br>Halog<br>0.025%, 0.1%<br>Halog-E 0.1%<br><br>Solution: 0.1% | See page 1453 for specific indications<br>Apply to affected area 2 to 4 times daily | Administration Issues:<br>For external use only; keep preparation away from the eyes, mouth, and mucous membranes; apply sparingly in a light film and rub in gently; do not use tight-fitting diapers or plastic pants on children treated with corticosteroids in the diaper area | ADRS:<br>Burning, itching, irritation, erythema, dryness, skin atrophy (especially with potent preparations), HPA axis suppression (especially with potent preparations)<br><br>Pharmacokinetics:<br>Systemic absorption through the skin depends on intrinsic properties of the drug itself, the vehicle used, the duration of exposure, and the surface area and condition of the skin involved; occlusive dressings | Contraindications:<br>Hypersensitivity to any component of the product; monotherapy in primary bacterial infections (i.e. impetigo)<br><br>Pregnancy Category: C<br><br>Lactation Issues:<br>Excretion in breast milk is unknown; use with caution in nursing mothers |

| | | | | |
|---|---|---|---|---|
| **Halobetasol Propionate**<br>Ultravate<br><br>Ointment: 0.05%<br><br>Cream: 0.05% | See page 1453 for specific indications<br><br>Apply to affected area 2 to 4 times daily | Administration Issues:<br>For external use only; keep preparation away from the eyes, mouth, and mucous membranes; apply sparingly in a light film and rub in gently; do not use tight-fitting diapers or plastic pants on children treated with corticosteroids in the diaper area; do not use occlusive dressings with very potent agents such as augmented betamethasone dipropionate, clobetasol, halobetasol propionate, and mometasone | greatly enhance skin penetration and drug absorption.<br><br>ADRS:<br>Burning, itching, irritation, erythema, dryness, skin atrophy (especially with potent preparations), HPA axis suppression (especially with potent preparations)<br><br>Pharmacokinetics:<br>Systemic absorption through the skin depends on intrinsic properties of the drug itself, the vehicle used, the duration of exposure, and the surface area and condition of the skin involved; occlusive dressings greatly enhance skin penetration and drug absorption. | Contraindications:<br>Hypersensitivity to any component of the product; monotherapy in primary bacterial infections (i.e. impetigo)<br><br>Pregnancy Category: C<br><br>Lactation Issues:<br>Excretion in breast milk is unknown; use with caution in nursing mothers |
| **Hydrocortisone**<br><br>Ointment<br>(0.5%, 1%, 2.5%)<br><br>Cream:<br>(0.5%, 1%, 2.5%)<br><br>Lotion: (0.25%, 0.5%, 1%, 2.5%)<br><br>Gel: (0.5%, 1%) | See page 1453 for specific indications<br><br>Apply to affected area 2 to 4 times daily | Administration Issues:<br>For external use only; keep preparation away from the eyes, mouth, and mucous membranes; apply sparingly in a light film and rub in gently; shake lotion and spray preparations prior to administration; hold spray 3 to 6 inches away from affected area while in use, spray for about 2 seconds to cover an area the size of your hand; do not use tight-fitting diapers or plastic pants on children treated with corticosteroids in the diaper area | ADRS:<br>Burning, itching, irritation, erythema, dryness, skin atrophy (especially with potent preparations), HPA axis suppression (especially with potent preparations)<br><br>Pharmacokinetics:<br>Systemic absorption through the skin depends on intrinsic properties of the drug itself, the vehicle used, the duration of exposure, and the surface area and | Contraindications:<br>Hypersensitivity to any component of the product; monotherapy in primary bacterial infections (i.e. impetigo)<br><br>Pregnancy Category: C<br><br>Lactation Issues:<br>Excretion in breast milk is unknown; use with caution in nursing mothers |

(continues on next page)

## 807. Corticosteroid Products  *continued from previous page*

| Drug and Dosage Forms | Usual Dosage Range | Administration Issues | Adverse Drug Reactions (ADRs) and Pharmacokinetics | Contraindications, Pregnancy Category, and Lactation Issues |
|---|---|---|---|---|
| **Hydrocortisone *cont.*** Solution: (1%) Aerosol/Pump Spray: 0.5% Pump Spray: (1%) | | | condition of the skin involved; occlusive dressings greatly enhance skin penetration and drug absorption. In some cases, generic "equivalents" have less vasoconstrictive activity compared to the name brand medication | |
| **Hydrocortisone Acetate** Ointment: (0.5%, 1%) Cortaid with Aloe, Lanacort-5, Maximum Strength Cortaid, Maximum, Anusol HC Cream: (0.5%, 1%) Corticaine, CaldeCort, Cortaid with Aloe, Lanacort | See page 1453 for specific indications Apply to affected area 2 to 4 times daily | Administration Issues: For external use only; keep preparation away from the eyes, mouth, and mucous membranes; apply sparingly in a light film and rub in gently; do not use tight-fitting diapers or plastic pants on children treated with corticosteroids in the diaper area | ADRS: Burning, itching, irritation, erythema, dryness, skin atrophy (especially with potent preparations), HPA axis suppression (especially with potent preparations)  Pharmacokinetics: Systemic absorption through the skin depends on intrinsic properties of the drug itself, the vehicle used, the duration of exposure, and the surface area and condition of the skin involved; occlusive dressings greatly enhance skin penetration and drug absorption. | Contraindications: Hypersensitivity to any component of the product; monotherapy in primary bacterial infections (i.e. impetigo)  Pregnancy Category:  C  Lactation Issues: Excretion in breast milk is unknown; use with caution in nursing mothers |
| **Hydrocortisone Valerate** Westcort | See page 1453 for specific indications Apply to affected area 2 to 4 times daily | Administration Issues: For external use only; keep preparation away from the eyes, mouth, and mucous membranes; apply sparingly in a light film | ADRS: Burning, itching, irritation, erythema, dryness, skin atrophy (especially with potent | Contraindications: Hypersensitivity to any component of the product; monotherapy in primary |

| | | | |
|---|---|---|---|
| Ointment: 0.2%<br><br>Cream: 0.2% | and rub in gently; do not use tight-fitting diapers or plastic pants on children treated with corticosteroids in the diaper area | preparations), HPA axis suppression (especially with potent preparations)<br><br>Pharmacokinetics:<br>Systemic absorption through the skin depends on intrinsic properties of the drug itself, the vehicle used, the duration of exposure, and the surface area and condition of the skin involved; occlusive dressings greatly enhance skin penetration and drug absorption. | bacterial infections (i.e. impetigo)<br><br>Pregnancy Category: C<br><br>Lactation Issues:<br>Excretion in breast milk is unknown; use with caution in nursing mothers |
| **Methylprednisolone Acetate**<br>Medrol Acetate Topical<br><br>Ointment: 0.25%, 1% | See page 1453 for specific indications<br>Apply to affected area 2 to 4 times daily<br><br>Administration Issues:<br>For external use only; keep preparation away from the eyes, mouth, and mucous membranes; apply sparingly in a light film and rub in gently; do not use tight-fitting diapers or plastic pants on children treated with corticosteroids in the diaper area | ADRS:<br>Burning, itching, irritation, erythema, dryness, skin atrophy (especially with potent preparations), HPA axis suppression (especially with potent preparations)<br><br>Pharmacokinetics:<br>Systemic absorption through the skin depends on intrinsic properties of the drug itself, the vehicle used, the duration of exposure, and the surface area and condition of the skin involved; occlusive dressings greatly enhance skin penetration and drug absorption. | Contraindications:<br>Hypersensitivity to any component of the product; monotherapy in primary bacterial infections (i.e. impetigo)<br><br>Pregnancy Category: C<br><br>Lactation Issues:<br>Excretion in breast milk is unknown; use with caution in nursing mothers |

(continues on next page)

| Drug and Dosage Forms | Usual Dosage Range | Administration Issues | Adverse Drug Reactions (ADRs) and Pharmacokinetics | Contraindications, Pregnancy Category, and Lactation Issues |
|---|---|---|---|---|
| **Mometasone Furoate**<br>Elocon<br><br>Ointment: 0.1%<br><br>Cream: 0.1%<br><br>Lotion: 0.1% | See page 1453 for specific indications<br>Apply to affected area 2 to 4 times daily | Administration Issues:<br>For external use only; keep preparation away from the eyes, mouth, and mucous membranes; apply sparingly in a light film and rub in gently; shake lotion and spray preparations prior to administration; do not use tight-fitting diapers or plastic pants on children treated with corticosteroids in the diaper area; do not use occlusive dressings with very potent agents such as augmented betamethasone dipropionate, clobetasol, halobetasol propionate, and mometasone | ADRS:<br>Burning, itching, irritation, erythema, dryness, skin atrophy (especially with potent preparations), HPA axis suppression (especially with potent preparations)<br><br>Pharmacokinetics:<br>Systemic absorption through the skin depends on intrinsic properties of the drug itself, the vehicle used, the duration of exposure, and the surface area and condition of the skin involved; occlusive dressings greatly enhance skin penetration and drug absorption. | Contraindications:<br>Hypersensitivity to any component of the product; monotherapy in primary bacterial infections (i.e. impetigo)<br><br>Pregnancy Category: C<br><br>Lactation Issues:<br>Excretion in breast milk is unknown; use with caution in nursing mothers |
| **Prednicarbate**<br>Dermatop<br><br>Cream: 0.1% | See page 1453 for specific indications<br>Apply to affected area 2 to 4 times daily | Administration Issues:<br>For external use only; keep preparation away from the eyes, mouth, and mucous membranes; apply sparingly in a light film and rub in gently; do not use tight-fitting diapers or plastic pants on children treated with corticosteroids in the diaper area | ADRS:<br>Burning, itching, irritation, erythema, dryness, skin atrophy (especially with potent preparations), HPA axis suppression (especially with potent preparations)<br><br>Pharmacokinetics:<br>Systemic absorption through the | Contraindications:<br>Hypersensitivity to any component of the product; monotherapy in primary bacterial infections (i.e. impetigo)<br><br>Pregnancy Category: C<br><br>Lactation Issues:<br>Excretion in breast milk is |

| Drug | Administration Issues | ADRs / Pharmacokinetics | Contraindications / Pregnancy / Lactation |
|---|---|---|---|
| (continued from previous) | | skin depends on intrinsic properties of the drug itself, the vehicle used, the duration of exposure, and the surface area and condition of the skin involved; occlusive dressings greatly enhance skin penetration and drug absorption. | unknown; use with caution in nursing mothers |
| **Triamcinolone Acetonide**<br><br>Ointment:<br>(0.025%, 0.1%, 0.5%)<br>Kenalog, Flutex, Aristocort, generics<br><br>Cream: (0.025%, 0.1%, 0.5%)<br>Kenalog, generics<br><br>Lotion: (0.025%, 0.1%)<br>Kenalog, generics<br><br>Aerosol: Kenalog | <u>See page 1453 for specific indications</u><br>Apply to affected area 2 to 4 times daily<br><br><u>Administration Issues:</u><br>For external use only; keep preparation away from the eyes, mouth, and mucous membranes; apply sparingly in a light film and rub in gently; shake lotion and spray preparations prior to administration; hold spray 3 to 6 inches away from affected area while in use, spray for about 2 seconds to cover an area the size of your hand; do not use tight-fitting diapers or plastic pants on children treated with corticosteroids in the diaper area | <u>ADRS:</u><br>Burning, itching, irritation, erythema, dryness, skin atrophy (especially with potent preparations), HPA axis suppression (especially with potent preparations)<br><br><u>Pharmacokinetics:</u><br>Systemic absorption through the skin depends on intrinsic properties of the drug itself, the vehicle used, the duration of exposure, and the surface area and condition of the skin involved; occlusive dressings greatly enhance skin penetration and drug absorption. In some cases, generic "equivalents" have less vasoconstrictive activity compared to the name brand medication | <u>Contraindications:</u><br>Hypersensitivity to any component of the product; monotherapy in primary bacterial infections (i.e. impetigo)<br><br><u>Pregnancy Category:</u> C<br><br><u>Lactation Issues:</u><br>Excretion in breast milk is unknown; use with caution in nursing mothers |

# 808. Corticosteroid Combinations

**Warnings about topical steroid products:** Topical corticosteroids have a repository effect; with continuous use, 1 to 2 applications per day may be as effective as 3 or more applications. Short term or intermittent therapy with high potency agents (i.e. every other day, 3 to 4 consecutive days per week) may be more effective and cause fewer adverse effects than continuous regimens using lower potency products. After long-term use or after using a potent agent, in order to prevent a rebound effect, switch to a less potent agent or alternative use of topical corticosteroids and emollient products. Treatment with very high potency topical corticosteroids should not exceed 2 consecutive weeks

| Drug and Dosage Forms | Usual Dosage Range | Administration Issues | Adverse Drug Reactions (ADRs) and Pharmacokinetics | Contraindications, Pregnancy Category, and Lactation Issues |
|---|---|---|---|---|
| **Hydrocortisone-Clioquinol**<br><br>Ointment:<br>1% hydrocortisone<br>3% clioquinol<br><br>Cream:<br>0.5% hydrocortisone<br>3% clioquinol | **Relief of inflammation associated with contact dermatitis, poison ivy, poison sumac, poison oak, eczema, insect bites, sunburn, and second-degree localized burns; adjunctive therapy in the treatment of psoriasis, seborrheic dermatitis, severe diaper rash, and chronic discoid lupus erythematosus**<br>Apply to affected area 2 to 4 times daily | Administration Issues<br>For external use only; keep preparation away from the eyes, mouth, and mucous membranes; apply sparingly and rub in gently; do not use tight-fitting diapers or plastic pants on children treated with corticosteroids in the diaper area | ADRs:<br>burning, itching, irritation, erythema, dryness<br><br>Pharmacokinetics:<br>systemic absorption through the skin depends on intrinsic properties of the drug itself, the vehicle used, the duration of exposure, and the surface area and condition of the skin involved; occlusive dressings greatly enhance skin penetration and drug absorption. In some cases, generic "equivalents" have less vasoconstrictive activity compared to the name brand medication | Contraindications:<br>Hypersensitivity to any component of the product; monotherapy in primary bacterial infections (i.e. impetigo)<br><br>Pregnancy Category:  C<br><br>Lactation Issues<br>Excretion in breast milk is unknown; use with caution in nursing mothers |
| **Hydrocortisone-Pramoxine**<br><br>Ointment:<br>1% hydrocortisone/<br>1% pramoxine<br>2.5% hydrocortisone/<br>1% pramoxine | See above for specific indications<br>Apply to affected area 2 to 4 times daily | Administration Issues:<br>For external use only; keep preparation away from the eyes, mouth, and mucous membranes; apply sparingly and rub in gently; shake lotion and spray preparations prior to administration; do not use tight-fitting diapers or plastic pants on | ADRs:<br>burning, itching, irritation, erythema, dryness<br><br>Pharmacokinetics:<br>systemic absorption through the skin depends on intrinsic | Contraindications<br>Hypersensitivity to any component of the product; monotherapy in primary bacterial infections (i.e. impetigo) |

| | | | |
|---|---|---|---|
| Cream:<br>1% hydrocortisone/<br>1% pramoxine<br><br>2.5% hydrocortisone/<br>2.5% pramoxine<br><br>Lotion:<br>1% hydrocortisone/<br>1% pramoxine<br><br>2.5% hydrocortisone/<br>1% pramoxine<br><br>Foam:<br>1% hydrocortisone/<br>1% pramoxine | See page 1470 for specific indications<br>Apply to affected area 2 to 4 times daily | children treated with corticosteroids in the diaper area<br><br>properties of the drug itself, the vehicle used, the duration of exposure, and the surface area and condition of the skin involved; occlusive dressings greatly enhance skin penetration and drug absorption | Pregnancy Category: C<br><br>Lactation Issues<br>Excretion in breast milk is unknown; use with caution in nursing mothers |
| **Hydrocortisone-Iodoquinol**<br>Vytone<br><br>Cream:<br>1% hydrocortisone/<br>1% iodoquinol | Administration Issues:<br>For external use only; keep preparation away from the eyes, mouth, and mucous membranes; apply sparingly and rub in gently; do not use tight-fitting diapers or plastic pants on children treated with corticosteroids in the diaper area | ADRs:<br>burning, itching, irritation, erythema, dryness<br><br>Pharmacokinetics:<br>systemic absorption through the skin depends on intrinsic properties of the drug itself, the vehicle used, the duration of exposure, and the surface area and condition of the skin involved; occlusive dressings greatly enhance skin penetration and drug absorption | Contraindications<br>Hypersensitivity to any component of the product; monotherapy in primary bacterial infections (i.e. impetigo)<br><br>Pregnancy Category: C<br><br>Lactation Issues<br>Excretion in breast milk is unknown; use with caution |

(continues on next page)

**808. Corticosteroid Combinations** *continued from previous page*

| Drug and Dosage Forms | Usual Dosage Range | Administration Issues | Adverse Drug Reactions (ADRs) and Pharmacokinetics | Contraindications, Pregnancy Category, and Lactation Issues |
|---|---|---|---|---|
| **Corticosteroid-Neomycin Combinations**<br><br>Ointment:<br>0.5% hydrocortisone/<br>0.5% neomycin<br>1% hydrocortisone/<br>0.5% neomycin<br><br>1% hydrocortisone/<br>0.5% neomycin/400 units<br>bacitracin zinc/gm<br>5000 units polymyxin B<br>sulfate/gm<br><br>Cream:<br>1% hydrocortisone/<br>0.5% neomycin<br><br>0.025% fluocinolone/<br>0.5% neomycin<br><br>0.1% dexamethasone/<br>0.5% neomycin<br><br>0.5% hydrocortisone/<br>0.5% neomycin/10,000 units<br>polymyxin B sulfate/gm | See page 1470 for specific indications<br>Apply to affected area 2 to 4 times daily | Administration Issues:<br>For external use only; keep preparation away from the eyes, mouth, and mucous membranes; apply sparingly and rub in gently; do not use tight-fitting diapers or plastic pants on children treated with corticosteroids in the diaper area | ADRs:<br>burning, itching, irritation, erythema, dryness<br><br>Pharmacokinetics:<br>systemic absorption through the skin depends on intrinsic properties of the drug itself, the vehicle used, the duration of exposure, and the surface area and condition of the skin involved; occlusive dressings greatly enhance skin penetration and drug absorption<br>In some cases, generic "equivalents" have less vasoconstrictive activity compared to the name brand medication | Contraindications:<br>Hypersensitivity to any component of the product; monotherapy in primary bacterial infections (i.e. impetigo)<br><br>Pregnancy Category:  C<br><br>Lactation Issues<br>Excretion in breast milk is unknown; use with caution in nursing mothers |

## Corticosteroid-Antifungal Combinations

**Ointment:**
Mycolog-II, various generics
0.1% triamcinolone acetonide
100,000 units nystatin/gm

**Cream:**
Mycolog-II, various generics
0.1% triamcinolone acetonide
100,000 units nystatin/gm

Lotrisone
0.05% betamethasone
dipropionate
1% clotrimazole

Fungoid-HC
0.5% hydrocortisone/triacetin

---

<u>See page 1470 for specific indications</u>
Apply to affected area 2 to 4 times daily

---

<u>Administration Issues:</u>
For external use only; keep preparation away from the eyes, mouth, and mucous membranes; apply sparingly and rub in gently; do not use tight-fitting diapers or plastic pants on children treated with corticosteroids in the diaper area

---

<u>ADRs:</u>
burning, itching, irritation, erythema, dryness

<u>Pharmacokinetics:</u>
systemic absorption through the skin depends on intrinsic properties of the drug itself, the vehicle used, the duration of exposure, and the surface area and condition of the skin involved; occlusive dressings greatly enhance skin penetration and drug absorption
In some cases, generic "equivalents" have less vasoconstrictive activity compared to the name brand medication

---

<u>Contraindications</u>
Hypersensitivity to any component of the product; monotherapy in primary bacterial infections (i.e. impetigo)

<u>Pregnancy Category:</u>  C

<u>Lactation Issues</u>
Excretion in breast milk is unknown; use with caution in nursing mothers

## 809. Miscellaneous Topical Products

| Drug and Dosage Forms | Usual Dosage Range | Administration Issues | Common Adverse Drug Reactions (ADRs) | Contraindications, Pregnancy Category, and Lactation Issues |
|---|---|---|---|---|
| **Aluminum Acetate Solution**<br><br>Solution:<br>Burow's Solution<br>480 ml<br><br>Tablet:<br>Domeboro Tablets<br>1 tablet in 1 pint of water<br>= 1:40 Burow's solution<br><br>Powder:<br>Domeboro Powder, Boropak Powder, Bluboro Powder<br>1 packet in 1 pint of water<br>= 1:40 Burow's solution | Astringent used for the relief of inflammation of the skin associated with insect bites, poison ivy, allergic reactions, and athlete's foot<br><br>Apply to affected area every 15 to 30 minutes for 4 to 8 hours<br><br>Do not use for > 7 days, if symptoms persists, seek medical attention | Administration Issues:<br>For external use only; keep preparation away from the eyes, mouth, and mucous membranes; apply as a wet dressing with a gauze pad saturated with solution<br><br>Drug Interactions:<br>Aluminum acetate solution may inhibit the effect of **collagenase;** remove aluminum acetate solution with repeated washings or normal saline before applying the enzyme ointment | ADRs:<br>irritation | |
| **Silver Sulfadiazine**<br>Silvadene, Thermazene, SSD Cream<br><br>Cream: 10 mg/g in a water miscible base | **Adjunct for prevention and treatment of sepsis in second and third degree burns**<br><br>Apply under sterile conditions once or twice daily to a thickness of approximately 1/16 inch to the clean and debrided wound. | Administration Issues:<br>For external use only. Re-apply immediately after hydrotherapy.<br><br>Drug Interactions:<br>Silver sulfadiazine may inactivate topical proteolytic enzymes. | ADRs:<br>Leukopenia, skin necrosis, erythema multiforme, skin discoloration, rashes<br><br>**Up to 10% of sulfadiazine may be absorbed. Use in patients with G-6-PD deficiency may be hazardous.** | Contraindications:<br>hypersensitivity, pregnant women at or near term, premature infants, infants <2 months<br><br>Pregnancy Category: B<br><br>Lactation Issues:<br>Sulfonamide derivatives can cause kernicterus; take into account risk to infant versus benefit to nursing mother |

## Sunscreens

Many products on market as lotions, creams and gels with the following SPFs: 2, 4, 6, 8, 10, 15, 16, 17, 18, 25, 29, 30, 40, 45, 46

<u>Waterproof formulas:</u>
maintain sunburn protection after being in the water up to 80 minutes

<u>Water resistant formulas:</u>
maintain sunburn protection after being in the water up to 40 minutes

<u>Sweat resistant formulas:</u>
maintain protection after ≤ 30 minutes of continuous heavy perspiration

<u>Lip Balm:</u>
SPFs 10, 15, 30, 45+

---

**Sunburn prevention**
Apply liberally to all exposed areas

**Do not use on infants < 6 months. Do not use SPFs as low as 2 or 3 on children < 2 years of age.**

**Any benefits that might be derived from using sunscreen with SPFs > 30 are negligible; an SPF of at least 15 for most individuals is recommended by the Skin Cancer Foundation**

---

<u>Administration Issues:</u>
Apply at least 30 minutes prior to sun exposure to allow penetration and binding to the skin; reapply after swimming or excessive sweating; for external use only; keep preparation away from the eyes, mouth, angles of nose, and mucous membranes; wash hands thoroughly after application; PABA containing sunscreens may cause permanent staining of clothes; wear protective eye coverings or sunglasses

---

<u>ADRs:</u>
contact dermatitis in PABA allergic patients

---

<u>Precautions</u>
Patients hypersensitive to PABA or its derivatives should avoid sunscreens containing PABA

# 900. URINARY TRACT PRODUCTS
## 901. Antispasmodics

| Drug and Dosage Forms | Usual Dosage Range | Administration Issues and Drug–Drug Interactions | Common Adverse Drug Reactions (ADRs) | Contraindications, Pregnancy Category, and Lactation Issues |
|---|---|---|---|---|
| **Flavoxate**<br>Uripas<br><br>Tablet:<br>100 mg | **Symptomatic relief of dysuria, urgency, frequency, and incontinence**<br><br>100 mg–200 mg 3 to 4 times daily; reduce dose when symptoms improve | Administration Issues:<br>Flavoxate may be given without regards to meals. Safety and efficacy in children <12 years has not been established | ADRs:<br>Nausea, vomiting, dry mouth, headache, drowsiness, blurred vision, vertigo | Contraindications:<br>Obstructive uropathies of the lower urinary tract<br><br>Pregnancy Category: C<br><br>Lactation Issues:<br>Excretion in breast milk is unknown; use with caution in nursing mothers |
| **Oxybutynin**<br>Ditropan, various generics<br><br>Tablet:<br>5 mg<br><br>Syrup:<br>5 mg/5 ml | **The relief of bladder instability symptoms (urgency, frequency, urinary leakage, urge incontinence, and dysuria) associated with voiding in patients with un-inhibited and reflex neurogenic bladder, treatment of primary nocturnal enuresis in children**<br><br>**Adults:** 5 mg 2 to 3 times daily; maximum dose is 20 mg daily<br><br>**Children > 5 years:** 5 mg bid; maximum dose is 15 mg daily<br><br>**Stress Urinary Incontinence**<br>2.5 to 5 mg tid | Administration Issues:<br>Periodic interruptions in therapy are recommended to assess continued need for drug. Tolerance has occurred in some patients.<br><br>Drug–Drug Interactions:<br>Increased anticholinergic side effects may occur with concurrent **phenothiazine, amantadine, tricyclic antidepressant** administration | ADRs:<br>Dry mouth, drowsiness, blurred vision, urinary hesitancy and retention, decreased GI motility | Contraindications:<br>Angle-closure glaucoma, myasthenia gravis, partial or complete gastric obstruction, severe colitis<br><br>Pregnancy Category: C<br><br>Lactation Issues:<br>Excretion in breast milk is unknown; use with caution in nursing mothers |

## 902. Cholinergic Stimulants

| Drug and Dosage Forms | Usual Dosage Range | Administration Issues and Drug–Drug Interactions | Common Adverse Drug Reactions (ADRs) and Pharmacokinetics | Contraindications, Pregnancy Category, and Lactation Issues |
|---|---|---|---|---|
| **Bethanechol Chloride**<br>Urecholine, various generics<br><br>Tablet:<br>5 mg, 10 mg,<br>25 mg, 50 mg | **Acute postoperative and postpartum treatment of nonobstructive urinary retention and neurogenic atony of the urinary bladder**<br><br>10 mg–50 mg 3 to 4 times daily; begin with 5 mg–10 mg initially and repeat dose every hour to a maximum of 50 mg or until satisfactory response | Administration Issues:<br>Take on an empty stomach (1 h before or 2 h after meals).<br><br>Drug–Drug Interactions:<br>**Quinidine and procainamide** may antagonize the cholinergic effects of bethanechol chloride. Additive cholinergic effects may occur with concurrent **cholinesterase inhibitor** use. A decrease in the cholinergic effects of bethanechol chloride may occur with concurrent **atropine, phenothiazine, or tricyclic antidepressant** administration | ADRs:<br>Abdominal cramping, nausea, hypotension, urinary urgency<br><br>Pharmacokinetics:<br>Onset of action usually in 30–90 minutes; duration of action usually 1 hour | Contraindications:<br>Patients with hyperthyroidism, peptic ulcer disease, latent or active bronchial asthma, coronary heart disease, mechanical obstruction of the GI or urinary tract, vagotonia, epilepsy, parkinsonism, obstructive pulmonary disease, bradycardia, and atrioventricular conduction defects<br><br>Pregnancy Category: C<br><br>Lactation Issues:<br>Excretion in breast milk is unknown; evaluate risk to infant versus importance of the drug to the mother |

## 903. Urinary Analgesics

For combination anti-infective/phenazopyridine products see Table 108.

| Drug and Dosage Forms | Usual Dosage Range | Administration Issues, Drug–Drug and Drug–Lab Interactions | Common Adverse Drug Reactions (ADRs) | Contraindications, Pregnancy Category, and Lactation Issues |
|---|---|---|---|---|
| **Phenazopyridine** Azo-Standard, Pyridium, various generics <br><br> <u>Tablet:</u> Azo-Standard 95 mg <br><br> Pyridium, various generics 100 mg, 200 mg | **Symptomatic relief of pain, burning, urgency, frequency, and other discomforts of the lower urinary tract usually associated with a UTI** <br><br> **Adults:** 200 mg tid after meals <br><br> **Children:** 6–12 years, 12 mg/kg/d divided tid | <u>Administration Issues:</u> Take after meals; may cause reddish-orange discoloration of the urine and may stain fabric. Staining of contact lenses has also occurred. <br><br> **Administration should not exceed two days when given with an antibiotic for the treatment of UTI. Do not use chronically to treat undiagnosed urinary tract pain.** <br><br> <u>Drug–Lab Interactions:</u> Phenazopyridine may interfere with urinalysis based on spectrometry or color reactions | <u>ADRs:</u> Headache, rash, itching | <u>Contraindications:</u> Hypersensitivity to phenazopyridine <br><br> <u>Pregnancy Category:</u> B <br><br> <u>Lactation Issues:</u> No information is available on phenazopyridine and lactation |
| **Pyridium Plus** <br><br> <u>Tablet:</u> 150 mg phenazopyridine 0.3 mg hyoscyamine 15 mg butabarbital | **Symptomatic relief of pain, burning, urgency, frequency, and other discomforts of the lower urinary tract usually associated with a UTI** <br><br> 1 tablet qid after meals and at bedtime | <u>Administration Issues:</u> Take after meals; may cause reddish-orange discoloration of the urine and may stain fabric. Staining of contact lenses has also occurred. <br><br> <u>Drug–Lab Interactions:</u> Phenazopyridine may interfere with urinalysis based on spectrometry or color reactions | <u>ADRs:</u> Headache, rash, itching | <u>Contraindications:</u> Hypersensitivity to phenazopyridine <br><br> <u>Pregnancy Category:</u> B <br><br> <u>Lactation Issues:</u> No information is available on phenazopyridine and lactation |

# 1000. MISCELLANEOUS AGENTS
## 1001. Agents for Impotence

| Drug and Dosage Forms | Usual Dosage Range | Administration Issues and Drug–Drug Interactions | Common Adverse Drug Reactions (ADRs) and Pharmacokinetics | Contraindications, Pregnancy Category, and Lactation Issues |
|---|---|---|---|---|
| **Alprostadil (PGE₁)** <br><br> <u>Lyophilized powder for injection</u> <br> Caverject <br> 11.9 mcg, 23.2 mcg <br><br> <u>Pellet</u> <br> Muse <br> 125 mcg, 250 mcg, 500 mcg, 1000 mcg | **Erectile dysfunction due to vasculogenic, psychogenic or mixed etiology:** <br><br> **Caverject** <br> <u>Treatment initiation:</u> Under medical care, administer 2.5 mcg. Partial response: titrate by 2.5 mcg, then by 5 to 10 mcg until produce erection suitable for intercourse but not exceeding 1 hour. No response to 2.5 mcg: titrate by 5 mcg, then by 5–10 mcg as above. Pt must stay in office until complete detumescence occurs <br><br> **Erectile dysfunction due to neurogenic etiology (spinal cord injury):** Treatment initiation: Under medical care, administer 1.25 mcg. Titrate by 1.25 mcg, then by 2.5–5 mcg as above. <br><br> **MUSE:** <br> Treatment Initiation: Titrate dose under supervision of physician to lowest dose sufficient for sexual intercourse. Onset of effect is 30–60 minutes. Do not use more than two systems/24 hour period | <u>Administration Issues:</u> <br> **Caverject:** <br> Reconstitute using 1 mL of diluent (bacteriostatic or sterile water for injection preserved with benzyl alcohol). 1 mL of solution = 10 or 20 mcg depending on vial strength. Do not change dose of alprostadil established in physician's office. <br> <u>Patient Instructions:</u> <br> – do not reuse needles/syringes <br> – Chose site of injection along side of the proximal third of the penis <br> – alternate injection sites <br> – avoid visible veins <br> – cleanse injection site with alcohol <br><br> **MUSE:** <br> Do not change dose of alprostadil established in physician's office. <br><br> <u>Drug–Drug Interactions:</u> <br> **Increased risk of bleeding:** anticoagulants (warfarin or heparin). Alprostadil may decrease **cyclosporine** concentrations. <br> **Unknown effect:** other vasoactive agents (do not use in combination) | <u>ADRs:</u> <br> **Caverject:** <br> <u>Local:</u> penile pain, prolonged erection (4–6 hrs), penile fibrosis, injection site hematoma or ecchymosis. <br> Other penile disorders (local): numbness, yeast infection, irritation, sensitivity, etc <br> Priapism (>6 hrs): occurs rarely (0.4% incidence) <br> <u>Systemic Effects:</u> upper respiratory infection, headache <br><br> **MUSE:** <br> <u>Local:</u> penile pain, urethral pain, urethral bleeding <br> <u>Systemic Effects:</u> upper respiratory infection, headache, dizziness, hypotension <br><br> <u>Pharmacokinetics:</u> <br> <u>Injection into corpora cavernosa/intraurethral:</u> systemic levels not significant | <u>Contraindications:</u> <br> Hypersensitivity; conditions predisposing patients to priapism (e.g., sickle cell anemia, multiple myeloma, leukemia); anatomical deformation of the penis; penile implants; females; pediatrics; use in men in whom sexual activity is contraindicated <br><br> <u>Other Considerations:</u> <br> Treat underlying causes of sexual dysfunction before using this agent <br><br> **Do not use alprostadil if female partner is pregnant unless the couple uses a condom barrier.** |

(continues on next page)

# 1001. Agents for Impotence  *continued from previous page*

| Drug and Dosage Forms | Usual Dosage Range | Administration Issues and Drug–Drug Interactions | Common Adverse Drug Reactions (ADRs) and Pharmacokinetics | Contraindications, Pregnancy Category, and Lactation Issues |
|---|---|---|---|---|
| **Sildenafil Citrate**<br>Viagra<br><br>Tablets:<br>25 mg, 50 mg, 100 mg | **Erectile dysfunction in males:**<br>50 mg, approximately 1 hour before sexual activity. Dose may be increased to 100 mg or decreased to 25 mg, based on efficacy and tolerability<br><br>Maximum recommended dosing frequency is once daily | Administration Issues:<br>Take no more frequently than once daily, as directed. Take tablet approximately 1 hour prior to sexual activity.<br><br>Drug–Drug Interactions:<br>**Increased effects:** nitrates (increased risk of hypotensive effects due to potentiation by sildenafil) | ADRs:<br>Blurred vision, headache, flushing, dyspepsia, nasal congestion, urinary tract infection, diarrhea, dizziness, rash<br><br>Pharmacokinetics:<br>$T_{1/2} = 4$ hr | Contraindications:<br>Hypersensitivity to sildenafil, patients receiving organic nitrates in any form |
| **Yohimbine**<br>Aphrodyne, Dayto Himbin, Yocon, Yohimex, various generics<br><br>Tablets: 5.4 mg | **NO FDA APPROVED INDICATIONS**<br><br>**Unlabeled Uses: Impotence (vascular or diabetic origins):**<br>5.4 mg tid | Drug–Drug Interactions:<br>**Increased adverse effects:** antidepressants (do not use together) | CNS:<br>Antidiuresis, nervousness, irritability, tremor, increased motor activity, dizziness, headache<br><br>Cardiovascular:<br>Elevated blood pressure, increased heart rate<br><br>Overdose:<br>Tachycardia, hypertension, paresthesias, incoordination, piloerection, rhinorrhea, tremulousness | Contraindications:<br>Hypersensitivity; renal disease, pregnancy, pediatrics<br><br>High-risk patients to avoid:<br>Geriatric, psychiatric, cardio-renal patients with history of gastric or duodenal ulcer |

## 1002. Agents for Obesity

For OTC agents used for obesity see Table 703 (Decongestants)

| Drug and Dosage Forms | Usual Dosage Range | Administration Issues and Drug–Drug Interactions | Common Adverse Drug Reactions (ADRs) and Pharmacokinetics | Contraindications, Pregnancy Category, and Lactation Issues |
|---|---|---|---|---|
| **Benzphetamine (CIII)**<br>Didrex<br><br>Tablets:<br>25 mg, 50 mg | **Short-term (8–12 weeks) adjunct in a regimen of weight reduction based on caloric restriction**<br><br>Initiate dosage with 25 to 50 mg qd; increase according to response; dosage range = 25 to 50 mg qd to tid | Administration Issues:<br>Anorexiant effects are temporary, seldom lasting more than a few weeks; tolerance may occur, therefore, long-term use is not recommended. To avoid insomnia, daily dose should be taken no later than 6 h before bedtime. Abrupt termination of therapy following prolonged high doses may result in GI distress, stomach cramps, trembling, weakness, mental depression. Physical and/or psychological dependence may occur with long-term use or abuse.<br><br>Drug Interactions:<br>Amphetamine elimination may be decreased by **acetazolamide, sodium bicarbonate.** Amphetamine elimination may be increased by **ammonium chloride** and **ascorbic acid.** Blood pressure effects may be increased by **furazolidone.** Amphetamines may decrease hypotensive effects of **guanethidine, guanadrel.** Hypertensive crisis and intracranial hemorrhage may occur when combined with **MAOIs** or **selegiline. Tricyclic antidepressants** may decrease effectiveness of amphetamines. | ADRs:<br>Restlessness, insomnia, palpitations.<br><br>Pharmacokinetics:<br>Readily absorbed; duration = 4 h | Contraindications:<br>Known hypersensitivity to sympathomimetic amines, angle-closure glaucoma, advanced arteriosclerosis, angina pectoris, severe cardiovascular disease, moderate to severe hypertension, hyperthyroidism, history of drug abuse, children <12<br><br>Cautious Use In:<br>Diabetes mellitus, elderly, psychosis<br><br>Pregnancy Category: X<br><br>Lactation Issues:<br>Safety has not been established |

*(continues on next page)*

## 1002. Agents for Obesity *continued from previous page*

| Drug and Dosage Forms | Usual Dosage Range | Administration Issues and Drug–Drug Interactions | Common Adverse Drug Reactions (ADRs) and Pharmacokinetics | Contraindications, Pregnancy Category, and Lactation Issues |
|---|---|---|---|---|
| **Diethylpropion (CIV)**<br>Tenuate, generics<br><br>Tablets: 25 mg<br><br>Tablets, sustained release: 75 mg | **Short-term (8–12 weeks) adjunct in a regimen of weight reduction based on caloric restriction**<br><br>Tablets: 25 mg tid, 1 h before meals, and in midevening if needed to overcome nighttime hunger<br><br>Sustained-release tablets: 75 mg qd, in midmorning | Administration Issues:<br>Sustained-release tablets should be swallowed whole and not chewed. Anorexiant effects are temporary, seldom lasting more than a few weeks; tolerance may occur, therefore, long-term use is not recommended. Abrupt termination of therapy following prolonged high doses may result in GI distress, stomach cramps, trembling, weakness, mental depression. Physical and/or psychological dependence may occur with long-term use or abuse.<br><br>Drug Interactions:<br>Amphetamine elimination may be decreased by **acetazolamide, sodium bicarbonate**. Amphetamine elimination may be increased by **ammonium chloride** and **ascorbic acid**. Blood pressure effects may be increased by **furazolidone.** Amphetamines may decrease hypotensive effects of **guanethidine, guanadrel**. Hypertensive crisis and intracranial hemorrhage may occur when combined with **MAOIs** or **selegiline. Tricyclic antidepressants** may decrease effectiveness of amphetamines. | ADRs:<br>Restlessness, insomnia, palpitations, ECG changes, decrease in seizure threshold in epileptics<br><br>Pharmacokinetics:<br>Readily absorbed; duration = 4 h, regular release; 10–14 h sustained release | Contraindications:<br>Known hypersensitivity to sympathomimetic amines, angle-closure glaucoma, advanced arteriosclerosis, angina pectoris, severe cardiovascular disease, moderate to severe hypertension, hyperthyroidism, history of drug abuse, children <12<br><br>Cautious Use In:<br>Diabetes mellitus, elderly, psychosis, epilepsy<br><br>Pregnancy Category: B<br><br>Lactation Issues:<br>Safety has not been established |

| | Administration Issues: | ADRs: | Contraindications: |
|---|---|---|---|
| **Fenfluramine (CIV)**<br>Pondimin<br><br>Tablets:  20 mg | **Short-term (8–12 weeks) adjunct in a regimen of weight reduction based on caloric restriction**<br><br>20 mg tid before meals; may increase at weekly intervals by 20 mg/d to max of 40 mg tid; max dosage = 120 mg/d | **Administration Issues:**<br>Administer on an empty stomach. Diarrhea may occur during first week of therapy. Anorexiant effects are temporary, seldom lasting more than a few weeks; tolerance may occur, therefore, long-term use is not recommended. Abrupt termination of therapy following prolonged high doses may result in GI distress, stomach cramps, trembling, weakness, mental depression. Physical and/or psychological dependence may occur with long-term use or abuse.<br><br>**Drug Interactions:**<br>Blood pressure effects may be increased by **furazolidone.** Hypertensive crisis and intracranial hemorrhage may occur when combined with **MAOIs** or **selegiline. Alcohol and other CNS depressants** may compound depressant effects. | **ADRs:**<br>Restlessness, insomnia, palpitations, dry mouth, diarrhea<br><br>**Pharmacokinetics:**<br>Readily absorbed; duration = 4 to 6 h | **Contraindications:**<br>Known hypersensitivity to sympathomimetic amines, angle-closure glaucoma, advanced arteriosclerosis, angina pectoris, severe cardiovascular disease, severe hypertension, hyper-thyroidism, history of drug abuse, children <12<br><br>**Cautious Use In:**<br>Mental depression, hypertension, diabetes mellitus, elderly<br><br>**Pregnancy Category:**  C<br><br>**Lactation Issues:**<br>Safety has not been established |
| **Mazindol (CIV)**<br>Mazanor, Sanorex<br><br>Tablets:<br>1 mg, 2 mg | **Short-term (8–12 weeks) adjunct in a regimen of weight reduction based on caloric restriction**<br><br>Initiate therapy at 1 mg qd and adjust to response. Usual dose is 1 mg tid, 1 h before meals or 2 mg qd, 1 h before lunch. | **Administration Issues:**<br>May take with meals to avoid GI discomfort. Anorexiant effects are temporary, seldom lasting more than a few weeks; tolerance may occur, therefore, long-term use is not recommended. Abrupt termination of therapy following prolonged high doses may result in GI distress, stomach cramps, trembling, weakness, mental depression. Physical and/or psychological dependence may occur with long-term use or abuse. | **ADRs:**<br>Restlessness, insomnia, palpitations, dry mouth, constipation<br><br>**Pharmacokinetics:**<br>Readily absorbed; duration = 8–15 h | **Contraindications:**<br>Known hypersensitivity to sympathomimetic amines, angle-closure glaucoma, advanced arteriosclerosis, angina pectoris, severe cardiovascular disease, moderate to severe hypertension, hyperthyroidism, history of drug abuse, children <12<br><br>**Cautious Use In:**<br>Diabetes mellitus, elderly, psychosis |

*(continues on next page)*

| Drug and Dosage Forms | Usual Dosage Range | Administration Issues and Drug–Drug Interactions | Common Adverse Drug Reactions (ADRs) and Pharmacokinetics | Contraindications, Pregnancy Category, and Lactation Issues |
|---|---|---|---|---|
| **Mazindol (CIV)** *cont.* | | Drug Interactions:<br>Amphetamine elimination may be decreased by **acetazolamide, sodium bicarbonate.** Amphetamine elimination may be increased by **ammonium chloride** and **ascorbic acid.** Blood pressure effects may be increased by **furazolidone.** Amphetamines may decrease hypotensive effects of **guanethidine, guanadrel.** Hypertensive crisis and intracranial hemorrhage may occur when combined with **MAOIs** or **selegiline. Tricyclic antidepressants** may decrease effectiveness of amphetamines. | | Pregnancy Category: C<br><br>Lactation Issues:<br>Safety has not been established |
| **Phentermine (CIV)**<br>Fastin, Ionamin, generics<br><br>Tablets: 8 mg, 30 mg, 37.5 mg<br><br>Capsules: 15 mg, 18.75 mg, 30 mg, 37.5 mg<br><br>Capsules, resin complex: 15 mg, 30 mg | **Short-term (8–12 weeks) adjunct in a regimen of weight reduction based on caloric restriction**<br><br>Take 8 mg tid, 30 minutes before meals, or 15 to 37.5 mg as a single daily dose before breakfast or 10 to 14 hours before bedtime | Administration Issues:<br>Anorexiant effects are temporary, seldom lasting more than a few weeks; tolerance may occur, therefore, long-term use is not recommended. Abrupt termination of therapy following prolonged high doses may result in GI distress, stomach cramps, trembling, weakness, mental depression. Physical and/or psychological dependence may occur with long-term use or abuse.<br><br>Drug Interactions:<br>Amphetamine elimination may be decreased by **acetazolamide, sodium** | ADRs:<br>Restlessness, insomnia, palpitations, hypertension, confusion, constipation<br><br>Pharmacokinetics:<br>Readily absorbed | Contraindications:<br>Known hypersensitivity to sympathomimetic amines, angle-closure glaucoma, advanced arteriosclerosis, angina pectoris, severe cardiovascular disease, moderate to severe hypertension, hyperthyroidism, history of drug abuse, children <12<br><br>Cautious Use In:<br>Diabetes mellitus, elderly, psychosis |

| | | | | Pregnancy Category: C<br><br>Lactation Issues:<br>Safety has not been established |
|---|---|---|---|---|
| | | bicarbonate. Amphetamine elimination may be increased by **ammonium chloride** and **ascorbic acid.** Blood pressure effects may be increased by **furazolidone.** Amphetamines may decrease hypotensive effects of **guanethidine, guanadrel.** Hypertensive crisis and intracranial hemorrhage may occur when combined with **MAOIs** or **selegiline. Tricyclic antidepressants** may decrease effectiveness of amphetamines | | |
| **Sibutramine (CIV)**<br>Meridia<br><br><u>Capsule:</u> 5 mg, 10 mg, 15 mg | **Management of obesity, including weight loss and the management of weight loss in conjunction with a reduced calorie diet**<br><br>Initial dose is 10 mg qd. If there is inadequate weight loss, dose may be titrated after 4 weeks to a dose of 15 mg qd. | <u>Administration Issues:</u><br>May be taken with or without food. It is recommended to take sibutramine in the morning. Routine monitoring of blood pressure should be done while taking this drug.<br><br><u>Drug Interactions:</u><br>Sibutramine should not be taken concomitantly with **MAOIs.** Drugs that raise blood **pressure,** such as **phenylpropanolamine, pseudoephedrine** or **ephedrine** should be avoided while taking sibutramine. **Ketoconazole** may decrease the clearance of sibutramine. | <u>ADRs:</u><br>Headache, back pain, flu syndrome, asthenia, abdominal pain, anorexia, constipation, increased appetite, nausea, dyspepsia, arthralgia, insomnia, dizziness, rhinitis, pharyngitis, rash, dysmenorrhea, increases in blood pressure<br><br><u>Pharmacokinetics:</u><br>Extensively metabolized, readily absorbed | <u>Contraindications:</u><br>Hypersensitivity to product, patients receiving MAOIs or other appetite suppressants, patients with anorexia nervosa, CAD, CHF, arrhythmias or stroke.<br><br><u>Cautious Use In:</u><br>Narrow angle glaucoma<br><br>Pregnancy Category: C<br><br><u>Lactation Issues:</u><br>Safety has not been established |

# 1003. Agents for Nicotine Withdrawal

| Drug and Dosage Forms | Usual Dosage Range | Administration Issues and Drug–Drug Interactions | Common Adverse Drug Reactions (ADRs) and Pharmacokinetics | Contraindications, Pregnancy Category, and Lactation Issues |
|---|---|---|---|---|
| **Bupropion**<br><br>Zyban<br><br>Tablets, sustained release:<br>100 mg, 150 mg | **An aid to smoking cessation:**<br>Begin dosing at 150 mg/d qd × 3 d, followed by a dose increase for most patients to the recommended dose of 300 mg/d. Do not give doses > 300 mg/d<br><br>Combination treatment:<br>Bupropion can be given in combination with nicotine transdermal system | Administration Issues:<br>Initiate treatment while patient is still smoking since 1 wk is required to reach steady state levels. Patients should set a "target quit date" within first 2 weeks of therapy, generally in the second week. Continue treatment for 7–12 wks.<br><br>Drug Interactions:<br>**Carbamazepine** may decrease bupropion levels; **levodopa, MAO inhibitors and ritonavir** may increase bupropion levels; **do not coadminister with MAOIs** | ADRs:<br>Abdominal pain, insomnia, anxiety, dizziness, myalgia, nervousness, nausea, dry mouth, arthralgia, constipation, diarrhea, rhinitis<br><br>Pharmacokinetics:<br>Extensively metabolized;<br>$T_{1/2}$ = 21 h | Contraindications:<br>Hypersensitivity to bupropion; coadministration with a MAOI; prior diagnosis of bulimia or anorexia nervosa, seizure disorder<br><br>Pregnancy Category:  B<br><br>Lactation Issues:<br>Bupropion is secreted in breast milk; due to potential serious adverse effects on the infant, decide whether to discontinue breastfeeding or discontinue drug, taking into account the importance of the drug to the mother |
| **Nicotine Transdermal System**<br><br>Patches:<br>Habitrol<br>21 mg/d, 14 mg/d, 7 mg/d<br><br>Nicoderm<br>21 mg/d, 14 mg/d, 7 mg/d<br><br>Nicotrol<br>15 mg/d, 10 mg/d, 5 mg/d | **As an aid for smoking cessation for the relief of nicotine withdrawal symptoms. Use as part of a comprehensive behavioral smoking-cessation program**<br><br>Apply 1 patch q 24 h by the following schedule:<br>**Habitrol, Nicoderm:** 21 mg/d × 6 wk, 14 mg/d × 2 wk, 7 mg/d × 2 wk. | Administration Issues:<br>Immediately after removing patch from protective container, apply to a nonhairy, clean, dry skin site. Always remove old patch before apply next patch. Dispose of old patches in a way that makes them inaccessible to children and pets. Follow written instructions in package.<br><br>Drug–Drug Interactions:<br>A decrease in theophylline dose may be required at cessation of smoking. | ADRs:<br>Erthyema, pruritus, local edema, rash<br><br>Pharmacokinetics:<br>75–90% absorbed through the skin; duration of action = 24 h;<br>$T_{1/2}$ = 1–2 h | Contraindications:<br>Hypersensitivity to nicotine, nonsmokers, immediate post-MI patients, serious arrhythmias, severe angina, pregnancy, nursing mothers<br><br>Cautious Use:<br>Hypertensive patients, hyperthyroidism, IDDM, hepatic or renal impairment, history of esophagitis, peptic ulcer disease |

| Drug / Dosage | Administration | ADRs / Pharmacokinetics | Contraindications / Pregnancy / Lactation |
|---|---|---|---|
| ProStep<br>22 mg/d, 11 mg/d<br><br>If weight <45 kg (100 lb.), smoke < 1/2 pack/d or have cardiovascular disease: 14 mg/d × 6 wk<br>**ProStep:** 22 mg/d × 4–8 wk, 11 mg/d × 2–4 wk; if weight <45 kg (100 lb.), smoke < 1/2 pack/d or have cardiovascular disease: 11 mg/d × 4–8 wk<br><br><u>Apply 1 patch q 16 h by the following schedule</u><br>**Nicotrol:** 15 mg/d × 4–12 wk, 10 mg/d × 2–4 wk | | | <u>Pregnancy Category:</u> D<br><br><u>Lactation Issues:</u><br>Nicotine passes freely into breast milk; weight risk of exposure of the infant to nicotine against risks associated with the mother's continued smoking |
| **Nicotine Polacrilex (Nicotine Resin Complex)**<br><br><u>Chewing Gum</u><br>2 mg/square<br>4 mg/square<br><br>**As an aid for smoking cessation for the relief of nicotine withdrawal symptoms. Use as part of a comprehensive behavioral smoking-cessation program**<br><br>Chew 1 piece of gum when patient has urge to smoke; may be repeated as needed; max for 2 mg = 30 pieces/d; max for 4 mg = 20 pieces/d | <u>Administration Issues:</u><br>Patients using the 2 mg strength should not exceed 30 pieces/day; those taking 4 mg strength should not exceed 20 pieces/day.<br><br>Follow written instructions in package.<br><br><u>Drug–Drug Interactions:</u><br>May increase the metabolism of caffeine and theophylline | <u>ADRs:</u><br>Headache, dizziness, lightheadedness, jawache, nausea, indigestion, sore mouth or throat, hiccups, irritation/tingling of tongue<br><br><u>Pharmacokinetics:</u><br>Approximately 90% of nicotine is absorbed over a 15–30 min period; rate of release is controlled by vigor and duration of chewing | <u>Contraindications:</u><br>Hypersensitivity to nicotine, nonsmokers, immediate post-MI patients, serious arrhythmias, severe angina, women with childbearing potential (unless effective contraception used)<br><br><u>Cautious Use:</u><br>Hypertensive patients, hyperthyroidism, IDDM, hepatic or renal impairment, history of esophagitis, peptic ulcer disease, patients with dentures<br><br><u>Pregnancy Category:</u> X<br><br><u>Lactation Issues:</u><br>Nicotine passes freely into breast milk; weight risk of exposure of the infant to nicotine against risks associated with the mother's continued smoking |

# 1100. VITAMINS, MINERALS, AND TRACE ELEMENTS
## 1101. Fat-Soluble Vitamins

*Source: Reproduced, by permission, from Williams, S.R. Nutrition and Diet Therapy, 8th ed. (1997, p. 177). St. Louis: Mosby.*

| Vitamin | Physiologic Functions | Results of Deficiency | Requirement | Food Sources |
|---|---|---|---|---|
| **Vitamin A**<br>Provitamin: beta-carotene | Production of rhodopsin and other light-receptor pigments | Poor dark adaptation, night blindness, xerosis, xerophthalmia | Adult male: 1000 µg or RE (5000 IU) | Liver, cream, butter, whole milk, egg yolk |
| Vitamin: retinol | Formation and maintenance of epithelial tissue | Keratinization of epithelium | Adult female: 800 µg or RE (4000 IU) | Green and yellow vegetables, yellow fruits |
| | Growth | Growth failure | Pregnancy: 1000 µg or RE (5000 IU) | Fortified margarine |
| | Reproduction | Reproductive failure | Lactation: 1200 µg or RE (6000 IU) | |
| | Toxic in large amounts | | Children: 400 µg or RE (2000 IU) to 800 µg or RE (4000 IU) | |
| **Vitamin D**<br>Provitamins: ergosterol (plants); 7-dehydrocholesterol (skin) | Calcitriol a major hormone regulator of bone mineral (calcium and phosphorus) metabolism | Faulty bone growth; rickets, osteomalacia | Adult: 5–10 µg cholecalciferol (200–400 IU) | Fortified milk |
| | | | | Fortified margarine |
| Vitamins D₂ (ergocalciferol) and D₃ (cholecalciferol) | Calcium and phosphorus absorption | | Pregnancy and lactation: 10–12.5 µg (400–500 IU) depending on age | Fish oils |
| | Toxic in large amounts | | Children: 10 µg (400 IU) | Sunlight on skin |
| **Vitamin E**<br>Tocopherols | Antioxidant | Anemia in premature infants | Adult: 8–10 mg α-TE | Vegetable oils |
| | Hemopoiesis | | Pregnancy and lactation: 10–11 mg α-TE | |
| | Related to action of selenium | | Children: 3–10 mg α-TE | |

1500

| Vitamin K | | | |
|---|---|---|---|
| K$_1$ (phylloquinone)<br>K$_2$ (menaquinone)<br>Analog: K$_3$ (menadione) | Activates blood-clotting factors (for example, prothrombin) by alpha-carboxylating glutamic acid residues<br><br>Toxicity can be induced by water-soluble analogs | Hemorrhagic disease of the newborn<br><br>Defective blood clotting<br><br>Deficiency symptoms are produced by coumarin anticoagulants and by antibiotic therapy | Adult: 70–140 µg<br><br>Children: 15–100 µg<br><br>Infants: 12–20 µg | Cheese, egg yolk, liver<br><br>Green leafy vegetables<br><br>Synthesized by intestinal bacteria |

## 1102. Water-Soluble Vitamins

*Source: Reproduced, by permission, from Williams, S.R. Nutrition and Diet Therapy, 8th ed. (1997, p. 196). St. Louis: Mosby.*

| Vitamin | Coenzymes:<br>Physiologic Function | Clinical Applications | Requirement | Food Sources |
|---|---|---|---|---|
| **Thiamin** | Carbohydrate metabolism<br><br>Thiamin pyrophosphate (TPP): oxidative decarboxylation | Beriberi (deficiency)<br><br>Neuropathy<br><br>Wernicke-Korsakoff syndrome (alcoholism)<br><br>Depressed muscular and secretory symptoms | 0.5 mg/1000 kcal | Pork, beef, liver, whole or enriched grains, legumes |
| **Riboflavin** | General metabolism<br><br>Flavin adenine dinucleotide (FAD)<br><br>Flavin mononucleotide (FMN) | Cheilosis, glossitis, seborrheic dermatitis | 0.6 mg/1000 kcal | Milk, liver, enriched cereals |

*(continues on next page)*

## 1102. Water-Soluble Vitamins *continued from previous page*

| Vitamin | Coenzymes: Physiologic Function | Clinical Applications | Requirement | Food Sources |
|---|---|---|---|---|
| **Niacin (nicotinic acid, nicotinamide)** | General metabolism<br><br>Nicotinamide-adenine dinucleotide (NAD)<br><br>Nicotinamide-adenine dinucleotide phosphate (NADP) | Pellagra (deficiency)<br><br>Weakness, anorexia<br><br>Scaly dermatitis<br><br>Neuritis | 6.6 NE/1000 kcal* | Meat, peanuts, enriched grains (protein foods containing tryptophan) |
| **Vitamin B₆ (pyridoxine, pyridoxal, pyridoxamine)** | General metabolism<br><br>Pyridoxal phosphate (PLP): transamination and decarboxylation | Reduced serum levels associated with pregnancy and use of oral contraceptives<br><br>Antagonized by isoniazid, penicillamine, and other drugs | 2 mg (men)<br><br>1.6 mg (women) | Wheat, corn, meats, liver |
| **Pantothenic acid** | General metabolism<br><br>CoA (coenzyme A): acetylation | Many roles through acyltransfer reactions (for example, lipogenesis, amino acid activation, and formation of cholesterol, steroid hormones, heme) | 4 to 7 mg | Liver, egg, milk |
| **Biotin** | General metabolism<br><br>N-Carboxybiotinyl lysine: $CO_2$ transfer reactions | Deficiency induced by avidin (a protein in raw egg white) and by antibiotics<br><br>Synthesis of some fatty acids and amino acids | 30 to 100 μg | Egg yolk, liver<br><br>Synthesized by intestinal microorganisms |
| **Folate (folic acid, folacin)** | General metabolism<br><br>Single-carbon transfer reactions (for example, purine nucleotide, thymine, heme synthesis) | Megaloblastic anemia | 200 μg (men)<br><br>180 μg (women) | Liver, green leafy vegetables |

*NE = niacin equivalents.

| | Functions | Deficiency/Conditions | RDA | Sources |
|---|---|---|---|---|
| **Cobalamin** | General metabolism<br><br>Methylcobalamin: methylation reactions (for example, synthesis of amino acids, heme) | Pernicious anemia induced by lack of intrinsic factor<br><br>Megaloblastic anemia<br><br>Methylmalonic aciduria<br><br>Homocystinuria<br><br>Peripheral neuropathy (strict vegetarian diet) | 2 $\mu$g | Liver, meat, milk, egg, cheese |
| **Vitamin C (ascorbic acid)** | Antioxidant<br><br>Collagen biosynthesis<br><br>General metabolism<br><br>Makes iron available for hemoglobin synthesis<br><br>Influences conversion of folic acid to folinic acid<br><br>Oxidation-reduction of the amino acids phenylalanine and tyrosine | Scurvy (deficiency)<br><br>Wound healing, tissue formation<br><br>Fevers and infections<br><br>Stress reactions<br><br>Growth | 60 mg | Fresh fruits, especially citrus<br><br>Vegetables such as tomatoes, cabbage, potatoes, chili peppers, and broccoli |

## 1103. Major Minerals

Source: *Reproduced, by permission, from Williams, S.R. Nutrition and Diet Therapy, 8th ed. (1997, p. 223). St. Louis: Mosby.*

| Mineral | Metabolism | Physiologic Functions | Clinical Applications | Requirements | Food Sources |
|---|---|---|---|---|---|
| **Calcium (Ca)** | Absorption according to body need; requires Ca-binding protein and regulated by vitamin D, parathyroid hormone, and calcitonin; absorption favored by protein, lactose, acidity<br><br>Excretion chiefly in feces; 70%–90% of amount ingested<br><br>Deposition-mobilization in bone tissue constant, regulated by vitamin D and parathyroid hormone | Constituent of bones and teeth<br><br>Participates in blood clotting, nerve transmission, muscle action, cell membrane permeability, enzyme activation | Tetany (decrease in serum Ca)<br><br>Rickets, osteomalacia<br><br>Osteoporosis<br><br>Resorptive hypercalciuria, renal calculuses<br><br>Hyperthyroidism and hypothyroidism | Adults: 800 mg (Premenopause: 1000 mg; Menopause: 1500 mg)<br><br>Pregnancy and lactation: 1200 mg<br><br>Infants: 400–600 mg<br><br>Children: 800–1200 mg | Milk, cheese<br><br>Green, leafy vegetables<br><br>Whole grains<br><br>Egg yolk<br><br>Legumes, nuts |
| **Phosphorus (P)** | Absorption with Ca aided by vitamin D and parathyroid hormone as for calcium; hindered by binding agents<br><br>Excretion chiefly by kidney according to serum level, regulated by parathyroid hormone<br><br>Deposition-mobilization in bone compartment constant | Constituent of bones and teeth, ATP, phosphorylated intermediary metabolites<br><br>Participates in absorption of glucose and glycerol, transport of fatty acids, energy metabolism, and buffer system | Growth<br><br>Recovery from diabetic acidosis<br><br>Hypophosphatemia: bone disease, malabsorption syndromes, primary hyperparathyroidism<br><br>Hyperphosphatemia: renal insufficiency, hypothyroidism, tetany | Adults: 800 mg<br><br>Pregnancy and lactation: 1200 mg<br><br>Infants: 300–500 mg<br><br>Children: 800–1200 mg | Milk, cheese<br><br>Meat, egg yolk<br><br>Whole grains<br><br>Legumes, nuts |

| Mineral | Absorption and excretion | Physiologic functions | Clinical applications | Requirements | Food sources |
|---|---|---|---|---|---|
| **Magnesium (Mg)** | Absorption according to intake load; hindered by excess fat, phosphate, calcium, protein<br><br>Excretion (regulated by kidney) | Constituent of bones and teeth<br><br>Coenzyme in general metabolism, smooth muscle action, neuromuscular irritability<br><br>Cation in intracellular fluid | Low serum level following gastrointestinal losses<br><br>Tremor, spasm in deficiency induced by malnutrition, alcoholism | Adults: 280–350 mg<br><br>Pregnancy and lactation: 290–355 mg<br><br>Infants: 40–60 mg<br><br>Children: 80–170 mg | Milk, cheese<br><br>Meat, seafood<br><br>Whole grains<br><br>Legumes, nuts |
| **Sodium (Na)** | Readily absorbed<br><br>Excretion chiefly by kidney, controlled by aldosterone | Major cation in extracellular fluid, water balance, acid-base balance<br><br>Cell membrane permeability, absorption of glucose<br><br>Normal muscle irritability | Losses in gastrointestinal disorders, diarrhea<br><br>Fluid-electrolyte and acid-base balance problems<br><br>Muscle action | Adults 500 mg<br><br>Infants: 120–200 mg<br><br>Children: 225–500 mg | Salt (NaCl)<br><br>Sodium compounds in baking and processing<br><br>Milk, cheese<br><br>Meat, eggs<br><br>Carrots, beets, spinach, celery |
| **Potassium (K)** | Readily absorbed<br><br>Secreted and resorbed in gastrointestinal circulation<br><br>Excretion chiefly by kidney, regulated by aldosterone | Major cation in intracellular fluid, water balance, acid-base balance<br><br>Normal muscle irritability<br><br>Glycogen formation<br><br>Protein synthesis | Losses in gastrointestinal disorders, diarrhea<br><br>Fluid-electrolyte, acid-base balance problems<br><br>Muscle action, especially heart action<br><br>Losses in tissue catabolism<br><br>Treatment of diabetic acidosis; rapid glycogen production reduces serum potassium level<br><br>Losses with diuretic therapy | Adults: 2000 mg<br><br>Infants: 500–700 mg<br><br>Children: 1000–2000 mg | Fruits<br><br>Vegetables<br><br>Legumes, nuts<br><br>Whole grains<br><br>Meat |

(continues on next page)

## 1103. Major Minerals  *continued from previous page*

| Mineral | Metabolism | Physiologic Functions | Clinical Applications | Requirements | Food Sources |
|---|---|---|---|---|---|
| **Chlorine (Cl)** | Readily absorbed<br><br>Excretion controlled by kidney | Major anion in extracellular fluid, water balance, acid-base balance, chloride-bicarbonate shift<br><br>Gastric hydrochloride—digestion | Losses in gastrointestinal disorders, vomiting, diarrhea, tube drainage<br><br>Hypochloremic alkalosis | Adults: 750 mg<br><br>Infants: 180–300 mg<br><br>Children: 350–750 mg | Salt (NaCl) |
| **Sulfur (S)** | Elemental form absorbed as such; split from amino acid sources (methionine and cystine) in digestion and absorbed into portal circulation<br><br>Excreted by kidney in relation to protein intake and tissue catabolism | Essential constituent of protein structure<br><br>Enzyme activity and energy metabolism through free sulfhydryl group (—SH)<br><br>Detoxification reactions | Cystine renal calculuses<br><br>Cystinuria | Diet adequate in protein contains adequate sulfur | Meat, eggs<br><br>Milk, cheese<br><br>Legumes, nuts |

## 1104. Trace Elements

Source: Reproduced, by permission, from Williams, S.R. Nutrition and Diet Therapy, 8th ed. (1997, p. 226). St. Louis: Mosby.

| Mineral | Metabolism | Physiologic Functions | Clinical Applications | Requirements | Food Sources |
|---|---|---|---|---|---|
| Iron (Fe) | Absorption controls bioavailability; favored by body need, acidity, and reduction agents such as vitamins; hindered by binding agents, reduced gastric HCl, infection, gastrointestinal losses<br><br>Transported as transferrin, stored as ferritin or hemosiderin<br><br>Excreted in sloughed cells, bleeding | Hemoglobin synthesis, oxygen transport<br><br>Cell oxidation, heme enzymes | Anemia (hypochromic, microcytic)<br><br>Excess: hemosiderosis, hemochromatosis<br><br>Growth and pregnancy needs | Adults: men—10 mg, women—15 mg<br><br>Pregnancy and lactation: 30 and 15 mg, respectively<br><br>Infants: 6–10 mg<br><br>Children: 10–12 mg | Liver, meat, eggs<br><br>Whole grains<br><br>Enriched breads and cereals<br><br>Dark green vegetables<br><br>Legumes, nuts<br><br>(Iron cookware) |
| Iodine (I) | Absorbed as iodides, taken up by thyroid gland under control of thyroid-stimulating hormone<br><br>Excretion by kidney | Synthesis of thyroxin, which regulates cell metabolism, basal metabolic rate | Endemic colloid goiter, cretinism<br><br>Hypothyroidism and hyperthyroidism | Adults: 150 µg<br><br>Infants: 40–50 µg<br><br>Children: 70–150 µg | Iodized salt<br><br>Seafood |
| Zinc (Zn) | Absorbed with zinc-binding ligand from pancreas<br><br>Transported in blood by albumin; stored in many sites<br><br>Excretion largely intestinal | Essential coenzyme constituent: carbonic anhydrase, carboxypeptidase, lactic dehydrogenase | Growth: hypogonadism<br><br>Sensory impairment: taste and smell<br><br>Wound healing<br><br>Malabsorption disease | Adults: 12–15 mg<br><br>Infants: 5 mg<br><br>Children: 10–15 mg | Widely distributed<br><br>Seafood, oysters<br><br>Liver, meat<br><br>Milk, cheese, eggs<br><br>Whole grains |

(continues on next page)

## 1104. Trace Elements continued from previous page

| Mineral | Metabolism | Physiologic Functions | Clinical Applications | Requirements | Food Sources |
|---|---|---|---|---|---|
| **Copper (Cu)** | Absorbed with copper-binding protein metallothionein<br><br>Transported in blood by histidine and albumin<br><br>Stored in many tissues | Associated with iron in enzyme systems, hemoglobin synthesis<br><br>Metalloprotein enzyme constituent | Hypocupremia: nephrosis and malabsorption<br><br>Wilson's disease, excess copper storage<br><br>Menke's syndrome, kinky hair, disordered copper metabolism | Adults: 1.5–3 mg<br><br>Infants: 0.4–0.7 mg<br><br>Children: 0.7–2.5 mg | Widely distributed<br><br>Liver, meat<br><br>Seafood<br><br>Whole grains<br><br>Legumes, nuts<br><br>(Copper cookware) |
| **Manganese (Mn)** | Absorbed poorly<br><br>Excretion mainly by intestine | Enzyme component in general metabolism | Low serum levels in diabetes, protein-energy malnutrition<br><br>Inhalation toxicity | Adults: 2–5 mg<br><br>Infants: 0.3–1.0 mg<br><br>Children: 1–5 mg | Cereals, whole grains<br><br>Legumes, soybeans<br><br>Leafy vegetables |
| **Chromium (Cr)** | Absorbed in association with zinc<br><br>Excretion mainly by kidney | Associated with glucose metabolism; improves faulty glucose uptake by tissues; glucose tolerance factor | Potentiates action of insulin in persons with diabetes<br><br>Lowers serum cholesterol, LDL-cholesterol*<br><br>Increases HDL* | Adults: 50–200 μg<br><br>Infants: 10–60 μg<br><br>Children: 20–200 μg | Cereals<br><br>Whole grains<br><br>Brewer's yeast<br><br>Animal protein |
| **Cobalt (Co)** | Absorbed as component of food source, vitamin $B_{12}$<br><br>Elemental form shares transport with iron<br><br>Stored in liver | Constituent of vitamin $B_{12}$, functions with vitamin | Deficiency associated only with deficiency of vitamin $B_{12}$ | Unknown; evidently minute | Vitamin $B_{12}$ source |

| Mineral | Absorption/Excretion | Functions | Deficiency/Toxicity | Requirements | Food Sources |
|---|---|---|---|---|---|
| **Selenium (Se)** | Absorption depends on solubility of compound form<br><br>Excreted mainly by kidney | Constituent of enzyme glutathione peroxidase<br><br>Synergistic antioxidant with vitamin E<br><br>Structural component of teeth | Marginal deficiency when soil content is low<br><br>Deficiency secondary to parenteral nutrition; malnutrition<br><br>Toxicity observed in livestock | Adults: 55–70 μg<br><br>Infants: 10–15 μg<br><br>Children: 20–50 μg | Varies with soil content<br><br>Seafood<br><br>Legumes<br><br>Whole grains<br><br>Low-fat meats and dairy products<br><br>Vegetables |
| **Molybdenum (Mo)** | Readily absorbed<br><br>Excreted rapidly by kidney<br><br>Small amount excreted in bile | Constituent of oxidase enzymes, xanthine oxidase | Deficiency unknown in humans | Adults: 75–250 μg<br><br>Infants: 15–30 μg<br><br>Children: 25–250 μg | Legumes<br><br>Whole grains<br><br>Milk<br><br>Organ meats<br><br>Leafy vegetables |
| **Fluoride (F)** | Absorption in small intestine; little known of bioavailability<br><br>Excreted by kidney—80% | Accumulates in bones and teeth, increasing hardness | Dental caries inhibited<br><br>Osteoporosis: may help control<br><br>Excess: dental fluorosis | Adults: 1.5–4 mg<br><br>Infants: 0.1–0.5 mg<br><br>Children: 0.5–2.5 mg | Fish<br><br>Fish products<br><br>Tea<br><br>Foods cooked in fluoridated water<br><br>Drinking water |

*LDL = low density lipoprotein; HDL = high-density lipoprotein.

# BIBLIOGRAPHY

American Hospital Formulary Service (AHFS). (1997). *Drug Information '97*. Bethesda, MD: American Society of Hospital Pharmacists.

Briggs, G. G., Freeman, R. K., Yaffe, S. J. (1994). *Drugs in Pregnancy and Lactation* (4th ed.). Baltimore: Williams and Wilkins.

*Drug Facts and Comparisons*. (1998). St. Louis: Facts and Comparisons.

Gelman, C. R., Rumack, B. H. (Eds.). (1998). *DrugDex Information System*. Denver: Micromedex.

Lacy, C., Armstrong, L. L., Ingrim, N. B., Lance, L. L., (Eds.). (1997–98). *Drug Information Handbook* (5th ed.). Hudson, OH: Lexi-Comp.

*Physician's Desk Reference* (51st ed.). (1997). Oradell, NJ: Medical Economics Co.

Shannon, M. T., Wilson, B. A., Stang, C. L. (Eds.). (1998). *Appleton & Lange's 1998 Drug Guide*. Stamford, CT: Appleton & Lange.

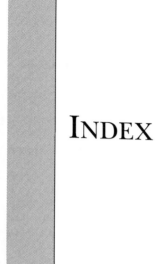

# INDEX

Note: Page references in boldface denote drug table entries. Page numbers followed by *f* or *t* indicate figures or tables, respectively.

A

**A-200, 1452**
**AA (Alcoholics Anonymous),** 787
**AA-HC, 1284–1285**
**Abortifacient,** 131*t*
**Absorption**
  adolescent, 183*t*, 185
  aging and, 199, 200*t*
  alterations, 17–18
  bioavailability and, 19, 19*f*
  children, 183*t*, 185
  completeness/extent, 16–17
  concentration gradient and, 17
  defined, 16
  in hepatic failure, 50
  intants/neonates, 182–184, 183*t*, 184
  interactions
    drug-drug, 18–19
    drug-nutrient, 107*t*–108*t*
  during pregnancy, 240, 240*t*
  presystemic metabolism and, 17, 18*f*
  rate
    contact time and, 17
    surface area and, 16
  in renal impairment, 50–51
**Acarbose, 1357**
  adverse events, 717
  for diabetes mellitus, 716–717
**Accidental poisonings, in elderly,** 202
**Accolate,** 1425

**Accupril,** 1052–1053
**Accutane,** 1429–1430
**Acebutolol,** 277*t*, **1060**
**ACE inhibitors.** *See* **Angiotensin converting enzyme inhibitors**
**Acephen.** *See* **Acetaminophen**
**Acetaminophen, 1088–1089**
  apparent volume of distribution, 23*t*
  for chronic pain, 230
  clearance, 29*t*
  combinations
    antacids, **1115**
    aspirin/caffeine, **1113**
    butalbital, **1119–1120**
    caffeine, **1114**
    caffeine/butalbital, **1119**
    codeine, **1100**
    codeine/caffeine/butalbital, **1102**
    dihydrocodeine/caffeine, **1106**
    dipenhydramine, **1183–1184**
    hydrocodone, **1104**
    magnesium/salicylate/pamabrom, **1114**
    oxycodone, **1108–1109**
    pamabrom, **1115**
    propoxyphene, **1111**
  metabolites, 23
  pediatric dosages, 190*t*
**Acetasol, 1280**
**Acetasol HC, 1280**
**Acetazolamide,** 29*t*, **1075, 1153**

**Acetic acid**
combinations
aluminum acetate, **1280**
burrow's solution/boric acid/propylene glycol, **1280–1281**
propylene glycol, 492
propylene glycol diacetate/benzethonium chloride/sodium acetate, **1280**
nonsteroidal anti-inflammatory agents, **1127–1131**
**Acetic Acid Otic, 1280**
**Acetoacetate, creatinine serum levels and,** 49t
**Acetophenazine, 1203**
**Acetylation,** 24
**Acetylcarbromal, 1178–1179**
**Acetylsalicylic acid.** See **Aspirin**
**Achromycin.** See **Tetracycline**
**Achromycin V.** See **Tetracycline**
**α-₁Acid glycoprotein,** 53
**Acid reducer ingredients, with OTC status,** 120t, 121t
**Acids,** 13, 14f
**Acitretin, 1430**
**Aclovate, 1453–1454**
**Acne**
neonatal, 576
from oral contraceptive usage, 272t
topical preparations, **1427–1429**
vulgaris
nonpharmacologic therapy, 577
pharmacotherapy, 576, 577–579
types, 576
**Acne lotion 10, 1435–1436**
**Acquired immunodeficiency syndrome.** See **HIV/AIDS**
**ACTH (adrenocorticotropic hormone),** 553
**Actidil, 1418**
**Actigall, 1305**
**Action potential,** 329
**Action potential duration (APD),** 329
**Activated charcoal,** 516
**Active immunity,** 151
**Actron,** 121t, **1124**
**Acular, 1129, 1274–1275**
**Acute otitis media (AOM),** 485, 487
**Acutrim.** See **Phenylpropanolamine**
**Acyclovir, 1002–1003, 1438**
for herpes genitalis, 873, 874, 874t
for infectious mononucleosis, 919
for varicella, 159, 583–584
**ADA (Americans with Disabilities Act),** 205
**Adalat.** See **Nifedipine**
**Adapin.** See **Doxepin**
**Adaptogen,** 131t
**Adenomyosis**
assessment/history taking, 854

nonpharmacologic therapy, 854
pharmacotherapy, 854–856
sites, 853–854
**AD/HD.** See **Attention deficit/hyperactivity disorder**
**Adherence (compliance)**
elderly and, 61, 201
family factors in, 74
health outcome and, 65–66
oral contraceptive, 276, 278–279, 278t
with pharmacotherapeutic regimen, 60–61
suboptimal, 60
**Adjuvant therapies, for burn injuries,** 597
**Administration, drug**
developmental stages and, neonate, 185–186
route, absorption and, 17
**Adolescents**
absorption, 183t, 185
administration of drugs and, 187
depression in, 748
**Adrenal cortex**
function, normal, 694–695
glucocorticoids, **1327–1333**
hyperfunction
aldosteronism, 699
Cushing's syndrome. See **Cushing's syndrome**
hirsuitism, 699, 700t
pharmacotherapy, 699–704, 702t
virilization, 699
hypofunction or insufficiency
Addison's disease, 696, 701t
hypoaldosteronism, 696–697
insufficiency, 696f
pharmacotherapy, 699, 700, 701–703
primary vs. secondary, 695, 697t
signs/symptoms, 697t
symptoms, 696
mineralocorticoids, **1334**
normal function, 694–695, 695f
**Adrenalin.** See **Epinephrine**
**Adrenergic receptors,** 35
**Adrenocorticotropic hormone (ACTH),** 553
**Adsorbocarpine, 1263**
**Adverse events, drug associated**
classification, 41, 41f, 98–99
defined, 97–98
in elderly, 201
evaluation, 98
predictable, 98
prevention, 104
reporting, 99, 100f–103f, 101
serious, 99, 101
unpredictable, 98–99
vaccine-related, reporting, 174
**Advertising, for over-the-counter drugs,** 113, 123

**Advil.** *See* **Ibuprofen**
**AeroBid.** *See* **Flunisolide**
**Aeroseb-Dex.** *See* **Dexamethasone**
**Affective disorders**
  depression.*See* **Depression**
  in traumatic head injury, 628–629
**Affinity,** 35
**African-Americans**
  as health care consumers, 66
  medication-taking behavior of, 68–69
**African ginger (ginger),** 132*f*
**Afrin,** 1404, 1406
**Aftate,** 1448–1449
**Age**
  absorption and, 18
  changes
    in elderly, 202
    in homeostatic mechanisms, 200–201
    in pharmacodynamics, 200
    in pharmacokinetics, 199–200, 200*t*
    ultraviolet light and, 592
  excretion and, 27
  of health care consumer, 66
  of onset, for disability, 206
**Agency for Health Care Policy and Research (AHCPR)**
  otitis classifications, 485
  pain management guidelines, 227, 228
**Aggression, in traumatic head injury,** 628
**Agitation**
  in dementia, 656
  in traumatic head injury, 628
**Agonist-antagonist,** 39
**Agonists**
  defined, 33
  full, 39, 40*f*
  partial, 39, 40*f*
  types, 39, 40*f*
**AHCPR.** *See* **Agency for Health Care Policy and Research**
***AHFS Drug Information***, 86*t*
**Airway**
  diameter, age-related, 394
  remodeling, in asthma, 394
**Akarpine,** 1263
**AKBeta,** 1261
**AK-Chlor.** *See* **Chloramphenicol**
**AK-Dex.** *See* **Dexamethasone**
**Akineton,** 1244–1245
**Akne-mycin.** *See* **Erythromycin**
**AK-Pred,** 1277–1278, 1332
**AK-Sulf,** 1268–1269, 1435
**AKTob,** 1269–1270
**Ak-Tracin,** 1264–1265, 1438
**AK-Zol.** *See* **Acetazolamide**
**Alanine aminotransferase (ALT),** 45

**Albumin**
  elimination by dialysis, 53
  in kidney disease, 51
  serum levels
    age-related changes, 199
    in hepatic dysfunction, 47
**Albuterol,** 26, **1395–1396**
**Alclometasone dipropionate, 1453–1454**
**Alcohol**
  interaction with drugs, 108–109
  preconception screening, 243–244
**Alcohol abuse,** 786–787
  assessment/history taking, 788–789
  incidence, 785
  nonpharmacologic therapy, 787
  patient/caregiver information, 788*t*, 789
  pharmacotherapy, 787
    drug selection, 788, 789
    follow-up, 790
    goals, 787
    initiation, time frame for, 787–788
    monitoring, 789–790
  withdrawal symptoms, 788
**Alcoholics Anonymous (AA),** 787
**Aldactone.** *See* **Spironolactone**
**Aldara,** 879, 1443
**Aldomet,** 611*t*, **1056**
**Aldosterone,** 694–695, 695
**Aldosteronism,** 699
**Alendronate, 1378**
  drug-food interactions, 107*t*
  for osteoporosis, 297, 547–548
**Alertness problems, herbal remedies,** 139–141
**Aleve.** *See* **Naproxen**
**Alka-Mints,** 1287
**Alka Seltzer/aspirin,** 1135–1136
**Allegra (fexofenadine),** 370, **1420**
**Allergan Ear Drops,** 1281
**Allergic responses,** 98–99
  defined, 914
  to drugs
    assessment, 916–917
    diagnosis, 915
    follow-up, 918
    monitoring of pharmacotherapy, 918
    patient/caregiver information, 917, 917*t*
    pharmacotherapy, 915–916, 915t, 917–918
    predisposing factors, 914–915
  prevention/treatment ingredients with OTC status, 121*t*
**Allergic rhinitis**
  assessment, 371
  forms, 370
  pathophysiology, 369
  patient/caregiver information, 371–372

Allergic rhinitis (*cont.*)
  pharmacotherapy, 370–371
    drug selection, 372–373
    goals, 371, 371*t*
    initiation, time frame for, 371
    monitoring, 373–374
  during pregnancy, 249–250, 249*t*
  prevention, 371*t*
  symptoms, 370
*Allium sativum* (garlic), 132*f*
Allopurinol, 554, 555, **1235–1236**
Aloe vera, 132*f*, 144
Alomide. *See* Lodoxamide
Alophen, 1312–1313
Alora, 1368
Alpha-adrenergic agonists, 812
Alpha$_2$-adrenergic agonists, 317
Alpha$_1$-adrenergic antagonists, 344
Alpha/beta adrenergic blocking agents,
    1059–1060
Alpha blockers, 317
Alpha-galactosidase preparations, 516
Alpha-glucosidase inhibitors, 716–717
Alpha$_1$-selective adrenergic receptor blockers,
    for benign prostatic hyperplasia, 827,
    829
Alprazolam, 1159–1160
  contraindications, 773
  for insomnia, 786*t*
Alprostadil, **1479**
Altace, **1053**
ALT (alanine aminotransferase), 45
Alterative, 131*t*
AlternaGEL, 1286–1287
Alternative therapies, 127. *See also* **Herbal**
    **remedies**
Aluminum acetate solution, **1474**
Aluminum carbonate gel, basic, **1286**
Aluminum hydroxide gel, 1286–1287
Aluminum magnesium hydroxide sulfate, **1288**
Alupent, **1397**
Alurate, **1397**
Alu-Tab, 1286–1287
Alzheimer's disease, 652–653
  agents for, **1234–1235**
  assessment, pretherapy, 654–655
  pharmacotherapy, 654, 655–657
Amantadine, **1016**, **1243**
  for influenza, 163, 377
  for Parkinson's disease, 666
  for pneumonia in pregnancy, 451–452
  toxicity monitoring, 378–379
Amaphen, **1119**
Amaryl. *See* **Glimepiride**
Amber (St. John's wort), 132*f*
Ambien. *See* **Zolpidem**

Amebicides, **931**
Amen. *See* **Medroxyprogesterone**
Amenorrhoea, 841–843
  assessment/history taking, 841–842
  etiology, 841
  nonpharmacologic therapy, 841
  patient/caregiver information, 842
  pharmacotherapy, 841, 842–843
  primary *vs.* secondary, 841
Americaine Otic. *See* **Benzocaine**
American Rheumatism Association, rheumatoid
    arthritis classification, 532*t*
Americans with Disabilities Act (ADA), 205
Amigesic, **1139**
Amiloride, **1079**
Aminoglycosides, 615*t*
Aminopenicillins, 962–965
Aminophylline, **1399**
Aminosalicylate, **994**
Amiodarone, 1037–1038
  for atrial fibrillation, 335
  drug-drug interactions, 106*t*
  thyroid function and, 685*t*
  for ventricular tachycardia, 338
Amipicillin/sulbactam, 881*t*
Amitriptyline, 1185–1186
  for chronic pain, 234
  combined with chlordiazepoxide, **1219**
  for depression, 667, 755
  interaction with oral contraceptives, 277*t*
  plasma protein binding, 21*t*
Amlodipine, **1067**
Amoxapine, 1186–1187
Amoxicillin, **962**
  apparent volume of distribution, 23*t*
  for chlamydia, 872*t*
  dosage calculations, pediatric, 188*t*
  for otitis media, 488, 489
  plasma protein binding, 21*t*
  for sinusitis, 380, 381
  for upper respiratory tract infections, 489*t*
  for urinary tract infections, 806*t*
Amoxicillin/clavulanate, 962–963
  dosage calculations, pediatric, 188*t*
  for otitis media, 489
  for pneumonia in pregnant women, 451
  for sinusitis, 382
  for upper respiratory tract infections, 489*t*
  for urinary tract infections, 806*t*
Amoxil. *See* **Amoxicillin**
Amphetamine, 28, 29*t*
Amphojel, 1286–1287
Amphotericin B, **1438**
Ampicillin, **964**
  clearance, 29*t*
  for upper respiratory tract infections, 489*t*

Anacin, 1115–1116
Anacin-3. *See* **Acetaminophen**
Anafranil. *See* **Clomipramine**
Analgesic agents
  for common colds, 376
  herbal, 131*t*
  ingredients with OTC status, 121*t*
  for low back pain, 558
  for osteoarthritis, 542
  urinary tract agents, **1478**
Anaphylactoid reactions, 98
Anaprox. *See* **Naproxen**
Anaspaz, 1294
Anaxinal. *See* **Hydroxyzine**
Androderm, 1336–1337
Androgen/estrogens combinations, 1376
Androgen inhibitors, 1337
Androgens, 695, 1335–1337
Android. *See* **Methyltestosterone**
Anemia
  classification, 606
  clinical presentation, 607
  defined, 606
  etiology, 606–607
  folate deficiency, 611–614
  iron deficiency, 607–611, 610*t*, 611*t*
  megaloblastic, 611–614
  pernicious, 614
  with renal failure, erythropoietin therapy for, 616, 616*t*
Angelica (*Angelica archangelica*), 132*f*
Angina pectoris, 346, 346*t*
Angiotensin
  blood pressure regulation and, 310
  hypertension and, 311
Angiotensin-converting enzyme inhibitors (ACE inhibitors), 1049–1053
  drug-drug interactions, 106*t*
  for heart failure, 325–326
  for hypertension, 315, 317–318
  for intermittent claudication, 343
Angiotensin II antagonists (inhibitors), 319, 328, 1054
Angiotensin II receptors, 319
Anoquan, 1120–1121
Anorectal/vasoconstrictor ingredients, with OTC status, 118*t*
Anorexia nervosa
  assessment/history taking, 778–779
  patient/caregiver information, 779, 779*t*
  pharmacotherapy, 776–777
    drug selection, 779–780
    monitoring, 780–781
  symptoms, 776
Ansaid, 1122–1123

Antacids, 1286–1291
  combinations, **1115, 1290–1291**
  for gastroesophageal reflux, 513
  herbal, 131*t*
  for peptic ulcer disease, 511
Antagonism, 39
Antagonists. *See also specific antagonists*
  competitive, 39
  defined, 33
  irreversible, 39
  noncompetitive, 39
  types, 39, 40*f*
Antazoline phosphate/naphazoline, 120*t*
Anterior uveitis, 482
Anthelmintic ingredients, with OTC status, 119*t*
Anthra-Derm, 1430–1431
Anthralin, 1430–1431
Antiabortive agents, 131*t*
Antiadrenergic agents, centrally and peripherally acting, 1055–1059
Antiallergic agents, ophthalmic, **1273**
Antianginal agents, 1034–1037
Antianxiety agents. *See also specific antianxiety agents*
  for insomnia, 786*t*
Antiarrhythmic agents, 1037–1042. *See also specific antiarrhythmic agents*
  for chronic pain, 235–236
Antiasthmatic agents, 131*t*
Antibiotics, 131*t*. *See also specific antibiotics*
  for acne vulgaris, 577–578
  aminopenicillins, **962–965**
  for bacterial endocarditis prophylaxis, 352, 353–354
  cephalosporins. *See* **Cephalosporins**
  for chronic obstructive pulmonary disease, 424
  for cystic fibrosis, 430–433, 432*t*
  for diarrhea, 501
  dosage calculations, pediatric, 188*f*–190*f*
  fluoroquinolones. *See* **Fluoroquinolones**
  interactions with oral contraceptives, 277*t*
  macrolide, **951–957**
  ophthalmic, **1264–1270**
  otic, **1279–1285**
  penicillins. *See* **Penicillin**
  for pharyngitis, 383
  for pneumonia, 451, 453
  sulfonamides. *See* **Sulfonamides**
  tetracyclines, **976–978**
  *in vitro* activity, in upper respiratory tract infections, 489*t*
Anticandidal ingredients, with OTC status, 120*t*, 121*t*
Anticaries gel ingredients, with OTC status, 118*t*

**Anticatarrhal agents,** 131*t*
**Anticholinergic agents, 1322–1324**
    for chronic obstructive pulmonary disease, 422
    combinations, **1296**
    for common colds, 376
    for flatus, 516
    gastrointestinal, **1291–1296**
    for Parkinson's disease, 666
    respiratory inhalants, **1389**
**Anticoagulant agents,** 1043
    for atrial fibrillation, 336–337, 336*t*, 337*t*
    interactions with oral contraceptives, 277*t*
    for thrombus formation prevention, 617–620,
        618*t*, 619*t*
**Anticonvulsant agents, 1153–1159**
    for alcohol abuse, 789, 790
    barbiturates.*See* **Barbiturates**
    benzodiazepines.*See* **Benzodiazepines**
    for bipolar disorder, 762
    for bulimia nervosa, 780
    for chronic pain, 235
    for eating disorders, 778
    efficacy, 672–673, 672*t*
    hydantoins, **1146–1149**
    interactions with oral contraceptives, 277*t*
    oxazolidinediones, **1150**
    selection, 671–672
    succinimides, **1151–1152**
    for traumatic head injury, 629
**Antidepressant agents, 1185–1202**
    adverse events, 234
    for anorexia nervosa, 780
    for anxiety disorders, 768, 771, 774
    for eating disorders, 778, 780
    for insomnia, 785
    monoamine oxidase inhibitors, **1198–1199**
    for pain management, 233–235
    selective serotonin reuptake inhibitors,
        **1199–1202**
    toxicity, 775
    tricyclic.*See* **Tricyclic antidepressants**
**Antidiabetic agents, 1352–1366**
    insulin.*See* **Insulin**
    interactions with oral contraceptives, 277*t*
    sulfonylureas, **1352–1357**
**Antidiarrheal agents, 1306–1308**
    ingredients with OTC status, 120*t*
    for irritable bowel syndrome, 520
**Antiemetic agents, with OTC status,** 119*t*
**Antiflatulent agents, 1320–1321**
**Antifungal agents, 979–985**
    ingredients with OTC status, 119*t*, 120*t*
    ophthalmic, **1270**
**Antihistamines**
    for allergic rhinitis, 370, 372–373, 374
    for anxiety disorders, 771

    for common colds, 375
    first generation, **1410–1418**
    ingredients with OTC status, 118*t*, 119*t*, 120*t*
    with OTC status, 120*t*
    relative costs, 917*t*
    second generation, **1419–1421**
    for sinusitis, 380
    topical preparations, **1437**
**Antihydrotic agents,** 131*t*
**Antihyperlipidemic agents, 1044–1048**
**Antihypertensive agents**
    ACE inhibitors.*See* **Angiotensin converting en-**
        **zyme inhibitors**
    alpha/beta adrenergic blocking agents,
        **1059–1060**
    angiotensin II antagonists, **1054**
    for anxiety disorders, 771
    beta-adrenergic blockers.*See* **Beta-adrenergic**
        **blocking agents**
    calcium channel blockers, **1067–1071**
    centrally and peripherally acting antiadrenergic
        agents, **1055–1059**
    follow-up, 319
    interactions with oral contraceptives, 277*t*
    monitoring, 316–319
    selection, 314–316
    vasodilators, **1071–1072**
**Antihypertensive and Lipid Lowering Heart**
    **Attack Prevention Trial (ALL-HAT),** 316
**Anti-infective agents**
    amebicides, **931**
    antibiotics.*See* **Antibiotics**
    antifungal.*See* **Antifungal agents**
    antimalarial, **985–993**
    anti-parasitics, **1023–1027**
    antituberculosis, **994–1001**
    antiviral.*See* **Antiviral agents**
    combinations, **1440–1441**
    ingredients with OTC status, 119*t*
    topical, **1438–1449**
    urinary, **1017–1023**
**Antimalarial agents, 985–993**
**Antiminth, 1026**
**Antimobility agents, for diarrhea,** 501–502
**Antineoplastic agents, drug-nutrient interac-**
    tions and, 108*t*
**Anti-parasitic agents, 1023–1027**
**Antiplatelet agents,** 343, **1072–1073**
**Antipruritic agents, with OTC status,** 118*t*, 120*t*
**Antipsoriatic agents, topical, 1430–1433**
**Antipsychotic agents, 1203–1220**
    atypical, **1216–1219**
    phenothiazines, **1203–1210**
    for psychosis, 628
        for Parkinson's disease, 667–668
    psychotherapeutic combinations, **1219–1220**

**Antipyretic agents,** 131*t,* 376
**Antipyrine/benzocaine otic,** 1281
**Antiseborrheic agents**
  combinations, **1436**
  topical, **1433–1436**
**Antiseptic agents,** 131*t*
**Antispasmodic agents,** 131*t,* **1291–1296**
  for irritable bowel syndrome, 520
  urinary tract, **1476**
**Antithrombotic therapy**
  for atrial fibrillation, 336–337, 336*t,* 337*t*
  for stroke prevention, 637
**Antithyroid agents,** 1381–1382
**Antituberculosis agents,** 994–1001
**Antitussive agents,** 1408–1409
  for common colds, 376
  ingredients with OTC status, 119*t,* 120*t*
**Antivert,** 651, 1323–1324
**Antiviral agents,** 1002–1017. *See also specific*
    *antiviral classes and/or drugs*
  interactions with oral contraceptives, 277*t*
  ophthalmic, **1271–1272**
  for pneumonia during pregnancy, 451–452
**Antrizine,** 1323–1324
**Ant stings,** 586
**Anturane,** 554, **1238**
**Anusol.** *See* **Hydrocortisone acetate**
**Anxiety disorders**
  after stroke, 641
  assessment/history taking, 771–772
  in dementia, 656
  herbal therapies, 129–131
  incidence, 766
  nonpharmacologic therapy, 770
  pathophysiology, 768–770
  patient/caregiver information, 772, 772*t*
  pharmacotherapy, 768–770
    drug selection, 770–771, 772–775
    follow-up, 775–776
    goals, 770
    initiation, time frame for, 770
    monitoring, 775
  symptoms, 766–767
  types, 767–768
**Anxiolytic agents,** 1159–1168. *See also*
    **Benzodiazepines**
**Aortic occlusive disease,** 340*t*
**APD (action potential duration),** 329
**Aphrodisiac,** 131*t*
**Aphrodyne,** 1480
**Apparent volume of distribution ($V_D$),** 23, 23*t*
*Applied Therapeutics: The Clinical Use of*
    *Drugs,* 86*t*
**Apraclonidine,** 1257
**Apresoline.** *See* **Hydralazine**
**Aprobarbital,** 1169

**Aquachloral Supprettes,** 1179
**Aquatensen,** 1084–1085
**Aralen,** 985–986
**Aralen phosphate/primaquine phosphate,**
    986–987
*Arctostaphylos uva ursi* **(bearberry),** 132*f*
**Area under the curve (AUC),** 8–9
**Argesic-SA,** 1139
**Aricept,** 1234
**Aristocort.** *See* **Triamcinolone**
**Armour Thyroid,** 1387
**Arousal, pharmacotherapy for,** 624, 626–628
**Arrhythmias.** *See also specific arrhythmias*
  conduction, 331*t*–332*t*
  nonpharmacologic therapy, 333
  outcomes management, 334–339, 336*t,* 337*t*
  pathophysiology, 328–329
  patient/caregiver information, 334
  pharmacotherapy, 329, 332–333. *See also*
      **Antiarrhythmic agents**
    assessment for, 333–334
    follow-up, 339
    goals, 333
    initiation, time frame for, 333
  supraventricular, 330*t*
  ventricular, 331*t*
**Artane,** 1251–1252
**Artane-Sequels,** 1251–1252
**Arterial disease, thrombus formation,** 617
**Artha-G,** 1139
**Arthritis**
  with psoriasis, 600
  rheumatoid.*See* **Rheumatoid arthritis**
**Arthropan,** 1136–1137
**Arthropod bites/stings,** 585–588
**ASA,** 1105
**Asacol,** 1318
**Ascorbic acid**
  creatinine serum levels and, 49*t*
  drug interactions, 615*t*
**Ascriptin,** 1135–1136
**Asendin.** *See* **Amoxapine**
**Asian-Americans, medication-taking behavior**
    **of,** 68
**Asiatic ginseng (ginseng),** 132*f*
**AskAdvice Patient Education software,** 94*t*
*Ask Rx,* 90*t*
**Aspartate aminotransferase (AST),** 45
**Aspergum.** *See* **Aspirin**
**Aspirin,** 1135
  buffered, **1135–1136**
  for chronic pain, 229–230
  combinations
    butalbital, **1121**
    caffeine, **1115–1116**
    caffeine/butalbital, **1120–1121**

Aspirin *(cont.)*
  combinations *(cont.)*
    codeine, **1101**
    codeine/caffeine/butalbital, **1103**
    dihydrocodeine/caffeine, **1107–1108**
    hydrocodone, **1105**
    meprobamate, **1116–1117**
    propoxyphene/caffeine, **1112–1113**
  for coronary heart disease, 350–351
  elimination, dose-dependent kinetics and, 31
  enteric-coated, absorption of, 17
  excretion, 29t
  ionization, 13
  plasma protein binding, 21t
  for rheumatoid arthritis, 534
  for stroke prevention, 638
**Aspirin Free Anacin PM Caplets, 1183–1184**
**Aspirin-Free Excedrin, 1115–1116**
**AST (aspartate aminotransferase),** 45
**Asteatotoic dermatitis (winter itch),** 589
**Astemizole,** 26, **1419**
**Asthma**
  adult, 394–395, 402t
  airway remodeling in, 394
  cystic fibrosis with, 444
  definition of, 394
  exacerbation, management of, 403
  herbal remedies, 133–134
  incidence, increase in, 393–394
  management, 394
  nonpharmacologic therapy, 396, 407
  pediatric, 402t, 405–406
  pharmacotherapy, 395, 413–414
    assessment for, 396, 396t–398t, 407, 408t, 415
    drug selection, 406, 408–412, 409t, 415–416
    efficacy monitoring, 403–404, 411, 416
    follow-up for, 405, 412–413, 416
    goals, 395–396, 406–407, 414
    inhaler usage for, 396–398
    initiation, time frame for, 396, 407, 414–415
    outcomes management, 408–413, 409t
    patient/caregiver information, 396–399,
      407–408, 415
    peak flow meter usage for, 398–399
    selection of agent for, 399–401, 400t, 403
    toxicity monitoring, 404–405, 411–412, 416
  in pregnancy, 413–416, 414t, 415t
    pharmacotherapy for, 413–416, 414t, 415t
  severity
    classification of, 399t
    drug selection and, 399–401, 400t, 408–412,
      409t
  "stop light" approach, 407, 407t
  triggers, 405
**Astringent,** 131t
**Atabrine, 991–992**

**Atarax.** *See* **Hydroxyzine**
**Ataxia, in multiple sclerosis,** 647
**Atenolol,** 35, **1061**
**Atherosclerosis**
  in coronary artery disease, 344–345
  lesions, classification of, 345
  occlusive disease and, 340t
  precursors, 355
  risk factors, 345
**Athlete's foot (tinea pedis),** 572, 575
**Ativan.** *See* **Lorazepam**
**Atopic dermatitis,** 589
**Atopy, asthma development and,** 405
**Atorvastatin,** 358–359, **1045**
**Atovaquone,** 107t, **1027**
**Atretol.** *See* **Carbamazepine**
**Atrial fibrillation**
  description/etiology, 330t
  duration, pharmacotherapy and, 334–335
  pharmacotherapy, 334–337, 336t
**Atrial flutter**
  description/etiology, 330t
  pharmacotherapy, 334–337, 336t
**Atrioventricular blocks**
  description/etiology, 331t–332t
  first-degree, 332t
  second-degree, 332t
  third-degree, 332t
**Atrioventricular dissociation,** 332t
**Atropine sulfate, 1291**
  combinations
    difenoxin, **1306**
    diphenoxylate, **1306–1307**
**Atrovent.** *See* **Ipratropium**
**Attapulgite,** 18, **1308**
**Attention, pharmacotherapy,** 624, 626–628
**Attention deficit/hyperactivity disorder
  (AD/HD)**
  background, 629
  differential diagnosis, 631
  DSM III-R criteria, 630–631, 630t
  nonpharmacologic therapy, 632–633
  patient/caregiver information, 633
  pharmacotherapy, 632
    assessment for, 633
    drug selection for, 633–634
    follow-up, 635
    initiation, time frame for, 633
    monitoring, 634–635
    toals for, 632
  treatment issues, 631
**AUC (area under the curve),** 8–9
**Augmented betamethasone dipropionate,
  1454–1455**
**Augmentin,** 34, **962–963**
**Auralgan, 1281**

Auranofin, 1252
Auro-Dri, 1282
Auro Ear Drops, 1283
Aurolate, 1253–1254
Aurothioglucose, 1253
Auroto, 1281
Auspitz's sign, 599
Autohaler, 397
Autonomic dysreflexia, in disabled individuals,
    211, 212t, 213
Ava (kava), 133
Aventyl. See Nortriptyline
Avonex, 645–646
Axid, 1300
Axotal, 1121
Aygestin. See Norethindrone
Azapirones. See also Buspirone
  for anxiety disorders, 771, 773
  toxicity, 775
Azatadine, 1410
Azathioprine, 1253
  monitoring, 530t
  for rheumatoid arthritis, 535–536
Azdone, 1105
Azelastine, 370
Azithromycin, 951–952
  for chlamydia, 872t
  dosage calculations, pediatric, 188t
  drug-food interactions, 107t
  for gonorrhea, 869
  for pharyngitis, 384–385
  for upper respiratory tract infections, 489t
  for urethritis, 821t
Azmacort. See Triamcinolone
Azo Gantanol, 1021
Azo Gantrisin, 1022
Azo-Standard. See Phenazopyridine
Azulfidine. See Sulfasalazine

B

Babinski's sign, 213
BAC, 1121
Bacampicillin, 964
Baciguent. See Bacitracin
Bacille Calmette-Guérin (BCG), 168, 169,
    460–461
Bacitracin, 1264–1265, 1438
Back pain, low
  etiology, 555
  incidence, 555
  nonpharmacologic therapy, 556
  patient/caregiver information, 557
  pharmacotherapy, 556
    assessment/history taking for, 557
    drug selection for, 558–559

follow-up, 559
  goals for, 556
  initiation, time frame for, 556
  monitoring, 559
Baclofen, 213, 559, 1224
Bacterial endocarditis, antibiotic prophylaxis,
    352, 353–354
Bacterial skin infections, 569
Bacterial vaginosis, 250–251, 251t, 888–890
Bacteruria, during pregnancy, 247, 248t
Bactocill, 968–969
Bactrim. See Trimethoprim-sulfamethoxazole
Bactroban, 836
Bancap, 1104, 1112–1120
Banthine, 1294–1295
Barbados aloe (aloe vera), 132f
Barbiturates, 1141–1143
  combined with nonnarcotic analgesics,
    1119–1121
  sedatives/hypnotics, 1169–1178
Barkley Side Effects Questionnaire (BSEQ),
    635
Barrier contraceptives. See Contraception, bar-
    rier methods
Barriers, health behavior, 69
Basal body temperature (BBT), 265
Basal cell carcinoma, 592
Basaljel, 1286
Bases, 13–14, 14f
Basic and Clinical Pharmacology, 86t
Baths, herbal, 130t
Bayer. See Aspirin
Bayer Select, 1114
Bayer Select Maximum Strength Menstrual
    Caplets, 1115
BBT (basal body temperature), 265
BCA (bichloroacetic acid), 879
BCG (bacille Calmette-Guérin), 168, 169,
    460–461
Bearberry, 132f, 145
Becloforte inhaler. See Beclomethasone
Beclomethasone, 1390, 1422
  for asthma, 400–401, 402t
  in pregnancy, 416
Beclovent. See Beclomethasone
Beconase. See Beclomethasone
Beepen VK, 961
Bee stings
  for multiple sclerosis, 646
  treating, 586
Behavior
  modification
    transtheoretical model of, 72–73
    for weight loss, 736
  problems, obesity and, 733, 735
Belladonna, 1292

Benadryl. *See* Diphenhydramine
Benazepril, 1049
Bendroflumethiazide, 1081
Benemid. *See* Probenecid
Benign paroxysmal positional vertigo (BPPV), 649, 650, 651
Benign prostatic hyperplasia (BPH)
  assessment/history taking, 827, 828*t*
  etiology, 825
  herbal remedies, 143
  incidence, 825
  patient/caregiver information, 827, 829*t*
  pharmacotherapy, 826–827
    drug selection, 827
    follow-up, 829
    goals, 827
    initiation, time frame for, 827
    monitoring, 828
  symptoms, 826
Bentoquatam, OTC status, 121*t*
Bentyl, 1293
Benylin. *See* Diphenhydramine
Benylin DM. *See* Dextromethorphan
Benzathine penicillin G, 866*t*
Benzethonium chloride/acetic acid/sodium acetate/propylene glycol diacetate, 1280
Benzocaine, 1282
  combinations
    antipyrine/phenylephrine/propylene glycol, **1281**
    antipyrin/glycerin, **1281**
    benzothonium chloride/glycerin/PEG 300, **1281**
Benzodiazepines (BZDs), 1143–1145
  for alcohol abuse, 789
  anxiolytic, 768, 770–771, 772–773, **1159–1165**
  for bipolar disorder, 763
  for chemotherapy-associated nausea/vomiting, 498–499
  hypnotics, 784
  for insomnia, 784, 785
  for seizures, 675
  toxicity, 775
  withdrawal syndrome, 770–771
Benzonatate, 1408
Benzoyl peroxide, 1427
Benzphetamine, 740, 1481
Benzthiazide, 1081–1082
Benztropine, 1243–1244
Bepridil, 1067
Beta-adrenergic agonists, 479
Beta₂-adrenergic agonists, selective, 743
Beta₂-adrenergic agonists, selective
  adverse events, 426*t*
  toxicity, 404
Beta₃-adrenergic agonists, selective, 743
Beta-adrenergic blocking agents, 1060–1066

Beta-adrenergic blocking agents (beta blockers)
  for alcohol abuse, 789, 790
  for anxiety disorders, 774–775
  cardioselective, 317
  for coronary heart disease, 349
  for heart failure, 327–328
  for hypertension, 317
  interactions with oral contraceptives, 277*t*
  for intermittent claudication, 343
  noncardioselective, 317
  stereoselectivity, 35–36, 36*f*
Betadine, 1433–1434
Betagan, 1261
Betamethasone, 1327
Betamethasone benzoate, 1455
Betamethasone dipropionate, 1456
Betamethasone valerate, 1456–1457
Betapace, 1065
Beta₂-receptor agonists, for chronic obstructive pulmonary disease, 422
Betaseron, 645
Betaxolol, 1061, 1257
Bethanechol chloride, 1477
Betoptic. *See* Betaxolol
Biaxin. *See* Clarithromycin
Bichloroacetic acid (BCA), 879
Bicillin
  C-R, 960–961
  dosage calculations, pediatric, 189*t*
  L-A, 959–960
Biguanides, 717–718
Bile acid sequestrants, 359, **1044–1047**
Bilirubin, 47
Biltricide, 1025
Bioavailability (F)
  absorption and, 19, 19*f*
  drug-nutrient interactions and, 107*t*–108*t*
Bioequivalence, 11–12, 12
Biologic membranes, 12–13
Biotransformation. *See* Metabolism
Biotransport
  defined, 12
  drug features and, 13
  mechanisms, 14–16, 15*f*
Biperiden, 1244–1245
Bipolar disorder
  assessment/history taking, 763
  classification, 759
  etiology, 762*t*
  incidence, 759
  nonpharmacologic therapy, 760–761
  patient/caregiver information, 763–764
  pharmacotherapy, 760
    algorithm, 761*f*
    drug selection, 762–763, 764–765
    follow-up, 766

goals, 760
  initiation, time frame for, 761–762
  monitoring, 765–766
  phases, 760
symptoms, 759–760
**Birth control pills.** *See* **Oral contraceptives**
**Bisacodyl,** 9
**Bismuth subsalicylate, 1306**
**Bisoprolol, 1061–1062**
**Bisphosphonates,** 547–548, **1378–1379**
**Bitolterol, 1396**
**Black cohosh,** 132*f*, 135–136
**Black currant (evening primrose oil),** 132*f*
**Black ginger (ginger),** 132*f*
**Blackheads,** 576
**Black snake root (black cohosh),** 132*f*, 135–136
**Black widow spider** *(latrodectus mactans),*
    585–586
**Bladder**
  dysfunction, in multiple sclerosis, 644, 647
  neurogenic, 209–210
  retraining, 293
**Bleph-10.** *See* **Sulfacetamide**
**Blepharitis,** 475, 476–477
**Blindness, glaucoma and,** 477
**Blocadren, 1066**
**Blockers (antagonists),** 33
**Blond psyllium (plantago seed),** 132*f*
**Blood-brain barrier,** 20
**Blood clotting, normal mechanism,** 617
**Blood flow**
  distribution and, 19–20
  hepatic, 46
  liver, 24
**Blood loss**
  anemia from, 606
  gastrointestinal, 608
**Blood pressure**
  elevated. *See* **Hypertension**
  regulation, 309–310
**Blood urea nitrogen (BUN),** 48
**Bluboro powder, 1474**
**"Blue balls,"** 875
**Body mass index (BMI)**
  calculation, 734*t*, 737
  morbidity and, 732
**Body oils, herbal,** 130*t*
**Body weight**
  loss
    noradrenergic agents for, 739–740
    serotonergic agents for, 740–741
  normal, 738*t*
  overweight, 731. *See also* **Obesity**
**Bone density measurements**
  for hormone replacement therapy monitoring, 301
  in menopause, 296
  for osteoporosis, 546

**Bone marrow, erythropoiesis,** 605–606
**Bone mineral density, estrogens and,** 298
**Bone resorption inhibitors**
  for menopause, 297
  for postmenopausal women, 300
**Bonine, 1323–1324**
**Borage seed oil (evening primrose oil),** 132*f*
*Bordetella pertussis,* 155
**Boric acid/ispropyl alcohol, 1282**
**Boropak powder, 1474**
**Bouchard's nodes,** 541
**Bowel**
  dysfunction, in multiple sclerosis, 644, 647
  neurogenic, 209–210
  training program, 210
**BPH.** *See* **Benign prostatic hyperplasia**
**BPPV (benign paroxysmal positional vertigo),**
    649, 650, 651
**Bradycardia, sinus,** 330*t*
**Brain injury, traumatic.** *See* **Traumatic brain in-**
    **jury**
**BRAT diet,** 500
**Breakthrough bleeding, from oral contracep-**
    **tive usage,** 272*t*
**Breast cancer**
  in menopause, risk factors for, 295*t*
  oral contraceptive usage and, 275
**Breast milk, drug transmission,** 242, 242*t*
**Breast tenderness**
  herbal remedies, 133, 141, 142–143
  in premenstrual syndrome, 849
**Breathing exercises, for cystic fibrosis,** 427
**Brethine, 1398–1399**
**Brevicon, 1339, 1345–1346**
**Bricanyl, 1398–1399**
**Bricker's intact nephron hypothesis,** 47
**Brochodilators**
  sympathomimetics, **1395–1399**
  xanthine derivatives, **1399–1402**
**Bromocriptine, 1245**
  for Parkinson's disease, 665
  for premenstrual syndrome, 849
**Bromphen, 1410–1411**
**Brompheniramine,** 118*t*, **1410–1411**
**Bronchial asthma.** *See* **Asthma**
**Bronchiolitis,** 416–417
  assessment, 418, 418*t*, 419*t*
  hospitalization, 419, 419*t*
  pharmacotherapy
    drug selection for, 417–419
    follow-up, 419–420
    goals, 418
    initiation, time frame for, 418
    monitoring, 419
    patient/caregiver information, 418
  respiratory synctial virus and, 416–417, 417*t*

**Bronchodilators**
for asthma, 401, 415
for bronchiolitis, 417
for cystic fibrosis, 429–430
interactions with oral contraceptives, 277*t*
in pregnancy, 415
**Bronchospasm, exercise-induced,** 400, 409–410
**Bronkaid Mist.** *See* **Epinephrine**
**Bronkosol.** *See* **Isoetharine**
**Brown recluse spider** *(loxosceles reculsa),*
585–586
**BSEQ (Barkley Side Effects Questionnaire),**
635
**Bubo, inguinal,** 875
**Bucindolol,** 327–328
**Bucladin-S Softabs,** 1322
**Buclizine,** 1322
**Budesonide,** 1390–1391
for asthma, 402*t*
intranasal, **1422**
for pediatric asthma, 406
**Buerger's disease (thromboangiitis obliterans),**
340*t*
**Buffalo hump,** 697
**Bufferin,** 1135–1136
**Buffex,** 1135–1136
**Bulimia nervosa**
assessment/history taking, 778–779
patient/caregiver information, 779, 779*t*
pharmacotherapy, 777
drug selection, 780
monitoring, 781
symptoms, 776
types, 776
**Bulk-forming agents,** 503–504
**Bullous impetigo,** 569–570
**Bumetanide,** 1077
**Bumex,** 1077
**BUN (blood urea nitrogen),** 48
**BUN:creatinine ratio,** 48
**Bupavicaine,** 21*t*
**Buprenorphine**
for chronic pain, 231
mechanism of action, 39
**Bupropion,** 1194, **1486**
for bipolar disorder, 763
for depression, 752, 756
for smoking cessation, 795
toxicity, 759
**Burns**
classification, 595
pharmacotherapy, 595–598
**Burow's Otic,** 1280
**Burow's solution,** 1474
**Bursitis,** 560–561
**BuSpar.** *See* **Buspirone**

**Buspirone,** 1165
for anxiety disorders, 773
for insomnia, 786*t*
toxicity, 775
**Butabarbital,** 1170
**Butace,** 1119
**Butalbital/acetaminophen/codeine/caffeine,**
1102
**Butalbital/aspirin/codeine/caffeine,** 1103
**Butisol sodium,** 1170
**Butoconazole,** 121*t*, 1438–1439
**Butorphanol,** 1099
**Butyrophenones,** 498
**BZDs.** *See* **Benzodiazepines**

C

**Cafatine,** 1241–1242
**Cafergot,** 1241–1242
**Caffeine**
combinations
acetaminophen/codeine/butalbital, **1102**
acetaminophen/dihydrocodeine, **1106**
aspirin/codeine/butalbital, **1103**
aspirin/dihydrocodeine, **1107–1108**
drug interactions, 611*t*
herbal preparations, 132*t*
preconception screening, 244
terminology, 132*f*
**CAGE questionnaire,** 788–789
**Caigua,** 132*f*, 145–146
**Caladryl.** *See* **Diphenhydramine**
**Calan.** *See* **Verapamil**
**Calcimar.** *See* **Calcitonin**
**Calcipotriene,** 601, **1431**
**Calcitonin,** 297, 548, **1380**
**Calcium carbonate,** 611*t*, **1287**
for osteoporosis, 546–547, 546*t*, 547*t*
for postmenopausal women, 300
for premenstrual syndrome, 847–848
**Calcium channel blockers,** 1067–1071
for atrial fibrillation, 336
for bipolar disorder, 763
for coronary heart disease, 349–350
drug-nutrient interactions, 107*t*
for heart failure, 328
for hypertension, 318
immediate-release, 11
for intermittent claudication, 343
L-type, 318
for Raynaud's disease, 343–344
T-type, 318
**Calcium pyrophosphate dihydrate (CPPD),** 549
**CaldeCort,** 1466
**Calmative,** 131*t*
**Calm-X,** 1323

*Camellia sinensis*, 132*t*
**Canadian Cardiovascular Society Classification System, for coronary heart disease**, 347*t*
*Candida albicans*, 885
**Candidiasis**
  congenital/neonatal, 574
  intertrigo, 573
  nonpharmacologic therapy, 574
  oral, 573
  paronychia onychia, 573
  pharmacotherapy, 574–576
  types, 573–574
  vulvovaginal, 251, 251*t*, 885–888
**Cannabinoids**, 498
**CAP.** *See* **Community-acquired pneumonia**
**CAPD (continuous ambulatory peritoneal dialysis )**, 54
**Capital/codeine, 1100**
**Capitrol, 1433**
**Capoten,** 107*t*, **1049–1050**
**Capreomycin, 460**
**Capsaicin**
  for osteoarthritis, 542
  for rheumatoid arthritis, 537
**Capsicum,** 141
**Capsium,** 132*f*
**Captopril,** 107*t*, **1049–1050**
**Carafate, 1201**
**Carbachol, 1258**
**Carbamazepine, 1153–1154**
  for bipolar disorder, 762–763, 764–765
  for chronic pain, 235
  clearance, 29*t*
  interactions
    drug-nutrient, 108*t*
    with oral contraceptives, 277*t*
  for seizures, 674
  thyroid function and, 685*t*
**Carbamide peroxide/alcohol/glycerin/polysorbate 20, 1283**
**Carbamide peroxide/anhydrous glycerin base, 1283**
**Carbamide peroxide/glycerin/propylene glycol/sodium stannate, 1282**
**Carbenicillin, 965**
**Carbidopa, 1246–1247**
**Carbidopa/levodopa,** 20, 626, **1246**
**Carbinoxamine, 1411**
**Carbohydrate digestion inhibitors, 743**
**Carbonic anhydrase inhibitors, 1075–1076**
**Carboptic, 1258**
**Carbuncles,** 570, 572
**Cardene, 1069**
**Cardiac arrhythmias.** *See* **Arrhythmias**
**Cardiac Arrhythmia Suppression Trial (CAST),** 338

**Cardiac glycosides,** 326–327, 326*t*, **1073–1074**
**Cardiac output**
  blood pressure and, 309–310
  decreased, 313
  hypertension and, 310
  increased, 313
**Cardioquin, 1041–1042**
**Cardiovascular system**
  complications from oral contraceptive usage, 271*t*, 273–275
  disease, 309
    arrhythmias.*See* **Arrhythmias**
    coronary heart disease.*See* **Coronary heart disease**
    heart failure.*See* **Heart failure**
    hyperlipidemia, 354–360, 356*t*–358*t*
    hypertension.*See* **Hypertension**
    in menopause, 292, 293–294, 295*t*
    mitral valve prolapse, 351–354
    peripheral vascular disease.*See* **Peripheral vascular disease**
**Cardizem.** *See* **Diltiazem**
**Cardura.** *See* **Doxazosin**
**Carisoprodol, 1224–1225**
**Carisoprodol/aspirin, 1230–1231**
**Carisoprodol/aspirin/codeine, 1231–1232**
**Carminative,** 131*t*
**Carotid stenosis,** 637
**Carrier-mediated transport,** 15–16, 15*f*
**Carteolol, 1062, 1258**
**Carvedilol,** 327, **1059**
*Cassia acutifolia* (senna), 132*f*, 135
*Cassia Angustifolia* (senna), 132*f*135
**CAST (Cardiac Arrhythmia Suppression Trial),** 338
**Castor oil, 1309–1310**
**Cataflam, 1127, 1274**
**Catapres.** *See* **Clonidine**
**Catheterization, clean intermittent,** 209
**Cayenne pepper (capsocum),** 132*f*
**CDC (Centers for Disease Control),** 93*t*
**CDD (direct-current cardioversion),** 334–335
**CD4+ T cell count, in HIV/AIDS,** 899, 900*t*
**Ceclor, 935**
**Cedax,** 189*t*, **941**
**Cefaclor, 935**
  dosage calculations, pediatric, 188*t*
  for upper respiratory tract infections, 489*t*
**Cefadroxil,** 188*t*, **933**
**Cefixime, 939**
  dosage calculations, pediatric, 188*t*
  for gonorrhea, 868, 869*t*
  for upper respiratory tract infections, 489*t*
  for urethritis, 821*t*
**Cefotetan,** 881*t*
**Cefoxitin,** 881*t*

Cefpodoxime proxetil, 940–941
  dosage calculations, pediatric, 189t
  for otitis media, 490
  for upper respiratory tract infections, 489t
Cefprozil, 937–938
  dosage calculations, pediatric, 189t
  for upper respiratory tract infections, 489t
Ceftibutin, 189t, 941
Ceftin, 936–937
Ceftriaxone, 941–942
  for epididymitis, 818t
  for gonorrhea, 868, 869t
  for urethritis, 821t
Cefuroxime axetil, 936–937
  dosage calculations, pediatric, 189t
  for upper respiratory tract infections, 489t
Cefzil, 937–938
Celestone, 1327
Cell membrane, 13, 13f
Cellulitis, 570, 572
Celontin Kapseals. See Methsuximide
Centers for Disease Control (CDC), 93t
Central analgesics, 1134
Centrax, 1164–1165
Cephalexin, 932
  apparent volume of distribution, 23t
  for urinary tract infections, 806t
Cephalosporins. See also specific cephalosporins
  creatinine serum levels and, 49t
  for cystic fibrosis, 432
  first-generation, 932–934
  second-generation, 935–942
  third-generation, for urinary tract infections, 806t
Cephradine, 933–934
Cephulac, 1317
Cerebrovascular accident
  defined, 635
  incidence, 635
  nonpharmacologic therapy, 636–637
  oral contraceptive usage and, 275
  patient/caregiver information, 638
  pharmacotherapy, 636
    for acute care, 639–640
    assessment for, 637–638
    contraindications, 641
    drug selection for, 637, 638
    follow-up, 641
    goals, 636
    initiation, time frame for, 637
    for poststroke symptoms, 640–641
    for prevention, 638–639
  risk factors, 635–636
  site, 635
Cerumenex drops, 1285
Cervical cancer, oral contraceptive usage and, 275

Cervical cap, 260
Cervical mucus, ovulation patterns and, 265–266
Cetamide. See Sulfacetamide
Ceta-Plus, 1104
Cetirizine, 370, 1419–1420
CF transmembrane conductance regulator
    (CFTR), 426
Chalazion, 475, 476–477
Chamomile, 132f, 136
Charcoal, 1320
Charcoal/simethicone, 1320
Charco Caps, 1320
Chaste berry (chaste tree berry), 132f, 142–143
CHD. See Coronary heart disease
Chemical antagonism, 39
Chemical conjunctivitis, 480
Chemical ntagonism, 39
Chemoreceptor trigger zone (CTZ), 498
Chemotherapy, nausea/vomiting associated
    with, 497–499
Chest x-rays
  for heart failure, 323–324
  for pneumonia monitoring, 441
Chibroxin. See Norfloxacin
Chickenpox. See Varicella-zoster virus
Children. See also Infants; Neonates
  absorption, 183t, 185
  allergic contact dermatitis, 589–590
  antibiotic dosage calculations, 188f–190f
  depression in, 748
  diabetic
    diagnosis of, 712
    self-management for, 712–713
  with disability, primary care for, 206
  distribution, 183t, 185
  drug safety/efficacy
    FDA and, 181
    historical aspects of, 181–182
  drug safety issues, 194t–195t
  families of, teaching tips for, 194t
  homeless, 221
  hyperactive.See Attention deficit/hyperactivity
      disorder
  hypothyroidism, levothyroxine for, 692, 692t
  pain relief for, 192–193, 195
  preschoolers, administration of drugs and,
      186–187
  prescribing medications for, 191–192, 193t
  pyelonephritis, 810
  school-age, administration of drugs and, 187
  selective serotonin reuptake inhibitors for, 755
  sunburn in, 595
  therapeutic disasters, 181
  therapeutic orphans, 182
  toddlers, administration of drugs and, 186
  urinary tract infections, 806t, 807t

Children's Kaopectate, 1308
Chile pepper (capsocum), 132*f*
Chirality, 35
Chlamydia
    assessment/history taking, 870–871, 871*t*
    pharmacotherapy, 870, 871–872, 872*t*
    during pregnancy, 252*t*
*Chlamydia pneumoniae* pneumonia, 438, 439*t*,
    448*t*, 451*t*
*Chlamydia trachomatis*, 870, 875
    conjunctivitis, 480
    lymphogranuloma venereum and, 875
    otitis media, 488
    pelvic inflammatory disease, 880–882, 881*t*
    pneumonia, in children, 447*t*
    sexually transmitted infections, 870–872, 871*t*,
      872*t*
Chlophedianol, 120*t*
Chloral hydrate, 104, **1179**
Chlorambucil
    monitoring, 531*t*
    for rheumatoid arthritis, 537
Chloramphenicol, 1028–1029, 1265, 1279
Chlorazepate, 786*t*
Chlordiazepoxide, 1160–1161
    for alcohol abuse, 789
    combined with amitriptyline, **1219**
    for insomnia, 786*t*
Chlormezanone, 1166
Chlorofon-F, 1232
Chloromycetin. *See* Chloramphenicol
Chloromycetin Otic. *See* Chloramphenicol
Chloroptic. *See* Chloramphenicol
Chloroquine, 29*t*, 985–986
Chloroquine phosphate/primaquine phosphate,
    986–987
Chlorothiazide, 1082
Chloroxine, 1433
Chlorphenesin carbamate, 1225
Chlorpheniramine, 1411–1412
    for allergic rhinitis, 372
    OTC status, 118*t*
    pediatric dosages, 190*t*
Chlorpromazine, 1204
Chlorpropamide, 1352
    apparent volume of distribution, 23*t*
    plasma protein binding, 21*t*
Chlorprothixene, 1211
Chlorthalidone, 1082–1083
Chlor-Trimeton. *See* Chlorpheniramine
Chlorzone Forte, 1232
Chlorzoxazone, 1225
    combined with acetaminophen, **1232**
    for low back pain, 558
Cholagogue, 131*t*
Cholchicine, 1236–1237

Cholecystographic agents, 685*t*
Cholecystokinetic ingredients, 120*t*
Cholecytokinase, 743
Choledyl. *See* Oxtriphylline
Cholera, 169
Cholesterol, serum levels, 357, 732
Cholestyramine, 1044
    drug interactions, 18
    drug-nutrient interactions, 108*t*
Choline magnesium trisalicylate, 29*t*
Cholinergic receptors, 35
Cholinergic stimulants, 1477
Choline salicylate, 29*t*, 1136–1137
Cholinesterase inhibitors, for dementia,
    655–656
Chronic obstructive pulmonary disease (COPD)
    assessment, 421
    characteristics, 420*t*
    drugs to avoid, 425
    in homeless population, 224–225
    nonpharmacologic therapy, 421
    pathogens, 424
    patient/caregiver information, 421–422
    pharmacotherapy, 422
      adverse reaction monitoring, 426*t*
      algorithm, 423*f*
      efficacy monitoring, 425
      follow-up for, 425
      goals, 420
      toxicity monitoring, 425
    risk factors, 420
    staging, 421*t*
Chronopharmacology, 7
Chronulac, 1317
Chrysanthemum parthenium (feverfew), 132*t*
Cibalith-S. *See* Lithium
Ciclopirox olamine, 1439
Cigarette smoking. *See* Smoking
Ciloxan. *See* Ciprofloxacin
Cimetidine, 1297–1298
    drug interactions, 26, 611*t*
    OTC status, 120*t*
*Cimicifuga racemosa* (black cohosh), 132
Cinobac. *See* Cinoxacin
Cinoxacin, 1017
Cipro. *See* Ciprofloxacin
Ciprofloxacin, 943–944, 1265–1266
    clearance, 29*t*
    for gonorrhea, 868, 869*t*
    interactions
      drug-food, 107*t*
      with tetracycline, 18
    for tuberculosis, 460
    for urethritis, 821*t*
Circadian rhythm theory of bipolar disorder,
    762*t*

**Cirrhosis**
  assessment, Pugh's criteria for, 47, 47*t*
  dosage regimen, 50
**Cisapride,** 19, 26, 106*t*, **1302**
**Citrate of Magnesia, 1311**
**Citrucel, 1311–1312**
**Citrucel Sugar Free, 1311–1312**
**Clarithromycin, 952–953**
  dosage calculations, pediatric, 189*t*
  drug-drug interactions, 106*t*
  for upper respiratory tract infections, 489*t*
**Claritin.** *See* **Loratadine**
**Clavulanic acid/amoxicillin,** 34, **962–963**
**Clearance**
  creatinine, 48–49
  drug, 29, 29*t*, 46
  inulin, 48
  total body drug, renal function and, 52, 52*f*
**Clemastine, 1412**
**Clemastine fumarate,** 120*t*
**Cleocin,** 881*t*, **1029**
**Cleocin T, 1427–1428**
**Clidinium bromide, 1292–1293**
**Climacteric,** 289. *See also* **Menopause**
**Climara, 1368**
**Clindamycin,** 881*t*, **1029**
**Clindamycin phosphate, 1427–1428**
*Clinical Pharmacology,* 90*t*
**Clinoril, 1130**
**Clioquinol, 1439**
**Clioquinol/hydrocortisone, 1470**
**Clistin.** *See* **Carbinoxamine**
**Clobetasol propionate, 1457**
**Clocortolone pivalate, 1458**
**Cloderm, 1458**
**Clofazimine,** 460, **994**
**Clomipramine,** 780, **1187**
**Clonazepam, 1143–1144**
**Clonidine, 1055**
  for attention deficit/hyperactivity disorder, 634
  for hypertension, 317
  for spasticity, 214
**Clorazepate dipotassium, 1144–1145, 1161**
**Cloroquine,** 170
**Closed-angle glaucoma,** 477
*Clostridium difficile* **pseudomembranous colitis,** 502
**Clotrimazole,** 120*t*, 121*t*, **979, 1439–1440**
**Clotting, normal mechanism,** 617
**Clove garlic (garlic),** 132*f*
**Cloxacillin sodium, 966**
**Cloxapen, 966**
**Clozapine, 1216–1217**
  for bipolar disorder, 763
  for Parkinson's disease, 667
**Clozaril.** *See* **Clozapine**

**Cluster headache,** 657, 658*t*, 659
**Coccidioidomycosis,** 452
**Codeine, 1408**
  combinations
    acetaminophen, **1100**
    acetaminophen/caffeine/butalbital, **1102**
    aspirin/caffeine/butalbital, **1103**
    fioricet, **1102**
    fiorinal, **1103**
    phenaphen, **1100**
  for common colds, 375
    efficacy monitoring, 377
    toxicity monitoring, 377
**Codeine sulfate, 1089–1090**
*Code of Federal Regulations,* 116
**Cogentin.** *See* **Benztropine**
**Co-Gesic, 1104**
**Cognex.** *See* **Tacrine**
**Cognitive impairments**
  in menopause, 290–291
  in multiple sclerosis, 643
  in traumatic head injury, 622, 628
**Coitus interruptus or withdrawal,** 266, 266t
**Colace, 1310–1311**
*Cola nitida* **(kola or cola;caffeine),** 132*f*
**ColBenemid, 1237–1238**
**Colchicine**
  combined with probenecid, **1237–1238**
  drug interactions, 615*t*
  for gout, 552
**Cold, common**
  assessment, 375–376
  etiology, 374
  herbal remedies, 134
  patient/caregiver information, 376
  pharmacotherapy, 375
    drug selection, 376–377
    goals, 375
    monitoring, 377
  prevention, 375*t*
  symptoms, 374–375
**Cold sores,** 579
**Colestid.** *See* **Colestipol**
**Colestipol,** 108*t*, **1044**
**Colistin M,** 430
**Colitis, herbal remedies,** 137, 144–145
**Colon motility stimulation,** 210
**Col-Probenecid, 1237–1238**
**Coly-Mycin S Otic, 1279**
**CoLyte, 1316–1317**
**Comedones,** 576
**Common cold.** *See* **Cold, common**
**Common nettle (nettle),** 132*f*
**Common warts,** 580
**Community-acquired pneumonia (CAP)**
  in adults and elderly, 434–436, 436

drug selection for, 437–440
goals for, 436
initiation of pharmacotherapy, time frame for, 436–437
mortality of, 434
nonpharmacologic therapy for, 436
pathogens in, 435–436, 435t
pretherapy assessment, 437, 437t–439t
risk for, 434–435
algorithm, 442f
pathogens, 435–436, 435t, 439t, 440t
pharmacotherapy
efficacy monitoring, 440–441
follow-up, 442–443
toxiicty monitoring, 441–442
**Community resources**
for homeless population, 225
for migrant workers, 225
**Comorbid illness**
with attention deficit/hyperactivity disorder, 631–632
with community-acquired pneumonia, 439–440
with obesity, 738
with stroke, 636
**Compazine, 1207–1208**
**Compliance.** See **Adherence**
**Compresses, herbal,** 130t
**Compulsive overeating,** 776
**Concentration gradient, absorption and,** 17
**Concentration problems, herbal remedies,** 139–141
**Condoms**
female, 258–259, 258t
male, 257–258, 258t
**Condylomata acuminata (genital warts),** 580, 583, 876–879
**Condylox, 1446**
**Congenital rubella syndrome,** 157–158
**Congestive heart failure**
ACE inhibitors for, 325–326
pharmacotherapy, in stroke management, 640
**Conjugated estrogens, 1366–1367**
combined with medroxyprogesterone acetate, **1373–1374**
for stress urinary incontinence, 815t
**Conjunctivitis,** 479–482, 480
**Constipation**
herbal remedies, 134–135
with neurogenic bowel, 209–210
from opioid usage, 232
pharmacotherapy, 502–504
during pregnancy, 249, 249t
**Contact dermatitis,** 589, 591
**Contact time, absorption and,** 17
**Contact urticaria,** 590
**Contemplation, in transtheoretical model of behavior change,** 72, 73

**Continuous ambulatory peritoneal dialysis (CAPD),** 54
**Contraception, implants, 1350–1351**
**Contraception.** See also **Oral contraceptives**
barrier methods, 257
cervical cap, 260
diaphragm, 259–260, 259t, 260t
female condoms, 258–259, 258t
intrauterine devices, 261–263, 262t–264t
male condoms, 257–258, 258t
spermicide, 260–261, 261t
sterilization, 263–265, 264t
coitus interruptus or withdrawal method, 266, 266t
defined, 255
for disabled women, 208
emergency or postcoital, 283–284
failure rates, 256t
fertility awareness methods, 264–265, 265t, 266t
future, 284
injections, **1351**
selection
factors in, 255–256, 256t
sexual history taking for, 256, 257t
sexually transmitted disease risk and, 256–257
**Control-L, 1452**
**Controlled-release transdermal systems,** 10f
**COPD.** See **Chronic obstructive pulmonary disease**
**Copolymer 1,** 646
**Cordarone.** See **Amiodarone**
**Cordran, 1463**
**Coreg, 1059**
**Corgard, 685t, 1063**
**Cornea**
abrasion, 473–475
nonpharmacologic therapy, 474
pharmacotherapy, 474–475
pretherapy assessment for, 473
functions, 473
**Coronary artery disease, risk factors,** 345
**Coronary heart disease (CHD)**
classification, 347t
coronary artery disease, atherosclerosis, 344–345
myocardial ischemia, 345–346
nonpharmacologic therapy, 346
obesity and, 732
outcomes management, 348–351
patient/caregiver information, 348
pharmacotherapy, 346
assessment for, 347–348
follow-up, 351
goals, 346
initiation, time frame for, 346–347
risk factors, 345
**Cortaid, 1466**

Cortef, 1466
Corticosporin otic suspension, 492
Corticosteroids
  for acne vulgaris, 578
  adrenal
    glucocorticoids, **1327–1333**
    mineralocorticoids, **1334**
  adverse events, 426*t*, 483, 591
  for allergic rhinitis, 370, 373, 374
  for asthma, 400–401
  for chemotherapy-associated nausea/vomiting, 498
  for chronic obstructive pulmonary disease, 424
  for chronic pain, 236
  combinations
    antifungal, **1473**
    neomycin, **1472**
  for croup, 386, 387
  for gout, 553
  half-life, 30
  for infectious mononucleosis, 919
  for inflammatory bowel disease, 507
  interactions with oral contraceptives, 277*t*
  for low back pain, 559
  monitoring, 531*t*
  for multiple sclerosis, 646
  onset of action, 38
  for osteoarthritis, 542–543
  for rheumatoid arthritis, 535
  topical, **1453–1473**
    for allergic rhinitis, 370
    combinations, **1470–1473**
    for psoriasis, 600
    for sinusitis, 380
    for vulvar dermatitis, 837
Corticotropin-releasing hormone (CRH), 696
Cortisol, 695
Cortisone, 1328
Cortisporin Otic, 1279
Cortone, 1328
*Corynebacterium diphtheriae*, 155
Cotazyme, 1304–1305
Cough suppressants
  for common colds, 375
  herbal, 135
Coumadin. *See* **Warfarin**
Counseling
  for drug therapy, 61
  lack of, for over-the-counter drugs, 116, 122
Counterirritation, for pain relief, 229
Covera-HS. *See* **Verapamil**
Cozaar, 1054
"Crabs," 882
Cradle cap, 590
Cranberry, 132*f*, 145
*Crataegus laevigata* (hawthorn), 132*f*
*Crataegus monogyna* (hawthorn), 132*f*

*Crataegus Oxyacantha* (hawthorn), 132*f*
Creatinine, serum levels, 49, 49*t*, 718
Creatinine clearance
  calculation, 48–49
  digoxin dosing and, 326–327, 326*t*
  glomerular filtration and, 26
  in renal impairment calculation, 441
Creon, 1304
CREST study, 264
M-Cresyl acetate/
        isopropanol/chlorbutanal/benzyl alco-
        hol/caster oil/propylene glycol, **1285**
Cresylate, **1285**
CRH (corticotropin-releasing hormone), 696
Crixavan, 1011
Crohn's disease
  agents for, **1318–1319**
  characteristics, 504–509
Crolom, **1273, 1393**
Cromolyn, **1273, 1393**
  for allergic rhinitis, 370, 372, 373, 374
  for asthma, 410
  intranasal, 370, 372
  OTC status, 121*t*
  toxicity, 412
Crotamiton, **1450**
Croup, 385–387
Crystodigin. *See* **Digitoxin**
CSA (Federal Controlled Substance Act), 79–80,
        80*t*
CTZ (chemoreceptor trigger zone), 498
Cultivate, **1463–1464**
Cultural factors, in medication-taking behavior,
        67–69
Cuprimine. *See* **Penicillamine**
Curaco aloe (aloe vera), 132*f*
Curretab. *See* **Medroxyprogesterone**
Cushing's syndrome
  ACTH-dependent, 697, 698*t*
  ACTH-independent, 697, 698*t*
  diagnostic algorithm, 698*f*
  signs/symptoms, 697, 699*t*
CVA. *See* **Cerebrovascular accident**
*Cyclanthera pedata* (caigua), 132*f*
Cyclizine, **1322**
Cyclobenzaprine, 558, **1225–1226**
Cyclophosphamide
  monitoring, 531*t*
  for multiple sclerosis, 646
  for rheumatoid arthritis, 537
Cycloserine, 460, **994–995**
Cyclosporin A
  drug-nutrient interactions and, 107*t*
  monitoring, 531*t*
  for rheumatoid arthritis, 537
Cyclothymia, 759

**Cycrin.** *See* **Medroxyprogesterone acetate**
**Cylert,** 635, **1223**
**Cyproheptadine, 1413**
  for anorexia nervosa, 780
  for eating disorders, 778
**Cystic fibrosis**
  with asthma, 444
  contraindicated drugs, 433, 434*t*
  drug selection, 429–433, 431*t*, 432*t*
  etiology, 426
  with heart disease, 444
  incidence, 425–426
  nonpharmacologic therapy, 427
  outcomes management, 429–434, 431*t*, 432*t*, 434*t*
  patient/caregiver information, 429
  pharmacotherapy, 427
    assessment for, 427, 428*t*, 429*t*
    efficacy monitoring, 433
    follow-up, 434
    goals for, 427
    initiation, time frame for, 427
    toxicity monitoring, 433–434
  with pneumonia, 444
  symptoms, 426–427
**Cystitis**
  asymptomatic *vs.* symptomatic, 802*t*
  incidence, 802–803
  pathogens, 801
  pharmacotherapy
    drug selection, 804–805, 806*t*
    follow-up, 807
    monitoring, 807
  during pregnancy, 247, 248*t*
  symptoms, 801
  uncomplicated *vs.* complicated, 802*t*
**Cystospaz-M, 1294**
**Cytochrome P-450 enzymes**
  acetylation differences, 24
  induction, 24
  inhibition, 24
  isoenzymes
    inducers of, 25*f*, 26
    inhibitors of, 25*t*–26*f*, 26
  phase I hepatic reactions, 46
  terminology, 24
**Cytomegalovirus, pharmacotherapeutic agents**
    **for,** 1015–1017
**Cytotec, 1299**
**Cytovene, 1015**
**Cytoxan.** *See* **Cyclophosphamide**

**D**

**DAI (diffuse axonal injury),** 621, 622
**Dalmane, 1175**
**Damason, 1105**

**Danazol**
  for adenomyosis, 855
  for endometriosis, 855
**Dantrium.** *See* **Dantrolene**
**Dantrolene, 1226–1227**
  for low back pain, 559
  for spasticity, 214
**Dapsone, 1027–1028**
**Daranide, 1075–1076**
**Daraprim, 990–991**
**Darvocet-N, 1111**
**Darvon, 1112–1113**
**DAW (dispense as written),** 12
**Daypro, 1126**
**Dayto Himbin, 1480**
**DCCT (Diabetes Control and Complications**
    **Trial** ), 710, 711
**ddI (didanosine),** 107*t*, **1005–1006**
**Debrox, 1282**
**Decadron.** *See* **Dexamethasone**
**Decadron phosphate, 1460–1461**
**Declomycin.** *See* **Demeclocycline**
**Decoctions, herbal,** 130*t*
**Decongestants**
  adverse effects, 9
  for allergic rhinitis, 370, 372, 373, 374
  for common colds, 375, 376, 377
  intranasal, 372
  with OTC status, 120*t*
  for sinusitis, 380
  topical, 9
**Deep vein thrombosis (DVT)**
  after stroke, 641
  characteristics, 341*t*
  oral contraceptive usage and, 274
**Defibrotide,** 343
**Dehydroepiandrosterone sulfate (DHEAS),** 695
**Delavirdine (DLV), 1009**
**Delsym.** *See* **Dextromethorphan**
**Delta-Cortef.** *See* **Prednisolone**
**Delta opioid receptor,** 231
**Deltasone,** 272*t*, **1331–1332**
**Delta-9-tetrahydrocannabinol (THC),** 105, 108
**Demadex, 1078**
**Demecarium, 1259**
**Demeclocycline, 976–977**
**Dementia**
  after stroke, 641
  Alzheimer's.*See* **Alzheimer's disease**
  assessment, pretherapy, 654–655
  clinical signs/symptoms, 652
  defined, 652
  etiology, 652–653, 653*t*
  nonpharmacologic therapy, 653–654
  in Parkinson's disease, 663
  patient/caregiver information, 655

Dementia (*cont.*)
  pharmacotherapy, 653
    drug selection for, 654, 655–657
    follow-up, 657
    goals, 653
    initiation, time frame for, 654
    monitoring, 657
    in Parkinson's disease, 667
**Demerol.** *See* **Meperidine**
**Demulcent,** 131*t*
**Demulen,** 1340
**Dental rinse ingredients, with OTC status,** 118*t*
**Depakene.** *See* **Valproic acid**
**Depakote,** 1158–1159
**Depen.** *See* **Penicillamine**
**Dephenhydramine,** 119*t*
**Depitol.** *See* **Carbamazepine**
**Depolarization,** 329, 329*t*
**Deponit,** 1036
**Depo-Provera (DMPA),** 280–282, 281*t*
**Depot injections,** 11
**Depot medroxyprogesterone acetate (DMPA),**
  280–282, 281*t*
**Depression**
  after stroke, 641
  assessment/history taking, 752–753
  atypical, 748
  in children/adolescents, 748
  herbal remedies.*See* **St. John's wort**
  incidence, 747
  manic.*See* **Bipolar disorder**
  in menopause, 290–291
  from oral contraceptive usage, 272*t*
  pathophysiology, 749, 751*t*
  patient/caregiver information, 753, 754*t*
  pharmacotherapy, 749
    algorithm, 750*f*
    drug selection, 751–752, 753–757
    efficacy monitoring, 757–758
    follow-up, 759
    goals, 749, 751
    initiation, time frame for, 751
    in Parkinson's disease, 667
    toxicity monitoring, 758–759
  resources, 755*t*
  symptoms, 747–748
  in traumatic head injury, 628–629
  types, 748
**Derma-Smoothe,** 1461–1462
**Dermatitis**
  pharmacotherapy, 590–592
  types, 589–590
  vulvar, 836–837
**Dermatologic disorders**
  arthropod bites/stings, 585–586, 587
  burns.*See* **Burns**

  dermatitis.*See* **Dermatitis**
  lice infestation, 587–589
  of migrant workers, 224
  pediculosis, 585
  pityriasis rosea, 599–601
  psoriasis, 598–601
  scabies, 584–585, 587–589
  skin infections.*See* **Skin infections**
  sunburn.*See* **Sunburn**
**Dermatop,** 1468–1469
**Dermatophytes,** 572–573
**Desenex,** 1448–1449
**DESI (Drug Efficacy Study Implementation),**
  114
**Designer estrogens,** 299–300
**Desipramine,** 1188
  adverse events, 635
  for anorexia nervosa, 780
  for depression, 755–756
**Desogen,** 1343
**Desogestrel**
  combined with ethinyl estradiol, **1343**
  in oral contraceptives, 268–269, 268*t*, 269*t*
**Desonide,** 1458–1459
**Desonide/acetic acid/propylene glycol,** 1283
**DesOwen,** 1458–1459
**Desoximetasone,** 1459
**Desyrel.** *See* **Trazodone**
**Desyrel Dividose.** *See* **Trazodone**
**Developmental factors, in drug metabolism,** 24
**DEXA (dual-energy x-ray absorptimetry),** 296,
  546
**Dexamethasone,** 1328–1329, 1391
  intranasal, **1422–1423**
  ophthalmic, **1276**
  topicall, **1460**
**Dexamethasone sodium phosphate,**
  1460–1461
**Dexatrim Pre-Meal.** *See* **Phenylpropanolamine**
**Dexbrompheniramine maleate,** 119*t*
**Dexchlorpheniramine,** 120*t*, **1413**
**Dexfenfluramine,** 739, 740
**Dextroamphetamine,** 626
**Dextromethorphan,** 375, 377, **1408–1409**
**Dextrorotary enantiomers,** 35
**DFA-TP (direct fluorescent antibody test-**
  *Treponema pallidum*)**,** 865
**DHA (dihydroxyacetone),** 596
**DHC Plus Capsules,** 1106
**DHEAS (dehydroepiandrosterone sulfate),** 695
**Diabeta.** *See* **Glyburide**
**Diabetes Control and Complications Trial**
  **(DCCT),** 710, 711
**Diabetes mellitus**
  assessment/history taking, 714–715, 715*t*
  classification, 709–710

clinical characteristics, 709
coronary artery disease risk and, 345
in homeless population, 224
nonpharmacologic therapy, 713
oral contraceptive usage and, 283
pharmacotherapy, 713–714, 715–716
  alpha-glucosidase inhibitors, 716–717
  biguanides, 717–718
  drug selection for, 711
  goals for, 710, 711–712, 714
  initation, time frame for, 714
  insulin.*See* **Insulin**
  meglitinides, 725
  open-loop, 710
  rationale for, 710–711
  sulfonylureas, 725–727
  thiazolidinediones, 727–728
pregnancy and, 721
self-management, 712–713
stroke risk and, 636
type 1, 709–710
  "honeymoon" period, 721
  insulin dosing for, 721
  insulin for, 719
  treatment goals for, 711
type 2, 710
  insulin dosing for, 721
  insulin for, 719–720
  treatment goals for, 711–712
**Diabetic ketoacidosis (DKA),** 725
**Diabinese.** *See* **Chlorpropamide**
**Dialose,** 1310
**Diamox,** 29*t*, **1075,** 1153
**DIAPERS,** 209
**Diaphoretic,** 131*t*
**Diaphragms, contraceptive,** 259–260, 259*t*,
  260*t*
**Diarrhea**
  classification, 499
  with neurogenic bowel, 209–210
  nonpharmacologic therapy, 500
  patient/caregiver information, 501
  pharmacotherapy, 499–500
    assessment/history taking for, 500–501
    drug selection for, 501–502
    efficacy monitoring, 502
    goals for, 500
    initiation, time frame for, 500
  traveler's, 170
**Diastolic dysfunction,** 321
**Diazepam,** 1145
  for anxiety disorders, 772–773, **1161–1162**
  apparent volume of distribution, 23*t*
  contraindications, 773
  GABA receptor binding, 38
  for insomnia, 786*t*

  for nonbacterial prostatitis, 824*t*
  plasma protein binding, 21*t*
  skeletal muscle relaxant, **1227**
  for spasticity, 213
**Dichlorphenamide, 1075–1076**
**Diclofenac, 1127, 1274**
**Dicloxacillin, 967**
**Dicyclomine, 1293**
**Didanosine (ddl),** 107*t*, **1005–1006**
**Didrex,** 740, **1481**
**Didronel.** *See* **Etidronate**
**Diet**
  creatinine serum levels and, 49*t*
  for diabetes mellitus, 713
  for hyperlipidemia, 356, 357
  lactose-free, 519–520
  modifications, for weight loss, 736
  for premenstrual syndrome, 847
**Dietary Supplement Health and Education Act,**
  128
**Diethylpropion, 739, 1482**
**Difenoxin/atropine sulfate, 1306**
**Diffuse axonal injury (DAI),** 621, 622
**Diflorasone diacetate, 1461**
**Diflucan.** *See* **Fluconazole**
**Diflunisal, 1137**
**Digestive enzymes, 1303, 1303–1305**
**Digitoxin, 1074**
**Digoxin, 1073–1074**
  absorption, 17
  apparent volume of distribution, 23*t*
  for atrial fibrillation, 336
  bioequivalence, 11
  clearance, 29*t*
  distribution in kidney disease, 51
  drug-food interactions, 107*t*
  for heart failure, 326–327, 326*t*
  pharmacologic effects, 37
  for renally impaired patient, 7
**Dihydrocodeine, combinations**
  acetaminophen/caffeine, **1106**
  aspirin/caffeine, **1107–1108**
**Dihydroxyacetone (DHA),** 596
**Dihydroxyaluminum sodium carbonate,**
  **1287–1288**
**Dilacor XR.** *See* **Diltiazem**
**Dilantin.** *See* **Phenytoin**
**Dilatrate-SR,** 1034
**Dilaudid.** *See* **Hydromorphone**
**Dilor.** *See* **Dyphylline**
**Diltiazem, 1067–1068**
  for atrial fibrillation, 336
  bioavailability, 19*t*
  drug interactions, 26
**Dimenhydrinate, 1323**
**Dimetabs, 1323**

Dimetane. *See* **Brompheniramine**
Dimetapp, 191*t*
Diovan, 1054
Dipenhydramine/acetaminophen, 1183–1184
Dipentum, 1318
Diphenhydramine
    antiemetic/antivertigo, 497, **1323**
    antihistamines, **1414, 1437**
    antitussives, **1409**
    for insomnia, 786*t*, **1183**
    OTC status, 119*t*
    for Parkinson's disease, **1247**
Diphenoxylate/atropine sulfate, 1306–1307
Diphenylan. *See* **Phenytoin**
Diphenylheptanes, 1095–1097
Diphtheria immunizations, 153*t*, 155–156
Dipivefrin, 1259
Diprolene, 1454–1455
Diprosone, 1456
Dipyridamole, 1072
Direct-current cardioversion (CDD), 334–335
Direct fluorescent antibody test-*Treponema*
        *pallidum* (DFA-TP), 865
Disability, individuals with, 216
    Americans with Disabilities Act and, 205
    autonomic dysreflexia in, 211, 212*t*, 213
    cognitive issues, 207
    heterotopic ossification, 211
    latex allergy and, 214–215
    mobility issues, 210–211
    neurogenic bowel/bladder issues, 209–210
    prescriptive considerations, 215
    primary health care issues for, 205–207
    sexuality issues, 207–208
    spasticity and, 213–214
    women, oral contraceptives for, 283
    women's health issues, 208
Disalcid, 1139
Disopyramide, 21*t*, 338, **1038**
Dissociation constant, 35
Distribution
    aging and, 199–200, 200*t*
    alterations, 21–22
    children, 183*t*, 185
    defined, 19
    drug-drug interactions, 22–23, 22*f*, 104–105
    factors in
        blood flow, 19–20
        plasma protein binding, 20–21, 20*f*, 21*t*
        special membrane barriers, 20
        tissue storage, 21
    infants, 183*t*, 184–185
    neonatal, 183*t*, 184
    during pregnancy, 240, 240*t*
    in renal impairment, 51
    volume, 23, 23*t*

Disulfiram
    for alcohol abuse, 790
    interaction with alcohol, 108
Ditropan, 209, **1476**
Diucardin, 1083–1084
Diurese, 1087
Diuretics
    carbonic anhydrase inhibitors, **1075–1076**
    defined, 131*t*
    for heart failure, 324–325
    for hypertension, 315, 316–317
    with laxative herbs, 742
    loop, **1077–1078**
    potassium-sparing, **1079–1080**
    for premenstrual syndrome, 849–850
    thiazide/thiazide-like, **1081–1087**
Diuril, 1082
Divalproex sodium, 1158–1159
Dizmiss, 1323–1324
Dizziness. *See also* **Vertigo**
    defined, 648
    from oral contraceptive usage, 272*t*
DKA (diabetic ketoacidosis), 725
DLV (delavirdine), 1009
DMPA (depot medroxyprogesterone acetate),
        280–282, 281*t*
Doan's pills, 1137–1138
Documentation, of drug therapy, 60
Docusate, 130–1311, 815*t*
Dolacte, 1104
Dolene. *See* **Propoxyphene**
Dolobid, 1137
Dolophine, 232, **1095–1096**
Domeboro tablets, 1474
Donepezil, 656, **1234**
Donnagel, 1308
Donnazyme, 1304
Donovanosis, 875–876
Dopamine, 20
Dopamine agonists, for Parkinson's disease,
        665–666
Dopamine blockers, thyroid function and, 685*t*
Dopar. *See* **Levodopa**
Doral, 1175–1176
Dorcol. *See* **Pseudoephedrine**
Doriden, 1181
Dormin Caplets. *See* **Diphenhydramine**
Dornase alfa, 1394
Doryx. *See* **Doxycycline**
Dorzolamide, 1259–1260
Dose-response relationships
    drug-receptor binding, 32–33, 33*f*
    ligands and, 33–35
Double depression, 748
Dovonex. *See* **Calcipotriene**
Down-regulation, 38

Doxazosin, **1058**
  for benign prostatic hyperplasia, 829*t*
  for nonbacterial prostatitis, 824*t*
Doxepin, **1166–1167, 1189, 1437**
  for depression, 755
Doxycycline, **976–977**
  for chlamydia, 871, 872*t*
  for epididymitis, 818*t*
  for granuloma inguinale, 876
  for lymphogranuloma venereum, 875
  for nonbacterial prostatitis, 824*t*
  for pelvic inflammatory disease, 881*t*
  for syphilis, 866*t*
  for urethritis, 821*t*
Doxylamine, 118*t*, 120*t*, **1182–1183**
Dramamine, **1323**
Dri/Ear, **1282**
Dristan. *See* Oxymetazoline
Dronabinol, 498, **1325**
Droperidol, 498
Drug abuse, 62–63, 785–786
Drug action. *See* Drug response
DrugDex CD-Rom, 89*t*
Drug Efficacy Study Implementation (DESI),
  114
*Drug Evaluations Annual*, 87*t*
*Drug Facts and Comparisons*, 86*t*
**Drug Facts and Comparisons CD-Rom**, 89*t*
**Drug information centers**, 92
**Drug Information Fulltext CD-Rom**, 89*t*
**Drug information web sites**, 92, 93*t*
*Drug Interaction Facts*, 86*t*, 90*t*
**Drug interactions**
  absorption alterations from, 18–19
  avoiding, 109
  clinical outcome, 109
  distribution, 22–23, 22*f*
  drug-disease, 105
  drug-drug, 104–105, 106*t*
    distribution, 104–105
    pharmacodynamic, 105
    pharmacokinetic, 104
  drug-food, 105, 107*t*–108*t*
  drug-social habit, 105, 108–109
  excretion, 28–29, 29*t*
  management, 109
  metabolism, 25*t*–26*t*, 26
  oral contraceptives, 276, 277*t*
  pharmacodynamic, 39–40
*Drug Interactions and Updates Quarterly*, 86*t*
**Drug Master Plus software**, 89*t*
*Drug Newsletter*, 89*t*
**Drug-receptor binding**, 32
**Drug response (action)**
  duration, 8, 8*f*
    half-life and, 30
  onset, 8, 8*f*
  phases, 7–8, 8*f*
  receptors and, 34–35, 34*f*
  termination, 8, 8*f*
  variability, 7–8, 8*f*
**Drugs.** *See also specific drugs*
  abuse of, 62–63
  C-II, filling prescriptions for, 81–82
  C-III, filling prescriptions for, 82
  C-IV, filling prescriptions for, 82
  controlled, schedules for, 79–80, 80*t*
  inappropriate, 62
  legend, 79
  misuse of, 61–62
  object, 104
  over-the-counter, 79
  plasma concentration, 8–9, 8*f*
  precipitant, 104
  regulatory control of, 79–83, 80*t*
  teratogenic, 241, 2424
  unnecessary, 62
*Drugs Available Abroad. A Guide to
    Therapeutic Drugs Available and
    Approved Outside the U.S.*, 87*t*
*Drugs in Pregnancy and Lactation*, 87*t*
**Dual-energy x-ray absorptimetry (DEXA)**, 296,
    546
**Ducolax**, 9
**Duocet**, 1104
**Duphalac**, 1317
**Duragesic**, 1094
**Duration.** *See* Oxymetazoline
**Durham-Humphrey Amendment**, 79,
    114
**Duricef**, 188*t*, **933**
**DVT.** *See* **Deep vein thrombosis**
**Dycill**, 967
**Dyclonine**, 119
**Dynacirc**, 1068
**Dynapen**, 967
**Dyphylline**, 1400
**Dyrenium**, 1080
**Dysfunctional uterine bleeding**, 843–844
**Dysmenorrhea**
  herbal remedies, 135–136
  from oral contraceptive usage, 272*t*
  pathophysiology, 851
  patient/caregiver information, 852, 852*t*
  pharmacotherapy, 852–853
  primary *vs.* secondary, 851–852
**Dyspareunia**, 856, 859
**Dyspepsia, from nonsteroidal antiinflammatory
    drugs**, 534
**Dysrhythmias.** *See* **Arrhythmias**
**Dysthymic disorder**, 748

E

**Ear disorders**
   middle ear inflammation.*See* **Otitis media**
   otitis externa, 491–492
**Ear-Dry, 1282**
**EarSol HC, 1284**
**Ear tubes, for otitis media,** 491
**Easprin.** *See* **Aspirin**
**Eating disorders**
   assessment/history taking, 778–779
   incidence, 776
   nonpharmacologic therapy, 777–778
   pathogenesis, 777
   patient/caregiver information, 779, 779*t*
   pharmacotherapy, 776–777
      drug selection, 778, 779–780
      follow-up, 781
      goals, 777
      initiation, time frame for, 778
      monitoring, 780–781
**ECG.** *See* **Electrocardiogram**
**Echinacea,** 132*f*, 134
**Echocardiogram,** 323
**Echothiophate,** 1260
**EC-Naprosyn.** *See* **Naproxen**
**Econazole nitrate,** 1441–1442
**Econopred Plus,** 1277–1278, 1332
**Ecotrin.** *See* **Aspirin**
**Ecthyma,** 570, 571–572
**Eczematous dermatitis,** 589
**Edecrin,** 1077
**Education**
   of health care consumers, 67
   patient, 61
**EEG (electroencephalogram),** 670
**Effective refractory period (ERP),** 329
**Effexor.** *See* **Venlafaxine**
**EIB (exercise-induced bronchospasm),** 400,
   409–410
**Elavil.** *See* **Amitriptyline**
**Eldepryl.** *See* **Selegiline**
**Elderberry (elder),** 132*f*, 134
**Elderly**
   accidental poisonings, 202
   with community-acquired pneumonia, 440
   compliance problems, 61
   with congestive heart failure, 61
   contraindicated drugs, 202*t*
   hypertension and, 314
   medication issues
      adherence, 201
      adverse drug events, 201
      polypharmacy, 201
**Electric fetal heart monitoring, for pregnant**
   **patient with pneumonia,** 450*t*

**Electrocardiogram (ECG)**
   arrhythmias, 334
   for heart failure, 323
   rheumatoid arthritis, 529
**Electroencephalogram (EEG),** 670
**Electrolyte theory of bipolar disorder,** 762*t*
**Electrophysiologic testing,** 334
**Eleuthero (Siberian ginseng),** 132*f*, 136
**Elimination, drug**
   by dialysis, 53–54
   dose-dependent kinetics, 31
   in hepatic impairment, 45
   by hepatic metabolism, 46, 46*t*
   in kidney disease, 51–52
   in renal impairment, 45
   steady state, 31, 31*f*
**Elimination half-life,** 29–30, 30*f*
**Elimite.** *See* **Permethrin**
**Elixophyllin.** *See* **Theophylline**
**Elocon,** 1468
**Emergency contraception,** 283–284
**Emetic,** 131*t*
**EMLA cream, pediatric usage,** 192–193
**Emmenagogue,** 131*t*
**Emollients**
   for constipation, 504
   defined, 131*t*
**Empirin.** *See* **Aspirin**
**Empirin/codeine,** 1101
**Emulsoil,** 1308
**Enalapril,** 23*t*, 1050
**Enantiomers**
   dextrorotary, 35
   levorotary, 35
**Encainide,** 1038–1039
**Endep.** *See* **Amitriptyline**
**End Lice,** 1452
**Endocrine system.** *See also* **Thyroid gland**
   adrenal cortex.*See* **Adrenal cortex**
   disorders, diabetes mellitus. *See* **Diabetes mellitus**
   function, 683
   hypothalamic-pituitary-thyroid axis, 683–684, 684*f*
**Endolor,** 1119
**Endometrial biopsy, in menopause,** 296
**Endometrial cancer, oral contraceptive usage**
   **and,** 275
**Endometriosis**
   assessment/history taking, 854
   nonpharmacologic therapy, 854–856
   pharmacotherapy, 854–856
   sites, 853–854
**End-stage renal disease (ESRD),** 50
   anemia of, 616, 616*t*
   dialysis, 53–54
**Enduron.** *See* **Methylclothiazide**
**Enemas,** 504, 1316–1317

**Enkaid.** *See* **Encainide**
**Enovid,** 1374–1375
**Enoxacin,** 107*t,* 944
**Enteral feedings, drug-nutrient interactions and,** 107*t*
**Enteric-coated preparations**
  gastrointestinal irritation and, 12
  plasma profiles, 9, 10*f*
**Enterohepatic recirculation (recycling),** 46
  excretion and, 27, 28*f*
  interruption, 29
**Entozyme,** 1304
**Environmental factors, in drug metabolism,** 24
**Environmental theory of bipolar disorder,** 762*t*
**Enzymes**
  cytochrome P-450.*See* **Cytochrome P-450 enzymes**
  for drug metabolism, 24
  hepatic, 45–46
    drug metabolizing, 46
  transmembranous, 38
*Ephedra* **(ma huang),** 128, 132*f,* 133–134, 741
**Ephedrine,** 1396, 1402–1403
  excretion, 29*t*
  OTC status, 118*t*
**Epididymitis**
  assessment/history taking, 816*t,* 817*t*
  nonsexually-transmitted, 815, 816–817, 818*t*
  pathogens, 813, 815
  patient/caregiver information, 818*t*
  pharmacotherapy, 815–817, 818*t*
  sexually-transmitted, 815, 816, 818*t*
  symptoms, 815
**Epifrin.** *See* **Epinephrine**
**Epilepsy**
  classification, 668–669, 668*t*
  development, after stroke, 640
  oral contraceptive usage and, 283
  seizures.*See* **Seizures**
**Epinephrine,** 1260–1261, 1397, 1403
  for allergic drug response, 915*t*
  nebulized racemic, for croup, 386, 387
**L-Epinephrine,** 386
**Epipen,** 916*t*
**Epitol.** *See* **Carbamazepine**
**Epivir,** 1006
**Epley maneuver,** 650
**Epson Salt,** 1311
**Epstein-Barr virus,** 918
**Equagesic tablets,** 1116–1117
**Equanil,** 771, **1168**
**Equilibrium dissociation constant ($K_D$),** 35
**Ercaf,** 1241–1242
**Erectile dysfunction**
  agents for, **1479–1480**
  assessment/history taking, 830, 831*t,* 832*t*

  etiology, 830, 830*t*
  incidence/prevalence, 830
  patient/caregiver information, 831–832
  pharmacotherapy, 830–831
    drug selection, 832
    follow-up, 833
    goals, 831
    initiation, time frame for, 831
    monitoring, 832–833
  terminology, 829–830
**Erection, penile,** 830
**Ergoloid mesylates,** 1234
**Ergostat,** 1239
**Ergotamine/caffeine,** 1241–1242
**Ergotamine tartrate,** 1239
**Ericaceae (bearberry),** 132*f*
**ERT.** *See* **Estrogen replacement therapy**
**Erysipelas,** 570
**Erythema infectiosum,** 582
**Erythrocin stearate.** *See* **Erythromycin stearate**
**Erythrodermic psoriasis,** 598
**Erythromycin,** 1266, 1428, 1442
  for acne vulgaris, 578
  apparent volume of distribution, 23*t*
  combinations, sulfisoxazole, 489*t*
  dosage calculations, pediatric, 189*t*
  for granuloma inguinale, 876
  interactions
    drug-drug, 106*t*
    with oral contraceptives, 277*t*
  for lymphogranuloma venereum, 875
  for nonbacterial prostatitis, 824*t*
  for pharyngitis, 383*t*
  for pneumonia, 445
  for syphilis, 866*t*
  for upper respiratory tract infections, 489*t*
**Erythromycin base,** 953–954
  for chlamydia, 872*t*
  drug-food interactions, 107*t*
  for urethritis, 821*t*
**Erythromycin estolate,** 384, **954–955**
**Erythromycin ethylsuccinate,** 956–957
  for chlamydia, 872*t*
  combinations
    acetyl sulfisoxazole, 189*t*
    sulfisoxazole, 189*t,* **973**
  dosage calculations, pediatric, 189*t*
  for pharyngitis, 384
  for urethritis, 821*t*
**Erythromycin stearate,** 107*t,* **955–956**
**Erythropoiesis,** 605–606
**Erythropoietin**
  for anemia with renal failure, 616, 616*t*
  elimination by dialysis, 53
  production, 605
  recombinant, 605

Eryzole, 189*t*, **973**
Eserine, **1262**
Esgic, **1119**
Esidrix, **1083**
Eskalith. *See* **Lithium**
Eskalith CR. *See* **Lithium**
Esophagitis, erosive, 12
ESRD. *See* **End-stage renal disease**
Essential fatty acids, drug-food interactions, 107*t*
Estazolam, 784, **1174**
Esterified estrogens, **1367**
Estinyl. *See* **Ethinyl estradiol**
Estolate, 383*t*
Estrace, **1368**
Estraderm, **1368**
Estradiol, **1368**
Estradiol transdermal system, **1368**
Estratab, **1367**
Estrates H.S., **1376**
Estratest, **1376**
Estrogen replacement therapy (ERT)
 contraindications, 294–295
 decision-making, 292–293
 follow-up, 301–302
 for hyperlipidemia, 360
 monitoring
  for efficacy, 300–301
  for toxicity, 301
 for osteoporosis, 547
 problems with, 299
 risks, 296–297
 selection of appropriate agent, 298–299
 short-term memory and, 291
 side effects, 297
 transdermal, 298–299, **1368**
Estrogens, **1366–1371**. *See also specific estrogens*
 for acne vulgaris, 578
 combinations
  androgens, **1376**
  progestins, **1373–1375**
 for dementia, 656
 designer, 299–300
 in menopause, 289
 for multiple sclerosis, 646
 in oral contraceptives, 267–268, 268*t*
 with progestin.*See* **Hormone replacement therapy**
 replacement therapy.*See* **Estrogen replacement therapy**
 serum levels
  in amenorrhea, 841
  for hormone replacement therapy monitoring, 301
 for stress urinary incontinence, 815*t*
 thyroid function and, 685*t*

Estropipate, **1368–1369**
Estrovis, **1370**
Ethacrynic acid, **1077**
Ethambutol, **995–996**
Ethanimate, **1180–1181**
Ethchlorvynol, **1180**
Ethinyl estradiol, **1369**
 combinations
  ethynodiol diacetate, **1340**
  levonorgestrel, **1344**
 in oral contraceptives, 267–268, 268*t*
Ethionamide, 460, **996**
Ethmozine, 338, **1040**
Ethnicity
 of health care consumer, 66–67
 medication-taking behavior and, 67–69
Ethopropazine, **1247–1248**
Ethosuximide, 676, **1151**
Ethotoin, **1146–1147**
Ethylsuccinate, 383*t*
Ethynodiol diacetate, in oral contraceptives, 268–269, 268*t*, 269*t*
Ethynodiol diacetate/ethinyl estradiol, **1340**
Etidronate, 107*t*, **1378–1379**
Etodolac, **1127–1128**
Etrafon. *See* **Perphenazine/amitriptyline**
Etretinate, 601, **1431–1432**
Eurax, **1450**
European angelica (angelica), 132*f*
European Working Party on Hypertension in the Elderly, 316
Euthyroid, **1385–1386**
Euthyroid hyperthroxinemia, 685*t*
Evac-Q-Mag, **1311**
Evac-U-Gen, **1312–1313**
Evac-U-Lax, **1312–1313**
*Evaluations of Drug Interactions*, 86*t*
Evening primrose oil, 132*f*, 141
Evista, 300, **1377**
Exanthema subitum (roseola), 582
Excedrin, **1113**
Excedrin PM, **1183–1184**
Excretion
 biliary, 26
 clearance, 29, 29*t*
 clinical implications of pharmacokinetics, 31–33
 defined, 26
 determining factors, 26–27, 28*f*
 drug interactions, 28–29, 29*t*
 enterohepatic recirculation and, 27, 28*f*
 infants, 183*t*, 185
 neonatal, 183*t*, 184
 during pregnancy, 240, 240*t*
 renal, 27*f*
Exelderm, **1447**

**Exercise**
absorption and, 17
creatinine serum levels and, 49*t*
for hyperlipidemia, 356
for hypertension, 312
training, for cystic fibrosis, 427
for weight loss, 736–737
**Exercise-induced bronchospasm (EIB),** 400,
409–410
**Ex-Lax, 1312–1313**
**Exna, 1081–1082**
**Expectancy-value theory,** 71
**Expectorants, 1424**
for chronic obstructive pulmonary disease, 424
for common colds, 375, 376
defined, 131*t*
**Experimental agents, for osteoarthritis,** 543
**Exsel, 1434–1435**
**Extracellular volume**
decreased, 313
increased, 313
**Extracts, herbal,** 130*t*
**Extra-Strenth Tylenol PM, 1183–1184**
**Eye**
disorders
conjunctivitis, 479–482
corneal abrasion, 473–475
glaucoma, 477–479, 478*t*
uveitis, 482–483
involvement, in rheumatoid arthritis, 529
patching, for corneal abrasion, 474
**Eyelid disorders,** 475–477

F

**F.** *See* **Bioavailability**
**Falls (accidental), preventing,** 545*f*
**Famciclovir,** 873, 874, 874*t*, **1003**
**Familial hemiplegia, migraine headache and,**
659
**Family**
adherence and, 74
teaching tips for, 194*t*
**Famotidine, 1298–1299**
OTC status, 120*t*
for peptic ulcer disease, 511
potency, 32–33
**FAMs (fertility awareness methods),** 264–265,
265*t*, 266*t*
**Famvir.** *See* **Famciclovir**
**Fansidar, 992–993**
**Fast channel,** 329
**Fastin.** *See* **Phentermine**
**Fatigue**
herbal remedies, 136
in multiple sclerosis, 647

**Fatty streak lesions,** 345
**FDA.** *See* **Food and Drug Administration**
**FDCA (Federal Food, Drug and Cosmetic Act),**
79, 114, 122
**Febrifuge,** 131*t*
**Federal Controlled Substance Act (CSA),** 79–80,
80*t*
**Federal Food, Drug and Cosmetic Act (FDCA),**
79, 114, 122
*Federal Register,* 116
**Feen-a-mint, 1312–1313**
**Felbamate, 1154–1155**
interaction with oral contraceptives, 277*t*
for seizures, 676
**Felbatol.** *See* **Felbamate**
**Feldene.** *See* **Piroxicam**
**Felodipine,** 328, **1068**
**Felty's syndrome,** 529
**Female orgasmic disorder,** 856
**Femcet, 1119**
**Femoral artery occlusive disease,** 340*t*
**Fempatch, 1368**
**Femstat, 1438–1439**
**Fenamates, 1132–1133**
**Fenfluramine,** 739, 740, **1483**
**Fenfluramine/phentermine,** 739, 740
**Fenoprofen, 1122**
**Fentanyl, 1094**
**Ferritin, serum,** 608
**Ferrous fumarate,** 609–610, 610*t*
**Ferrous gluconate,** 609–610, 610*t*
**Ferrous sulfate,** 609–610, 610*t*
**Fertility awareness methods (FAMs),** 264–265,
265*t*, 266*t*
**Fertility control.** *See* **Contraception**
**Fetal alcohol syndrome (FAS),** 244
**Fever blisters,** 579
**Feverfew,** 132*f*, 137–138
**Fexofenadine,** 370, **1420**
**Fexofenadine/pseudoephedrine,** 370
**Fiber, dietary,** 742
**Fiberall, 1313**
**FiberCon, 1313**
**Fibric acids,** 360
**Fibrillation, ventricular,** 331*t*
**Fibrinogen, in thrombus formation,** 617
**Fibrous plaque lesions,** 345
**Filtration,** 14–15, 15*f*
**Finasteride,** 827, 828–829, 829*t*, **1337**
**Fiorgen PF, 1120–1121**
**Fioricet, 1119**
**Fioricet/codeine, 1102**
**Fiorinal, 1120–1121**
**Fiorinal/codeine, 1103**
**First-degree burn,** 595
**First-order kinetics,** 31

First-pass metabolism, 17, 19*t*
Five-fingers (ginseng), 132*f*
Five-leafed ginseng (ginseng), 132*f*
"The Five Toos," 99
Flagyl. *See* Metronidazole
Flarex, 1276–1277
Flatulence
    herbal remedies, 136
    pharmacotherapy, 515–516
Flat warts, 580
Flavoxate, 1476
Flecainide, 335, 1039
Fleet, 1311
    bisacodyl, 1316
    flavored castor oil, 1308
    mineral oil, 1316
    phospha-soda, 1314
    therevac, 1316
Flexaphen, 1232
Flexeril, 558, 1225–1226
Flonase. *See* Fluticasone
Floppy mitral valve. *See* Mitral valve prolapse
Florinef, 1334
Florone, 1461
Flovent. *See* Fluticasone
Floxin, 948
FLQN. *See* Fluoroquinolones
Fluconazole, 887, 888, 979–981
5-Flucytosine, 49*t*
Fludrocortisone, 1334
Flumadine. *See* Rimantadine
Flunisolide, 402*t*, 1391, 1423
Fluocinolone acetonide, 1461–1462
Fluocinonide, 1462–1463
Fluonex, 1462–1463
Fluonid, 1461–1462
Fluorometholone, 1276–1277
Fluor-Op. *See* Fluorometholone
Fluoroquinolones (FLQN), 943–950
    absorption, in renal impairment, 50
    for community-acquired pneumonia, 438
    for cystitis, 806*t*
    drug-food interactions, 107*t*
    drug interactions, 611*t*
    for prostatitis, 824, 824*t*
Fluoxetine, 1199–1200
    for anorexia nervosa, 780
    apparent volume of distribution, 23*t*
    clearance, 30
    for depression, 754
    for eating disorders, 778
    plasma protein binding, 21*t*
    for weight loss, 740–741
Fluoxymesterone, 1335
Fluphenazine, 1204–1205
Flurandrenolide, 1463

Flurazepam, 784, 1175
Flurbiprofen, 1122–1123, 1274
Flu remedies, herbal, 134
Flutex, 1469
Fluticasone, 1391–1392
    for asthma, 402*t*
    intranasal, 1423
    topical, 1463–1464
Fluvastatin, 1045
Fluvoxamine, 754, 1200–1201
FML, 1276–1277
Focal cortical contusion, 621, 622
Folic acid (folate)
    deficiency, 611–614
        nonpharmacologic therapies, 613
        pharmacotherapy, 613–614
        pregnancy and, 612–613
    drug-food interactions, 107*t*
    supplementation, 612–614
Follicle-stimulating hormone (FSH)
    in amenorrhea, 841–842
    in menopause, 296
    suppression, 267
Folliculitis
    characteristics, 570
    drug selection for, 572
    vulvar, 835–836
Food, interaction with drugs, 105, 107*t*–108*t*
Food and Drug Administration (FDA)
    approval process for over-the-counter drugs, 114, 115*t*
    Federal Food, Drug and Cosmetic Act and, 79
    herbal remedies and, 128
    MedWatch program, 99, 100*f*–101*f*
    pregnancy risk classification, 240–241, 241*t*
    safety and efficacy of pediatric drugs, 181
    web site, 93*t*
Food contamination, diseases associated with, 169–170
Fortovase, 1013–1014
Fosamax. *See* Alendronate
Fosinopril, 1050–1051
Fostex Medicated Cleansing, 1436
Free thyroxine, 686*t*
Free thyroxine index (FT₄I), 686*t*
Frei test, 875
FSH. *See* Follicle-stimulating hormone
FT₄I (free thyroxine index ), 686*t*
Fulvicin P/G, 982
Fulvicin U/F, 981
Functional antagonism, 39
Fungal infections
    conjunctivitis, 480
    of skin, 572–573
Fungizone, 1438

**Fungoid-HC, 1473**
**Furacin.** *See* **Nitrofurazone**
**Furadantin.** *See* **Nitrofurantoin**
**Furazolidone, 1029–1030**
**Furosemide,** 23*t,* **1078**
**Furoxone, 1029–1030**
**Furunculosis,** 570, 572

G

**Gabapentin, 1155–1156**
   dosage adjustments in kidney disease, 52, 53*f*
   for seizures, 675
**GABA receptor binding,** 38
**Gabatril, 1157**
**GAD (generalized anxiety disorder),** 767–768
**Galactogogue,** 131*t*
**Galenicals, herbal,** 130*t*
**Ganciclovir, 1015**
**Gantanol, 970–971**
**Gantrisin, 971, 1269**
**Garamycin.** *See* **Gentamicin**
**Garden angelica (angelica),** 132*f*
**Garlic,** 132*f,* 138
**Gastric-emptying inhibitors,** 743
**Gastric ulcers, herbal remedies,** 136–137
**Gastritis, herbal remedies,** 137, 144–145
**Gastrocrom.** *See* **Cromolyn**
**Gastroesophageal reflux,** 513–515
**Gastrointestinal agents**
   antacids, **1286–1291**
   anticholinergics/antispasmodics, **1291–1296**
   antidiarrheals, **1306–1308**
   antiflatulents, **1320–1321**
   for Crohn's disease, **1318–1319**
   digestive enzymes, **1303–1305**
   enemas, **1316–1317**
   laxatives, **1309–1315**
   stimulants, **1302–1303**
   for ulcerative colitis, **1318–1319**
   for ulcers/GERD, **1297–1301**
**Gastrointestinal anticholinergic combinations,**
   **1296**
**Gastrointestinal reflux disease (GERD), agents**
   **for, 1297–1301**
**Gastrointestinal system (GITS),** 12
**Gastrointestinal tract**
   absorption, in neonates, 182–183, 183*t*
   disorders
     constipation, 502–504
     diarrhea, 499–502
     flatus, excessive, 515–516
     gastroesophageal reflux, 513–515
     hemorrhoids, 516–517
     hepatitis, 517–519
     inflammatory bowel disease, 504–509

     irritable bowel syndrome, 519–521
     nausea, 495–499, 496*t*
     peptic ulcer disease, 509–513
     vomiting, 495–499, 496*t*
**Gas-X, 1321**
**Gated channels,** 38
**Gelpirin, 1113**
**Gemfibrozil, 1047**
**Gender, of health care consumer,** 66
**Gender differences, in drug distribution,** 21–22
**Generalized anxiety disorder (GAD),** 767–768
**Generic drugs.** *See also specific generic drugs*
   bioequivalence, 11–12
**Genetic factors**
   coronary artery disease risk and, 345
   in drug metabolism, 24, 99
   in obesity, 735
   in osteoarthritis, 539–540
   in rheumatoid arthritis, 527
**Genetic theory of bipolar disorder,** 762*t*
**Genital herpes,** 580
**Genital warts (condylomata acuminata),** 580
**Genoptic.** *See* **Gentamicin**
**Genora, 1338–1339**
**Genpril.** *See* **Ibuprofen**
**Genprin.** *See* **Aspirin**
**Gensan, 1115–1116**
**Gentacidin.** *See* **Gentamicin**
**Gentak.** *See* **Gentamicin**
**Gentamicin, 1266–1267, 1442**
   apparent volume of distribution, 23*t*
   clearance, 29*t*
   intravenous, 16
   for pelvic inflammatory disease, 881*t*
**Gen-Xene, 1144–1145**
**Geocillin,** 965
***Geriatric Dosage Handbook,*** 88*t*
**German Americans, medication-taking behav-**
   **ior of,** 67
**German measles (rubella),** 582
**German or Hungarian chamomile (chamomile),**
   132*f*
**Gestodene, in oral contraceptives,** 268–269,
   268*t,* 269*t*
**GFR (glomerular filtration rate),** 26, 27*f,* 48–49
**Ginger,** 132*f,* 142
**Gingivostomatitis, herpetic,** 579
***Ginkgo biloba* (maidenhair tree),** 132*f,* 139–140
**Ginseng,** 132*f,* 140–141
**Glaucoma, ophthalmic agents for, 1257–1264**
**Glaucon.** *See* **Epinephrine**
**Glia,** 20
**Glimepiride,** 727, **1353–1354**
**Glipizide,** 21*t,* **1353**
**Glomerular filtration rate (GFR),** 26, 27*f,*
   47–48

**Glomerulus,** 47
**Glucocorticoids, 1327–1333**
  for bronchiolitis, 417
  excessive, in Cushing's syndrome, 697
  function, 694
  thyroid function and, 685*t*
**Glucophage,** 717–718, **1358**
**Glucose**
  intolerance, oral contraceptive usage and, 274
  plasma levels
    in diabetes mellitus, 709
    optimal, for insulin therapy, 721, 722*t*
**Glucotrol,** 21*t,* **1353**
**Glucuronidation,** 24
**Glutethimide, 1181**
**Glyburide, 1354–1355**
**Glycerin, 1311**
**Glycerin/carbamide peroxide/propylene gly-**
    **col/sodium stannate, 1282**
**Glycerites,** herbal, 130*t*
**Glycopyrrolate, 1293**
*Glycyrrhiza glabra* **(licorice),** 132*f*
*Glycyrrhiza uralensis Fisch.* **(licorice),** 132*f*
**Glynase Pres Tab.** *See* **Glyburide**
**Glyset.** *See* **Miglitol**
**GnRH.** *See* **Gonadotropin-releasing**
    **hormone**
**GnRH agonists (gonadotropin-releasing hor-**
    **mone agonists),** 850
**Goatweed (St. John's wort),** 132*f*
**Goldenrod,** 132*f,* 145
**Gold sodium thiomalate, 1253–1254**
**Gold therapy**
  monitoring, 530*t*
  for rheumatoid arthritis, 536
**GoLYTELY, 1316–1317**
**GoLYTLY, 1316–1317**
**Gonadorelin acetate, 1388**
**Gonadotropin measurements,** in menopause di-
    agnosis, 295–296
**Gonadotropin-releasing hormone agonists**
    **(GnRH agonists),** 850
**Gonadotropin-releasing hormone (GnRH),**
    **1388**
  for adenomyosis, 855
  for endometriosis, 855
  in premenstrual syndrome, 845
**Gonococcal conjunctivitis,** 479
**Gonorrhea**
  assessment/history taking, 867–868
  etiology, 867
  pharmacotherapy, 867–870, 869*t*
  during pregnancy, 252*t*
  symptoms, 867
**Goody's Extra Strength Powders, 1113**
**Goserelin acetate implant,** 855

**Gout**
  clinical manifestations, 549
  epidemiology, 549
  nonpharmacologic therapy, 550
  pathogenesis, 550, 550*t*
  patient/caregiver information, 551–552
  pharmacotherapy, 550
    agents for, **1235–1238**
    assessment/history taking for, 551
    drug selection for, 552–554
    follow-up for, 555
    goals for, 550
    for hyperuricemia, 554–555
    initiation, time frame for, 550–551
    monitoring, 555
    prophylactic, 553–554
  stages, 551 .*See also* **Gouty arthritis;**
      **Hyperuricemia**
**Gouty arthritis,** 549, 551
**G proteins,** 38
**Granisetron,** 498, **1326**
**Granuloma inguinale,** 875–876
**Graves' disease**
  etiology, 686–687
  patient/caregiver information, 691*t*
  pharmacotherapy, 692–693
**Great stinging nettle (Nettle),** 132*f,* 137, 143
**Grepafloxacin, 945**
**Grifulvin V, 981**
**Grisactin, 981**
**Grisactin ultra, 982**
**Griseofulvin,** 575
  interactions
    drug-nutrient, 108*t*
    with oral contraceptives, 277*t*
  microsize, **981**
  ultramicrosize, **982**
**Gris-PEG, 982**
**Group A beta-hemolytic streptococci**
  antibiotic susceptibility, 489*t*
  carriers, drug choice for pharyngitis, 385
**Guaifenesin,** 190*t,* **1424**
**Guanabenz, 1055**
**Guanadrel, 1056–1057**
**Guanethidine, 1057**
**Guanfacine, 1056**
**Guiatuss,** 190*t,* **1424**
**Guttate psoriasis,** 598, 600–601
**Gyne-Lotrimin.** *See* **Clotrimazole**


**H**


**Habitrol.** *See* **Nicotine, transdermal system**
*Haemophilus influenzae*
  antibiotic susceptibility, 489*t*
  beta-lactamase-producing strains, 488

cellulitis, 570
otitis media, 485
type B, immunizations, 158–159, 162
*Haemophilus influenzae* **pneumonia**
diagnosis, 439*t*
in pregnant women, 451*t*
**Hair growth ingredients, with OTC status,** 121*t*
**Halazepam,** 786*t*, **1162–1163**
**Halcinonide, 1464–1465**
**Halcion, 1177–1178**
**Haldol, 1212**
**Haldol Deconate, 1212**
**Half-life ($t_{1/2}$),** 29–30, 30*f*, 49
**Halobetasol propionate, 1465**
**Halog, 1464–1465**
**Haloperidol,** 498, **1212**
**Haloprogin,** 119*t*, **1442**
**Halotestin.** *See* **Fluoxymesterone**
**Halotex, 1442**
**Halotussin, 1424**
**Haltran.** *See* **Ibuprofen**
*Hamamelis vernalis* **(witch hazel),** 132*f*
*Hamamelis virginiana* **(witch hazel),** 132*f*
**Hand**
osteoarthritis of, 540, 541*t*
tinea of, 573
*Handbook of Nonprescription Drugs*, 86*t*
**Hashimoto's thyroiditis,** 686–687, 690*t*
**Hawthorn,** 132*f*, **138–139**
**Hay fever, herbal remedies,** 137
**HbA1c (glycated hemoglobin),** 711, 712, 716
**HBIG (hepatitis B immune globulin),** 518
**H$_2$ blockers, for cystic fibrosis,** 432–433
**HCA (hydroxycitric acid), for weight loss,** 742
**HDCV (human diploid cell vaccine),** 167, 168
**Headache**
assessment, 660–661
diagnosis, 657–659, 658*t*
herbal remedies, 137
incidence, 657
menstrual, 849
nonpharmacologic therapy, 660
from oral contraceptive usage, 272*t*
patient/caregiver information, 661
pharmacotherapy, 659–660
drug selection for, 660, 661
follow-up, 661–662
goals, 660
initiation, time frame for, 660
monitoring, 661
**Head injury**
pathophysiology, 621
traumatic.*See* **Traumatic brain injury**
**Head & Shoulders Intensive Treatment**
**Dandruff Shampoo, 1434–1435**
**Head & Shoulders shampoo, 1434**

**Health belief model (HBM),** 69–70
**Health care consumer**
demographics, 66–69
education of, 111–112
sophistication of, 111–112
**Health care costs, over-the-counter drug usage**
**and,** 113
**Health care plans, over-the-counter drug usage**
**and,** 113–114
**Health maintenance organizations (HMOs),**
**over-the-counter drug usage and,** 114
**Hearald patch,** 599
**Heartburn, during pregnancy,** 248–249
**Heart disease, cystic fibrosis with,** 444
**Heart failure**
activity limitation and, 319–320
classification, 322*t*
compensatory mechanisms, 320, 320*f*
definition of, 320
nonpharmacologic therapy, 322
outcomes management, 324–328, 326*t*
pathophysiology, 320–321, 320*f*
patient/caregiver information, 324
pharmacotherapy, 321
assessment for, 322–324
follow-up, 328
goals, 321–322
initiation, time frame for, 322
monitoring of, 324–328, 326*t*
selecting agent for, 324
types, 321
**Heart rate, blood pressure and,** 309–310
**Heberden's nodes,** 541
**Height-weight tables, normal,** 738*t*
*Helicobacter pylori* **ulcers,** 511–512
**HELIX,** 93*t*
**Hematocrit,** 606*t*
**Hemodialysis,** 53–54
**Hemoglobin,** 606*t*, 607
**Hemolysis,** 606
**Hemorrhoids,** 138, 516–517
**Hemostatic,** 131*t*
**Heparin**
low-dose *vs.* high-dose, 618, 618*t*
low molecular weight *vs.* standard unfractionated,
618, 618*t*
**Hepatitis,** 517–519
**Hepatitis A immunization,** 165–166, 169
**Hepatitis B immune globulin (HBIG),** 518
**Hepatitis B immunizations,** 161–162, 246
**Herbal remedies,** 132*t*. *See also specific herbs*
alertness problems, 139–141
anti-anxiety, 129–131
benign prostate enlargement, 143
for breast tenderness, 133, 141, 142–143
for bronchial asthma, 133–134

Herbal remedies (*cont.*)
  cold/flu, 134
  colitis, 137, 144–145
  concentration problems, 139–141
  constipation, 134–135
  dangers, 129
  dosage forms, 129, 130*t*
  dysmenorrhea, 135–136
  effectiveness, 127, 128–129
  fatigue, 136
  flatulence, 136
  in foreign countries, 128
  in future, 145–146
  gastric ulcers, 136–137
  gastritis, 137, 144–145
  harmful, 128
  hay fever, 137
  headaches, 137
  hemorrhoids, 134–135, 138
  historical aspects, 127
  hyperlipidemia, 138
  insomnia, 138–139
  irritable bowel syndrome, 134–135, 136, 139
  laryngitis, 144–145
  memory problems, 139–141
  menopausal symptoms, 135–136, 141, 142–143
  motion sickness, 142
  mouth ulcers, 136, 141
  muscle/joint pain and inflammation, 141–142
  nausea, 142
  obesity, 142
  premenstural symptoms, 135–136, 141, 142–143
  quality, 128–129
  regulation, 128
  safety, 127, 128–129
  skin problems, 141, 144
  sore throat, 144–145
  stress-relieving, 129–131
  under study, 145–146
  terminology, 130*t*, 131*t*
  urinary infection/inflammation, 145
  for weight loss, 741–742
**Herd immunity,** 152
**Herpes genitalis**
  assessment/history taking, 873
  etiology, 872
  pharmacotherapy, 872–874, 874*t*
**Herpes simplex virus (HSV)**
  drug selection for, 582
  pharmacotherapy, 583, **1002–1004**
  during pregnancy, 252*t*
  signs/symptoms, 579–580
**Herpes zoster virus (HZV)**
  pharmacotherapy, **1002–1004**
  shingles, 581
**Herpetic whitlow,** 579–580

**Herplex.** *See* **Idoxuridine**
**Heterotopic ossification, in disabled individuals,** 211
**Hexadrol.** *See* **Dexamethasone**
**High-flux membranes,** 54
**Hip osteoarthritis,** 540, 541*t*
**Hiprex, 1018**
**Hirsutism,** 272*t*, 699, 700*t*
**Hismanal.** *See* **Astemizole**
**Hispanic-Americans**
  as health care consumers, 66
  medication-taking behavior of, 68
**Histamine receptors,** 35
**HIV/AIDS,** 897
  assessment/history taking, 900, 901*t*–903*t*
  in children, 906–907
    assessment, 912
    classification of, 906–907, 907*t*, 908*t*
    drug selection, 912–913
    drug treatment, 907, 911*t*
    initiation of therapy, time frame for, 910–911
    monitoring of pharmacotherapy, 913–914
    nonpharmacologic therapy, 909–910
    patient/caregiver information, 912
    prevention, 908–909
  in homeless population, 221
  illness spectrum, 898*t*
  nonpharmacologic therapy, 898, 899*t*
  pathogenesis, antiviral action on, 897, 898*t*
  patient/caregiver information, 900
  pharmacotherapy, 900*t*
    drug selection, 903–905, 904*t*
    follow-up, 906
    goals, 898
    initiation, time frame for, 899, 900*t*
    monitoring, 905–906
    for opportunistic infections, 904–905, 905*t*
    rationale, 897–898
  postexposure prophylaxis, 920
  prevention, 898
  symptoms, 899, 899*t*, 906*t*
**Hivid, 1007**
**HLA antigens, psoriasis and,** 598
**HMOs (health maintenance organizations), over-the-counter drug usage and,** 114
**HMS, 1277**
**Hold.** *See* **Dextromethorphan**
**Homatropine,** 474
**Homeless population**
  community resource implications, 225
  continuity of care issues, 225
  demographics, 220
  health problems, 220–221
  lifestyle factors contributing to disease, 221–222
  medication/treatment considerations, 222–225, 223*t*

Homeostatic mechanisms, age-related changes, 200–201

Hordeolum (stye), 475, 476–477

Horehound, 132f, 135

Hormonal factors, in osteoporosis, 544

Hormone replacement therapy (HRT)
  decision-making, 292–293
  follow-up, 301–302
  monitoring, 300–301
  for osteoporosis, 547
  problems with, 299
  risks, 296–297
  selection of appropriate agent, 298–299
  side effects, 297

Hornet stings, 586

Hospitalization
  for bronchiolitis, 419, 419t
  for eating disorder, 777
  for urinary tract infections, 806t–807t

Hot flashes (flushes), 290, 293

H₂-receptor antagonists
  for gastroesophageal reflux, 513
  for peptic ulcer disease, 511

HRIG (human rabies immune globulin), 168

HRT. See Hormone replacement therapy

HSD (hypoactive sexual desire), 856

HSV. See Herpes simplex virus

Humalog, 723t, 1360–1361

Human diploid cell vaccine (HDCV), 167, 168

Human immunodeficiency virus. See HIV/AIDS

Human papillomavirus (HPV)
  assessment/history taking, 877
  nonpharmacologic therapy, 877
  pharmacotherapy, 876–879
  during pregnancy, 252t
  types, 876
  warts, 580

Human rabies immune globulin (HRIG), 168

Humatin, 931

Humibid, 1424

Humilin L, 1363

Humilin R, 1361–1362

Humorsol, 1259

Humulin, 1364–1365

Humulin 70/30, 1364–1365

Humulin N, 1362–1363

Humulin U Ultralente, 1363–1364

Hydantoins, 1146–1149

Hydergine, 1234

Hydralazine, 327, 1071

Hydrocet, 1104

Hydrochlorothiazide (HCTZ), 316, 1083

Hydrocil, 1313

Hydrocodone, combinations
  acetaminophen, 1104
  aspirin, 1105

Hydrocortisone, 1329–1330
  combinations
    acetic acid glacial/propylene glycol diacetate/ sodium acetate/benzothonium chloride/citric acid, 1284–1285
    acetic acid/propylene glycolol diacetate/ sodium aceta/benzethionium chloride, 1284
    alcohol/propylene glycol/dermprotective factor/ yerba santa/benzyl benzoate, 1284
    clioquinol, 1470
    iodoquinol, 1471
    neomycin, 1279
    neomycin/polymyxin B, 1279
    polymyxin B, 1279
    pramoxine, 1470–1471
  OTC status, 118t, 120t
  topical, 1465–1466

Hydrocortisone acetate, 1466

Hydrocortisone valerate, 1466–1467

Hydrodiuril, 1083

Hydroflumethiazide, 1083–1084

Hydrogenated soybean oil/lecithin, 120t

Hydromorphone, 1090–1091

Hydromox, 1086–1087

Hydrophilic drugs, 13, 14f

Hydroxychloroquine, 987–988
  monitoring, 530t
  for Parkinson's disease, 1254–1255
  for rheumatoid arthritis, 535

Hydroxycitric acid (HCA), 742

Hydroxyzine, 786t, 1167, 1414–1415

Hygroton, 1082–1083

Hylorel, 1056–1057

Hymenoptera, 586

L-Hyoscyamine sulfate, 1294

HyperDOC, 93t

Hyperglycemia, drug-induced, 728t

Hypericum perforatum. See St. John's wort

Hyperlipidemia
  blood lipids and, 354–355
  herbal remedies, 138
  nonpharmacologic therapy, 356
  patient/caregiver information, 357–358
  pharmacotherapy, 355
    assessment for, 356–357
    follow-up, 360
    goals, 355–356
    initiation, time-frame for, 356, 356t, 357t
    monitiorng, 358–360
    selection of appropriate agent for, 358, 358t

Hypertension
  blood pressure regulation and, 309–310
  coronary artery disease risk and, 345
  diagnosis, 312–314, 313t
  elderly and, 314
  etiology, 310–311

Hypertension (*cont.*)
  in homeless population, 224
  isolated systolic, 311
  nonpharmacologic therapy, 311–312, 312*t*
  from oral contraceptive usage, 273
  outcomes management, 314–319
  patient/care giver information, 314
  pharmacotherapy, 311, 312*t* .*See also*
    **Antihypertensive agents**
    assessment for, 312–314, 313*t*
    contraindications, 315
    follow-up, 319, 320*t*
    goals, 311
    initiation, time frame for, 312
    monitoring, 316–319
    selection of appropriate agent, 314–316
    in stroke management, 639–640
  severity categories, 313*t*, 315–316
  stroke risk and, 635–636
**Hyperthyroidism**, 686–687
  assessment/history taking, 690
  causes, 689*t*
  patient/caregiver information, 690, 691*t*
  pharmacotherapy, 688–689, 692–693
    adverse effects, 685*t*
    efficacy monitoring, 693
    follow-up, 694
    goals, 689
    initiation, time frame for, 690
    toxicity monitoring, 694
  signs/symptoms, 688–689, 689*t*
**Hypertriglyceridemia**, 358
**Hyperuricemia**, 551, 554–555
**Hypnotics**, 784–785
**Hypoactive sexual desire (HSD)**, 856
**Hypoalbuminemia, in hepatic dysfunction**, 47
**Hypoaldosteronism**, 696–697
**Hypoestrogenemia, coronary artery disease**
    **risk and**, 345
**Hypoglycemia**
  drug-induced, 728*t*
  from insulin therapy, 724
  nocturnal, 724
  risk, diabetic control and, 711
  sulfonylurea-induced, 727
  treating, 724, 724*t*
  in type 2 diabetes mellitus, 710
**Hypothalamic-pituitary-adrenal axis**, 695*f*
**Hypothalamic-pituitary-thyroid axis**, 683–684, 684*f*
**Hypothyroidism**
  assessment/history taking, 690
  causes, 688*t*
  patient/caregiver information, 690, 690*t*
  pharmacotherapy, 687–688
    adverse effects, 685*t*
    drug selection for, 691–692

    efficacy monitoring, 693
    follow-up, 694
    goals, 689
    initiation, time frame for, 689690
    toxicity monitoring, 693–694
  signs/symptoms, 688*t*
**Hypoxic-ischemic injury**, 621–622
**Hytrin.** *See* **Terazosin**
**Hytuss**, 1424

I

**IBD.** *See* **Inflammatory bowel disease**
**IBS.** *See* **Irritable bowel syndrome**
**Ibuprofen**, 1123
  hepatic extraction, 46*t*
  OTC status, 119*t*, 120*t*
  pediatric dosages, 191*t*
  plasma protein binding, 21*t*
  suspension for pediatric use, 120*t*
**Idiosyncratic reactions**, 98
**Idoxuridine**, 1271
**Iliac artery occlusive disease**, 340*t*
**Illicit drug use**
  preconception screening, 244
  treatment, 785–786
  types, 62–63
**Ilotycin.** *See* **Erythromycin**
**Imazodan**, 328
**Imdur**, 1034–1035
**Imipramine**, 1190
  bioavailability, 19*t*
  clearance, 29*t*
  plasma protein binding, 21*t*
  SR, for stress urinary incontinence, 815*t*
**Imiquimod**, 879, 1443
**Imitrex**, 1240–1241
**Immediate-release preparations**, 9, 10*f*, 12
**Immigrants, as health care consumers**, 67
**Immobilization, of disabled individuals**, 210–211
**Immune globulins**, 151, 156
**Immune system, disorders**
  allergic responses.*See* **Allergic responses**
  HIV/AIDS.*See* **HIV/AIDS**
  infectious mononucleosis, 918–920
  postexposure prophylaxis, 920
**Immunity**
  active, 151
  herd, 152
  passive, 151
  principles, 151–152
**Immunization**
  adverse event reporting, 174
  childhood
    diphtheria, 155–156
    *Haemophilus influenzae* type B, 158–159

hepatitis B, 161–162
measles, 156–157
mumps, 158
pertussis, 153*t*, 154–155
poliomyelitis, 152–154
rubella, 157–158
schedule for, 153*t*
tetanus, 153*t*, 156
varicella, 159–161
decision-making, 171, 172*f*, 173*f*, 174
future improvements, 174–175
hepatitis A, 165–166
influenza, 162–164
Japanese encephalitis, 170
malaria, 170
meningococcal disease, 166–167, 170
plague, 170
pneumococcal disease, 164–165
poliomyelitis, 170–171
during pregnancy and lactation, 245–246
rabies, 167–168
rate improvement, programs for, 175
schedules
adult, 173*f*
catch-up for children, 172*f*
for HIV-positive children, 910*t*
for travelers, 169–171
tuberculosis, 168–169
yellow fever, 170
**Imodium,** 1307
**Impetigo,** 569–572
**Impotence.** *See* **Erectile dysfunction**
**Imuran.** *See* **Azathioprine**
**Incontinence, urinary**
after stroke, 640
in menopause, nonpharmacologic therapy for, 293
stress.*See* **Stress urinary incontinence**
**Indapamide,** 1084
**Inderal.** *See* **Propranolol**
**Indian plantago seed (plantago seed),** 132*f*
**Indigestion, during pregnancy,** 248–249
**Indinavir,** 1011
**Indochron E-R,** 1128
**Indocin,** 1128
**Indomethacin,** 1128
**Induction, cytochrome P-450 enzymes,** 24
**Infants**
absorption, 183*t*, 184
administration of drugs and, 186
antibiotic dosage calculations for, 188*f*–190*f*
distribution, 183*t*, 184–185
excretion, 183*t*, 185
metabolism, 183*t*, 185
newborn.*See* **Neonates**
over-the-counter drug doses, 190*t*–191*t*
prescribing medications for, 191–192, 193*t*

pyelonephritis, 810
therapeutic disasters, 181
**Infectious mononucleosis,** 918–920
**Inflammatory bowel disease (IBD)**
nonpharmacologic therapy, 505
outcomes management, 506–509
patient/caregiver information, 506
pharmacotherapy, 504
assessment/history taking for, 506
efficacy monitoring, 508
follow-up, 509
goals for, 504
initiation, time frame for, 505–506, 507–508
toxicity monitoring, 508–509
**Influenza**
antigen types, 162–163
immunizations, 162–164
pharmacotherapy, 377–380
symptoms, 163
type A pneumonia, in pregnant women, 451*t*
**Infusions, herbal,** 130*t*
**Inhalers, asthma therapy,** 396–398
**Injectable polio vaccine (IPV),** 152, 153*t*, 154
**Insomnia**
assessment/history taking, 786
defined, 781
in dementia, 657
etiology, 781–782
herbal remedies, 138–139
incidence, 781
nonpharmacologic therapy, 782–783, 783*t*
patient/caregiver information, 786
pharmacotherapy, 782
drug selection, 783–785
follow-up, 785
goals, 782
initiation, time frame for, 783
monitoring, 785
primary *vs.* secondary, 781
**Insulin,** 1360–1366
blood glucose levels and, 721, 722*t*
in diabetes mellitus, 710
interaction with oral contraceptives, 277*t*
physiologic secretion, 719*f*
preparations, 719
administration, 723–724
for cystic fibrosis, 433
for diabetes mellitus, 718–719
dosing, 721, 723*t*
duration of action, 719–721, 720*f*
immediate therapy, situations requiring, 725
injectables, 723
intermediate-acting, 720–721, 720*f*
long-acting, 720*f*, 721
Regular, 723*t*, **1361–1362**
short-acting, 720, 720*f*

Insulin (*cont.*)
　　side effects, 724–725
　　storing, 723
　　zinc suspension, **1363**
　　extended, **1363–1364**
　regimens, 722–723, 722*t*
**Intal.** *See* **Cromolyn**
**Interferon beta-1a,** 645–646
**Interferon beta-1b,** 645
**Intermediate uveitis,** 482
**Intermittent claudication,** 339, 340*t*, 343
**Internal analgesic/antipyretic ingredients, with**
　　　**OTC status,** 119*t*, 120*t*
**International Pharmaceutical Abstracts (IPA),**
　　90*t*
**Intracellular receptors,** 38
**Intranasal medications, for allergic rhinitis,** 372
**Intrauterine devices (IUDs),** 261–263, 262*t*–264*t*
**Intrinsic factor,** 614
**Inulin clearance,** 48
**Invirase,** 1013–1014
**Iodine and iodine products,** 1383
**Iodoquinol,** 931
**Iodoquinol/hydrocortisone,** 1471
**Ionization,** 13, 14*f*
**Ion trapping (pH partitioning),** 16
**Iopidine,** 1257
**Iouiuds,** 232–233
**IPA (International Pharmaceutical Abstracts),**
　　90*t*
**Ipratropium,** 1389
　adverse events, 426*t*
　for allergic rhinitis, 370–371, 373
　intranasal, 370–371, 375, 377
**Irish Americans, medication-taking behavior of,**
　　67
**Iron**
　absorption, during pregnancy, 608–609
　daily loss, normal, 608
　drug-food interactions, 107*t*
　stores, of infants, 608
　supplements
　　drug interactions, 611, 611*t*
　　for iron deficiency anemia, 609–610, 610*t*
　　monitoring, 611
　　prenatal, 245, 245*t*
　　side effects, 610
**Iron deficiency anemia,** 607–608
　nonpharmacologic therapy, 609
　patient/caregiver information, 610
　pharmacotherapy, 608
　　assessment/history taking for, 609
　　drug selection for, 609–610, 610*t*
　　goals, 609
　　initiation, time frame for, 609
　prevention in pregnancy, 608–609

**Irritable bowel syndrome (IBS)**
　herbal remedies, 134–135, 136, 139
　pharmacotherapy, 519–521
**Ismelin,** 1057
**ISMO,** 1034–1035
**Isocom,** 1242
**Isoetharine,** 1397
**Isometheptene mucate/dichloralphenazone/ac-**
　　　**etaminophen,** 1242
**Isoniazid (INH),** 996–997
　combination with rifampicin, **998**
　for tuberculosis, 456–457, 458, 460
**Isopap,** 1242
**Isophane insulin suspension (NPH),** 1362–1363
**Isophane insulin suspension/Regular insulin,**
　　1364–1366
**Isoptin.** *See* **Verapamil**
**Isopto Carbachol,** 1258
**Isopto Carpine,** 1263
**Isordil,** 19*t*, 327, **1034**
**Isosorbide dinitrate,** 19*t*, 327, **1034**
**Isosorbide mononitrate,** 1034–1035
**Isotretinoin,** 1428–1429
**Isradipine,** 1068
**Italian Americans, medication-taking behavior**
　　**of,** 68
**Itraconazole,** 982–983
　for candidiasis, 575
　drug-drug interactions, 106*t*
**IUDs (intrauterine devices),** 261–263, 262*t*–264*t*
**Ivermectin,** 884

J

**Janimine.** *See* **Imipramine**
**Japanese encephalitis,** 170
**Jarisch-Herxheimer reaction,** 867
**JCAHO (Joint Commission on Accreditation of**
　　　**Hospital Organizations),** 99
**Jenest-28,** 1339, 1345–1346
**Jet lag,** 785
**JNC (Joint National Committee),** 312, 314–315
**Jock itch (tinea cruris),** 573, 575
**Johnswort (St. John's wort),** 132*f*
**Joint Commission on Accreditation of Hospital**
　　　**Organizations (JCAHO),** 99
**Joint disorders, herbal remedies,** 141–142
**Joint National Committee (JNC),** 312, 314–315
*Journal Watch,* 89*t*

K

**Kanamycin sulfate,** 1030
**Kantrex,** 1030
**Kaolin/pectin (Kaopectin),** 18, **1307–1308**
**Kappa opioid receptor,** 231

**Kava,** 132*f*, 133

**K$_D$ (equilibrium dissociation constant),** 35

**Kefauver-Harris Amendment,** 114

**Keflet.** *See* **Cephalexin**

**Keflex.** *See* **Cephalexin**

**Keftab.** *See* **Cephalexin**

**Kegal exercises,** 293

**Kemadrin,** 1249–1250

**Kenacort.** *See* **Triamcinolone**

**Kenalog,** 1469

**Kerlone (Betaxolol),** 1061, 1257

**Ketoconazole,** 19, 983–984

   for candidiasis, 575

   drug-drug interactions, 106*t*

   topical, **1443**

**Ketoprofen,** 121*t*, **1124**

**Ketorolac,** 1129, 1274–1275

**Kidney**

   disease

      absorption of drugs and, 50–51

      dialysis, 53–54

      distribution of drugs and, 51

      dosing issues, 50–54, 52*f*–54*f*, 55

      elimination of drugs and, 51–53, 53*f*, 54*f*

   drug clearance, 29*t*

   elimination, 200, 200*t*

   excretion, drug-induced alteration of, 105

   functional assessment, 47–49, 49*t*

   toxicity, of nonsteroidal antiinflammatory drugs, 534–535

**Klamath weed (St. John's wort),** 132*f*

*Klebsiella* pneumonia, 439*t*

**Klonapin,** 1143–1144

**Knee osteoarthritis,** 540, 541*t*

**Koebner's phenomenon,** 599

**KOH slide test (potassium hydroxide slide test),** 885

**Kondon's Nasal.** *See* **Ephedrine**

**Kondremul Plain,** 1312

**Koplik's spots,** 581

**Kutrase,** 1303

**Ku-Zyme,** 1303

**Kwell,** 1450–1451

**Kytril,** 1326

L

**Label instructions, for over-the-counter drugs,** 122

**Labetalol,** 1059–1060

   bioavailability, 19*t*

   clearance, 29*t*

   stereoselectivity, 36

**Laboratory tests, diagnostic**

   for arrhythmias, 334

   for asthma, 397*t*, 408, 408*t*

   drug plasma concentrations, drug interaction and, 22–23

   for gout, 551

   for heart failure, 323–324

   for hypertension, 313

   for osteoarthritis, 541

   for osteoporosis, 545–546

   for peripheral vascular disease, 342

   for prostatitis, 823*t*

   for urinary tract infections (UTIs), 804*t*

**Labrynthitis, meningogenic,** 488–489

**Lactation**

   drug therapy during, 241–243, 242*t*, 243*t*

   immunizations during, 245–246

**Lactose-free diet,** 519–520

**Lactulose,** 1317

**Lamictal,** 674, **1156**

**Lamisil,** 985, **1447**

**Lamivudine,** 912, **1006**

**Lamotrigine,** 674, **1156**

**Lamprene,** 994

**Lanacort.** *See* **Hydrocortisone**

**Laniazid.** *See* **Isoniazid**

**Lanorinal,** 1120–1121

**Lanoxicaps.** *See* **Digoxin**

**Lanoxin.** *See* **Digoxin**

**Lansoprazole,** 511, **1299**

**Larium,** 988–989

**Larodopa.** *See* **Levodopa**

**Laryngitis, herbal remedies,** 144–145

**Lasix,** 1078

**Latanoprost,** 1261

**Latex allergy, disabled individuals and,** 214–215

*Latrodectus mactans* **(black widow spider),** 585–586

**Lavender,** 146

**Laxative combinations,** 1315

**Laxatives,** 131*t*, **1309–1314**

**LDL (low density lipoprotein),** 354–355, 356, 356*t*

**Leg**

   cramps, nocturnal, 344

   lower occlusive disease, 340*t*

**Legatrin,** 992

**Legend drugs,** 79, 81

*Legionella* pneumonia, 439*t*

**Lemon balm (melissa),** 132*f*

**Lente Iletin,** 1363

**Lente L,** 1363

**Leptin, recombinant,** 743

**Leptin agonist,** 743

**Lescol,** 1045

**Leukotriene modifiers,** 401, 405

**Leukotriene receptor antagonists,** 1425

**Leukotriene receptor inhibitors,** 1426

Leuprolide acetate, 855
Levaquin, 945–946
Levatol, 1063–1064
Levlen, 1344, 1347
Levobunolol, 1261
Levocabastine, 370, 1273
Levodopa, 1246
    blood-brain barrier, 20
    carrier-mediated transport, 16
    drug interactions, 611t
    for Parkinson's disease, 666–667
    thyroid function and, 685t
Levo-Dromoran, 1091
Levofloxacin, 945–946
Levonorgestrel, 1350–1351
    with ethinyl estradiol, 1344, 1347
    implant, 282–283, 282t
    in oral contraceptives, 268–269, 268t, 269t
Levora, 1344, 1347
Levorotary enantiomers, 35
Levorphanol, 1091
Levothyroxine, 1384
    for hypothyroidism, 691–692
    patient/caregiver information, 690t
    pediatric dosing, 692, 692t
Levsin, 1294
Levsinex, 1294
LGV (lymphogranuloma venereum), 875–876
LH. See Luteinizing hormone
Lhermitte's sign, 642t
Libido
    decreased, drug-induced, 858t
    testosterone for, 859
Libritabs. See Chlordiazepoxide
Librium. See Chlordiazepoxide
Lice, 587–589
Lichen sclerosus, 839–840
Licorice, 132f, 135, 136–137
Lidex, 1462–1463
Lidocaine
    bioavailability, 19t
    clearance, 29t
    plasma protein binding, 21t
Lidocainel, 46t
Lifestyle, coronary artery disease risk and, 345
Ligands, 33
Limbitrol DS, 1219
Lindane, 884, 1450–1451
Lioresal (Baclofen), 213, 559, 1224
Liothyronine, 1384–1385
Liotrix, 1385–1386
Lipase inhibitors, 742
Lipids
    abnormal, obesity and, 732
    metabolism, oral contraceptive usage and, 273
Lipitor (atorvastatin), 358–359, 1045

Lipoatrophy, insulin-induced, 724–725
Lipophilic drugs, 13
Liquid supplements, for cystic fibrosis, 433
Lisinopril, 1051
Lispro, 723t, 1360–1361
Lithane. See Lithium
Lithium, 1221–1222
    apparent volume of distribution, 23t
    for bipolar disorder, 764
    drug-drug interactions, 106t
    for eating disorders, 778
    patient/caregiver information, 763–764
    thyroid function and, 685t
    toxicity, 765–766
Lithobid. See Lithium
Lithotabs. See Lithium
Liver
    blood flow, 24
    disease
        dosing issues, 49–50, 54–55
        drug elimination and, 45
    drug clearance, 29t, 46
    drug elimination, 45–47, 46t
    drug metabolism, 23–24
    functional assessment, 45–47
    metabolism
        age-related changes, 200
        enzyme inhibition of, 104–105
Liver function tests, 45–47, 728
Livostin, 370, 1273
llex paraguariensis, 132t
Lobac, 1232
Lodine, 1127–1128
Lodosyn, 1246–1247
Lodoxamide, 1273
Loestrin, 1339, 1345–1346
Lomefloxacin, 107t, 946–947
Lomotil, 1306–1307
Lonamin. See Phentermine
Loniten, 1071–1072
Loop diuretics, 1077–1078
    for heart failure, 324–325
    monitoring, 316
Lo/Ovral, 1342, 1348
Loperamide, 120t, 1307
Lopid, 1047
Lopressor. See Metoprolol
Loprox, 1439
Lorabid, 938
Loracarbef, 938
    dosage calculations, pediatric, 190t
    for upper respiratory tract infections, 489t
Loratadine, 1421
Lorazepam, 1163
    contraindications, 773
    for insomnia, 786t

Lorcet, 1104
Lortab, 1104, 1105
Losartan, 1054
Lotensin, 1049
Lotrimin. *See* Clotrimazole
Lotrisone, 1473
Lovastatin, 108*t*, 1046
Low density lipoprotein (LDL), 356, 356*t*
Loxapine, 1213
Loxitane, 1213
*Loxosceles reculsa* (brown recluse spider), 585–586
Lozol, 1084
Lubricants, vaginal, 859
Ludiomil, 1194–1195
Lufyllin, 1400
Lugol's Solution. *See* Iodine
Lurline, 1115
Luteinizing hormone (LH)
    in amenorrhea, 841–842
    in menopause, 296
    suppression, 267
Lutrepulse, 1388
Luvox (Fluvoxamine), 754, 1200–1201
Lymphogranuloma venereum (LGV), 875–876

M

Maalox Anti-Diarrheal, 1307
McCoy cell culture, 870–871
Macrobid, 1020–1021
Macrocytosis, 607
Macrodantin, 1020–1021
Macrolide antibiotics, 438, **951–957**. *See also specific macrolide antibiotics*
Magaldrate, 1288
Magan, 1137–1138
Magnesium, for premenstrual syndrome, 847–848
Magnesium citrate, 1311
Magnesium hydroxide, 1288–1289
Magnesium oxide, 1289
Magnesium salicylate, 1137–1138
Magnesium salicylate/phenyltoloxamine, 1118
Magnesium sulfate, 1311
Mag-Ox 400 mg, 1289
Magsal, 1118
Ma huang (ephedra), 128, 132*f*, 133–134, 741
Maintenance, in transtheoretical model of behavior change, 73
Major depressive disorder (MDD), 748
Malabsorptive disorders, oral drug absorption and, 18
Malaria, 170
Malathion, 1451–1452
Male condoms, 257–258, 258*t*

Mammography, in menopause, 296
Mandelamine, 1018–1019
Mania
    pharmacotherapy algorithm, 761*f*
    in traumatic head injury, 628–629
Manic-depression. *See* Bipolar disorder
Manic episode, 760. *See also* Bipolar disorder
Mantaux skin test (PPD), 453, 454, 454*t*, 455, 456
Manufacturer's sales representatives (MSRs), 92
MAOIs. *See* Monoamine oxidase inhibitors
Maolate, 1225
Maprotiline, 1194–1195
Marezine, 1322
Margesic No. 3, 1100
Marijuana, interaction with drugs, 105, 108
Marinol, 1325
Marmine, 1323
Marrubium (horehound), 132*f*
*Marrubium vulgare* (horehound), 132*f*
*Martindale: The Extra Pharmacopoeia*, 87*t*
*Matricaria recutia* (chamomile), 132*f*
Matrix forms, 12
Maxair, 1398
Maxaquin, 946–947
Maxidex. *See* Dexamethasone
Maxiflor, 1461
Maximal efficacy, 32
Maximum Pain Relief Pamprin, 1114
Maximum Strength Mylanta Gas, 1321
Maxivate, 1456
May bush or tree (hawthorn), 132*f*
Mazanor, 1483–1484
Mazindol, 739, 1483–1484
MCA (middle cerebral artery), 635
MDD (major depressive disorder), 748
Mdibfradil, 350
MDR-TB (multiple-drug resistant tuberculosis), 457
Mean corpuscular hemoglobin concentration (MCHC), 606*t*, 607
Mean corpuscular volume (MCV), 606*t*, 607
Measles-mumps-rubella immunization, 245–246
Measles (rubeola), 581–582
    immunizations, 157
    symptoms, 156–157
Mebaral, 1141
Mebendazole, 1023–1024
Mechanical obstruction, 499
Meclizine, 651, 1323–1324
Meclofenamate, 1132
Meclomen, 1132
Medicaid coverage, for over-the-counter drugs, 114
*The Medical Letter*, 89*t*

Medical oophorectomy, 855
*The Medical Sciences Bulletin*, 88t
**Medicare, for over-the-counter drugs,** 114
**Medication Management Module for
   Schizophrenic Patients,** 61
**Medication-taking behavior**
   implications for practice, 74–75
   of minority ethnic groups, 68–69
   prediction models, integration of, 71–72, 72f
   psychosocial factors, 69–74, 72f
   of white ethnic groups, 67–68
*The Medication Teaching Manual: The Guide to
   Patient Drug Information,* **6th edition,**
   94t
**Medihaler Ergotamine, 1239**
**MEDLINE CD-Rom,** 89t
**MED (minimal erythemal dose),** 596
**MedPulse,** 93t
**Medrol.** *See* **Methylprednisolone**
**Medrol acetate topical, 1467**
**Medroxyprogesterone acetate (MPA),** 299,
   **1351, 1372**
   for endometriosis/adenomyosis, 855
   for perimenopause, 298
   for stress urinary incontinence, 815t
**Medrysone, 1277**
**MedTeach software,** 94t
**MedWatch program,** 99, 100f–101f
**Mefenamic acid, 1132–1133**
**Mefloquine, 988–989**
**Megace.** *See* **Megastrol**
**Megastrol, 1372**
**Meglitinides,** 725
**Meibomian glands,** 475
**Melacortin,** 743
*Melaleuca alternifolia* **(tea tree oil),** 132f
**Melancholic depression,** 748
**Melanomas,** 592
**Melatonin,** 785, 786, 849
**Melissa,** 132f, 144
*Melissa officinalis* **(melissa),** 132f
**Mellaril,** 40, **1209**
**Membrane barriers, distribution and,** 20
**Memory problems**
   in dementia, 652
   herbal remedies, 139–141
**Menadol.** *See* **Ibuprofen**
**Menest, 1367**
**Meni-D, 1323–1324**
**Meniere's disease,** 649–651
**Meningococcal disease immunization,** 166–167,
   170
**Menopause**
   changes in, 289
   conditions associated with, 290–292
   definition of, 289

   nonpharmacologic therapy, 293–294
   pharmacotherapy, 289–290, 292–293
      contraindications, 294–295
      counseling/client information for, 296–297
      drug classes for, 294t
      efficacy monitoring, 300–301
      goals, 293
      history-taking for, 294–295
      initiation, time frame for, 294
      laboratory tests, 295–296
      physical examination for, 294–295
      risk factors, 295t
      selection of appropriate agent for, 297–299
   symptoms, herbal remedies, 135–136, 141,
      142–143
**Menstruation**
   disorders, 840–841
      adenomyosis, 853–856
      amenorrhea, 841–843
      dysfunctional uterine bleeding, 843–844
      dysmenorrhea, 851–853, 852t
      endometriosis, 853–856
      from oral contraceptive usage, 272t
      premenstrual syndrome.*See* **Premenstrual
         syndrome**
   heavy, from oral contraceptive usage, 272t
   menopause and, 289
   migraine headache and, 659
**Mental illness**
   in homeless population, 221
   treatment, 747
*Menthax piperita* **(peppermint),** 132f
**Mepergan Fortis, 1110–1111**
**Meperidine, 1094–1095**
   bioavailability, 19t
   clearance, 29t
   drug-drug interactions, 106t
   hepatic extraction, 46t
   metabolites, 52
   plasma protein binding, 21t
**Meperidine promethazine, 1110–1111**
**Mephenytoin, 1147–1148**
**Mephobarbital, 1141, 1171**
**Meprobamate,** 771, **1168**
**Mepron,** 107t, **1027**
**Meprospan,** 771, **1168**
**Meridia, 1485**
**Mesalamine,** 507–508, **1318**
**Mesantoin, 1147–1148**
**Mesoridazine, 1205–1206**
**Mestranol**
   combined with norethynodrel, **1374–1375**
   in oral contraceptives, 268, 268t
**Metabolism (biotransformation)**
   age-related changes, 200, 200t
   alterations, 24
   defined, 23–24

drug interactions, 26
enzyme activity and, 24
first-pass, drugs susceptible to, 19t
infants, 183t, 185
liver blood flow and, 24
neonatal, 183t, 184
oral contraceptive usage and, 271t, 273–275
during pregnancy, 240, 240t
**Metabolites, active,** 23
**Metahydrin, 1087**
**Metamucil, 1313**
**Metaprel, 1397**
**Metaproterenol, 1397**
**Metaxalone, 1227–1228**
**Metered dose inhaler,** 397, 401
**Metformin,** 717–718, **1358**
**Methadone,** 232, **1095–1096**
**Methantheline bromide, 1294–1295**
**Methazolamide, 1076**
**Methdilazine, 1415**
**Methenamine hippurate, 1018**
**Methenamine mandelate, 1018–1019**
**Methimazole, 1381**
for hyperthyroidism, 692–693
patient/caregiver information, 691t
**Methocarbamol, 1228**
**Methocarbamol/aspirin, 1229–1230**
**Methotrexate, 1255**
adverse events, 601
monitoring, 530t
for multiple sclerosis, 646
for psoriasis, 601
for rheumatoid arthritis, 536–537
**Methsuximide, 1151–1152**
**Methylcellulose, 1311–1312**
**Methylclothiazide, 1084–1085**
**Methyldopa,** 611t, **1056**
**Methylene blue, 1030–1031**
**Methylphenidate, 1222–1223**
for attention deficit/hyperactivity disorder,
633–635
for traumatic head injury, 626
**Methylprednisolone, 1330–1331, 1467**
**Methyltestosterone, 1335–1336**
**Methysergide maleate, 1239–1240**
**Metipranolol, 1262**
**Metoclopramide, 1302–1303**
for chemotherapy-associated nausea/vomiting, 498
drug interactions, 19
for eating disorders, 778
for gastroesophageal reflux, 513
**Metolazone, 1085**
**Metoprolol, 1062–1063**
bioavailability, 19t
for heart failure, 327
interaction with oral contraceptives, 277t

**MetroGel.** *See* **Metronidazole**
**Metronidazole, 1031–1032, 1429**
for bacterial vaginosis, 889–890
clearance, 29t
for inflammatory bowel disease, 508
interaction with alcohol, 108
for pelvic inflammatory disease, 881t
during pregnancy, 250–251, 251t
for *Trichomonas vaginalis,* 891–892
**Mevacor,** 108t, **1046**
**Mexiletine, 1040**
excretion, 29t
for ventricular tachycardia, 338
**Mexitil.** *See* **Mexiletine**
*Meyler's Side Effects of Drugs (SEDBASE),* 90t
**Miacalcin.** *See* **Calcitonin**
**Mibefradil, 1069**
**Micatin.** *See* **Miconazole nitrate**
**Miconazole nitrate,** 119t, 120t, 121t, **1443–1444**
**Microcytosis,** 607
**Micronase, 1354–1355**
**Micronor.** *See* **Norethindrone**
**Microsomal enzymes,** 24, 46. *See also*
**Cytochrome P-450 enzymes**
**Midamor, 1079**
**Middle cerebral artery (MCA),** 635
**Middle ear inflammation.** *See* **Otitis media**
**Midol IB.** *See* **Ibuprofen**
**Midol Maximum Strength,** 1114, 1115
**Midrin, 1242**
**Miglitol, 1359**
**Migraine headache**
agents for, **1239–1242**
diagnosis, 657–659, 658t
pharmacotherapy, 497
**Migrant workers**
community resource implications, 225
continuity of care issues, 225
health problems, 219–220
lifestyle factors contributing to disease, 220
medication/treatment considerations, 222–225,
223t
population size, 219
**Migratine.** *See* **Isometheptene mucate/dichlo-
ralphenazone/acetaminophen**
**Milkinol, 1312**
**Milontin Kapseals.** *See* **Phensuximide**
**Miltown, 1152**
**Miltown 600, 1152**
**Mineralocorticoids,** 694, **1334**
**Mineral oil,** 504, **1312**
**Minerals, 1492–1494**
for preconception period, 244–245, 245t
**Minimal erythemal dose (MED),** 596
**Minipill,** 279–280, 280t
**Minipress.** *See* **Prazosin**

Minitran, 1036
Minocin, 977–978
Minocycline, 977–978
Minority ethnic groups, medication-taking behavior of, 68–69
Minoxidil, 121t, 1071–1072
Mintezol, 1026–1027
Mint (peppermint), 132f
Mirapex. See Pramipexole
Mirtazapine, 752, 757, 1195–1196
Misoprostol, 1299
Misuse of medications, 61–62
Mite infestation, 584–585, 587–589
Mitral valve prolapse
    nonpharmacologic therapy, 352
    patient/caregiver information, 353
    pharmacotherapy, 352
        assessment for, 353
        goals, 352
        initiation, time frame for, 352–353
        selection of appropriate agent for, 353–354
    symptoms, 351
Mitran. See Chlordiazepoxide
Mitrolan, 1313
Mixed-function oxidases. See Cytochrome P-450 enzymes
Moban, 1213–1214
Mobidin, 1137–1138
Mobigesic, 1118
Modicon, 1339, 1345–1346
Moexipril, 1052
Molindone, 1213–1214
Mometasone furoate, 1468
Monamine reuptake inhibitors, 742
Moniliasis. See Candidiasis
Monistat-Derm. See Miconazole nitrate
Monitoring, pharmacotherapeutic, 59–60. See also under specific disorders
Monoamine oxidase inhibitors (MAOIs), 1198–1199
    for anxiety disorders, 774
    for bipolar disorder, 763
    co-administration with SSRIs, 755
    for depression, 752, 757
    dietary information for patients, 754t
    drug-drug interactions, 106t
    drug-nutrient interactions and, 108t
    toxicity, 759
Monoket, 1034–1035
Monopril, 1050–1051
Monosodium urate crystals, in synovial fluid, 551
Monospot test, 919
Montelukast, 1425
    for asthma, 401, 403, 404
    for chronic obstructive pulmonary disease, 424–425

Mood disorders
    bipolar. See Bipolar disorder
    depression. See Depression
    dysthymia, 748
    incidence, 747
    in multiple sclerosis, 647–648
    resources, 755t
Mood-stabilizing agents, for bipolar disorder, 762, 764–765
Moon face, 697
Moraxella catarrhalis
    antibiotic susceptibility, 489t
    beta-lactamase-producing strains, 488
    otitis media, 485
Moricizine, 338, 1040
Morning sickness
    nonpharmacologic therapy, 496
    pharmacotherapy, 497
Morphine, 1091–1092
    bioavailability, 19t
    for chronic pain, 231–232
    clearance, 29t
    hepatic extraction, 46t
Mortality rates, obesity and, 732–733
Motility disorders, 499
Motion sickness, herbal remedies, 142
Motofen, 1306
Motrin. See Ibuprofen
Mouth ulcers, herbal remedies, 136, 141
MS. See Multiple sclerosis
MSIR. See Morphine
MSRs (manufacturer's sales representatives), 92
Mucolytics
    for chronic obstructive pulmonary disease, 424
    for sinusitis, 380
Mucus liquifying agents, for cystic fibrosis, 430
Multiinfarct dementia, 655
Multiple-drug resistant tuberculosis (MDR-TB), 457
Multiple Risk Factor Intervention Trial, 316
Multiple sclerosis (MS)
    clinical signs/symptoms, 642–643, 642t
    diagnosis, 643, 643t
    incidence, 641–642
    nonpharmacologic therapy, 643–644
    pathophysiology, 642
    patient/caregiver information, 645
    pharmacotherapy, 643
        assessment for, 645
        drug selection for, 644–645
        for exacerbation prevention, 645–646
        follow-up, 648
        goals, 643
        initiation, time frame for, 644
        for symptomatic treatment, 646–648

Mumps immunizations, 158
Mu opioid receptor, 231
Mupirocin, **1444**
Murine Ear, **1283**
Muscle relaxants, for low back pain, 558–559
Musculoskeletal disorders
    bursitis, 560–561
    gout.*See* **Gout**
    herbal remedies, 141–142
    incidence, 527
    low back pain.*See* **Back pain, low**
    osteoarthritis, 539–543
    osteoporosis.*See* **Osteoporosis**
    rheumatoid arthritis.*See* **Rheumatoid arthritis**
    sprains, 560–561
    strains, 560–561
    tendinitis, 559–561
Mus-Lax, **1232**
Myambutol, 995–996
Mycelex. *See* **Clotrimazole**
Mycifradin, **1032**
Myciguent, **1445**
Mycitracin, **1440–1441**
*Mycobacterium avium*, 905*t*
*Mycobacterium tuberculosis*, 168, 905*t*
Mycobutin. *See* **Rifabutin**
Mycolog-II, **1473**
*Mycoplasma pneumoniae* **pneumonia**
    in children/adolescents, 448*t*
    diagnosis, 439*t*
    in pregnant women, 451*t*
Mycostatin. *See* **Nystatin**
Mykrox, **1085**
Mylanta, **1287**
Mylanta Gas, **1321**
Mylicon, **1321**
Myocardial infarction
    oral contraceptive usage and, 274–275
    pharmacotherapy in stroke management, 640
Myocardial ischemia, 345–346
Myochrisine, **1253–1254**
Myringotomy (ear tubes), 491
Mysoline. *See* **Primidone**

N

Nabilone, 498
Nabumetone, **1129–1130**
Nadolol, 685*t*, **1063**
NAEPP. *See* **National Asthma Education and
    Prevention Program**
Nafarelin acetate, 855, **1388**
Nafcillin, 967–968
Naftifine, **1445**
Naftin, **1445**
Na+,K+-ATPase, 37

Nalfon, **1122**
Nalidixic acid, **1019**
Naloxone
    mechanism of action, 231
    opioid receptor blockade, 39
Naltrexone
    for alcohol abuse, 789, 790
    mechanism of action, 231
Naphazoline, **1403**
Naprelan. *See* **Naproxen**
Napron X. *See* **Naproxen**
Naprosyn. *See* **Naproxen**
Naproxen, 9, **1124–1125**
    formulations, 9
    OTC status, 120*t*
Naqua, **1087**
Narcotic agonists
    diphenylheptanes, **1095–1097**
    phenanthrenes, **1089–1093**
    phenylpiperidines, **1094–1095**
Narcotic agonists-antagonists combinations,
    **1097–1099**
Narcotics combinations, **1100–1113**
Nardil, 108*t*, **1198**
Nasacort. *See* **Triamcinolone**
Nasalcrom. *See* **Cromolyn**
Nasal decongestants, **1402–1407**
    with OTC status, 118*t*, 119*t*
Nasalide. *See* **Flunisolide**
Nasolacrimal obstruction, 182
Natacyn, **1270**
Natamycin, **1270**
National Asthma Education and Prevention
    Program (NAEPP)
    asthma management recommendations, 394, 395
    asthma severity classification, 399–400, 399*t*
    "stop light" approach, 407, 407*t*
National Cholesterol Education Program
    (NCEP), 356
National Institutes of Health web site, 93*t*
Native-Americans, medication-taking behavior
    of, 69
Naturetin, **1081**
Nausea
    herbal remedies, 142
    nonpharmacologic therapy, 496, 496*t*
    from oral contraceptive usage, 272*t*
    patient/caregiver information, 497
    pharmacotherapy, 495
        assessment and history taking for, 496–497
        drug selection for, 497–499
        efficacy monitoring, 499
        goals, 495
        initiation, time frame for, 496
    during pregnancy, 248
Navane, **1215**

**NCEP (National Cholesterol Education Program),** 356
**NDMA,** 122
**Nebulizer therapy,** 410
**NebuPent,** 1033
**Nedocromil,** 373, 374, **1393–1394**
**NEE (norethindrone/ethinyl estradiol),** 1339, 1345–1346
**Nefazodone,** 752, 756–757
**NegGram,** 1019
*Neisseria gonorrhoeae*
    gonorrhea, 867, 868
    pelvic inflammatory disease, 880–882, 881*t*
*Neisseria meningitidis,* 166
**Nelfinavir,** 1012
**Nelova,** 1338–1339, 1345–1346
**Nelova 10/11,** 1339, 1345–1346
**Nembutal,** 1171–1172
**Neomycin sulfate,** 1032, 1445
**Neonatal conjunctivitis,** 481
**Neonatal herpes simplex,** 580
**Neonates**
    administration of drugs and, 185–186
    antibiotic dosage calculations for, 188*f*–190*f*
    drug absorption, 182–184, 183*t*
    over-the-counter drug doses, 190*t*–191*t*
    therapeutic disasters, 181
**Neoplasms, oral contraceptive usage and,** 275
**Neosporin,** 1440–1441
**Neo-Synephrine,** 118*t*, **1404–1405**
**Neptazane.** *See* **Methazolamide**
**Nervine,** 131*t*
**Nettle,** 132*f*, 137, 143
**Neuramate (meprobamate),** 771, **1168**
**Neurobehavioral rating scale,** 624, 625*f*–626*f*
**Neurogenic bladder,** 209
**Neurogenic bowel,** 209–210
**Neuroleptics, for dementia,** 656
**Neurologic disorders**
    attention deficit/hyperactivity disorder.*See*
        **Attention deficit/hyperactivity disorder**
    dementia.*See* **Dementia**
    headache.*See* **Headache**
    multiple sclerosis.*See* **Multiple sclerosis**
    Parkinson's disease.*See* **Parkinson's disease**
    seizures.*See* **Seizures**
    stroke.*See* **Cerebrovascular accident**
    traumatic brain injury.*See* **Traumatic brain injury**
    vertigo.*See* **Vertigo**
**Neurologic manifestations, rheumatoid arthritis,** 529
**Neurontin.** *See* **Gabapentin**
**Neuropathic pain,** 228
**Neuropeptide Y antagonist,** 743
**Neuroprotective agents,** 664–665

**Neurosyphilis,** 865, 866*t*
**Neurotransmitter theory of bipolar disorder,** 762*t*
**Neutrogena T/Gel,** 1433
**Nevirapine,** 277*t*, **1010**
**Niacin,** 359, **1048**
**Nicardipine,** 1069
**Niclocide,** 1024
**Niclosamide,** 1024
**Nicobid Tempules,** 1048
**Nicoderm,** 1486–1487
**Nicotine**
    abuse.*See* **Smoking**
    chewing gum, 793
    for chronic obstructive pulmonary disease, 424
    nasal spray, 793–795
    transdermal system, 17, 793, **1486–1487**
        OTC status, 121*t*
    for ulcerative colitis, 505
    withdrawal, agents for, **1486–1487**
**Nicotine polacrilex,** 121*t*, **1487**
**Nicotinex,** 1048
**Nicotinic acid,** 359, **1048**
**Nicotrol.** *See* **Nicotine, transdermal system**
**Nifedipine,** 1069–1070
    apparent volume of distribution, 23*t*
    bioavailability, 19*t*
    extended-release, 12
    immediate-release, 11
**Nilstat,** 984, 1445
**Nimodipine**
    for stroke prevention, 639
    for vertigo, 651
**Nisaval,** 1416
**Nisoldipine,** 1070
**Nitrates,** 348–349
**Nitro-Bid,** 1035–1036
**Nitrocine Timecaps,** 1035
**Nitrodisc,** 1036
**Nitro-Dur,** 1036
**Nitrofurantoin,** 1019–1020
    adverse effects, 9
    drug-nutrient interactions and, 108*t*
    excretion, 29*t*
    macrocrystals, **1020–1021**
**Nitrofurazone,** 1432
**Nitrogard,** 1037
**Nitroglycerin**
    absorption, 17
    hepatic extraction, 46*t*
    sublingual, **1035**
    sustained release, **1035**
    topical, **1035–1036**
    transdermal, **1036**
    translingual, **1036–1037**
    transmucosal, **1037**

Nitroglyn, 1035
Nitrol, 1035–1036
Nitrolingual, 1036–1037
Nitrong, 1035
Nitrostat, 1035
Nix 1%. *See* **Permethrin**
Nizatidine, 1300
　OTC status, 121*t*
　for peptic ulcer disease, 511
Nizoral. *See* **Ketoconazole**
NKHH (non-ketosis hyperglycemic, hyperosmo-
　sis ), 725
NMDA (Nonprescription Drug Manufacturers
　Association), 112, 113
Nociceptive pain, 228
Noctec, 104, **1179**
Nocturnal leg cramps, 344
Nodules, rheumatoid, 529
Nolahist, 1415–1416
Nonbullous impetigo, 569
Noncompliance (nonadherence), 60, 65
Nonketosis hyperglycemic, hyperosmosis
　(NKHH), 725
Nonnarcotic analgesic combinations,
　1113–1118
　with barbiturates, **1119–1121**
Nonnucleoside reverse transcriptase inhibitors,
　1009–1010
Nonnucleoside transcriptase inhibitors, for
　HIV/AIDS, 903
Nonprescription Drug Manufacturers
　Association (NMDA), 112, 113
*Nonprescription Products: Lists for Patients*
　*with Special Needs*, 88*t*
Nonsteroidal antiinflammatory drugs (NSAIDs)
　acetic acids, 1127–1131
　adverse effects, 534
　central analgesics, **1134**
　chemical classes, 533*t*
　for chronic pain, 229–230
　drug-drug interactions, 106*t*
　for dysmenorrhea, 852, 853
　fenamates, **1132–1133**
　for gout, 552–553
　for low back pain, 558
　monitoring, 530*t*
　for nonbacterial prostatitis, 824*t*
　ophthalmic, **1274–1275**
　for osteoarthritis, 542
　oxicams, **1133**
　for premenstrual syndrome, 849
　propionic acids, **1122–1126**
　for rheumatoid arthritis, 532–535, 533*t*
Noradrenergic agents
　monitoring, 743
　for weight loss, 739–740

Nordette, 1344, 1347
Norethin, 1338–1339
Norethindrone, 299, **1349**, **1373**
　combinations
　　ethinyl estradiol, **1339**, **1345–1346**
　　mestranol, **1338–1339**
　in oral contraceptives, 268–269, 268*t*, 269*t*
Norethynodrel, in oral contraceptives, 268–269,
　268*t*, 269*t*
Norflex, 1228–1229
Norfloxacin, 947, 1267
Norgesic, 1233
Norgesic Forte, 1233
Norgestimate, in oral contraceptives, 268–269,
　268*t*, 269*t*
Norgestimate/ethinyl estradiol, 1342, 1348
Norgestrel, 1349–1350
　combined with ethinyl estradiol, **1341**
　in oral contraceptives, 268–269, 268*t*, 269*t*
Norinyl, 1338–1339, 1341
Normodyne. *See* **Labetalol**
Noroxin, 947
Norpace, 21*t*, 388, **1038**
Norplant, 282–283, 282*t*, **1350–1351**
Norpramin. *See* **Desipramine**
Nor-QD. *See* **Norethindrone**
Nortriptyline, 1191
　bioavailability, 19*t*
　plasma protein binding, 21*t*
Norvasc, 1067
Norvir, 1013
Novolin 70/30, 1365
Novolin L, 1363
Novolin N, 1362–1363
Novolin R, 1361–1362
NPH Iletin, 1361–1362
NPH-N, 1361–1362
NSAIDs. *See* **Nonsteroidal antiinflammatory**
　**drugs**
Nucleoside analogues, for HIV/AIDS, 903
Nucleoside reverse transcriptase inhibitors,
　1005–1008
Nummular dermatitis, 591
Nummular eczema, 590
Numorphan. *See* **Oxymorphone**
Nuprin. *See* **Ibuprofen**
Nutritional supplements, for alcohol abuse, 789
Nystatin, 984, 1445
Nytol. *See* **Diphenhydramine**


O

Obesity
　agents for, **1481–1485**
　assessment, 737–738, 738*t*
　causes, 733, 735

Obesity (*cont.*)
  comorbid disease states, 738
  defined, 731
  herbal remedies, 142
  incidence, 731
  nonpharmacologic therapy, 736–737
  patient/caregiver information, 738
  pharmacotherapy, 735
    contraindications, 738
    drug selection for, 739–743
    follow-up, 743–744
    goals, 735–736
    herbal products, 741–742
    initiation, time frame for, 737
    investigational agents, 742–743
    monitoring, 743–744
  prevalence, 731–732
  risks, 732–733
  surgical therapy, 737
**Obsessive-compulsive disorder (OCD),** 767, 768
**Occipital cephalagia,** 560
**Occupational allergic contact dermatitis,** 589
**OCD (obsessive-compulsive disorder),** 767, 768
**Ocufen,** 1122–1123, 1274
**Ocuflox.** *See* **Ofloxacin**
**Ocular vasoconstrictor ingredients, with OTC status,** 119t
**Ocupress,** 1062, 1258
**Ocusert Pilo,** 1263
**Ocusulf-10,** 1268–1269
**Odansetron,** 498
*Oenothera biennis* **(evening primrose oil),** 132f
**Office of Alternative Medicine,** 127
**"Off-label" drug use,** 182
**Ofloxacin,** 948, 1267–1268
  for chlamydia, 872t
  drug-food interactions, 107t
  for epididymitis, 818t
  for pelvic inflammatory disease, 881t
  for urethritis, 821t
**Ogen,** 1368–1369
**Olanzapine,** 1217
**Olsalazine,** 1318
**OM.** *See* **Otitis media**
**OME.** *See* **Otitis media, with effusion**
**Omeprazole,** 511, 1300
**Omnipen.** *See* **Ampicillin**
**Ondansetron,** 1326
**Onychomycosis, of toenails,** 573
**Oophorectomy, medical,** 855
**Open-angle glaucoma,** 477
**Ophthalmic preparations,** 1257–1278
  antiallergic agents, **1273**
  antibiotics, **1264–1270**
  antifungal agents, **1270**

antihistamine/decongestant ingredients with OTC status, 120t
  antiviral agents, **1271–1272**
  for glaucoma, **1257–1264**
  nonsteroidal anti-inflammatory agents, **1274–1275**
  solutions/suspensions
    administration, 478t
    selection, for glaucoma, 478–479
  steroidal agents, **1276–1278**
**Opioid receptors,** 231
**Opioids**
  administration, 233
  for chronic pain, 230–233
  classifcations, 231
  physical dependence, 231
  tolerance, 231, 232
**Opportunistic infections, in HIV/AIDS,** 904–905, 905t
  nonpharmacologic therapy, 909–910
  prevention in children, 909
  treatment in children, 913
**Optimine.** *See* **Azatadine**
**Optipranolol.** *See* **Metipranolol**
**Optivite,** 848
**Oral anesthetic ingredients, with OTC status,** 119t
**Oral contraceptives**
  for acne vulgaris, 578
  activity, 270t
  adverse events, 271t
    ACHES warning signs, 270
    cardiovascular, 271t, 273–275
    management of, 269–270, 272t
    metabolic, 271t, 273–275
    neoplastic, 275
  biphasic, **1345**
  compliance, 276, 278–279, 278t, 279t
  components, 267
  contraindications, 273t
  for diabetics, 283
  for disabled women, 283
  drug interactions, 276, 277t
  for epileptics, 283
  formulations, current, 267, 268t
  initiation of therapy, 276
  mechanism of action, 267
  missed scheduled pills, 278–279, 279t
  monophasic, **1338–1344**
  for perimenopausal period, 296, 298
  popularity, 266–267
  progestin-only, **1349–1350**
    long-acting, 280–283, 281t, 282t
    minipill, 279–280, 280t
  risks/benefits of, 270–271, 273
  selection, 270t, 271t, 276
  triphasic, **1346–1348**

**Oral hypoglycemic agents,** 277*t*, 725–727. *See also specific oral hypoglycemic agents*
**Oral polio vaccine (OPV),** 152, 153*t*, 154*t*
**Orap,** 1214–1215
**Orasone,** 277*t*, 1331–1332
**Oretic,** 1083
**Oreton Methyl,** 1335–1336
**Orgasm prevention, drug-induced,** 858*t*
**Orinase,** 21*t*, 1356–1357
**Orphenadrine citrate,** 1228–1229
**Orphenadrine citrate/aspirin/caffeine,** 1233
**Orphengesic,** 1233
**Ortho-Cept,** 1343
**Ortho-Cyclen,** 1342, 1348
**Ortho-Est,** 1368–1369
**Ortho-Novum,** 1339
**Ortho-Novum 7/7/7,** 1346
**Ortho-Novum 10/11,** 1345
**Ortho Tri-Cyclen,** 1342, 1348
**Orudis,** 121*t*, 1124
**Orudis KT,** 121*t*, 1124
**Oruvail,** 121*t*, 1124
**Osteoarthritis**
    incidence, 539
    nonpharmacologic therapy, 540–541
    pathogenesis, 540
    patient/caregiver information, 542
    pharmacotherapy, 540
        assessment/history taking, 541
        drug selection, 542–543
        follow-up, 543
        goals, 540
        initiation, time frame for, 541
        monitoring, 543
    risk factors, 539–540
**Osteocalcin (calcitonin),** 297, 548, **1380**
**Osteoporosis**
    agents for, **1377–1380**
    categories, 543
    menopause and, 292, 295*t*
    nonpharmacologic therapy, 544–545
    pathology, 543–544
    patient/caregiver information, 545*f*, 546
    pharmacotherapy, 544
        assessment/history taking for, 545–546
        drug selection for, 546–549
        follow-up, 549
        goals for, 544
        initiation, time frame for, 545
        monitoring, 549
    prevention
        nonpharmacologic, 293
        pharmacologic, 297
    risk factors, 295*t*
**OTCs.** *See* **Over-the-counter drugs**
**Otic Domeboro,** 1280

**Otic preparations,** 1279–1285
**Otic Tridesilon,** 1283
**Otitis externa (OE)**
    defined, 485
    outcomes management, 492
    pharmacotherapy, 491–492
**Otitis media (OM),** 485–486
    antibiotic therapy
        absorption of, 487–488
        alternative initial, 489–490
        first-line, 489
        follow-up, 491
        goals, 486–487
        indications for, 486
        monitoring for efficacy, 490–491
        resistance to, 485
        selection of, 488–490, 489*t*
        time frame for, 487
        toxicity monitoring, 491
    assessment, 487–488
    ear tube placement for, 491
    with effusion, 485, 487*t*, 490
    history, 487–488
    incidence, 485
    nonpharmacologic therapy, 487*t*
    pathogens, 485
    patient/caregiver information, 487–488
    during pregnancy, 250, 250*t*
    risk, 485–486
**Otobiotic Otic,** 1279
**Otocain.** *See* **Benzocaine**
**Otocalm,** 1281
**Otosporin,** 1279
**Otrivin,** 118*t*, 1407
**Ovarian cancer, oral contraceptive usage and,** 275
**Ovcon,** 1339, 1345–1346
**Over-the-counter drugs (OTC)**
    accessibility, 113
    advertising, 113
    categories, 116
    consumer knowlege about, 111–112
    defined, 79
    pediatric doses, 190*t*–191*t*
    problems
        delay in obtaining needed treatment, 122–123
        improper use, 116
        labeling concerns, 122, 124
        lack of counseling for, 116, 122
        product-line extensions, 112, 113*t*
    reclassification to prescription status, 116–117, 117*f*, 118*t*–121*t*
    regulation
        drug review process, 114, 116
        FDA approval process, 114, 115*t*
    self-care movement and, 111

Over-the-counter drugs (OTC) (*cont.*)
  usage
    demographics of, 112–113, 112*t*
    health care costs and, 113
    health care plans and, 113–114
  usage guidelines, 123–124
**Ovide, 1451–1452**
**Ovral, 1341**
**Ovrette, 1349–1350**
**Ovulation,** 265–266
**Oxacillin, 968–969**
**Oxaprozin, 1126**
**Oxazepam,** 786*t*, **1164**
**Oxazolidinediones, 1150**
**Oxfloxacin,** 868, 869*t*
**Oxicams, 1133**
**Oxiconazole nitrate, 1446**
**Oxistat, 1446**
**Oxtriphylline, 1400–1401**
**Oxybutynin,** 209, **1476**
**Oxycodone, 1092–1093**
**Oxycodone/acetaminophen, 1108–1109**
**OxyContin, 1092–1093**
**Oxygen therapy, for chronic obstructive pulmonary disease,** 424
**Oxymetazoline, 1404**
  adverse effects, 9
  OTC status, 118*t*, 119*t*
**Oxymorphone, 1093**

P

**Pabalate-Enteric Coated Tablets, 1117**
**Pain**
  acute, *vs.* chronic, 227–228
  AHCPR management guidelines, 227, 228
  assessment, 228
  in burn management, 597
  chronic
    acetaminophen for, 230
    antiarrhythmics for, 235–236
    anticonvulsants for, 235
    antidepressants for, 233–235
    aspirin/salicylates for, 229–230
    corticosteroids for, 236
    nonpharmacologic analgesic therapies for, 228–229
    nonsteroidal antiinflammatory drugs, 229–230
    opioids for, 230–233
    *vs.* acute, 227–228
  nociceptive *vs.* neuropathic, 228
**Pamelor.** *See* **Nortriptyline**
**Pamprin, Multi-Symptom, 1115**
**Panadol.** *See* **Acetaminophen**
**Panasal, 1105**
***Panax ginseng* (ginseng),** 132*f*

***Panax quinquefolius* (ginseng),** 132*f*
**Pancrease, 1304–1305**
**Pancreatic enzymes,** 430, 431*t*. *See also specific pancreatic enzymes*
**Pancreatin, 1304**
**Pancrelipase, 1304–1305**
**Panic disorder**
  pharmacotherapy, 768, 769*f*
  symptoms, 767
**Panuveitis,** 482
**Panwarfarin.** *See* **Warfarin**
**PAOM (persistent acute otitis media),** 485
**Para-aminosalicylic acid (PAS),** 460
**Paradione, 1150**
**Paraflex, 1232**
**Parafon Forte DSC, 1232**
**ParaGard Copper T380A,** 261–262, 262*t*
**Paramethadione, 1150**
**Parasites, intestinal**
  drugs for, **1023–1027**
  infestations, characteristics of, 502
**Parasympathomimetics,** 479
**Parents, teaching tips for,** 194*t*
**Pargen Fortified, 1232**
**Parkinson's disease**
  agents for, **1243–1252**
  assessment, 663
  clinical signs/symptoms, 662
  etiology, 662, 662*t*
  incidence, 662
  nonpharmacologic therapy, 663
  patient/caregiver information, 663–664
  pharmacotherapy, 662
    algorithm, 664, 664*f*, 682
    amantadine, 666
    anticholinergics, 666
    for dementia, 667
    for depression, 667
    dopamine agonists, 665–666
    follow-up, 668
    goals, 663
    initiation, time frame for, 663
    levodopa, 666–667
    neuroprotective agents, 664–665
    for psychosis, 667–668
**Parlodel.** *See* **Bromocriptine**
**Parnate.** *See* **Tranylcypromine**
**Paromomycin, 931**
**Paronychial candidia,** 575
**Paroxetine,** 754, **1201–1202**
**Paroxysmal supraventricular tachycardia (PSVT)**
  description/etiology, 330*t*
  nonpharmacologic therapy, 333
  pharmacotherapy, 337–338
**Parsidol, 1247–1248**
**PAS (para-aminosalicylic acid),** 460

Passive diffusion, 16
Passive immunity, 151
Passive reabsorption, 27, 27f
Pathocil, 967
Patient
 decision-making capabilities, 112
 education programs, 61
 medication information, 92
*Patient Drug Facts*, 94t
*Paullinia cupana. See* **Caffeine**
Paxarel, 1178–1179
Paxil, 1201–1202
Paxipam, 1162–1163
PBO (prescribed brand only), 12
PBZ (tripelennamine), 1417
PCOS (polycystic ovarian syndrome), 841–842
PDD (premenstrual dysphoric disorder), 845,
  845t, 846t
Peak expiratory flow (PEF), 394, 403
*Pediatric Dosage Handbook*, 88t
Pediazole, 189t, 973
Pediculocides, 1452
 ingredients with OTC status, 120t
 topical, **1450–1452**
Pediculosis
 head, 585, 587, 588
 pubic, 252t, 585, 587, 588, 882–884
Peganone, 1146–1147
Pehnurone, 1156–1157
Pelamine, 1417
Pelvic examinations, for disabled individuals, 208
Pelvic inflammatory disease (PID), 880–882, 881t
Pemoline, 635, **1223**
Penbutolol, 1063–1064
Pender Model, 71–72, 72f
Penetrex, 944
Penicillamine, 1255–1256
 drug interactions, 611t
 monitoring, 530t
 for rheumatoid arthritis, 536
Penicillin, 958–961
 aminopenicillins, **962–965**
 for community-acquired pneumonia, 438–439
 excretion, 27
 interaction with oral contraceptives, 277t
 penicillinase-resistant, **966–969**
 for pharyngitis, 384
 for syphilis, 866–867, 866t
Penicillin-allergic patients, 488
 gonorrhea treatment, 869
 pharyngitis treatment, 384
 syphilis treatment, 866t
Penicillinase-resistant penicillins, 966–969
Penicillin G
 absorption, 17
 drug-food interactions, 107t

Penicillin G benzathine, 959–960
 combined with procaine, 960–961
 for pharyngitis, 383t, 384
Penicillin G potassium, 958
Penicillin G procaine, 958–959
Penicillin V, 961
 dosage calculations, pediatric, 190t
 for pharyngitis, 383t, 384
Pentamidine, 1033
Pentasa, 1318
Pentazocine/acetaminophen, 1099
Pentazocine/aspirin, 1098
Pentazocine/naloxone, 1097
Pentids, 958
Pentoxifylline, 343
Pen-Vee K, 961
Pepcid/Pepcid AC, 1298–1299
PEPI trials, 299
Peppermint, 132f, 139
Peptic ulcer disease
 nonpharmacologic therapy, 510
 patient/caregiver information, 510
 pharmacotherapy, 509–510
  assessment/history taking for, 510
  drug selection for, 510–512
  efficacy monitoring, 512
  follow-up, 512–513
  goals for, 510
  initiation, time frame for, 510
  toxicity monitoring, 512
Pepto-Bismol, 1306
Pepto Diarrhea Control, 1307
Perceived behavioral control, 70
Percocet, 1108–1109
Perdiem Fiber, 1313
Perforated tympanic membrane (PTM),
  485
Performance anxiety
 pharmacotherapy, 773
 symptoms, 767
Pergolide, 665, **1248**
Periactin. *See* **Cyproheptadine**
Perimenopause, 289. *See also* **Menopause**
Peripheral vascular disease (PVD)
 nonpharmacologic therapy, 339, 342
 occlusive, 339, 340t–341t
 outcomes management, 342–344
 patient/caregiver information, 342
 pharmacotherapy, 339
  assessment for, 342
  follow-up, 344
  goals, 339
  initiation, time frame for, 342
  monitoring, 343
  selecting appropriate agent for, 342
 venous, 339, 341t

**Peripheral vascular resistance, hypertension and,** 310–311
**Peristalsis,** 12
**Peritoneal dialysis,** 54
**Permax.** *See* **Pergolide**
**Permethrin, 1451**
   OTC status, 120*t*
   for pubic lice, 884
   for scabies, 883–884
**Permitil, 1204–1205**
**Pernicious anemia,** 614
**Perphenazine, 1206–1207**
**Perphenazine/amitriptyline, 1220**
**Persantine, 1072**
**Persistent acute otitis media (PAOM),** 485
**Personality, coronary artery disease risk and,** 345
**Pertussin CS.** *See* **Dextromethorphan**
**Pertussis (whooping cough)**
   immunizations, 153*t*, 154–155
   signs, 447*t*
**PET (peak expiratory flow),** 394, 403
**Petrolatum, liquid,** 504
**Pharmaceutical companies, medication information resources,** 92–93
**Pharmaceutical process,** 4
**Pharmaceuticals, defined,** 4*t*
**Pharmaceutic phase (rate-limiting step),** 9
**Pharmaceutics**
   clinical implications, 12
   defined, 4*t*, 7
   drug action and, 8*f*
**Pharmacodynamics**
   age-related changes, 200
   agonists and, 39
   antagonists and, 39
   defined, 4*t*, 7
   drug action and, 8*f*
   drug-drug interactions, 105
   drug interactions, 39–40, 108*t*
   drug-receptor binding, 32
      dose-response relationships and, 32–33, 33*f*
      ligands, 33–34
      receptors, 34–35, 34*f*
   intracellular receptors, 38
   mechanisms of action, 32
   process, 4
   receptor-effector coupling, 36–37
   response variability, 38–39
   signal transduction, 37, 37*f*
   structure-activity relationships, 35–36, 36*f*
**Pharmacodynanics, clinical implications,** 42
**Pharmacogenetics, defined,** 7
**Pharmacognosy, defined,** 4*t*
**Pharmacokinetics**
   absorption.*See* **Absorption**
   age-related changes, 199–200, 200*t*

   clinical implications, 31–33
   defined, 4*t*, 7
   distribution.*See* **Distribution**
   drug action and, 8*f*
   drug-drug interactions, 104
   excretion.*See* **Excretion**
   metabolism.*See* **Metabolism**
   pediatric variations, 182
      neonatal, 182–184, 183*t*
      *vs.* adult, 183*t*
   phase, 16
   during pregnancy, 239–240, 240*t*
   process, 4
**Pharmacologic, defined,** 4*t*
**Pharmacological, defined,** 4*t*
**Pharmacologic effects, unwanted.** *See* **Adverse events**
**Pharmacology, defined,** 4*t*, 7
**Pharmacotherapeutics**
   defined, 7
   process, 4
   regimen
      compliance, 60–61
      monitoring, 59–60
      selection, 5
**Pharmacotherapy.** *See also under specific disorders*
   decisions, 3–4
   defined, 4*t*
   library, suggested minimum, 93, 94*f*
   planning for, 4–5
   requirements, 5
   resources, printed, 85, 86*t*–90*t*, 90–91
***Pharmacotherapy: A Pathophysiologic Approach,*** 86*t*
**Pharmacy**
   biennial inventory, 83–84
   defined, 7
   filling prescriptions, 82–83
   prescription filing, 83
   registration, 83–84
**PharminfoNet,** 93*t*
**Pharyngitis**
   pathogenesis, 382
   pharmacotherapy, 383–385, 383*t*
   during pregnancy, 250, 250*t*
**Phase I reactions,** 24, 46, 50
**Phase II reactions,** 24, 46, 50
**Phazyme/ Maximum Strength Phazyme, 1321**
**Phenacemide, 1156–1157**
**Phenanthrenes, 1089–1093**
**Phenaphen/codeine, 1100**
**Phenazopyridine, 1478**
   combined with sulfamethoxazole, **1021**
   for cystitis, 806*t*
**Phendimetrazine,** 739

**Phenelzine**, 108*t*, **1198**
**Phenindamine**, **1415–1416**
**Pheniramine maleate/naphazoline**, 120*t*
**Phenobarbital**, **1142**, **1172–1173**
    excretion, 29*t*
    hepatic extraction, 46*t*
    interaction with oral contraceptives, 277*t*
    plasma protein binding, 21*t*
    for seizures, 674–675
**Phenolphthalein**, **1312–1313**
**Phenothiazines**, 498
**Phenoxine**. *See* **Phenylpropanolamine**
**Phenoxybenzamine**, 39
**Phensuximide**, **1152**
**Phentermine**, 739, 740, **1484–1485**
**Phentermine/fenfluramine**, 739, 740
**Phentobarbital**, **1171–1172**
**Phenylephrine**, 118*t*, **1404–1405**
**Phenylpiperidines**, **1094–1095**
**Phenylpropanolamine**, **1405**
    OTC status, 118*t*
    for stress urinary incontinence, 815*t*
    for weight loss, 739
**Phenytoin**, **1148–1149**, 1149
    for alcohol abuse, 789, 790
    drug-nutrient interactions, 108*t*
    elimination by dialysis, 53
    hepatic extraction, 46*t*
    interaction with oral contraceptives, 277*t*
    with phenobarbital, **1149**
    plasma protein binding, 21*t*
    during pregnancy, folate deficiency and, 612–613
    for seizures, 673–674
    therapeutic range, in kidney disease, 51
    thyroid function and, 685*t*
**Phillips' Milk of Magnesia**, **1288–1289**
**Phosphate fluoride**, 118*t*
**Phospholine**, **1260**
**Photoaging**, 592
**Photoallergic dermatitis**, 590
**Photosensitivity, St. John's wort and**, 130–131
**pH partitioning (ion trapping)**, 16
**Phrenilin**, **1119–1120**
**Phrenilin Forte**, **1119–1120**
*Phthirus pubis*, 882
**Physical activity, for weight loss**, 736–737
*Physician's Desk Reference*, 87*t*
*Physician's Desk Reference Generics*, 87*t*
*Physician's Desk Reference-OTC*, 87*t*
**Physostigmine**, **1262**
**PID (pelvic inflammatory disease)**, 880–882, 881*t*
**Pilocar**, **1263**
**Pilocarpine**, **1263**
**Pilocarpine ocular therapeutic system**, **1263**
**Piloptic**, **1263**
**Pilostat**, **1263**

**Pimozide**, **1214–1215**
**Pindolol**, **1064**
**Pinocytosis**, 15, 15*f*
**Pin-Rid**, **1026**
**Piperazine**, **1025**
*Piper methysticum* (kava), 132*f*
**Pirbuterol**, **1398**
**Piroxicam**, **1133**
**Pityriasis rosea**, 599–601
**Placental transfer, of drugs**, 240
**Placidyl**, **1180**
**Plague immunization**, 170
**Planned behavior, theory of**, 70
**Planning/preparation, in transtheoretical
    model of behavior change**, 72, 73
**Plantago seed/husk**, 132*f*, 134–135
**Plantar warts**, 580, 583
**Plaque, atherosclerotic**, 345
**Plaquenil**, **987–988**
**Plaque psoriasis, chronic**, 598
**Plasma compartment**, 20*f*
**Plasma profile**, 8–9, 8*f*
**Plasma protein binding**
    competition, 22–23, 22*f*
    in liver disease, 50
**Platelets, in thrombus formation**, 617
**Plendil**, **1068**
**PMS Escape**, 848
**Pneumococcal disease immunization**, 164–165
*Pneumocystis carinii* pneumonia, 452, 905*t*
**Pneumonia**
    in children/adolescents, 443
        clinical signs, 446*t*–448*t*
        diagnosis, 445*t*, 446*t*–448*t*
        drug selection for, 444–445
        efficacy monitoring, 448
        follow-up, 449
        goals, 443
        initiation of pharmacotherapy, time frame for,
          443
        nonpharmacologic therapy, 443
        pathogens, 446*t*–448*t*
        patient/caregiver information for, 444
        pretherapy assessment, 443–444, 444*t*
        toxicity monitoring, 449
    community-acquired.*See* **Community-acquired
        pneumonia**
    cystic fibrosis with, 444
    pneumococcal, 164
    in pregnancy, 449
        contraindicated drugs, 452
        drug selection for, 450–452, 451*t*, 452*t*
        efficacy monitoring, 453
        follow-up for, 453
        initiation of pharmacotherapy, time frame for,
          449–450

Pneumonia (*cont.*)
  in pregnancy (*cont.*)
    nonpharmacologic therapy, 449
    pathogens, 449
    patient/caregiver information, 450
    pretherapy assessment, 450, 450t
    therapeutic goals, 449
    toxicity monitoring, 453
*Pocket Guide to Evaluations of Drug*
    *Interactions*, 88t
*Pocket Version-Drug Facts and Comparisons*,
    88t
**Podcon-25**, 1446–1447
**Podofilox**, 879, 1446
**Podofin**, 1446–1447
**Podophyllin (podophyllin)**, 878–879, **1446–1447**
**Poison control center**, 92–93
**Poisonings, accidental**, 28, 202
**Poison ivy agents**, 121t, 589
**Poison oak**, 589
**Poison Prevention Act**, 82
**Poison sumac**, 589
**Poladex**, 1413
**Polaramine**, 1413
**Polarity**, 13, 14f
**Poliomyelitis**
  childhood immunizations, 152–154, 153t
  immunization, 170–171
  nonparalytic, 152
  paralytic, 152
  vaccine-associated paralytic, 152–153
**Polish Americans, medication-taking behavior**
    **of**, 67
**Poltices, herbal**, 130t
**Polycarbophil**, 1313
**Polycillin.** *See* **Ampicillin**
**Polycystic ovarian syndrome (PCOS)**, 841–842
**Polyethylene glycol-electrolyte solution**,
    1316–1317
**Polymox.** *See* **Amoxicillin**
**Polymyxin B**, 1268
  combinations
    hydrocortisone, **1279**
    neomycin/hydrocortisone, **1279**
**Polypharmacy**, 201
**Polysporin**, 1440–1441
**Polythiazide**, 1086
**Pondimin.** *See* **Fenfluramine**
**Ponstel**, 1132–1133
**Popliteal artery occlusive disease**, 340t
**Posicor**, 1069
**Postcoital contraception**, 283–284
**Posterior uveitis**, 482
**Postexposure prophylaxis**, 920
**Postpartum depression**, 748
**Postpolio syndrome**, 152

**Post-traumatic stress disorder (PTSD)**, 767–769
**Potassium hydroxide slide test (KOH slide test)**,
    885
**Potassium-sparing diuretics**, 1079–1080
  drug-drug interactions, 106t
  for heart failure, 325
  monitoring, 316–317
**Potassium supplements, drug interactions**, 106t,
    615t
**Potency of drug, *vs.* efficacy**, 32
**Povidone-iodine**, 1433–1434
  sponge, OTC status, 119t
**PPD test**, 455, 456
**Practitioners, drug prescribing**, 81
**Pramipexole**, 1249
**Pramoxine/hydrocortisone**, 1470–1471
**Prandin.** *See* **Repaglinide**
**Pravachol.** *See* **Pravastatin**
**Pravastatin**, 1046
**Prazepam**, 786t, 1164–1165
**Praziquantel**, 1025
**Prazosin**, 1058
  drug interactions, 40
  irreversible antagonism, 39
  plasma protein binding, 21t
**Preconception period**
  care
    defined, 243
    substance use/abuse screening, 243–244
  drug use guidelines for, 244
  vitamins/supplements for, 244–245, 245t
**Precontemplation, in transtheoretical model of**
    **behavior change**, 72, 73
**Precose.** *See* **Acarbose**
**Pred Forte**, 227t, 1331–1332
**Pred Mild**, 227t, 1331–1332
**Prednicarbate**, 1468–1469
**Prednisolone**, 1277–1278, 1332
**Prednisone**, 277t, **1331–1332**
**Pregnancy**
  accidental, 255, 255t
  asthma therapy, 413–416, 414t, 415t
  diabetes mellitus and, 721
  discomforts, management of
    allergic rhinitis, 249–250, 249t
    constipation, 249, 249t
    indigestion/heartburn, 248–249
    nausea, 248, 248t
    otitis media, 250, 250t
    pharyngitis, 250, 250t
    sinusitis, 250, 250t
    tension headache, 246–247
    upper respiratory infections, 249–250, 249t
    urinary tract infection, 247, 248t
    vaginitis, 250–251, 251t
    vomiting, 248, 248t

drug therapy, guidelines for, 240–241, 241*t*

excretion and, 27

folate deficiency and, 612–613

gonorrhea treatment, 869, 869*t*

immunizations during, 245–246, 245*t*

iron deficiency anemia prevention in, 608–609

pharmacokinetics during, 239–240, 240*t*

physiologic changes during, 239

placental transfer of drugs, 240

sexually transmitted diseases during, 251–252, 252*t*

teratogenesis and, 241

urinary tract infections, pylonephritis, 808

urinary tract infections during, 802, 805, 806*t*, 807*t*

pyelonephritis, 809, 810

**Prelone, 1277–1278, 1332**

**Premarin.** *See* **Conjugated estrogens**

**Premarketing process, deficiencies in,** 99

**Premature beats**

atrial, 330*t*

ventricular, 331*t*, 338

**Premenstrual dysphoric disorder (PDD),** 845, 845*t*, 846*t*

**Premenstrual syndrome (PMS)**

assessment/history taking, 848–849

etiology, 845–846

herbal remedies, 135–136, 141, 142–143

incidence/prevalence, 844–845

nonpharmacologic therapy, 847–848

patient/caregiver information, 849

pharmacotherapy, 846

drug selection, 849–851

goals, 847

intitation, time frame for, 848

monitoring, 850

symptoms, 844, 845, 845*t*, 846*t*

**Premphase, 1373–1374**

**Prempro, 1373–1374**

**Premsyn PMS, 1115**

**Prenatal vitamins,** 245

**Preschoolers, administration of drugs and,** 186–187

**Prescribers, of legend drugs,** 81

*Prescriber's Letter,* 88*t*

**Prescriptions**

for disabled individuals, 215

dispensing guidelines, 82

for elderly, 202–203

elements of, 80–81

filing, 82

filling, 81–82

refill information, 82

writing, for pediatric patients, 191–192, 193*t*

**Presystemic metabolism, absorption and,** 17, 18*f*

**Pretz-D.** *See* **Ephedrine**

**Prevacid, 1299**

**Prevalite.** *See* **Cholestyramine**

**Prilosec, 1300**

**Primaquine phosphate, 989**

**Primatene Mist.** *See* **Epinephrine**

**Primidone, 1142–1143**

interaction with oral contraceptives, 277*t*

for seizures, 675

**Principen.** *See* **Ampicillin**

**Prinivil, 1051**

**Prinzmetal angina,** 346*t*

**Privine.** *See* **Naphazoline**

**Probalan.** *See* **Probenecid**

**Pro-Banthine, 1295**

**Proben-C, 1237–1238**

**Probenecid, 1237**

combined with colchicine, **1237–1238**

drug interactions, 28

excretion, 29*t*

for hyperuricemia, 554

**Probucol,** 360

**Procainamide, 1041**

hepatic extraction, 46*t*

for ventricular tachycardia, 338

**Procaine penicillin G,** 866*t*

**Procaine/penicillin G benzathine, 960–961**

**Procan SR.** *See* **Procainamide**

**Procardia.** *See* **Nifedipine**

**Prochlorperazine, 1207–1208**

**Procyclidine, 1249–1250**

**Prodrugs,** 23

**Profenal, 1275**

**Progestasert,** 261, 262*t*

**Progesterone,** 850

**Progestin only contraceptives, 1349–1350**

**Progestins, 1372–1373**

for adenomyosis, 855

combined with estrogens, **1373–1375**

for endometriosis, 855

in menopause, 289

in oral contraceptives, 267, 268–269, 268*t*, 269*t*

for perimenopause, 298

**Prokinetic agents**

drug interactions, 18–19

for gastroesophageal reflux, 513

**Prolactin,** 842

**Prolixin, 1204–1205**

**Proloid.** *See* **Thyroglobulin**

**Prolonged-release preparations**

crushing or chewing, 12

intramuscular injectable.*See* **Depot injections**

matrix or reservoir systems, 10*f*, 11

plama profiles, 10*f*, 11

terminology, 11

**Proloprim, 1023**

**Promazine, 1208–1209**
**Pronestyl.** *See* **Procainamide**
**Propacet, 1111**
**Propafenone, 1041**
   for atrial fibrillation, 335
   for ventricular tachycardia, 338
**Propagest.** *See* **Phenylpropanolamine**
**Propantheline bromide, 1295**
**Propine.** *See* **Dipivefrin**
**Propionic acids, 1122–1126**
**Propoxyphene,** 51, **1096–1097**
**Propoxyphene/acetaminophen, 1111**
**Propranolol, 1064–1065**
   absorption, 51
   antagonist effect, 33–34
   bioavailability, 19*t*
   clearance, 29*t*
   hepatic extraction, 46*t*
   for insomnia, 786*t*
   interaction with oral contraceptives, 277*t*
   plasma protein binding, 21*t*
   receptor affinity, 35
   thyroid function and, 685*t*
**Propulsid (cisapride),** 19, 26, 106*t*, **1302**
**Propylene glycol/carbamide peroxide /glyc-**
   **erin/sodium stannate, 1282**
**Propylene glycol diacetate/acetic acid/ben-**
   **zethonium chloride/sodium acetate, 1280**
**Propylthiouracil (PTU), 1382**
**Proscar.** *See* **Finasteride**
**Pro Som, 1174**
**Prostadynia, 825**
**Prostaglandin E₁**
   deficiency, 848
   for intermittent claudication, 343
**Prostaglandin I₂,** 343
**Prostaphlin, 968–969**
**Prostate enlargement, benign.** *See* **Benign pros-**
   **static hyperplasia**
**Prostatitis**
   assessment/history taking, 823*f*
   bacterial, 820, 821*t*, 822
   defined, 821*t*
   etiology, 820, 821*t*, 822
   nonbacterial, 821*t*
   patient/caregiver information, 822
   pharmacotherapy, 822–825, 824*f*
**Prostatodynia, 821*t***
**ProStep.** *See* **Nicotine, transdermal system**
**Protease inhibitors,** 903–904, **1011–1014**
**Protein binding**
   age-related changes, 199
   changes, in kidney disease, 51
   interactions, 104
**Protein receptors, 34**
**Prothrombin time (PT),** 47, 619

**Proton pump inhibitors,** 513–514
**Protostat.** *See* **Metronidazole**
**Protriptyline,** 755, **1191–1192**
**Proventil, 1395–1396**
**Provera.** *See* **Medroxyprogesterone acetate**
**Provider/patient relationship,** 71, 73–74
**Prozac.** *See* **Fluoxetine**
**Pseudoephedrine, 1406**
   adverse effects, 9
   combined with fexofenadine, 370
   OTC status, 118*t*, 119*t*
   pediatric dosages, 191*t*
   for stress urinary incontinence, 815*t*
**Pseudohypertension, 311**
**Pseuodgout (calcium pyrophosphate dihydrate**
   **;CPPD), 549**
**Psittocosis, 440**
**Psoralen plus ultraviolet (PUVA),** 600
**Psorcon, 1461**
**Psoriasis,** 598–601
**PSVT.** *See* **Paroxysmal supraventricular tachy-**
   **cardia**
**Psychological functioning, in menopause,**
   290–291
**Psychological methods, for pain relief,** 229
**Psychosis**
   pharmacotherapy, in Parkinson's disease, 667–668
   in traumatic head injury, 628
**Psychosocial factors**
   in medication-taking behavior, 69–74, 72*f*
   in rheumatoid arthritis, 538–539
**Psychotherapeutic agents, 1221–1223**
   antipsychotic combinations, **1219–1220**
**Psychotherapy, for bipolar disorder,** 760
**Psychotic depression,** 748, 749
**Psyllium,** 504, **1313**
*Pthirus pubis,* **585**
**PTM (perforated tympanic membrane),** 485
**PT (prothrombin time),** 47, 619
**PTSD (post-traumatic stress disorder),** 767–769
**PTU (propylthiouracil),** 692, 693
**Pugh's criteria for cirrhosis assessment,** 47, 47*t*
**Pulmicort Turbuhaler.** *See* **Budesonide**
**Pulmoonary embolism, oral contraceptive**
   **usage and,** 274
**Pulmozyme, 1394**
**Purgative,** 131*t*
**Pustular psoriasis,** 598
**PVD.** *See* **Peripheral vascular disease**
**Pyelonephritis**
   assessment/history taking, 803*t*, 804*t*
   complicated *vs.* uncomplicated, 802*t*
   incidence, 808
   nonpharmacologic therapy, 805*f*, 808
   pathogens, 808
   patient/caregiver information, 805*t*, 809

pharmacotherapy, 808
   drug selection, 806*t*–807*t,* 809
   follow-up, 810
   goals, 808
   initiation, time frame for, 809
   monitoring, 809–810
  prevalence, 808
  symptoms, 807–808
**Pygeum,** 132*f,* 143–144
**Pyrantel,** 1026
**Pyrantel pamoate,** 119*t*
**Pyrazinamide,** 460, **998–999**
**Pyrethrins,** 884
**Pyridium.** *See* **Phenazopyridine**
**Pyridium plus,** 1478
**Pyridoxine (vitamin B₆),** 847
**Pyrilamine,** 1416
**Pyrimethamine, 990–991**
**Pyrithione zinc,** 1434

Q

**Q fever,** 440
**Quarzan, 1292–1293**
**Quazepam,** 784, **1175–1176**
**Questran.** *See* **Cholestyramine**
**Questran Light.** *See* **Cholestyramine**
**Quetiapine, 1217–1218**
**Quibron-T.** *See* **Theophylline**
*Quick Look Drug Book*, 88*t*
**Quinacrine, 991–992**
**Quinaglute Dura-Tabs, 1041–1042**
**Quinamm,** 992
**Quinapril, 1052–1053**
**Quinestrol,** 1370
**Quinethazone, 1086–1087**
**Quinidex, 1041–1042**
**Quinidine, 1041–1042**
   excretion, 29*t*
   plasma protein binding, 21*t*
**Quinine,** 29*t,* **992**
**Quinolone antibiotics, drug-drug interactions,**
   106*t*

R

**Rabies immunization,** 167–168
**Race**
   drug acetylation and, 24
   of health care consumer, 66–67
**Race ginger (ginger),** 132*f*
**Radioiodine,** 692, 693
**Raloxifene,** 300, **1377**
**Ramipril,** 1053
**Rantidine,** 1301
   OTC status, 121*t*
   potency, 32–33

**Rapid eye movement sleep (REM), in**
   **menopause,** 291
**Rate-limiting step (pharmaceutic phase),** 9
**Rattleweed (black cohosh),** 132*f,* 135–136
**Rattlewood (black cohosh),** 132*f*135–136
**Raxar,** 945
**Raynaud's disease,** 341*t*
**Raynaud's phenomenon,** 343–344
**R&C,** 1452
**RDW (red blood cell width),** 606*t*
**Receptor-effector coupling,** 32, 36–37
**Receptors,** 34–35, 34*f,* 38
**Recombinant erythropoietin,** 605
**Recombinant leptin,** 743
**Rectal administration,** 18
**Recurrent herpes labialis,** 579
**Red blood cells (RBCs)**
   count, normal values, 606*t*
   life cycle, 606
   production, 605–606
   size, 607
**Red blood cell width (RDW),** 607
*Red Book*, 88*t*
**Red pepper (capsicum),** 132*f*
**Reflex sympathetic dystrophy, after stroke,**
   640–641
**Refractory period,** 329
**Reglan.** *See* **Metoclopramide**
**Regular Iletin,** 723*t,* **1361–1362**
**Regular insulin,** 723*t,* **1361–1362**
**Regutol, 1310–1311**
**Reinfection,** 802*t*
**Relafen, 1129–1130**
**Relapse,** 802*t*
**Relative refractory period,** 329
**Remeron, 1195–1196**
**Remular-S.** *See* **Chlorzoxazone**
**Renal impairment.** *See* **Kidney, disease**
**Renese,** 1086
**Renin**
   blood pressure regulation and, 310
   hypertension and, 311
**Renin-angiotensin system,** 695
**Repaglinide,** 725, **1359**
**Repan,** 1119
**Repolarization,** 329, 329*t*
**Reposans-10.** *See* **Chlordiazepoxide**
**Reproductive choice, factors affecting,** 255–256,
   256*t*
**Requip,** 1250
**Rescriptor,** 1009
**Reserpine,** 317, **1057**
**Reservoir systems,** 12
**Resistribution phenomenon,** 19–20
**Resources**
   computer-based, 89*t*–90*t,* 91
   on-line, 91–92

**Respiratory agents**
 brochodilators
  sympathomimetics, **1395–1399**
  xanthine derivatives, **1399–1402**
 inhalants, **1389–1394**
  anticholinergics, **1389**
 nasal decongestants, **1402–1407**
**Respiratory depression, from opioid usage,**
  232–233
**Respiratory inhalants, corticosteroids,**
  **1390–1392**
**Respiratory syncytial virus immune globulin**
  **(RSVIG),** 417, 418–419
**Respiratory syncytial virus (RSV),** 416–417, 417*t,*
  446*t*
**Respiratory tract**
 disorders, lower
  asthma.*See* **Asthma**
  bronchiolitis, 416–420, 417*t*–419*t*
  chronic obstructive pulmonary disease,
   420–425, 420*t,* 421*t,* 423*f*
  cystic fibrosis.*See* **Cystic fibrosis**
  pneumonia.*See* **Pneumonia**
  tuberculosis.*See* **Tuberculosis**
 manifestations, of rheumatoid arthritis, 529, 532
**Response variability,** 38–39
**Resting membrane potential,** 329
**Restoril,** 1176–1177
**Reticulocytes,** 606
**Reticulocytosis,** 614
**Retin-A,** 1429
**Retrovir.** *See* **Zidovudine**
**Reverse transcriptase inhibitors, for HIV/AIDS,**
  903
**Rezulin.** *See* **Troglitazone**
**Rheumatism.** *See also specific rheumatic*
  *disorders*
 agents for, **1252–1256**
**Rheumatoid arthritis**
 classification, 532*t*
 etiology, 527–528
 extraarticular manifestations, 529, 532
 incidence, 527
 nonpharmacologic therapy, 528
 outcomes management, 532–539, 533*t,* 538*t*
 patient/caregiver information, 532
 pharmacotherapy, 528
  approach for, 537–538, 538*t*
  assessment/history taking for, 528–529, 532
  drug selection for, 532–538, 533*t,* 538*t*
  efficacy monitoring, 538–539, 539*t*
  follow-up, 539
  goals, 528
  initiation, time frame for, 528
  monitoring, 530*t*–531*t*
  toxicity monitoring, 539

**Rheumatoid factor,** 529
**Rheumatology Attitudes Index (RIA),** 538–539
**Rheumatrex Dose Pack.** *See* **Methotrexate**
**Rhindecon.** *See* **Phenylpropanolamine**
**Rhinitis, allergic.** *See* **Allergic rhinitis**
**Rhinocort.** *See* **Budesonide**
**Rhinocort Turbuhaler.** *See* **Budesonide**
*Rhus* **contact dermatitis,** 589
**RIA (Rheumatology Attitudes Index),** 538–539
**RICE,** 560–561
**RID,** 1452
**Ridaura,** 1281
**Rifabutin,** 999
**Rifadin.** *See* **Rifampin**
**Rifamate,** 998
**Rifampin,** 999–1001
 combined with isoniazid, **998**
 interaction with oral contraceptives, 277*t*
 for tuberculosis, 460
**Rimactane,** 998
**Rimantadine,** 163, 377–379, **1016–1017**
**Rimexolone,** 1278
**Riopan,** 1288
**Risperidone (Risperdal),** 763, **1218–1219**
**Ritalin.** *See* **Methylphenidate**
**Ritonavir,** 277*t,* 1013
**RMS.** *See* **Morphine**
**Robaxin,** 1228
**Robaxisal,** 1229–1230
**Robinul/Robinal Forte,** 1293
**Robitussin,** 112, 113*t,* 1424
**Robitussin Pediatric,** 626
**Rocephin,** 941–942
**Rolaids,** 1287–1288
**Ropinirole,** 1250
**Roseola (exanthema subitum),** 582
**Rotavirus,** 175
**Rowasa,** 1318
**Roxanol.** *See* **Morphine**
**Roxicet,** 1108–1109
**Roxicodone,** 1092–1093
**Roxicodone intensol,** 1092–1093
**RSVIG (respiratory syncytial virus immune**
  **globulin ),** 417, 418–419
**RSV (respiratory syncytial virus),** 416–417, 417*t,*
  446*t*
**RT₃U (triiodothyronine resin uptake),** 686*t*
**Rubefacient,** 131*t*
**Rubella (German measles),** 582
 immunization, 157–158, 245–246
 treatment, 584
**Rubeola (measles),** 581–582, 584
**RuVert-M,** 1323–1324
**RxList,** 93*t*
**RxTriage software,** 89*t*
**Rythmol.** *See* **Propafenone**

S

*Sabal serrulata* (saw palmetto), 132
SAD (seasonal affective disorder), 130, 748
Safety issues
  compliance, 60–61
  misuse of medications, 61–62
  patient education/counseling, 61
St. John's wort
  common/scientific names, 132*t*
  dosage, 133
  with ephedra, 741
  for stress/anxiety, 129–131
St. Josephs Cough Suppressant. *See*
      Dextromethorphan
Saleto, 1113
Salflex, 1139
Salicylates, 1135–1140
  for chronic pain, 229–230
  combinations, **1138**
  monitoring, 530*t*
  nonacetylated, for rheumatoid arthritis, 534
  thyroid function and, 685*t*
Salicylic acid, 583
Saline laxatives, 504
Salmeterol, 1398
Salmonine. *See* Calcitonin
Salsalate, 29*t*, 1139
Salsitab, 1139
Salt of drug, plasma profiles, 10*f*
Saluron, 1083–1084
*Sambucca canadensis nigra* (elder), 132*f*
Sampson root (echinacea), 132*f*
Sani-Supp, 1311
Sanorex, 1483–1484
Sansert, 1239–1240
Santmyer swallow reflex, 185–186
Saquinavir, 1013–1014
*Sarcoptes scabiei*, 882
Saw palmetto, 132*f*, 143
Scabicides, topical, 1450–1452
Scabies
  etiology, 584–585
  pharmacotherapy, 587–589, 882–884
  during pregnancy, 252*t*
Scopolamine
  adverse events, 652
  for morning sickness, 497
  transdermal, **1324**
Seasonal affective disorder (SAD), 130, 748
Sebizon, 1435
Seborrheic dermatitis, 590, 591
Secobarbital, 1173
Seconal Sodium Pulvules, 1173
Second-degree burn, 595
Second messengers, 38

Sectral, 277*t*, **1060**
Sedapap-10, 1119–1120
Sedatives/hypnotics
  barbiturates, **1169–1178**
  nonbarbiturates, **1178–1182**
Seizures
  from antidepressant usage, 234
  assessment, 670–671
  in epilepsy, 668–669, 668*t*
  nonpharmacologic therapy, 669–670
  patient/caregiver information, 671
  pharmacotherapy, 629, 669
    acting on calcium channels, 676
    acting on GABAa receptors, 674–676
    acting on glutamate receptors, 676
    acting on sodium channels, 673–674
    drug selection for, 670, 671–672, 673–676
    efficacy monitoring, 672–673, 672*t*
    follow-up, 676
    goals, 669, 669*t*
    initiation, time frame for, 670
    in stroke management, 640
    toxicity monitoring, 673
  types, 668–669, 668*t*
Seldane. *See* Terfenadine
Selective estrogen receptor modulators
      (SERMs), 299–300, **1377**
Selective serotonin reuptake inhibitors (SSRIs),
      **1199–1202**
  for anxiety disorders, 774
  co-administration with MAOIs, 755
  for depression, 751, 754–755
  for premenstrual syndrome, 850
  toxicity, 758, 775
Selegiline, **1251**
  adverse events, 665
  for Parkinson's disease, 665
Selenium sulfide, 575, **1434–1435**
Self-care movement, 111, 112*t*
  over-the-counter drugs and. *See* **Over-the-
      counter drugs**
Self-efficacy, 70
Selsun, **1434–1435**
Selsun Blue shampoo, **1434–1435**
Semont maneuver, 650
Senna, 132*f*, 135, **1313–1314**
Senokot, **1313–1314**
Sensitization theory of bipolar disorder, 762*t*
Septra. *See* Trimethoprim-sulfamethoxazole
Serax, 766*t*, **1164**
*Serenoa epens* (saw palmetto), 132*f*
Serentil, **1205–1206**
Serevent, **1398**
SERMs (selective estrogen receptor modula-
      tors), 299–300, **1377**
Serological tests, for syphilis, 865

Seromycin pulvules. *See* Cycloserine
Seroquel, 1217–1218
Serotonergic agents, for weight loss, 740–741, 743–744
Serotonin antagonists, for chemotherapy-associated nausea/vomiting, 498
Serotonin deficiency, in premenstrual syndrome, 846
Serotonin selective reuptake inhibitors (SSRIs)
    for affective disorders, in traumatic head injury, 629
    drug-drug interactions, 106*t*
Serotonin syndrome, 758
Serpentine receptors, 34, 34*f*
Sertraline, 1202
    for depression, 754
    in pregnancy, 754
    for premenstrual syndrome, 850
    for weight loss, 741
Sex. *See* Gender
Sexual dysfunction
    female
        assessment/history taking, 858
        classification, 856
        nonpharmacologic therapy, 857
        patient/caregiver information, 858
        pharmacotherapy, 856–859, 858*t*
    male.*See* Erectile dysfunction
Sexual history taking, 256, 257*t*
Sexuality
    after stroke, 641
    menopause and, 291–292
Sexually transmitted diseases (STDs)
    assessment/history taking, 804*t*
    chlamydia, 870–872, 872*t*
    gonorrhea.*See* Gonorrhea
    granuloma inguinale, 875–876
    herpes genitalis, 872–874, 874*t*
    human papillomavirus, 876–879
    infestations, 882–884
    lymphogranuloma venereum, 875–876
    pelvic inflammatory disease, 880–882, 881*t*
    during pregnancy, 251–252, 252*t*
    risk, contraceptive choice and, 256–257
    syphilis.*See* Syphilis
    vaginitis.*See* Vaginitis
SHEP (Systolic Hypertension in the Elderly Program), 312, 315–316, 317
Shingles, 581
Short-acting preparations, plasma profiles, 10*f*
Shoulder-hand syndrome, 640–641
Sialogogue, 131*t*
Siberian ginseng (eleuthero), 132*f*, 136
Sibutramine, 1485
Sick sinus syndrome, 331*t*
Signal transduction, 37, 37f

Sildenafil citrate, 1480
Silvadene, 595, 1474
Silver sulfadiazine, 595, 1474
Simethicone, 516, 1321
Simvastatin, 1047
Simvastin, 21*t*
Sinemet, 1246
Sinequan. *See* Doxepin
Sinex, 1404
Singulair. *See* Montelukast
Sinus arrhythmias, 330*t*
Sinusitis, 250, 250*t*, 379–382
Skelaxin, 1227–1228
Skeletal muscle relaxants, 1224–1229
    combinations, 1229–1233
Skelex, 1232
Skelid, 1379
Skin
    infections.*See* Skin infections
    problems, herbal remedies for, 141, 144
    tanning response, 592
    type, 593*t*
Skin cancer
    incidence, 592
    ultraviolet B exposure and, 592
Skin-fold thickness, 737–738, 739*t*
Skin infections
    acne, 576–579
    bacterial, 569
        nonpharmacologic therapy for, 571
        pharmacotherapy for, 570–572
        primary, 569–570
        secondary, 570
    fungal/yeast, 572–573
        candidiasis, 573–576
        dermatophytes, 572–573
    viral, 579
        exanthems, 581–582
        herpes simplex, 579–580
        herpes zoster, 581
        pharmacotherapy, 582–584
        varicella, 580–581
        warts, 580
Skin salves, herbal, 130*t*
Sleep Aid. *See* Diphenhydramine
Sleep aids
    ingredients with OTC status, 118*t*, 119*t*
    nonprescription, 1182–1184
Sleep deprivation, headaches and, 660
Sleep-eze 3. *See* Diphenhydramine
Sleep-wake cycle, 782
Slippery elm, 132*f*, 144–145
Slo-bid. *See* Theophylline
Slo-Niacin, 1048
Slo-Phyllin. *See* Theophylline
Slow channel, 329

Smoking, 786
  assessment/history taking, 793
  cessation
    agents, with OTC status, 121*t*
    for peripheral vascular disease, 339
    programs for, 791
  coronary artery disease risk and, 345
  interaction with drugs, 105
  nonpharmacologic therapy, 791
  patient/caregiver information, 793, 794*t*
  pharmacotherapy, 791
    algorithm, 792*f*
    drug selection, 792, 793–795
    follow-up, 795
    goals, 791
    initiation, time frame for, 791–792
    monitoring, 795
  risks, 790–791
  screening, preconception, 244
Social cognitive theory, 71
Social habits, interaction with drugs, 105, 108–109
Social phobia
  pharmacotherapy, 768
  symptoms, 767
Socioeconomic status, compliance and, 60–61
Soda Mint, 1289
Sodium, hypertension and, 310
Sodium acetate/acetic acid/benzethonium chloride/propylene glycol diacetate, 1280
Sodium bicarbonate, 1289
Sodium biphosphate/sodium phosphate, 1314
Sodium fluoride
  for osteoporosis, 548
  OTC status, 118*t*
Sodium P.A.S., 994
Sodium phosphate/sodium biphosphate, 1314
Sodium-potassium pump, hypertension and, 310
Sodium salicylate, 1139–1140
Sodium salicylate/aminobenzoate, 1117
Sodium stannate/carbamide peroxide /glycerin/propylene glycol, 1282
Sodium Sulamyd, 1268–1269, 1435
Sodol Compound, 1230–1231
Sofarin. *See* Warfarin
Solfoton. *See* Phenobarbital
Solganal, 1253
*Solidago* (goldenrod), 132*f*, 145
Soma, 1224–1225
Soma Compound, 1230–1231
Soma Compound w/ Codeine, 1231–1232
Sominex. *See* Diphenhydramine
Sorbitrate, 1034
Sore throat, herbal remedies, 144–145
Soriatane, 1430

Sotalol, 335, 1065
Sparfloxacin, 949
Sparine, 1208–1209
Spasticity
  after stroke, 640
  in disabled individuals, 213–214
  in multiple sclerosis, 647
Spectazole, 1441–1442
Spectinomycin, 869*t*
Spectrobid, 964
Spermicide, 260–261, 261*t*
Spina bifida, 214
Spinal cord injury
  autonomic dysreflexia and, 211, 212*t*, 213
  cognitive issues, 207
  sexuality issues, 207–208
Spinal manipulation, for low back pain, 556
Spironolactone, 1079–1080
Split-virus vaccine (subvirion; purified-surface-antigen), 163
Sporanox, 982–983
Sprains, musculoskeletal, 560–561
S-P-T (pork thyroid), 1387
Squamous cell carcinoma, 592
Squawroot (bearberry), 132*f*
SSD cream, 1474
SSRIs. *See* Selective serotonin reuptake inhibitors
Stable angina, 346*t*, 350
Stadol NS, 1099
*Staphylococcus aureus* otitis media, 488
*Staphylococcus pneumoniae*
  pneumonia
    in children, 447*t*
    in children/adolescents, 448*t*
    diagnosis, 439*t*
    in infants, 446*t*
    in pregnant women, 451*t*
  resistant strains, 488
Star Otic, 1280–1281
Statins, for hyperlipidemia, 358–359
*STAT!-Ref*, 90*t*
Status epilepticus, 669
Stavudine, 1006
Steady state, 31, 31*f*
Stelazine, 1209–1210
Stereoselectivity, 35–36, 36*f*
Sterilization, 263–265, 264*t*
Steroids. *See also* Corticosteroids
  for cystic fibrosis, 432
  inhaled, for asthma in pregnancy, 415
  intranasal, **1422–1423**
  ophthalmic, **1276–1278**
  oral, toxicity of, 404–405, 412
  for uveitis, 483
Stiff neck syndrome, 560

Stimulant, 131*t*
Stimulants
    cholinergic, **1477**
    gastrointestinal, **1302–1303**
Stinging nettle (nettle), 132*f*
Stomachic, 131*t*
Stool softeners, 504
STOP-Hypertension (Swedish Trial in Old
        Patients with Hypertension), 316
"Stop light" approach, for asthma, 407, 407*t*
Strains, musculoskeletal, 560–561
Streptococcal pharyngitis, 382, 384
*Streptococcus pneumoniae*, 905*t*
    antibiotic susceptibility, 489*t*
    otitis media, 485
Streptomycin, **1001**
    for tuberculosis, 460
Stress
    headache, 659
    herbal therapies, 129–131
    management, for low back pain, 556
Stress urinary incontinence (SUI)
    assessment/history taking, 813*t*, 814*t*
    defined, 810
    nonpharmacologic therapy, 811–812
    patient/caregiver information, 814*t*
    pharmacotherapy, 811
        drug selection, 812
        follow-up, 812–813
        goals, 811
        initiation, time frame for, 812
        monitoring, 812
    prevalence, 811
    risk factors, 811
    symptoms, 810–811
Stroke. *See* Cerebrovascular accident
Stroke volume, blood pressure and, 309–310
Style (hordeolum), 475, 476–477
Substance abuse
    alcohol.*See* Alcohol abuse
    drug abuse, 62–63, 785–786
    in homeless population, 221
    nicotine.*See* Smoking
Subvirion (purified-surface-antigen), 163
Sucralfate, **1301**
    drug-drug interactions, 106*t*
    drug-food interactions, 107*t*
    for peptic ulcer disease, 511
Sucrets. *See* Dextromethorphan
Sudafed. *See* Pseudoephedrine
Sudden death, ventricular fibrillation and, 333
SUI. *See* Stress urinary incontinence
Sular, **1070**
Sulf-10, **1268–1269**, **1435**
Sulfacetamide, **1268–1269**, **1435**

Sulfadiazine, **969–970**
Sulfadoxine/pyrimethamine, **992–993**
Sulfa drugs, adverse events, 579
Sulfamethoxazole, **970–971**
    dosage calculations, pediatric, 190*t*
    plasma protein binding, 21*t*
Sulfasalazine, **1256**, **1318–1319**
    for inflammatory bowel disease, 507
    monitoring, 530*t*
    for rheumatoid arthritis, 535
Sulfinpyrazone, 554, **1238**
Sulfisoxazole, **971**, **1269**
Sulfisoxazole/phenazopyridine, **1022**
Sulfonamides, **969–972**
    combinations, **973–975**
    multiple, **972**
Sulfonylureas, **1352–1357**
    adverse events, 727–728
    for diabetes mellitus, 725–727
Sulfur preparations, 884, **1435–1436**
Sulindac, **1130**
Sumatriptan, **1240–1241**
Sumycin. *See* Tetracycline
Sunburn
    nonpharmacologic therapy, 594–595, 594*t*
    pharmacotherapy, 595–598
    prevention, 592
    sunscreen prevention, 592–593
Sunscreens, 592–595, **1475**
    chemical, 593
    efficacy monitoring, 597–598
    physical, 593
    SPF values, 594, 594*t*
Suprax, **939**
Suprofen, **1275**
Surface area, absorption and, 16–17
Surfak, **1310**
Surmontil, **1416–1417**
Suspensions, 12
Sustained-release preparations (prolonged),
        plasma profiles, 10*f*
Sweat gland infection, 570
Swedish Trial in Old Patients with
        Hypertension (STOP-Hypertension), 316
Sweet licorice (licorice), 132*f*
Sweet wood (licorice), 132*f*
Swimmer's ear. *See* Otitis externa
Symadine. *See* Amantadine
Symmetrel. *See* Amantadine
Sympathomimetics, brochodilators, **1395–1399**
Symptothermal method, 265, 266
Synalar, **1461–1462**
Synalogos-DC, **1107–1108**
Synarel, **855**, **1388**
Syndrome X, 346*t*, 350–351
Synthroid. *See* Levothyroxine

**Syphilis**
   assessment/history taking, 864–866
   congenital, 863
   etiology, 863
   latent, 865–866
   nonpharmacologic therapy, 864
   pharmacotherapy, 863
      drug selection, 866–867, 866t
      goals, 864
      initiation, time frame for, 864
   during pregnancy, 252t
   primary, 864–865, 866t
   risk factors, 863
   secondary, 865, 866t
**Systolic dysfunction,** 321
**Systolic Hypertension in Europe (SYST-EUR),**
   316
**Systolic Hypertension in the Elderly Program
   (SHEP),** 312, 315–316, 317

T

**Tacaryl.** *See* **Methdilazine**
**Tachycardia**
   paroxysmal supraventricular, 330t, 333, 337–338
   sinus, 330t
   ventricular, 331t, 338–339
**Tacrine,** 655–656, **1234–1235**
**Tagamet.** *See* **Cimetidine**
**Talacen Caplets,** 1099
**Talwin Compound Caplets,** 1098
**Talwin NX,** 1097
**Tambocor,** 1039
**Tamoxifene,** 300
*Tanacetum parthenium* **(feverfew),** 132f
**Tanning, skin,** 592
**Tao,** 957
**Tapazole.** *See* **Methimazole**
**Tapiramate,** 676
**Taractan,** 1211
**Tar containing products,** 1432
**Tar derivative shampoos,** 1433
**TASS (Ticlopidine Aspirin Stroke Study),** 639
**Tavist,** 1412
**TBI.** *See* **Traumatic brain injury**
**TCA (trichloracetic acid),** 879
**Teas, herbal,** 129, 130t
**Tea tree oil,** 144
**Tea tree oil (***Melaleuca alternifolia***, tea tree),**
   132f
**Tebamide,** 1324–1325
**Tegison,** 1431–1432
**Tegopen,** 966
**Tegretol.** *See* **Carbamazepine**
**Tegrin Medicated Shampoo,** 1433
**Temaril,** 1416–1417

**Temazepam,** 784, **1176–1177**
**Temor, in multiple sclerosis,** 647
**Temovate,** 1457
**Tempra.** *See* **Acetaminophen**
**Tendinitis,** 559–561, 560
**Tenex,** 1056
**Tenormin,** 1061
**Tension headache**
   characteristics, 659
   during pregnancy, 246–247, 247t
**Tension neck syndrome,** 560
**TENS (transcutaneous electrical nerve stimula-
   tion ),** 556
**Tenuate,** 1482
**Teratogenesis,** 241, 242t
**Teratogens,** 241, 242t
**Terazol,** 1447–1448
**Terazosin,** 1058–1059
   for benign prostatic hyperplasia, 829t
   for nonbacterial prostatitis, 824t
**Terbinafine,** 985, **1447**
**Terbutaline,** 1398–1399
**Terconazole,** 1447–1448
**Terfenadine,** 1421
   for allergic rhinitis, 370
   combined with pseudoephedrine, 370
   drug-drug interactions, 106t, 372
**Terpin hydrate,** 1424
**Tessalon Perles,** 1408
**Testoderm,** 1336–1337
**Testosterone**
   for libido, 859
   in menopause, 289
   transdermal system, **1336–1337**
**Testred,** 1335–1336
**Tetanus immunizations,** 153t, 156
**Tetracycline,** 976–978, **1448**
   adverse events, 579
   for community-acquired pneumonia, 438
   interactions
      with ciprofloxacin, 18
      drug-drug, 611t
      drug-food, 107t
      with oral contraceptives, 277t
   plasma protein binding, 21t
   for syphilis, 866t
**Tetrahydrolipstatin,** 742
**Tetrahydrozoline,** 1407
**Thalitone,** 1082–1083
**THC (delta-9-tetrahydrocannabinol),** 105, 108
*Theobroma cacao* **(cocoa; caffeine),** 132f
**Theo-Dur.** *See* **Theophylline**
**Theolair.** *See* **Theophylline**
**Theophylline,** 1401–1402
   adverse events, 426t
   apparent volume of distribution, 23t

Theophylline (*cont.*)
　for chronic obstructive pulmonary disease, 422–423
　clearance, 29*t*
　hepatic extraction, 46*t*
　interactions
　　drug-drug, 106*t*
　　drug-food, 107*t*
　　with oral contraceptives, 277*t*
　for pediatric asthma, 410–411
　thyroid function and, 685*t*
**Therapeutic effects, excessive,** 42
**Therapeutic orphan,** 182
**Therapeutic range,** 8, 45
**Therevac-SB, 1316**
**Thermazene, 1474**
**Thermogenic agents,** 743
**Thiabendazole, 1026–1027**
**Thiamine,** 789
**Thiazide diuretics**
　drug-drug interactions, 106*t*
　for hypertension, 315, 316–317
**Thiazolidinediones,** 727–728
**Thioridazine,** 40, **1209**
**Thiothixene, 1215**
**Third-degree burn,** 595
**Thorazine, 1204**
**Thorn-apple tree (hawthorn),** 132*f*
**Thrombin, in thrombus formation,** 617
**Thromboangiitis obliterans (Buerger's disease),** 340*t*
**Thrombolytic agents,** 639
**Thrombophlebitis,** 341*t*
**Thrombus formation**
　normal, 617
　pathologic, 616–617
　pharmacotherapy, 617–620, 618*t*, 619*t*
**Thrush,** 573
**Thyrar, 1387**
**Thyro-Block.** *See* **Iodine**
**Thyroglobulin, 1386**
**Thyroid desiccated thyroid USP, 1387**
**Thyroid function tests,** 684–686, 686*t*
**Thyroid gland**
　disorders. *See also* **Hyperthyroidism; Hypothyroidism**
　　classification of, 685–686
　　diagnostic algorithm for, 687*f*
　　subclinical, 685
　function
　　adverse effect of drugs on, 685*t*
　　normal, 683
**Thyroid hormones, 1384–1387.** *See also specific thyroid hormones*
　drug interactions, 611*t*
　for weight loss, 743

**Thyroid-stimulating hormone.** *See* **Thyrotropin**
**Thyroid strong, 1387**
**Thyrolar, 1385–1386**
**Thyrotropin-releasing hormone (TRH),** 683, 684*f*, 685*t*
**Thyrotropin (thyroid-stimulating hormone; TSH),** 685*t*
　in amenorrhea, 842
　normal values, 686*t*
　in thyroid disorders, 686*t*
**Thyroxine (T$_4$),** 683–684, 684*f*
**Tiagabine, 1157**
**TIA (transient ischemic attack),** 636
**TIBC (total iron-binding capacity),** 608
**Ticlid,** 638–639, **1072–1073**
**Ticlopidine,** 638–639, **1072–1073**
**Ticlopidine Aspirin Stroke Study (TASS),** 639
**Tigan, 1324–1325**
**Tilade, 1393–1394**
**Tiludronate sodium, 1379**
**Time, patient perception of,** 74
**Timolol, 1066, 1263–1264**
**Timoptic, 1066, 1263–1264**
**Tinactin, 1448–1449**
**Tinctures**
　belladonna, **1292**
　herbal, 130*t*
**Tindal, 1203**
**Tinea infections,** 572–573
　of beard/moustache, 573
　capitis, 573, 575
　corporis, 575
　cruris, 573, 575
　of hand, 573
　pedis, 572, 575
　versicolor, 575
**Tioconazole,** 119*t*, 121*t*, **1448**
**Tissue compartment,** 20*f*
**Tissue plasminogen activator,** 639
**Tissue storage, distribution and,** 21
**TMP-SMX.** *See* **Trimethoprim-sulfamethoxazole**
**Tobacco**
　dependence.*See* **Smoking**
　usage screening, preconception, 244
**Tobramycin,** 430, **1269–1270**
**Tobrex, 1269–1270**
**Tocainide,** 338, **1042**
**Toddlers, administration of drugs and,** 186
**Tofranil.** *See* **Imipramine**
**Tolazamide, 1355–1356**
**Tolbutamide,** 21*t*, **1356–1357**
**Tolectin, 1131**
**Tolinase, 1355–1356**
**Tolmetin, 1131**
**Tolnaftate, 1448–1449**

**Tonic,** 131*t*
**Tonocard,** 1042
**Topamax,** 1157–1158
**Topical preparations,** 1474–1475
   acne, **1427–1429**
   antihistamine-containing, **1437**
   anti-infective, **1438–1449**
   antipsoriatic, **1430–1433**
   antiseborrheic, **1433–1436**
   corticosteroids, **1453–1473**
   nitroglycerin, **1035–1036**
   pediculocides, **1450–1452**
   scabicides, **1450–1452**
   sunscreens, **1475**
   vaginal, **1438–1449**
**Topicort,** 1459
**Topiramate,** 674, **1157–1158**
**Toprol XL.** *See* **Metoprolol**
**Toradol,** 1129, **1274–1275**
**Tornalate,** 1396
**Torsemide,** 324–325, **1078**
**Totacillin.** *See* **Ampicillin**
**Total iron-binding capacity (TIBC),** 608
**Total thyroxine**
   normal values, 686*t*
   in thyroid disorders, 686*t*
**Tourette's syndrome,** 631–632
**Toxicity, plasma concentration and,** 8
**Toxicology, defined,** 7
*Toxoplasma gondii,* 905*t*
**Trace elements,** 1495–1497
**Training programs,** 61
**Tramadol,** 1134
**Trancopal Caplets,** 1166
**Trandate.** *See* **Labetalol**
**Trandserm-Scop,** 1324
**Transcobalamin,** 614
**Transcutaneous electrical nerve stimulation**
   **(TENS),** 556
**Transdermal systems**
   controlled-release, plasma profiles of, 10*f*
   estradiol, 298–299, **1368**
   estrogen replacement, 298–299
   nicotine.*See* **Nicotine, transdermal system**
   nitroglycerin, **1036**
   patches, 12
   scopolamine, **1324**
   testosterone, **1336–1337**
**Transderm-Nitro,** 1036
**Transient ischemic attack (TIA),** 636
**Transmembranous enzymes,** 38
**Transtheoretical model of behavior change,**
   72–73
**Tranxene,** 1144–1145
**Tranxene-SD,** 1144–1145
**Tranylcypromine,** 108*t*, **1198–1199**

**Traumatic brain injury (TBI)**
   deficits in, 622, 623*t*
   defined, 621
   nonpharmacologic therapy, 623
   outcomes management, 624, 626–629
   pathophysiology, 621–622
   patient/caregiver information, 624
   pharmacotherapy, 622, 627*t*
      for affective disorders, 628–629
      for agitation/aggression, 628
      assessment for, 624, 625*f*–626*f*
      for attention/arousal, 624, 626–628
      for cognition, 628
      contraindicated drugs, 623*t*
      drug selection for, 623–624, 623*t*
      goals, 622–623
      initiation, time frame for, 623
      for psychosis, 628
      for seizures, 629
   prognosis, 622
**Traveler's diarrhea,** 499, 501
**Traveler's immunizations,** 169–171
**Trazodone,** 1196–1197
   for bulimia nervosa, 780
   for depression, 752, 756
**Trecator-SC,** 996
*Treponema pallidum,* 863, 865
**Tretinoin,** 1429
**TRH (thyrotropin-releasing hormone),** 683,
   684*f*, 685*t*
**Triacetin,** 1449
**Triamcinolone,** 1333, 1392
   for asthma, 400–401, 402*t*
   intranasal, **1423**
   topical, **1469**
**Triaminic,** 191*t*
**Triamterene,** 1080
**Triaprin,** 1119–1120
**Triavil,** 1220
**Triazolam,** 784, **1177–1178**
**Tri-Chlor,** 1449
**Trichloracetic acid (TCA),** 879
**Trichlormethiazide,** 1087
**Trichloroacetic acid,** 1449
*Trichomonas vaginalis,* 251, 251*t*, 890–892
**Tricyclic antidepressants (TCAs),** 1185–1193
   adverse events, 756
   for anxiety disorders, 774
   for bulimia nervosa, 780
   for dementia, 656
   for depression, 751–752, 755–756
   drug-drug interactions, 106*t*
   interactions with oral contraceptives, 277*t*
   toxicity, 758–759, 775
**Tridesilon,** 1458–1459
**Tridione,** 1150

Triethanolamine polypeptide oleate-condensate/ chlorobutanol/propylene glycol, 1285
Trifluoperazine, 1209–1210
Trifluridine, 1271–1272
Triglycerides
    formation, 354–355
    pharmacotherapy, 356, 357t
Trihexy-2, 1251–1252
Trihexy-5, 1251–1252
Trihexyphenidyl, 1251–1252
Triiodothyronine resin uptake (RT₃U), 686t
Triiodothyronine (T₃), 683–684, 684f
Trilafon, 1206–1207
Tri-Levlen, 1344, 1347
Trilisate, 1138
Trimazide, 1324–1325
Trimeprazine, 1416–1417
Trimethadione, 1150
Trimethobenzamide, 1324–1325
Trimethoprim, 190t, 1023
Trimethoprim-sulfamethoxazole (TMP-SMX), 974–975
    adverse effects, 441–442
    for cystitis, 806t
    for diarrhea, 502
    drug-drug interactions, 106t
    for pneumonia, 439–440
    for prostatitis, 824, 824t
    for sinusitis, 380, 381, 382
    for upper respiratory tract infections, 489t
Trimipramine, 1192–1193
Trimox. See Amoxicillin
Trimpex, 1023
Tri-Norinyl, 1339, 1345–1346
Tripelennamine, 1417
Triphasil, 1347
Triple sulfa No. 2, 972
Triprolidine, 119t, 1418
Triptone Caplets, 1323
Troandomycin, 277t
Troglitazone, 1359–1360
    for diabetes mellitus, 727
    interaction with oral contraceptives, 277t
Troleandomycin, 957
Trovafloxacin, 949–950
Trovan, 949–950
Trusopt, 1259–1260
TSH. See Thyrotropin
T₃ (triiodothyronine), 683–684, 684f
Tuberculosis
    drug-resistant, 457–458
    drug selection
        for children, 461
        for pregnant women, 461
    in homeless population, 221

immunization, 168–169
incidence, 453
multiple-drug-resistant, 454
nonpharmacologic therapy, 455
pharmacotherapy, 454–455, 454t, 459t
    algorithm, 458f
    assessment for, 455–456
    drug selection for, 456–458, 457t, 460–461
    efficacy monitoring, 461–462
    follow-up, 463
    goals, 455
    initiation, time frame for, 455
    patient/caregiver information, 456
    prophylactic, 458–459, 459t
    toxicity monitoring, 462–463
prophylaxis
    for children, 461
    for pregnant women, 461
risk, 454t
Tubular secretion, 16, 26–27, 27f
Tums, 1287
Tums, Extra Strength, 1287
Tums Ultra, 1287
Turbuhaler, for asthma, 397, 402t
Tusstat. See Diphenhydramine
Twilite. See Diphenhydramine
Tylenol. See Acetaminophen
Tylenol, Extra Strength Headache Plus Caplets, 1115
Tylenol w/Codeine, 1100
Tylox, 1108–1109
Tympagesic, 1281
Tympanic membrane, in otitis media, 487
Typhoid fever, 169–170
Tyzine, 1407

U

Ulcerative colitis, 504–509
    agents for, 1318–1319
Ulcers, agents for, 1297–1301
Ulmus fulva (slippery elm), 132f
Ulmus rubra Muhl (slippery elm), 132f
Ultralente U, 720f, 721, 1363–1364
Ultram, 1134
Ultrasound, for pregnant patient with pneumonia, 450t
Ultravate, 1465
Ultraviolet light
    protection against, 594–595, 594t
    skin cancer and, 592
Unipen, 967–968
Uniphyl. See Theophylline
Unisom Nighttime Sleep-Aid, 1182–1183
United States Pharmacopeia, 94t
Univasc, 1052

**Unstable angina,** 346*t,* 350
**Upper extremity pain, after stroke,** 640–641
**Upper respiratory disorders**
  allergic rhinitis.*see* **Allergic rhinitis**
  antibiotic *in vitro* activity, 489*t*
  common cold.*see* **Cold, common**
  croup.*see* **Croup**
  influenza.*see* **Influenza**
  pharyngitis.*see* **Pharyngitis**
  during pregnancy, 249–250, 249*t*
  prevention, 375*t*
  sinusitis.*see* **Sinusitis**
**Up-regulation,** 38
**Urea (blood urea nitrogen),** 48
**Urecholine.** *See* **Bethanechol chloride**
**Urethritis**
  gonoccal, 818
  gonococcal, 821*t*
  male, 817–820
    assessment/history taking, 819*t,* 820*t*
    pathogens, 818
    patient/caregivern information, 819, 820*t*
    pharmacotherapy, 818–820
  nongonoccal, 818
  nongonococcal, 821*t*
  symptoms, 801
**Urex, 1018**
**Urinalysis,** 804*t*
**Urinary retention, after stroke,** 640
**Urinary tract agents**
  analgesics, **1478**
  antispasmodics, **1476**
  cholinergic stimulants, **1477**
**Urinary tract infections (UTIs)**
  assessment/history taking, 803, 803*t,* 804*t*
  herbal remedies, 145
  lower
    incidence, 801
    pathogens, 801
    prevalence, 801
  male
    epididymitis, 813, 815–817, 816*t,* 817*t*
    urethritis, 817–820
  patient/caregiver information, 804, 805*t*
  pharmacotherapy, 803
    drug selection, 804–805, 806*t*–807*t*
    follow-up, 807
    goals, 803
    initiation, time frame for, 803
    monitoring, 805, 807
  during pregnancy
    diagnosis of, 247
    drug management of, 247, 248*t*
  reinfection, 802*t,* 805, 807
  relapse, 802*t,* 805, 807
  upper.*See* **Pyelonephritis**

**Urine pH, drug excretion and,** 28, 29*t*
**Uripas,** 1476
**Urogenital atrophy, in menopause,** 291
**Urolene Blue,** 1030–1031
**Uro-Mag,** 1289
**Ursodiol,** 1305
*Urtica diocia* **(nettle),** 132*f*
**USP DI,** *Volume I, Drug Information for the*
        *Health Care Professional,* 87*t,* 90*t*
**Uterine bleeding, dysfunctional,** 290, 843–844
**Uticort,** 1455
**UTIs.** *See* **Urinary tract infections**
*Uva-ursi* **(bearberry),** 132*f*
**Uveitis,** 482–483

V

**Vaccine Adverse Event Reporting System**
        **(VAERS),** 99, 102*f*–103*f,* 174
**Vaccine-associated paralytic poliomyelitis**
        **(VAPP),** 152–153
**Vaccine Injury Compensation Program (VICP),**
        174
**Vaccines**
  adverse event reporting, 174
  development, 175
  hepatitis, 517–518, 519
  hepatitis A, 165–166, 169
  hepatitis B, 161–162
  historical aspects, 151
  injection procedures, for children, 192
  measles, 157
  meningococcal, 166–167
  mumps, 158
  pertussis, 155
  rabies, 167–168
  split-virus; subvirion; purified-surface-antigen, 163
  typhoid fever, 169–170
*Vaccinium macrocarpon (cranberry),* 132*f*
**VAERS (Vaccine Adverse Event Reporting**
        **System),** 99, 102*f*–103*f,* 174
**Vagal nerve stimulator,** 669–670
**Vaginal agents, anti-infective topical,**
        **1438–1449**
**Vaginal Creams and Ring.** *See* **Vaginal estro-**
        **gens**
**Vaginal cytology, for hormone replacement**
        **therapy monitoring,** 301
**Vaginal dryness, nonpharmacologic therapy,**
        293
**Vaginal estrogens,** 1370–1371
**Vaginal lubricants,** 859
**Vaginal yeast infections, over-the-counter drug**
        **use for,** 123
**Vaginismus,** 856, 859
**Vaginitis, during pregnancy,** 250–251, 251*t*

Vaginosis, bacterial, 888–890
Vagistat-1, 1448
Valacyclovir, 873, 874, 874*t*, **1004**
Valerian, 132*f*, 133, 139
Valisone, 1456–1457
Valium. *See* Diazepam
Valmid Pulvules. *See* Ethanimate
Valproic acid (Valproate), 1158
    adverse events, 766
    for bipolar disorder, 762–763, 764
    plasma protein binding, 21*t*
    for seizures, 675
Valrelease. *See* Diazepam
Valsartan, 1054
Valtrex. *See* Valacyclovir
Vancenase. *See* Beclomethasone
Vanceril. *See* Beclomethasone
Vancocin, 1033
Vancomycin, 1033
    clearance, 29*t*
    elimination by dialysis, 53
Vantin, 940–941
VAPP (vaccine-associated paralytic po-
        liomyelitis ), 152–153
Variant angina, aspirin for, 350
Varicella-zoster immune globulin (VZIG), 159
Varicella-zoster virus
    immunizations, 159–161, 246
    pharmacotherapy, 580–581, 583–584
    pneumonia, in pregnancy, 451*t*, 452, 452*t*
Varicose veins, 341*t*, 342
Varivax, 159–160
Vascor, 1067
Vascular resistance, 313
Vasoconstriction, hypertension and, 310
Vasodilators, 1071–1072
    for heart failure, 327
    for hypertension, 310, 318–319
    for intermittent claudication, 343
Vasomotor instability, in menopause, 290
Vasotec, 23*t*, **1050**
Veetids, 961
Velosef, 933–934
Velosulin Human, 1361–1362
Venlafaxine, 752, 754, 757, **1197**
Venous thromboembolism, oral contraceptive
        usage and, 274
VentEase, 401
Ventolin, 1395–1396
Ventolin Rotocaps, 1395–1396
Ventricular arrhythmias, 338–339
Ventricular block, 332*t*
Ventricular fibrillation, sudden death and, 333
Verapamil, 1070–1071
    for atrial fibrillation, 336
    bioavailability, 19*t*
    for bipolar disorder, 765
    clearance, 29*t*
    hepatic extraction, 46*t*
    plasma protein binding, 21*t*
Vermox, 1023–1024
Verrucae (warts), 580
Vertigo
    defined, 648
    etiology, 648–649, 648*t*
    nonpharmacologic therapy, 650
    patient/caregiver information, 651
    pharmacotherapy, 649
        assessment for, 650–651
        drug selection for, 650, 651
        follow-up, 652
        goals, 650
        initiation, time frame for, 650
        monitoring, 651–652
Very low-density lipoproteins (VLDLs),
        354–355
Vesicular tinea pedis, acute, 572–573
Vestibulitis, vulvar, 838–839
Vexol. *See* Rimexolone
Viagra. *See* Sildenafil citrate
Vibramycin. *See* Doxycycline
Vibra-Tabs. *See* Doxycycline
Vicks 44. *See* Dextromethorphan
Vicks Vatronol. *See* Ephedrine
Vicodin, 1104
VICP (Vaccine Injury Compensation Program),
        174
Vidarabine, 1272
Videx, 1005–1006
Vigabatrin, 675–676
Vinegars, herbal, 130*t*
Vioform, 1439
Viokase, 1304–1305
Vira-A. *See* Vidarabine
Viracept, 1012
Viral conjunctivitis, 479–480, 481
Viramune, 1010
Virilization, 699
Virilon, 1335–1336
Viroptic, 1271–1272
Visken, 1064
Vistaril. *See* Hydroxyzine
Vitamins, 1488–1491
    A, 107*t*, **1488**
    B$_6$, 847, **1490**
    B$_{12}$
        deficiency, 606, 614–616, 615*t*
        drug interactions, 615*t*
    C, 375, 377, **1491**
    D, 546–547, **1488**
    E, 848, **1488**
    K, **1489**

Biotin, **1490**
Cobalamin, **1491**
for cystic fibrosis, 430, 431*t*
fat-soluble, 107*t*
Folate, **1490**
Niacin, **1490**
for preconception period, 244–245
prenatal, 245
Riboflavin, **1489**
Thiamin, **1489**
***Vitex agnus-castus* (chaste tree berry)**, 132*f*
***Vitex* (chase tree berry)**, 132*f*
**Vivactil**, 1191–1192
**Vivelle**, 1368
**VLDLs (very low-density lipoproteins)**, 354–355
**VolSol**, 1280
**Voltaren**, 1127, 1274
**Volume of distribution, in hepatic failure**, 50
**Vomiting**
nonpharmacologic therapy, 496, 496*t*
from oral contraceptive usage, 272*t*
patient/caregiver information, 497
pharmacotherapy, 495
assessment and history taking for, 496–497
drug selection for, 497–499
efficacy monitoring, 499
goals, 495
initiation, time frame for, 496
postoperative, 499
during pregnancy, 248, 248*t*
self-induced, 495
**VoSol HC**, 1280
**Vulvar conditions**, 835
dermatitis, 836–837
dystrophies, 839
folliculitis, 835–836
vestibulitis, 838–839
vulvodynia.*See* **Vulvodynia**
**Vulvodynia**
defined, 837
lichen sclerosus and, 839–840
vulvar vestibulitis and, 838–839
**Vulvovaginal candidiasis**, 251, 251*t*, 885–888
**Vytone**, 1471
**VZIG (varicella-zoster immune globulin)**, 159

W

**Waist:hip ratio (WHR)**, 732
**Walking, for peripheral vascular disease**, 339
**Warfarin**, 1043
adverse effects, 619
apparent volume of distribution, 23*t*
for atrial fibrillation, 336–337, 336*t*, 337*t*
contraindications, 617–618
hepatic extraction, 46*t*

indications, 619*t*
interactions
drug-drug, 106*t*, 619*t*
drug-nutrient, 108*t*, 619*t*
with oral contraceptives, 277*t*
length of treatment, 619*t*
for mitral valve prolapse, 354
plasma protein binding, 21, 21*t*
for stroke prevention, 639
**Warts**, 580, 582, 583
**Wasp stings**, 586
**Water contamination, diseases associated with**, 169–170
**Weight change, from oral contraceptive usage**, 272*t*
**Wellbutrin.** *See* **Bupropion**
**Wesprin buffered**, 1135–1136
**Westcort**, 1466–1467
**Wheezing, in infants/children**, 405, 406
**White ethnic groups, medication-taking behavior of**, 67–68
**Whiteheads**, 576
**Whitehorn (hawthorn)**, 132*f*
**Whooping cough (pertussis) immunizations**, 154–155
**WHR (waist:hip ratio)**, 732
**Wigraine**, 1241–1242
**Wild cucumber (caigua)**, 132*f*
**Willow bark**, 141–142
**Witch hazel**, 132*f*, 138
**Withdrawal bleeding**
from oral contraceptive usage, 272*t*
progestin challenge and, 842
**Wolff-Chaikoff paradoxical effect**, 693
**Wolff-Parkinson-White syndrome**, 335
**Women's health issues, for individuals with a disability**, 208
**Wonder-of-world (ginseng)**, 132*f*
**World Health Organization (WHO)**
adverse drug reaction definition, 97–98
web site, 93*t*
**Wounds, cleansing/protecting**, 597
**Wyamycin stearate.** *See* **Erythromycin stearate**
**Wycillin**, 958–959
**Wymox.** *See* **Amoxicillin**
**Wytensin**, 1055

X

**Xalatan**, 1261
**Xamaterol**, 328
**Xanax.** *See* **Alprazolam**
**Xanthine derivative brochodilators**, 1399–1402
**Xylocaine.** *See* **Lidocaine**
**Xylometazoline**, 118*t*, **1407**

## Y

Yellow fever, 170
Yocon, 1480
Yodoxin, 931
Yohimbine, 1480
Yohimex, 1480

## Z

Zafirlukast, 1425
    for asthma, 401, 404
    for chronic obstructive pulmonary disease, 424–425
    toxicity, 405
Zagam, 949
Zalcitabine, 1007
Zantac, 1301
Zarontin, 1151
Zaroxolyn, 1085
Zebeta, 1061–1062
Zerit, 1006
Zero-order kinetics, 31
Zestril, 1051
Zetran. See Diazepam
Zidovudine (AZT; ZDV), 1007–1008
    drug-food interactions, 107t
    for HIV/AIDS in children, 912

for postexposure prophylaxis, 920
Zileutin, 1426
Zileuton
    for asthma, 401, 404
    for chronic obstructive pulmonary disease, 424
    toxicity, 405
Zinc
    deficiency, in postmenopausal women, 300
    drug interactions, 611t
Zinc gluconate, 375, 377
Zincon, 1434
Zingiber officinale Rosc. (ginger), 132f
Ziradryl. See Diphenhydramine
Zithromax. See Azithromycin
Zocor, 1047
Zofran, 1326
Zollinger-Ellison syndrome, 511, 512
Zoloft. See Sertraline
Zolpidem, 1181–1182
    for insomnia, 785
Zonalon. See Doxepin
Zovirax. See Acyclovir
Zyban. See Bupropion
Zyflo, 1426
Zyloprim, 1235–1236
Zyprexa, 1217
Zyrtec, 1419–1420